VASCULAR AND ENDOVASCULAR SURGERY

A Comprehensive Review

Eighth Edition

VASCULAR AND ENDOVASCULAR SURGERY

A Comprehensive Review

Eighth Edition

Wesley S. Moore, MD
Professor and Chief Emeritus
David Geffen School of Medicine
University of California–Los Angeles
Vascular Surgeon
University of California–Los Angeles
Center for the Health Sciences
Los Angeles, California

With 695 illustrations

ELSEVIER
SAUNDERS

ELSEVIER
SAUNDERS

1600 John F. Kennedy Blvd.
Suite 1800
Philadelphia, PA 19103-2899

VASCULAR AND ENDOVASCULAR SURGERY ISBN: 978-1-4557-4601-9

Notices

Knowledge and best practice in this field are constantly changing. As new research and experience broaden our understanding, changes in research methods, professional practices, or medical treatment may become necessary.

Practitioners and researchers must always rely on their own experience and knowledge in evaluating and using any information, methods, compounds, or experiments described herein. In using such information or methods they should be mindful of their own safety and the safety of others, including parties for whom they have a professional responsibility.

With respect to any drug or pharmaceutical products identified, readers are advised to check the most current information provided (i) on procedures featured or (ii) by the manufacturer of each product to be administered, to verify the recommended dose or formula, the method and duration of administration, and contraindications. It is the responsibility of practitioners, relying on their own experience and knowledge of their patients, to make diagnoses, to determine dosages and the best treatment for each individual patient, and to take all appropriate safety precautions.

To the fullest extent of the law, neither the Publisher nor the authors, contributors, or editors, assume any liability for any injury and/or damage to persons or property as a matter of products liability, negligence or otherwise, or from any use or operation of any methods, products, instructions, or ideas contained in the material herein.

Library of Congress Cataloging-in-Publication Data or Control Number
Vascular and endovascular surgery : a comprehensive review / [edited by] Wesley S. Moore. – 8th ed.
    p. ; cm.
    Includes bibliographical references and index.
    ISBN 978-1-4557-4601-9 (hardcover : alk. paper)
    I. Moore, Wesley S.
    [DNLM: 1. Vascular Surgical Procedures.   2. Vascular Diseases–surgery. WG 170]
    617.4′13–dc23
                                                                    2012036620

Acquisitions Editor: Michael Houston
Senior Content Development Specialist: Arlene Chappelle
Publishing Services Manager: Catherine Jackson
Senior Project Manager: Rachel E. McMullen
Design Direction: Steve Stave

Printed in the United States of America

Last digit is the print number: 9 8 7 6 5 4 3 2 1

The eighth edition of this book is dedicated to the next generation of vascular surgeons. The effort that has gone into this book by the editor and chapter contributors is directed primarily to the education of our trainees. The future of our specialty will be in their capable hands. In addition, and in recognition of the importance of continuing medical education, the size and scope of this book provides an ideal text for vascular surgeons who are preparing for certification and recertification in our specialty. The editor and chapter authors have also directed their efforts to meet this objective, and we wish our colleagues well in their certification efforts.

CONTRIBUTORS

Christopher J. Abularrage, MD
Assistant Professor of Surgery, Division of Vascular
    Surgery and Endovascular Therapy, Johns Hopkins
    University School of Medicine, Baltimore, Maryland
    56: Prosthetic Graft Infection

Justin S. Ahn, MD
Medical Student, University of Texas Southwestern,
    Dallas, Texas
    *31: Thoracic Outlet Syndrome and Vascular Disease
    of the Upper Extremity*

Samuel S. Ahn, MD, FACS, MBA
Founder and Partner, University Vascular Associates,
    Los Angeles, California; DFW Vascular Associates,
    Dallas, Texas
    *31: Thoracic Outlet Syndrome and Vascular Disease
    of the Upper Extremity*
    63: Building an Outpatient Intervention Suite

George Andros, MD
Los Angeles Vascular Specialists, Medical Director,
    Amputation Prevention Center, Valley Presbyterian
    Hospital, Van Nuys, California
    59: The Diabetic Foot

Niren Angle, MD, RVT, FACS
Vascular and Endovascular Surgery, The Vascular
    Center, Mission Regional Medical Center
    Mission Viejo, California
    *33: Thrombolysis for Arterial and Graft Occlusions:
    Technique and Results*
    56: Prosthetic Graft Infection

Margaret W. Arnold, MD
Assistant Professor of Surgery, Division of Vascular
    Surgery and Endovascular Therapy, Johns Hopkins
    University School of Medicine, Baltimore, Maryland
    *58: Management of Complications After Endovascular
    Abdominal Aortic Aneurysm Repair*

Enrico Ascher, MD
Division of Vascular Services, Maimonides Medical
    Center, Brooklyn, New York
    *26: Surgical Management of Femoral, Popliteal, and
    Tibial Arterial Occlusive Disease*

Amir F. Azarbal, MD
Assistant Professor of Surgery, Division of Vascular
    Surgery, Oregon Health and Science University,
    Portland, Oregon
    *32: Natural History and Nonoperative Treatment of
    Chronic Lower Extremity Ischemia*

Ali Azizzadeh, MD, FACS
Associate Professor, Program Director in Vascular
    Surgery, Department of Cardiothoracic and Vascular
    Surgery, University of Texas Medical School at
    Houston; Director of Endovascular Surgery,
    Memorial Hermann Heart and Vascular Institute,
    Houston, Texas
    *34: Descending Thoracic and Thoracoabdominal Aortic
    Aneurysms: General Principles and Open Surgical Repair*

J. Dennis Baker, MD
Professor Emeritus of Surgery, Division of Vascular
    Surgery, David Geffen School of Medicine,
    University of California–Los Angeles, Los Angeles,
    California
    14: The Noninvasive Vascular Laboratory

Jeffrey L. Ballard, MD
Staff Vascular Surgeon, Division of Vascular Surgery,
    St. Joseph Hospital, Orange, California
    4: Anatomy and Surgical Exposure of the Vascular System

Wiley F. Barker, MD
Professor Emeritus of Surgery and Vascular Surgery,
    University of California–Los Angeles, Los Angeles,
    California
    1: A History of Vascular Surgery

Jonathan Bath, MD
Fellow in Vascular Surgery, University of Pittsburgh
    Medical Center, Pittsburgh, Pennsylvania
    *12: Medical Management of Vascular Disease Including
    Pharmacology of Drugs Used in Vascular Disease
    Management*

Ronald Belczyk, DPM
Consultant Physician, Amputation Prevention Center,
    Valley Presbyterian Hospital, Van Nuys, California
    59: The Diabetic Foot

Michael Belkin, MD
Chief, Division of Vascular and Endovascular Surgery,
  Brigham and Women's Hospital, Boston,
  Massachusetts
21: Surgical Management of Aortoiliac Occlusive Disease

Ramon Berguer, MD, PhD
Professor of Surgery, Medical School, Professor of
  Biomedical Engineering, College of Engineering,
  University of Michigan Health System, Ann Arbor,
  Michigan
*19: Surgical Reconstruction of the Supra-Aortic Trunks
and Vertebral Arteries*

Todd L. Berland, MD
Assistant Professor, Division of Vascular Surgery,
  New York University Langone Medical Center,
  New York, New York
*41: Open Surgical and Endovascular Management of
Ruptured Abdominal Aortic Aneurysm*

John D. Bisognano, MD, PhD
Professor of Medicine, Division of Internal
  Medicine, Cardiology Division, University
  of Rochester Medical Center, Rochester,
  New York
*62: Carotid Sinus Stimulation: Background, Technique,
and Future Directions*

W. Austin Blevins, Jr., MD[†]
*20: Endovascular Repair of Extracranial Cerebrovascular
Lesions*

Luke P. Brewster, MD
Assistant Professor of Surgery, Division of Vascular
  Surgery, Department of Surgery, Emory University
  School of Medicine, Atlanta, Georgia
*16: Vascular Grafts: Characteristics and Rational
Selection*

Ruth L. Bush, MD, MPH
Professor of Surgery, Texas A&M Health Science
  Center College of Medicine, Round Rock, Texas;
  Chief, Vascular Surgery, Central Texas Healthcare
  System, Temple, Texas
*22: Angioplasty and Stenting for Aortoiliac Disease:
Technique and Results*

Catherine Cagiannos, MD
Assistant Professor, Division of Vascular Surgery,
  Michael E. De Bakey Department of Surgery,
  College of Medicine, Baylor University,
  Waco, Texas
*42: Laparoscopic Aortic Surgery for Aneurysm and
Occlusive Disease: Technique and Results*

Danielle N. Campbell, MD
Integrated Vascular Surgery Resident, Section
  of Vascular Surgery, Department of Surgery,
  University of Michigan, Ann Arbor, Michigan
47: Venous Thromboembolic Disease

Neal S. Cayne, MD, FACS
Director of Endovascular Surgery, Division of Vascular
  Surgery, New York University School of Medicine,
  New York, New York
*26: Surgical Management of Femoral, Popliteal, and
Tibial Arterial Occlusive Disease*
*41: Open Surgical and Endovascular Management of
Ruptured Abdominal Aortic Aneurysm*

Kristofer M. Charlton-Ouw, MD
Assistant Professor, Department of Cardiothoracic and
  Vascular Surgery, University of Texas Medical School
  at Houston, Houston, Texas
*34: Descending Thoracic and Thoracoabdominal
Aortic Aneurysms: General Principles and Open
Surgical Repair*

Zulfiqar F. Cheema, MD
Assistant Professor, Division of Vascular Surgery and
  Endovascular Therapy, University of Texas Medical
  Branch, Galveston, Texas
46: Endovascular Approach to Vascular Trauma

Charlie C. Cheng, MD
Assistant Professor, Division of Vascular Surgery and
  Endovascular Therapy, University of Texas Medical
  Branch, Galveston, Texas
*17: Arterial Access; Guidewires, Catheters, and Sheaths;
and Balloon Angioplasty Catheters and Stents*
46: Endovascular Approach to Vascular Trauma

Jae S. Cho, MD
Professor of Surgery and Cardiothoracic Surgery, Chief
  of Vascular Surgery and Endovascular Therapy,
  Stritch School of Medicine, Loyola University,
  Maywood, Illinois
35: Endovascular Repair of Thoracic Aortic Aneurysm

Lorraine Choi, MD
Assistant Professor, Department of Vascular Surgery
  and Endovascular Therapy, University of Texas
  Medical Branch, Galveston, Texas
46: Endovascular Approach to Vascular Trauma

Anthony J. Comerota, MD, FACS, FACC
Director, Jobst Vascular Center, The Toledo Hospital,
  Toledo, Ohio; Adjunct Professor of Surgery,
  University of Michigan, Ann Arbor, Michigan
*48: Thrombolysis for Deep Venous Thrombosis and
Pulmonary Embolism*

Rachel C. Danczyk, MD
Resident, Division of Vascular Surgery, Oregon Health
  and Science University, Portland, Oregon
5: Hemostasis and Thrombosis

[†]Deceased.

Ralph G. DePalma, MD
Professor, Norman Rich Department of Surgery,
Uniformed Services University of the Health
Sciences, Bethesda, Maryland; Special Operations
Office, Office of Research and Development, U.S.
Department of Veterans Affairs, Washington, DC
*6: Atherosclerosis: Pathology, Pathogenesis, and Medical
Management*
9: Vasculogenic Erectile Dysfunction

Brian G. DeRubertis, MD
Assistant Professor in Residence, Division of Vascular
Surgery, University of California–Los Angeles
Medical Center, Los Angeles, California
*28: Infrainguinal Endovascular Reconstruction: Technique
and Results*

Matthew J. Eagleton, MD
Associate Professor of Surgery, Department of Vascular
Surgery, Cleveland Clinic Lerner College of
Medicine, Cleveland, Ohio
*37: Branched and Fenestrated Grafts for Endovascular
Thoracoabdominal Aneurysm Repair*

James M. Edwards, MD
Chief of Surgery, Portland Veterans Affairs Medical
Center, Professor of Surgery, Division of Vascular
Surgery, Oregon Health and Science University,
Portland, Oregon
7: Nonatherosclerotic Vascular Disease

Christian Eisenring, MSN, ACNP-c
Division of Cardiothoracic Surgery, Department of
Cardiothoracic Surgery, David Geffen School of
Medicine, University of California–Los Angeles,
Los Angeles, California
27: Endoscopic Harvesting of the Saphenous Vein

Sharif H. Ellozy, MD
Associate Professor of Surgery, Radiology, and Medical
Education, Division of Vascular Surgery, Mount Sinai
Medical Center, New York, New York
*58: Management of Complications After Endovascular
Abdominal Aortic Aneurysm Repair*

Anthony L. Estrera, MD, FACS
Professor, University of Texas Medical School at
Houston, Houston, Texas
*34: Descending Thoracic and Thoracoabdominal Aortic
Aneurysms: General Principles and Open Surgical Repair*

Ronald M. Fairman, MD
Professor of Surgery, University of Pennsylvania School
of Medicine, Chief of Vascular Surgery and
Endovascular Therapy, Hospital of the University of
Pennsylvania, Philadelphia, Pennsylvania
*40: Endovascular Repair of Juxtarenal (Chimney),
Infrarenal, and Iliac Artery Aneurysms*

Steven Farley, MD
Assistant Clinical Professor, Department of Vascular
Surgery, University of California–Los Angeles,
Los Angeles, California
60: The Wound Care Center and Limb Salvage

D. Preston Flanigan, MD
Director, Vascular Services, Director, Vascular
Laboratory, St. Joseph Hospital, Vascular and
Interventional Specialists of Orange County Inc.,
Orange, California
44: Aneurysms of the Peripheral Arteries

Julie Ann Freischlag, MD
Professor and Chair, Department of Surgery,
Johns Hopkins University School of Medicine,
Baltimore, Maryland
56: Prosthetic Graft Injection

Brian Funaki, MD
Professor of Radiology, Section Chief, Vascular and
Interventional Radiology, University of Chicago,
Chicago, Illinois
*23: Diagnosis and Surgical Management of the Visceral
Ischemic Syndromes*

Nitin Garg, MBBS, MPH
Assistant Professor of Surgery and Radiology, Division
of Vascular Surgery, Medical University of South
Carolina, Department of Surgery, Ralph H. Johnson
VA Medical Center, Charleston, South Carolina
49: Surgical Management of Chronic Venous Obstruction

Nicholas J. Gargiulo, MD
Associate Professor of Surgery, Hofstra School of
Medicine, North Shore–LIJ Health System,
New York, New York
*26: Surgical Management of Femoral, Popliteal, and
Tibial Arterial Occlusive Disease*

Hugh A. Gelabert, MD
Professor of Clinical Surgery, Division of Vascular
Surgery, University of California, Los Angeles
Medical Center, Los Angeles, California
*10: Primary Arterial Infections and Antibiotic
Prophylaxis*
52: Portal Hypertension

Bruce L. Gewertz, MD
Surgeon-in-Chief, Chair, Department of Surgery, Vice
President, Interventional Services; Vice Dean,
Academic Affairs, Cedars-Sinai Health System,
Los Angeles, California
*23: Diagnosis and Surgical Management of the Visceral
Ischemic Syndromes*

Racheed J. Ghanami, MD
24: Management of Renovascular Disease

David L. Gillespie, MD, RVT, FACS
Professor of Surgery, Chief, Division of Vascular
Surgery, University of Rochester, School of Medicine
and Dentistry, Rochester, New York
45: Vascular Trauma

Peter Gloviczki, MD
Joe M. and Ruth Roberts Professor of Surgery,
Consultant and Chair Emeritus, Division of Vascular
and Endovascular Surgery, Mayo Clinic, Rochester,
Minnesota
8: Vascular Malformations
*30: Thoracic and Lumbar Sympathectomy: Indications,
Technique, and Results*
49: Surgical Management of Chronic Venous Obstruction

Jerry Goldstone, MD
Professor of Surgery, Case Western Reserve University
School of Medicine, Chief Emeritus, Vascular
Surgery and Endovascular Therapy, University
Hospital Case Medical Center, Cleveland, Ohio
39: Aneurysms of the Aorta and Iliac Arteries

Antoinette S. Gomes, MD
Professor of Radiology and Medicine, Department of
Radiological Sciences/Med-Cardio, David Geffen
School of Medicine, University of California–
Los Angeles, Los Angeles, California
15: Principles of Imaging in Vascular Disease

Roy K. Greenberg, MD
Professor of Surgery and Biomedical Engineering,
Director, Endovascular Research, Department of
Vascular Surgery, Cleveland Clinic Hospital Systems,
Cleveland, Ohio
*37: Branched and Fenestrated Grafts for Endovascular
Thoracoabdominal Aneurysm Repair*

Howard P. Greisler, MD
Professor of Surgery, Professor of Cell Biology,
Neurobiology, and Anatomy, Loyola University
Medical Center, Maywood, Illinois; Research Service
and Surgical Service, Hines Veterans Affairs Hospital,
Hines, Illinois
*16: Vascular Grafts: Characteristics and Rational
Selection*

Eric Hager, MD
Assistant Professor of Surgery, Department of Vascular
Surgery, University of Pittsburgh Medical Center,
Pittsburgh, Pennsylvania
35: Endovascular Repair of Thoracic Aortic Aneurysm

Kimberley J. Hansen, MD
Professor of Surgery, Chief, Department of Vascular
and Endovascular Surgery, Division of Surgical
Sciences, Wake Forest University, Winston-Salem,
North Carolina
24: Management of Renovascular Disease

Peter K. Henke, MD
Professor of Surgery, University of Michigan,
Ann Arbor, Michigan
47: Venous Thromboembolic Disease

Kim J. Hodgson, MD
David Sumner Professor and Chairman of Vascular and
Endovascular Surgery, Southern Illinois University
School of Medicine, Springfield, Illinois
25: Endovascular Treatment of Renovascular Disease

Douglas B. Hood, MD
Associate Professor of Surgery, Southern Illinois
University School of Medicine, Springfield, Illinois
25: Endovascular Treatment of Renovascular Disease

Glenn C. Hunter, MD
Professor of Clinical Surgery, University of Arizona,
Tucson, Arizona
57: Noninfectious Complications in Vascular Surgery

Karl A. Illig, MD
Professor of Surgery, Director, Division of Vascular
Surgery, Department of Surgery, University of South
Florida College of Medicine, Tampa, Florida
*62: Carotid Sinus Stimulation: Background, Technique,
and Future Directions*

Juan Carlos Jimenez, MD, FACS
Assistant Professor of Surgery, Gonda (Goldschmied)
Vascular Center, David Geffen School of Medicine,
University of California, Los Angeles Medical
Center; Attending Surgeon Ronald Reagan Medical
Center, Olive View Medical Center, Santa Monica
Hospital, University of California, Los Angeles
Medical Center, Los Angeles, California
27: Endoscopic Harvesting of the Saphenous Vein
*38: Acute and Chronic Aortic Dissection: Medical
Management, Surgical Management, Endovascular
Management, and Results*
54: Hemodialysis and Vascular Access

Kenneth K. Kao, MD
General Surgery Resident, Division of Vascular
Surgery, University of California, Los Angeles
Medical Center, Los Angeles, California
*51: Etiology and Management of Chronic Venous
Insufficiency: Surgery, Endovenous Ablation, and
Sclerotherapy*

Vikram S. Kashyap, MD, FACS
Professor of Surgery, Case Western Reserve University;
Chief, Division of Vascular Surgery and Endovascular
Therapy; Co-Director, Harrington Heart and
Vascular Institute, University Hospitals Case Medical
Center, Cleveland, Ohio
*33: Thrombolysis for Arterial and Graft Occlusions:
Technique and Results*

Hwa Kho, PhD, MBA
Executive Vice President, Vascular Management
  Associates, Los Angeles, California
63: Building an Outpatient Intervention Suite

Melina R. Kibbe, MD
Co-Chief, Peripheral Vascular Service, Jesse Brown
  Veterans Administration Medical Center; Associate
  Professor and Vice Chair of Research, Division of
  Vascular Surgery, Northwestern University, Chicago,
  Illinois
55: Neointimal Hyperplasia

Jordan Knepper, MD
Integrated Vascular Surgery Resident, Section of
  Vascular Surgery, University of Michigan, Ann Arbor,
  Michigan
47: Venous Thromboembolic Disease

Brian S. Knipp, MD, LCDR
Vascular Fellow, School of Medicine and Dentistry;
  Naval Reserve Officer Training Command,
  Rochester University, Rochester, New York
45: Vascular Trauma

Ted R. Kohler, MD, MSc
Chief, Division of Peripheral Vascular Surgery, Puget
  Sound Health Care System; Professor of Surgery,
  Division of Vascular Surgery, University of
  Washington Medical School, Seattle, Washington
*3: Anatomy, Physiology, and Pharmacology of
the Vascular Wall*
55: Neointimal Hyperplasia

Ralf Kolvenbach, MD, PhD, FEBVS
Chief, Department of General and Vascular Surgery,
  Augusta Hospital; Professor of Vascular Surgery,
  University of Dusseldorf, Dusseldorf, Germany
*42: Laparoscopic Aortic Surgery for Aneurysm and
Occlusive Disease: Technique and Results*

Toshifumi Kudo, MD
*31: Thoracic Outlet Syndrome and Vascular Disease
of the Upper Extremity*

Andrew K. Kurklinsky, MD
Assistant Professor of Medicine, Division of
  Cardiovascular Medicine, Mayo Clinic, Jacksonville,
  Florida
53: Lymphedema

Mario Lachat, MD, FECTS, FEBVS
Professor and Head of Vascular Surgery, Clinic for
  Cardiovascular Surgery, University Hospital of
  Zurich, Zurich, Switzerland
*41: Open Surgical and Endovascular Management of
Ruptured Abdominal Aortic Aneurysm*

Gregory J. Landry, MD
Associate Professor of Surgery, Division of Vascular
  Surgery, Oregon Health and Science University,
  Portland, Oregon
7: Nonatherosclerotic Vascular Disease
*32: Natural History and Nonoperative Treatment of
Chronic Lower Extremity Ischemia*

Peter F. Lawrence, MD
Professor and Chief, Division of Vascular Surgery,
  University of California–Los Angeles, Los Angeles,
  California
60: The Wound Care Center and Limb Salvage

Wesley Kwan Lew, MD
Vascular Surgeon, Kaiser Foundation Hospital–Sunset,
  Kaiser Permanente Medical Group, Los Angeles,
  California
*36: Combined Endovascular and Surgical (Hybrid)
Approach to Aortic Arch and Thoracoabdominal Aortic
Pathology*

Timothy K. Liem, MD
Associate Professor of Surgery, Division of Vascular
  Surgery; Vice-Chair for Quality, Department of
  Surgery, Oregon Health and Science University,
  Portland, Oregon
5: Hemostasis and Thrombosis

Evan C. Lipsitz, MD
Associate Professor of Surgery; Chief, Division of
  Vascular and Endovascular Surgery, Department of
  Cardiovascular and Thoracic Surgery, Montefiore
  Medical Center and the Albert Einstein College of
  Medicine, Bronx, New York
*26: Surgical Management of Femoral, Popliteal, and
Tibial Arterial Occlusive Disease*

Michel S. Makaroun, MD
Co-Director, UPMC Heart and Valve Institute;
  Professor and Chair, Division of Vascular Surgery,
  University of Pittsburgh School of Medicine,
  Pittsburgh, Pennsylvania
35: Endovascular Repair of Thoracic Aortic Aneurysm

Tara M. Mastracci, MD
Assistant Professor of Surgery, Department of
  Vascular Surgery, Cleveland Clinic Foundation,
  Cleveland, Ohio
*37: Branched and Fenestrated Grafts for Endovascular
Thoracoabdominal Aneurysm Repair*

Jon S. Matsumura, MD
Professor and Chair, Division of Vascular Surgery,
  Department of Surgery, University of Wisconsin
  School of Medicine and Public Health, Madison,
  Wisconsin
*40: Endovascular Repair of Juxtarenal (Chimney),
Infrarenal, and Iliac Artery Aneurysms*

David S. Maxwell, MD[†]
2: Embryology of the Vascular System

Dieter Mayer, MD, FEBVS, FAPWCA
Assistant Professor of Vascular Surgery, Clinic for
 Cardiovascular Surgery, University Hospital of
 Zurich, Zurich, Switzerland
*41: Open Surgical and Endovascular Management of
Ruptured Abdominal Aortic Aneurysm*

James F. McKinsey, MD
*23: Diagnosis and Surgical Management of the Visceral
Ischemic Syndromes*

Louis M. Messina, MD
Professor and Chief, Division of Vascular Surgery;
 Vice-Chair, Department of Surgery, University of
 Massachusetts Medical School, UMass Memorial
 Health Care, Worcester, Massachusetts
43: Splanchnic and Renal Artery Aneurysms

Charles C. Miller III, PhD
Professor and Chair, Department of Biomedical
 Sciences, Paul L. Foster School of Medicine, Texas
 Tech University, El Paso, Texas
*34: Descending Thoracic and Thoracoabdominal Aortic
Aneurysms: General Principles and Open Surgical Repair*

Joseph L. Mills, Sr., MD
Professor of Surgery; Chief, Division of Vascular and
 Endovascular Surgery; Co-Director, Southern
 Arizona Limb Salvage Alliance, Department of
 Surgery, University of Arizona Health Sciences
 Center, Tucson, Arizona
*29: Endovascular Therapy for Infrapopliteal Arterial
Occlusive Disease*

Erica L. Mitchell, MD
Associate Professor of Surgery; Program Director for
 Vascular Surgery, Division of Vascular Surgery;
 Associate Medical Director for VirtuOHSU, Surgical
 Simulation, Oregon Health and Science University,
 Portland, Oregon
*32: Natural History and Nonoperative Treatment of
Chronic Lower Extremity Ischemia*

Gregory L. Moneta, MD
Professor and Chief, Division of Vascular Surgery,
 Oregon Health and Science University, Portland,
 Oregon
*32: Natural History and Nonoperative Treatment of
Chronic Lower Extremity Ischemia*

Wesley S. Moore, MD
Professor and Chief Emeritus, Division of Vascular
 Surgery, University of California, Los Angeles
 Medical Center, Los Angeles, California
*18: Extracranial Cerebrovascular Disease:
The Carotid Artery*
55: Neointimal Hyperplasia

Matthew M. Nalbandian, MD
Clinical Assistant Professor of Surgery and
 Orthopedics, New York University, Langone Medical
 Center, New York, New York
*61: Spine Exposure: Operative Techniques for the Vascular
Surgeon*

William B. Newton III, MD
24: Management of Renovascular Disease

Tina T. Ng, MD
*23: Diagnosis and Surgical Management of the Visceral
Ischemic Syndromes*

Andrea Obi, MD
Resident in Surgery, Department of General Surgery,
 University of Michigan, Ann Arbor, Michigan
47: Venous Thromboembolic Disease

Jessica B. O'Connell, MD
Associate Director, Surgical and Perioperative Careline;
 Co-Chief, Vascular Surgery Service VA Greater Los
 Angeles Healthcare System; Assistant Clinical
 Professor, University of California–Los Angeles
 Gonda (Goldschmied) Vascular Center, Los Angeles,
 California
*12: Medical Management of Vascular Disease Including
Pharmacology of Drugs Used in Vascular Disease
Management*

Christopher D. Owens, MD
Assistant Professor, Department of Vascular and
 Endovascular Surgery, University of California–
 San Francisco, San Francisco, California
21: Surgical Management of Aortoiliac Occlusive Disease

Madhukar S. Patel, MD
Orange, California
54: Hemodialysis and Vascular Access

Charles M. Peterson, MD, MBA
Senior Scientist, Telemedicine and Advanced
 Technology Research Center, U.S. Army Medical
 Research and Tateriel Command, Potomac,
 Maryland
*11: Influence of Diabetes Mellitus on Vascular Disease and
Its Complications*

William J. Quiñones-Baldrich, MD
Professor of Surgery, Division of Vascular Surgery;
 Director, UCLA Aortic Center, University of
 California, Los Angeles Medical Center,
 Los Angeles, California
*33: Thrombolysis for Arterial and Graft Occlusions:
Technique and Results*
*36: Combined Endovascular and Surgical (Hybrid)
Approach to Aortic Arch and Thoracoabdominal Aortic
Pathology*

[†]Deceased.

Seshadri Raju, MD
Professor Emeritus of Surgery; Director, The Rane
Center, River Oaks Hospital, Jackson, Mississippi
50: Endovascular Repair of Chronic Venous Obstruction

John Rectenwald, MD, MS
Associate Professor of Surgery, Department of Surgery,
Section of Vascular Surgery, University of Michigan,
Ann Arbor, Michigan
47: Venous Thromboembolic Disease

Todd D. Reil, MD
Associate Professor of Surgery; Director of
Endovascular Surgery, Department of Surgery
University of Minnesota, Minneapolis, Minnesota
*12: Medical Management of Vascular Disease Including
Pharmacology of Drugs Used in Vascular Disease
Management*

David A. Rigberg, MD
Associate Clinical Professor of Surgery, Division of
Vascular Surgery, University of California–
Los Angeles Medical Center, Los Angeles, California
*51: Etiology and Management of Chronic Venous
Insufficiency: Surgery, Endovenous Ablation, and
Sclerotherapy*
52: Portal Hypertension

Lee C. Rogers, DPM
Co-Director, Amputation Prevention Center, Valley
Presbyterian Hospital, Los Angeles, California
59: The Diabetic Foot

Thom W. Rooke, MD
Professor of Vascular Medicine, Gonda Vascular
Center, Mayo Clinic, Rochester, Minnesota
53: Lymphedema

Carlos A. Rueda, MD
Vascular Surgeon, Colorado Cardiovascular Surgical
Associates, Denver, Colorado
*22: Angioplasty and Stenting for Aortoiliac Disease:
Technique and Results*

Hazim J. Safi, MD
Professor and Chairman, Department of Cardiothoracic
and Vascular Surgery, University of Texas Medical
School at Houston, Houston, Texas
*34: Descending Thoracic and Thoracoabdominal Aortic
Aneurysms: General Principles and Open Surgical Repair*

Peter A. Schneider, MD
Chief, Division of Vascular Therapy, Kaiser Foundation
Hospital, Kaiser Permanente Medical Group,
Honolulu, Hawaii
*17: Arterial Access; Guidewires, Catheters, and Sheaths;
and Balloon Angioplasty Catheters and Stents*
*20: Endovascular Repair of Extracranial Cerebrovascular
Lesions*
*28: Infrainguinal Endovascular Reconstruction: Technique
and Results*

Lewis B. Schwartz, MD
Section of Vascular Surgery and Endovascular Therapy,
University of Chicago, Chicago, Illinois
*23: Diagnosis and Surgical Management of the Visceral
Ischemic Syndromes*

Michael B. Silva, Jr., MD
The Fred J. and Dorothy E. Wolma Professor in
Vascular Surgery; Chief and Program Director,
Division of Vascular Surgery and Endovascular
Therapy; Director, Texas Vascular Center Professor
in Radiology, University of Texas Medical Branch,
Galveston, Texas
*17: Arterial Access; Guidewires, Catheters, and Sheaths;
and Balloon Angioplasty Catheters and Stents*
46: Endovascular Approach to Vascular Trauma

Daniel Silverberg, MD
Senior Consultant, Department of Vascular Surgery,
The Chaim Sheba Medical Center, Tel Hashomer,
Israel
*58: Management of Complications After Endovascular
Abdominal Aortic Aneurysm Repair*

James C. Stanley, MD
Professor of Surgery; Director, Cardiovascular Center,
University of Michigan Medical School, Ann Arbor,
Michigan
43: Splanchnic and Renal Artery Aneurysms

D. Eugene Strandness, Jr., MD†
13: Hemodynamics for the Vascular Surgeon

Gale L. Tang, MD
Assistant Professor, Division of Vascular Surgery,
University of Washington, Puget Sound Veterans
Administration Medical Center, Seattle, Washington
*3: Anatomy, Physiology, and Pharmacology of
the Vascular Wall*

Frank Vandy, MD
Integrated Vascular Surgery Resident, Section of
Vascular Surgery, University of Michigan Health
System, Ann Arbor, Michigan
47: Venous Thromboembolic Disease

Frank J. Veith, MD
Professor of Vascular Surgery, New York University
Medical Center; Professor of Surgery, William J. von
Liebig Chair in Vascular Surgery, Cleveland Clinic,
Riverdale, New York
*26: Surgical Management of Femoral, Popliteal, and
Tibial Arterial Occlusive Disease*
*41: Open Surgical and Endovascular Management of
Ruptured Abdominal Aortic Aneurysm*

†Deceased.

Thomas W. Wakefield, MD
Professor of Surgery; Head, Section of Vascular
  Surgery, University of Michigan Medical School,
  Ann Arbor, Michigan
  47: Venous Thromboembolic Disease

Grace J. Wang, MD
Assistant Professor of Surgery, Division of Vascular
  Surgery and Endovascular Therapy, Hospital of
  the University of Pennsylvania, Philadelphia,
  Pennsylvania
  *40: Endovascular Repair of Juxtarenal (Chimney),
  Infrarenal, and Iliac Artery Aneurysms*

Alex Westerband, MD
Vascular Surgery, Northwest Allied Physicians, Tucson,
  Arizona
  57: Noninfectious Complications in Vascular Surgery

Matthew L. White, MD
Vascular Surgeon, Division of Vascular Surgery,
  The Iowa Clinic, West Des Moines, Iowa
  *29: Endovascular Therapy for Infrapopliteal Arterial
  Occlusive Disease*

Samuel E. Wilson, MD
Professor, Department of Surgery, University of
  California–Irvine, Orange, California
  54: Hemodialysis and Vascular Access

Gerald B. Zelenock, MD
Professor and Chairman, Department of Surgery,
  University of Toledo College of Medicine, Toledo,
  Ohio
  43: Splanchnic and Renal Artery Aneurysms

R. Eugene Zierler, MD
Professor of Surgery, University of Washington School
  of Medicine, Medical Director, D.E. Strandness Jr.
  Vascular Laboratory, University of Washington
  Medical Center and Harborview Medical Center,
  Seattle, Washington
  13: Hemodynamics for the Vascular Surgeon

PREFACE TO THE EIGHTH EDITION

The eighth edition has been completely revised and the chapters have been organized under sections. These sections include general principles, arterial occlusive disease, arterial aneurysm disease, venous disease, complications, and miscellaneous topics. The signature chapters, organized under sections, remain. The signature chapter authors have fully updated their material. In recognition of the continuing expansion of endovascular technology as well as medical management, new chapters have been added. These include medical management of vascular disease, endoscopic harvest of saphenous veins, endovascular repair of infrapopliteal arteries, nonoperative treatment of lower extremity ischemia, endovascular repair of thoracic aneurysm, the hybrid appoach to aortic arch and thoracoabdominal aneurysm, fenestrated and branched endograft repair, management of acute and chronic aortic dissection, the use of chimney in endovascular repair of aneurysms, open and endovascular repair of ruptured aneurysm, laparoscopic aortic surgery, endovascular management of vascular trauma, surgical management of chronic venous obstruction, endovascular repair of chronic venous obstruction, complications of endovascular surgery, the diabetic foot, management of hypertension with carotid sinus stimulation, and finally a new chapter describing the building and operation of an outpatient interventional suite.

In summary, we have a completely revised and up-to-date volume directed to the comprehensive management of patients with vascular disorders.

Wesley S. Moore, MD

PREFACE TO THE FIRST EDITION

During the past 20 years of rapid growth and development in vascular surgery, many graduates of general surgery programs found that their training in vascular surgery represented a valuable new resource for their hospital and practice communities. That training in vascular surgery often provided an important edge in establishing a new practice and led to the widespread use of the term general and vascular surgery on the community announcements and business cards of new surgeons.

Yet in 1969, a survey conducted by a committee composed of James A. DeWeese, F. William Blaisdell, and John H. Foster discovered that among the 83 residents graduating from the 22 general surgery training programs surveyed, only 19 had performed more than 40 arterial reconstructive procedures during the course of their training, and more than half of the graduating residents had performed fewer than 20 arterial reconstructive procedures. The DeWeese committee, which had been established in 1969 to develop a document on optimal resources in vascular surgery, thus concluded that there was considerable suboptimal vascular surgery being performed in the United States, owing to a combination of both inadequate training and continued deficiencies in vascular surgery experience following training. A survey of the frequency of vascular operations in 1143 hospitals across the United States had revealed that in over 75% of these hospitals, fewer than 10 aneurysm resections and 10 femoropopliteal arterial reconstructions were conducted annually. This discovery led to the unfortunate conclusion that many surgeons were performing only occasional vascular operations, often leading to poor results.

The substance of the DeWeese report was reviewed by the two national vascular societies and their responsible leadership. This paved the way for, among other things, the definition of adequate training in vascular surgery and the recommendation that physicians who wish to practice vascular surgery spend an additional year of training to guarantee adequate experience in the speciality. To ensure prospective candidates that a given fellowship program in vascular surgery would provide a broad and responsible experience, the vascular societies established a committee for program evaluation and endorsements from which program directors could request review. Programs reviewed and found to meet the criteria of appropriate education as established by the committee would be announced annually.

Program evaluation by the joint council of the two national vascular societies was taken on as a temporary responsibility because the role would ultimately become the purview of the Residency Review Committee and the Liaison Committee for Graduate Medical Education. It was recognized that once adequate training programs were developed, the certification of candidates successfully completing training rested with the American Board of Surgery.

After approximately 10 years of experience, debate, and review, the American Board of Medical Specialties approved an application by the American Board of Surgery to grant "Certification of Special Competence in General Vascular Surgery." The first examination for certification was given to qualified members of the American Board of Surgery and Thoracic Surgery in June 1982. The second written examination was held in November 1983 in several centers across the United States.

The intent of this textbook is to provide a comprehensive review of vascular surgery, together with the related medical and basic science disciplines. This edition of the text has been developed to accompany a postgraduate course designed to help candidates prepare for the examination leading to certification in general vascular surgery. Accordingly, a list of questions designed to aid the reader in self-examination completes each chapter. All question sets simply represent the authors' opinion, a fair and adequate survey of the material covered, as none of the chapter authors is a member of the American Board of Surgery (this would be a conflict of interest).

Although chapter outlines were suggested by an editorial committee, the final chapter test represents, in the opinion of its authors, core material in each subject. Particular effort to identify and separate generally accepted concepts from new or controversial material was made. Although this book was designed as a comprehensive review to prepare for an examination, it is also in view of its organization and content, a comprehensive text of vascular surgery.

Wesley S. Moore, MD

Contents

VIDEO CONTENTS

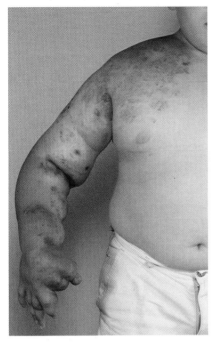

PLATE 8-6 ■ Diffuse extratruncular venous malformation involving the right arm. (Courtesy David J. Driscoll, MD, Mayo Foundation).

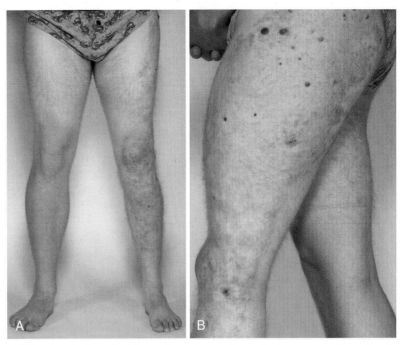

PLATE 8-10 ■ In Servelle-Martorell syndrome, the typical venous malformation is extratruncular and diffuse. The affected extremity is shorter, there are phleboliths present on plain radiographs, and there is no arteriovenous shunting. Spontaneous bone fracture and osteopenia is frequent. Usually there are no port-wine stains. (Courtesy David J. Driscoll, MD, Mayo Foundation).

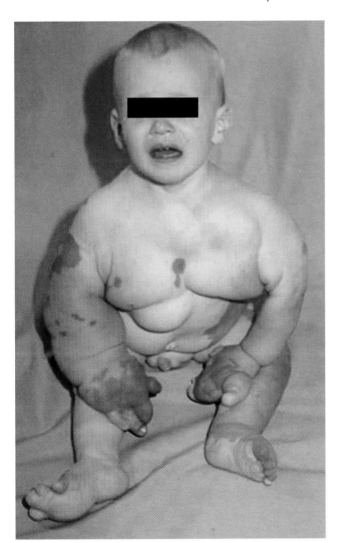

PLATE 8-11 ■ Patient with Proteus syndrome consisting of disproportionate overgrowth of multiple tissues, vascular malformations, and connective tissue or linear epidermal nevi. The patient had multiple lipomas and hyperostosis. (Courtesy David J. Driscoll, MD, Mayo Foundation).

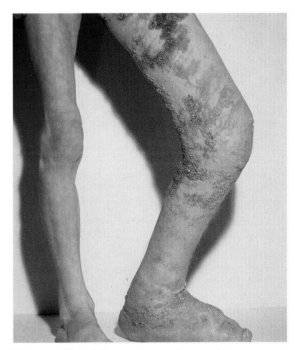

PLATE 8-12 ■ Klippel-Trenaunay syndrome with overgrowth of the left lower extremity by 12 cm.

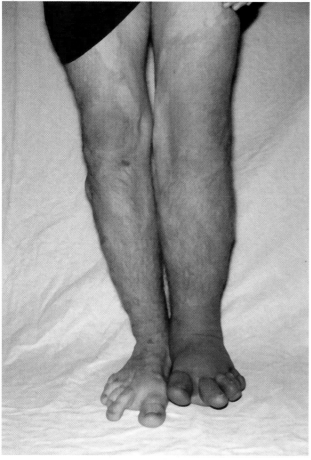

PLATE 8-13 ■ Klippel-Trenaunay syndrome with involvement of both lower extremities. Note the port-wine stain and digital anomalies.

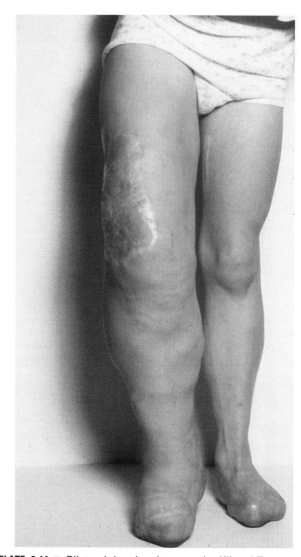

PLATE 8-14 ■ Bilateral leg involvement in Klippel-Trenaunay syndrome. Bilateral transmetatarsal amputations were needed because of digital anomalies.

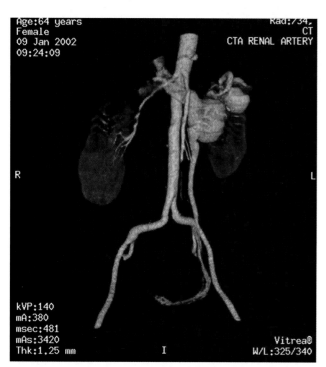

PLATE 8-18 ■ Three-dimensional computed tomographic reconstruction of a venous malformation involving the left renal vein and the hilum of the left kidney. (Courtesy Terri J. Vrtiska, MD, Mayo Foundation).

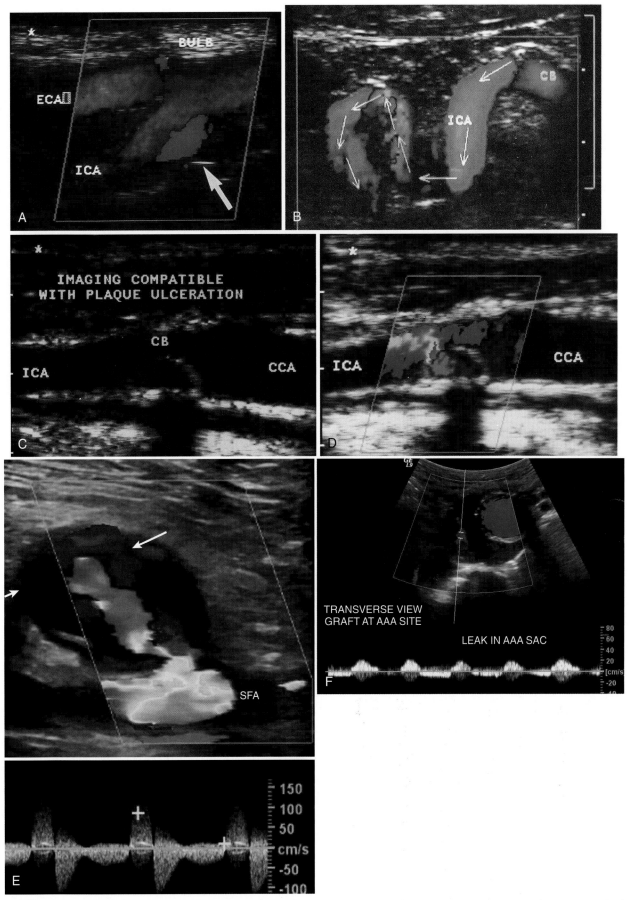

PLATE 14-5 ■ **A,** Advantages of using color duplex scanning. Normal carotid bifurcation, illustrating the reverse flow occuring in the bulb during peak systole *(arrow)*. **B,** Marked tortuosity of internal carotid artery *(ICA)* is easily demonstrated with color scan. **C,** Conventional gray-scale image does not provide clear identification of large ulcer. **D,** Blood flow within plaque confirms the ulcer. **E,** Pseudoaneurysm originating from the superficial femoral artery *(SFA)* resulting from catheterization. Note the bidirectional flow recorded in the neck. **F,** Type 2 endoleak with flow detected in the aneurysm sac outside of prosthesis.

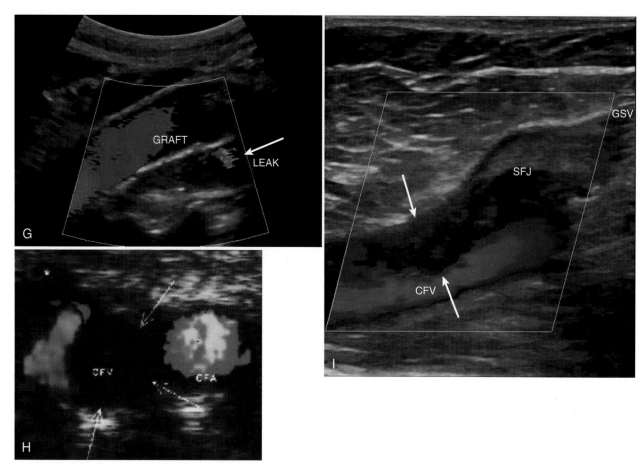

PLATE 14-5, cont'd ■ **G,** Longitudinal view of same aorta showing leak is posterior to graft. **H,** Blood flow around partial occluding thrombus. **I,** Thrombus extending into common femoral vein, seen 2 days after endovascular ablation of great saphenous vein.

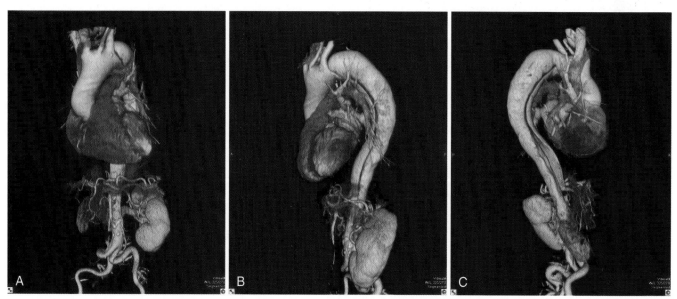

PLATE 15-13 ■ Multidetector row helical computed tomography angiography of acute aortic dissection on 16-row multislice computed tomography CT scanner. Three dimensional volume rendered images of type B aortic dissection showing the intimal flap and the true and false lumens. Note the clear delineation of the origins of the major branch vessels.

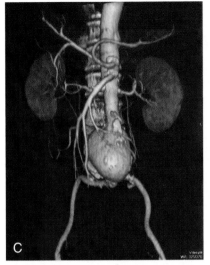 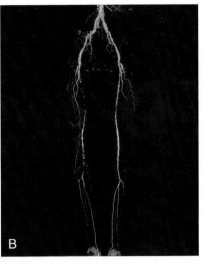 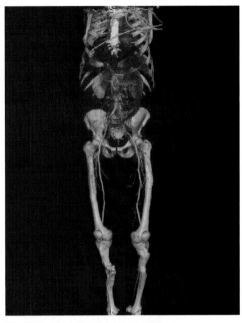

PLATE 15-14 ■ Multidetector row helical computed tomography angiography of infrarenal abdominal aortic aneurysm. **C,** Partial removal of bone shows the renal arteries and superior mesenteric artery branches.

PLATE 15-18 ■ Multidetector row helical computed tomography angiography of peripheral runoff. **B,** Three-dimensional volume rendering may also be performed.

PLATE 15-19 ■ Total-body magnetic resonance angiography. Imaging of the entire body is possible using 16- or 64-row MDCT scanners. Extensive postprocessing is required to remove bone and soft tissue.

Quick Endotheliazation and Gradual Absorption

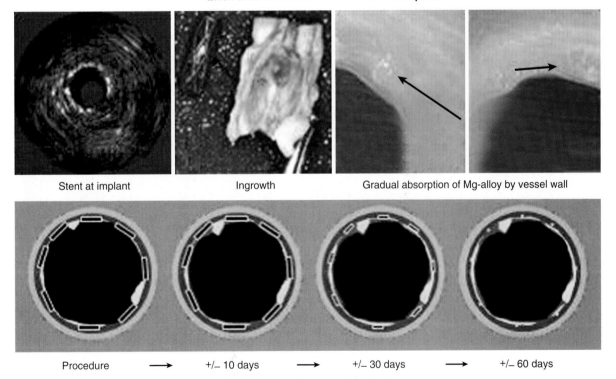

Stent at implant   Ingrowth   Gradual absorption of Mg-alloy by vessel wall

Procedure → +/− 10 days → +/− 30 days → +/− 60 days

PLATE 17-29 ■ Biodegradable stent.

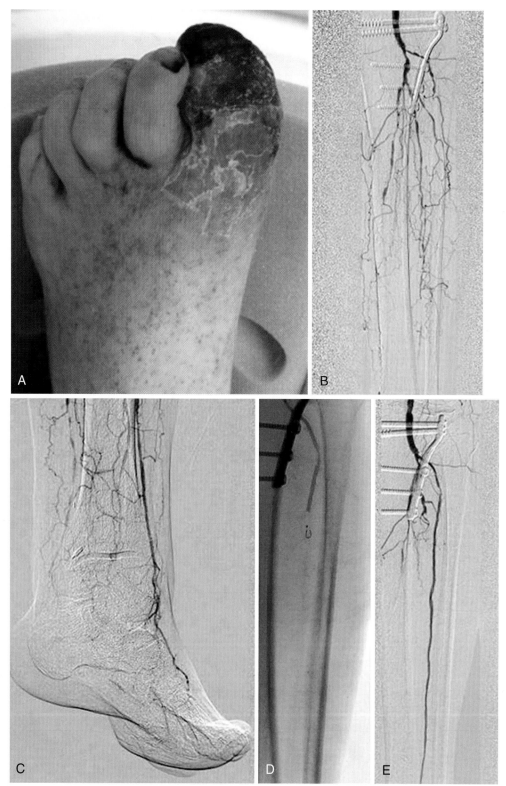

PLATE 29-2 ■ A 77-year-old high-risk patient with diabetes and great toe gangrene. **A,** Critical limb ischemia with ankle-brachial index (ABI) of 0.39. **B,** Three-vessel long-segment (>25 cm) tibial artery occlusions, with **(C)** distal anterior tibial artery reconstitution. **D,** Subintimal angioplasty of long-segment occlusion. **E,** Anterior tibial artery after long-segment subintimal angioplasty with ABI improved to 0.81. Toe amputation healed and the vessel remains patent 6 months after intervention.

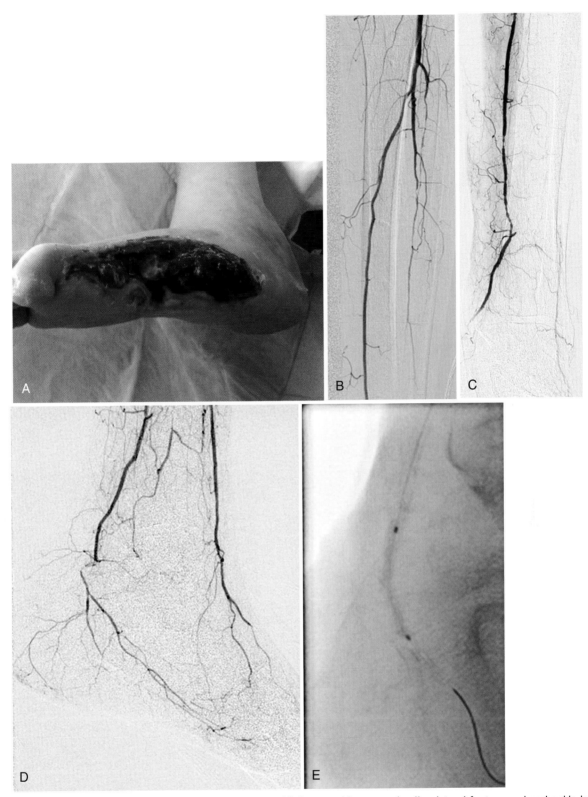

PLATE 29-3 ■ **A,** A 67-year-old frail patient with diabetes; renal failure; and large, nonhealing lateral foot wound and ankle-brachial index (ABI) of 0.71 after angioplasty of the superficial femoral artery owing to long-segment tibial disease. **B,** Angiogram with catheter placed in popliteal artery shows patent posterior tibial artery proximally. **C,** Multiple distal posterior tibial artery stenoses. **D,** Calcified, total inframalleolar posterior tibial artery occlusion and severe angulation. **E,** 2 mm × 2 cm balloon angioplasty of tibial occlusion.

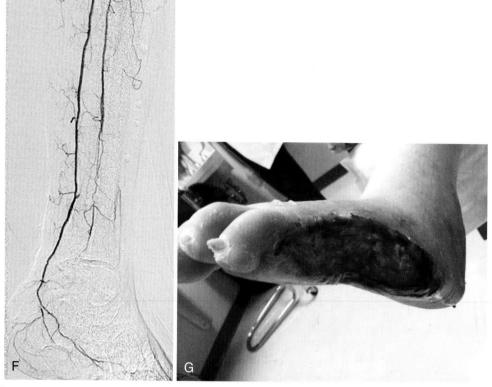

PLATE 29-3, cont'd ■ **F,** Posterior tibial artery with continuous flow into the foot after 2.5 mm angioplasty of the distal posterior tibial artery and 2 mm angioplasty of the inframalleolar posterior tibial occlusion. **G,** ABI improved to 1.01 with good wound granulation after repeated debridement.

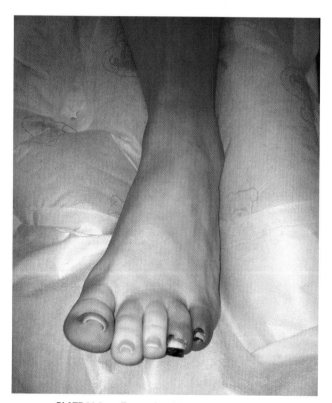

PLATE 34-3 ■ Example of blue toe syndrome.

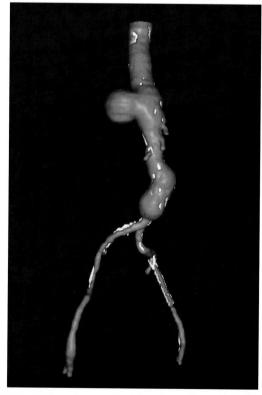

PLATE 34-4 ■ Three-dimensional reconstruction of saccular thoracoabdominal aortic aneurysm extent V before repair. Note the aneurysm proximity to the celiac artery, the presence of a left iliac stent, and a synchronous infrarenal abdominal aortic aneurysm.

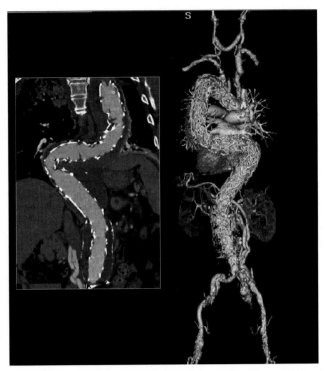

PLATE 36-1 ■ Type II thoracoabdominal aortic aneurysm with partial aortic arch debranching and visceral debranching. The aortic stent graft spans nearly the entire aorta, from distal to the innominate artery to above the aortic bifurcation.

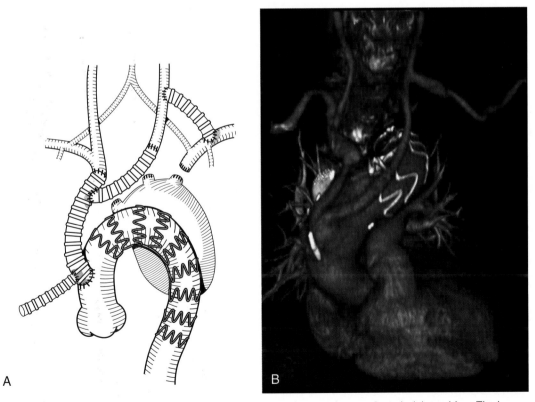

A

B

PLATE 36-5 ■ Schematic **(A)** and three-dimensional **(B)** reconstruction of a complete aortic arch debranching. The bypass graft originates off the ascending aorta to right innominate and left carotid artery. A left carotid to subclavian artery bypass can also be seen. In the schematic there is a conduit off the ascending aortic graft.

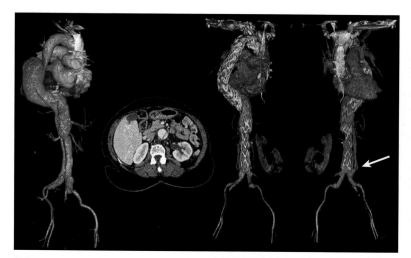

PLATE 36-8 ■ Aneurysmal degeneration of a type B dissection resulting in a type I thoracoabdominal aortic aneurysm *(left)*. The infrarenal aorta is not aneurysmal *(middle)*, allowing for replacement of the infrarenal aorta with an aortoiliac graft onto which a bypass graft *(arrow)* originates and provides the distal endograft seal zone *(right)*.

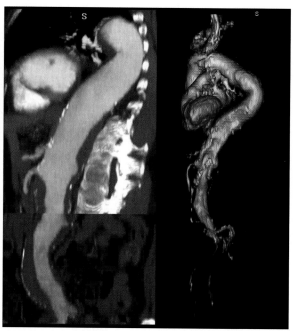

PLATE 36-9 ■ Type II thoracoabdominal aneurysm. Entire aorta is aneurysmal without a spared segment for a hybrid repair.

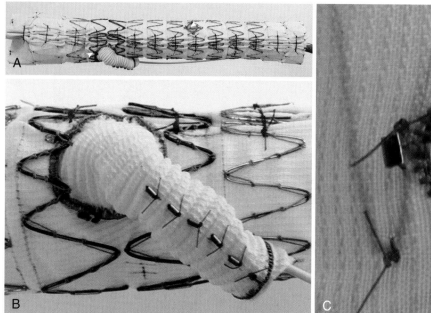

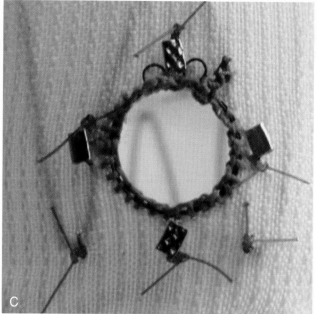

PLATE 37-2 ■ **A,** Custom-designed main body device tethered to the delivery system demonstrating branch fenestrations for the renal arteries and a helical branch providing antegrade perfusion of the celiac artery. **B,** The helical branch is an 8-mm polyester graft sewn to the aortic prosthesis above the target vessel. These directional branches provide long regions (2 cm) of overlap, allowing mating of a self-expanding stent-graft (Fluency) sized to the visceral vessel. The helical branch construct provides a more secure seal into both the mating vessel and the aortic component given the extensive potential for overlap with both sealing regions, resulting in a reduced tendency to develop endoleaks or component separation. **C,** The fenestrated branch is a nitinol-reinforced opening in the main body device that is sized and aligned with the target vessel ostium. This is mated with a balloon-expandable stent-graft lumen, and the aortic portion is subsequently flared with a compliant balloon to achieve a seal around the fenestration. (From Soltesz EG, Greenberg RK: Endovascular repair of thoracoabdominal aortic aneurysms with fenestrated-branched stent-grafts. Operative Techniques Thorac Cardiovasc Surg 15:86–99, 2010.)

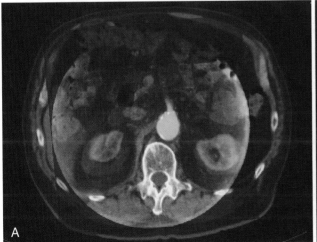

PLATE 37-4 ■ Accurate planning and construction of the custom-designed branched thoracoabdominal stent-graft require detailed computerized three-dimensional modeling to provide a 360-degree view of the aortoiliac and visceral branch anatomy. Centerline-of-flow analysis allows the surgeon to generate a straightened image of the aorta and assess the precise angle of visceral branches as well as the distance between branches **(A)**. Orthogonal slices through the centerline-of-flow provide measurements that are then used for branched stent-graft construction. These reference points are usually described as a location from the origin as noted on a clock face **(B, C)**. *SMA,* Superior mesenteric artery. (From Soltesz EG, Greenberg RK: Endovascular repair of thoracoabdominal aortic aneurysms with fenestrated-branched stent-grafts. Operative Techniques Thorac Cardiovasc Surg 15:86–99, 2010.)

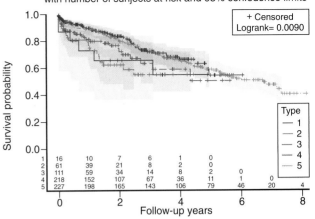

Product-limit survival estimates
with number of sunjects at risk and 95% confedence limits

+ Censored
Logrank= 0.0090

1	16	10	7	6	1	0		
2	61	39	21	8	2	0		
3	111	59	34	14	8	2	0	
4	218	152	107	67	36	11	1	0
5	227	198	165	143	106	79	46	20	4

CCF categories	Baseline	1m	6m	1y	2y	3y	4y	5y	6y
Type 1	16	14	14	10	9	6	1	0	0
Type 2	61	58	50	42	25	13	3	0	0
Type 3	111	109	90	68	50	21	11	4	1
Type 4	218	212	189	164	129	85	51	20	4
Fen repair	227	190	180	166	148	117	88	58	22

PLATE 37-6 ■ Life table analyses with 95% confidence intervals were constructed for each type of aneurysm treated (type I, II, III, IV, and juxtarenal). *Curve 5* indicates the survival curve for juxtarenal aneurysms. *CCF,* Cleveland Clinic Foundation. (From Greenberg RK, Eatleton MJ, Mastracci TM: Branched endografts for thoracoabdominal aneurysms. J Thorac Cardiovasc Surg 140:S171–S178, 2010.)

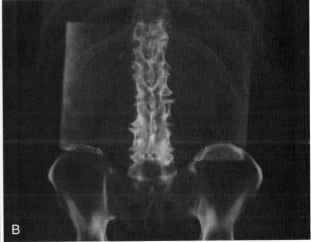

PLATE 37-5 ■ Images depicting the fusion of the cone-beam computed tomography (CBCT) performed before stent-graft introduction. The colored images represent those of the preoperative multidetector computed tomography (MDCT), and the grayscale images are the ones obtained from the CBCT. The images are aligned in multiple planes including axial **(A)**, anterior **(B)**, and lateral (not shown). Once the scans are registered, or fused, with each other, the images from the MDCT can be overlaid on the live fluoroscopic image. (From Dijkstra ML, Eagleton MJ, Greenberg RK, et al. Intraoperative C-arm cone-beam computed tomography in fenestrated aortic endografting: a preliminary experience. J Vasc Surg 53:583–590, 2011.)

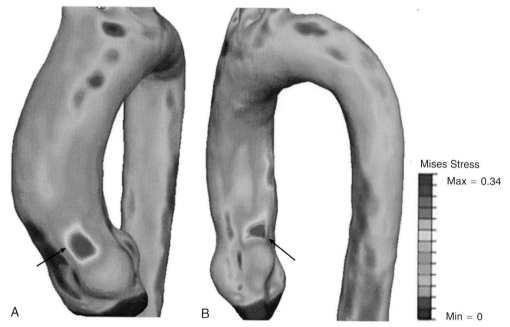

PLATE 38-3 ■ Three-dimensional wall stress distribution for the normal ascending aorta. The black arrows indicate maxima of stress on the convex **(A)** and concave **(B)** sides of the ascending aorta. (From Nathan DP, Xu C, Gorman III JH, et al: Pathogenesis of acute aortic dissection: a finite element stress analysis. Ann Thorac Surg 91:458–464, 2011.)

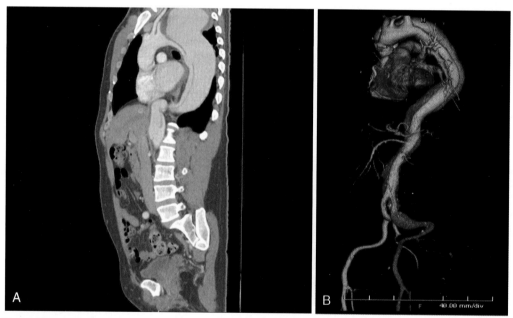

PLATE 38-4 ■ Three-dimensional reconstruction following computed tomography for aortic dissection delineates the complex anatomy of this disease process.

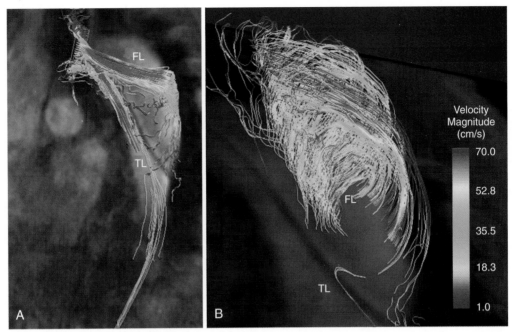

PLATE 38-5 ■ Streamline visualization shows **(A)** parasagittal view of blood flow in the true and false lumen and **(B)** a double-oblique view of blood flow in the false lumen distal to the primary entry. (From Müller-Eschner M, Rengier F, Partovi S, et al: Tridirectional phase-contrast magnetic resonance velocity mapping depicts severe hemodynamic alterations in a patient with aortic dissection type Stanford B. J Vasc Surg 54:559–562, 2011.)

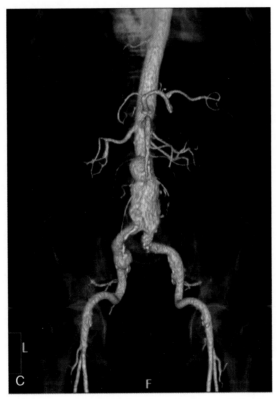

PLATE 39-3 ■ **C,** Three dimensional reconstruction, anteroposterior view, showing only the flow channel. Note the irregular aneurysm shape.

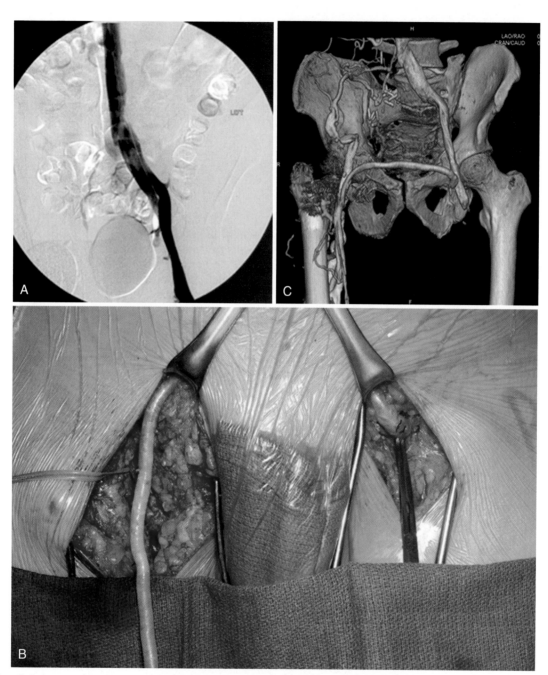

PLATE 49-1 ■ Palma procedure in a 38-year-old male with postthrombotic syndrome. **A,** Chronic right iliofemoral obstruction after multiple failed attempts at endovenous recanalization. **B,** A right-to-left femoral vein bypass with left GSV (Palma procedure). **C,** Follow-up computed tomographic venogram at 2 months. (**A-C,** From Garg N, Gloviczki P, Karimi KM, et al: Factors affecting outcome of open and hybrid reconstructions for nonmalignant obstruction of iliofemoral veins and inferior vena cava. J Vasc Surg 53:383–393, 2011.)

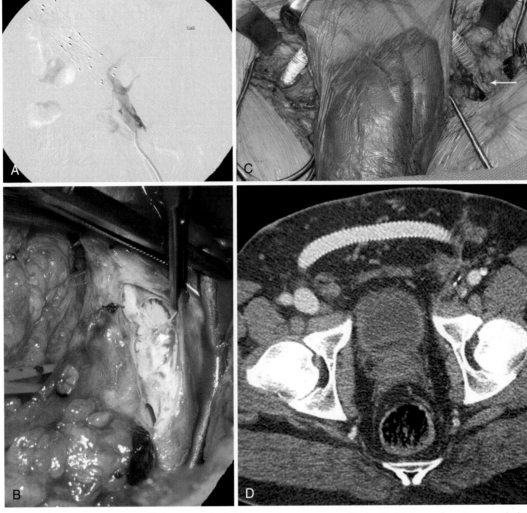

PLATE 49-2 ■ Femoro-femoral crossover (Palma prosthetic) bypass in a young patient with history of posttraumatic left iliofemoral deep venous thrombosis and chronic venous ulceration. **A,** Venogram demonstrating occluded venous stent that could not be recanalized. **B,** Chronic scarring and postthrombotic changes in the left CFV. **C,** Left-to-right femoral vein bypass with 12 mm externally supported polytetrafluoroethylene (prosthetic Palma procedure), with a left SFA to graft AV fistula *(arrow)*. **D,** Computed tomographic venogram preformed at 1 year demonstrated a patent bypass. (**A to D,** From Garg N, Gloviczki P, Karimi KM, et al: Factors affecting outcome of open and hybrid reconstructions for nonmalignant obstruction of iliofemoral veins and inferior vena cava. J Vasc Surg 53:383–393, 2011.)

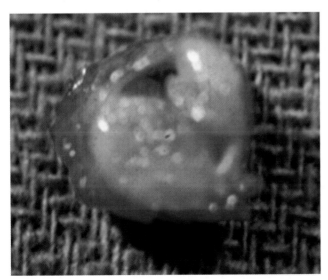

PLATE 50-7 ■ Transverse section of a postthrombotic vein. The guidewire is threaded through these small channels in the trabeculated vein during the recanalization procedure.

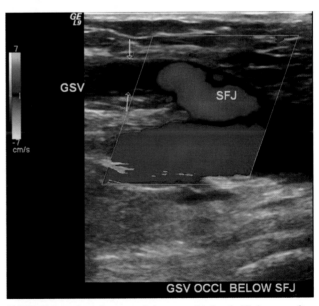

PLATE 51-1 ■ An ultrasound image obtained 48 hours after endovenous ablation of the great saphenous vein (GSV) is shown. The GSV is occluded, as evidenced by the lack of color flow. The saphenofemoral junction is patent, and clearly there is no involvement with the common femoral vein (blue flow on scan).

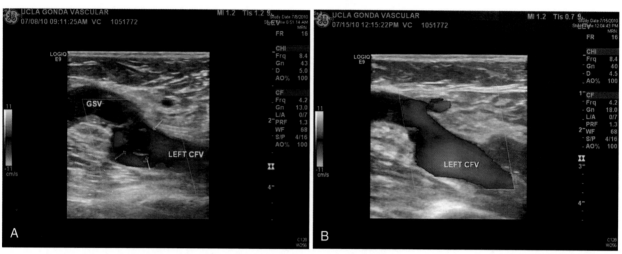

PLATE 51-3 ■ **A,** Initial scan after radiofrequency ablation demonstrates thrombus extending into the common femoral vein. This patient was given enoxaparin (Lovenox), and the scan was repeated 1 week later. **B,** Note the complete retraction of the thrombus and patency of the epigastric vein on the follow up scan. Lovenox was stopped after the second scan demonstrated an appropriate level of closure. Of note, most patients with level 4 and 5 closures do not have postprocedure symptoms that differ from patients with closure levels of 3 or less.

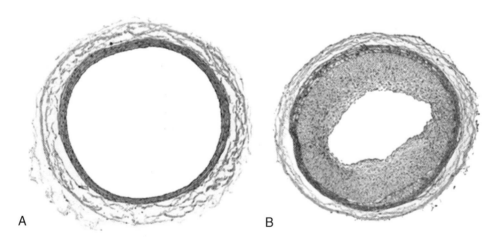

PLATE 55-2 ■ **A,** Cross-section of a rat carotid artery. **B,** Cross-section of a rat carotid artery two weeks after ballon injury.

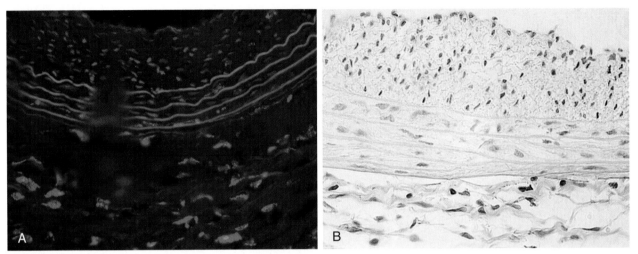

PLATE 55-6 ■ Arterial cross sections of immunohistochemical staining for (**A**) monocytes/macrophages *(red staining)* and (**B**) lymphocytes *(brown staining)* two weeks after arterial balloon injury in the rat carotid artery. Note that the majority of infiltrates are found in the adventitia.

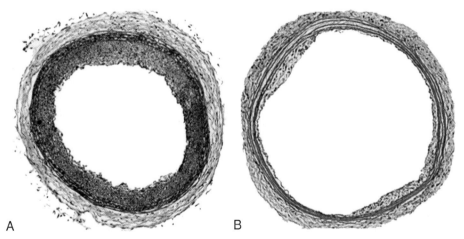

PLATE 55-8 ■ The nitric oxide donor PROLI/NO applied to the periadventitial surface of the rat carotid artery after balloon injury inhibits the development of neointimal hyperplasia at two weeks. **A,** Rat carotid artery cross section after balloon injury; **B,** rat carotid artery cross section after balloon injury and application of PROLI/NO.

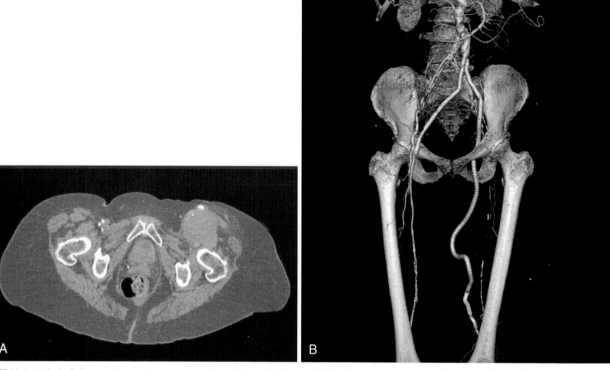

PLATE 56-8 ■ **A,** Left femoral pseudoaneurysm *(arrow)* due to late graft infection and anastomotic rupture in a patient who previously had an aortobifemoral bypass and left femoropopliteal bypass for rest pain. At the time of surgery, the left limb of the aortobifemoral graft was approached from a retroperitoneal incision and was found to be well incorporated. **B,** Therefore an obturator bypass was performed from the left limb of the aortobifemoral bypass to the distal aspect of the previous femoropopliteal bypass with immediate excision of the infected segments.

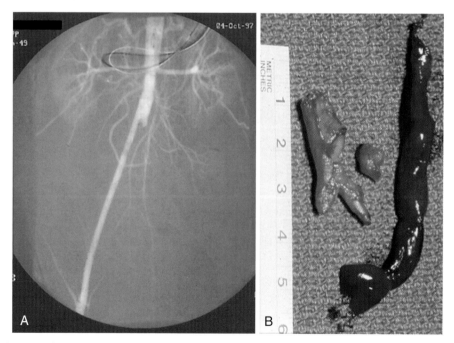

PLATE 57-8 ■ **A,** Angiogram of the occluded limb of an aortofemoral graft. **B,** The operative specimen demonstrating the thrombus and plaque removed from the proximal superficial femoral and profunda femoris arteries.

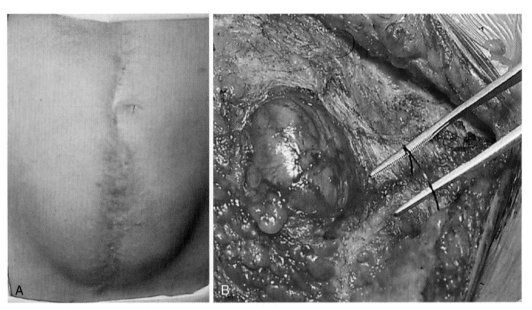

PLATE 57-13 ■ **A,** Photograph demonstrating a large abdominal incisional hernia in a patient after repair of an abdominal aortic aneurysm. **B,** Operative photograph demonstrating the intact sutures adjacent to the fascial defect *(arrow).*

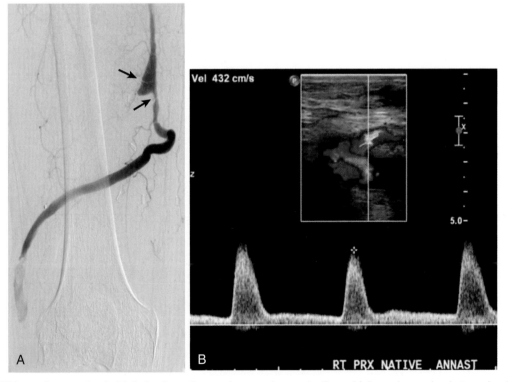

PLATE 57-21 ■ Vein graft stenosis. **A,** Digital subtraction angiogram demonstrating a high-grade proximal stenosis of an arm vein femoropopliteal graft. **B,** Duplex scan demonstrating increased velocities at the origin of the graft.

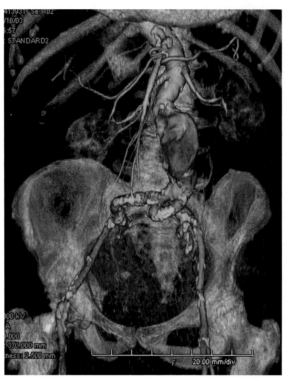

PLATE 58-1 ■ Challenging iliac access vessels. Note the calcification and severe tortuosity. (From Moore WS, Ahn SS: Endovascular surgery, ed 4, Philadelphia, 2011, Saunders.)

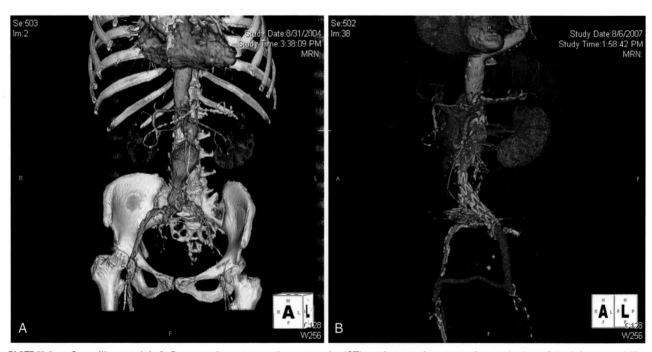

PLATE 58-2 ■ Open iliac conduit **A,** Preoperative computed tomography (CT) angiogram demonstrating occlusion of the left external iliac artery, with tortuosity, stenosis, and calcification seen on the right. **B,** Follow-up CT angiogram after repair with an aorto-uniiliac device delivered via a left common iliac conduit. The conduit was then anastomosed to the left common femoral artery, and a femoro-femoral bypass was performed. (From Moore WS, Ahn SS: Endovascular surgery, ed 4, Philadelphia, 2011, Saunders).

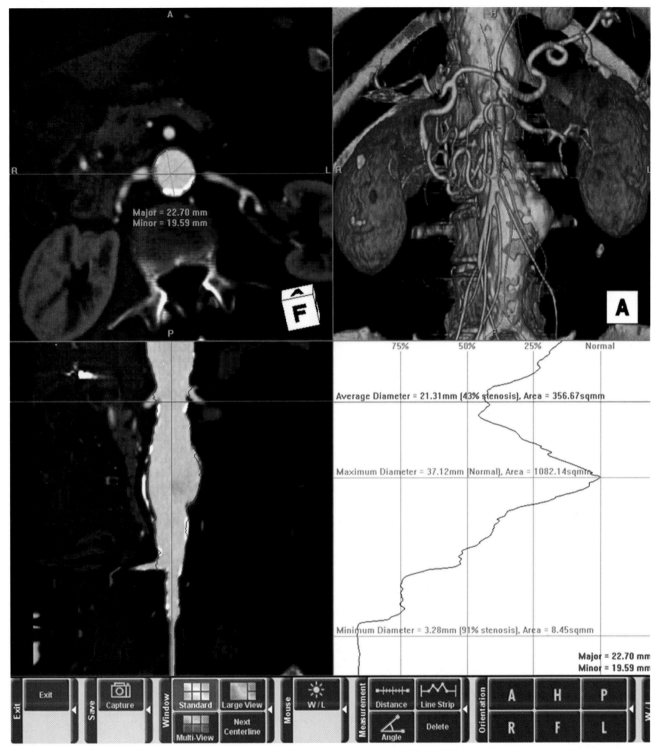

PLATE 58-5 ■ Three-dimensional computed tomographic reconstruction showing orthogonal, shaded surface, and stretched views of the abdominal aorta. (From Moore WS, Ahn SS: Endovascular surgery, ed 4, Philadelphia, 2011, Saunders.)

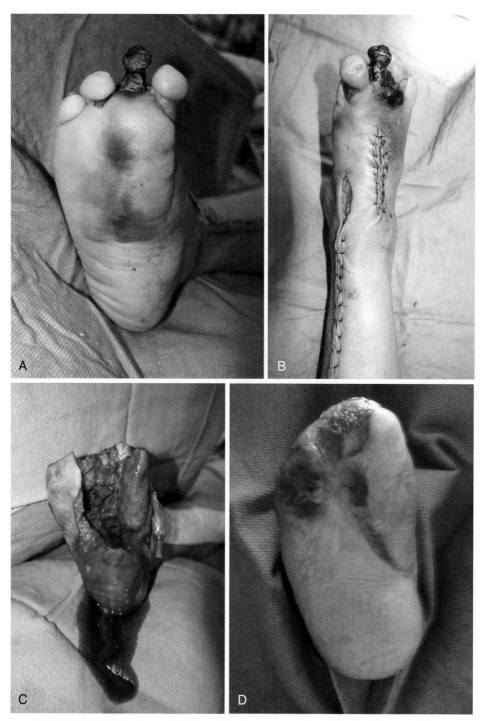

PLATE 59-9 ■ Clinical example illustrating team approach and typical interventions.

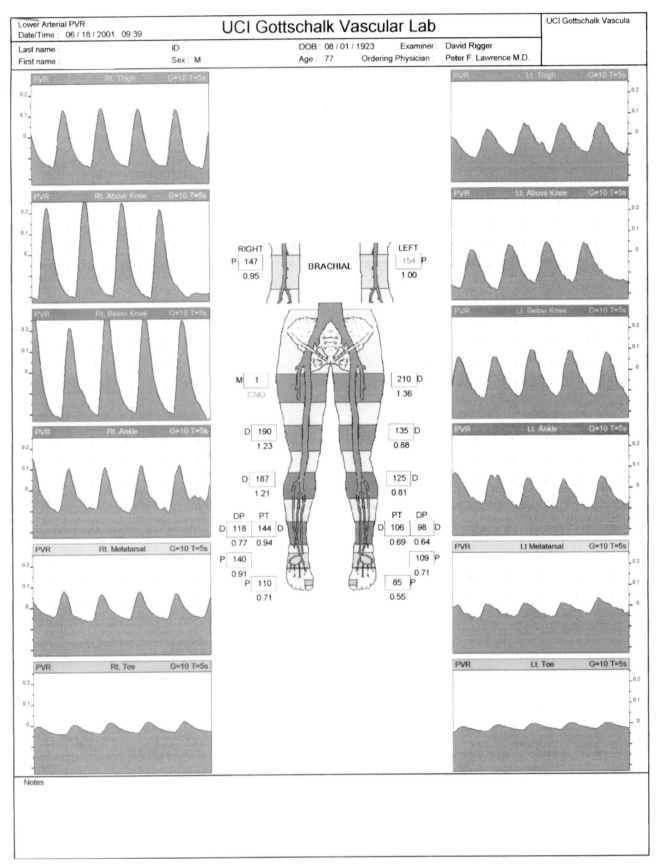

PLATE 60-5 ■ Physiologic studies of the lower limb are useful to determine the likelihood of wound healing. An ankle-brachial index (ABI) greater than 0.6 and biphasic or triphasic Doppler waveforms suggests a high likelihood of healing, whereas an ABI less than 0.4 and monophasic waveforms makes the likelihood of healing low.

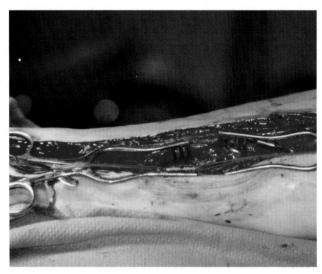

PLATE 60-9 ■ Incisions that are made in the distal part of an ischemic limb are at significant risk for wound complications of infection or dehiscence. An alternative is to harvest a more proximal vein and tunnel it distally.

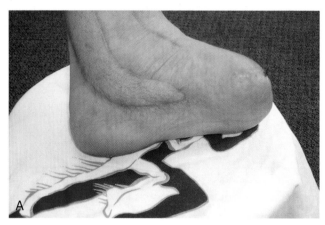

PLATE 60-10 ■ The use of a flow-through flap provides an autogenous conduit for bypass with skin and fat to cover a wound with a large skin defect. This patient received a radial flow-through flap to cover a large medial ankle wound. The bypass was from the mid-calf posterior tibial artery to the inframalleolar posterior tibial artery. A transmetatarsal amputation was also performed.

SECTION 1

INTRODUCTION

A HISTORY OF VASCULAR SURGERY

Wiley F. Barker

History is not a precise record, for it is only that which has been remembered or written down. Inevitably, there is much personal interpretation of that original material. In addition, interpreting events from the past is often difficult, and history sometimes changes as new information becomes available. It is often hard for an observer to see recent events in proper perspective, especially when the observer is close to or involved with those events.

In the last few years, there have been immense developments in molecular biology and in the techniques of minimally invasive surgery and interventional endovascular procedures. The value of these developments remains difficult to assess, despite their incalculable promise for the future. As Mao Zedong reportedly replied when asked about the effect of the French Revolution on the revolution in China, "It is much too soon to tell."

This chapter is presented in sections that can be considered as a series of scenes and acts. As with many modern stage plays, different actors appear in different scenes in different roles, and many scenes take place concurrently and must be observed from different points of view, depending on the subject at hand. Ultimately, the whole fits together.

PROLOGUE

Although some might argue that Guy de Chauliac or Ambroise Paré should properly be called the sires of surgery, John Hunter is the prototype of the modern vascular surgeon. He was an unbelievably productive and tireless worker, cut from the same Scottish mold as his brother William, who was 10 years older. John was largely unlettered, whereas William had become sophisticated through his education at Glasgow, yet they shared a frenetic capacity for work and an incurable curiosity.

To place the Hunters in a clear perspective in regard to nonmedical history, one should note that they were contemporaries of George Washington and Benjamin Franklin. William Hunter was born in Scotland in 1718, his brother John was born 10 years later; William died in 1783, and John died in 1793.[1,2] John was even made a member of the American Philosophical Society, although he never attended a meeting.

William Hunter preceded John to London, where he soon established a busy medical practice and interested himself in many subjects, including aneurysms. In fact, William proposed the concept that a lancet used carelessly during bloodletting might enter both artery and vein, and after healing, the two channels might be connected. He thus imagined an arteriovenous fistula. He soon found just such a patient and described the clinical manifestations with great accuracy.[3] William's primary activity, however, was focused on obstetrics and on the teaching of anatomy. John became his assistant in this latter project.

John Hunter is remembered for many things, but especially for his studies of the dynamics and efficiency of collateral arterial circulation, which he described in the vessels feeding the antlers of a stag after he had interrupted the major arteries in its neck. More renown came from his ligation of the femoral artery in its subsartorial course at a distance above a popliteal aneurysm—in Hunter's canal.[1,2]

To be sure, others had preceded him in performing proximal ligation of arteries to treat aneurysms. In the third century, a Roman surgeon named Antyllus had described proximal and distal ligation of the artery, followed by incision of the aneurysm and removal of its contents—a formidable operation without either anesthesia or asepsis.[4] In 1680, Purmann, faced with a large aneurysm in the antecubital space, performed ligation of the vessels and excision of the aneurysmal mass.[5] In 1714, Anel described an operation in which he placed one ligature on the artery at the proximal extent of the aneurysm. Hunter, however, had found that the ligature would sometimes cut through the artery when it was placed too close to the popliteal aneurysm; therefore he chose a site that was more remote, but was easily reached by the surgeon and would preserve collaterals. Most of Anel's patients suffered from false aneurysms caused by bloodletting in otherwise healthy arteries. The femoropopliteal aneurysms treated by Hunter were due to degenerative processes, probably a mixture of syphilis and trauma.[1,6]

Many other surgeons were ligating aneurysms in various anatomic sites at this time. Cooper, one of John Hunter's students, was soon established as one of the early vascular surgeons when he ligated the carotid artery for an aneurysm in 1805,[7] as well as the aorta for an iliac artery aneurysm.[8] Only these few important events occurred before the latter part of the nineteenth century.

At the time, ligation was virtually the only procedure available to surgeons for the management of arterial problems, and those problems were limited to the control of hemorrhage and the treatment of aneurysms. Hallowell in Newcastle-on-Tyne performed one arterial repair of an artery torn during bloodletting. The laceration was a short one, and at the suggestion of Lambert, he placed a short ($\frac{1}{4}$ inch) steel pin through the edges of the wound and looped a ligature around it in a figure-of-eight pattern, approximating the edges of the wound with apparent success. Hallowell wrote to William Hunter concerning this operation in 1761, foreseeing that if this were a successful technique, "we might be able to cure wounds of some arteries that would otherwise require amputation, or be altogether incurable."[9] That Hallowell wrote to William instead of John is probably due to William's published work on arteriovenous fistulas secondary to inept bloodletting. Twelve years later in 1773, Asman reviewed the Newcastle repair, attempted some experiments of his own that were disastrous, and concluded that such a procedure could not work and that Lambert and Hallowell's efforts had probably failed as well.[10] After Asman's criticism, the matter of arterial repair rested quietly for nearly another 100 years.

John Hunter's less widely known contributions are scattered throughout the immense museum he left to the Royal College of Surgeons of England, and they hint at an understanding of arterial pathology that would not be general knowledge for half a century. They include dissections of several atherosclerotic aortic bifurcations (specimens P.1177 and P.1178), showing the atheromatous lesion at the aortic bifurcation that Leriche would describe 150 years later; a carotid bifurcation with an ulcerated atheroma from a patient who died of a ruptured syphilitic thoracic aneurysm (specimen P.1171); and an extracranial internal carotid aneurysm (specimen P.282) in a patient whose neatly described symptoms are almost typical of what today are recognized as classic transient ischemic episodes.[11] Regrettably, most of Hunter's notes did not survive to provide more than this fragmentary view of his understanding of vascular disease. To cap it all, in a postmortem specimen, Hunter had dissected the atheromatous layers (although the term atheroma had not yet come into use) from the remaining intact wall of an atherosclerotic terminal aorta (specimen P.1176), foreshadowing dos Santos by 150 years.

Both Hunter and Cooper seemed to hold with the teleologic belief of the times that when senile or spontaneous gangrene occurred in older persons, thrombosis of the major vessels supervened so that the patient would not bleed to death when the gangrenous part separated.[12] It was Cruveilhier who first clearly stated that the phrase "gangrene due to obstruction of the arteries" by thickening and by thrombosis should replace the terms spontaneous and senile gangrene,[13] but he attributed the concept to Dupuytren.

The recognition that arterial obstruction causes functional disability that limits the use of the affected part may have arisen in the veterinary world. Bouley described the clinical picture in a horse in 1831.[14]

Four years later in 1835, a nearly anonymous physician on the ward of a Professor Louis provided the first clear description of human claudication. Barth's patient was a 51-year-old woman who died of heart failure resulting from mitral valvular disease. His report described her incidental history of claudication in terms that we would recognize today.[15] In the postmortem report, he noted thrombosis of the terminal aorta and included a sketch suggesting that the lesion was a thrombosed hypoplastic terminal aorta, a contracted atherosclerotic lesion, or a combination of both. Barth also repeated Hunter's observation that the obstructing material could be separated easily from the residual intact arterial wall. Barth was never identified further, not even by an initial.

Charcot is often erroneously given credit for recognizing the syndrome of intermittent claudication caused by arterial insufficiency in humans.[16] Charcot described, just as Bouley had done, the vanishing pulses, the cold extremity, and what is now recognized as the loss of sympathetic tone in a horse in the throes of a spasm of severe claudication; he reported a human case as well. Homans liked to joke that Charcot observed the former because he spent so much time at the horse races.

As a neurologist, Charcot was familiar with intermittent claudication in humans caused by various neurologic processes. The patient Charcot described, however, suffered claudication in one leg secondary to an old gunshot wound that resulted in occlusion of the iliac artery and an aneurysm proximal to the occlusion. The aneurysm, which was adherent to and in communication with the jejunum, gave rise to a series of small gastrointestinal hemorrhages before the final fatal episode. Charcot thus deserves credit for identifying the herald hemorrhages that often presage major bleeding from an aortoenteric fistula. (Charcot credited both Bouley and Barth with their prior observations regarding claudication.)

SUCCESSFUL ARTERIAL SUTURE

Such information was of little utility to surgeons, however, until arterial repair became a reality. Consistent with the observations of Asman, several German masters had deemed arterial repair (as opposed to ligation) to be impossible. Langenbeck stated in 1825 that, because the primary requirement for healing is perfect rest, an arterial incision could never heal as long as the pulsatile movements of the arterial wall continued.[17] Heinecke was certain that the patient would bleed to death through the suture holes and the apposed edges of the arterial wall.[18]

Repair of small injuries to veins, however, was becoming an established procedure. The lateral ligature, in which a clamp is placed on the defect in the venous wall and a ligature is tied around the puckered wall, had been performed in 1816.[19] The first lateral suture of a venous defect (an erosion of the common jugular vein from an infected neck wound) was undertaken by Czerny in 1881, but the patient died of sepsis and hemorrhage.[20] Jassinowsky[19] credits Schede[21] with the first successful repair of a large venous injury (to the common femoral vein) by lateral sutures.

Going beyond the stage of venous repair, Eck reported the experimental creation of a portocaval fistula in dogs.[22] The original description hints that he had little to confirm his success. Among a series of eight dogs, one died within 24 hours, six lived 2 to 6 days, and the one survivor "tired of life in the laboratory and ran away after 2 months." The doctoral dissertation of Jassinowsky, written in 1889 and based purely on library research, reviewed the published information on arterial suture and concluded that it could not be successful at that time, but that there might be hope in the future.[19]

Only 2 years later, however, Jassinowsky himself succeeded. In 1891, he reported his successful animal experiments involving arterial suture.[23] The suture he described was passed carefully only two thirds of the way through the media; he tried to avoid penetrating the intima, except in very thin-walled vessels. This effort should be recognized for its intrinsic difficulty using even the finest milliner's needles, because without sutures swaged onto needles, two pieces of suture have to be dragged through the arterial wall. Dörfler modified Jassinowsky's method and passed the suture through all thicknesses of the arterial wall.[24] He also recognized that the arterial suture exposed in the lumen of the vessel did no harm if uninfected. He observed that it soon became covered with a glistening membrane. Shortly thereafter in 1896, Jaboulay and Briau described successful end-to-end carotid arterial anastomoses in animals using an everting U-shaped suture.[25]

Jaboulay was one of the surgeons in Lyon, France, under whom Carrel studied. When Sadi Carnot, the president of the Republic of France, was wounded by an assassin and died because no one dared to try to repair his portal vein, Carrel was highly critical, because he believed that blood vessels could be sutured as well as any other tissue.[26] He soon undertook experimental arterial anastomoses; some of the earliest of these were arteriovenous communications in which the high-flow system ensured patency. Carrel's contributions to technical arterial surgery included methods that vascular surgeons routinely use today.[27,28] He devised the triangulation suture to facilitate end-to-end anastomosis, described the patch technique to anastomose a small vessel to the side of a larger one (as in replantation of an inferior mesenteric artery), and pioneered the use of vessel grafts and organ transplantation. His work, however, was not fully accepted in the United States for many years. In part, this stemmed from disputes that arose between him and Guthrie, who was his coworker for 1 year.[29]

In contrast, European surgeons not only accepted Carrel's work but also began to follow his lead. In 1906, Goyanes of Madrid, Spain, resected a popliteal aneurysm, then restored arterial continuity with an in situ venous graft using the popliteal vein, which was probably the first successful clinical vascular replacement.[30]

Surgeons in the United States were beginning to perform vascular surgery in their own way. In New Orleans in 1888, Matas described a landmark operation.[31] He stumbled onto the surgical procedure for which he is commonly remembered, endoaneurysmorrhaphy, when an aneurysm for which he had ligated only the proximal brachial artery, with apparent initial success, began to pulsate again 10 days later. Reportedly, it was a medical student who called this to the professor's attention. He chose to reoperate and to ligate the brachial artery distally. Even after this distal ligation, the aneurysm continued to pulsate, and he was forced to open the aneurysm, clean out the sac (the operation performed by Antyllus), and oversew the other arteries feeding the aneurysm from inside the sac. This foreshadowed the problems with endoleaks that confound vascular surgeons who place endovascular aortic prostheses today.

Matas's operation differed from that of Antyllus, in that Matas used a suture within the aneurysmal sac to obliterate the feeding vessels instead of ligating them outside the sac. The extensive dissection that would have been required outside might have damaged the collateral circulation and other adherent anatomic structures. It was many years before Matas performed another endoaneurysmorrhaphy, because most patients were treated successfully by simple proximal ligation.[32] Matas ultimately expanded the descriptions of his technique to include "restorative" and "reconstructive" modifications, and he reported an approach to the arteriovenous fistula through the venous component,[33] as had been proposed by Bickham.[34]

Murphy, of Chicago, performed a series of experiments on animals in which he successfully restored continuity by invagination of the proximal into the distal vessel. In 1897, he presented a successful human case.[35] Edwards briefly revived this anastomotic technique of invagination when he recommended the use of the first braided nylon grafts.[36]

Murphy's invagination techniques were reflected in other nonsuture methods of anastomosis: Nitze[37] and Payr[38] used small metal or ivory rings through which the vessel was drawn, everted, and tied in place; this unit was then inserted into the mouth of the distal vessel, and another ligature secured it there. This is substantially the Blakemore tube,[39] used during World War II, albeit without signal success.[40]

During his tenure at Johns Hopkins Hospital, W.S. Halsted had an abundance of traumatic and syphilitic aneurysms commanding his attention. In the early 1900s, Carrel visited Halsted and described his own technical experiments, including his early arteriovenous anastomoses. As a result, Halsted almost made history in 1907 when he faced the dilemma of a patient whose popliteal artery and vein had been sacrificed during an en bloc dissection of a sarcoma of the popliteal space.[41] Halsted went to the other leg, took the saphenous vein, reversed it, and anastomosed the distal saphenous vein to the proximal femoral artery. For his distal anastomosis, however, he chose the popliteal vein. Although the graft pulsated for 40 minutes, it soon thrombosed. It is possible that Halsted was pursuing the chimera of reversal of arterial flow through the venous bed. One can only imagine what a dramatic leap forward vascular surgery would have made if Halsted, with his superb supporting cast of talented surgeons, had chosen the popliteal artery for the distal anastomosis and had achieved a truly successful arterial reconstruction in the pattern of the modern vascular surgeon.

There is considerable literature on attempts to revascularize ischemic extremities via arteriovenous anastomoses. San Martín[42] and A. E. Halsted[43] attempted to improve the distal circulation using arteriovenous anastomoses.

Meanwhile, German surgeons such as Höpfner,[44] Lexer,[45,46] and Jeger[47] had become familiar with the use of short (<10 cm) vein grafts. Höpfner described the bypass procedure, which was illustrated in an encyclopedic book by Jeger. Jeger's book, republished posthumously in 1937, included a foreword that described

Jeger's replantation of the completely severed arm of a German soldier, which he had performed in 1914. One year later, Jeger came to an untimely death from typhus while on the Russian front.

Lexer collected and reported on 65 vein transplants, 13 of which were his personal cases.[45] In 8 of these 13 cases, Lexer had obtained a distal pulse. This report prompted a Polish surgeon, Weglowski, to present his own personal series of 51 vein grafts, mostly for trauma, operated on between 1914 and 1921; in 40 patients he could document good distal pulses and normal arterial tracings.[48] Yet all this seemed to be forgotten for the next 25 years as Germany suffered the agonies of the interbellum years, and as the forceful and charismatic personality of Leriche appeared on the scene (Leriche's role is described in a later section).

ABDOMINAL AORTIC ANEURYSMS

Beyond the management of trauma to the arteries, the aneurysm is clearly one of the great surgical challenges. The previous section detailed early attempts to treat peripheral aneurysms, but these were sporadic and lacked a continuing series.

Vesalius is said to have been the first to describe an abdominal aneurysm.[49] The successful management of the abdominal aneurysm is certainly one of vascular surgery's major accomplishments. The technical maneuvers described previously concerning the ligation of aneurysms in various anatomic sites usually involved aneurysms of the peripheral vessels; aneurysms of the trunk were sacrosanct, because proximal control was not feasible. Cooper had continued many of Hunter's studies, including evaluation of collateral arterial supplies. In 1805, he had ligated the common carotid artery for an aneurysm,[7] but he opened the door for even wider surgical applications when, in 1818, he ligated the abdominal aorta to control external hemorrhage from an aneurysm of the external iliac artery that had eroded to the surface of the skin of the flank, bleeding openly at that site.[9]

Interest in the treatment of major vessel aneurysms lagged for almost a century. Eventually Colt, at the end of the nineteenth century, used wire to pack an aneurysm and then heated the wire.[50] Blakemore and King revived interest in this technique in 1938,[51] and many surgeons undertook modifications of the wiring technique, largely without success. Meanwhile, more direct attempts were being made by the major actors in the next scene: Matas of New Orleans and Halsted of Baltimore. Their interest in the management of vessel trauma, and in the management of late sequelae of such trauma, provided material for the fertile imaginations of the many surgeons who were emboldened to follow in their footsteps. Reid reported the experience of the Johns Hopkins Hospital (headed by Halsted) with aneurysms in 1926.[52] The aneurysms treated included many varieties, both anatomic and etiologic, but treatment of abdominal aneurysms was substantially a failure. These operations were only preparation for the end of ligation as a treatment for aneurysms of the abdominal aorta.

Matas finally accomplished a successful aortic ligation (just below the renal arteries) for an aneurysm at the bifurcation of the aorta. He reported it first in 1925 and then again in 1940.[53,54] In the issue of *Annals of Surgery* that contained Matas's second report was a similar paper by Elkin,[55] as well as a hint of the coming era of vascular reconstruction in a report by Bigger of Virginia.[56] Bigger had ligated the neck of an abdominal aneurysm using fascia that he expected to loosen gradually and allow restoration of flow. With the protection of this temporary control, he performed a plication of the aneurysm, restoring the aorta to its proper caliber. The patient had a protracted survival without recurrence of the aneurysm and also with restoration of femoral pulses.

About this time, however, cardiac surgery began to emerge. During the first decade of the twentieth century, Jeger had proposed valved venous grafts between the left pulmonary veins and the left ventricle to bypass mitral stenosis, and a valved venous graft from the left ventricle to the innominate artery to bypass aortic stenosis.[47] In the mid 1920s, Cutler and colleagues[57] had attempted to treat mitral stenosis surgically, but with minimal success. A valvulotome was used through a ventricular approach.

Nonetheless, the influence of these attempts led Gross to the successful ligation and, 5 years later, division of the patent ductus arteriosus.[58,59] In Baltimore, Blalock and Taussig[60] began their series of pioneering surgical procedures for various cardiac anomalies, the first and most dramatic of which was the "blue baby" operation—the creation of a systemic shunt from the subclavian artery to the pulmonary artery in patients with congenital pulmonic stenosis.

Crafoord and Nylin[61] reported the successful end-to-end anastomosis of the aorta after resection of an aortic coarctation at the same time that Gross and Hufnagel[62] carried out their first case. This last operation demonstrated that lesions of the thoracic and abdominal segments of the aorta were amenable to a surgical approach.

Development of Vascular Prostheses

Although arterial homografts functioned fairly well in the aorta (discussed later), they were difficult to obtain, harvest, sterilize, and store. Grafts other than those of the aorta fared poorly. Homografts of smaller vessels containing a higher proportion of smooth muscle were even less satisfactory. The development of an artificial arterial substitute would allow the expansion of arterial reconstruction.

Following the experience in the laboratory reported by Abbe,[63] Tuffier had used rigid tubes of metal and of paraffined glass to try to replace small- to medium-size arteries during World War I, without success.[64] Similar tubes were used in World War II, but the results were no better than those obtained by immediate ligation of the artery.[40] Hufnagel chose a more inert surface, methylmethacrylate, as well as a tube with a better hemodynamic design.[65] Hufnagel's tubes functioned remarkably well in animal experiments, except for the difficulty in securing them within a major artery such as the aorta without the risk of ultimate erosion. Eventually the use of pliable plastic fabrics virtually eliminated the rigid tube.

In 1947, Hufnagel reported on the use of rapid freezing for the preservation of arterial homografts and suggested their utility in the repair of long aortic coarctations.[66] Gross, who at first feared that frozen vessels could not survive, published a laboratory and clinical report on his experiences with homografts preserved in electrolyte solutions for use in various cardiac operations, but particularly for the management of coarctation of the aorta.[67] Swan soon used a homograft for a thoracic aneurysm associated with a coarctation.[68]

The arterial homograft initially seemed to be a good substitute for the thoracic or abdominal aorta. At first, fresh grafts were used; then they were preserved in Tyrode's solution. Improvements in the preservation of grafts by freezing[69] and then lyophilization[70] facilitated the development of arterial graft banks. Early successes were soon erased by late failures of the homografts, however, and a truly satisfactory aortic substitute was sorely needed.

In 1952, Voorhees and colleagues observed that fabric threads in a chamber of the heart soon became covered with endothelium.[71] Dörfler had made a similar gross observation 60 years earlier, but had not carried the observation to its conclusion.[64] Voorhees and associates at Columbia pursued experiments not only with Vinyon-N, but also with parachute silk and other materials. Many fabrics were tried, and most were quickly discarded. Braided and crimped nylon tubes were introduced by Edwards and Tapp,[36] but it was soon discovered that nylon rapidly lost strength and was unsatisfactory.[72] Both Orlon[73] and Teflon[74] were used. Szilagyi and colleagues[75] and Julian and colleagues[76] introduced various fabrications of Dacron. The transcripts of the vascular surgery meetings of the late 1950s might be mistaken for a textile journal, as various weaves, deniers, calenderizing, and the advantages of braid versus knit versus taffeta weaves were discussed. The summation of the principles of vascular grafting by Wesolowski and coworkers had enunciated the importance of porosity,[77,78] but the substantially nonporous Teflon undercut that thesis.

The knitted Dacron introduced by DeBakey and colleagues placed a generally successful graft in the hands of every surgeon.[79] Subsequent modifications by the addition of velour to the surface by Sauvage[80] and also by Cooley[81] refined this outstanding contribution. Wesolowski and colleagues' concept[78] that the fabric tube would become "encapsulated" and might develop a firm new endothelial surface has been pursued as a goal but has not been achieved in humans.

The immediate porosity of the grafts has been troublesome on occasion, especially in patients who require heparinization or in whom even minor blood loss from a weeping graft is intolerable. Impregnation with either collagen[82] or albumin[83] was a useful advance. Teflon in the form of an extruded tube (Gore-Tex) rather than as a woven or knitted fabric was introduced clinically by Soyer,[84] and it has achieved great popularity. Introduced first for use as a venous substitute, it came to be used extensively in arterial reconstructions as a second choice after autologous vein,[85] although Quiñones-Baldrich and colleagues[86] expressed a preference for Gore-Tex in femoral anastomoses above the knee, preserving the vein for more distal reconstructions if such become necessary.

Biological substitutes other than the arterial homograft have also been suggested. Rosenberg and associates used bovine carotid arteries that had been subjected to enzymatic treatment to remove all the tissue-specific protein, except the basic structural collagen of the bovine artery.[87] Sawyer and colleagues[88] attempted to modify the bovine heterograft by inducing a negatively charged lining in an effort to inhibit thrombosis. Dardik and coworkers[89] used treated umbilical vein grafts supported with a mesh of Dacron as a peripheral arterial substitute.

The world turns, however, and there is currently renewed interest in the use of cryopreserved (frozen but not lyophilized) arterial homografts, especially in infected aortic sites. Experience is limited, and this topic deserves to be in a clinical area rather than a historic one.

Modern Management of Aortic Aneurysms

The grave risk posed by abdominal aneurysms was exposed in a timely paper by Estes in 1951.[90] Other experiences with the aorta were preparing the way for present-day management of abdominal aneurysms. Alexander and Byron[91,92] had resected a thoracic aneurysm associated with coarctation of the aorta and successfully oversewn the ends of the vessel, although the patient ultimately died of renovascular hypertension. Swan had used a homograft to replace a thoracic aneurysm.[68]

Various attempts were made to use either reactive cellophane[93] or the tissue-irritating plasticizer dicetyl phosphate[94] as a means of inducing sclerosis that might restrain the dilatation of the aneurysm. These attempts to control the growth of the aneurysm were not rewarding.

Oudot[95] set the stage for other forms of aortic replacement when he used a homograft to restore circulation in a patient with Leriche syndrome. Dubost is recognized as the pioneer who first successfully replaced an abdominal aneurysm with a homograft on March 19, 1951.[96] Schaffer and Hardin[97] actually preceded Dubost by 4 weeks, but their publication appeared considerably later and focused on the use of a polythene shunt to maintain distal circulation during the operation rather than on the priority of resecting the aneurysm itself. It appears that Wylie actually accomplished a successful endarterectomy of an abdominal aneurysm on January 13, 1951. Similarly, Freeman and Leeds treated three patients, two successfully, with inlay grafts of the patient's own iliac veins beginning on February 12, 1951. Wylie's and Freeman's operations were not graft replacements, however, but rather modifications of Bigger's procedure.[56]

Dubost's operation was soon followed by those of Julian,[98] Brock,[99] DeBakey,[100] and Bahnson.[101] It is a curious twist of fate to find that Dubost had left the practice of colorectal surgery to become a cardiac surgeon after he saw Blalock and Bahnson perform dramatic cardiac operations while they were visiting France in the late 1940s. Szilagyi's[102] classic study of the benefits of the operation in 1966 provided confirmation and justification of the thesis Estes had presented in 1950.

The complicated abdominal aneurysm still posed a major problem. Ellis was one of the first to implant the renal arteries into the graft when the aneurysm was found to include their orifices.[103] Etheredge[104] extended this operation to resect a major thoracoabdominal aortic aneurysm. He used a heparinized plastic shunt of the type described in Schaffer's resection and replacement of an abdominal aneurysm with a homograft in March 1951. Etheredge established the shunt, divided the aorta, and performed the proximal anastomosis; he then moved the clamp down the graft after each successive visceral anastomosis was completed and finished with the lower aortic anastomosis to the graft.

DeBakey and colleagues[105] reported in 1956 a series of complicated abdominal and thoracoabdominal aneurysms that were resected with a technique similar to that later used by Shumacker.[106] In 1973, Stoney and Wylie[107] popularized the long thoracoabdominal incision for the approach to this lesion. The great advance in the management of these complicated lesions was made by Crawford,[108] who introduced a direct approach to the aneurysm in which the aorta is clamped above and below and then opened throughout the length of the aneurysm. A fabric graft is sewn into the proximal aorta; the major groups of arteries, including the lower intercostals when possible, are sewn into the wall of the fabric tube using the expeditious Carrel patch method of anastomosis; then the distal anastomosis is completed. This direct method has greatly simplified the approach to these challenging lesions.

The placement of a graft within the lumen of an aneurysm—whether abdominal, thoracic, or peripheral—was logically extended by a technique that allows one to place the graft within the aneurysm from a distance through a short arteriotomy in either the femoral or the external iliac artery. The evolution of this method stems circuitously from Dotter and coworkers.[109] In 1983, they attempted to improve the results of simple arterial dilatation or to maintain the patency of a graft with small endarterial spiral coils. After several generations of devices that did not gain wide acceptance, Palmaz and associates[110] introduced a metal mesh stent that can be expanded by balloon dilatation, which secures the stent in place. Introduced originally to maintain the patency of a segment of artery that had undergone percutaneous dilatation, this method was at first used in occlusive disease, but Parodi and colleagues[111] modified the technique to secure a fabric graft that had been placed within an aneurysm. Although initially used as a tube graft, modifications soon allowed the placement of bifurcation grafts.[112,113] The anticipated decrease in morbidity and mortality accompanying this method led to its widespread use, although not all aneurysms are amenable. The need for prolonged follow-up versus the security of a one-time operation has raised the clinical question of the ultimate role of the endovascular repair of aneurysms. Here the narrative becomes so contemporaneous as to require clinical rather than historical description.

PERIPHERAL ARTERIAL ANEURYSMS

The peripheral arterial aneurysm was one of the first arterial lesions treated by surgeons, but its importance paled beside the advances made in the management of the aortic aneurysm. The early history of treatment by ligation was described earlier.

In 1949, Linton used Leriche's concept of arteriectomy and sympathectomy for the management of 14 patients who had popliteal aneurysms—an ingenious approach that resulted in no amputations in his series.[114] The patients received a preliminary sympathectomy; shortly afterward, or sometimes at the same operation, the aneurysm was resected, with ligation of the artery above and below it.

The ability to replace vessels of the size of the popliteal artery brought to the fore the concept that the popliteal aneurysm had a risk-benefit pattern similar to that of the abdominal aneurysm. If operations were done electively, the results were excellent, but once thrombosis occurred, the risk to the limb was grave, as Wychulis and associates demonstrated.[115] Wylie (in the discussion of Wychulis[115]) and Edwards[116] introduced the procedure of excluding the aneurysm and restoring flow through a bypass technique.

OCCLUSIVE ARTERIAL DISEASE

As mentioned earlier in this chapter, it was not until the middle of the nineteenth century that the relationship between arterial occlusion and gangrene was clearly established. Repair of acute injuries had been accomplished, but management of more chronic arterial obstructions had hardly been considered a surgical problem. Recognition of the clinical symptoms of less severe ischemia came to surgery by way of veterinary medicine.[14] The association between the sympathetic nervous system and the arteries was recognized in the early twentieth century, especially during World War I.

Leriche, born in 1879, had been educated and trained at Lyon, where he had known Jaboulay and Carrel. Shortly after Leriche completed his training, World War I broke out, and Leriche acquired considerable experience with wounds of the extremities. After he was demobilized, Leriche continued to work in a trauma hospital in Lyon for several years. There he saw many patients with posttraumatic neuralgias, and he developed his concepts of the role of the sympathetic nervous system and the possible treatment by periarterial sympathectomy, about which he had first written in 1917.[117] Then, seeing patients with arterial thrombosis caused by artérite (a nonspecific term used by French surgeons to describe arterial disease and occlusion in general), Leriche concluded that if the patient was seen before the occluding thrombosis was too widespread, local resection of the thrombosed artery provided relief. Because many patients did well after this simple procedure and soon developed relatively warm feet, he concluded that the collateral circulation in these patients must have been satisfactory and that the coldness of the extremity was due to vasospasm rather than insufficient arterial flow. He therefore applied the principle of sympathectomy, first as a periarterial operation, then as an arteriectomy (excising the obstructed segment), and then as a division of the sympathetic rami.[118]

Diez,[119] dissatisfied with the results of periarterial sympathectomy, modified that operation into the lumbar ganglionectomy. At nearly the same time, Royle[120] and Hunter[121] introduced the same fruitless operation for the management of spasm in striated muscle. Use of this operation for the management of pain syndromes and ischemic extremities remains controversial.

It seems likely that the forcefulness of Leriche's personality led European surgical thought to diverge from the known techniques of vascular grafting. This is not to say that Leriche actively spoke against the use of grafts; in fact, it was noted by some of his former trainees that he often said that it would be ideal to connect the two ends of a severed artery by a graft, but the risk of infection and the distance to be bridged always seemed too great. Instead, he offered arterial excision and sympathectomy, an approach that seemed to be beneficial and posed less risk.

One of Leriche's most important early observations was the definition of the syndrome that now bears his name, the atherosclerotic obliteration of the terminal aorta and the iliac arteries. He described this in 1923, during the period when he was beginning to evaluate arteriectomy.[122] It would be 17 years, however, before he found a suitable case in which he could perform resection of the aortic bifurcation and lumbar sympathectomy.[123] Leriche's surgical clinic became famous, and he attracted a long line of surgeons who came to learn: DeBakey, Learmonth, dos Santos, and Kunlin, to name a few.

The possibility of effective arterial suture anastomosis had been developed through the ideas of Jaboulay[25] and Carrel[27] at Lyon. After World War I, another surgeon from Lyon assumed a major role in vascular surgery.

In 1909, Murphy removed an embolus from the common iliac artery and restored flow into the femoral system. Although locally successful, distal thrombosis required a distal amputation.[124] Two years later, Labey (as cited by Mosny and Dumont[125]) removed an embolus from the artery of a patient, with complete success. Embolectomy was thereafter performed with occasional success worldwide, but it did not become a fully satisfactory procedure because of the need to operate hastily, before extensive distal thrombosis supervened. After the clinical introduction of heparin by Murray,[126] it became possible to extend the indications for embolectomy and to extend the time limit for undertaking the procedure and thus improve the results.

Surgeons such as João Cid dos Santos and his father, Reynaldo, used heparin to prevent thrombosis after performing the nearly forgotten Matas endoaneurysmorrhaphy.[127] The younger dos Santos believed that with the protection of heparin, he might be able to remove chronically adherent arterial emboli and their associated thrombus and achieve healing without rethrombosis. After finding such a patient with advanced renal disease and a seriously ischemic extremity, dos Santos removed the clot and reestablished flow. He was chided by the pathologist for having removed the intima as well. After another successful case, in which he removed a chronic thrombosis of the subclavian, axillary, and brachial arteries secondary to scalenus anticus syndrome, he sent his report to Leriche. Leriche presented the work in the name of dos Santos to the French Academy of Surgery[128] and introduced endarterectomy to the surgical world. It is interesting to note that neither of these patients suffered primarily from the usual forms of atherosclerotic thrombosis.

Subsequently, Freeman and colleagues,[129,130] Wylie and associates,[131] and others adopted the operation, using the open technique that was championed primarily by Bazy and coworkers.[132] In September 1951, Wylie described endoaneurysmectomy and endarterectomy of the aorta. At the time, my colleagues and I had undertaken six procedures without success, but in the summer of 1951, Wylie had visited us, and in October 1951 we performed the first successful endarterectomy in our series.[133] The operation consisted of a combination of the Matas endoaneurysmorrhaphy and the dos Santos endarterectomy (or the technique as revised by Reboul): an abdominal aneurysm was endarterectomized, tailored to a proper size, and wrapped with fascia lata, and an endarterectomy in continuity was performed throughout the length of the left iliofemoropopliteal system. In fact, these operations were only extensions of the aneurysm repair performed by Bigger in 1940.[56]

Cannon and Barker later introduced the long, closed endarterectomy using intraluminal strippers,[134] which was a modification of the original method of dos Santos. Several similar varieties of endarterectomy loops were devised by Butcher[135] and by Vollmar and Laubaeh,[136] among others. A period of early success was followed by disenchantment owing to the difficulty of the operation in comparison with the increasingly popular grafting procedures.

Leriche and his close associate Kunlin had not had great technical success with endarterectomy, especially in the femoral artery system. Kunlin revived the use of the vein graft in the form of a long venous bypass.[137] His first patient had already undergone arteriectomy and sympathectomy, thus justifying the then-unorthodox procedure.

Veins had been used for short (4 to 8 cm) replacements on rare occasions during the prior 40 years. This technique has persisted as the basic method of arterial reconstruction ever since.

Saphenous vein grafting was useful only in the femoral and iliofemoral systems, however, and it remained for Oudot to perform a comparable reconstructive operation on the aorta using an aortic homograft,[95] which thoracic and cardiac surgeons were already using to replace segments of the thoracic aorta. Oudot was presented with a 51-year-old patient with claudication as a result of proximal iliac and distal aortic occlusion. Oudot's operation is commonly described as a simple bifurcation graft, common iliac to common iliac, but it was actually a much more complicated procedure. He approached the bifurcation extraperitoneally through a left flank incision and resected the bifurcation. The patient's internal iliacs were found to be thrombosed and were ligated. The external iliac arteries of the graft were very small, but the graft's internal iliacs were large; Oudot therefore anastomosed the graft's internal iliacs to the patient's external iliacs. However, he did the left-sided anastomosis first and then found that the repaired vessel obstructed his view and hindered manipulations of the right-sided anastomosis. This difficult anastomosis thrombosed promptly. Oudot made the best of a bad situation and pointed out that he had done a perfect experiment, as there was still some discussion from Leriche's camp about whether grafting at this level would be worthwhile. On the right side, Oudot had performed substantially nothing more than an arteriectomy; on the left, he had reconstituted the lumen. The right side was warm but pulseless and still fatigued easily, whereas the left side had a pulse and did not tire. Six months later, Oudot reoperated on the patient, who was still complaining of right-sided claudication; he performed an iliac-to-iliac "extraanatomic" bypass, as had been suggested by Kunlin in 1951.

A few months later, Oudot climbed Annapurna with the French team. Shortly after his return to France, he was killed in an automobile crash at the age of 40.

The saga of the treatment of arterial disease continues with the development and then the failure of artery banks and the introduction of the plastic prosthesis, but by 1952 the stage was set for nearly everything that is done today. Linton's espousal of the reversed saphenous vein in 1952 confirmed the approach of Kunlin and established the procedure of choice for peripheral reconstruction for many years.[138]

Endarterectomy did not die out completely; it persists in carotid operations, but only occasionally is it used in the aorta and as part of local tailoring procedures elsewhere. Edwards made one important attempt to use it in the femoral artery by means of a long patch; the procedure worked well unless the patch was so wide that it created a stagnant column of blood in the femoral artery.[139] Femoropopliteal endarterectomy fell from favor because of its limited applicability to reconstructions that ended proximal to the distal portion of the popliteal artery. The full open repair was tedious, and most surgeons had limited success in restoring flow.

In recent years, however, closed endarterial procedures have become commonplace. Dotter and Judkins began in 1956 by using a stiff dilator,[140] a procedure that was not widely accepted. Gruntzig and Hopff modified this method by using a balloon that could distend and fracture the stenotic plaque.[141]

Endarterial procedures have been extended to include not only dilatation and placement of emboli of several kinds in bleeding arteries, but also removal of atherosclerotic lesions by endarterial manipulations through a percutaneous route. A major requirement for endarterial procedures was believed to be endarterial visualization, beyond that provided by contrast radiography. Visualization began effectively with the work of Greenstone and others.[142]

Actual removal of plaque by several mechanical means followed: Simpson and associates[143] used a side-biting forceps in a catheter, Kensey and coworkers[144] used a catheter through which a rapidly rotating auger-like tip was passed, and Ahn and colleagues[145] advocated a high-speed rotary bur. Others have used various forms of laser energy to destroy plaque.[146] In one procedure, the laser recognizes the difference between plaque and normal arterial wall.[147] In another, the laser-heated probe "melts" the atheroma.[148] Further mechanical dilatation often

accompanies these initial coring methods. Appraisal of these methods, however, belongs in the clinical rather than the historical section of this volume; they appear to achieve only limited removal of the atheromatous material and much less satisfactory results than the classic techniques of endarterectomy, albeit without requiring a major operative procedure.

Dotter and others[109] proposed the addition of intraluminal stents to maintain graft patency, as well as the patency of vessels that had been dilated. In the surgical literature, this maneuver was largely ignored until Palmaz and associates[110] introduced balloon-expandable stents, which were first used to maintain patency in dilated arteries. The use of percutaneous arterial dilatation and endarterectomy has suffered from inadequate and inconstant reporting standards in the hands of many nonsurgeons, but the technique appears to have reached a level of acceptance that requires the definition of its historical role.

Parodi and coworkers[111] hybridized the technique of endarterial placement of these stents and added the placement of fabric grafts, a technique described previously in the section on aneurysms.

Two other important extensions of distal femoral reconstruction came on the scene. The first was introduction of the graft to the infrapopliteal artery. In 1960, Palma[149] published descriptions of vein graft insertions into the tibial arteries. Later information from Palma (personal communication, 1990) indicates that these were performed as early as 1956. McCaughan described the exposure of the "distal popliteal artery" (more commonly known as the *tibioperoneal trunk*) and anastomoses to it in 1958,[150] but his work went unrecognized because of his unconventional terminology. In that article, McCaughan[151] described a successful graft into the tibial vessels in July 1957, using an exposure in the upper third of the calf. He presented six additional patients with grafts into the tibial segment in 1960. In 1966, McCaughan[152] went one step further when he reported four grafts in which the distal insertion of the graft was into the posterior tibial artery at the ankle. Morris and coworkers[153] and Tyson and DeLaurentis[154] were other contemporary pioneers in the development of various configurations of infrapopliteal procedures.

The second extension of distal femoral reconstruction was application of the in situ vein graft, with destruction of valvular competence within the vein, by Hall.[155] The procedure did not receive much attention until it was revitalized by Leather and associates in 1981.[156] Many variations on the theme of the distal bypass have been introduced, combining free grafts and in situ methods.

Dardik and associates introduced the use of tanned human umbilical vein and then added a distal arteriovenous fistula.[157] The fistula was not a revival of earlier attempts by Carrel and others to revascularize an extremity through the veins, rather it was an attempt to provide sufficient outflow for a long graft to ensure its patency, with some of the graft flow still directed through the distal arterial tree. DeLaurentis and Friedman introduced a method of sequential multiple bypasses in the extremity,[158] and Veith and associates[159] carried this to extremes with bypasses from one tibial artery to another, and even with bypasses beginning and ending below the malleolus. Nehler's group[160] applied this small vessel bypass technique to the management of small vessel disease in the distal upper extremity.

A different approach to the ischemic lower limb was advocated by Oudot and Cormier[161] when they observed how frequently the superficial femoral artery was occluded, but the profunda femoris remained patent. Martin and coworkers described an extended form of profundaplasty, particularly as the site of insertion of a graft from above.[162]

None of these advances in reconstructive surgery has been helpful in the management of the frustrating syndrome of thromboangiitis obliterans, or Buerger's disease. It is likely that von Winiwarter[163] was describing the pathologic process of thromboangiitis obliterans, but his description and clinical correlation are ambiguous. Certainly, Buerger described the clinical picture,[164] although neither he nor von Winiwarter noted the association with tobacco or the involvement of the upper extremities.

One other major contribution rounds out this section. In 1963, Fogarty and coworkers devised one of the most useful methods for managing occlusive arterial disease—the balloon embolectomy catheter for the extraction of clot in the treatment of embolization.[165] This technique has been modified for use in many other arterial and venous operations and has even been adapted to many general surgical uses.

The development of endarterial stenting and grafting has already been mentioned. These methods have undoubtedly improved the results of arterial dilatation, but the lack of standardized methods of reporting in the nonvascular literature and the overenthusiastic promotion of the method still cloud its value. Furthermore, the application of these techniques has become a point of conflict among radiologists, cardiologists, and surgeons over whose "turf" it should be. Some areas are obviously suitable for treatment by an interventional radiologist or cardiologist, but in many instances the presence and active participation of a surgeon in the operating room are mandatory. In any event, comparison of methods and results should be made possible by accurate and standardized methods of analysis. Here again, current clinical choices supersede historical interpretation.

ARTERIAL TRAUMA

Arterial injuries have always been a challenge to surgeons. Trauma was the source of Hallowell's first arterial repair. During the years after the Civil War, Mitchell described the syndrome of burning pain ("causalgia") that followed many arterial injuries[166]; it was this lesion that had intrigued Leriche and led to his interest in the sympathetic nervous system.[118] Halsted had remarked on surgeons' fascination with arterial injuries. During World War I, Makins[167] surveyed the injuries to blood vessels incurred by the British forces. DeBakey and Simeone[168] provided a similar service for U.S. forces after World War II and noted almost no benefit from the vascular surgical techniques then available because of the

incidental and associated surgical complications and the problem of delay.

Few arterial injuries were treated definitively, except for ligation of the artery, until the Korean War. Before that time, the main interest in arterial injuries seemed to be estimating the likelihood of survival of the limb and selecting the appropriate level for ligation of the artery. Generations of anatomy students learned the "site of election" for ligation of various arteries.

During the Korean War, however, Jahnke and Howard,[169] Hughes,[170] and Spencer and Grewe[171] participated in a program in which acute vascular injuries were treated with fresh vein grafts. Whelan and coworkers[172] and Rich and Hughes[173] continued using these techniques of arterial repair in Vietnam. The Registry of Vascular Injuries from Vietnam, as maintained at the Walter Reed Army Medical Center under the direction of Rich, has continued to yield a monumental body of information concerning acute vascular repair. Civilian medical centers have continued to apply these techniques to the everyday patterns of vessel injuries.

The arteriovenous fistula is one sequela of trauma to the major vessels that poses a special challenge to surgeons. Its acute effects on the distal circulation, its systemic effects as a major left-to-right shunt, and its local changes, which result in increased blood flow through the feeding arterial supply, are all intriguing examples of the body's adaptability—or lack thereof.

The arteriovenous fistula was first described by Hunter.[3] The lesion did not become common until the end of the nineteenth century, as weapons (i.e., high-speed projectiles) and the injuries they caused changed. Volumes have been written in an attempt to interpret the diverse physiologic parameters involved in this lesion, but as early as 1913, Soubbotitich[174] noted that simple ligation of the proximal artery should never be done. Not long after, Lexer introduced the "ideal" operation,[45] consisting of resection of the aneurysmal sac and restoration of flow through the artery with a short venous graft if the ends of the artery could not be brought back together. Reconstruction of the vein was desirable but not mandatory. Bickham suggested approaching the arterial repair through the venous component of the sac, with repair of the vein if possible[34]—a modification of the Matas endoaneurysmorrhaphy.

For the most part, however, until the Korean War era in the 1950s and later, the most common form of surgical management was quadruple ligation and excision of the sac and fistula. Such an operation depended on the development of sufficient collateral circulation to the distal limb to allow the limb to survive after arterial interruption, but it had to be done before the extra load placed on the heart by a left-to-right shunt caused serious cardiac disability; timing was thus a matter of delicate clinical judgment. Holman,[175] whose lifelong interest in the arteriovenous fistula began during his training at Johns Hopkins, was the most eminent contributor to the understanding of the physiology of the arteriovenous fistula. With the advent of prompt exploration and repair of acute arterial injuries, it was anticipated that the number of late arteriovenous fistulas would be greatly reduced, but this has not been the case. The current ability to reconstruct the artery diminishes the need to delay to allow the development of collateral circulation, as was once necessary.

EXTRACRANIAL CEREBROVASCULAR ARTERIAL OCCLUSIONS

The critical nature of the blood flow to the brain through the great arteries of the neck was recognized by the ancient Greeks, who named the carotid artery after the symptoms that followed its occlusion—asphyxia, or stupor. The clinical importance of carotid artery stenosis and obstruction was only slowly accepted by the neurologic community in general, however, despite the fact that eminent neurologists such as Savory,[176] Hunt,[177] and Fisher[178,179] had observed the relationship between arterial lesions and atheroembolic phenomena many years before surgical treatment became accepted.

The first elective attempt to restore flow to the ischemic brain was made by Carrea and associates in 1951 but not reported until 1955.[180] The proximal portion of the diseased internal carotid artery was excised, and flow was restored by an anastomosis of the unusually large proximal external carotid artery to the cut end of the distal internal carotid. A slightly different reconstruction of the carotid bifurcation, necessitated by a gunshot wound, was accomplished by Lefèvre in 1918.[181] He resected the carotid bulb, ligated the common trunk, and anastomosed the distal ends of the internal and external carotid arteries to provide the brain with the arterial supply from the rich anastomoses of the external carotid artery.

The most widely acclaimed early carotid reconstruction and the one that truly began the modern reconstructive era was the resection of the carotid bifurcation and restoration of carotid flow by anastomosis of the common carotid to the internal carotid by Eastcott and colleagues in 1954.[182] It now appears that others, including Cooley and colleagues,[183] Roe,[184] and DeBakey,[185] were among the first to successfully perform true carotid endarterectomies. As was the case with Estes[90] and his paper justifying the approach to abdominal aneurysms, so the report to the National Research Council of Great Britain by Yates and Hutchinson[186] indicated the importance of occlusive disease of the carotid and vertebral arteries.

Whisnant and associates[187] in Rochester, Minnesota, identified the risk of stroke in the presence of transient ischemic attacks and provided the solid basis for operation on the carotid artery to prevent major strokes. Hollenhorst[188] called attention to the bright cholesterol emboli seen in the eye grounds that are pathognomonic of atherosclerotic embolization, but Julian and associates[189] and Moore and Hall[190] clearly demonstrated that embolization was the major cause of transient cerebral ischemic symptoms, rather than simple hemodynamics. Further landmark studies of the morphology of carotid plaque and its evolution were presented by Imparato and coworkers[191] and Lusby and associates.[192] Moore and Hall[193] and others among Wylie's group called attention to the role of carotid back-pressure in identifying patients whose brains needed protection from ischemia during the period of operative occlusion.

Operation for symptomatic patients was soon relatively well accepted, but operation to prevent stroke in asymptomatic patients whose carotid stenosis manifests as a bruit or a measurable change in retinal artery pressure or some other noninvasive laboratory test remains controversial. Work by Thompson and colleagues[194] is the predominant authoritative source, despite criticism concerning its lack of perfect controls. Dixon and associates[195] provided further evidence of the role of large, asymptomatic ulcerations of the carotid bifurcation. Berguer and coworkers[196] showed that many "asymptomatic" patients with carotid lesions actually demonstrate multiple small cerebral infarcts that are not clearly reflected in the patient's symptoms.

In 1992, Moore summarized several early multicenter, randomized trials that were performed to compare carotid endarterectomy with nonsurgical methods.[197] These trials revealed carotid endarterectomy to be so highly effective that many early criticisms of the operation were quieted. An immense body of controversial literature exists concerning the role of anticoagulant or antiplatelet agents to prevent thrombosis or thromboembolization, but these modalities remain an adjunct to carotid endarterectomy performed by trained surgeons. Continuing comparisons of several different modalities continue to define appropriate clinical measures.

The surgeon's inability to clear the totally occluded bifurcation safely and effectively has been addressed by the use of microsurgical techniques. Yasargil and associates[198] first popularized this technique. Many neurosurgeons have become skillful in the performance of extracranial-to-intracranial bypass. A randomized study cast serious doubts about the value of this technique in preventing strokes,[199] and its true role remains to be clarified.

VISCERAL VASCULAR OCCLUSIONS

One of the most important lesions in relatively small arteries is the occlusive lesion in the coronary arteries. Longmire and colleagues[200] performed a few successful coronary endarterectomies in 1958. The difficulties associated with endarterectomy in small vessels led others to use the vein graft, first as a replacement by Favoloro[201] in 1968 and then as a bypass by Johnson and associates[202] in 1969.

Renal arterial insufficiency has been treated successfully for many years. Goldblatt and coworkers[203] recognized the importance of renal ischemia as a cause of arterial hypertension, and others explained the details of the deranged physiology. Freeman and associates[129] were among the first to treat this lesion successfully, leading to the surgical management of renovascular hypertension. DeCamp and coworkers,[204] Poutasse,[205] and Foster and associates[206] were leaders in the perfection of these techniques.

Recognition of several forms of fibromuscular hyperplasia in the renal artery was followed by its identification in the internal carotid artery by Connett and Lansche.[207]

Ehrenfeld and associates put the surgical management of this lesion on a firm footing.[208]

Occlusive disease is much less common in the mesenteric vessels than in most other visceral beds, but it is frequently lethal when it does occur. It was commonly recognized only when it had reached an advanced stage and caused extensive intestinal necrosis. Dunphy[209] in 1936 related the progression of symptoms of mesenteric ischemia to frank intestinal infarction. Fifteen years later, Klass[210] removed an embolus from the superior mesenteric artery successfully, although the patient died of his primary cardiovascular disease. Barker and Cannon[133] included in their first endarterectomy series a patient who underwent a superior mesenteric endarterectomy at the same time as an aortoiliac procedure. In 1957, Shaw and Rutledge[211] performed an embolectomy of the superior mesenteric artery without concomitant bowel resection. The following year, Shaw and Maynard[212] identified two patients with both malabsorption and mesenteric ischemia who were treated successfully by endarterectomy. In the meantime, Mikkelsen and Zaro[213] reported similar experiences from California, and they clarified the useful term intestinal angina.

The meandering mesenteric collaterals so well described by Kountz and associates[214] provided a radiographic sign suggesting the presence of serious stenosis of the celiac axis and superior mesenteric vessels. Recognition of this sign has become cause for careful evaluation of the mesenteric vessels, whether found in the radiology suite or the operating room.

One of the important nonsurgical lesions that mimics obstructive mesenteric vascular disease is the nonocclusive form of mesenteric vascular insufficiency identified by Heer and associates.[215] This condition occurs in forms of cardiogenic shock in which the cardiac output is low and the mesenteric vascular resistance is high.

The extrinsic compression syndrome of the celiac axis is a subject capable of generating considerable discussion. Marable and associates first described this as compression by the arcuate ligament of the diaphragm.[216] Some authors believe that other anatomic structures, such as the neural components of the celiac ganglion, may also be involved. Many support the existence of this lesion, whatever its anatomic cause, as a source of serious symptoms; others forcefully deny its existence.[217]

EXTRAANATOMIC BYPASS AND VASCULAR INFECTIONS

There are many technical and mechanical advances that cannot properly be placed in any of the previously described compartments of the history of vascular surgery. One of these is the concept of extraanatomic bypass. The term itself is controversial. It has been suggested that the term implies a bypass outside the body instead of outside the classic anatomic routes, but its usage is so well established that it is retained here. It was proposed as a possibility by Kunlin[137] and actually carried out as an ilioiliac bypass by way of the prevesical space by Oudot in 1951. Although rerouting of flow through short shunts had been done by many surgeons for various reasons, the first

dramatic step was taken by Blaisdell and colleagues,[218] who led a graft from the thoracic aorta extraperitoneally to the femoral artery. Shortly thereafter, this anatomic arrangement was modified as the axillofemoral and then the axillobifemoral graft in 1963 by Blaisdell and Hall.[219]

The axillofemoral bypass was first advised as a means of establishing flow to the extremity in the presence of an infected aortic reconstruction that had to be removed. Similarly, in 1966, Mahoney and Whelan[220] introduced the obturator bypass to avoid an established infection in the groin. Vetto[221] introduced a slightly different anatomic variant—the femorofemoral bypass—in 1962, 11 years after Oudot's ilioiliac operation. Today the pattern of unusual anatomic configurations seems limited only by the patient's needs and the surgeon's ingenuity.

One of the important indications for replacement of the classic aortic prosthesis is the development of an aortoenteric fistula. These lesions have plagued surgeons since the first aortic grafts were performed. Elliott and coauthors[222] contributed one of the first important papers toward the understanding of this problem. Later, Busuttil and associates[223] defined the common primary role played by the false aneurysm at the aortic suture line and clarified the management.

VENOUS SURGERY

The history of venous surgery is in one sense older and in another sense newer than that of arterial surgery. Venous repairs were undertaken before arterial repairs were generally successful. Most of the first generation of arterial surgeons learned about the vagaries of the venous system as their first experiences in vascular surgery. Varicose veins, venous thrombosis, pulmonary embolism, and the postphlebitic extremity were the four major topics.

Although operations on the veins were the major procedures that vascular surgeons were called on to perform in the first half of the twentieth century, venous surgery was overshadowed by the more glamorous arterial reconstructions until recently, when the American Venous Forum was established to study the management of problems involving the veins. Phlebology never lost its major role in Europe, and the Venous Forum has returned venous surgery to prominent status in the United States.

The earliest modern operations for varicosities consisted of little more than local excision of the varix, and it was probably Trendelenburg who introduced the physiologically useful ligation of the long saphenous vein in the upper leg.[224,225] Trendelenburg's interruption of the saphenous vein was carried out in the midthigh. Although Trendelenburg's operation introduced and was directed at the concept of reversal of flow in the diseased saphenous system, the collaterals at the saphenous bulb allowed prompt return to a pattern of saphenous flow toward the foot. Homans[226] is generally credited with defining the importance of interrupting the saphenous vein flush with the femoral vein and dividing its major collateral trunks in the first few centimeters below that junction.

Babcock devised techniques to strip or avulse veins by means of extraluminal strippers,[227] and for many years the Mayo external stripper has been a useful instrument to facilitate dissection of the vein.[228]

Radical stripping of the major saphenous trunks has become less common in the last quarter century, once the importance of preserving a nonvaricose vein for possible later use as an arterial conduit became an important consideration.

Pulmonary embolism has long been a major problem for physicians in all areas of medical practice. In 1908, Trendelenburg introduced the operation of pulmonary embolectomy.[229] This operation was undertaken infrequently and was usually unsuccessful, but its rare successes have continued to challenge surgeons. It is an operation that can be applied more frequently today because of the ability to support the patient's cardiovascular system until the operation can be performed. The role of direct operation may be lessened by the ability to place catheters in the pulmonary artery and dissolve the clot with thrombolytic agents.[230]

In 1934, the true relationship between deep venous thrombosis of the leg veins and pulmonary embolism was clarified by Homans,[231,232] who matched the ends of a thrombus taken from the pulmonary artery at autopsy with a residual clot in the popliteal vein, showing that this must have been the source of the embolus. Homans recognized that the great venous sinuses in the soleal veins were capable of returning large quantities of blood during exercise, but at rest, blood might be stagnant there. Thus, given the other factors of Virchow's triad (stagnant flow, endothelial injury, and increased coagulability), one might anticipate spontaneous thrombosis at that site. In fact, subsequent studies with radioiodinated fibrinogen showed an alarming rate of thrombosis there. Fortunately, only a small proportion of these thromboses yields thrombi that propagate into the mainline channels and produce serious clinical problems.

The next step in the management of patients with venous thrombosis was also made by Homans,[233] who introduced ligation of the superficial femoral vein where it joins the deep femoral system in the groin. The introduction of this procedure must be viewed in the context of the times, when there was no practical anticoagulant commonly in use. Allen,[234] Veal,[235] and others quickly took up this operation.

Homans experienced disappointment over the outcome of a patient whose superficial femoral vein he and I had ligated. A clot propagated through the deep femoral system and into the common femoral vein, causing an embolism and the patient's death, despite the interruption of the superficial femoral vein.

The preferred level of venous ligation was moved upward because of other similar failures of superficial femoral vein interruption. First, the common femoral and then the iliac veins were ligated bilaterally. These operations could be performed under local anesthesia through groin incisions, but it was soon recognized that bilateral ligation of the iliac veins was preferred to the common femoral site. Vena caval interruption soon became the procedure of choice. It is hard to identify who first ligated the vena cava for pulmonary embolism, but Northway and Buxton,[236] O'Neill,[237] and Collins and coworkers[238] are all credited with early reports.

It seems unfortunate that once anticoagulants became readily available—first warfarin (Coumadin) and then heparin—their combination with ligation was not common; ligation and anticoagulation were used on an either-or basis by most physicians. Simple ligation without anticoagulant therapy was often associated with extension of thrombosis in the stagnant systems below the ligature, which led to severe postphlebitic symptoms. Anlyan and colleagues,[239] Bowers and Leb,[240] and others seriously criticized interruption, giving rise to a school that treated venous thrombosis primarily with increasingly large doses of heparin.[241] The extent of postphlebitic syndrome, however, seems to be more clearly related to the extent of the inflammatory thrombophlebitic process and its destruction of the valves in the leg than to ligation or the level of ligation.[242] The successful use of large doses of heparin has greatly diminished the need for venous interruption.

Spencer[243] introduced another approach to caval interruption, however, to maintain some flow through the cava but still prevent the passage of emboli to the lungs by plication of the cava with sutures. Other extraluminal occlusive devices were suggested by Moretz and associates,[244] Miles and colleagues,[245] and Adams and DeWeese.[246] Mobin-Uddin's invention of a transvenous umbrella[247] and Greenfield's transvenous wire trap[248] reduced the need for major venous interruption by open surgical methods even further.

The problems of the postphlebitic extremity remain. This syndrome was well described by Homans,[249] but his contributions to its treatment were not particularly fruitful, except that they represent the culmination of the best forms of nonoperative management. Trout,[250] Linton,[251] and Dodd and Cockett[252] separately advocated methods that accomplish subfascial interruption of the communicating veins in the lower leg; this procedure remains a surgical standard.

The re-creation of a venous drainage channel that is protected from regurgitant flow offered a new approach to this old problem. Kistner demonstrated a technique of converting an incompetent valve into a competent one.[253] Venous transposition, redirecting flow through a competent vein and around an area of venous incompetence, is another approach used by Dale[254] and Palma and Esperoti.[255]

Taheri and coworkers[256] published the results of a free graft of a valved segment of the axillary vein into the diseased femoral system. Taheri and others[257] went even farther, attempting to develop prosthetic venous valves.

HIGHLIGHTS IN DIAGNOSTIC MODALITIES

The diagnosis of both arterial and venous diseases has long depended on the use of contrast radiography. One of the first to use this technique successfully in a living patient was Brooks,[258] who injected sodium iodide to demonstrate the lesions of Buerger's disease in digital vessels. Moniz described "arterial encephalography" for neurologic lesions in 1927.[259] His presentation was not only a seminal paper; it also defined the technical needs of the radiographer in terms that are pertinent nearly 80 years later.

In the audience at Moniz's presentation was dos Santos (the elder). He and his colleagues soon published the basic technical approach to arteriography of the vessels of the abdomen and their branches.[260] Each of these authors foresaw the great advances that would accompany the development of rapid cassette changers and less toxic contrast media, but the techniques of image enhancement and subtraction by electronic means are recent and highly effective contributions.

One of the major technical advances for the angiographer was Seldinger's technique,[261] which, instead of using a single needle to inject contrast material, used a catheter that was passed over a wire that had been introduced through the primary vessel puncture. The guidewire was first advanced to the desired site, then the appropriate catheter was advanced over the wire. Wire and catheter could be alternated so that injections could be made at different sites and at different rates. With this method, a catheter can be placed and injection can be achieved at almost any intravascular site in the body. The culmination of these technical advances is the clarification and modification of the radiographic image by subtraction, digitization, enhancement, and various electronic manipulations.

A totally different field of radiology was signaled by the work of Dotter and Judkins,[140] who used a rigid dilator passed through a large needle under fluoroscopic guidance to dilate narrowed arteries in 1956. Dotter's contributions were followed by those of Gruntzig.[141] This percutaneous intravascular technique evolved into the burgeoning field of interventional rather than purely diagnostic radiology.

The growth of vascular surgery in recent years has been almost synonymous with the development of methods of noninvasive diagnosis of peripheral vascular disease. This is an outgrowth of those methods commonly taken for granted, which had their humble beginnings in the stethoscope, the sphygmomanometer,[262] and the ophthalmoscope.

The measurement of many physiologic parameters in the laboratory was extended to the patient by such physicians as Winsor,[263] whose definition of pressure gradients remains a critical basis for the clinical estimation of the severity of arterial obstruction. Combined with a sphygmomanometer and a Doppler sensor, evaluation of segmental arterial pressures became a useful means of evaluating peripheral arterial disease and identifying segmental pressure differences, just as Winsor had done with less accurate sensing methods.

Other common measurements performed in the early vascular diagnostic laboratories included digital and segmental plethysmography and skin temperature and resistance, both before and after sympathetic blockade.

Pachon[264] introduced a modification of the sphygmomanometer and the segmental plethysmograph; the oscillometer provided a rough measure of the volume of the distensile arterial pulse wave. The values obtained bore no physiologic definition, but comparisons at different levels in one extremity, of comparable levels in opposite extremities, or at one site on successive occasions provided the surgeon with some objective evidence of change. Although the stethoscope is used by all physicians, its role

in the evaluation of murmurs over the peripheral arteries was clarified and codified by Edwards and Levine[265] and then by Wylie and McGuiness[266] at a surprisingly late date. The usefulness of inexpensive auscultation has diminished as electronic assessment has become readily available.

One of the interesting early techniques was that of Baillart,[267] who used the ophthalmoscope and concurrent ophthalmodynamometry to evaluate lesions of the eye and thus estimate retinal arterial pressures, which were assumed to reflect pressure and hence flow through the internal carotid artery. Operator sensitivity and reproducibility, critical aspects of many such techniques, were such that the method's utility was not great. Kartchner[268] and Gee[269] and their respective colleagues introduced a recording device to reproduce relative pressure curves within the ocular globe or to compare the peak time of the retinal artery pulse wave, which is reflected in the globe's pressure, with the arrival of the pulse wave in the earlobe; this enabled estimation of the severity of obstruction in the carotid system. Gee and associates developed a method to evaluate the back-pressure in the stenotic carotid artery to predict the necessity of a shunt during operative carotid occlusion. Their method, however, is actually of greater value in evaluating the forward pressure beyond the stenotic carotid artery; it provides more precise measurement of the pressures but does not provide time relationships, as Kartchner's system does. These subtle physiologic evaluations of the intraocular arterial pressure as an indirect reflection of the intracranial carotid flow have been supplanted by more direct physiologic studies of the extracranial arteries in the neck.

Ultrasonography has become one of the most popular modalities in its many ramifications. Leopold and associates[270] used classic ultrasonic imaging (B-mode) techniques to outline the aorta and identify aneurysmal changes there.

Use of the ultrasonic flow detector was soon modified by Brockenbrough to determine the direction of flow through the supraorbital artery,[271] which is reversed in the presence of high-grade obstruction of the ipsilateral carotid artery. Machleder and Barker dramatized the technique,[272] but extreme operator sensitivity limits its use.

Imaging of the crude Doppler signal was introduced by Thomas and coworkers,[273] who simply mounted a Doppler probe on a scanning device. Increased sophistication of these scanning methods ultimately led to duplex scanning techniques.

Ultrasonography in another form (i.e., either the continuous or the gated Doppler mode that measures the shift in frequency of the ultrasonic signal reflected from moving red blood cells) was introduced by Strandness and colleagues[274] and by Sumner and Strandness.[275] Here, ultrasonic B-mode scanning defines the anatomy and obtains a reference point to be combined with pulsed, "gated" Doppler reflections to show blood flow patterns and velocities at the designated site within the lumen. Use of these studies is limited to vessels that can be "reached" by the Doppler signal.[276] This method became widely used to evaluate the carotid bifurcation, but its application has now been extended as a monitor in peripheral arterial sites, vertebral arteries,[277] mesenteric vessels,[278] and at the operating table.[279] Evaluation of the circle of Willis is also possible, but is not consistently reliable.[280]

Carotid angiography has been shown to contribute a major proportion of the morbidity and mortality associated with carotid surgery in many randomized trials. As a result, duplex imaging has rapidly replaced it as the primary diagnostic tool for carotid artery disease. It provides highly accurate anatomic as well as physiologic data, although arteriography is still necessary in some patients.

A new twist on computed tomography was introduced by Kalender and associates.[281] Use of this form of spiral computed tomography has become more common, and although its images may lose some of the detail obtained by other methods, it provides a superb overall picture of the course and collaterals of an arterial segment, and its software allows manipulation so that the three-dimensional image can be visualized from many different angles. Magnetic resonance imaging has become a useful evaluation tool, especially of the aorta, and magnetic resonance angiography also shows promise,[282] but these techniques are at the stage of clinical rather than historical evaluation at the moment.

Evaluation of the venous side of the circulation beyond classic physical examination has not yielded such exact information. Cranley and coworkers[283] introduced "phleborheography," which evaluates changes in venous pulse, outflow, and respiratory excursions to diagnose deep venous disease of the legs. Wheeler's impedance plethysmography[284] is less sophisticated and easier to handle, but perhaps less informative.

The Doppler velocity probe, despite some drawbacks related to operator sensitivity, remains a useful method for identifying lesions in the major superficial veins, such as in the groin, the popliteal space, and the axilla. It can also be used in the postphlebitic extremity to identify both regurgitant flow in superficial channels and flow from communicating veins. It can be used even in the presence of brawny edema, which otherwise obscures much of the venous system from sight and palpation.

Just as the duplex scan in carotid surgery has become popular, color-assisted duplex imaging is an important part of the evaluation of the venous system,[285] where its use was first popularized.

VASCULAR ACCESS SURGERY

Kolff's introduction of hemodialysis in the mid 1950s revolutionized nephrology,[286] but it also added to the number of difficult procedures that vascular surgeons are asked to perform, including providing and maintaining access to the vascular system, often on an emergency basis. Vascular access surgery lacks the glamour of much of the rest of vascular surgery, but it constitutes a significant portion of vascular surgical practice. The construction and maintenance of a well-functioning access site demand both surgical skill and judgment.

The first approaches involved the use of silicone tubing as an external shunt between the arterial and venous systems in the arm.[287] The natural progression by Brescia and his team was to use a direct arteriovenous fistula, usually in the arm.[288] The fistula results in dilated veins suitable for recurrent punctures. The addition of an autologous vein graft to allow a better fistula and better access to the vein[289] was soon followed by the use of other materials as shunts, both biologic and plastic.[290]

THORACIC OUTLET SYNDROMES

The problems and care of the varied thoracic outlet syndromes are shared by vascular surgeons, orthopedists, neurosurgeons, and physiotherapists. Although first treated surgically as an exostosis of the first rib in 1861,[291] clear anatomic understanding was achieved through the works of Murphy,[292] Adson and Coffey,[293] and Ochsner and coworkers.[294] It appeared to early authors that a cervical rib was the offending anatomic structure, but Adson and Coffey introduced the concept of entrapment of the brachial plexus and accompanying artery by the anterior scalene muscle and the highest rib. Naffziger and Grant confirmed the mechanical origins of the syndrome and demonstrated the anterior supraclavicular approach.[295] One of the illustrations, however, taking an anatomist's point of view from inside the chest, showed the anatomy that Roos would subsequently use in his transaxillary approach.[296] Falconer and Li[297] proposed resection of the first rib to relieve the costoclavicular compression of the vessels. Edwards offered a thesis that consolidated the anatomic and evolutionary origins of these syndromes, pointing out that the human is one of the few animals in which there is a descent of the heart and great vessels in relation to the shoulder girdle, which leads to draping of the great vessels over the highest rib, whatever its number might be.[298]

The surgical approaches to this area have been varied: paraspinal and anterior supraclavicular and transaxillary. The latter involves no major muscle division and provides a better cosmetic result. It is especially helpful in muscular athletes, who are prone to symptoms from compression.

The most common form involves pressure on the nerves and arteries, but a slightly different anatomic arrangement is responsible for the variations in Paget-Schroetter syndrome, in which obstruction of the venous system is the major problem. McLeery and coworkers[299] defined the anatomic basis of intermittent venous obstruction from the subclavian and anterior scalene muscles.

BIBLIOGRAPHY

Bigger IA: Surgical treatment of aneurysm of the aorta: Review of the literature and report of two cases, one apparently successful. Ann Surg 112:879–894, 1940.

Blaisdell FW, Hall AD: Axillary-femoral artery bypass for lower extremity ischemia. Surgery 54:563–568, 1963.

Blalock A, Taussig HB: The surgical treatment of malformations of the heart in which there is pulmonary stenosis or pulmonary atresia. JAMA 128:189–202, 1945.

Buerger L: Thromboangiitis obliterans: A study of the vascular lesions leading to presenile spontaneous gangrene. Am J Med Sci 136:567–580, 1908.

Carrel A: The surgery of blood vessels, etc. Johns Hopkins Hosp Bull 190:18–28, 1907.

Charcot JM: Obstruction artérielle et claudication intermittente dans le cheval et dans l'homme. Mem Soc Biol 1:225–238, 1858.

Crafoord C, Nylin G: Congenital coarctation of the aorta and its surgical treatment. J Thorac Surg 14:347–361, 1945.

DeBakey ME, Cooley SA, Crawford ES, et al: Clinical application of a new flexible knitted Dacron arterial substitute. Arch Surg 77:713–724, 1958.

DeCamp P, Snyder CH, Bost RB: Severe hypertension due to congenital stenosis of artery to solitary kidney: Correction by splenorenal anastomosis. Arch Surg 75:1026–1030, 1957.

Dobson J: John Hunter, Edinburgh, 1969, E & S Livingstone.

dos Santos JC: Sur la désobstruction des thromboses artérielles anciennes. Mem Acad Chir 73:409–411, 1947.

dos Santos R, Lamas A, Caldas P: L'artériographie des membres, de l'aorte et des ses branches abdominales. Bull Mem Soc Natl Chir 55:587–601, 1929.

Dubost C, Allary M, Oeconomos N: Resection of an aneurysm of the abdominal aorta: Reestablishment of the continuity by a preserved human arterial graft, with result after five months. Arch Surg 64:405–408, 1952.

Dunphy JE: Abdominal pain of vascular origin. Am J Med Sci 92:109–113, 1936.

Eastcott HHG, Pickering GW, Rob C: Reconstruction of internal carotid artery in a patient with intermittent attacks of hemiplegia. Lancet 2:994–996, 1954.

Edwards WS, Tapp JS: Chemically treated nylon tubes as arterial grafts. Surgery 38:61–76, 1955.

Fogarty TJ, Cranley JJ, Krause RJ, et al: A method of extraction of arterial emboli and thrombi. Surg Gynecol Obstet 116:241–244, 1963.

Gross RE: Complete surgical division of the patent ductus arteriosus. Surg Gynecol Obstet 78:36–43, 1944.

Holman E: Clinical and experimental observations on arteriovenous fistulae. Ann Surg 112:840–878, 1940.

Homans J: Thrombosis of the deep veins of the lower leg causing pulmonary embolism. N Engl J Med 211:993–997, 1934.

Homans J: The late results of femoral thrombophlebitis and their treatment. N Engl J Med 235:249–253, 1946.

Jaboulay M, Briau E: Recherches expérimentales sur la suture et la greffe artérielles. Bull Lyon Med 81:97–99, 1896.

Jahnke EJ, Jr, Howard JM: Primary repair of major arterial injuries. Arch Surg 66:646–649, 1953.

Jassinowsky A: Die Arteriennaht: Eine experimentelle Studie [dissertation], Dorpat, Estonia, 1889, University of Tartu.

Julian OC, Dye WS, Javid H, et al: Ulcerative lesions of the carotid artery bifurcation. Arch Surg 86:803–809, 1963.

Kistner RL: Surgical repair of the incompetent vein valve. Arch Surg 110:1336–1342, 1975.

Kolff WJ: The first clinical experience with the artificial kidney. Ann Intern Med 62:608–619, 1965.

Kunlin J: Le traitement de l'ischemie artéritique par la greffe veineuse longue. Rev Chir 70:207–235, 1951.

Leriche R: Des oblitérations artérielles hautes (oblitération de la terminasion de l'aorte) comme causes des insuffisances circulatoires des membres inférieures. Bull Mem Soc Chir (Paris) 49:1404–1406, 1923.

Longmire WP, Jr, Cannon JA, Kattus HA: Direct-vision coronary endarterectomy for angina pectoris. N Engl J Med 259:993–999, 1958.

Marrangoni AC, Cecchini LP: Homotransplantation of arterial segments by the freeze-drying method. Ann Surg 134:977–983, 1951.

Matas R: Traumatic aneurism of the brachial artery. Med News 53:462–466, 1888.

Moore WS, Hall AD: Carotid artery back pressure: A test of cerebral tolerance to temporary carotid artery occlusion. Arch Surg 99:702–710, 1969.

Murphy JB: Resection of arteries and veins injured in continuity … end to end suture … experimental and clinical research. Med Rec 51:73–88, 1897.

Murray GDW: Heparin in thrombosis and embolism. Br J Surg 27:567–576, 1940.

Ochsner A, Gage M, DeBakey ME: Scalenus anticus (Naffziger) syndrome. Am J Surg 28:669–693, 1935.

Parodi J, Palmaz JC, Barone HD: Transfemoral intraluminal graft implantation for abdominal aortic aneurysms. Ann Vasc Surg 5:491–499, 1991.

Strandness DE, Schultz RD, Sumner DS, et al: Ultrasonic flow detection: A useful technique in the evaluation of peripheral vascular disease. Am J Surg 113:311–320, 1967.

Thompson JE, Patman RD, Talkington CM: Asymptomatic carotid bruit. Ann Surg 188:308–316, 1978.

Voorhees AB, Jr, Jaretzki A, III, Blakemore AH: Use of tubes constructed of Vinyon-"N" cloth in bridging arterial defects. Ann Surg 135:332–336, 1952.

Winsor T: Pressure gradients: Influence of arterial disease on the systolic blood pressure gradients of the extremity. Am J Med Sci 220:117–126, 1950.

References available online at expertconsult.com.

QUESTIONS

1. Implantation of a small artery into the side of a larger one by the patch technique was described by whom?
   a. Linton
   b. W. Hunter
   c. DeBakey
   d. Carrel
   e. Hufnagel

2. The first treatment of arterial obstruction in the leg by an endarterial approach was reported by whom?
   a. Homans
   b. Cannon
   c. Wylie
   d. Dotter
   e. Leriche

3. The chronic burning pain described by Mitchell is known as what?
   a. Artérite
   b. Thromboangiitis
   c. Causalgia
   d. Peripheral neuritis
   e. Postherpetic neuralgia

4. The first successful coronary artery reconstruction for angina was performed by whom?
   a. May
   b. DeBakey and Cooley
   c. Cooley and Morris
   d. Edwards and Lyons
   e. Longmire and Cannon

5. Who is commonly credited with interrupting major draining veins in the leg to treat deep venous thrombosis?
   a. Holman
   b. Hall
   c. Homans
   d. Allen
   e. Trendelenburg

6. The duplex scan was introduced to evaluate what?
   a. Flow in the venous system
   b. Carotid stenosis
   c. Size and progression of abdominal aneurysms
   d. Raynaud's syndrome
   e. Pulmonary embolism

7. The possibility of an extraanatomic bypass of an obstructed artery was first proposed by _____ and carried out by _____.
   a. J. Hunter and Cooper
   b. Wylie and Moore
   c. DeBakey and Morris
   d. Kunlin and Oudot
   e. Linton and Darling

8. John Hunter's famous operation to cure popliteal aneurysm consisted of what?
   a. Ligation of the popliteal artery above and below the aneurysm
   b. Sympathectomy and excision of the aneurysm
   c. Sympathectomy and ligation of the common femoral artery
   d. Sympathectomy and external compression (using the Massachusetts General compressor) of the popliteal artery
   e. Ligation of the "superficial" femoral artery in the subsartorial region

9. Murray's introduction of heparin to clinical use led which surgeon to attempt delayed arterial embolectomy?
   a. Homans
   b. Osler
   c. Kunlin
   d. J. dos Santos
   e. Matas

10. Although not described in the exact words, the principle behind the concept of endoleaks following operation for aneurysm was described by whom?
   a. Vesalius
   b. J. Hunter
   c. Holman
   d. Matas
   e. Parodi

ANSWERS

1. **d**
2. **d**
3. **c**
4. **e**
5. **c**
6. **a**
7. **d**
8. **e**
9. **d**
10. **d**

CHAPTER 2

EMBRYOLOGY OF THE VASCULAR SYSTEM

David S. Maxwell

It is quite evident that the vascular apparatus does not independently and by itself "unfold" into the adult pattern. On the contrary, it reacts continuously in a most sensitive way to the factors of its environment, the pattern in the adult being the result of the sum of the environmental influences that have played upon it throughout the embryonic period. We thus find that this apparatus is continuously adequate and complete for the structures as they exist at any particular stage as the environmental structures progressively change; the vascular apparatus also changes and thereby is always adapted to the newer conditions. Furthermore, there are no apparent ulterior preparations at any time for the supply and drainage of other structures which have not yet made their appearance. For each stage it is an efficient and complete going-mechanism, apparently uninfluenced by the nature of its subsequent morphology.

GEORGE L. STREETER (1918)

This observation made more than 80 years ago exemplifies the finest tradition of the working scientist: years of attention to the most minute details of a subject, which eventuate in the broadest and most comprehensive view of the fundamental issues. In this statement, Streeter summarizes all that needs to be said and virtually all that can be said about the development of the vascular system, save for some specific details that would only embellish the theme he has laid out.

The story of the development of the vascular system encompasses the life span of the organism. This system retains the ability to grow, change, regenerate, and add on in response to the changing needs of the tissues, from the earliest stages of embryonic life to the final breath. Thus, it supports normal growth, wound healing, and revascularization of tissues endangered by restricted flow in existing vessels, just as it supports the new growth of tumors and transiently develops a highly efficient transport and exchange system through the uteroplacental circulation during pregnancy. All this is accomplished by the opening and enlarging of preexisting vessels and the budding of new vascular growth from preexisting stem vessels. That it may eventually fail to respond to adequately supply the myocardium or the central nervous system is not as remarkable as the fact that it responds so well for so long. It seems likely that, in the embryonic and fetal history of the vascular system, there would be clues to the mysteries that surround this responsiveness throughout life. Furthermore, in the prenatal unfolding of the vascular system lie the origins of the various cardiovascular malformations to which the human organism is subject. We do not yet know whether the mechanisms of growth and the stimuli to vascularization of the embryo and fetus are the same as those that encourage and sustain the responsiveness of the vasculature in the postnatal organism.

This chapter does not attempt to review the enormous literature on the subject, and many exciting details are omitted in the interest of providing a simple narrative exposition of the high points. The organizational scheme first discusses a short history of the heart, which is simply a greatly modified blood vessel, followed by descriptions of the development of the large arteries and veins. The chapter concludes with some comments on the growth of small vessels, which, like acorns, must appear and flourish first to produce the mighty trunk and branches of the vascular tree.

EARLY HISTORY

An organism of a cubic millimeter or so in volume (depending on the surface area and other factors related to the effectiveness of diffusion) may thrive without a vascular system. The human embryo enjoys the elaboration of a vascular system from its earliest stages, almost as if it can anticipate that its bulk will soon require a highly sophisticated transport system. As the embryonic disk becomes recognizable, blood islands rapidly accumulate around the periphery of the disk. These isolated "puddles" begin to coalesce and communicate with one another until the embryo resembles a bloody sponge. Most prominent is the precephalic region, where the seemingly random coalescence of blood islands forms a network in the region soon to be identified as the cardiogenic plate (Figure 2-1A).

In these earliest stages of development, the vascular system manifests some of its greatest mysteries: to what extent is the developmental pattern dictated by tissue needs and demands (possibly through the release of angiogenic factors or through stimuli provided by metabolic products), and to what extent is it dictated by factors

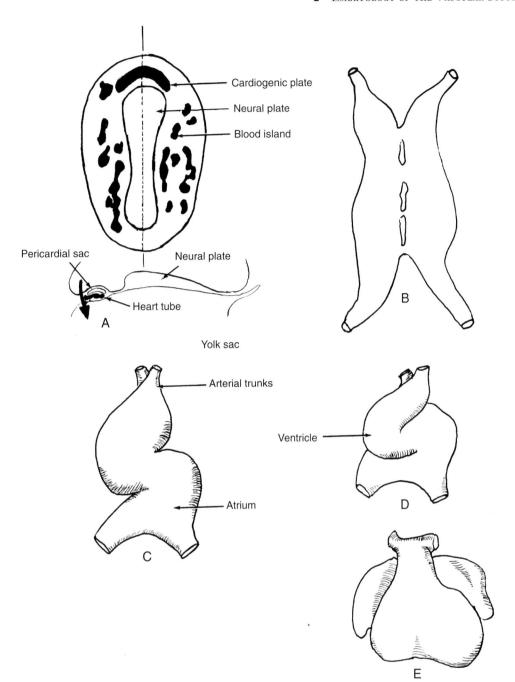

FIGURE 2-1 ■ **A,** Embryonic disk from above, with the head of the embryo facing upward. The *dotted line* indicates the plane of the longitudinal section below, with the cranial end to the left. In the section, the pericardial sac is above the heart tube, but as the head folds under the forebrain (direction of the *large arrow*), the positions of the heart and sac will be reversed, with the heart invaginating from above the pericardial sac. **B,** The two parallel primitive heart tubes (dorsal view) fuse in the midline to form a single heart tube and a single-chambered heart. **C-E,** Successive stages of the folding of the heart tube, viewed from the front. The venous end of the tube swings posteriorly to form the atria, whereas the arterial end (ventricles) remains anterior. This represents the loop stage. (Adapted from Moore KL: The developing human, ed 3, Philadelphia, 1982, WB Saunders, 1982; and Rushmer RF: Cardiovascular dynamics, ed 2, Philadelphia, 1961, WB Saunders.)

such as extravascular pressures restricting flow in one set of possible blood channels and forcing the enlargement of adjacent alternative routes of blood flow? To what extent is the overall pattern dictated genetically? The similarity of the vascular tree from one individual to another favors the speculation that there is a detailed genetic code. The variability from one to another—each pattern seemingly equally efficient in supporting tissues

and organs—argues for development according to need and use and based on mechanical and other adventitious factors.

In the case of the heart, a detailed genetic code is surely the guiding factor. Here, curiously, we begin with a parallel pair of cardiac tubes that fuse into one large tube; the latter then divides internally into the right and left hearts. At first glance, this seems inefficient. Why not simply have each original tube of the pair form a right or left heart? The reason is clear when examining the details of internal division of the heart, in which the single outflow tract is divided in such a way as to connect the right heart to the primitive vessels supplying the pulmonary circuit and to connect the remaining members of the branchial arch arteries to the left heart.

HEART

Our interest in the development of the heart in this chapter is restricted to its bearing on the origins of the great vessels. The heart is simply a highly modified artery from both histologic and embryologic viewpoints. Histologically, it resembles a muscular artery because it has three layers to its walls: adventitia (epicardium), tunica media (myocardium), and tunica intima (endocardium). At the beginning, the heart tubes are simply a parallel pair of vessels, seemingly little different from the other components of the random network of primitive blood vessels. Nonetheless, the fusion of these two tubes and the development of a feeble myocardial investment around the endothelium quickly lead to irregular contractions of the musculature, with feeble and inefficient ejection of blood. Subsequent events include the development of septa, dividing the single-chambered heart into right and left halves, and the appearance of valves that dictate unidirectional flow. The heart is beating with increasing regularity and with an efficiency-improving peristalsis and force as the myocardial element thickens and cytodifferentiates. Presumably from these first feeble, sporadic beats there is a stirring of the blood contents of the primitive vessels, perhaps providing some benefit to the growing tissues around them and perhaps beginning to stimulate the enlargement of those channels that will survive into later embryonic stages. Beginning to channel blood through preferred pathways leads to closure and disappearance of less satisfactory routes and enlargement of the more successful channels into definitive blood vessels that are soon worthy of names recognizable in terms of the adult circulatory pattern. Channel formation from blood islands might be influenced simply by the choice of the lowest resistance among the available pathways.

The now-fused heart tube (see Figure 2-1*B*) begins to invaginate the presumptive pericardial cavity, acquiring its visceral and parietal layers of pericardium while still a single-chambered heart configured as a simple, relatively straight tube. As the somites begin to appear in the neck and trunk region, the heart tube begins to fold on itself, first bulging ventrally, further invaginating the pericardial sac. The heart that is now swinging ventrocaudally comes to lie in front of the head and will continue its descent down the front of the neck and into the anterior chest. The ventrally directed bulge created by the U-shaped fold of the heart characterizes the loop stage.[1] The ventral limb of the U is the arterial outflow path, and the dorsal limb of the U will become the venous inflow tract (see Figure 2-1*C* to *E*). By the 10-somite stage, approximately 3 weeks' ovulation age, the heart has begun to fold in a coronal plane as well, directing the

ventricular region to the left and forming a recognizable outflow tract, now termed the *bulbus cordis*, whose distal part is called the *truncus arteriosus* (see Figure 2-1*C*). At this stage, the heart is still a single-chambered structure innocent of valves but completely enclosed in a pericardial sac and demonstrably beating, albeit irregularly. There is no single primordium, no segment of the primitive heart tube, that can be identified as leading to a specific cardiac cavity in the early postloop stage. Instead, there are microscopically and experimentally identifiable zones, each of which gives rise to a specific anatomic region of a definitive cardiac cavity. These primordia are most accurately termed *primitive cardiac regions;* therefore referring to segments of the heart tube as forerunners of the chambers of the fully formed heart is misleading.[1] The folds in the heart tube and the peristaltic nature of myocardial contraction lead to a predetermined direction of flow out through the bulbus cordis, the folds acting as inefficient valves to direct the flow. Such early vitality is not surprising, because the cardiovascular system is the earliest to attain form and function among the organ systems of the body. The heart is disproportionately large for the size of the embryo at this stage, and this disproportion remains until birth, with only a modest decline in heart-to-body ratio toward birth. Obviously, this occurs because the heart must support not only the growing tissue of the organism but also the embryo's share of the enormous placental circulation.

It is worth digressing here to emphasize the functional problems faced by the developing heart. It is required to form and to function in such a way as to maintain and support the growth of the developing organism in an intrauterine (aquatic) environment; that is, it must support an organism incapable of independent gas exchange and dependent on the placenta for oxygen and nutriments and for other metabolic exchange. The lungs are developed rather late and require only to be supplied with enough blood to support their growth. To perfuse the embryonic lungs with a rate of blood flow commensurate with an air-breathing existence would be energetically inefficient and perhaps an impediment to their growth and development, but during the early stages of development of the cardiovascular system, the lungs are simply not sufficiently developed to be called anything other than *buds*, volumetrically incapable of containing any significant quantity of blood. As a result, the heart must develop a mechanism whereby it can support the organism in an aquatic environment with extensive exchange across the placenta and provide adequate distribution of blood throughout the growing body of the embryo; however, it must simultaneously develop a configuration that will enable it to shift its mode of function instantly at birth to support the organism by way of pulmonary gas exchange. Simply put, in fetal and embryonic life, the two sides of the heart function as two pumps operating in parallel, with the output of both ventricles distributed to the placenta and to the growing tissues of the body, and with no interdependence of the output. However, the two hearts must have the means to shift from functioning in parallel to functioning in tandem at birth, wherein the outflow of one heart becomes the inflow of the other, and blood is obligated to perfuse the pulmonary circuit, return to the heart, and then perfuse the systemic circuit, and so on. One emphasis of this chapter is to focus on the development of features that render the heart capable of these sequential and different modes of function.

ARTERIES

During the early folding of the heart, and with identification of a bulbus cordis and truncus arteriosus as an outflow tract, the aortic arches are beginning to form. The truncus arteriosus is continuous with a ventral aorta. This large, single-channeled artery is connected to a pair of dorsal aortas through a series of branchial (pharyngeal) arch arteries. The developing pharynx passes through a period in its development when it is said to mimic the development of the gill apparatus of fish. Outpouchings of the pharyngeal wall grow as pockets toward the surface, where they are met or at least approached by corresponding infoldings of the ectodermal surface. Normally these outpouchings and infoldings neither meet nor coalesce to form gill slits or fistulas. The supporting tissue on both sides of the pouches is endowed with a cartilaginous supporting bar, a nerve, and a blood vessel, respectively known as the *branchial arch (pharyngeal) cartilage, branchial arch nerve,* and *branchial arch artery.* The first such cartilaginous bar is Meckel's cartilage, in front of the first pharyngeal pouch; the second, Reichert's cartilage, lies between the first and second pouches. The pharynx is supported by six arch complexes, surrounding and intervening between the pharyngeal pouches. The arteries of these arches are the connectives from the ventral aorta to the dorsal aortas, and they appear in sequence from cranial to caudal. Rarely are more than three such arch arteries identifiable at one time; in this case, as elsewhere in the embryo, the cranial development leads or precedes that occurring more caudally. As the fourth arch artery appears, the first is being transformed into its successor structures and ceases to be identifiable as an arch artery. In humans, there are five such arch arteries, numbered 1, 2, 3, 4, and 6, in recognition of the dropping out in phylogeny of the fifth arch artery, which has no significant role in human development (the fifth pharyngeal pouch fuses with the fourth at its opening into the pharynx; its rudimentary arch between the fourth and fifth pouches contributes to the formation of the larynx). In contrast to the constancy of innervation of the derivatives of the pharyngeal arches, the vascular supply to the arches is subject to later, often extensive modification. The motor nerve to an arch persists throughout phylogeny and throughout ontogenetic development in supplying the derivatives of that arch (first arch, mandibular nerve; second arch, facial nerve; third arch, glossopharyngeal nerve; fourth through sixth arches, recurrent and superior laryngeal nerves and vagal pharyngeal nerve). The geometric representation of the arch artery pattern and the fate of those arteries are summarized in Figure 2-2. The paired dorsal aortas sweep posteriorly and fuse in the midline to form a single dorsal aorta (see Figure 2-2, *inset*) posterior to entry points of the arch arteries.

The lungs begin their development as a ventrally directed outgrowth from the pharynx, and the single tube that will become the trachea descends into the presumptive chest cavity, where it branches into a pair of lung buds. These buds receive a small blood supply from branches of the sixth aortic arch arteries (see Figure 2-2A). Clearly the sixth arch arteries will have a role in the development of the pulmonary arterial tree. The developmental problem posed here is that the sixth arch arteries are initially part of the systemic circulation, simply representing the most caudal of the branchial arch arteries springing from the truncus arteriosus and uniting with the dorsal aortas. In the division of the heart tube into right and left hearts, some provision must be made for joining the right ventricular outflow tract to the sixth arch arteries and joining the remainder of the great branchial arch system and aortas with the left ventricle. The rationale for fusion of the primitive heart tubes into a single channel and subsequent division is now clarified by this need to divide the bulbus cordis and truncus arteriosus into a pulmonary artery and an aortic artery. The manner of that division solves the problem of connecting the right ventricle and the developing pulmonary artery to the lungs and connecting the remainder of the arch arteries to the systemic circulation and the left ventricle. The interested reader is encouraged to examine the article by Congdon[2] for further clarification of this point.

The heart is divided into four chambers that compose two separate hearts, with provision for a parallel mode of function before birth and a tandem mode after birth. The umbilical veins (after the sixth week, a single left umbilical vein) return blood to the fetal heart by their union with the inferior vena cava. This return route sees the umbilical vein enter the liver, where a shunt, the ductus venosus, bypasses the complex hepatic circulation and shunts the blood directly into the inferior vena cava. Thus, the right atrium receives a supply of freshly oxygenated blood, in contrast to the adult condition. Before separation of the right and left atria, that placental return is into the single atrial chamber, which is diagrammatically depicted in Figure 2-3A. The single chamber undergoes a constriction in the plane of the atrioventricular orifices and the atrioventricular sulcus on the exterior of the heart. From the margins of this constriction, endocardial cushions grow inward to begin the formation of the tricuspid and mitral valves. The single atrium begins its separation into halves by downgrowth from the dorsocranial wall of a filmy crescentic curtain—the septum primum (see Figure 2-3B). The leading invaginated edge of the crescent grows down toward the floor of the single atrium; that floor forms by virtue of the growth of the atrioventricular valve primordia. Figure 2-3B shows the septum primum from the right side as it progresses toward complete closure of the single atrial chamber in its midline. In addition, just before the foramen primum closes, a group of perforations forms in the dorsocranial part of the partition (see Figure 2-3B) and then coalesces into a foramen secundum (see Figure 2-3C). This process is necessary because throughout this developmental sequence, the heart is pumping blood to and returning it from the placenta, and the returning blood must be shunted from the right side of the heart into the left

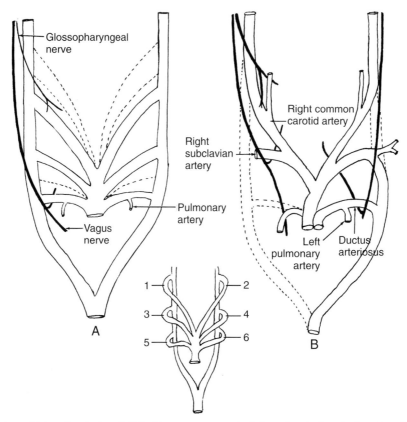

Glossopharyngeal
nerve

Right common
carotid artery

Right
subclavian
artery

Pulmonary
artery

Vagus
nerve

Left
pulmonary
artery

Ductus
arteriosus

1   2
3   4
5   6

A   B

FIGURE 2-2 ■ Fate of the branchial arch arteries. **A,** Primitive arrangement of six arch arteries. Arches 1 and 2 have formed and have been accommodated into the vessels of the head (dotted lines indicate arteries that are no longer arches—that is, 1, 2, and 5). Arches 3, 4, and 6 connect the ventral aorta (aortic sac and truncus arteriosus) with the paired dorsal aortas. The latter fuse posteriorly to form a single dorsal aorta. **B,** Subsequent disposition of these vessels. The *dotted lines* indicate vessels that normally disappear, including the right sixth arch beyond the right pulmonary artery. The glossopharyngeal nerve (motor to the third arch) and the recurrent laryngeal nerve (motor to the sixth arch derivatives) are shown. The recurrent laryngeal nerve is a branch of the vagus "recurring" around the sixth arch in **A;** in **B,** these nerves recur around the ductus arteriosus and around the right subclavian. **Inset,** The first three aortic arch arteries from the front (ventral) view during the branchial period. At no time are all arch arteries evident at the same time. The paired dorsal aortas unite into a single dorsal aorta posterior to the entry of the arch arteries. The postbranchial period, when the heart descends from the branchial region into the chest, is characterized by modification of the arch system into the adult disposition of the derived arteries.

atrium in large volume to sustain the systemic circulation. Therefore at no point in fetal life may the right and left atria be functionally separate. During the time that the placental circulation is intact, the pressure in the right atrium exceeds that in the left atrium, and a right-to-left shunt will be operative. As a result, the foramen secundum opens just in time to continue that shunt as the foramen primum closes. Next, on the right side of the septum primum, a much more robust and rigid septum secundum begins its downgrowth, following the same pattern as that of the septum primum (see Figure 2-3C); a crescent-shaped leading edge grows down from above toward the endocardial cushions that will finally separate the atria from the ventricles. This downgrowth of the septum secundum comes to overlie the orifice of the foramen secundum. Fortunately, the septum secundum is sturdy and relatively unyielding, whereas the septum primum is thin and curtainlike. As long as the free lower edge of the septum secundum fails to reach the floor of the atrium, thus forming the foramen ovale, the elevated pressure in the right atrium pushes blood through the ovale, deflecting the septum primum and allowing blood

to pass through the foramen secundum into the left atrium and permitting continuation of the obligatory right-to-left shunt. Inasmuch as the downgrowth of the septum secundum is arrested, leaving a fixed foramen ovale, such a shunt operates throughout the intrauterine life of the organism. The orifice of the foramen ovale is just above and medial to the orifice of the inferior vena cava (see Figure 2-3D), so that inferior caval (i.e., placental) blood is preferentially directed into that foramen, and then into the left atrium, with remarkably little mixing of this oxygenated blood with the oxygen-poor blood returning via the superior vena cava.

The division of the ventricles and the single aortic outflow path are both simpler to understand and more critically complex. The ventricle begins to divide by the upward growth of a muscular partition of myocardium from the cardiac apex toward the truncus arteriosus (Figure 2-4A); this will form the muscular part of the interventricular septum. At the same time, a pair of ridges (the spiral ridges) grow toward each other as outgrowths of the walls of the truncus arteriosus. These ridges will fuse to form a spiral septum, dividing the septum from

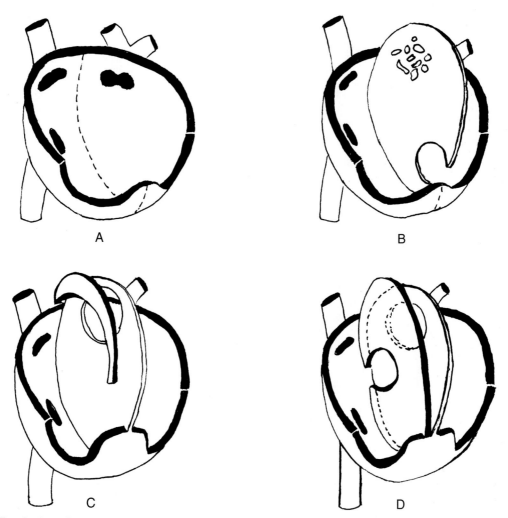

FIGURE 2-3 ■ The single early atrium is represented as a hollow sphere, from an anterolateral view. The atrioventricular canals are the lower part of the cutaway sphere. **A,** The *dotted line* indicates the plane of division into right and left atria. The entry of the superior and inferior venae cavae (right atrial segment of the sphere) and the pulmonary arteries (left segment of the sphere) is indicated by entering tubes. **B-D,** Successive stages in development of the interatrial septum. In **B,** the septum primum grows downward, leaving a free margin as the ostium primum. As this ostium prepares to close, holes appear in the upper posterior part of the septum, which in **C** have coalesced into an ostium secundum. In **C,** the septum secundum begins to grow downward to the right of the septum primum, covering the ostium secundum on that side. The free margin of the septum secundum does not close over in **D,** leaving the foramen ovale open. The right atrial contents flow into the left atrium via the foramen ovale and ostium secundum. (Adapted from Tuchmann-Duplessis H, David HG, Haegel P: Illustrated human embryology, New York, 1972, Springer-Verlag.)

above downward. The lower ends of the spiral ridges contribute to the formation of the final septal closure (see Figure 2-4*B*). This phenomenon is extraordinarily complex, involves early histologic changes, and is probably initiated by hemodynamic influences and is subsequently controlled by genetic factors (see the analysis by Fanapazir and Kaufman[3]). The membranous interventricular septum is formed where the three cushions meet. Figure 2-4*C* and 2-4*D* schematically depict the spiral arrangement of the division of the truncus arteriosus whereby the single outflow tract is divided into pulmonary and aortic tubes, each connected to its corresponding ventricular cavity. The complexity of the closure lies in the precise pitch of the spiral septum; its lower end must be aligned with the upthrusting muscular cushion so as to meet accurately in a single plane. Interference in the fusion of these cushions into a complete membranous septum will lead to a membranous interventricular septal defect. Misalignment of the spiral ridges may result in failure of the great arteries to form and function independently through the accident of a pulmonary aortic fistula. Misalignment of the lower end of the dividing arteries and asymmetry in the positioning of the spiral ridges could lead to such errors as an overriding aorta, with the right ventricular contents partially ejected into the aorta. The features of the tetralogy of Fallot can be readily interpreted as a result of such misalignment in the truncus division. The tetralogy consists of an overriding aorta, pulmonary stenosis, membranous septal defect (presumably due to asymmetrical division of the proximal truncus arteriosus), and right ventricular hypertrophy (secondary to the right-to-left shunt through the overriding aorta and to the stenotic pulmonary artery).

A superbly illustrated and classic account of early experimental findings, as well as an excellent historical review of the anatomy and physiology of fetal circulation,

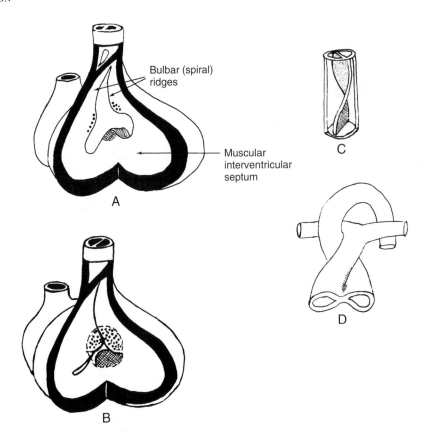

Bulbar (spiral)
ridges

Muscular
interventricular
septum

FIGURE 2-4 ■ Stages in the division of the ventricle and formation of the great arteries from the truncus arteriosus and bulbus cordis. **A,** The ventricle has begun to divide, with formation of the muscular part of the interventricular septum by means of growth of the ventricular wall musculature. The bulbus cordis is dividing into two vessels, beginning with the growing together of two spiral ridges. **B,** The two spiral ridges meet and fuse to divide the bulbus cordis into two outflow tracts: the pulmonary artery and the ascending aorta. The ridges at their lower extremities *(stippled cushions)* meet a muscular cushion derived from the muscular interventricular septum *(hatched)* to form the membranous part of the interventricular septum (outlined by *dotted lines*). The spiral character of the arterial division connects the sixth arch arteries to the right ventricle and connects the left ventricle to the other arch arteries and their derivatives. **C,** Spiral septum shown diagrammatically, in a cutaway cylinder representing the single bulbus cordis. The hatched surface of the septum represents the aortic side of the division, and the stippled side represents the pulmonary surface of the septum. The two resulting arteries must spiral around each other, as in **D**. Derived from a single tube, they are constrained to remain wrapped in a single pericardial sleeve. (Adapted from Tuchmann-Duplessis H, David HG, Haegel P: *Illustrated human embryology,* New York, 1972, Springer-Verlag; and Moore KL: *The developing human,* Philadelphia, 1982, WB Saunders.)

can be found in the book by Barclay and associates.[4] More recent summaries can be obtained in standard works by Arey,[5] Clemente,[6] Hamilton and Mossman,[7] Moore,[8] Sabin,[9] and Tuchmann-Duplessis and associates.[10]

The original plan of five pairs of aortic arch arteries (see Figure 2-2) becomes modified by incorporation of the first two arch arteries into the internal carotid system, dropping out of the paired dorsal aortas between the third and fourth arches, and participation in the formation of the common carotid arteries by the third arches. Caudal to the lost segments of dorsal aortas, the fourth arches become the roots of the subclavian arteries; the right sixth arch is lost distal to its pulmonary branch, and the left sixth arch becomes the left pulmonary artery, with the segment distal to the pulmonary "branch" serving as the ductus arteriosus (see Figure 2-2B). This arterial shunt vessel develops specialized muscle in its tunica media, which is stimulated to contract and shut down the shunt vessel after birth. It is believed that abnormal migration of some of this specialized smooth muscle into the aortic wall accounts for aortic stenosis, the stricture

developing in the aorta at the site of this ectopic ductus muscle after birth.

The closure of this right-to-left shunt on the arterial side at birth results in a great increase in pulmonary blood flow (the resistance of pulmonary vessels drops dramatically with inflation of the lungs and elongation of helicine arteries). On the venous side, the rise in left atrial pressure and loss of umbilical venous return arrest the interatrial right-to-left shunt. Elevated left atrial pressure results in the two interatrial septa operating as a flap valve, closing the foramen ovale by applying the curtainlike septum primum against the left one (see Figure 2-3D).

Certainty in the derivation of the arteries of the head is not easy to achieve. The arteries form from a loose network of interconnected vessels in which it is often impossible to distinguish between arteries and veins.[11] The artery of the first arch becomes a part of the internal carotid artery, which also forms in part from persistence of the rostral parts of the dorsal aortas. The second arch artery appears in the form of the stapedial artery. This artery of the tympanic cavity passes through the annulus (obturator foramen) in the stapes, and in some mammals it persists in this form. In humans, this form of stapedial artery may remain into adulthood as a surgically troublesome vascular anomaly. This artery of the second arch for a time supplies three branches (supraorbital, infraorbital, and mandibular), distributed with the divisions of the trigeminal nerve. An anastomosis between the infraorbital and mandibular branches of the stapedial artery and the external carotid artery is said to give rise to the maxillary artery and its middle meningeal branch. It is further argued that the orbital anastomotic branch of the middle meningeal artery is the remnant of the original supraorbital branch of the stapedial artery. Some information is indicated in the phylogenetic history of the artery. In most mammals, the originally small external carotid artery, as it grows forward, taps the origin of the stapedial artery and appropriates its branches, which at one stroke reduces the size and causes the disappearance of the original stapedial artery and extends the distribution of the external carotid. As Romer said, "the process is analogous to 'stream piracy,' whereby one river taps the headwaters of another."[12] Padget offers a detailed discussion and critical appraisal of the literature of the general mammalian stapedial artery and of the human artery, and her discussion is recommended to the interested reader.[13]

The third arch artery forms the common carotid arteries and the first segments of the internal carotid arteries. Thus, it is probable that portions of the first three arches all contribute to the external carotid arteries. The left fourth arch forms the arch of the aorta, and the left dorsal aorta distal to the point of union of this arch forms the descending aorta, along with the single dorsal aorta more caudally (see Figure 2-2B). The entirety of the right dorsal aorta is lost. The right horn of the aortic sac forms the brachiocephalic artery, from which the right common carotid and subclavian arteries spring.

The sixth arches are associated with the pulmonary blood supply, first as the source of the small twigs to the lung buds. Those twigs and their parent stems from the truncus arteriosus become the definitive pulmonary arteries. At this point it should be clear why the complex twist of the spiral septum dividing the truncus arteriosus is necessary. In dividing the truncus, it is essential to connect the right ventricle to the origins of the sixth arches from the truncus, leaving the more rostral arch arteries connected to the part of the truncus connected to the left ventricle. The arch arteries spring from a single vessel, the truncus, and must end as arteries arising from separate arteries—the sixth arising from the pulmonary artery, and the first through fourth from the aortic component of the truncus. The twisting division of the truncus also accounts for the intertwined course of the pulmonary artery and the ascending aorta; their derivation from a single vessel, the truncus, accounts for these great arteries being wrapped in a single pericardial sleeve (see Figure 2-4D).

The branchial arches develop nerve supplies along with their vascular supplies, and it is an axiom of anatomy that nerve supply is never lost once it is established. The motor nerves of the branchial arches supply the structures derived from those arches, no matter what developmental events ensue. In Figure 2-2, the position of the

glossopharyngeal nerve as the motor nerve of the third arch, and the recurrent laryngeal branch of the vagus as the motor nerve of the sixth arch, can be seen as these nerves are drawn caudally by the descent of the heart and growth of the branchial arch system. The recurrent branch of the vagus is in fact the motor nerve derived from the nucleus ambiguus of the brainstem, which happens to distribute by way of the vagus, having emerged from the brainstem as the cranial root of the spinal accessory nerve (cranial nerve XI). The recurring course of the nerve is accounted for by its inherited requirement of lying caudal to the sixth arch artery. The distal part of the left sixth arch artery becomes the ductus arteriosus (the ligamentum arteriosum after birth); thus arises the asymmetry in the courses of the two recurrent laryngeal nerves. The left nerve is constrained to maintain its original relationship to its arch artery as that artery is drawn down into the chest by the descent of the heart. The right nerve loses that constraint as the sixth arch drops out distal to the origin of the pulmonary artery. The only persisting arch to prevent the nerve's remaining in the neck as the heart descends is the fourth arch on the right side (the right subclavian artery), around which the nerve recurring in the adult human is found (see Figure 2-2B). If, during thyroid surgery, the surgeon finds that the right recurrent nerve does not come up around the subclavian artery, he or she should take that as a warning that a developmental abnormality in the formation of the right subclavian artery might be expected (e.g., a retroesophageal right subclavian). In that event, the right subclavian forms from the right seventh intersegmental artery and part of the right dorsal aorta, the right fourth arch artery, and right dorsal aorta having involuted cranial to the origin of the seventh intersegmental artery.[8]

The developing embryo in its earliest stages is supported by a yolk sac of nutriment, sustaining growth until the placenta is sufficiently developed to assume those duties. The embryo lies on the surface of the yolk sac, with the interior of the latter in continuity with the developing gastrointestinal tract. The digestive tract cranial to the yolk sac is termed the *foregut*, that caudal to the yolk sac is termed the *hindgut*, and that directly connected to the yolk sac is termed the *midgut*. Three aortic branches, midline and unpaired, arise to supply each of these segments of the digestive tract, and these arteries remain the source of arterial blood for those portions of the tract and their derivatives. Thus, the celiac artery is the artery of the foregut and the derivatives of the foregut, including the liver and spleen. The artery of the midgut is the superior mesenteric artery; the artery of the hindgut is the inferior mesenteric artery. During development, the digestive tract outgrows the room available for it in the abdominal cavity and temporarily herniates out into the umbilical cord. Its return from this extraabdominal sojourn is accompanied by a rotation that accounts for the disposition of the stomach, the duodenum, and the bowel in the adult. The axis of rotation around which this reentry into the abdomen occurs is the superior mesenteric artery.[14]

The kidneys begin their development in the pelvis and migrate cranially to their final position on the posterior abdominal wall. The pelvic kidneys derive their arterial blood supply from the iliac system; as they ascend, the previous arterial supply drops out and new vessels from the aorta are established. The ascent and the history of the previous blood supply can be seen in the sources of small vessels supplying the ureter, their origins indicating the stems of vessels formerly supplying the kidney. Should the ascent of the kidney be arrested, the blood supply at the time remains the supply into adulthood. Thus, the ascent of the horseshoe kidney is arrested by the overhanging inferior mesenteric artery, and the horseshoe

kidney has arterial blood supplied from common iliac vessels or the aorta at a level lower than the origin of the normal renal arteries. In addition, accessory renal arteries usually arise below the renal arteries and enter the inferior pole of the kidney, attesting to a previous source of blood that did not entirely disappear with ascent to the final renal destination.

The limbs seem to be organized around a central arterial stem, so that from the beginning an axial artery is identifiable. Figure 2-5 depicts the changes in circulatory

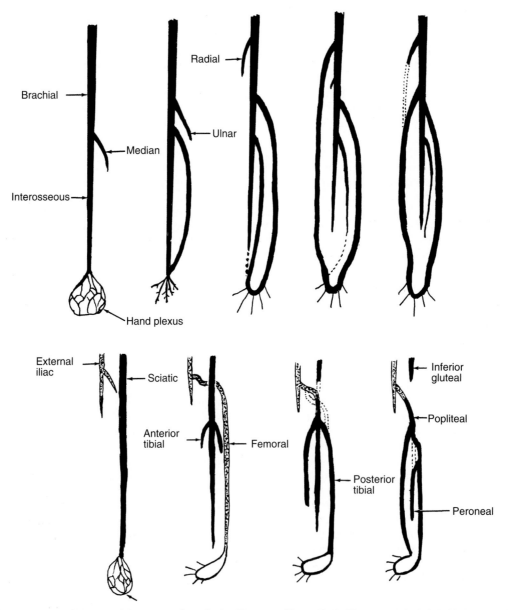

FIGURE 2-5 ■ Development of the arterial pattern of the limbs. **Top row,** Upper limb. The upper limb is initially organized around a single axial artery—the brachial and its interosseous continuation—terminating in a hand plexus. The hand plexus will develop into the palmar arches. The stem artery gives rise in succession to the median, ulnar, and radial arteries. The median artery normally has an evanescent existence as a major vessel, losing its connection with the hand plexus, which it usurped from the axial vessel. **Bottom row,** Lower limb. The axial vessel for the lower limb is the sciatic, which remains in the adult as the inferior gluteal, and portions of the popliteal and peroneal arteries. The femoral artery arises from the external iliac and appropriates the distal part of the sciatic to dominate the vascular distribution of the limb. The anterior tibial artery arises as a branch of the popliteal; the posterior tibial is developed from the union of the femoral and the popliteal. Notice in the third figure from the left that an upper segment of the femoral artery is lost, allowing the popliteal to become interposed. (Adapted from Arey LB: Developmental anatomy, ed 7, Philadelphia, 1965, WB Saunders.)

pattern for the two limbs. Generally, the axial artery in large part disappears and certainly ceases to be the principal source of limb blood.

In the upper limb, the axial artery passes down the core of the limb to the hand plexus. It is a continuation of the subclavian and axillary systems, already established in the 5-mm embryo, and is the forerunner of the brachial artery and, more distally, the interosseous artery. The upper limb axial artery sprouts a median branch and an ulnar arterial branch on the medial side of the stem artery. The median branch temporarily joins with the ulnar branch in the volar arch. A radial sprout follows on the preaxial side of the limb, and this new branch usurps the median's connection with the volar arch. The distal axial artery persists as the anterior interosseous artery. This pattern is completed before the end of the second month, and the early dominance of the axial and median arteries is permanently lost. The median artery persists as a branch of the anterior interosseous artery, serving as the nutrient artery of the median nerve. It may persist in an enlarged form as an anomaly, accompanying the median nerve into the palm and retaining its connection with and contribution to the palmar arterial arches.

Figure 2-5 shows the steps by which the adult pattern of arterial supply to the lower limb is derived from the axial artery of the limb bud. The axial vessel is the sciatic artery, a direct branch of the umbilical; it is the primary source of the blood for the limb bud in the 9-mm embryo. The major stem artery for the limb becomes the femoral artery, as the latter continues the course of the external iliac. The femoral artery annexes the foot plexus of the sciatic artery and the origin of this axial vessel. The remaining proximal "stump" of the once-dominant sciatic artery persists as the inferior gluteal artery. A branch of the latter, the artery of the sciatic nerve, is all that remains of the former glory of the sciatic artery. The distal parts of the sciatic stem, appropriated by the femoral artery near its origin from the external iliac, give rise to the anterior tibial artery, which connects with the plantar arch distally. The newer, more distal femoral artery establishes a new connection to the distal sciatic so that it and the plantar arch come to branch from the sciatic. The most distal segment of the sciatic shifts its origin to the posterior tibial as the peroneal, and the adult pattern is established. The remnants of the sciatic persist (from above downward) as the inferior gluteal with its small artery of the sciatic nerve, the popliteal artery, and the peroneal artery. In the adult arterial plan, these persisting segments of the original sciatic artery no longer have continuity with one another in any significant way.

The umbilical arteries, carrying blood to the placenta for gas and metabolite exchange, appear as large branches of the internal iliac arteries and persist unmodified throughout gestation. These arteries develop robust branches to the upper surface of the urinary bladder. At birth, the segments of the umbilical arteries distal to the origin of the arteries to the bladder are obliterated and remain as fibrous cords—the medial umbilical ligaments. The stem of these arteries and the branches to the bladder are henceforth known as the *superior vesicle arteries*.

VEINS

As the arterial distribution system develops, appropriate return pathways arise simultaneously. The venous system is extensively interconnected, with a great capacity for collateral routes of venous return, and arteries are generally accompanied by corresponding veins. The short review of the venous system in this section focuses only on the great systems of veins that arise early in embryonic life and give rise to the major collecting pathways recognizable in the normal adult. As a result, even such important but developmentally simple systems as the pulmonary venous system are not discussed here.

A passing comment on venous valves is appropriate here, to draw attention to a provocative analysis and comparative study of superficial veins in the limbs of primates.[15] The number and spacing of venous valves are dictated genetically and are relevant to the need to maintain optimum pressures within capillary beds to ensure a balanced fluid exchange in tissues. The distance between venous valves in the limbs is sufficient to provide the transcapillary pressure gradients required for an equilibrium in fluid efflux and return to the vascular bed; it is not, as previously supposed, an adaptation to counter the effects of gravity in the bipedal posture.

The veins of the embryo fall into three major groups: vitelline (omphalomesenteric) veins, umbilical veins, and the cardinal system of veins. The coalesced blood islands that give rise to undifferentiated blood networks develop a venous side, as they do an arterial side, as directions of blood flow become established through them. Preferential pathways emerge on the venous side, giving rise to larger and more dominant veins that undergo modification as regional or organ-specific changes occur. Many of the venous channels developed in support of fetal life disappear as the need for them vanishes through subsequent development.

The vitelline veins are the veins of the yolk sac. They pass through the intestinal portal of the umbilical cord, alongside the (at first) wide channel of communication between the sac and the midgut region of the alimentary canal. A vitelline plexus is formed of communicating venous channels between the vitelline veins in the septum transversum. As the liver develops in the septum, it infringes on the vitelline plexus, separating it into hepatic sinusoids. Despite this encroachment, the vitelline pathway from the septum transversum into the heart persists as hepaticocardiac channels. The right channel of this return persists as the terminal segment of the inferior vena cava (Figure 2-6). The vitelline plexus also surrounds the duodenum during the stage of hepatic growth, and the plexus is further distorted when the herniated midgut returns in a spiraling motion into the abdominal cavity. It is this rotation during the return that brings the duodenum into its transverse position and fixes this position by peritonealization. This position forces the blood in the surrounding plexus to shunt from the right to the left vitelline vein, which is the segment of the vitelline system lying just caudal to the transversely oriented duodenum. The left vitelline vein then sends its blood directly across to the liver by way of its dorsal

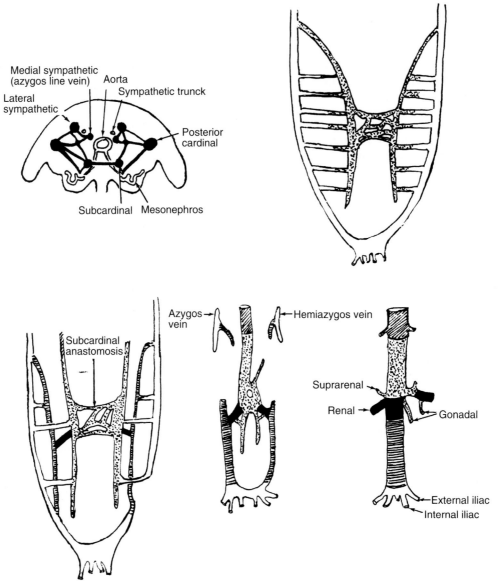

FIGURE 2-6 ■ Development of the large veins. **Upper left,** Schematic cross section of the embryo shows the relative positions and extensive interconnections of the major body wall veins. **Upper right** and **lower row** (left to right), Succession of stages in the development of the inferior vena cava and the related body wall veins. The key in the lower row identifies the component veins making up the inferior vena cava (lower right). For simplicity, the azygos and hemiazygos veins are depicted as if they arise from the lateral sympathetic veins, but in fact they arise as derivatives from the parallel medial sympathetic (azygos line) veins. (Adapted from Williams PL, Wendell-Smith CP, Treadgold S: Basic human embryology, ed 2, Philadelphia, 1969, JB Lippincott; and Hollinshead WH, Rosse L: Textbook of anatomy, ed 4, Philadelphia, 1985, Harper and Row.)

anastomosis with the persistent cranial end of the right vitelline vein.

The portal vein thus formed does not spiral around the duodenum, as commonly described and illustrated; instead, it is short and straight, with the duodenum spiraling around it. The ease with which these changes occur can be understood if two basic facts are appreciated: (1) the essentially plexiform nature of the embryonic vascular system, and (2) the natural tendency for blood to seek the most direct route of flow because of hydrodynamic factors. (Refer to the clear sequence of illustrations of this development in Hamilton and Mossman,[7] page 274.)

The umbilical veins, entering the abdominal cavity by way of the umbilicus, must also traverse the septum transversum to arrive at the heart, and their septal segments within the septum also become enmeshed with the vitelline veins in the hepatic plexus of sinusoids. In the 5-mm embryo, the umbilical veins communicate extensively with the vitelline plexus in the liver. Two days later, the right umbilical vein undergoes atrophy, and all placental blood returns to the fetal heart via the left vein. The left vein's channel through the liver enlarges to accommodate this enhanced flow and forms the ductus venosus, a direct channel through the liver between the left umbilical vein and the inferior vena cava. This channel obliterates at birth with cessation of flow through the umbilical system, and the intrahepatic shunt is replaced by the ligamentum venosum. There is a sphincter in this shunt that regulates umbilical flow, which is a particularly important feature to prevent overloading of the fetal heart during uterine contractions. This sphincter's closure at birth contributes to the prompt obliteration of the shunt. The course of the left umbilical vein caudal to the liver is in the free margin of the ventral mesentery. The obliterated umbilical vein between the umbilicus and liver is the ligamentum teres hepatis of the adult, lying in the free margin of the falciform ligament; the latter is the adult counterpart of the ventral mesentery between the liver and the anterior abdominal wall.

The cardinal veins are the body wall veins of the embryo and fetus. There are several sets designated by distinguishing names. The anterior cardinal veins (also termed *precardinal veins*) drain the cranial region of the early embryo. The posterior cardinal veins drain the caudal portion and arise slightly later than the anterior cardinals. The subcardinal veins appear shortly after the posterior cardinal veins and are derived in conjunction with the rapidly growing progenitor of the kidney, the mesonephros. The term *supracardinal veins* is sometimes used to designate lateral sympathetic or thoracolumbar line veins or paraureteric veins. To limit the number of cardinal veins requiring attention, in discussing the veins of the posterior body wall anterior to the segmental vessels, the term *lateral sympathetic veins* is used instead.

The primary head vein of the embryo evolves into the complex system of dural sinuses and venous pathways of the head, and the reader is referred to the classic accounts of Streeter[16] and Padget,[11,13] whose illustrations amply clarify the changes leading to the adult pattern. The anterior and posterior cardinal veins unite behind the heart to form the common cardinal veins, or ducts of Cuvier (right and left). The union of the ducts of Cuvier is the ductus venosus at the venous end of the heart. Part of the ductus venosus becomes incorporated into the walls of the atria, most notably the right atrium.

The posterior cardinal veins are the first of a series of caudal longitudinal body wall veins, which form an interconnected system (see Figure 2-6), giving rise to the caudal body wall venous drainage and to the inferior vena cava and azygos system of veins.

The subcardinal veins appear soon after the posterior cardinal veins as a pair of veins along the medial side of the urogenital folds. They are associated with the mesonephros and probably arise as a series of longitudinal anastomoses for the plexuses of the mesonephroi. They drain the mesonephroi and the germinal epithelium and terminate cranially and caudally by connecting with the posterior cardinal veins (see Figure 2-6). The subcardinal veins unite with each other and, along their lengths, with the posterior cardinal veins through anastomoses; the multiple transverse anastomoses of these veins are probably their most distinctive feature. One of these anastomoses is the intersubcardinal anastomosis between the two veins ventral to the aorta. The right subcardinal vein establishes a communication with the liver sinusoids, and that segment becomes the hepatic segment of the inferior vena cava (see Figure 2-6). The preaortic anastomosis

comes into play in the establishment of the vena cava inferior to that segment.

The lateral sympathetic veins appear soon after the hepatic segment of the inferior vena cava, anterior to the segmental vessels. They appear first as a plexus but quickly become a longitudinal trunk, ending cranially in the posterior cardinal vein and anastomosing posteriorly with the subcardinal vein, especially strongly on the right side. The part caudal to that latter anastomosis persists, and most of the remainder of the lateral sympathetic veins regresses; the persisting right caudal segment survives as the infrarenal part of the inferior vena cava (see Figure 2-6). As the lateral sympathetic veins appear, a medial pair (medial sympathetic or azygos line veins) also arises, but medial to the sympathetic trunk in the abdominal wall. These veins link across the midline and, with the loss of an intermediate segment on the left side, form the azygos system of veins.

The adult pattern is completed by the emerging dominance of the right common cardinal vein. The left upper intercostal spaces drain into the remainder of the left common cardinal vein, which connects with the left brachiocephalic vein after the lateral part of the left common cardinal is lost. The left superior intercostal vein is formed in part by the left posterior and anterior cardinal veins. The potential communication between the two may persist as a left superior vena cava; the latter's position may be identified in the normal adult as the oblique cardiac vein (of Marshall), which can be traced to the left superior intercostal vein as a reminder of that origin.

The inferior vena cava has a complex origin. The hepatic segment, as noted previously, is derived from the cranial segment of the right vitelline vein and the hepatic sinusoids. A prerenal segment forms distal to this as an anastomosis between the hepatic segment and the right subcardinal vein. This latter vein forms the prerenal segment (down to the junction of the renal veins). A renal segment is formed from a renal collar (note the preaortic anastomosis between the subcardinals described previously). The renal collar is an anastomosis involving this preaortic anastomosis and anastomoses between the right subcardinal and lateral sympathetic veins. A postrenal segment forms from the lumbar part of the right lateral sympathetic vein down to the level of the common iliac veins. The common iliacs join with the lower part of the inferior vena cava as the postcardinal veins degenerate, forcing the iliacs to find this secondary route of venous return to the heart. As the kidneys come to rest in the adult position, the definitive renal veins are formed as connections to the inferior vena cava through anastomoses between the subcardinal and lateral lumbar veins. On the left side, the longer path to the inferior vena cava is accomplished through recruitment of this anastomosis between the subcardinal veins. On the right, this anastomosis is incorporated into the formation of the renal segment of the inferior vena cava, and the situation is less complex.

The multiple sources incorporated into the inferior vena cava, including anastomoses across the midline, can lead to some bizarre malformations. Most dramatic of these is the rare retrocaval ureter, which is clearly not a malformation of the ureter or a misguided path of ascent of the kidney; rather, it must be interpreted as incorporation of unusual components of the renal collar into the inferior vena cava. Accounts in the literature agree on this interpretation of a caval rather than a ureteric malformation.[17-19]

GROWTH OF NEW VESSELS

It would be helpful to know whether the development of new blood vessels in the fetus and during postnatal growth is a model for vascular proliferation under other circumstances. It is likely that this is so, although the factors that stimulate and direct such growth might be quite different. The central nervous system (CNS) provides a model that has been studied by a variety of means. The relative maturity of the brain at birth provides an existing and fully functional vascular tree that can be used as a model of a relatively mature vascular system. The further growth and development of the CNS dictate the need for postnatal neovascularization to support further maturation of the tissue.

Examination of the vascularization of the CNS addresses a fundamental issue in vascular growth during development: To what extent is development of a vascular bed a permissive condition for the subsequent onset of function; that is, to what extent is it anticipatory of and necessary for function? Or, conversely, to what extent is the development of a vasculature the response to the greater metabolic demands of a tissue as it increases or begins to achieve the functional levels expected of it at full maturation?

Studying CNS regions at the time of onset of measurable function (e.g., the auditory system) reveals that vascular sprouting parallels such events in their time courses (Skolnik and Maxwell, unpublished observations). Such observations cannot distinguish cause and effect, and perhaps they must go hand in hand—functional and vascular maturation identically timed or responsive to some common signal from yet another source. Greater temporal resolution would have to be applied than we have been able to achieve to date.

It is possible to describe the manner of new vessel growth in the CNS and to derive some quantitative information. Rowan and Maxwell[20] studied the postnatal rat cerebral cortex, which is structurally and cytologically quite immature at birth and undergoes a remarkable degree of maturation in the first 3 weeks after birth. CNS blood vessels are the only CNS tissue elements to display alkaline phosphatase activity. Using a simple histochemical procedure, it is possible to visualize small vessels by light and electron microscopy, relying on the enzyme reaction to label vessels—and those cells in the process of becoming vessels through cytodifferentiation—with no ambiguity whatsoever.[21] It has been widely accepted that new vessels in the CNS and perhaps elsewhere begin as a proliferation of solid cords of cells that later canalize (i.e., develop lumens). Yet such a mechanism seems improbable on purely mechanistic grounds, and this does not seem to be the case in the CNS. In this tissue, postnatal growth of new vessels seems to occur by budding from preexisting vessels; the buds are recognizable by

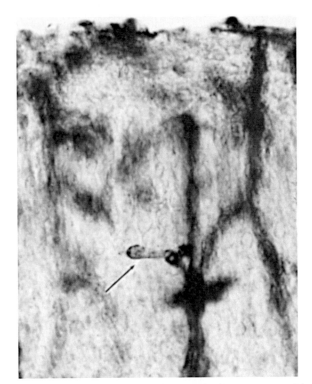

FIGURE 2-7 ■ Light micrograph of rat cerebral cortex, reacted for alkaline phosphatase. A vascular sprout *(arrow)* is seen in the superficial cortex 2 days after birth. The cortical surface is at the top (∞1548). (Courtesy Dr. R. Rowan.)

their enzyme content and by the presence of lumens, although they are collapsed and empty. The lumens are not identifiable by light microscopy; therefore the interpretation of solid cords of cells is understandable. The buds or sprouts have characteristic cytoplasmic protuberances, or fingers, that "explore" in advance of growth of the sprout, seeming to seek the most appropriate path or perhaps sensing the direction where vessel growth will best satisfy the perceived need. Figures 2-7 through 2-10 show a series of such sprouts from the rat cerebral cortex. These sprouts presumably link with a venous channel, establishing hemodynamics, which should serve to open the lumen as a capillary link. Figure 2-11 is an electron micrograph of such a sprout, in which the unopened state of the lumen is evident. Because CNS arteries prominently display alkaline phosphatase activity, and because sprouts at their earliest detectable stages also display this enzyme, it is likely that postnatal vascularization proceeds by arteriolar sprouting, with subsequent linkage to the venous bed. An excellent historical review of the study of growth and differentiation of blood vessels and a statement of the status of the field can be found in Eriksson and Zarem's chapter in *Microcirculation.*[22]

The factors that induce an arteriole to sprout may be multiple, and possibly legion. An enormous literature on angiogenic factors is available for the CNS and other tissues, including tumors. Attention must be drawn, however, to a series of papers announcing a major achievement by Vallee's group at Harvard.[23-25] These investigators isolated and analyzed an angiogenic factor from

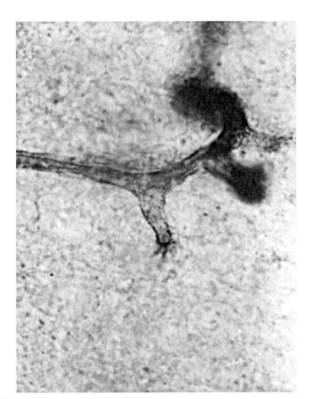

FIGURE 2-8 ■ Light micrograph of rat cerebral cortex, reacted for alkaline phosphatase. A vascular sprout is seen in the middle third of the rat cortex 7 days after birth. Delicate exploratory fingers, or pseudopodia, are seen at the tip of the sprout (∞3148). (Courtesy Dr. R. Rowan.)

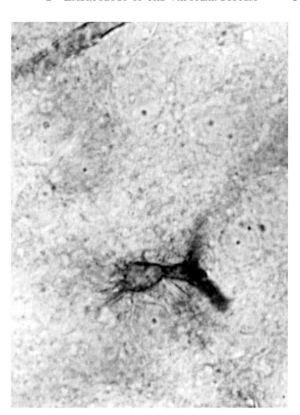

FIGURE 2-9 ■ Light micrograph of rat cerebral cortex, reacted for alkaline phosphatase. A vascular sprout is seen in the middle third of the cortex 8 days after birth. Pseudopodia are evident at the tip (∞3148). (Courtesy Dr. R. Rowan.)

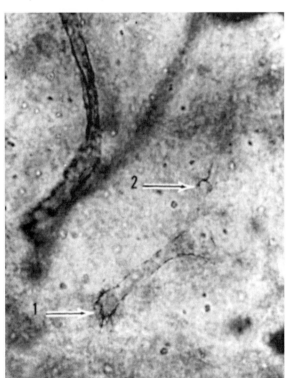

FIGURE 2-10 ■ Light micrograph of rat cerebral cortex, reacted for alkaline phosphatase. A branched sprout with two tips *(arrows)* is evident. The larger tip (*1*) extends down and to the left of the stem vessel; the smaller tip (*2*) extends upward. The parent sprout and the two sprout tips are much less intensely stained than are the mature vessels dominating the upper and left parts of the micrograph (∞3148). (Courtesy Dr. R. Rowan.)

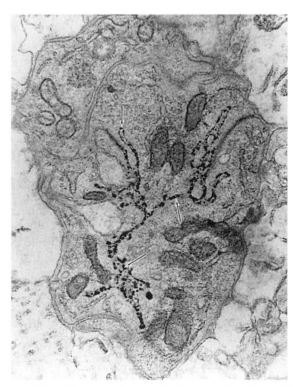

FIGURE 2-11 ■ Electron micrograph of a sprout in the middle third of the rat cortex 8 days after birth. The unopened lumen *(arrows)* is delicately outlined by the deposition of enzyme (alkaline phosphatase) reaction product (∞42,200). (Courtesy Dr. R. Rowan.)

human carcinoma cells, marking the first time that an angiogenic factor was isolated, its amino acid sequence determined, and its genetic code identified. Curiously, this factor (angiogenin) is remarkably similar in its amino acid sequence to a ribonuclease, and the unraveling of the biologic meaning of this similarity and possible relationship will be fascinating to watch in the literature. This is not to say that only one angiogenic protein is the cause of neovascularization. There may be many, perhaps different ones, operating in the embryo and fetus, in the adult during wound healing, and in neoplasms. There is abundant evidence that tissue metabolites are capable of stimulating vascular development (e.g., high carbon dioxide and low oxygen content in tissue fluids). A complex list of possibilities will have to be sorted to determine which factors act to stimulate the production or release of specific angiogenic factors from cells (and which cells) and which are sufficient factors in their own right, acting directly on preexisting vessels.

It might not be satisfying to conclude with a dismaying array of unanswered questions. It is compelling evidence, however, that the questions are there and that the vigorous activity taking place in laboratories around the world will eventually yield some answers. The control of neovascularization, of which the embryo is such a master, may allow us to apply these concepts to a wide spectrum of problems afflicting adults in our clinics and hospitals.

References available online at expertconsult.com.

SECTION 2

GENERAL PRINCIPLES

CHAPTER 3

Anatomy, Physiology, and Pharmacology of the Vascular Wall

Gale L. Tang • Ted R. Kohler

NORMAL ANATOMY

The primary purpose of the vascular system is to serve as a nonthrombogenic conduit for blood flow, which is critical for delivery of oxygen, nutrients, hormonal signals, and cellular components throughout the body. The cellular elements of blood vessels, (endothelial cells, smooth muscle cells, fibroblasts, and niche progenitor cells) are similar throughout the vasculature. However, structure and function varies throughout the vascular tree to allow for the dynamic regulation of blood flow, primarily regulated by changes in arteriolar resistance and venous capacitance. In addition, the vasculature regulates the cellular and molecular trafficking between the intravascular and extravascular space, as well as into and out of the vessel wall. As discussed later in this chapter, the normal adaptive responses of the endothelium and smooth muscle cells to inflammation and injury may account for some of the abnormal properties of vessels undergoing atherosclerotic change or thickening after transplantation (transplant atherosclerosis).

The organization of the cellular elements and extracellular matrix components varies dramatically throughout the vasculature, accounting for its distinctive anatomic and physiologic features at various levels. Vessels larger than capillaries possess three distinct layers or tunics, called the *intima*, the *media*, and the *adventitia*. These layers are generally thicker and better defined in arteries than in veins. In arteries, the intima is composed of a sheet of endothelial cells lining the luminal surface and a subendothelial extracellular matrix. It is divided from the media by an internal elastic lamina. Rare inflammatory cells and smooth muscle cells may be found within the normal intima, although larger populations can be seen, generally as a reaction to injury or as a result of atherosclerotic disease. The media contains circular smooth muscle fibers embedded in a matrix of collagen, elastin, and proteoglycans and is divided from the adventitia by an external elastic lamina. Although the media is composed mostly of smooth muscle cells, there is increasing evidence that smooth muscle cell progenitors reside in niche populations within the media.[1] Both the internal and external elastic laminae are visualized as bright white lines using B-mode ultrasonography, allowing a measurement of intima-media thickness, which can be used as a surrogate marker for atherosclerosis.[2] The adventitia, which serves as the strength layer supporting endarterectomy, is composed primarily of loose connective tissue and fibroblasts. Inflammatory cells, nerve fibers, niche progenitor cells,[1] and a nutrient microcirculation, known as the *vasa vasorum*,[3] also reside within the adventitia.

Veins, as befitting their role as capacitance vessels under low-pressure conditions,[4] are larger and thinner walled than arteries. The subendothelial layer of the intima is missing entirely, and an internal elastic lamina is apparent only in the larger veins. The medial layer contains few smooth muscle cells, collagen, and elastin. Thin bicuspid valves, consisting of two layers of endothelium sandwiched around a layer of connective tissue, are present in larger numbers in peripheral extremity veins, and rarely in central veins. The contractile state of both venules and veins is largely controlled by sympathetic adrenergic activity.

The arterial tree can be divided into three separate categories: large elastic arteries, medium muscular arteries, and small arteries. The aorta and its major branches are classified as large elastic arteries, the distributing arteries to major organs comprise the muscular arteries, and the arteries within organs compose the small arteries. From small arteries, blood flow travels through arterioles to capillary beds, postcapillary venules, and small veins and returns to the heart via larger veins. Collateral arteries are a special class of muscular arteries that traverse from one artery to another rather than feeding into arterioles. Normally there is little flow through collateral arteries and low shear stress. However, when the main conduit artery is obstructed, collateral artery flow and shear stress increase substantially as a compensatory mechanism, which after adaption eventually can restore up to one third of the normal conduit artery blood flow (Figure 3-1).

The aortic media is composed of well-defined lamellar units; each unit consists of a concentric plate of elastin and a circumferentially oriented layer of smooth muscle cells surrounded by a network of type III collagen fibrils embedded in a matrix of basal lamina. Finer elastin fibers compose a network between lamellae as do bundles of interstitial type I collagen.[5] As the aorta traverses away from the heart, the percentage of collagen increases and that of elastin decreases, such that while the thoracic aorta and its major branches have more elastin than collagen, the abdominal aorta has more collagen than elastin. When thoracic aortic segments from multiple

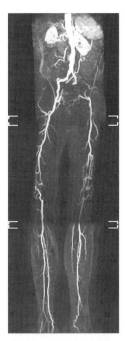

FIGURE 3-1 ■ Magnetic resonance angiogram demonstrating abundant collaterals from the bilateral profunda femoris arteries reconstituting the above knee popliteal arteries. Note that the collaterals traverse between two muscular arteries and that they have both dilated and elongated, resulting in a characteristic corkscrew appearance.

mammalian species across a wide range of body sizes were analyzed, the number of lamellar units was found to be proportional to the radius of the aorta, regardless of the wall thickness. The tangential tension on the artery wall can be roughly estimated with Laplace's law (tension is proportional to the product of the radius and the pressure), which results in a remarkably constant average wall tangential tension per lamellar unit across different species.[6] The upper two thirds of the thoracic aorta, which is thicker than 28 lamellar units, also contains a medial vasa vasorum.[3] The dependence of the abdominal aortic wall on luminal nutrition may explain its increased propensity to aneurysm formation.

In contrast to elastic arteries where collagen and elastin comprise approximately 60% of the dry weight of the media, muscular arteries contain proportionally more smooth muscle cells and less collagen and elastin, allowing them to alter their diameter rapidly through vasodilation or vasoconstriction. In addition, their ratio of media to lumen is higher, contributing to their function as resistive arteries (Figure 3-2). Elastin is further lost as arteries become smaller, and the internal and external elastic lamellae become discontinuous and fragmented. The smallest arteries (arterioles) consist of only an endothelium, a layer of smooth muscle cells, and a filamentous collagenous adventitia. At the capillary level, only the endothelium remains, supported by an occasional contractile connective tissue cell known as a *pericyte*.[7]

The differentiation of the three types of arteries has pathologic significance, as each class of vessel is subject to particular types of disease.[8] Atherosclerosis affects the elastic and muscular arteries, whereas medial calcific

sclerosis is confined to muscular arteries. Small arteries are subject to diffuse fibromuscular thickening and hyalinization.

REGULATION OF LUMINAL AREA

The basic structural components described previously combine together to allow for the vasculature to dynamically regulate blood flow by changing luminal area and wall thickness, both in acute reaction (e.g., increased blood flow induced by exercise, vascular injury, temperature, and pain) and in chronic structural changes to the structural wall induced by ongoing stimuli (hypertension, increased or decreased inflow or outflow, and pathologic inflammation). These alterations require changes within the individual cellular elements and cell-cell interactions, which allow the fully formed vessel to function as an integrated organ.

Blood flow within the vasculature creates unique patterns of biomechanical forces on the vessel walls at different levels through the vascular tree. These biomechanical forces are pressure and shear stress. Pressure is created by the hydrostatic force created by cardiac contraction with the addition of the hydrostatic pressure created by gravity. It is a compressive force and also creates wall tension, as described by the law of Laplace. The greatest wall tension occurs in the large elastic vessels. Wall tension is distributed across all three layers of the vessel wall and determines wall thickness. Shear stress primarily affects the endothelium and is a result of drag caused by the tangential flow of viscous blood over the intimal surface. Endothelial cells align with the direction of this shear stress, which in laminar flow conditions is directly proportional to blood flow and fluid viscosity and inversely related to the cube of the radius.[9] Shear stress is normally maintained in mammals at a constant between 10 and 20 dynes/cm[2] at all levels of the arterial tree.[10]

Both developing and mature vessels respond to changes in hemodynamic forces by adjusting their diameters to maintain a constant level of shear stress. Acutely, this occurs by altering vasomotor tone.[11] Vessels subjected to chronic changes in blood flow remodel by altering their structure in order to regain an appropriate level of shear stress and return vasomotor tone to normal.[11] For example, during embryonic development, higher-volume flow leads to vessel enlargement, whereas lower-volume flow leads to vessel regression. Similarly, in adult vessels, an artery proximal to an arteriovenous fistula will enlarge and can eventually become aneurysmal.[12] Conversely, an artery carrying less flow, either from proximal obstruction or a decrease in outflow (e.g., following amputation or paralysis) will adapt by decreasing its diameter.[11,13,14]

Diseased vessel segments also adapt to alterations in blood flow. A coronary artery with an enlarging atherosclerotic plaque is subject to increased blood flow velocity in the area of luminal stenosis. The coronary artery acutely responds by vasodilating and chronically undergoes a process known as outward remodeling to preserve luminal diameter (Glagov's phenomenon). This adaptive process works to preserve a normal luminal diameter as

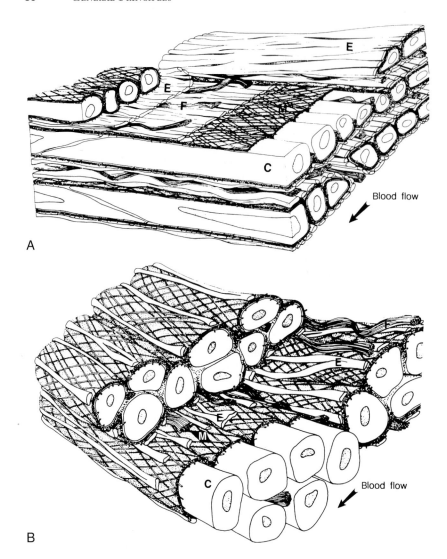

A

B

Blood flow

Blood flow

FIGURE 3-2 ■ Schematic representation of the lamellar organization of elastic *(A)* and muscular *(B)* arteries. Each unit is composed of a group of commonly oriented smooth muscle cells *(C)* surrounded by matrix *(M)* consisting of basal lamina and a fine meshwork of collagen and surrounded by elastic fibers *(E)* oriented in the same direction as the long axes of the cells. Wavy collagen bundles *(F)* lie between the elastic fibers. The elastic lamellae are much better defined in the elastic arteries *(A)* than in the muscular arteries *(B)*. (From Clark JM, Glagov S: Transmural organization of the arterial media: the lamellar unit revisited. Arteriosclerosis 5:19, 1985.)

long as the intimal lesion does not exceed 40% of the area within the internal elastic lamina, at which point pathologic narrowing begins.[15] This process is dependent on an intact endothelium to translate the biomechanical information from shear stress to biochemical signals which regulate vessel diameter. Vessels denuded of endothelium in general do not respond to changes in flow.[16]

Pharmacologic agents regulating vasodilation and vasoconstriction affect vasomotor tone, and can be classified as endothelial and nonendothelial-dependent.[17] Relaxation of the isolated rabbit aorta and other arteries induced by acetylcholine and other muscarinic receptor agonists was initially demonstrated to be dependent on the presence of endothelial cells by Furchgott and Zawadzki in 1980.[18] In the absence of endothelial cells, acetylcholine causes contraction of the arterial wall instead of relaxation. In addition to acetylcholine, multiple other pharmacologic agents produce endothelial-dependent relaxation of vessels including arachidonic acid, adenosine triphosphate, adenosine diphosphate, bradykinin, histamine, norepinephrine, serotonin, thrombin, and vasopressin. The endothelial-dependence of these agents results from their ability to stimulate endothelial nitric oxide synthase (eNOS) to convert L-arginine

to the soluble gas nitric oxide (NO; previously known as *endothelial-derived relaxation factor* and identified in 1987).[19] NO stimulates guanylate cyclase in vascular smooth muscle cells leading to an increase in cyclic guanosine monophosphate and vasodilation. Nitric oxide is the most potent of the endothelial-derived relaxation factors; however, prostacyclin and endothelium-derived hyperpolarizing factors can also be demonstrated to be endothelial-derived vasodilators.[20] In contrast, other pharmacologic agents such as adenosine, adenosine monophosphate, papaverine, isoproterenol, and nitrovasodilators (e.g., sodium nitroprusside) cause vasodilation even in the absence of endothelial cells.

In addition to releasing vasodilating factors, under different conditions the endothelium can also produce vasoconstricting factors in response to arachidonic acid, hypoxia, and in some isolated cerebral vessels by stretch.[17,21] Arachidonic acid is metabolized by cyclooxygenase (COX) into endoperoxides, which are vasoconstrictors, and further metabolized by other enzymes to thromboxane, prostacyclin, and other prostaglandins, all of which can result in vasoconstriction. Reactive oxygen species, formed as by-products of COX generation of prostanoids, also stimulate vasoconstriction.[21]

Endothelin and angiotensin II are both peptide vasoconstrictors, which have been isolated from cultured endothelial cells. Increases in shear stress suppress endothelin gene expression and increase the production of eNOS by endothelial cells; endothelin promotes smooth muscle growth, whereas NO suppresses it.

It is likely that these endothelium-derived relaxing and constricting factors contribute to long-term vascular adaptation in response to changes in blood flow. Flow patterns also affect the expression of receptors involved in leukocyte recruitment, including intercellular adhesion molecule 1, vascular cell adhesion molecule 1, and monocyte chemoattractant protein-1.[22] Missing or abnormal endothelium can contribute to certain pathologic conditions associated with acute and chronic vasospasm, such as atypical angina from coronary vasospasm and cerebrovasospasm after cerebral hemorrhage. In addition, endothelial dysfunction, as measured by abnormal flow-mediated vasodilation of the brachial or radial artery in response to reactive hyperemia, can be detected in the presence of most major cardiovascular risk factors, including hypertension, tobacco exposure (either active or passive), dyslipidemia, aging, diabetes mellitus, obesity, hyperhomocysteinemia, and chronic inflammation.[20]

REGULATION OF MEDIAL AND INTIMAL THICKENING

As described previously, arterial wall thickness is initially determined by tangential tension. Wall thickening is a prominent feature of most pathologic processes. Hypertension causes arterial medial thickening in both humans and animals. Atherosclerosis, hypercholesterolemia, and reaction to injury such as endothelial denudation cause intimal thickening.[23-26] Exactly how these responses are regulated is not clear, although it is certain that in each instance smooth muscle cells proliferate and drive accumulation of extracellular matrix.[24,27] In addition, hypercholesterolemia promotes the accumulation of lipids and lipoproteins, followed by lipid-filled macrophages into the intimal lesion.[24]

Because smooth muscle accumulation is a central feature of most forms of vascular wall thickening, it is worth discussing the currently understood mechanisms of smooth muscle growth control.[27,28] Although smooth muscle cell proliferation is an essential process during growth and development, these cells are predominantly quiescent in adult vessels. In the adult rat, smooth muscle cells turn over at a rate of 0.06% per day, which is barely detectable by available methods.[29] Vascular smooth muscle cells can be stimulated by various pathologic conditions to undergo a phenotypic switch to a synthetic phenotype. In this state, they undergo high levels of proliferation, migration into the intimal layer, and generation of significant amounts of extracellular matrix components. A recent theory suggests that resident or perhaps bone marrow derived progenitor cells, rather than quiescent mature smooth muscle cells, are the primary cells contributing to vascular remodeling in response to arterial injury or disease.[1,30] Regulation of the contractile and synthetic phenotypic states is

incompletely understood, but appears to occur at the transcriptional level; this regulation clearly is critical to the problems of arterial wall remodeling in reaction to primary hypertension as well as local susceptibility to atherosclerotic change.

Because of the importance of vascular smooth muscle cells in pathologic processes, including atherosclerosis and restenosis in response to arterial and vein grafts as well as balloon angioplasty and stenting, many in vivo models of smooth muscle cell growth and proliferation have been developed. Perhaps increasingly relevant is a model using an angioplasty balloon catheter in the rat carotid artery, with or without stent implantation. In this model, significant intimal hyperplasia is only observed when the internal elastic lamina is ruptured.[31,32] The best characterized model, however, is the balloon injury model, in which smooth muscle cell proliferation is stimulated by the passage of an inflated balloon catheter along an artery.[33,34] The passage of the inflated balloon both stretches the arterial wall as well as denudes the endothelium. Immediately following balloon passage, platelets adhere to the denuded wall, spread, and degranulate, releasing numerous growth factors, chemotactic factors, and vasoactive substances.

Endothelial denudation and platelet adherence are followed 1 to 2 days later by the stimulation of medial smooth muscle proliferation and migration across the internal elastic lamina to form a neointima.[29] This response can be dramatic, as illustrated by the marked increase in thymidine incorporation index (a measure of DNA replication, and therefore proliferation) in the ballooned rat carotid artery (Figure 3-3). Smooth muscle

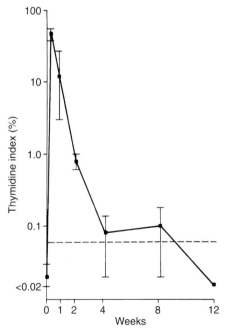

FIGURE 3-3 ■ Smooth muscle cell proliferation rates following balloon catheter injury of the rat carotid artery, as measured by the percentage of cells that incorporate thymidine. Proliferation is greatest at 48 hours and falls rapidly thereafter. (Adapted from Clowes AW, Reidy MA, Clowes MM: Kinetics of cellular proliferation after arterial injury. I. Smooth muscle growth in the absence of endothelium. Lab Invest 49:327, 1983.)

cells commit to proliferation early after injury; this response can be blocked by giving heparin during the first few days after injury. Heparin blocks entry in the cell cycle, significantly reducing both the number of dividing cells and the eventual mass of neointima.[35] Not all smooth muscle cells respond equally to mitogenic stimuli, probably because of the differing phenotypes of smooth muscle cells that can be derived from either the mesoderm or the ectoderm as well as the presence or absence of progenitor cells.[30,36]

The initial proliferative response of smooth muscle cells occurs in the media of the injured artery and does not lead to an increase in wall thickness. Rather, the wall thickens only after the smooth muscle cells migrate into the intima and proliferate there. This process persists for approximately 2 weeks and spontaneously subsides regardless of whether endothelium reappears at the luminal surface. Intimal thickness is further increased by the accumulation of extracellular matrix synthesized by the smooth muscle cells (Figure 3-4).[37]

Several lines of evidence suggest that platelet degranulation stimulates smooth muscle cell proliferation and migration.[25,38-42] Many growth factors, including platelet-derived growth factor (PDGF), transforming growth factor-β, and an epidermal growth factor–like protein, are found within platelet granules.[38] Of these, PDGF appears to be the dominant growth factor affecting vascular smooth muscle cells after injury, as evidenced by work using anti-PDGF antibodies or infusion of PDGF after balloon injury.[39,42] Injured arteries in thrombocytopenic animals show little intimal thickening.[41] This effect occurs despite no measurable change in smooth muscle cell proliferation, suggesting that platelets are more important in stimulating migration rather than cell proliferation.[40] However, it remains unknown where soluble growth factors and other platelet-derived granular proteins go after being released from the platelet. An attractive hypothesis is that they accumulate within the arterial wall and stimulate subsequent smooth muscle growth and migration.

Despite intensive study, the mechanisms that start or stop the intimal thickening process are still poorly understood. Several interesting and potentially important observations about the process have been made. First, the surface of the injured artery will only accumulate a single layer of platelets. Fibrin and microthrombi are seen at the luminal surface only when the artery that has already undergone intimal thickening is injured again or when small craters have been formed in the luminal surface in association with adherent macrophages in hypercholesterolemic animals.[43] Therefore active fulminant thrombosis is not a usual reaction to injury; when it occurs, it must represent a major aberration of vessel function.

Second, in models in which reendothelialization occurs early or partial deendothelialization occurs without medial injury, intimal thickening does not

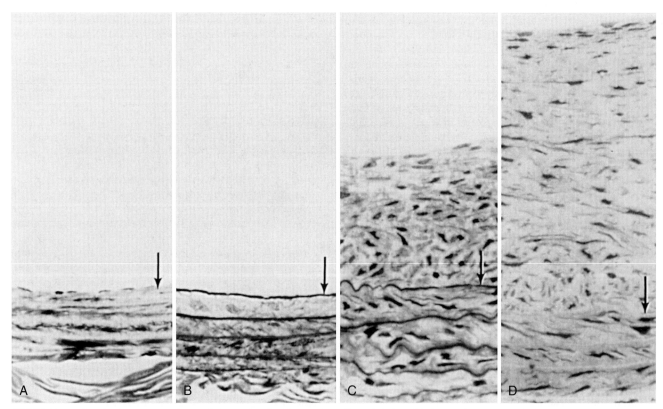

FIGURE 3-4 ■ Histologic cross-sections of the region lacking endothelium in injured left carotid arteries. **A,** Normal vessel. Note the single layer of endothelium in the intima. **B,** Denuded vessel at 2 days. Note the loss of endothelium. **C,** Denuded vessel at 2 weeks. The intima is now markedly thickened because of smooth muscle proliferation. **D,** Denuded vessel at 12 weeks. Further intimal thickening has occurred. The internal elastic lamina is indicated by the *arrow*. The lumen is at the top. (From Clowes AW, Reidy MA, Clowes MM: Kinetics of cellular proliferation after arterial injury. I. Smooth muscle growth in the absence of endothelium. Lab Invest 49:327, 1983.)

develop although one or two rounds of medial smooth muscle cell proliferation may occur. This observation suggests that the endothelium normally suppresses smooth muscle proliferation and migration from the media into the intima. This suggestion is supported by the isolation of smooth muscle growth inhibitors from the vessel wall. In addition, the endothelium can synthesize a heparin-like molecule that inhibits in vitro smooth muscle cell growth; heparin suppresses both proliferation and migration of smooth muscle cells in vitro and in vivo.[44] The endothelium also releases NO in a flow-dependent manner; NO is a growth inhibitor for smooth muscle cells.[45,46] These findings suggest that an intact, functional endothelium actively maintains the medial smooth muscle cells and smooth muscle progenitor cells in a quiescent state instead of the quiescent state being attributable to the lack of growth factors. These findings also support the more general concept that the cells of the vascular wall communicate with each other and regulate each other's function.

Third, the process of atherosclerosis appears to first require intimal thickening. The hypothesis that atherosclerosis results as a cellular response to endothelial injury was first proposed by Ross and Glomset in 1973.[47] This theory has been modified and refined over the last 30 years, with a more recent recognition of the importance of the role of inflammation and inflammatory cells.[48,49] In its current state, the theory proposes that injury leads to endothelial cell dysfunction, which changes endothelial permeability, adhesive characteristics, and responses to various growth factors. The changes in endothelial permeability allow inflammatory cells such as activated platelets, monocytes, and T lymphocytes to infiltrate into the arterial wall. The subsequent cell-cell interaction between endothelial cells, smooth muscle cells, and inflammatory cells create a fibroproliferative response, which eventually leads to the formation of atherosclerotic plaque.

CELL-CELL COMMUNICATION WITHIN THE VASCULAR WALL

The importance of cell-cell communication within the vascular wall has now been introduced three times, once in regard to chronic vasodilation in response to increased flow, second in regard to control of vascular smooth muscle cell proliferation and migration, and third in regard to the initiation of the atherosclerotic plaque. The following section will explore the participants and kinds of messages in more detail, especially as they pertain to growth control and maintenance of the antithrombotic state. Cell-cell communication can be direct by means of intercellular junctions or can occur at a distance through paracrine and hormonal communication by molecules secreted into the extracellular space.

Direct cell-cell communication across gap junctions has been demonstrated in monolayers of endothelium[50] and in mixed cell populations between endothelial and smooth muscle cells.[51] Gap junctions have been demonstrated morphologically between endothelial cells as well as between endothelial and smooth muscle cells in vitro

and in vivo. The significance of these direct links has not been well defined; although in culture, pericytes and smooth muscle cells can inhibit endothelial cell growth when the cells are in contact with one another.[51] Plasma membrane preparations from confluent large vessel endothelium also actively inhibit growing endothelial cells.[52] In vivo, endothelial proliferation occurs in the absence of pericytes; this growth ceases when pericytes become associated with the endothelium.[53] Some aspects of vasodilation are likely translated from the endothelium to smooth muscle cells by gap junctions. In addition, direct intercellular links may help to regulate endothelial proliferation and endothelial-mediated vascular relation in collateral vessels by propagating signals from one cell to the next upstream from a large vessel occlusion to a downstream vessel. These intercellular links provide a mechanism for a local response by the vessel wall in the absence of release and wide dissemination of potent vasoactive or growth-regulating substances.

Cell-cell communication over distances is mediated by secreted soluble factors. As previously mentioned, platelets, which are nonnucleated fragments of megakaryocytes, carry granules bearing an array of potent mitogens. Platelets are clearly involved in wound healing, atherogenesis, angiogenesis, and vascular remodeling.[54] This is evidenced by the observation that whole blood serum contains much more growth-promoting activity than does serum lacking platelets (plasma-derived serum); this observation led to the isolation of PDGF from platelet α-granules and more recently has led to work demonstrating platelet-progenitor cell interactions.[55] PDGF is a basic dimeric protein with a molecular weight of approximately 30 kD and acts as a potent smooth muscle cell mitogen at active concentrations of nanograms per milliliter.[56] In addition, its mitogenic activity, it also stimulates smooth muscle cell migration, contraction, and extracellular matrix synthesis and serves as a chemotactic factor for other inflammatory cells. This last activity is likely responsible for its in vivo activity of stimulation of granulation tissue when placed in a subcutaneously implanted wound chamber[57] and has been exploited as the topical agent Regranex (becaplermin or recombinant human PDGF-BB) for use in assisting wound healing.

In 1983, the structure of the oncogene v-sis, a gene associated with cellular transformation by the simian sarcoma virus, was found to be almost identical to the PDGF gene structure.[58,59] This discovery, coupled with the finding that a variety of both normal and oncogenic cells synthesize and secrete active PDGF, raised the possibility that only subtle changes in gene regulation separate normal wound healing from malignant, unregulated growth of tumor cells. In terms of vascular wall components, endothelium, smooth muscle cells, and leukocytes, including macrophages, have been demonstrated to express the PDGF gene (c-sis) both in vitro and in vivo.[56] All the activities of PDGF within the vascular wall are incompletely characterized; however, as previously discussed, its primary role in animals undergoing balloon-catheter carotid injury appears to be to stimulate smooth muscle cell migration rather than proliferation.[39,42] Recently, PDGF also has been found to be

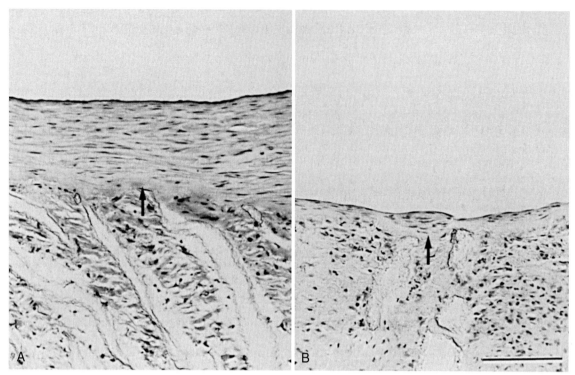

FIGURE 3-5 ■ Cross-sections of polytetrafluoroethylene grafts 3 months after placement in the aortoiliac circulation in baboons. **A,** Control side with normal flow. **B,** Experimental side with a distal arteriovenous fistula causing increased flow. The *arrows* indicate the junction of the graft and neointima. Scale bar, 100 μm. (From Kohler TR, Kirkman TR, Kraiss LW, et al: Increased blood flow inhibits neointimal hyperplasia in endothelialized vascular grafts. Circ Res 69:1557, 1991.)

upregulated—along with acidic fibroblast growth factor, basic fibroblast growth factor (bFGF), and vascular endothelial growth factor—within developing collateral arteries.[60]

In contrast, smooth muscle cell proliferation is likely to be primarily stimulated by intracellular mitogens released from injured medial smooth muscle cells. Hydrostatic distention models of arterial injury that do not cause significant endothelial injury lead to significant smooth muscle cell proliferation without migration, presumably because of a lack of platelet degranulation in this model.[61] In addition, when the endothelium is injured using a fine nylon loop that does not damage the media, very little smooth muscle cell proliferation is observed.[62,63] The principal mitogen responsible for smooth muscle cell proliferation after injury appears to be bFGF. Both bFGF messenger RNA and protein are found in the uninjured vessel wall.[64] Infusion or local administration of bFGF after arterial injury causes a marked increase in smooth muscle cell proliferation and intimal thickening, whereas infusion of antibodies against bFGF causes a significant reduction in smooth muscle cell proliferation.[64-66] Interestingly, bFGF is not mitogenic for smooth muscle cells in uninjured vessels, suggesting that other products of injury are required to induce mitogenesis. When smooth muscle cells are cultured from injured media, they produce up to fivefold more PDGF than do cells cultured from uninjured arteries.[67] Smooth muscle cells derived from injured media also express messenger RNA for insulin-like growth factor[68] and transforming growth factor-β,[69] both of which are mitogenic

for smooth muscle cells in vitro. Thus, injury to smooth muscle cells may stimulate cell growth in a paracrine fashion by releasing a number of mitogens.

The rate of blood flow, which as previously discussed affects the diameter of developing and mature arteries, also influences intimal hyperplasia in injured vessels and vascular grafts. Wall thickening of vein and synthetic grafts is increased in areas of reduced flow[70,71] and is reduced by high flow (Figure 3-5).[72,73] Increased flow causes regression of intima in endothelialized expanded polytetrafluoroethylene grafts implanted into baboons.[74] These changes are presumably the result of the endothelial response to changes in shear stress, resulting in the release of factors that regulate the arterial diameter and wall structure. For example, reduced flow causes an increase in PDGF expression in rat carotid arteries.[75] High flow upregulates NOS in synthetic grafts; this effect can be blocked by the local infusion of a NOS inhibitor.[76] Interestingly, flow also appears to affect intimal hyperplasia in balloon-injured rat carotid arteries, even though the endothelium is denuded in this model.[77] This finding implies that surface smooth muscle cells can respond to flow in a manner similar to that of endothelium. Finally, restoration of eNOS activity by gene transfer into the denuded wall of injured rat carotid arteries suppresses intimal hyperplasia and increases vessel reactivity.[78]

Growth control of the vascular wall must involve a complex interaction between endothelial cells, vascular smooth muscle cells, inflammatory cells, progenitor cells, and the extracellular matrix. Tissue culture media conditioned with endothelial cells in vitro is growth-promoting for smooth muscle cells; a portion of this activity is due to PDGF-like proteins and perhaps other characterized factors such as bFGF. Production of PDGF is increased when cells are exposed to endotoxin or phorbol esters and decreased when cells are exposed to oxidized low-density lipoproteins.[79] Activated smooth muscle cells in vitro also make PDGF, specifically those derived from neonatal as opposed to adult aorta and those from injury-induced intimal thickening as opposed to quiescent media.[28] Stimulated macrophages also increase their production of PDGF. Lastly, as previously mentioned, injured vascular wall cells release intracellular mitogens (e.g., bFGF). In addition to growth factors, platelets also release chemotactic factors for progenitor and inflammatory cells (e.g., stromal-cell derived factor-1), whereas endothelial cells can upregulate adhesion molecules and chemotactic factors that also attract inflammatory cells. These fragmentary results support the concept that activated vascular wall cells can amplify the initial stimulus (perhaps an influx of platelet-derived factors) by producing PDGF, PDGF-like proteins, and other growth-promoting factors that further act on vascular wall cells. These and other factors might also act to regulate the traffic of leukocytes and progenitor cells in and out of the wall; the activated leukocytes and progenitors could then reciprocate by producing additional factors to affect the function of the vascular wall cells. These findings support the theory that there is a great deal of cross-talk between the cells within the vascular wall and those within the blood, with many complex feedback loops.[80,81]

POSSIBLE THERAPIES FOR PREVENTION OF RESTENOSIS

New therapeutic possibilities for preventing restenosis are emerging from the increasing understanding of the cellular and molecular events surrounding the formation of intimal hyperplasia. A complete listing of therapeutic strategies is beyond the scope of this chapter, but therapies that are already in clinical practice are worth noting. We have previously emphasized the importance of the platelet in triggering activation of the vascular cell wall in response to injury. Multiple antiplatelet drugs are commonly used in clinical practice, including aspirin (irreversible COX inhibitor); dipyridamole (phosphodiesterase and thromboxane synthase inhibitor); cilostazol (phosphodiesterase-3 inhibitor); thienopyridines such as ticlopidine, clopidogrel, and prasugrel (adenosine diphosphate receptor inhibitors); and abciximab (chimeric human-murine monoclonal antibody blocking the glycoprotein IIb/IIIa receptor). Interestingly, although vein graft patency was not improved by the addition of clopidogrel to aspirin in a recent randomized trial, prosthetic bypass patency was improved.[82] Although cilostazol is more commonly used for its vasodilatory properties in improving symptoms of intermittent claudication, recent evidence suggests it also has a role in suppressing intimal hyperplasia after angioplasty and stenting procedures.[83-85] Lastly, abciximab reduces the incidence of repeated procedures, death, and myocardial infarction after coronary angioplasty.[86] A single dose was able to improve clinical results 3 years out from the procedure, suggesting either that platelet blockade can abort the initiation of the intimal hyperplastic response or that the drug affects smooth muscle cell proliferation and migration.[87]

Of the various strategies for local control of smooth muscle cell proliferation following vascular injury, drug eluting stents have had the most success, primarily in the coronary circulation,[88] whereas local delivery of radiation and antisense oligonucleotides to inhibit cell cycle regulatory proteins lack clinical efficacy.[89,90] The first generation of drug-eluting stents provides local delivery of the potent cell-cycle inhibitors sirolimus and paclitaxel via a permanent polymer coating.[88] However, there have been several reports of delayed stent thrombosis (up to 5 years after implantation), generally after cessation of dual antiplatelet therapy. When examined histologically, drug-eluting stents show delayed endothelialization, which has been theorized to result from inflammation and hypersensitivity to the permanent polymers used to coat the stent and allow drug delivery. Second-generation drug-eluting stents elute zotarolimus and everolimus and are coated with new polymers that cause less inflammation. Third-generation drug-eluting stents—which feature biodegradable polymers, are polymer-free, or are completely biodegradable, thus avoiding the problems incited by late stent fracture—are under development.[91] Studies of drug-eluting stents and balloons in the peripheral arterial system are underway. The ideal device would inhibit intimal hyperplasia while encouraging positive outward remodeling and early reendothelialization.

REGULATION OF THROMBOSIS BY THE ENDOTHELIUM

The normal artery with a functional endothelium is resistant to thrombosis, even with complete cessation of blood flow for a prolonged period. However, blood within a damaged vessel clots readily. This empirical observation led to the theory that the endothelium must produce one or more antithrombotic or anticoagulant molecules, which has been borne out by the isolation of these molecules. Teleologically, the endothelium must also be capable of expressing an extensive array of procoagulant functions as well; these molecules have also been isolated and determined to be regulated by messages from the blood or from neighboring cells.[92]

On the anticoagulation side of the balance, the endothelium synthesizes several membrane-associated proteins that have extracellular heparan sulfate moieties, which, like heparin, increase the affinity of antithrombin III for thrombin.[93] This interaction occurs at the level of the endothelial surface and causes rapid inactivation of circulating thrombin and other activated serine proteases in the clotting cascade, including factors VII, IX, and X. As previously observed, heparan sulfate also impedes smooth muscle cell proliferation; this in conjunction with its anticoagulant properties helps to impede two aspects of the response to injury.[44] In addition, endothelial cells synthesize and secrete thrombomodulin, which acts as a cell surface receptor for thrombin. Thrombin bound to thrombomodulin loses it proteolytic activity for fibrinogen and activates protein C instead. Activated protein C binds protein S on the endothelial surface, and as a complex degrades factors Va and VIIIa to inhibit the clotting cascade. The importance of this pathway is amply demonstrated by the prothrombotic tendencies of patients with genetic protein C and S deficiencies, and patients with factor V Leiden, in which a point mutation renders factor V resistant to activated protein C cleavage. Endothelial cells synthesize tissue factor pathway inhibitor. Heparin increases its release into the plasma, where it quenches the activity of tissue factor bound factor VII. Lastly, endothelial cells synthesize and secrete tissue plasminogen activator, as well as binding sites to colocalize tissue plasminogen activator and plasminogen on the endothelial surface and enhance fibrinolytic activity at the blood vessel wall.[94]

On the procoagulation side, endothelial cells synthesize and secrete von Willebrand factor, which supports platelet adhesion, fibronectin, which stabilizes fibrin clot by cross-linking fibrin monomers, and thrombospondin, which promotes platelet aggregate stabilization and depresses fibrinolysis. In addition, under certain pathologic conditions such as exposure to inflammatory mediators (e.g., endotoxin, interleukin-1, tumor necrosis factor) from the blood or possibly also from resident macrophages, the endothelium downregulates its antithrombotic properties by internalizing thrombomodulin and decreasing production of heparan sulfate proteoglycans. The endothelium also upregulates several prothrombotic pathways, including expression of tissue factor, release of P-selectin, generation of platelet-activating factor, secretion of plasminogen activator inhibitor, and exposure of factor IX/Xa binding sites.[94] In addition, endothelial cells also synthesize and express interleukin-1, which could affect the underlying smooth muscle cells.[95]

Only 0.2% of the total thrombin released during the process of thrombosis is generated during the initiation phase. The vast majority of thrombus-associated thrombin is formed after clotting is complete and continues to be released by the mural thrombus. After endothelial injury, thrombin can come into contact with the subendothelial smooth muscle cells. Thrombin is a mitogen for vascular smooth cells in vitro. Furthermore, antithrombin agents can block the increase in PDGF gene expression that is the normal response to injury; it can also limit the smooth muscle cell proliferation following injury. In addition to thrombomodulin, thrombin also binds to a class of protease activated receptors. In normal vessels, thrombin receptors are primarily expressed in the endothelium; however, significant expression is found both in smooth muscle cells in atherosclerotic plaques as well as those reacting to vascular injury. Likewise, thrombomodulin production by smooth muscle cells is rapidly upregulated in response to endothelial denudation or damage; this appears to reduce the mitogenic effect of thrombin on smooth muscle cells. Vasodilatory prostaglandins negatively regulate the expression of thrombin protease activated receptors and upregulate the transcription of thrombomodulin.[96] The derangements of the normal antithrombotic endothelial surface associated with atherosclerotic plaques as well as the significant inflammatory component within the plaque presumably have a direct bearing on the thrombotic complications associated with end-stage atherosclerosis.

SUMMARY

The vasculature should not be regarded as a passive conduit for blood flow, but as an organ with integrated endothelial, smooth muscle, and progenitor cells that can respond to physical and chemical stimuli in the blood by adjusting vascular diameter and thickness acutely and over time. Vascular wall cells participate in local and systemic inflammatory reactions and communicate among themselves to express factors regulating cell proliferation and coagulation.

References available online at expertconsult.com.

QUESTIONS

1. In normal arteries, most of the smooth muscle cells are found in which area?
   a. Intima
   b. Media
   c. Adventitia
   d. None of the above

2. Arteries respond to an increase in blood flow by doing which of the following?
   a. Contracting
   b. Dilating
   c. Intermittently contracting
   d. Intermittently dilating

3. Endothelial cells synthesize and secrete substances that cause what?
   a. Vasodilatation
   b. Vasoconstriction
   c. Both vasodilatation and vasoconstriction
   d. None of the above

4. What causes injured arteries to thicken?
   a. Medial smooth muscle hyperplasia
   b. Intimal smooth muscle hyperplasia
   c. Intimal endothelial hyperplasia
   d. None of the above

5. The reaction-to-injury hypothesis was proposed to explain the initial stages of atherosclerosis. Which element of this hypothesis has not been proved?
   a. Smooth muscle cells are important components of plaque.
   b. Thrombus can accumulate on atherosclerotic lesions.
   c. Platelets contain potent growth factors.
   d. Growth factors released from platelets stimulate smooth muscle growth in vivo.

6. Platelet-derived growth factor (PDGF) is found in which cells?
   a. Platelets
   b. Smooth muscle cells
   c. Endothelium
   d. All of the above

7. Smooth muscle cells respond to PDGF by doing which of the following?
   a. Proliferating
   b. Synthesizing matrix
   c. Migrating
   d. All of the above

8. Based on in vitro studies, endothelial cells appear to express molecules that regulate the behavior of the blood at the luminal surface. Which of the following endothelium-derived molecules act to sustain the anticoagulant state? (There may be more than one correct answer.)
   a. Heparan sulfate
   b. Von Willebrand factor
   c. Plasminogen activator inhibitor
   d. Thrombomodulin
   e. Prostacyclin

9. Which of the following molecules are procoagulants? (There may be more than one correct answer.)
   a. Heparan sulfate
   b. Von Willebrand factor
   c. Plasminogen activator inhibitor
   d. Thrombomodulin
   e. Prostacyclin

10. In general, inflammatory mediators (e.g., interleukin-1) cause endothelial cells to express which of the following?
   a. Increased procoagulant activities
   b. Increased anticoagulant activities
   c. Increased endothelium-derived relaxing factor
   d. None of the above

ANSWERS

1. **b**
2. **b**
3. **c**
4. **b**
5. **d**
6. **d**
7. **d**
8. **a, d, e**
9. **b, c**
10. **a**

CHAPTER 4

ANATOMY AND SURGICAL EXPOSURE OF THE VASCULAR SYSTEM

Jeffrey L. Ballard

A well-planned surgical exposure facilitates even the most difficult operative procedure. Awareness of the relationship between surface anatomy and underlying vascular structures allows precise incision placement as well as percutaneous access, which minimizes tissue trauma and reduces the likelihood of wound infection. Detailed knowledge of vascular anatomy helps to prevent injury to adjacent vital structures within the operative field. In this chapter, anatomic relationships and variations that may be encountered during common vascular exposures are highlighted. Several alternative surgical approaches are also described. Exposure of the carotid bifurcation is discussed first and is followed by a systematic discussion of the anatomy and surgical exposure of the peripheral vascular system, ending with commonly used approaches for the arterial circulation in the leg and foot.

EXPOSURE OF THE CAROTID BIFURCATION

The common carotid artery bifurcates approximately 2.5 cm below the angle of the mandible. Normally, the sternocleidomastoid muscle, the posterior belly of the digastric muscle, and the omohyoid muscle bound the carotid bifurcation. Thus, a skin incision placed along the anterior border of the sternocleidomastoid muscle facilitates exposure of the carotid sheath.

The surgeon must be aware of the location of important cranial and somatic nerves during carotid endarterectomy. The mandibular ramus of the facial nerve is vulnerable to injury during this operation. Nerve damage by retraction or surgical dissection can cause temporary or permanent dysfunction. Turning the head toward the opposite side draws the mandibular ramus well below the mandible and increases the possibility of facial nerve injury.

The great auricular nerve (C-2 and C-3 dermatomes) should be protected in its location on the sternocleidomastoid muscle just anterior to and below the ear. Damage to this nerve results in numbness of the posterior aspect of the auricle and may cause distressing ipsilateral occipital headaches.

The common facial vein comes into view as the incision is deepened. This vessel courses superficially to the carotid bifurcation to join the internal jugular vein. It serves as an important landmark during the dissection. Several small vessels coursing toward the sternocleidomastoid muscle are nutrient branches from the superior thyroid artery and vein. These vessels should be ligated and divided to avoid troublesome postoperative bleeding. In the typical carotid dissection, the common carotid artery should be exposed above the level of the omohyoid muscle. Once this vessel is isolated, further distal dissection along its medial aspect facilitates exposure of the superior thyroid and external carotid arteries. Dissection in the V of the carotid bifurcation should be avoided, because this area is extremely vascular. It is wise to encircle the internal carotid artery well above the level of gross atherosclerotic disease. This dissection is usually 1 to 2 cm above the bifurcation and thereby avoids the highly vascular carotid sinus tissue.

The descending branch of the hypoglossal nerve (ansa cervicalis) is located anterior and parallel to the sternocleidomastoid muscle. If this branch is followed upward, the main hypoglossal nerve trunk can be located. Division of the descending branch of the hypoglossal nerve near its origin allows the main nerve trunk to be displaced upward and forward, thus providing higher exposure of the internal carotid artery. A nutrient vein and artery associated with the sternocleidomastoid muscle course in immediate relation to this nerve at this level. Care should be taken to avoid injury to the underlying hypoglossal nerve when these vessels are ligated and divided. This maneuver allows the nerve to retract superomedially and out of harm's way. Division of this artery-vein "sling" about the hypoglossal nerve facilitates exposure of the internal carotid artery under the posterior belly of the digastric muscle.

The surgeon must also maintain an awareness of the location of the vagus nerve and its branches. It lies within the carotid sheath between the common carotid artery and the internal jugular vein. Normally, it is directly behind the internal carotid artery at its origin. Care must be taken to prevent injury to the nerve at this vulnerable location. Additional care is required to prevent vagus nerve injury during repeated carotid exposure, because the nerve, which may be encased in scar tissue, frequently courses anterior to the carotid bifurcation. The superior laryngeal nerve arises from the vagus nerve above the carotid bifurcation, passes behind the internal carotid artery, and descends medial to the superior thyroid artery. Care must be taken during mobilization of this vessel not to injure the superior laryngeal nerve or its external branch (Figure 4-1). The external branch of the superior laryngeal nerve sometimes passes between the branches of the superior thyroid artery or is adherent to

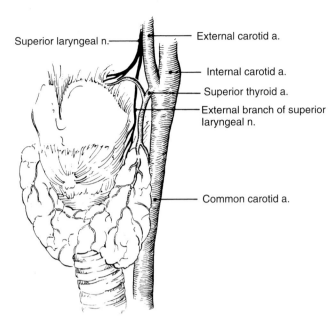

Superior laryngeal n.

External carotid a.

Internal carotid a.

Superior thyroid a.

External branch of superior laryngeal n.

Common carotid a.

FIGURE 4-1 ■ Note the vulnerable location of the external branch of the superior laryngeal nerve to the superior thyroid artery.

it. Table 4-1 lists the locations and the tests for function of the important nerves encountered during exposure of the carotid bifurcation.

A carotid arteriotomy should be created proximal to the carotid bulb and lateral to the carotid flow divider in the typical endarterectomy scenario. This incision is then lengthened distally through the diseased internal carotid artery under direct vision to a point where there is normal-appearing intima. It is critical not to make this arteriotomy on the anterior aspect of the internal carotid artery near the carotid sinus, because this is a relatively fixed area that is difficult to reapproximate without creating a focal narrowing that is at risk for restenosis. It is wise to find the correct endarterectomy plane at the level of the carotid bulb. Endarterectomy then proceeds proximally first, and the specimen is excised sharply with Potts scissors at the level of the common carotid artery. Everting the external carotid artery into the carotid bulb facilitates endarterectomy at this level. Next, the transition point between the atherosclerotic plaque to be removed and the remaining nondiseased internal carotid artery is located. This step is critical in the performance of a technically sound carotid endarterectomy; if it is done correctly, tacking sutures are rarely required. Meticulous care is then taken to ensure that no loose areas of media

---

TABLE 4-1 Regional Nerves Encountered during Exposure of the Carotid Bifurcation

Nerve Branch	Location Encountered	Test for Function	Remarks
Mandibular ramus of facial nerve (cranial nerve VII)	Deep to platysma muscle; can be 5-10 mm below inferior margin of mandible	Ask patient to show teeth; check for paralysis of lower lip	Use gentle retraction of mandible; nerve is pulled down when head is rotated to opposite side
Great auricular nerve (C2, C3)	Anteromedial surface of SCM muscle anterior to and below ear	Anesthesia of ear and adjacent scalp	May cause ipsilateral occipital headache when damaged
Cutaneous cervical nerve (C2, C3)	Subcutaneous on deep fascia	Anesthesia of skin below mandible	Warn patient preoperatively about possible sensory loss
Glossopharyngeal nerve (cranial nerve IX)	Between external and internal carotid arteries; branch is the carotid sinus nerve, also known as the *nerve of Hering*	Loss of ability to swallow	Manipulation of branch nerve may cause bradycardia or hypotension; IV atropine or local infiltration of the nerve with lidocaine relieves circulatory changes
Vagus nerve (cranial nerve X)	Within carotid sheath; between IJV and CCA; directly behind proximal ICA	Indirect laryngoscopy for vocal cord function	Dissect "right on" distal CCA and ICA to avoid injury, avoid past-pointing with occluding clamp tips
External branch of superior laryngeal nerve (branch of cranial nerve X)	Adjacent and medial to superior thyroid artery	Loss of function of cricothyroid muscle	Inability to produce high tones
Hypoglossal nerve (cranial nerve XII)	Main nerve trunk crosses ICA and ECA 1-2 cm above bifurcation, SCM artery and vein branches sling around nerve, dividing these branches improves distal ICA exposure	Extended tongue deviates to side of injured nerve	Visualize descending branch first and follow it to main nerve trunk; carefully ligate "sling" vessels to maintain dry operative field

IV, Intravenous; *IJV,* internal jugular vein; *CCA,* common carotid artery; *ICA,* internal carotid artery; *ECA,* external carotid artery; *SCM,* sternocleidomastoid.

remain through the endarterectomized surface. In the author's practice, Bovine patch angioplasty reapproximates the arteriotomy, and intraoperative duplex ultrasound scanning completes the procedure. The reader is referred to *Wylie's Atlas of Vascular Surgery* for color illustrations of the steps used to perform a classic carotid endarterectomy.[1]

For eversion endarterectomy, the carotid artery is obliquely transected at the transition between the proximal internal carotid artery and the carotid bulb. Plaque control with forceps and gentle eversion of the internal carotid artery enable one to establish an appropriate endarterectomy plane of dissection. This maneuver enables visualization of a distal break point that will allow the plaque to feather away from the mid to distal internal carotid artery without the need for tacking sutures. Proximally, angled Potts scissors can be used to create a longitudinal arteriotomy, which opens the carotid bulb and common carotid artery similar to a standard endarterectomy. This move facilitates endarterectomy at the level of the carotid bulb and external carotid artery. The transected internal carotid artery can be shortened if necessary and then reattached using a continuous Prolene suture. Appropriate alignment of the internal carotid artery to the carotid bulb frequently requires a longitudinal incision of the medial aspect of the artery with Potts scissors.

The value of cranial nerve protection during carotid surgery cannot be overemphasized. Despite this admonition, cranial nerve injury (CNI) remains a significant postoperative complication of carotid endarterectomy.[2-6] Sajid and colleagues[3] reviewed the incidence of CNI after carotid endarterectomy over a 25-year period of time. This metaanalysis included 10,847 patients in 31 studies and compared results that were published before 1995 (15 publications) with those published after 1995 (16 publications). The overall incidence of CNI was 9.4% (1020 injured nerves), and the incidence was higher in publications that occurred before 1995 (10.6% versus 8.3%). Not surprisingly, there was a significant range in the incidence of CNI among different vascular centers, which varied from 1.35% to 31%. The hypoglossal nerve, vagus nerve, and its branches and facial nerves were most often injured, whereas glossopharyngeal and spinal accessory nerve injuries occurred less frequently. Fortunately, almost all (99%) CNIs were transient, and nerve function returned within 3 months with conservative therapy only. Permanent and often disabling CNI occurs with an incidence of 0.5% to 1% after carotid endarterectomy.

In a single-center study published in 1999, Ballotta and colleagues[5] reviewed 200 consecutive carotid endarterectomies in Italy. There were 25 cranial nerve injuries (12.5%) in 24 patients, distributed as follows: hypoglossal (11), recurrent laryngeal (8), superior laryngeal (2), marginal mandibular (2), greater auricular (2). Fortunately, the deficits were transient, with all but four resolving by 6 months. The mean recovery time was 5.8 months, with a range of 1 week to 37 months. Forssell and associates[6] reviewed 663 consecutive carotid endarterectomy patients in Malmö, Sweden, who were examined preoperatively and postoperatively at the Department of Phoniatrics to determine cranial nerve function. Seventy-five carotid operations (11.4%) resulted in one or more cranial nerve injuries. These injuries included 70 hypoglossal, 8 recurrent laryngeal, 2 glossopharyngeal, and 2 superior laryngeal injuries. Only two nerve injuries (0.30%) were permanent. The frequency of injury increased with a junior surgeon, shunt use, and patch closure.

In summary, cranial nerve injuries are usually caused by direct trauma such as stretch, retraction, clamping, or transection. Nerve transection should be rare in experienced hands. Reapproximating the epineurium primarily with a fine suture at the time of injury is the best way to repair a transected cranial nerve. Most cranial nerve injuries are transient, with full recovery within 3 to 6 months, on average.

EXPOSURE OF THE DISTAL INTERNAL CAROTID ARTERY

One of the most difficult surgical exposures is that of the distal internal carotid artery. The surgeon must contend with many vital structures within a confined space. This exposure is frequently made more difficult by the presence of a space-occupying vascular lesion or a vascular injury with hemorrhagic staining and displacement of the tissues. Structures that overlie the distal internal carotid artery in the neck include the facial nerve, parotid gland, ramus of the mandible, and mastoid and styloid processes. The hypoglossal nerve, glossopharyngeal nerve, digastric and stylohyoid muscles, and occipital and posterior auricular arteries cross the distal internal carotid artery. The distal cervical internal carotid artery courses progressively deeper to enter the petrous canal of the temporal bone.

Exposure routinely begins at the level of the common carotid artery proximal to the carotid bifurcation. The omohyoid muscle serves as a landmark for the proximal extent of this exposure. The dissection continues distally, protecting the vagus nerve, which lies immediately behind the internal carotid artery. The hypoglossal nerve is exposed, and the descending branch is divided to displace the hypoglossal nerve forward. The digastric and stylohyoid muscles are divided to facilitate this exposure. In addition, the styloid process and the stylohyoid ligament are excised. The glossopharyngeal and superior laryngeal nerves must be identified and preserved. One is now working in a progressively narrowing triangle, with inadequate space to perform any major vascular reconstructive procedure.

Anatomic dissection in human cadaver specimens demonstrates that division of the posterior belly of the digastric muscle facilitates exposure of the internal carotid artery to the middle of the first cervical vertebra. Anterior subluxation of the mandible improves exposure to the superior border of the first cervical vertebra. The addition of styloidectomy to the maneuvers described previously extends the exposure cephalad, approximately 0.5 cm.[7]

Fisher and associates described a unique technique of wire fixation of the mandible to hold its subluxed position

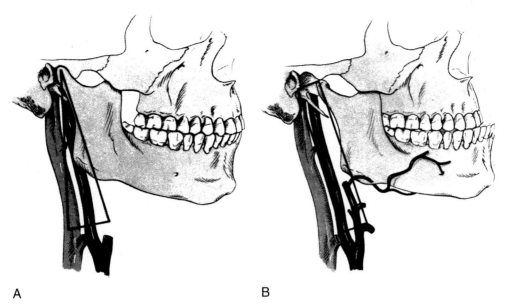

A   B

FIGURE 4-2 ■ The narrow triangle of exposure **(A)** for the high internal carotid artery is expanded to a narrow rectangle **(B)** by anterior subluxation of the condyle of the mandible. (From Fisher DF, Jr, Clagett GP, Parker JI, et al: Mandibular subluxation for high carotid exposure. J Vasc Surg 1:727, 1984.)

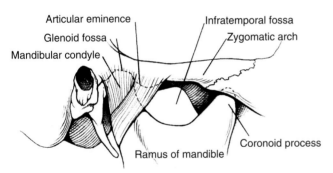

FIGURE 4-3 ■ Anterior subluxation moves the condyle of the mandible to the articular eminence but not to the infratemporal fossa, as would occur with dislocation of the mandible. (From Fisher DF, Jr, Clagett GP, Parker JI, et al: Mandibular subluxation for high carotid exposure. J Vasc Surg 1:727, 1984.)

during the operative procedure.[8] The 12 to 15 mm of space obtained converts the triangle described earlier into a narrow rectangle (Figure 4-2). It is important to avoid dislocation of the mandible, because serious injury can occur to the temporomandibular joint and even to the contralateral internal carotid artery. In the discussion of Fisher and associates' paper,[8] Stanley suggested that a towel clip placed on the angle of the mandible through two small stab incisions would allow the subluxation to be fixed by minimal retraction. Dossa and associates[9] also suggested that temporary mandibular subluxation can be accomplished in a safe and expeditious manner using diagonal, interdental Steinmann pin wiring. Figure 4-3 shows a diagram of the relationship of the mandibular condyle to the auricular eminence and infratemporal fossa.

In situations requiring more room for vascular reconstruction, transection of the mandibular ramus with either translocation or temporary removal of the condyle and ramus fragment affords wider exposure. Wylie and

associates[10] described this approach and provided detailed color illustrations of the involved anatomy.

Following induction of anesthesia, arch bars and wires immobilize the mandible. The usual carotid endarterectomy incision is extended posteriorly to a point behind the ear. The carotid bifurcation and internal carotid artery are exposed as described previously. The mandibular ramus of the facial nerve is protected. The angle of the mandible is exposed, and the periosteum is elevated toward the mandibular notch anteriorly and posteriorly. The mandibular ramus is divided vertically using a power saw posterior to the foramen of the inferior alveolar artery and nerve. The posterior bone fragment is gently rotated out and upward as the pterygoid muscles are divided, allowing the fragment's removal. The bone fragment is preserved in chilled lactated Ringer solution until it is replaced after arterial reconstruction.

Once the mandibular ramus is removed, the digastric and stylohyoid muscles are divided, and the dissection is continued to the skull base. Care should be taken to protect the hypoglossal, glossopharyngeal, and vagus nerves, which are in immediate relation to the distal internal carotid artery. The mandibular fragment is returned to its anatomic location after completion of the internal carotid artery reconstruction, and interrupted nonabsorbable sutures close the temporomandibular joint capsule. A thin titanium plate is used to fix the mandibular fragment in place. The cervical fascia and platysma muscle are closed in layers, followed by routine skin closure.

EXPOSURE OF AORTIC ARCH BRANCHES AND ASSOCIATED VEINS

The most widely accepted direct route for the surgical exposure of the innominate and proximal left common

Skin incision

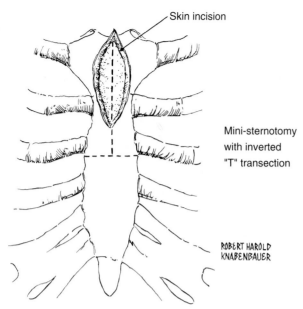

Mini-sternotomy
with inverted
"T" transection

ROBERT HAROLD
KNABENBAUER

FIGURE 4-4 ■ Skin incision and mini-sternotomy sternal division. (From Sakopoulos AG, Ballard JL, Gundry SR: Minimally invasive approach for aortic branch vessel reconstruction. J Vasc Surg 31:200, 2000.)

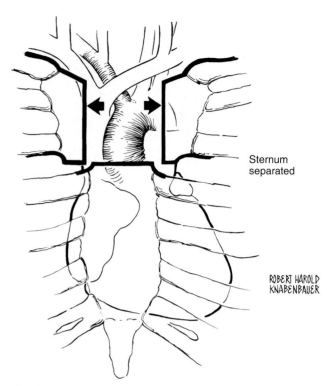

Sternum
separated

ROBERT HAROLD
KNABENBAUER

FIGURE 4-5 ■ The upper sternum is divided and separated, exposing the ascending aorta and arch vessels. (From Sakopoulos AG, Ballard JL, Gundry SR: Minimally invasive approach for aortic branch vessel reconstruction. J Vasc Surg 31:200, 2000.)

carotid arteries, as well as the superior vena cava and its confluent brachiocephalic veins, is through a full median sternotomy. Although this approach is certainly appropriate in the trauma setting, elective aortic arch branch vessel exposure can be performed with a limited approach. Mini sternotomy is a less invasive surgical exposure for the direct treatment of aortic arch branch vessels and associated major veins.[11] Similar to a median sternotomy, this surgical approach provides excellent exposure of the aortic arch branch vessels, with the exception of the left subclavian artery. The first portion of the left subclavian artery is not readily accessible from either anterior approach, because the aortic arch passes obliquely posterior and to the left after its origin from the base of the heart.

Mini sternotomy is performed by first making a limited skin incision measuring 7 to 8 cm in the midline. This incision should extend from the sternal notch to just past the angle of Louis. The manubrium and upper sternum are divided in the midline down to the third intercostal space with a narrow blade mounted on a redo sternotomy oscillating saw (Stryker, Kalamazoo, Mich.). The sternum is then transected transversely at the third intercostal space, creating an upside-down T incision (Figure 4-4). Care is taken not to injure the internal mammary arteries, which are adjacent to the sternum. After accurate hemostasis along the periosteal edges, a Rienhoff or similar pediatric sternal retractor is placed to open the upper sternum. The skin incision can be extended upward along the anterior border of either sternocleidomastoid muscle, with division of the strap muscles to expose the proximal right common carotid artery or the more distal left common carotid artery. This extension can also be used to expose the carotid bifurcation.

The two lobes of the thymus gland are separated in the midline, and if the surgeon carefully observes the pleural bulge during positive-pressure inspiration, entry into either pleural space can be avoided. Nutrient vessels to the thymus gland are carefully ligated and divided, keeping a dry field for visibility. These vessels arise from the internal thoracic artery and drain into the internal thoracic or brachiocephalic veins. The upper pericardium is then opened vertically, and the edges are sewn to the skin with silk suture.

The left brachiocephalic vein can be visualized in the upper portion of the wound. A thymic vein may join this vessel inferiorly, and an inferior thyroid vein may require ligation and division as it joins the brachiocephalic vein superiorly. After complete mobilization of the left brachiocephalic vein, the anterior surface of the aortic arch can be visualized, as well as the origin of the innominate artery. The base of the heart and the innominate and left common carotid arteries are thus exposed (Figure 4-5). The recurrent laryngeal nerve must be protected during exposure of the distal innominate artery. It courses from the vagus nerve anteriorly around the origin of the subclavian artery to return in the tracheoesophageal groove to its termination in the larynx.

Innominate or left common carotid artery endarterectomy, patch angioplasty, or bypass can then be performed in the usual fashion (Figure 4-6). After the procedure, a 19 French Blake drain (Johnson and Johnson, Cincinnati,

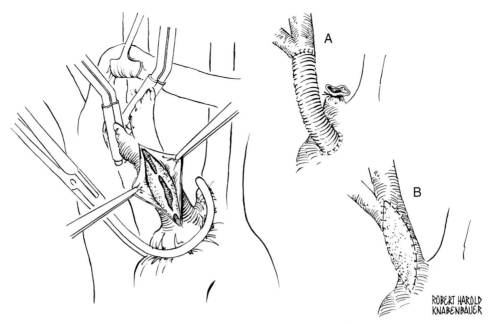

FIGURE 4-6 ■ Surgical exposure of an innominate artery with visible atherosclerotic stenosis. **A,** Repair by proximal exclusion and ascending aorta–to–innominate artery bypass. **B,** Repair by endarterectomy and patch angioplasty. (From Sakopoulos AG, Ballard JL, Gundry SR: Minimally invasive approach for aortic branch vessel reconstruction. J Vasc Surg 31:200, 2000.)

Ohio) is placed in the mediastinum and brought out laterally through one of the intercostal spaces. This drain is connected to a Heimlich valve grenade suction device. Chest tubes are not used. Two wires are used to bring the upper and lower sternal edges of the T together, and two more are placed in the manubrium. If necessary, another wire placed as a figure eight at the level of the second intercostal space completely rejoins the divided upper sternum. After approximating the muscular and subcutaneous planes in two layers, the skin is closed in a subcuticular fashion.

EXPOSURE OF THE ORIGIN OF THE RIGHT SUBCLAVIAN ARTERY AND VEIN

The origin of the right subclavian artery is exposed through a sternotomy incision with extension above and parallel to the clavicle. The right sternohyoid and sternothyroid muscles are divided, followed by exposure of the scalene fat pad. Branches of the thyrocervical trunk are divided, and the dissection is deepened to expose the anterior scalene muscle. The phrenic nerve should be identified and protected as it courses from lateral to medial across the surface of the anterior scalene muscle to pass into the superior mediastinum. The proximal right subclavian artery comes into view with division of the anterior scalene muscle just above its insertion on the first rib.

Traumatic vascular injury at the confluence of the subclavian artery and internal jugular and subclavian veins is difficult to manage solely through a supraclavicular approach. Ideally, sternotomy for proximal vascular control should be followed by supraclavicular extension of the incision. However, in the event that the injury is

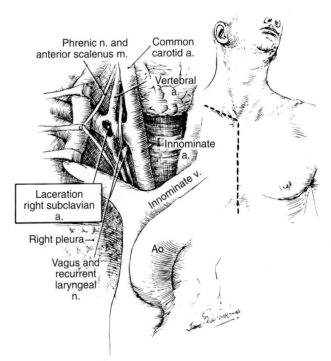

FIGURE 4-7 ■ Exposure of the anterior aortic arch branches through a median sternotomy incision. Note the location of the phrenic, vagus, and recurrent laryngeal nerves, which must be identified and protected. *Ao,* Aorta. (From Ernst C: Exposure of the subclavian arteries. Semin Vasc Surg 2:202, 1989.)

exposed without proximal control, the incision should be promptly extended via a sternotomy while an assistant maintains compression of the vessels against the undersurface of the sternum to temporarily control hemorrhage (Figure 4-7). Alternatively, temporary percutaneous balloon occlusion of the distal innominate artery from a femoral or brachial artery approach can be lifesaving and greatly facilitates this exposure.

EXPOSURE OF THE ORIGIN OF THE LEFT SUBCLAVIAN ARTERY

The left subclavian artery arises from the aortic arch posteriorly and from the left side of the mediastinum; therefore it cannot be adequately exposed for vascular reconstruction through a sternotomy incision. Traumatic injuries and aneurysms of the proximal left subclavian artery should be approached through the left side of the chest. The preferred exposure is an anterolateral thoracotomy through the fourth intercostal space or the bed of the resected fourth rib.

If the vascular injury or aneurysm is extensive, it is wise to prepare the left upper extremity for inclusion in the operative field so that it can be positioned for a second supraclavicular incision. This allows ready access to the second portion of the subclavian artery to gain distal vascular control. Anterolateral exposure of the left side of the chest also facilitates partial occlusion of the aortic arch for lesions involving the origin of the subclavian artery. The phrenic and vagus nerves must be identified and preserved after the pleura is opened and before the dissection of the first portion of the subclavian artery.

In situations in which there is exigent bleeding into the pleural space from a traumatic injury of the proximal left subclavian artery and percutaneous balloon occlusion is not possible, prompt vascular control can be obtained an anterior thoracotomy in the third or fourth intercostal space. This exposure facilitates placement of a vascular clamp across the origin of the bleeding subclavian artery (Figure 4-8). An inframammary incision is preferred in women, with the breast mobilized superiorly for the exposure just described.

EXPOSURE OF THE SUBCLAVIAN AND VERTEBRAL ARTERIES

Exposure of the second portion of the subclavian artery is accomplished through a supraclavicular incision beginning over the tendon of the sternocleidomastoid muscle and extending laterally for 8 to 10 cm. The platysma muscle is divided, and the scalene fat pad is mobilized superolaterally. Thyrocervical vessels are ligated and divided as encountered, with exposure of the anterior surface of the anterior scalene muscle. The phrenic nerve can be seen coursing in a lateral to medial direction over this muscle and should be gently mobilized and preserved. The thoracic duct must also be protected at its termination with the confluence of the internal jugular, brachiocephalic, and subclavian veins. Unrecognized injury can result in a lymphocele or lymphocutaneous fistula.

The anterior scalene muscle is divided just above its point of insertion on the first rib to facilitate exposure of the subclavian artery. Division of this muscle should be done under direct vision and without cautery, because the brachial plexus is immediately adjacent to the lateral aspect of the anterior scalene muscle. The origin of the left vertebral artery arises from the medial surface of the subclavian artery medial to the anterior scalene muscle and behind the sternoclavicular joint. The internal thoracic artery, which originates from the inferior surface of the subclavian artery opposite the thyrocervical trunk, should be protected as the subclavian artery is dissected free of surrounding tissue. Figure 4-9 depicts the essential anatomy of this exposure.

Resection of subclavian artery aneurysms and emergency exposure for vascular injury involving the second and third portions of this vessel require wide exposure. This can be accomplished by resecting the clavicle, including the periosteum. The latter structure, when preserved, results in reossification of a deformed clavicle.

The surgical exposure of the distal vertebral artery is described in detail in Chapter 19 of this text and in the surgical literature.[12] Injury to the intraosseous portion of the vertebral artery with associated hemorrhage is best

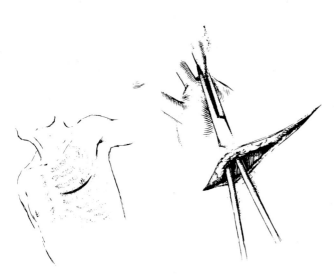

FIGURE 4-8 ■ Anterior thoracotomy with placement of an occluding vascular clamp for control of exigent bleeding from the proximal left subclavian artery. (From Trunkey D: Great vessel injury. In Blaisdell F, Trunkey D, editors: Trauma management, vol 3, Cervicothoracic trauma, New York, 1986, Thieme, p 255.)

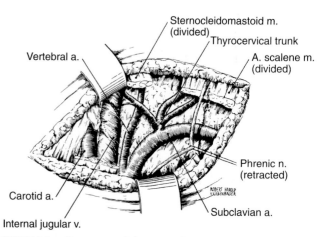

Sternocleidomastoid m. (divided)
Thyrocervical trunk
Vertebral a.
A. scalene m. (divided)
Carotid a.
Phrenic n. (retracted)
Internal jugular v.
Subclavian a.

FIGURE 4-9 ■ Exposure of the second portion of the left subclavian artery via a supraclavicular incision. Note that both the lateral head of the sternocleidomastoid muscle and the anterior scalene muscle are divided for this exposure.

managed by embolic occlusion proximal and, if possible, distal to the area of injury.

EXPOSURE OF THE AXILLARY ARTERY

The proximal axillary artery is exposed by a short incision made between the clavicular and sternal portions of the pectoralis major muscle. Branches of the thoracoacromial vessels are divided to expose the axillary vein first and then the axillary artery above and posterior to the vein. Dissection medial to the pectoralis minor muscle provides appropriate exposure of the axillary artery for axillofemoral bypass graft origin. If additional exposure is required laterally, a portion of the pectoralis minor muscle can be divided near its insertion into the coracoid process of the scapula.

The second portion of the axillary artery is more difficult to expose because it lies directly behind the pectoralis major muscle. Extension of the previously mentioned incision continues across the distal portion of the pectoralis major muscle at the anterior axillary fold and out onto the midline of the proximal medial surface of the arm (Figure 4-10). The tendinous portion of the muscle is divided near its insertion to expose the axillary contents. The pectoralis minor muscle can also be divided if more medial exposure is desired.

EXPOSURE OF THE THORACIC OUTLET

Either a supraclavicular or a transaxillary approach facilitates surgical exposure of the thoracic outlet. Roos described the transaxillary approach for first rib resection

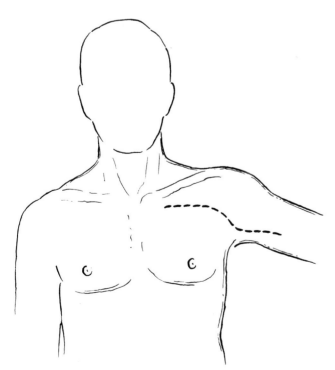

FIGURE 4-10 ■ Incision used for exposure of the axillary artery.

in the management of thoracic outlet syndrome.[13] However, current treatment approaches for thoracic outlet syndrome favor supraclavicular exposure of the neurovascular structures within the superior thoracic aperture. Essential anatomic elements of this approach have been detailed in *Wylie's Atlas of Vascular Surgery*.[14]

A transverse supraclavicular incision based 1.5 cm above the medial half of the clavicle is deepened to develop subplatysmal flaps and to expose the scalene fat pad. Reflection of the fat pad superolaterally facilitates exposure of the anterior scalene muscle. This exposure also requires ligation and division of the transverse cervical artery and vein and resection of the omohyoid muscle.

Identification and careful manipulation of the phrenic nerve are essential to avoid excessive traction or injury. Complete removal of the anterior scalene muscle begins at the level of the first rib and ends at the transverse processes of the cervical vertebrae. Subtotal removal of the middle scalene muscle in a plane parallel to and just inferior to the long thoracic nerve exposes all five roots and three trunks of the brachial plexus.

This unencumbered exposure of the brachial plexus facilitates neurolysis and complete mobilization of the nerve roots. Additional myofibrous bands or bony anomalies are removed at this time. If the course of the lower trunk and C8 to T1 nerve roots are deviated by the first rib, the rib should be partially or totally removed to free the path.

Incision of the Sibson fascia and displacement of the dome of the pleura inferiorly help to fully expose the inner aspect of the first rib. Gentle anteromedial retraction of the plexus ensures adequate posterior division of the first rib near the T1 nerve root. Anteriorly, the rib is transected distal to the scalene tubercle. This approach is useful for rib resection in association with axillosubclavian vein thrombosis. A counterincision just below the clavicle can be used to facilitate anterior transection of the first rib, but this counterincision is rarely needed in the usual dissection. Final removal of the first rib requires division of intercostal muscle attachments to the second rib and division of any other soft tissue.

The scalene fat pad can be wrapped around the plexus if split in a sagittal plane. Repositioning of the fat pad decreases dead space and may help to prevent incorporation of the brachial plexus into the healing scar tissue. The wound is closed in layers after secure hemostasis and reapproximation of the lateral head of the sternocleidomastoid muscle.

EXPOSURE OF THE DESCENDING THORACIC AND PROXIMAL ABDOMINAL AORTA

No single approach is better for extensive exposure of the thoracic and abdominal aorta than a properly positioned thoracoabdominal incision. After pulmonary artery and radial artery line placement and dual-lumen tracheal intubation, the patient is placed in a modified right lateral decubitus position, with the hips rotated 45 degrees from horizontal. This position allows exposure of both groins if needed. A beanbag device is helpful to support the patient's position on the operating table. The free left upper extremity should be passed across the upper chest and supported on a cushioned Mayo stand. In this way, thoracoabdominal aortic exposure is gained by unwinding the torso, as described by Stoney and Wylie.[15]

The extent of thoracic aorta to be exposed will determine which rib interspace to enter. The fourth or fifth intercostal space is used when the entire thoracoabdominal aorta from the subclavian artery origin through the abdominal aorta is to be exposed, whereas the seventh or eighth intercostal space allows mid to terminal thoracic aortic exposure plus wide abdominal aortic visualization. Dividing the respective lower rib posteriorly facilitates this exposure. The thoracic incision is continued across the costal margin in a paramedian plane to the level of the umbilicus (Figure 4-11). If the terminal aorta and iliac vessels are to be exposed, the incision is extended to the left lower quadrant.

With the left lung deflated, the origin of the left subclavian artery and proximal descending thoracic aorta can be dissected free of surrounding tissue to facilitate aortic cross-clamping. The vagus and recurrent laryngeal nerves are densely adherent to the aorta just proximal to the subclavian artery, and meticulous care should be taken not to injure these structures. Division of the inferior pulmonary ligament exposes the middle and distal descending thoracic aorta. The diaphragm is radially incised toward the aortic hiatus, and the left diaphragmatic crus is divided to expose the terminal descending thoracic aorta. Alternatively, just the central tendinous portion of the diaphragm can be divided, or it can be incised circumferentially at a distance of approximately 2.5 cm from the chest wall.

The left retroperitoneal space is developed in a retronephric extraperitoneal plane, because surgical exposure of the thoracoabdominal aorta is greatly facilitated by forward mobilization of the left kidney. Division of the median arcuate ligament and lumbar tributary to the left renal vein allows further medial rotation of the abdominal viscera and left kidney. Clearing the posterolateral surface of the thoracoabdominal aorta facilitates aortotomy. With this exposure, the origins of the left renal artery, celiac axis, and the superior mesenteric artery can then be visualized and dissected free of surrounding tissue, as indicated by the disease process present (Figure 4-12). Dissection over the anterior aorta just distal to the left renal artery and underneath the medially rotated left renal vein will bring the right renal artery into view. Alternatively, the origin of this vessel can be readily identified from within the aorta if it is too scarred across the anterior portion of the abdominal aorta or if the aneurysm is too large to safely perform the maneuver described previously.

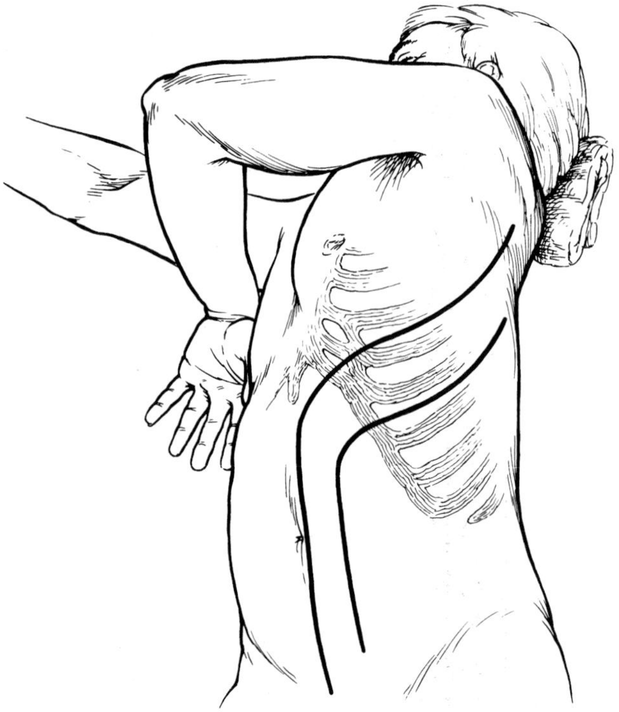

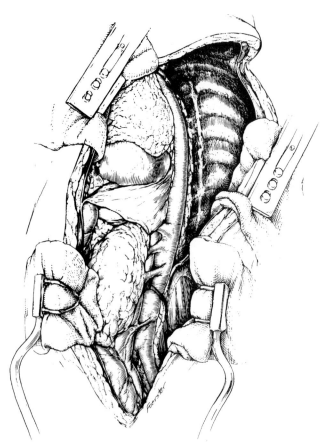

FIGURE 4-11 ■ Incision options for thoracoabdominal aortic procedures are based on the extent of thoracic aorta to be exposed and the desire to stay in an extraperitoneal plane. (From Rutherford RB: Thoracoabdominal aortic exposures. In Rutherford RB, editor: Atlas of vascular surgery: basic techniques and exposures, Philadelphia, 1993, WB Saunders, p 223.)

FIGURE 4-12 ■ Thoracoabdominal aortic exposure from the origin of the left subclavian artery to the common iliac arteries. (From Rutherford RB: Thoracoabdominal aortic exposures. In Rutherford RB, editor: Atlas of vascular surgery: basic techniques and exposures, Philadelphia, 1993, WB Saunders, p 233.)

Preservation of the blood supply to the spinal cord is critical in this extensive operation. Brockstein and associates[16] stressed the importance of the arteria radicularis magna (artery of Adamkiewicz) in providing circulation to the anterior spinal artery (Figure 4-13). This vessel is a branch of either a distal intercostal or a proximal lumbar artery. It has been identified as proximal as T5 and as distal as L4. However, the artery generally arises at the T8 to L1 level; therefore it is unwise to ligate any large intercostal or proximal lumbar artery until the aorta has been opened so that an assessment of arterial backbleeding can be made under direct vision. This important topic is discussed further in Chapter 34.

Exposure of the distal infrarenal aorta and iliac arteries is improved by ligation and division of the inferior mesenteric artery flush with the abdominal aorta. Encircling either the distal common iliac artery or the external and internal iliac arteries individually, depending on presenting pathology, will allow transection of the vessel of vascular reconstruction interest so that end-to-end grafting can be performed. This graft-to-vessel configuration facilitates the actual construction of the anastomosis and also improves surgical exposure within the pelvis, as the vessel can be clamped distal with a baby Cooley clamp and turned toward the surgeon.

Closure of this extensive aortic exposure begins by reapproximating the diaphragm with Prolene suture. A posterior (28 or 32 French) chest tube is placed under direct vision, and the ribs are reapproximated with an interrupted Vicryl suture. Occasionally, a segment of the cartilaginous costal arch is excised to provide stable rib approximation. Thoracic musculature is reapproximated in layers with Vicryl suture. In the abdomen, the posterior rectus sheath is reapproximated, and the anterior rectus sheath is closed with a running PDS suture. Finally, the skin is reapproximated with a running subcuticular suture or with staples.

RETROPERITONEAL EXPOSURE OF THE ABDOMINAL AORTA AND ITS BRANCHES

Transperitoneal exposure is generally regarded as the standard operative approach to the abdominal aorta; however, retroperitoneal exposure has gained wide acceptance among vascular surgeons because it affords a more direct route to the aorta and facilitates complex aortic reconstruction above the level of the renal arteries. Several investigators have demonstrated that in comparison to transperitoneal aortic exposure, the retroperitoneal approach is associated with decreased perioperative morbidity, earlier return of bowel function, fewer respiratory complications, shorter intensive care and hospital stay, and lower overall cost.[17-19]

For this aortic exposure, the patient is positioned on the operating table with the kidney rest at waist level. After pulmonary artery and radial artery line placement and tracheal intubation, the patient is turned to the right lateral decubitus position, with the pelvis rotated posteriorly to allow exposure of both groins. Although not necessary, the kidney rest can be elevated and the operating table gently flexed to open the space between the left anterior superior iliac spine and the costal margin (Figure 4-14). The free left upper extremity is positioned as described earlier.

The incision begins over the lateral border of the rectus muscle approximately 2 cm below the level of the umbilicus and is carried laterally toward the tip of the twelfth rib. This decreases the chance of injury to the main trunk of the intercostal nerve within the eleventh intercostal space. In males, resection of a significant

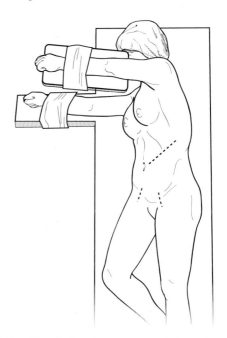

FIGURE 4-14 ■ Positioning for exposure of the retroperitoneal aorta. The patient is positioned right lateral decubitus with the hips rotated open with respect to the OR table, and the left arm is passed across the chest on a Mayo stand. This position unwinds the torso, for greater exposure of the right lower quadrant and bilateral groins as well as the left flank.

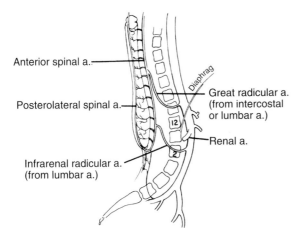

FIGURE 4-13 ■ Diagram of the great and infrarenal radicular arteries supplying the anterior spinal artery. (From Szilagy DG, Hageman JH, Smith RF, et al: Spinal damage in surgery of the abdominal aorta. Surgery 83:38, 1979.)

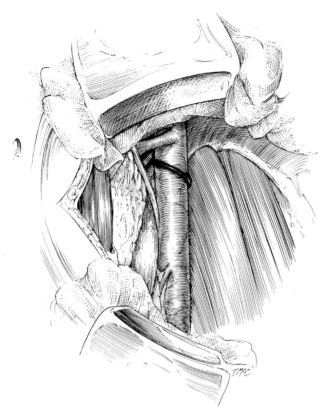

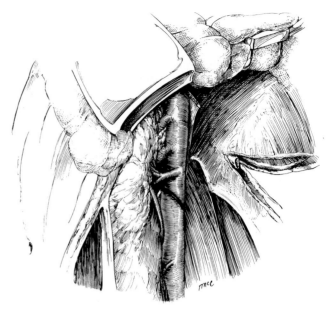

FIGURE 4-16 ■ Division of the median arcuate ligament and left diaphragmatic crus facilitates suprarenal and supraceliac exposure. (From Rutherford RB: Thoracoabdominal aortic exposures. In Rutherford RB, editor: Atlas of vascular surgery: basic techniques and exposures, Philadelphia, 1993, WB Saunders, p 207.)

FIGURE 4-15 ■ The left renal artery serves as a landmark for this dissection. Note the iliolumbar venous tributary just distal to the left renal artery. (From Rutherford RB: Thoracoabdominal aortic exposures. In Rutherford RB, editor: Atlas of vascular surgery: basic techniques and exposures, Philadelphia, 1993, WB Saunders, p 201.)

portion of this rib facilitates retroperitoneal aortic exposure. However, in females, twelfth rib resection is not always required. The anterior rectus sheath is incised to allow medial retraction of the left rectus abdominis muscle. The incision is carried laterally through the external and internal oblique muscle fibers. Careful incision of the most lateral aspect of the posterior rectus sheath facilitates development of an extraperitoneal plane. The remaining posterior sheath is divided toward the midline, and laterally, transversus abdominis muscle fibers are split toward the twelfth rib.

The peritoneum is gently swept off the posterior rectus sheath, the transversus abdominis fibers, and the diaphragm to allow safe entry into the left retroperitoneal space. This space is best entered inferolaterally. The peritoneum and its contents are swept medially off the psoas muscle toward the diaphragm, along with the Gerota fascia and the contained left kidney. With careful manual control of the left kidney and peritoneal contents and countertraction upward on the diaphragm, further medial rotation of the left kidney and viscera will expose the abdominal aorta from the left diaphragmatic crus to its bifurcation. The Omni-Tract retraction system (Omni-Tract Surgical, Minneapolis, Minn.) is critical for maintaining this exposure.

The left renal artery is readily identified and serves as the main landmark for suprarenal and infrarenal aortic exposure (Figure 4-15). Just above this level, division of

the median arcuate ligament and left diaphragmatic crus facilitates exposure of the supraceliac aorta (Figure 4-16). The celiac axis and superior mesenteric artery can be dissected free of surrounding neural tissue for a significant length distal to their origins to enable vascular reconstruction. The distal thoracic aorta is readily accessible if the dissection is carried proximally between the crura and in an extrapleural plane. This extended exposure facilitates repair of suprarenal aortic disease and transaortic renal or mesenteric endarterectomy, as well as antegrade bypass to these vessels.

EXPOSURE OF THE VISCERAL AND RENAL ARTERIES

The left flank approach is ideal for visceral and renal artery exposure. The celiac axis and proximal aspects of its major branches are readily accessible. In addition, the splenic artery can be mobilized off the posterior aspect of the pancreas to facilitate extraanatomic splenorenal bypass. Hepatorenal bypass requires a right retroperitoneal approach. There are no major branches that emanate from the superior mesenteric artery for a distance of up to 5 cm distal to its origin. Therefore, bypass or endarterectomy of the superior mesenteric artery well beyond its origin is possible without ever entering the peritoneal space. The first major branch of the superior mesenteric artery is usually the middle colic artery, which arises from the anterior and right lateral surface of the vessel as it emerges from the pancreas. This branch is the usual site for an embolus to lodge. It is important to remember that in addition to a possible replaced right hepatic artery, the common hepatic artery occasionally arises from the superior mesenteric artery.[20] In both circumstances, the replaced artery arises from the proximal aspect of the superior mesenteric artery just past its origin and courses back toward the right upper quadrant.

Dissection at the origin of the left renal artery and along the posterolateral aspect of the infrarenal aorta exposes the large communicating vein connecting the renal to the hemiazygos vein. Once this venous tributary (often two tributaries are encountered) is divided, the left renal vein can be elevated off the infrarenal aorta to enable safe cross-clamping. This maneuver facilitates right renal artery exposure as the origin of this vessel comes into view with superolateral retraction of the left renal vein. This retroperitoneal surgical exposure also allows dissection of either renal artery to its branch vessels in preparation for endarterectomy or bypass.

To perform transaortic renal endarterectomy with direct visualization of a clean end point, it is necessary to dissect the renal arteries well beyond their respective origins. In addition, the segment of aorta to be isolated must be mobilized completely, with control of any adjacent lumbar arteries; this eliminates troublesome back-bleeding that can obscure vision after creation of an aortotomy. Proximal exposure of the suprarenal aorta should include at least the origin of the superior mesenteric artery so that an aortic clamp can be placed above this level. This is particularly important if there is little distance between the origins of the renal arteries and mesenteric vessels. Transaortic endarterectomy is accomplished either by transecting the aorta below the level of the renal arteries or by making a longitudinal aortotomy posterolateral to the left renal artery or superior mesenteric artery, or both.[21] Aortotomy can also be carried to the supraceliac aorta to facilitate visceral endarterectomy. Alternatively, any of these visceral vessels can be transected well beyond the disease process to facilitate direct end-to-end bypass.[22] The ability to extensively mobilize the renal and mesenteric arteries is a major advantage of this retroperitoneal surgical exposure.

The inferior mesenteric artery is the primary blood supply to the left colon and is located by carrying the infrarenal dissection inferiorly along the posterolateral aspect of the aorta. In some large aneurysms, the thickened wall of the aorta obscures the actual origin of the inferior mesenteric artery. Division of this mesenteric vessel flush with the aorta is generally well tolerated. However, its inadvertent division distal to the left colic branch may result in sigmoid colon infarction. This complication is much more likely to occur when there is atherosclerotic occlusion of the marginal artery of Drummond.[23] In patients with visceral artery occlusive disease, the left colic artery communicates with the left branch of the middle colic artery to become the meandering mesenteric artery (also known as the *central anastomotic artery*). This artery provides collateral circulation between the superior and inferior mesenteric arteries, and vice versa (Figure 4-17).[20]

Beyond the pelvic brim, the left common, external, and internal iliac arteries are readily accessible for vascular control. Ligation and division of the inferior mesenteric artery flush with the aorta facilitates exposure of the distal anterolateral surface of the aorta and the right

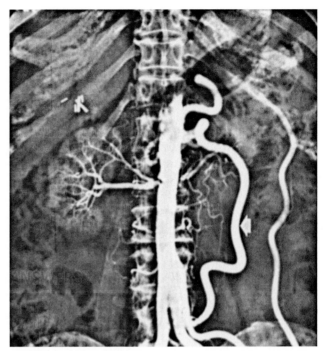

FIGURE 4-17 ■ Angiogram from a patient with occlusion of the celiac and superior mesenteric arteries. Note the large inferior mesenteric artery with a central anastomotic artery *(arrow)* and a large marginal artery (lateral position) providing collateral circulation.

common, external, and internal iliac arteries. It is wise to remember that the common iliac veins and vena cava are adherent to the posteromedial aspect of the left common iliac artery and the posterolateral aspect of the right common iliac artery. Vascular control of these vessels is safest after gently elevating them off their respective underlying major veins. This maneuver also facilitates transection of the distal common iliac artery under direct vision so that end-to-end aortoiliac reconstruction can be accomplished. If the iliac artery anastomosis cannot be performed at this level, it is wise to graft end-to-end to the internal iliac artery and then jump a separate graft to the external iliac artery. With this graft configuration, even an aneurysmal internal iliac artery can be simultaneously excluded (by opening it) and bypassed to the level of its first branch vessel, which helps to maintain vital pelvic perfusion.

Wound closure is accomplished in layers using Vicryl suture for the posterior rectus sheath, transverse fascia, transversus abdominis, and internal oblique muscle layers. The anterior rectus sheath and external oblique muscle aponeurosis are closed with PDS suture. Subcuticular or staple skin closure completes this multilayer wound closure.

ALTERNATIVE EXPOSURE OF THE RENAL ARTERY

The distal right renal artery can be exposed through a right-sided flank incision, which is a mirror image of the

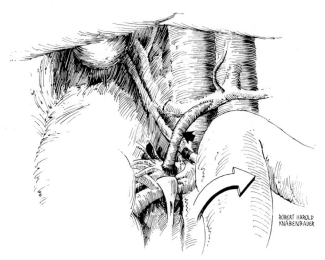

FIGURE 4-18 ■ Hepatic–to–right renal artery bypass. The duodenum is kocherized *(open arrow)* for exposure. The reverse saphenous vein bypass is identified *(solid arrow)*. Note the retraction of the right renal vein for exposure.

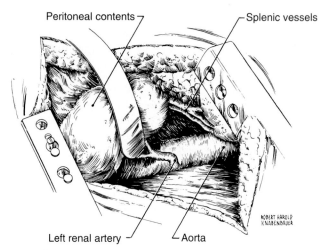

FIGURE 4-19 ■ Flank exposure of the left renal artery.

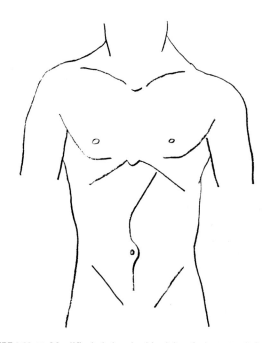

FIGURE 4-20 ■ Modified abdominal incision for greater left upper quadrant exposure during transperitoneal medial visceral rotation. (From Deiparine MK, Ballard JL: Transperitoneal medial visceral rotation. Ann Vasc Surg 9:607, 1995.)

incision described in the section on retroperitoneal exposure of the aorta. With the patient on the operating table in a modified left lateral decubitus position, the retroperitoneal space is entered laterally after division of the abdominal wall muscles. The peritoneum and contents are gently mobilized anteriorly and medially, including the right kidney enclosed in the Gerota fascia. The renal artery is palpated distally and carefully dissected free of surrounding tissue toward the abdominal aorta. The inferior vena cava is also identified and mobilized after ligation of two or three paired lumbar veins. The vena cava can be elevated to expose the right posterolateral aspect of the infrarenal aorta. Partial aortic occlusion with a side-biting vascular clamp is used for anastomosis of the proximal bypass graft. Thereafter, a distal end-to-end anastomosis completes renal artery revascularization.

Moncure and associates[24] described an extraanatomic revascularization procedure for the right kidney. This exposure uses a right subcostal incision extending into the right flank. The hepatic flexure of the colon is mobilized and rotated to the left. The duodenum is kocherized toward the midline to expose the right kidney. The renal artery is located behind and just above the right renal vein. Next, the hepatic artery is palpated in the hepatoduodenal ligament, and the gastroduodenal artery is identified. The common hepatic artery proximal to the gastroduodenal artery is dissected free. An end-to-side anastomosis of the bypass graft to the hepatic artery is constructed first. The bypass graft is then routed over the hepatoduodenal ligament and anastomosed to the transected end of the renal artery to revascularize the kidney. Figure 4-18 demonstrates the essential anatomy and a side-to-side distal anastomosis. However, end-to-end reconstruction is recommended and easier to accomplish.

The left renal artery can be exposed peripherally for extraanatomic bypass by using the same incision described earlier in the section on retroperitoneal exposure of the abdominal aorta. Once the pararenal aorta is exposed, the tail of the pancreas is separated from the left adrenal gland to expose the splenic artery for bypass to the left renal artery (Figure 4-19).[24] Inflow can also be obtained from the aorta proximal or distal to the renal artery. This bypass can originate from the side of the aorta, with a destination to the transected left renal artery.

ALTERNATIVE EXPOSURE OF THE ABDOMINAL AORTA AND ITS BRANCHES

Modification of the standard midline abdominal incision can be used to expose the proximal abdominal aorta without entering the chest as illustrated in Figure 4-20.

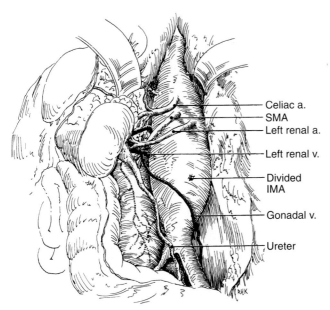

FIGURE 4-21 ■ Transperitoneal medial visceral rotation, with the left kidney rotated forward, for repair of a supraceliac aortic aneurysm. *IMA,* Inferior mesenteric artery; *SMA,* superior mesenteric artery. (From Ballard JL: Management of renal artery stenosis in conjunction with aortic aneurysm. Semin Vasc Surg 9:221, 1996.)

Celiac a.
SMA
Left renal a.
Left renal v.
Divided IMA
Gonadal v.
Ureter

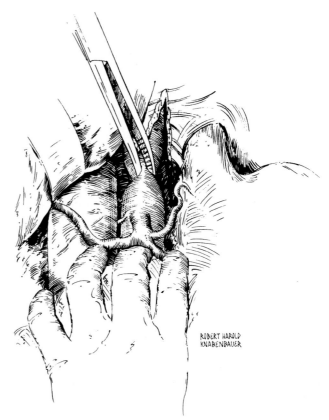

FIGURE 4-22 ■ Exposure of the abdominal aorta at the diaphragm.

An inverted hockey-stick incision is used, beginning at the left midcostal margin. The left rectus muscle is transected, and the oblique and transversus abdominis muscles are divided in the direction of the skin incision. The incision is continued down the linea alba to the symphysis pubis. The left side of the colon is mobilized by incising the peritoneum along the white line of Toldt from the pelvis to the lateral peritoneal attachments of the spleen. The spleen is mobilized and brought forward toward the midline by incising the splenorenal and splenophrenic ligaments.

Dissection is continued by forward mobilization of the spleen, pancreatic tail, and splenic flexure of the colon between the mesocolon and the Gerota fascia, with care not to damage the adrenal gland medially or the adrenal vein at its junction with the left renal vein. This left-to-right transperitoneal medial visceral rotation affords excellent exposure of the supraceliac and visceral aorta, including the renal arteries (Figure 4-21). This exposure is facilitated by forward displacement of the left kidney along with the rest of the mobilized viscera. Division of the median arcuate ligament and diaphragmatic crura exposes the distal thoracic aorta without entering the left chest.

TRANSPERITONEAL EXPOSURE OF THE ABDOMINAL AORTA AT THE DIAPHRAGMATIC HIATUS

Exposure of the supraceliac aorta at the diaphragmatic hiatus is lifesaving for early control of exigent hemorrhage in the case of a ruptured abdominal aortic aneurysm. It is also useful for temporary control of the aorta during repair of an aortocaval or aortoenteric fistula and for proximal control outside an infected aortic graft field. Less frequently, this exposure is suitable for revascularization of the celiac axis and its proximal branches or the superior mesenteric artery.

Supraceliac aortic exposure through the lesser sac is facilitated by downward retraction of the stomach and lateral retraction of the esophagus. The aortic pulse is palpated, and the arching fibers of the diaphragm at the aortic hiatus are divided directly over the aorta. The periaortic fascia is opened, and the index and middle fingers are passed medially and laterally to the aorta. Gentle blunt finger dissection between the diaphragmatic fibers and the aorta creates space on either side of the aorta. This maneuver is critical, because any overlying muscle fibers would allow a vascular occluding clamp to slide up and off the aorta. No effort is made to completely encircle the aorta in this circumstance because inadvertant avulsion of an intercostal artery or proximal lumbar artery or vein can result in troublesome bleeding. At this point, a partially opened aortic clamp is advanced over the dorsal hand and fingers that have been appropriately positioned to cross-clamp the aorta and interrupt blood flow. This exposure is illustrated in Figure 4-22.

Celiac axis reconstruction requires more exposure. A generous incision is made in the posterior parietal peritoneum, and the diaphragmatic crura are completely divided. The inferior phrenic arteries should be isolated, ligated, and divided. The aortic branch to the left adrenal gland is also usually visualized and sacrificed. Dissection is continued distally to expose the celiac axis, which can be palpated at its origin from the anterior surface of the aorta. Dense fibers of the median arcuate ligament are divided, along with the neural elements forming the celiac plexus. This tissue is quite vascular; thus, stick ties and cautery are useful for hemostasis. Once the celiac axis has been exposed, the common hepatic artery is dissected free of surrounding tissue as it courses toward the liver hilum. Sympathetic nerve fibers can be seen to entwine on the surface of this vessel. There is usually a 3- to 4-cm segment of the hepatic artery that is free of branches and thus useful as a site for vascular anastomosis. The splenic artery is palpable at the superior border of the pancreas and courses to the left toward the splenic hilum. Here again, there is a 4- to 5-cm segment that is free of branches and can be used for placement of a vascular anastomosis. The left gastric artery is the smallest of the three main branches of the celiac axis. It courses anteriorly to follow the lesser curvature of the stomach and should be protected during this exposure.

The supraceliac aorta can also be used as the bypass origin for superior mesenteric artery reconstruction. The proximal anastomosis is constructed on the anterior surface of the aorta after the aortic hiatus is opened as described earlier. Using careful finger dissection, a tunnel must then be created behind the pancreas. The bypass graft is passed through the tunnel and anastomosed to the distal patent superior mesenteric artery. Kinking of the bypass graft, which can occur with retrograde aorta–to–superior mesenteric artery bypass during replacement of bowel, is unlikely in this tunneled position.

Anterior exposure of the superior mesenteric artery inferior to the transverse mesocolon requires opening the posterior parietal peritoneum lateral to the third and fourth portions of the duodenum (Figure 4-23). The left renal vein is identified and mobilized as described previously for exposure of the renal arteries. The left renal vein is retracted downward, and the dissection is carried upward on the aorta until the superior mesenteric artery origin can be palpated. It usually arises from the left side of the anterior surface of the aorta. The artery is immediately encased by the superior mesenteric sympathetic nerve plexus, which must be incised for exposure. Cautery and suture ligatures are used to control bleeding from the vascular plexus tissue. The overlying transverse mesocolon and pancreas significantly limit this exposure.

TRANSPERITONEAL EXPOSURE OF THE INFRARENAL ABDOMINAL AORTA

A midline abdominal incision from the xiphoid to the symphysis pubis is commonly used for anterior exposure of the infrarenal abdominal aorta. One disadvantage of this approach is incomplete visualization of the proximal abdominal aorta or renal artery origins. Proximally extending the midline incision around the xiphoid process and completely mobilizing the third and fourth portions of the duodenum improve this potential lack of exposure. The dissection continues through the posterior peritoneum just lateral to the duodenum and medial to the

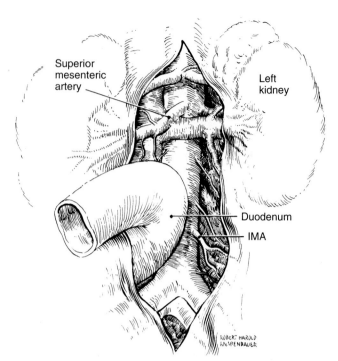

FIGURE 4-23 ■ Infracolic exposure of the superior mesenteric artery. The pancreas and transverse colon are not shown, but are retracted upward and forward. *IMA,* Inferior mesenteric artery.

inferior mesenteric vein to avoid damaging the arterial circulation to the left or sigmoid colon. This is particularly important in the case of ruptured abdominal aortic aneurysms, when landmarks are frequently obscured by an extensive retroperitoneal hematoma. The duodenum can nearly always be visualized and used as a landmark during this exposure.

It is wise to palpate the aortic bifurcation and expose the common iliac arteries from the midline, thereby avoiding injury to the ureters. Fibers of the sympathetic nerves arch over the left common iliac artery in males, and damage to these sympathetic fibers can result in erectile dysfunction and retrograde ejaculation. Figure 4-24 shows the relationship of the infrarenal sympathetic nerve fibers to the terminal aorta and iliac arteries. Incising along the white line of Toldt and mobilizing the sigmoid or proximal ascending colon toward the midline can readily identify the external iliac arteries. Graft limbs coursing out to this level should be passed under both the colon mesentery and the respective ureter.

TRANSPERITONEAL EXPOSURE OF THE RENAL ARTERIES

The left main renal artery originates from the posterolateral surface of the aorta. Usually this location is at the level of the upper border of the left renal vein, where it crosses over the abdominal aorta. The right renal artery often arises at a slightly lower level. Anterior exposure of either renal artery origin involves incision of the posterior parietal peritoneum just lateral to the fourth portion

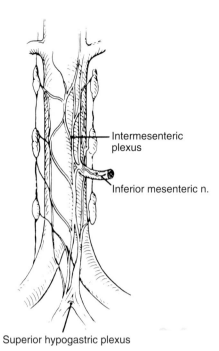

FIGURE 4-24 ■ Relationship of the infrarenal sympathetic nerves to the aorta and iliac arteries. Note the condensation of nerve elements coursing over the left common iliac artery origin. (From Weinstein MH, Machleder HI: Sexual function after aortoiliac surgery. Ann Surg 181:787, 1975.)

of the duodenum. Additional exposure is obtained by continuing this incision along the distal third portion of the duodenum.

The left renal vein is identified and carefully mobilized. Frequently, there is a small parietal vein that terminates in the inferior margin of the left renal vein over the aorta. Otherwise, there are two major venous tributaries to be identified, ligated, and divided. The first is located by following the inferior margin of the left renal vein laterally to the termination of the left gonadal vein. Next, the dissection is carried laterally along the superior surface of the left renal vein until the confluence of the left adrenal vein is identified. This vein should be ligated flush with the renal vein and divided. The entire left renal vein can then be mobilized on a Silastic vascular loop.

Cautious dissection is advisable in this area, because there is an important large communicating vein arising from the posterior surface of the proximal left renal vein. This vein communicates with the adjacent lumbar vein and then to the hemiazygos system and superior vena cava. The presence of this venous collateral allows acute ligation of the left renal vein without significant impairment of renal function. This lumbar venous communication should be preserved, if possible, during this anterior transperitoneal approach.

Once the left renal vein is mobilized, attention should be directed to exposing the left lateral surface of the aorta above and below the level of the left renal vein. The left renal artery arising from the posterolateral surface of the aorta is thus exposed. Autonomic nerve elements are encountered adjacent to the renal artery but can be divided without concern. Gentle placement of a vein retractor under the left renal vein with upward retraction

by an assistant greatly facilitates this exposure. A Silastic loop placed about the renal artery origin aids in the mobilization and dissection of this vessel.

The right renal artery is more difficult to expose because it passes directly behind the inferior vena cava on its course to the renal hilum. The origin of this artery is palpated as it emerges from the right posterolateral aspect of the aorta. Care should be taken not to injure the right adrenal branch, which arises 5 to 10 mm from the origin of the right renal artery. The size of this vessel may be 2 to 3 mm when renal artery stenosis is present because it becomes an important collateral to the distal right renal artery via capsular branches. In the event that the entire right renal artery and its branches must be exposed, the surgeon must completely mobilize the vena cava above and below the artery by carefully ligating and dividing all adjacent lumbar veins.

The subhepatic space is then entered, and the duodenum is kocherized to allow exposure of the right renal vein as it joins the inferior vena cava. The renal vein is mobilized from surrounding tissue to aid in identifying the main renal artery lying beneath the vein. Exposure of the right renal artery is complete when this distal dissection joins the medial exposure already described.

EMERGENCY EXPOSURE OF THE ABDOMINAL AORTA AND VENA CAVA

Vascular exposure of injured vessels within the abdomen is best performed through a generous midline abdominal incision. Location of the hematoma determines the exposure to be used. Because the abdominal circulation arises in a retroperitoneal location, the overlying viscera need to be rotated medially or elevated superiorly to expose the aorta and its major branches and the caval and portal venous circulation.

Kudsk and Sheldon divided the retroperitoneal space into three zones (Figure 4-25).[25] The presence of a central hematoma (zone 1) indicates injury to the aorta, the proximal renal or visceral arteries, the inferior vena cava, or the portal vein. An expanding zone 1 retroperitoneal hematoma with extension to the left indicates a proximal aortic or adjacent major branch vessel injury. Transperitoneal left-to-right medial visceral rotation swiftly and widely exposes the aorta from the diaphragm to its bifurcation. Exposure can be facilitated by division of the left rectus muscle transversely in the left upper quadrant or by the modified abdominal incision described earlier. The splenic flexure is mobilized, including the spleen and the left kidney, with rotation of these viscera to the right. The origins of the celiac axis and the superior mesenteric and renal arteries are similarly exposed (Figure 4-26).

The presence of a zone 1 retroperitoneal hematoma with extension into the right flank is indicative of major caval, portal venous, or proximal injury to a major arterial branch in the right upper quadrant. Incising the peritoneum lateral to the ascending colon and reflecting this structure medially, followed by duodenal kocherization, gains exposure. This right-to-left medial visceral rotation exposes the entire vena cava from the iliac confluence to the liver (Figure 4-27).

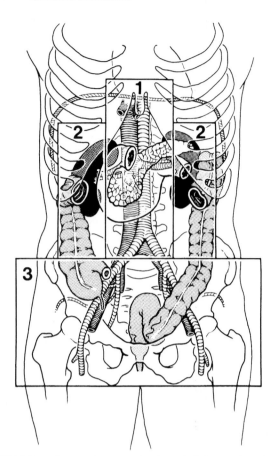

FIGURE 4-25 ■ Anatomic zones (*1*, *2*, and *3*) for exploration of retroperitoneal hematomas. (From Kudsk KA, Sheldon GF: Retroperitoneal hematoma. In Blaisdell FW, Trunkey DD, editors: Trauma management, vol 1, ed 2, New York, 1993, Thieme Medical Publishers, p 400.)

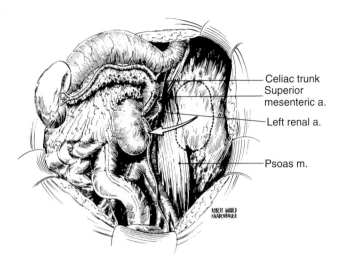

FIGURE 4-26 ■ Rotation of the intraabdominal contents, including the left kidney, to the right for complete visualization of the abdominal aorta. The kidney is rotated forward and to the right *(arrow)* from the renal fossa *(dotted outline)*. (From Smith LL, Catalano RD: Exposure of vascular injuries. In Bongard FS, Wilson SE, Perry MO, editors: Vascular injuries in surgical practice, Norwalk, Conn, 1991, Appleton and Lange, p 18.)

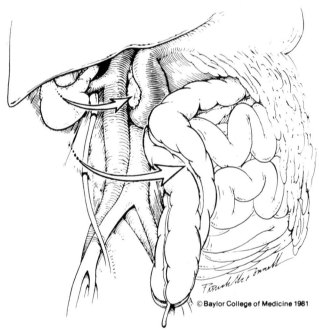

FIGURE 4-27 ■ Rotation of the intraabdominal viscera to the left by mobilization of the right colon and kocherization of the duodenum. The right kidney can also be mobilized to inspect the posterior surface of the vena cava if necessary. (Courtesy M. Dohrmann, the original illustrator.)

Incising the hepatoduodenal ligament above the duodenum exposes the portal vein. The common bile duct is retracted laterally, and the hepatic artery is palpated and isolated for inspection. Thereafter, retracting the hepatic artery toward the midline facilitates examination of the portal vein. The right side of the aorta, as well as the proximal right renal artery, can be inspected if rotation and mobilization of the overlying bowel are continued to the midline.

Lateral hematomas (zone 2) indicate injury to distal visceral and renal vessels. Despite their lateral location, it is wise not to enter a large hematoma to control exigent hemorrhage until central aortic exposure has been secured for possible cross-clamping. Retroperitoneal pelvic hematomas (zone 3) usually indicate torn branches of the iliac vessels associated with pelvic fractures. These might not require exploration unless the hematoma is expanding or there is evidence of large vessel injury demonstrated by angiography.

EXTRAPERITONEAL EXPOSURE OF THE ILIAC ARTERIES

This exposure begins with an oblique incision in the lower quadrant of the abdomen on the side of involved iliac artery occlusive disease. It is good practice to start the incision near the pubic tubercle, with extension obliquely lateral, staying medial to the anterior superior iliac spine of the pelvis. The external oblique aponeurosis is opened in the direction of its fibers, and the incision is continued into the fleshy portion of this muscle. The internal oblique and transversus abdominis muscles are

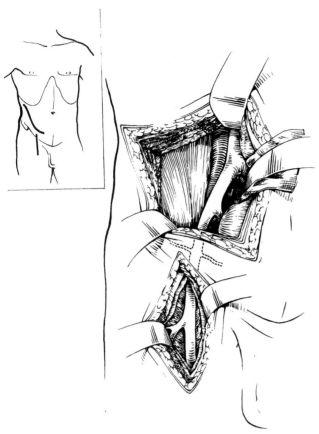

FIGURE 4-28 ■ Extraperitoneal exposure of the distal common and external iliac arteries. Counterincision at the groin facilitates iliofemoral reconstruction.

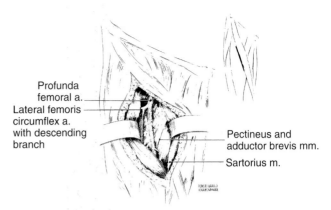

FIGURE 4-29 ■ Lateral approach to the deep femoral artery. *Upper right,* The incision is lateral to the sartorius muscle. *Lower left,* Exposure of the deep femoral vessel.

divided in the direction of the incision to enter the preperitoneal space. The peritoneum is gently rotated medially to expose the external iliac artery. The ureter, which is adherent to the peritoneum and usually retracts with the peritoneal contents, is vulnerable to injury as it courses across the iliac bifurcation. Exposure of the common iliac artery requires extension of the incision proximally and laterally into the flank region.

Care should be taken not to injure the ilioinguinal or genitofemoral nerves during exposure or retraction. Their location on the anterior surface of the psoas muscle is vulnerable. Combination of this incision with a curvilinear incision over the common femoral artery permits exposure from the terminal common iliac artery to the proximal superficial or deep femoral arteries (Figure 4-28). The iliac artery exposed in this extraperitoneal fashion is particularly appealing as an inflow source in cases in which there is extensive scarring at the groin from previous peripheral vascular procedures and this exposure is commonly used to place a conduit for thoracic aortic endograft procedures.

EXPOSURE OF THE COMMON FEMORAL ARTERY

A curvilinear incision placed directly over the palpable pulse, with extension above and below the groin crease,

provides excellent exposure of the common femoral artery and its branches. An incision made just medial to the midpoint of the inguinal ligament suffices in the absence of a palpable pulse. Frequently the diseased artery can be rolled beneath the index finger, and this guides the plane of deeper dissection. It is important to remember to check for posterior branches, because an aberrant medial femoral circumflex artery can arise anywhere along the posterior surface of the common femoral artery. Failure to control this vessel can result in troublesome bleeding when the common femoral artery is opened.

Gentle dissection about the origin of the deep femoral artery is important. The lateral femoral circumflex artery arises from the lateral side of the deep femoral artery, and this vessel can be easily injured. Care should also be taken to identify the lateral femoral circumflex vein, which courses from lateral to medial across the origin of the deep femoral artery. Division of this vein facilitates arterial mobilization and distal dissection. This maneuver is paramount if the proximal deep femoral artery is to be used as an inflow source, and it provides excellent exposure for eversion endarterectomy.

EXPOSURE OF THE DEEP FEMORAL ARTERY

The deep femoral artery is located 1.5 cm medial to the femur and lies on the pectineus and adductor brevis muscles. In cases in which the deep femoral artery is being exposed as an initial procedure, the dissection is aided by flexion and external rotation of the thigh to relax the involved muscles. Colborn and associates[26] described the surgical anatomy of the deep femoral artery, and the reader is well advised to consult their excellent and well-illustrated article.

The deep femoral artery can be a useful inflow or outflow source in a patient with a hostile groin after previous surgical exposures. Nuñez and associates[27] described a practical approach to the middle and distal thirds of this artery that avoids a scarred femoral bifurcation. This surgical dissection begins lateral to the sartorius muscle. Figure 4-29 demonstrates the incision over the lateral aspect of the sartorius muscle and branches of the lateral femoral circumflex artery. These branches are followed medially to the deep femoral artery after the incision is deepened between the vastus medialis and adductor longus muscles. Complete mobilization of the artery at this level requires division of overlying venous tributaries to the deep femoral vein. This dissection can then be safely extended distally or, if needed, proximally to the femoral bifurcation.

Alternatively, the distal third of the deep femoral artery can be exposed by a surgical plane of dissection that is posterior to the adductor longus muscle in the medial thigh.[28] This exposure is deepened between the gracilis and adductor longus muscles to the medial aspect of the deep femoral artery. Knee flexion relaxes the involved muscles and aids in this exposure.

EXPOSURE OF THE POPLITEAL ARTERY

The popliteal artery is typically exposed from a medial approach, with few exceptions. The proximal and distal portions of this vessel are readily exposed. However, the medial head of the gastrocnemius muscle and the tendinous insertions of the long adductor muscles obscure the midportion of the artery at the joint space of the knee. A posterior approach to the midpopliteal artery is useful for isolated disorders such as popliteal entrapment or cystic adventitial disease and some trauma situations.

The proximal popliteal artery is exposed through an incision placed in the groove between the vastus medialis and sartorius muscles. The greater saphenous vein lies just posterior to this incision, and care must be taken to preserve it during the dissection. The sartorius muscle is retracted posteriorly, and the investing fascia is incised longitudinally, preserving the saphenous nerve, which is usually seen lying on the deep fascial surface. Once the fascia is opened, the popliteal artery can be palpated in its location under the adductor magnus tendon.

Although not usually necessary, additional exposure can be obtained distally by dividing the tendon of the medial head of the gastrocnemius muscle. Gentle insertion of the left index finger behind its tendinous origin aids in isolating this structure and protecting the underlying neurovascular bundle. Should additional distal exposure be necessary, the tendinous insertions of the sartorius, semimembranous, semitendinous, and gracilis muscles can be divided. It is wise to mark these tendons with identifying sutures to aid in their subsequent repair.

The terminal popliteal artery and tibioperoneal trunk are exposed through an incision placed approximately 1.5 cm posterior to the medial margin of the tibia. The surgeon must be aware of the greater saphenous vein and protect it in its subcutaneous location. The thick muscular fascia overlying the gastrocnemius muscle is incised to enter the popliteal space. The popliteal vein is usually encountered first within the neurovascular sheath. Gentle downward retraction of the vein facilitates dissection of the popliteal artery, which lies superolateral to the vein. The origin of the anterior tibial artery arises anteriorly and laterally from the terminal popliteal artery. Further exposure of the tibioperoneal trunk and proximal

peroneal and posterior tibial arteries requires the division of the soleus muscle fibers arising from the medial margin of the tibia. Division of overlying venous tributaries between the often paired popliteal veins facilitates this exposure.

LATERAL EXPOSURE OF THE POPLITEAL ARTERY

A lateral approach to the popliteal artery can be used when previous medial exposure has resulted in dense tissue scarring, making repeated procedures difficult. The incision for the above-knee popliteal artery is placed between the iliotibial tract and the biceps femoris muscle as described by Veith and associates.[29] The dissection is deepened through the fascia lata posterior to the junction of the lateral intramuscular septum and the iliotibial tract to enter the popliteal space. The popliteal vein is encountered first within the vascular sheath. It can be mobilized and retracted posteriorly to allow exposure of the popliteal artery. The tibial and peroneal nerves are also posterior and loosely adherent to the hamstrings, and they naturally fall out of harm's way with retraction of the biceps femoris, semimembranous, and semitendinous muscles.

The lateral approach to the below-knee popliteal artery begins with an incision over the head and proximal one fourth of the fibula. As the incision is deepened, care must be taken to preserve the common peroneal nerve as it courses around the neck of the fibula (Figure 4-30). The biceps femoris tendon is divided. The ligamentous attachments to the head of the fibula are also divided, and the proximal fibula is removed. The entire below-knee popliteal artery, anterior tibial artery origin, and tibioperoneal trunk are accessible after removal of the bone fragment (Figure 4-31). The proximal posterior tibial and

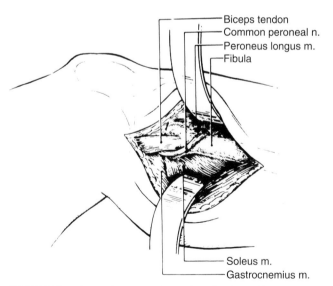

FIGURE 4-30 ■ Lateral approach to the distal popliteal artery. Note the common peroneal nerve coursing around the neck of the fibula. (From Veith F, Ascer E, Gupta S: Lateral approach to the popliteal artery. J Vasc Surg 6:119, 1987.)

peroneal arteries can be exposed if more of the distal fibula is resected.

EXPOSURE OF THE TIBIAL AND PERONEAL ARTERIES

Management of lower extremity ischemic vascular disease requires accurate knowledge of the arterial and venous

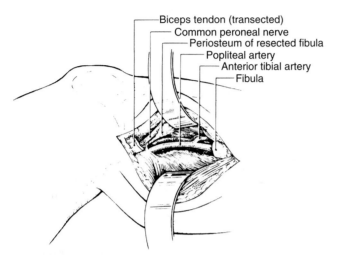

FIGURE 4-31 ■ Lateral approach to the distal popliteal artery after removal of the proximal fibula. Note the transected tendon of the biceps muscle and the intact common peroneal nerve. (From Veith F, Ascer E, Gupta S: Lateral approach to the popliteal artery. J Vasc Surg 6:119, 1987.)

circulation of the leg. It is important to keep in mind the relationship of the three major leg arteries to the tibia and fibula as well as the compartments of the leg. Figure 4-32 demonstrates these important relationships. Note the anterior tibial vessels lying on the interosseous membrane in the anterior compartment. The peroneal artery, which is adjacent to the medial margin of the fibula in the deep posterior compartment, lies in close proximity to the transverse crural intermuscular septum. The posterior tibial vessels are medial to the peroneal artery and veins, but also above the intermuscular septum and in the deep posterior compartment of the leg.

Surgical exposure of the crural vessels requires patience and great care. There are numerous small muscular branches, and each artery has two accompanying veins with their respective tributaries to protect. Careless dissection leads to bleeding that obscures the operative field and increases the likelihood of injury to these delicate vascular structures.

Anterior Tibial Artery

This vessel travels between the anterior tibial and extensor digitorum longus muscles in the proximal portion of the anterior compartment of the leg. The extensor hallucis longus muscle crosses over the artery, laterally to medially, in the distal leg above the level of the flexor retinaculum. Surgical exposure of the anterior tibial artery is best accomplished either in the proximal leg or just above the flexor retinaculum proximal to the ankle.

A skin incision made approximately 2.5 cm lateral to the anterior border of the tibia facilitates proximal

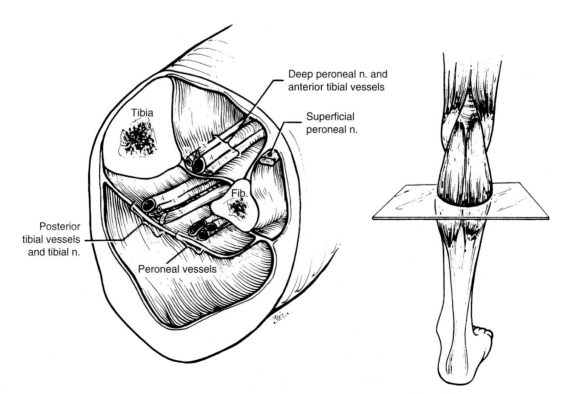

FIGURE 4-32 ■ Cross section of the leg showing the location of the anterior tibial artery in the anterior compartment of the leg and the posterior tibial and peroneal arteries in the deep posterior compartment. (From Briggs S, Seligson D: Management of extremity trauma. In Richardson D, Polk H, Flint M, editors: Trauma: clinical care and pathophysiology, Chicago, 1987, Year Book Medical, p 544.)

exposure of the anterior tibial artery. Deepening the dissection between the two muscle bellies assists this surgical exposure. Dorsiflexion and internal rotation of the foot aid in identifying the groove between these two muscles. The muscles are gently separated down to the anterior tibial artery, which lies between its two accompanying veins and anterior to the deep peroneal nerve on the interosseous membrane.

Alternatively, a dissection course that passes between the extensor hallucis longus and extensor digitorum longus laterally and the anterior tibial muscle medially exposes the artery just above the flexor retinaculum.[28] The upper portion of the flexor retinaculum can be divided to improve distal exposure; however, complete division is not recommended. If the anterior tibial artery is unsuitable for vascular reconstruction at this level, the dissection should skip down to the dorsal pedal artery below the inferior portion of the retinaculum.

Posterior Tibial Artery

Extending the incision described earlier for medial exposure of the tibioperoneal trunk facilitates proximal exposure of the posterior tibial artery. This exposure requires incising the origin of the soleus muscle from the medial border of the tibia. Tributary veins traveling through this muscle origin can cause troublesome bleeding. These veins should be ligated to keep the operative field dry. Immediately deep to the soleus fibers, the posterior tibial vessels can be observed coursing between the posterior tibial and flexor digitorum longus muscles. The tibial nerve, which crosses the artery posteriorly from medial to lateral, must be protected. This exposure can be challenging, because there is a dense network of venous tributaries overlying the origin of the posterior tibial artery.

Exposure of the middle aspect of the posterior tibial artery is best achieved distal to the lower edge of the soleus muscle fibers in the medial calf.[28] This dissection into the deep posterior compartment of the leg continues above the intermuscular septum to expose the neurovascular bundle. The artery must be carefully dissected free from its accompanying paired veins and tibial nerve.

Peroneal Artery

The proximal and middle aspects of the peroneal artery can be exposed using the same medial leg incisions described for exposure of the posterior tibial artery. Once this latter artery is exposed, the dissection continues on the intermuscular septum to a deeper level. The peroneal artery is located adjacent to the medial border of the fibula. This exposure is deep and therefore more difficult in a large leg.

Resecting a short segment of the fibula through a lateral incision over this bone can also expose the peroneal artery. This incision should be placed below the entrance of the peroneal nerve into the anterior compartment of the leg. The peroneal vessels lie just deep to the medial border of the fibula. Once this short segment of bone is removed, the vessels are exposed. Careful division and removal of the fibula are essential, because the accompanying venous plexus that surrounds the peroneal

artery is easy to disturb and can cause significant bleeding. Surprisingly little postoperative morbidity is associated with this exposure.

EXPOSURE OF THE PEDAL ARTERIES

A detailed understanding of the pedal arterial circulation is important because distal bypass sites in the foot are often used for limb-threatening ischemic vascular disease. Ascer and associates[30] described various surgical approaches and the results of these distal lower extremity bypass procedures. Figure 4-33 shows the branches and distribution of the distal anterior and posterior tibial arteries in the foot.

Distal Posterior Tibial Artery and Plantar Branches

Exposure of the terminal posterior tibial artery, with its concomitant veins and tibial nerve, is accomplished by a retromalleolar incision. Division of the flexor retinaculum continues the dissection distally. The neurovascular bundle is surrounded by fatty tissue, and the artery is usually superior to the nerve. Further dissection may require sequential incisions to accurately follow the course of the terminal posterior tibial artery into the plantar surface of the foot. Small self-expanding retractors facilitate this exposure, as the plantar tissue is thick and rigid. The plantar aponeurosis and the flexor digitorum brevis muscle can be incised to expose the medial and lateral plantar arteries (Figure 4-34). This latter vessel continues distally into the foot to form the deep plantar arch.

Dorsal Pedal Artery and Lateral Tarsal Branch

The dorsal pedal artery and lateral tarsal branch are approached through a longitudinal incision lateral to the

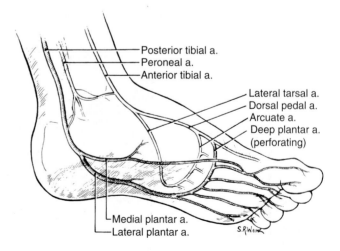

FIGURE 4-33 ■ Anatomy of the arterial circulation of the foot. (From Ascer E, Veith F, Gupta S: Bypasses to plantar arteries and other tibial branches: an extended approach to limb salvage. J Vasc Surg 8:434, 1988.)

extensor hallucis longus tendon. The inferior extensor retinaculum is partially incised just distal to the ankle joint to expose the proximal dorsal pedal artery and lateral tarsal branch. The lateral tarsal artery usually arises at the level of the navicular bone and beneath the extensor digitorum brevis muscle. This artery communicates with the arcuate artery in the midfoot; therefore it is an important collateral blood supply to the dorsum of the foot. Division of the inferior extensor retinaculum is not required for more distal exposure of the dorsal pedal artery. It is necessary to protect the distal deep peroneal nerve coursing medially to this artery.

Deep Plantar Artery

The deep plantar artery is the main continuation of the dorsal pedal artery at the level of the metatarsal bones. It is best approached through a curvilinear incision over the dorsum of the foot lateral to the extensor hallucis longus tendon. The artery is followed distally until it divides into the first dorsal metatarsal and deep plantar branches. The latter vessel descends between the two heads of the first dorsal interosseous muscle to collateralize with the lateral plantar branch, forming the deep plantar arch of the foot (Figure 4-35).

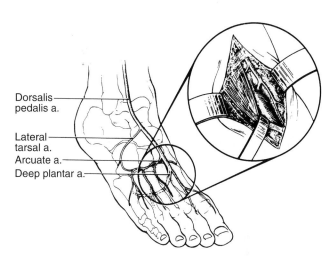

FIGURE 4-35 ■ Diagram of the arterial circulation on the dorsum of the foot. The inset shows the origin of the deep plantar branch as it courses between the two heads of the first dorsal interosseous vessel. (From Ascer E, Veith F, Gupta S: Bypasses to plantar arteries and other tibial branches: an extended approach to limb salvage. J Vasc Surg 8:437, 1988.)

FIGURE 4-34 ■ Exposure of the terminal left posterior tibial artery using a retromalleolar incision. The terminal branches of this vessel are shown; the larger is the lateral plantar branch. (From Ascer E, Veith F, Gupta S: Bypasses to plantar arteries and other tibial branches: an extended approach to limb salvage. J Vasc Surg 8:436, 1988.)

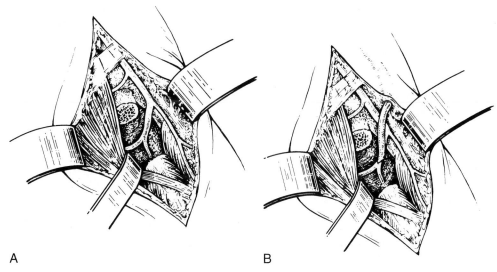

A   B

FIGURE 4-36 ■ **A,** Deep plantar arch branch following resection of a portion of the second metatarsal bone. **B,** Distal anastomosis of a bypass to this vessel. (From Ascer E, Veith F, Gupta S: Bypasses to plantar arteries and other tibial branches: an extended approach to limb salvage. J Vasc Surg 8:437, 1988.)

Adequate exposure of the deep plantar branch requires retraction of the extensor hallucis brevis muscle. The periosteum of the second metatarsal bone is then carefully elevated, and a portion of the bone is removed by a rongeur to provide adequate exposure for distal arterial anastomosis (Figure 4-36). This exposure requires delicate dissection, because injury to adjacent arterial branches and venous tributaries may obscure the operative field or create ischemia to marginally viable tissue.

BIBLIOGRAPHY

Ascer E, Veith F, Gupta S: Bypasses to plantar arteries and other tibial branches: an extended approach to limb salvage. J Vasc Surg 8:434, 1985.

Ballard JL, Abou-Zamzam AM, Jr, Teruya TH: Type III and IV thoracoabdominal aortic aneurysm repair: results of a trifurcated/two-graft technique. J Vasc Surg 36:211, 2002.

Brockstein B, Johns L, Gewertz BL: Blood supply to the spinal cord: anatomic and physiologic correlations. Ann Vasc Surg 8:394, 1994.

Colborn GL, Mattar SG, Taylor B, et al: The surgical anatomy of the deep femoral artery. Am Surg 61:336, 1995.

Effeney DJ, Stoney RJ: Disorders of the extremities. In Effeney DJ, Stoney RJ, editors: Wylie's atlas of vascular surgery, Philadelphia, 1992, JB Lippincott, p 210.

Mock CN, Lilly MP, McRae RG, et al: Selection of the approach to the distal internal carotid artery from the second cervical vertebra to the base of the skull. J Vasc Surg 13:846, 1991.

Moncure A, Brewster D, Darling R, et al: Use of the splenic and hepatic arteries for renal revascularization. J Vasc Surg 3:196, 1986.

Rutherford RB: Exposure of lower extremity vessels. In Rutherford RB, editor: Atlas of vascular surgery: basic techniques and exposures, Philadelphia, 1993, WB Saunders, p 112.

Sakopoulos AG, Ballard JL, Gundry SR: Minimally invasive approach for aortic branch vessel reconstruction. J Vasc Surg 31:200, 2000.

Uflacker R: Abdominal aorta and branches. In Uflacker R, editor: Atlas of vascular anatomy: an angiographic approach, Baltimore, 1997, Williams & Wilkins, p 405.

References available online at expertconsult.com.

QUESTIONS

1. Which of the following nerves has the highest incidence of injury during carotid endarterectomy?
   a. Recurrent laryngeal nerve
   b. Hypoglossal nerve (cranial nerve XII)
   c. Superior laryngeal nerve
   d. Glossopharyngeal nerve (cranial nerve IX)

2. Structures contributing to thoracic outlet compression syndrome include all of the following except:
   a. Subclavius muscle
   b. First rib or congenital cervical rib
   c. Anterior scalene muscle
   d. Sternocleidomastoid muscle

3. Which of the following statements regarding lower extremity circulation is true?
   a. The deep femoral artery is accessible only by an approach that is lateral to the sartorius muscle.
   b. It is not possible to expose the popliteal artery above or below the knee by a lateral approach.
   c. The lateral tarsal artery is the largest distal branch of the posterior tibial artery.
   d. The deep plantar arch is formed by the deep plantar artery and the lateral plantar artery.

4. During repair of an infrarenal abdominal aortic aneurysm, all of the following statements are true except:
   a. Autonomic nerve fibers crossing the left common iliac artery should be protected to preserve erectile function.
   b. A large anastomotic artery appearing on arteriography between the superior and inferior mesenteric arteries indicates satisfactory perfusion of the left colon with little risk of ischemia if the inferior mesenteric artery is ligated.
   c. A large lumbar artery near the renal arteries should be preserved, if possible, because this may represent a significant contribution to the anterior spinal artery.
   d. The left renal vein may be safely ligated and divided to facilitate aortic exposure if the lumbar and adrenal tributaries are maintained for collateral circulation.

5. Patients with celiac and superior mesenteric artery occlusive disease would be expected to have all the following except:
   a. A large central anastomotic artery
   b. Retrograde filling of the superior mesenteric artery
   c. A large marginal artery of Drummond
   d. A low incidence of left colon ischemia following inferior mesenteric artery ligation

6. Which of the following statements about renal artery reconstruction is true?
   a. It may be performed via a left or right retroperitoneal approach.
   b. It may be difficult in an obese or previously operated patient if an anterior transabdominal approach is used.
   c. It is facilitated in a high-risk patient by using splenic artery–to–left renal artery bypass or hepatic artery–to–right renal artery bypass.
   d. All of the above

7. Regarding carotid artery exposure, all the following are true except:
   a. The distal internal carotid artery is crossed anteriorly by the hypoglossal nerve (cranial nerve XII).
   b. The vagus nerve (cranial nerve X) passes posterolateral to the carotid bifurcation.
   c. Distal exposure is safely facilitated by anterior dislocation of the mandible.
   d. Distal exposure may be facilitated by division of the posterior belly of the digastric muscle and the stylohyoid muscle.

8. Regarding trauma to the great vessels, which of the following is true?
   a. Exposure of the proximal left subclavian artery is best accomplished via sternotomy.
   b. Temporary right third interspace thoracotomy can be used to control exigent hemorrhage from the innominate artery.
   c. Exposure of either common carotid artery origin is best accomplished via a sternal splitting incision extended along the anterior border of the appropriate sternocleidomastoid muscle.
   d. Right subclavian exposure via a simple supraclavicular incision is adequate for most traumatic injuries in this area.

9. Exposure of the infrapopliteal arteries is best described by which of the following anatomic relationships?
   a. The anterior tibial artery passes posterior to the interosseous membrane.
   b. Lateral exposure of the peroneal artery requires segmental fibular resection.
   c. The tibial nerve crosses the posterior tibial artery anteriorly.
   d. The posterior tibial artery lies deep to the transverse crural intermuscular septum.

10. Which of the following statements regarding the arteria radicularis magna (artery of Adamkiewicz) is true?
   a. It may provide up to two thirds of the spinal cord blood supply.
   b. It appears as a branch of either a distal intercostal or a proximal lumbar artery.
   c. It is rarely identified preoperatively via standard arteriography.
   d. All of the above

ANSWERS

1. **b**
2. **d**
3. **d**
4. **b**
5. **d**
6. **d**
7. **c**
8. **c**
9. **b**
10. **d**

CHAPTER 5

HEMOSTASIS AND THROMBOSIS

Rachel C. Danczyk • Timothy K. Liem

Most of the bleeding that occurs during surgery or in association with trauma is mechanical and usually can be controlled. Occasionally, bleeding is caused or accelerated by congenital or acquired defects of the hemostatic mechanisms. The vascular surgeon must understand the hemostatic system sufficiently to arrest bleeding or restore hemostasis, or both, according to the patient's needs.

There is increasing evidence that a significant number of acute arterial and venous thrombotic disorders are associated with congenital and acquired hypercoagulable states. Therefore the vascular surgeon should also be able to recognize and manage common thrombophilic states and restore arterial and venous blood flow by both mechanical and pharmacologic means.

HEMOSTASIS

Components of Hemostasis

Hemostasis is the process by which bleeding from injured tissue is controlled. Although hemostasis is a dynamic process, it can be divided into four components: vessel response to injury, platelet activation and aggregation, activation of coagulation with clot stabilization, and coagulation inhibition. Each component has numerous modulatory mechanisms.

Vessel Response

When a vessel is injured, the interaction of humoral, neurogenic, and myogenic systems leads to temporary vasoconstriction in the muscular arteries and arterioles. Mechanisms for vasoconstriction remain poorly understood, but may include the release of thromboxane A_2 (TXA_2) by activated platelets, endothelin by endothelial cells, bradykinin, and fibrinopeptide B. Vasoconstriction has less of a role in obtaining hemostasis in veins and venules.

In normal vessels, endothelial cells cover the luminal surface, forming a monolayer with tight cell-cell interaction.[1] Once regarded as a passive barrier between the blood and the underlying thrombogenic subendothelium, the endothelium is now recognized as a biologically active organ that participates in and modulates various physiologic processes, including hemostasis and thrombosis.

In their quiescent state, endothelial cells are actively antithrombotic (Box 5-1). They synthesize and secrete several modulators that lead to vasodilation, decreased platelet aggregation, decreased levels of thrombin, factors Va and VIIIa, and factors IXa and Xa by which an antithrombotic state is promoted. Specifically, prostacyclin and nitric oxide are potent vasodilators and inhibitors of platelet aggregation. Heparan sulfates accelerate the activity of antithrombin (AT), thereby inactivating thrombin. Thrombomodulin (TM) also inactivates thrombin[2] by forming the thrombomodulin-thrombin complex, a potent activator of protein C,[3] which with the help of cofactor protein S inactivates factors Va and VIIIa, leading to decreased thrombin and factor Xa levels. Tissue factor pathway inhibitor (TFPI), which is bound to the endothelial surface, strongly inhibits the external coagulation pathway after heparin administration.[4,5] Tissue-type plasminogen activator (t-PA) and urokinase are synthesized, which bind fibrinogen and fibrin, increase plasmin, and promote fibrinolysis.

The endothelium also possesses substantial procoagulant activity and acts as a scaffold for hemostasis when stimulated after vessel injury (see Box 5-1). Tissue factor (thromboplastin, factor III) is a lipoprotein that is constitutively expressed by most cells; however, endothelial cells only express tissue factor when stimulated by agonists such as thrombin or endotoxin. Vessel injury causes endothelial denudation and activation, which result in exposure of tissue factor to low circulating levels of activated factor VII in blood to form complexes that catalyze the conversion of factor IX to IXa and factor X to Xa, leading to thrombin formation.

Endothelial cells also synthesize and secrete von Willebrand factor (vWF), which is necessary for platelet adhesion to the vessel wall. This factor has binding sites for collagen, platelet glycoproteins (GPs) Ib and IIb/IIIa, and factor VIII. Factor VIII and vWF circulate together as a complex. Endothelial cells, in addition to the liver, synthesize factor V. Factors V and VIII are cleaved by thrombin into their activated states (Va and VIIIa) and then become integral components of membrane-bound complexes that accelerate the formation of thrombin and factor Xa (Figure 5-1). Endothelial cells also synthesize plasminogen activator inhibitor (PAI-1), which rapidly inactivates circulating t-PA.

Platelet Activation

Platelets are small, discoid-shaped, anuclear cells with an average circulatory life span of 8 to 12 days. There are usually 200,000 to 400,000 platelets/mm³ in human blood. Platelets are released as cytoplasmic fragments of megakaryocytes within bone marrow.

BOX 5-1	Endothelial Cell as Modulator of Hemostasis

FUNCTION EFFECT

Thrombogenic

- Profound loss of NO and PGI$_2$ after injury
- Loss of vasodilating stimulus
- Von Willebrand factor synthesis: ↑Platelet adhesion
- Factor V synthesis: ↑Thrombin
- Expression of tissue factor: ↑Thrombin
- Binding of factors VIIa and IXa: ↑Thrombin
- Surface membrane site for prothrombinase complex: ↑Thrombin
- Plasminogen activator inhibitor synthesis: ↑Thrombin

Antithrombotic

- NO and PGI$_2$ synthesis
- Vasodilating stimulus
- PGI$_2$ synthesis and granule release: ↓Platelet aggregation
- Thrombomodulin synthesis: ↓Factors Va and VIIIa
- Protein S synthesis: ↓Factors Va and VIIIa
- Heparan sulfate synthesis: ↓Thrombin
- t-PA and urokinase synthesis: ↓Plasmin
- Tissue factor pathway inhibitor: ↓Factors IXa and Xa

NO, Nitric oxide; *PGI$_2$*, prostaglandin I2; *t-PA*, tissue plasminogen activator.

The platelet membrane is composed of a phospholipid bilayer, glycoproteins, and proteins. Circulating proteins interact with the carbohydrate moieties of the glycoproteins. Several surface receptors are known to exist. Some of the more common receptors bind thrombin, adenosine diphosphate (ADP), TXA$_2$, fibrinogen, collagen, and vWF.[6] Platelets contain three types of storage granules: (1) dense granules, which contain serotonin, ADP, adenosine triphosphate (ATP), and calcium; (2) α-granules, which contain coagulation proteins (high-molecular-weight kininogen [HMWK], fibrinogen, fibronectin, factor V, vWF, platelet factor 4), growth factors, and adhesion proteins (fibronectin, thrombospondin, P-selectin); and (3) lysosomes.

The initial stage of hemostasis, consisting of vasoconstriction and platelet plug formation, is termed *primary hemostasis*. Immediately after vascular injury, platelets adhere to the subendothelial matrix via proteins, such as collagen and vWF. VWF binds primarily to the GP Ib-IX-V complex and the GP IIb-IIIa complex, whereas collagen binds via the GP Ia-IIa complex and GP IV. Collagen-induced platelet activation results in platelet shape change and release of prothrombotic α- and dense granule contents. Granule release reactions further amplify platelet activation and aggregation via several proteins including vWF, fibrinogen, and ADP.

Platelet activation is associated with numerous downstream signals, including protein kinase C activation, inositol triphosphate formation, intracellular calcium mobilization, and generation of arachidonic acid. Arachidonic acid is then converted by cyclooxygenase-1 (COX-1) to prostaglandin endoperoxides (PGG$_2$, PGH$_2$). PGG$_2$ is converted to TXA$_2$ by thromboxane synthetase. PGG$_2$, PGH$_2$, and TXA$_2$ stimulate further aggregation and platelet granule release.[7]

Regardless of the agonist, the final common pathway for platelet aggregation involves a conformational change in the GP IIb-IIIa complex that leads to the reversible exposure of binding sites for fibrinogen, which allows fibrinogen to form bridges between adjacent platelets.[8]

Numerous medications inhibit platelet function at several steps in the pathway above. Aspirin irreversibly inhibits platelet COX-1, inhibiting TXA$_2$-mediated platelet aggregation for the life of the platelet. Ticlopidine and clopidogrel inhibit ADP-mediated platelet activation and aggregation.[9,10] Novel GP IIb-IIIa inhibitors prevent platelet aggregation by blocking the binding of fibrinogen.[11]

Coagulation Activation

The platelet plug, which is required for normal hemostasis, de-aggregates unless thrombin is generated and fibrin stabilization of the plug occurs; this is known as *secondary hemostasis*. The formation of fibrin requires the interaction of platelet aggregates, endothelial cells, and plasma coagulation proteins.

Thirteen plasma coagulation proteins have been designated by the Roman numerals I through XIII (the letter a follows the Roman numeral when the factor has been activated). Most of these factors are synthesized in the liver. The hepatic synthesis of factors II, VII, IX, and X is vitamin K dependent. When vitamin K is not available, these factors are synthesized and released, but are not biologically active.

The sequence of enzymatic events leading to thrombin formation is the coagulation cascade (see Figure 5-1). The intrinsic pathway is activated when plasma is exposed to a negatively charged surface such as subendothelium, collagen, or endotoxin. Factor XII is activated to XIIa by the interaction of HMWK, prekallikrein, and the negatively charged surface; however, the physiologic significance of factor XII activation is unclear because deficiencies in factor XII, HMWK, and prekallikrein are not associated with any clinical bleeding diatheses.

The extrinsic pathway is the more physiologic route for the generation of thrombin and fibrin. It is initiated by the exposure of tissue factor, which binds to low levels of circulating factor VIIa in the presence of calcium (TF-VIIa).[12,13] This complex activates factor X and factor IX.[14] Factor Xa alone does not generate thrombin efficiently; however, factors Xa and thrombin together can activate factors VII, V, and VIII. Factors Va and VIIIa are critical components of the prothrombinase and tenase complexes (see Figure 5-1), respectively, which are 10^5-fold to 10^6-fold more active at generating thrombin than their serine protease factors acting independently.[13]

Thrombin proteolytically cleaves peptides from the fibrinogen molecule, resulting in the polymerization of fibrin monomers to form a gel. Thrombin also activates factor XIII in a reaction that is greatly accelerated (>80-fold) by the presence of fibrin.[15] Factor XIIIa covalently cross-links adjacent fibrin monomers, forming a stable clot that is more resistant to lysis by plasmin.

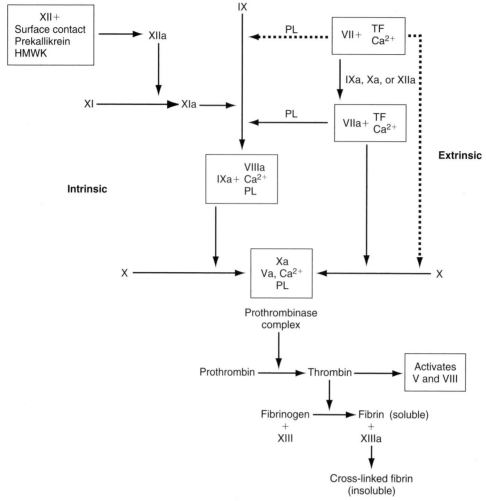

FIGURE 5-1 ■ The intrinsic and extrinsic pathways of coagulation. The intrinsic pathway is initiated by surface contact; the extrinsic pathway is initiated by the release of tissue factor (TF) from tissues injured during surgery or trauma. Factor VIIa possesses an activity 100-fold greater than that of factor VII. The pathways are interrelated and operate in tandem to achieve hemostasis. *HMWK,* High-molecular-weight kininogen; *PL,* phospholipid from activated platelet or endothelial membranes.

Coagulation Inhibition

Several mechanisms have evolved to control the rate of thrombin and fibrin formation (Figure 5-2). Antithrombin is a serine protease inhibitor that is synthesized in the liver and endothelial cells. AT inhibits numerous coagulation factors, but its most important targets are thrombin and factor Xa. AT activity is enhanced at least 1000-fold whenever it binds to circulating heparin or endothelial-bound heparin-like molecules. After the AT–heparin complex binds to an activated coagulation factor, the heparin dissociates and continues to act as a catalyst for the formation of other AT–serine enzyme complexes.

TFPI is an enzyme inhibitor synthesized by the endothelium and megakaryocytes.[16,17] It binds to the TF-VIIa-Xa complex and inhibits the further activation of factors X and IX.[18] TFPI is constitutively expressed on the endothelium, and its activity and antigen levels increase dramatically after the administration of heparin.

Thrombomodulin (TM) is a proteoglycan expressed on the surface of most endothelial cells[2] that binds thrombin, causes a conformational change in the substrate binding site, and renders the thrombin molecule incapable of binding active coagulation factors. TM also accelerates the inactivation of thrombin by AT.[19,20]

Protein C and protein S are synthesized by the liver, but protein S has also been found in endothelium and platelets.[21,22] Activated protein C binds to protein S on the endothelial or platelet surface and cleaves several peptide bonds in factors Va and VIIIa, resulting in decreased formation of the prothrombinase and tenase complexes.

Heparin cofactor II is another specific thrombin inhibitor that forms a stable 1 : 1 complex with thrombin. Heparin, heparan-like molecules, and dermatan sulfate accelerate the activity of heparin cofactor II. Unlike AT, heparin cofactor II cannot inhibit other coagulation factors. The plasma concentration of heparin cofactor II (70 µg/L) is much lower than that of AT (150 mg/L), and it is unlikely that heparin cofactor II has a major role in the regulation of hemostasis.

Fibrinolysis. Plasminogen, an inactive precursor synthesized in the liver, can be converted to plasmin by

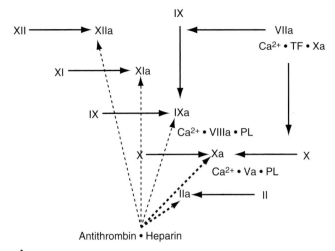

A

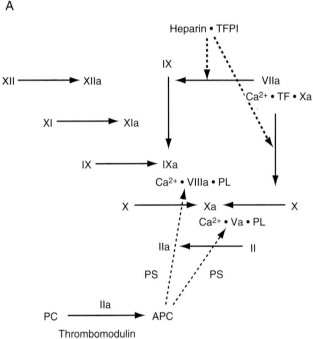

B

FIGURE 5-2 ■ Sites of activity for natural anticoagulants. *Dotted lines* indicated inhibitory activity. *APC,* Activated protein C; *AT,* antithrombin; *PS,* protein S; *TF,* tissue factor; *TFPI,* tissue factor pathway inhibitor.

several plasminogen activators. Circulating t-PA does not activate plasminogen efficiently; however, both t-PA and plasminogen have high affinity for fibrin, which acts as a template for accelerated plasminogen activation (>1000-fold).[23,24] Thus, the primary role for t-PA–activated plasmin is the formation of fibrin degradation products. Alternatively, exogenously administered t-PA may also activate plasminogen, which is bound to one of the fibrin degradation by-products, resulting in the release of free plasmin.[25,26] This release can lead to the limited break-down of fibrinogen, factor V, and factor VIII and to a systemic fibrinolytic state.

t-PA is commercially available in several forms. Recombinant human t-PA is the most widely used agent

for peripheral vascular applications. t-PA has a half-life of less than 5 minutes, but it has less specificity for thrombus-bound plasminogen. Tenecteplase is a recombinant variant of t-PA with amino acid substitutions at three sites, resulting in a longer half-life and a higher affinity for thrombus-bound plasminogen. Reteplase is another variant that contains 355 of the 527 amino acids of human t-PA, also resulting in a longer half-life of 13 to 16 minutes.

Three types of urokinase plasminogen activator (u-PA) have been studied. The precursor, pro-urokinase (single-chain u-PA), has a low level of enzymatic activity and no affinity for fibrin, but it demonstrates specificity against fibrin-bound plasminogen. Single-chain u-PA is readily converted by plasmin or kallikrein to the more active two-chain u-PA, which has a high-molecular-weight and a low-molecular-weight form. Commercially produced urokinase is composed primarily of the low-molecular-weight variant. Two-chain u-PA activates circulating plasminogen and fibrin-bound plasminogen equally well, resulting in a more pronounced systemic fibrinolysis.[27]

Each step within the plasminogen activation system has a known inhibitor. PAI-1 is released by endothelial cells, platelets, and hepatocytes. This inhibitor efficiently inactivates t-PA and two-chain u-PA and performs other functions, including the inhibition of thrombin and smooth muscle cell migration. PAI-2 is a less potent inhibitor of t-PA and two-chain u-PA, but its role in physiologic hemostasis remains uncertain. α_2-Antiplasmin inactivates circulating plasmin more readily than it does fibrin-bound plasmin, thus decreasing overall systemic fibrinolysis.

Preoperative Evaluation

Clinical Evaluation

A thorough history and physical examination will detect the majority of bleeding disorders preoperatively. Laboratory testing is warranted if a bleeding disorder is present or suspected. Careful questioning should distinguish a congenital bleeding disorder from an acquired one. Determining the pattern of inheritance can further aid in identifying a congenital deficiency. A history of bleeding problems beginning in childhood or at the beginning of menses implies an inherited bleeding disorder. A history of postoperative or spontaneous bleeding in a family member is important, because many patients with inherited disorders do not experience serious bleeding until challenged by an operative procedure or trauma. All patients should be asked about bleeding after tooth extraction, minor trauma, circumcision, and other surgical procedures.

An acquired hemostatic disorder should be suspected in adults who bleed during or after surgery or trauma, but who have no previous history of bleeding disorders; however, some patients with congenital disorders, such as von Willebrand disease, may not demonstrate a bleeding diathesis until challenged. Patients with liver disease are at increased risk for developing a coagulopathy during surgery, after trauma, and after massive transfusion. A detailed history of drug use is also important, because many drugs alter platelet function and predispose patients to bleeding complications.

Physical examination should include a thorough inspection for ecchymoses, petechiae, purpura, hemangiomas, jaundice, hematomas, and hemarthroses. Petechiae, ecchymoses, and mucocutaneous bleeding (epistaxis, gastrointestinal or genitourinary bleeding, menorrhagia) are more commonly associated with defects in primary hemostasis. Bleeding into deep tissues (hemarthroses, muscle and retroperitoneal hematomas) tends to occur with defects in coagulation. Signs of hepatic insufficiency should be noted, because these patients may have decreased production of coagulation proteins. Patients with myeloproliferative disorders, some malignant neoplasms, collagen disorders, or renal insufficiency are at increased risk for bleeding complications.

Laboratory Screening

Screening laboratory tests include prothrombin time (PT), activated partial thromboplastin time (aPTT), platelet count, and mixing tests. The PT assesses the extrinsic pathway and is prolonged by deficiencies of prothrombin, fibrinogen, and factors V, VII, and X. The PT is also useful in monitoring patients being prescribed anticoagulant therapy such as warfarin.

The aPTT is prolonged by deficiencies of factors in the intrinsic pathway, including VIII, IX, XI, and XII. To a lesser extent, aPTT detects factor deficiencies in the common pathway: V, X, prothrombin, and fibrinogen. The aPTT is also prolonged by heparin and is used to monitor patients receiving heparin anticoagulation therapy.

Platelet count is a key component in evaluating the patient with suspected thrombocytopenia; however, this test does not offer information regarding platelet function. Platelet function analyzers (PFA-100) are used to quantify congenital and acquired platelet dysfunction and von Willebrand disease. They are also helpful when preoperatively screening those with a positive family history of bleeding disorders, or those with liver or renal disease. The PFA-100 can be used to identify possible causes for intraoperative or postoperative bleeding, monitor treatment for von Willebrand disease, and identify those high-risk patients resistant to aspirin therapy. Essentially the PFA-100 measures how fast platelets adhere, activate, and aggregate into a platelet plug onto a collagen coated membrane in the presence of either epinephrine or ADP. In the presence of epinephrine, the cartridge (CEPI) allows for the detection of aspirin-induced defects and in the presence of ADP, the cartridge (CADP) allows for detection of more severe platelet defects.[28]

In those patients with elevated aPTT, the presence of platelet inhibitors may be suspected. A useful test in determining the presence of platelet inhibitors is the mixing study. In a mixing study, normal plasma is added in a 1:1 ratio to a patient's plasma. If the aPTT corrects to normal, a specific factor deficiency (factors VIII, IX) is suspected. If the aPTT does not correct with the addition of normal plasma to the sample, the test is suggestive of the presence of a specific or nonspecific factor inhibitor in the patient's sample. The abnormal mix then can be incubated at 37°C for 30 to 60 min and reassessed. If there is no change in the aPTT, the patient likely has a nonspecific inhibitor such as lupus anticoagulant. If the aPTT increases after incubation, the patient likely has a specific factor inhibitor such as anti–factor VIII antibodies. Mixing studies are sensitive but not specific and should be used only as a screening test. If lupus anticoagulant or other factor inhibitors are suspected, further testing is required to confirm the diagnosis.[28] The common causes of elevated PT and aPTT are shown in Table 5-1.

Platelet Disorders

Hemorrhagic complications can occur because of quantitative or qualitative platelet disorders that are acquired or congenital in origin. Thrombocytopenia and qualitative platelet defects are among the most common causes of bleeding in surgical patients. Spontaneous bleeding can occur when platelet counts fall to less than 20,000/mm^3. Platelet counts between 30,000 and 50,000/mm^3 are adequate to ensure hemostasis, provided that there are no associated functional platelet or coagulation disorders. Platelet counts of 50,000 to 100,000/mm^3 are required to restore hemostasis during bleeding.

Thrombocytopenia

Thrombocytopenia can occur from increased platelet destruction, abnormal production, dilution, or temporary sequestration (usually in the spleen). Increased destruction can occur via nonimmune or immune mechanisms. Non–immune-mediated thrombocytopenia occurs in hemolytic-uremic syndrome, thrombotic thrombocytopenic purpura, disseminated intravascular coagulation (DIC), and some vasculitides. In these syndromes, platelets are stimulated to aggregate within the microcirculation, often affecting the brain, kidneys, heart, lungs, and adrenal glands.[29] Early plasmapheresis and plasma transfusion (platelet-poor fresh frozen plasma [FFP], cryoprecipitate-poor plasma), along with high-dose glucocorticoid administration, can reverse most cases of thrombotic thrombocytopenic purpura.[30,31] Platelet transfusions should be used only for intracerebral or other life-threatening hemorrhagic complications. The treatment for hemolytic-uremic syndrome varies considerably but may include hemodialysis, heparin therapy, and plasma exchange, depending on the duration and severity of the illness. GP IIb-IIIa inhibitors may become a useful adjunct in hemolytic-uremic syndrome.[32]

Immune-mediated platelet destruction can occur with certain collagen vascular diseases (lupus erythematosus), immune thrombocytopenic purpura (ITP), and lymphoproliferative disorders (chronic lymphocytic leukemia, non-Hodgkin lymphoma), or it may be drug induced. Acute ITP is a postinfectious thrombocytopenia that occurs predominantly in children and is usually self-limited. Chronic ITP is idiopathic and results when autoimmune antibodies are generated against the platelet membrane. Initial therapy for the chronic form consists of corticosteroids followed by splenectomy in nonresponders. Severely thrombocytopenic patients with major

TABLE 5-1 Common Causes of Elevated PT and aPTT in the Presence and Absence of Bleeding

Bleeding				No Bleeding
Increased aPTT/ Increased PT	Increased aPTT/ Normal PT	Normal aPTT/ Increased PT	Normal aPTT/ Normal PT	Increased aPTT/ Increased PT
Inherited				
Deficient Factors I, II, V, X Dysfibrinogenemia	Deficient Factors VIII, IX, XI von Willebrand disease	Factor VII deficiency Dysfibrinogenemia	Platelet function disorders Von Willebrand disease Factor XIII deficiency α_2-antiplasmin deficiency PAI-1 deficiency	Deficient Factors XI, XII, kininogen, prekallikrein Dysfibrinogenemia Factor VII deficiency
Acquired				
Factor inhibitors II, V, X DIC Liver disease Vitamin K deficiency Paraproteinemia Amyloidosis Heparin therapy	Factor inhibitors VIII, IX, XI Heparin therapy	Warfarin therapy Liver disease Vitamin K deficiency DIC Paraproteinemia Specific inhibitors Factor VII	Platelet inhibitors Thrombolytic agents von Willebrand syndrome	Lupus anticoagulant Heparin therapy Warfarin therapy or vitamin K deficiency Liver disease Dysfibrinogenemia Specific inhibitor factor V

DIC, Disseminated intravascular coagulation.

hemorrhagic complications and patients requiring urgent surgery can be treated with platelet transfusions, intravenous (IV) gamma globulin, and plasmapheresis.

Some drugs (e.g., quinidine, quinine, sulfonamides, penicillins, valproic acid, heparin) can induce thrombocytopenia via the formation of antigen-antibody complexes on the platelet surface, increasing platelet destruction. In general, discontinuation of the drug reverses the thrombocytopenia within 2 to 5 days. Adjuvant therapy for active bleeding may include corticosteroids, platelet transfusions, and, in some cases, IV gamma globulin. Heparin-induced thrombocytopenia is a prothrombotic condition that is discussed later in the section on thrombosis.

Impaired platelet production may be caused by aplastic anemia, megakaryocytic aplasia, radiation, myelosuppressive drugs, viral infections, vitamin B_{12} and folate deficiencies, and several other drugs (ethanol, estrogens, interferon, thiazides). Thrombocytopenia also has been described in association with numerous congenital disorders (Fanconi aplastic anemia, sex-linked recessive thrombocytopenia, Alport syndrome).

Thrombocytopenia commonly occurs after massive transfusions of banked blood. Only 10% of platelets remain viable in blood held in cold storage for longer than 24 hours. In general, the replacement of one blood volume decreases the platelet count by one third to half.[33] Nevertheless, abnormal bleeding is uncommon, and the routine administration of platelets following massive transfusion is not warranted unless hemorrhage is ongoing.[34] Hypothermia (body temperature less than 32°C) also may cause thrombocytopenia, but the mechanism remains unclear, although it is known that sequestration of platelets during hypothermia occurs. Platelets appear to activate, release α-granule products, aggregate, and sequester in the portal circulation. Rewarming can

cause a significant portion to return to the circulation. Cold-induced coagulopathy is best prevented by transfusing warmed blood products and maintaining the core body temperature greater than 32°C.

The centrifugation of one unit of whole blood yields 8 to 10×10^{10} platelets. Approximately 4 to 8 units of whole blood are required to yield enough platelets for administration in the average adult. Current apheresis techniques can yield 2.5 to 10×10^{11} platelets from a single donor (over 1 to 2 hours). One unit of single-donor platelets usually increases the platelet count by 10,000/ mm^3 per square meter of body surface area.

Qualitative Disorders of Platelet Function

Qualitative platelet disorders should be suspected when bleeding occurs in patients with normal coagulation studies and platelet counts. Qualitative disorders may be congenital or acquired; acquired disorders are much more common. Disturbances of platelet adherence and aggregation rarely cause bleeding spontaneously but certainly exacerbate bleeding secondary to surgery and trauma. Congenital qualitative disorders of platelet function include von Willebrand disease, Bernard-Soulier syndrome, Glanzmann thrombasthenia, storage pool diseases, and diseases of platelet activation.

Von Willebrand disease is the most common inherited bleeding disorder, characterized by a deficiency or defect in vWF. It has been classified into six subtypes (1, 2A, 2B, 2M, 2N, 3), with type 1 being the most common (70%).[35] Type 1 von Willebrand disease is usually transmitted as an autosomal dominant trait with incomplete penetrance. In general, patients manifest epistaxis, ecchymoses, menorrhagia, and posttraumatic or postsurgical bleeding. Decreased platelet adherence causes prolongation of the bleeding time. The aPTT also may be elevated, because most patients with this disease have concomitant decreases in factor VIII coagulation activity (VIII:C). Ristocetin agglutination of platelets is impaired, but can be corrected with the addition of vWF-rich cryoprecipitate.

Treatment of von Willebrand disease can consist of replacement (cryoprecipitate, purified factor VIII concentrates, platelet transfusions) or nonreplacement (vasopressin, antifibrinolytic agents) therapy. Approximately 80% of patients with type 1 disease respond to desmopressin acetate (1-deamino-8-D-arginine vassopressin, DDAVP) with increased vWF:Ag and VIII:C (within 60 minutes), which can last for 4 to 6 hours. Unfortunately, response to therapy cannot be predicted without trial administration. Repeated administration of DDAVP (every 12 hours) may be required in patients with type 1 disease who undergo surgical procedures. Most type 2 and type 3 patients do not respond to DDAVP. Antifibrinolytic agents (ε-aminocaproic acid, tranexamic acid) have been used for the treatment of mucocutaneous bleeding and for prophylaxis during oral surgical procedures.[36] Patients who are unresponsive to DDAVP may require replacement therapy during the perioperative period. Until recently, cryoprecipitate (rich in vWF, factors VIII and XIII, and fibronectin) was the treatment of choice. More recently, some purified factor VIII concentrates, which contain large quantities of multimeric vWF, and a newly formulated vWF concentrate have been used successfully.[37] There are no clear guidelines regarding the amount and frequency of administration; replacement therapy is largely empirical. The bleeding time and factor VIII levels are used to monitor response to replacement therapy.

Bernard-Soulier syndrome is transmitted as an autosomal recessive trait and is characterized by a deficiency in the GP Ib-IX-V complex (primary binding site for vWF). These patients have prolonged bleeding times (>20 minutes), mild to moderate thrombocytopenia, and absent ristocetin-induced platelet agglutination. Heterozygous patients have half the normal amount of GP Ib-IX-V, but demonstrate normal platelet responses. Platelet transfusions are the mainstay of therapy, but they are limited by the development of antibodies to human leukocyte antigens (HLAs) (alloimmunization) and to the GP Ib-IX-V complex. The use of HLA crossmatched and leukocyte-depleted platelets should minimize alloimmunization. Other unproved therapies include DDAVP and corticosteroids.

Glanzmann thrombasthenia is a rare autosomal recessive trait in which platelet membranes lack GP IIb-IIIa receptors, leading to failure of platelet aggregation regardless of the initial stimulus. These patients have normal platelet counts, markedly prolonged bleeding times, deficient clot retraction, and normal ristocetin-induced agglutination. Patients who are heterozygous exhibit normal platelet aggregation responses. As with Bernard-Soulier syndrome, platelet transfusions are the primary form of therapy. Again, the use of HLA crossmatched and leukocyte-depleted platelets is optimal.

Storage pool diseases are a group of rare hereditary disorders characterized by deficiencies in platelet granules, their contents, or both. These deficiencies include α-granule contents (gray platelet syndrome), δ-granule storage diseases (Wiskott-Aldrich syndrome, Hermansky-Pudlak syndrome, Chédiak-Higashi syndrome), and αδ-granule storage diseases.[38] Cryoprecipitate and platelet transfusions can be used in the perioperative period. DDAVP also has been used to decrease the requirement for transfusions.

Acquired qualitative platelet abnormalities can be caused by certain drugs, uremia, cirrhosis, myeloproliferative disorders, and dysproteinemias. Aspirin irreversibly acetylates platelet cyclooxygenase-1, inhibiting thromboxane- and endoperoxide-mediated platelet activation for the life of the platelet. The effect of aspirin on the bleeding time is variable and may depend largely on the technique used to perform the test.[39,40] Nonsteroidal anti-inflammatory drugs (e.g., indomethacin, phenylbutazone, ibuprofen) reversibly inhibit cyclooxygenase. Numerous antibiotics, including some β-lactams, cephalosporins, and nitrofurantoin, impair platelet aggregation and prolong the bleeding time. Mechanisms can include inhibition of agonist binding to the membrane receptor and inhibition of intracellular signal transduction. Platelet GP IIb-IIIa inhibitors (e.g., abciximab, eptifibatide, tirofiban) block the binding of fibrinogen to the GP IIb-IIIa receptor and effectively prevent platelet aggregation in a dose-dependent fashion. Correction of bleeding can be accomplished with platelet transfusions.

Uremia causes defective platelet adherence and aggregation, resulting in a prolonged bleeding time. Clinical manifestations can include petechiae, ecchymoses, and mucocutaneous bleeding. The pathophysiology remains unclear, but may involve impaired thromboxane and calcium metabolism or defective platelet-subendothelial adhesion (via vWF). DDAVP has been shown to shorten bleeding times preoperatively in uremic patients.[41] Intravenous DDAVP, 0.3 to 0.4 μg/kg over 15 to 30 minutes, shortens the bleeding time in most patients within 1 hour. Hemodialysis, peritoneal dialysis, and infusions of cryoprecipitate and conjugated estrogens have been used with some success.[42]

Coagulation factor deficiencies, DIC, dysfibrinogenemias, impaired thrombopoiesis, platelet sequestration, and impaired platelet aggregation all contribute to the hemostatic defects associated with liver failure. Therapy is nonspecific but can include DDAVP and platelet transfusions for severe thrombocytopenia.

Disorders of Secondary Hemostasis

Congenital Disorders

Congenital disorders of coagulation usually involve a single factor. Preoperative transfusion of the appropriate factor is necessary and may be required during surgery and postoperatively as well. Deficiencies of factor XII, HMWK, and prekallikrein cause prolongation of the aPTT but do not cause significant bleeding diatheses. Deficiencies of the remaining factors can result in serious bleeding after surgery or trauma.

Hemophilia A (factor VIII deficiency) is the most common of the inherited coagulation defects, with a prevalence of 1 in 10,000 males. Hemophilia B

(Christmas disease, factor IX deficiency) has a prevalence of approximately 1 in 50,000 males. Both are X-linked recessive disorders that are clinically indistinguishable. The severity of these disorders depends on the levels of factor VIII or IX that are present. Severely affected individuals (factor levels < 1%) manifest spontaneous hemarthroses and deep tissue hematomas during infancy or early childhood. Patients with mild to moderate hemophilia (factor levels > 5%) may develop hemorrhagic complications only after surgery or trauma.

Patients with hemophilia A who require major surgery should receive factor VIII replacement to achieve 100% of normal activity just before the procedure. For each unit per kilogram of body weight infused, the factor VIII level is increased by approximately 0.02 U/mL (normal activity is 1 U/mL).[43] Levels should be monitored postoperatively, and replacement therapy should be repeated every 12 hours to maintain at least 50% of normal activity until all wounds are healed.[44] Factor VIII levels can be restored using donor-directed cryoprecipitate, virus-inactivated factor VIII concentrate, or recombinant factor VIII. DDAVP (which increases factor VIII levels) and ε-aminocaproic acid may be used as adjunctive therapies in patients with mild hemophilia to reduce or avoid the need for replacement therapy during oral or minor surgical procedures.

Patients with hemophilia B should have at least 50% of normal activity before major surgery and for the first 7 to 10 days postoperatively. Factor IX can be replaced with prothrombin complex concentrates (containing factors II, VII, IX, and X), purified factor IX, or recombinant factor IX. Replacement therapy may be limited by several factors. Prothrombin complexes are associated with the development of arterial or venous thromboses in some patients. In addition, therapy with recombinant factor IX may not achieve as much activity as purified factor IX. This may be due to the need for posttranslational modifications (γ-carboxylation) that are not present in recombinant factor IX. In addition, replacement therapy for hemophilia A and B is complicated by the development of inhibitors to factors VIII and IX in approximately 15% of patients. Alternative strategies include the use of high-dose factor VIII or recombinant factor VIIa and attempts to induce immune tolerance.

Rare coagulation factor deficiencies of factors II, V, VII, and X occur with a prevalence of 1:500,000 to 1:1,000,000. They are usually transmitted with an autosomal recessive pattern. The most severe complications occur with deficiencies of factors II and X.[45] In general, only low levels of factor activity (10% to 20% of normal) are required for normal hemostasis. Replacement therapy for factors II and X can be accomplished with fresh frozen plasma or factor concentrates. Factor IX concentrates contain significant amounts of factors II and X and can be used for their replacement. The short half-life of factor VII requires a more frequent replacement schedule using factor VII concentrates. Recombinant factor VIIa also can be used for factor VII deficiencies. Factor V deficiencies can be treated with fresh frozen plasma, because factor V concentrates are not yet commercially available.

Abnormalities of fibrinogen and fibrinolysis are also heritable. Afibrinogenemia is a rare disorder transmitted as an autosomal recessive trait; hypofibrinogenemia can occur in heterozygous individuals. Clinical manifestations include gastrointestinal and mucous membrane bleeding, hemarthroses, intracranial hemorrhage, and recurrent fetal loss. The PT and aPTT, which are markedly prolonged, usually correct when mixed with normal plasma. Replacement therapy with cryoprecipitate is usually reserved for active bleeding, the perioperative period, and prophylaxis during pregnancy. The level of fibrinogen necessary for hemostasis ranges between 50 and 100 mg/dL. Each unit of cryoprecipitate usually increases the fibrinogen level by approximately 10 mg/dL.[46]

Dysfibrinogenemias are a heterogeneous group of disorders that can cause defective fibrin formation, polymerization, cross-linkage, or impaired fibrinolysis. Patients may manifest mild to moderate bleeding diatheses (30%) or recurrent thromboses (20%).[47] The PT and aPTT usually are prolonged. Functional assays for fibrinogen are abnormal, whereas antigenic assays are normal. Cryoprecipitate is indicated for hemorrhage, but contraindicated for acute thrombotic episodes.

Congenital hyperfibrinolytic states can result in delayed bleeding. The congenital hyperfibrinolytic states include heterozygous and homozygous α2-antiplasmin deficiencies and functionally abnormal or deficient PAI-1.[48] The whole blood clot lysis time and the euglobulin clot lysis time are characteristically shortened. Antifibrinolytic agents (ε-aminocaproic acid or tranexamic acid) are recommended for the management of active bleeding.[49]

Acquired Disorders

Patients develop coagulation disorders because of deficiencies of coagulation proteins, synthesis of nonfunctioning factors, and consumption or inadequate replacement of coagulation proteins.

Hepatic insufficiency can cause decreased plasma levels of several coagulation factors (including factors II, V, VII, IX, X, XIII, and fibrinogen) because of a decreased synthetic capacity, defective posttranslational modification (γ-carboxylation), and increased breakdown of activated factors (because of subclinical DIC). Thrombocytopenia can also occur because of increased splenic sequestration; however, levels of factor VIII and vWF may be elevated because they are synthesized in extrahepatic locations. Correction of the coagulation factor deficits and the thrombocytopenia is accomplished with fresh frozen plasma and platelet transfusions, respectively. Vitamin K administration alone does not completely reverse the coagulopathy.

Vitamin K deficiency can cause a bleeding diathesis as a result of the synthesis of nonfunctional forms of the vitamin K–dependent coagulation factors II, VII, IX, and X. Normal sources of vitamin K include dietary intake (e.g., leafy green vegetables, soybean oil) and vitamin K synthesis by normal intestinal flora. Vitamin K deficiency can be caused by poor dietary intake, decreased intestinal absorption of vitamin K, decreased production by the gut flora, and liver failure. This situation more commonly arises in patients receiving antibiotic bowel preparations or long-term parenteral nutrition (without vitamin K supplementation). Vitamin K deficiency also occurs in patients who have a prolonged recovery after intestinal surgery and in those with intrinsic bowel diseases (e.g., Crohn disease, celiac sprue, ulcerative colitis), as well as in patients with obstructive jaundice. Vitamin K should be administered preoperatively to patients with hepatic insufficiency, obstructive jaundice, malabsorption states, or malnutrition. Patients with an intact enterohepatic circulation can receive vitamin K orally (2.5 to 5 mg), with normalization of the PT within 24 to 48 hours. Slow IV administration should be used in patients with biliary obstruction or malabsorption. Patients who require urgent correction of the PT should receive slow IV vitamin K and replacement therapy (fresh frozen plasma or prothrombin concentrates).

DIC is characterized by the systemic generation of fibrin, often resulting in the thrombosis of small- and medium-sized blood vessels. The consumption of clotting factors and platelets also results in impaired coagulation and hemorrhagic complications. DIC is mediated by several cytokines (including tumor necrosis factor-α and interleukin-6), which result in the systemic generation of TF, thrombin, and fibrin.[50] Fibrinolytic activity, which is initially increased via the release of t-PA, becomes depressed in response to elevated PAI-1.[50,51] DIC can develop in association with bacterial infections (grampositive and gram-negative infections), trauma, malignancy, obstetric complications, hemolytic transfusion reactions, giant hemangiomas (Kasabach-Merritt syndrome), and aortic aneurysms. A compensated DIC (present in more than 80% of patients who undergo major surgery), in which coagulation factors and platelets are replaced as they are consumed, may be asymptomatic or may appear with ecchymoses and petechiae. Surgery, trauma, hypotension, or transfusion reactions can exacerbate the coagulopathy and hypofibrinolysis, leading to excessive bleeding and intravascular thrombosis.

A combination of laboratory tests may help to confirm the clinical diagnosis of DIC. These tests include detection of thrombocytopenia or a rapidly decreasing platelet count, prolongation of the PT and aPTT, and the presence of fibrin degradation products (D-dimer assay, latex agglutination for fibrous degradation products). Extrinsic pathway coagulation proteins (factors II, V, VII, and X) and physiologic coagulation inhibitors (AT, protein C) usually are depressed, whereas vWF and factor VIII levels may be increased.[52] The fibrinogen level is variably affected by DIC.

The first goal of management is elimination of the cause of DIC. When this is possible, the intravascular coagulation ceases with the return of normal hemostasis. In severe DIC, with ongoing blood loss, patients are best managed by replacing deficient blood elements using fresh frozen plasma (up to 6 units per 24 hours) and platelets while the precipitating cause of DIC is eliminated.[50] Administration of AT and protein C concentrates may retard the consumption of coagulation factors, although this remains to be proved. Some trials have demonstrated a benefit with the administration of heparin or low-molecular-weight heparin (LMWH).[53,54] Given that patients with DIC already have a coagulopathy, heparin should be used cautiously (lower IV doses of 300 to 500 units/hour) and with careful clinical observation and laboratory monitoring. Direct thrombin inhibitors (hirudin, recombinant TM), activated protein C, and extrinsic pathway inhibitors (recombinant TFPI) are under investigation as well.

Management of Anticoagulation

Given the increasing number of patients taking anticoagulants prior to surgery, it is wise to consider how to manage these complicated patients in the face of active hemorrhage and during the perioperative period.

Active Hemorrhage

Controlled clinical studies have shown that treatment with vitamin K antagonists (VKAs) increases the risk of major bleeding by 0.5% per year and the risk of intracranial hemorrhage by 0.2% per year.[55] Risk factors associated with hemorrhage in patients treated with VKAs include target international normalized ratio (INR) greater than 3,[56] patient age, cytochrome P450 CYP2C9 polymorphisms that decrease VKA metabolism,[57] and renal and hepatic insufficiency. The addition of antiplatelet therapy and nonsteroidal antiinflammatory medications in the setting of VKA therapy also increases the risk of major bleeding 2.5-fold greater than normal and increases the risk of gastrointestinal bleeding 11-fold, respectively.[58-60]

In the face of bleeding, the reversal of VKA therapy is critical and varies depending on the INR and clinical status of the patient. To reverse VKA therapy, vitamin K replacement is often the first line of therapy in clinically stable patients with minimum signs of hemorrhage. Vitamin K replacement can be administered orally, but the INR usually takes 24 hours to normalize in this case. IV vitamin K can normalize INR within 12 to 16 hours. Intramuscular and subcutaneous routes should be avoided because absorption can be unpredictable and delayed.[61] The recommended dose for vitamin K replacement varies depending on the INR. If INR is less than 7, 2.5 to 5 mg of vitamin K is effective. If the INR is greater than 7, 5 to 10 mg of vitamin K is required.

Factor replacement including the use of FFP, prothrombin complex concentrates (PCCs), and recombinant factor VIIa can be considered when active hemorrhage is apparent and rapid correction of INR is necessitated. When administered, FFP elicits a 2% to 4% rise in factor activity per unit infused. Large volumes of FFP are often required to correct an elevated INR, and there is an associated risk of transfusion-related acute lung injury (TRALI), anaphylaxis, and transmission of viral infections with FFP administration. In addition, FFP must be thawed before infusion and needs to be crossmatched to assure ABO compatibility limiting the rapidity of INR correction and hemorrhage cessation. Because of the variability of vitamin K–dependent clotting factors in FFP, others have studied the effect of clotting factor concentrates on the INRs of anticoagulated patients who require rapid correction. Makris and colleagues[62] found that patients given FFP did not normalize their INR, whereas those treated with clotting factor concentrates did, largely in part to increased factor

TABLE 5-2   **Risk Stratification and Recommendations for Perioperative Arterial or Venous Thromboembolism**

	Indication for Antithrombotic Therapy			Recommended Management of Antithrombotic Therapy
Risk	Mechanical Heart Valve	Atrial Fibrillation	VTE	
High	Any MVR, older aortic valve, recent CVA or TIA (<6 mo)	CHADS2 score, 5-6; recent CVA or TIA (<3 mo)	VTE within 3 mo; severe thrombophilia; ProtC, ProtS, AT deficiency; antiphospholipid antibody; multiple abnormalities	Bridging anticoagulation: therapeutic-dose SC LMWH or IV heparin (grade 1C). Suggest LMWH over IV heparin (grade 2C)
Moderate	Bileaflet AVR plus one of: atrial fibrillation, prior CVA or TIA, HTN, DM, CHF, or age >75 yr	CHADS2, score 3-4	VTE 3-12 mo ago; nonsevere thrombophilia; factor V Leiden; prothrombin mutation; recurrent VTE; active cancer	Bridging anticoagulation: therapeutic-dose SC LMWH, IV heparin, or low-dose SC LMWH (grade 2C); suggest therapeutic dose SC LMWH over others (grade 2C)
Low	Bileaflet AVR without other CVA risk factors	CHADS2, score 0-2	VTE >12 mo ago and no other risk factors	Bridging anticoagulation: low-dose SC LMWH; no bridging anticoagulation (grade 2C)

From Douketis JD, Berger PB, Dunn AS, et al: The perioperative management of antithrombotic therapy: American College of Chest Physicians Evidence-Based Clinical Practice Guidelines (8th Edition). Chest 133(6 Suppl):299S–339S, 2008.
VTE, Venous thromboembolism; *MVR,* mitral valve replacement; *CVA,* cerebrovascular accident; *TIA,* transient ischemic attack; *CHADS2,* classification system: congestive heart failure, hypertension, age ≥75 years, diabetes, stroke; *ProtC,* protein C; *ProtS,* protein S; *AT,* antithrombin; *SC,* subcutaneous; *LMWH,* low-molecular weight heparin; *IV,* intravenous; *AVR,* aortic valve replacement; *HTN,* hypertension; *DM,* diabetes mellitus; *CHF,* congestive heart failure.

IX levels in the clotting factor concentrate compared to the factor IX levels found in FFP.

Recombinant factor VII (rVIIa) replacement can also be used to correct INR and halt hemorrhage in patients taking VKAs. The rVIIa contains hamster proteins, bovine IgG, and mouse IgG. The mechanism of action for rVIIa is that it complexes with tissue factor to activate factors IX and X, initiating the clotting cascade while bypassing the activation of factors VIII and IX. A typical dose of rVIIa is 5 to 16 µg/kg IV.[63] A comparison of rVIIa to PCC (Octaplex, Octapharma AG, Lachen, Switzerland) showed that although both rVIIa and PCC corrected INR, only PCC restored endogenous thrombin generation, which is the key endpoint in restoring hemostasis.[64]

PCCs are lyophilized concentrates of a standardized amount of factor IX and different amounts of factors II, VII, and X that vary by manufacturer. PCCs are currently approved in Europe, Australia, and Canada for use in patients with factor IX deficiency or for rapid reversal of VKA therapy, whereas PCCs are approved by the U.S. Food and Drug Administration (FDA) only for factor IX deficiency. Although many PCCs are poor in factor VII, they are virally inactivated, undergo prion reducing processes, are lyophilized rather than frozen, and are administered in small volumes (40 to 80 mL). Should PCCs be approved by the FDA for use in patients taking VKAs, it should be noted that the use of PCCs is indicated specifically for those patients exhibiting major bleeding or requiring urgent surgical procedures (<6 hours). PCCs are not recommended for VKA reversal in the elective setting, for elevated INR without bleeding or an urgent need for surgery, for use in massive transfusions, coagulopathy of liver disease, patients with a recent history of thrombosis, ischemic stroke or DIC, or patients with a history of heparin-induced thrombocytopenia. Complications of PCC use include thrombosis, DIC, hemorrhage, and viral transmission.[65]

Perioperative Management

Patients who are being treated with VKAs before surgery must be assessed to determine the best mode of anticoagulation management for that patient to decrease the risk of bleeding and thrombosis. The general options for managing these patients in the perioperative period include continuing anticoagulation, decreasing warfarin dosage, or discontinuing warfarin and administering bridging therapy with LMWH or unfractionated heparin using the American College of Chest Physicians (ACCP) guidelines published in 2008.[66] Currently, the ACCP guidelines are most frequently referred to as the standard of care for these complex patients; however, there is some evidence supporting the continuation of anticoagulation therapy or decreasing the dose perioperatively to reduce the risk of bleeding while maintaining adequate anticoagulation to prevent arterial thrombosis.

Table 5-2 shows the risk stratification for patients receiving anticoagulation therapy for three common indications, including mechanical heart valves, atrial fibrillation, and venous thromboembolism. Table 5-2 also shows the recommended management of anticoagulation therapy by risk stratification. Generally, in patients deemed to be at high risk, bridging anticoagulation with therapeutic-dose LMWH or IV heparin is recommended (grade 1C) and LMWH is recommended over IV heparin (grade 2C).

In patients with moderate risk, bridging anticoagulation with therapeutic-dose LMWH, IV heparin, or low-dose LMWH are recommended (grade 2C), where therapeutic-dose LMWH is recommended over other agents and doses (grade 2C). Low-risk patients can be bridged with low-dose LMWH or without bridging therapy (grade 2C).[66]

Given that these recommendations are grade 2C, the lowest level, a randomized controlled trial has been designed and is underway to examine whether bridge therapy prevents arterial thromboembolism in patients with atrial fibrillation who require interruption of VKA therapy. It also aims to compare the safety of bridging therapy with no bridging therapy on the rate of major bleeding in patients requiring interruption of their VKA therapy. This study, sponsored by the National Heart, Lung, and Blood Institutes is aptly named "*B*ridging Anticoagulation in Patients who *R*equire Temporary *I*nterruption of Warfarin Therapy for an Elective Invasive Proce*D*ure or Sur*GE*ry" (BRIDGE) and will be completed in 2013.[67]

Some authors advocate for continuing VKA therapy throughout the perioperative period, citing relatively low rates of hematoma or bleeding during or immediately after surgery (4%).[68,69] The range of INR in these studies was broad (1.1 to 4.9). Larson and colleagues[70] have suggested decreasing the dose of warfarin perioperatively to achieve a goal INR of 1.5 to 2 on the day of surgery; they show a relatively low risk of bleeding complications (4% major, 2% minor) when warfarin doses were decreased to a target INR of 1.5 to 2. The mean INR at the time of surgery was 1.77, and the one patient who died after cerebrovascular accident had failed to increase his warfarin dose appropriately postoperatively while at home. The authors also note that considerable effort, including the need for repeated blood testing, was necessary to assure a safe INR before surgery.

THROMBOSIS

In 1856, Virchow suggested that thrombus formation was the result of an interaction among an injured surface, stasis, and the hypercoagulability of blood.[70a] One or more components of Virchow's triad can be invoked when determining the cause of in vivo thrombosis. Hypofibrinolysis is the only major process not recognized by Virchow that contributes to intravascular thrombosis.

Most of the inherited thrombophilic conditions, with the exception of congenital hyperhomocysteinemia, are more closely associated with venous than with arterial thromboembolism. Acquired conditions such as the presence of antiphospholipid antibodies and heparin-associated antibodies have a well-recognized association with both arterial and venous thromboses. The more common inherited and acquired hypercoagulable states are discussed later, as are the indications for testing and the optimal timing for the performance of these assays. The more commonly used antithrombotic agents, as well as alternative agents, are discussed briefly in regard to the management of established thromboses and prophylaxis against thromboembolism.

Prothrombotic Conditions

Inherited Prothrombotic Conditions

Activated protein C (APC) resistance is most commonly caused by a mutation in the factor V gene, during which Arg506 is replaced with Gln (factor V Leiden), making activated factor V resistant to degradation by APC.[71] It is the most common inherited hypercoagulable condition, occurring in approximately 12% to 33% of patients with venous thromboembolism.[72-75] In contrast, it has a prevalence of 3% to 6% in control populations.[73-75] The white population is affected more commonly than black, Asian, or Native American populations. Individuals who are heterozygous for the factor V mutation have a 2.7-fold to sevenfold increased risk for venous thromboembolism, whereas homozygous patients may have an 80-fold increased risk.[74,75] A small percentage of patients with APC resistance do not have the Leiden mutation. Other factor V mutations (factor V Cambridge, factor V HR2 haplotype) can also cause APC resistance.[76,77]

Functional APC resistance can be detected by performing the aPTT in the presence and absence of purified APC. In general, an aPTT ratio (aPTT with APC/aPTT without APC) of less than 2 is considered a positive study (normal is 2.4 to 4.0). Numerous factors can affect the accuracy of the aPTT ratio, including protein C deficiency, the presence of anticoagulants, and antiphospholipid antibodies. Modifications to this functional assay have improved its sensitivity and specificity.[78] DNA testing using the polymerase chain reaction to amplify the factor V Leiden mutation is standard. The optimal management of patients with APC resistance remains to be defined. APC-resistant individuals in high-risk situations (e.g., pregnancy, surgery) should receive thrombosis prophylaxis. Patients with prior thrombotic episodes may benefit from long-term warfarin therapy. This is especially true for patients with multiple prior episodes, thromboses in unusual locations, and multiple inherited thrombophilic mutations.

Prothrombin 20210A is a mutation (G to A substitution) in the prothrombin gene at nucleotide 20210, resulting in increased levels of plasma prothrombin.[79] The prothrombin 20210A mutation is present in 18% of selected patients with strong family histories of venous thromboembolism, 6.2% of unselected patients with a first episode of thrombosis, and 2.3% of healthy controls. The prevalence is even higher in southern European whites.[80] A significant number of patients have more than one congenital thrombophilic condition, further increasing their risk for venous thromboembolism.[79,81]

AT deficiency was the first reported congenital thrombophilic condition.[82] It is transmitted with an autosomal dominant pattern and has a prevalence of 1:5000 in the population.[83] AT deficiency has been detected in approximately 1% of patients with venous thromboses, conferring a risk that may be as high as 50-fold greater than normal.[84,85] The lifetime risk for developing a thrombotic episode ranges between 17% and 50%.[86] Although thromboembolism may occur spontaneously, it is usually associated with a precipitating event such as surgery, trauma, or pregnancy. Arterial thromboses, although less common than venous thromboses, also occur. AT levels may be reduced to less than 80% of normal in other conditions, including hepatic insufficiency, DIC, acute venous thrombosis, sepsis, and nephrotic syndrome, and in patients receiving heparin or estrogen supplementation.

The mainstay of therapy in AT-deficient patients with venous thromboembolism is still heparin anticoagulation, although supranormal dosages may be required.[87] AT concentrates may be appropriate in patients who do not achieve adequate anticoagulation with heparin alone. The minimum level of AT necessary to prevent thrombosis is unknown; however, it is suggested that levels be adjusted to greater than 80% of normal activity. Antithrombin can be replaced with AT concentrate (1 U/kg increases the AT activity by 1% to 2%) or fresh frozen plasma. Asymptomatic patients should receive thrombosis prophylaxis during high-risk situations such as prolonged immobilization, surgery, or pregnancy; however, long-term warfarin therapy is usually reserved for AT-deficient patients who have experienced thrombotic events.

Protein C and protein S deficiencies account for a number of disorders. Congenital protein C deficiency may be transmitted as an autosomal dominant or recessive trait and has a prevalence of 1:200 to 1:500.[88,89] The incidence of thrombosis varies, depending on the population in question. Studies identifying protein C deficiency in healthy blood donors demonstrate a low prevalence of venous thrombosis, whereas studies that screen patients with venous thromboembolism find a higher prevalence of protein C deficiency compared with controls.[84,88-90] Overall, inherited protein C deficiency is associated with an approximately sevenfold increased risk for developing a first venous thromboembolic event.[90] Common sites for venous thromboses include the lower extremities, mesenteric veins, and cerebral venous sinuses. Functional and immunologic assays are available to establish the diagnosis of protein C deficiency. Healthy adults have protein C antigen levels ranging from 70% to 140% of normal. Patients with antigen levels less than 55% are likely to have heterozygous protein C deficiency.

Approximately 60% of the total protein S circulates bound to C4b complement-binding protein.[91] Deficiency states can occur with decreased total protein S, decreased free protein S, and decreased functional protein S activity (with total and free protein S concentrations in the normal range). Histories of patients with congenital protein S deficiencies are similar to those of patients with protein C deficiency, although arterial thromboses also have been described in patients with protein S deficiency. Protein S can be measured with functional assays, which assess the ability to catalyze the inhibition of factor Va by APC, or immunologic assays.

Both protein C and protein S are vitamin K–dependent proteins synthesized in the liver. Consequently, plasma levels may be decreased in patients with hepatic insufficiency. Acquired protein C and protein S deficiencies can also occur with warfarin administration, vitamin K deficiency (malabsorption, biliary obstruction), sepsis, DIC, and acute thromboses and in patients receiving some chemotherapeutic medications. Because C4b is also an acute-phase reactant, inflammatory conditions can increase C4b levels, causing a decrease in free protein S and an increased tendency toward thrombosis.[92]

Heparin is the first line of therapy in the management of acute thromboembolic episodes in patients with known protein C and S deficiencies. Because warfarin-induced skin necrosis is more likely to occur in patients with protein C deficiency, heparin therapy should overlap with the first 4 or 5 days of warfarin therapy, and large loading dosages of warfarin should be avoided. Longer-term treatment with warfarin is effective in the prevention of recurrent venous thromboembolic episodes in patients with protein C and protein S deficiencies. FFP occasionally may be required to restore functional levels of protein C and protein S.

Abnormalities of fibrinogen and fibrinolysis include dysfibrinogenemias, which may impair any of the steps involved in the generation and cross-linkage of fibrin. These anomalies have been reported in association with bleeding diatheses (30%) and venous thromboembolism (20%). Therapeutic alternatives have been described earlier.

Elevated factor XI is a mild risk factor for the development of venous thrombosis.[93,94] Factor XI levels in the 90th percentile or greater confer a 2.2-fold relative risk for the development of venous thrombosis. Even lower factor XI levels demonstrate a linear dose-response relationship with thrombotic risk. The underlying cause for elevated factor XI levels remains to be determined.

Acquired Prothrombotic Conditions

Many clinical disorders predispose to thrombosis by activating the coagulation system or causing platelet aggregation. Soft tissue trauma, thermal injuries, and operative dissection all predispose to thrombosis through the release of tissue factor and activation of the extrinsic coagulation pathway.

Sepsis predisposes to thrombosis via multiple mechanisms. Gram-positive bacteria may directly cause platelet aggregation and subsequent thrombosis. Gram-negative bacterial endotoxin may stimulate platelet aggregation but may also, through interaction with leukocytes and endothelial cells, cause TF-like activation of the coagulation system. Endotoxin is known to be a major stimulus for the development of DIC.

As many as 11% of patients with malignancies have venous thromboembolic complications.[95] Pancreatic, prostate, gastrointestinal, and lung cancers have a particularly strong association with thrombosis. Conversely, patients with idiopathic venous thromboembolism are more likely to be diagnosed with cancer (up to 7.6%).[96] Aggressive screening for occult malignancies in patients with venous thromboembolism has not been shown to be cost effective or to result in improved long-term survival.

Pregnancy is associated with a fourfold increased risk for venous thromboembolism.[85,97] The risk may be threefold to fivefold greater in the immediate postpartum period. Oral contraceptives are also associated with an approximately threefold increased risk, which is conferred immediately and is reversible.[98] Dinger and colleagues[99] performed a case-control study evaluating newer preparations with lower doses of ethinylestradiol, but found similar rates of venous thromboembolism (VTE) between patients using low-dose and standard-dose combined oral contraceptives.[99] Although the exact mechanism is unclear, women taking oral contraceptives demonstrate increased levels of thrombin and fibrinogen, with decreased levels of protein S and plasminogen activators.

Antiphospholipid antibodies, including lupus anticoagulants and anticardiolipin antibodies, are immunoglobulin (Ig) G, IgM, or IgA, which are directed against phospholipid-binding proteins (prothrombin and β_2-GP I). These antibodies interfere with in vitro phospholipid-dependent clotting assays, such as aPTT, kaolin clotting time, and the dilute Russell viper venom time. In vivo, antiphospholipid antibodies may promote thrombosis by interfering with the activation of protein C.[100] The presence of antiphospholipid antibodies is associated with a ninefold increased risk for venous thrombosis. Clinical manifestations of the antiphospholipid syndrome may include venous and arterial thromboses (coronary, cerebral) and recurrent fetal loss. Lupus anticoagulants are also associated with arterial thrombosis. As many as 50% of patients who are positive for lupus anticoagulants and undergo vascular surgical procedures develop thrombotic complications.[101] Patients with thrombotic episodes should receive heparin and warfarin anticoagulation. Long-term warfarin therapy (at higher intensity, international normalized ratio greater than 3) has been shown to reduce the recurrence of thrombosis.[102] Warfarin may be discontinued when the IgM or IgG immunoglobulins are no longer detectable.

Heparin-associated antibodies (HAAbs) and heparin-induced thrombocytopenia (HIT) are important considerations for patients receiving anticoagulation therapy. HAAbs IgG and IgM target the heparin–platelet factor 4 complex. These immune complexes bind to the $Fc\gamma$-RII platelet receptor, causing pathophysiologic platelet activation, aggregation, and thrombocytopenia. The incidence of HAAb formation varies widely, depending on the indications for heparin, the type of heparin used, and the tests used to detect HAAbs. LMWHs are associated with a significantly decreased incidence of HAAb formation and HIT.[103] Up to 20% of patients who undergo vascular surgical procedures develop HAAbs, which are associated with a greater than twofold increased risk for thrombotic complications.[104] The incidence of HIT ranges between 2% and 9%, depending on the type of heparin used, the route of administration, and the definition of thrombocytopenia used.[105,106] Most authors use a platelet count of less than 100,000/mm^3 to define HIT-associated thrombocytopenia. However, thrombocytopenia is not a prerequisite for the development of thrombotic complications.

The diagnosis of HIT can be made according to the following criteria:
1. The development of thrombocytopenia or a significantly decreased platelet count while receiving heparin
2. Resolution of thrombocytopenia after cessation of heparin
3. Exclusion of other causes for thrombocytopenia
4. A positive HAAb assay (two-point platelet aggregation assay, serotonin release assay, enzyme-linked immunosorbent assay)

Patients who develop HIT or thrombosis in the setting of a positive HAAb assay should discontinue heparin immediately. Most patients require continued anticoagulation with alternative agents such as argatroban or recombinant hirudin. Long-term antithrombotic therapy with warfarin remains effective.

Hyperhomocysteinemia can be caused by inborn errors of metabolism (cystathionine β-synthase deficiency, methylene tetrahydrofolate reductase variant) or, more commonly, by acquired deficiencies in vitamin B$_6$, vitamin B$_{12}$, and folic acid. Elevated homocysteine is an independent risk factor for myocardial infarction, stroke, and peripheral arterial atherothrombosis[107]; it is also an independent inherited risk factor for venous thrombosis, with an odds ratio of approximately 2 to 2.5.[108-110] The risk may be much higher in patients with combined hyperhomocysteinemia and other thrombophilic conditions.[111,112] Homocystinemia can be detected using fasting plasma levels or after methionine loading (100 mg/kg). Elevated homocysteine levels can be effectively reduced with folate, vitamin B$_6$, and vitamin B$_{12}$ supplementation.[113] Despite this association, two randomized placebo-controlled trials have failed to show a reduction in VTE after correction of hyperhomocysteinemia.[114,115] The underlying link between hyperhomocysteinemia and increased VTE risk has yet to be elucidated.

Surgery and trauma are strong risk factors for the development of venous thrombosis. Venous thromboembolism occurs in up to 25% of patients undergoing general surgical procedures without thrombosis prophylaxis. Orthopedic procedures (hip and knee replacement, hip fracture repair) are associated with an even greater risk for venous thromboembolism (45% to 61%). The incidence of venous thromboembolism in trauma patients depends on the severity of injury. Multisystem trauma is associated with a greater than 50% incidence.[116]

Myeloproliferative diseases (polycythemia vera, chronic myelogenous leukemia, myeloid metaplasia, essential thrombocytosis), hypergammaglobulinemia, and hyperfibrinogenemia may predispose to thrombosis by causing a hyperviscous state. At clinical presentation, patients manifest cerebral (arterial and venous), coronary, pulmonary, and peripheral arterial and venous thromboemboli. Hemolytic-uremic syndrome and thrombotic thrombocytopenic purpura cause microvascular thromboses and thrombocytopenia.

Indications and Timing for Thrombophilia Screening

Before 1993, inherited prothrombotic conditions were detected in less than 10% to 15% of patients with venous thromboembolism. Since the discovery of factor V Leiden and the prothrombin 20210A mutation, the number of patients with detectable thrombophilia has increased significantly.

Currently, the *American Society of Hematology Education Program Book* suggests that testing for thrombophilia for patients with VTE is indicated for patients in the following clinical settings[117]:
1. Idiopathic first event
2. Secondary, non-cancer-related first event and age less than 50 years, including thrombosis on contraceptives or postmenopausal hormones

3. Recurrent idiopathic or secondary, non–cancer events
4. Thrombosis at an unusual site

Most authorities include cerebral, renal, portal, or hepatic vein thrombosis as unusual sites. However, the association with upper-extremity thrombosis or retinal vein thrombosis is less certain. Testing usually includes evaluations for activated protein-C resistance (a screening assay for factor V Leiden), prothrombin 20210A gene variant, testing for antithrombin, protein C, and protein S deficiency, factor VIII activity, fasting homocysteine, and testing for anticardiolipin antibodies and lupus anticoagulant. In patients with visceral vein thrombosis, testing for paroxysmal nocturnal hemoglobinuria (PNH) and myeloproliferative syndrome should be performed. PNH is screened for with a flow cytometry assay, and myeloproliferative syndromes are detected with DNA testing for the JAK2 mutation. Timing for the performance of these tests varies widely. In addition, patients who develop arterial or venous thrombosis while receiving heparin or LMWH should be tested for heparin-associated antiplatelet antibodies.

Acute thrombosis, inflammation, and a large thrombus burden can cause transient depression of antithrombin, protein C and protein S levels. Concomitant administration of oral vitamin K antagonists also decreases protein C and protein S activity. If abnormal results are obtained under these conditions, then repeated testing should be performed once the acute thrombosis has resolved and after discontinuation of the vitamin K antagonist. To avoid the need for repeated blood testing, many clinicians do not perform the thrombophilia testing until after 6 months of warfarin therapy, waiting 4 weeks after the vitamin K antagonists have been discontinued. It is also important to remember that many antiphospholipid antibodies are transient, and the official criteria for antiphospholipid antibody syndrome require two positive test results at least 12 weeks apart.

Management of Established Thrombosis

Unfractionated heparin, low-molecular-weight heparin, and warfarin are the most commonly used antithrombotic agents. Numerous other drugs have been made available by the FDA for limited indications. These drugs include recombinant hirudin, argatroban, fondaparinux, dabigatran, clopidogrel, and several GP IIb-IIIa receptor antagonists. Although numerous other agents are in development or in clinical trials (e.g., recombinant TFPI, GP Ib inhibitors, other factor IIA inhibitors), they are not discussed in this chapter.

Unfractionated and Low-Molecular-Weight Heparins

Unfractionated bovine lung and porcine intestinal heparin have been the mainstay of therapy for episodes of acute arterial (coronary, cerebral, peripheral arterial) and venous (deep venous) thromboses for the past several decades. Unfractionated heparins are glycosaminoglycans composed of repetitive disaccharide units (uronic acid and glucosamine) with molecular weights ranging from 4000 to 40,000 Da. LMWHs are derived from the enzymatic or alkaline degradation of unfractionated heparin purified from porcine intestinal mucosa. The average molecular weight of the various preparations ranges from 3000 to 6000 Da.[118]

Unfractionated heparin and LMWH bind to AT via a specific pentasaccharide sequence that is present in only 30% of molecules. This binding causes a conformational change in the AT molecule, exposing an active site for the neutralization of numerous activated coagulation factors. Factor Xa is inactivated via this mechanism. In contrast, factor IIa (thrombin) inactivation requires the formation of a ternary complex in which thrombin and AT bind to heparin molecules with at least 18 to 20 saccharide units. Only 25% to 50% of LMWH molecules contain this critical length, thus reducing their anti-IIa activity while maintaining anti-Xa activity. Unfractionated heparin and LMWH also cause a twofold to sixfold increase in TFPI via release from the endothelial surface. TFPI forms a complex with factors VIIa, Xa, and TF, inhibiting the conversion of factor IX to IXa and factor X to Xa.

Unfractionated heparin binds to numerous plasma proteins (platelet factor 4, vitronectin, fibronectin), platelet glycoprotein receptors, and vascular endothelium. This may be responsible for the variable bioavailability and anticoagulant response. Heparin is cleared via the reticuloendothelial cells (saturable) and kidneys (nonsaturable), resulting in a dose-dependent half-life that ranges from 45 to 150 minutes. LMWHs demonstrate less binding to plasma proteins and endothelium, resulting in a greater bioavailability and a more predictable therapeutic response. As a result, weight-adjusted doses may be administered without therapeutic monitoring. LMWHs are cleared primarily via the kidneys, with plasma half-lives that are twofold to fourfold longer than that of unfractionated heparin.

LMWHs are rapidly absorbed after subcutaneous injection. The dose varies according to the commercial preparation used. Some preparations with longer half-lives require only daily dosing. LMWH is at least as effective as, and is perhaps safer than, unfractionated heparin for some treatment indications (e.g., venous thromboembolism).[119] The primary advantage of LMWH is the convenience of infrequent subcutaneous dosing without the need for therapeutic monitoring assays, which may allow outpatient treatment in many cases. The lower incidence of HIT and osteoporosis is another advantage of LMWH. Disadvantages of LMWH include expense and the need for monitoring in certain patients, including those with advanced renal failure, morbid obesity, and pregnant patients.

Pentasaccharides

Fondaparinux is the only synthetic pentasaccharide currently available in the United States. It binds to and increases the activity of antithrombin, thereby inhibiting factor Xa, but it has no activity against factor IIa. It is indicated for VTE prophylaxis in orthopedic and high-risk general surgical patients and treatment of DVT and pulmonary embolism in medical or surgical patients. One of the major advantages of fondaparinux is the substantially lower risk of HIT compared with LMWH or unfractionated heparin. Fondaparinux is renally excreted and is not recommended for use in patients with renal failure or insufficiency.[120]

Direct Thrombin Inhibitors

Indirect thrombin inhibitors (unfractionated heparin and LMWH) have a limited ability to neutralize fibrin-bound thrombin and are dependent on adequate levels of AT. In contrast, direct thrombin inhibitors are capable of inhibiting thrombin on established thrombi and do not require the presence of antithrombin in order to exert anticoagulant effects.[121] Direct thrombin inhibitors are based on the naturally occurring anticoagulant produced in the salivary gland of the medicinal leech (Hirudo medicinalis). Hirudin derivatives (lepirudin and desirudin) and bivalirudin (a hirudin analog) are bivalent direct thrombin inhibitors. Univalent direct thrombin inhibitors include argatroban and ximelagatran.

Hirudin forms a stoichiometric complex with thrombin, blocking the catalytic site, substrate groove, and anion binding site, thus preventing the formation of fibrin and factors Va, VIIIa, and XIIIa.[122] Hirudin also inhibits thrombin-induced platelet activation and aggregation. It is excreted via the kidneys and has a half-life ranging from 1 to 2 hours. Patients with renal insufficiency or failure and patients weighing more than 110 kg require significant dose adjustments. Hirudin may also be administered subcutaneously.

Hirudin is currently approved for the management of HIT complicated by thrombosis.[123] However, the rate of adverse events still remains significant (up to 30%), probably reflecting the severity of illness in HIT patients. Numerous clinical trials have compared hirudin with heparin in the treatment of patients undergoing coronary angioplasty and coronary thrombolysis and patients with unstable angina. Hirudin was associated with a decreased risk for ischemic events compared with heparin therapy. Some trials also demonstrated an increased incidence of major hemorrhage, although this complication usually occurred when hirudin was given in conjunction with thrombolytic agents.[124] As with heparin, hirudin has the potential to cause an immunologic reaction with resulting anaphylaxis. Approximately 40% of patients develop detectable antihirudin antibodies; however, unlike heparin antibodies, they are not associated with the development of any resistance to therapy or with thromboembolic or bleeding complications.[125]

Bivalirudin is a synthetic, 20–amino acid polypeptide analog of hirudin that reversibly binds to thrombin. When compared with hirudin, it has several advantages, including the ability to administer the medication intravenously or subcutaneously. Bivalirudin also has a shorter half-life, a nonrenal route of metabolism, and decreased immunogenicity. Currently it is approved in the United States as an anticoagulant in patients with unstable angina who undergo angioplasty.[126]

Argatroban is a synthetic univalent direct thrombin inhibitor that reversibly binds to thrombin.[121] It is approved for use as an anticoagulant for prophylaxis or treatment of thrombosis in patients with HIT. It is also approved as an anticoagulant in patients undergoing percutaneous coronary intervention who are at risk for HIT. Argatroban has a short half-life of 39 to 51 minutes and reaches a steady state with IV infusion at 1 to 3 hours. The level of anticoagulation may be monitored with the aPTT or activated clotting time. Argatroban is metabolized primarily by the liver and is excreted in the feces via biliary secretion; therefore doses should be decreased in patients with hepatic impairment. When treating suspected or established HIT in vascular surgical patients, argatroban tends to be preferred over recombinant hirudin; this is likely related to the higher prevalence of renal insufficiency and lower prevalence of liver disease in our patient population.

The direct oral thrombin inhibitor dabigatran was approved in September 2010 as an alternative anticoagulant for patients with atrial fibrillation. Connolly and colleagues[127] showed that a twice per day dose of 110 mg of dabigatran was as effective as warfarin in reducing the risk of stroke and systemic embolism in patients with atrial fibrillation, with lower rates of hemorrhage, compared with warfarin. When given at 150 mg orally twice per day, dabigatran was associated with lower rates of stroke and systemic embolism and lower rates of bleeding, when compared with warfarin. The oral dose of 150 mg twice per day was approved by the FDA rather than the oral dose of 110 mg twice per day because although the bleeding risk was less in the 110-mg dose group (4.4/100 patient-years versus 5.1/100 patient-years), the stroke risk was slightly higher when compared with the 150-mg dose group (1.9/100 patient-years versus 1.4/100 patient-years). It is thought that the FDA believed that stroke was a worse outcome than bleeding and chose to approve the 150-mg dose instead of the 110-mg dose. An additional benefit to dabigatran is that its use does not require titration or serial laboratory INR monitoring.

Dabigatran also has been shown to be effective in the treatment of VTE when a 150-mg dose is taken twice daily.[128] Specifically, dabigatran was shown to be as effective as warfarin for the treatment of acute VTE, has a similar safety profile as warfarin, and does not require INR monitoring. The half-life of dabigatran ranges from 12 to 17 hours, and it is eliminated via renal excretion; therefore the dosing should be decreased to 75 mg by mouth twice per day if the patient has moderate to severe renal impairment.

Warfarin

Coumarin derivatives, including warfarin, block the vitamin K–dependent factors II, VII, IX, and X and proteins C and S. This blocking results in decreased coagulation factor biological activity by more than 95%. An antithrombotic state depends on the replacement of functional coagulation factors present in the circulation with the altered coagulation proteins. Although warfarin may prolong the PT within 24 hours, owing to factor VII depletion, an antithrombotic state is usually not attained for 2 to 4 days.

Warfarin is rapidly absorbed and reaches a maximum plasma concentration within 2 to 12 hours. Ninety-seven

BOX 5-2	Common Drug Interactions with Oral Anticoagulants

POTENTIATE	ANTAGONIZE
Acetaminophen	Barbiturates
Anabolic steroids	Carbamazepine
Cephalosporins	Chlordiazepoxide
Chloral hydrate	Cholestyramine
Cimetidine	Dicloxacillin
Ciprofloxacin	Griseofulvin
Clofibrate	Nafcillin
Cotrimoxazole	Rifampin
Disulfiram	Sucralfate
Erythromycin	Vitamin K
Fluconazole	
Isoniazid	
Itraconazole	
Metronidazole	
Omeprazole	
Phenylbutazone	
Phenytoin	
Piroxicam	
Propafenone	
Propoxyphene	
Propranolol	
Quinidine	
Sulfinpyrazone	
Tamoxifen	
Tetracycline	

From Hirsh J, Dalen JE, Anderson DR, et al: Oral anticoagulants: mechanism of action, clinical effectiveness, and optimal therapeutic range, Chest 114(Suppl):445S–469S, 1998; and Wells PS, Holbrook AM, Crowther NR, et al: The interaction of warfarin with drugs and food: a critical review of the literature, Ann Intern Med 121:676–683, 1994.

percent of warfarin circulates bound to albumin, with the unbound portion being responsible for the anticoagulant effect. The amount of warfarin required to cause a prolongation of the PT depends on the amount of dietary vitamin K, the age of the patient, and comorbid conditions (liver failure, obstructive jaundice, starvation). Numerous medications have been found to potentiate or interfere with the activity of warfarin (Box 5-2). Patients receiving long-term oral anticoagulation who begin or stop a medication that may interfere with or potentiate warfarin activity should be monitored with more frequent PT measurements.

Warfarin therapy is initiated by the oral intake of 5 to 7.5 mg once per day. Reduced doses should be given to older patients and those with liver disease or vitamin K deficiency as a result of malnutrition or long-term parenteral feeding. Because factor II and factor X depletion might not be effective for 2 to 4 days, heparin or an alternative agent should be administered during the first few days of warfarin therapy for patients who require immediate anticoagulation. The PT assay is most commonly used to monitor warfarin therapy.

The primary complication of warfarin therapy is hemorrhage, which occurs in 3% to 12% of patients.[129] Less common complications include alopecia, urticaria, dermatitis, fever, nausea, diarrhea, abdominal cramping, and

hypersensitivity reactions. Dermal gangrene is a rare complication (0.01% to 0.1% of patients receiving warfarin) caused by the rapid depletion of protein C before depletion of factors II, IX, and X.[130] This risk increases to approximately 3% in patients with protein C deficiency.[131] Concomitant administration of unfractionated heparin or LMWH should decrease the risk of this complication.

Direct Factor Xa Inhibitors

Rivaroxaban is an orally administered direct factor Xa inhibitor that does not require antithrombin as a cofactor. It has a half-life that ranges from 5 to 9 hours, and it is eliminated via renal excretion, fecal excretion, and hepatic metabolism. Rivaroxaban was approved by the FDA in July 2011 as a prophylaxis against deep vein thrombosis (DVT) and pulmonary embolism in patients who undergo knee or hip replacement surgery (at a dose of 10 mg by mouth daily). Rivaroxaban (at a dosage of 15 mg by mouth twice per day for 3 weeks, followed by 20 mg by mouth daily) also has been shown not to be inferior to subcutaneously administered therapeutic enoxaparin in combination with orally administered warfarin in patients with acute symptomatic DVT.[132] Although rivaroxaban results in a dose-dependent prolongation of the PT, aPTT, and factor Xa activity, these assays and the INR have not been tested as an accurate method to monitor anticoagulation.

Thromboembolism Prophylaxis

Venous Thromboembolism Prophylaxis

The annual incidence of DVT is between 69 and 139 cases per 100,000 people in the general population.[133] The prevalence of VTE in hospitalized patients is approximately 350 cases per 100,000 admissions and is a cause of death in approximately 250,000 people per year.[134,135] Pulmonary embolism contributes to or causes up to 12% of all deaths in hospitalized patients.[136] DVT poses an immediate threat to life because of the potential for pulmonary embolism and may also lead to long-term impairment owing to resultant venous insufficiency. The 20-year cumulative incidence rate is 26.8% and 3.7% for the development of venous stasis changes and venous ulcers, respectively, after an episode of DVT.[137]

General risk factors for VTE include blood flow stasis, endothelial damage, and hypercoagulability. Relative hypercoagulability appears to be most important in the majority of cases of spontaneous DVT, whereas stasis and endothelial damage are more important in DVT following surgery or trauma. Specific risk factors include prior history of VTE, age, surgery, malignancy, obesity, trauma, varicosities, cardiac disease, hormones, immobilization or paralysis, pregnancy, venous catheterization, and hypercoagulable states.[96,97,136,138-145] In one population-based study, more than 90% of patients hospitalized for VTE had more than one risk factor.[136] In surgical patients, the risk of VTE is dependent on the type of operation and the presence of one or more risk factors.[146] Without prophylaxis, patients undergoing surgery for intraabdominal malignancy have a 25% incidence of DVT; orthopedic patients undergoing hip fracture surgery have a 40% to 50% incidence of DVT in the postoperative period. Those at highest risk are older patients undergoing major surgery or those with previous VTE, malignancy, or paralysis.

The incidence of venous thrombosis and pulmonary embolism may be reduced by limiting venous stasis, administering drugs to inhibit coagulation, or a combination of these approaches. Stasis is reduced by ambulation and pneumatic compression of the lower extremities.

Intermittent pneumatic compression (IPC) devices reduce lower extremity venous stasis, enhance fibrinolytic activity, and increase plasma levels of TFPI.[147] Elastic stockings also decrease stasis and increase venous flow velocities. Both devices appear to decrease the incidence of DVT in patients who undergo general, urologic, and gynecologic surgical procedures. The incidence of DVT in control patients ranges from 20% to 27%, whereas the use of IPC is associated with a DVT incidence of 10% to 18%.[139,148] IPC devices also decrease the incidence of DVT in patients undergoing hip or knee replacement; however, mechanical prophylaxis alone is not sufficient in patients undergoing total hip replacement and should be supplemented with either LMWH or adjusted-dose unfractionated heparin or warfarin.[116] The effectiveness of IPC devices is limited by a lack of compliance among patients and nursing staff. Intermittent pneumatic foot compression devices can improve patient acceptance; however, these devices are less effective than other forms of DVT prophylaxis.[149]

Subcutaneous heparin is used to decrease the incidence of VTE. Unfractionated heparin decreases the overall incidence of venous thrombosis to approximately 8%.[116] The incidence of pulmonary embolism is reduced as well. This regimen is probably adequate in moderate- and high-risk general surgical patients. Two large meta-analyses have demonstrated that LMWH confers no additional protection in this population and may be associated with an increased risk of hemorrhagic complications.[150,151]

It should be noted that fixed low-dose unfractionated heparin prophylaxis is not as effective in patients with hip fractures or in those undergoing total hip or knee replacement. Orthopedic and very high-risk general surgical patients should receive more effective DVT prophylaxis such as LMWH, adjusted-dose warfarin, adjusted-dose unfractionated heparin, or combination prophylaxis with IPC. The aPTT does not require monitoring in patients receiving fixed-dose unfractionated heparin or LMWH prophylaxis. Platelet counts should be monitored for the detection of HIT.

LMWH produces fewer thromboembolic complications than unfractionated heparin does. Early use of LMWH for VTE prophylaxis is contraindicated in patients with intracranial bleeding, spinal hematoma, ongoing and uncontrolled hemorrhage, or uncorrected coagulopathy. Patients who undergo major orthopedic procedures without DVT prophylaxis are at high risk for thromboembolic complications (45% to 61%). Depending on the preparation, LMWH decreases the incidence significantly (15% to 31%) compared with fixed-dose

unfractionated heparin (27% to 42%).[116,152] Preoperative initiation of LMWH (versus beginning postoperatively) can decrease the overall incidence of DVT in patients undergoing hip replacement (10% preoperative versus 15.3% postoperative) without increasing the incidence of hemorrhage.[153] There is also evidence that longer durations of prophylaxis are more effective. Several randomized trials have found a significantly lower rate of thrombosis with 21 to 35 days of LMWH administration.[154-156]

Numerous randomized trials have compared various LMWH preparations (enoxaparin, certoparin, dalteparin, nadroparin, parnaparin, reviparin, tinzaparin) against unfractionated heparin as DVT prophylaxis in general surgical patients. Only 4 of 29 trials identified a significant improvement with LMWH.[157] Although the dosing regimens varied widely among trials, there was a tendency toward superior prophylaxis with LMWH when higher doses were used. Very high-risk patients who undergo general surgical procedures (multiple risk factors, malignancy, thrombophilia) may benefit most from LMWH prophylaxis. The optimal timing for the first prophylactic dose of LMWH remains in question. General surgical patients who receive the first dose before surgery do not appear to experience any additional hemorrhagic complications.[157]

Fondaparinux is a chemically synthesized agent that binds and activates antithrombin, which then selectively inhibits factor Xa. It does not act against thrombin. Because fondaparinux is chemically synthesized, it does not contain any animal products. It is specific to antithrombin and does not bind to platelets, thereby minimizing the risk of HIT. The results of a randomized, double-blinded trial comparing fondaparinux and LMWH for the prevention of VTE after elective hip replacement surgery showed no statistical difference between the two groups in the incidence of VTE.[158] The incidence of VTE was 6% in the fondaparinux group and 8% in the enoxaparin group. There was also no difference in the incidence of major bleeding complications. Fondaparinux is indicated for VTE prophylaxis in orthopedic patients and treatment of VTE and pulmonary embolism in medical and surgical patients.

Warfarin has been established in several studies as efficacious prophylaxis against VTE. Sevitt and Gallagher[159] found that the incidence of clinical venous thrombosis in patients with hip fractures decreased from 28.7% in the control group to 2.7% in the group treated with oral anticoagulation. At autopsy, the incidence of thrombosis in the two groups was 83% and 14%, respectively.[159] In other studies, oral anticoagulants with an INR range of 2 to 3 were effective in preventing venous thrombosis in patients undergoing orthopedic and gynecologic surgery.[160,161]

Very high-risk patients, such as those undergoing major orthopedic procedures, should receive either LMWH or adjusted-dose warfarin. LMWH may be more effective than warfarin, but the difference is probably small. If warfarin is selected, it should be started preoperatively or immediately after surgery. The dose should be adjusted to achieve a target INR between 2 and 3.[116] With warfarin, the duration of prophylaxis can be extended easily in patients who continue to have risk factors for VTE (e.g., immobility, malignancy, a history of previous venous thrombosis).

Arterial Thromboembolism Prophylaxis

Arterial thrombosis occurs in regions with disturbed flow or disrupted endothelial coverage (as with plaque rupture or endarterectomy). Subendothelial collagen and vWF initiate platelet adhesion and activation, whereas TF activates the coagulation cascade, leading to the generation of thrombin and fibrin. Arterial thrombi contain relatively higher concentrations of platelets. As a result, most long-term arterial antithrombotic regimens focus on the inhibition of platelet function.

Aspirin acetylates platelet COX1, blocking the conversion of arachidonic acid to the prostaglandin endoperoxides PGH_2 and PGG_2; this effectively inhibits the synthesis of TXA_2 for the lifespan of the platelet. Aspirin also inhibits prostacyclin synthesis by endothelial cells; however, endothelial cells have nuclei and can synthesize new prostacyclin synthetase, reversing the effects of aspirin.

Aspirin is the most widely used antithrombotic agent, and there is considerable evidence supporting its efficacy in reducing the relative risk of serious vascular events (nonfatal myocardial infarction, nonfatal stroke, vascular death) in patients at high risk for these complications. The Antithrombotic Trialists' Collaboration (ATTC) reviewed 287 studies encompassing more than 135,000 patients and noted absolute reductions in serious vascular events in patients with recent or remote myocardial infarction, stroke or transient ischemic attack, stable angina, peripheral arterial disease, and atrial fibrillation.[162] Nonfatal myocardial infarction risk was reduced by 33%, nonfatal stroke was reduced by 25%, and vascular death was reduced by 16%. Of note, the risk of hemorrhagic complications outweighs the benefits of aspirin therapy in patients at low risk for cardiovascular events.[119,124,163] In general, lower doses of aspirin (75 to 150 mg/day) are effective. The ATTC concluded that aspirin (75 to 150 mg/day) is recommended routinely for all patients without contraindications and who are at high or intermediate risk for vascular events (>2% per year risk), regardless of whether they have had a prior vascular event. Aspirin is also efficacious in maintaining vascular graft patency after lower extremity revascularization. The Seventh Antithrombotic Consensus Conference, the American Heart Association, and the American College of Cardiology recommend aspirin (80 to 325 mg/day) for prosthetic or saphenous vein peripheral bypass grafts and after carotid endarterectomy.[164,165]

Ticlopidine and clopidogrel are thienopyridine derivatives that irreversibly inhibit ADP-mediated platelet activation. Both are rapidly absorbed after oral administration and are highly bound to plasma proteins. Ticlopidine may alter platelet function within 24 to 48 hours, but maximum inhibition is not achieved for 8 to 11 days. Clopidogrel induces a more rapid, dose-dependent inhibition of platelet aggregation within 2 hours.

Ticlopidine significantly improves the patency of femoropopliteal and femorotibial saphenous vein grafts (66% versus 51% at 2 years) compared with placebo.[166] Compared with aspirin, ticlopidine also is associated with a decreased risk of stroke (10% versus 13%).[167] Other studies have demonstrated a decreased risk of myocardial infarction in patients with unstable angina and improved walking distance in patients with claudication; however, no studies have demonstrated that ticlopidine is superior to aspirin in improving lower extremity vascular graft patency.[168,169] In addition, widespread use of ticlopidine is limited by the potentially severe side effects of pancytopenia and neutropenia.[170]

Clopidogrel has been advocated as an antiplatelet agent with an efficacy superior to that of aspirin. The Clopidogrel versus Aspirin in Patients at Risk of Ischaemic Events (CAPRIE) study evaluated more than 19,000 patients with a history of recent ischemic stroke, recent myocardial infarction, or symptomatic atherosclerotic peripheral vascular disease.[171] Clopidogrel was associated with a relative risk reduction of 8.7% for future ischemic events, representing an absolute reduction of only 0.5% (5.32% with clopidogrel, 5.83% with aspirin); however, subgroup analyses demonstrated that patients with peripheral vascular disease received the greatest degree of risk reduction.

Clopidogrel may be more beneficial as a combination therapy agent, because aspirin and clopidogrel inhibit platelet function via different signal transduction pathways (TXA_2 and ADP inhibition). Some evidence for this comes from the more recent Clopidogrel in Unstable Angina to Prevent Recurrent Events (CURE) trial, involving more than 12,500 patients.[172] Patients receiving clopidogrel and aspirin had a decreased incidence of cardiovascular death, myocardial infarction, or stroke when compared with those receiving aspirin alone (9.3% versus 11.4%, representing a 20% relative risk reduction). The incidence of neutropenia and pancytopenia with clopidogrel is similar to the incidence with aspirin or placebo.

Glycoprotein IIb-IIIa inhibitors have been evaluated for stroke prevention in clinical trials. Fibrinogen binds to the platelet GP IIb-IIIa receptor via the amino acid sequence Arg-Gly-Asp (RGD), representing the final common pathway for platelet aggregation regardless of the platelet agonist. The first GP IIb-IIIa inhibitor to be developed was abciximab, the antigen-binding fragment of a monoclonal anti-GP IIb-IIIa antibody. The primary indication for the use of GP IIb-IIIa receptor antagonists is for acute coronary syndromes. GP IIb-IIIa inhibitors have no role in the long-term prevention of stroke or complications related to peripheral vascular disease.

Warfarin has an established role in the prevention of thromboembolism in selected patients with atrial fibrillation and prosthetic heart valves. Other possible indications for long-term warfarin therapy include the prevention of myocardial ischemia and the prevention of systemic embolism after acute myocardial infarction.[173]

Several studies also indicate that warfarin may improve the patency of lower extremity bypass grafts. In a randomized trial involving 130 patients who underwent femoropopliteal vein bypass surgery, Kretschmer and colleagues[174,175] found improved patency, limb salvage, and overall survival in patients receiving phenprocoumon (a coumarin derivative). Flinn and colleagues[176] also found that warfarin improved patency in patients with infrageniculate prosthetic grafts. More recent studies involving patients at high risk for failure (e.g., suboptimal vein, poor outflow, redo procedures) have confirmed an improved patency with warfarin plus aspirin compared with aspirin alone.[177] Long-term warfarin therapy is a reasonable option for most patients with prosthetic infrainguinal or axillofemoral bypass grafts, suboptimal venous conduit, or poor outflow tracts (e.g., isolated popliteal arteries). Patients who are treated with warfarin should receive overlapping unfractionated heparin, LMWH, or IV heparin until the therapeutic INR is achieved (target INR, 2 to 3).

BIBLIOGRAPHY

Almeida JI, Coats R, Liem TK, et al: Reduced morbidity and mortality of the heparin-induced thrombocytopenia syndrome. J Vasc Surg 27:309–314, 1998.

Antiplatelet Trialists' Collaboration: Collaborative overview of randomised trials of antiplatelet therapy. I. Prevention of death, myocardial infarction, and stroke by prolonged antiplatelet therapy in various categories of patients. BMJ 308:81–106, 1994.

Eriksson H, Wahlander K, Gustafsson D, et al: A randomized, controlled, dose-guiding study of the oral direct thrombin inhibitor ximelagatran compared with standard therapy for the treatment of acute deep vein thrombosis: THRIVE I. J Thromb Haemost 1:41–47, 2003.

Hiatt WR: Preventing atherothrombotic events in peripheral arterial disease: the use of antiplatelet therapy. J Intern Med 251:193–206, 2002.

Hirsh J, Dalen J, Guyatt G: The sixth (2000) ACCP guidelines for antithrombotic therapy for prevention and treatment of thrombosis: American College of Chest Physicians. Chest 119:1S–370S, 2001.

Lowe GDO: State of the art 2003: XIX Congress of the International Society on Thrombosis and Haemostasis. J Thromb Haemost 1: 1335–1670, 2003.

Manco-Johnson MJ, Riske B, Kasper CK: Advances in care of children with hemophilia. Semin Thromb Hemost 29:585–594, 2003.

Midathada MV, Mehta P, Waner M, et al: Recombinant factor VIIa in the treatment of bleeding. Am J Clin Pathol 121:124–137, 2004.

Ridker PM, Goldhaber SZ, Danielson E, et al: Long-term, low-intensity warfarin therapy for the prevention of recurrent venous thromboembolism. N Engl J Med 348:1425–1434, 2003.

Warkentin TE: Management of heparin-induced thrombocytopenia: a critical comparison of lepirudin and argatroban. Thromb Res 110:73–82, 2003.

References available online at expertconsult.com.

QUESTIONS

1. Which of the following statements regarding antiplatelet therapy is true?
   a. Lower dosages of aspirin (75 to 150 mg/day) are not as effective as higher dosages (325 mg/day) for the prevention of cerebrovascular ischemic events.
   b. Ticlopidine is associated with a small but significant incidence of neutropenia.
   c. Compared with aspirin, clopidogrel is associated with a significantly greater incidence of neutropenia.
   d. For the prevention of ischemic events, combination therapy with clopidogrel and aspirin is no better than aspirin alone.

2. Regarding the management of heparin-induced thrombocytopenia (HIT), which of the following is true?
   a. Unfractionated heparin and low-molecular-weight heparin have a similar incidence of heparin-associated antibody formation.
   b. Low-molecular-weight heparin can be administered safely in patients with established HIT.
   c. The platelet count must be less than 100,000/mm³ to be diagnosed with HIT.
   d. Antihirudin antibodies develop in approximately 40% of patients receiving hirudin, but resistance to therapy is uncommon.

3. Which of the following statements regarding von Willebrand disease is false?
   a. Defects of primary hemostasis commonly cause petechiae and ecchymoses.
   b. Hemophilic disorders commonly cause hemarthroses and deep tissue hematomas.
   c. Von Willebrand disease is the most common inherited bleeding disorder.
   d. Type 1 von Willebrand disease is usually unresponsive to DDAVP.
   e. Cryoprecipitate and some factor VIII concentrates are rich in vWF.

4. Which of the following statements regarding thrombophilic conditions is true?
   a. Elevated homocysteine levels are associated with arterial and venous thromboses.
   b. The prothrombin 20210A mutation results in resistance to antithrombin.
   c. Warfarin is ineffective in patients with antiphospholipid syndrome.
   d. Activated protein C resistance may be due to a defect in protein C or protein S.
   e. Antithrombin concentrates are the mainstay of therapy for antithrombin-deficient patients with venous thromboembolism.

5. Following major surgical procedures in patients with hemophilia A, factor VIII:C plasma activity should be at least:
   a. 5% of normal
   b. 25% of normal
   c. 50% of normal
   d. 75% of normal
   e. 100% of normal

6. Which of the following statements regarding low-molecular-weight heparin (LMWH) is false?
   a. LMWHs demonstrate less binding to plasma proteins and endothelium.
   b. LMWHs preferentially inactivate factor Xa over factor IIa.
   c. LMWH thrombosis prophylaxis is superior to unfractionated heparin prophylaxis in orthopedic surgery patients.
   d. LMWH is clearly superior to unfractionated heparin for routine general surgical procedures.

7. Which of the following statements regarding danaparoid, hirudin, and argatroban is true?
   a. There is no significant cross-reactivity between danaparoid and heparin in patients with heparin-associated antibodies.
   b. Hirudin is a direct thrombin inhibitor, preventing the formation of fibrin.
   c. Hirudin therapy does not have to be adjusted in patients with renal failure.
   d. Argatroban dosing should be adjusted in patients with hepatic insufficiency.
   e. Hirudin therapy may be monitored with the aPTT, and argatroban may be monitored with the PT.

8. Which of the following statements regarding the risk associated with pregnancy and hormonal therapy is false?
   a. The risk of venous thrombosis decreases after delivery.
   b. The thrombosis risks associated with oral contraceptives are immediate and reversible.
   c. Oral contraceptives are associated with a two- to fourfold increased risk for venous thrombosis.
   d. LMWHs have been shown to be safe and effective in pregnant patients with venous thromboembolism.

9. Which of the following is not a vitamin K–dependent coagulation factor?
   a. Factor II
   b. Factor V
   c. Factor VII
   d. Factor IX
   e. Factor X

10. Which of the following is not a major regulator of the coagulation cascade?
    a. Antithrombin
    b. Protein C
    c. Protein S
    d. Tissue factor pathway inhibitor
    e. Heparin cofactor II

ANSWERS

1. **b**
2. **d**
3. **d**
4. **a**
5. **c**
6. **d**
7. **d**
8. **a**
9. **b**
10. **e**

CHAPTER 6

ATHEROSCLEROSIS: PATHOLOGY, PATHOGENESIS, AND MEDICAL MANAGEMENT

Ralph G. DePalma

Vascular surgeons commonly treat patients with the complications of atherosclerosis. Currently, more precise lesion classification and imaging, a better understanding of atherogenesis, and increasingly effective medical treatment before and after vascular interventions promise improved long-term results. A better understanding of atherosclerosis and technical advances for its treatment now provide scientifically based prevention and management strategies. The pivotal role of lipids in the pathogenesis of atherosclerosis has been delineated, along with the effects of treatment on plaques and the recognition of the crucial role of inflammatory and immune responses which affect arterial plaques. Novel risk factors for late progression, independent of conventional risk factors, have been identified; these comprise elevated blood levels of biomarkers such as inflammatory cytokines, metalloproteinases, and smooth muscle growth factors including glucose and insulin. Advanced imaging can detect unstable plaques that are prone to rupture, thrombosis, and downstream embolization. Prospective randomized trials using drugs, micronutrients, and other interventions continue to provide therapeutic guidelines. Coronary thrombosis or stroke, the main causes of death in patients with peripheral arterial disease,[1] require active management strategies to improve survival and enhance long-term reconstructive results.

Vascular surgeons must be familiar with the location and natural history of individual lesions and, in considering various interventions, distinguish primary prevention from secondary treatment. When active intervention is required, vascular surgeons will use strategies geared toward the pathology of a specific vascular lesion in particular arterial sites. For example, a stenotic lesion composed of smooth muscle and well-organized collagen, although producing some degree of distal ischemia, is a much safer lesion than a plaque containing an unstable core of atheromatous debris beneath a tenuous cap. The smooth stenosis of an adductor hiatus plaque in the femoral artery, causing stable claudication, is clearly not as threatening as unstable carotid or coronary plaques characterized by soft cores beneath friable caps; these lesions have differing vulnerabilities based on differing composition and morphology.[2] It is now recognized that operative or endovascular treatment of segmental lesions does not prevent the progression of systemic atherosclerosis elsewhere. Medical treatment is required to ensure long-term results.

Variations in patterns and rates of progression of atherosclerosis have critical clinical implications for the timing and choice of treatment.[3,4] Considering the atherosclerotic process as a single disease leads to oversimplification. With considerable lesion diversity and clinical presentations, atherosclerosis can be viewed as a polypathogenic process comprising a group of closely related vascular disorders.[5,6] Multiple risk factors promoting atherosclerosis and its complications include dyslipidemia, smoking, diabetes, hypertension, and proinflammatory factors. This multiplicity of disease-promoting factors make a single-disease–single-etiology view difficult to reconcile. This chapter considers atherosclerosis as though it were a single entity, at the same time recognizing its variable pathology and differing clinical presentations. Despite the complexity of this process, new concepts for treatment have resulted in increasingly favorable outcomes. This progress is based on advances in surgical approaches and effective medical therapy based on a better understanding of the pathology and pathogenesis of this disease.

Theories of pathogenesis can be understood relative to their usefulness for predicting and controlling the disease; each, in part, is relevant in devising treatment strategies. Particular elements of various pathogenetic theories are more or less applicable in formulating treatment approaches. For example, direct interventions combined with medical treatment for symptomatic unstable carotid and coronary atheromas are needed. In contrast, medical treatment often suffices for quiescent plaques in stable claudicants.

PATHOLOGY

General Concepts

The term *atheroma* derives from the Greek *athere*, meaning "porridge" or "gruel"; *sclerosis* means "induration" or "hardening." A gruel-like color and consistency and induration or hardening exist to various degrees in different plaques, different disease stages, and different individuals. In 1755, von Haller[7] first applied the term *atheroma* to a common type of plaque that, on sectioning, exuded a yellow, pultaceous content from its core.[7] Figure 6-1 illustrates a typical fibrous plaque containing a central atheromatous core with a fibrous or fibromuscular cap, macrophage accumulation, and round cell

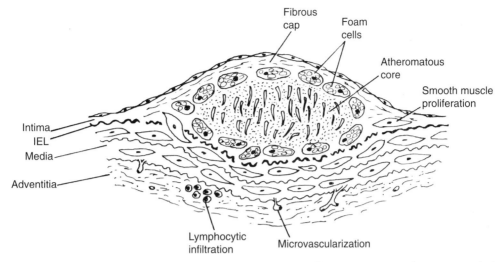

FIGURE 6-1 ■ Typical atheroma or type IV lesion. Note the central lipid core, fibrous cap, macrophage accumulation, and zone of synthetically active smooth muscle at the "shoulders" of the core. Note too the tendency of the lesion to bulge outward, neovascularization, and adventitial lymphocyte infiltration. *IEL*, Internal elastic lamina. (Modified from DePalma RG: Pathology of atheromas. In Bell PRF, Jamieson CW, Ruckley CV, editors: Surgical management of vascular disease, London, 1992, WB Saunders, p 21.)

adventitial infiltration. A past, generic definition of atherosclerotic plaque as "a variable combination of changes in the intima of arteries consisting of focal accumulation of lipids, complex carbohydrates, blood and blood products, fibrous tissue and calcium deposits"[8] failed to encompass the spectrum of atherosclerotic lesions. Advanced plaques invade the media, and at certain stages produce bulging or even enlarged arteries. Round cell infiltration, medial changes, and neovascularization characterize advanced atherosclerotic lesions. The atherosclerotic process ultimately involves the entire arterial wall. The process is complex and variable and, although all atherosclerotic lesions may not evolve in the same way, certain patterns of its progression are more common than others.

The development and expansion of the lipid atherosclerotic core and its relationship to an overlying cap have been recognized as causes of plaque complications. The observation of a lipid "core," developing early in atherosclerosis and accumulating in the deep aspects of early lesions before actual fibrous plaque formation begins, is a key insight.[9] Another important insight is the recognition of the role of inflammation and immune reactions in the early and late stages of atherogenesis.[10,11] The inflammatory cascade includes the appearance of proinflammatory cytokines such as interleukin-6 (IL-6), tumor necrosis factor (TNF) α, and antiinflammatory cytokines such as IL-10 within arterial tissue and in the bloodstream. Lipid accumulation appears to attract inflammatory cells that produce cytokines locally, whereas cytokines or biomarkers derived from a variety of tissues appear systemically in atherosclerotic subjects. For example, in atherosclerotic claudicants, plasma levels of inflammatory cytokines TNF-α and IL-6 are elevated, whereas antiinflammatory IL-10 levels are reduced.[12] Elevated levels of cytokines such as TNF-α and its receptors have also been shown to affect the arterial wall.[13-15] The atherosclerotic plaque contains leukocytes, of which

approximately 80% are monocytes or monocyte-derived macrophages. Lymphocytes, predominantly memory T cells,[16] constitute 5% to 20% of this cell population. Inflammation, size, and composition of the lipid core determine plaque instability or "vulnerability," promoting sudden expansion, rupture, release of distal emboli, and vascular occlusion.

Fatty Streaks

The first stages of atherosclerosis, fatty streaks, minimally raised yellow lesions, develop in characteristically vulnerable segments of the arterial tree. These lesions contain lipids deposited intracellularly in macrophages and in smooth muscle cells. Stary and colleagues[17] defined initial fatty streaks and intermediate lesions of atherosclerosis as follows: type I lesions in children are early microscopic lesions, consisting of an increase in intimal macrophages and the appearance of foam cells. Type II fatty streak lesions are grossly visible; in contrast to type I lesions, type II lesions stain with Sudan III or IV. Foam cells and lipid droplets appear in intimal smooth muscle cells and heterogeneous droplets of extracellular lipids characterize type II fatty streaks. Type III lesions are intermediate lesions, considered to be the bridge between the fatty streak (Figure 6-2) and the prototypical atheromatous fibrous plaque, the type IV plaque (see Figure 6-1).[17] Type III lesions occur in plaque-prone locations in the arterial tree[19] at sites exposed to forces (particularly low-shear stress) promoting increased low-density lipoprotein (LDL) influx.[20]

The fatty streak type II lipids are chemically similar to those of plasma.[21] Plasma lipids can enter the arterial wall in several ways. As described in a review of pathogenesis,[22] LDL accumulation can occur because of (1) alterations in the permeability of the intima; (2) increases in the intimal interstitial space; (3) poor metabolism of LDL by vascular cells; (4) impeded transport of LDL from the

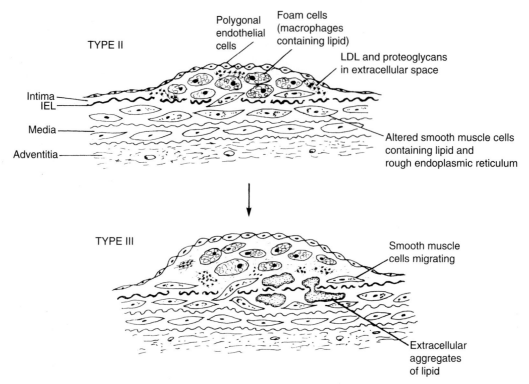

FIGURE 6-2 ■ Type II fatty streak lesions with foam cells. Note the low-density lipoprotein (LDL) particles in the matrix and altered smooth muscle cells, with developed rough endoplasmic reticulum also containing lipid particles. Note too the evolution to an intermediate, more advanced lesion (type III) containing extracellular aggregates or pools of lipid deep in the intima and extending into the media. *IEL,* Internal elastic lamina. (From DePalma RG: Atherosclerosis: theories of etiology and pathogenesis. In Sidawy AN, Sumpio BE, DePalma RG, editors: Basic science of vascular disease, Armonk, NY, 1997, Futura Publishing, pp 319-332.)

intima to the media; (5) increased plasma LDL concentrations; or (6) specific binding of LDL to connective tissue components, particularly proteoglycans in the arterial intima. Experimental studies show that LDL cholesterol accumulates in the intima even before lesions develop and in the presence of intact endothelium. These observations comport with classic descriptions of lesion formation by Aschoff[23] in the early twentieth century and Virchow[24] in the mid nineteenth century.

A second event in early atherogenesis, as shown in animal experiments, is binding of monocytes to the endothelial lining, with their subsequent diapedesis into the subintimal layer to become tissue macrophages.[25-27] Fatty streaks are populated mainly by monocyte-derived macrophages. These lipid-engorged scavenger cells mainly become the foam cells characterizing fatty streaks and more advanced lesions. LDL is altered by oxidation or acetylation to be taken up by the macrophages to form foam cells.[28] Oxidized LDL itself is a powerful chemoattractant for monocytes. Another aspect of this theory suggests that the endothelium modifies LDL to promote foam cell formation. In either case, oxidative reactions are seen as enhancing atheroma development.

The initial interactions of plasma LDL with the arterial wall and macrophage appear as the basis for earliest lesion formation. LDL traverses the endothelium mostly through receptor-independent transport, possibly also through cell breaks.[29] Endothelial cells,[30] smooth cells,[31] and macrophages[32] are capable of promoting oxidation of

LDL. The oxidized LDL, in turn, further attracts monocytes into the intima to promote their transformation into macrophages. Macrophages produce cytokines, which initiates the cytokine inflammatory cascade. Oxidized LDL also induces gene products that are ordinarily not expressed in normal vascular tissue. A notable example is tissue factor, the cellular initiator of the coagulation cascade abundantly expressed by atheroma monocytes and foam cells.[33] Expression of tissue factor requires the presence of bacterial lipopolysaccharide, suggesting that hypercoagulability in atherosclerosis might be enhanced by infectious factors.

Large numbers of macrophages and T lymphocytes in the plaques suggest cellular immune responses; oxidized lipoproteins, heat shock proteins, and microorganisms are possible antigens. A study analyzing endarterectomy specimens by immunohistochemistry and reverse transcription polymerase chain reaction showed proinflammatory T cell cytokines, IL-2, and interferon-7 in a large proportion of plaques, indicating that a helper T cell 1–type cellular immune response likely occurs in the atherosclerotic plaque.[34]

Endothelium

Animal studies reveal that endothelial cells tend to be oriented away from the direction of flow; these cells show increased stigmata or stomata, increased proliferation, and a decrease in microfilament bundles.[25,26] In humans and animals, endothelial cells become polyhedral or rounded; in humans, increased formation of multinucleated cells and cilia occurs. Animal studies reveal increased proliferation and cell death, with retraction and exposure of subendothelial foam cells. The endothelium becomes more permeable to macromolecules in experimental models; in humans, it exhibits increased tissue factor expression and mural thrombus formation. Leukocyte adherence increases with the expression of a monocyte adhesion molecule (VCAM-1). Endothelium-derived relaxing factor and prostacyclin release are decreased and vasoconstriction is enhanced.

Media

The smooth muscle shows increased proliferation, with increased rough endoplasmic reticulum, phenotypic changes, and increased production of altered intracellular and extracellular matrices. In humans, these matrices include increased expression of type I and type III collagen, dermatan sulfate, proteoglycan, and stromelysin. The smooth muscle cells produce cytokines, including macrophage colony-stimulating factor, TNF, and monocyte chemoattractant protein-1. Myocytes accumulate native and modified lipoproteins by both native receptor pathways and nonspecific phagocytosis. These cells also express increased lipoprotein lipase activity; experimentally they display a scavenger receptor similar to that of foam cells.

Macrophages

Macrophages proliferate and express monocyte chemoattractant protein-1, macrophage colony-stimulating factor, TNF, IL-1 and other interleukins, and platelet-derived growth factor (PDGF), along with CD immune antigens and, as previously described, tissue factor.[33] Plaque macrophages contain increased free and esterified cholesterol and increased acetyl coenzyme A, cholesterol acyltransferase, and acid cholesterol ester hydrolase. Neutral cholesterol ester hydrolase is decreased. These altered cells also express the scavenger receptor 15-lipoxygenase and exhibit increased lipoprotein oxidation products in humans and in animal models. These extensive changes indicate the complexity of the morphologic, functional, biochemical, and genetic expressions of the arterial wall in early atherosclerosis. The reader is referred to an original report for comprehensive details,[17] with references for the cellular alterations given.

Gelatinous Plaques

Intimal gelatinous lesions may, less commonly, be considered atheroma precursors. Haust described these lesions in 1971,[35] first noted in 1856 by Virchow[24] as potential progenitors of advanced atherosclerosis. Smith later described their identification and composition.[36] Gelatinous plaques are translucent and neutral in color, with central grayish opaque areas. Most plaques are characterized by finely dispersed, perifibrous lipid along with collagen strands around the lesions. Grossly, gelatinous lesions feel soft. With gentle lateral pressure, these

plaques "wobble." Gelatinous plaques can be the gelatinous material separates easily from the underlying arterial wall without entering a conventional endarterectomy plane. Gelatinous plaques appear in the aorta as extensive areas of flat, translucent thickenings, particularly in its lower abdominal segment. These lesions have a low lipid and high fluid content. In some plaques, numerous smooth muscle cells are present while the lesions contain substantial amounts of cross-linked fibrin.

Fibrous Plaques

Figure 6-1 typifies the most common prototypical atherosclerotic lesion: fibrous or type IV plaque. These lesions are composed of large numbers of smooth muscle cells and connective tissue, which form a fibrous cap over an inner yellow (atheromatous) core. This soft core contains cholesterol esters, mainly cholesteryl oleate, likely derived from disrupted foam cells. A second type of particle contains both free cholesterol and cholesterol linoleates. The early core is associated with vesicular lipids that are rich in free cholesterol.[9] These particles are likely derived directly from LDL, possibly by modification of LDL by specific lipolytic enzymes capable of hydrolyzing LDL cholesterol esters. Lipoprotein aggregation and fusion are thought to be the chief pathway of cholesterol ester accumulation. Fibrous plaques contain large numbers of smooth muscle cells, connective tissue cells, and macrophages. Almost 2 decades ago, the composition and integrity of the atheromatous cap were underscored, as this structure stabilizes the atheroma, preventing intraluminal rupture of its soft core.[37]

Fibrous plaques appear later than fatty streak and often in similar locations. Fibrous plaques likely evolve from fatty streaks or from areas of fatty streak involvement. Gelatinous plaques, injured arterial areas, or thrombi less commonly may lead to fibrous plaque formation. Mural thrombi can be converted into atheromas, as demonstrated by experimental intraarterial catheter implantation.[38]

Fibrous plaques protrude into the arterial lumen in fixed cut sections; however, when arteries are fixed at arterial pressure, they produce an abluminal or external bulge. For example, coronary plaques in vivo must occupy at least 40% of the arterial wall before angiographic detection is possible,[39] and within limits, atheroma growth is compensated by arterial enlargement.[40] Compensatory remodeling of coronary arteries in subhuman primates and humans has been stressed as a protective response.[41] However, with lesion growth, ulceration, rupture, or overlying thrombosis, the arterial lumen suddenly becomes compromised, which is a sequence seen in coronary atheromas. A unique adaptive response involving dilatation, with atheromatous involvement of the entire arterial wall and participation of inflammatory cells and immunologically active T lymphocytes, and elastolysis may predispose to aneurysm formation.

During the early stages of evolution from fatty streak to fibrous plaque, cholesterol esters appear in the form of ordered arrays of intracellular lipid crystals. In intermediate type III and fibrous plaques, the lipids assume isotropic forms and occur extracellularly.[42] Cholesterol esters and oxysterols are highly irritating, causing severe inflammatory reactions in the connective tissue[43]; they probably behave similarly within the arterial wall to promote inflammation, fibrosis, and lymphocytic infiltration. Advancing neovascularization from the adventitia characterizes intermediate fibrofatty and fibrous plaque lesions. Atherosclerotic lesions contain immunoglobulin (Ig) G in large quantities, as well as other immunoglobulins and complement components. The IgG recognizes epitopes characteristic of oxidized LDL, indicating that immunologic processes characterize more advanced atherosclerotic plaques.[44] This process is associated with systemic effects; for example, patients with carotid atherosclerosis have higher antibody ratios of antioxidized LDL and IgM than do comparable nonatherosclerotic controls.[45]

Experiments in complement-deficient rabbits suggest that the chronic inflammation of atherosclerosis is driven mainly by activation of the complement and monocyte-macrophage systems.[46] In this sequence, enzymatic degradation, not oxidation, is considered to be the central predisposing process.

Complicated Plaques

Fibrous plaques become complicated by calcification, ulceration, intraplaque hemorrhage, or necrosis. These later developments cause the clinical complications of stroke, gangrene, and myocardial infarction. Aneurysm formation can represent a unique genetic or immune interaction with atherosclerosis. Alternatively, aneurysms have been viewed as nonspecific, inflammatory, degenerative, or purely mechanical arterial responses. Patients harboring aortic aneurysms have a high prevalence of risk factors for atherosclerosis and concurrent atherosclerotic involvement of other arteries, suggesting a unique response to atherosclerosis involving this arterial segment in certain individuals.[47]

As with early plaque evolution,[17] advanced atherosclerotic lesions have been described and classified in a separate report.[18] The type IV lesion, or atheroma, is potentially symptom producing. Extracellular lipid is the precursor of the core that characterizes type IV lesions. Lesions that contain a thick layer of fibrous connective tissue are characterized as type V lesions, whereas those with fissures, hematoma, or thrombus are characterized as type VI lesions. Type V lesions have been further described as largely calcified (type Vc) or consisting mainly of connective tissue with little or no lipid or calcium (type Vb). This definition of advanced disease includes atherosclerotic aneurysms, though aneurysm formation may follow other distinct sequences.

THEORIES OF ATHEROGENESIS

Lipid Hypothesis

Virchow believed that the cellular changes characterizing atherosclerosis were simply reactive responses to lipid infiltration.[24] Later, Aschoff remarked, "From plasma of low cholesterin content no deposition of lipids will occur even though mechanical conditions are favorable."[24] As

can be seen from fatty streak to fibrous plaque evolution, lipids, particularly LDL cholesterol, have a pivotal role in lesion morphology, composition, and evolution. Early experiments by Anitschkow with cholesterol-fed rabbits appeared to validate a simple "lipid filtration hypothesis."[48] However, the atherosclerotic process was soon appreciated to be pathogenetically much more complex. Atherosclerosis develops in various species in proportion to the ease with which an experimental regimen displaces the normal lipid pattern toward hypercholesterolemia, particularly hyperbetalipoproteinemia. At the same time, arterial susceptibility and inflammatory responses vary among locations, species, and individuals. Enhanced inflammatory responses, genetically determined by toll-like receptors, are known to influence atherogenesis.[49,50]

Canine and subhuman primate (rhesus and cynomolgus monkey) models develop atherosclerosis in response to dietary manipulation[50-60] and demonstrate plaque regression in response to serum cholesterol lowering. However, lesion production in susceptible species is not a result of simple dietary cholesterol overload. Any diet that causes hypercholesterolemia induces atherosclerosis. The presence of excess, or even any, cholesterol is not necessary in atherogenic diets. In developmental subhuman primate feeding experiments, reduction of cholesterol content to 0.5% combined with sugar and eggs produced rapidly progressive plaques, whereas high cholesterol addition (up to 7% by weight) did not.[53,54] In rabbits, a variety of semipure, purified cholesterol-free diets with various amino acid compositions induces hypercholesterolemia and atherosclerosis.[60]

Epidemiologic observations provide important circumstantial evidence linking hyperlipidemia to atherosclerosis.[61] The genetically determined hyperlipidemias provide compelling evidence that elevated LDL cholesterol is a prime etiologic factor in atherosclerosis, despite objections that highly cellular lipid-laden atheromas may be different lesions in these patients.[62] These metabolic disorders are most often caused by a lack or abnormality of LDL receptors on hepatocytes, which causes an ability to internalize and metabolize LDL, an important observation that earned Brown and Goldstein a Nobel Prize.[63] Serum cholesterol levels are markedly elevated early in life; individuals with the homozygous condition die prematurely from atherosclerosis, rarely living beyond the age of 26 years. Unfortunately, the heterozygous condition is not uncommon, with total cholesterol levels ranging up to 350 mg/dL. These individuals account for 1 in 500 live births[64] and develop atherosclerosis during early middle age. The atheromas of these patients are similar in morphology to those seen in individuals with acquired hyperlipidemia or premature atherosclerosis associated with heavy smoking.

This unfortunate natural experiment is powerful evidence that elevated LDL cholesterol is a relentless factor in plaque inception and the rapid progression of atherosclerosis to lethal consequences. Liver transplantation has been successful in retarding the progress of this type of atherosclerosis.[65] Familial hypercholesterolemias are autosomal dominant disorders produced by at least 12 different molecular defects of the LDL receptors. Familial abnormalities of high-density lipoprotein (HDL), a negative risk factor for atherosclerosis, also exist. In addition to LDL and HDL metabolism, surface proteins of the lipoprotein complex or apoproteins also appear to be relevant to pathogenesis. With the availability of effective therapy, a need for childhood screening for these disorders has been endorsed recently.[66]

Thrombogenic Hypothesis

In the mid nineteenth century, von Rokitansky postulated that fibrinous substances deposited on the arterial intimal surface as a result of abnormal hemostatic elements in the blood could undergo metamorphosis into atheromatous masses containing cholesterol crystals and globules.[67] This theory held that atheromatous lesions resulted mainly from degeneration of blood proteins (i.e., fibrin deposited in the arterial intima). Duguid[68] resurrected this theory in 1946 with the observation that in rabbits, indwelling arterial catheters or arterial injury caused cholesterol accumulation and arterial lesions in the absence of dietary cholesterol.

Mesenchymal Hypothesis: Hemodynamic Effects

Active smooth muscle cells with connective tissue production by these cells have been considered as primary, even crucial steps, in atherogenesis.[69-71] Proteoglycan, a ubiquitous arterial wall element, can trap infiltrated LDL, even when LDL is not elevated in the blood. Collagen is the other space-filling component of advanced atherosclerotic lesions. Hauss and colleagues[72] viewed the migration of smooth muscle cells from the media to the intima, with proliferation and production of connective tissue, as a nonspecific arterial reaction to any injury; atherosclerosis simply reflects a generic arterial response. Chisolm and colleagues[22] called this the "nonspecific" mesenchymal hypothesis. These scenarios are similar to wound-healing responses to injury. In part, this theory attempts to explain why physical factors such as shear stress, vasoactive agents, and repetitive injuries eventually lead to atheroma formation.

In one view, "Atherosclerosis constitutes the degenerative and reparative process consequent upon the hemodynamically induced engineering fatigue of the blood vessel wall."[63] This theory postulates that "the vibrations consisting of the pulsations associated with cardiac contractions and the vortex shedding generated in the blood vessels at branchings, unions, curvatures, and fusiform dilatations (carotid sinus) over a lifetime are responsible for fatigue failure after a certain, but individually variable, number of vibrations."[63] Atherosclerosis, a process of wear and tear, therefore becomes an inexorable (and unavoidable) process associated with aging. In support of this concept, hypertension[73] and tachycardia induced in experimental animals receiving atherogenic feeding caused accelerated plaque development, whereas bradycardia induced by sinoatrial node ablation in monkeys reduced coronary and carotid atherosclerosis.[74,75]

Monoclonal Hypothesis: Smooth Muscle Proliferation

The morphologic similarity of smooth muscle proliferation in some atherosclerotic lesions to uterine smooth muscle myomas led to the suggestion that atherosclerotic lesions are derived from a singular or, at most, a few mutated smooth muscle cells that, like tumor cells, proliferate in an unregulated fashion.[70] This theory is based on the finding of only one allele for glucose-6-phosphate dehydrogenase in lesions from heterozygotes. A homology exists between the β chain of human PDGF and the protein product of the v-sis oncogene, which is a tumor-causing gene derived from simian sarcoma virus. Tumor-forming cells in culture express the genes for one or both of the PDGF chains and secrete PDGF into a culture medium. This hypothesis, once again, considers events causing smooth muscle cell proliferation to be a critical atherogenic factor. Actions of other growth factors, which might either stimulate or inhibit cell proliferation, depend on circumstances as well as on macrophage-derived cytokine activity. For example, the finding of transforming growth factor (TGF)-β receptors in human atherosclerosis provides evidence of an acquired resistance to apoptosis.[76] Resistance to apoptosis can lead to proliferation of resistant cell subsets associated with progression of lesions.

Response-to-Injury Hypothesis

Ross and Glomset[77] initially postulated two pathways for the promotion of atheroma formation. In the first pathway (e.g., in hypercholesterolemia), monocyte and macrophage migration occurs without endothelial denudation. In some instances, endothelial loss occurs, with platelets carpeting bare areas. In this event, platelets would stimulate proliferation of smooth muscle by releasing PDGF.

In the second pathway, the endothelium itself was postulated to release growth factors, stimulating smooth muscle proliferation. Experimental rabbit arterial balloon injury shows that regrowing endothelium induces myointimal proliferation beneath its advancing edges, stimulating accumulation of collagen[78] and glycosaminoglycans.[79] Stimulated smooth muscle itself then releases growth factors, leading to a continued autocrine proliferative response. In the initial iteration of this theory, the second pathway was postulated to be relevant to atheroma stimulated by diabetes, possibly in relation to insulin-derived growth factors, cigarette smoking, or hypertension. Hypertension causes endothelial injury, but striking differences exist between the behavior of smooth muscle cells in atherosclerosis and hypertension. Atherosclerosis stimulates an overt smooth muscle proliferative response. In most instances, pure hypertension causes thickening of the arterial wall by virtue of increased protein synthesis, without an increase in cell number.[80]

Arterial trauma, such as clamping or balloon injury, produces stenoses and vascular injuries (ranging from minor to severe) and initiates both myointimal hyperplasia and atheromas. This mode of atherogenesis invokes a response to injury hypothesis. In this scenario, physical or chemical agents cause endothelial denudation, followed by platelet adherence and subsequent release of PDGF,[81] triggering smooth muscle migration proliferation and lipid accumulation. This sequence applies to specific arterial wall injuries, particularly when the internal elastic lamina is disrupted.

Injury as a global theory of atherogenesis is unsupported by subsequent observations of early atherogenesis. Arterial denudation is a rare finding in early atherogenesis in humans and animals, although endothelial cells may be injured or dysfunctional while remaining in place.[82] It is known that systemic endothelial dysfunction exists in atherosclerosis.[83] Endothelial dysfunction exerts profound effects on systemic vasodilatation and the upregulation of endothelial receptors facilitating entry of cells and blood components through an apparently intact endothelium. Because all arterial wall cells secrete growth factors that are similar if not identical to PDGF and its derivatives, postulating physical endothelial disruption and platelet deposition is unnecessary.

The responses of the arterial wall after injury remain of considerable practical interest in both atherogenesis and intimal hyperplasia. With injury, early medial smooth muscle proliferation is the first step, influenced primarily by basic fibroblast growth factor.[84] Migration and production of an extracellular matrix are the second and third stages of injury. These mechanisms are relevant to trauma-provoked atheromas, which occur as a result of clamping or balloon injuries in the presence of modestly elevated levels of LDL cholesterol.[85] Angiotensin II also causes smooth muscle to proliferate and induces expression of growth factors.[86,87] One of these growth factors, TGF-β, exerts either stimulatory or inhibitory effects, depending on circumstances. Injury also induces medial angiotensinogen gene expression and angiotensin receptor expression.[88] Other smooth muscle antigens include thrombin, catecholamine, and possibly endothelin. As a result, atheromas developing in a setting of injury (mechanical, immunologic, or infectious) are influenced by trauma-induced growth factors in varying degrees and sequences. However, plasma LDL elevation accentuates neointimal hyperplasia[89,90] without actual atheroma formation.

Lesion Arrest or Regression

The potential for plaque regression and stabilization of vulnerable plaques is key in the consideration of prevention and treatment of atherosclerosis. Regression of atherosclerosis in response to lowered serum cholesterol has been demonstrated in autopsy studies of starved humans dating back to World War I,[23] in many animal models,[91] and in pioneering clinical angiographic trials combining cessation of smoking with lipid reduction.[92] In humans, trials of vascular end points have shown some impressive examples of regression in coronary arteries; more commonly, minimal anatomic regression is seen, along with slowing of progression, but with drastic reductions in coronary events.[93] Importantly, magnetic resonance imaging has documented favorable longitudinal changes in carotid plaque composition, with reduction of the lipid core and increased fibrous tissue.[94]

As atherosclerotic plaques in experimental animals regress, plaque bulk is reduced mainly by lipid egress. This has been shown convincingly in experiments using hypercholesterolemic dogs[52,53] and monkeys.[54-57] The exact mechanisms of lesion regression, particularly the roles of inflammatory and immune responses, are incompletely understood. Regression has been demonstrated using serial observations of decreased bulk of individual plaques; reduced luminal encroachment, as shown by edge defects on sequential angiography; and decreased plaque lipid and altered fibrous protein content measured histologically and chemically.[57] An important technical aspect of this research was the confirmation of regressive changes using immediate autopsy or surgical observation and biopsy. Grossly or histopathologically, plaque change correlated with observed regressive angiographic changes.[58,59] Stary[95] described regression of advanced lesions in atherosclerotic rhesus monkeys, clearly documenting disappearance of macrophages, macrophage-derived foam cells, lymphocytes, and extracellular lipids, as a result of drastic reduction of blood cholesterol for 42 months. Arterial wall calcium deposits, however, did not regress, and as might be expected, calcification is a definite limiting factor in regression and also important while planning endovascular interventions.

Correlative sequential plaque observations are not readily obtained in humans, but angiography and ultrasonography are currently used to assess treatment effects. Experimentally, decreased luminal intrusion on sequential angiography coincided with decreased plaque size and reduced lipid content. In some instances, it has been found that plaque fibrous protein increased during regression.[57] Although residual fibrosis might limit plaque bulk reduction, fibrosis may convert a soft atheromatous plaque into a more stable lesion. Active lesions, particularly in the coronary arteries, are not necessarily the most occlusive ones. Although angiographic edge changes appear to be minimal, the reduction in coronary events in response to lipid-lowering treatment likely relates more to plaque stabilization than to bulk reduction. To produce regression consistently, total serum cholesterol must be reduced to approximately 150 mg/dL. Modest serum cholesterol elevations exist above which lesions inevitably progress.[59] Antiplatelet treatment does not appear to retard plaque progression; combinations of antiplatelet agents, high-dose aspirin, and dipyridamole in the rhesus model caused rapid, dramatic plaque progression during hypercholesterolemia.[60] Favorable lipid thresholds for human regressive responses approximate a total serum cholesterol level of 150 to 170 mg/dL and an LDL level of 100 mg/dL or less, levels that Roberts cited in populations in which atherosclerosis is virtually absent.[96] This observation led him to conclude that elevated lipid levels are the single etiologic risk factor in atherogenesis. However, in extrapolating this concept to secondary treatment, inflammatory responses need to be considered. These responses likely contribute to plaque instability leading to atherosclerotic complications, as often occurs, in the absence of hyperlipidemia.

MEDICAL MANAGEMENT

General Considerations

Populations free of coronary disease generally exhibit total cholesterol levels less than 150 mg/dL and LDL cholesterol levels less than 100 mg/dL. This observation questions the primacy of other atherosclerotic risk factors that commonly manifest in these relatively disease free populations.[96] In examining the usefulness of the lipid hypothesis for treatment rather than prevention, considerable positive evidence has accumulated to support an energetic approach to overall lipid reduction. The Heart Protection Study—a randomized, placebo-controlled trial using simvastatin in more than 20,000 individuals—showed a reduction of adverse cardiovascular events and prolongation of life when this agent was used for primary and secondary prevention, even in individuals without elevated lipid levels.[97] Statins have antiinflammatory effects, as shown by decreased C-reactive protein levels,[98] occurring independently of LDL reduction.[99,100] Overall, many more individuals are candidates for treatment to achieve recently revised goals of the National Cholesterol Education Project of total cholesterol less than 150 mg/dL and LDL less than 100 mg/dL.[101] These stringent lipid target levels can seldom be achieved with diet alone. The Heart Protection Study has recently addressed the issue of baseline C-reactive protein (CRP) in statin therapy, to report, once again, that allocation to simvastatin therapy, proved significantly effective regardless of baseline levels of CRP and in participants with normal lipid levels.[102] Empirically a statin, along with low-dose aspirin, clopidogrel (an antiplatelet agent), and angiotensin-converting enzyme (ACE) inhibitors are recommended for patients with peripheral arterial disease.[103]

Complications and deleterious clinical events associated with atherosclerosis are neither singular nor univariate, but multiple and interactive. In the late stages, the instability of the fibrous plaques involves more than lipid dynamics. More than 4 decades ago, Holman and colleagues[104] pointed out that "a sharp line of distinction exists between atherogenesis and the subsequent evolution of lesions that may or may not precipitate clinical disease, for the factors involved in the evolution of lesions beyond the stage of fatty streaks may be entirely different from the factors that initiate fatty streaks." Among these factors are inflammatory and immune mechanisms, altered fibrous proteins, accumulation of blood elements, and cap rupture. Among interventions intended to produce plaque stabilization or regression, decreasing LDL cholesterol promotes favorable changes in atheromas and improved outcomes. The antiinflammatory statin effect, as judged by biomarkers, also presents as an important synchronous effect. The effect of cigarette smoking, a crucial promoter of complications of atherosclerosis, might be viewed as a contributor to inflammation, which cannot be overcome solely by lipid reduction.

In angiographic regression trials, the most favorable plaque changes in terms of arrest or regression relate to the degree and duration of blood lipid reduction. In peripheral arteries, regression and stabilization were 1.5-fold to twofold more common in treated subjects than in those receiving placebos.[92] Although angiographic studies show plaque regression trends, wall change or plaque reduction is usually modest compared with what is believed to be stabilization of vulnerable lesions. Intravascular ultrasound is an important tool to visualized plaque relationships to the arterial wall in response to treatment. Serial angiography has been used to describe favorable clinical results among patients randomly assigned to an experimental group consuming a 10% fat, 12-mg cholesterol diet and undergoing smoking cessation, stress management training, and exercise.[104] After 1 year, 82% of the treated group showed regressive changes in coronary artery plaques that depended, in some degree, on the amount of initial lesion encroachment.

Treatment aims to improve the arterial lesions and improve survival. Increased fibrous protein synthesis produces a stable, fibrotic plaque as opposed to a soft, friable plaque containing an unstable, atheromatous core covered by a tenuous cap. However, a densely sclerotic, highly occlusive lesion can also cause distal ischemia. In evaluating these hypotheses with a view toward better prediction and control, ameliorating the atheroma itself and providing quantifiable evidence of favorable changes has correlated mostly with effective, even drastic, blood lipid reduction.

Atherosclerosis is often segmental; bypassing or removing symptomatic arterial lesions in selected arterial segments minimizes the deleterious effects of dangerous lesions. These observations, made more than 40 years ago, were uniquely surgical insights and brought life- and limb-saving interventions to many patients.[3] Arterial interventions, which include endovascular approaches, evolved as highly effective means of treating patients with advanced, symptomatic atheromas, including specific patterns of coronary involvement, high-grade carotid lesions, and aortic disease. However effective, surgical or endovascular treatment of one arterial segment does not prevent disease progression in other segments—life expectancy remains shortened. Continued smoking after reconstruction make matters worse, particularly after ill-advised infrainguinal or aortic reconstruction for stable claudicants. Aspirin, urokinase, and anticoagulants can prevent or minimize superimposed embolic phenomena and clotting, but underlying plaques continue to progress. Modification of inflammatory responses provoked by cytokine-derived or immune-modulating factors has potential and may now be practical, given the current ability to monitor blood levels for biomarkers such as inflammatory cytokines and CRP, which predict cardiovascular complications and mortality.[105,106]

Apparently insignificant or small plaques, particularly in coronary or cerebral arteries provoke arterial spasm. Atherosclerotic plaques impair the normal action of endothelium-derived relaxing factor,[107-109] impairing vasodilator responses in coronary and cerebral arteries.[108] Dietary treatment of experimental atherosclerosis restores endothelium-dependent relaxation responses,[110] whereas long-term inhibition of nitric oxide synthesis by feeding promotes experimental atherosclerosis.[111]

Clinical Management

All individuals with two or more risk factors or any form of vascular disease require a lipid profile and a fasting blood glucose sample. Fasting blood samples measure HDL cholesterol levels. The LDL cholesterol level is calculated as follows: LDL cholesterol = Total cholesterol − HDL cholesterol + (Triglycerides/5). This formula holds for fasting patients with triglycerides less than 400 mg/dL. Serum cholesterol levels must be obtained with patients on a regular diet outside the hospital. Acute illnesses cause sudden, inexplicable decrements in total serum cholesterol.

The National Cholesterol Education Program recommends dietary approaches as a first step for patients with atherosclerotic vascular diseases.[101] The patient's age and sex are considered when choosing treatment. The initial emphasis is on physical activity and weight loss. It recommended that clinicians supply hyperlipidemic patients with information on diet and routinely recommend exercise in the form of walking. Drug treatment is delayed in patients with a low risk of coronary heart disease (e.g., no smoking, diabetes, or hypertension) in men younger than 45 years and women younger than 55 years. Emphasis has been placed on high levels of HDL cholesterol, a powerful negative risk factor, but selectively increasing HDL levels is difficult to accomplish. Although these guidelines apply to primary prevention, virtually all patients with vascular disease are candidates for drug therapy, usually with statins.

Drug Therapy for Hyperlipidemia

Currently available drugs include cholestyramine and colestipol (bile acid sequestrants), nicotinic acid (a B-complex vitamin), and the widely used statin drugs. Statins are 3-hydroxy-3-methylglutaryl coenzyme A–reducing agents that include pravastatin, lovastatin, simvastatin, atorvastatin, and fluvastatin. These agents inhibit hepatic cholesterol biosynthesis. Gemfibrozil, a fibric acid derivative, is used to treat hypertriglyceridemia. Recent trials have shown that vitamin C and E supplements have no effect in preventing coronary heart disease events or in improving outcomes in established coronary heart diease.[112,113] Treatment that both lowers LDL cholesterol and raises HDL cholesterol is considered desirable. The dramatic results of intensive LDL lowering in the 2004 REVERSAL trial support the concept of "the lower the better" for treatment of patients with coronary artery disease.[114,115] A higher dose of atorvastatin (80 mg) was more effective than a lower dose of pravastatin (40 mg) in reducing LDL to 79 mg/dL, significantly reducing C-reactive protein while producing a significant reduction in atheroma volume and preventing the progression of coronary lesions. Statin drugs, combined with niacin in nondiabetics, have achieved dramatic reductions in coronary events, possibly related to nonlipid actions affecting endothelial function, inflammatory response, plaque stability, and thrombus formation.[116] The side effects of niacin, such as flushing, can be difficult to tolerate, and raising HDL levels remains less practical than lowering LDL levels.

Control of Associated Risk Factors

Cigarette Smoking

Cigarette smoking is a powerful risk factor for atherosclerotic disease, promoting its clinical complications even when lipids are normal. This addiction relates directly to limb amputation, high mortality owing to ischemic heart disease, and failure of aortic and femoropopliteal grafts.[117-119] The mechanisms by which cigarette smoking promotes atherosclerosis and graft thrombosis are incompletely understood. Carbon monoxidemia can predispose to endothelial injury, producing increased plasma flux and entry of LDL and other proteins. Cigarette smoking is associated with increased platelet reactivity, peripheral vasoconstriction, and lowered HDL levels.[120] From the standpoint of pathogenesis, lipid abnormalities are clearly important, but from the standpoint of clinical interventions for established disease, smoking cessation is critical in preventing amputation, myocardial infarction, and stroke.

At a minimum, clinical practice guidelines should include routine institutional identification of and intervention with all tobacco users at every visit. Clinicians should ask about and record the tobacco use status of every patient. All smokers should be offered smoking cessation treatment at every office visit—nicotine replacement therapy short term, and bupropion long term to treat depression.[121] The latter drug offers prosexual benefits over other antidepressants. Cessation advice, even as brief as 3 minutes, is useful. But formal clinician-delivered support and life skills training are important treatment components for smoking cessation. The more intense the treatment, the more effective it will be in achieving long-term abstinence. In addition, elective interventions in smokers for claudication alone should be avoided, because graft occlusion often occurs making eventual amputation more likely.

Hypertension

Control of hypertension prolongs life and reduces coronary mortality.[122] Chronic hypertension accelerates atherosclerosis in experimental hyperlipidemic animals.[123] Paradoxically, as with cigarette smoking, Asian and Caribbean populations exhibit hypertension with a low incidence of atherosclerotic disease in the absence of hyperlipidemia. In affluent societies, however, prospective studies show that hypertension is related to the risk of premature atherosclerotic disease independently of the risk factors of hyperlipidemia and cigarette smoking.[124] Hypertension may be linked with risk factor clustering, including glucose intolerance, hyperinsulinemia, and dyslipidemia promoted by abdominal obesity,[125] comprising the metabolic syndrome, or syndrome X. Weight loss, exercise, and combined drug treatment for hypertriglyceridemia require consideration. Treatment of hypertension with thiazide diuretics alone was not advantageous in terms of coronary outcome in a subgroup of men in the Multiple Risk Factor Intervention Trial,[126] likely owing to inadequate control of lipid levels when total cholesterol in the intervention group remained greater than 200 mg/dL before the availability of statins. The current goal for blood pressure is 120/80 mm Hg using lifestyle changes, weight loss, and blood pressure medications based on patient age, race, and presence or absence of diabetes. Drugs with specific benefits include ACE inhibitors, diuretics, and beta blockers. Lifestyle alterations include weight reduction, reduced dietary sodium intake, reduced alcohol intake, increased physical activity, and possibly increased calcium intake.[127]

Exercise

Regular exercise decreases total serum cholesterol, LDL, and fasting triglycerides and has variable effects on HDL.[128] The preventive effects of exercise have been amply documented; a sedentary lifestyle is an important risk factor for coronary disease.[129] No study, however, has shown that exercise has a direct effect on established atherosclerotic plaques; experimental and clinical data have demonstrated arrest or regression of plaques with lipid reduction. Strenuous unsupervised exercise can be dangerous in the presence of preexisting coronary disease.[130] Exercise does not compensate for persistent uncorrected hyperlipidemia or continued cigarette smoking. This is an important message for patients with vascular disease. Exercise is not sufficient to offset the effects of elevated total cholesterol and LDL, nor should it be considered a replacement for treatment of hypertension. Weight loss and drugs are probably more effective.[131]

Beneficial effects of exercise in peripheral vascular disease (i.e., increased walking distance) relate to improved skeletal muscle oxidative metabolism.[132] Exercise is important secondary therapy. Exercise programs can be more effective for claudication over the long term than surgical or endovascular intervention, particularly in infrainguinal atherosclerosis. In patients with coronary atherosclerosis, exercise prescriptions must be carefully structured. Before prescribing strenuous exercise, stress testing or monitoring to detect silent ischemic heart disease is recommended, and strenuous intermittent exercise is unadvisable. Recently, exercise has been shown to reduce CRP levels, demonstrating a favorable effect on this biomarker of inflammation.[133]

Diabetes

Diabetes, an increasingly prevalent risk or pathogenetic factor, promotes atherosclerosis. Most patients with peripheral arterial disease who are nonsmokers are diabetic. In its singular form, diabetes is associated with severe infracrural and coronary atherosclerosis. One diabetes control trial showed a reduction in microvascular complications with "tight control" using insulin; unfortunately, this trial was not designed to study end points of macrovascular atherosclerotic complications.[134] Causes of enhanced atherogenesis in diabetes include abnormalities in apoproteins and lipoprotein particle distribution, particularly elevated levels of lipoprotein(a),[135] an independent thromboatherosclerotic risk factor. In poorly controlled diabetes, a procoagulant state exists. Increased glucose levels are associated with accelerated platelet aggregation in vitro, and accompanying hypertriglyceridemia enhances thrombogenic factors V, II, and X.

Glycooxidation and oxidation contribute to LDL entry into macrophages, and glycation of proteins and plasma in the arterial wall contributes to accelerated atherosclerosis. Hormones, growth factors, cytokine-enhanced smooth muscle cell proliferation, and increased foam cell formation may relate to the pathogenesis of atherogenesis in diabetes mellitus.[136]

Both hyperinsulinemia and insulin resistance are associated with atherosclerosis,[137] and both occur in type 2 diabetes. Both insulin and glucose stimulate the growth of diabetic infragenicular smooth muscle cells.[138] A possible mechanism accounting for atherogenesis in diabetes is impaired vasoactivity; troglitazone, an insulin-action enhancer, corrects impaired brachial artery vasoactivity in patients with occult impaired glucose tolerance.[139]

Consistent control of blood glucose is advisable as described in Chapter 11 in this volume. A recent trial studying the effectiveness of intensive versus standard blood glucose control on cardiovascular events showed no significant effects upon cardiovascular events, death or microvascular complications except for the progression of albuminuria.[140] For any given level of LDL, coronary heart disease risk is increased threefold to fivefold in diabetics compared with nondiabetics.[141] Elevated triglyceride levels most commonly accompany severely elevated cholesterol levels in diabetics; this particular combination greatly increases the risk of adverse coronary events. Diabetics exhibit particular lipid abnormalities, including chylomicronemia, increased very-low-density lipoprotein (VLDL) levels, increased VLDL and chylomicron remnants, and triglyceride-rich LDL and HDL concentrations. Mamo and Proctor[142] emphasized the pathogenicity of these remnants. Glycosylation of lipoproteins and collagen relates directly to levels of glucose, contributing to increased binding of LDL by collagen, and glycosylated lipoproteins are taken up avidly by macrophages to transform them into foam cells. Extensive clinical experience documents the efficacy of bariatric surgery in diabetics with body mass index exceeding 35.[143] Target goals for treatment of diabetics include fasting glucose less than 110 mg/dL, hemoglobin A1c less than 7%, blood pressure less than 130/80 mm Hg, LDL less than 100 mg/dL, and triglycerides less than 150 mg/dL. The use of an ACE inhibitor with a statin should be considered in all cases.

Antioxidants and Oxidative Stress

Treatment with antioxidants is based on the concept that oxidative stress related to reactive oxygen species promotes oxidized LDL to form foam cells and activate macrophages, which release inflammatory cytokines and growth factors that stimulate smooth muscle proliferation. Not all cytokines provoke the inflammatory response; IL-10, an antiinflammatory cytokine, prevents atherosclerotic events in vitro and in vivo.[144] Conversely, plaque components such as metalloproteinases, inflammatory cytokines, and high-sensitivity C-reactive protein appear in the systemic circulation, presumably as markers of disease severity.[11,145] Biomarkers are characteristics that can be measured and evaluated as indicators of normal or pathogenic responses as well as pharmacologic responses to treatment. Determination of the exact relationships between biomarkers and plaque change requires both observational and outcome studies. Ideally, improved plaque morphology linked to improved outcomes provides the strongest evidence of validity of a particular biomarker. While oxidation is recognized as an important disease promoting mechanism,[146,147] results of randomized trials with antioxidant vitamins have proved disappointing.[113] Vitamins C and E, at a molecular level, theoretically might function as prooxidants promoting formation of reactive oxidative species.

Elevated blood levels of homocysteine, earlier proposed as a thromboatherosclerotic risk factor,[148] have not shown promise. Elevated levels can be reduced by folic acid intake, but recent trial data from a 5-year study demonstrated no effect on cardiovascular outcomes, although folic acid levels were effectively reduced.[149]

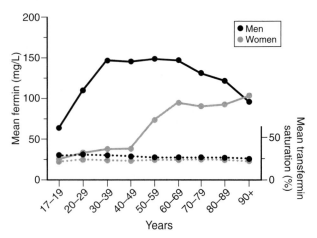

FIGURE 6-3 ■ Mean ferritin and transferrin levels versus age in men and women. (Adapted from Zacharski L, Woloshin S. Schwartz LM: Association of age, sex and race with body iron stores in adults: analysis of NHANES III data. Amer Heart J 140:98–104, 2000.)

Iron Hypothesis

Sullivan first postulated the delay in heart risk in women after menopause related to total body iron stores, with iron accumulating particularly in men and in women after menopause.[150] Iron in its ferrous form is a powerful inflammatory and oxidizing agent promoting progressive inflammatory diseases.[151] Recent studies show that iron balance is regulated by the hormone hepcidin. Its action is relevant in that high hepcidin levels promote iron retention in macrophages, in turn relating to increased intralesional iron content and inflammation.[151,152] The effect of deliberate reduction of iron stores was investigated in a single blinded clinical trial, the Iron and Atherosclerosis Study (FeAST), which tested the effects of clinical outcomes of reducing iron stores by phlebotomy to levels approximating those of menstruating women.[153] Participants were 1277 mainly male veterans with stable peripheral arterial disease, cancer free at the time on entry, and with an average age of 67 years. The primary outcome was all cause mortality, and secondary outcomes combined death plus nonfatal myocardial infarction and stroke. Overall results did not show a difference in outcomes related to phlebotomy, but the study did demonstrate strikingly significant, age-related, favorable outcomes, with improvement related to iron reduction occurring in younger participants (age 43 to 61 years). This effect diminished with increasing age.[154] Overall, lower ferritin levels strongly predicted outcomes regardless of randomization with ferritin level threshold benefits less than 76 to 78 ng/mL. Improved outcomes occurred upon removal of the amount of iron in one to two units of blood, the latter approximating annual blood loss in menstruating women. Figure 6-3 shows average ferritin levels, a marker of iron status in stable individuals, in men and women over time. Note the sharp increase of ferritin at the time of menopause in women and its continued increase in men over time. Increased ferritin levels are associated with increased incidence of cardiovascular disease.

Substudies carried out in FeAST participants at the Veterans' Administration (VA) Sierra Nevada Health Care System in Reno, Nevada, demonstrated inflammatory cytokine signatures in atherosclerotic participants compared with individuals apparently free of disease,[12] determined biomarker relationships to statin administration at baseline[155] and, upon completion of the 6-year study, demonstrated significant correlations between mortality, ferritin levels, and inflammatory biomarkers, particularly IL-6 and CRP.[156] Mortality and inflammatory cytokine levels related to ferritin rather than to lipid levels, regardless of participant allocation to control or phlebotomy groups.

Another line of evidence supporting the unfavorable health consequences of iron accumulation relates to regular blood donors, some of whom maintain protective ferritin levels characteristic of premenopausal women.[157] Studies of blood donors in the United States and Finland[158-160] showed reduced risk of myocardial infarction in regular blood donors; however, a 2001 report[161] did not support this effect. Divergent outcomes could relate to the need to achieve significantly lowered ferritin levels which range for 17-25 ng/mL in premenopausal women. A later study of frequent blood donors achieving an average ferritin level of 17 ng/mL demonstrated that significantly improved flow mediated brachial artery dilatation and reduced oxidative stress markers compared with infrequent blood donors' levels of average ferritin of 52 ng/mL.[162] Blood donation has also been reported to improve glucose control and insulin sensitivity in type 2 diabetics.[163]

An additional set of observations, ultrasound longitudinal observation of carotid plaques, provided plaque observations relating changes to iron stores (ferritin levels) and to favorable outcomes in the study group.[164] These investigators concluded that the iron effect on carotid plaques related synergistically with elevated lipid levels suggesting that iron excess promoted higher levels of oxidized LDL. Ultimately, studies relating outcomes to plaque morphology in response to treatment provide the strongest evidence supporting specific intervention strategies.

Another line of evidence compared iron parameters and oxidative markers in older men living in Crete and exhibiting lower disease risk compared with men of similar age living in Zutphen, the Netherlands.[165] This cohort study provides biologic support to the link between iron levels and oxidative stress. Markers of oxidative stress were significantly lower in the healthier Cretan men together with a twofold lower mean ferritin level (mean 69.8 ng/mL) in Crete compared with men from Zutphen ($p < 0.0001$). The Mediterranean diet is low in iron content[166]; combined with other favorable characteristics, this might contribute to the difference between the two populations. Excess iron storage can be avoided by eating less red meat while avoiding iron supplements that appear ubiquitously in Western industrialized diets. A rigorous definition of optimal iron stores, the relationship of ferritin levels to oxidative stress, and outcome trials with robust continuous iron reduction are needed to provide mainstream recommendations for iron reduction as a means of clinical intervention.

Antiplatelet and Anticoagulant Therapy

Antiplatelet therapy does not produce regressive effects on established lesions, although antiinflammatory effects may occur. Favorable therapeutic effects relate mainly to the prevention of superimposed thrombosis on advanced plaques, as described in detail later. Generally, smaller rather than larger doses of aspirin are advantageous. The Physicians' Health Study showed that 325 mg of aspirin on alternate days reduced subsequent need for peripheral vascular surgery.[167] Aspirin doses ranging from 74 to 159 mg daily have been found to be as effective as larger doses. Aspirin is recommended as an adjunct, not an alternative, to managing accompanying cardiovascular risk factors.[168] Reports concerning the possible promotion of intraplaque hemorrhage in carotid lesions in patients receiving aspirin are conflicting.

Results of a long-term study of the effects of clopidogrel indicate a statistical advantage of this therapy over aspirin therapy alone. This population included patients with recent myocardial infarction, recent stroke, or established peripheral arterial disease.[167] The largest relative risk reduction for clopidogrel, compared with aspirin, was in fatal and nonfatal myocardial infarction—19.2%.[169,170] Antiplatelet therapy and oral anticoagulants on review appear to reduce the risk of graft occlusion and ischemic events after infrainguinal bypass surgery.[171] Oral anticoagulant therapy is the more effective treatment in high-risk patients. Evidence of the beneficial effects of antiplatelet and oral anticoagulant therapy was based on a small number of trials; there is no proof as to which modality is most effective in preventing graft occlusion and ischemic events.

The end point of epidemiologic and clinical studies of atherosclerosis usually involves a thrombotic episode.[172] A prospective study of hemostatic function and cardiovascular death showed that elevated levels of factors VIIc and VIIIc and fibrinogen, in addition to elevated plasma cholesterol levels, appeared to be important predisposing factors.[173] Elevated fibrinogen, a major risk factor for coronary artery disease, is associated with peripheral arterial disease in men[172]; leukocyte levels may be elevated in both disease states.[175] Continued low-dose aspirin therapy, as described previously, is the therapeutic mainstay of antiplatelet therapy,[167] although resistance to its antithrombotic effects might be present in a significant proportion of individuals.[176]

Vasoactive Drugs

Nonlipid strategies, beyond cholesterol reduction, include the use of β-adrenergic receptor blocking agents to reduce catecholamine release, calcium channel blockers to reduce wall stress and inhibit lipid intake, nitrates to relax vascular smooth muscle by nitric oxide release, and ACE inhibitors to block atherogenic effects on angiotensin II. The Heart Outcome Prevention Evaluation (HOPE) study showed that ACE inhibitors improved the primary end points of myocardial infarction, stroke, and death from cardiovascular causes.[177] The use of perioperative beta blockade for patients undergoing non cardial has been brought into question as a result of the Perioptic Ischemic Evaluation (POISE) trial demonstrating increased postoperative risks of perioperative metoprolol administration.[178] Current Surgical Complications Improvement Project (SCIP) guidelines recommend that patients receiving preoperative β-blockers continue to receive β-blockade postoperatively. When a clear indication for β-blockade exists, it appears best to begin this step well before operative intervention. In another separate issue concerning vasodilators, the drug cilostazol has been reported to be effective in improving walking distance.[179]

Atherosclerosis and Infection

Cytomegalovirus (CMV) and *Chlamydia pneumoniae* infections have been associated with atherosclerosis. Comprehensive reviews, summarizing biologic evidence supporting relationships between infection and atherosclerosis included CMV, is a ubiquitous virus.[180,181] Seropositivity was reported to be associated with a high rate of restenosis after coronary bypass.[182]

The organism *C. pneumoniae* and its DNA have been detected in atherosclerotic plaques with some frequency.[183] Chlamydial heat shock protein colocalizes in plaques with *C. pneumoniae*–specific antigen,[181,184] leading to the hypothesis that *C. pneumoniae*–infected macrophages, upon entering the intima, mediate inflammatory and autoimmune responses by producing chlamydial heat shock proteins.[185,186] In addition to *C. pneumoniae* and CMV, *Helicobacter pylori* and herpesvirus have been suggested in the pathogenesis of atherosclerotic plaques. The deleterious effects of infection presumably relate to inflammation and bacterial heat shock proteins inciting arterial inflammatory and autoimmune reactions. While the molecular mechanisms inciting arterial wall reactions are of pathogenic interest, the results of recent large, randomized prospective trials assessing the efficacy of antibiotics to prevent cardiovascular events have been negative.[187]

Observations linking periodontal disease epidemiologically to atherosclerosis[188] might be related to atherogenesis by increasing circulating inflammatory cytokine levels, possibly promoting a proatherogenic endothelial cell phenotype with loss of antithrombotic, growth inhibitory, and vasodilator properties.[189] Subjects with periodontal disease, along with diabetics, show impaired brachial artery dilatation.[190] Oral infection in an experimental model with the periodontal pathogen *Porphyromonas gingivalis* has been shown to increase IL-6 levels and accelerate atherosclerosis.[191] Recently a protocol for a single randomized trial of periodontal treatment examining brachial flow measurements, inflammatory biomarkers, and other surrogates in individuals with periodontal disease and atherosclerosis has been registered.[192] As mentioned previously, the outcome results of this and other interventions will serve as gold standards.

SUMMARY

Effective medical therapy for atherosclerosis ideally induces plaque stabilization, reduces adverse clinical events, and prolongs life. Recommendations derive from a broad base of pathologic evidence, imaging observations, and randomized trials. For stable claudicants with infrainguinal atherosclerosis and patients after vascular reconstruction, secondary prevention methods include cessation of smoking; aspirin (preferably 81 mg daily), clopidogrel, or both; lipid reduction of total cholesterol to less than 150 mg/dL and LDL less than 100 mg, best achieved with statins, which also offer antiinflammatory benefits; walking briskly for 30 to 60 minutes daily; and addition of ACE inhibitors for diabetics, even with normal blood pressure. These medical measures should not cause a delay direct arterial interventions in the presence of life- or limb-threatening lesions. The provocative question in medical rather than surgical treatment of specific lesions (e.g., asymptomatic, stable carotid plaques)[193] requires highly reliable imaging and outcome studies to identify truly stable lesions and the best choices for individuals. Comparative effectiveness research, focusing on evidence to provide the best decisions for all stakeholders, will likely inform future treatment choices for ageing patients with atherosclerotic disease.[194] Vascular specialists, intervening at crucial times and in specific ways during the course of this complex chronic disease, need to understand opportunities and challenges implicit in assessing comparative effectiveness of selected treatments for individual patients with variable disease patterns.

BIBLIOGRAPHY

DeBakey ME, Lawrie GM, Glaeser DH: Patterns of atherosclerosis and their surgical significance. Ann Surg 201:115, 1985.

DePalma RG: Patterns of peripheral atherosclerosis: implications for treatment. In Shepard J, editor: Atherosclerosis: Developments, Complications and Treatment, New York, 1987, Elsevier, p 161.

DePalma RG, Bellon EM, Manalo PM, et al: Failure of antiplatelet treatment in dietary atherosclerosis: a serial intervention study. In Gallo LL, Vahouny GV, editors: Cardiovascular Disease: Molecular and Cellular Mechanisms, Prevention, Treatment, New York, 1987, Plenum Press, p 407.

DePalma RG, Hayes VW, Chow B, et al: Ferritin levels, inflammatory biomarkers, and mortality in peripheral arterial disease: a substudy of the Iron (Fe) and Atherosclerosis (FEAST) trial. J Vasc Surg 51:1498, 2010.

DePalma RG, Hubay CA, Insull W, Jr, et al: Progression and regression of experimental atherosclerosis. Surg Gynecol Obstet 131:633, 1970.

Heart Protection Study Group: MRC/BHF heart protection study group of cholesterol lowering with simvastatin in 20,536 high-risk individuals: a randomized placebo controlled trial. Lancet 360:7, 2002.

Ridker PM, Hennekens CH, Buring JE, et al: C reactive protein and other markers of inflammation in the prediction of cardiovascular disease in women. N Engl J Med 342:836, 1990.

Ross R: Atherosclerosis is an inflammatory disease. Am Heart J 138:S419, 1999.

Stary HC, Chandler AB, Dinsmore RE, et al: A definition of advanced types of atherosclerotic lesions and a histological classification of atherosclerosis. A report from the Committee on Vascular Lesions of the Council on Arteriosclerosis, American Heart Association. Arterioscler Thromb Vasc Biol 15:1512, 1995.

Stary HC, Chandler AB, Glagov S, et al: A definition of initial fatty streak and intermediate lesions of atherosclerosis. A report from the Committee on Vascular Lesions of the Council on Atherosclerosis. Arterioscler Thromb Vasc Biol 14:840, 1994.

References available online at expertconsult.com.

QUESTIONS

1. Type IV (fibrous plaques) usually evolve:
   a. In areas of fatty streak involvement
   b. From thrombotic clots
   c. In areas of endothelial shedding
   d. From gelatinous plaque progression
   e. From hypertrophic smooth muscle cells

2. Atherosclerotic plaque regression or stabilization is characterized by:
   a. Decreased fibrosis
   b. Lipid egress
   c. Less calcification
   d. Thrombolysis
   e. Activated macrophages

3. In atherosclerosis, macrophages in plaques produce all of the following except:
   a. Lipoproteins
   b. Interleukin-1
   c. Metalloproteinases
   d. Growth factors
   e. Interleukin-10

4. Examples of inflammatory or cytokines include all except:
   a. Interleukin (IL) 1
   b. IL-2
   c. IL-6
   d. Tumor necrosis factor α
   e. IL-10

5. Evidence-based medical management for patients with peripheral arterial disease usually includes:
   a. Folic acid supplements
   b. Statin administration
   c. Antioxidant vitamin C and E supplements
   d. Aspirin and dipyridamole
   e. Beta blockade

6. Characteristics of unstable or vulnerable plaques include:
   a. A thin fibrous cap
   b. A prominent lipid core
   c. Intense round cell infiltration
   d. Variable degrees of luminal intrusion
   e. All of the above

7. Which of the following statements about genetic disorders promoting increased levels of low-density lipoprotein cholesterol and atherosclerosis is true?
   a. They are exceedingly rare.
   b. They are associated with type 1 diabetes.
   c. They occur in about 1 in 500 live births.
   d. They relate to surface defects in a high-density lipoprotein protein moiety.
   e. They can be treated with diet in most cases.

8. In stable patients, low ferritin levels are most commonly seen in:
   a. Hemachromatosis
   b. Middle-aged men
   c. Menstruating women
   d. Northern Europeans
   e. Postmenopausal women

9. Immediate preoperative management for patients undergoing vascular intervention may include all except:
   a. Aspirin administration
   b. Initiating beta blockade
   c. Prophylactic antibiotic administration
   d. Reinforcing smoking cessation advice
   e. Central line placement

10. Most recently accepted concepts of atherogenesis include:
    a. Intimal lipid infiltration
    b. Endothelial denudation
    c. Excess platelet derived growth factor
    d. Core lipid accumulation and inflammation
    e. Smooth muscle hypertrophy

ANSWERS

1. **a**
2. **b**
3. **a**
4. **e**
5. **b**
6. **e**
7. **c**
8. **c**
9. **b**
10. **d**

CHAPTER 7

Nonatherosclerotic Vascular Disease

Gregory J. Landry • James M. Edwards

Although the majority of arterial abnormalities of interest to vascular surgeons are caused by atherosclerosis, a significant number result from inflammatory, acquired, congenital, and developmental abnormalities. This chapter briefly describes the pathogenesis, symptoms, diagnosis, and treatment of a variety of nonatherosclerotic vascular diseases. Topics covered include vasospastic disorders, the vasculitides, heritable arteriopathies, anatomic anomalies, homocystinemia, and a variety of other uncommon disease processes that may be encountered by vascular surgeons.

VASOSPASTIC DISORDERS

Raynaud syndrome (RS), variant angina, and migraine headache are the most frequent vasospastic disorders seen in clinical practice. RS is by far the most common vasospastic condition referred to vascular surgeons and is considered in detail here.

Raynaud Syndrome

Since the initial description by Maurice Raynaud in 1862, episodic digital ischemia (or RS) has remained an enigmatic clinical entity. The digital ischemia in patients with this condition traditionally manifests as tricolor changes—white, blue, and red—although one or more of these color changes may be absent. The affected digits return to normal 10 to 15 minutes after removal of the precipitating stimulus (usually environmental cold or emotional stress), and the fingers remain normal between attacks.

The prevalence of RS in the general population varies with climate and, probably, ethnic origin. In cool, damp climates such as the Pacific Northwest, Scandinavia, and Great Britain, the prevalence approaches 20% to 25%.[1] It is not known whether the lower prevalence in warm, dry climates is due to a decreased occurrence of the syndrome or merely lack of patient complaints. RS occurs most frequently in young women.[2] The median age of onset of RS is 14 years, with only 27% of cases beginning after age 40.[3] Approximately one quarter of patients have a family history of RS in a first-degree relative.[4]

The mechanism of vasoconstriction in RS has been the subject of intense debate for more than a century. Raynaud speculated that sympathetic nervous system hyperactivity was responsible, a proposition disproved by Lewis in the 1920s when he demonstrated that blockade of digital

nerve conduction did not prevent vasospasm.[5] Lewis then proposed the theory of a local vascular fault, the nature of which remains undefined.

In recent years, the focus in RS pathophysiology has been on alterations in peripheral adrenoceptor activity. Increased finger blood flow was noted in patients following α-adrenergic blockade with drugs such as reserpine. Oral and intraarterial reserpine was the cornerstone of medical management of RS for several years, but it is no longer available.[6] Angiograms of an RS patient before and after cold exposure and before and after intraarterial reserpine are shown in Figure 7-1.

Research in human vessel models demonstrated increased α_2 receptor sensitivity to cold exposure.[7] α_2 Adrenoceptors appear to have a major role in the production of the symptoms of RS. α_2 Receptors are present in a pure population on human platelets. Receptor levels in circulating cells appear to mirror tissue levels. Owing to the difficulty of obtaining digital arteries from human subjects, some researchers have measured levels of platelet α adrenoceptors, and an increased level of platelet α_2 adrenoceptors in patients with RS has been demonstrated.[8-10] Possible mechanisms of α_2-adrenergic–induced RS include an elevation in the number of α_2 receptor sites, receptor hypersensitivity, and alterations in the number of receptors exposed at any one time.[11,12]

The response of subcutaneous resistance vessels to acetylcholine has been shown to be diminished in patients with RS compared with controls, indicating a possible endothelium-dependent mechanism.[13] The possible roles of the vasoactive peptides endothelin, a potent vasoconstrictor, and calcitonin gene-related peptide (CGRP), a vasodilator, have also been investigated. Serum endothelin levels increased significantly with cold exposure in patients with RS compared with controls.[14,15] Depletion of endogenous CGRP may also contribute, because increased skin blood flow in response to CGRP infusion has been demonstrated in patients with RS compared with that in controls.[16]

Based on observations primarily at the Mayo Clinic 70 years ago by Allen and Brown,[17] patients with Raynaud symptoms have traditionally been classified as having either Raynaud disease or Raynaud phenomenon, depending on the presence or absence of an associated systemic disease process. However, Raynaud phenomenon may precede the development of an associated disease by years. In addition, this system does not address the underlying palmar and digital artery disease that may be

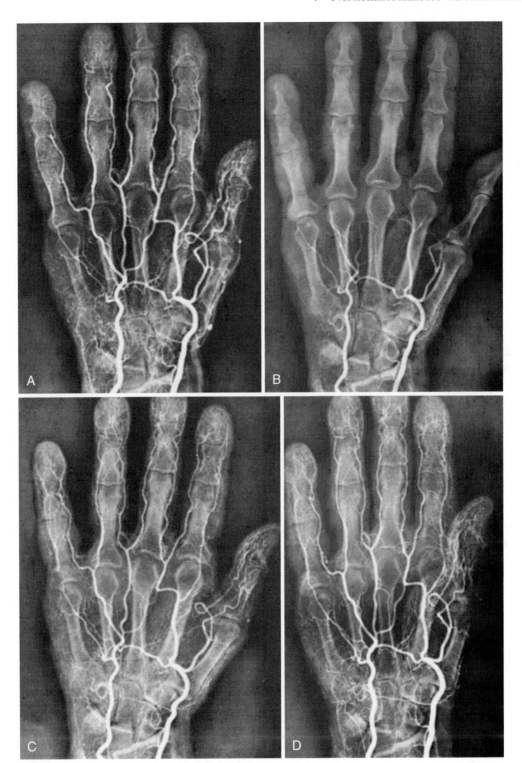

FIGURE 7-1 ■ Hand angiograms of a Raynaud syndrome patient before and after cold exposure and before and after administration of intraarterial reserpine. A marked vasospastic response to cold exposure, which is blocked by reserpine administration, is demonstrated. **A,** Before cold, before reserpine. **B,** After cold, before reserpine. **C,** Before cold, after reserpine. **D,** After cold, after reserpine.

present. Patients with cold- or stress-induced digital ischemia are referred to as having RS, thus avoiding the semantic conflict of *disease* versus *phenomenon*.

We have found it useful to subdivide patients with RS into two distinct pathophysiologic groups: obstructive and vasospastic, based on the presence or absence of

arterial occlusive disease. Patients with vasospastic RS have patent digital arteries and normal digital artery pressures at room temperature. These patients have an abnormally forceful vasoconstrictive response to cold exposure or emotional stress, leading to digital arterial closure and episodic digital ischemic symptoms. Patients with obstructive RS have significant obstruction of either the palmar and digital arteries or the proximal arm arteries, with a concomitant reduction in resting digital arterial pressure. In these patients, a normal vasoconstrictive response to cold appears to be sufficient to cause digital arterial closure with resultant episodic digital ischemia.

In patients with obstructive RS, the mechanism of the obstructive process is variable. Patients with connective tissue disease typically have an autoimmune vasculitis, which is probably the mechanism underlying the widespread digital and palmar artery occlusions. Patients who work with vibrating tools have a similar process and frequently develop a peculiar fibrotic form of palmar and digital artery obstruction, presumably associated with injury from repeated shear stress.[18] Hypercoagulable states may appear with digital artery occlusions, as can emboli from various sources, including valvular heart disease and subclavian, axillary, and ulnar aneurysms. Atherosclerosis involving the upper extremities is rarely seen in the younger age group, but is frequently observed in older patients, especially men.

A number of diseases have been recognized in association with RS, among which the connective tissue diseases are the most frequent; scleroderma is the most common. Associated diseases recognized in patients with RS are shown in Table 7-1.[19] Estimates of the percentage of patients with RS and an associated disease range from 30% to 80%.[1,20-24] It is important to note that the data from most series come from tertiary-care referral centers; therefore they might not reflect the actual incidence in the general population and may overestimate the actual prevalence of associated diseases. Clearly, most individuals with RS view the condition as a nuisance and do not seek medical advice.

The diagnosis of RS is made by history and physical examination. Noninvasive vascular laboratory testing is used to differentiate obstructive from vasospastic RS. Symptoms are typically described as coldness, numbness, or mild discomfort. Significant pain during attacks is conspicuously absent. Classically, both hands are involved, with frequent sparing of the thumbs. The lower extremities are infrequently involved. Most episodes are induced by cold; however, the cold threshold varies from patient to patient. Emotional stimuli can induce attacks in some patients. Episodes typically commence with blanching of one or several fingers extending as far as the metacarpophalangeal joint, rarely involving the palm or extending proximally to the wrist. This phase corresponds to vasoconstriction with the absence of blood in digital arteries. After rewarming, the first blood to reach the skin is desaturated, leading to finger cyanosis. Finally, reactive hyperemia leads to digital rubor. Episodes usually last as long as the cold stimulus is present and resolve within 10 to 15 minutes of rewarming. The hands and fingers are normal between attacks.

A history suggestive of an associated connective tissue disease should be sought, including arthralgias, dysphagia, sclerodactyly, xerophthalmia, or xerostomia, as well as any prior history of large vessel occlusive disease, malignancy, hypothyroidism, frostbite, trauma, use of vibrating tools, and drug use. More than half of patients with carpal tunnel syndrome can have coexistent RS.[25] The examiner should carefully evaluate the pulses and assess the digits for evidence of active or healed ulceration, sclerodactyly, telangiectasia, and calcinosis. The optimal serologic evaluation has not been defined. It is common to obtain a complete blood cell count, erythrocyte sedimentation rate, antinuclear antibody titer, and rheumatoid factor. Patients who exhibit sudden-onset digital ischemia should be evaluated for hypercoagulable states. Tests for specific connective tissue diseases are obtained based on clinical suspicion. Importantly, the physical examination in patients with RS is frequently normal, and the diagnosis relies on history and noninvasive tests.

Routine vascular laboratory testing consists of digital photoplethysmography and digital blood pressures. The digital photoplethysmographic recording provides qualitative information on the character of the arterial waveform.[26] Normal digital blood pressure is within 30 mm Hg of brachial pressure. Patients with obstructive RS have blunted waveforms, whereas patients with vasospastic RS have either normal waveforms or a "peaked pulse." The peaked pulse pattern, first described by Sumner and Strandness,[27] appears to reflect increased vasospastic arterial resistance.

The utility of cold provocation testing remains controversial. Tests involving immersion of patients' hands in ice water are not clinically useful because of low specificity and reproducibility.[28,29] Of greater clinical utility is a digital hypothermic cold challenge test described by Nielson and Lassen.[30] This test is performed with a liquid-perfused cuff placed on the proximal phalanx of the target finger. The cuff is inflated to suprasystolic

TABLE 7-1 Associated Diseases in Raynaud Syndrome Patients: Oregon Health Sciences University Series

Disease	No. of Patients
Autoimmune disease	**290**
Scleroderma	95
Undifferentiated connective tissue disease	24
Mixed connective tissue disease	23
Systemic lupus erythematosus	17
Sjögren's syndrome	16
Rheumatoid arthritis	9
Positive serology	106
Other diseases or conditions	**300**
Atherosclerosis	46
Trauma	44
Hematologic abnormalities	42
Carpal tunnel syndrome	35
Frostbite	32
Buerger disease	28
Vibration	21
Hypersensitivity angiitis	18
Hypothyroidism	13
Cancer	13
Erythromelalgia	8
No associated disease	**498**
Total	**1088**

From Landry G, Edwards JM, McLafferty RM, et al: Long-term outcome of Raynaud's syndrome in a prospective analyzed cohort. J Vasc Surg 23:76–86, 1996.

pressure for 5 minutes while it is perfused with cold water. The pressure at which blood flow is detected on deflation of the cuff is recorded. A control finger on the same hand is tested at room temperature. The test is repeated at several temperatures, and the result is expressed as the percentage drop in finger systolic pressure with cooling. This test has an overall sensitivity and accuracy of approximately 90%.[31]

Duplex scanning does not appear to have a major role in the diagnosis of RS, although it can be used to search for proximal arterial obstructive or aneurysmal disease. Laser Doppler imaging is a promising new modality that quantifies digital microvascular blood flow and may have future diagnostic applications in RS.[32,33] Angiography was used extensively in the past, particularly in the evaluation of patients with obstructive RS. Patients with an underlying systemic disease process and bilateral palmar and digital arterial obstructive disease documented by vascular laboratory testing do not require angiography to confirm digital artery occlusive disease. Patients with unilateral disease, particularly those who have only one or two digits of one arm involved, should be considered for angiography to determine both the presence of bilateral disease and the presence of any proximal arterial disease. Avoidance of triggering stimuli, such as cold or emotional stress, is the hallmark of conservative treatment.[34] We advise all patients with RS to avoid tobacco use, although a multicenter epidemiologic study suggested that RS is not strongly influenced by tobacco consumption.[35] Medications that have been associated with the causation of RS symptoms, such as ergot alkaloids and β-blockers, should be avoided if appropriate alternative therapies exist. More than 90% of patients with RS respond adequately to these simple conservative measures and require no additional treatment. The small number of patients who develop digital ulcers in association with obstructive RS can also be managed conservatively. A healing rate of 85% has been achieved with simple treatment consisting of soap and water scrubs, antibiotics as selected by culture, and conservative debridement.[36] Calcium channel blockers are the most widely used pharmacologic agent for the treatment of RS. As a rule, patients with vasospastic RS respond more favorably to medical therapy than do those with occlusive RS. The dihydropyridine calcium channel blockers are most effective, and nifedipine has been the most studied, with a significant decrease in attack frequency and severity in numerous trials.[37] Potential side effects include headache, ankle swelling, pruritus, and, rarely, severe fatigue. Other calcium channel blockers include nicardipine, amlodipine, and felodipine.[38] Second-line medications with proven efficacy include α-blockers (prazosin),[39] angiotensin II receptor blockers (losartan),[40] serotonin reuptake inhibitors (fluoxetine),[41] phosphodiesterase 5 inhibitors (sildenafil, tadalafil),[42,43] and topical nitrates.[44]

Active research continues in the treatment of RS with the prostaglandins: PGE_1, PGE_2, and prostacyclin, (PGI_2). Intravenous iloprost, a stable analog of PGI_2, has been shown to be effective in the treatment of RS associated with systemic sclerosis.[45] In placebo-controlled, double-blind studies, intravenous iloprost was associated with both decreased frequency of Raynaud episodes and increased frequency of ulcer healing.[46] Several multicenter clinical trials have examined the efficacy of oral forms of iloprost. Although some groups have detected modest improvements in patients with RS, particularly if associated with systemic sclerosis,[47] others have found no benefit when compared with placebo.[48,49] Endothelin receptor antagonists (bosentan) have also shown benefit in preventing and treating digital ulcers,[50] but has a high rate of liver toxicity and is approved by U.S. Food and Drug Administration only for treatment of pulmonary hypertension. Temperature biofeedback, in which patients are taught hand warming through behavioral techniques, was initially believed to reduce symptom frequency in patients with vasospastic RS.[51] However, a randomized trial showed no improvement in symptoms after 1 year compared with a control technique.[52] Transcutaneous electrical nerve stimulation, which has been described as causing vasodilatation, resulted in only mild increases in skin temperature; it caused no improvements in digital plethysmography or transcutaneous partial pressure of oxygen in test hands and had a negligible effect on symptoms.[53] Acupuncture has also been suggested as a possible treatment alternative, with a significant reduction in frequency and severity of attacks.[54]

Several small case series have demonstrated decreased frequency of attacks and improved ulcer healing with chemical sympathectomy using an interdigital injection of botulinum toxin.[55,56] Surgical cervicothoracic sympathectomy has not been shown to have a lasting benefit in most series, with recurrence rates as high as 82% at 16 months' follow-up.[57] In a large series of patients undergoing thoracoscopic sympathectomy, increased digital artery perfusion was maintained out to 5 years' follow-up, although symptom recurrence occurred in 28% of patients.[58] In contrast to upper extremity sympathectomy, excellent results have been achieved with lower extremity sympathectomy, with long-term symptomatic relief noted in more than 90% of patients undergoing this procedure.[59] Lumbar sympathectomy remains a viable option in the rare patient with severely symptomatic lower extremity vasospasm, and it is amenable to minimally invasive laparoscopic techniques.[60]

Periarterial neurectomy is performed by removing the adventitia of the radial, ulnar, palmar, or common digital arteries. Several modifications of this technique have been published, generally characterized by increasing the length of adventitial stripping to facilitate more distal sympathectomy.[61,62] Results have been mixed, with some series reporting improved quality of life and ulcer healing, although complication rates are as high as 37%[63]; therefore widespread use is generally discouraged.

A minority of patients with RS have an identifiable proximal cause of upper extremity arterial insufficiency demonstrated on angiogram. Patients with subclavian, axillary, or brachial artery obstruction from atherosclerosis, emboli, proximal arterial aneurysms, or other causes are appropriate surgical candidates and can expect excellent results from operative intervention. Reconstruction of the palmar arch and direct microvascular bypass of occluded segments of palmar and digital arteries have been successful in a small number of patients.[64,65] Arteriovenous reversal at the wrist has been advocated as a

TABLE 7-2   Long-Term Outcome of Raynaud's Syndrome Patients Based on Classification at Initial Presentation: Oregon Health Sciences University Series

Initial Classification	Initial Presence of Connective Tissue Disease (%)	Final Presence of Connective Tissue Disease (%)	Presence of Digital Ulceration (%)	Requirement for Digital or Phalangeal Amputation (%)
Spastic, negative serology	0.0	2.0	5.2	1.6
Spastic, positive serology	48.6	57.0	15.5	1.4
Obstructive, negative serology	0.0	8.5	48.2	19.0
Obstructive, positive serology	72.9	81.2	55.6	11.6

From Landry G, Edwards JM, McLafferty RM, et al: Long-term outcome of Raynaud's syndrome in a prospective analyzed cohort. J Vasc Surg 23:76–86, 1996.

method of providing retrograde arterial perfusion to ischemic hands for limb salvage.[66] These procedures, however, are applicable to only a few carefully selected patients.

The long-term outcome of patients with RS is not known with certainty, although epidemiologic studies have shown that up to one third of patients with RS can experience symptom resolution over time.[67] We reviewed our experience with more than 1000 RS patients followed for up to 23 years and found RS to be a relatively benign condition in the majority of patients.[19] We divided the patients into four groups at presentation to determine whether this classification scheme provided prognostic information: vasospastic RS with negative serologies, vasospastic RS with positive serologies, obstructive RS with negative serologies, and obstructive RS with positive serologies. Patients with no evidence of an associated disease or arterial obstruction did extremely well, with minimal risk of severe finger ischemia or development of an associated disease; those with obstruction and positive serologies were most likely to develop worsening finger ischemia and ulceration. A summary is presented in Table 7-2. Patients without a diagnosable connective tissue disorder, but with one or more clinical signs or laboratory tests suggesting such a disease, are much more likely to receive a diagnosis of connective tissue disorder at a later date. Current estimates of progression range from 2% to 6% in patients with initially negative serologic tests to 30% to 75% in patients with positive serologic tests at presentation.[1,22,23,68] Although fingertip debridement and occasional distal phalanx amputation are required to aid ulcer healing, we have performed major interphalangeal finger amputations in only 2 of the more than 1000 RS patients we have evaluated and treated.

SYSTEMIC VASCULITIS

Vasculitis has a deceptively simple definition—inflammation, often with necrosis and occlusive changes of the blood vessels—but its clinical manifestations are diverse and complex.[69] The term *arteritis* has been used to describe many of these syndromes, but *vasculitis* is a more precise term, because many of the entities involve veins as well as arteries. Vasculitis can be generalized or localized. Knowledge of this condition is incomplete, and the currently used classification systems are filled with exceptions and overlapping syndromes. The most useful classification system is based on the size of the vessels

---

BOX 7-1   Vasculitides with Potential Vascular Surgical Importance

LARGE VESSEL VASCULITIS
- Giant cell (temporal) arteritis
- Takayasu disease
- Radiation-induced arterial damage

MEDIUM VESSEL VASCULITIS
- Polyarteritis nodosa (classic)
- Kawasaki disease
- Drug abuse arteritis
- Behçet disease
- Cogan syndrome
- Vasculitis associated with malignancy

SMALL VESSEL VASCULITIS
- Hypersensitivity vasculitis
- Henoch-Schönlein purpura
- Essential cryoglobulinemic vasculitis
- Vasculitis of connective tissue diseases

(small, medium, large) involved by the vasculitic process (Box 7-1).[70] Medium and small vessel vasculitis is further subdivided by the presence or absence of antineutrophil cytoplasmic antibodies (ANCAs), a group of autoantibodies formed against enzymes found in primary granules of neutrophils. The most common ANCA-positive vasculitides include Wegener granulomatosis, microscopic polyangiitis, and Churg-Strauss syndrome, which are rarely encountered by vascular surgeons.[71]

The cause and pathogenesis of most vasculitides are complex and are currently either unknown or incompletely understood. Earlier attempts to associate vasculitis with a single mechanism of immune complex-induced injury have not been substantiated in the majority of vasculitides.[72] The basic pathologic mechanism of vasculitis implicates immune-mediated injury, which can include recognition of a vascular structure as antigen, deposition of immune complexes in a vessel wall with complement activation and injury, direct deposition of antigen in a vessel wall, or a delayed hypersensitivity reaction.

The majority of vasculitides are associated with a cellular immunoreaction involving the production of soluble mediators including cytokines, arachidonic acid metabolites, and fibrinolytic and coagulation by-products. The production of cytokines results in neutrophilic, eosinophilic, monocytic, and lymphocytic interactions at the inflammatory site. Endothelial cells express cell membrane receptors specific for many of these inflammatory cells. Binding of inflammatory cells to the endothelial cell triggers intracellular production of additional endothelial cytokines that affect the local inflammatory environment. Complement binding is thought to aid the attachment of leukocytes to endothelial cells. Platelet interactions with both intact and injured endothelium can contribute to the inflammatory process through activation of coagulation pathways and release of cytokines capable of stimulating and modifying immune responses.[72,73]

The vascular surgeon attends to the sequelae of vasculitic injury in these diseases. Thrombosis, aneurysm formation, hemorrhage, or arterial occlusion may all follow or accompany transmural damage created by inflammatory reactions on the vascular wall. An abbreviated list of the vasculitides that have potential significance to vascular surgeons is presented in Box 7-1 and is considered in this section.

Large Vessel Vasculitis

Giant Cell Arteritis Group

The two conditions included in the giant cell arteritis group are systemic giant cell, or temporal, arteritis and Takayasu disease. Although they have fairly distinctive clinical patterns (Box 7-2), the two entities likely represent different manifestations of the same disease process. The microscopic pathologic findings of the two conditions are similar, and it is often impossible to clearly categorize individual tissue sections as one or the other. Both conditions consist of localized periarteritis with inflammatory mononuclear infiltrates and giant cells, along with disruption and fragmentation of the elastic fibers of the arterial wall. The arterial inflammation begins and is most pronounced in the media. In both conditions, the intensity of the cellular infiltrate and the number of giant cells are variable. Histologically, giant cells are pathognomonic but not essential to make the diagnosis of giant cell arteritis.

BOX 7-2	Clinical Patterns in Giant Cell Arteritis	
	TEMPORAL ARTERITIS	**TAKAYSU'S DISEASE**
Age, sex	Elderly, white women	Young females
Pathology	Inflammatory cellular infiltrates Giant Cells	Same
Area of involvement	Usually branches of carotid; may involve any artery	Aortic arch and branches; pulmonary artery
Complications	Blindness	Hypertension, stroke
Response to steroids	Excellent	Unpredictable, unproved

Both giant cell arteritis and Takayasu disease have a propensity for the insidious development of aneurysms of the thoracic and abdominal aorta, which may be accompanied by dissection. Both may be associated with slowly progressive occlusive lesions of the upper extremity, carotid, visceral, and renal arteries. The main differences between these two disease entities are the age and sex of afflicted individuals.[74]

Systemic Giant Cell Arteritis (Temporal Arteritis). Systemic giant cell arteritis (GCA) is essentially limited to patients older than 50 years; it occurs twofold to sixfold more frequently in women as in men and is more prominent in whites. The annual incidence in white women older than 50 years is 15 to 25 cases per 100,000.[75] Polymyalgia rheumatica, a clinical syndrome of aching and stiffness of the hip and shoulder girdle muscles lasting 4 weeks or longer and associated with an elevated erythrocyte sedimentation rate, is present in 50% to 75% of patients with temporal arteritis.[76]

GCA can involve any large artery of the body, although it has a propensity to affect branches of the carotid artery. The clinical history usually begins with a febrile myalgic process involving primarily the back, shoulder, and pelvic regions. Headache, malaise, anorexia, weight loss, and jaw claudication are common. The most characteristic complaint is severe pain along the course of the temporal artery, accompanied by tenderness and nodularity of the artery and overlying skin erythema. The involvement is frequently bilateral. Visual disturbances occur in more than 50% of patients. The mechanism of the visual alterations may be ischemic optic neuritis, retrobulbar neuritis, or occlusion of the central retinal artery. Unilateral blindness occurs in as many as 17% of patients with GCA, followed by contralateral, usually permanent, blindness in one third of these patients within 1 week.[77] Amaurosis fugax is an important warning sign that precedes visual loss in 44% of patients.[78]

GCA is of concern to cardiac and vascular surgeons, because it can cause aneurysms or stenoses of the aorta or its main branches. Both true thoracic aortic aneurysms and dissecting aneurysms can occur. Patients with GCA have a 17-fold increased risk of thoracic aortic aneurysms and a 2.4-fold increased risk of abdominal aortic aneurysms compared with age-matched controls.[79] Classic arteriographic findings of GCA include smooth, tapering stenoses of subclavian, axillary, and brachial arteries (Figure 7-2). Aortic involvement is best visualized with computed tomography (CT) or magnetic resonance angiography (MRA), in which aortic wall thickening is demonstrated.[80] Klein and associates[81] found that 14% of patients with GCA had evidence of symptomatic large artery involvement. Symptomatic subclavian-axillary occlusion is a frequent presenting symptom of GCA.[82] Although rare, lower extremity involvement has also been described.[83] Laboratory findings supporting a diagnosis of GCA include an elevated erythrocyte sedimentation rate. The diagnostic criteria of the American College of Rheumatology include an erythrocyte sedimentation rate of at least 50 mm/hour.[84] However, up to 25% of patients with GCA have a normal sedimentation rate at the time of diagnosis,[85] and this finding should not

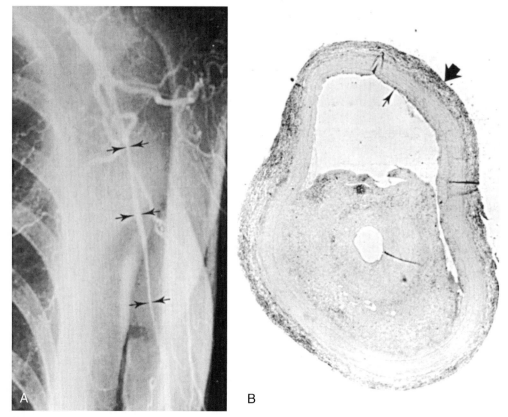

FIGURE 7-2 ■ **A,** Typical giant cell arteritis with smooth tapering of the axillary artery *(arrows)*. **B,** Photomicrograph of an axillary artery involved with giant cell arteritis showing transmural inflammation *(large arrow)* and an inner zone of fibrosis *(small arrow)*. (From Rivers SP, Baur GM, Inahara T, et al: Arm ischemia secondary to giant cell arteritis. Am J Surg 143:554–558, 1982.)

preclude treatment if clinical suspicion is high. C-reactive protein may be a more sensitive indicator of disease activity than the sedimentation rate.[86]

Temporal artery biopsy remains the gold standard of diagnosis in patients suspected of having GCA. Because of skip lesions, a specimen at least 2 cm long should be obtained. When possible, temporal artery biopsy should be performed before corticosteroid treatment; however, histologic evidence of arteritis may be found after up to 2 weeks of treatment.[87] Bilateral sequential temporal artery biopsies are frequently performed if the results of unilateral biopsy are inconclusive, but in 97% of cases, the two specimens show the same findings.[88] Characteristic findings on color-flow duplex scans have been described, typically a hypoechoic halo around the artery corresponding with associated periarterial inflammation, with a sensitivity of 75% and specificity of 83% compared with temporal artery biopsies.[89]

The importance of a precise and early diagnosis lies in the early initiation of steroid therapy. Prompt steroid therapy frequently results in restoration of pulses and prevention of lasting visual disturbances. Typical treatment consists of initial high-dose intravenous steroids followed by a gradual oral taper. Most patients require at least 1 year of treatment, although some require lifelong therapy.[90,91] Although corticosteroids remain the cornerstone of medical therapy, cytotoxic agents (e.g., methotrexate), immunosuppressants (e.g., azathioprine,

cyclosporin), and antitumor necrosis factor monoclonal antibody (infliximab) are used occasionally.[92,93] However, trials of steroid-sparing drugs have had conflicting results. With the exception of those with aortic dissections, the life expectancy of patients with GCA is the same as that of the general population.[94]

Takayasu Disease. Takayasu disease frequently affects the aorta and its major branches and, in contrast to GCA, the pulmonary artery. The majority of patients are Asian, about 85% are female, and the median age at onset is between 25 and 41 years.[95] The disease has two recognized stages. The first stage is characterized by fever, myalgia, and anorexia in approximately two thirds of patients. In the second stage, these symptoms may be followed by multiple arterial occlusive symptoms, with manifestations dependent on disease location.

The cardiovascular areas of involvement have been characterized as types I, II, III, and IV and are shown in Figure 7-3. Type I is limited to involvement of the arch and arch vessels and occurs in 8.4% of patients. Type II involves the descending thoracic and abdominal aorta and accounts for 11.2% of cases. Type III involves the arch vessels and the abdominal aorta and its branches and accounts for 65.4% of cases. Type IV consists primarily of pulmonary artery involvement, with or without other vessels, and accounts for 15% of patients.[96] Most of the lesions are stenotic, although localized aneurysms have

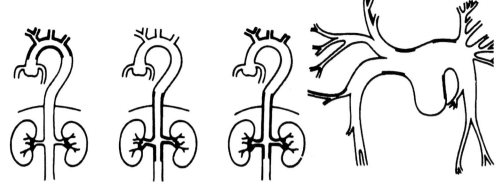

FIGURE 7-3 ■ Diagrammatic representation of the recognized types of Takayasu arteritis. The areas of arterial involvement are shown in heavy lines. (From Lupi-Herrera E, Sanchez-Torres G, Marcustiamer J, et al: Takayasu arteritis: clinical study of 107 cases. Am Heart J 93:94–103, 1977.)

been reported. Arteriography has traditionally been the imaging modality of choice.[97] However, color-flow duplex scanning,[98] CT,[99] magnetic resonance imaging (MRI),[100] and positron emission tomography scanning[101] have emerged as important alternatives, providing information about both luminal and mural involvement in affected vessels.

Cardiovascular findings include diminished peripheral arterial pulsations and hypertension. The hypertension may be due to aortic coarctation or renal artery stenosis. The possible relationship of this disease to the middle aortic, or abdominal coarctation, syndrome is described in a subsequent section. Neurologic symptoms can result from hypertension or central nervous system ischemia associated with large artery occlusion or stenosis. Coronary artery involvement in Takayasu disease is rare. The cardiac pathologic feature most frequently found is nonspecific and appears to result from heart failure associated with systemic and pulmonary hypertension.

Available information suggests that a conservative surgical approach is best for these patients. A poor long-term outcome is predicted by the presence of major complications (retinopathy, hypertension, aortic insufficiency, aneurysm formation) and a progressive disease course.[102] Surgical intervention is generally reserved to treat symptomatic stenotic or, less commonly, aneurysmal lesions resulting from chronic Takayasu arteritis. Surgical intervention is best performed with the disease in a quiescent state. Restenosis rates in the presence of active disease are approximately 45%, compared with 12% restenosis rates with quiescent disease.[103] Successful surgical management requires bypass graft implantation into disease-free arterial segments and continuation of corticosteroid therapy.[104] Excellent long-term survival rates of up to 75% at 20 years have been reported in large operative series.[105] Owing to its inflammatory nature, endarterectomy has resulted in early failure and is generally not recommended.

Percutaneous transluminal angioplasty and stenting has had mixed success, with high early success rates of up to 90%[106]; however, high rates of in-stent restenosis have been reported.[107] In general, surgical intervention remains a more durable option.

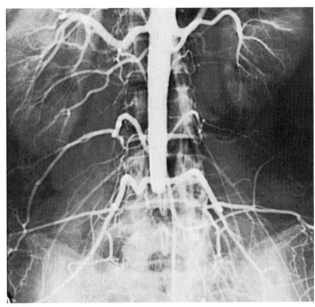

FIGURE 7-4 ■ Radiation arteritis. Arteriogram in a 40-year-old woman who had received extensive internal and external irradiation for treatment of carcinoma of the cervix. There is a typical absence of atherosclerotic disease of the infrarenal aorta.

Radiation-Induced Arterial Damage

Radiation given for the treatment of regional malignancy causes well-recognized changes in arteries within the irradiated field. The primary changes consist of intimal thickening and proliferation, medial hyalinization, proteoglycan deposition, and cellular infiltration of the adventitia. Normal endothelium has a slow rate of turnover, and following irradiation, endothelial cells do not proliferate. Pleomorphic endothelial cells can develop as a result of irradiation, with exposure of the basement membrane leading to thrombosis of small vessels.[108] Post-irradiation changes in large arteries often resemble atherosclerosis (Figure 7-4).

Of considerable importance is the tendency for arteries in an irradiated area to show stenosis years later, thought to be due to chronic oxidative stress with upregulation of matrix metalloproteinases, proinflammatory cytokines, smooth muscle cell proliferation and apoptosis, with downregulation of nitric oxide.[109] There is an unusually high incidence of carotid artery stenosis in patients years after neck irradiation, along with an increased likelihood of stroke.[110] The lesions vary from diffuse scarring to areas of typical atheromatous narrowing, with a preponderance of the latter. Patients who have had regional irradiation, especially of the cervical region, should have careful vascular follow-up, including noninvasive vascular laboratory examinations. Stenoses of the subclavian and axillary arteries have been demonstrated in patients undergoing radiation therapy for breast cancer and Hodgkin lymphoma, and aortoiliac involvement has been noted in patients undergoing abdominal or pelvic radiation therapy.

Vascular surgery on irradiated arteries can be performed using standard techniques. Prosthetic and autogenous bypass grafts, as well as endarterectomy, have all been performed satisfactorily.[111] Prudence suggests avoidance of a prosthetic graft in a field in which infection may be expected, such as a radical neck dissection after irradiation, and autologous vein reconstruction is preferred. Late graft infections occurring 2 to 5 years after surgery have been described.[112] The treatment of carotid artery stenosis in irradiated areas with percutaneous angioplasty and stenting has been reported, with excellent results,[113,114] although rates of restenosis and reintervention are significantly higher than in nonirradiated arteries and historical surgical controls. Although data are limited, endovascular treatment of other arterial beds appears to be safe and effective in selected cases.[115]

Medium Vessel Vasculitis

Polyarteritis Nodosa

Polyarteritis nodosa (PAN) is a disseminated disease characterized by focal necrotizing lesions involving primarily medium-size muscular arteries. This is a rare disorder with a population of 2 to 16 per 1 million, a male-female preponderance of 2-4:1, and a peak incidence in the 40s.[116] The clinical manifestations of PAN are varied. It can involve only one organ or multiple organs simultaneously or sequentially over time. The most frequent manifestations of PAN include a characteristic crescent-forming glomerulonephritis, polyarteritis, polymyositis, and abdominal pain. A cutaneous form also exists, presenting with subcutaneous nodules, livedo reticularis, and cutaneous ulcers.[117]

The essential pathologic feature of PAN is focal transmural arterial inflammatory necrosis. The process begins with medial destruction, followed by a sequential acute inflammatory response, fibroblastic proliferation, and endothelial damage. Immune complexes do not appear to be involved in the endothelial degeneration. The vascular injury is resolved by intimal proliferation, thrombosis, or aneurysm formation, all of which may culminate in luminal occlusion, with consequent organ ischemia and infarction.[118]

The erythrocyte sedimentation rate, C-reactive protein, and factor XIII–related protein, all nonspecific serologic markers of inflammation, are elevated in PAN. Positive hepatitis B serologies are common in adults with PAN.[119] Mild anemia and leukocytosis are frequent. ANCAs have been detected in patients with systemic vasculitis, including PAN, Wegener granulomatosis, Churg-Strauss syndrome, temporal arteritis, and Kawasaki disease.[120]

The hallmark of PAN is the formation of multiple saccular aneurysms associated with inflammatory destruction of the media, with the most frequently involved organs being the kidney, heart, liver, and gastrointestinal tract. Rupture of intraabdominal PAN aneurysms has been well described and may represent a surgical emergency.[121] Coil embolization of ruptured visceral aneurysms in PAN has also been described and represents an alternative to surgical intervention.[122] Curiously, these aneurysms have been documented to regress on occasion after vigorous steroid and cyclophosphamide therapy, which should be recommended for all asymptomatic visceral aneurysms.[123] An arteriogram of a patient with PAN showing the typical visceral and renal artery aneurysms is shown in Figure 7-5. Visceral PAN lesions can also lead to visceral artery narrowing incident to the inflammatory process, which can progress to occlusion. The visceral ischemia can manifest as cholecystitis, appendicitis, enteric perforation, gastrointestinal hemorrhage, or ischemic stricture formation with bowel obstruction.[124]

The routine use of steroid therapy has improved 5-year survival from 15% to the current 50% to 80%.[125] Cyclophosphamide can be added to the steroid regimen in acute, severe cases.[126] It has been suggested that prognosis can be determined by the absence or presence of creatinemia, proteinuria, cardiomyopathy, and gastrointestinal or central nervous system involvement at the time of presentation. Five-year mortality with zero, one, or two or more of these signs was 12%, 26%, and 46%, respectively.[127] During the acute phase of PAN, renal and gastrointestinal lesions account for the majority of deaths, whereas cardiovascular and cerebral events account for mortality in chronic cases.

To date, little vascular surgical experience with PAN has been reported. The multiplicity of diseased areas renders elective vascular repair of all lesions impossible, and there is no accurate way to recognize the dangerous ones. The role of vascular surgery in intestinal revascularization in PAN is presently undefined.

Kawasaki Disease

In the 1960s, an unusual febrile exanthematous illness swept Japan. Kawasaki observed 50 cases in the Department of Pediatrics at the Japan Red Cross Medical Center and termed the disease the *mucocutaneous lymph node syndrome*.[128] Over the next decade, the spread of the disease was noted worldwide, and it became known as Kawasaki disease. The disease is not limited to those of Asian descent and occurs in all ethnic groups, although children of Japanese or mixed Japanese ancestry appear to be most susceptible. The annual incidence in Japan is 140 cases per 100,000 children younger than 5 years,[129] compared

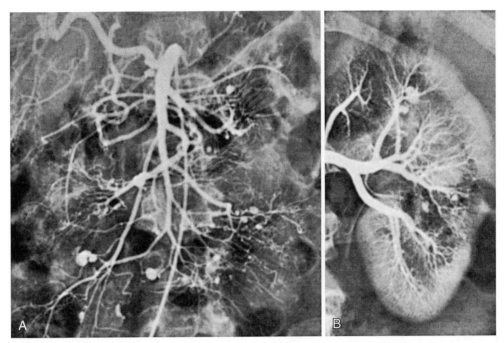

FIGURE 7-5 ■ **A,** Arteriogram showing multiple visceral aneurysms in a patient with polyarteritis nodosa. **B,** Multiple renal artery aneurysms in the same patient.

with the incidence in the United States of approximately 17 cases per 100,000 children.[130] The vasculitis associated with Kawasaki disease has a propensity to affect the coronary arteries, making it the most common cause of acquired heart disease in children in the developed world.[131]

As the disease has become better known, strict clinical criteria have evolved for diagnosis: (1) high fever present for 5 days or more; (2) bilateral congestion of ocular conjunctiva; (3) changes in the mucous membranes of the oral cavity, including erythema, dryness, and fissuring of the lips or diffuse reddening of the oropharyngeal mucosa; (4) changes in the peripheral portions of the extremities, including reddening and induration of the hands and feet and periungual desquamation; (5) polymorphous exanthem; and (6) acute nonsuppurative swelling of the cervical lymph nodes. The presence of a prolonged high fever and any four of the five remaining criteria, in the absence of concurrent evidence of bacterial or viral infection, establishes the diagnosis.[132]

Kawasaki disease has a unimodal peak incidence at 1 year of age; it has not been described in neonates and is rarely observed for the first time in those older than 5 years. The acute symptoms can persist for 7 to 14 days before improvement occurs as the fever subsides. Notable laboratory features include elevation of the erythrocyte sedimentation rate and C-reactive protein, thrombocythemia, and elevated levels of von Willebrand factor.[133]

The etiology of Kawasaki disease is likely multifactorial. An infectious cause has long been assumed, given the self-limited nature of the disease, its seasonal incidence, and geographic outbreaks. However, no single infectious agent has been demonstrated. An immunologic defect has also been postulated, as there appears to be an altered immunoregulatory state in these patients, with decreased

numbers of T cells and an increased proportion of activated helper T4 cells. Genetic susceptibility also appears to have a role pathogenesis.[134] The most serious disease manifestation is coronary arteritis, which is likely present in all children with this disease. The spectrum of documented coronary artery pathologic changes consists of active arteritis, thrombosis, calcification, and stenosis, although the distinguishing feature of Kawasaki disease is the formation of diffuse fusiform and saccular coronary artery aneurysms.

Routine echocardiography in patients with Kawasaki disease has demonstrated coronary artery dilatation or aneurysms in 25% to 50%, with the aneurysms typically appearing in the second week of illness and reaching a maximum size from the third to eighth week after the onset of fever.[135] Echocardiography may show dilatation of the right, left, or anterior descending coronary arteries, while the circumflex coronary artery is rarely involved.[136]

Serial arteriographic studies have shown a considerable capacity for all types of coronary arterial lesions to evolve. The aneurysms may regress, leaving a patent arterial lumen, or the arterial segment may become stenotic. Most stenotic lesions regress, with maintenance of a patent lumen, but a few progress to occlusion. Stenotic lesions demonstrated by coronary angiography are most frequently seen in the left anterior descending artery. Patients older than 2 years with fever lasting longer than 14 days and pericardial effusion and those not treated with anticoagulant agents appear to have a higher incidence of aneurysm formation.[135] Patients treated with immune globulin have shown a decreased incidence of aneurysm formation. New coronary arterial lesions occur infrequently after 2 weeks. Regression of the lesions occurs over a 2-month period, although some

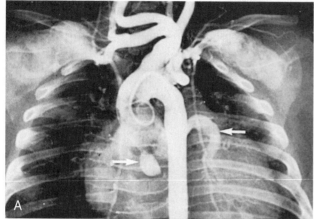

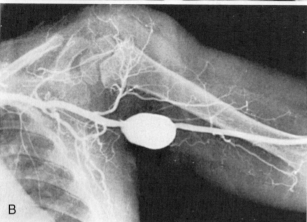

FIGURE 7-6 ■ **A,** Arteriogram of an infant with Kawasaki disease showing coronary artery aneurysms *(white arrows)* and massive subclavian artery aneurysms. **B,** Arteriogram of a 2-year-old child showing a large axillary artery aneurysm resulting from Kawasaki disease.

lesions remain unchanged for more than 1 year before regression.[137]

Systemic arteritis also occurs in Kawasaki disease, with iliac arteritis as prevalent as coronary arteritis. Aneurysm formation is far less frequent in the systemic arteries than in the coronary arteries, with one report identifying systemic arterial aneurysms (axillary and iliac) in 3.3% of 662 patients with Kawasaki disease and coronary artery aneurysms.[138] The healing process in the systemic arterial lesions can lead to focal arterial stenosis or aneurysm formation, just as in the coronary arteries. The coexistence of peripheral arterial involvement (subclavian and axillary arteries) and coronary artery aneurysms is shown in Figure 7-6.

Thrombosis of coronary artery aneurysms is the overwhelming cause of death in the early stages of Kawasaki disease, causing acute myocardial infarction or arrhythmia. Coronary aneurysm rupture has also been described. With the initiation of aspirin and immune globulin therapy in the acute phase, the mortality from Kawasaki disease has decreased to 1.1%, and among patients with no cardiac sequelae does not differ from the general population.[139] Intravenous gamma globulin is typically given as a single-infusion high dose of 2 g/kg. Aspirin is given orally at a dose of 80 mg/kg per day until the child

is afebrile, then continued in low-dose form (3 to 5 mg/kg per day) for an additional 6 to 8 weeks.[131] Approximately 10% to 15% of patients are refractory to standard therapy,[140] and corticosteroids or other immunosuppressant agents (e.g., infliximab, cyclosporin) are considered in these patients.[141]

Coronary artery bypass grafting was first used in Kawasaki disease in 1976.[142] The first procedure used the saphenous vein as a conduit; however, concerns over its potential to grow with the child have been raised. This concern led to the use of the internal mammary artery (unilateral or bilateral)[143] and the right gastroepiploic artery[144] for coronary revascularization in patients with Kawasaki disease. Five- and 15-year patency rates of internal mammary grafts are 91% in children older than 12 years of age, but only 73% and 65%, respectively, in patients younger than 12.[145] Percutaneous angioplasty of anastomotic lesions, however, has improved 10-year patency rates in this group to 94%.[146] Primary catheter based interventions, such as stent implantation[147] and coronary rotational ablation,[148] have also had excellent results in selected cases of focal coronary artery stenosis. Cardiac transplantation for severe ischemic heart disease as a sequela of Kawasaki disease is considered in patients who are not candidates for revascularization because of distal coronary stenosis or aneurysms and those with severe irreversible myocardial dysfunction.[149]

Aneurysms of the abdominal aorta and iliac, axillary, brachial, mesenteric, and renal arteries have been observed as late sequelae of systemic vasculitis. When these lesions become symptomatic from occlusion, expansion, or embolization, most surgeons proceed with standard repair techniques using interposition grafting. Although experience is limited, surgical repair of the aneurysms has been accomplished safely.[150]

Drug Abuse Arteritis

Intravenous drug abuse, particularly the use of methamphetamines or cocaine, is associated with a panarteritis similar in presentation and appearance to PAN,[151] with combinations of renal failure, central nervous system dysfunction, and localized intestinal necrosis and perforation. Isolated cerebral angiitis has also been reported in the setting of methamphetamine and cocaine abuse.[152,153] No medical therapy has proved effective for this condition. Necrotizing renal vasculitis secondary to oral methamphetamines ("ecstasy") has also been described.[154]

A second type of arterial obstruction has been reported in drug abuse patients following the accidental intraarterial injection of drugs during attempted intravenous injection. The drugs most commonly involved are parenteral barbiturates, in which case arterial injury and thrombosis appear to result from chemical damage, perhaps related to the low pH of the injectant.[155] Another pattern of arterial damage results from the accidental injection of drug preparations intended for oral use. The practice of dissolving tablets in water for intravenous injection is enormously harmful because of the large number of substances (e.g., silica, tragacanth) in tablets. When this material is accidentally injected intraarterially, significant

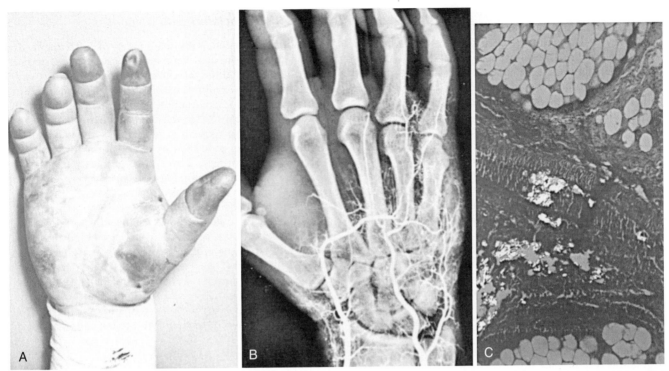

FIGURE 7-7 ■ **A,** Photograph of the hand of a 22-year-old man who injected a pentazocine tablet dissolved in tap water into his radial artery. The hand was severely ischemic, with gangrenous changes of the radial side. **B,** Arteriogram showing massive arterial obstruction of the common and proper digital arteries to the thumb, index, and long fingers. **C,** Slide from amputation specimen under polarized light showing bright refractile silica particles in the hand arteries.

distal ischemia can result from obstruction of the small arteries by the inert materials (Figure 7-7).[156]

No convincing evidence has demonstrated the value of any specific treatment in these patients. A number of therapeutic efforts have been tried, including anticoagulation, regional sympathetic block, and the administration of vasodilators, without proof of efficacy. The outcome appears to be determined at the time of injection by the quantity and concentration of injectant reaching the distal arterial bed. Nonetheless, heparin anticoagulation is favored if the patient is seen acutely and has no contraindications to this treatment. Compartment syndrome requiring fasciotomy is an infrequent but reported sequela.[157]

Behçet Disease

In 1937, Behçet described three patients with iritis and associated oral and genital mucocutaneous ulcerations, an association subsequently termed *Behçet disease*.[158] More than half of these patients have joint involvement. The underlying pathologic lesion is a vasculitis, which results in both venous thromboses and specific arterial lesions. Venous thrombosis is the most frequent vascular disorder in Behçet disease, representing approximately 70% of vascular lesions and affecting up to one third of patients.[159] Arterial lesions are distinctly less frequent, occurring in 1% to 7% of patients, and include occlusive and aneurysmal disease.[159] This systemic disease largely affects individuals from the Mediterranean area and East Asia and is more common in men.

The pathogenesis of vascular damage in Behçet disease appears to be an immune-mediated destructive process. A humorally mediated cause has been suggested by the identification of enhanced neutrophil activity and circulating immune complexes in affected patients.[160] Specific T cell subsets have also been identified in high concentrations at the sites of vascular involvement, indicating a cellular-mediated process.[161] Activation of complement within the vessel wall can lead to destruction of the media and subsequent aneurysm formation. Vasa vasorum occlusion can then lead to transmural necrosis of the large muscular arterial walls, with perforation and pseudoaneurysm formation and injury to adjacent tissues.[162]

Behçet disease may have a genetic component, because there is an increased incidence of the HLA-B51 allele among patients with the disease, with resultant abnormalities in tumor necrosis factor (TNF)-α expression.[163] Both viral and bacterial causes have been proposed, although definitive evidence is lacking.[164]

Large artery involvement is an uncommon but serious complication of Behçet disease. Arterial aneurysms, although distinctly less common than the mucocutaneous, ophthalmic, or arthritic lesions, are the most frequent cause of death in patients with Behçet disease.[165] Aneurysms have been described in numerous arteries, including the carotid, popliteal, femoral, iliac, pulmonary, and subclavian, but the aorta is the most frequent site of aneurysm formation in this disease.[159] Curiously, the aneurysms frequently appear phlegmonous, suggesting acute bacterial infection, although cultures are invariably negative. The arterial aneurysms are frequently multiple and may be metachronous. Unfortunately, interposition bypass grafts have a high incidence of thrombosis, in addition to the propensity to develop anastomotic pseudoaneurysms, which tend to occur within the first 18 months in up to 13% of cases.[166] Owing to the recognized difficulties of surgical aneurysm repair in Behçet disease, endovascular repair is emerging as the treatment of choice. The focal, saccular nature of these lesions makes them ideally suited to endovascular treatment. Excellent patency rates of endovascular treatment have been reported, but the fragile nature of the arteries puts patients at risk for pseudoaneurysm formation at seal zones, and aggressive stent oversizing is discouraged. Long-term immunosuppressive therapy is recommended after endovascular repair to limit pseudoaneurysm formation.[167]

Venous involvement is prominent, and lower extremity superficial or deep vein thrombosis occurs in 12% to 34% of patients, frequently alone or in association with arterial disease.[159] Thrombosis of the superior or inferior vena cava or of intracerebral veins occurs less frequently but can be fatal. Lifelong anticoagulation is recommended in patients with Behçet disease who develop venous thrombosis, but the role of prophylactic anticoagulation is uncertain.

Immunosuppressive agents, including azathioprine, corticosteroids, TNF-α antagonists (infliximab) and interferon-α, have been used with some success for nonarterial symptoms.[168] Although corticosteroids may prevent blindness and limit discomfort associated with the mucocutaneous disease, they do not appear to alter the progression or course of the underlying vascular disease. Currently, no uniformly satisfactory therapy exists for Behçet disease; however, early diagnosis and meticulous reconstructive management of identified arterial aneurysms have provided long-term limb salvage in some patients, despite the well-recognized propensity for arterial graft complications.[169] Vigilant follow-up is required once large artery disease is recognized.

Cogan Syndrome

Cogan syndrome is a rare condition consisting of interstitial keratitis and vestibuloauditory symptoms. It is a disease primarily of young adults, with the mean age of onset in the third decade. It is occasionally associated with a systemic vasculitis similar to PAN. Aortitis with subsequent development of clinically significant aortic insufficiency occurs in 10% of patients with Cogan syndrome.[170] Mesenteric vasculitis and thoracoabdominal aneurysms have also been described in association with Cogan syndrome.[171,172]

Daily administration of high-dose corticosteroids has been successful in reversing the visual and auditory components of Cogan syndrome, although deafness may be irreversible. The response of the aortitic component to steroids used singly or in combination with cyclosporine is less well established.[173] Surgical therapy, including aortic valve replacement, mesenteric revascularization, and thoracoabdominal aortic aneurysm repair, is occasionally indicated and can be performed safely.

Vasculitis Associated with Malignancy

Vasculitis associated with malignancy is infrequent. A strong association has been made between a systemic necrotizing vasculitis resembling PAN and hairy cell leukemia. The vasculitis in this situation presents after the diagnosis of leukemia and is indistinguishable from classic PAN. An immune-mediated mechanism is postulated. More frequently, vasculitides involving small vessels have been described in association with lymphoproliferative disorders. These have primarily cutaneous manifestations and minimal visceral involvement and are often referred to as *paraneoplastic vasculitides*.[174]

Vasculitis associated with solid tumors is rare, but resolution with tumor excision has been reported.[175] RS has been reported in association with carcinoma and lymphoproliferative malignancies. These cases were characterized by cold-induced ischemia, which frequently led to digital artery occlusion and ischemic ulcerations. The symptoms of finger ischemia preceded the diagnosis of malignancy, and several of these patients experienced marked improvement of their hand lesions after removal of the tumor.

Small Vessel Vasculitis

Hypersensitivity Vasculitis Group

The entities in the hypersensitivity vasculitis group include classic hypersensitivity vasculitis, mixed cryoglobulinemic vasculitis, and Henoch-Schönlein purpura. These conditions appear to result from antigen exposure followed by antigen-antibody immune complex deposition in small arteries and arterial damage. Hypersensitivity vasculitis usually has prominent skin involvement. In some conditions, a drug, an environmental chemical, or the hepatitis B virus may be implicated as the inciting antigen, but no causative agent is identified in more than half of cases. Henoch-Schönlein purpura is a self-limiting disease that occurs primarily in children and affects the skin, gastrointestinal tract, and kidneys. The disease course and findings are similar in cryoglobulinemic vasculitis, which may be associated with a hematologic malignancy or hepatitis B or C infection.[176]

The clinical syndromes typically associated with this group of diseases include skin rash, fever, and evidence of organ dysfunction, none of which specifically concerns vascular surgeons. It is clear, however, that some of these syndromes can manifest with arteritic involvement substantially limited to the hands and fingers. In these patients, the clinical picture is typically that of severe and widespread palmar and digital arterial occlusions and digital ischemia. The vasculitis can be treated with steroids, with the occasional use of immunosuppressive agents or plasmapheresis. The treatment of hand lesions can otherwise follow the approach outlined later in this chapter for Buerger disease.[177]

Vasculitis of Connective Tissue Diseases

The connective tissue diseases often are complicated by vasculitis. These diseases have associated immunologic

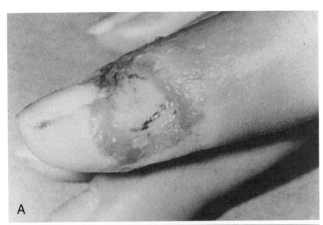

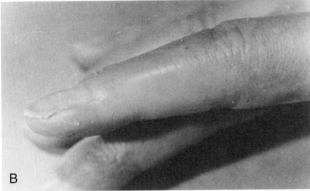

FIGURE 7-8 ■ Photographs of a patient with scleroderma and a digital ulcer. **A,** Digital ulcer. **B,** Healed ulcer following conservative management.

abnormalities, and the occurrence of vasculitis in these patients likely results from immune-mediated damage, as described for other vasculitides.[178] Vasculitis frequently accompanies scleroderma, rheumatoid arthritis, and systemic lupus erythematosus.

Scleroderma is a generalized disorder of connective tissue, microvasculature, and small arteries. It is characterized by progressive scarring and small vessel occlusion in the skin, gastrointestinal tract, kidneys, lungs, and heart. CREST syndrome (calcinosis, Raynaud syndrome, esophageal dysmotility, sclerodactyly, and telangiectases) describes a variant of scleroderma with limited cutaneous involvement. The vasculitis associated with scleroderma results in fibrinoid necrosis and concentric thickening of the intima, with deposition of layers of mucopolysaccharide.

Scleroderma is the most frequent connective tissue disease recognized in our patients with RS, as well as those with digital ulceration (Figure 7-8).[19] Approximately 80% to 97% of patients with scleroderma have symptoms of RS. In our experience, the RS usually begins as vasospastic and progresses to the obstructive type.

The vasculitis associated with rheumatoid arthritis involves primarily small arteries with a predilection for vasa nervorum and the digital arteries. Intimal proliferation, medial necrosis, and progression to fibrosis with vessel occlusion occur. Symptoms of mononeuritis multiplex are common following involvement of small arteries. Cutaneous lesions are often present and include digital ulcers, nail fold infarcts, and palpable purpura.[179] Rarely, there is coronary, mesenteric, or cerebral artery involvement. Patients with rheumatoid arthritis who have positive ANCAs or higher titers of rheumatoid factor have a more aggressive disease course with a more frequent incidence of rheumatoid vasculitis.[180,181] The presence of vasculitis portends a poor prognosis for patients with rheumatoid arthritis.

The vasculitis of systemic lupus erythematosus is believed to be due to deposition of immune complexes.[182] The most frequent clinical vascular problem in lupus is RS, which can affect 80% of patients. Other vasculitic manifestations include palpable purpura and mononeuritis multiplex. Thrombotic disorders of the arterial and venous system occur in patients with lupus and appear to be related to the lupus anticoagulant, not vasculitis. IgA anti–double-stranded DNA antibodies and anti–endothelial cell antibodies are markers of more virulent vasculitic involvement.[183] In addition to small vessel vasculitis, patients with systemic lupus erythematosus are clearly prone to premature large vessel atherosclerosis.[184]

Management of the vasculitides associated with the connective tissue diseases consists primarily of steroid therapy.[182] Steroids appear to have little or no role in the treatment of the occlusive vascular lesions of scleroderma. Immunosuppressive therapy with cyclophosphamide has also been shown to have modest benefit in selected patients.[185] The treatment of RS associated with lupus or scleroderma is as described earlier.

BUERGER DISEASE

Buerger disease, also known as *thromboangiitis obliterans*, is a clinical syndrome characterized by the occurrence of segmental thrombotic occlusions of small- and medium-sized arteries in the lower and frequently the upper extremities, accompanied by a prominent arterial wall inflammatory cell infiltration.[186] Buerger disease is a discrete pathologic entity and is clinically distinct from either atherosclerosis or immune arteritis. Affected patients are predominantly young male smokers (mean age, 34 years); they usually exhibit distal limb ischemia, frequently accompanied by localized digital gangrene.

Buerger disease appears to be on the decline in North America, although there has been an increase in the incidence in women. Women currently constitute up to 20% of patients in certain series.[187] It is unclear whether there is a true decline in incidence or simply more uniform application of strict diagnostic criteria. A large volume of patients continue to be reported from East and Southwest Asia. In patients with peripheral vascular disease, the reported incidence of Buerger disease is 0.75% in North America, 3.3% in Eastern Europe, and 16.6% in Japan.[188]

Approximately 40% to 50% of patients with Buerger disease have a history of superficial migratory thrombophlebitis, RS, or both.[187] The arterial lesions of Buerger disease usually occur in the distal portions of both the upper and the lower extremities and may be accompanied by digital gangrene, especially of the toes. Although there have been rare, well-documented reports, both arteriographically and pathologically, of iliac[189] and visceral artery involvement,[190] in the overwhelming majority of patients with thromboangiitis obliterans, disease is limited to the arteries distal to the elbow and knee. In North America, approximately 50% of patients with Buerger disease have isolated lower extremity involvement, 30% to 40% have upper and lower extremity involvement, and approximately 10% have isolated upper extremity involvement.[187]

The cause of Buerger disease remains unknown. Although a strong association with tobacco use has been recognized clinically, a causal relationship has not been conclusively demonstrated.[187] Most patients are heavy cigarette smokers, although cases of Buerger disease in users of smokeless tobacco[191] and cannabis[192] have also been reported. An increased cellular response to tobacco antigen has been noted in patients with Buerger disease, as well as in healthy smokers compared with nonsmokers. Tobacco is currently considered at least a permissive factor and likely a causative factor.

The major histocompatibility complex, specifically HLA-A9, -B5, -DR4, and -DRw6, has been implicated in Buerger disease, but its role is unclear.[187,193] Considerable evidence indicates that an autoimmune process is central to the illness. Several independent investigators have identified elevated levels of anticollagen antibodies[194] and antiendothelial antibodies[195] in patients with Buerger disease. Immunohistochemical analysis of the arterial wall of patients with Buerger disease demonstrates accumulation of immunoglobulins and complement in the intimal layer, with sparing of the medial and adventitial layers.[196]

The acute lesion of Buerger disease is a nonnecrotizing inflammation of the vascular wall with a prominent component of intraluminal thrombosis. In contrast to both atherosclerosis and immune arteritis, the internal elastic lamina remains intact in Buerger disease; therefore Buerger disease is not a true vasculitis, because it lacks vascular wall necrosis. Both T and B cell–mediated activation of macrophages or dendritic cells in the intima have been implicated in the pathogenesis of Buerger disease.[197] The chronic phase of Buerger disease includes a decline in hypercellularity, with the production of perivascular fibrosis and frequent recanalization of the luminal thrombus. Adjacent veins and nerves are frequently involved in the perivascular inflammatory process.

Currently, well-established diagnostic criteria exist to make the diagnosis of Buerger disease (Box 7-3).[187] The major criteria are essential for diagnosis, whereas the minor criteria are supportive. Central to the diagnosis is the onset of symptoms before the age of 45 years, a uniform exposure to tobacco, and absence of arterial lesions proximal to the knee or elbow. It is essential to exclude other frequent causes of limb ischemia in young adults. In North America, atherosclerosis is much more prevalent than Buerger disease, and major atherosclerotic risk factors such as hyperlipidemia, diabetes, and hypertension must be absent. Proximal sources of emboli (cardiac, proximal arterial occlusive, or aneurysmal disease), underlying autoimmune disease, hypercoagulable states, trauma, and local lesions (popliteal

---

BOX 7-3 | **Criteria for the Diagnosis of Buerger Disease**

MAJOR CRITERIA

- Onset of distal extremity ischemic symptoms before age 45 years
- Tobacco use
- Exclusion of the following:
  - Proximal embolic source (cardiac, thoracic outlet syndrome, arteriosclerosis obliterans, aneurysms)
  - Trauma and local lesions (entrapment, adventitial cyst)
  - Autoimmune disease
  - Hypercoagulable states
  - Atherosclerosis
  - Atherosclerotic risk factors (diabetes, hypertension, hyperlipidemia)
- No evidence of arterial disease proximal to popliteal or distal brachial arteries
- Objective documentation of distal occlusive disease by one of the following: plethysmography, histopathology, or arteriography

MINOR CRITERIA

- Migratory superficial phlebitis
- Raynaud syndrome
- Upper extremity involvement
- Instep claudication

From Mills JL, Porter JM: Buerger disease: a review and update. Semin Vasc Surg 6:14–23, 1993.

---

entrapment, adventitial cystic disease) must also be excluded. We recognize that these criteria are so restrictive that some patients with Buerger disease will be excluded, but we believe that these strict criteria are essential to eliminate the diagnostic uncertainty obvious in many publications of purported Buerger disease. Similar clinical diagnostic criteria were reported by Shionoya from Japan: (1) smoking history, (2) onset before the age of 50 years, (3) infrapopliteal arterial occlusion, (4) either upper limb involvement or phlebitis migrans, and (5) absence of other atherosclerotic risk factors.[198]

After the clinical criteria have been met, objective confirmation of distal occlusive disease limited to small- and medium-sized vessels is required. This confirmation can be done with four-limb digital plethysmography, distinct histopathologic findings when available, or arteriography. The arteriographic findings reveal that the extremity arteries proximal to the popliteal and distal brachial levels are normal, proximal atherosclerosis and vascular calcification are absent, and there is an abrupt transition from a normal, smooth proximal vessel to an area of occlusion.[187] Involvement tends to be segmental rather than diffuse and is commonly symmetrical. In the upper extremity, the ulnar or radial artery is frequently occluded, and extensive digital and palmar arterial occlusion is uniformly present. In the lower extremity, the infrageniculate vessels are extensively diseased, with diffuse plantar arterial occlusion. Tortuous "corkscrew" collaterals frequently reconstitute patent distal arterial segments and,

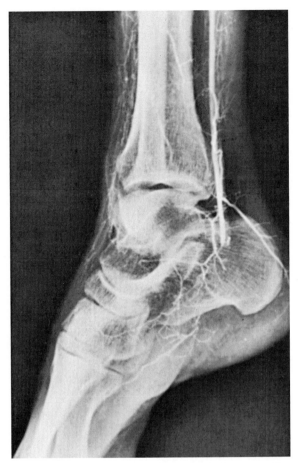

FIGURE 7-9 ■ Arteriogram of patient with Buerger disease showing occlusion of the posterior tibial artery at the ankle, total occlusion of the anterior tibial artery, and numerous small collateral vessels.

although not pathognomonic, are suggestive of Buerger disease (Figure 7-9).

Arteriography, although desirable, is not essential for the diagnosis of every case of Buerger disease.[187] Arteriography may be omitted when a patient's history is typical of Buerger disease, there are no associated atherogenic risk factors, the serologic tests for autoimmune disease and hypercoagulable states are negative, and vascular laboratory examination reveals diffusely abnormal digital plethysmographic tracings in all four extremities accompanied by a conspicuous absence of proximal large artery occlusive disease.

Digital plethysmography frequently provides especially important diagnostic information. In the typical patient with Buerger disease, obstructive arterial waveforms are present in all digits, providing objective evidence of widespread digital arterial occlusion or stenosis. Patients with unilateral digital plethysmographic abnormalities should undergo arteriography to rule out a proximal, potentially correctable arterial lesion causing the digital ischemia. In addition, patients with symptoms and objective findings localizing their disease to the distal feet and toes and who have normal hand and finger plethysmography should undergo arteriography to rule out a proximal embolic source for the ischemia.

The cornerstone of treatment for Buerger disease is complete tobacco abstinence. All other forms of treatment are palliative. The disease typically undergoes remissions and relapses that correlate closely with the cessation and resumption of cigarette smoking with patients sustaining no further tissue loss following cessation of smoking.[187] Unfortunately, prolonged tobacco abstinence is the exception rather than the norm. Persistent efforts on the part of the physician and family members may ultimately result in smoking cessation. In a report from Japan, an impressive 50% of patients were able to quit smoking.[199]

We use a prolonged, conservative local treatment program for areas of finger ulceration and gangrene, with the primary goal being a clean, dry digit.[200] Ischemic ulcer debridement, often including nail removal, is used frequently, accompanied by minimal rongeur removal of exposed phalangeal bone as needed. Any associated infection is treated with antibiotics. Proximal finger amputations are rarely required, and wrist or forearm amputations have never been necessary in our patients with Buerger disease. Prolonged conservative management is usually rewarded by healing with preservation of maximal digital length, provided that smoking has been discontinued. We have found thoracic sympathectomy ineffectual, and we find no convincing evidence that this procedure is of any significant benefit in these patients.

The course of lower-extremity Buerger disease stands in marked contrast to that observed with upper extremity involvement. Ischemic rest pain can be severe, and narcotic analgesics are frequently required. Several large series reported a 12% to 31% incidence of major leg amputation over a 5- to 10-year period.[201,202] Overall quality of life and the ability to continue working are directly related to limb loss, which is related to continued smoking.[203] Lumbar sympathectomy for refractory Buerger disease has been advocated by some, but results have been equivocal, with 50% ulcer healing rates at 6 months.[204] Anecdotal reports of improved lower-extremity symptoms with the use of an implantable spinal cord stimulator are encouraging,[205] but the device has not yet been subjected to clinical trials.

Arteriography should be performed in all patients with threatened limb loss. If arteriography reveals a patent distal vessel and if autogenous vein is available, a distal arterial bypass may be considered. The use of autogenous vein is mandatory. Distal bypass is seldom feasible because of the diffuse nature of the arterial occlusive disease process. In our experience and that of others, the long-term results of reconstruction are mediocre. However, published data suggest that acceptable primary (30% to 49%) and secondary (47% to 63%) 5-year patency rates can be achieved in lower extremity bypasses, including inframalleolar bypasses, in patients with Buerger disease.[206,207] A novel operative approach developed in India involves a pedicled omental transfer to the lower extremity for limb-threatening ischemia.[208] In 62 patients treated, 94% experienced relief of pain, and none required amputation.

Many medications have been recommended for the treatment of Buerger disease, including corticosteroids, PGE_1, vasodilators, hemo-rheologic agents, antiplatelet agents, and anticoagulants. There is no evidence that any are effective. A randomized European trial comparing the oral prostacyclin analog iloprost with placebo demonstrated improved pain control with iloprost, but no improvement in wound healing.[209] Preliminary results of gene therapy with intramuscular injection of vascular endothelial growth factor have been promising in promoting ulcer healing and limb salvage, but they remain investigational.[210,211]

Although lower-extremity Buerger disease portends a significantly worse prognosis for limb salvage than does atherosclerotic occlusive disease, life expectancy for patients with Buerger disease approaches that of an age-matched population. This is likely due to a lack of coronary artery involvement in the disease process. Reported survival is 97% at 5 years, 94% at 10 years, and 85% at 25 years.[201-203]

HERITABLE ARTERIOPATHIES

Hereditary disorders of the arterial wall account for a minute fraction of the problems encountered by vascular surgeons. These disorders affect the structure or stability of collagen or elastin, resulting in weakness of the arterial wall. These patients may possess characteristic phenotypic features, but they are often not recognized until the patient exhibits a catastrophic vascular complication. The heritable arteriopathies discussed in this chapter include Marfan syndrome, Ehlers-Danlos syndrome, Loeys-Dietz syndrome, cystic medial necrosis, and pseudoxanthoma elasticum. Arteriomegaly is also included in this section, although it is not strictly a heritable disease and there are no distinguishing phenotypic features.

Marfan Syndrome

Marfan syndrome is an inherited disorder of connective tissue characterized by abnormalities of the skeletal, ocular, and cardiovascular systems, with variable phenotypic expression.

Classic Marfan syndrome is caused by mutations in the fibrillin gene on chromosome 15.[212] Fibrillin, a large glycoprotein (350 kD), is one of the structural components of the elastin-associated microfibrils. Both a reduction in fibrillin formation and abnormalities in the fibrillin molecule have been identified.[213]

The incidence of Marfan syndrome is estimated to be 1 in 5000, and there has been no identified race or sex preference.[214] Inheritance is by an autosomal dominant pattern, although nearly 25% of all cases are the result of spontaneous genetic mutations. In its classic form, the syndrome is easily recognizable and consists of abnormalities of the eye (subluxation of the lens), skeleton (arachnodactyly, extreme limb length, pectus excavatum or carinatum, and joint laxity), and cardiovascular system (aortic dilatation and aortic valvular incompetence). The diagnosis is established on the basis of clinical manifestations in most cases. However, some patients have only one or a few of the characteristic features. Prenatal diagnosis can be accomplished using chorionic villus sampling.[215]

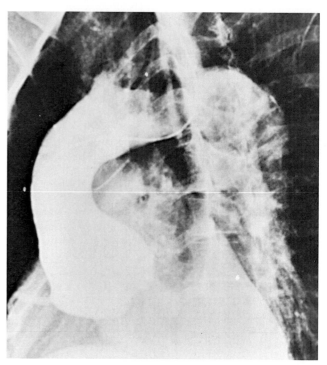

FIGURE 7-10 ■ Thoracic aortogram of a patient with Marfan syndrome showing massive aortic dilatation and associated aortic insufficiency.

Patients with Marfan syndrome develop progressive dilatation of the aortic root, with a resultant ascending aortic aneurysm and aortic valve incompetence (Figure 7-10). A significant number have mitral valve prolapse and mitral insufficiency. Mild aortic isthmus coarctation may be associated with this syndrome, predisposing the patient to ascending aortic dissection. Less frequently, aneurysmal dilatation and dissection involve the pulmonary, coronary, carotid, and splenic arteries and the infrarenal aorta.

If Marfan syndrome is untreated, life expectancy is approximately 40 years, with 95% of deaths related to cardiovascular causes. Progressive aortic root dilatation leading to aortic dissection or aortic valvular insufficiency accounts for 80% of fatal complications. The remainder of deaths are due to congestive heart failure.[216]

Histopathologic evaluation of aortic segments from patients with Marfan syndrome has revealed cystic medial necrosis, with disruption of collagen fibers and fibrosis of the media.[217] Immunohistochemical analysis has revealed an upregulation of matrix metalloproteinases and abnormalities in elastin synthesis, leading to increased susceptibility to degradation by matrix metalloproteinases.[218] Compared with normal subjects, Marfan syndrome patients have decreased aortic distensibility and increased aortic stiffness indices in both the ascending and abdominal aortic regions, regardless of the aortic diameter.[219]

In view of the predictably progressive nature of the aortic dilatation, all patients with Marfan syndrome should be followed from childhood with annual echocardiograms to detect aortic dilatation.[220] There is evidence that β-blocker therapy initiated before the development of aortic incompetence can retard the onset of incompetence and perhaps retard aneurysmal degeneration,[216,221,222] and this remains the current standard of care with the goal of a resting heart rate less than 60 beats/min. Other potential medical therapies include angiotension converting enzyme inhibitors and angiotension II receptor blockers.[223]

Elective repair of the aortic valve and ascending aorta should be accomplished prophylactically before severe aortic insufficiency compromises left ventricular function or the ascending aorta exceeds 6 cm in diameter, at which point the risk of dissection and rupture increases. Surgical intervention typically includes graft replacement of the ascending aorta, with concomitant aortic valve replacement, with 30-day mortality as low as 1.5% and 20-year survival of 59%.[224] Equally good results have been achieved with valve sparing aortic root reconstruction.[225] As endovascular technology continues to improve, less invasive options for treatment of aortic arch pathology will surely emerge. Thoracic aortic stenting for chronic descending aortic dissection in Marfan patients has been described, but progressive aortic root dilatation is frequently noted.[226]

Ehlers-Danlos Syndrome

Ehlers-Danlos syndrome includes a group of diseases first clearly described by van Meekeren in 1682 and later by Ehlers and Danlos, characterized by hyperextensible skin, hypermobile joints, fragile tissues, and a bleeding diathesis primarily related to fragile vessels.[227-229] Ehlers-Danlos syndrome is the most frequent of the heritable connective tissue disorders and occurs in autosomal dominant, autosomal recessive, and sex-linked patterns, with an incidence of approximately 1 in 5000 births.[230] Eleven different types of Ehlers-Danlos syndrome have been described, each with variable clinical signs and symptoms. The specific biochemical defects are known in types IV, VI, VII, and XI and involve defects in collagen production.[231]

The extreme fragility of tissues in many patients with Ehlers-Danlos syndrome leads to problems of surgical importance. The skin and soft tissues are easily disrupted, tend to fragment and tear with manipulation, and hold sutures and heal poorly. Wound dehiscence is common when surgery is required.[232] In addition to these significant problems incident to any surgery, a number of patients with Ehlers-Danlos syndrome are prone to arterial disorders that may require surgical intervention.

Ehlers-Danlos syndrome types I, III, and IV frequently have arterial complications. Type IV represents only 4% of all cases of Ehlers-Danlos syndrome but causes the most severe arterial complications. These patients produce little or no type III collagen, which is of major structural importance in vessels, viscera, and skin. Patients are prone to spontaneous rupture of major vessels, aneurysm formation, and acute aortic dissections.[233] Other complications include spontaneous lacerations, false aneurysms, and arteriovenous fistulas. Bleeding or easy bruising occurs in two thirds of patients with type IV disease. Hemorrhage can be life threatening despite normal platelet function and coagulation proteins.

Defective type III collagen appears to facilitate bleeding by failing to stimulate platelets exposed to subendothelial connective tissue. The media of the arterial wall is thin and disorganized, with fragmented elastic fibers on microscopic examination. Treatment of spontaneous arterial rupture in patients with Ehlers-Danlos syndrome should be nonoperative, consisting of compression and transfusion whenever possible. If operation for major arterial disruption is required, the therapeutic objective should be ligation to control bleeding if this procedure can be accomplished without tissue loss. Gentle dissection, proximal vessel control with external tourniquets or internal balloon catheters, and the use of carefully applied heavy ligatures reinforced with fine vascular sutures are the keys to success. Arteriography carries special risks of vessel laceration and hemorrhage in these patients and should be avoided if possible. Despite the many pitfalls, major arterial reconstruction can be accomplished in patients with Ehlers-Danlos syndrome. In a recent Mayo Clinic series, perioperative mortality was low, but the morbidity was 46% and delayed graft complications occurred in 40% of arterial reconstructions, with only 68% of patients surviving to age 50.[234] Slightly better results were noted in a recent series from Johns Hopkins, in which survival free of any complications at 5 years was 85% and 54% following endovascular and open repairs respectively, although not all patients in this series had vascular Ehlers-Danlos syndrome.[235]

Cystic Medial Necrosis

Cystic medial necrosis is a condition associated with aortic dissection; it manifests pathologically with uniform hyaline degeneration of the media and replacement by a mucoid-appearing basophilic substance. Erdheim[236] believed that the disease was the result of medial replacement by overproduction of mucoid ground substance. Subsequently, numerous studies have shown that the pathologic changes of cystic medial necrosis, with the resultant clinical problems of aortic dissection, spontaneous arterial rupture, and disseminated aneurysm formation, result from a variety of metabolic conditions and syndromes affecting the composition and structure of collagen, elastin, and mucopolysaccharide ground substance. Thus, Marfan syndrome, Ehlers-Danlos syndrome, any of the mucopolysaccharidoses, and occasionally neurofibromatosis can all manifest with the typical arterial lesions and pathologic changes identified as cystic medial necrosis. Although the specific biochemical alterations for some of these syndromes have been discovered, others remain obscure.

Although most patients with cystic medial necrosis have an identifiable clinical syndrome, most commonly Marfan syndrome or Ehlers-Danlos syndrome, a distinct subpopulation of patients with aortic root disease and histologic findings consistent with cystic medial necrosis fail to show the classic phenotypes of either syndrome. These patients often seek treatment at an older age and with more advanced vascular disease. Ninety-four percent of the deaths in this patient group are related to cardiovascular disease, with the majority owing to aortic dissection, rupture, or sudden death.[237]

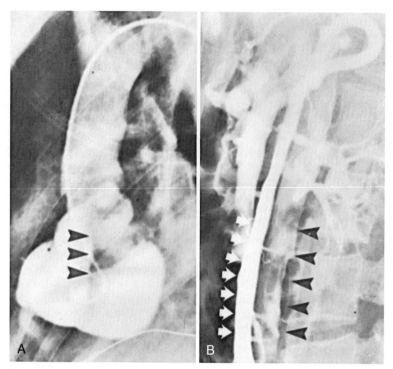

FIGURE 7-11 ■ **A,** Cystic medial necrosis with aortic root dissection. The junction of the true and false lumen is outlined *(black arrows).* **B,** Lateral aortogram of the same patient showing the outline of a double-lumen abdominal aorta *(white* and *black arrows).*

The most frequent arterial condition resulting from cystic medial necrosis is aortic dissection, the treatment of which is discussed elsewhere in this text. Although unusual, cystic medial necrosis has also been reported to involve the pulmonary arteries and the superficial temporal artery.[238] Cystic medial necrosis has also been implicated as a cause of abdominal aortic aneurysms in children.[239] Rarely, patients have a rapidly progressive syndrome of disseminated arterial dissection, spontaneous arterial rupture, and aneurysm formation in which the only discernible lesion is cystic medial necrosis.[240] The angiograms of such a patient are shown in Figure 7-11.

Loeys-Dietz Syndrome

Initially described in 2005, the Loeys-Dietz syndrome is an autosomal dominant connective tissue disorder caused by a defect in the transforming growth factor β gene.[241] Features of the clinical syndrome include hypertelorism, blue sclerae, bifid uvula, cleft palate, and arterial tortuosity and aortic aneurysm formation. Patients are particularly prone to ascending aorta dilatation and dissection, the main source of death in affected individuals.[242] Aneurysm formation occurs at a younger age than Marfan and Ehlers-Danlos syndrome, and in general surgical results are better. Women are susceptible to pregnancy complications and uterine rupture. Preventive therapy with β-blockers and angiotensin receptor blockers may slow the progression of disease.[243]

Neurofibromatosis

Neurofibromatosis, first described by von Recklinghausen in 1882, is an autosomal dominant mutation of chromosome 17 with variable clinical expression, including café-au-lait spots, neurofibromas, axillary or inguinal freckling, bone lesions, optic gliomas and iris lesions (Lisch nodules). Vascular lesions are also common, but likely underreported. Up to 25% of patients have hypertension related to renal artery stenosis or middle aortic syndrome.[244] Arterial aneurysms involving multiple arteries have also been reported, including renal, aortic, iliac, subclavian, visceral, popliteal, and radial. Surgical treatment of symptomatic lesions is indicated, although operations can be difficult because of associated vessel fragility and arteriovenous malformations.

Pseudoxanthoma Elasticum

Pseudoxanthoma elasticum is an inherited disorder of elastic tissue manifested clinically by loose, baggy skin with multiple creases and small, yellow-orange cutaneous papules in intertriginous areas. These patients also have changes in the eye (angioid streaks) and distinct vascular abnormalities. The prevalence of pseudoxanthoma elasticum is 1 in 70,000 to 160,000.[245] Studies have demonstrated an autosomal recessive inheritance in the majority, although there is also an autosomally dominant form.[246]

The basic pathologic change is degeneration of medial elastic fibers, with calcification, fragmentation, and secondary proliferation of the intima leading to luminal narrowing and obstruction. This change results in a markedly abnormal pulse contour owing to loss of the elastic recoil and distensibility of vessels and may be demonstrated plethysmographically. Arterial stenoses, occlusions, or both are the end results of this pathologic process and may involve the cerebral, coronary, visceral, and peripheral arteries. Radiography frequently reveals extensive arterial calcification in a young patient without obvious risk factors for atherosclerosis. Arterial occlusive disease occurs at an early age, usually presenting in the 20s or 30s.[247] With careful examination, decreased peripheral pulses and evidence of peripheral arterial occlusive disease can be found in 24% to 80% of these patients.[248] Symptoms include intermittent claudication, periodic abdominal pain, and angina.[249] Gastrointestinal hemorrhage is frequent and is believed to originate from the widespread arterial degeneration. Hypertension is common in these patients and is usually ascribed to extensive vascular calcification, although renovascular hypertension has been reported.

Standard techniques of vascular surgery, including autogenous vein bypass and endarterectomy, have been used with success in patients with pseudoxanthoma elasticum.[248] Anecdotal benefit from pentoxifylline for the relief of ischemic pain has been reported.[250] The indications for surgery in these patients are the same as for patients with arteriosclerotic occlusive disease.

Arteria Magna Syndrome

Leriche was the first to describe patients with arteria magna syndrome, which is characterized by extreme arterial dilatation, elongation, and tortuosity, which he termed *dolicho et méga-artère*.[251] Since then, many such patients have been recognized, and the terms *arteria magna*, *arteria dolicho et magna*, and *arteriomegaly* have all been used to describe this condition. Pathologic study reveals that the arterial media of these patients has a striking loss of elastic tissue.[252]

Angiography in patients with this syndrome reveals characteristic changes. They have arterial widening and tortuosity (100% of patients), extremely slow arterial flow velocity (100% of patients), and multiple aneurysms (66% of patients; Figure 7-12).[253] The slow arterial flow present in patients with this condition makes arteriography difficult. Large amounts of contrast must be used, and visualization of distal vessels may require multiple injections and special timing sequences with delayed filming.

The propensity to form arterial aneurysms at multiple sites results in the frequent need for surgical correction. Because of the generalized arterial dilatation in these patients, standard criteria for determining the size of aneurysms to be repaired may not be useful. All patients with arteria magna should undergo annual examinations of all pertinent sites (aorta and iliac, femoral, and popliteal arteries), together with ultrasound imaging of nonpalpable or questionable areas. Any aneurysm that reaches twofold to 2.5-fold the size of the parent vessel or becomes symptomatic should be repaired. Arterial occlusions in these patients are almost always thrombotic or embolic complications of aneurysmal disease.

The relationship of arteria magna to typical atherosclerosis is uncertain. The syndrome occurs, albeit rarely, in young people with no evidence of atherosclerosis, and it has been reported in children. Lawrence and colleagues[254] reported a 36% familial incidence among first-degree relatives. Clinical experience suggests that most patients in the United States with arteria magna have significant associated atherosclerosis along with the usual

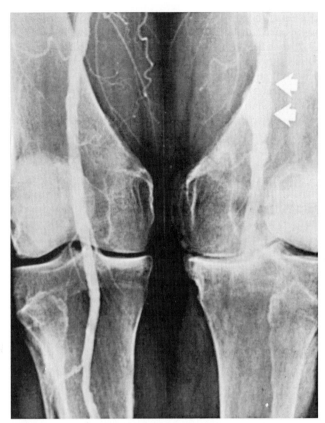

FIGURE 7-12 ■ Arteriogram of a 68-year-old man showing very dilated popliteal arteries and a left popliteal aneurysm *(arrows)*. This patient's arterial dilatation extended throughout his body, a condition termed *arteria magna syndrome*.

risk factors, including tobacco use. In these patients, however, the atherosclerosis is typically nonocclusive, and dilatation predominates.

CONGENITAL CONDITIONS AFFECTING THE ARTERIES

Abdominal Coarctation

Coarctation of the aorta below the diaphragm is a rare but well-recognized condition. Quain[255] described a stricture of the abdominal aorta in 1847 that he believed to be congenital in origin. In 1952, Glenn and coworkers[256] reported the first successful surgical repair, which consisted of bypassing the coarctation with a splenic artery graft. Since that time, the surgical treatment and clinical courses of a large number of patients have been reported.[257] Abdominal coarctation is usually discovered during an evaluation for hypertension. Most patients with abdominal coarctation become symptomatic during their teens with complaints associated with hypertension, including headache, fatigue, shortness of breath, and palpitations. The hypertension is mediated through the renin-angiotensin system.[258] Severe leg ischemia is distinctly unusual,[259] but moderate claudication is often present. Involvement of the superior mesenteric artery occurs frequently, although symptoms of visceral ischemia have not been reported.

Physical findings in these patients include reduced or absent lower extremity pulses, with a noticeable radial or femoral pulse delay. All patients have prominent abdominal systolic bruits, and many have systolic bruits in the lumbar region or lower posterior thoracic area. The natural history of untreated abdominal coarctation is severe hypertension, with death from either renal or cardiac failure within a few years of the onset of symptoms.[260]

Multiple variants of abdominal coarctation have been described, with the variable factors being the precise location and length of the aortic involvement and the number of visceral branches affected. The origins of the visceral arteries may be involved even when they originate from an area of relatively uninvolved aorta. Stenosis or occlusion of the visceral arteries usually does not extend beyond a few millimeters from the origin, implicating a process that is primarily aortic.[257]

Two primary pathogenetic theories have been presented. The first proposes a congenital anomaly representing a failure of normal fusion of the two dorsal aortas of the embryo, resulting in aortic narrowing. The existence of multiple renal arteries in a number of these patients supports this theory, because the formation of a single renal artery is a developmental step that coincides in both location and timing with fusion of the dorsal aortas. The congenital origin of abdominal coarctation in some of these patients may be related to intrauterine injury, because the anomaly has been reported in association with the maternal rubella syndrome.[261] In patients in whom the lesion is congenital, the involved vessels are hypoplastic, without gross or microscopic inflammatory reaction.

The second proposed cause of abdominal coarctation is inflammation. In this group of patients, microscopic examination of involved arteries reveals pronounced inflammatory changes. This lesion is sometimes referred to as the *middle aortic syndrome* to emphasize its acquired rather than congenital nature.[262] This inflammatory middle aortic narrowing is probably a variant of Takayasu arteritis and appears to occur with a frequency reflecting the primarily Asian distribution of that disease.[263] Although this arteritis can be treated successfully with corticosteroids during the acute stage, the diagnosis is usually made later, when the chronic fibrotic and stenotic lesions are amenable only to surgical treatment.

Arteriography is necessary to define the extent of the lesion and to plan treatment (Figure 7-13). Lateral and oblique views are helpful in detecting the extent of visceral vessel involvement. Renovascular hypertension is assumed, and renin studies or split renal function studies are not necessary unless the potential viability of a poorly visualized kidney is questionable (to determine the need for nephrectomy versus revascularization).

Many authors have reported successful surgical treatment of abdominal coarctation by a variety of methods, including aortoaortic bypass, iliac or femoral bypass, prosthetic patch aortoplasty, and splenoaortic anastomosis.[257,264,265] In contrast to thoracic coarctation, prosthetic bypass grafting from the descending thoracic aorta to an

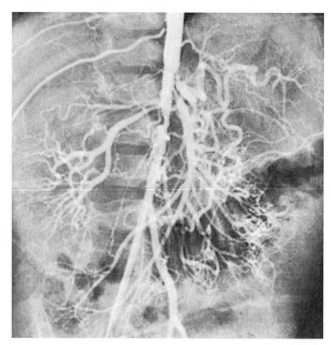

FIGURE 7-13 ■ Abdominal aortic coarctation in a 2-year-old child with infrarenal aortic narrowing and high-grade stenoses at the origins of the celiac, superior mesenteric, and right renal arteries and nearly total occlusion of the left renal artery.

uninvolved area of the infrarenal aorta or the iliac or femoral arteries has traditionally been the procedure of choice, although autologous repair with extensive aortic patching is often preferred if feasible.[257] When possible, a single abdominal operative incision is preferable, using medial visceral rotation to allow optimal exposure of the supraceliac aorta. Alternatively, this operation can be performed through a thoracoabdominal incision or through separate laparotomy and thoracotomy incisions. Complete revascularization has been reported as a staged procedure.[265] However, single-stage repair is recommended because most of these patients are young and tolerate extensive procedures well.[266] Results of surgical treatment of abdominal coarctation have been good. Stanley and associates[257] reviewed the results of 53 cases and found no operative mortality with either primary or secondary interventions, and overall graft patency of 97% at 5 years and 76% at 10 years.[257] In very small children, operation may be delayed until age 5 to 6 years, at which time increased vessel size allows a greater chance of successful repair, as long as cardiac and renal function can be preserved by medical management of hypertension. Successful repair of middle aortic coarctation with stent implantation has been reported, although long-term durability is unknown.[267,268]

Persistent Sciatic Artery

In the embryo, the axial sciatic artery arises from the umbilical artery and supplies blood to the lower limb, following a dorsal course to the popliteal area and then proceeding through the midcalf to the ankle. As development proceeds, this artery is replaced in its upper part by the femoral artery developing from the external iliac artery. By the third month of gestation, the femoral artery predominates, and the vestiges of the sciatic artery remain only as the inferior gluteal artery, the distal popliteal artery, and the peroneal artery.[269]

Rarely, all or part of the sciatic artery persists into postnatal life as a large artery originating from the internal iliac artery, exiting the pelvis through the sciatic notch near the sciatic nerve and following a course through the buttock and posterior thigh to join the popliteal artery in the popliteal fossa. The artery may coexist with a normal superficial femoral artery, or the superficial femoral artery may be hypoplastic. In some patients, the entire superficial femoral artery is absent, with the sciatic artery being the only vessel in the limb in continuity with the popliteal artery. The incidence of persistent sciatic artery is reportedly 0.03% to 0.06% in large series of femoral arteriograms, with one third of all cases being bilateral.[270]

The anomalous lower extremity blood supply usually remains undetected until later life (mean age of detection, 51 years). Patients eventually exhibit with claudication or more severe lower extremity ischemic symptoms, pulsatile buttock masses,[271] or, rarely, sciatic neuropathy.[272] The anomalous artery has a proclivity for aneurysmal degeneration; up to 50% of detected sciatic arteries have been found to be aneurysmal.[273] Vascular surgeons are involved in treating both the aneurysmal and the ischemic manifestations. Although the traditional treatment is surgical ligation, endovascular coiling or covered stent placement is emerging as the procedure of choice.[274] Arterial reconstruction for lower extremity ischemia is typically performed with either femoropopliteal or iliopopliteal bypass.[275]

Popliteal Entrapment Syndromes

Stuart in 1879 was the first to describe the anatomic abnormality associated with popliteal entrapment,[276] and Hamming in 1959 reported the first successful treatment of the condition.[277] Love and Whelan[278] coined the term *popliteal artery entrapment syndrome* in 1965. The anatomic basis of this syndrome lies in the anomalous embryonic development of two independent structures, the popliteal artery and the gastrocnemius muscle.[279] Below the knee, the embryonic sciatic artery gives rise to the popliteal and tibial vessels. The femoral artery arises later as the amalgamation of a capillary plexus connecting branches of the external iliac artery proximally and branches of the sciatic artery distally. Both the femoral and sciatic arteries contribute to the popliteal artery. The femoral artery becomes dominant as the proximal sciatic artery regresses.

During this period of femoral maturation and sciatic regression, the heads of the gastrocnemius muscles develop. The anlage of the gastrocnemius muscle develops as a single muscle migrating cephalad from its origin on the calcaneus. As the gastrocnemius matures, it divides into larger medial and smaller lateral heads that gain their final attachments on the femoral epicondyles. The medial head of the gastrocnemius migrates from its lateral origin toward the medial epicondyle at the same developmental stage at which the mature popliteal artery is developing from the femoral and sciatic arteries.

A simplified classification system of popliteal entrapment recognizes four main variants based on the anomalous relationship of the popliteal artery and surrounding musculature (Figure 7-14).[280,281] In type 1, accounting for approximately 50% of cases, the popliteal artery deviates medial to the normally placed medial head of the gastrocnemius muscle. Type 2 lesions (25% of cases) involve an abnormal attachment of the medial head of the gastrocnemius, with the popliteal artery passing medially but with less deviation than in type 1. In type 3 (6% of cases), the normally situated popliteal artery is compressed by muscle slips of the medial head of the gastrocnemius. Type 4 lesions have associated fibrous bands of the popliteus or plantar muscles compressing the popliteal artery. Type 5 lesions, in which the popliteal vein accompanies the artery in its abnormal course, and type 6 or functional entrapment, which occurs in symptomatic patients without identifiable anatomic abnormalities, have also been described.[282] The true incidence of popliteal artery entrapment syndrome is unknown. The reported incidence is increasing coincidentally with the development of more sophisticated diagnostic tests. A review of 20,000 patients screened with routine vascular laboratory testing identified verifiable popliteal artery entrapment syndrome in less than 1%.[280] However, in an autopsy series, Gibson and colleagues[283] found an incidence of 3.5% in 86 postmortem examinations. Interestingly, all the patients were older than 60 years when they died, and the popliteal arteries showed no histologic abnormalities. Clearly, not all entrapped popliteal arteries become symptomatic. Approximately 90% of reported cases have occurred in men; more than half these patients became symptomatic before age 30 years. The defect is bilateral in 20% of patients.[279]

Symptoms are due to obstruction of the popliteal artery with gastrocnemius contraction. Histopathologic changes distinct from typical atherosclerosis have been identified.[284] Repeated microtrauma leads to inflammatory cell infiltration and vessel wall disruption, which ultimately causes fibrosis and collagen scar formation. Thrombosis, embolism, or aneurysm formation may ensue. Symptomatic patients may have acute ischemia owing to popliteal artery occlusion (10%) or progressive intermittent claudication. Calf claudication in patients younger than 40 years is sufficiently infrequent that its presence should suggest the possibility of popliteal artery entrapment.

Diagnosis of popliteal artery entrapment syndrome is difficult, because most patients are asymptomatic at rest. Symptomatic patients may have normal, reduced, or absent pulses of the lower leg. Ankle dorsiflexion or plantar flexion or knee extension may diminish or occlude distal pulses. Continuous-wave Doppler, photoplethysmography, and arterial duplex scanning have been used with these leg maneuvers to provide objective confirmation of popliteal artery entrapment.[285] However, these noninvasive tests and physical findings are nonspecific, as maneuver-induced pulse diminution can occur in normal individuals.

Arteriography demonstrating midpopliteal artery compression or medial deviation with the leg in a position of stress had been the gold standard for the diagnosis

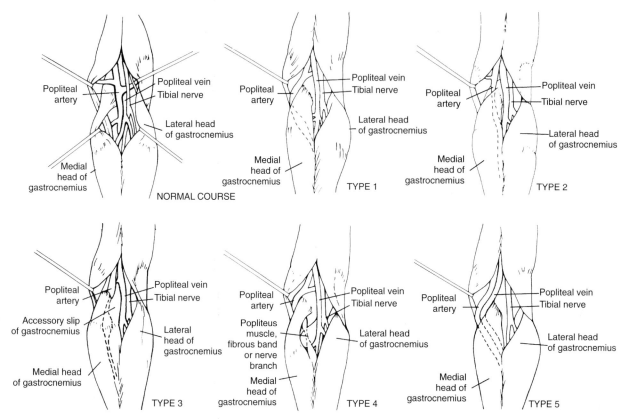

FIGURE 7-14 ■ Diagram of the types of popliteal artery entrapment. (From Rich NM, Collins G Jr, McDonald PT, et al: Popliteal vascular entrapment: its increasing interest. Arch Surg 114:1377–1384, 1979.)

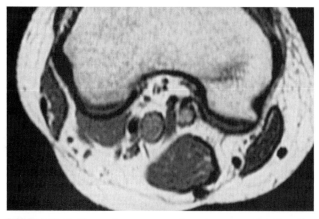

FIGURE 7-15 ■ Magnetic resonance imaging scan showing the abnormal insertion of the medial head of the gastrocnemius muscle between the popliteal artery and vein. The popliteal artery ends up medial to the medial head of the gastrocnemius muscle.

of popliteal artery entrapment syndrome during plantar flexion. The current gold standard for defining the popliteal anatomy at rest is MRI, which provides superior soft tissue definition and does not require the use of intravenous contrast to localize the vascular structures or define their patency status (Figure 7-15).[286]

Treatment of this condition is surgical if the syndrome is diagnosed early and if minimal arterial changes are present; myotomy of the medial gastrocnemius head may

be sufficient. Bypass grafting is required in patients with significant arterial stenosis, occlusion, or aneurysm formation.[287] Autogenous vein is the favored conduit for grafts across the knee. The original descriptions of the surgical technique for this condition favored a posterior approach to the popliteal fossa. Later, a medial approach was emphasized to expose the entire length of the popliteal artery, ensure total division of the medial head of the gastrocnemius, and act as a safeguard against iatrogenic popliteal artery entrapment. To date, similar results have been obtained with both techniques. Almost all patients are able to return to normal activity and have excellent long-term graft patency.[288,289]

Functional popliteal entrapment remains a controversial clinical entity. These patients have clinical findings of popliteal entrapment with normal popliteal fossa musculotendinous anatomy. Proposed mechanisms include popliteal artery compression due to gastrocnemius muscle hypertrophy, compression by the soleal sling, or against the lateral condyle of the tibia. Surgical gastrocnemius debulking and release of the soleal sling have been performed with successful relief of symptoms.[290] Intraoperative duplex with provocative maneuvers has been used to determine adequacy of surgical debulking.[291]

Fibromuscular Dysplasia

Fibromuscular dysplasia (FMD) is a nonatherosclerotic, noninflammatory vascular disease most frequently involving the renal arteries of young white women. Detailed

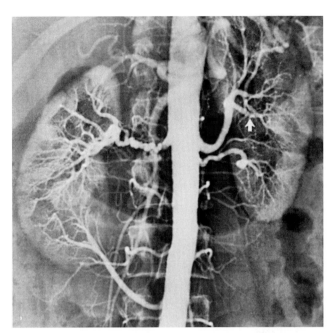

FIGURE 7-16 ■ Fibromuscular dysplasia (FMD). The superior right renal artery shows typical involvement extending beyond the primary branching. Moderate left kidney segmental artery FMD is present *(white arrow)*.

histologic studies have resulted in the recognition of at least four distinct pathologic types: intimal fibroplasia, medial fibroplasia, medial hyperplasia, and perimedial dysplasia.[292]

The first report of FMD by Leadbetter and Burkland[293] in 1938 described a patient with renal artery involvement. Approximately 75% of cases involve the renal artery, with the carotid and iliac arteries representing distant second and third areas of involvement.[292] Rarely, femoral, popliteal, mesenteric, subclavian, axillary, forearm, vertebral, and coronary arteries may be involved. Ninety percent of adult patients with FMD are women. With renal involvement, 70% of patients display bilateral disease. The more severe disease almost always occurs on the right side. Lesions affecting the left renal artery alone occur in less than 10% of these patients. The lesions of medial fibroplasia have the classic "string of beads" morphology on angiography (Figure 7-16).

Medial fibroplasia accounts for 85% of FMD, perimedial dysplasia for 10%, and intimal fibroplasia for 5%. The types are distinguished from one another by which vessel wall layer is primarily affected and by the tissue components that predominate. An increase of fibrous connective tissue, collagen, and ground substance within the media is characteristic of medial fibroplasia. The smooth muscle cell is multipotential and appears to be the source of the proliferative changes in FMD. The cause of FMD is unknown. Several theories have been advanced, including (1) arterial stretching, (2) mural ischemia secondary to an abnormal distribution of vasa vasorum, (3) estrogenic (or other hormonal) effects on the arterial wall, (4) immunologic insult, and (5) anomalous embryologic development. A familial prevalence of 11% has been noted.[294] Symptoms produced by FMD are generally secondary to the associated arterial stenoses

and are indistinguishable from those caused by atherosclerosis. The two most frequently seen clinical syndromes are renovascular hypertension and transient cerebral ischemic attacks. Duplex scanning of the renal arteries has proved useful in the diagnosis of renovascular FMD. As opposed to atherosclerotic renal artery stenosis, which typically involves the orifice or proximal renal artery, FMD lesions have a predilection for the middle and distal renal artery.[295] Duplex scanning not only identifies the lesions but also provides useful information about parenchymal resistance, which has predictive value in determining response to treatment.[296] MRA and CT angiography are also emerging as imaging modalities, although they have not been systematically compared with contrast arteriography, which remains the gold standard for diagnosis.[297]

Treatment is recommended for arterial stenotic lesions only when they produce significant symptoms. Renovascular hypertension caused by FMD has responded more favorably to surgery than has that caused by atherosclerosis.[298-300] Technical success of surgical procedures ranges from 89% to 97%, with cured or improved hypertension in 67% to 93%.[298-300] Results of surgical management of children with renovascular FMD have been particularly encouraging, with cured or improved hypertension in 96% after up to 16 years' follow-up.[301] Percutaneous transluminal angioplasty has emerged as the primary treatment modality, with technical success rates of 94% to 100% and cured or improved hypertension in 74% to 88%,[302-304] although the duration of follow-up has not been as long as that of surgical series. FMD of the renal artery may be associated with the formation of renal artery aneurysms and renal artery dissection.

Cerebrovascular FMD causes symptoms identical to atherosclerotic lesions. Unlike atherosclerotic disease, fibromuscular disease typically involves the distal extracranial internal carotid artery and stops before the internal carotid artery enters the base of the skull. Duplex ultrasonography, CT, MRA, and contrast arteriography all have a role in diagnosis. Less than 1% of patients undergoing carotid arteriography have FMD. Ten percent to 51% of patients with FMD of the internal carotid artery harbor intracranial aneurysms.[305]

Treatment of cerebrovascular FMD is generally reserved for symptomatic patients. Before the widespread application of percutaneous revascularization, surgical repair was the favored approach. Multiple techniques have been described, including open graduated internal dilatation, patch angioplasty, and interposition grafting, depending on the location and extent of involvement.[306] However, percutaneous angioplasty has become the preferred treatment.

Adventitial Cystic Disease

Adventitial cystic disease is a rare condition that must always be considered in the differential diagnosis of claudication in a young patient. Single or multiple synovial-like cysts in the subadventitial layer of the arterial wall compressing the arterial lumen cause arterial stenosis. The cysts typically contain mucinous degenerative debris or clear, gelatinous material similar to that found in ganglia. Eighty percent of patients with this condition are men, and the median age at presentation is 42 years.[307] The first case report describing operative management was in 1954.[308] The popliteal artery is by far the most commonly involved artery, with the femoral and iliac arteries being the next most frequent areas of involvement.

The cause of adventitial cystic disease is unknown. The once-popular theory that it was caused by repeated arterial microtrauma has largely been abandoned. A direct communication with the adjacent knee joint, similar to a true ganglion, has been demonstrated in selected cases.[309,310] Currently, the most widely accepted theory is that the cysts result from the presence within the arterial wall of mucin-secreting cell rests derived embryologically from the synovial anlage of the knee joint.[311] On examination, the finding of a popliteal bruit and the absence of palpable pulses with knee flexion have been noted in a number of patients with adventitial cystic disease involving the popliteal artery. Diagnosis is possible using ultrasonography, CT, and MRI.[312] Intravascular ultrasonography has also emerged as a helpful imaging modality.[313] Arteriography may demonstrate segmental popliteal arterial occlusion or may show a "scimitar" sign of luminal encroachment by the cyst in a normally placed vessel that has no other signs of occlusive disease.[314]

Several methods of treatment have been described. Although spontaneous resolution has been reported,[315] for most patients, percutaneous or surgical treatment is required. Arteries with a small cyst have been successfully treated with CT- or ultrasound-guided needle aspiration or cyst enucleation,[316] although approximately 10% recur following this treatment. In more severely affected patients, segmental arterial replacement may be required. Patients with popliteal occlusion require bypass grafting with an autogenous conduit. Treatment has been successful in more than 90% of reported cases.[307]

External Iliac Endofibrosis

In the 1980s, thigh claudication symptoms in competitive cyclists was initially described, and the term *external iliac endofibrosis* was proposed.[317] Although this disorder is likely related to repetitive shear stress, it is not clear why specific individuals are affected, while the vast majority of competitive athletes are not at risk. Histologically, the process is distinctly different from atherosclerosis, with loosely packed collagen, no calcification, and minimal cellularity.[318] Primarily competitive cyclists are affected, but rare cases in other athletes, such as long distance runners, have also been reported.[319]

Duplex ultrasound of the external iliac artery is often used as a diagnostic test, although a postexertional evaluation is often more illuminating because patients are often normal at rest.[320] MRI and contrast arteriography are also useful; however, findings are often subtle, with mild luminal narrowing over the length of the external iliac artery without focal stenoses. Conservative therapy should be the initial therapeutic recommendation, as patients are typically only symptomatic with extreme levels of activity. For patients who wish to continue with competitive athletics, surgical options are available. Endofibrosectomy with saphenous vein patching is most frequently performed.[321] Typically, the entire length of the external iliac artery needs to be treated because of the diffuse nature of the disease. Prosthetic bypass should be avoided because of the typically young age of affected individuals. The majority of patients are eventually able to return to competitive athletic activities.

COMPARTMENT SYNDROME

Compartment syndrome occurs whenever tissue pressure within a confined space becomes sufficiently elevated to impair perfusion. If untreated, diminished nutritive blood flow results in limb dysfunction secondary to ischemic muscle contracture. The first clinical description of this syndrome was by von Volkmann more than a century ago in a report on contracture involving the arm following trauma. He attributed the deformity to a prolonged interruption of the vascular supply to the muscle.[322] In 1926, Jepson[323] reported successful experimental reproduction of the syndrome and demonstrated that early compartment decompression may prevent ischemic muscle paralysis and contracture.

The multiple clinical causes of compartment syndrome have been well documented.[324] Any loss of vascular integrity, such as occurs following prolonged ischemia or reperfusion injury, leads to increased edema within a compartment. This edema then compromises venous outflow and increases venous and capillary pressures, leading to increased compartment pressure and decreased perfusion pressure. Pivotal to the development of the syndrome, whether from external compression or internal tissue swelling, is the production of sufficient intracompartment pressure to impair blood flow to the tissues.

The capillary leak following ischemia and reperfusion is believed to be mediated through inflammatory mediators and oxygen-derived free radicals.[325] The return of oxygenated blood to the microcirculation of ischemic tissue causes activation of inflammatory mediators locally and systemically. Neutrophil adherence to endothelium leads to oxidant release (H_2O_2, O_2, and OH^-), which damages the endothelium. Animal models suggest that treatment with free radical scavengers may mitigate the damage in compartment syndrome.[326] Experimentally blocking neutrophil adherence has also been shown to decrease reperfusion injury.[327]

There is no absolute pressure above which compartment syndrome invariably occurs, although tissue blood flow diminishes rapidly as intracompartment pressure approaches the level of the diastolic blood pressure. In addition, conditions such as hypotension or vasoconstriction may lead to the syndrome's occurrence at lower intracompartment pressures. In addition to the absolute and relative intracompartment pressures, the duration of ischemia is an important factor. Nerve tissue appears to be most susceptible to ischemia, with symptoms occurring within minutes and permanent damage at 2 hours or less. Muscle death begins at approximately 4 hours. Maximal muscle contracture appears to require approximately 12 hours of ischemia.[324] Skin and subcutaneous tissues are capable of tolerating periods of ischemia that are not tolerated by skeletal muscle or peripheral nerves.[328]

In patients with acute interruption of arterial blood flow, the incidence of compartment syndrome averages 8%.[329] The need for fasciotomy following revascularization is increased if the duration of ischemia was more than 6 hours or if there was a substantial period of shock in association with the arterial injury. Other circumstances increasing the need for fasciotomy include the occurrence of a tight swelling of the extremity preoperatively or intraoperatively, the combination of arterial and venous injury, and the presence of concomitant soft tissue crush injury. Compartment syndrome can develop in up to 30% of all extremities after combined fracture and arterial injury. Thrombolytic therapy for acute arterial occlusion must be recognized as a possible mode of reperfusion injury.[330]

In the lower leg, compartment syndrome most frequently occurs in the anterior compartment, followed by the lateral, deep posterior, and superficial posterior compartments. The quadriceps compartment in the thigh and the gluteal compartment in the buttock may be involved. In the upper extremity, the volar forearm compartment is most frequently involved, but involvement of the dorsal forearm, biceps, deltoid, and hand interosseous muscle compartments has also been reported.

The accurate diagnosis of compartment syndrome leading to successful treatment is based on recognition of the early signs and symptoms of increased compartment pressure. Diminished function of the extremity precedes nerve and muscle necrosis by several hours. Clinical signs include fullness and tenderness of the compartment, pain disproportionate to the physical findings, paresthesias of the compartment nerves, and weakness of the involved muscles. The palpable pulse status and Doppler pressures are unreliable reflections of intracompartment pressure. With compression of postcapillary venules and a continued fall in the arteriovenous perfusion gradient, tissue damage can occur despite continued arterial inflow and palpable pulses.[331]

In questionable clinical situations or when the patient is unable to communicate adequately, objective data reflecting either intracompartment pressure or nerve function may be monitored. Continuous or intermittent pressure determinations may be made by the Wick catheter technique, in which a plastic catheter is placed percutaneously into the compartment and connected to a pressure transducer.[332] A solid-state transducer that fits within a catheter tip in a hand-held unit, the "solid-state transducer in catheter" monitor, eliminates the artifacts inherent to pressure lines.[333] Surgical decompression is generally recommended for patients who have a compartment pressure of 40 mm Hg or greater or for those whose compartment pressure is greater than 30 mm Hg for 4 hours. Others argue that intervention based on fixed pressure is inappropriate and that critical intracompartment pressures occur within 30 mm Hg of the mean arterial pressure or 20 mm Hg of the diastolic pressure.[334]

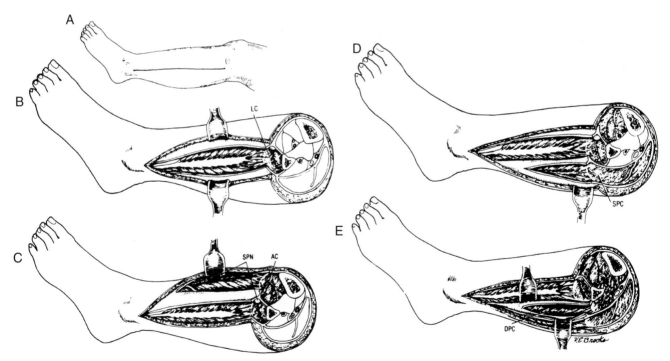

FIGURE 7-17 ■ Parafibular decompression of all four compartments of the leg. **A,** The skin incision runs the length of the fibula. **B,** The lateral compartment (LC) is opened directly beneath the skin incision. **C,** The anterior compartment (AC) is exposed by retracting the anterior skin flap and is opened over the entire length. Care is taken to preserve the superficial peroneal nerve (SPN). **D,** The superficial posterior compartment (SPC) is exposed by retracting the posterior skin flap and is opened over its entire length. **E,** The lateral compartment is retracted anteriorly, and the superficial posterior compartment is retracted posteriorly after the fibular origin of the soleus muscle is released (not shown). This exposes the deep posterior compartment (DPC), which is opened over its entire length. (From Matsen FA, Winquist RA, Krugmire RB: Diagnosis and management of compartmental syndromes. J Bone Joint Surg 62:286–291, 1980.)

Once compartment syndrome occurs, the time delay before treatment becomes the critical factor in determining outcome. Twelve hours appears to be the point beyond which significant residual dysfunction will likely occur despite adequate surgical decompression.[335] All circumferential bandages or casts should be removed at the first suspicion of increased compartment pressure to allow a complete examination of the extremity. The extremity should be placed at the level of the heart and not elevated, because elevation may further jeopardize ischemic compartment components. If physical examination, pressure measurements, or nerve conduction studies suggest a compartment syndrome, immediate surgical decompression is indicated. A frequently used decompressive technique is shown in Figure 7-17.

Untreated compartment syndrome results in direct neurologic dysfunction or the development of contractures following fibrous replacement of myonecrosis. Symptomatic severity ranges from mild to critical, and amputation may be required. Frequent examination of the blood from patients with compartment syndrome may reveal elevated levels of creatinine phosphokinase as well as hyperkalemia. Subsequently, there may be myoglobinuria and renal failure.[336] In such patients, restoration of normal hemodynamics, the administration of mannitol to enhance urine flow and improve intrarenal blood distribution, and alkalinization of the urine to prevent precipitation of myoglobin within the renal tubules are specific therapeutic measures.[336] Prevention of the reperfusion syndrome has been shown in selected patients after the administration of hypertonic mannitol, presumably as a result of its free radical scavenging.[337]

Deep muscle infections are uncommon but potentially life-threatening sequelae.

A rare but well-described form of compartment syndrome is exertional compartment syndrome seen in highly trained athletes.[338] As with other forms, the antero-lateral compartments are most frequently affected. The diagnosis can be made by measuring compartment pressures at the point of exertional pain in affected individuals, with pressures in excess of 25 mm Hg consistent with the diagnosis. Turnipseed[339] described his experience of 276 patients with documented exertional compartment syndrome undergoing surgical treatment with open fasciectomy. Ninety-two percent of patients had complete relief of symptoms and return to normal activities.

BIBLIOGRAPHY

Espinosa G, Font J, Tassies D, et al: Vascular involvement in Behçet's disease. Am J Med 112:37–43, 2002.

Gio HVL, Greene PS, Alejo DE, et al: Replacement of the aortic root in patients with Marfan's syndrome. N Engl J Med 340:1307–1313, 1999.

Miyata T, Sato O, Koyama H, et al: Long-term survival after surgical treatment of patients with Takayasu's arteritis. Circulation 108:1474–1480, 2003.

Olin JW: Current concepts: thromboangiitis obliterans (Buerger's disease). N Engl J Med 343:864–869, 2000.

Salvarani C, Cantini F, Boiardi L, et al: Polymyalgia rheumatica and giant-cell arteritis. N Engl J Med 347:261–271, 2002.

Slovut DP, Olin JW: Current concepts: fibromuscular dysplasia. N Engl J Med 350:1862–1871, 2004.

Turnipseed WD: Popliteal entrapment syndromes. J Vasc Surg 35:910–915, 2002.

Wigley F: Raynaud's phenomenon. N Engl J Med 347:1001–1008, 2002.

References available online at expertconsult.com.

QUESTIONS

1. Which group with Raynaud syndrome has the lowest risk of developing a connective tissue disease?
   a. Vasospastic, negative serologies
   b. Vasospastic, positive serologies
   c. Obstructive, negative serologies
   d. Obstructive, positive serologies
   e. Obstructive, unknown serologies

2. Vasculitis is a central feature in all of the following syndromes except:
   a. Kawasaki disease
   b. Cogan syndrome
   c. Behçet disease
   d. Takayasu disease
   e. Gilbert disease

3. The majority of patients with temporal arteritis are encompassed in which of the following groups?
   a. 50 years, male, white
   b. 50 years, female, nonwhite
   c. 50 years, male, nonwhite
   d. 50 years, male and female, nonwhite
   e. 50 years, female, white

4. What is the optimal initial treatment for subacute upper extremity ischemia caused by temporal arteritis?
   a. Steroids
   b. Endarterectomy
   c. Saphenous vein bypass
   d. Thrombolytic therapy
   e. Warfarin anticoagulation

5. Which of the following is of greatest benefit in the treatment of patients with Buerger's disease?
   a. Sympathectomy
   b. Oral vasodilators
   c. Arterial reconstructive surgery
   d. Warfarin anticoagulation
   e. Cessation of tobacco use

6. Extensive vascular calcification in a young patient with normal parathyroid function suggests which of the following?
   a. Hyperlipidemia
   b. Hurler syndrome
   c. Pseudoxanthoma elasticum
   d. Marfan syndrome
   e. Ehlers-Danlos syndrome

7. Abdominal coarctation is most frequently discovered during evaluation for which symptom?
   a. Claudication
   b. Blue toe syndrome
   c. Weight loss
   d. Hypertension
   e. Abdominal pain

8. Calf claudication in a nonsmoker younger than 30 years is most commonly caused by which disorder?
   a. Popliteal entrapment syndrome
   b. Atherosclerosis
   c. Polyarteritis nodosa
   d. Takayasu disease
   e. Homocystinemia

9. The early objective diagnosis of anterior compartment syndrome is best made by which finding?
   a. Absent dorsal pedal pulse
   b. Footdrop
   c. Tense swelling
   d. Localized compartment pain
   e. Compartment pressure measurement with Wick or the "solid-state transducer in catheter" monitor

10. Which of the following regarding popliteal artery entrapment is true?
    a. Usually associated with abnormal relationship between popliteal artery and lateral head of gastrocnemius muscle
    b. Frequently seen in association with persistent sciatic artery
    c. Equally affects males and females
    d. Can occur with normal popliteal anatomy
    e. Predisposes affected individuals to anterior collateral ligament injury

ANSWERS

1. **a**
2. **e**
3. **e**
4. **a**
5. **e**
6. **c**
7. **d**
8. **a**
9. **e**
10. **d**

CHAPTER 8

Vascular Malformations

Peter Gloviczki

Vascular malformations (VMs) are developmental abnormalities of the vascular system. They should be differentiated from vascular tumors or hemangiomas, because they have different etiology, growth patterns, treatment and outcome. Malformations can involve any segment of the vascular tree: arteries, capillaries, veins, or lymphatics. High-flow arteriovenous malformations are associated with shunting of large amount of arterial blood into the venous system. These lesions can have alarming hemodynamic manifestations, such as venous engorgement, distal limb ischemia, and high output cardiac failure. Patients with low-flow venous malformations are seen most commonly at vascular clinics; most have a benign clinical course and require no special treatment. In one series the ratio of venous versus arteriovenous malformations was 4:1.[1] Most VMs are mixed and some complex malformations like Klippel-Trenaunay syndrome or Parkes-Weber syndrome are associated with developmental abnormalities of other tissues, such as bone and soft tissue overgrowth or digital abnormalities.[2,3]

HISTORICAL NOTES

Birthmarks and congenital deformities afflicting mankind have been described by historians and depicted by painters for centuries. Slowing of the heart rate after compression of a high-shunt congenital arteriovenous malformation was first described by Nicoladoni in 1875.[4] This so-called bradycardia sign of arteriovenous fistulas was observed later by Branham in a patient with acquired arteriovenous fistula.[5] Malan and Puglionisi[6] presented a detailed classification of VMs (angiodysplasia), although the first practical guidelines for clinical classification and treatment were given by Szilagyi et al.[7,8] Rutherford,[9] summarized the state of the art of VMs. Of the multiple classifications published on VMs, the Hamburg classification, in a revised form, is the one used most frequently.[9-12] Although surgical excision has been recommended for local lesions, it is selective catheterization and embolotherapy, as well as percutaneous sclerotherapy, with absolute alcohol and most recently with foam, that have changed the multidisciplinary management of VMs in the last decades.[1,12-14]

DEFINITION OF VASCULAR MALFORMATIONS AND VASCULAR TUMORS

Vascular malformations are localized errors of angiogenic development, whereas hemangiomas are vascular tumors.

Mulliken and Glowacki[15-17] defined the endothelial characteristics and cell biology of VMs and vascular tumors. The term *hemangioma* should be reserved for vascular tumors alone; during the proliferative phase, they undergo growth and then undergo resolution. The proliferative phase occurs during the first year, and spontaneous involution of hemangiomas is observed in 95% by the age of 7 years. The female-to-male ratio is 5:1. Thirty percent of the hemangiomas are present at birth, and the rest develop within the first 3 months of life. Endothelial hyperplasia is evident on biopsy specimens obtained from hemangiomas; these cells grow in tissue culture. In the proliferative phase, they incorporate [^{3}H]-thymidine and have an increased mast cell count.[15] Most patients with hemangiomas require no treatment at all.

In contrast, VMs are developmental, congenital abnormalities. There is increasing evidence that aberrant signaling at the molecular level results in dysfunction of normal proliferation, differentiation, maturation, and apoptosis of the vascular cells.[18-20] Localized superficial, mostly venous or capillary VMs ("birthmarks" of the skin and the mucosa) are the most frequent, but VMs also occur in the skeletal muscles, pelvis, chest, visceral organs such as the lungs, gastrointestinal system, and brain. The abnormal vascular channels are lined by a continuous endothelium and surrounded by abnormal complement of mural cells. Ninety percent of these cells are present at birth, and the male-to-female ratio is 1:1. VMs show no endothelial proliferation, no cell growth is observed in tissue culture, the cells do not incorporate [^{3}H]-thymidine, and no mast cells have been observed in biopsy specimens.[15-17] Clinically, no proliferation or spontaneous involution has been observed in VMs. The growth of the malformation is usually commensurate with the growth of the child, although hemodynamic factors (arteriovenous shunting, venous stasis) can accelerate growth and morbidity. Most low-flow VMs have a benign course, although complications such as bleeding, thrombophlebitis, skin changes, or infection may need treatment. High-flow arteriovenous malformations usually have a more ominous course and a worse prognosis. Treatment of these lesions is frequently needed.

DEVELOPMENT OF THE VASCULAR SYSTEM

The classification, clinical presentation, and prognosis of VMs are largely dependent on the point at which there is an arrest or abnormality in the development of the vascular system; therefore it is worthwhile to review briefly the normal development of the vascular tree of the limbs. Primitive vascular channels first appear in the third week of gestation. During its development, the vascular system undergoes differentiation through multiple stages.[21] Stage 1 is the undifferentiated stage with only a capillary network being present. Stage 2 is the retiform stage when large plexiform structures can be seen. In stage 3, by the third week of gestation, the maturation stage includes development of large channels, arteries, and veins.

Vascular endothelial growth factor (VEGF) secreted by keratinocytes has been found to be responsible for inducing penetration of capillary vessels into the avascular epidermis.[22] This invasion and the subsequent arterial differentiation are also guided by VEGF originating from sensory nerves.[23] A defective migratory response of endothelial cells to VEGF is the consequence of abnormal signaling of VEGF receptors. Malformations develop if the differentiation is abnormal and there is an arrest in the development of normal vascular tissue. It is, indeed, the persistence of the normal embryonic vascular system and any additional abnormal development that result in VMs.

CLASSIFICATION

Classification has been difficult because of the complex presentation and frequently mixed nature of VMs. Malan and Puglionisi[6] attempted to separate VMs based on anatomic appearance and the presence or absence of arteriovenous shunting. The classification by Szilagyi and colleagues[7,8] was based primarily on Woollard's stages of embryologic development: capillary malformations develop when there is an arrest in stage 1 (Figure 8-1).

Although Szilagyi named them hemangiomas, these are not tumors, but capillary or cavernous VMs. Microfistulous or macrofistulous arteriovenous malformations develop if there is an arrest in stage 2 (see Figure 8-1). Persistence of large embryonic veins that develop in stage 3 is seen in patients with persistent sciatic vein (Figure 8-2) or in those with large lateral veins of the leg (Figure 8-3). There are many mixed VMs owing to involvement of several segments of the vascular system (capillaries, veins, lymphatics).

Forbes and colleagues[24] distinguished VMs based on hemodynamic and contrast angiographic appearance. Depending on the amount of blood supplying the malformation, high-flow and low-flow lesions are distinguished. There are high-shunt and low-shunt lesions; the size of the shunts is determined by the volume of blood that enters the feeding vessels. High-shunt lesions correspond with macrofistulous arteriovenous malformations, whereas microfistulous arteriovenous malformations are low-shunt lesions. A whole spectrum of malformations can be found between these two extremes.

The most recent and widely used classification is the 1988 Hamburg classification, with modifications by Rutherford, Lee, and Gloviczki (Table 8-1).[9-12,25] Malformation is classified by the predominant vascular defect (e.g., arterial, venous, arteriovenous, capillary, lymphatic, and combined); it is further classified for most categories into truncular or extratruncular form depending on the involvement of major axial vessels or branches of major arteries or veins.

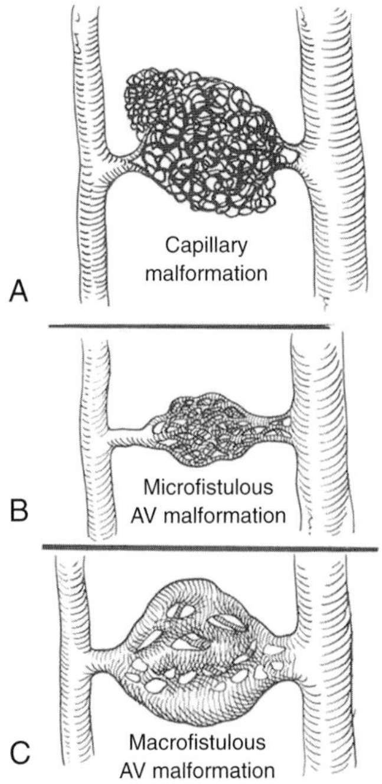

FIGURE 8-1 ■ **A,** Capillary malformation. **B,** Microfistulous arteriovenous malformation. **C,** Macrofistulous arteriovenous malformation.

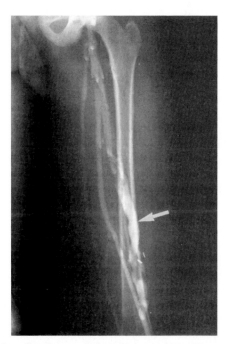

FIGURE 8-2 ■ Persistent sciatic vein *(arrow)* in a 12-year-old girl. Surgical resection of the painful vein through a posterior approach resulted in excellent clinical result at 7 years. The dilated vein contained no valves. (From Cherry KJ, Gloviczki P, Stanson AW: Persistent sciatic vein: diagnosis and treatment of a rare condition. J Vasc Surg 23:490–497, 1996.)

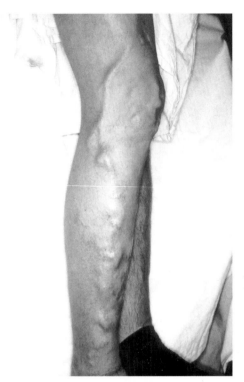

FIGURE 8-3 ■ Persistent lateral embryonic veins in a 19-year-old male with Klippel-Trenaunay syndrome. (From Noel AA, et al: Surgical treatment of venous malformations in Klippel-Trenaunay syndrome. J Vasc Surg 32:840–847, 2000.)

TABLE 8-1	Hamburg Classification of Vascular Malformations (Revised)
Affected Segment of the Vascular System	**Anatomic Forms**
Arterial malformations	Truncular forms
	Aplasia or obstruction
	Dilatation
	Extratruncular forms
	Infiltrating
	Limited
Venous malformations	Truncular forms
	Aplasia or obstruction
	Dilatation
	Extratruncular forms
	Infiltrating
	Limited
Arteriovenous malformations (with shunting)	Truncular forms
	Deep AV fistula
	Superficial AV fistula
	Extratruncular forms
	Infiltrating
	Limited
Capillary malformations	
Lymphatic malformations	Truncular forms
	Aplasia or obstruction
	Dilatation
	Extratruncular forms
	Infiltrating
	Limited
Combined vascular malformations	Truncular forms
	Arterial and venous
	Hemolymphatic
	Extratruncular forms
	Infiltrating hemolymphatic
	Limited hemolymphatic

AV, Arteriovenous.

The truncular forms of arterial VMs include aplasia or obstruction, stenosis, coarctation, dilation, or aneurysms. These forms include malformations such as the persistent sciatic artery or an aberrant left subclavian artery that runs behind the esophagus and causes the typical syndrome of dysphagia lusoria.[26] Thoracic or abdominal aortic coarctation (Figure 8-4),[27,28] anomalies of the aortic arch or persistence of embryonic mesenteric vessels, are additional examples of these malformations. The extratruncular forms can be diffuse or localized.

Venous malformations may also be truncular; these include aplasia or obstruction, stenosis or hypoplasia, dilations, and aneurysms. Many patients with Klippel-Trenaunay syndrome have persistence of large embryonic veins or hypoplasia, dilation or aneurysmal dilatation of the deep veins of the limb (Figure 8-5).[29,30] The estimated prevalence of deep venous anomalies in patients with predominantly venous malformations was 47% in one study.[31] Phlebectasia was the most frequent (36%), followed by aplasia or hypoplasia of the deep venous trunks (8%) and venous aneurysms (8%).

Extratruncular venous VMs are the most frequent malformations, and they can be diffuse (Figure 8-6; see color plate) and localized. Most venous malformations are localized defects of vascular morphogenesis that manifest as single or multiple bluish-purple lesions, mainly in the skin and the mucosa.[32] Biopsy specimens show enlarged endothelial-lined veinlike channels with abnormal smooth-muscle cells.

Arteriovenous malformations are divided into truncular and extratruncular lesions, both can be localized and diffuse. Lesions with clinical or angiographic evidence of arteriovenous communications on the limbs (Parkes-Weber–type malformations) or pelvis are those most frequently seen by a vascular surgeon. Low shunt (Figure 8-7) and high shunt malformations (Figure 8-8) are distinguished. The hereditary arteriovenous VMs in the lung and sometimes in the brain and gut are part of hereditary hemorrhagic teleangiectasia (HHT) syndrome.[32] Arteriovenous malformations are perhaps most frequent in the central nervous system, and vascular surgeons performing carotid arteriography and stenting should recognize and be familiar with arteriovenous VMs and high-flow arteriovenous fistulas of the brain.

Capillary malformations, or port-wine stains, are frequent. These cutaneous lesions appear as a red macular stain that darkens over years (Figure 8-9). Capillary malformations are typical in patients with Sturge-Weber syndrome, Klippel-Trenaunay syndrome, and Parkes Weber syndrome.[3,12]

Lymphatic malformations have been found frequently in some series. The truncular form includes obstruction or hypoplasia causing congenital lymphedema,[33,34] or dilation leading to valvular incompetence and rupture of lymphatics causing chylous effusions or chylocutaneous fistulas owing to reflux of the chyle.[35,36] Most lymphatic

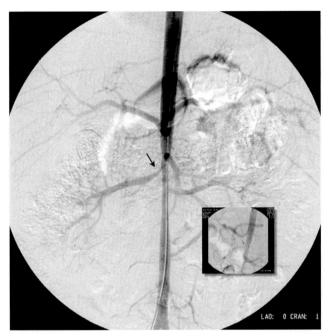

FIGURE 8-4 ■ Abdominal aortic coarctation associated with renal and mesenteric artery stenosis in a 9-year-old boy with reno-vascular hypertension. The *arrow* indicates right renal artery stenosis; the *arrow* in the *insert* shows superior mesenteric stenosis. (From West CA et al: Middle aortic syndrome: surgical treatment in a child with neurofibromatosis, renovascular hypertension, superior mesenteric artery stenosis and intermittent claudication. J Vasc Surg 42(6): 1236, 2005.)

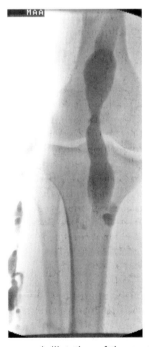

FIGURE 8-5 ■ Aneurysmal dilatation of the popliteal vein with a bandlike narrowing associated with atypical lateral varicosity in a 19-year-old male with Klippel-Trenaunay syndrome. (From Noel AA et al. Surgical treatment of venous malformations in Klippel-Trenaunay syndrome. J Vasc Surg 32:840–847, 2000.)

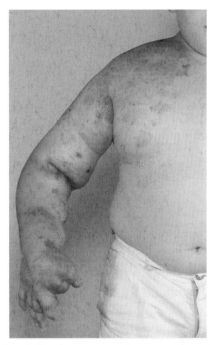

FIGURE 8-6 ■ Diffuse extratruncular venous malformation involving the right arm. (Courtesy David J. Driscoll, MD, Mayo Foundation). See Color Plate 8-6.

cysts and lymphangiomas are lymphatic malformations, and many venous malformations contain lymphatic tissue.

More than 70% of the VMs are mixed, and these frequently complex abnormalities can include arterial, capillary, venous, or lymphatic elements as well. Although the Hamburg classification discourages the use of eponyms, some terms are named after physicians who first described the conditions; these have been widely accepted and used. The list of clinical syndromes of vascular malformation includes Parkes-Weber, Klippel Trenaunay, Servelle-Martorell (Figure 8-10; see color plate), Sturge-Weber, Rendu-Osler-Weber, von Hippel-Lindau, Kasabach-Merritt, Proteus (Figure 8-11; see color plate), and Maffucci syndromes (Table 8-2.)[12,13,30,37,38]

GENETICS

Genetic information on VMs has greatly increased in recent years.[39] Most VMs are sporadic, but autosomal dominant inheritance has also been described. Genetic studies of families have resulted in the identification of mutated genes[18,40-42] that have an important role in angiogenesis. These mutated genes in some patients encode tyrosine kinase receptors and intracellular signaling molecules.[18] Vikkula and colleagues[18] identified the endothelial-specific angiopoietin receptor TIE2/TEK, located on 9p21, as the cause of familial mucocutaneous VMs. Glomuvenous malformations (venous malformations with glomus cells, or glomangiomas) are similar to VMs; most of these lesions are inherited, and Boon and colleagues[43] identified the gene glomulin, a novel locus on the short arm of chromosome 1.[43]

Port-wine stains have also been observed in families, and a genetic susceptibility for capillary malformations

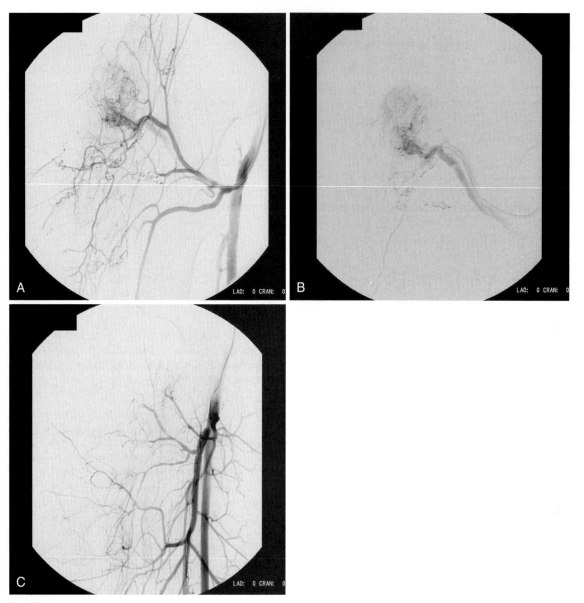

FIGURE 8-7 ■ **A,** Low shunt arteriovenous malformation supplied mainly by branches of the lateral circumflex femoral artery. **B,** Selective catheterization of the feeding vessel was performed, and the lesion was treated with absolute ethanol injection. **C,** Completion arteriography shows no filling of the lesion. (Courtesy Michael A. McKusick, MD, Mayo Foundation.)

was suggested. Eerola and colleagues[40] identified a large locus, CMC1, on chromosome 5q. These authors used genetic fine mapping to identify a positional candidate gene, RASA1; heterozygous inactivating RASA1 mutations were detected in families manifesting capillary malformations. Of interest, arteriovenous malformation, arteriovenous fistula, or Parkes-Weber syndrome were also documented in all the families with this mutation.

Arteriovenous malformations in the lungs, brain, or gut may be part of hereditary hemorrhagic telangiectasia (HHT).[44] Two genes encoding transforming growth factor beta receptor–associated proteins have been identified causing HHT1 and HHT2.

Primary congenital lymphedema can be hereditary (Milroy disease), whereas late onset primary lymphedema was also observed in multiple members of the same families (Meige disease).[45,46] Congenital lymphedema

has been linked to chromosome 5q35.3, where the VEGFR3 gene (vascular endothelial growth factor receptor 3) is located. It is likely that congenital lymphedema is caused by lack of sufficient signaling via the VEGFR3 receptor.[18]

INCIDENCE

VMs occur in approximately 1.5% of the population.[31] Published series of VMs seen at referral centers suggest that predominantly venous malformations are the most common vascular anomalies; they are estimated to occur in between 1/5000 and 1/10,000 childbirths.[18] Venous malformations are certainly the most frequent that require medical attention.[13] Still, it is likely that capillary malformations or port-wine stains of the skin and mucosa

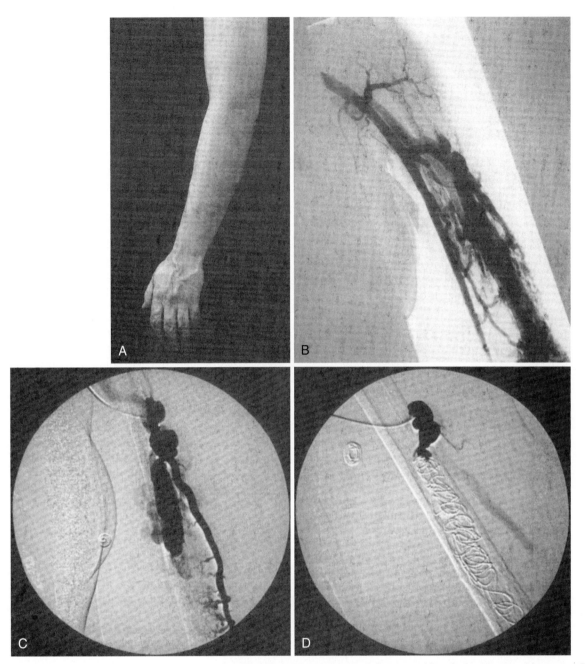

FIGURE 8-8 ■ **A,** High-shunt, high-flow arteriovenous malformation involving the left arm and hand of a 26-year-old woman. **B,** Left arm arteriogram reveals extensive arteriovenous malformation with involvement of the bone and soft tissue. **C,** Selective injection of the deep brachial artery reveals involvement of the interosseous branches of the humerus as well. **D,** The large arteriovenous fistula in the medullary cavity of the humerus was embolized using numerous coils and three strands of no. 2 silk sutures. Almost complete occlusion of the arteriovenous fistula in the humerus was noted. (Courtesy A.W. Stanson, MD, Mayo Foundation.)

are the most frequent VMs, occurring in 0.3% of child-births.[40] Among 797 patients with VMs reported by Lee and colleagues,[1] 40% had predominantly lymphatic malformations. Arteriovenous shunts in this series occurred in 9.5%.

CLINICAL PRESENTATIONS

Patients with VMs are frequently asymptomatic, and a birthmark of the skin or the mucosa is a cosmetic deformity only. However, patients who seek consultations by

vascular surgeons may have a complex presentation or juvenile varicosity, and the limbs or pelvis may have extensive involvement by the malformation. Clinical presentations include varicose veins (see Figure 8-3), limb edema or overgrowth (Figure 8-12; see color plate), port-wine stain or digital anomalies (Figures 8-13, 8-14; see color plate). The affected limb or pelvis may harbor a mass that is pulsatile and may have a systolic-diastolic bruit and a palpable thrill. The varicose veins are usually atypical, lateral or suprapubic, although occasionally varicosity may involve the great saphenous vein and its tributaries. Bleeding or leakage of lymph fluid from VMs is not infrequent. Thrombophlebitis, cellulitis and lymphangitis, skin lesions, induration, pigmentation, and ulcerations can be signs of chronic venous insufficiency. Many of the patients with mixed lesions have associated lymphedema. Patients with pelvic involvement may exhibit hematuria and rectal bleeding. Any patient with

varicose veins or port-wine stains with a longer or shorter limb could also have an underlying vascular malformation. Patients with primary or secondary lymphedema have limbs of identical length.

EVALUATION

The diagnostic tests should focus on evaluation of the type and extent of the malformation. The presence or absence of any arteriovenous shunting must also be established. Physical examination of limb and pelvic lesions should be complemented by segmental systolic limb pressure measurement and establishment of the ankle-brachial index. Pulse volume recording is helpful in patients with arteriovenous shunting (Figure 8-15). Placement of a tourniquet on a limb with a high-flow, high-shunt arteriovenous malformation and occlusion of the fistula will increase systolic blood pressure, which is followed by slowing of the heart rate because of a vagal response in the baroreceptors in the aorta and carotid arteries (bradycardia sign). Duplex scanning will confirm other hemodynamic consequences (Figure 8-16) of an arteriovenous shunt, such as low-resistance waveform in the arteries and pulsatile flow in the veins. Duplex scanning will also establish patency of the superficial and deep veins and other abnormalities including aneurysm or dilation, hypoplasia, or valvular incompetence of the superficial or deep veins.

Of the diagnostic test to document arteriovenous shunting labeled microspheres are useful. ^{99m}Tc-Labeled human albumin microspheres are injected into the artery proximal to an arteriovenous shunt, and the radioactivity in the lungs is measured. Normally less than 3% of the microspheres pass through a normal capillary bed. The percent of the shunted material is calculated based on

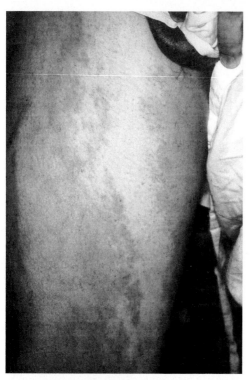

FIGURE 8-9 ■ Port-wine stain (capillary malformation) on affected extremity of patient with Klippel-Trenaunay syndrome. Note also large lateral embryonic vein of the thigh. (From Noel AA et al: Surgical treatment of venous malformations in Klippel-Trenaunay syndrome. J Vasc Surg 32:840–847, 2000.)

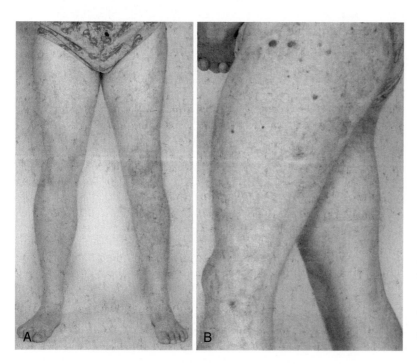

FIGURE 8-10 ■ In Servelle-Martorell syndrome, the typical venous malformation is extratruncular and diffuse. The affected extremity is shorter, there are phleboliths present on plain radiographs, and there is no arteriovenous shunting. Spontaneous bone fracture and osteopenia is frequent. Usually there are no port-wine stains. (Courtesy David J. Driscoll, MD, Mayo Foundation). See Color Plate 8-10.

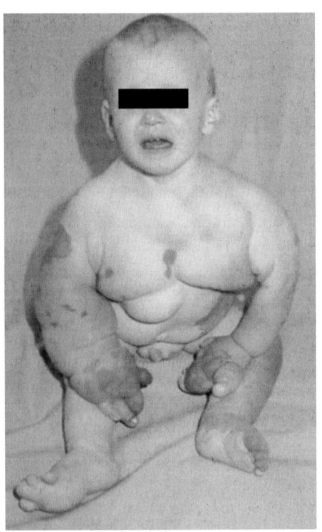

FIGURE 8-11 ■ Patient with Proteus syndrome consisting of disproportionate overgrowth of multiple tissues, vascular malformations, and connective tissue or linear epidermal nevi. The patient had multiple lipomas and hyperostosis. (Courtesy David J. Driscoll, MD, Mayo Foundation). See Color Plate 8-11.

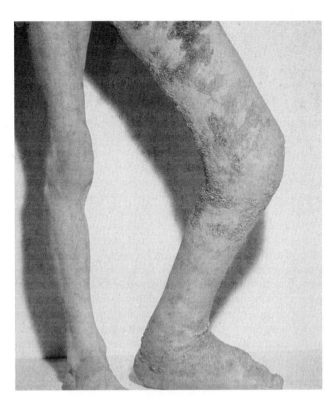

FIGURE 8-12 ■ Klippel-Trenaunay syndrome with overgrowth of the left lower extremity by 12 cm. See Color Plate 8-12.

radioactivity in the lungs measured after a separate injection of the colloid in a vein of the body.[9]

Contrast echocardiography is also useful to establish arteriovenous shunting. It can detect the appearance of indocyanine green on the venous side after intraarterial injection. The test was used by Pritchard and colleagues[47] to determine residual shunts after surgical excision.

IMAGING STUDIES

Scanograms are performed to document any length discrepancy between the limbs. Scanograms are long bone radiographs that provide the most accurate measurement of the length of the different long bones of the upper and lower limbs (Figure 8-17).

Computed tomography (CT) scans and three-dimensional CT arteriography and venography have progressed rapidly in recent years; they provide excellent

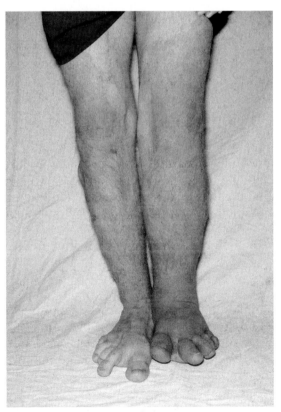

FIGURE 8-13 ■ Klippel-Trenaunay syndrome with involvement of both lower extremities. Note the port-wine stain and digital anomalies. See Color Plate 8-13.

TABLE 8-2   Clinical Syndromes Associated with Vascular Malformations

Syndrome	Inheritance	Type	Location	Characteristic Features	Treatment	Prognosis
Parkes-Weber	Somatic mutations	AVM (intraosseal or close to epiphyseal plate), port-wine stain	Extremities, pelvis	Soft tissue and bony hypertrophy; varicosity (atypical); capillary and high-flow, high-shunt AVM	Observation, elastic support, embolization ± excision (localized lesions only)	Deep diffuse lesions have poor prognosis
Klippel-Trénaunary	Somatic mutations	No or low-shunt AVM, venous or lymphatic, port-wine stains	Extremities, pelvis, trunk	Soft tissue and bone hypertrophy; varicosities (lateral lumbar to foot pattern); capillary or venous vascular malformation, lymphatic malformation	Elastic support Seldom: epiphyseal stapling or selective excision of ablation of varicose veins	Usually good
Rendu-Osler-Weber (hereditary hemorrhagic telangiectasia)	Autosomal dominant	Punctate angioma, telangiectasia, GI tract AVM	Skin, mucous membranes, liver, lungs, kidneys, brain, spinal cord	Epistaxis, hematemesis, melena, hematuria, hepatomegaly, neurologic symptoms	Transfusions; embolization vs. laser treatment ± excision	Good of bleeding can be controlled and no CNS manifestations
Sturge-Weber (encephalotrigeminal angiomatosis)	No	Port-wine stains	Trigeminal area, leptomeninges, choroid, oral mucosa	Convulsions, hemiplegia, ocular deformities, mental retardation, glaucoma, intracerebral calcification	Anticonvulsants, neurosurgical procedure	Guarded; depends on intracranial lesion
von Hippel-Lindau (oculo cerebellar hemangioblastomatosis)	Autosomal dominant	Hemangioma	Retina, cerebellum	Cysts in cerebellum, pancreas, liver, adrenals, kidneys	Excision of cysts	Depends on intracranial lesion
Blue rubber bleb nevus	Autosomal dominant	Cavernous venous malformation	Skin, GI tract, spleen, liver, CNS	Bluish, compressible rubbery lesions; GI bleeding; anemia	Transfusions, electrocoagulation, excision	Depends on CNS and GI involvement
Kasabach-Merritt	Autosomal dominant	Larger cavernous malformation	Trunk, extremities	Thrombocytopenia, hemorrhage, anemia, ecchymosis, purpura	Compression; transfusion of blood, platelets	Death from hemorrhage or infection
Maffucci (dyschondroplasia with vascular hamartoma)	Probably autosomal dominant	AVM, cavernous lymphangioma	Fingers, toes, extremities, viscera	Enchondromas; spontaneous fractures; deformed, shorter extremity; vitiligo	Orthopedic management	Chance of malignancy 20%

AVM, Arteriovenous malformation; CNS, central nervous system; GI, gastrointestinal.
Adapted from Gloviczki AA, Noel AA, Hollier LH: Arteriovenous fistulas and vascular malformations. In Ascher E, editor: Haimovici's vascular surgery, ed 5, Malden, Mass, 2004, Blackwell, pp 991–1014.

pictures of the malformation (Figure 8-18; see color plate). CT will show the extent of involvement, but arteriovenous malformations might not always be distinguished from venous malformations. Because intravenous contrast is required, appropriate timing of the imaging is needed depending on the amount of blood shunted in the vascular malformation.

MR (magnetic resonance) scan, MRA (magnetic resonance arteriography) and MRV (magnetic resonance

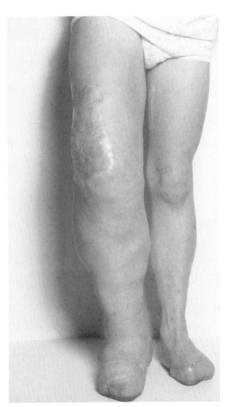

FIGURE 8-14 ■ Bilateral leg involvement in Klippel-Trenaunay syndrome. Bilateral transmetatarsal amputations were needed because of digital anomalies. See Color Plate 8-14.

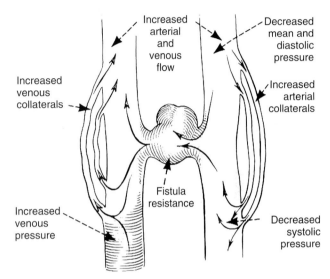

FIGURE 8-16 ■ Hemodynamic consequences of an arteriovenous fistula. (With permission from the Mayo Foundation.)

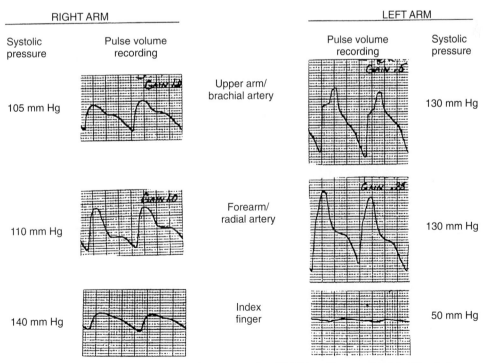

FIGURE 8-15 ■ Systolic limb pressures (SLP) and pulse volume recording (PVR) in a 13-year-old girl with arteriovenous malformation of the left hand. Increased brachial systolic pressure proximal to the fistula and decreased pressure of the index finger distal to the fistula was recorded. The PVR shows sharp, high systolic peaks and slightly decreased anacrotic notches proximal to the fistula. (From Rutherford RB, Anderson BO, Durham JD: Congenital VMs of the extremities. In Moore WS, editor: Vascular surgery: a comprehensive review, ed 5, Philadelphia, 1998, WB Saunders, pp 191–202.)

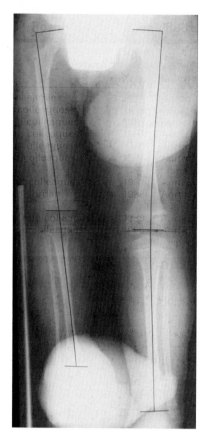

FIGURE 8-17 ■ Long bone films (scanogram) confirms leg length discrepancy in bilateral Klippel-Trenaunay syndrome.

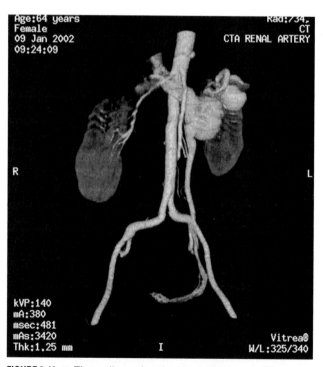

FIGURE 8-18 ■ Three-dimensional computed tomographic reconstruction of a venous malformation involving the left renal vein and the hilum of the left kidney. (Courtesy Terri J. Vrtiska, MD, Mayo Foundation). See Color Plate 8-18.

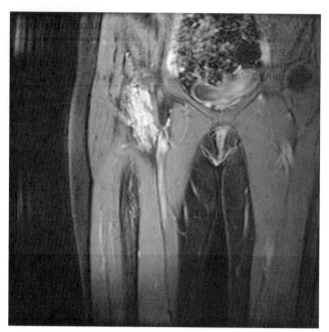

FIGURE 8-19 ■ Sagittal magnetic resonance image of an arteriovenous malformation involving the head of the right femur.

venography) have multiple advantages. MR can differentiate between muscle, bone, fat, and vascular tissue, without the need for radiation or intravenous contrast, which can be deleterious to the kidneys. Axial, coronal, and sagittal images (Figure 8-19) can be generated, and gadolinium enhancement provides high-quality angiography. High-flow and low-flow fistulas can be distinguished. Dynamic contrast-enhanced MR imaging has emerged as an excellent imaging technique of VMs.[48]

Contrast arteriography is reserved only for patients who are potential candidates for arterial embolization (Figures 8-20, 8-21). Arteriovenous shunting is confirmed by contrast arteriography, which also delineates the feeding arteries and excludes any vascular tumor (see Figure 8-8). The size of the feeding arteries can be measured, and the size of the arteriovenous shunts (2 mm in large shunts, 100 to 200 μm in small shunts) can be estimated on the basis of appearance time of contrast in the vein. The flow volume is determined by the size and rate of opacification of the feeding arteries, whereas the shunt volume can be estimated with acceptable accuracy by the time and appearance of contrast medium in the veins.

Contrast venography is reserved for patients who are potential candidates for venous intervention (see Figure 8-5). Contrast venography is frequently done through multiple injections in the limb, with the use of tourniquet or Esmarque bandage to visualize the deep system and with direct injection into the malformation, before or after ethanol sclerotherapy.

TREATMENT

Indications

There are absolute and relative indications for treatment of VMs. The absolute indications include hemorrhage,

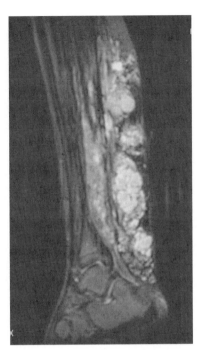

FIGURE 8-20 ■ Magnetic resonance image of a predominantly venous malformation involving the superficial and deep compartments of the distal calf.

ischemia, refractory ulcers, and congestive heart failure. Bleeding from malformations can occur through defects in the skin or mucosa, or the patient can have intramuscular or retroperitoneal hematoma, hematuria, rectal bleeding, hematemesis, hemoptysis, or intracerebral or intraspinal bleeding. Relative indications for treatment include pain, claudication, functional impairment, limb asymmetry, and cosmetic reasons. A multidisciplinary approach in the evaluation and treatment of VMs provides the best chance for the patient. The team may include a pediatrician; pediatric, orthopedic, plastic, and vascular surgeons; an interventional radiologist; a cardiologist or vascular internist; and a physical therapy physician. Conservative treatment is used for most patients. Laser therapy has been used effectively for capillary malformations (port-wine stains). Effective and minimally invasive percutaneous techniques include transcatheter embolization and percutaneous or transcatheter sclerotherapy. Surgical excision is reserved for the minority of patients with localized superficial lesions or for those patients who have symptomatic juvenile varicose veins or localized venous malformations.

Conservative Treatment

Treatment of VMs is most frequently conservative. Elastic garment or bandage, local wound care, compression dressings, special orthopedic footwear, and life style modification may be required to manage daily life and improve limb function. Lymphedema is frequently managed using elastic garments, intermittent compression treatment, or lymphatic massage treatment by physical therapists.[49] The psychological problem caused by a visible deformity should not be underestimated. Long-term antibiotic therapy may be needed for recurrent cellulites, and patients who had recurrent deep vein thrombosis are treated life-long with anticoagulants.

Embolization

Embolization with selective catheterization has emerged as the primary therapy of arteriovenous malformations. Materials for embolization include polyvinyl alcohol particles (100 to 500 μm), absolute ethanol, stainless steel coils (Figures 8-8 and 8-21), usually with tufted Dacron, absorbable gelatin pledgets, powder coils, and cyanoacrylate adhesives. Each of these agents acts at different levels in the arterial system. Coils are equivalent to surgical ligation, although the tufted Dacron and the addition of thrombin will generate more extensive arterial thrombosis than ligation alone. Coils occlude medium to small arteries. Liquid agents and the smaller diameter particles occlude at the arteriolar level or the capillary bed.[50]

New detachable coils permit using a double catheter technique to deliver the first coil as a filter to assure accurate location of the others, while final detachment of the first coil is done at the end of the procedure. Size selection is important to avoid embolization through large fistulas. For very large fistulae or a single communication, the use of vascular plugs can be considered. Particulate agents used for embolotherapy include gel foam, polyvinyl alcohol particles (100 to 500 μm), spherical embolics, or absorbable gelatin pledgets.

Liquid and sclerosing agents permanently occlude or destroy the endothelium of the feeding vessels or the malformation. Their use for high-flow arteriovenous malformations is more difficult because they can pass through the shunts to the venous side.

Glue can be used for those lesions that will be excised or for those in the pelvis; however, most of them can be used for low-shunt lesions. Absolute ethanol is used most frequently; other liquid agents include tissue adhesives such as cyanoacrylate or onyx, a liquid embolic agent.[51] Sclerosing agents can cause endothelial damage owing to osmotic effect, such as hypertonic saline, or they are detergents such as sodium morrhuate, sodium tetradecyl sulfate (STS), or polidocanol. The use of foam detergents have progressed tremendously in all areas of VMs.[52]

Each of these agents acts at different levels in the arterial system. Coils are equivalent to surgical ligation, although the tufted Dacron and the addition of thrombin will generate more extensive arterial thrombosis than will ligation alone. Coils occlude medium to small arteries; liquid agents and the smaller diameter particles occlude at the arteriolar level or the capillary bed (see Figure 8-9).

Jacobowitz and colleagues[53] reported on transcatheter embolization of pelvic arteriovenous malformations in 35 patients. A mean of 2.4 embolization procedures (range, 1 to 11 procedures) were needed over a mean period of 23.3 months (range, 1 to 144 months), using rapidly polymerizing acrylic adhesives most frequently. More than one procedure was performed in 53% of the patients. Adjunctive surgical excision was performed in only five patients (15%). Eighty-three percent of patients were

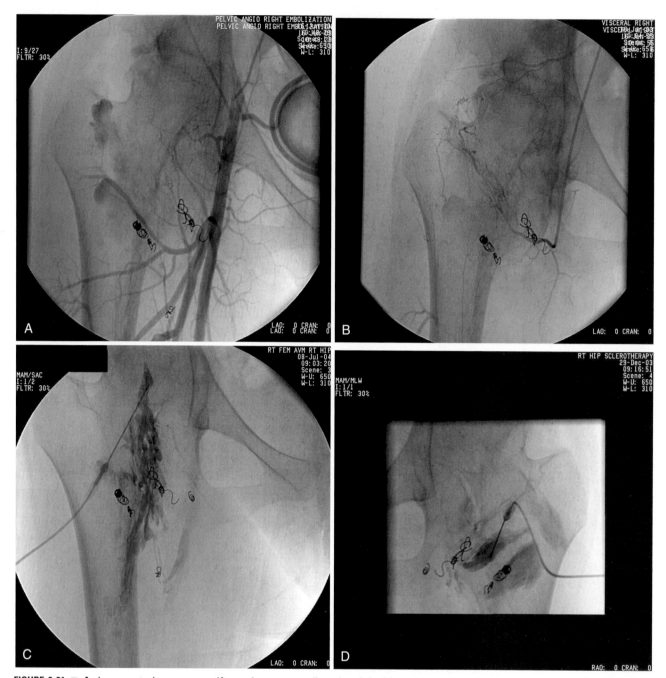

FIGURE 8-21 ■ **A,** Large arteriovenous malformation surrounding the right hip, with partial destruction of the hip joint. Previous embolization of the feeding vessels with coils was performed. **B,** Repeated embolization with ivalon particles and with absolute alcohol was performed through selective catheterization of the lateral circumflex femoris artery. **C** and **D,** Additional ethanol sclerotherapy with direct percutaneous injections of absolute alcohol into the lesion. (Courtesy Michael A. McKusick, MD, Mayo Foundation.)

asymptomatic or significantly improved at a mean follow-up of 84 months (range, 1 to 204 months).

Rockman and colleagues[54] reviewed results of transcatheter embolization therapy for VMs in the upper and lower extremities in 50 patients. The most common presenting symptoms included pain (80%), swelling (68%), ulceration or distal ischemia (18%), and hemorrhage (6%). Arteriovenous and arterial lesions were treated by embolization via the arterial branch feeding vessels with cyanoacrylate. Sixteen patients (32%) underwent more

than one embolization procedure. Adjunctive surgical procedures were performed in three cases (6%). Ninety-two percent of patients remained asymptomatic or improved at a mean follow-up of 56 months. There was one case of limb loss (2%).

In another group of 31 patients with high-flow VMs treated at Duke University, 8 (25.8%) were managed conservatively, 8 (25.8%) were treated with transcatheter arterial embolization, 6 (19.4%) required embolization followed by sclerotherapy, and 5 (16.1%) were resected.[55] Treatment with embolization resulted in improvement in seven (87.5%) patients, while combination therapy resulted in improvement in six (100.0%), and surgical resection led to improvement in four (80%). Complications occurred in two (7.4%) patients treated with embolization or combination therapy.

Sclerotherapy

Absolute ethanol induces denaturation of tissue protein, precipitating protoplasm and destroying the endothelial cells. It is delivered through selective arterial catheterization for arteriovenous malformations and through direct percutaneous injections into lesions in patients with predominantly venous malformations (see Figures 8-7, 8-21). Unfortunately, alcohol sclerotherapy causes significant pain; therefore general anesthesia and pain control are required. Absolute ethanol can also cause significant side effects. Treatment should be performed selectively and by a physician with expertise and knowledge of the dose- and toxicity-related complications.

For large arteriovenous malformations, pulmonary artery catheter and arterial pressure line monitoring is suggested by Coldwell and colleagues[50] and Yakes and colleagues,[56] who also recommend giving dexamethasone sodium phosphate (3 to 10 mg) intravenously before the procedure. The maximum dose should not exceed 1 mL/kg body weight. Pulmonary hypertension should be monitored when large doses are given, and nitroglycerine can be used to treat pulmonary vasospasm. Yakes and colleagues[56] reported on a complication rate that ranged from 10% to 30%, depending on their years of experience. Tissue necrosis, sloughing of the skin and pulmonary hypertension are the most frequent side effects, followed by deep vein thrombosis, motor nerve injury, and sensory nerve injury.

One of the largest experiences using ethanol sclerotherapy of venous or arteriovenous malformations was compiled by Lee and colleagues and reported in a consensus document[57] and in other publications.[58] In 87 patients who underwent 399 sessions of sclerotherapy treating VMs, Lee and colleagues[57] reported on an initial success rate in 95% of the sessions. The mean follow-up was 24 months, and 71 of the 87 patients (82%) showed no recurrence of the treated lesion. Minor to major complications, mostly skin damage, developed after 47 sessions (12%) in 24 patients (28%). There was one permanent facial nerve palsy and one peroneal nerve palsy. The authors concluded that absolute ethanol sclerotherapy can deliver excellent results to patients with diffuse venous malformation with a 25% rate of early and 3% rate of permanent complications. The low complication rate in this series was remarkable; most authors report complication rates between 10% and 30%. Complication rates in predominantly venous malformations are significantly less than in patients who have arteriovenous shunting. The benefits and potential major complications of absolute alcohol sclerotherapy was emphasized by Villavicencio[59] and by Burrows and Mason.[51]

Other materials that have been used for sclerotherapy include sotradecol and polydocanol foam.[52,60-62] The advantage of foam detergent solutions is that smaller amounts can be used to achieve thrombosis. Polidocanol is less allergic and produces less pain and inflammatory response than other sclerosing solutions. Tessari and colleagues[63] use 1% polidocanol for duplex-guided foam sclerotherapy: two syringes are attached by a three-way stopcock; one is filled with polidocanol, the other with air.[63] The foam is obtained by mixing the contents of the two syringes. Five to 10 mL of the foam is injected under duplex and venographic guidance into the venous malformation. Foam has been used with increasing frequency and with good results for venous malformations.[52,60-62] Although longer follow-up is required, early complications are less than with ethanol sclerotherapy; foam could have great promise in the treatment of venous malformations.

Lidsky and colleagues[55] recently reported on results of sclerotherapy used for low-flow VMs in 38 patients, using sodium tetradecyl sulfate, polidocanol, or ethanol. An additional 18 patients' malformations were surgically resected, and 8 were managed with a combination of modalities. Response to sclerotherapy resulted in improvement in 32 (84.2%) patients, surgical resection resulted in improvement in 16 (88.9%) patients, and combination therapy resulted in improvement in all 8 (100%) patients. Complications were observed in six (6.8%) patients treated for LFVMs (zero with sodium tetradecyl sulfate or polidocanol, four with ethanol, two with resection).

Laser Treatment

Cutaneous capillary malformations (port-wine stains) were initially treated with argon lasers, with good results in many patients, but with scarring that has been reported to occur in 5% to 24% of the cases.[64] The best results were obtained in adults, with purple, well-vascularized lesions. Scarring has become less frequent with the introduction of the yellow light lasers.[65,66] The best results are achieved with the flashlamp-pumped pulsed dye laser. The 585-nm wavelength achieves deep tissue penetration while maintaining vascular specificity.[65,70] Both pale and dark skins can be treated with minimal intraoperative discomfort and low chance of postoperative epidermal damage or pigmentary change. Lasers have revolutionized the treatment of superficial vascular lesions, especially port-wine stains and facial teleangiectasias.[65,67] In a series of 56 patients with venous malformations the success rate of laser treatment was 93%; 4% had minimal scarring and deformity, and no long-term complications were noted.[68]

Surgical Excision

Surgical excision of arteriovenous malformation is rarely curative. In a classic series by Szilagyi, only 18 of 82 patients underwent surgical treatment. Improvement was documented in 10 patients only. Surgical attempts at excision can result in significant blood loss, and ligation of a major feeding vessel is not a good option, because it prevents later use of selective catheterization and embolotherapy. Excision of venous malformation, if they are localized, can be done with a higher rate of success.

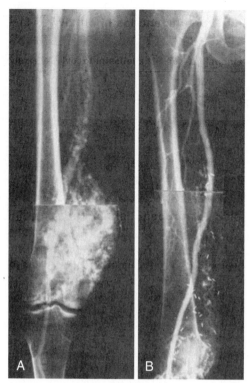

FIGURE 8-22 ■ **A,** Large macrofistulous arteriovenous malformation of the right thigh. **B,** Arteriogram 5 months after surgical resection, that was preceded with multiple embolization of the lesion. (From Gloviczki AA, Noel AA, Hollier LH: Arteriovenous fistulas and VMs. In Ascher E, editor: Haimovici's vascular surgery, ed 5, Malden, Mass, 2004, Blackwell.)

Exsanguinations of the limb with an elastic (Esmarque) bandage and the use of a proximal tourniquet will greatly decrease blood loss and makes the operation technically easier.[69] If excision is decided, preoperative sclerotherapy or embolization should be considered to minimize bleeding (Figure 8-22). The use of rapid cell saver is mandatory. In high-flow, high-shunt lesions, the only operation that can be performed in some patient is amputation. For these patients, however, amputation may mean cure and a prosthesis brings hope for functional recovery.

In 73 procedures performed in 41 patients with VMs treated with open surgical resection, Maftei and colleagues[70] investigated factors leading to major intraoperative bleeding. Significantly higher blood loss was associated with debulking surgery ($p = 0.006$) and with previous history of major hemorrhage during VM surgery ($p = 0.041$). Blood loss was higher in lesions where proximal tourniquet application was not possible ($p = 0.093$). Interestingly, high-flow lesions were not strongly associated with major blood loss ($p = 0.288$). Major blood loss (≥ 2L) occurred in 16 (20.8%) procedures performed on 11 (26.2%) patients, but this did not prolong hospital stay.

COMPLEX MALFORMATIONS

For vascular surgeons, management of complex clinical syndromes with VMs deserves separate discussions. The most frequently encountered problem of these rare malformations is the Klippel-Trenaunay syndrome.

KLIPPEL-TRENAUNAY SYNDROME

First described by Klippel and Trenaunay at the turn of the century, the clinical triad of this mixed malformation includes capillary malformations (port-wine stain), soft tissue and bone hypertrophy, atypical, usually lateral varicosity, and venous and lymphatic malformations (see Figures 8-3, 8-5, 8-12, 8-13).[71,72] The deep veins are frequently affected. The most frequent deep venous anomalies include ectasia or aneurysm, external compression, hypoplasia, aplasia, or persistent sciatic veins.[73] Klippel-Trenaunay syndrome is clearly a mixed vascular malformation that includes predominantly venous, lymphatic, and capillary elements, but no arteriovenous shunting. Many patients have lymphedema and some have cavernous lymphatic malformations.

In a review of 252 patients with Klippel-Trenaunay syndrome, 246 (98%) had capillary malformations, 236 (94%) had soft tissue or bone hypertrophy, and 182 (72%) had varicosities or venous malformations.[71] The lower extremities were involved in 70%, and the malformation was bilateral in 19%. The upper extremity was involved in 74 of the 252 patients (29%). Symptoms of patients with Klippel-Trenaunay syndrome included swelling (70%), pain (7%), and bleeding (43/252; 17%). Thirty-nine patients (15%) had a history of superficial phlebitis, 4% had a history of deep vein thrombosis, and 4% had pulmonary embolism, which was fatal in one. Lateral varicose veins were frequent (56%). One percent had suprapubic varicosities owing to iliac vein agenesis or aplasia, and 19% of the patients had medial varicosities.

The management of Klippel-Trenaunay syndrome has been largely conservative, using elastic garment or treatment of any cellulitis or lymphangitis. Most patients who undergo surgical treatment do so because of overgrowth of one limb: these patients are managed with epiphiseodesis, with good results.[71] Vascular interventions must be preceded by careful evaluation of the patency of the deep venous system. Ablation of the symptomatic incompetent superficial veins can be performed if the deep venous system is patent. Symptomatic, predominantly venous malformations can be managed by percutaneous sclerotherapy while localized capillary malformations of the skin responds to laser therapy. Large, subcutaneous lateral embryonic veins can be treated well with invagination stripping or occasionally with endovenous thermal ablation, and ambulatory mini phlebectomy. In a series of 20 patients with Klippel-Trenaunay syndrome, all had varicosities with lateral distribution, although 65% had medial varicosities as well.[73] Stripping and avulsion was performed in all patients; avulsion of varicose veins and excision of superficial venous malformations were done usually with the help of a thigh tourniquet. Additional, concomitant, or staged procedures included release of the constricted popliteal veins, deep vein reconstruction, perforator ligation, and excision of an incompetent, persistent sciatic vein. Mean follow-up was 64 months. The results were excellent or good in 18 patients and no improvement was noted in only 2 patients. Twelve percent had developed hematoma that required drainage, but no deep vein thrombosis, pulmonary embolism, or nerve injury was observed in this group of patients. The improvement was excellent in patients with varicosities, although some recurrence was noted in half of the patients. Clinical severity score significantly decreased in the entire group from 4.3 to 3.1, documenting significant clinical benefit. In patients with a history of deep vein thrombosis, preoperative placement of a vena cava filter should be considered.

Venous malformations and varicose veins can also be treated effectively, in multiple sessions, using ethanol sclerotherapy or foam. In addition, endovenous thermal ablations with radiofrequency or laser have been used selectively for patients with Klippel-Trenaunay syndrome.[74] Long-term results with endothermal ablations are not well known because of the small number of patients treated in single centers. Because of the rarity of this disorder and the presence of a mixed malformation, a multidisciplinary management of patients with Klippel-Trenaunay syndrome, just like with other complex VMs, is clearly warranted.

CONCLUSIONS

Improved imaging of the vascular system with duplex scanning, MR, or CT angiographies has changed evaluation and treatment of patients with VMs in recent years. Most vascular malformations are still managed conservatively, but treatment options have increased in numbers and effectiveness and they are less invasive. Treatment should be individualized, offering a combination of open surgery, sclerotherapy, embolization, laser or radiofrequency ablations. Complex VMs should be treated in specialized multidisciplinary centers.

BIBLIOGRAPHY

Gloviczki P, Driscoll DJ: Klippel-Trenaunay syndrome: current management. Phlebology 22(6):291–298, 2007.

Lee BB, Bergan J, Gloviczki P, et al: Diagnosis and treatment of venous malformations. Consensus document of the International Union of Phlebology (IUP)-2009. Int Angiol 28(6):434–451, 2009.

Lee BB, Do YS, Yakes W, et al: Management of arteriovenous malformations: a multidisciplinary approach. J Vasc Surg 39(3):590–600, 2004.

Lee BB, Kim I, Huh S, et al: New experiences with absolute ethanol sclerotherapy in the management of a complex form of congenital venous malformation. J Vasc Surg 33:764–772, 2002.

Vikkula M, Boon LM, Mullikan JB: Molecular genetics of VMs. Matrix Biology 20:327–335, 2001.

References available online at expertconsult.com.

QUESTIONS

1. Which of the following lesions is not a vascular malformation?
   a. Juvenile hemangioma
   b. Port wine stain
   c. Persistent sciatic vein
   d. Congenital arteriovenous fistula
   e. Lymphangiectasia

2. What type of vascular malformation is seen most frequently at vascular clinics?
   a. Capillary
   b. Arterial
   c. Venous
   d. Arteriovenous
   e. Lymphatic

3. Which of the following statements is not true for vascular malformations?
   a. They have a proliferative phase and then undergo resolution.
   b. The male to female ratio is 1 : 1.
   c. They are developmental anomalies.
   d. There is no cell growth in tissue culture.
   e. They do not contain mast cells in biopsy specimen.

4. Microfistoulos arteriovenous malformations have an arrest in the development of which stage?
   a. Undifferentiated
   b. Retiform
   c. Syncytial
   d. Maturational

5. Which of the following classes are not part of the modified Hamburg classification used currently for vascular malformations?
   a. Arterial
   b. Hemangiomatous
   c. Venous
   d. Arteriovenous
   e. Lymphatic

6. In young patients with lateral varicose veins preoperative evaluation must establish:
   a. Incompetence of the superficial veins
   b. Incompetence in the deep veins
   c. A normal saphenous system
   d. A patent deep venous system
   e. Leg length discrepancy

7. Which of the following findings are not typical for Klippel Trenaunay Syndrome?
   a. Port wine stain
   b. Lateral varicosity
   c. Thrill with machinery murmur
   d. Deep vein anomalies
   e. Limb length discrepancy

8. A large cavernous low flow venous malformation involves the left thigh and buttock in a 22-year-old woman. What is the most useful imaging study in this patient?
   a. CT venogram
   b. Duplex scan to exclude deep vein thrombosis
   c. Intravascular ultrasound
   d. MR imaging and MR venogram
   e. Plethysmography

9. The best treatment for this patient with symptoms of pain and frequent bleeding is:
   a. Surgical excision with skin graft
   b. Radiofrequency ablation
   c. Staged sclerotherapy
   d. Transcatheter embolization with coils
   e. Conservative management

10. Which of the following statement is true for sclerotherapy of venous malformations?
   a. Absolute alcohol injection is not painful.
   b. The advantage of foam over liquid sclerotherapy is that smaller amounts of the detergent can be used to achieve venous thrombosis
   c. Ethanol sclerotherapy has significantly lower complication rates than foam sclerotherapy
   d. Venous malformations are best managed by transfemoral embolization of the feeding arteries
   e. Skin necrosis with ethanol sclerotherapy is very rare.

ANSWERS

1. **a**
2. **c**
3. **a**
4. **b**
5. **b**
6. **d**
7. **c**
8. **d**
9. **c**
10. **b**

CHAPTER 9

VASCULOGENIC ERECTILE DYSFUNCTION

Ralph G. DePalma

Impotence, or male erectile dysfunction (ED), is the persistent or repeated inability to attain and maintain an erection sufficient for satisfactory performance in the absence of an ejaculatory disorder.[1] ED, now better understood and more effectively treated than in the past, is important in the diagnosis and treatment of vascular disease. Progress in this field includes comprehension of normal erectile physiology, understanding of stimuli promoting cavernous sinus smooth muscle relaxation,[2] and development of effective treatments for ED.[3] Vascular surgeons will be mainly concerned with prevention of ED and other sexual dysfunction in relation to aortoiliac interventions. They should be able to delineate the varying etiologies of ED as well as vasculogenic ED, and recognize that aortoiliac reconstruction itself can cause ED by failing to perfuse the internal iliac arteries or by damaging autonomic genital nerves.[4] Techniques of concern for vascular surgeons are those that minimize or completely avoid damage to the pelvic nerves and restore or maintain internal iliac artery perfusion. Familiarity with these techniques can prevent sexual dysfunction and, in some instances, restore potency after aortoiliac interventions.[5,6]

This chapter describes surgical approaches for the prevention of postoperative ED during aortoiliac interventions. Vasculogenic ED owing to small vessel disease, cavernous smooth muscle dysfunction, and primary ED are also common disorders. The vascular specialist should also be aware of evolving approaches to medical and surgical treatment of male sexual function[7] and recognize female sexual dysfunction (FSD) caused by vascular disease, following aortoiliac surgery[8] and after radical hysterectomy.[9] Nerve-sparing and revised operative techniques are available to prevent or minimize these effects.[10,11] Indications for and results of microvascular procedures are summarized along with medical treatment for ED, which is a rapidly expanding area of interest. More than 16,500 citations about ED appeared in PubMed since the 1940s, and more than 180 reports were published within the first quarter of 2011.

PHYSIOLOGY OF ERECTION

Penile erection requires adequate arterial inflow and closure of cavernosal outflow, mediated by a complex interplay between neural and local factors.[12,13] Erection results primarily through relaxation of the smooth muscle of the corporal bodies. Endothelial-mediated relaxation responses stimulated by neural mechanisms function to open the penile cavernous spaces.[14] Nitric oxide (NO) as the chemical mediator[15] and increasing arterial blood flow with oxygenation of the cavernous smooth muscle[16] promote the erectile process. As intracavernosal flow increases, a greater amount of oxygen stimulates additional NO synthesis by cavernosal nerves and endothelium. Cavernosal oxygenation promotes penile erection, whereas hypoxemia is inhibitory. Testosterone, in addition to its central effects, stimulates NO synthase activity in corporal tissues,[17] thus enhancing sensitivity to cavernosal nerve stimulation. NO, in turn, activates conversion of guanosine triphosphate to cyclic guanosine monophosphate (GMP). The latter provides the message leading to relaxation of the smooth muscle within the corpora cavernosa.[18] Agents inhibiting hydrolysis of cyclic GMP increase messenger cyclic GMP, thus facilitating smooth muscle relaxation, which promotes penile erection.[19] Cyclic nucleotide phosphodiesterase (PDE) isoenzymes increase hydrolysis of cyclic GMP; among these, PDE-5 and PDE-6, which are specific for the substrate in human cavernosal tissue.[20] Inhibition of PDE-5 is a key means of treatment for ED. As corporal arterial pressure increases, draining emissary veins are compressed against the tunica albuginea causing venous outflow occlusion. During full erection, cavernosal artery flow virtually ceases. During flaccidity, a constant venous leak balances baseline penile inflow and outflow. With insufficient arterial inflow, the corpora fail pressurize adequately, and secondary venous leakage occurs. Intracavernous pressure increases from 10 to 15 mm Hg to levels ranging from 80 to 90 mm Hg in the erect state. Intracavernous pressures higher than systemic pressure, generated by perineal muscle contraction,[13] contribute to penile rigidity.

INVESTIGATION OF THE COMPLAINT OF ERECTILE DYSFUNCTION

Box 9-1 summarizes general factors contributing to erectile dysfunction; the complaint of ED occuring preoperatively and, of more concern, postoperatively. In screening 1023 men with the chief complaint of impotence, 461 demonstrated an arterial inflow problem, based on noninvasive criteria using the penile brachial index and pulse volume recordings.[21,22] However, many men exhibited other contributing factors, including diabetes, neuropathy (approximately 20%), antihypertensive medication, and cavernous dysfunction, including Peyronie disease. Older men with multiple factors contributing to ED are

- Vasculogenic
- Neurogenic
- Endocrine
- Drug induced
- Psychogenic

| BOX 9-2 | Classification of Vasculogenic Erectile Dysfunction |

- Arterial
- Large vessel aorta and branches to internal iliac artery
- Small vessel anterior division of internal iliac artery and penile arteries
- Combined atheroembolism from aortoiliac segment
- Cavernosal
- Fibrosis postpriapic, drug injection, idiopathic with aging
- Peyronie's disease deformity; venous leakage
- Refractory states hormonal, diabetic, blood pressure medication
- Venous
- Acquired various patterns; dorsal vein, crural, spongiotic
- Congenital cavernous spongiosis leak

generally not candidates for vascular surgical intervention for this complaint alone. Approximately 6% to 7% of the men investigated for ED ultimately became candidates for vascular interventions. In this experience, only 15.6% of men with decreased arterial perfusion were found to have large vessel disease. Imposing a selective screening sequence for surgical case selection yields a sharp funnel effect that minimizes candidacy for vascular intervention for ED.[22] Although proportionate vascular involvement is not high, for young men with small vessel disease or trauma or macrovascular disease, vascular intervention is a logical first step for those failing medical therapy and for those who do not desire prosthetic implantation.[23]

Box 9-2 offers an updated classification of vasculogenic ED. Some type of small vessel, cavernosal, or arteriolar cause is present in 43.3% of men exhibiting abnormal penile perfusion. An additional 41.1% of men with the primary complaint of impotence exhibit a combination of large and small vessel involvement, as ascertained by noninvasive and physical criteria. Most men with the primary complaint of ED are more likely to have small vessel or cavernosal disorders than macrovascular disease. Importantly, the complaint of impotence is associated with occult aortoiliac occlusive or aneurysmal disease.

In men with Leriche syndrome,[24,25] impotence as a sentinel complaint sometimes precedes the onset of claudication. Atheroembolism from ulcerated plaques or occult aneurysms can cause sudden onset of erectile dysfunction.[21] Men younger than 55 years are often potent before reconstruction for aneurysm; an accurate history of their sexual activity must be obtained. Despite the best surgical techniques to preserve sexual function, ED and other sexual disabilities continue to occur after reconstructions for aneurysms and occlusive disease. Therefore, before intervention, the surgeon must make careful inquiries into the patient's sexual function and, when necessary, assess preoperative penile artery perfusion. A detailed history and noninvasive testing are particularly important when postoperative sexual function is an expressed concern of the patient.

HISTORY AND PHYSICAL FINDINGS IN ERECTILE DYSFUNCTION

A history of gradual erectile failure, in the absence of traumatic life events occuring with intermittants claudication, suggests large vessel arteriogenic ED. In these men, both the intensity and the duration of atherosclerotic risk factors, mainly cigarette smoking, hypertension, diabetes, and hypercholesterolemia, contribute to vascular disease. This pattern signals patients who have involvement of the aorta or the iliac system. As mentioned, abrupt onset of erectile failure can be due to emboli from abdominal aneurysms or ulcerated aortoiliac disease.[21] Perineal injury and pelvic fractures can cause arteriogenic impotence. The immediate onset of erectile failure after urologic, vascular, or rectal operations suggests neurovascular damage. Although either neural or vascular interruption can cause ED, periaortic, sympathetic, or hypogastric neural interruption can cause ejaculatory disorders. Alcohol and drug abuse contribute to progressive erectile failure, including drugs used to treat hypertension, some antiinflammatories, and sedatives. Hormonal disorders, such as hypogonadism, rarely cause ED. Our group detected two prolactinomas during the screening of approximately 1400 men; these men exhibited dramatic responses to medical therapy.

Decreased femoral pulses or bruits or palpation of an abdominal aortic aneurysm in those whose waists measure less than 38 to 40 inches confirm aortoiliac involvement. Sensory testing of the extremities, perineum, or glans may reveal neuropathies associated with diabetic impotence. However, these abnormalities are most reliably quantified by neurovascular testing, using pudendal evoked potentials and measurement of bulbocavernosus reflex times.[26,27] Currently, neurologic screening is initially deferred; medical treatment with vasoactive agents is often effective, even with associated neuropathy. In cases of postoperative or posttraumatic dysfunction, neurologic testing documetnting a deficit guides decision making, particularly in recommending prompt prosthetic implantation as a treatment option.

The prostate should be examined, and nodular abnormalities should be investigated. Prostate-specific antigen determinations should routinely be obtained before the prostate examination. Methodical palpation of the corpora cavernosa for Peyronie plaques and estimation of testicular size complete the examination. In most men with primary ED, the results of a physical examination are completely normal.

At this point, the erectile mechanism can be tested in the clinic by intracavernous injection of Prostaglandin E1 (10 to 20 μg).[28] Rigid erection sufficient for intercourse demonstrates adequate arterial inflow and venoocclusive mechanisms. Provided that aneurysmal disease has been ruled out by sonography, initial treatment is with oral, injectable, or intra-uretheral vasoactive agents, which may be effective in up to approximately 60% of cases depending on population demographics and underlying patterns of disease.

ED is a symptom, not a single disease. The factors summarized in Box 9-1 help to guide approaches to the diagnosis and treatment of sexual dysfunction and, in some respects, are relevant to both sexes. An important area has been the study of FSD, which appears in women with diabetes[29,30] and cardiovascular disease[31] and in postmenopausal women as disordered sexual arousal,[32] failure to achieve orgasm, and dyspareunia with failure to lubricate. Feminine arousal and vaginal lubrication are difficult to measure, whereas penile erection can be readily seen and quantified. Progress in understanding the cause, physiology, and treatment of FSD continues.[33] Recently, variable results of aortic surgery in women have been described.[34,35] Treatment of FSD with PDE-5 inhibitors is not recommended; however topical alprostadil has been proved effective in a recent randomized trial.[36] From the standpoint of aortic reconstruction, the potential benefits of nerve-sparing dissections with preserved internal iliac flow for both sexes should be recognized.

No universally accepted approach for diagnosis and management of ED exists; as mentioned, ED is a symptom rather than a single disease. Ideally, correction of the underlying condition should be attempted. In current practice, the patient's goals tend to direct therapy. In the absence of aneurysmal disease, further treatment will depend on the initial response to medical therapy.[37] When oral medication with PDE-5 inhibitors fails, more elaborate investigations can be considered.[38] Should the intracavernous administration of vasoactive agents fail and vacuum constrictor devices prove ineffective, and if vascular intervention is an option, evaluation may progress to more elaborate invasive tests to delineate more subtle anatomic vascular abnormalities. Depending on circumstances, treatment might also progress directly to prosthetic implantation.

NEUROVASCULAR TESTING

Neurovascular testing, initially used for all patients by our group[22] to screen candidates for reconstructive procedures,[23] was found useful in determining an initial dose for intracavernous injection of vasoactive agents. Patients with neurologic deficits were discovered to be exquisitely sensitive to injection of intracavernosal agents with a heightened risk of priapism. With availability of orally administered PDE-5 agents, such testing was less frequently needed. Comprehensive testing is useful for the investigation of postoperative onset and ED owing to perineal trauma, and occasionally to resolve legal issues.

The penile brachial index (PBI), the ratio between systolic pressure detected by a Doppler probe placed distal to a penile cuff and systemic or brachial arm pressure, is a convenient, easily accomplished perfusion measure.[39] A plethysmographic cuff of 2.5 cm, used for an average-size penis, is inflated, then deflated. The reappearance of Doppler signals in the dorsal artery branch proximal to the corona signals reflow. Normally, this pressure approaches systemic pressure. A PBI greater than 0.75 suggests that no major obstacle exists between the aorta and the distal measurement point. Generally, PBIs less than 0.6 relate to major vascular obstructions in the aortoiliac system, while PBIs between 0.6 and 0.75 are considered abnormal.

Penile pulse volume characteristics are then recorded using a pneumoplethysmographic cuff (Buffington) with a contained transducer. This test, as with PBI, is performed with the penis in the flaccid state. Measures observed include crest time, waveform, and the presence or absence of a dicrotic notch as conventionally used for lower extemity recordings. This technique measures the total pulsation of all penile arteries as the cuff compresses the cavernous tissues. The measurements are taken with the cuff inflated to mean arterial pressure and are calculated as diastolic pressure plus one third of systemic pulse pressure. Waveforms on a polygraph with a chart speed of 25 mm/s and a sensitivity setting of 1 demonstrate in normal patients that the upstroke of the waveform is completed by 0.2 seconds, whereas normal waveform amplitudes vary from 5 to 30 mm in height. Waveforms might be abnormal with small vessel disease or cavernosal disorders, whereas PBI is normal.

These noninvasive tests have limited sensitivity and specificity. The combination of PBI and pulse volume recording predicts an abnormal arteriogram with a sensitivity of 85% and a specificity of 70%. In suspected cases of venogenic impotence (i.e., normal arterial noninvasive tests), 23% of men examined with normal noninvasive studies had associated arterial lesions demonstrated angiographically.[40] Therefore, before microvascular interventions are performed for those failing medical therapy,[18] both pudendal arteriography and dynamic infusion cavernosography are required for proper case selection.

PBI detects inadequate arterial inflow from large arteries, but does not detect vasculogenic impotence caused by venous leak, Peyronie disease, or cavernosal fibrosis. In these instances, color-flow duplex scanning after an intracavernous injection to produce erection or tumescence has been used mainly by urologists, sometimes in combination with visual erotic stimulation, to measure deep cavernosal and dorsal blood flow velocity at intervals after the injection of a vasodilator.[41] Based on these studies, ED can be classified as arterial, venous, or mixed vascular. Studies of local blood flow dynamics yield little information about aortoiliac anatomy. Nocturnal penile tumescence and rigidity monitoring, using noninvasive strain gauge techniques, are performed in a sleep laboratory over several nights. Home monitoring devices are available. A normal rigid erection observed during sleep rules out organic impotence.[42]

CAVERNOSOMETRY AND CAVERNOSAL ARTERY OCCLUSION PRESSURE

Invasive studies provide quantitative information about arterial inflow and venoocclusive mechanisms.[43] A calibrated pump provides a flow of warm, heparinized saline via 20-gauge needles inserted into the corpora. During maximal erection, intracavernous pressure at some point equilibrates with arterial inflow pressure, and flow in the deep cavernosal artery stops. This value is called *cavernosal artery occlusion pressure;* it is measured with Doppler insonation at the point of full erection. Normal pressure is greater than 90 mm Hg. A pressure gradient from brachial levels greater than 30 mm Hg suggests arterial inflow occlusion. Dynamic infusion cavernosography measures the flow required to maintain erection. This value is normally 40 mL or less after intracavernous injection of a standard papaverine-phentolamine mixture. Nonionic dilute contrast is injected to visualize venous leaks. Spot filming in various obliquities identifies specific abnormal or leaking veins when cavernosography is positive. As mentioned previously, failure of erection can be caused by an excess of venous leakage over inflow. Venous leakage also can be a seondary effect of arterial insufficiency. Therefore selective pudendal arteriography should be done before venous ablation.

AORTOILIAC RECONSTRUCTION PRINCIPLES

Given the standard indications for large vessel aortoiliac reconstruction (i.e., aneurysm or occlusive disease), the procedure, whether endovascular[44,45] or open,[46,47] should be planned to provide perfusion of both internal iliac arteries whenever possible. Flushing of debris into the internal iliacs should be avoided, and endovascular repair should attempt to maintain internal iliac flow—at least to one internal iliac artery.[17] The dissection in open cases must spare the neural fibers about the aorta and the iliac arteries (which are especially rich on the left side) and about the inferior mesenteric artery. In all these cases, a specific history of preoperative sexual activity must be sought. If an elderly person manifests no interest in sexual activity, complicated preoperative testing is unnecessary. However, when sexual interest exists, preoperative PBI and pulse volume recordings are helpful for later postoperative blood flow assessment.

OPERATIVE TECHNIQUES

Operative techniques to spare autonomic nerves and to preserve or restore internal iliac blood flow have been published.[46,47] The two basic principles described previously apply equally to endovascular and open procedures. Open aortoiliac reconstruction can be accomplished by dissecting the aortoiliac segment from the right and sparing the nerves and inferior mesenteric artery. In cases of aortoiliac aneurysm, perfusion of the internal iliac is ensured by an inlay technique (Figure 9-1). Again, the aneurysmal sac is incised well to the right, avoiding

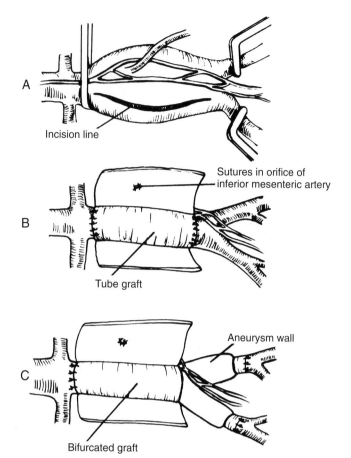

FIGURE 9-1 ■ Inlay nerve-sparing techniques for aneurysm repair. Note the incision on the right side of the aneurysm. (From DePalma RG: Prevention of sexual dysfunction in aortoiliac surgery. In Jamieson CW, editor: Current operative surgery, Eastbourne, East Sussex, United Kingdom, 1985, Bailliere-Tindall, pp 781–788.)

interruption of a dominant left periaortic nerve plexus. The inferior mesenteric artery is sutured from within the aneurysmal sac. Figure 9-2 shows techniques of exposure for endartectomy or bypass for occlusive disease. In men with buttock claudication and impotence related to local disease in the arterial distribution of the internal iliac artery, an extraperitoneal approach with endarterectomy or bypass is not a difficult procedure, although endovascular interventions have been used. The open approach uses a longitudinal incision along the edge of the rectus muscle, with reflection of the peritoneum medially (Figure 9-3). In renal transplant patients, end-to-side renal artery anastomosis to the external iliac artery avoids division of the internal iliac artery. The efficacy of this procedure to prevent ED has been judged to be more effective by some groups than by others.[48-50]

Fredberg and Mouritzen[51] described sexual dysfunction resulting from conventional aortoiliac operations.[51] In their series, 55% of men (11 of 20) with aneurysms were preoperatively impotent, whereas 95% (19 of 20) were postoperatively impotent. Among those with occlusive disease, 31% (15 of 48) were preoperatively impotent, and 60% (29 of 48) were postoperatively impotent. Miles and colleagues[52] found that about 22% (17 of 76)

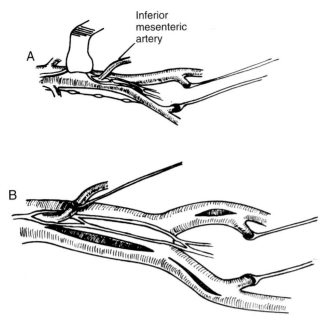

Inferior
mesenteric
artery

A

B

FIGURE 9-2 ■ Dissection of infrarenal aorta for endarterectomy or bypass. **A,** Aorta exposed without mobilization, and inferior mesenteric artery spared along with neural fibers. **B,** Internal iliacs controlled, and common or external iliacs clamped with minimal mobilization. (From DePalma RG: Prevention of sexual dysfunction in aortoiliac surgery. In Jamieson CW, editor: Current operative surgery, Eastborne, East Sussex, United Kingdom, 1985, Bailliere-Tindall, pp 781–788.)

patients receiving conventional aortoiliac operations reported preoperative sexual dysfunction; an additional 30% of those operated on for aneurysm or occlusive disease were rendered impotent.[52] Postoperative impotence was twice as common in men reporting unspecified preoperative "minor dysfunction." It seems unlikely that prospective trials comparing conventional aortic reconstructions with nerve-sparing, internal iliac revascularization techniques will surface, given that attention to the details of these procedures imposes little additional surgical burden or risk. However, comparison with endovascular repair is of considerable interest and will be considered later.

Rich interconnections of the vegetative nervous system about the aortoiliac vessels and the inferior mesenteric artery include both sympathetic and parasympathetic fibers that promote normal ejaculatory function. Damage to these fibers also causes other types of sexual dysfunction: retrograde ejaculation with or without erection and orgasm, anejaculation, failure of emission, and, rarely, normal erection with failure to achieve either ejaculation or orgasm. Ejaculatory disorders, reportedly the most prevalent sexual dysfunction, occur in nearly 40% of men.[53] This primary complaint is more likely encountered in urology[54] or fertility practices, but can occur after open aortoiliac dissection with disruption of autonomic nerve plexi. Ejaculatory disorders should be differentiated from ED, although the psychological consequences of ejaculatory disorders can interfere with erection.

Women were said to be less susceptible to sexual dysfunction after aortoiliac surgery.[55] In this author's experience, three women regained arousal, lubrication,

and orgasm after aortoiliac surgery using nerve-sparing aortoiliac reconstructions that provided internal iliac flow. In this limited case series, operations were performed using the same technique as in men. The approach was chosen out of habit, with no intention of influencing sexual function; these women later reported durable favorable effects. Data are scant; few women in their sexually active years require aortoiliac reconstruction, and methodic measurement of female arousal preoperatively and postoperatively is difficult to assess. Based on questionnaires, Hultgren and coworkers[8] described sexual dysfunction in women before and after aortoiliac operations.[8] They underscored the possibility of iatrogenic nerve damage as a cause of postoperative sexual dysfunction.

Several reports indicated that up to 25% of men regained erectile function after aortoiliac reconstructions using open repairs in patients of varying ages for obstructive disease or aneurysms.[56-64] The prevalence and exact cause of preoperative ED in various series are difficult to assess with accuracy. Erectile function depends on age; comorbid factors, including the use of drugs; and methods of subjective or objective documentation available to clinicians. Flanigan and coworkers[57] stated that, with planning to avoid the diversion of pelvic blood flow, nerve-sparing aortoiliac dissections, and selective use of indirect methods, iatrogenic impotence can be minimized, and a significant proportion of patients can regain normal sexual function postoperatively. In their series of 110 patients using direct and indirect aortoiliac revascularization, 45% of patients with preoperative vasculogenic impotence regained normal sexual function postoperatively, no patients with normal preoperative sexual function were rendered impotent, and two men developed retrograde ejaculation.

A series of men operated on by the author using techniques previously described were followed for at least 3 years using direct interrogation and penile plethysmography. Of 126 men who underwent operation for aortoiliac disease, 4 became impotent as a result of emergency operations or the presence of internal iliac aneurysms. In all the instances of ED, penile plethysmography showed flat-line recordings, and PBIs were well below 0.5. Fifty-three men, average age 64.6 years, were impotent both preoperatively and postoperatively; 30 men, average age 57 years (range, 39 to 71), were potent both preoperatively and postoperatively; 39 men, average age 58.0 years (range, 38 to 69), were impotent preoperatively and regained function postoperatively. Thus, among 126 men undergoing aortoiliac surgery, approximately 3% were rendered impotent, commonly in emergency settings. Overall, function was restored or maintained in 54% of men requiring aortoiliac surgery. The data from this experience, as with all surgical case series, are necessarily retrospective and nonconcurrent. However, longitudinal individual measurements of blood flow along with direct interrogation postoperatively provide advantages over the use of questionnaires in assessing sexual function, particularly as surgical techique evolves.

A randomized trial in the Veterans Administration compared immediate elective repair to imaging surveillance of abdominal aortic aneurysms measuring 4.0 to

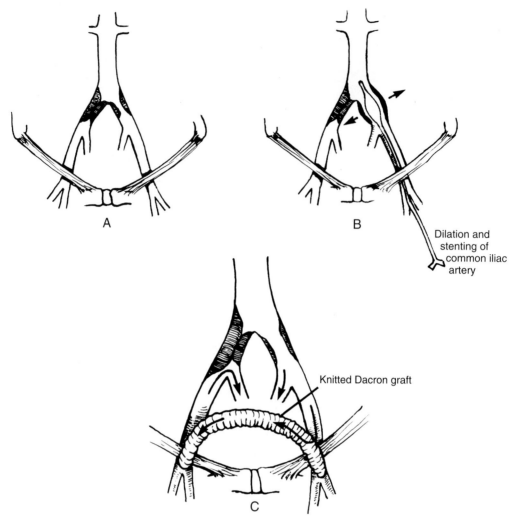

FIGURE 9-3 ■ Femorofemoral bypass with transluminal angioplasty and stenting. **A,** Initial lesion. **B,** Left iliac angioplasty. **C,** Femorofemoral bypass using dilated left iliac donor limb. (From DePalma RG: Prevention of sexual dysfunction in aortoiliac surgery. In Jamieson CW, editor: Current operative surgery, Eastborne, East Sussex, United Kingdom, 1985, Bailliere-Tindall, pp 781–788.)

Within figure: Dilation and stenting of common iliac artery; Knitted Dacron graft

5.5 cm in men aged 50 to 79 years.[65] Quality of life, impotence, and activity level were later assessed using the SF-36 health status instrument in men followed from 3.5 to 8 years (mean, 4.9 years). For most measures and times, there was no difference between the randomized groups, but overall, significantly more men became impotent after immediate repair than after surveillance ($p < 0.03$). A higher prevalence of impotence in the surgical group was found more than 1 year after randomization, paradoxically associated with an improved perception of health during the first 2 years. The data suggest that open intervention for small abdominal aortic aneurysms carries a finite risk of sexual dysfunction, and decreasing potency with age does not appear to be related to patient perception of health status. Possibly, the loss of erectile function was not considered important by many of these older men. Schiavi and colleague[66] showed that age-related changes in frequency, duration, and degree of nocturnal penile tumescence correlated with desire, arousal, and coital frequency. Age of the patient preoperatively and normal postoperative aging contribute to

diminished sexual function. An age-related decrement in function does not appear to be linearly related to compromised arterial inflow.

A retrospective questionnaire study of 90 men showed that sexual orgasmic and erectile function deteriorated after open aneurysm repair compared with endovascular repair.[67] My experience with endovascular interventions for ED directed toward the common or external iliac arteries has been favorable.[45] Others have described selective dilatation of the internal iliac arteries, with modest success.[68,69] Procedures attempting endovascular intervention below this level—that is, in the pudendal arteries—have failed.[70] Lin and associates[71] reported severe pelvic ischemia and erectile dysfunction with internal iliac embolization associated with endovascular repair.[1] The severity of ischemia related to both bilateral embolization and the presence of disease in the deep femoral arteries. Endovascular repair may require occlusion of the orifice of one or both internal iliac arteries to achieve safe and adequate landing sites. Bilateral internal iliac occlusion is associated with a finite risk of pelvic ischemia; adequate hypogastric flow, through at least one of these vessels, relates to normal sexual function. The risk of internal iliac occlusion is not absolute. Femoral collaterals sometimes compensate for internal iliac occlusion, and femoral artery branches have been shown to provide significant collateral circulation to the penis in the face of hypogastric artery occlusion.[72] Internal iliac collateral flow in the presence of acute hypogastric artery ligation is more dependent on the ipsilateral external iliac artery than it is on the contralateral internal iliac artery, even though abundant collateralization between the left and right internal iliac arteries is common in chronic ischemia.[73,74] The variability of responses to internal iliac embolization before endovascular repair has been emphasized.[75] Buttock or thigh claudication and late ischemic complications, seen in 3 of 10 patients after 6 months, led the investigators to suggest limiting bilateral internal iliac embolization before endovascular repair to only those patients considered unfit for open aortic repair.

The Dutch Randomized Endovascular Aneurysm (DREAM) Trial prospectively assessed function during the first postoperative year to compare the effects of elective EVAR or open repair.[35] This group evaluated 153 patients, 141 of them men with a mean age 71 years randomly allocated to endovascular aortic aneurism repair (EVAR) or open repair. No immediate significant difference in sexual function between the two groups was observed; postoperatively, the proportion of patients (including women) rose to 79% in the open repair group and 82% in the EVAR group. Given expectations of sexual function at an average age of 71 years in the DREAM trial, this endeavor, though well done should not be counted upon to answer the question of whether EVAR is to be favored with regards to sexual function. With increasing experience, other reasons to consider EVAR exist; these notably include reduced mortality and morbidity short term.[76,77]

Femorofemoral bypass combined with intraluminal dilatation of donor external or common iliac arteries is an excellent choice for certain candidates with occlusive disease (Figure 9-4). The procedure completely avoids aortoiliac dissection, and patency remains durable. Objective information from pulse volume recordings before and after femorofemoral bypass correlates with improved patterns of penile plethysmography and pressures after reconstruction.[78] Common iliac artery transluminal dilatation is both practical and useful. Transluminal dilatation of the external iliac arteries can also improve penile perfusion by relieving steal via the internal iliac and gluteal arteries. Although transluminal dilatation of the common iliac arteries is effective, the internal iliac arteries can be difficult to dilate. A report in the Italian literature describes three successful cases among 25 men treated with endovascular interventions for ED.[69] Transluminal dilatation of the distal pudendal and penile arteries was plagued by restenosis.[79]

MICROVASCULAR PROCEDURES

Small vessel reconstructions initially used direct arterialization of the corpus cavernosum, but this approach was

Extraperitoneal incision, lateral border of rectus sheath

FIGURE 9-4 ■ Iliac artery endarterectomy. **A,** Incision for retroperitoneal exposure. **B,** Incision for isolated plaque of internal iliac artery. **C,** Linear incision when the external iliac artery is also involved. (From DePalma RG: Prevention of sexual dysfunction in aortoiliac surgery. In Jamieson CW, editor: Current operative surgery, Eastborne, East Sussex, United Kingdom, 1985, Bailliere-Tindall, pp 781–788.)

soon abandoned. These procedures induced priapism or thrombosis due to fibrosis at the anastomosis between the artery and the corpus cavernosum. Although interest in small vessel reconstruction persists,[80] a 1996 metaanalysis by a urology guidelines panel stated that the chances of success with venous or arterial surgery did not justify its routine use.[81] These procedures are applicable to men who fail to respond to medical therapy and who do not wish to have prostheses. With the availability of effective vasoactive drugs, these procedures are rarely performed. Two types of microvascular bypasses have been used: bypass into the dorsal artery and arterialization of the deep dorsal vein. The inferior epigastric artery is a readily available inflow source, behaving much like the internal mammary artery. Some use a vein graft originating from the femoral artery. Use of the inferior epigastric artery with microvascular arterial anastomosid to the dorsal artery is preferred when possible.

PATIENT AND PROCEDURE SELECTION

Candidates for microvascular correction of ED must be selected rigorously. They must have failed to respond to lifestyle alterations, maximal oral PDE-5 inhibitors, and other measures including cavernosal or intraurethral injection therapy and vacuum erection devices. The options, risks, and benefits of prosthetic insertion should be explored with these patients. Candidates for microvascular surgery are young men with a history of trauma or localized disease.[21,23] Some exhibit diffuse distal penile lesions of unknown origin. Candidates should be free of neural, hormonal, and medication-induced causes of impotence. All patients require selective pudendal arteriography. Communication between the dorsal penile artery and the cavernosal artery requires detailed visualization of individual penile vessels after intracavernous injection of a vasoactive agent to produce tumescence. As previously described, a full erection masks inflow into the cavernosal artery and is not appropriate for evaluation of the penile microvasculature. Anatomy permitting, the inferior epigastric artery, dissected in continuity, is turned down for microvascular anastomosis to the appropriate dorsal artery.

Deep Dorsal Vein Arterialization

Candidates for deep dorsal vein arterialization are younger men with small vessel disease whose dorsal arteries are not suitable for direct bypass. A microvascular anastomosis is done between the inferior epigastric artery and the deep dorsal vein. The rationale of this operation was postulated to be reverse flow via emissary veins into the corpus cavernosum. However, the author's arteriographic observations and those of others indicate that flow is largely by the circumflex veins into the spongiosum. Follow-up data at 12 to 84 months (average, 34.5 months) showed that 33% of these men attained spontaneous erections, 47% responded to intracavernous injections, and 21% remained impotent.[21] Glans hyperperfusion is a serious, specific complication of venous arterialization. Venous hypertension, heralded by urinary spraying owing to urethral edema, ultimately progresses glans ulceration and necrosis. To minimize this complication, the anastomosis should be performed proximally under the arch of the pubis, and the dorsal vein is ligated proximally and distally, sparing the circumflex veins, which provide outflow. This complication, which can occur late, urgently requires further distal penile vein ligation or ligation of the inflow source.

Venous Interruption

Reported success rates for venous ligation vary considerably, and opinions about this procedure range from advocacy to qualified reservation to condemnation. This variability probably relates to patient selection and failure to evaluate all factors, including arterial supply or prior penile trauma that can cause venous leakage. At follow-up ranging from 12 to 100 months (average, 48 months), 33% of men functioned spontaneously, 44% used intracavernous injection, and the remainder were impotent.[21,23] Venous ligation requires direct ligation and excision of the veins in cases selected by dynamic infusion cavernosography. These procedures are confined to excision of the dorsal vein without approaching the crural veins directly.[82] Other draining veins can be occluded using coils inserted by an invasive radiologist. At times, an introducing catheter inserted via the deep dorsal vein is useful. Yu and associates[83] recommend routine dynamic cavernosography and cavernosometry at 3 months in all cases of venous ligation to rule out sham effect.[83] At this time, embolization for recurrent leaks can be done; with these procedures, apprximately 70% of men can regain erectile function and are able to function with supplemental intracavernous injection. Interest in correction of venous leakage continues; Virag and Paul[84] recently used CT to delineate abnormal venous drainage to improve results of venous occlusion for treatment of ED.[84]

MEDICAL TREATMENT

Once aneurysms, large vessel disease, and uncontrolled diabetes have been ruled out, the branched logic sequence shown in Figure 9-5 can be used. Treatment begins with control of risk factors such as cigarette smoking, hyperlipidemia, and obesity. It is possible to minimize the necessity for antihypertensive treatment by weight control or exercise or to minimize the sexual effects of such treatment by changing drugs to angiotensin-converting enzyme inhibitors, angiotensive receptor blockers, and calcium channel blockers, which appear to have no relevant effect on erectile function.[85] Some men improve after one or two intracavernous injections have produced artificial erection, and they then resume spontaneous function.

Specific medical therapy and risk factor modification are done synchronously with initial oral therapy using selected PDE-5 inhibitors widely available in oral form. With dose titration, sildenafil was effective in 59% of individuals, compared with 20% in the placebo group.[86] Administration of nitrates or α-blockers is a specific contraindication to PDE-5 therapy. The PDE-5 class of drugs has been discovered to be useful in treatment of pulmonary hypertension[87,88] and Raynaud phenomenon,[89,90] using daily doses for benign prostatic hypertrophy[89] and as adjuncts to reduce cell resistance to chemotherapy.[91] PDE-5 inhibitors will be used more frequenly and for wider indications in the future over and above their utility as first line treatment for erectile dysfunction.

SUMMARY

The first task of the vascular surgeon is to understand the basic techniques for open and endovascular aortoiliac interventions that prevent or relieve ED associated with large vessel disease. They need to be familiar with the causes of ED and collaborate with urologists and other experts in treating men with primary ED. They will be called upon to deal with this complication should it occur postoperatively. After screening and a trial of medical treatment, some individuals become candidates for vascular surgical intervention for the sole purpose of treating a sexual disability. Those with macrovascular disease, occult aneurysms, and poorly controlled diabetes require the particular attention of vascular specialists. Treating men, and less commonly women, with sexual disabilities requires a unique sensitivity to individual needs. Outcomes of medical treatment and surgical interventions continue to improve in concert with more accurate diagnosis, advances in surgical technique, patient selection, and availability of effective drug therapy.

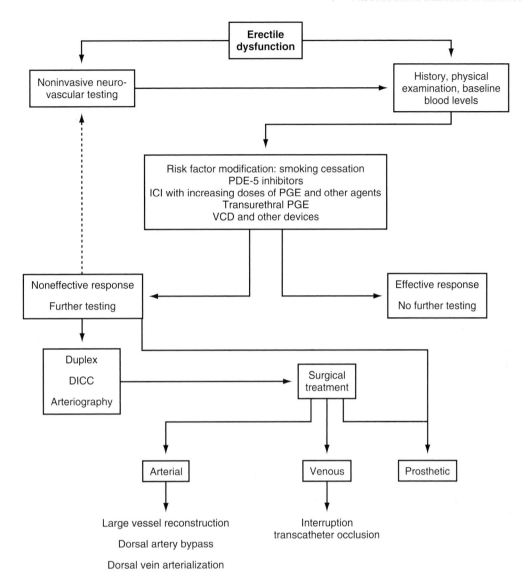

FIGURE 9-5 ■ Algorithm for erectile dysfunction. *DICC,* Dynamic infusion cavernosometry and cavernosography; *ICI,* intracavernous injection; *PGE,* prostaglandin E₁; *VCD,* vacuum erection constrictor device.

BIBLIOGRAPHY

DePalma RG, Levine SB, Feldman S: Preservation of erectile function after aortoiliac reconstruction. Arch Surg 113:958, 1978.

DeTejada IS, Goldstein I, Azadzoi K, et al: Impaired neurogenic and endothelium-mediated relaxation of penile smooth muscle from diabetic men with impotence. N Engl J Med 32:1025, 1989.

Flanigan DP, Schuler JJ, Keifer T, et al: Elimination of iatrogenic impotence and improvement of sexual dysfunction after aortoiliac revascularization. Arch Surg 117:544, 1982.

Goldstein I, Lue TF, Padma-Nathan H, et al: Oral sildenafil in the treatment of erectile dysfunction. N Engl J Med 338:1397, 1998.

Harris JD, Jepson RP: Aorto-iliac stenosis: a comparison of two procedures. Aust J Surg 34:211, 1965.

Leriche R, Morel A: The syndrome of thrombotic obliteration of the aortic bifurcation. Ann Surg 127:193, 1948.

Merchant RF, Jr, DePalma RG: Effects of femorofemoral grafts on postoperative sexual function: correlation with penile pulse volume recordings. Surgery 90:962, 1981.

Rajfer J, Aronson WJ, Bush PA, et al: Nitric oxide as a mediator of the corpus cavernosum in response to nonadrenergic noncholinergic neurotransmission. N Engl J Med 326:90, 1992.

References available online at expertconsult.com.

QUESTIONS

1. During full penile erection:
   a. Deep cavernosal artery flow increases.
   b. Venous valves close.
   c. Perineal muscles relax.
   d. Cavernosal smooth muscle relaxes.
   e. Glandular hypertension occurs.

2. Men with erectile dysfunction most often exhibit which of the following?
   a. Decreased dorsal arterial flow
   b. Severe psychoneurosis
   c. Occult aneurysms
   d. Neurologic abnormalities
   e. Normal physical examination

3. Which of the following statements about endovascular aortoiliac procedures is true?
   a. They may require bilateral internal iliac artery occlusion.
   b. They may result in buttock ischemia.
   c. They may result in more ED postoperatively.
   d. They spare periaortic nerves.
   e. They may be more effective in women.

4. When does the penile brachial index (PBI) indicate aortoiliac occlusive disease?
   a. PBI between 0.6 and 0.75
   b. PBI 0.6 or less
   c. PBI 0.8 or less
   d. PBI 0.8, accompanied by flattened pulse volume waves
   e. PBI 0.75, accompanied by abnormally shaped pulse waves

5. Women with female sexual dysfunction may have which of the following?
   a. Failure to lubricate
   b. Dyspareunia
   c. Aortoiliac occlusive disease
   d. Arousal failure
   e. All of the above

6. When a sexually active man expresses concern about possible erectile dysfunction before aneurysm repair, what should the surgeon do?
   a. Assure the patient and spouse that this is preventable.
   b. Refer the patient to a psychiatrist.
   c. Measure baseline levels of testosterone and prolactin.
   d. Obtain preoperative penile brachial index and pulse volume recordings.
   e. Perform preoperative selective pudendal arteriography.

7. Useful techniques in preventing sexual dysfunction after aortic surgery include all except:
   a. Preservation of flow into internal iliac arteries
   b. Suturing of the inferior mesenteric artery within the aortic sac
   c. Minimial disruption of periaortic nerve plexi
   d. Retrograde flushing of the internal iliac arteries
   e. Careful dissection of the branches of the inferior mesenteric artery

8. Age-related decline in sexual activity reported on postoperative surveys may relate to:
   a. Decreased arterial penile perfusion
   b. Autonomic neuropathy
   c. Perineal fibrosis
   d. Progressive venous leakage
   e. Lack of interest

9. Microvascular penile revascularization is most applicable for:
   a. Men failing initial medical treatment
   b. Men with generalized atherosclerosis
   c. For ED occurring after aortoiliac reconstruction
   d. After removal of a penile prosthesis
   e. Young men with perineal or pelvic trauma

10. Initial medical treatment for erectile dysfunction most often requires which of the following?
    a. PDE-5 inhibitors
    b. Cavernosometry
    c. Arteriography
    d. Psychotherapy
    e. Intra-uretheral prostadil

ANSWERS

1. **d**
2. **e**
3. **d**
4. **b**
5. **e**
6. **d**
7. **e**
8. **e**
9. **e**
10. **a**

CHAPTER 10

Primary Arterial Infections and Antibiotic Prophylaxis

Hugh A. Gelabert

PRIMARY ARTERIAL INFECTIONS

A primary arterial infection is a condition in which an infectious agent invades and destroys the wall of an artery, resulting in disruption of the normal arterial architecture and pseudoaneurysm formation. Ultimately these lesions can result in symptoms resulting from sepsis, compression, erosion, embolization, thrombosis, or hemorrhage. The essential features include the destruction of the arterial wall by an infectious process, septic illness, and rapid onset of pseudoaneurysm formation. The presentation varies from indolent to cataclysmic. Successful management requires familiarity with the processes involved and the ability to make prompt decisions at the time of surgery. The goal of this chapter is to review primary arterial infections in terms of their pathophysiology, diagnosis, and treatment.

Historical Perspective

In the nineteenth century, Rokitansky[1] and Koch[2] recognized an association between arterial infection and aneurysm formation. In 1885, Osler[3] presented the first comprehensive description of this relationship. In addressing the Royal College of Physicians, he described a 30-year-old man who had died from fever, chills, and pneumonia. At autopsy, the patient was found to have endocarditis involving the aortic valve, as well as multiple aneurysms of the thoracic aorta. Based on carefully described pathologic findings, Osler proposed a causal relationship between infection of the aortic wall and subsequent aneurysm formation. Because of a similarity between the beaded appearance of these aneurysms and fungal vegetations, he introduced the term *mycotic aneurysm* and thus the concept of primary arterial infection.

Definitions

There is no universally accepted definition of primary arterial infection. Moreover, there continues to be confusion regarding the general classification of infections that involve the native arterial tree. Although the term *mycotic aneurysm* initially signified an infected aneurysm found in association with bacterial endocarditis, it has come to denote an infected aneurysm of any type. Another problem is that there is considerable disparity among the several definitions that have been proposed. Finally, it should be recognized that, with the exception of a secondarily infected arterial aneurysm, most of these lesions are actually infected pseudoaneurysms. Most lesions arise by means of the local destruction of the arterial wall and the fibrous encapsulation of an expanding hematoma; therefore these lesions do not have the histologic components of an arterial wall.

For practical purposes, *primary arterial infection* can be defined as the direct invasion of a pathogen into the wall of a native artery, irrespective of the preexisting state of the underlying artery or source of the pathogen. The term *mycotic aneurysm* is used to denote both true aneurysms and false aneurysms that are associated with infection of the arterial wall.

Pathogenesis

Five basic mechanisms have been implicated in the development of primary arterial infections. They can be grouped broadly as (1) oslerian mycotic aneurysms, (2) microbial arteritis with aneurysm formation, (3) infected aneurysms, (4) arterial injury with contamination, and (5) arteritis from contiguous spread.

Oslerian Mycotic Aneurysms: Embolization of Infected Cardiac Vegetations

Osler, in coining the term *mycotic aneurysm*, both named the condition and described what would be the most prevalent cause of primary arterial infection in the pre-antibiotic era. As he described it, a mycotic aneurysm is limited to the unique clinical condition characterized by bacterial endocarditis with septic embolization from valvular vegetations. These septic emboli lodge within the arterial wall, where a suppurative infection develops. The arterial wall is destroyed by the infection, and the resultant pseudoaneurysm is recognized as a mycotic aneurysm.

Considerable confusion has arisen because the term *mycotic aneurysm* has been expanded and applied to various types of infected aneurysms. Crane[4] attempted to classify mycotic aneurysms as primary and secondary types. He introduced the term *primary mycotic aneurysm* to refer to infected aortic aneurysms not associated with endocarditis or an infectious focus; secondary types were those that formed as a result of preceding endocarditis. Ponfick[5] and Eppinger[6] were among the first to characterize the anatomic features of these aneurysms pathologically. Ponfick[5] proposed that the initial insult to the arterial wall was a mechanical injury inflicted by the embolization of septic material. Eppinger in 1887 provided further support for the theory of septic emboli by culturing the same strain of bacteria from both vegetative lesions and the wall of an aneurysm in a patient with endocarditis. He applied the term *embolomycotic* to describe the combination of infectious and embolic components that led to the formation of mycotic aneurysms.[6]

Microbial Arteritis with Aneurysm Formation: Hematogenous Seeding

The second mechanism of arterial infection involves hematogenous microbial seeding of arteries during an episode of bacteremia. Microbial arteritis with aneurysm formation occurs when a normal or atherosclerotic artery becomes infected and the weakened artery becomes aneurysmal.

In 1906, the German pathologist Weisel[7] described distinctive pathologic changes in arterial walls that occurred during the course of an infectious disease, but were not related to cardiac valve vegetation emboli.[7] Lewis and Schrager[8] and Cathcart[9] presented case reports of infected peripheral aneurysms that developed in normal arteries of patients with osteomyelitis and typhoid fever, respectively. Despite these reports, nearly 30 years passed before consideration was given to the mechanism by which bacteremia led to arterial infection. Crane[4] described an infected aneurysm in a patient with hypoplasia of the aorta, but no associated bacterial endocarditis or other identifiable source of infection.[4] He proposed that the combination of the "force of the blood stream" and abnormal development of the aorta allowed bacteria to invade that portion of the aorta. This resulted in an arterial infection, disruption of the aortic wall, and an infected pseudoaneurysm. Revell extended the concept of aortic bacterial seeding one step further and proposed that the route of infection was through the aortic vasa vasorum.[10] Hawkins and Yeager,[11] acknowledging the resistance of arterial intima to infection, suggested that an intimal defect such as that produced by arteriosclerosis allowed bacterial localization and infection.

Infected Aneurysms

The term *infected aneurysm* refers to an infection of a preexisting aneurysm, most often by hematogenous microbiologic seeding of the aneurysm. The original aneurysm is most commonly atherosclerotic; however, it may also be the result of trauma or arteritis. The diseased artery becomes host to bacterial pathogens when these lodge within the intramural thrombus and arteriosclerotic intima.

Arterial Injury with Contamination

Another cause of arterial infections is mechanical arterial injury by contaminated instruments. This type of infection can occur after an inadvertent arterial puncture with a contaminated needle in a drug abuser, as an accidental contamination during radiologic procedures, during placement of hemodynamic monitoring catheters, or as

a result of traumatic injury. The combination of mechanical disruption of the intima and seeding of the arterial lesion with pathogenic bacteria leads to the formation of suppurative arteritis and destroys a portion of the arterial wall. This subsequently becomes an infected arterial pseudoaneurysm.

Arteritis from Contiguous Spread

Arterial infections can also develop through the spread of infection from a contiguous focus. Contiguous infections that have been recognized as potential sources of bacteria include lesions such as osteomyelitis, infected lymph nodes, tuberculous lymph nodes, and abscesses from narcotic injection.[12] Bacteria, and less commonly mycobacteria or fungi, invade the artery either by direct extension or via lymphatics. They subsequently produce a necrotizing invasive infection of the arterial wall, with eventual destruction of the wall.

Other Forms of Arterial Infection

There are three other, less common forms of infected aneurysms: syphilitic aortitis, true fungal aneurysms, and primary (spontaneous) aortoenteric fistulas. Because of significant differences in the pathogens and pathogenesis of these lesions, they merit separate discussion.

Syphilitic aneurysms are a rarely encountered complication of advanced syphilis. These lesions occur in approximately 10% of patients with the tertiary form of the disease.[13] These aneurysms commonly arise in the ascending aorta, frequently involve the aortic valve, and are secondary to treponemal invasion of the vasa vasorum. The reasons why *Treponema* species prefers this portion of the aorta remain unclear. After spirochete penetration, an infiltrate develops within the vessel wall consisting of plasma cells, epidermal cells, and giant cells. This infiltrate results in destruction of the elastic and muscular components of the tunica media, replacement of the normal wall with fibrous tissue, and dilatation and subsequent formation of saccular aneurysms.

Fungal arterial infections are also extremely rare and occur most often in patients who are immunosuppressed. Common risk factors include diabetes, immunosuppressive medications, and chronic hematologic disorders such as leukemia or lymphoma. The species most often implicated are *Histoplasma capsulatum*, *Aspergillus fumigatus*, *Candida albicans*, and *Penicillium* species. These lesions most commonly result from either colonization of a preexisting aneurysm or infection of a damaged artery.

HIV-related vasculitis can result in aneurysmal degeneration of the arterial wall. Radiologic appearance may be identical to that which results from a bacterial arterial infection. The distinction is noted in the pathologic evaluation of the affected arterial wall, which demonstrates acute and chronic adventitial inflammatory changes. Secondary bacterial infections may be present, and cultures may be positive in a minority of these patients. There appears to be a predilection toward carotid and femoral arteries; however, the aorta may also be involved.[14-16]

Spontaneous or "primary" aortoenteric fistulas (AEFs) arise as a consequence of progressive aneurysmal

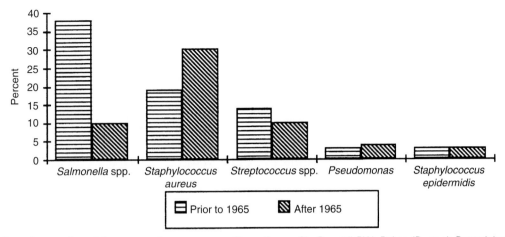

FIGURE 10-1 ■ Organisms cultured from mycotic aneurysms. (From Brown SL, Busuttil RW, Baker JD, et al: Bacteriologic and surgical determinants of survival in patients with mycotic aneurysms. J Vasc Surg 1:541, 1984.)

enlargement, with gradual erosion into an adjacent segment of the gastrointestinal tract. The erosion is thought to be facilitated by the indurated, atherosclerotic artery pressing against a tethered portion of bowel. The most common location for this erosion is the third portion of the duodenum. In their 1951 review of a series of 16,633 autopsies, Hirst and Affeldt[17] reported the incidence of this type of fistula to be 0.05%. Because the majority of patients with aortic aneurysms now undergo elective operation before they can progress to develop a primary aortoenteric fistula, the incidence of these lesions is thought to be considerably lower today. Patients with spontaneous AEFs may have an initial or "herald" bleed, which represents the initial hemorrhage of blood into the duodenum. In this presentation, the initial hemorrhage may abate then later resume in a more prolonged and dramatic manner. Presumably, clot within the AEF is responsible for the intermittent nature of the bleeding episodes. This condition is considerably different from that associated with aortic graft infection, or secondary AEF. Secondary AEF is more common, more dangerous, and more difficult to manage.

Graft excision and remote reconstruction are the standard management of secondary AEF. In contrast, significant evidence exists that primary AEF can be managed by closure of the duodenal rent, debridement of the aorta, and in situ reconstruction with an arterial prosthesis. The prerequisites of this approach are the absence of purulence at the fistula site, a small defect in the duodenum, and a relatively healthy patient. It should be noted that the management of primary aortic infections (mycotic aneurysms) is similar to that of primary AEF, in that the absence of gross infection along with adequate debridement may allow in situ graft reconstruction of the aorta.[18]

Causative Organisms

The organism most commonly associated with microbial aortitis is *Salmonella*. This is followed, in order of frequency, by *Streptococcus* species, *Bacteroides* species, *Arizona hinshawii*, *Escherichia coli*, and *Staphylococcus aureus*.[18] Studies that focus on subpopulations such as intravenous

(IV) drug abusers or those with femoral mycotic aneurysms tend to identify a predominance of gram-positive bacteria such as staphylococci and streptococci, along with gram-negative organisms such as *E. coli* and *Pseudomonas* species.

The bacteriology of primary arterial infections has undergone considerable transformation since its original description in the mid 1800s (Figure 10-1). Brown and colleagues[19] suggested that the reason for this change is antibiotic selective pressure leading to bacterial adaptation. Also, there has been a change in the relative incidence of pathogenic mechanisms with the more common use of invasive diagnostic modalities, as well as the increased illicit use of IV drugs. The majority of arterial infections during the preantibiotic era were oslerian mycotic aneurysms; that is, they were related to bacterial endocarditis. The bacteriology of arterial infections during this period, therefore, was similar to that of endocarditis. Stengal and Wolferth[20] in the 1920s and Revell[10] in the 1940s reported that the predominant organisms were nonhemolytic streptococci, staphylococci, and pneumococci. Magilligan and Quinn,[21] in a 1986 review, subdivided 91 patients with bacterial endocarditis into two groups: those known to be IV drug abusers (36 patients) and those who were not (55 patients). Of the first group, the most common organisms were *S. aureus* (36%), *Pseudomonas* species (16%), polymicrobial organisms (15%), *Streptococcus faecalis* (13%), and *Streptococcus viridans* (11%). Organisms in the second group (non-IV drug abusers) were *S. viridans* (22%), *S. aureus* (20%), *S. faecalis* (14%), and *Staphylococcus epidermidis* (11%). The declining incidence of rheumatic fever and the adoption of early, appropriate antibiotic treatment have resulted in a significant decrease in bacterial endocarditis. This in turn has resulted in a decline in the incidence of oslerian mycotic aneurysms in recent decades.

Concurrent with the declining incidence of oslerian mycotic aneurysms has been an increase in various other types of primary arterial infections. Principal among these are microbial arteritis and infected aneurysms. This may be due, in part, to the increasing age of the population and the simultaneous increase in the prevalence of

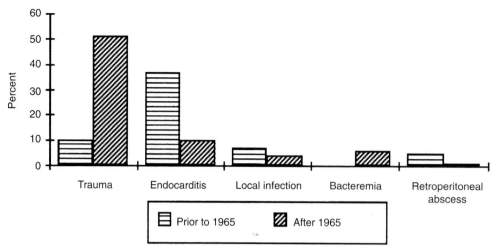

FIGURE 10-2 ■ Causes of mycotic aneursyms. (From Brown SL, Busuttil RW, Baker JD, et al: Bacteriologic and surgical determinants of survival in patients with mycotic aneurysms. J Vasc Surg 1:541, 1984.)

atherosclerosis. The bacteriology of these arterial infections is different from that of oslerian mycotic aneurysms. The microorganisms most commonly associated with microbial arteritis are *Salmonella* species, *Staphylococcus* species, and *E. coli*. *Salmonella* species, in particular, have a striking propensity for invading diseased (atherosclerotic) aortas. In selected series, the involvement of *Salmonella* species has been reported to be as high as 50%. The most virulent species, *Salmonella choleraesuis* and *Salmonella typhimurium*, account for more than 60% of the reported cases of *Salmonella arteritis*.[22] Less commonly reported organisms associated with microbial arteritis include fungi and anaerobic organisms. Among the latter, *Bacteroides fragilis* has been reported in association with supraceliac aortic aneurysms.

The bacteriology of infected aneurysms is similar to that of both mycotic aneurysms and microbial arteritis. Despite this, some variation exists among reported series. Although Bennett and Cherry[23] reported a 66% incidence of *Salmonella* infections, Jarrett and associates[24] described a predominance of gram-positive cocci (59%), with *S. aureus* representing 41%. In two prospective studies of patients undergoing aneurysmectomy, cultures obtained from both the aneurysm wall and the bowel bag revealed a predominance of gram-positive organisms.[24,25] Both of these series are thought to represent cases of bacterial colonization. Despite the relative infrequency of gram-negative organisms observed in Jarrett's series, the distinction between gram-negative and gram-positive cultures proved clinically important. Patients with gram-negative bacteria demonstrated a greater likelihood of aortic rupture than did those with gram-positive organisms. Specifically, the rupture rate associated with gram-negative bacterial isolates was 84%, whereas that associated with gram-positive bacterial cultures was 10%.

According to Brown and associates,[19] the most common infected aneurysms since 1965 are those that occur as a result of mechanical arterial injury with contamination of the vessel wall. The organism most frequently implicated in this type of arterial infection is *S. aureus*, which Brown's group cultured in as many as 30% of cases. Reddy and

associates,[26] in a series of infected femoral false aneurysms, reported a 65% incidence of *S. aureus* and a 33% rate of polymicrobial infection.[26] Although arterial infections secondary to contiguous spread are most commonly bacterial, mycobacterial and fungal infections may also occur in these lesions. As with microbial arteritis, *Salmonella* organisms are the predominant pathogen, and *Staphylococcus* organisms are second in frequency (Figure 10-2).

The increased number of immunosuppressed patients in certain settings has resulted in an increase of reports indicating opportunistic infections. Patients with cancer, prolonged steroid use, transplantation and other immunosuppressive conditions may present with infections. In these populations, infections from opportunistic agents are more prominent. Specifically noted are infections from *Campylobacter* species, *Listeria* species, and *Mycobacterium tuberculosis*.[27]

Anatomic Distribution

The anatomic distribution of primary arterial infections varies somewhat, depending on the pathologic type. True oslerian mycotic aneurysms most often involve the larger muscular and elastic arteries. In retrospective reviews, both Lewis and Schrager[8] and Brown and colleagues[19] found the most common sites of infection to be the abdominal aorta and the femoral and superior mesenteric arteries (Figure 10-3). The predisposition for aortic involvement is thought to be related to the higher incidence of underlying atherosclerotic aneurysms in this location compared with other anatomic sites.

Microbial arteritis with aneurysm formation occurs when a pathogen localizes at the site of an arterial lesion such as an atherosclerotic plaque. As one would anticipate, the arteries most commonly involved are the ones that demonstrate advanced atherosclerotic changes—namely, the distal aorta and the femoral, iliac, and popliteal vessels. In theory, infected aneurysms can occur at any site within the arterial tree where there is a preexisting aneurysm. It is curious that all series in the literature

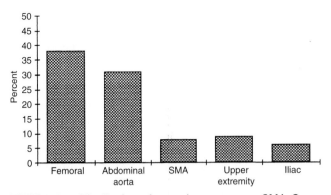

FIGURE 10-3 ■ Distribution of mycotic aneurysms. *SMA,* Superior mesenteric artery. (From Brown SL, Busuttil RW, Baker JD, et al: Bacteriologic and surgical determinants of survival in patients with mycotic aneurysms. J Vasc Surg 1:541, 1984.)

demonstrate a strong propensity for involvement of the abdominal aorta. Involvement of this artery has been reported in up to 79% of cases. Whether this represents a tendency of the bacteria to infect aortic aneurysms or a study bias toward aortic aneurysms is not clear. Certainly, aortic aneurysms have been subjected to closer scrutiny than have other peripheral arterial aneurysms. This may account, in part, for this reported predilection.

Arterial infections due to mechanical injury with contamination most commonly involve arteries that have minimal soft tissue coverage. There are three main causes: accidental drug injection, vascular access, and trauma. Because these causes are related to the accessibility of the arteries and their superficial locations, these infections most commonly involve the femoral or brachial arteries. These locations also have an important effect on the presentation of these lesions, because femoral and brachial artery aneurysms are usually identified by the pulsatile mass, erythema, and tenderness of the aneurysm itself rather than by symptoms of arterial sepsis.

Clinical Presentation

The most common clinical presentation in patients with primary arterial infection is fever, leukocytosis, and tenderness over the affected artery. Patients may have a wide range of signs and symptoms, depending on the pathophysiology, bacteriology, and location of the infected artery or arteries. Most components of the clinical presentation can be assigned to one of two general groups: signs and symptoms resulting from infection or bacteremia, and signs and symptoms occurring secondary to local arterial involvement or aneurysm formation. Night sweats, general malaise, arthralgias, and increased fatigability in conjunction with fever and leukocytosis occur as a consequence of the recurrent bacteremias associated with sepsis from the arterial infections. In patients with oslerian mycotic aneurysms, the clinical signs and symptoms of bacterial endocarditis may be difficult to distinguish from those associated with the arterial infection. Similarly, symptoms in patients with arterial lesions that

developed by spread from a contiguous suppurative source may derive from either infectious focus.

The second group of signs and symptoms occurs as a result of inflammation and aneurysmal dilatation of the infected artery. Localized tenderness is the most readily recognized symptom related to the inflammatory destruction of the arterial wall. Characteristics such as abdominal or peripheral bruits, neurologic defects from nerve compression, or pulsatile masses may also be present.

Thrombosis and thromboembolization are common sequelae of such arterial aneurysms. When they appear, they elicit associated symptoms such as ischemic digital or limb pain. Initially, these embolic presentations may be indistinguishable from similar events in uninfected aneurysms. If the embolic material is infected and causes a secondary arterial infection, the mycotic nature of the lesion may be revealed. Other findings of arterial infection include petechial skin lesions and septic arthritis.

Arterial rupture is common in cases of infected arterial aneurysms. This presentation is identical to that of any arterial rupture. If the damaged artery is contained and supported by a capsule of fibrous connective tissue, it may progress to form a pseudoaneurysm, and the principal symptom would be pain. If the rupture is uncontrolled, the presentation is that of hypotensive shock. If the rupture is in a superficial artery that erodes through the skin, the presentation is that of evident life-threatening hemorrhage.

Periarterial gas formation signals the presence of a gas-producing organism and should be a clear signal that urgent treatment is needed. Although this is not a common presentation, it should be considered in any patient who has unexplained periaortic gas and symptoms suggestive of sepsis.

Diagnostic Testing

The diagnosis of a primary arterial infection is based on elements of the clinical presentation, along with appropriate testing. The primary factor in making such a diagnosis is a high clinical suspicion, followed by a search for evidence to support the diagnosis of a primary arterial infection. The choice and use of diagnostic tests are of singular importance in identifying and substantiating the presence of an arterial infection. Because of the potentially fulminant course of these infections and the fatal outcome of improperly managed cases, diagnostic speed and accuracy are crucial. The basic elements of diagnostic testing include bacteriologic sampling and radiologic imaging.

Blood Cultures

The demonstration of bacterial organisms in association with an arterial lesion is central to the diagnosis of an arterial infection. The bacteria may be detected by either blood cultures or cultures of the arterial wall itself. Blood cultures, by virtue of their availability, are frequently one of the first tests done in patients suspected of having a significant infection. If the patient is floridly bacteremic, the blood culture may detect the circulating bacteria. However, several problems limit the usefulness of blood cultures. The incidence of negative blood cultures testifies to the fact that they are helpful in only a fraction of symptomatic patients; many patients with arterial infections never have positive blood cultures. In the review by Brown and associates,[19] only 60% of patients had positive preoperative blood cultures. In addition, blood cultures might not detect the infectious organism until several days or weeks have elapsed, limiting the test's effect on clinical management.

The presence of bacteria in the blood may be an important early clue to an arterial infection, but the information from such tests must be evaluated in the proper clinical context. Most bacteremic patients have an evident source of bacteremia that should be identified and treated. Patients with positive blood cultures and no clinical evidence of a concurrent infection should be examined for possible arterial lesions. The significance of a positive blood culture in an otherwise asymptomatic patient is difficult to determine without considering the patient's underlying problems and risk factors. It should also be noted that patients who are relatively asymptomatic (no systemic manifestations of sepsis) tend to have fewer positive blood cultures. As a result, in a study of patients undergoing clean arterial procedures, only 2% of blood cultures were positive, whereas 12% of arteries and 14% of periarterial adipose tissues harbored bacteria.[28] Obvious clues, such as a recently noted aneurysm or a history of drug abuse, may promote further investigation.

The type of organism identified in blood cultures may suggest a source of the infection. If a blood culture reveals *Salmonella* species in a patient with an aneurysm, an arterial infection should be seriously considered. Although *Staphylococcus* organisms are a common pathogen in arterial infections, their ubiquitous presence on skin often confuses the diagnosis and calls into question the results of the blood culture.

The importance of the preoperative blood culture is difficult to understate. It represents the earliest reliable clue to the presence of an arterial infection. Even in the event of a delayed result, such as when several days are required before the blood culture can identify the bacteria, the information provided may be invaluable in managing the patient.

Arterial Cultures

Arterial wall cultures may also help secure the diagnosis of an arterial infection. In any circumstance in which the diagnosis of an infectious aneurysm is entertained, arterial cultures should be attempted. The principal drawback to arterial wall cultures is the time required before any information about the infection is available. Patient management must therefore depend on other factors, such as the clinical setting, the index of suspicion, the presence of prior blood culture data, and the results of angiographic studies.

Because clinical decisions cannot always be based on arterial culture results, other techniques such as intraoperative Gram staining and frozen section of the arterial tissue are often considered. Unfortunately, these methods might not provide significant improvement in the

detection of bacteria. In the study by Brown and associates,[19] although 60% of patients had positive preoperative blood cultures, only 20% of intraoperative Gram stains were positive. Arterial wall frozen sections have not seen widespread use, but they may prove helpful. Histologic findings of inflammation and bacterial invasion are strong evidence supporting the diagnosis of arterial infection.

When obtaining blood or arterial wall cultures, it should be noted that the type of organism can affect the yield of the tests. Brown and associates[19] noted that 60% of arterial wall cultures were negative. Approximately 25% of their cultures failed to detect any organism at all. Presumably, these were difficult organisms to collect and culture. *S. epidermidis* may be difficult to culture without sonicating the specimen. *Treponema pallidum* may require darkfield examination for identification. *Mycobacterium tuberculosis* is a fastidious organism that is difficult to grow. These considerations should prompt the special attention of the pathology laboratory and the collection of adequate specimens.

Molecular Diagnosis of Arterial Infection

Molecular biology technique allows the evaluation of biological specimens for the detection of bacterial nucleic acids. This has been applied to the detection of bacteria within arterial samples. The application of techniques such as polymerase chain reaction (PCR) may allow the detection and amplification of genetic material from the bacteria within the arterial wall. These techniques diagnose the presence of microbiological organisms, identify the organism, and may identify the presence of resistant strains allowing for direction of antimicrobial therapy.

Da Silva and colleagues reported use of PCR for detection of bacterial ribosomal nucleic acid (RNA) in specimens of normal aortic tissue removed at the time of surgical repair.[29] Using universal eubacteria primers to amply 16SrRMA, they were able to identify the RNA from a wide variety of bacteria in the arterial specimen, thus demonstrating the potential of the technique. Their report is striking in its ability to detect bacteria that are ordinarily difficult to culture. Dickinson and colleagues[30] reported the application of this technique in the case of a 72-year-old man with a suspected mycotic femoral artery aneurysm and blood cultures that showed *S. pneumoniae*. Arterial wall samples subjected to routine culture technique yielded no microorganisms. The same samples analyzed with pneumococcal primers for PCR were able to identify the presence of *S. pneumoniae*.

Dickinson used PCR to confirm the presence of a suspected pathogen, whereas da Silva used PCR to identify a wide spectrum of bacteria which were present in arterial tissue. Although widely available, these molecular techniques are not commonly used; they are costly, and interpretation of the test results might not be intuitive because they can detect both pathogenic and symbiotic bacteria. Still, these techniques could prove beneficial in the diagnosis of organisms that are notoriously difficult to culture, such as slow-growing organisms (e.g., mycobacteria) or those that produce biofilms (e.g., *S. epidermidis*). These techniques would likely allow improved diagnosis of bacteria present in the approximately 20%

to 60% of suspected mycotic aneurysms that fail to yield bacterial growth on culture examination.

Nuclear Imaging: Tagged White Blood Cell Scans

Nuclear imaging has become an important tool in the identification of arterial graft infections, but it has not played as important a role in identifying primary arterial infections. The technique is based on the ability of various radioisotope markers to be linked to white blood cells, which then become involved in an inflammatory process. The advantages of these tests are their relatively low risk to the patient and the facility of their application. The principal drawback is that the tests may detect many inflammatory lesions, not just those that are the result of an arterial infection. The interpretation of the results of a nuclear scan must account for many clinical issues. Although the usefulness of these tests has been debated, in the absence of recent trauma or infection, the use of radiolabeled indium or gallium as markers may allow localization of an arterial infection.

Computed Tomography and Magnetic Resonance Imaging

The success of techniques such as computed tomography (CT) and MRI in identifying primary arterial infections depends largely on their ability to resolve the characteristic anatomic features of the lesions. Because of the detailed anatomic data these scans present, they have become popular in the evaluation of intraabdominal vascular lesions. There are some significant limitations, however, in regard to their ability to secure the diagnosis of an arterial infection.

The essential diagnostic characteristics of arterial infections include the presence of a focal defect in the wall of the aorta, the saccular shape of the aneurysm, and the tissue edema that accompanies the inflammatory reaction. Routine two-dimensional reconstruction of CT images does not readily allow recognition of the diagnostic features of mycotic aneurysms. A three-dimensional reconstruction does allow their recognition, but such reconstruction is not routinely performed and must be specifically requested.

MRI represents an improvement over CT scanning because current computer analysis allows a more flexible assemblage of the data and facilitates the recognition of essential diagnostic characteristics. MRI may not require intravascular contrast agents, which are frequently needed with CT. Finally, MRI is able to detect tissue differences with regard to certain molecular constituents. Another advantage of MRI is its ability to detect the accumulation of water in tissues; this tissue edema is frequently the hallmark of an inflammatory process and may identify an arterial infection.

Angiography

Angiography is the most widely used technique for the investigation and definition of arterial infections (Figure 10-4). Historically, it was the first method by which the characteristics of primary arterial infections were

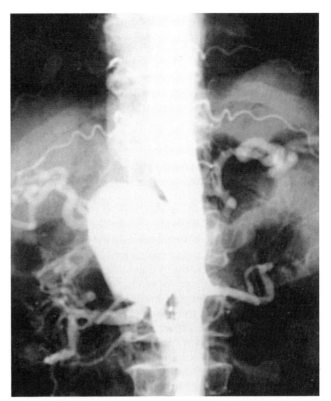

FIGURE 10-4 ■ Angiogram of mycotic aortic aneurysm.

identified. Angiography served to define the characteristics of these lesions. Angiography is clearly superior in areas such as the intestinal mesentery and the visceral vessels, where the size of the arterial lesion may be less than the resolution of computed techniques. In the case of aortic mycotic aneurysms, the angiogram usually provides excellent definition of the defect in the aortic wall, the saccular pseudoaneurysm, and the contiguous arterial anatomy. Finally, the arteriogram offers the best definition of the relationship between the visceral vessels and the arterial defect—an essential step in planning patient management.

The role of arteriography in the management of a peripheral arterial infection has been questioned. Because some peripheral arterial infections can be managed with ligation and debridement without reconstruction, an angiogram might not be necessary. However, there is a benefit to assessing the native circulation before attempting arterial ligation. Should the limb require urgent revascularization after arterial ligation, an angiogram obtained before the ligation would be helpful in planning the revascularization. For this reason, an arteriogram of the involved vessels is strongly advised in all but emergent cases.

Hybrid Positron Emission Tomography and Computed Tomographic Scan

Positron emission tomography (PET) is a technique in which positron emissions from a biomarker are detected and displayed in an image. The PET scan relies on the ability of fludeoxyglucose, a glucose analog which has a positron-emitting radioactive isotope, to be taken up by high–glucose-using cells. In the setting of infections, these cells are macrophages, leucocytes, granulocytes, and inflammatory cells. The positron emission may then be detected by the PET scanner.

New "fusion technology" allows the images acquired from both a CT scanner and a PET scanner to be taken sequentially in the same session and combined into a single superposed or co-registered image. This allows combining the metabolic information of the PET scan with the spatial information of the CT scan. The technique may provide greater sensitivity and specificity in the detection and localization of an infection. Fukuchi and colleagues[31] described their initial experience with this technique when applied to suspected vascular graft infections in 2005.[31] They observed that this technique may be of particular benefit in patients who might have an infection; however, the presentation is not clinically evident or severe. Their experience indicated that the PET/CT had a high sensitivity and that in several instances this resulted in false-positive scans. In addition, the PET techniques suffer the general limitation of requiring the production of radiopharmaceuticals for the scan—a process that is highly specialized, requires significant infrastructure, and is expensive. This technique is still far from general clinical application.

Timing of Diagnosis

The diagnosis of a primary arterial infection may be made preoperatively, intraoperatively, or postoperatively. Should the diagnosis be suspected before surgery, preoperative antibiotics may be commenced, and the patient can be better informed about potential problems. Plans can also be drawn for contingencies that might require alternative reconstructions. The diagnosis may be established or confirmed by the findings at surgery. The presence of gross purulence, engorged lymph nodes, and inflamed tissues helps to establish the diagnosis conclusively. Adjunctive tests such as the Gram stain and bacterial cultures may be performed. The intraoperative findings help to determine the mode of arterial reconstruction. Gross infection, abscess, and pus should be taken as indications for debridement and remote reconstruction, whereas minimal evidence of infection may suggest reasonably good results from in situ reconstruction. If the diagnosis is confirmed in the postoperative period by positive bacterial cultures, a prolonged course of antibiotics and graft surveillance is advisable.

Natural History

Given the pathogenesis of a primary arterial infection—bacterial invasion, colonization, and destruction of an artery—the sequence of events after this initial insult is predictable and inexorable. Destruction of the arterial wall leads to either the development of an arterial pseudoaneurysm and life-threatening hemorrhage. Which of these two events occurs is probably related to the rate of progression of the infection, its location, and the subsequent development of an inflammatory response. If the destruction of the arterial wall is gradual and

accompanied by a vigorous inflammatory response, the arterial infection may produce a pseudoaneurysm. If the process of arterial infection leads to a rapid loss of arterial integrity, the arterial infection can result in hemorrhage.

Complications of arterial infections include those common to all aneurysms: embolization, thrombosis, and rupture. The high rupture rate is reflected in both the virulent course (rapid expansion and progression to rupture) and the high mortality of these lesions. For these reasons, mycotic aneurysms are urgent cases that should be repaired as soon as possible. One final complication, which is significantly increased in cases of primary arterial infection, is the rate of infection of the vascular reconstruction. Although the anticipated incidence of graft infection in "clean" cases is less than 1% or 2%, the incidence of graft infection after remote (extraanatomic) reconstruction in cases of primary arterial infection may be as high as 15%. In older series, when in situ reconstruction was performed in the face of a purulent infection and without concurrent antibiotics, the reinfection rate approached 100%.

Principles of Management

Two elemental principles form the basis of therapy in primary arterial infections: control of sepsis and arterial reconstruction.

Control of Sepsis

Antibiotic therapy and surgical débridement represent the primary treatment modalities for the control of sepsis in arterial infections. All infected arterial tissue must be debrided. It is important that the arterial resection encompass all inflamed tissues and continue to the point where the arterial tissue is normal and healthy. This helps to prevent recurrence of the infection and disruption of the arterial suture line.

Soft tissues adjacent to the infected artery that appear to be involved are also debrided. Major structures such as the vena cava and ureters are left intact. Retroperitoneal tissues that appear to be involved are resected as well. Once all infected tissues have been removed, the wound is thoroughly irrigated with an antibiotic solution—ideally, one that contains antibiotic directed toward the suspected pathogens (as detected by preoperative blood cultures). Surgical drains are useful when there is clear evidence of purulence or abscess. When collateral circulation allows, the excision may be accompanied by proximal and distal ligation and no effort to reconstruct the artery.

The use of antibiotics is mandatory in these situations. Broad-spectrum antibiotics must be initiated as soon as a strong clinical suspicion of arterial infection has been established. Blood cultures should be obtained before the initiation of antibiotics. When positive, these cultures are then used to select an antibiotic regimen with the highest therapeutic value and the fewest side effects. Negative cultures should not preclude the institution of broad-spectrum antibiotics when arterial infection is suspected. The use of high-dose preoperative antibiotics is directed toward sterilizing the aneurysm and adjacent tissues in order to minimize bacteremia and local contamination during surgical manipulation of infected tissues. Antibiotics must be continued until the source of the bacteremia has been corrected either surgically or medically. Similarly, the primary source of bacteremia or local bacterial invasion must be controlled as a mainstay of therapy in all types of primary arterial infections. In patients with SBE-related mycotic aneurysms, specific consideration must be given to sterilization of cardiac valvular vegetations. When possible, a period of preoperative antibiotic administration is associated with improved outcome.

The duration of antibiotic treatment is somewhat controversial, and several competing regimens have been proposed. Several authors suggest that IV antibiotics be initiated before surgery and extended for no less than 6 weeks postoperatively.[32-34] In addition, these authors recommend that patients with prosthetic reconstructions, especially in situ prosthetic reconstructions, be prescribed lifelong oral regimens of suppressive antibiotics. Typically, oral trimethoprim-sulfamethoxazole (Bactrim), a sulfa drug, or a first-generation cephalosporin or penicillin is the agent of choice.

Important technical points include the use of monofilament suture material in ligation and oversewing of the arteries. This recommendation is based on the superiority of monofilaments over braided suture in resisting recurrent infection. Whenever possible, the resected arterial stump should be covered with a pedicle of healthy, viable tissue to further reduce the possibility of a recurrent infection and to accelerate healing of the arterial segment. In the abdomen, this tissue pedicle is frequently the omentum. A flap of fascia from the prevertebral fascia and ligaments can be used to reinforce the aortic suture line. In the periphery, muscle transposition is the preferred means of obtaining tissue coverage. In the femoral region, this is most readily accomplished by rotating the head of the sartorius.

Nonoperative Therapy

Nonoperative therapy for arterial infections has been proposed by Kaufman and coworkers[35] for high-risk or debilitated patients. This treatment modality, although effective anecdotally, remains controversial, and further investigation is necessary. Hsu and colleagues[36] reported a series of 22 cases of infected aortic aneurysms treated with antibiotics only and without surgery.[6] The in-hospital mortality was 50%. The event-free survival at 1 year was 32%. The authors noted that these results compared poorly to standard surgical approaches.

Arterial Reconstruction

Restoration of arterial continuity is necessary both to control hemorrhage and to provide for perfusion of the distal arterial beds. This can be accomplished with open surgical approaches or by endovascular approaches. Currently, open surgical technique with extraanatomic reconstruction is considered the most conservative approach; however, new reports suggest that this may be changing as familiarity with endovascular technique progresses.

The open surgical management of mycotic aneurysms includes debridement of infected tissues (including the infected artery), along with extraanatomic reconstruction or in situ arterial reconstruction. Reconstruction of the infected arterial tree presents the problem of material interaction with the infectious organisms. Several materials are available for reconstruction: synthetic graft (Dacron), autologous veins, and human cryopreserved arterial allografts.

The material used for reconstruction of the arterial tree in the face of infection represents a significant choice that could influence the outcome of surgery. This is particularly true when the consideration is in situ reconstruction of an infected artery. Reconstruction alternatives include prosthetic grafts, autogenous veins, and cadaveric allografts. Prosthetic grafts are readily available and inexpensive, but present an increased risk of reinfection. Biological grafts are thought to have a better ability to resist infection than do prosthetic grafts. Autologous femoral vein grafts require a time-consuming dissection for graft procurement and may be accompanied by complications related to this dissection. Arterial allograft reconstructions are expensive, are not commonly available, and may be subject to aneurysmal degeneration.

Antibiotic-Impregnated Grafts. Experimental and clinical evidence suggests that in situ reconstruction with antibiotic-impregnated prosthetic grafts is feasible. Bandyk and colleagues[37] reported 27 patients operated on with rifampin-impregnated grafts as treatment for a variety of arterial infections. At least four recurrent infections were reported, including two that resulted in death. They concluded that in situ replacement using a rifampin-bonded prosthetic graft was most effective for low-grade staphylococcal arterial infection. An added caveat was that in the presence of virulent and antibiotic-resistant bacterial strains, this therapy usually failed. A more recent experience of 27 patients with both graft infections and mycotic aneurysms managed with silver-coated polyester grafts was published by Batt and associates.[38] There were 7 perioperative deaths and 20 long-term survivors. Of the long-term (actuarial period, 24 months) survivors, one developed a recurrent infection. Rifampin may be more readily available rather than the silver-coated polyester grafts. Rifampin has been shown to have a significant effect in reducing in situ graft reinfection in experimental settings.[39] This approach has been reported from a number of authors who note a low rate of recurrent infections (0% to 8%) involving the reconstruction graft when placed in situ.[40-43]

Vein Grafts. Aortoiliac reconstruction with autogenous veins has been performed with both saphenous and femoral veins. An initial experience using femoral veins for aortic and iliac reconstruction was reported by Schulman and associates.[44] The use of superficial femoral and popliteal veins has been advocated by Clagett and associates[45] for a number of infectious indications, including primary aortoiliac arterial infections has been termed the *NAIS procedure*. In their series of 38 patients with aortofemoral infections who underwent successful reconstruction with autogenous superficial femoral vein, the long-term primary patency was 85% at 5 years.[45]

Human Allografts. In situ reconstruction with human allografts for infected aneurysms in the aortoiliac region has been reported with good results: low mortality and good durability. Reinfection rates after prolonged administration of culture-directed antibiotics are generally low. The most common problem associated with allograft reconstruction is the eventual degradation of the allograft, which is subject to aneurysmal degeneration.

Kieffer and associates[46] reported their experience with 43 patients with infected infrarenal aortic prosthetic grafts who underwent in situ replacement using preserved allografts obtained from cadavers. In the early postoperative period, there were five septic complications, including two pseudoaneurysm ruptures; two cases of septic shock; and one instance of peritonitis from colon perforation. In follow-up, one late death may have been related to persistent infection. A report focusing on mycotic aortic aneurysms was published by Leseche and associates.[47] They reported a series of 28 patients operated on for a variety of vascular infections, including five mycotic aneurysms. There were five perioperative deaths, two from sepsis and two from multisystem organ failure. The long-term outcomes were good. There were no recurrent infections and only three instances of aneurysmal degeneration of the allograft. More recent reports of cryopreserved human allograft indicate that the incidence of late aneurysmal degeneration may be further reduced by changes in cryopreservation processing.[48-50]

Extraanatomic Reconstruction

Extraanatomic reconstruction of the arterial tree has become a standard approach to management of graft infection and has been widely advocated for arterial infection in general.[51] In a review of spontaneous abdominal aortic infections, Ewart and associates[52] demonstrated a 23% to 63% reoperation rate for graft infection after immediate in situ reconstruction and a 7% recurrent infection rate when patients were initially treated with arterial debridement and remote reconstruction.[52]

In a review of 51 cases of mycotic aneurysms, Brown and associates[19] noted that the mortality of local graft reconstruction was 32%, whereas extraanatomic reconstruction was associated with a 13% mortality rate.[19] Still, the authors advocated in situ reconstruction in selected cases; they proposed that if no gross purulence was encountered intraoperatively, and if the result was gram-negative, in situ reconstruction using prosthetic material (Dacron) could be performed safely. This approach is predicated on the recommendation that postoperative antibiotics be continued for a minimum of 6 to 8 weeks. Brown and associates[19] demonstrated 63% survival and 19% reinfection rates for aneurysms treated with this approach. In comparison, the rate of infection of extraanatomic bypasses following repair of mycotic aortic aneurysms was as high as 13%.

In Situ Reconstruction. The benefits of the in situ reconstruction are reduced length of surgery, improve graft patency, and simpler technical management of the case. The risk associated with this reconstruction is that the new arterial prosthesis may become infected.

In Situ Reconstruction with Graft. Experience with in situ reconstruction for primary aortoduodenal fistulas has encouraged some authors to proceed with in situ graft reconstruction of the aorta when there is minimal contamination, no pus, and little extent of the infectious process.[18] Approximately 70% of aneurysms associated with primary aortoduodenal fistulas are not due to arterial infection; the majority of the remaining aneurysms are thought to be infectious in origin.[30] In the case of a primary mycotic aortoduodenal fistula, extensive debridement and extraanatomic bypass graft are recommended for significant infection and obvious involvement of the arterial bed. In situ graft replacement has been performed successfully in cases in which the level of contamination was mild. When the aneurysm is not of infectious origin, in situ reconstruction has been advised by a number of authors.[53,54]

A recent report by Lee and colleagues compares in-situ versus extra-anatomic reconstructions for infected infrarenal aortic aneurysms.[55] Their series consisted of 28 patients: 15 who underwent extraanatomic bypass and 13 who underwent in situ reconstruction. Early graft infection was noted in one extraanatomic reconstruction and none of the in situ reconstructions. The authors noted that survival was similar in patients who underwent in situ and extraanatomic reconstruction. Late complications were significantly more common in the extraanatomic reconstruction patients. All told, five of the extraanatomic graft patients suffered graft thrombosis, and two of these had graft infections. None of the in situ grafts suffered late infection or other complication. These results are surprising in that in situ reconstructions would be anticipated to have more frequent graft infections. The retrospective nature of the report as well as the limited sample size may partially account for the unexpected findings.

In Situ Reconstruction with Biological Grafts. Currently, no large series allograft reconstruction done for mycotic aortic aneurysms exists. All reports are series that combine both primary (mycotic aneurysms) and secondary (aortic graft infection, aortic stent infection, aortic stent graft) infections.

Brown and associates[49] report the use of arterial allograft in the form of cryopreserved arteries (CPA) is compared to extraanatomic reconstruction using Dacron grafts or autogenous tissues.[49] This series compared 18 aortic homograft reconstructions and 18 axillofemoral reconstructions done for a variety of aortic infections (both primary 7, and secondary 29 infections). They noted that the in situ cryopreserved aortic homograft group suffered fewer complications (amputation, amputations, death), and no recurrent infections. Although follow-up was limited to a mean of 25 months, no late aneurysmal degeneration was noted in the aortic allograft group. They observed that anastomosis of a cryopreserved allograft to a remnant prosthetic graft in a leg may present a risk of re-infection and graft disruption. They concluded that cryopreserved human aortic allografts represent a viable alternative to reconstruction of the aorta in the presence of an infection. They also caution that this is an early experience and that larger numbers of patients and longer follow-up are required.

Bisdas and associates[50] reported a series of 57 aortic cryograft reconstructions. They report a 30-day mortality of 9%. The actuarial survival at 3 years was 81% and at 5 years was 64%. With a median follow-up of 36 months, they noted one graft occlusion, one graft aneurysmal degeneration, one fistula between a limb of the homograft and duodenum, one postoperative hemorrhage. The authors note that none of the original infections recurred. They noted that the results from their study suggest aortic cryografts are safe and effective. Cryografts suffer the drawbacks of being costly and at risk of degeneration, and the availability of these grafts is limited.

McCready and associates[56] present a series of 51 aortic reconstructions using cryopreserved arterial homografts. Of these, 15 were primary aortic infections, 28 were aortic graft infections and 8 were peripheral infections. They report a mean follow-up of 46 months. No aneurysmal degeneration was noted during this period. They did observe 10 graft failures, of which 7 occurred in patients with aortoenteric or bronchial fistulas. They note that the long-term complications of a CPA are uncommon. Finally, they caution that patients with aortoenteric or bronchial fistulas have a high mortality rate.

In Situ Reconstruction: Endovascular Repair. The ongoing development of endovascular technique and familiarity with endovascular repair has led to the gradual adoption of endovascular technique to the management of mycotic aneurysms. Endovascular repair (EVAR) offers the advantages of rapid control of hemorrhage, with reduced surgical morbidity and reduced mortality. When coupled with use of antibiotics, endovascular repair offers an effective means of treating mycotic aneurysms with perioperative and intermediate survival, which is comparable to open repair. A significant concern is that it places a graft in direct proximity to the infection and does not afford the opportunity to debride the infected tissue. This appears to be particularly significant when there may be a source of ongoing contamination such as an aerodigestive aortic fistula, osteomyelitis of the spine, or a psoas abscess. Management of the ongoing infection is critical.

The reports of endovascular treatment indicate that, in combination with prolonged antibiotic administration and the use of drainage, some patients may achieve resolution of the arterial infection, with no infection of the endoprosthesis.[57,58] In 2002, Berchtold and colleagues[57] reported a case of *Salmonella*-associated mycotic infrarenal aortic aneurysm managed with an endovascular graft and prolonged antibiotics. After a 4-year follow-up period, repeated CT scans demonstrated resolution of the aneurysm and no sign of residual infection. More recently, Koeppel and associates[58] reported successful endovascular repair of a mycotic aneurysm of the infrarenal aorta associated with a retroperitoneal abscess. The aneurysm was treated with an endoprosthesis, and the abscess was drained percutaneously. Antibiotics were continued for 6 months. A CT scan done 1 year after implantation revealed no sign of retroperitoneal inflammation. These investigators noted that endovascular repair was particularly attractive in critically ill patients who might not be able to tolerate an open surgical repair.

These observations are highlighted by Kan and colleagues in two reviews.[59,60] In 2007, they reviewed the use of EVAR in thoracic and abdominal infected aneurysms. They reported 48 cases that accrued an 89% 30-day survival and an 82% 2-year survival.[59] They noted that fever, age over 65 years, and rupture of the aneurysm were predictors of persistent infection. They concluded that EVAR should be considered a temporary measure in patients who present with fever and rupture. They also noted that the preoperative use of antibiotics for 1 week was a protective measure that appeared to reduce persistence of infection.

In 2010, Kan and associates[60] reviewed the efficacy of EVAR in infected abdominal aortic aneurysms. They reported a series of 41 cases who underwent either EVAR or conventional surgery. They noted that early postoperative mortality was similar in both groups. Late mortality, however, was greater in the conventional surgery group (10% versus 25%). An actuarial analysis indicated that the aneurysm-related event-free survival was the same in both the open and EVAR-treated groups. Factors that predisposed toward poor outcomes included age, *Salmonella* infection, aortoenteric fistula, and shock.

In a similar note, Forbes and Harding[61] noted that *Salmonella*-infected aneurysms may be at risk for late recurrence of the infection. They detailed two cases of *Salmonella* aortic infections that were managed with endovascular aneurysm repair. Recurrence sepsis was noted at 5 months and at 3 years following EVAR.[61] The authors conclude that EVAR should be used with caution in patients with *Salmonella* infections. They suggest that the EVAR in these circumstances may be used as an intermediary to top hemorrhage and allow later definitive reconstruction in a more stable patient.

Lew and associates[62] identified the presence of an aerodigestive fistula in association with a mycotic aneurysm as a significant risk factor for ongoing sepsis and death.[62] They presented a series of nine patients with mycotic aneurysms treated with endovascular stent grafts. Of these, seven were associated with aerodigestive fistulas. They noted a mortality of 67% within the period of hospitalization. Furthermore, they noted that reoperation for infection of the endograft was required in one of the three long-term survivors. They conclude that EVAR serves to temporize patients with aerodigestive fistulas, but given the ongoing source of infection, other more lasting reconstruction should be attempted.

In the absence of aerodigestive fistula or virulent organisms, endovascular repair may be definitive. Vallejo and associates[63] recently presented a series of 19 patients with primary mycotic aneurysms of the thoracic and abdominal aorta. The focus of their report is to detail changes on management of these aneurysms resulting from the endovascular approach. All mycotic aneurysms were managed with TEVAR, EVAR, and hybrid reconstruction (for aneurysms involving the visceral aorta). They reported three perioperative deaths (17%) from sepsis, cardiac arrest, and bowel ischemia. The median follow up was 30 months. Three late deaths were noted to result from myeloma, bowel ischemia, and gastrointestinal hemorrhage. They concluded that endovascular repair is effective, but reconstruction of the visceral aortic segment still requires an open surgical hybrid approach.[63]

Management of Mycotic Aneurysms According to Location

Thoracic Aneurysms

While not common, thoracic aortic infections may appear with hemoptysis because of a fistula between the mycotic aneurysm and the bronchial tree. In these instances, uncontrolled hemorrhage can lead to asphyxia or secondary pneumonia. Management consists of controlling the hemorrhage and repair of the aneurysm. EVAR offers the most rapid means of controlling the hemorrhage in most instances. Because of the ongoing contamination from the fistula, infection of the aortic endograft is likely. A secondary procedure must be planned to close the fistula, resect the endoprosthesis, and reconstruct the aorta. Given the frequent comorbidities of these patients, these secondary operations are accompanied by considerable morbidity and may present a considerable risk for the patients.[40,55,62,63]

Suprarenal Aneurysms

Because of their unique anatomic characteristics, arterial infections of the paravisceral and suprarenal aorta almost always require immediate in situ arterial reconstruction. It is nearly impossible to bypass the visceral vessels without traversing the bed of the infected paravisceral aorta. Experience gained from the repair of suprarenal mycotic aneurysms has given credence to the concept of in situ repair with adjunctive lifelong antibiotic therapy.

When combined with debridement of grossly infected tissue and appropriate use of antibiotics, most series reporting this type of reconstruction have demonstrated acceptable morbidity and mortality rates. Chan and associates[32] reported a series of 22 patients with mycotic aneurysms of the thoracic and abdominal aorta. Of these, 13 had involvement of the paravisceral aorta, all of which required in situ reconstruction. Twelve of the 13 patients survived surgery and were given lifelong suppressive antibiotics. None had clinical recurrence of the infection. In the overall series, three patients died; two of the deaths were attributed to multisystem organ failure and one to aspiration pneumonia. The authors concluded that in situ reconstruction, along with surgical debridement and lifelong antibiotics, offers the best chance of survival in these patients who are difficult to treat patients. It should be noted that although this form of therapy (in situ reconstruction) is inescapable in the reconstruction of infected paravisceral aneurysms, its application to arterial infections at other sites (e.g., infrarenal aorta or femoral artery) is less well established and should be approached with caution.

Infected Femoral Pseudoaneurysms

Infections of the vessels of the femoral region are the most common type of arterial infection. In the review by Brown and colleagues,[19] these lesions accounted for 38% of all arterial infections. The most common manifestation is an inflamed, tender, pulsatile inguinal mass. The more common complications include erosion through the skin with hemorrhage, embolization, compression of adjacent structures (femoral vein and nerve), and thrombosis. Of these, erosion and hemorrhage are the most feared complications.

The debate regarding reconstruction is of particular interest in the subset of patients with infected pseudoaneurysms of the femoral bifurcation that are the result of IV drug abuse. Because of the tendency to reuse femoral sites for drug administration, the arterial reconstruction may be in jeopardy of recurrent infection. If the reconstruction required prosthetic material, the resultant reinfection would be all the more complicated and dangerous. Finally, the incidence of graft infection after immediate reconstruction is sufficient by itself to warrant hesitation in such reconstructions. Because of these concerns, some authors have advocated simple arterial ligation and resection of the infected tissues. The problem is that simple ligation of the femoral arteries at the level of the arterial bifurcation can result in a subsequent amputation rate approaching 33%.[26,64]

An alternative approach is to proceed with biological graft reconstruction. The reconstruction should be performed with autogenous tissue if possible. In the course of these reconstructions, the infected arteries and adjacent tissues should be debrided and the reconstruction should be coursed through uninfected tissues.[65]

A third option is to resect, debride, and observe. The artery is ligated, but no reconstructions are performed in the initial setting. The limb is observed for signs of severe ischemia. If the limb appears viable with collateral perfusion alone, no effort is made to reconstruct. If the limb appears severely ischemic, revascularization is attempted. Femoral artery reconstruction should be performed either with in situ saphenous vein interposition grafting or through an extraanatomic approach, such as a transobturator bypass.

Infection and pseudoaneurysm of the common femoral (above the bifurcation), superficial femoral, and deep femoral arteries do not appear to suffer a similar fate. These vessels stand a far better chance of tolerating simple ligation without requiring reconstruction. Wright and Shepard[66] reported a low incidence of amputation following ligation and resection in this circumstance. In a series of 39 patients with such infections, they noted an amputation rate of 5%; these amputations occurred in two patients who had impaired collateral circulation from prior (contralateral) common femoral artery ligation. In the absence of these two cases, the amputation rate in this group of patients was 0%.

Mesenteric Artery Infections

Mesenteric artery infections tend to appear as pseudoaneurysms within the mesentery of the intestine. These lesions may be asymptomatic, but the more common presentation is abdominal pain. These lesions may develop as a consequence of IV drug abuse. Pathophysiologically, they are considered to be the result of mycotic embolization. Because of this, it is necessary to consider the source of the emboli as well as the possibility of other embolic targets. In practical terms, this means that these patients should be screened for both cardiac vegetations and other arterial lesions. Preoperative angiography is recommended if possible. Postoperative angiography should be considered if a preoperative study was not obtained.

Mesenteric artery infections tend to develop rapid expansion and intramesenteric hemorrhage. Alternatively, these aneurysms may result in thrombosis and infarction of the intestine. Management of these vessels is related to the location of the lesion, the available collateral circulation, and the presence and extent of intestinal infarction. Lesions of the proximal mesenteric arteries frequently require reconstruction with autogenous tissues. More distally located pseudoaneurysms can often be managed by simple excision. If a small area of intestinal ischemia develops, a limited bowel resection may also be necessary. In instances of extensive intestinal ischemia, a second-look celiotomy may be advisable after restoration of intestinal perfusion.

Arterial Infections of the Upper Extremity

Infections of the arteries of the upper extremities are fairly rare. Collectively, they represented approximately 10% of arterial infections in the review by Brown and colleagues.[19] Frequently, these lesions are associated with trauma. Like other infections of peripheral vessels, these lesions develop in a number of ways, with the most common presentation being an inflamed, tender, pulsatile mass. In the upper extremities, careful inspection should detect evidence of digital embolization, splinter hemorrhages, and ischemic lesions.

Because of the extensive collateral blood supply to the upper extremities, arterial infections there can often be treated with simple ligation and excision. This is particularly true when the involved segment is between the thyrocervical trunk and the subscapular artery or distal to the deep brachial artery. Reconstruction, when required, should be accomplished with a saphenous vein graft or similar autogenous tissues. As with all mycotic aneurysms, preoperative and postoperative antibiotics should be given for a prolonged period.

Conclusions

Primary arterial infections are relatively rare, but they are frequently lethal. They often follow a rapidly progressive course toward expansion and rupture. Astute diagnosis and correct management can improve a patient's chance of survival. The diagnosis is established by a high index of suspicion, along with identification of risk factors and appropriate testing. Once an arterial infection is identified, management must be tailored to the organism involved and the site and severity of the infection, as well as the condition of the patient. Surgical excision is almost always necessary in the course of management. Long-term (6 weeks) IV antibiotics are almost always required, and the use of lifelong oral antibiotic suppression is strongly recommended for these patients. Optimal care

can reduce the mortality of these lesions from nearly 100% to less than 10% to 15%.

PROPHYLACTIC ANTIBIOTIC THERAPY

Although infections of implanted vascular prostheses are relatively uncommon, when they do occur, they are associated with significant morbidity and mortality. Complications of graft infection include pseudoaneurysm, anastomotic disruption, hemorrhage, fistula formation, and sepsis. Infection of a vascular graft almost always requires partial or complete graft removal, which is associated with a high incidence of amputation. Vascular graft infection leads to the patient's death in one fourth to half of cases in contemporary series. These dire consequences have prompted laboratory and clinical investigation into the role of antibiotics in the prevention of vascular graft infection. The widespread use of prophylactic antibiotics in vascular surgery has significantly altered the microbiology and clinical presentation of graft infections. New insights have been gained into the pathogenesis of this process, and alternative methods of antibiotic delivery have been developed in animal models. This section presents the bacteriology and current understanding of the pathogenesis of graft infection, a historical overview of the development of antibiotic prophylaxis in vascular surgery, current recommendations for prophylaxis, and new directions in antibiotic delivery.

Clinical Significance of Graft Infection

The reported incidence of infection after the placement of vascular prostheses ranges from 1% to 6%. This relatively low rate of infection has remained stable over time, despite improvements in technique and the introduction of routine preoperative antibiotic prophylaxis. Two early series, from Hoffert and colleagues[67] in 1965 and Fry and Lindenauer[68] in 1967, reported graft infection rates of 6.0% (12 of 201) and 1.34% (12 of 890), respectively. In 1972, Szilagyi and colleagues[69] reported a large series of 3397 cases in which the graft infection rate was 1.9%. Later reports detailed similar findings. The series of Lorentzen and coauthors from[70] 1985 described graft infections in 62 of 2411 patients, a rate of 2.6%. Although the overall incidence of infection has not changed significantly, the use of antibiotic prophylaxis has clearly changed the clinical presentation of most vascular graft infections. Suppurative infections appearing in the first few weeks after graft implantation have given way to more insidious, low-grade, chronic infections.[71,72]

Infection in prosthetic grafts remains a critical issue in vascular surgery. Reported mortality rates from graft infection range from 25% to 75% (Table 10-1).[67,68,71,73-75] Mortality is greatest for proximal grafts, with almost uniform lethality reported in aortic stump sepsis.[68,69,73,76] Despite attempts to reduce mortality in aortic graft infection, it remains relatively high at 24% to 43%.[78-82] Peripheral graft infections are generally associated with lower mortality rates (as low as 6%).[82] Amputation rates are similar for survivors of aortic and peripheral graft infections, ranging from 22.5% to 43%.[69,74,84] In more

TABLE 10-1　Influence of Graft Site on Incidence and Outcome of Graft Infection

Author	Year	Type of Graft	Patients	Rate (%)*	Rate (%)†	Rate (%)
Hoffert and colleagues[67]	1965	Aortoiliac	84	0	NA	NA
		Aortofemoral	30	0	NA	NA
		Iliofemoropopliteal	83	13.0	75	25
Szilagyi and colleagues[69]	1972	Aortoiliac	418	0.7	0	66
		Aortofemoral	1244	1.6	21	53
		Iliofemoropopliteal	270	3.0	40	7
Bouhoutsos and colleagues[93]	1974	Aortoiliac/aortofemoral	412	1.5	0	50
		Iliofemoropopliteal	108	7.4	25	0
Liekweg and Greenfield[74]	1977	Aortoiliac	NR	NR	3	8
		Aortofemoral	NR	NR	11	47
		Iliofemoropopliteal	NR	NR	30	13
Yashar and colleagues[76]	1978	Aortoiliac	300	1.0	0	33
		Aortofemoral	210	2.9	33	50
		Iliofemoropopliteal	65	4.6	67	0
Casali and colleagues[144]	1980	Aortoiliac	NR	NR	0	50
		Aortofemoral	NR	NR	25	67
		Iliofemoropopliteal	NR	NR	33	33
Lorentzen and colleagues[70]	1985	Aortoiliac	515	0.0	NA	NA
		Aortofemoral	1497	3.0	22	29
		Iliofemoropopliteal	489	3.5	53	18
Edwards and colleagues[84]	1987	Aortic/aortoiliac	769	0.0	NA	NA
		Aortofemoral	1060	0.47	20	40
		Iliofemoropopliteal	583	2.9	12	18

*Primary graft infections only; excludes aortoenteric fistulas.
†Amputation rate among survivors.
NA, Not applicable; *NR*, not reported.

recent series, reported amputation rates range from 24% to 27%.[81-83]

Principles of Antibiotic Prophylaxis

The goal of prophylactic antibiotic therapy is to prevent infection after surgery. The most important indication for antibiotic prophylaxis in vascular reconstructive surgery is the use of prosthetic materials. Synthetic materials provide a protective substrate for bacterial colonization and proliferation. Experimental studies have demonstrated that the presence of a foreign body increases the infectivity of *Staphylococcus aureus* 10,000-fold.[85] In light of the potentially catastrophic consequences of vascular graft infection, prophylactic antibiotics are recommended in patients undergoing procedures in which prosthetic materials are used.

The ideal prophylactic antibiotic should be bactericidal for the most common pathogens causing postoperative infection and adequately concentrated in serum and at the site of surgery. It should be present in adequate concentrations throughout the surgical procedure and nontoxic to the patient. In addition, its cost should be reasonable enough to justify its routine use.

Most vascular graft infections are caused by relatively few specific bacteria; therefore broad-spectrum antibiotic prophylaxis is unnecessary. Selecting an antibiotic with the narrowest spectrum of activity that includes the most common pathogens involved in graft infection will limit the emergence of resistant organisms. Antibiotics that are the principal line of therapy in difficult infections (such as vancomycin in the treatment of *Staphylococcus*

epidermidis infections) should generally be reserved for that indication and not used in prophylaxis.

Bacteriology of Graft Infection

Gram-positive cocci, the predominant flora of the skin and dermal appendages, are most often responsible for vascular graft infections. Although the bacteriology of graft infection varies somewhat by anatomic site, when all sites are considered together, approximately 60% to 65% of reported cases are currently due to gram-positive organisms. The remaining 35% to 40% are largely due to gram-negative rods, which account for approximately half of all infections in intraabdominal (aortic, aortoiliac) grafts. Although *S. aureus* has historically been the most frequently cultured pathogen, the introduction of routine antibiotic prophylaxis and improved culture techniques have led to the emergence of *S. epidermidis* and other coagulase-negative staphylococci as the most frequent cause of vascular graft infection (Table 10-2). The most commonly cultured gram-negative rod is *E. coli*, followed by *Proteus* species, *Pseudomonas* species, and *Klebsiella* species.

In early reports from the 1960s and 1970s, *S. aureus* was identified as the predominant pathogen in vascular graft infections. In 1965, Hoffert and colleagues[67] reported that *S. aureus* was cultured in 67% (8 of 12) of aortic, femoral, and popliteal reconstructions.[67] Likewise, in a series of 890 aortic grafts from Fry and Lindenauer,[68] *S. aureus* was cultured in 67% (8 of 12) of cases. In 1967, Smith and colleagues[86] reported on nine cases of femoropopliteal graft infection, eight of which were due to

TABLE 10-2 Effect of Antibiotic Prophylaxis on the Microbiology of Graft Infection

Author	Year	Type of Graft	Antibiotics	Cultured Organisms (%)				Culture Negative (%)
				S. aureus	S. epidermidis	E. coli	Other GNRs	
Hoffert and colleagues[67]	1965	Aortic and distal	No	67	17	8	25	17
Fry and Lindenauer[68]	1967	Aortic	No	67	0	25	8	8
Goldstone and Moore[71]	1974	Aortic and distal	In some cases†	41	26	15	11	7
Liekweg and Greenfield[74]	1977	Aortic and distal	No	50	4	13	18	NR
Bandyk and colleagues[72]	1984	Aortofemoral	Yes	10	60	13	23	10
Yeager and colleagues[82]	1985	Aortic	Yes	0	50	0	0	33
		Distal	Yes	14	14	0	29	43
Quiñones-Baldrich and colleagues[88]	1991	Aortic	Yes	13	21	18	45	21

*Expressed as the percentage of cases from which each organism was cultured.
†Prophylaxis administered in 10 of 27 cases of graft infection.
GNR, Gram-negative rod; *NR,* not reported.

S. aureus. In a review of 108 published cases of vascular graft infection reported between 1959 and 1974, Liekweg and Greenfield[74] noted that *S. aureus* was responsible for 50% of cases. The next most common pathogens were gram-negative rods (30.5%) and streptococci (8.5%); only 3.6% of cases were due to *S. epidermidis.*

Goldstone and Moore[71] were among the first to note the effects of antibiotic prophylaxis on the presentation and bacteriology of graft infection. They retrospectively reviewed the incidence of graft infection before and after the initiation of routine antibiotic prophylaxis. During the preantibiotic prophylaxis period (1959 to 1966), the vascular graft infection rate was 4.1% (9 of 222). From 1966 to 1973, when prophylactic antibiotic use became routine, the graft infection rate dropped to 1.5% (5 of 344). Of all staphylococcal infections treated at the author's institution between 1959 and 1973, 14 of 18 (78%) occurred before the routine use of prophylactic antibiotics.

Reviews of graft infection since the advent of routine antibiotic prophylaxis demonstrate an increasing incidence of late infections resulting from fastidious organisms such as *S. epidermidis* and other coagulase-negative staphylococci. Bandyk and colleagues[72] presented a report of 30 patients treated for aortofemoral graft infections from 1972 to 1982; 60% of these infections were due to *S. epidermidis.* The time of presentation influenced the microbiology of graft infection. Four of five early (<4 months) infections were due to gram-negative rods. Late infections (>4 months) were much more common, totaling 25; of these, 15 (60%) were due to *S. epidermidis.*

In 1985, Yeager and associates[82] reported a 9-year experience in which they managed 14 aortic and 11 peripheral graft infections. Whereas peripheral graft infections appeared an average of 8 months after surgery, aortic graft infections appeared an average of 5 years afterward. Of five primarily infected aortic grafts (not graft-enteric fistulas or erosions) with positive cultures, four were due to *S. epidermidis.* A wide range of organisms was cultured from peripheral grafts, including coagulase-positive and -negative staphylococci, gram-negative rods, anaerobic streptococci, and diphtheroids.

Edwards and associates[87] reported on 24 infections from a series of 2614 aortofemoropopliteal grafts over a 10-year period from 1975 to 1986; the majority (29%) were due to *S. aureus.* The authors noted, however, that prophylactic antibiotics were administered according to the departmental protocol in only 7 of 24 cases. This observation is supported by the fact that 63% of these infections appeared within 3 months of implantation. In addition, cultures were negative in 21% of patients, suggesting that the presence of fastidious organisms such as *S. epidermidis* may have been underestimated. In 1991, Quiñones-Baldrich and colleagues[88] reported an 18-year experience (1970 to 1988) with 45 aortic graft infections. Culture results were available for 38 of 45 patients. Gram-negative organisms, most commonly *Pseudomonas* species (21%) and *E. coli* (18%), were cultured from 24 patients (63%). Gram-positive cocci, most frequently *S. epidermidis* (21%), were cultured from 21 patients (55%). Of note is the fact that cultures grew multiple organisms in 39% of cases. There were eight (21%) negative cultures, again suggesting that the incidence of infection owing to fastidious organisms may have been underestimated.

Pathogenesis of Graft Infection

Although there is no definitive explanation of how graft infection occurs, the two principal routes of infection are thought to be direct contamination (bacteria present in the surgical wound) and hematogenous or lymphatogenous seeding. It is generally thought that most graft infections are caused by direct intraoperative contamination of the prosthesis. Potential sources of infecting organisms include the patient's skin, breaks in aseptic technique, adjacent active infections, transudation of bowel flora into the peritoneal space, and the diseased arterial tree itself, which may become colonized with pathogenic bacteria.

TABLE 10-3 Positive Arterial Wall Cultures: Incidence and Significance

Author	Year	Culture Source	Positive Cutures (%)	Associated with Subsequent Infection?	Frequency of S. epidermidis among Positive Cultures (%)
Ernst and colleagues[25]	1977	Aortic aneurysms	15	Yes	53
Scobie and colleagues[94]	1979	Aortic aneurysms	23	No	71
Macbeth and colleagues[101]	1984	Femoropopliteal specimens	43	Yes	71
McAuley and colleagues[145]	1984	Aortic thrombus	14	No	NR
Buckels and colleagues[100]	1985	Aortic aneurysms	8	Yes	30
Durham and colleagues[102]	1987	Aortofemoropopliteal specimens	44	Yes	56
Schwartz and colleagues[146]	1987	Aortic aneurysms	10	No	54
Ilgenfritz and Jordan[147]	1988	Aortic aneurysms and atrial septal defects	20	No	55
Brandimarte and colleagues[148]	1989	Aortic aneurysms	31	No	NR
Wakefield and colleagues[28]	1990	Aortofemoropopliteal specimens	12	No	60

NR, Not reported.

Skin Flora

The normal skin flora is the most important source of bacteria. Accordingly, preoperative skin preparation influences subsequent infection rates. Kaiser and coworkers[89] noted a higher rate of infection with a hexachlorophene-ethanol preparation compared with povidone-iodine. Close and colleagues[90] reported that hexachlorophene is more effective alone than when used in combination with ethanol. In a prospective study, Cruse demonstrated that preoperative hexachlorophene showering can be effective in reducing wound infection rates, and overzealous shaving may actually increase the risk of infection.[91] Wooster and colleagues[92] demonstrated that vascular grafts routinely become contaminated with skin organisms intraoperatively and suggested that careful attention to aseptic technique can significantly reduce this occurrence.

Groin incisions appear to have special significance in the development of vascular graft infections. Grafts involving an inguinal wound have a higher incidence of infection than do those that avoid this region.[69,71,93] Jamieson and colleagues[73] reported that the presence of a groin incision increased the risk of graft infection 3.5-fold; the presence of a groin complication such as a seroma or hematoma increased the risk of infection ninefold over patients without groin complications. Up to 33% of groin incisions with hematomas may develop infections.[76] Lorentzen and associates[70] reported that the highest incidence of infection was in patients who underwent aortobifemoral grafting for abdominal aortic aneurysms (5.9%), whereas there were no infections in 425 patients who underwent aortoiliac bypass for aneurysms (213) and occlusive atherosclerosis (212).

Gastrointestinal Flora

The gastrointestinal tract is a potential source of contamination during aortic reconstruction. Cultures of intestinal bag fluid have been reported by some investigators to yield enteric bacteria[74] and skin organisms such as coagulase-negative staphylococci.[25] In a report of 109 bowel bag cultures from abdominal aortic

reconstructions, Scobie and colleagues[94] found positive cultures in 14% of patients. *S. epidermidis* was the single most common organism isolated (n = 11), whereas enteric flora were cultured in 12.

The impact of concomitant gastrointestinal surgery in the development of vascular graft infection is unclear. In separate series, DeBakey and colleagues,[95] Stoll,[96] and Hardy and colleagues[97] reported a total of 670 patients who underwent aortic graft placement and simultaneous gastrointestinal procedures, with no episodes of graft infection. These authors concluded that such coincident procedures can be undertaken safely. Other investigators, however, described the development of graft infection in patients undergoing simultaneous appendectomy,[71] cholecystectomy and gastrostomy,[98] and anterior resection.[92]

Arterial Colonization

The native arterial tree may harbor bacteria. The presence of pathogenic bacteria, particularly coagulase-negative staphylococci, in vascular tissues not previously operated on has been widely documented (Table 10-3). Lalka and colleagues[99] postulated that transient bacteremias resulting from breaks in the skin or mucous membranes may lead to arterial colonization. Bacterial contamination of vascular prostheses may therefore be inevitable in some cases. It is not yet clear, however, to what extent the presence of positive arterial wall cultures influences the likelihood of subsequent graft infection.

The 1977 report by Ernst and associates[25] of abdominal aortic aneurysmal wall cultures was one of the first to highlight the presence of pathogenic organisms in the native aorta. The overall incidence of positive cultures was 15%, and cultures were more likely to be positive when atherosclerotic disease was more advanced. Asymptomatic aneurysms were less likely to be culture positive (9%) than were symptomatic (13%) or ruptured aneurysms (35%). *S. epidermidis* was the most frequently isolated organism. The late graft sepsis rate was 10% in the culture-positive group versus 2% in the culture-negative group. In a similar report, Buckels and coauthors[100] described an 8% (22 of 275) incidence of positive cultures from aortic aneurysm contents. The incidence of graft sepsis was 32% (7 of 22) in patients with positive cultures, compared with 2.4% (6 of 253) in the culture-negative group.

Similar data suggest that lower extremity arteries can also become infected. In 1984, Macbeth and colleagues[101] reported on cultures of arterial wall specimens from 88 clean, elective lower extremity revascularization procedures. Control cultures were taken from adjacent adipose or lymphatic tissue. Although all control cultures were negative, arterial wall cultures were positive in 43% of cases (38 of 88). Of these, 71% (27 of 38) grew *S. epidermidis*. The authors described three graft infections in 335 cases (0.9% infection rate), all of which had positive arterial wall cultures. Also included in this report was a retrospective review of 22 cases of graft infection for which arterial and graft culture data were available. Of the patients with positive arterial cultures, 57% (8 of 14) had suture line disruption, whereas there were no disruptions in the culture-negative group. Durham and colleagues[102] reported a series of 102 patients undergoing vascular reconstruction with a 74% (75 of 102) incidence of positive arterial wall cultures.[102] *S. epidermidis* accounted for 56% of the cultured organisms. Six infections (3.5%) occurred over 18 months; all these patients had prior positive arterial cultures. No patients with negative arterial cultures developed graft infection. The greatest risk for graft infection appeared to be in patients with positive arterial wall cultures undergoing reoperation.

Hematogenous and Lymphatogenous Seeding

Hematogenous seeding of vascular prostheses is another potential source of graft infection. Anecdotal reports implicate urinary tract infection,[70,71] abdominal sepsis,[71,76,94] and other infections[69] in the development of vascular graft infections. Laboratory models demonstrate that bacteremia reliably produces prosthetic graft infections.[103-105]

Other Local and Systemic Factors

Open wounds on the distal lower extremities can be a source of contaminating bacteria. Hoffert and colleagues[67] noted that 75% of patients with graft infections (9 of 12) had open, infected lesions on the distal lower extremity at the time of graft implantation. Liekweg and Greenfield[74] reported that 33% of inguinal infections (20 of 60) occurred proximal to open foot infections. Bunt and Mohr[106] described the presence of bacteria cultured from a distally infected extremity in the inguinal lymph nodes of two patients undergoing lower extremity revascularization; both patients developed graft infection.

Prior vascular surgery has been implicated as a risk factor for vascular graft infection. Dense scar tissue, increased bleeding, and lymphatic leak may all contribute to this phenomenon. Goldstone and Moore[71] noted that 45% of patients (12 of 27) with graft infections had undergone one or more revisions of the original graft before developing an infection in the same region.[71] In 8 of the 12 patients, the infection was in the groin. In the series by Edwards and coworkers,[87] 9 of 18 patients (50%) had undergone a previous vascular surgery at the site of the graft infection. Similarly, a report from Reilly and colleagues[80] described a history of multiple previous vascular procedures at the site of graft infection in 40% of cases. Johnson and associates[107] found that prior vascular procedures were not a significant risk factor for graft infection; however, only 12 of 135 patients in this series had prior operations at the site of infection.

The immunologic status of patients with vascular disease may also have an impact on the development of graft infection. Systemic disease, malnutrition, and medical debility may suppress the host response to invading microorganisms. Kwaan and colleagues[108] reported on 12 patients with advanced, fulminating graft infections, all of whom had critical deficiencies in immune status as determined by serum albumin, hemoglobin, immunoglobulin, and lymphocyte assays and by response to standard skin test antigens. Eight of 12 patients who received total parenteral nutrition had significant enhancement of immune response and accelerated recovery from the graft infection. Of the four patients who did not receive nutritional support, two had a prolonged convalescence, and two subsequently died from complications of graft infection.

Experimental Investigations

The suggestion that prophylactic antibiotic therapy may be effective in the prevention of surgical infections was first made 50 years ago.[109-113] In the early 1960s, Alexander and colleagues[114,115] demonstrated the efficacy of penicillin prophylaxis in experimental wound infections.

Lindenauer and associates[75] reported an experimental demonstration of the importance of antibiotics in preventing graft infection. Three groups of dogs underwent femoral arteriotomy with primary, Teflon patch, or vein patch closure. A fourth group received sham operation alone. Wounds were contaminated with 10,000 to 100,000 *S. aureus* organisms. All subjects, except controls, received intramuscular procaine penicillin. Among control animals, the infection rate was 94% (8 of 9 shams, 3 of 3 arteriotomies, 3 of 3 Teflon patches, 3 of 3 vein patches). In animals treated with penicillin, the infection rate was 0% (15 shams, 5 arteriotomies, 5 Teflon patches, 5 vein patches). As a result, antibiotic therapy may sterilize a contaminated wound even in the presence of a prosthetic arterial patch.

Moore and colleagues[116] tested the utility of antibiotic prophylaxis in a canine model of hematogenous aortic graft contamination. Thirty minutes before laparotomy, dogs were infused intravenously with 10 million *S. aureus* organisms and then underwent placement of a Dacron infrarenal aortic graft. The experimental group received an IV dose of cephalothin (25 mg/kg), which was started just before the skin incision and continued for 30 minutes after the procedure. Experimental animals then received intramuscular cephalothin three times a day for 5 days; control animals received no antibiotics. Control animals experienced a significantly increased rate of positive cultures (72%) compared with animals that received perioperative cephalothin (24%).

Clinical Investigations

Early Experience

Until the mid 1970s, the use of antibiotics in vascular reconstruction with synthetic materials was largely based on personal preference. It is notable that in the series of Szilagyi and colleagues,[69] the graft infection rate among 2145 cases in which prophylactic antibiotics were not administered was 1.5%. Fry and Lindenauer[68] reported an incidence of 1.34% in 890 cases in which no antibiotics were used. These infection rates were comparable with, and often lower than, those reported in series in which prophylactic antibiotics were used.[73] Noting the preponderance of *S. aureus* in vascular graft infections, particularly in cases involving an inguinal incision, Szilagyi and colleagues[69] suggested a clinical trial of an antibiotic directed at this organism in reconstructions that required an inguinal anastomosis.

In 1974, Goldstone and Moore[71] published a review of the San Francisco Veterans Administration Hospital experience with vascular prosthetic infection. This series of 566 aortofemoropopliteal reconstructions was divided into two time periods: 1959 to 1965, when antibiotics were administered only postoperatively; and 1966 to 1973, when prophylaxis included preoperative, intraoperative, and postoperative antibiotics. The incidence of graft infection in the former group was 4.1% (9 of 222), compared with 1.5% (5 of 344) in the latter. Although the investigators conceded that greater experience and skill may have contributed to the lower incidence of infection, they maintained that the major factor responsible was the more appropriate use of antibiotics in the second group of patients. The following year, Perdue[117] published a similar retrospective review that suggested that the institution of routine antibiotic prophylaxis reduced the incidence of wound infections and other nosocomial infections in patients undergoing major arterial reconstructive procedures.

Prospective Trials

The first large, prospective, randomized, blinded clinical study of antibiotic prophylaxis in vascular reconstructive surgery was published by Kaiser and colleagues in 1978.[89] In that series, 462 patients undergoing aortofemoropopliteal reconstruction were randomized to receive either 1 g of cefazolin or a saline placebo. There were no graft infections among 225 patients who received cefazolin, compared with 4 of 237 placebo recipients (1.7%). When superficial skin infections and subcutaneous skin infections were considered in the analysis (Szilagyi classes I and II), the overall infection rates were 0.9% in the cefazolin group and 6.8% in the placebo group. Given no adverse drug reactions and no noted cefazolin resistance, the authors strongly recommended a short course of cefazolin prophylaxis in patients undergoing arterial reconstructive surgery.

In 1980, Pitt and colleagues reported the results of a controlled study of cephradine prophylaxis in vascular procedures involving groin incisions in which topical, systemic, and topical plus systemic administration were compared.[118] Of 205 patients, 52 had prosthetic grafts placed, whereas the remainder received vein grafts. Infection rates were equivalent in these two groups. Wound infection rates were 0% for those receiving topical administration alone and systemic administration alone, 5.9% for patients receiving both, and 24.5% for controls. No distinction was made between graft (Szilagyi class III) and isolated wound (Szilagyi classes I and II) infections. Minimum follow-up was 4 weeks, but the mean length of follow-up was not indicated. Patients in whom synthetic graft material was used did not experience a higher incidence of wound infection. The authors concluded that topical and systemic prophylaxes were equally efficacious and that combined prophylaxis was unnecessary. The follow-up interval in this study, however, was not long enough to make conclusive statements.

The benefit of a short course of systemic cephalosporin prophylaxis in vascular reconstructive surgery was subsequently confirmed in a number of other prospective, randomized trials. In 1983, Salzmann[119] reported a trial of cefuroxime (a second-generation agent) and later cefotaxime (a third-generation agent) versus placebo in 300 patients undergoing aortofemoropopliteal reconstruction. The prophylaxis regimen was changed from cefuroxime to cefotaxime midway through the study because the latter was found to be more effective in vitro against the most common graft infection pathogens at the author's institution. Graft infection rates were 2.4% for the placebo group and 0.8% for the prophylaxis group. The incidence of wound infection was 15.1% in the placebo group and 3.0% in the prophylaxis group. No differences in infection rate were noted between the two antibiotics, and the author concluded that either agent could be used effectively in the prophylaxis of postoperative infection.

Addressing the question of duration of treatment for antibiotic prophylaxis, Hasselgren and colleagues[120] compared 1- and 3-day courses of cefuroxime versus placebo in lower extremity arterial reconstruction. There was only one graft infection in this small cohort of 110 patients, and it occurred in the placebo group. The wound infection rate was 16.7% for patients receiving placebo, compared with 3.8% in the 1-day and 4.3% in the 3-day prophylaxis groups. The investigators recommended that prophylactic antibiotic therapy be limited to a short-term course.

Bennion and colleagues[121] examined the utility of antibiotic prophylaxis in patients with chronic renal insufficiency undergoing placement of a prosthetic arteriovenous shunt for hemodialysis. Patients were randomized to receive cefamandole or placebo just before placement of a PTFE graft, followed by two subsequent doses. The wound infection rate for the cefamandole group was 10.5% (2 of 19), with 1 graft (Szilagyi class III) infection. The wound infection rate in the placebo group was 42.1% (8 of 19), with 3 graft infections. This high rate of infection is not uncommon in renal failure patients, and the study emphasized the importance of perioperative antibiotic prophylaxis.

Robbs and associates reported a trial of cloxacillin plus gentamicin versus cefotaxime in infrainguinal arterial reconstruction.[122] This group had adopted a 48-hour course of cloxacillin plus gentamicin as their routine prophylaxis owing to the predominance of *S. aureus* and gram-negative infections at their institution. Length of follow-up ranged from 6 to 20 months. The wound infection and graft infection rates for patients receiving cloxacillin plus gentamicin were 5.4% (7 of 129 wounds) and 1.5% (1 of 63 grafts), respectively. The rates for patients receiving cefotaxime were 6.3% (8 of 127 wounds) and 3.3% (2 of 61 grafts). The differences were not statistically significant. The authors concluded that the multiagent 2-day regimen conferred no advantage over the shorter, single-agent regimen.

Comparisons of Antibiotic Regimens

Because it has become evident that a short course of a cephalosporin antibiotic is the ideal prophylaxis for vascular reconstructive procedures, several studies have focused on whether the most widely used cephalosporin, cefazolin, is the best choice. A large number of graft infections, particularly in abdominal grafts, are due to gram-negative rods. A theoretical disadvantage of first-generation cephalosporins such as cefazolin is that they are more vulnerable to gram-negative beta-lactamase than are second- and third-generation agents. Gram-negative activity is thus limited to *E. coli*, *Proteus* species, and *Klebsiella* species, and many hospital-acquired strains of these organisms are cefazolin resistant. It has also been demonstrated that other cephalosporins, such as the second-generation agent cefamandole, have greater in vitro activity against coagulase-negative staphylococci, which have been found to colonize the native arterial wall in a large number of patients. It is clear from previous studies by Salzmann,[119] Hasselgren and colleagues,[120] and Robbs and colleagues[122] that second- and third-generation cephalosporins can be used effectively in vascular surgery prophylaxis.

In 1989, Lalka and colleagues examined this issue in a prospective study of arterial wall microbiology and antibiotic penetration.[99] Forty-seven patients undergoing aortofemoropopliteal reconstruction were randomized to receive perioperative cefazolin or cefamandole, 1 g every 6 hours for nine doses. Serial samples of serum, subcutaneous fat, thrombus, atheroma, and arterial wall were obtained for culture and assay of drug levels by high-performance liquid chromatography. Serum and tissue levels of cefazolin were significantly higher than those of cefamandole at almost all time points. Positive arterial wall cultures were obtained in 41.4% of patients, and 68.8% of bacterial isolates were coagulase-negative staphylococci (half of these were slime producers). At times, the arterial wall concentration of both antibiotics fell below the geometric mean minimal inhibitory concentration for all organisms combined, but this occurred significantly more often with cefamandole. The investigators concluded that both antibiotics needed to be administered in larger doses (cefazolin, 1.5 g every 4 hours; cefamandole, 2 g every 3 hours) and that the antibiotics were essentially equal in efficacy if administered appropriately. This study corroborated the findings of Mutch and colleagues,[123] who noted that serum antibiotic levels did not correlate well with aortic tissue

concentrations of bioactive antibiotic, and it suggested that arterial tissue levels rather than serum levels should be the standard for comparison of antibiotic efficacy.

Edwards and colleagues[124] reported a prospective trial of cefazolin versus the more β-lactamase–stable second-generation cephalosporin cefuroxime in patients undergoing aortic and peripheral vascular reconstruction. Prior studies had suggested that some failures of cefazolin prophylaxis were due to this agent's susceptibility to staphylococcal β-lactamase and that other cephalosporins might provide better protection in cardiac surgery.[89,125,126] Antibiotics were administered just before surgery, redosed intraoperatively, and continued every 6 hours postoperatively for 24 hours. Dosage and administration schedules were based on a prior pharmacokinetic study. The infection rate in the cefazolin group was 1% (3 of 287), versus 2.6% (7 of 272) in the cefuroxime group. This difference was not statistically significant. Cefuroxime exhibited lower trough concentrations than did cefazolin, and the length of the operative procedure was found to be a risk factor for infection only in the cefuroxime group. The investigators concluded that despite its lower resistance to β-lactamase, cefazolin provides better perioperative prophylaxis because of its greater antistaphylococcal potency and superior pharmacokinetic profile.[124] Data from this and other studies[89] suggest that intraoperative redosing of cefazolin should be more frequent in prolonged procedures than in routine therapeutic administration—that is, every 4 hours rather than every 6 hours.

Current Status of Antibiotic Prophylaxis

Antibiotic Selection

Cefazolin is currently the antibiotic of choice for routine vascular surgery prophylaxis. It is relatively inexpensive, has negligible toxicity and a low incidence of severe allergic reactions, and is active against many of the bacteria commonly implicated in graft infection (Tables 10-4, 10-5). Its pharmacokinetic profile is ideal for this indication, with reliably high peak serum concentrations and a long half-life of elimination compared with other cephalosporins.[124,127] It penetrates arterial tissue well, with drug concentrations exceeding the minimal inhibitory concentration of common graft infection pathogens in most instances.[99] Cefazolin is active against *S. aureus* (including penicillinase-producing strains), some strains of *S. epidermidis*, and the more commonly encountered gram-negative rods *E. coli*, *Proteus* species, and *Klebsiella* species. Most other gram-negative rods are resistant, including indole-positive *Proteus vulgaris*. Cephalothin, the other first-generation agent in common clinical use, is somewhat more resistant to staphylococcal β-lactamase, but it is less active against gram-negative organisms. More important, it is cleared from plasma fourfold to fivefold as rapidly as cefazolin.[127]

Later-generation cephalosporins have greater gram-negative activity and the potential benefit of increased resistance to staphylococcal β-lactamase; however, in vitro and in vivo activity against gram-positive cocci is reduced. Many investigators have tailored their choice of

TABLE 10-4 **Wound Infections among Patients Receiving Cefazolin or Placebo Prophylaxis**

Prophylaxis	No. of Infections	No. of Patients	Infected (%)	Class I Infections (%)	Class II Infections (%)	Class III Infections (%)
Cefazolin	2	225	0.9*	0	2	0
Placebo	16	237	6.8*	4	8	4
Total	18	462	3.9	4	10	4

*Difference is significant at $p < 0.001$. Brachiocephalic procedures are not included.
From Kaiser AB, Clayson KR, Mulherin JL, et al: Antibiotic prophylaxis in vascular surgery. Ann Surg 188:283, 1978.

TABLE 10-5 **Antibacterial Spectrum of Selected Antibiotics**

	Antibacterial Activity (MIC-90 in μg/mL)*				
Antibiotic	S. aureus	S. epidermidis	E. coli	Klebsiella spp.	Pseudomonas spp.
Cefazolin	1.0	0.8	5.0	6.0	R
Cephalothin	1.0	0.5	5.0	32.0	R
Cefamandole	1.0	2.0	4.0	8.0	R
Cefuroxime	2.0	1.0	4.0	R	R
Cefotaxime	2.0	8.0	0.25	0.25	32.0
Vancomycin	1.0	3.0	R	R	R
Penicillin V	ALP+: >25.0 ALP–: 0.03	0.02†	R	R	R
Oxacillin	0.25	0.2†	R	R	R
Gentamicin	0.6	2.0†	4.0	1.0	2.0
Ciprofloxacin	0.5	0.25	0.03	0.125	0.5
Rifampin	0.015	0.015	16.0	32.0	64.0

*MIC-90 is the minimal inhibitory concentration for 90% of strains. MIC > 64 μg/mL is considered resistant. Values are approximate and may vary among institutions.
†Many strains are resistant.
ALP, Alkaline phosphatase; R, resistant.
Data from Mandell RGD, editor: Principles and practice of infectious diseases, ed 3, New York, 1989, Churchill Livingstone.

antibiotic to the predominant organisms responsible for graft infection at their particular institutions. Cefamandole,[99] cefuroxime,[128] and cefotaxime[122] have all been used effectively as prophylactic agents in prospective trials. However, cefamandole has fallen out of favor for routine use owing to an association with hypoprothrombinemia and bleeding, particularly in elderly patients and those with renal insufficiency. Cefuroxime has been shown to have antistaphylococcal potency and pharmacokinetic properties inferior to those of cefazolin.[124] Third-generation agents such as cefotaxime have broad anti–gram-negative activity but are generally less active against staphylococci. Moreover, the later-generation cephalosporins are, in most instances, significantly more expensive than the first-generation agents. As a result, cefazolin remains the antibiotic of choice, except in specific instances when in vitro testing has revealed that another agent more adequately covers the principal pathogens of graft infection.

A potential disadvantage of cefazolin prophylaxis is the inconsistent activity of this agent against the organism that is currently responsible for the greatest number of graft infections, S. epidermidis. It has been shown that during hospitalization, patients acquire multiply resistant strains of this bacterium.[129,130] Up to 75% of S. epidermidis

isolates at some institutions are now cefazolin resistant. Vancomycin is highly active against both S. epidermidis and S. aureus; resistance in these organisms is rarely encountered. Vancomycin, however, provides no gram-negative coverage. It is the drug of choice for prophylaxis in patients with a history of anaphylaxis to β-lactam antibiotics, often in combination with an aminoglycoside in procedures in which there is significant risk of gram-negative infection, such as aortic reconstruction. Vancomycin is also considered the antibiotic of choice for the prophylaxis of prosthetic hemodialysis access grafts and for patients known to be colonized with methicillin-resistant S. aureus. It is excreted primarily by glomerular filtration and therefore persists in high serum concentrations in patients with end-stage renal disease.

The broad antibacterial spectrum, excellent tissue penetration, and low toxicity of the fluoroquinolones make them potentially ideal agents for the prophylaxis of surgical infections. Limited data are available concerning the use of fluoroquinolones for this indication, but there are reports of efficacy equal or superior to that of cephalosporin antibiotics in the prophylaxis of colorectal,[131,132] biliary,[131,133] and urologic surgery.[134-136] Auger and coauthors[137] reported a randomized study of pefloxacin, a nalidixic acid analog, and cefazolin in patients undergoing cardiac surgery. Of 111 patients, 14 receiving pefloxacin developed bacterial colonization at culture sites, compared with 11 in the cefazolin group. One patient who received cefazolin developed mediastinitis from a cefazolin-resistant strain of *S. epidermidis*. As yet, there are no published clinical trials of a fluoroquinolone versus a cephalosporin in the prophylaxis of peripheral vascular surgery procedures.

Resistant Bacteria

The contemporary use of antibiotics has resulted in further progression of bacterial resistance so that methicillin-resistant species of *Staphylococcus* are encountered more frequently. Institutional bacteriologic analysis may reveal an increased incidence of resistant species such as MRSA. In recent reports, as many as 20% to 30% of vascular surgical site infections may be MRSA related.[138,139]

Measures that have been proposed to help address the risk of MRSA infections include surveillance of patients by nasal swab screening to identify high-risk patients, decolonization of carriers, and attention to host factors (nutritional support, control of hypothermia, and blood glucose regulation). The Centers for Disease Control and Prevention has offered guidelines that are directed at reducing surgical site infections. Attention to patient preparation, skin cleansing, hand disinfection, surgical site care, and sterile technique are emphasized. In addition, recommendations for the selection and use of antibiotics are proposed.[140]

In keeping with these recommendations, antibiotic prophylactic regimens must be adapted to these conditions to include agents directed at MRAS in high-risk populations. The use of daptomycin (a bactericidal cyclic lipopeptide) with cefazolin has been advocated. An alternative regimen is the use of vancomycin and cefazolin.[141] Other authors have reported the use of vancomycin alone for prophylaxis. In a report of 6465 patients undergoing cardiac procedures, Garey and colleagues[142] noted that the use of vancomycin resulted in reduction of the incidence of surgical site infections and a reduction in the incidence of coagulase-negative *Staphylococcus* species and MRSA infections. It should be emphasized that these recommendations for first-line use of vancomycin or daptomycin are directed at institutions where there is a high incidence of methicillin-resistant *Staphylococcus* bacteria.

Antibiotic Administration

Prophylactic antibiotics are administered just before surgery and again intraoperatively during long procedures. Pharmacokinetic studies suggest that prophylactic antibiotics should be administered more frequently and in higher doses during surgery than is recommended for routine therapeutic indications (e.g., cefazolin 1.5 g every 4 hours).[89,125,143] Prophylaxis is usually continued postoperatively for up to 24 hours, and possibly longer when there is a theoretical risk of postoperative bacteremia from indwelling venous catheters, arterial lines, bladder catheters, and endotracheal tubes. The advantage of continuing coverage beyond the operating room, however, has not been clearly demonstrated. In the absence of these risk factors, there is clearly no advantage in extending antibiotic prophylaxis for longer than 24 hours.

Regimens of prophylaxis should be tailored to the type of vascular reconstruction undertaken. Cefazolin prophylaxis is recommended in all procedures involving the placement of prosthetic materials. It is probably not necessary in "clean" vascular procedures of the neck and upper extremities that do not involve the use of synthetic grafts. In contrast, the marked colonization and favorable bacterial environment of the lower abdomen and groin necessitate the use of antibiotic prophylaxis in all aortofemoropopliteal vascular procedures. The risk of gram-negative infection in aortic reconstruction may necessitate the addition of an aminoglycoside, particularly in institutions with a high degree of cefazolin resistance among gram-negative isolates. Alternatively, a second- or third-generation cephalosporin with broader anti–gram-negative activity may be substituted, as this obviates the risk of aminoglycoside-associated nephrotoxicity.

Cephalosporins should be avoided in patients with a history of anaphylaxis to β-lactam antibiotics. Patients with a history of minor allergic reactions to penicillin antibiotics can be given a cephalosporin test dose to determine whether cross-reactivity is present. Reduced dosing of cefazolin and most other cephalosporins is recommended in renal insufficiency, based on the calculated creatinine clearance.

There is evidence that remote bacteremia may be implicated in vascular graft infection. Accordingly, oral prophylaxis for procedures that are highly associated with bacteremia, such as tooth extraction, cystoscopy, and colonoscopy, is recommended. Wooster and colleagues[92] demonstrated in 200 vascular surgery patients undergoing cystoscopy that the incidence of bacteremia was 64% among inpatients and 8% among outpatients. For procedures such as tooth extraction and colonoscopy, prophylaxis must be tailored to the most common normal flora of the traumatized site. Penicillins are appropriate choices for major dental procedures, whereas broader gram-negative and anaerobic coverage may be warranted in colonoscopy. It should be emphasized, however, that the true risk of graft infection after procedures associated with bacteremia is unclear, and there is currently no consensus on the role of antibiotic prophylaxis in this setting.

References available online at expertconsult.com.

QUESTIONS

1. True or false: Arterial trauma is involved in the pathogenesis of most primary arterial infections.

2. When should prosthetic grafts be used to replace excised mycotic aneurysms?
   a. If the surgical field is laved with antibiotics
   b. In the upper extremities
   c. Only in carefully selected instances
   d. In fungal arterial infections
   e. Never

3. Since 1965, what organism is most commonly associated with microbial aortitis?
   a. *Salmonella* species
   b. Fungi
   c. Mycobacteria
   d. *Pseudomonas* species
   e. *Staphylococcus aureus*

4. In the management of a mycotic mesenteric aneurysm located in the distal arterial arcade (adjacent to the intestine), what is the recommended management?
   a. Reconstruction with a Dacron graft
   b. Reconstruction with a PTFE graft
   c. Reconstruction with an umbilical vein graft
   d. Reconstruction with a vein graft
   e. Ligation and excision without reconstruction

5. True or false: The recommended management of an infrarenal mycotic aneurysm involves the use of antibiotics, debridement of infected tissues, and reconstruction through a remote (extraanatomic) uninfected field.

6. What is the average reported incidence of prosthetic graft infection?
   a. 1% to 6%
   b. 6% to 10%
   c. 10% to 15%
   d. Greater than 15%
   e. 0% to 1%

7. True or false: The study by Pitt and colleagues revealed that intravenous antibiotics were much more effective than antibiotic irrigation.

8. Risk factors for prosthetic graft infection include which of the following?
   a. Multiple reoperations
   b. Inguinal incisions
   c. Open, infected wounds on the extremities
   d. Prior graft infections
   e. Positive arterial wall cultures
   f. All of the above

9. Avenues of infection include which of the following?
   a. Skin
   b. Arterial wall
   c. Open wounds on the distal limb
   d. Intestinal transudate accumulated during aortic bypass
   e. Foley catheter
   f. All of the above

10. What are the most common organisms found in prosthetic graft infections?
    a. *Proteus* species
    b. *Escherichia coli*
    c. *Staphylococcus aureus*
    d. *Streptococcus viridans*
    e. *Staphylococcus epidermidis*

ANSWERS

1. **true**
2. **c**
3. **a**
4. **e**
5. **true**
6. **a**
7. **false**
8. **f**
9. **f**
10. **e**

CHAPTER 11

INFLUENCE OF DIABETES MELLITUS ON VASCULAR DISEASE AND ITS COMPLICATIONS

Charles M. Peterson*

Diabetes mellitus is a heterogeneous collection of syndromes characterized by hyperglycemia. It is described in the Ebers Papyrus, an Egyptian text dating to approximately 1550 BC. Nevertheless, despite being recognized for four millennia, the disease in many ways remains poorly undefined. It is estimated to affect approximately 26 million inhabitants of the United States with total estimated costs in the United States in 2007 of $174 billion. More than 60% of nontraumatic lower-limb amputations occur in people with diabetes.[1] With new criteria for diagnosis,[2] the prevalence of diabetes may be even higher. Owing to the high prevalence of diabetes mellitus in patients with peripheral arterial disease, screening for this disorder is recommended for all patients in vascular wards who do not already carry the diagnosis.[3]

Insulin-dependent diabetes mellitus (IDDM), or type 1 diabetes, accounts for approximately 10% of diabetic patients; the majority have non–insulin-dependent diabetes mellitus (NIDDM), or type 2 diabetes. Other types of diabetes include gestational diabetes mellitus, (occurs de novo during pregnancy), a type that can occur from toxins or trauma to the insulin-secreting cells (β cells) of the pancreatic islets of Langerhans, or secondary diabetes mellitus owing to another disease that impairs pancreatic function or induces insulin resistance, such as occurs in iron overload syndromes, acromegaly, or Cushing disease.

IDDM, or the type characterized by low or undetectable insulin secretion and a need for insulin administration to sustain life, is generally accepted as primarily autoimmune in etiology.[4] The genetic vulnerabilities and the environmental insults that elicit IDDM are under intense study but remain poorly characterized. The complexity of these interactions is illustrated by the fact that less than 50% of monozygotic twins of a diabetic proband develop IDDM. NIDDM is a highly concordant genetic disease, with nearly 100% of monozygotic twins of a diabetic proband acquiring the disease. The concordance for first- and second-degree relatives increases given the challenge of obesity. NIDDM subjects tend to have insulin levels in the normal to high range yet remain insulin resistant, with an inadequate ability to secrete insulin in a manner sufficient to lower blood glucose into the normal range.[5]

Clinical practice guidelines are published yearly by the American Diabetes Association.[1] These guidelines define diabetes as an AIC level (glycated hemoglobin) greater than 6.5%, a fasting glucose higher than 126 mg/dL, a 2-hour glucose greater than 200 mg/dL on an oral glucose tolerance test (or at random in a symptomatic patient). Prediabetes is defined as a fasting glucose level of 100 to 125 mg/dL.

Persons with either IDDM or NIDDM tend to be at especially high risk for the development of vascular disease, in part because they have glucose toxicity as a result of elevated blood glucose levels, insulin toxicity as a result of elevated insulin levels from peripheral insulin injection (IDDM and some NIDDM) or elevated endogenous insulin secretion (most NIDDM), and a persistent inflammatory state. The nature of these toxicities is described in some detail later. This chapter also emphasizes the importance of minimizing these two toxicities through therapeutic approaches that target normal glucose levels without unduly raising insulin levels or promoting hypoglycemia.[6]

The recognition of vascular disease as an obligatory concomitant of diabetes mellitus occurred during the twentieth century. Osler noted in 1908 that "the thickening of the arteries in . . . diabetes . . . may be due to the action on the blood vessels of poisons retained within the system."[7] In the 1945 edition of his textbook, 20 years after the use of insulin had become common, Joslin noted that "arteriosclerosis in the form of gangrene of the lower extremities has decreased while at the same time it has increased in the heart as coronary disease and in the brain as apoplexy."[8]

It is now generally agreed that diabetes mellitus accelerates the initiation and propagation of vascular disease. At present, 84% of diabetic subjects who live longer than 20 years after diagnosis have some form of vascular

---

*This chapter was written in the author's private capacity. The views expressed in the chapter do not necessarily represent the views of the U.S. Department of Defense.

disease, and 75% of persons with diabetes die of vascular disease or its complications, primarily myocardial infarction and stroke.[9] Thus persons with diabetes, regardless of type, have an increased risk for disease of the large and small vessels. In addition, the distribution of large vessel disease is more diffuse.

Diabetes remains problematic for the vascular surgeon for several reasons. The clinical diagnosis of vascular disease in a person with diabetes may be confounded by the presence of sensorimotor polyneuropathy and multiple sites of disease, which may mask typical pain or pulse patterns. The outcome of surgical intervention tends to be less favorable in persons with diabetes because the hospital stay is generally longer, the risk for infection is greater, and the probability of an adverse outcome is higher than in persons without diabetes. In the 1960s, mortality rates in diabetic patients who had surgery were reported to be 3.6% to 13.2%.[10] In 1983, Hjortrup and colleagues[11] studied morbidity in diabetic and nondiabetic patients who had major vascular surgery and found that there were no deaths in either group and comparable morbidity. Although their theories were unproved, the authors hypothesized that the improvement in statistical outcome in the intervening 20 years was due to improvements in diabetes care. A recent study of the 25-year cumulative incidence of lower extremity amputations in people with type 1 diabetes would appear to confirm the hypotheses raised previously. The cumulative incidence within the Wisconsin Epidemiologic Study of Diabetic Retinopathy participants (n = 943) was still high at 10.1%. Being male, heavy smoking, hypertension, diabetic retinopathy, neuropathy, and higher hemoglobin (Hb) A_{1c} were independently associated with the incidence of lower extremity amputation. Thus increased attention to the modifiable factors of smoking, blood pressure, and glucose control is warranted.[12]

There appears to be little doubt that diabetes care enhances the outcome of perioperative infection. From 1990 to 1995, Golden and coworkers[13] at Johns Hopkins evaluated 411 adults with diabetes who underwent coronary artery surgery, conducting glucose surveillance six times per day. After adjusting for age, sex, race, underlying comorbidity, acute severity of illness, and length of stay in the surgical intensive care unit, patients with higher mean glucose readings were at increased risk of developing infections. Thus the investigators concluded that in patients with diabetes who undergo coronary artery surgery, postoperative hyperglycemia is an independent predictor of short-term infectious complications.

This chapter reviews the epidemiologic data and the mechanisms behind the factors that make individuals with diabetes vulnerable to the initiation and propagation of vascular disease, with an emphasis on the effects on the large vessels. The chapter also details protocols that have proved useful for the control of glucose in patients with IDDM and NIDDM. In view of the increasing evidence that both acute and chronic risk can be modified by intensive glucose control protocols, these approaches should be part of the therapeutic armamentarium of surgical teams and specialists in diabetes care.

CEREBROVASCULAR, CARDIOVASCULAR, AND PERIPHERAL VASCULAR DISEASE AND DIABETES

There are now several large studies across multiple cultures that attest to the adverse effect of elevated glucose levels on the various forms of large vessel disease. Elevated glucose not only accelerates the appearance of vascular disease but also predicts vascular events and prognosis once a vascular event has occurred. This section reviews the major large studies because they address the issues of stroke, cardiovascular disease (CVD), and peripheral vascular disease.

A number of studies documented that the glucose level at the time of hospital admission is a predictor of outcome and extent of neurologic deficit in persons with acute stroke. For example, Toni and associates[14] attempted to identify predictors and possible pathogenic mechanisms of early neurologic deterioration in patients with acute ischemic strokes and to evaluate their effect on clinical outcome. They studied a continuous series of 152 patients with first-ever ischemic hemispheric strokes who were hospitalized within 5 hours of onset, evaluated according to the Canadian Neurological Scale, and assessed with a computed tomography (CT) scan. The initial subset of 80 patients also underwent angiography. A repeated CT scan or autopsy was performed within 5 to 9 days of a patient's stroke. Progressing neurologic deficit was defined as a decrease of 1 point or more in the global neurologic scale score during hospitalization compared with the score at entry. Those whose condition deteriorated had been hospitalized earlier and had higher serum glucose levels at admission.

The Oslo Study also found that diabetes and the level of nonfasting glucose predicted the outcome of stroke.[15] That study, started in 1972, included 16,209 men aged 40 to 49 years. Of these, 16,172 had no previous history of stroke and 151 were known to have diabetes. Five diabetic and 80 nondiabetic subjects died of stroke during the 18 years of follow-up, giving a rate ratio of 7.87 (95% confidence interval [CI], 2.48 to 19.14) for diabetic subjects. The rate of mortality for all causes in diabetic subjects was more than fivefold that of those who were not diabetic. Nonfasting serum glucose was a predictor of fatal stroke in all participants (diabetic subjects included) without a history of stroke in age-adjusted univariate analysis. The relative risk (RR) was 1.13 (95% CI, 1.03 to 1.25) by an increase of 1 mmol/L (18 mg/dL) of serum glucose, according to results of proportional hazards regression analysis.

Similar observations were made in Scotland, where women were found to be more vulnerable to the effects of glucose than were men.[16] Sex-specific CVD, ischemic heart disease, and stroke mortality rates and relative risks for asymptomatic hyperglycemic subjects (top 5%) were compared with those of normoglycemic individuals (bottom 95%) during a mean follow-up of 11.6 years (range, 10 to 14 years) of 4696 men and 5714 women in western Scotland aged 45 to 64 years at entry. Univariate analysis showed that asymptomatic hyperglycemia was associated with increased risk of all causes of CVD, ischemic heart disease, and stroke mortality in both men and women. The degree of this association was greater in women than in men. Using multiple logistic regression analysis to take into account differences in age, systolic and diastolic blood pressure, serum cholesterol, body mass index (BMI), and cigarette smoking, a high causal blood glucose level was still a significant risk factor for CVD mortality in both men and women.

Within the diabetic population, the level of complications such as retinopathy, preexisting nephropathy, and coronary and peripheral vascular disease, in addition to age, is a predictor of outcome.[17] In a cohort of 2124 diabetic persons identified at multiphasic health checkups from 1979 through 1985, 56 suffered a nonembolic ischemic stroke during the follow-up period, which extended through 1991. For each case subject, one diabetic control subject, matched by sex and year of birth, was selected from the same cohort of diabetic subjects. The estimated relative risk of stroke in diabetic subjects with retinopathy was 2.8 (95% CI, 1.2 to 6.9). After adjusting for age, sex, smoking, use of insulin, average systolic blood pressure, and average random glucose level, the estimated relative risk was 4.0 (95% CI, 1.0 to 14.5). The relative risk of stroke in diabetic subjects with retinopathy remained elevated after the exclusion of those with complications other than retinopathy.

The Honolulu Heart Program also confirmed a poorer prognosis for vascular disease associated with hyperglycemia.[18] This study examined the association between a variety of baseline lifestyle and biologic factors in a middle-aged cohort of Japanese American men and the 20-year incidence rates of total atherosclerotic end points and each of the initial clinical manifestations of this disease, including fatal and nonfatal coronary heart disease, angina pectoris, thromboembolic stroke, and aortic aneurysm. Japanese American men (n = 2710) between the ages of 55 and 64 years at the time of the initial clinical examination (1965 through 1968) who had no evidence of coronary heart disease, cerebrovascular disease, cancer, or aortic aneurysm were studied. Among these men, 602 atherosclerotic events developed during the 23-year follow-up period (1965 through 1988). After adjusting for each of the baseline characteristics examined, significant positive associations between quartile cutoffs of BMI, systolic blood pressure, serum glucose levels, cholesterol, triglycerides, and uric acid, as well as cigarette smoking, and the occurrence of any atherosclerotic end point were noted.

Within the diabetic population, nonfatal or small infarction, especially with multiple occurrences, is a feature of cerebrovascular disease complicating diabetes mellitus and correlates with elevated blood glucose and blood pressure.[19] Asymptomatic cerebral infarction is not rare in diabetic subjects and can now be pathologically and clinically evaluated with accuracy using magnetic resonance imaging.

The Wisconsin Epidemiologic Study also confirmed the finding of elevated risk for vascular disease in the diabetic population.[20] The association of glycemia with cause-specific mortality in a diabetic population was studied in a cohort design based in a primary care setting. All participants (n = 1210) had diabetes, were taking insulin, and received a diagnosis when they were younger than 30 years. They were compared with a random sample of diabetic persons with a diagnosis at 30 years or older (n = 1780). Thus, both IDDM and NIDDM were studied, although the National Diabetes Data Group criteria for diagnosis were not used.[21] Glycosylated hemoglobin levels were obtained at baseline examinations. Median follow-up was 10 years in patients with an earlier onset and 8.3 years in those with a later onset. The main outcome measure was cause-specific mortality determined from death certificates. In the early-onset group, after controlling for other risk factors in proportional hazard models and considering the underlying cause of death, the glycosylated hemoglobin level as an index of average glucose control was significantly associated with mortality from diabetes (hazard ratio [HR] for a 1% change in glycosylated hemoglobin, 1.25; 95% CI, 1.13 to 1.38) and ischemic heart disease (HR, 1.18; 95% CI, 1.00 to 1.40). In the later-onset group, glycosylated hemoglobin was significantly associated with mortality from diabetes (HR, 1.32; 95% CI, 1.21 to 1.43), ischemic heart disease (HR, 1.10; 95% CI, 1.04 to 1.17), and stroke (HR, 1.17; 95% CI, 1.05 to 1.30), but not cancer (HR, 0.99; 95% CI, 0.88 to 1.10). The authors concluded that "these results suggest . . . benefit to the control of glycemia with respect to death due to vascular disease and diabetes."[21]

The Copenhagen Stroke Study also found that diabetes is a risk factor for stroke and that diabetes influences the nature of stroke.[22] The study evaluated stroke type, stroke severity, prognosis, and the relation between admission glucose levels and stroke severity and mortality. This community-based study included 1135 acute stroke patients, of whom 233 (20%) had diabetes. All patients were evaluated until the end of rehabilitation by weekly assessment of neurologic deficits (Scandinavian Stroke Scale) and functional disabilities (Barthel index). A CT scan was performed in 83% of stroke cases. The diabetic stroke patient was 3.2 years younger than the nondiabetic stroke patient ($p < 0.001$) and had hypertension more frequently (48% vs. 30%; $p < 0.0001$). Intracerebral hemorrhages were six times less frequent in diabetic patients ($p = 0.002$). Initial stroke severity, lesion size, and site were comparable between the two groups; mortality was higher in diabetic patients (24% vs. 17%; $p = 0.03$), and diabetes independently increased the relative death risk by 1.8 (95% CI, 1.04 to 3.19). Outcome was comparable in surviving patients with and without diabetes, but patients with diabetes recovered more slowly. Mortality increased with higher glucose levels on admission in nondiabetic patients, independent of stroke severity (odds ratio [OR], 1.2 per 1 mmol/L; 95% CI, 1.01 to 1.42; $p = 0.04$). Thus, diabetes influences stroke in terms of age, subtype, speed of recovery, and mortality. The authors concluded that "the effect of reducing high admission glucose levels in nondiabetic stroke patients should be examined in future trials."[22]

A Finnish study, although of short duration, confirmed the excess risk of elderly diabetic women for acute stroke.[23] The study examined whether NIDDM, its metabolic control and duration, and insulin level predict stroke. Cardiovascular risk factors, including glucose tolerance, plasma insulin, and glycosylated hemoglobin, were determined in a Finnish cohort of 1298 subjects aged 65 to 74 years, and the effects of these risk factors on the incidence of both fatal and nonfatal stroke was investigated during 3.5 years of follow-up. Of 1298 subjects participating in the baseline study, 1069 did not have diabetes and 229 had NIDDM. During the 3.5-year follow-up, 3.4% (n = 36) of nondiabetic subjects and 6.1% (n = 14) of NIDDM subjects had a nonfatal or fatal stroke. The incidence of stroke was significantly higher in diabetic women compared with nondiabetic women (OR, 2.25; 95% CI, 1.65 to 3.06). In multivariate logistic regression analyses including all study subjects, fasting and 2-hour glucose ($p < 0.01$ and $p < 0.05$, respectively), glycosylated Hb A_{1c} ($p < 0.01$), atrial fibrillation ($p < 0.05$), hypertension ($p < 0.05$), and previous stroke ($p < 0.01$) predicted stroke events. In diabetic subjects, fasting and 2-hour glucose ($p < 0.01$ and $p < 0.05$, respectively), glycosylated Hb A_{1c} ($p < 0.05$), duration of diabetes ($p < 0.05$), and atrial fibrillation ($p < 0.05$) were the baseline variables predicting stroke events. Finally, fasting insulin ($p < 0.05$), hypertension ($p < 0.05$), and previous stroke ($p < 0.01$) were associated with stroke incidence in nondiabetic subjects.

The longer-term Honolulu Heart Program confirmed that, for men, diabetes confers extra risk of thromboembolic stroke but not hemorrhagic stroke.[24] The goal of this study was to determine whether glucose intolerance and diabetes increase the risk of thromboembolic, hemorrhagic, and total stroke, independent of other risk factors. Among the 7549 Japanese American men aged 45 to 68 years and free of coronary heart disease and stroke from 1965 to 1968, a total of 374 thromboembolic, 128 hemorrhagic, and 36 type-unknown strokes occurred. The incidence of thromboembolic but not hemorrhagic stroke increased with the worsening glucose tolerance category. Compared with the low-normal (glucose <151 mg/dL) group, subjects in the high-normal (151 to 224 mg/dL), asymptomatic high (≥225 mg/dL), and known diabetes groups all had significantly elevated age-adjusted relative risks of thromboembolic stroke. After adjusting for other risk factors, relative risks remained significantly elevated for the asymptomatic high and known diabetes groups (RR, 1.43 and 2.45; 95% CI, 1.00 to 2.04 and 1.73 to 3.47, respectively). Associations were the same in hypertensive and nonhypertensive subjects and similar but slightly stronger in younger (45 to 54 years) than in older (55 to 68 years) men.

The Northern Manhattan Stroke Study found that an admission blood glucose level greater than 140 mg/dL was an important predictor of mortality in stroke.[25] Ethanol abuse (RR, 2.5), hypertension requiring discharge medications (RR, 1.6), and elevated blood glucose within 48 hours of index ischemic stroke (RR, 1.2/50 mg/dL) were found to be independent predictors of recurrence.

This review emphasizes that the relationship between glucose and vascular disease appears to hold across various cultures and genetic backgrounds. In a study in Taiwan of 479 NIDDM patients 40 years or older from four community primary care health centers, cholesterol, high-density lipoprotein cholesterol, plasma glucose, and Hb A_{1c} were studied.[26] The duration of diabetes was associated with the development of stroke, with an RR of 1.063 for every 1-year increment ($p < 0.07$). Significant risk factors were serum cholesterol and Hb A_{1c} levels. For every 1-mg/dL increase in mean total cholesterol level, the relative risk of developing vascular disease increased 1.016-fold ($p < 0.04$). For every 1% (approximately 35 mg/dL) increase in Hb A_{1c}, the relative risk of developing vascular disease increased 1.170-fold ($p < 0.01$). Female diabetic subjects had a higher relative risk than male subjects did. The risk of CVD is therefore twofold to threefold higher in diabetic than nondiabetic subjects. There is a gender difference; the incidence is twofold higher in diabetic men and threefold times higher in diabetic women.[27-30]

In the nondiabetic group in the Honolulu Heart Program, there was a dose-response relation between glucose intolerance at baseline and coronary heart disease incidence, coronary heart disease mortality, and total mortality. This risk was independent of other risk factors in this cohort of 8006 middle-aged and older Japanese American men.[31] Therefore, even in the normal range, glucose levels predict risk for vascular disease. A more recent study confirms these conclusions.[32] The Atherosclerosis Risk in Communities (ARIC) also documented that Hb A_{1c} levels in the normal range predict diabetes incidence, heart disease events, stroke, and death over more than a decade in both African Americans and white adult subjects.

Persons with diabetes have shorter life spans. Approximately 75% of increased mortality in men and 50% in women is caused by CVD. Kleinman and colleagues[27] found that the RR of mortality from ischemic heart disease was 2.8 for men and 2.5 for women after controlling for other confounding variables of hypertension, obesity, age, serum cholesterol, and smoking. In a Utah population, CVD accounted for 48% of all-cause mortality in diabetic subjects.[28] Diabetic subjects do not have only an increased mortality from acute myocardial infarction; they also have an increased rate of congestive heart failure, cardiogenic shock, and dysrhythmias, not necessarily correlated with the size of the infarct.[30,33] It is thought that the increased rate of congestive heart failure is secondary to hypocontractility, which may be due to microvascular disease, the metabolic effects of diabetes leading to cardiomyopathy, and autonomic dysfunction.[33]

Disease of the large vessels in one area of the vascular tree appears to predict disease in other areas. Associations of vascular disease are also found with perturbations in coagulation and inflammation.[34] Heinrich and coworkers investigated the vessel status of coronary and peripheral arteries and those arteries supplying the brain in 929 consecutive male patients admitted to a coronary rehabilitation unit.[34] The severity of coronary atherosclerosis was scored using coronary angiography. Changes in extracranial brain vessels and manifest CVD were determined by B-mode ultrasound and Doppler examination. Peripheral arterial disease was diagnosed using baseline and stress oscillography. There was a significant increase in plasma fibrinogen, plasminogen, D-dimer, and C-reactive protein with increasing severity of coronary heart disease. Compared with men who had unaffected arteries, men with three diseased coronary arteries had 58% greater D-dimer concentrations. Patients with cerebrovascular disease and peripheral vascular disease also had significantly higher fibrinogen, D-dimer, and C-reactive protein concentrations.

Many of the vascular lesions may also be asymptomatic, emphasizing the potential role of prophylactic screening for vascular lesions in other parts of the vascular tree when an index lesion is identified in a diabetic subject.[34] In a prospective population-based study of Dutch white inhabitants between 50 and 75 years of age, 2484 subjects were screened with respect to glucose tolerance. A group of 173 people with diabetes and a representative age- and sex-stratified sample of 288 nondiabetic subjects were studied in the vascular laboratory. Carotid artery disease was investigated with duplex scanning, and arm and leg artery obstructions were evaluated with real-time frequency analysis of continuous-wave Doppler signals and indirect blood pressure measurements. Comparing diabetic with nondiabetic subjects, the authors found significantly more obstructions of the carotid arteries (8.7% vs. 2.8%), arm arteries (2.3% vs. 0%), and leg arteries (31.8% vs. 18.4%). This was also true only if crural artery obstructions were compared (23.7% vs. 16.0%). More than half the subjects with carotid artery obstructions also had leg artery obstructions.[35]

The same group investigated the cross-sectional association between peripheral arterial disease and glycemic level, age, sex, and glucose tolerance.[36] The prevalence rates of ankle-brachial index (ABI) less than 0.90 were 7.0%, 9.5%, 15.1%, and 20.9% in normal glucose-tolerant, impaired glucose-tolerant, NIDDM, and known diabetic subjects under treatment, respectively (chi-square test for linear trend, $p < 0.01$). Prevalence rates of any peripheral arterial disease (ABI < 0.90, at least one monophasic or absent Doppler flow curve, or vascular surgery) were 18.1%, 22.4%, 29.2%, and 41.8% in these categories (chi-square test for linear trend, $p < 0.0001$). Logistic regression analyses showed that any arterial disease was significantly associated with Hb A_{1c}, fasting, and 2-hour postload plasma glucose after correction for cardiovascular risk factors (OR, 1.35, 1.20, and 1.06, respectively; 95% CI, 1.10 to 1.65, 1.06 to 1.36, and 1.01 to 1.12, respectively). These authors did not find an association between insulin levels and vascular disease.

Diabetes-related peripheral vascular disease remains a huge public health problem.[37] Although rates of lower extremity amputation and arterial reconstruction declined from 1983 to 1992, by 1996, the rate of major amputation had increased 10.6% since 1979. The earlier 12-year decline was positively correlated with reductions in the prevalence of smoking, hypertension, and heart disease, but not diabetes.[38]

Diabetic subjects with peripheral vascular disease are more likely to have small vessel disease of the foot, as well as large vessel disease elsewhere.[39] These findings may contribute to the higher risk for the development of chronic foot ulcers in diabetic patients with peripheral vascular disease. Other independent predictors of amputation include sensory neuropathy and foot ulcers.[40]

Doppler studies using the ABI appear to be as useful in diabetic as in nondiabetic populations for identifying vascular disease, as documented by the Cardiovascular Health Study of 5084 participants.[41] Risk factors associated with an ABI of less than 1.0 in multivariate analysis included smoking (OR, 2.55), history of diabetes (OR, 3.84), increasing age (OR, 1.54), and nonwhite race (OR, 2.36). In the 3372 participants free of clinical coronary vascular disease, other noninvasive measures of subclinical CVD, including carotid stenosis by duplex scanning, segmental wall motion abnormalities by echocardiogram, and major electrocardiographic abnormalities, were inversely related to the ABI (all $p < 0.01$). Therefore, the lower the ABI, the greater the increase in CVD risk; however, even those with modest, asymptomatic reductions in the ABI (0.8 to 1.0) had an increased risk of coronary vascular disease. The ABI Collaboration confirmed these earlier observations.[42] This metaanalysis of 16 cohort populations comprised 24,955 men and 24,339 women. A low ABI (<0.90) predicted vastly increased risks of 10-year cardiovascular mortality in both genders.

The risk for amputation in diabetic subjects appears to parallel the risk for vascular disease in general.[43] A case-control study was conducted among 10,068 patients from a large health maintenance organization at a multiphasic health checkup between 1964 and 1984, with an average length of follow-up after baseline of 13.2 years. Case patients were 150 cohort members with a first nontraumatic lower extremity amputation after baseline. Control subjects were 278 cohort members who did not experience an amputation during follow-up, matched to patients by age, sex, and year of baseline. Level of glucose control ($p < 0.0001$), duration of diabetes ($p = 0.04$), and baseline systolic blood pressure ($p = 0.004$) were independent predictors of amputation, as were microvascular complications (retinopathy, neuropathy, and nephropathy). The observation that type of diabetes (or genetic background) did not predict amputation but that glycemia was predictive lends credence to the "glucose toxicity" hypothesis of vascular risk.

CLINICAL STUDIES OF INTERVENTION

As noted earlier, there seems to be a consensus that there is a relationship between glucose levels and cardiovascular events that shows a dose response within both normal and diabetic populations.[44] There have been several intervention studies that tested the glucose toxicity hypothesis, as well as studies of blood pressure control and lipid control in patients with diabetes mellitus. Table 11-1 summarizes the results of prospective glucose-lowering trials and CVD in people with diabetes mellitus. As can be seen, a significant risk reduction was demonstrated in seven of the eight published trials in type 1 and type 2 diabetes.

A Stockholm study provided convincing evidence that control of glycemia prevents microvascular complications in IDDM.[45] The Diabetes Control and Complications Trial (DCCT) clearly confirmed that tight control decreased the incidence of microvascular complications in IDDM.[46] The DCCT showed a trend of decreased

TABLE 11-1 Glucose-Lowering Trials and Cardiovascular Disease in Diabetes Mellitus

Study	Duration of Trial (yr)	Hb A$_{1c}$ Intense (%)	Hb A$_{1c}$ Control (%)	Treatment	Outcome	Relative Risk Reduction (%)
UKPDS[48]	10	7.0	7.9	Insulin and sulfonylurea	MI	16
UKPDS[49]	10.7	7.4	8.0	Metformin	MI	39
Kumamoto[49a]	6.0	7.1	9.4	Insulin	CV events	46
VACSDM[49b]	2.3	7.1	9.3	Insulin and sulfonylurea	CV events	−40
DIGAMI[47,49c]	1.0	7.1	7.9	Insulin	Mortality	29
Type 1 DM metaanalysis[46]	2-7	7.6	8.7	Insulin	Any event	45
Type 1 DM metaanalysis[46]	2-7	7.6	8.7	Insulin	First event	28

Hb, Hemoglobin; *UKPDS,* United Kingdom Prospective Diabetes Study; *MI,* myocardial infarction; *CV,* cardiovascular; *VACSDM,* Veterans Affairs Cooperative Study on Glycemic Control and Complications in NIDDM; *DIGAMI,* Diabetes and Insulin Glucose Infusion in Acute Myocardial Infarction; *DM,* diabetes mellitus.

TABLE 11-2 Lipid-Lowering Trials and Cardiovascular Disease in Type 2 Diabetes Mellitus

Study	No. of Patients	Follow-up (yr)	Decreased LDL (%)	First Treatment	Outcome	Relative Risk Reduction (%)
Helsinki Heart[54a]	135	5.0	10	Gemfibrozil	CHD death, nonfatal MI	69
WOSCOPS[54b]	76	4.9	26	Pravastatin	CHD death, nonfatal MI	NA
AF/Tex CAPS[54c]	155	5.2	25	Lovastatin	CHD death, nonfatal MI, angina	37
Metaanalysis of primary prevention trials above						55
4S[55]	202	5.5	34	Simvastatin	CHD death, nonfatal MI	55
CARE[56]	586	4.9	27	Pravastatin	CHD death, nonfatal MI	13
LIPID[57]	782	6.1	25	Pravastatin	CHD death, nonfatal MI	19
Metaanalysis of secondary prevention studies above[58]						29

LDL, Low-density lipoprotein; *CHD,* coronary heart disease; *MI,* myocardial infarction; *WOSCOPS,* West of Scotland Primary Prevention Study; *NA,* not available; *AF/Tex CAPS,* Air Force/Texas Coronary Atherosclerosis Prevention Study; *4S,* Scandinavian Simvastatin Survival Study; *CARE,* Cholesterol and Recurrent Events; *LIPID,* Long-Term Intervention with Pravastatin in Ischemic Disease.

incidence of CVD, but the result was not statistically significant. The DCCT was not designed primarily to test the hypothesis that blood glucose control would influence the risk for CVD. The patients were too young and it was too early in the course of their diabetes to expect significant cardiovascular event rates. Nevertheless, 17 initial major cardiovascular events were recorded: 14 in the conventional treatment group and 3 in the intensive treatment group.[47] Total major cardiovascular and peripheral vascular events numbered 40 in the conventional group, compared with 23 in the intensive group. Thus, with intensive treatment, the risk for cardiac events was reduced by 78%, and the risk for combined cardiac and peripheral vascular events was reduced by 42%. As noted earlier, these risk differences did not achieve the defined limits for statistical significance. In contrast, a metaanalysis published in 1999 clearly shows that intervention with intensive glucose control has a beneficial effect on the incidence of the first and any cardiovascular event in type 1 patients (see Table 11-1).[48]

As summarized in Table 11-1,[41-54] the results in persons with type 2 diabetes are even more convincing. Of particular note is the Diabetes and Insulin Glucose Infusion in Acute Myocardial Infarction study, which documented that acute management with intense insulin treatment at the time of myocardial infarction with subsequent insulin therapy has a significant effect on mortality at 1 year. The 1998 publication of the United Kingdom Prospective Diabetes Study reinforced the clinical goal of obtaining Hb A$_{1c}$ values equal to or less than 7% in these patients.

Earlier studies of peripheral vascular risk in IDDM show that an intensive program of glucose control documented by glycosylated hemoglobin and multiple daily blood glucose self-monitoring measures can reverse lesions of the red blood cell, polymorphonuclear leukocyte, platelet, and fluid phase of coagulation associated with diabetes.[55-59] In addition, basement membrane thickening, nerve conduction, and the ABI were found to improve after an 11-month program of intensive glucose control and exercise. In view of the association between the ABI and the risk in diabetic subjects noted earlier, these studies still provide some of the most compelling evidence for programs of glucose control and exercise in persons with diabetes to avoid or even facilitate the reversal of large vessel disease. The goal is to aggressively treat elevated blood glucose and blood pressure and abnormal lipid profiles.

Table 11-2 summarizes the major lipid-lowering trials in patients with type 2 diabetes.[60-63] There are three primary randomized trials for primary prevention and an equal number for secondary prevention of CVD.

TABLE 11-3 **Blood Pressure–Lowering Trials and Cardiovascular Disease in Type 2 Diabetes Mellitus**

Study	Duration of Trial (yr)	BP Intervention (mm Hg)	BP Control (mm Hg)	First Treatment	Outcome	Relative Risk Reduction (%)
UKPDS[49]	9.0	144/82	154/87	Captopril/atenolol	CVD	29
					Stroke	20
					MI	42
SHEP[54c]	4.5	145/70	155/70	Chlorthalidone	CVD	45
					Stroke	26
Syst-Eur[54c]	2.0	153/78	162/82	Nitrendipine	CVD	62
					Stroke	69
HOT[54c]	3.8	140/81	144/85	Felodipine	CVD + stroke	51
ABCD[54c]	5.6	130/80	135/85	Nisoldipine/ enalapril	MI	−12
Overall primary prevention[54c]						38
Cochrane primary prevention[54c]	5.0			Various	CVD mortality and morbidity	30
Cochrane secondary prevention[54c]	>1			Various	CVD mortality and morbidity	11

BP, Blood pressure; *UKPDS,* United Kingdom Prospective Diabetes Study; *CVD,* cardiovascular disease; *MI,* myocardial infarction; *SHEP,* Systolic Hypertension in the Elderly; *Syst-Eur,* Systolic Hypertension in Europe Trial; *HOT,* Hypertension Optimal Treatment; *ABCD,* Appropriate Blood Pressure Control in Diabetes.

Metaanalysis of these trials shows an overall relative risk reduction of 55% for primary prevention and 29% for secondary prevention. The Scandinavian Simvastatin Survival Study also documented the cost-effectiveness of lipid lowering. In persons with coronary heart disease with normal fasting glucose levels, simvastatin reduced the average cost of CVD-related hospitalization by $3585, which offset 60% of the cost of drug. For those with impaired fasting glucose levels, average CVD-related hospitalization costs were reduced by $4478, which offset 74% of the drug cost. For diabetic subjects, there was a net cost savings of $1801 per subject. Current American Diabetes Association guidelines recommend low-density lipoprotein cholesterol targets of less than 2.59 mmol/L (100 mg/dL) for diabetic subjects with one additional cardiovascular risk factor and an intervention level of 3.36 mmol/L (130 mg/dL), with a target of 2.59 mmol/L for all other subjects with diabetes.[56] As shown by the Long-Term Intervention with Pravastatin in Ischemic Disease Study, patients appear to benefit from statin therapy over a wide range of initial lipid levels.

Table 11-3 summarizes the trials of blood pressure lowering in persons with type 2 diabetes.[64-66] As emphasized in a 1998 Cochrane Library review, primary intervention trials indicate a treatment benefit for coronary vascular disease, but not for total mortality in people with diabetes.[66a] For both short- and long-term secondary prevention, there is a benefit for total mortality in persons with diabetes. Most of the published data from randomized, controlled trials of antihypertensive therapy in diabetes for all-cause mortality and CVD outcomes are taken from hypertension trials that are not specific to diabetes.

It has been suggested that it is cost-effective to treat all patients with type 2 diabetes with angiotensin-converting enzyme inhibitors.[65] This approach is reinforced by the publication of the Heart Outcomes Prevention Evaluation, a placebo-controlled study of more than 9000 subjects that indicated that ramipril substantially lowers the risk of death, heart attack, stroke, coronary revascularization, heart failure, and complications related to diabetes mellitus in a high-risk group of patients with preexisting vascular disease. The results are remarkable both for the magnitude of the treatment effect (an overall reduction of 22% in the primary outcome of myocardial infarction, stroke, or death from cardiovascular causes) and for the rather small reduction (3.2 mm Hg) in blood pressure. The authors also noted a marked reduction in the incidence of complications related to diabetes and new cases of diabetes in those taking ramipril.

There has been less enthusiasm for calcium channel blockers in persons with diabetes.[66] Nevertheless, there is evidence that they can be effective as well, as shown in Table 11-3.

Subsequent trials in patients with type 2 diabetes have been designed to examine the role of intensive glycemic control on cardiovascular outcomes have focused on optimal targets of Hb A_{1c}, including levels less than 7%. The Veterans Affairs Diabetes Trial (VADT showed significant reductions in albuminuria with median Hb A_{1c} of 6.9% compared with standard glycemic control in retinopathy and neuropathy.[67,68] The Action in Diabetes and Vascular Disease Preterax and Diamicron Modified Release Controlled Evaluation (ADVANCE) study of intensive versus standard glycemic control in type 2 diabetes found a statistically significant reduction in albuminuria with a target Hb Q_{1c} of 6.5%.[69] The Action to Control Cardiovascular Risk in Diabetes (ACCORD) trial showed lower rates of microvascular complications in the intensive arm compared with the standard arm.[70,71] Early reports from ACCORD of a potential increase in mortality in the intensive care subgroup that could not meet target A1c goals have generated controversies that have yet to be resolved. In the interim, an Hb A_{1c} target of 7% remains the consensus.[72]

EVIDENCE FOR THE INFLUENCE OF GLUCOSE ON THE PATHOPHYSIOLOGY OF VASCULAR DISEASE

Hyperglycemia is associated with vascular disease, as documented earlier. The reasons for this association remain speculative. Box 11-1 documents some of the hypothesized means by which glucose might influence pathologic vascular changes. These factors are discussed here in some detail.

Glycation and Advanced Glycation End Products, or Early and Late Maillard Reactions

In 1976, it became clear that a minor hemoglobin component, Hb A_{1c}, resulted from a posttranslational modification of hemoglobin A by glucose and that there was a clinical relationship between Hb A_{1c} and fasting plasma glucose, the peak on the glucose tolerance test, the area under the curve on the glucose tolerance test, and mean glucose levels over the preceding weeks.[73-76] It soon became apparent that an improvement in ambient blood glucose levels resulted in correction of Hb A_{1c} levels and that these nonenzymatic glycosylation reactions might provide a hypothesis that could explain a number of the pathologic sequelae of diabetes mellitus via toxicity arising from glucose adduct formation with proteins or nucleic acids.[77]

As early as 1912, Maillard[78] suggested that the chemical reactions that now bear his name might play a role in the pathologic changes associated with diabetes mellitus. The ability of reducing sugars to react with the amino

groups of proteins is now widely recognized, as is the natural occurrence of many nonenzymatically glycosylated proteins.

The initial step (or early Maillard reaction) involves the condensation of an amino moiety with the aldehyde form of a particular sugar. Only a small fraction of most common sugars is normally present in the aldehyde form.[78,79] A number of transformations are possible after the addition of an amine to a sugar carbonyl group. Considerable evidence supports the involvement of an Amadori-type rearrangement for the adduct of glucose with the N-terminal of the β chain of hemoglobin. The labile Schiff base aldimine adduct is transformed into a relatively stable ketoamine adduct via the Amadori rearrangement.

Because hemoglobin circulates in its red blood cell for approximately 120 days, there is little opportunity in this cell for late Maillard reactions, or nonenzymatic browning, to occur. In these late Maillard reactions, the Amadori product is degraded into deoxyglucosones that react again with free amino groups to form chromophores, fluorophores, and protein cross-links.[80,81] In tissues that are longer lived, these reactions may be important mediators of diabetic changes as well as the aging process. Although the structure of a large number of nonenzymatic browning products has been elucidated, few have been obtained under physiologic conditions, thus making detection in vivo difficult and their pathologic role uncertain.[82] Box 11-2 summarizes some of the observations and hypotheses whereby glycation might promote pathologic changes in persons with elevated blood glucose.

The Maillard reaction is ubiquitous in nature. The accumulation of advanced glycation end products (AGEs) in tissues in the human body has been implicated in the complications of diabetes, aging, and renal failure. The links between these reactions and the pathogenesis of nephropathy, macroangiopathy, microangiopathy, and cataracts in diabetic subjects are increasingly strong.[83,84] There is a growing body of evidence supporting a connection between circulating and tissue-accumulated AGEs, their receptors, and diabetic complications.

Coagulation Factors

The coagulation cascade has been implicated in diabetes-related complications through disorders of the platelet, fluid phase, and vascular components of clotting. The following sections briefly review the abnormalities in glucose metabolism and their relationship to these factors.

Platelet

The platelet, when obtained from patients with diabetes mellitus, has long been recognized as showing abnormal behavior in in vitro and in vivo studies.[58,59] In general, the correction of hyperglycemia is associated with an improvement in platelet behavior and release. The potential role of the platelet in vascular disease in general is discussed elsewhere in this book. The lesion of the platelet associated with hyperglycemia appears to be related to a hypersensitivity to stimuli. Thus, platelet aggregation in vitro may occur spontaneously by stirring in

---

BOX 11-1   Glucose Toxicity Hypothesis: Hyperglycemia Initiates or Propagates Vascular Disease by Multiple Mechanisms

- Glycation of proteins and genetic material leading to dysfunctional or toxic products
- Interference with the fluid, vascular, and platelet phases of coagulation
- Perturbations in oxidation-reduction pathways
- Production of abnormal lipid metabolism
- Vascular volume shifts associated with changes in glycemia, or intracellular osmotic shifts associated with alternative metabolic pathways invoked when glucose is elevated, are toxic to the vascular tree
- Abnormal insulin or proinsulin levels in response to hyperglycemia contribute to vascular disease
- Perturbations in the immune system, including lymphokine production and polymorphonuclear leukocyte function, contribute to vascular disease

BOX 11-2	Hypotheses Regarding the Potential Role of Nonenzymatic Glycation and Browning in the Pathologic Changes Associated with Diabetes Mellitus

I. Structural proteins
   A. Collagen: decreased turnover, flexibility, solubility, strength; increased aggregating potential for platelets; binding of immunoglobulins; cross-linking; and immunogenicity
   B. Lens crystallina and membrane: opacification, increased vulnerability to oxidative stress
   C. Basement membrane: increased permeability, decreased turnover, increased thickness
   D. Extracellular matrix: changes in binding to other proteins
   E. Hemoglobin: change in oxygen binding
   F. Fibrin: decreased enzymatic degradation
   G. Red blood cell membrane: increased rigidity
   H. Tubulin: cell structure and transport
   I. Myelin: altered structure and immunologic recognition
II. Carrier proteins
   A. Lipoproteins: alternative degradative pathways and metabolism by macrophages and endothelial cells, increased immunogenicity
   B. Albumin: alteration in binding properties for drugs and in handling by the kidney
   C. IgG: altered binding
III. Enzyme systems
   A. Copper-zinc superoxide dismutase: altered redox defense
   B. Fibrinogen: altered coagulation
   C. Antithrombin III: hypercoagulable state
   D. Purine nucleoside phosphorylase: aging of erythrocytes
   E. Alcohol dehydrogenase: substrate metabolism
   F. Ribonuclease A: loss of activity
   G. Cathepsin B: loss of activity
   H. N-acetyl-D-glucosaminidase: loss of activity
   I. Calmodulin: decreased calcium binding
IV. Nucleic acids
   A. Age-related changes, congenital malformations
   B. Epigenetic responses
V. Potentiation of other diseases of postsynthetic protein modification
   A. Carbamoylation-associated disorders in uremia
   B. Steroid cataract formation
   C. Acetaldehyde-induced changes in alcoholism

plasma obtained from persons with Hb A$_{1c}$ greater than 10%, with concomitant release of vasoactive substances including serotonin, adenosine diphosphate, and prostaglandins. The increased functional properties of diabetic platelets result in part from the primary release of larger platelets with enhanced thromboxane formation capacity and increased numbers of the functional glycoprotein (GP) receptors GP Ib and GP IIb/IIIa, which are synthesized in megakaryocytes.[85] Insulin exerts an antiaggregating effect, but that effect is diminished in obese patients and in subjects with NIDDM.[86] Increased platelet aggregation to arachidonic acid has also been linked to reduced antioxidant properties seen in persons with diabetes.[87]

Platelet-rich or fibrin clots are less amenable to lysis in patients with diabetes than in controls.[88] Furthermore, the release of platelet plasminogen activator inhibitor-1 (PAI-1) in whole blood has been found to be increased in NIDDM subjects.[89] PAI-1 levels have been noted to decrease with the lowering of blood glucose in NIDDM[90]; therefore the platelet contributes not only to a prethrombotic state in persons with diabetes, but also to problems of clot lysis in hyperglycemic subjects.

The Evaluation of Platelet IIb/IIIa Inhibitor for Stenting Trial substudy is the most extensive evaluation of stenting and platelet IIb/IIIa blockade in persons with diabetes and provides additional evidence for the role of the platelet in the morbidity and mortality of heart disease and the associated processes in diabetes.[91] The trial involved 491 diabetic patients who were divided into three groups: the first group received both a stent and abciximab, the second group underwent balloon angioplasty and also received the drug, and the third group had a stent implanted but received only a placebo. The reblockage rate was cut in half in the patients who received both the stent and the drug. Those patients had an 8.1% reblockage rate in the 6 months after the procedure, which was about half that of the other two groups. Ongoing trials of eptifibatide and tirofiban should help to determine whether platelet IIb/IIIa receptor blockers should be used routinely to reduce restenosis after stenting in diabetic subjects, as well as the role of activated platelets and endothelium in pathologic conditions. These agents will become more attractive, in part because of the report of thrombotic thrombocytopenic purpura associated with ticlopidine in the setting of coronary artery stents.[92]

Fluid Phase of Coagulation

Fibrinogen is increasingly recognized as a potential cardiovascular risk factor.[93-95] Fibrinogen levels generally have been found to be elevated in diabetes. Fibrinogen synthesis is increased in part because of increased turnover and feedback to the liver with fragment D and because insulin increases fibrinogen synthesis.[96]

Early studies of fibrinogen kinetics in diabetic subjects documented a reversible disorder associated with hyperglycemia that was corrected with normal glucose levels or heparin administration, consistent with a lesion of antithrombin III activity in hyperglycemic subjects.[97,98] These findings were confirmed by the PLAT Group study.[99]

Oxidative stress, which is accentuated in diabetic subjects, has been linked to thrombin activation, and a correlation between markers of oxidative stress and fibrinogen has been reported in diabetic subjects. Thus, oxidative stress, which is mediated by hyperglycemia and compounded by glycation, may represent an additional link between diabetes and hyperfibrinogenemia.[100-102]

Endothelial Phase of Coagulation

Studies indicate that elevated glucose levels can be toxic to vascular endothelial cells through multiple mechanisms.[103] Having observed that glucose levels mimicking diabetic hyperglycemia induce in vitro endothelial cell overexpression of extracellular matrix molecules, decreased replication, and increased levels of transforming growth factor-β (TGF-β) messenger RNA (mRNA), Cagliero and colleagues[103] examined whether the effects of high glucose are mediated by autocrine TGF-β. Whereas the inhibitory effect of high glucose levels on endothelial cell replication was reversible, that of TGF-β was not. Both perturbations induced upregulation of fibronectin expression, but the effects were additive. Thus, there are growth-inhibitory effects of high glucose levels that are independent of TGF-β, and high glucose levels and TGF-β exert their effects through distinct pathways and at different loci.

Pieper and coworkers[104] attempted to evaluate the relative roles of hyperglycemia and insulin lack on endothelial cell dysfunction in diabetes. Rats were continuously infused with glucose or saline for 72 hours to achieve peak plasma glucose concentrations of approximately 25 mM. Plasma insulin rose by twelvefold in glucose-infused rats. Blood pressure was not altered by this intervention. Aortic rings taken from control rats relaxed to the administration of the endothelium-dependent vasodilators acetylcholine and A-23187 and the endothelium-independent vasodilator nitroglycerin. Relaxation to acetylcholine but not to A-23187 or nitroglycerin was impaired in glucose-infused rat aortic rings. Incubation in vitro with either indomethacin or superoxide dismutase did not restore the impaired relaxation to acetylcholine in rings taken from glucose-infused rats. Thus, hyperglycemia with hyperinsulinemia selectively impairs receptor-dependent, endothelium-dependent relaxation. These studies are consistent with the idea that elevated glucose may be a common pathway leading to endothelial dysfunction in IDDM and NIDDM.

Baumgartner-Parzer and associates[105] showed that adhesion molecule gene expression can be modulated by ambient glucose levels as well. These authors found an increase in intercellular adhesion molecule-1, but not platelet endothelial cell adhesion molecule expression in response to a high glucose level in human umbilical vein endothelial cells. These findings are also consistent with the specific abnormalities in endothelial dysfunction occurring in diabetes.

In vivo–generated nitric oxide circulates in plasma mainly as an adduct of serum albumin. Compared with free nitric oxide, this nitric oxide adduct is relatively long-lived and exhibits vasodilating and platelet inhibitory properties. Farkas and Menzel[106] documented that proteins lose their nitric oxide–stabilizing function after advanced glycosylation, thus providing another mechanism by which AGE-modified proteins can potentially promote vascular disease.

Lipids

Hyperlipidemia is a normal concomitant of hyperglycemia. As discussed earlier, both triglyceride and cholesterol levels tend to improve with normalization of blood glucose levels, as documented by ambient glucose levels and glycated hemoglobin levels and glycation of low-density lipoproteins and modification by AGEs leads to

a more atherogenic pattern of lipid metabolism. The presence of renal failure accelerates the pathologic changes associated with the presence of AGEs.[107,108] Thus, improvement in glycemia corrects at least some of the perturbations of lipid metabolism unique to the individual with diabetes.

Oxidation-Reduction Pathways

Both the metabolism of excess glucose and the Amadori rearrangement product resulting from excess glycation can promote prooxidant activity.[109,110] Lipid peroxides are thought to be formed by free radicals and could have an important role in the development of atheromatous vascular disease.

Vascular Volume Shifts

In studies of fibrinogen turnover, it became apparent that it was important to correct for vascular volume shifts induced by changes in glucose. When blood glucose was elevated from 100 to 300 mg/dL, a rise in vascular volume of 8% was documented by double-labeling techniques.[95] The implications for these types of recurrent volume shifts and the resultant stresses on the vascular tree have not been studied. Nevertheless, recent studies confirmed that AIC variability is an independent risk factor for microalbuminuria in 1232 persons with type 1 diabetes.[111]

Insulin Levels

In NIDDM there is thought to be an increased atherogenic potential related to the presence of insulin resistance, hyperinsulinemia, central obesity, and dyslipidemia. This syndrome, formerly known as *syndrome X* or *metabolic syndrome*,[110] was previously called CHAOS (coronary artery disease, hypertension, NIDDM, obesity, stroke) or the "deadly quartet" of upper body obesity, glucose intolerance, hypertriglyceridemia, and hypertension. All were associated with the early development of coronary artery disease. Because of these syndromes, insulin resistance with hyperinsulinemia has been studied as a risk factor for CVD. Perhaps these various entities are best subsumed under the term *prediabetes*.

Immunologic Mechanisms

There are multiple potential interactions of the immune system in the genesis of vascular disease. A number of the cytokine-lymphokine perturbations induced by glycation were discussed earlier. Immune perturbations specific to diabetes and the development of vascular disease have not yet been identified. Because diabetes is heterogeneous and exhibits similar vascular changes despite the cause or the phenotype, it is unlikely that a particular genetic lesion of the immune system will be linked to the accelerated vascular disease seen in diabetes.[112]

One lesion in the immune system of importance to the surgeon is that of the polymorphonuclear leukocyte. The polymorphonuclear leukocyte functions abnormally in a person with hyperglycemia, with decreased adherence, migration, chemotaxis, and killing.[55,113] The lesion of the polymorphonuclear leukocyte reverses within a marrow transit time of 14 days.[55] Therefore the optimal surgical candidate is one who has had normoglycemia for 2 weeks before surgery.

Inflammatory Processes

The Atherosclerosis Risk in Communities study found a role for inflammation and endothelial dysfunction in the pathogenesis of type 2 diabetes.[112,114] It also appears that circulating inflammatory factors such as tumor necrosis factor-α and interleukin-6 may cause insulin resistance and obesity.[112,115] Unlike the polymorphonuclear leucocyte, the macrophage is activated during hyperglycemia. Even modest hyperglycemia is a potent stimulator of monocyte activity even without chemokines.[116]

Smoking

The Speedwell study among others emphasized the critical role of smoking in the genesis of vascular disease, especially in persons with diabetes.[117] Systolic blood pressure, fasting plasma glucose, triglycerides, and white blood cell count were all independently associated with the development of intermittent claudication, angina, and death, but the most striking association was with smoking.

OTHER RISK FACTORS FOR DIABETES- OR HYPERGLYCEMIA-ASSOCIATED VASCULAR DISEASE

Physical Inactivity and Obesity

Over the last few decades, the importance of physical activity for disease prevention and health maintenance has been recognized increasingly. The benefits of exercise and increased physical activity include enhanced insulin sensitivity and glucose effectiveness, decreased risk for hypertension, improved plasma lipids and lipoproteins, decreased obesity and improved body fat distribution, enhanced immunologic function, decreased anxiety and depression, improved sleep, improved psychological characteristics in both normal and psychiatric patients, and disease prevention.[118] As a consequence, new guidelines advocate both cardiovascular and resistance exercise for all persons with diabetes tailored to need.[2]

Obesity and an unfavorable body fat distribution, with increased abdominal fat, are well-established risk factors for diabetes, confounded by ethnicity and family history.[111-121] For obese individuals, the rates of diabetes are higher in Hispanics than in African Americans, and the rates in African Americans are higher than those in whites. Up to 50% of obese Native Americans develop diabetes.[122] Data from the Second National Health and Nutrition Examination Survey revealed that 24.2% of men and 27.1% of women aged 20 to 74 years were overweight (BMI = 27.8 kg/m[2] for men and BMI = 27.3 kg/m[2] for women). It is estimated that there are 34 million overweight adults in the United States, 12.5 million of whom are "severely overweight."[123] Current North American obesity prevalence estimates were compared with estimates from the 1988-1994 NHANES and the 1986-1992 Canadian Heart Health Surveys (CHHS). In both countries, the prevalence of obesity rose significantly since these earlier surveys, and the magnitude of the increases were fairly similar in the two countries. The prevalence rose by approximately 10 percentage points in Canadian men, and the prevalence rose by 12 percentage points among men in the United States. Among women, the increase was approximately 8 percentage points in Canada and approximately 10 percentage points in the United States.[124-131] The obesity epidemic shows little signs of abating along with a concomitant increase in the prevalence of diabetes.

In a study of 8715 men (mean age, 42 years) followed for an average of 8.2 years, the age-adjusted death rate increased with higher levels of fasting glucose, and fit men had a lower age-adjusted all-cause death rate compared with unfit men regardless of glycemic status.[132] Fit men with a fasting blood glucose (FBG) less than 6.4 mM had the lowest age-adjusted death rate (21.4 per 10,000 person-years). Within each class of glycemic status (FBG < 6.4 mM; FBG = 6.4 to 7.8 mM; FBG $\geq$ 7.8 mM, or diagnosed NIDDM), those who were fit had lower mortality rates than those who were unfit. Men who were fit but in the highest glycemic status group had an age-adjusted all-cause mortality rate (45.9 per 10,000 person-years) similar to that of men who were unfit but in the lowest glycemic status group. The data suggest that the risk of death for fit men with an FBG of 7.8 mM or with NIDDM is similar to that of men who are unfit with a normal FBG. The authors suggested that because cardiorespiratory fitness can be improved by regular physical activity, using exercise to improve fitness could be a "cornerstone to the effective management of patients with abnormal blood glucose profiles or NIDDM."[133-135]

No primary prevention projects for NIDDM have used increased physical activity or exercise as the sole intervention for the prevention or deferment of disease.[132-134] Nevertheless, there is evidence of an association between exercise and diabetes from societies that have abandoned a traditional active lifestyle for a more sedentary, modern lifestyle. There is a dramatic increase in NIDDM in people who become more sedentary. Conversely, physically active societies have lower rates of NIDDM than do more sedentary societies.[136-141]

Ethnicity

Ethnic minority populations in the United States have high rates of impaired glucose tolerance (IGT) and are at higher risk for NIDDM.[142] Minorities are especially afflicted with obesity, notably minority women. The age-adjusted percentages of overweight and severely overweight individuals are 24.6% and 9.6%, respectively, for white women, 45.1% and 19.7% for African American women, and 41.5% and 16.7% for Mexican American women. It is acknowledged that although some races tend to be generally heavier than others, without adverse health effects, and that perhaps the norms and standards need to be adjusted for different races, maintaining a normal weight according to the overall population norm was associated with a 23% lower risk of mortality compared with being persistently overweight.

Results from the National Health and Nutrition Examination Survey Epidemiologic Follow-up Study suggest that the higher rate of lower extremity amputations in black compared with white Americans with diabetes is not attributable to biological causes, but rather to a combination of social and environmental factors, including obesity.[142] The findings included an analysis of more than 14,000 people who participated, 2240 of whom had diabetes at baseline or developed it during the study. The authors found that during 20 years of follow-up, the age-adjusted rate of all lower extremity amputations was 2.8-fold higher in black than in white subjects. Diabetes and its duration were strong predictors of risk, as were hypertension, smoking, low educational level, and low socioeconomic status.[143]

The Diabetes Prevention Program (DPP) was a major multicenter clinical research study aimed at discovering whether modest weight loss through dietary changes and increased physical activity or treatment with the oral diabetes drug metformin (Glucophage) could prevent or delay the onset of type 2 diabetes in study participants. At the beginning of the DPP, participants were all overweight and had blood glucose in the prediabetes range. The DPP found that participants who lost a modest amount of weight through dietary changes and increased physical activity sharply reduced their chances of developing diabetes. Taking metformin also reduced risk, although less dramatically.[144]

PROTOCOLS TO IMPROVE GLUCOSE CONTROL BEFORE, DURING, AND AFTER SURGERY

The rationale for maintaining near-normal glucose levels was established earlier. Another consideration for a patient with diabetes who faces surgery is the possibility of hemodynamic instability during anesthesia owing to dehydration and osmotic shifts. In addition, as noted earlier and in a 1999 review,[145] a diabetic patient is more prone to infection,[146] as slower wound healing,[147] and may have increased free fatty acids, the metabolism of which requires greater myocardial oxygen consumption. This section provides guidelines for various situations encountered preoperatively, perioperatively, and postoperatively.

Preparation for Elective Surgery

Ideally, all patients with diabetes should have attained good glucose control before elective surgery. Good glucose control is defined as the glycemic level that provides the optimal setting for elective surgery, minimizes the risk of infection, facilitates healing, and prevents thrombogenesis. The ideal targets for glucose control are 80 to 100 mg/dL before meals and no higher than 180 mg/dL 1 hour after meals. Maintenance of these

glucose targets achieves an Hb A_{1c} level that is associated with the lowest risk of diabetic complications (<7%). Current recommendations for hospitalized patients including those in surgical intensive care units include a blood glucose level target a blood glucose range of 140 to 200 mg/dL.[148,149]

Standing Insulin Orders: Improving Glucose Control in the Hospital

There are now many approaches to maintaining glucose levels during surgery and in the surgical intensive care unit. Many of these are relatively "high tech," with continuous glucose monitoring and insulin infusion systems. The following is intended as a potential approach for the clinician who does not have some of these latter methods available and has been found to be useful in attaining the above target levels of glucose over time.

When a patient with diabetes is admitted to the hospital, the usual outpatient dose of insulin is not appropriate. First, the patient is generally put to bed, with a resultant decrease in insulin requirements of 10% to 20%, depending on his or her usual daily activity level. Second, there is an increased insulin requirement associated with the psychological and physical stress (i.e., infection, trauma, inflammation, surgery) of hospitalization. Therefore the patient's usual dose of insulin generally needs to be adjusted. The only way to arrive at an appropriate dose of insulin is to measure the blood glucose frequently and adjust as needed. Alternatively, the admitting orders could be written to start with a prescription that is near the estimated needs and allow the staff to automatically adjust each insulin dose based on the blood glucose response to that dose.

In the following discussion, a long-acting insulin, neutral protamine Hagedorn (NPH), insulin, and regular insulin are emphasized because of clinicians' long-term familiarity with them. Those interested in newer insulins may wish to consult a 2005 review.[150] Short-acting insulins such as insulin lispro can be substituted for regular insulin; their advantages include a rapid onset of action and peak effect, with less delayed hyperinsulinemia and hypoglycemia.

The protocol for standing insulin orders was designed to go hand in hand with a 40% carbohydrate diet consisting of three meals and three snacks. The diet is generally calculated based on body weight. A general guideline is 30 kcal/kg for malnourished adults, 25 kcal/kg for persons of ideal body weight, and 18 kcal/kg for obese patients.

Calculating the 24-Hour Insulin Requirement

The insulin requirements for increasingly stressful states are listed in Box 11-3. Standing orders (Figure 11-1) start with a default calculation of 0.6 unit/kg per 24 hours in persons who are given nothing by mouth (NPO) orders. This dose is safe and is generally an undercalculation. If, however, it is clear to the admitting physician that 0.6 unit/day is too little, the standing orders state that all handwritten orders will be followed. Thus, it is possible to override the standing orders by writing in

BOX 11-3	Increased Insulin Requirements for Stress

The 24-hour insulin requirement (BIG I) is calculated based on the degree of stress the patient is experiencing:

I = −0.6 units × the patient's weight in kilograms for a person who is healthy and physically active

I = −0.7 units × the patient's weight in kilograms for a person who is premenstrual or is placed on bed rest or who is mildly stressed (whether infectious, physical trauma, or psychological stress)

I = −0.11 to 2.0 units × the patient's weight in kilograms for a person who is moderately to severely stressed. Note that stress doses of steroids may require 1 to 2 units/kg.

Patient's weight: _____ kg
Constant chosen for BIG I: _____
Thus, I = _____ units/24 hr
BIG I is then fractioned into
4/9 I = prebreakfast NPH = _____ units of NPH
2/9 I = prebreakfast reg = _____ units of reg
1/6 I = predinner reg = _____ units of reg
1/6 I = 11 pm NPH = _____ units of NPH

NPH, Neutral protamine Hagedorn (insulin); *reg,* regular insulin.

a higher constant when calculating the 24-hour insulin requirement.

Frequency of Monitoring and Charting Glucose

To ensure that the peak response to insulin and the peak postprandial response to food are monitored, eight blood glucose tests are required each day: before and 1 hour after each meal, before bed, and at 3 AM. These blood glucose levels are charted on the insulin worksheet illustrated in Figure 11-2. The initial calculations of such insulin requirements are written on the worksheet, as are all subsequent insulin changes.

The standing orders allow the nurses to adjust each of the injections daily. The percentage change for the sliding scale is 3% of the total insulin requirement. The sliding scale is adjusted as a percentage of the total dose, because these orders apply to small children as well as obese adults. A 2-unit change to correct for the following day is included to make orders slightly easier to follow, but if a patient is very small or very large, it may be necessary to override the orders and rewrite them, making smaller or larger changes for the subsequent dose.

Automatic Adjustments by Standing Orders

Each dose of insulin is changed as outlined in the established orders (see Figure 11-1) by the nursing staff. The morning dose of NPH insulin is adjusted according to the predinner blood sugar. For example, if the predinner blood sugar is too low, the following morning NPH insulin dose will be decreased by 2 units.

The NPH insulin dose at bedtime requires three blood glucose checks before it can be safely adjusted. The NPH insulin dose before bed is designed to "fix the fasting" or conquer the wake-up blood glucose for the

following morning. Other forces come into play, however, that could make the interpretation of a high fasting blood glucose difficult. There are six ways to acquire a high fasting blood glucose level:

1. Go to bed with a high glucose level because of a persisting high dinner level and stay elevated all night long. The cause is either not enough regular insulin at dinner or too much food at dinner.
2. Go to bed with a normal blood glucose level but have a bedtime snack, which then produces a high wake-up glucose level. This can be avoided by having a smaller bedtime snack.
3. Go to bed with a normal blood glucose level but "drift up" throughout the night because the NPH insulin dose at bedtime was inadequate.
4. Go to bed with a normal blood glucose level, become hypoglycemic in the middle of the night, and wake up with a high level because of the counterregulatory hormonal response to the low blood glucose. The cause is too much bedtime NPH insulin or an inadequate bedtime snack.
5. Go to bed with a high glucose level but still have a hypoglycemic reaction in the middle of the night, mount a counterregulatory response, and wake up with a high glucose level. In this case, the cause is not enough regular insulin at dinner (or too much food at dinner) and too much bedtime NPH insulin.
6. Have a normal bedtime glucose level that stays normal until after 3 AM, when the blood glucose level rises with increasing insulin needs (the dawn phenomenon). More bedtime insulin is needed.

Thus, the adjustment of the bedtime dose of NPH requires all three readings: bedtime, 3 AM, and wake-up blood glucose levels.

If the wake-up blood glucose level is low (<70 mg/dL), decrease the bedtime NPH insulin dose by 2 units. If the wake-up level is high and if the previous night's bedtime and 3 AM levels were also high, the 11 PM NPH insulin dose should be increased by 2 units. If the 3 AM glucose reading is low, no matter what the bedtime or the wake-up blood glucose is, reduce the bedtime dose of NPH insulin. In this case, the physician would need to write separate orders to indicate whether the quantity of food at dinner or at the bedtime snack should be adjusted. The established orders (see Figure 11-1) would also increase the NPH insulin dose before bedtime if the wake-up blood glucose level is high but the bedtime and 3 AM blood glucose levels are normal, because there is room for a little more bedtime NPH insulin to conquer the fasting hyperglycemia.

The 3 AM Touch-up Insulin Dose

One additional order that can speed the normalization process is to prescribe regular insulin at 3 AM. If the blood glucose level is high at 3 AM, it will definitely be high at 7:30 AM because of the dawn-associated rise in counterregulatory hormones. Therefore a convenient and worthwhile addition to these orders is a sliding scale for regular insulin at 3 AM, which is generally the same as the lunchtime touch-up:

☐ 1. Routine: NPH plus regular schedule.

Nursing will calculate and administer the starting dose of insulin as outlined below:

I = 0.6 × weight kg/24 hours divided so that 4/9 of dose is NPH given before breakfast and 1/6 of dose is NPH given before bedtime.

Regular insulin is given before breakfast as 2/9 of dose and before dinner as 1/6 of dose. The regular insulin is titrated on the blood glucose.

0730: NPH = 4/9 dose = _____.

Check last predinner BS:

If the predinner BS is <70, then decrease the AM NPH by 2 units.
If the predinner BS is 71–120, then no change in the AM NPH.
If the predinner BS is >120, then increase the AM NPH by 2 units.

Regular = 2/9 dose =_____ to be adjusted according to the following scale:

BS < 70 =_____ = (2/9 I dose) − 3% of the total insulin requirement.
71–100 =_____ = 2/9 I dose.
101–140 =_____ = (2/9 I dose) + 3% of I.
>141 =_____ = (2/9 I dose) + 6% of I.

If the BS 1 hour after the meal is <110, then decrease the corresponding next-day mealtime regular insulin by 2 units.
If the BS 1 hour after the meal is 111–150, no change in the corresponding next-day mealtime regular insulin.
If the BS 1 hour after the meal is >151, then increase the corresponding next-day mealtime regular insulin by 2 units.

1130 prelunch: Regular insulin is given based on the following scale:

BS < 120 = 0 insulin.
121–140 = 1/181 =_____.
141–180 = 1/181 + 2 units =_____.
>181 = 1/181 + 4 units =_____.

1700 predinner: Regular is 1/6 dose =_____ and based on the following scale:

BS < 70 =_____ = (1/6 I dose) − 3% of I.
71–100 =_____ = 1/6 I dose.
101–140 =_____ = (1/6 I dose) + 3% of I.
>141 =_____ = (1/6 I dose) + 6% of I.

If the BS 1 hour after the meal is <110, then decrease the corresponding next-day mealtime regular insulin by 2 units.
If the BS 1 hour after the meal is 111–150, no change in the corresponding next-day mealtime regular insulin.
If the BS 1 hour after the meal is >151, then increase the corresponding next-day mealtime regular insulin by 2 units.

2330 bedtime NPH: Give 1/6 dose =_____.

If the prebreakfast BS is <70, then decrease the bedtime NPH by 2 units.
If the prebreakfast BS is 71–120, then no change in the bedtime NPH.
If the prebreakfast BS is >121, then check the last HS and 3 AM BS:

If the HS, 3 AM, and prebreakfast BS are >121, then increase the bedtime NPH by 2 units.
If the 3 AM BS is <70 (regardless of the HS or prebreakfast BS), decrease the bedtime NPH by 2 units.
If the HS and the 3 AM BS are 70–120, but the prebreakfast is >121, then increase the bedtime NPH by 2 units.

NOTE: ALL ORDERS CHECKED OR HANDWRITTEN WILL BE FOLLOWED

Physician's signature   Date   Time

FIGURE 11-1 ■ Standing orders for insulin for hospitalized diabetic patients. *BS,* Blood sugar; *HS,* hour of sleep; *NPH,* neutral protamine Hagedorn.

- BS < 120 = 0
- BS 121 to 140 = 1/18 I
- BS 141 to 180 = 1/18 I + 2 units
- BS > 181 = 1/18 I + 4 units

where *BS* is blood sugar and *I* is total insulin dose per 24 hours.

It is worth noting that bedtime regular insulin is dangerous. Between the hours of 11 PM and 3 AM, patients are more sensitive to regular insulin because of low levels of counterregulatory hormones. It is generally preferable to leave a high bedtime glucose level untreated, but wake the patient at 3 AM and give regular

DATE											
0300 Blood glucose											
BREAKFAST	AC Basal NPH insulin										
	AC Regular insulin										
	<70 =										
	71–100 =										
	101–140 =										
	>140 =										
	AC Blood glucose	AC	PC	AC	PC	AC	PC	AC	PC	AC	PC
LUNCH	AC Regular insulin										
	<120 =										
	121–140 =										
	141–180 =										
	>180 =										
	AC Blood glucose	AC	PC	AC	PC	AC	PC	AC	PC	AC	PC
DINNER	AC Regular insulin										
	<70 =										
	71–100 =										
	101–140 =										
	>140 =										
	AC Blood glucose	AC	PC	AC	PC	AC	PC	AC	PC	AC	PC
2330 Blood glucose											
2330 Basal NPH insulin											
COMMENTS											
INITIALS											

FIGURE 11-2 ■ Insulin worksheet for charting blood glucose levels. *AC,* Before meal; *PC,* after meal; *NPH,* neutral protamine Hagedorn.

insulin at that time if the blood glucose is still elevated.

Hypoglycemia Prevention

Although the standing orders for insulin begin with 0.6 unit/kg per 24 hours, which is most likely an undercalculation, it is always best to pair this protocol with a protocol for hypoglycemia. Suggested hypoglycemia orders are given in Box 11-4.

Deriving the "Personal Lag Time" for Insulin Action

At times, the health care professional may actually create brittle diabetes. All that may be needed is an injection of

BOX 11-4	Standing Orders for Hypoglycemia

Routine: nursing staff will carry out the protocol outlined below:

1. For BS < 60 mg/dL:
   Give 8 oz milk and recheck BS in 15 min.
2. For symptomatic BS < 60 mg/dL:
   Give 8 oz milk and recheck BS in 15 min.
   If BS is still <60 mg/dL, give another 8 oz milk and recheck BS in 15 min.
   If BS is still <60 mg/dL, give 8 oz orange juice and a slice of bread.
3. If the patient is unable to take fluids, lethargic, or argumentative:
   Give 0.15 mg glucagon SC and recheck BS in 10 min.
   If BS is still <60 mg/dL, give another 0.15 mg glucagon SC and recheck BS in 10 min.
   Once BS is >60 mg/dL but <120 mg/dL and patient is able to hear, give 8 oz milk.
4. When patient is unresponsive:
   Give 1.0 mg glucagon IM and call the physician.
   Check BS in 10 min. If patient is still unresponsive, start IV catheter line of 1000 mL D_{10} to run wide open.
   Recheck BS in 10 min; turn down IV catheter to 100 mL/hr when BS is >80 mg/dL.

BS, Blood sugar; D_{10}, 10% dextrose in water; *IV,* intravenous; *SC,* subcutaneous.

regular insulin at the moment the meal is ingested. The simple sugars in foods peak as sugar in the bloodstream in 15 to 20 minutes. Complex carbohydrates peak as sugar in the bloodstream in 60 minutes.

Regular insulin injected under the skin requires approximately 45 minutes before an effect can be documented in terms of a decrement in blood glucose. The hypoglycemic action of the injected insulin does not peak for 2 to 3 hours. The result is that after an injection of insulin given at the same time as a meal with a fairly large percentage of calories as carbohydrate, blood glucose peaks approximately 1 hour after the start of the meal, and the patient is hypoglycemic at 3 hours, concomitant with the peak in insulin action. Such an occurrence might be referred to as *iatrogenic reactive hypoglycemia.* Counterregulatory hormones secreted (and extra food ingested) in response to the hypoglycemia lead to a marked rise in glucose (usually 250 to 350 mg/dL) approximately 3 hours later, which in turn prompts the need for additional insulin.

To convert this type of brittle diabetes into a smoother glycemic profile, it is necessary to change the timing of the injection of regular insulin in relationship to the meal. Increasing the lag time between the insulin injection and the ingestion of food can dampen glycemic excursions despite no change in meal plan or dose of insulin. The usual optimal lag time for abdominal injections is 30 to 40 minutes. The usual lag time for leg injections of regular insulin is 40 to 50 minutes. The use of shorter acting insulins have markedly decreased the need for a lag time calculation.

Several approaches can shorten the lag time between insulin injection and action. First, insulin lispro has a rapid peak and rapid disposal compared with regular insulin. Thus, it can be given when food arrives or even after ingestion of a meal, with calculation of the ingested carbohydrate. Second, the warmer the skin temperature, the faster the insulin is absorbed. A hot washcloth placed over the injection site accelerates absorption. Third, muscle activity at the site of injection shortens lag time. Thus, exercise can speed insulin absorption.

Suggested Sliding Scale for Insulin

A simple way to think about insulin action is to assume that hypoglycemia increases insulin sensitivity and hyperglycemia increases insulin resistance. Therefore, a premeal sliding scale for regular insulin might include not only a scale of graded doses of insulin but also a scale of lag times for beginning the meal after the injection. In practice, it is often prudent on a busy inpatient ward to await the arrival of food before injecting insulin, to avoid hypoglycemia. As noted earlier, the use of insulin lispro obviates the problem.

Nothing by Mouth Orders

Compliance with NPO orders might be simpler if all patients used an insulin infusion pump; then the patient merely skips the breakfast bolus and maintains the basal infusion of insulin. However, this advice presupposes that the patient is on a perfectly calculated basal infusion of insulin (the dose of insulin that keeps the patient normoglycemic during fasting). Unfortunately, the basal infusion rate is often adjusted higher than the basal need in order to provide extra insulin to cover extra calories or foods that convert slowly to glucose (e.g., protein and high-fiber carbohydrates). Thus, even well-controlled patients using a pump may need to be instructed to decrease the basal infusion rate by 20% for as long as they are NPO or to adjust the calculated basal infusion to 0.25 unit/kg per 24 hours, whichever is lower. A good starting point is 0.3 unit/kg per 24 hours as a basal constant infusion. The blood glucose is measured before bed, at 3 AM, at 7 AM, and every 2 hours thereafter. These frequent checks allow one to increase or decrease the basal rate or to "touch up" with insulin, intravenous (IV) glucose, or glucagon, as needed.

If a patient is on an NPH insulin system, the doses during the fasting period are calculated (0.1 × Weight [kg]) to be given every 8 hours that the patient is NPO. The blood glucose should be measured at midnight, 3 AM, 8 AM, and then every 2 hours until the operation. If the blood glucose is elevated, touch-up doses of regular insulin, similar to the ultralente insulin protocol, may be given.

If the patient is hospitalized and an IV catheter is started, hypoglycemia and hyperglycemia can be avoided with IV infusions at 2 mL/kg per hour based on blood glucose checks every hour (during the procedure and recovery) or every other hour. The guidelines for maintaining normoglycemia on IV infusion are outlined in Table 11-4.

TABLE 11-4 **Guidelines for Intravenous Infusion Based on Blood Glucose Values**

Blood Glucose (mg/dL)	Infusion at 2 mL/kg/hr
<70	D_{10}
70-120	D_5
>120	Normal saline
>150	Use touch-up IV insulin (0.02 unit) while normal saline is continued at 2 mL/kg/hr and adjust rate based on hourly readings

D_5, 5% Dextrose in water; D_{10}, 10% dextrose in water; *IV*, intravenous.

These algorithms for the maintenance of normoglycemia during periods of fasting are essentially the same as those used to prescribe a true basal insulin dose or the dose of insulin that maintains normal blood glucose levels in a person with IDDM when he or she does not eat. Extra insulin may be needed during periods of increasing stress, such as surgery. Nevertheless, these guidelines and the surveillance system provide a relatively simple and safe approach to managing insulin doses during fasting for patients with IDDM or NIDDM.

Enteral and Parenteral Nutrition in Diabetic Patients

Given a severely stressful situation, or after the administration of high-dose corticosteroids, the population estimated to be frankly hyperglycemic rises to more than 25% (referred to as *stress-induced diabetes*). Furthermore, when highly concentrated glucose solutions are given intravenously during stressful situations, the percentage of hyperglycemic individuals rises to more than 50%.[151] It can be seen that a significant number of surgical patients require additional attention to enteral and parenteral nutrition because of elevated blood glucose values if optimal glucose levels are to be maintained.

Enteral Route

There are multiple formulas for tube feeding. They differ by protein concentration and composition, density, fat, and carbohydrate percentage. These basic formulas contain 45% to 60% carbohydrates. The elemental formulas contain low residue and thus are completely absorbed from the jejunum. These elemental diets have more than 70% carbohydrates and sugars. Corn syrup is usually the carbohydrate used. There are two formulas with a low percentage of carbohydrates: one is for pulmonary patients to help lower the respiratory quotient (28% carbohydrates); the other is designed for diabetic patients, with 38% high-fiber carbohydrates. The carbohydrate content of the formula directly affects the blood glucose level achieved; the lower the carbohydrate content of a formula, the lower the resultant blood glucose level. If hyperglycemia is documented by blood glucose determinations every 4 hours, insulin can be given as a constant IV infusion or subcutaneously. One

BOX 11-5 | **Enteral Nutrition: Normal Fasting for Patients with Normal Glucose Tolerance and for Patients with Non–Insulin-Dependent Diabetes Mellitus and Normal Fasting Glucose without Insulin**

1. Monitor fingerstick blood glucose every 6 hours for 2 days. If all glucose levels remain <180 mg/dL, the frequency of monitoring may be decreased to once a day.
2. If hyperglycemia occurs, continue to monitor blood glucose every 6 hours and proceed to Step 3.
3. Begin insulin as a continuous infusion while the enteral nutrition is being infused: 1 unit of regular insulin for every 10 g of carbohydrate in the feeding.
4. Based on the blood glucose level every 6 hours, change the insulin dose for tomorrow as follows:
   ≤80: decrease ratio (0.5 unit/10 g carbohydrate)
   81-180: no change in ratio (1.0 unit/10 g carbohydrate)
   ≥181: increase ratio (1.5 units/10 g carbohydrate)

unit of regular insulin per 10 g of carbohydrate is given over 24 hours in the formula. Box 11-5 summarizes the protocol for blood glucose monitoring and initiating insulin therapy in a nondiabetic patient.

If a patient with known NIDDM has a normal fasting blood glucose level before the enteral infusion is started, the patient can be given insulin with the enteral infusion at a dose of 1 unit of regular insulin for every 10 g of carbohydrate given over 24 hours (Figure 11-3). Most severely stressed NIDDM patients have fasting hyperglycemia even if their interim fasting glucose levels are normal. In the majority of cases, NIDDM patients require both a 24-hour basal insulin infusion, calculated as 0.3 units of regular insulin multiplied by the patient's weight in kilograms, and the meal requirement, which is 1 unit of regular insulin for every 10 g of carbohydrate in the formula (Box 11-6).

IDDM patients who require enteral nutrition may also be given insulin for their basal and formula-related needs (see Box 11-6). If the patient is severely ill or is also taking glucocorticoids, the basal insulin dose can be calculated as 1 unit/kg body weight, and the formula-related insulin dose can start at 1 unit per 10 g carbohydrate. The blood glucose should be checked every 4 to 6 hours; if it is elevated, additional regular insulin can be given subcutaneously by the floor nursing staff, using the following scale:

- BS < 180 = no extra regular insulin
- BS 181 to 240 = 6 units regular insulin
- BS 241 to 300 = 8 units regular insulin
- BS ≥ 301 = 10 units regular insulin

If the blood glucose level is between 80 and 180 mg/dL, no change in the carbohydrate ratio is necessary. If the blood glucose level is less than 80 mg/dL, the ratio may be decreased to 0.5 unit regular insulin per 10 g carbohydrate. If the blood glucose level is greater than

ENTERAL NUTRITION ORDER

DATE AND TIME			
	1. FEEDING TUBE:		
	☐ Nasogastric ☐ Nasoduodenal ☐ Gastrostomy ☐ Jejunostomy		
	Feeding tube: Type _____ French Size _____		
	☐ Abdominal x-ray to confirm tube placement and termination point prior to		
	feeding initiation.		
	2. FORMULA:	**DESCRIPTION**	**INDICATIONS**
	ISOTONIC (1 kcal/mL)		
	☐ Jevity	Contains fiber	Normal bowel function
	☐ Glucerna	Low carbohydrate	Abnormal glucose tolerance
	☐ Osmolite HN	High nitrogen	Low intestinal residue
	HYPERTONIC (1.5 kcal/mL)		
	☐ Ensure Plus	High calorie	Increased caloric needs, volume restriction
	☐ Pulmocare	High fat/Low carbohydrate	Respiratory failure
	ELEMENTAL (1 kcal/mL)		
	☐ Vital HN	Hydrolyzed	Impaired GI function
	OTHER:		
	3. DELIVERY:		
	METHOD: ☐ Continuous Other:		
	STRENGTH: ☐ Full ☐ 3/4 ☐ 1/2 Other:		
	RATE/FEEDING SCHEDULE: ☐ 25 mL/hr ☐ 50 mL/hr Other: _____ mL/hr		
	Increase rate to _____ mL/hr after _____ hrs		
	Other feeding schedule:		
	ADDITIONAL WATER: Total additional water volume, including		
	flushes/medications, to be _____ mL/24 hr.		
	Briskly irrigate tubing with 30 mL water BEFORE and AFTER		
	medication administration or if feeding is interrupted for more		
	than 5 minutes.		
	4. MONITORING:		
	GASTRIC RESIDUALS: Check residuals every _____ hrs. If greater than _____ mL,		
	hold feeding for _____ hr(s). Recheck residual. Restart		
	feeding at _____ mL/hr, when residual less than _____ mL.		
	EXAMPLE: For 50 mL/hr, check residual q 4 hr and hold if 200 mL.		
	WEIGHT: ☐ Weigh patient on intiation of feeding and M/W/F.		
	5. LABORATORY: ☐ CHEM 20 AND TRANSFERRIN NOW AND WEEKLY		
	OTHER LABORATORY:		
	DATE TIME SIGNATURE		
	NOTE: ALL ORDERS CHECKED OR HANDWRITTEN WILL BE FOLLOWED		

FIGURE 11-3 ■ Enteral nutrition order form for diabetic patients.

180 mg/dL, the insulin-carbohydrate ratio should be increased to 1.5 units per 10 g carbohydrate (Box 11-7).

Intravenous Parenteral Nutrition

Most normal, healthy persons become hyperglycemic if they are given IV solutions with a concentration of 20% dextrose (D_{20}) or more. For a person with normal glucose tolerance, only the dextrose load needs to be covered with insulin, at a dose of 1 unit regular insulin per 10 g dextrose. For example, if 500 g of dextrose is infused over 24 hours (usually 2.5 L of a 20% dextrose solution),

50 units of regular insulin may be placed in the dextrose solution to be infused over 24 hours. The blood glucose should be checked every 4 to 6 hours and extra regular insulin should be given as detailed earlier. The dose of insulin for the following day can be adjusted based on blood glucose levels: if the blood glucose level is 80 to 180 mg/dL, no change in the ratio of 1 unit regular insulin per 10 g dextrose is necessary; if the blood glucose is less than 80 mg/dL, the ratio can be decreased to 0.5 units per 10 g dextrose; if the blood glucose level is greater than 180 mg/dL, the ratio may be increased to 1.5 units per 10 g dextrose. If a patient remains

BOX 11-6	Enteral Nutrition for Patients with Known Non–Insulin-Dependent Diabetes and Elevated Fasting Glucose

1. Monitor blood glucose every 6 hours.
2. Begin enteral nutrition and insulin infusion at the same time.
3. Insulin infusion is calculated as the sum of the basal and carbohydrate-related need.
   Basal need is dependent on stress level and weight:

STRESS LEVEL	UNITS OF REGULAR INSULIN
Mild	0.3 × Weight (kg)
Moderate	0.5 × Weight (kg)
Severe	1.0 × Weight (kg)
Steroid therapy (maximum doses) regardless of degree of illness	1.0 × Weight (kg)

   Carbohydrate-related need: 1 unit regular insulin for every 10 g carbohydrate in enteral nutrition.
4. Adjustment for tomorrow's dose: the insulin-carbohydrate ratio is changed based on today's blood glucose levels:
   ≤80: decrease ratio (0.5 unit/10 g carbohydrate)
   81-180: no change in ratio (1.0 unit/10 g carbohydrate)
   ≥181: increase ratio (1.5 units/10 g carbohydrate)

BOX 11-7	Intravenous Nutrition for Patients with Normal Glucose Tolerance and Patients with Non–Insulin-Dependent Diabetes Mellitus and Normal Fasting Blood Glucose

1. Monitor blood glucose every 6 hours for 2 days and then twice per day as long as blood glucose remains normal.
2. If hyperglycemia occurs, continue to monitor every 6 hours.
3. Regular insulin may be given SC every 6 hours for the immediate treatment of hyperglycemia:
   ≤180: 0 units
   181-240: 6 units
   241-300: 8 units
   ≥301: 10 units
4. Begin with an IV solution containing 1 unit of regular insulin for every 10 g of dextrose in the bag.
5. Adjust tomorrow's insulin dose based on today's blood glucose levels, as follows:
   ≤80: decrease ratio (0.5 unit/10 g carbohydrate)
   81-180: no change in ratio (1.0 unit/10 g carbohydrate)
   ≥181: increase ratio (1.5 units/10 g carbohydrate)

SC, Subcutaneous; *IV*, intravenous.

hyperglycemic while receiving 500 g of dextrose over 24 hours despite 50 units of insulin, the insulin dose may be increased to 75 units of regular insulin for 500 g dextrose (1.5 units per 10 g dextrose; Box 11-8 and Figure 11-4).

For the patient with fasting hyperglycemia before parenteral nutrition is started, a basal insulin need must be added to the dextrose-insulin–related need. The basal dose depends on body weight, severity of illness, and the administration of steroids. Boxes 11-7 and 11-8 list the incremental increase in insulin response with increasing need in NIDDM. The dextrose-related need must be added to the basal need for all diabetic patients.

The parenteral solutions may have both the basal insulin need and the dextrose need placed in the bottles to be infused over 24 hours. The three-in-one bags contain an entire day's nutritional needs in one bag. In addition, the day's insulin requirement (basal plus dextrose-related needs) can all be put in one bag.

There is a product available for peripheral nutrition that substitutes dextrose with glycerol. Because glycerol does not require insulin for metabolism, this product (ProcalAmine, B Brawn and Co., Inine, CA) does not raise the blood glucose level of diabetic patients.

In summary, prevention and treatment of hyperglycemia in up to 50% of all patients given parenteral or enteral nutrition is necessary to optimize care in the severely ill patient. The protocols outlined here are designed to monitor and avoid potentially dangerous iatrogenic hyperglycemia.

BOX 11-8	Intravenous Nutrition for Patients with Insulin-Dependent Diabetes Mellitus and Patients with Non–Insulin-Dependent Diabetes Mellitus and Fasting Hyperglycemia

1. Monitor blood glucose every 6 hours.
2. Begin intravenous solution and insulin together in the same bag.
3. Insulin dose is calculated as the sum of the basal and the dextrose-related insulin needs.
   Basal need is dependent on stress level and weight:

STRESS LEVEL	UNITS OF REGULAR INSULIN
Mild	0.3 × weight (kg)
Moderate	0.5 × weight (kg)
Severe	1.0 × weight (kg)
Steroid therapy (maximum doses) regardless of degree of illness	1.0 × weight (kg)

   Dextrose-related need: 1 unit regular insulin for every 10 g dextrose in the infusion solution.
4. Adjustment for tomorrow's dose: the insulin-carbohydrate ratio is changed based on today's blood glucose levels:
   ≤80: decrease ratio (0.5 unit/10 g carbohydrate)
   81-180: no change in ratio (1.0 unit/10 g carbohydrate)
   ≥181: increase ratio (1.5 units/10 g carbohydrate)

TOTAL PARENTERAL NUTRITION ORDER FORM

ADMINISTER OVER 24 HOURS: ALL TPN SOLUTIONS WILL BEGIN AT 1800 HOURS DAILY.
ALL CHANGES, ADDITIONS, OR DELETIONS <u>MUST</u> BE RECEIVED BY 1400 HOURS.

1. Select One Only:

☐ **Custom** FORMULA AND RATE   **or**   ☐ **Standard** FORMULA (SET RATES DO NOT CHANGE)

CUSTOM: PER DAY

Usual requirements:	
Total daily kcals:	25%–35 kcal/kg/day
Protein: 1–2 g/kg or	10%–15% of total kcal
Dextrose:	45%–55% of total kcal
Lipids:	25%–35% of total kcal

PROTEIN: (4 kcal/g)	g/day
DEXTROSE: (3.4 kcal/g)	kcal/day
LIPIDS: (10 kcal/g)	kcal/day

RATE: (for custom only) _____ mL/hr

Start at _____ mL/hr for 4 hours, then increase to rate above.

NOTE: TPN typically requires 2–3 liters.
Call pharmacy at ext. XXXX for LEAST POSSIBLE
VOLUME, or assistance.

STANDARD: PER DAY

☐ PERIPHERAL	2.4 L	1652 kcal
Protein 3.5%	84 g	336 kcal
Dextrose 10%	240 g	816 kcal
Lipids 20% 250 mL	50 g	500 kcal
Total Volume = 2400 mL	**Rate: 100 mL/hr**	

☐ CENTRAL	2 L	1564 kcal
Protein 3.5%	70 g	280 kcal
Dextrose 13%	260 g	884 kcal
Lipids 20% 200 mL	40 g	400 kcal
Total Volume = 2000 mL	**Rate: 83 mL/hr**	
*** for 50-kg patient (30 kcal/kg)		

☐ CENTRAL	2.4 L	2214 kcal
Protein 4.25%	102 g	408 kcal
Dextrose 16%	384 g	1306 kcal
Lipids 20% 250 mL	50 g	500 kcal
Total Volume = 2400 mL	**Rate: 100 mL/hr**	
*** for 70-kg patient (30 kcal/kg)		

☐ Delete lipids
☐ Start at 50 mL/hr for 4 hr

2. Select Additives FOR ALL TPN
(BOTH CUSTOM AND STANDARD)

ADDITIVES: PER DAY

mark this box for standard additives ⟶			Custom and/or additional orders
Item	Range	☐ ⟵	
NaCl	60–150	20	mEq/day
Na Acetate		50	mEq/day
Na Phosphate	10–25 mM	12	mM/day
K Phosphate		✕	mM/day
K Acetate		✕	mEq/day
KCl	40–80	40	mEq/day
MgSO$_4$	15–30	10	mEq/day
Ca Gluconate	9–18	9	mEq/day
Vitamins [MVI–12]	10 mL	10	mL/day
Trace elements	3 mL	3	mL/day
Reg insulin 1 U/10 g or 3 U/100 kcal dextrose (if diabetic add 0.3 U/kg)		✕	U/day
Heparin 1000 U/L	2–3000 U	✕	U/day
Folic acid	1 mg	✕	mg/day
Vit. K 10 mg Monday to MWF	1–3x wk	✕	mg/day every Monday
OTHER:_____			

3. MONITORING:

☐ Glucose monitoring Q6H × 5D, then BID.
☐ Renal panel, phosphorus, and magnesium
  ordered daily × 3, then MWF.
☐ Serum transferrin, CHEM 20
  ordered now and 1 week after start of TPN.
☐ Triglycerides now and 48 hrs after start of TPN.
☐ Daily weights.
☐ Other:_____

NOTE HOSPITAL POLICY:

• Dextrose 10% will replace TPN during
  interruptions at same rate.
• Nutrition Support Team (NST) will provide
  basic assessment and monitoring.
• For new orders received by pharmacy after 1800,
  Standard Peripheral TPN formula will be used until
  1800 the following day per physician approval. Rate
  and additives will remain as ordered.

_____   _____
Physician signature   Date

FIGURE 11-4 ■ Intravenous parenteral nutrition order form for diabetic patients.

Matching Insulin to Food

The correlation of postprandial glucose to percentage carbohydrate in a fixed caloric meal is excellent for the dinner meal and quite good for breakfast and lunch. The amount of insulin required to cover carbohydrate in the evening meal is approximately 1.0 unit per 10 g carbohydrate and for breakfast, about 1.5 units per 10 g carbohydrate. The amount of insulin required to cover lunch usually falls between that required to cover breakfast and dinner. Nevertheless, the above ratios are approximations. An insulin-to-carbohydrate ratio for each meal is ideally established for each patient. The advantage in developing the skill of matching insulin and carbohydrate lies in the freedom to vary meal composition. It is useful not only for persons on an insulin pump, but also for patients on a fixed meal plan if they choose to eat out or vary the meal plan. If an individual knows that an ingested meal is going to exceed the normal carbohydrate quota for a meal, an upward adjustment in the insulin dose may be made by calculating the extra insulin needed from the number of grams of carbohydrate to be ingested above the established quota of the prescribed diet. The approach is equally useful when calories and carbohydrate are eliminated from a meal or diet as might occur in a weight-loss program. Out patient management protocols are being updated continually by the American Diabetes Association.[2]

References available online at expertconsult.com.

QUESTIONS

1. Which of the following statements most accurately reflects the course of diabetic patients following the discovery of insulin?
   a. Life expectancy is longer.
   b. Mortality from coma and sepsis is decreased.
   c. Mortality from vascular disease is increased.
   d. Control of glucose prevents microvascular and macrovascular disease.
   e. All of the above.

2. Abnormal glucose tolerance or diabetes is found more frequently in which of the following?
   a. Relatives of a person with diabetes
   b. Hispanic and black minorities
   c. Women with a history of gestational diabetes
   d. The obese and unfit
   e. All of the above

3. Which statement is most accurate?
   a. Diabetes is a single known genetic disease.
   b. Diabetes is characterized by low insulin levels.
   c. A person with diabetes may be at excess risk for vascular disease because of both increased insulin levels and increased glucose levels.
   d. Diabetes in pregnancy does not increase the risk of eye disease.

4. Which of the following statements is not true?
   a. Diabetic patients tend to have a higher prevalence of stroke, myocardial infarction, and peripheral vascular disease.
   b. Diabetic patients tend to have more diffuse large vessel disease.
   c. The most likely cause of death in a person with diabetes is vascular disease.
   d. Most cardiovascular deaths in persons with diabetes are the result of microvascular disease.

5. Which of the following statements regarding stroke is not true?
   a. Nonfasting serum glucose predicts outcome, including speed of recovery and mortality.
   b. Women are less vulnerable to the increased vascular risk associated with hyperglycemia than men.
   c. Systolic and diastolic blood pressures predict risk in diabetic patients.
   d. Cholesterol and body mass index are risk factors for stroke.
   e. Glycosylated hemoglobin predicts risk.
   f. Persons with diabetes are at increased risk for thrombotic but not hemorrhagic stroke.

6. Which statement is not true?
   a. The risk of cardiovascular disease is twofold to threefold higher in persons with diabetes than in nondiabetic subjects.
   b. The risk of vascular disease associated with diabetes is secondary to obesity, lipid disorders, and increased blood pressure, but not diabetes per se.
   c. The increased prevalence of congestive heart failure in diabetic patients with coronary artery disease has been attributed to microvascular disease and autonomic dysfunction.
   d. Large vessel disease in one area of the vascular tree predicts disease in other areas as well.
   e. Many vascular lesions in persons with diabetes are asymptomatic.

7. Which of the following statements is not true?
   a. The ABI is not a good screening tool for persons with diabetes.
   b. Intervention studies in persons with diabetes have shown improvement in the ABI after 9 months of normoglycemia and exercise.
   c. The prevalence of foot ulcers in diabetic patients with peripheral vascular disease is increased in part by problems with the microcirculation and neuropathy.
   d. Glucose control, blood pressure, and duration of diabetes are all independent predictors of amputation.

8. Which of the following probably contributes to vascular disease in hyperglycemic subjects?
   a. Glycation and advanced glycation end products
   b. Perturbations in the fluid phase of coagulation
   c. Increased reactivity of the platelet
   d. Endothelial cell dysfunction
   e. Increased oxidative stress
   f. Vascular volume shifts
   g. All of the above

9. Which of the following statements is most accurate regarding the indications for vascular reconstruction in a diabetic patient?
   a. It should be performed primarily for limb salvage rather than claudication.
   b. It should be avoided in subjects with severe neuropathy.
   c. It should be performed less frequently because of poorer outcome statistics.
   d. It should be performed for the same indications in diabetic and nondiabetic patients.

10. Physiologic blood glucose control with careful glucose monitoring before, during, and after surgery is important for which of the following reasons?
    a. To minimize the risk of infection
    b. To increase wound healing and strength
    c. To avoid hypoglycemia
    d. To minimize the risk of a prothrombotic state
    e. All of the above

ANSWERS

1. **e**
2. **e**
3. **c**
4. **d**
5. **b**
6. **b**
7. **a**
8. **g**
9. **d**
10. **e**

CHAPTER 12

MEDICAL MANAGEMENT OF VASCULAR DISEASE INCLUDING PHARMACOLOGY OF DRUGS USED IN VASCULAR DISEASE MANAGEMENT

Jessica B. O'Connell • Jonathan Bath • Todd D. Reil

Arterial disease is the leading cause of death and significant morbidity in the United States and throughout the world. The American Heart Association estimates that 80 million (36.3%) Americans have cardiovascular disease, leading to 864,500 deaths annually.[1a] Patients with peripheral arterial disease (PAD) compose a significant proportion of this group, including 795,000 Americans who will have strokes each year. Stroke itself is the third leading cause of death in the United States, with an estimated 143,600 patients dying each year. Those who survive often have significant neurologic deficits that can become major social and economic burdens to the patients and their families.

PAD is a significant public health issue because of the need for extensive long-term care for patients with these serious disabilities and because much of atherosclerosis and therefore PAD is preventable or diminishable by avoiding tobacco, fatty foods, and taking medications regularly to control hypertension, diabetes, and hyperlipidemia. Although we now have excellent diagnostic modalities that can help to identify patients at risk for atherosclerosis, along with well-planned preventative strategies, patients are often still reluctant to make the necessary lifestyle modifications. It is estimated that for 2009, the total direct and indirect cost of cardiovascular diseases and stroke in the United States was $475.3 billion.[1a]

In this chapter, we will discuss the risk factors for development of atherosclerosis and the clinical relevance of the disease, discuss preventative modalities and evolving medical treatments, and review the pharmacologic agents used in vascular disease management.

ATHEROSCLEROSIS BASIC PRINCIPLES AND MEDICAL MANAGEMENT

Risk Factors for Atherosclerotic Disease and Modification Strategies

This chapter reviews the traditional cardiovascular risk factors that have been proved and established over a body of literature spanning the past half-century and examines the contribution that each risk factor brings to an individual patient's cardiovascular disease risk. Novel or emerging risk factors will be discussed. These promising new biochemical correlates have been experimentally linked to atherosclerotic cardiovascular disease; however, their clinical applicability is in many cases yet to be determined, thus limiting their utility as predictors of individual cardiovascular risk.

Many theories and causes of atherogenesis have been postulated and studied, and they have led to a handful of clear risk factors for atherosclerosis. These risk factors have long been recognized as the framework for a preventative strategy for cardiovascular diseases. The identification of specific cardiovascular risk factors that led to the concept of risk factor modification arose from the findings of the Framingham Heart Study of the 1960s.[14] A risk factor can be defined simply as an entity that can be identified early in the disease course of an individual or group of individuals and confers an increased risk of disease development. An essential part of disease prevention in the context of identification of risk factors is the ability for modification of that specific risk factor, usually in the form of behavioral or pharmacologic manipulation.

Cardiovascular disease is increasingly recognized as the largest growing burden of disease for health care systems.[15] Though progress in treatment regimens and surgical outcomes once atherosclerotic disease is established has improved morbidity and mortality from cardiovascular complications, there has been a shift in emphasis toward the development of effective clinical guidelines for prevention and modification at an earlier stage in the disease process. Box 12-1 lists the most common risk factors for atherosclerotic cardiovascular disease.

Smoking

Smoking is the greatest contributor to atherosclerotic cardiovascular disease and is the number one cause of preventable deaths in the United States annually.[16] There has been an increase in the number of smokers despite extensive antismoking campaigns, and smoke-related

---

BOX 12-1 Risk Factors for Atherosclerotic Cardiovascular Disease

WELL-ESTABLISHED

- Smoking
- Diabetes mellitus
- Hypertension
- Dyslipidemia
- Physical inactivity
- Advanced age
- Family history of early cardiovascular disease

EMERGING

- High sensitivity C-reactive peptide
- Lipoprotein (a)
- Fibrinogrn and fibrin-degradation products
- Homocysteine

BOX 12-2 Current Target Guidelines for Diabetic Patients

- Fasting blood glucose <110 mg/dL
- Hemoglobin A_{1c} <7%
- Blood pressure <130/80 mm Hg (combination HCTZ/ACE inhibitor as first-line therapy)
- LDL < 100 mg/dL (<70 mg/dL considered if established coronary artery disease)
- Triglyceride level <150 mg/dL

HCTZ, Hydrochlorothiazide; *ACE,* angiotensin-converting enzyme; *LDL,* low-density lipoprotein.

---

deaths continue to rise particularly in the developing world.

A dose-related phenomenon has been described for cigarette-smoking that correlates with increased rates of coronary events, ischemic strokes, and peripheral vascular disorders.[9] Despite this dose effect, complete smoking cessation has been demonstrated to be the only significantly effective approach to reducing health risks associated with smoking. Smoking cessation remains a pivotal part of cardiovascular disease prevention. However, initiatives aimed at improving public awareness of the deleterious effects of ischemic heart disease, peripheral vascular disease including amputation, and cerebrovascular events have met with limited success. As much as one third of cardiovascular mortality can be prevented by abstinence from smoking, an effect that has not yet been realized by pharmaceutical risk-factor management.[17]

Attitudinal approaches to smoking cessation have been well described in the addiction literature and can be classified into five main stages: precontemplation, contemplation, preparation, action, and maintenance. These five stages are often referred to within the construct of the transtheoretical model of health behavior change.[18]

Effective holistic treatment plans exist for patients who are motivated to cease smoking, such as nicotine replacement by transdermal patch or chewable gum, behavioral modification, and antidepressant therapy. However, many physicians do not routinely document smoking behavior or pursue smoking cessation at every clinical encounter, an endeavor that should form part of the standard of care for any patient who endorses an active or recent history of smoking.

Diabetes Mellitus

Coronary artery disease is the principal cause of death in diabetic patients and rivals smoking in contribution to cardiovascular mortality.[19] The rate of coronary and peripheral arterial disease approximately doubles in patients with a diagnosis of diabetes.[20] The length of time and severity of diabetic control are strong predictors of atherosclerotic events and have been correlated with the degree of peripheral arterial disease experienced by patients. The microvascular complications of diabetes are beyond the scope of this chapter but diabetic nephropathy, heralded by microalbuminuria, exacerbates large vessel changes imposed by insulin resistance and hyperglycemia.[21] Atherosclerosis can be shown experimentally to be induced by insulin resistance preceding the development of a clinical diagnosis of diabetes and has been diagnosed in adolescents and teenagers as part of the metabolic syndrome.

Significant improvements in the glycemic profile and reduction in diabetic complications with prolongation of life expectancy can be achieved through behavioral modification of diabetes. Level 1 data from large, randomized national trials of monitored lifestyle modification demonstrate up to 30% reduction in frank diabetes with associated reduction in cardiovascular events. The addition of effective glycemic agents such as metformin, sulfonylureas, and thiazolidinediones further contributes to cardiovascular risk reduction. Current glucose targets for diabetic patients are listed in Box 12-2. A causal relationship has been described for long-term blood glucose control as assessed by the hemoglobin A1c (HbA_{1c}) in the national United Kingdom Prospective Diabetes Study (UKPDS) with an increase in the risk of adverse cardiovascular events for each percentage point above an HbA_{1c} level of 6.2%. The UKPDS recommendations for metabolic control of diabetic patients also focus on other parameters that are known to interact deleteriously with diabetes to increase cardiovascular risk such as hypertension and hyperlipidemia.[22] Physicians now recognize the need for aggressive management of patients with the constellation of diabetes, hypertriglyceridemia, hypertension, and obesity, some of which will fit the definition of the metabolic syndrome.

Hypertension

The prevalence of hypertension in the United States is estimated at one in three individuals and rising steadily. Part of the difficulty in managing hypertension is the racial disparity in prevalence, response to antihypertensive medications, and associated exacerbating factors such as renal disease and diabetes. High-risk groups include African Americans, those older than 60 years, and women.[23] A dose phenomenon has been described for hypertension. In general, an elevation in blood pressure of 20 mm Hg systolic from a theorized normal of 120 mm Hg systolic confers a cardiovascular risk double that of the normotensive population. A working definition of *hypertension* is a systolic blood pressure greater than 140 mm Hg or a diastolic pressure greater than 90 mm Hg. *Prehypertension* can be defined further as blood pressure ranging between 120 and 139 mm Hg systolic and 80 to 89 mm Hg diastolic.[24] Traditional views of hypertension primarily focused on diastolic dysfunction and elevation as more significant than the systolic component; however, this perspective has been shifted with more recent data indicating a greater risk for cardiovascular events and mortality in the face of systolic hypertension. Pulse pressure increases for a given systolic blood pressure have also received more attention as markers of impairment of vascular receptive relaxation and predictors of coronary risk over normal controls. Although hypertension is an independent risk factor for the development of coronary disease, it should be noted that it is much more potent when considered alongside other commonly associated risk factors, such as triglyceride profile, diabetes, and obesity. Almost two thirds of patients with hypertension have at least one other risk factor for cardiovascular disease; therefore treatment of hypertension should be ideally managed using therapies that are multivariate in effect, such as dietary modification or pharmacologic agents with benefits for both triglyceride and blood pressure profile.

The 2003 Joint National Committee on Prevention, Detection, Evaluation and Treatment of High Blood Pressure (JNC-7) panel published guidelines that summarize management goals for the treatment of hypertension-associated risk factors.[24] For example, hyperlipidemia may be more difficult to control when a combination of diuretic and β-blocking agents is used because of slight alterations in lipid metabolism as a side-effect of these medications. In the presence of diabetes, calcium-channel blockers, angiotensin-converting enzyme (ACE) inhibitors, and β-blockers are recommended. Lifestyle modifications are clearly identified with the following JNC-7 guidelines: weight reduction or maintenance of body mass index between 18.5 and 24.9 kg/m^2; the Dietary Approaches to Stop Hypertension eating plan consisting of a diet rich in fruits, vegetables, low-fat dairy products, low sodium (ideally less than 100 mmol or 6 g of sodium chloride per day), reduced fat content, moderate alcohol consumption with less than 2 drinks per day for men and 1 drink per day for women and lighter weight individuals; and regular aerobic activity for at least 30 minutes most days of the week.

Dyslipidemia

Low-density lipoprotein (LDL) is firmly established in cardiovascular risk profiling as the major contributor to atherosclerotic disease and is found in abundance in atherosclerotic plaque. Higher serum levels of LDL correlate to a higher risk of cardiovascular disease—data borne of clinical studies that indicate LDL as the main risk factor for coronary disease.[25] The Post-Coronary Artery Bypass Graft trial examined this relationship further and attempted to define a threshold target level for LDL.[26] From this work, guidelines were established supporting

intensive LDL treatment to a level less than 100 mg/dL to influence a favorable change in atherosclerotic plaque morphology (see Box 12-2).

Although LDL has been identified as a target for cardiovascular risk reduction, other lipid and lipoprotein abnormalities have been recognized in contributing to the overall risk of atherosclerotic disease. Elevated levels of very-low-density lipoprotein (VLDL), apolipoprotein B, and decreased high-density lipoprotein (HDL) are adverse markers for cardiovascular risk.[27] Clinical evidence for the involvement of these lipoproteins is found in the acceleration of atherosclerotic build-up seen in patients suffering from inherited forms of dyslipidemia, such as familial hypercholesterolemia.

First-line therapies for reducing cholesterol, LDL, and VLDL and increasing HDL involve behavioral modification in the form of dietary changes.[28] Animal fat, including meats and egg yolks, is a significant source of cholesterol, and goal strategies focus on reduction of cholesterol-rich products by at least 50%. Simply reducing body weight toward a goal body mass index will produce significant reductions in LDL levels and reduce the overall cardiovascular risk profile.

The main pharmacologic modality used to impair cholesterol metabolism is the hydroxymethylglutaryl coenzyme A (HMG-CoA) reductase inhibitors (or statin medications). The mechanism of statin action occurs at the hepatocellular level to inhibit cholesterol synthesis in the liver. Statins are powerfully effective in reducing total body LDL levels (from 30% to 60% depending on dosage). Not surprisingly, these medications have become first-line drug therapy for patients with elevated lipid profiles in the absence of drug contraindications. Myopathy, heralded by a rise in creatine kinase, and transient elevation of hepatic aminotransferases are the most commonly quoted side effects of statin use. These derangements usually resolve with discontinuation of the medication.[28] Statins along with four other medications used in the treatment of dyslipidemias (ezetimibe, niacin, fibric acid derivatives, and bile acid sequestrants) will be discussed.

Metabolic Syndrome

Over the past half century, a constellation of metabolic derangements has been seen more frequently occurring in association. Hypertension, diabetes mellitus, obesity, and dyslipidemia are the four entities most commonly described as part of the metabolic syndrome or colloquially known as *syndrome X*.[29] According to the definition established by the 2001 Adult Treatment Panel-III of the National Cholesterol Education Program metabolic syndrome is diagnosed when three of the following criteria are present[27]:

1. Central obesity; waist circumference >102 cm (males) or >88 cm (females)
2. Fasting plasma glucose >6.1 mmol/L
3. Hypertension ≥135/85 mm Hg or the presence of antihypertensive medications
4. Dyslipidemia including triglycerides ≥1.7 mmol/L, HDL cholesterol <1.0 mmol/L (males) or <1.3 mmol/L (females).

The metabolic syndrome for many of the reasons highlighted earlier in this chapter is strongly associated with the development of cardiovascular disease portending an approximately 2.5 times risk of fatal cardiovascular events in the population. The single most effective treatment for the metabolic syndrome is loss of body weight either by nonsurgical or surgical means, which in almost all cases of dramatic weight loss leads to amelioration of all individual components.[30]

Emerging Novel Risk Factors

Although the well-established risk factors have been strongly linked to the development of cardiovascular disease, there remains a significant proportion of the atherosclerotic population that does not possess these described risk factors. Searches for other contributing factors have focused on molecular biomarkers as diverse as homocysteine levels, high-sensitivity C-reactive protein (CRP) (hs-CRP), fibrin-degradation products, and microalbuminuria.

Elevated plasma homocysteine levels have been cited as a defined risk factor for the development of atherosclerotic coronary arterial disease in epidemiologic and clinical research studies.[31] On a molecular basis, high levels of homocysteine have been demonstrated to occur with disruption of normal methionine metabolism. Homocysteine and related metabolites can be detected in abnormally high levels in the blood and have been linked to an increased risk of stroke, owing to carotid plaque buildup, as well as cardiovascular disease.[32] Endothelial damage in association with an alteration of the normal coagulation balance has led to the hypothesis that elevated homocysteine levels directly influence atherogenesis in large vessels. Therapeutic options for individuals diagnosed with homocystinemia have centered on replacement of vitamin B_{12} and folic acid as a primary treatment with additional restriction of dietary intake of methionine in patients insensitive to vitamin B_{12}. However, studies have not shown that lowering homocysteine levels decreases the risk of cardiovascular disease in these patients.[33]

Inflammatory markers such as hs-CRP and fibrin-degradation products have been deemed to be associated with risk of cardiovascular disease; although they were originally thought to have a role as potential serum biomarkers of cardiovascular disease, they have been only weakly associated with risk stratification and burden of atherosclerotic disease. The relative lack of specificity of these markers dilutes their clinical effect, because many unassociated noncardiovascular conditions can cause elevations of either marker. As a result, the clinical applicability of these markers has been limited, and their use in the setting of cardiovascular risk reduction is yet to be elucidated.

Hs-CRP has recently been the subject of much attention with the results of the Justification of the Use of Statins in Prevention: an Intervention Trial Evaluating Rosuvastatin (JUPITER) trial, which was a large multinational, double-blind, placebo-controlled trial of more than 17,000 people.[34] The trial was designed to observe the effect that treatment with a statin (rosuvastatin) had on individuals with normal lipid profiles but elevated hs-CRP levels. The study arose from the observation that statins have an antiinflammatory property and decrease hs-CRP levels in an effect that is independent from their cholesterol-lowering ability. The JUPITER trial demonstrated a reduction in both LDL and hs-CRP levels to around half of pretreatment and was terminated prematurely on the basis of this beneficial result. However, the benefit of a normal hs-CRP has not yet been firmly established as a treatment goal in cardiovascular risk profiling and is additionally confounded by the possible benefit of statin therapy in the face of normal lipid profile in certain populations. Nevertheless, hs-CRP remains an active and controversial area of cardiovascular risk-modification research, and its clinical role is yet to be formally determined.[35]

Microalbuminuria is a sensitive predictor of mortality and is highly associated with specific adverse cardiovascular events. Diabetic and hypertensive nephropathy can be diagnosed reliably by evidence of proteinuria, which is also associated with an increase in cardiovascular risk profile. Microalbuminuria is similarly associated with an elevated risk of coronary disease, independent of proteinuria; therefore it could have clinical use in patients who do not have a diagnosis of hypertension or diabetes as a screening tool for atherosclerotic disease. Treatment strategies based on the detection of microalbuminuria are therefore likely to take the form of existing risk-reduction strategies for well-established cardiovascular risk factors.

Surveillance and Secondary Prevention

Given the focus on prevention of atherosclerotic disease, increased surveillance for the development of signs of atherosclerotic disease in those with established risk factors should be included in the routine health care maintenance and follow-up of patients. Regular carotid duplex evaluation for older patients with one or more risk factors for atherosclerosis in addition to at least annual physical examinations is a relatively inexpensive and highly effective screening tool for carotid disease. Similarly, screening aortic ultrasonography, physical examination, and ankle-brachial pressure indices should be considered for at-risk patients in the primary care setting. Electrocardiography, two-dimensional echocardiography, and stress echocardiography are procedures that are best used as diagnostic rather than screening tools; however, their utility is as a prediction tool for those at the highest risk of cardiovascular disease and may act as the gateway to more invasive diagnostic and treatment options, such as angiographic interventions or cardiac surgery.

For patients who progress to severe or acute cardiovascular disease, secondary prevention guidelines are well documented and rigorously studied. Many cardiovascular centers have established protocols for treating patients with established disease. One such example is the University of California–Los Angeles Cardiac Hospitalization Atherosclerosis Management Program (CHAMP) which focuses on using secondary prevention measures while patients are in the hospital in order to improve clinical outcomes.[36] This program arose through the observation that although evidence-based guidelines for secondary risk prevention are widely disseminated, they are consistently underutilized. The CHAMP guidelines are summarized as follows:

1. Aspirin should be initiated (81 to 162 mg daily). In the presence of contraindications to aspirin, other platelet agents should be considered, such as clopidogrel. Combination therapy can be recommended in the setting of acute coronary syndromes or post-revascularization therapy.
2. Statin therapy should be initiated in all patients in the absence of contraindications and in all diabetic patients regardless of their lipid profile. Target levels of LDL should be <70 mg/dL, HDL >40 mg/dL, and triglycerides <150 mg/dL.
3. ACE inhibitors or angiotensin-receptor blockers should be commenced in the absence of contraindication regardless of the blood pressure or cardiac ejection fraction.
4. Beta blockade should be prescribed for all patients in the absence of contraindication.
5. Fish oil or omega-3 fatty acids should be commenced with dietary instruction for all patients.
6. Aerobic exercise programs that involve 30 to 60 minutes of moderately intense exercise at least five times per week should be prescribed.
7. Smoking cessation should be pursued including access to formal smoking cessation programs.
8. Before hospital discharge and at 6-week follow-up, cardiovascular lipid profile and liver enzymes should be checked and routinely thereafter at future follow-up appointments.

PHARMACOLOGY OF DRUGS USED IN THE MANAGEMENT OF VASCULAR DISEASE

Anticoagulants (Table 12-1)

Heparin

Structure and Mechanism of Action. Heparin is an anticoagulant composed of a heterogeneous group of straight-chain glycosaminoglycans with molecular weights ranging from 5 to 30 kD (mean, 15 kD).[1] It is strongly acidic secondary to its high content of sulfate and carboxyl groups. Heparin is a naturally occurring substance excreted by mast cells and basophils in the process of clot formation. Standard, unfractionated heparin is derived commercially from porcine gut mucosa or bovine lung tissue. Heparin acts at multiple points within the coagulation system. Its major anticoagulant effect is via interaction with antithrombin III, leading to the inactivation of factor Xa and subsequent inhibition of the conversion of prothrombin to thrombin.[2,3] Heparin further inhibits coagulation by inactivating thrombin, preventing the conversion of fibrinogen to fibrin.[4] Heparin also prevents stable fibrin clot formation through the inhibition of fibrin stabilization factor. Heparin has no fibrinolytic activity and therefore does not lyse existing clots.

Heparin's onset of action is immediate with intravenous injection. It can also be administered subcutaneously. Response to heparin is monitored by measuring the activated partial thromboplastin time (aPTT) and activated clotting time (ACT). An aPTT 1.5- to 2.5-fold greater than normal has been shown to prevent recurrent thromboembolism.[5] Weight-adjusted nomograms have been shown to be useful in dosing.[6]

The anticoagulant activity of heparin varies greatly among patients. The heterogeneous clinical response is primarily due to nonspecific binding of heparin to variable concentrations of plasma and cellular proteins, limiting heparin's bioavailability. This leads to marked variability of the anticoagulant response.[2] There also appears to be natural inhibitors of heparin that can be released by sites of active thrombus.[7] Furthermore, the biophysical limitations of the large heparin–antithrombin III complex can block receptors on thrombin to heparin cofactor 2, limiting heparin's effectiveness.[7]

Clinical Use. Heparin is indicated for intraoperative anticoagulation in vascular and cardiac surgery, for the prophylaxis and treatment of deep venous thrombosis, for the prevention of pulmonary embolism in surgical patients, and in patients with atrial fibrillation and embolization.[2]

Adverse Reactions. Heparin therapy is associated with increased risk of bleeding. It also can cause skin lesions, including papules, plaques, and necrosis.[8] Heparin therapy can lead to hypoaldosteronism,[9] priapism,[10] and osteoporosis.[11] Thrombocytopenia is a known complication of heparin administration. Heparin-induced thrombocytopenia (HIT) can lead to thromboembolic complications, including skin necrosis, extremity gangrene, myocardial infarction, pulmonary embolism, and stroke.[2]

Heparin-Induced Thrombocytopenia. Two major forms of HIT are recognized. Type I HIT is an early-onset, benign, reversible thrombocytopenia with no associated platelet antibodies. It is not immune mediated and is usually self limited without complications.[12] Type II HIT is a more serious immune-modulated thrombocytopenia.[13] It is caused by platelet immunoglobulin G antibodies that target platelet factor 4, a heparin binding protein, leading to platelet activation.[14,15] Activation of platelets and endothelium and neutralization of heparin all contribute to a highly thrombogenic state.[2] Patients with type II HIT have a high risk of developing thrombotic complications.[2] Fortunately, most patients who develop HIT antibodies do not develop thrombocytopenia or thrombosis. Furthermore, almost all patients who develop mild to moderate thrombocytopenia during the first 4 days of heparin treatment do not have antibodies. Type II HIT should be considered a clinicopathologic syndrome with a combination of thrombocytopenia and associated clinical events, including thrombosis and confirmation of platelet antibodies.[2] The management of HIT is aimed at preventing thromboembolic complications. All heparin should be discontinued and an alternative anticoagulant initiated.

TABLE 12-1 Anticoagulant Dress Used in the Management of Vascular Disease

Medication	Examples	Mechanism of Action	Metabolized	Half-Life	Side Effects	Dosage
Anticoagulants						
Unfractionated heparin	Heparin	Interacts with antithrombin III, which inactivates factor Xa and subsequent conversion of prothrombin to thrombin. Inactivates thrombin preventing conversion of fibrinogen to fibrin. Inhibits fibrin stabilization factor. Varied response owing to binding of plasma and cellular proteins	Liver	1.5 hour	Bleeding, thrombocytopenia (type I and II HIT), skin lesions, hypoaldosteronism, priapism, osteoporosis	VTE prophylaxis 5000 units SC q8-12h; VTE treatment: bolus 80 units/kg IV once, then 18 units/kg/h and adjust dose to aPTT based on nomogram
Low-molecular-weight heparin	Enoxaparin (Lovenox)	Inactivate factor Xa by binding to antithrombin III. Reduced ability to inactivate thrombin owing to molecular size compared with unfractionated heparin. Decreased nonspecific protein binding. Decreased platelet binding (reduces risk of HIT)	Liver	4.5-7 hour	Bleeding, ecchymosis, thrombocytopenia, decreased risk of HIT compared to standard heparin	VTE prophylaxis: 30-40 mg SC q12h; VTE/PE treatment: 1 mg/kg SC q12h; Adjust dose for renal impairment
Warfarin	Coumadin	Inhibits vitamin K dependent clotting factors (II, VII, IX, X) and the anticoagulant protein C and protein S. Response is variable based on genetic factors, drug interactions, various disease states, and diet	Liver	20-60 hour	Bleeding, skin necrosis or gangrene, purple toe syndrome	Start 2-5 mg PO daily for 2-4 days, adjust dose based on INR; Overlap treatment 4-5 days when switching from heparin
Direct thrombin inhibitors	Lepirudin (IV; Refludan)	Inhibits thrombin directly to prevent conversion of fibrinogen to fibrin	Unknown	1.3 hour	Hemorrhage, epidural/spinal hematoma, anemia	0.15 mg/kg IV, monitor aPTT*
	Desirudin (SC; Iprivask)		Renal	3 hour		15 mg SC q12h*
	Bivalirudin (IV; Angiomax)		Plasma	25 min		02.-0.3 mg/kg/h IV, monitor ACT*
	Argatroban (IV)		Liver	39-51 min		2 µg/kg/min IV, monitor aPTT
	Dabigatran (PO; pradaxa)		Liver	12-17 hour		150 mg PO bid, no routine monitoring*
Factor X inhibitors	Fondaparinux (SC; Arixtra)	Binds to antithrombin III resulting in inactivation of factor X but does not mediate the inactivation of thrombin by antithrombin III	Unknown	17-21 hour	Hemorrhage	VTE prophylaxis: 2.5 mg SC q24h; DVT/PE Tx: 7.5 mg SC q24h†; VTE prophylaxis: 10 mg PO q24h†
	Rivaroxaban (PO; Xarelto)		Liver	7-11 hour	Anemia, thrombocytopenia	

Antiplatelet Agents

		Mechanism	Metabolism	Half-life	Side effects	Dose
Aspirin	Bayer aspirin, Ecotrin	Blocks prostaglandin metabolism and synthesis of thromboxane A2, a potent platelet aggregator. The effect on the platelet is permanent, with the platelet lifespan approximately 10 days	Gut and plasma acetyl salicylic acid(ASA), liver (salicylate)	20 min	Bleeding, GI irritation, angioedema, bronchospasm, pancytopenia	75-325 mg PO q24h; 75-150 mg of aspirin appears to be as effective as higher doses with fewer side effects
Thienopyridines	Clopidogrel (Plavix)	Inhibit P2Y receptor, an adenosine diphosphate receptor, which results in platelet aggregation	Liver	8 hour	Bleeding, diarrhea skin rash, neutropenia; clopidogrel has fewer side effects than ticlopidine	75 mg PO q24h
	Ticlopidine (Ticlid)		Liver	7.9-12.6 hour		250 PO bid
	Prasugrel (Effient)	Prodrug that must undergo hydrolysis to active metabollite	Liver	7 hour		5-10 mg PO q24h
Glycoprotein IIb/IIIa inhibitors	Abciximab (Reopro) Eptifibatide (Integrilin)	Binds to IIb/IIIa receptors, inhibiting aggregation of platelets	Unknown	10-30 min / 2.5 hour	Thrombocytopenia, bleeding	0.125-10 µg/kg/min IV; µg/kg/min IV*
	Tirofiban (Aggrastat)			2 hour		1-2 µg/kg/min IV*

Medication Treatment of Claudication

		Mechanism	Metabolism	Half-life	Side effects	Dose
Pentoxifylline	Trental	Lowers blood viscosity, decreasing platelet adhesiveness, and improves erythrocyte flexibility which increases flow in the microcirculation	Liver	0.4-16 hour	Arrhythmia, dyspepsia, nausea, vomiting	Conflicting data regarding benefits and is not currently recommended: 400 mg PO tid; Cr Cl 10-50, dose q24h to bid; Cr Cl < 10, give once daily
Cilostazol	Pletal	Type III phosphodiesterase inhibitor that inhibits platelet aggregation and promotes vasodilation	Liver	11-13 hours	Contraindicated with CHF; Bleeding; Anemia; Thrombocytopenia; Agranulocytosis	100 mg BID PO; 50 mg BID if on CYP3A4 inhibitors

*Adjust dose for renal impairment.

†Use with caution CrCl 30-50; avoid is less than 30.

HIT, Heparin-induced thrombocytopenia; VTE, venous thromboembolism; SC, subcutaneous; IV, intravenous; aPTT, activated partial thromboplastin time; PO, by mouth; INR, international normalized ratio; ACT, activated clotting time; GI, gastrointestinal; DVT, deep venous thrombosis (DVT); PE, pulmonary embolism (PE); Tx, treatment; Cr Cl, creatine clearance.

From Epocrates Online Drugs, 2011, San Mateo, Calif, Epocrates. Available at http://www.epocrates.com. Accessed July 19, 2011.

Protamine

Structure and Mechanism of Action. Protamine is composed of a heterogeneous group of low-molecular-weight proteins. These proteins are rich in arginine and are strongly basic. They occur naturally in the sperm of salmon and certain other fish species. The mechanism of action for heparin reversal is through electrostatic bonding. Heparin is highly acidic and forms a strong bond with the highly basic protamine molecules, forming an inactive complex.[16]

Clinical Use. Protamine is used clinically as a heparin antidote. When administered alone, protamine has an anticoagulant effect similar to that of heparin. However, in the presence of heparin, it forms a stable salt, and the anticoagulant activity of both is lost. Protamine has a rapid onset of action; it begins to neutralize heparin within 5 minutes of administration.

Adverse Reactions. Too rapid administration can have serious side effects, including hypotension and anaphylaxis.[17] Decreased blood pressure, pulmonary hypertension, shortness of breath, flushing, and urticaria have all been associated with rapid administration.[18] Protamine should be administered slowly over 10 minutes, with a goal of 1 mg of protamine to neutralize every 90 units of heparin. Further dosing should be guided by coagulation studies.[16] Severe allergies have been well documented causing transient systemic hypotension, anaphylaxix and severe pulmonary vasoconstriction. Patients with risk factors for a protamine reaction include those with fish allergies, vasectomy, and prior protamine exposure, including protamine insulin-dependent diabetics.[19,20]

Low-Molecular-Weight Heparins

Structure and Mechanism of Action. Low-molecular-weight heparins (LMWHs) are collections of heparin molecules that have significantly lower molecular weights than standard, unfractionated heparin.[21] LMWHs are derived from unfractionated heparin via chemical or enzymatic depolymerization. This produces fragments one third the size of heparin, with mean molecular weights of 4 to 5 kD (range, 1 to 10 kD). Similar to unfractionated heparin, LMWHs are heterogeneous in terms of both molecular size and anticoagulant activity.[22] The LMWHs have distinct differences from standard heparin. LMWHs have reduced ability to catalyze the inactivation of thrombin, because the smaller fragments cannot bind to thrombin. However, LMWHs retain the ability to inactivate factor Xa. There is a reduction in nonspecific protein binding and subsequent improved predictability in dose-response relationships.[22] LMWHs have an increased half-life compared with standard heparin. This is thought to be secondary to reduced macrophage binding. Similarly, there is reduced binding to platelets and a decrease in the incidence of HIT.[22] LMWHs also have been associated with a reduction in bone loss compared with standard heparin.

Clinical Use. The LMWHs have been examined extensively in the prevention of deep venous thrombosis in patients undergoing major abdominal surgery or knee and hip replacement surgery and in patients with restricted mobility.[21] LMWHs have also been investigated for the treatment of acute deep venous thrombosis and pulmonary embolism.[21] LMWHs are used in patients with acute coronary syndromes and unstable angina.[23] The advantages of LMWHs over standard heparin are longer plasma half-life and a more predictable anticoagulant response, allowing for simple dosing and decreasing the need for laboratory monitoring.[22] LMWHs are also commonly used to bridge patients to oral warfarin therapy.

Adverse Reactions. Adverse reactions to LMWHs are similar to those associated with standard heparin. Bleeding, ecchymosis, and thrombocytopenia can all occur with LMWH administration. The incidence of HIT is decreased compared with standard heparin, but LMWHs can cause HIT, and patients should be monitored for this complication.[24]

Warfarin

Structure and Mechanism of Action. Warfarin is a coumarin derivative that produces an anticoagulant effect through the inhibition of vitamin K–dependent coagulation factors (II, VII, IX, X) and the anticoagulant proteins C and S. Warfarin interferes with the conversion of vitamin K to 2,3-epoxide.[25] Vitamin K is an essential cofactor for postribosomal synthesis of clotting factors, acting through the carboxylation of glutamine residues in the protein.[26] Carboxylation promotes binding of vitamin K–dependent coagulation factors to phospholipid surfaces.[25] Coumarins specifically block vitamin K epoxide reductase, preventing the carboxylation of the factors rendering them inactive.[27] The vitamin K antagonists also inhibit carboxylation of the regulatory anticoagulant proteins C and S.[27]

Warfarin is a racemic mixture of two optically active isomers.[25] Absorption from the gastrointestinal tract is rapid, reaching maximal plasma levels within 90 minutes. Warfarin has a half-life of 36 to 42 hours. Response is variable owing to certain genetic factors, drug interactions, various disease states, and diet. The anticoagulant effect can be overcome by low doses of vitamin K_1, because vitamin K_1 bypasses vitamin K epoxide reductase.[25] Warfarin anticoagulation is monitored via measurement of the prothrombin time (PT). The PT reflects the depression of the vitamin K–dependent factors. PT measurement is laboratory dependent, and physicians should be aware of the specific method used to measure it at their institutions.

Clinical Use. Warfarin is indicated for the prophylaxis or treatment of venous thrombosis and thromboembolism. It is also indicated for the prophylaxis or treatment of the thromboembolic complications associated with atrial fibrillation and cardiac valve replacement. Warfarin has been shown to reduce the risk of death, recurrent myocardial infarction, and thromboembolic events such as stroke or systemic embolization after myocardial infarction.[25]

Warfarin has been studied in terms of its usefulness in promoting the patency of infrainguinal bypass grafts.[28-31] Although some studies suggest improved patency of infrainguinal bypass grafts with warfarin or a combination of warfarin and aspirin, the *American College of Chest Physicians 8th Edition Guidelines for Antithrombotic Therapy for Peripheral Artery Occlusive Disease* recommends against long-term anticoagulation in general for extremity reconstructions. The guidelines recommend vitamin K antagonists (VKAs) to not be routinely used for infrainguinal vein bypass, except in those patients at high risk of bypass occlusion and limb loss where VKAs plus aspirin is recommended. For infrainguinal prosthetic bypass, VKAs are not recommended to be used routinely.[32] These conclusions are based on small improvements in patency in the face of relatively high rates of bleeding complications.

Adverse Reactions. Warfarin therapy is associated with an increased risk of hemorrhagic complications. It also can cause necrosis and gangrene of skin or other tissues. It should be used with caution in patients with HIT, because it can lead to increased thrombotic complications early in the treatment of HIT.[33]

Direct Thrombin Inhibitors

The direct thrombin inhibitors are small molecules that act directly at the active site of thrombin, without the use of an intermediate such as antithrombin III with heparin. There are five direct thrombin inhibitors currently available for clinical use: lepirudin, desirudin, bivalirudin, argatroban, and dabigatran.

Thrombin is the central enzyme in hemostasis. It is a serine protease that catalyzes the conversion of fibrinogen to fibrin. In addition, thrombin serves many other roles, including the activation of various coagulation factors, platelets, smooth muscle cells, fibroblasts, and endothelium.[34] Thrombin is chemotactic, stimulates secretion of vasoactive proteins from platelets and inflammatory cells, and plays a role in angiogenesis and restenosis.[34]

Antithrombin III, the major regulator of thrombin, forms an irreversible complex with thrombin to block its active site.[22] For years, this has been the main target for thrombin inhibition and anticoagulation via heparin. However, the use of heparin is limited by several major factors: (1) the development of HIT; (2) heparin's inability to penetrate clot, leading to the release of active thrombin from clots; and (3) the variable anticoagulant response, owing to heparin's propensity to bind to plasma proteins.[35] The rationale for the development of direct thrombin inhibitors was to create a small molecule with site-specific thrombin inhibition.[35] With an increased understanding of the detailed molecular structure of thrombin, site-specific agents have been developed with a high specificity for thrombin.[36]

Clinical Use. Direct thrombin inhibitors have been studied in the treatment of HIT with thrombosis, the treatment of acute coronary events, and the prevention and treatment of deep venous thrombosis, pulmonary embolism, and stroke.[34,36]

Hirudin. Hirudin, the first direct thrombin inhibitor, was originally isolated from the salivary gland of the medicinal leech Hirudo medicinalis after it was noted that leech saliva had anticoagulant properties.[36] It is now produced via recombinant technology as lepirudin and desirudin. It is a 65– to 66–amino acid polypeptide. The amino terminus forms a tight bond with thrombin's active site, and the carboxy terminus binds to the thrombin exosite-1 (fibrinogen binding site).[37] Peak plasma levels are reached after parenteral administration in 20 to 30 minutes. Hirudin is rapidly cleared by the kidneys, having a half-life of 1 to 3 hours. Some hepatic excretion also occurs, but is not clinically significant. Hirudin should not be used in patients with renal failure, because no specific antidote exists should overdose occur.

Bivalirudin. Bivalirudin is a recombinant protein based on hirudin. It is a 20–amino acid peptide that interacts with the active site of thrombin.[34] It has a short half-life of 25 minutes. In contrast to hirudin, renal excretion is not the major route of excretion.[36]

Argatroban. Argatroban is a synthetic, small-molecule arginine derivative that interacts only with the active site of thrombin.[34,36] It is metabolized by the liver, with a half-life of 45 minutes. Dose reduction may be necessary in patients with liver dysfunction. The anticoagulant effect can be monitored with the aPTT or ACT.

Ximelagatran (Melagatran). There is great interest in the development of oral direct thrombin inhibitors. Ximelagatran is a prodrug of melagatran, a synthetic active-site direct inhibitor of thrombin. Initial studies were promising for the use of ximelagatran, but it has been removed from clinical investigation because of significant hepatotoxicity.

Dabigatran

Structure and Mechanism of Action. The oral direct thrombin inhibitor most recently approved by the U.S. Food and Drug Administration (FDA) is dabigatran etexilate. It is a synthetic, nonpeptide, direct thrombin inhibitor which inhibits both circulating and clot-bound thrombin and lowers thrombin-stimulated platelet aggregation.[37] It is rapidly absorbed from the gut. Peak concentrations occur approximately 1 hour after oral administration, but slows to approximately 3 hours when taken with a high-fat meal. The drug is mainly renally excreted and has a half-life of 12 to 17 hours. Renal impairment can increase serum concentrations of dabigatran. The anticoagulation effect is quite stable[40] and monitoring is not required, which makes this drug a potential alternative to warfarin. Unlike warfarin, however, there is no effective antidote, although it is dialyzable. Coadministration of dabigatran with other P-glycoprotein transporter substrates, such as rifampin decreases serum concentrations of dabigatran and may lower its effectiveness. P-glycoprotein inhibitors such as ketoconazole may increase serum concentrations.[41]

Clinical Use. Dabigatran has been initially approved by the FDA for prevention of thromboembolic stroke in patients with nonvalvular atrial fibrillation. The Randomized Evaluation of Long-Term Anticoagulation Therapy (RE-LY) trial studied 18,113 patients with atrial fibrillation considered high risk for stroke. Over a median 2-year of follow-up, they found a decrease in the rate per year of stroke or systemic embolism with dabigatran compared with warfarin (1.54% versus 1.71%; $p < 0.05$).[42] Since 2008, dabigatran has been used in Canada for prevention of thromboembolism in orthopedic surgery patients undergoing knee or hip replacement. In two studies, dabigatran was noted to be as effective as enoxaparin in preventing venous thromboembolism (VTE) after surgery, with no significant hepatotoxicity and a similar incidence of major bleeding. Administration of both 150 and 220 mg dabigatran was as safe and effective as enoxaparin (40 mg) in preventing VTE and all-cause mortality in both the RE-NOVATE and RE-MODEL trials.[41,43] In the RE-NOVATE trial, although 24% of patients studied were not available for assessment for the primary efficacy outcome, in those that could be assessed, results showed similar efficacy with both doses of dabigatran and enoxaparin. However, in another trial evaluating VTE, the RE-MOBILIZE study, dabigatran failed to show equivalence to a higher dose of enoxaparin (60 mg).[44] For prevention of VTE, clinical investigation continues for dabigatran.

Adverse Reactions. Dyspesia and gastritis were more common with dabigatran compared to warfarin. In the RE-LY trial, overall major bleeding rates were similar to warfarin, although major gastrointestinal bleeding was higher with dabigatran.[45,46]

Factor X Inhibitors

Fondaparinux

Fondaparinux is a pentasaccharide that activates antithrombin III in a manner similar to heparin, leading to inactivation of factor X.[47] It differs in one major respect from heparin, in that the pentasaccharide is unable to mediate the inactivation of thrombin by antithrombin III.[47] It is administered subcutaneously and does not require laboratory monitoring. It is renally excreted and is contraindicated in patients with renal failure. Fondaparinux has been evaluated in multiple trials for preventing deep venous thrombosis in patients undergoing major hip fracture and knee replacement surgery.[48-51] It also has been evaluated in the treatment of deep venous thrombosis[52] and acute coronary syndromes.[53]

Rivaroxaban

Structure and Mechanism of Action. Rivaroxaban is an oral oxazolidinone derivative that binds directly to factor Xa. Rivaroxaban has a high bioavailability of 80% to 100%. Peak serum concentration occurs in 2 to 4 hours, and it has a half-life of 7 to 11 hours. One third of the active metabolite is renally excreted, and two thirds

is hepatically metabolized by the cytochrome P450 pathway. Strong inhibitors or inducers of the cytochrome P450 pathway can therefore alter serum concentrations. Rivaroxaban (10 mg) can be administrated orally, once or twice daily, without any monitoring or need for dose adjustment. It is contraindicated in severe liver insufficiency and not recommended in patients with severe renal impairment.

Clinical Use. Rivaroxaban received FDA approval in 2011 for prevention of VTE in hip and knee arthroplasty. A series of phase III trials of rivaroxaban evaluated almost 10,000 patients undergoing elective knee or hip arthroplasty (RECORD 1, 2, and 3 trials).[54-56] Results from these studies showed the superior efficacy of rivaroxaban compared with enoxaparin. In a study of 2531 patients undergoing knee arthroplasty, the composite primary end point (any deep vein thrombosis [DVT], nonfatal pulmonary embolism [PE], or death from any cause) after 10 to 14 days of therapy was noted in 9.6% of patients taking rivaroxaban compared with 18.9% of patients receiving enoxaparin; major bleeding occurred in 0.6% and 0.5% of patients, respectively.[55] In 3153 hip arthroplasty patients, after 36 days of therapy the same primary endpoint was noted in 1.1% of patients on rivaroxaban and in 3.7% of patients taking enoxaparin. Major bleeding occurred in 0.3% of patients with rivaroxaban and in 0.1% with enoxaparin ($p > 0.05$).[54]

In all three trials, rivaroxaban and enoxaparin had comparable safety profiles and low rates of major bleeding. A pooled analysis from REgulation and Congulation in ORthopedic Surgery to Frequent Deep Venous Thrombosis and Pulmonary Embolism (RECORD) 1, 2, and 3 showed that compared with enoxaparin, rivaroxaban decreases the composite of symptomatic VTE and all-cause mortality after elective total hip or knee arthroplasty, with a small increase in bleeding, no evidence of hepatotoxicity, and fewer serious adverse events.[57] Furthermore, rivaroxaban has been shown to have a significantly lower rate of recurrent DVT than warfarin-treated patients in the EINSTEIN DVT study.[58] And rivaroxaban has been found to be as effective as warfarin for preventing stroke in patients with atrial fibrillation in the Rivaroxaban-Once daily, oral, direct factor Xa inhibition Compared with vitamin K antagonism for prevention of stroke and Embolism Trial in Atrial Fibrillation (ROCKET-AF) study. Throughout all these studies, rivaroxaban has maintained a slightly better safety profile.[59]

Adverse Reactions. Adverse reactions with rivaroxaban are related to bleeding, although they may in fact be lower than with other anticoagulants. Hepatotoxicity has not been noted.

Apixaban

Apixaban is an investigational oral Xa inhibitor in the United States. It is approved for knee and hip arthroplasty in Europe. It is excreted 25% by the kidneys and 75% via the biliary route. Apixaban has been shown in several trials to be equivalent or superior to enoxaparin in VTE prevention for knee and hip arthroplasty.[60,61] It has also shown promising results in stroke prevention in atrial fibrillation.[62,63]

Antiplatelet Agents

Aspirin

Structure and Mechanism of Action. Aspirin inhibits platelet aggregation by irreversibly acetylating prostaglandin synthase, inhibiting its cyclooxygenase activity. This blocks prostaglandin metabolism and, most importantly, the synthesis of thromboxane A_2, a potent stimulator of platelet aggregation.[64,65] There are two isoforms of the cyclooxygenase (COX) enzyme: COX-1 and COX-2.[66] COX-1 is constitutively expressed in many cell types, including platelets, whereas COX-2 is present only in inflammatory cells. Aspirin is fiftyfold to 100-fold more potent in inhibiting COX-1 than COX-2; therefore lower doses are required to obtain antiplatelet compared with antiinflammatory effects.[66] Several other mechanisms for platelet inhibition have been proposed, including inhibiting neutrophil activation of platelets[67] and interfering with prostacyclin synthesis by endothelium.[68] There are also data suggesting an antioxidant role for aspirin[69,70] and the improvement of endothelial cell function by aspirin.[71] It is primarily the antiplatelet and antithrombotic effects of aspirin that result in cardiovascular benefits. Aspirin is rapidly absorbed by the upper gastrointestinal tract, with measurable platelet effects within 1 hour.[66] Enteric coating significantly impairs its absorption, taking up to 4 hours to reach peak plasma levels. Although the plasma half-life is only 20 minutes, the effect on COX-1 and the platelet is permanent, as the anucleate platelet cannot synthesize new enzyme. The life span of a platelet is approximately 10 days. After a single dose of aspirin and with normal platelet turnover of approximately 10% per day, it may take 10 days for renewal of the platelet population. However, data suggest that as little as 20% of platelets with normal COX enzyme activity is required for normal hemostasis.[66,72]

Clinical Use. The benefit of aspirin therapy is determined largely by the patient's absolute risk of vascular events. Those at high risk and those with unstable angina or prior myocardial infarction or stroke derive the most benefit.[73]

Primary Prevention. Aspirin for primary disease prevention has been carefully evaluated in multiple clinical trials.[74-79] The combined data demonstrated a significant reduction in myocardial infarction with aspirin but did not demonstrate a decrease in overall mortality. There was a slightly increased risk of bleeding complications with aspirin; therefore the benefits and risks must be balanced. Generally, the greater the thrombotic risk, the greater the benefits of aspirin for primary prevention.[73]

Secondary Prevention. The benefits of aspirin in preventing cardiovascular disease complications have been clearly demonstrated in several large clinical trials.[80] The Antiplatelet Trialists Committee published a metaanalysis that included 287 trials with more than 300,000 patients.[76,81] In high-risk patients—those with a history of myocardial infarction, angina, or stroke—long-term therapy with aspirin significantly decreased the risk of nonfatal myocardial infarction, nonfatal ischemic stroke, and vascular death.[76,77]

Aspirin is also recommended in patients undergoing prosthetic inguinal bypass grafting or carotid endarterectomy and those with asymptomatic and recurrent carotid stenosis.[31] Aspirin has been demonstrated to improve long-term vessel patency in patients undergoing lower extremity angioplasty with or without stenting.[31]

Adverse Reactions. The most significant adverse reactions associated with aspirin therapy include bleeding and gastrointestinal irritation. These side effects appear to be dose related. Aspirin dosing varied widely in the Antiplatelet Trialists Committee overview, and there was no significant benefit associated with higher doses.[81] Daily dosing of 75 to 150 mg of aspirin appears to be as effective as higher doses for long-term treatment.[76] Because of the increased side effects with higher doses and the lack of any conclusive data favoring higher doses, the concept of lower dosing is supported.[82]

Thienopyridines: Clopidogrel, Ticlopidine, and Prasugrel

Structure and Mechanism of Action. Adenosine diphosphate (ADP) plays a central role in platelet aggregation and activation. ADP released from activated platelets induces further platelet activation and adhesion through binding to the ADP receptor on the platelet surface. The ADP receptor is a membrane-bound, G-protein–coupled receptor.[83,84] There are two main types of ADP receptors, $P2Y_1$ and $P2Y_{12}$.[83] The overall effect of platelet ADP receptor binding is increased platelet activation and aggregation.[83]

Ticlopidine and clopidogrel are selective antiplatelet agents that inhibit the $P2Y_{12}$ receptor. Their chemical structures are similar, with clopidogrel having an extra carboxymethyl side group. Both parent compounds are quickly metabolized in the liver to active metabolites that covalently bind to the ADP receptor. Clopidogrel is sixfold more potent than ticlopidine. The effect is permanent over the life span of the platelet, and overall platelet function generally recovers within 7 to 10 days after stopping the drug.[83] Prasugrel is a thienopyridine prodrug that must undergo hydrolysis by intestinal esterases and oxidation by CYP3A4 and CYP2B6 to be converted to its active metabolite. The active metabolite then binds to the P2Y12 ADP receptor, causing irreversible inhibition of platelet activity.[83]

Clinical Use. Ticlopidine has been evaluated in several clinical trials in patients with peripheral arterial disease and has been associated with a reduction in the risk of myocardial infarction, stroke, and vascular death.[84-87] However, the clinical usefulness of ticlopidine is limited by the potential for severe hematologic side effects, particularly neutropenia.[88,89]

Clopidogrel, which has fewer side effects than ticlopidine, has been approved for use in patients with recent myocardial infarction, stroke, or established peripheral vascular disease for the reduction of thrombotic events.

The FDA has also approved clopidogrel for use in patients with non-ST elevation acute coronary syndromes and percutaneous coronary interventions. A landmark study of clopidogrel was the Clopidogrel versus Aspirin in Patients at Risk of Ischemic Events (CAPRIE) trial.[91] This randomized, prospective, double-blinded trial compared the efficacy of aspirin and clopidogrel in reducing the risk of ischemic stroke, myocardial infarction, or vascular death. The study of nearly 20,000 patients with atherosclerotic disease (those with recent stroke, myocardial infarction, or established peripheral arterial disease) found that clopidogrel resulted in an 8.7% relative risk reduction in vascular death, ischemic stroke, or myocardial infarction compared with aspirin. Remarkably, this was not a placebo comparison but a comparison with a known effective antiplatelet agent already proved to confer a 25% risk reduction.[81-92] Subset analyses of CAPRIE showed an even greater benefit in high-risk patients, diabetics, and those with previous vascular interventions.[92]

The newest thienopyridine, prasugrel, has been compared to clopidogrel in the TRial to access Improvement in Therapeutic Outcomes by optimizing platelet inhibitioN with prasugrel Thombolysis In Myocardial Infarction 38 (TRITON-TIMI 38) study, in which 13,608 patients with acute coronary syndrome undergoing percutaneous coronary intervention (after coronary anatomy was defined) were randomized to prasugrel or clopidogrel, in addition to aspirin, for up to 15 months. The primary endpoint (cardiovascular death, nonfatal myocardial infarction [MI], or nonfatal stroke) was noted in 9.9% of patients taking prasugrel compared to 12.1% with clopidogrel ($p < 0.001$). This lower incidence was mainly due to a reduction in MI, with no difference stroke rate or cardiovascular death. Coronary stent thrombosis was seen in 2.4% of patients treated with clopidogrel and 1.1% of those with prasugrel.[94-96]

Thienopyridines have been used in vascular surgery practice as antithrombotic therapy for carotid artery and lower extremity balloon angioplasty and stenting. This has not yet been examined in randomized clinical trials; therefore there are insufficient data to recommend thienopyridine use in this setting.[31] Ticlopidine (Ticlid) has been demonstrated to improve the patency of infrainguinal bypass grafts, but its clinical use has been superseded by clopidogrel's significantly fewer adverse effects.[31,97] Currently, there are no controlled trials specifically examining clopidogrel or prasugrel and infrainguinal graft patency; therefore it cannot be recommended at this time.

Adverse Reactions. Side effects of clopidogrel include gastrointestinal complaints and skin rash. Bleeding complications are similar to those associated with aspirin. Neutropenia is a rare complication with clopidogrel, but is much more frequent with ticlopidine.[90,98] Neutropenia can be severe and has resulted in fatalities; it generally occurs within 3 months after instituting therapy, and strict hematologic monitoring is recommended.[83] Diarrhea and skin rashes are also common with ticlopidine.[83] Thrombotic thrombocytopenic purpura is a recognized complication of thienopyridine treatment, with an incidence between 1:1600 and 1:5000 patients.[99] With the widespread use of clopidogrel, there has been a subgroup of patients noted to be poor responders to the drug because of genetic polymorphisms of the cytochrome P450 enzyme CYP2C19.[100] At least one of the associated genetic polymorphisms has been found to occur in 15% of Caucasians, 17% of African Americans, and 30% of Asians.[101] At this time there are no clear recommendations for genetic testing for these variants before induction of clopidogrel therapy[102]; however, if clinical concern exists, genetic testing is available, or patients who are taking clopidogrel could have functional platelet aggregation assays to evaluate whether the drug is being activated. Another alternative is to switch to prasugrel, although these same polymorphisms may also affect conversion of prasugrel to its active form by CYP2B6.[103] Another nuance in clopidogrel therapy is the finding that proton pump inhibitors may interfere with clopidogrel activation and decrease the antiplatelet effect, increasing the risk of cardiovascular events. A review of four randomized trials has noted that a metabolic drug-drug interaction does appear to exist between clopidogrel and omeprazole, but not between clopidogrel and pantoprazole.[104]

It is important to note that prasugrel appears to have a significantly higher risk of bleeding compared with clopidogrel. In TRITON-TIMI 38, more patients taking prasugrel had major bleeding than with clopidogrel (2.4% versus 1.8%; $p = 0.03$), life-threatening bleeding, and a small, but significant, increase in fatal bleeding (0.4% versus 0.1%; $p = 0.002$). Among the 4% of patients with ST-elevation MI who required coronary artery bypass graft surgery, major bleeding occurred in 18.8% of prasugrel-treated patients compared with 2.7% of clopidogrel-treated patients ($p = 0.003$).[96]

Glycoprotein IIb/IIIa Receptor Inhibitors

Structure and Mechanism of Action. The glycoprotein (GP) receptor is an integrin found in high concentrations on the platelet membrane. The GP receptor (GP IIb/IIIa) represents a final common pathway to platelet aggregation and subsequent thrombus formation.[105] Once activated, the receptor undergoes a conformational change that permits the binding of fibrinogen. This allows cross-linking of platelets and aggregation, with the formation of the hemostatic platelet plug.[106] Selective inhibition of the GP IIb/IIIa receptor is a logical target for more specific antiplatelet therapy. There are three main inhibitors approved for clinical use: abciximab (ReoPro), eptifibatide (Integrilin), and tirofiban (Aggrastat).

Abciximab. Abciximab was the first GP IIb/IIIa receptor inhibitor developed. It is a macromolecule composed of the Fab fragment of the chimeric human murine monoclonal antibody c7E3.[107] It has a high binding affinity for the GP IIb/IIIa receptor, which accounts for its prolonged antiplatelet effect after cessation of infusion, with up to 10 days of low-level receptor blockade.[107] Platelet aggregation is almost completely inhibited by 2 hours after infusion, with recovery evident 48 hours after discontinuing the drug. However, platelet-bound drug can still be detected for up to 10 days.[108]

Tirofiban. Tirofiban is a small, nonpeptide antagonist of the GP IIb/IIIa receptor.[108] It is a tyrosine derivative with a molecular weight of 495 kD. At standard doses, platelet function is inhibited as early as 5 minutes after infusion, with bleeding time and platelet aggregation normalizing within 3 to 8 hours after discontinuation.[108]

Eptifibatide. Eptifibatide is a nonimmunogenic, cyclic heptapeptide that inhibits the GP IIb/IIIa receptor. It is derived from the structure of barbourin from the venom of a species of rattlesnake.[109] It has a short plasma half-life of 15 minutes, with peak platelet effects within 15 minutes of infusion; platelet function returns to 50% of baseline by 4 hours after terminating the infusion.[110]

Clinical Use. The GP IIb/IIIa receptor antagonists have been shown to reduce cardiac event rates in patients with acute coronary syndromes treated by medicine alone or in combination with percutaneous coronary intervention.[111] Evidence supporting their use in percutaneous coronary interventions is good. It confers significant long-term mortality benefits and decreases ischemic events.[105,106,112-114] There are currently no large, randomized clinical trials of GP IIb/IIIa inhibitors specifically in vascular surgery patients.

Adverse Reactions. Bleeding is the principal adverse effect of all the GP inhibitors. Nearly all trials demonstrate an increase in serious bleeding rates. Fatal bleeding is rare (<0.1%), which is similar to the rate with combined heparin and aspirin therapy.[108] Thrombocytopenia is also associated with GP inhibition. Abciximab causes severe thrombocytopenia (<20,000/µL) in 0.7% of patients, and eptifibatide and tirofiban in 0.2% of patients.[108]

The optimal patients to receive GP inhibitors are those with acute coronary syndrome who undergo percutaneous coronary intervention and are at high risk for early failure. The value of GP inhibition in other vascular interventions is not yet established.[108]

Medical Treatment of Claudication

Pentoxifylline

Structure and Mechanism of Action. Pentoxifylline is an antithrombotic agent whose exact mechanism of action is unknown. It is thought to improve blood flow by increasing red cell deformity, decreasing platelet adhesiveness, and decreasing blood viscosity, leading to increased flow in the microcirculation.[115-117]

Clinical Use. Multiple clinical trials of pentoxifylline have demonstrated conflicting results in the treatment of claudication. Some suggested improved walking distance with pentoxifylline,[118-123] whereas others showed little benefit compared with placebo.[124-127] Based on such conflicting data, it is currently not recommended for use in claudication.

Cilostazol

Structure and Mechanism of Action. Cilostazol is a type III phosphodiesterase inhibitor that increases cellular cyclic adenosine monophosphate and acts to inhibit platelet aggregation and thrombus formation. It is also a direct vasodilator.[31] Cilostazol has been shown to improve claudication symptoms, but the exact mechanism is unknown. It is absorbed after oral administration and extensively metabolized by hepatic cytochrome P-450 enzymes, with two main active metabolites being produced.[11] Excretion is predominantly urinary.

Clinical Use. Cilostazol was approved in 1999 by the FDA for the treatment of intermittent claudication, based on randomized clinical trials that demonstrated increased walking distance and quality of life.[128-130] Compared with those given placebo, patients taking cilostazol experienced significant increases in walking distance. The effect was apparent as early as 2 to 4 weeks after initiating therapy. Cilostazol is more effective than pentoxifylline in improving claudication.[11] Current recommendations are that cilostazol should be used only by those with moderate to severely disabling claudication and who are not revascularization candidates.[31] Cilostazol has weak antiplatelet effects, but there are no clinical data to support its use as an antiplatelet agent.[31]

Adverse Reactions. Because cilostazol is a phosphodiesterase inhibitor, it should not be used in patients with congestive heart failure. The only adverse effect in study patients leading to discontinuation of the drug was headache, likely secondary to its vasodilatory effects. Other more common side effects include palpitations and diarrhea.

Agents to Prevent Contrast-Induced Nephropathy

Contrast nephropathy (CN) is the third leading cause of acute renal failure in hospitalized patients.[131,132] Most cases of CN are reversible and nonoliguric; however, up to 25% to 30% of patients who develop CN have a permanent decline in renal function.[133] In addition, patients who develop acute renal failure have increased morbidity and mortality.[134] The main risk factors for developing CN are underlying renal insufficiency and diabetes.[135] The exact mechanism behind the development of CN remains unknown, but is likely a combination of direct renal tubule epithelial cell toxicity and renal medullary ischemia.[135,136]

The use of low volumes of low-osmolar and iso-osmolar contrast agents appears to reduce the risk of CN compared with the use of high-osmolar contrast agents.[137-139] Multiple trials have demonstrated that saline hydration is also beneficial in preventing CN.[140,141]

Sodium Bicarbonate

Intravenous infusion of isotonic sodium bicarbonate has been demonstrated to be somewhat superior to isotonic sodium chloride (saline) in preventing CN in high-risk patients.[142] This protocol used an infusion of 3 mL/kg/h for 1 hour before and 1 mL/kg/h for 6 hours after the procedure. Although additional studies are needed, particularly given the low risk for adverse reactions, this study suggests that sodium bicarbonate may be effective in high-risk patients.

N-Acetylcysteine

Structure and Mechanism of Action. N-Acetylcysteine (NAC) is the acetylated form of the amino acid L-cysteine. NAC has been in clinical use for more than 40 years, mostly as a mucolytic.[143] NAC is an antioxidant and a free radical scavenger. It can stimulate glutathione synthesis and has vasodilatory properties through its effects on nitric oxide.[144]

Clinical Use. Clinical data on the value of NAC in preventing CN are mixed. NAC initially demonstrated a significant reduction in CN in patients with preexisting renal insufficiency.[145] The frequency of CN in patients receiving hydration plus NAC was 2%, compared with 22% in those receiving hydration alone. Other studies conducted later demonstrated similar protective effects of NAC[146,147]; however, subsequent trials have not demonstrated a clear benefit in the prevention of CN.[148,149] Proponents of NAC argue that its ease of administration, relatively low cost, and limited side effects make it an appealing agent in high-risk patients.

Fenoldopam

Structure and Mechanism of Action. Fenoldopam is a selective dopamine-1 agonist that increases both cortical and medullary renal blood flow. Unlike dopamine, fenoldopam does not stimulate the α- and β-adrenergic receptors or the dopamine-2 receptors, which can produce vasoconstriction.[150,151] Fenoldopam has been shown to increase the glomerular filtration rate and induce diuresis.[150]

Clinical Use. Early retrospective studies suggested that fenoldopam reduced the incidence of CN.[151-153] However, more recent prospective, randomized trials have not shown that it offers any protection against CN.[154,155] As a result, fenoldopam cannot be recommended for the prevention of CN.

Theophylline

Structure and Mechanism of Action. Theophylline blocks adenosine receptors in the kidney. Adenosine is an important intrarenal mediator that can cause a decrease in glomerular filtration rate through vasoconstriction of afferent arterioles and vasodilatation of efferent arterioles and mesangial cell contraction.[156] It also induces cortical vasoconstriction and increases free radical generation in the tubular cells.[156] Animal studies suggest a benefit of adenosine receptor blockade in the renal vascular response to contrast media.[156]

Clinical Use. Initial clinical trials suggested a benefit of theophylline in the prevention of CN.[157,158] Another study demonstrated that theophylline offered no additional protection compared with hydration alone.[159] Thus, with no convincing clinical data, theophylline

cannot currently be recommended for the prevention of CN.

Other Agents

Prostaglandin E₁

Prostaglandin E_1 has vasodilatory effects that may be beneficial in preventing CN.[135] One randomized trial suggested protection in patients receiving prostaglandin E_1, but this was not statistically significant.[160] Further trials are needed.

Endothelin Antagonists

Endothelin-1 is an endogenous vasoconstrictor; it has been examined as a possible cause of CN.[131] Blockade of the endothelin-1 receptor with endothelin-α antagonists has been shown in animal models to reduce the incidence of nephropathy.[161] However, a clinical trial actually demonstrated decreased renal function after radiocontrast with endothelin receptor antagonism.[162] There are currently no data to support endothelin receptor blockade in the prevention of CN.

Calcium Channel Blockers

Calcium channel blockers prevent the influx of calcium into smooth muscle cells, causing a vasodilatory effect in all vascular beds, including the kidney. They also offer some cytoprotective effects.[163] Animal studies have shown that calcium channel blockade confers protection against CN,[163] but there is no consensus among clinical trials.[164-168] Large-scale clinical trials of calcium channel blockers are required.

Dopamine

Dopamine has variable effects, depending on dose. Low-dose dopamine activates DA-1 and DA-2 receptors. Medium doses activate β-adrenergic receptors, and high doses activate α receptors.[169] The DA-1 receptor causes renal vasodilatation, and low-dose dopamine has been investigated in regard to preventing CN.[131] There are conflicting data regarding dopamine and protection against CN[169-172]; therefore dopamine is not currently recommended for the prevention of CN.

Diuretics

Furosemide and mannitol have had disappointing results when examined for the prevention of CN. The majority of the evidence is against their use, as they may exacerbate renal dysfunction.[140,173]

Statins

Statin therapy has been demonstrated to reduce cardiovascular morbidity and mortality in multiple patient populations.[174-178] Although the primary mechanism of action is to reduce cholesterol levels, the benefits of statin therapy appear to extend beyond that effect.[179]

Structure and Mechanism of Action. Statins decrease cholesterol levels through inhibition of the HMG-CoA reductase enzyme, the rate-limiting step through which cells synthesize cholesterol. Inhibition of cholesterol synthesis leads to increased hepatocyte expression of LDL receptors, with increased cellular uptake of LDL and a reduction in plasma LDL and cholesterol levels.[179] Statins also reduce the rate at which apolipoprotein B particles are secreted by the liver.[179]

Clinical Use. There are considerable data to support the use of statins in patients with cardiovascular disease. The Scandinavian Simvastatin Survival Study clearly established that lipid-lowering therapy was safe, and it reduced morbidity and mortality in patients with ischemic heart disease who had elevated cholesterol levels.[175] Statin treatment reduced major coronary events, coronary mortality, and overall mortality. Multiple subsequent studies of patients with elevated cholesterol demonstrated a significant reduction in cardiovascular events and overall mortality with statin therapy.[176,180,181] Statins are also beneficial in patients with cardiovascular disease who have normal lipid levels.[174,178,181,182] In addition, statin therapy is associated with a reduction in the risk of stroke in patients with cardiovascular disease.[183,184]

Besides lowering cholesterol, statins are thought to have significant so-called pleiotropic effects.[179] Statins can improve endothelial cell function[185,186] and reduce inflammation and thrombosis, leading to plaque stabilization.[179,182,187,188] The majority of studies support the aggressive use of statins in patients at high risk for coronary or cerebrovascular events, particularly in those with established disease, irrespective of their baseline cholesterol levels.

Specific studies focusing on vascular surgery patients are few. Subgroup analysis of patients with peripheral vascular disease in the major statin trials demonstrated a significant decrease in myocardial infarction and cardiovascular events.[189] The Scandinavian Simvastatin Survival Study trial found that the incidence of new-onset or worsening intermittent claudication was reduced 38% with statin therapy.[175] Statin treatment in patients undergoing noncardiac vascular surgery has been shown to reduce cardiac morbidity and mortality.[190-192] Statins also improve vein graft patency.[193]

Adverse Reactions. High-dose statin therapy leads to hepatic necrosis in animal models.[194] In clinical trials, statins have not been demonstrated to cause significant liver enzyme elevations compared with controls.[195] Current recommendations are to monitor hepatic enzymes for 4 to 6 weeks after initiating treatment. In high-risk patients or those taking certain medications, closer monitoring may be warranted. The most serious risks associated with statin therapy are myositis and rhabdomyolysis.[194,196] Cerivastatin was withdrawn from the market owing to deaths from such complications.[197] Risks for rhabdomyolysis are increased with small body size, advanced age, renal or hepatic

dysfunction, diabetes, and hypothyroidism.[197] Patients receiving statins should be monitored closely for symptoms of myopathy.

Fish Oil

Long-chain, highly unsaturated omega-3 fatty acids, found in cold-water fish and now widely commercially available in capsules, can decrease fasting triglyceride concentrations 20% to 50% by reducing hepatic triglyceride production and increasing triglyceride clearance.[198] With long-term intake, they have been shown to increase HDLs, enhance the antiplatelet activity of aspirin and clopidogrel, improve heart failure, and improve vascular function in diabetes.[198] A large, randomized, 5-year trial in more than 18,000 hypercholesterolemic patients already treated with statins showed a significant reduction in major coronary events when eicosapentaenoic acid was added.[199] A subanalysis of the JELIS trial demonstrated that specifically in patients with peripheral arterial disease, the incidence of coronary artery disease (CAD) was higher than in controls, and that eicosapentaenoic acid markedly reduced the occurrence of CAD in those patients.[200] Fish oil benefits the vascular surgical patient through stabilization of the overall cardiovascular system.

Other Lipid-Lowering Agents

Ezetimibe

Ezetimibe is a cholesterol transport inhibitor that acts primarily on the small intestine to reduce cholesterol absorption. Ezetimibe is most effective when combined with statin medications and has been shown to have a synergistic effect on lipid reduction in this setting.[201,202]

Niacin (Nicotinic Acid)

Niacin has been demonstrated to be beneficial in both reducing VLDL and LDL, in addition to increasing levels of HDL. Flushing, diarrhea, and a mild diabetogenic effect are all recognized side-effects of niacin use and form the majority of reasons for discontinuation of the medication.[203,204]

Fibric Acid Derivatives

Fibric acid derivatives such as gemfibrozil and fenofibrate have limited applicability in the primary risk reduction strategy for dyslipidemia as their effect on LDL levels are marginal. However, are of marked benefit in patients with pancreatitis associated with hypertriglyceridemia owing to their selective reduction in triglycerides.[205,206]

Bile Acid Sequestrants

Bile acid sequestrants are weak cholesterol and LDL lowering medications and act by interrupting the enterohepatic recirculation of bile acids via inhibition of small intestinal bile acid reabsorption.[207]

CONCLUSIONS

Cardiovascular disease continues to be the most significant cause of mortality in the United States and similarly developed countries. The detection of modifiable risk factors for atherosclerosis continues to remain one of the most promising areas of research in the field of cardiovascular medicine. As the population ages and becomes more obese, there will be a rise in the number of patients with cardiovascular disease. Aggressive risk-factor modification can only occur if there is vigilance and attention to the detection and subsequent treatment of such conditions as diabetes, obesity, dyslipidemia, smoking, and renal disease. Although there are many effective strategies for risk-reduction, including an array of pharmacologic agents, once these conditions have been diagnosed, there is a growing body of epidemiologic evidence that indicates greater health outcomes when the predisposing factors for these diseases are addressed early, before full-blown disease diagnosis.

Preventing individuals from becoming smokers rather than focusing on smoking cessation, educating individuals about diet and exercise strategies to prevent obesity, and modulation of cholesterol intake to reduce hyperlipidemia are all paradigms for reducing the exposure of the population to cardiovascular risk factors. Unfortunately patients have not embraced these preventative strategies, and public health measures have not been successful in a cost-effective and widespread manner.

Despite advances in pharmacologic treatment of identified risk factors, effective behavioral modification strategies are limited. Attitudes toward health and cultivation of risk factor avoidance have been difficult to implement; however, it is these very attributes that are most likely to reduce the burden of cardiovascular disease most significantly. These core health traits must be adopted by individuals and supported by education and demonstration of identifiable health benefit before prevention of cardiovascular disease can be entertained at a population level.

BIBLIOGRAPHY

Antithrombotic Trialists' Collaboration: Collaborative meta-analysis of randomised trials of antiplatelet therapy for prevention of death, myocardial infarction, and stroke in high risk patients. BMJ 324:71–86, 2002.

Becker RC, Fintel DJ, Green D, editors: Antithrombotic Therapy, ed 2, West Islip, New York, 2002, Professional Communications, pp 63–76.

Cox CD, Tsikouris JP: Preventing contrast nephropathy: what is the best strategy? A review of the literature. J Clin Pharmacol 44:327–337, 2004.

Dawson DL, Cutler BS, Hiatt WR, et al: A comparison of cilostazol and pentoxifylline for treating intermittent claudication. Am J Med 109:523–530, 2000.

Fonarow GC, Gawlinski A, Moughrabi S, et al: Improved treatment of coronary heart disease by implementation of a Cardiac Hospitalization Atherosclerosis Management Program (CHAMP). Am J Cardiol 87(7):819–822, 2001.

Frangos SG, Chen AH, Sumpio B: Vascular drugs in the new millennium. J Am Coll Surg 191:76–92, 2000.

Hiatt WR: Pharmacologic therapy for peripheral arterial disease and claudication. J Vasc Surg 36:1283–1291, 2002.

Kam PC, Nethery CM: The thienopyridine derivatives (platelet adenosine diphosphate receptor antagonists), pharmacology and clinical developments. Anaesthesia 58:28–35, 2003.

Kaplan KL: Direct thrombin inhibitors. Expert Opin Pharmacother 4:653–666, 2003.

Poldermans D, Bax JJ, Kertai MD, et al: Statins are associated with a reduced incidence of perioperative mortality in patients undergoing major noncardiac vascular surgery. Circulation 107:1848–1851, 2003.

Randomised trial of cholesterol lowering in 4444 patients with coronary heart disease: The Scandinavian Simvastatin Survival Study (4S). Lancet 344:1383–1389, 1994.

Sobel M, Verhaeghe R: Antithrombotic therapy for peripheral artery occlusive disease: American College of Chest Physicians Evidence-Based Clinical Practice Guidelines (8th Edition). Chest 133(6 Suppl):815S–843S, 2008.

References available online at expertconsult.com.

QUESTIONS

1. Which of the following risk factors has not been reproducibly demonstrated to confer a reduction in cardiovascular risk when modified?
   a. Smoking
   b. Homocysteine levels
   c. HDL, LDL, and triglyceride levels
   d. HbA_{1c} level
   e. Diastolic blood pressure

2. Which of the following targets is not part of the guidelines for the management of diabetic patients?
   a. Triglyceride level <150 mg/dL
   b. HbA_{1c} level <7%
   c. Fasting blood glucose <110 mg/dL
   d. Blood pressure <140/90 mm Hg
   e. LDL <100 mg/dL

3. Which of the following is a well-established side-effect of use of HMG-CoA reductase inhibitors (statins)?
   a. Thrombocytopenia
   b. Stroke
   c. Myositis
   d. Hepatitis
   e. Deep vein thrombosis

4. Which of the following provides the most durable reduction in cardiovascular risk in patients with the metabolic syndrome?
   a. Weight loss
   b. Tight glucose control
   c. Blood pressure <130/80
   d. Tight lipid control
   e. Euthyroidism

5. Which of the following is not part of the Cardiac Hospitalization Atherosclerosis Management Program (CHAMP) guidelines:
   a. Antiplatelet agents
   b. β-Blockade
   c. ACE inhibition
   d. HMG-CoA reductase inhibitors
   e. Calcium-channel blockade

6. Which of these therapies has clearly been shown to prevent contrast-induced nephropathy?
   a. High-osmolar contrast agents
   b. Intravenous hydration
   c. Fenoldopam
   d. Theophylline
   e. Lasix

7. True or false: Argatroban, being renally excreted, needs to be dosed carefully in patients with renal failure.

8. Which antigen is thought to be associated with the development of heparin-induced thrombocytopenia?
   a. Platelet factor 4
   b. Von Willebrand factor
   c. Factor X
   d. Platelet ADP receptor

9. Patients with a history of fish allergy may have an increased risk of reaction to which of the following?
   a. Protamine
   b. Heparin
   c. Argatroban
   d. Tirofiban
   e. Clopidogrel

10. Which of the following has clear indications for use in the treatment of intermittent claudication?
    a. Ticlopidine
    b. Clopidogrel
    c. Cilostazol
    d. Pentoxifylline
    e. Tirofiban

ANSWERS

1. **b**
2. **d**
3. **c**
4. **a**
5. **e**
6. **b**
7. **False**
8. **a**
9. **a**
10. **c**

CHAPTER 13

Hemodynamics for the Vascular Surgeon

R. Eugene Zierler • D. Eugene Strandness, Jr.

Blood flow in human arteries and veins can be described in terms of hemodynamic principles. Although the elements of hemodynamics are derived from engineering, mathematics, and physiology, these principles also form the theoretical foundation for the treatment of vascular disease.

The major mechanisms of arterial disease are obstruction of the lumen and disruption of the vessel wall. Arterial obstruction or narrowing can result from atherosclerosis, emboli, thrombi, fibromuscular dysplasia, trauma, or external compression. The clinical significance of an obstructive lesion depends on its location, severity, and duration, as well as on the ability of the circulation to compensate by increasing cardiac output and developing collateral pathways. Open surgical or endovascular treatment requires the identification and correction of arterial lesions associated with significant hemodynamic disturbances. Disruption of the arterial wall occurs with ruptured aneurysms or trauma. The tendency of aneurysms to rupture is determined by arterial wall characteristics, intraluminal pressure, and size. In this situation, the role of surgical intervention is to prevent rupture or to reestablish arterial continuity after rupture occurs.

On the venous side of the circulation, the major hemodynamic mechanisms of disease are obstruction and valvular incompetence. These are generally the sequelae of thrombosis in the deep venous system, and they produce venous hypertension distal to the involved venous segment. The clinical consequences of venous hypertension are the signs and symptoms of the postthrombotic syndrome: pain, edema, subcutaneous fibrosis, pigmentation, stasis dermatitis, and ulceration. Treatment of this condition involves elevation, external compression, venous interruption, and, rarely, direct venous interventions.

This chapter begins with a discussion of the hemodynamic principles and vessel wall properties that govern arterial flow. The hemodynamic alterations produced by arterial stenoses and their effect on flow patterns in human limbs are considered next. These principles are then related to the treatment of arterial obstruction. Finally, the hemodynamics of the venous system are briefly reviewed and related to the pathophysiology and treatment of venous disease.

BASIC PRINCIPLES OF ARTERIAL HEMODYNAMICS

Fluid Pressure

The pressure in a fluid system is defined as force per unit area (in dynes per square centimeter). Intravascular arterial pressure (*P*) has three components: (1) the dynamic pressure produced by contraction of the heart, (2) the hydrostatic pressure, and (3) the static filling pressure. Hydrostatic pressure is determined by the specific gravity of blood and the height of the point of measurement above a specific reference level. The reference level in the human body is considered to be the right atrium. The hydrostatic pressure is given by the following equation:

$$P \text{ (hydrostatic)} = -\rho g h \qquad [1]$$

where ρ is the specific gravity of blood (approximately 1.056 g/cm^3), g is the acceleration due to gravity (980 cm/s^2), and h is the distance in centimeters above or below the right atrium. The magnitude of hydrostatic pressure may be large. In a man 5 feet 8 inches tall, this pressure at ankle level is approximately 89 mm Hg.[1]

The static filling pressure represents the residual pressure that exists in the absence of arterial flow. This pressure is determined by the volume of blood and the elastic properties of the vessel wall, and it is typically in the range of 5 to 10 mm Hg.

Fluid Energy

Blood flows through the arterial system in response to differences in total fluid energy. Although pressure gradients are the most obvious forces involved, other forms of energy drive the circulation.[2] Total fluid energy (*E*) can be divided into potential energy (E_p) and kinetic energy (E_k). The components of potential energy are intravascular pressure (*P*) and gravitational potential energy.

The factors contributing to intravascular pressure have already been mentioned. Gravitational potential energy represents the ability of a volume of blood to do work because of its height above a specific reference level. The formula for gravitational potential energy is the same as that for hydrostatic pressure (see Equation 1) but with an opposite sign: $+\rho g h$. Because the gravitational potential energy and hydrostatic pressure usually cancel each other out and the static filling pressure is relatively low, the predominant component of potential energy is the dynamic pressure produced by cardiac contraction. Potential energy can be expressed as follows:

$$E_p = P + (\rho gh) \qquad [2]$$

Kinetic energy represents the ability of blood to do work on the basis of its motion. It is proportional to the specific gravity of blood and the square of blood velocity (v), in centimeters per second:

$$E_k = \frac{1}{2}\rho v^2 \qquad [3]$$

By combining Equations 2 and 3, an expression for the total fluid energy per unit volume of blood (in ergs per cubic centimeter) can be obtained:

$$E = P + \rho gh + \frac{1}{2}\rho v^2 \qquad [4]$$

Fluid Energy Losses

Bernoulli's Principle

When fluid flows from one point to another, its total energy *(E)* along any given streamline is constant, provided that flow is steady and there are no frictional energy losses. This is in accordance with the law of conservation of energy and constitutes Bernoulli's principle:

$$P_1 + \rho gh_1 + \frac{1}{2}\rho v_1^2 = P_2 + \rho gh_2 + \frac{1}{2}\rho v_2^2 \qquad [5]$$

This equation expresses the relationships among pressure, gravitational potential energy, and kinetic energy in an idealized fluid system. In the horizontal diverging tube shown in Figure 13-1, steady flow between point 1 and point 2 is accompanied by an increase in cross-sectional area and a decrease in flow velocity. Although the fluid

A₁ = 1 cm²   A₂ = 16 cm²

V₁ = 80 cm/sec   V₂ = 5 cm/sec

P₁ = 100 mm Hg   P₂ = 102.5 mm Hg

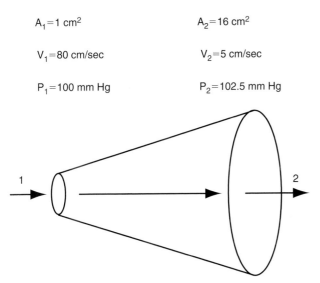

FIGURE 13-1 ■ Effect of increasing cross-sectional area on pressure in a frictionless fluid system. While pressure increases, total fluid energy remains constant as a result of a decrease in velocity. (Redrawn from Sumner DS: The hemodynamics and pathophysiology of arterial disease. In Rutherford RB, editor: Vascular surgery, Philadelphia, 1977, WB Saunders.)

moves against a pressure gradient of 2.5 mm Hg and therefore gains potential energy, the total fluid energy remains constant because of the lower velocity and a proportional loss of kinetic energy. In other words, the widening of the tube results in the conversion of kinetic energy to potential energy in the form of pressure. In a converging tube, the opposite would occur; a pressure drop and increase in velocity would result in potential energy being converted to kinetic energy.

The situation depicted in the preceding example is not observed in human arteries because the ideal flow conditions specified in the Bernoulli relationship are not present. The fluid energy lost in moving blood through the arterial circulation is dissipated mainly in the form of heat. When this source of energy loss is accounted for, Equation 5 becomes the following:

$$P_1 + \rho gh_1 + \frac{1}{2}\rho v_1^2 = P_2 + \rho gh_2 + \frac{1}{2}\rho v_2^2 + \text{Heat} \qquad [6]$$

Viscous Energy Losses and Poiseuille's Law

Energy losses in flowing blood occur either as viscous losses resulting from friction or as inertial losses related to changes in the velocity or direction of flow. The term viscosity describes the resistance to flow that arises because of the intermolecular attractions between fluid layers. The coefficient of viscosity (η) is defined as the ratio of shear stress (τ) to shear rate (D):

$$\eta = \frac{\tau}{D} \qquad [7]$$

Shear stress is proportional to the energy loss owing to friction between adjacent fluid layers, whereas shear rate is the relative velocity of adjacent fluid layers. Fluids with particularly strong intermolecular attractions offer a high resistance to flow and have high coefficients of viscosity. For example, motor oil has a higher coefficient of viscosity than water.[3] The unit of viscosity is the poise, which equals 1 dyne-s/cm². Because it is difficult to measure viscosity directly, relative viscosity is often used to relate the viscosity of a fluid to that of water. The relative viscosity of plasma is approximately 1.8, whereas the relative viscosity for whole blood is in the range of 3 to 4.

Because viscosity increases exponentially with increases in hematocrit, the concentration of red blood cells is the most important factor affecting the viscosity of whole blood. The viscosity of plasma is determined largely by the concentration of plasma proteins. These constituents of blood are also responsible for its non-Newtonian character. In a Newtonian fluid, viscosity is independent of shear rate or flow velocity. Because blood is a suspension of cells and large protein molecules, its viscosity can vary greatly with shear rate (Figure 13-2). Blood viscosity increases rapidly at low shear rates, but approaches a constant value at higher shear rates. In most of the arterial circulation, the prevailing shear rates place the blood viscosity on the asymptotic portion of the curve. Thus, for arteries with diameters greater than approximately 1 mm, human blood resembles a constant-viscosity, or Newtonian, fluid.

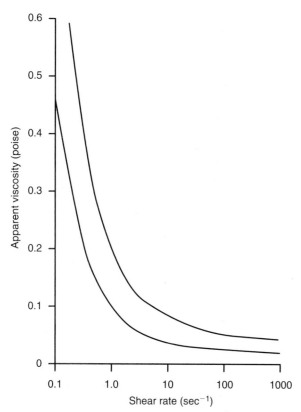

FIGURE 13-2 ■ Viscosity of human blood as a function of shear rate. Values range between the two lines. (From Strandness DE, Sumner DS: Hemodynamics for surgeons, New York, 1975, Grune and Stratton.)

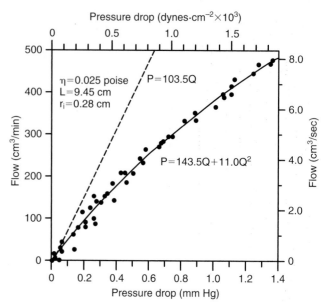

FIGURE 13-3 ■ Pressure drop across a 9.45-cm length of canine femoral artery at varying flow rates. The experimental data line *(solid)* has both linear and squared terms, corresponding to viscous and inertial energy losses. The pressure-flow curve predicted by Poiseuille's law *(dashed line)* depicts much lower energy losses than those actually observed. (From Sumner DS: The hemodynamics and pathophysiology of arterial disease. In Rutherford RB, editor: Vascular surgery, Philadelphia, 1977, WB Saunders.)

Poiseuille's law describes the viscous energy losses that occur in an idealized flow model. This law states that the pressure gradient along a tube ($P_1 - P_2$, in dynes per square centimeter) is directly proportional to the mean flow velocity ($\bar{V}$, in centimeters per second) or volume flow (Q, in cubic centimeters per second), the tube length (L, in centimeters), and the fluid viscosity (η, in poise), and is inversely proportional to either the second or fourth power of the radius (r, in centimeters):

$$P_1 - P_2 = \bar{V}\frac{8L\eta}{r^2} = Q\frac{8L\eta}{\pi r^4} \qquad [8]$$

When this equation is simplified to Pressure = Flow × Resistance, it is analogous to Ohm's law of electrical circuits.

The strict application of Poiseuille's law requires the steady, laminar flow of a Newtonian fluid in a straight, rigid, cylindrical tube. Because these conditions seldom exist in the arterial circulation, Poiseuille's law can only estimate the minimum pressure gradient or viscous energy losses that may be expected in arterial flow. Energy losses owing to inertial effects often exceed viscous energy losses, particularly in the presence of arterial disease.

Inertial Energy Losses

Energy losses related to inertia (ΔE) are proportional to a constant (K), the specific gravity of blood, and the square of blood velocity:

$$\Delta E = K \tfrac{1}{2}\rho v^2 \qquad [9]$$

Because velocity is the only independent variable in this equation, inertial energy losses result from the acceleration and deceleration of pulsatile flow, variations in lumen diameter, and changes in the direction of flow at points of curvature and branching. The combined effects of viscous and inertial energy losses are illustrated in Figure 13-3. When the pressure drop across an arterial segment is measured at varying flow rates, the experimental data fit a line with both linear (viscous) and squared (inertial) terms. The viscous energy losses predicted by Poiseuille's law are considerably less than the total energy loss actually observed.

Vascular Resistance

Hemodynamic resistance (R) can be defined as the ratio of the energy drop between two points along an artery ($E_1 - E_2$) to the mean blood flow (Q):

$$R = \frac{E_1 - E_2}{Q} \cong \frac{P_1 - P_2}{Q} \qquad [10]$$

Because the kinetic energy term ($\tfrac{1}{2}\rho v^2$) is typically a small component of the total fluid energy, and the artery is usually assumed to be horizontal so that the gravitational potential energy terms (ρgh) cancel, Equation 4 can be used to express resistance as the simple ratio of pressure drop ($P_1 - P_2$) to flow. Thus, Equation 10 becomes a rearranged version of Poiseuille's law

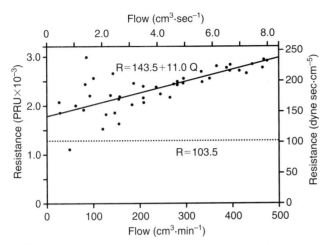

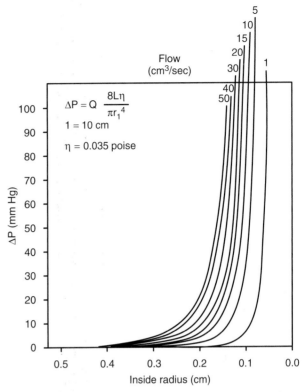

FIGURE 13-4 ■ Resistance derived from the pressure-flow curve in Figure 13-3. The resistance increases with increasing flow. Constant resistance predicted by Poiseuille's law is shown by the dotted line. *PRU,* Peripheral resistance unit. (From Sumner DS: The hemodynamics and pathophysiology of arterial disease. In Rutherford RB, editor: Vascular surgery, Philadelphia, 1977, WB Saunders.)

FIGURE 13-5 ■ Relationship of pressure drop to inside radius of a cylindrical tube 10 cm in length at various rates of steady laminar flow. Flow rates are comparable to those in the human iliac artery. (From Strandness DE, Sumner DS: Hemodynamics for surgeons, New York, 1975, Grune and Stratton.)

(Equation 8), and the minimum resistance or viscous energy losses are given by the resistance term:

$$R = \frac{8L\eta}{\pi r^4} \qquad [11]$$

The hemodynamic resistance of an arterial segment increases as the flow velocity increases, provided that the lumen size remains constant (Figure 13-4). These additional energy losses are related to inertial effects and are proportional to $\frac{1}{2}\rho v^2$.

According to Equation 11, the predominant factor influencing hemodynamic resistance is the fourth power of the radius. The relationship between radius and pressure drop for various flow rates along a 10-cm vessel segment is shown in Figure 13-5. For a wide range of flow rates, the pressure drop is negligible until the radius is reduced to approximately 0.3 cm; for radii less than 0.2 cm, the pressure drop increases rapidly. These observations may explain the frequent failure of femoropopliteal autogenous vein bypass grafts less than 4 mm in diameter.[4]

The calculation of total resistance (R_t) depends on whether the component resistances ($R_1...R_n$) are arranged in series or in parallel. This is also analogous to electrical circuits.

$$R_t \ (series) = R_1 + R_2 + ... R_n \qquad [12]$$

$$\frac{1}{R_t \ (parallel)} = \frac{1}{R_1} + \frac{1}{R_2} + ... + \frac{1}{R_n} \qquad [13]$$

The standard physical units of hemodynamic resistance are dyne-seconds per centimeter to the fifth power. A more convenient way of expressing resistance is the peripheral resistance unit (PRU), which has the dimensions of millimeters of mercury per cubic centimeter per minute. One PRU is approximately 8×10^4 dyne-s/cm.[5]

In the human circulation, approximately 90% of the total vascular resistance results from flow through the arteries and capillaries, whereas the remaining 10% results from venous flow. The arterioles and capillaries are responsible for more than 60% of the total resistance, whereas the large- and medium-sized arteries account for only about 15%.[2] Thus, the arteries that are most commonly affected by atherosclerotic occlusive disease are normally vessels with low resistance.

Blood Flow Patterns

Laminar Flow

In the steady-state conditions specified by Poiseuille's law, the flow pattern is laminar. All motion is parallel to the walls of the tube, and the fluid is arranged in a series of concentric layers, or laminae, like those shown in Figure 13-6. While the velocity within each lamina remains constant, the velocity is lowest adjacent to the tube wall and increases toward the center of the tube. This results in a velocity profile that is parabolic in shape (Figure 13-7). As discussed previously, the energy expended in moving one lamina of fluid over another is proportional to viscosity.

Turbulent Flow

In contrast to the linear streamlines of laminar flow, turbulence is an irregular flow state in which velocity varies

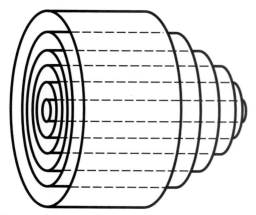

FIGURE 13-6 ■ Concentric laminae of fluid in a cylindrical tube. Flow is from left to right. The center laminae move more rapidly than those near the periphery, and the flow profile is parabolic. (From Strandness DE, Sumner DS: Hemodynamics for surgeons, New York, 1975, Grune and Stratton.)

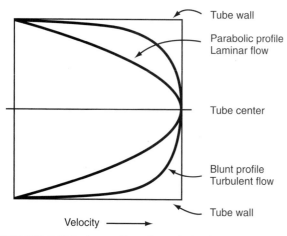

FIGURE 13-7 ■ Velocity profiles of steady laminar and turbulent flow. Velocity is lowest adjacent to the tube wall and maximal in the center. (From Sumner DS: The hemodynamics and pathophysiology of arterial disease. In Rutherford RB, editor: Vascular surgery, Philadelphia, 1977, WB Saunders.)

rapidly with respect to space and time. These random velocity changes result in the dissipation of fluid energy as heat. The point of transition between laminar and turbulent flow depends on the tube diameter (*d*, in centimeters), the mean velocity, the specific gravity of the fluid, and the fluid viscosity. These factors can be expressed as a dimensionless quantity called the Reynolds number (*Re*), which is the ratio of inertial forces to viscous forces acting on the fluid:

$$Re = \frac{d\overline{V}\rho}{\eta} \qquad [14]$$

In flowing blood at Reynolds numbers greater than 2000, inertial forces may disrupt laminar flow and produce fully developed turbulence. With values less than 2000, localized flow disturbances are damped out by viscous forces. In the normal arterial circulation, Reynolds numbers are usually less than 2000, and true turbulence is unlikely to occur; however, Reynolds numbers greater than 2000 can be found in the ascending aorta, where

small areas of turbulence develop.[3] Although turbulent flow is uncommon in normal arteries, the arterial flow pattern is often disturbed.[5] The condition of disturbed flow is an intermediate state between stable laminar flow and fully developed turbulence. It is a transient perturbation in the laminar streamlines that disappears as the flow proceeds downstream. Arterial flow may become disturbed at points of branching and curvature.

When turbulence is the result of a stenotic arterial lesion, it generally occurs immediately downstream from the stenosis and may be present only over the systolic portion of the cardiac cycle when the critical value of the Reynolds number is exceeded. Under conditions of turbulent flow, the velocity profile changes from the parabolic shape of laminar flow to a rectangular or blunt shape (see Figure 13-7). Because of the random velocity changes, energy losses are greater for a turbulent or disturbed flow state than for a laminar flow state. Consequently, the linear relationship between pressure and flow expressed by Poiseuille's law cannot be applied. This deviation from Poiseuille's law in arterial flow is shown in Figure 13-3.

Boundary Layer Separation

In fluid flowing through a tube, the portion of fluid adjacent to the tube wall is referred to as the *boundary layer*. This layer is subject to both frictional interactions with the tube wall and viscous forces generated by the more rapidly moving fluid toward the center of the tube. When the tube geometry changes suddenly, such as at points of curvature, branching, or variations in lumen diameter, small pressure gradients are created that cause the boundary layer to stop or reverse direction. This change results in a complex, localized flow pattern known as an *area of boundary layer separation* or *flow separation*.[6]

Areas of boundary layer separation have been observed in models of arterial anastomoses and bifurcations.[7,8] In the carotid artery bifurcation shown in Figure 13-8, the central rapid flow stream of the common carotid artery is compressed along the inner wall of the carotid bulb, producing a region of high shear stress. An area of flow separation has formed along the outer wall of the carotid bulb that includes helical flow patterns and flow reversal. The region of the carotid bulb adjacent to the separation zone is subject to relatively low shear stresses. Distal to the bulb, in the internal carotid artery, flow reattachment occurs, and a more laminar flow pattern is present.

The complex flow patterns described in models of the carotid bifurcation have also been documented in human subjects by pulsed Doppler studies.[9,10] As shown in Figure 13-9, the Doppler spectral waveform obtained near the inner wall of the carotid bulb is typical of the forward, quasi-steady flow pattern found in the internal carotid artery. However, sampling of flow along the outer wall of the bulb demonstrates lower velocities with periods of both forward and reverse flow. These spectral characteristics are consistent with the presence of flow separation and are considered to be a normal finding, particularly in young individuals.[10] Alterations in arterial distensibility with increasing age make flow separation less prominent in older individuals.[11]

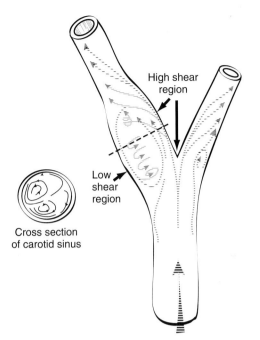

FIGURE 13-8 ■ Carotid artery bifurcation showing an area of flow separation adjacent to the outer wall of the bulb. Rapid flow is associated with high shear stress, whereas the slower flow of the separation zone produces a region of low shear. (From Zarins CK, Giddens DP, Glagov S: Atherosclerotic plaque distribution and flow velocity profiles in the carotid bifurcation. In Bergan JJ, Yao JST, editors: Cerebrovascular insufficiency, New York, 1983, Grune and Stratton.)

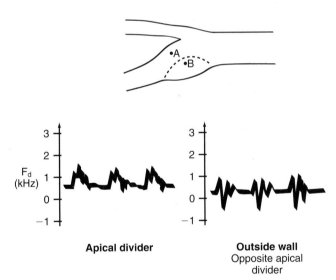

FIGURE 13-9 ■ Flow separation in the normal carotid bulb shown by pulsed Doppler spectral analysis. The flow pattern near the apical divider *(A)* is forward throughout the cardiac cycle, but near the outside wall *(B)* the spectrum contains both forward (positive) and reverse (negative) flow components. The latter pattern indicates an area of flow separation. F_d, Doppler shift frequency, in kHz. (Courtesy J.F. Primozich, BS, and D.J. Phillips, PhD.)

The clinical importance of boundary layer separation is that these localized flow disturbances may contribute to the formation of atherosclerotic plaques.[12] Examination of human carotid bifurcations, both at autopsy and during surgery, indicates that intimal thickening and

atherosclerosis tend to occur along the outer wall of the carotid bulb, whereas the inner wall is relatively spared.[8] These findings suggest that atherosclerotic lesions form near areas of flow separation and low shear stress. It is not known whether flow separation represents a true causative factor or simply promotes the development of previously existing lesions.

Pulsatile Flow

In a pulsatile system, pressure and flow vary continuously with time, and the velocity profile changes throughout the cardiac cycle. The hemodynamic principles already discussed are based on steady flow, and they are not adequate for a precise description of pulsatile flow in the arterial circulation; however, as previously stated, they can be used to determine the minimum energy losses occurring in a specific flow system.

The complex interactions of cardiac contraction, arterial wall characteristics, and blood flow are extremely difficult to define rigorously. For example, estimation of the inertial energy losses in pulsatile flow requires a value for the velocity term (see Equation 9); however, in pulsatile flow, velocity varies with both time and position across the flow profile, and skewing of the velocity profile can occur as a result of curvature or branching. The resistance term of Poiseuille's law (see Equation 11) estimates viscous energy losses in steady flow, but it does not account for the inertial effects, arterial wall elasticity, and wave reflections that influence pulsatile flow. The term vascular impedance is used to describe the resistance or opposition offered by a peripheral vascular bed to pulsatile blood flow.[3]

Pulsatile flow appears to be important for optimal organ function. For example, when a kidney is perfused by steady flow instead of pulsatile flow, a reduction in urine volume and sodium excretion occurs.[13] The critical effect of pulsatile flow is probably exerted on the microcirculation. Although the exact mechanism is unknown, transcapillary exchange, arteriolar tone, and lymphatic flow are all influenced by the pulsatile nature of blood flow.

Bifurcations and Branches

The branches of the arterial system produce sudden changes in the flow pattern that are potential sources of energy loss. However, the effect of branching on the total pressure drop in normal arterial flow is relatively small. Arterial branches commonly take the form of bifurcations. Flow patterns in a bifurcation are determined mainly by the area ratio and the branch angle. The area ratio is defined as the combined area of the secondary branches divided by the area of the primary artery.

Bifurcation flow can be analyzed in terms of pressure gradient, velocity, and transmission of pulsatile energy. According to Poiseuille's law, an area ratio of 1.41 would allow the pressure gradient to remain constant along a bifurcation. If the combined area of the branches equals the area of the primary artery, the area ratio is 1.0, and there is no change in the velocity of flow.[14] For efficient transmission of pulsatile energy across a bifurcation, the vascular impedance of the primary artery should equal that of the branches, a situation that occurs with an area ratio of 1.15 for larger arteries and 1.35 for smaller arteries.[15] Human infants have a favorable area ratio of 1.11 at the aortic bifurcation, but there is a gradual decrease in the ratio with age. In the teenage years, the average area ratio is less than 1.0; in the 20s, it is less than 0.9; and by the 40s, it drops below 0.8.[16] This decline in the area ratio of the aortic bifurcation leads to an increase in both the velocity of flow in the secondary branches and the amount of reflected pulsatile energy. For example, with an area ratio of 0.8, approximately 22% of the incident pulsatile energy is reflected in the infrarenal aorta. This mechanism may play a role in the localization of atherosclerosis and aneurysms in this arterial segment.[17]

The curvature and angulation of an arterial bifurcation can also contribute to the development of flow disturbances. As blood flows around a curve, the high-velocity portion of the stream is subjected to the greatest centrifugal force; rapidly moving fluid in the center of the vessel tends to flow outward and be replaced by the slower fluid originally located near the arterial wall. This can result in complex helical flow patterns, such as those observed in the carotid bifurcation.[9] As the angle between the secondary branches of a bifurcation is increased, the tendency to develop turbulent or disturbed flow also increases. The average angle between the human iliac arteries is 54 degrees; however, with diseased or tortuous iliac arteries, this angle can approach 180 degrees.[3] In the latter situation, flow disturbances are particularly likely to develop.

Physical Properties of the Arterial Wall

Composition

Blood vessels are viscoelastic tubes. In this context, *viscosity* refers to the resistance of a material to shear, and *elasticity* describes the tendency of a material to return to its original shape after being subjected to a deforming force. As blood proceeds from the large arteries of the thorax and abdomen to the medium-sized arteries of the extremities, the relative amount of elastic tissue in the vessel wall decreases as the amount of collagen and smooth muscle increases. At the level of the arterioles, the wall consists almost entirely of smooth muscle. Thus, the viscoelastic properties of an artery depend primarily on the elastin-to-collagen ratio. Elastin is the predominant component of the thoracic aorta that allows energy to be stored during cardiac systole and returned to the system in diastole. Because collagen is much less extensible than elastin, the more distal arteries, such as the brachial and femoral, do not store much of the pulsatile energy but serve mainly as conduits for blood. The function of the muscular arterioles is to control blood pressure and flow by actively altering the lumen diameter.

As the structure of the arterial wall changes, each successive branching also increases the total cross-sectional area of the arterial tree. The cross-sectional area at the arteriolar level is approximately 125-fold that of the aorta; at the capillary level, it has increased approximately 800 times.[3] The reduced elastin-to-collagen ratio and

increased stiffness of the peripheral arteries result in a more rapid pulse wave velocity and a high vascular impedance. Although the impedance of the thoracic aorta must be low to minimize cardiac work, the impedance of peripheral arteries should match the high arteriolar impedance to decrease the reflected components of the pulse wave.

TANGENTIAL STRESS AND TENSION

The tangential stress (τ) within the wall of a fluid-filled cylindrical tube can be expressed as follows:

$$\tau = P\frac{r}{\delta} \qquad [15]$$

where P is the pressure exerted by the fluid (in dynes per square centimeter), r is the internal radius (in centimeters), and δ is the thickness of the tube wall (in centimeters). Stress (τ) has the dimensions of force per unit area of tube wall (dynes per square centimeter). Thus, tangential stress is directly proportional to pressure and radius but inversely proportional to wall thickness.

Equation 15 is similar to Laplace's law, which defines tangential tension (T) as the product of pressure and radius:

$$T = Pr \qquad [16]$$

Tension is given in units of force per tube length (dynes per centimeter). The terms *stress* and *tension* have different dimensions and describe the forces acting on the tube wall in different ways. Laplace's law can be used to characterize thin-walled structures such as soap bubbles; however, it is not suitable for describing the stresses in arterial walls.

Arterial Wall Properties in Specific Conditions

Aging and Atherosclerosis. Arterial walls become less distensible with age. This increase in stiffness cannot be explained on the basis of atherosclerosis alone.[3] Alterations in the elastin fibers and elastic lamellae, together with an increase in wall thickness, probably account for this increase in arterial stiffness. Changes associated with aging include fragmentation of elastic lamellae and deposition of collagen between the elastin layers. This tends to maintain the elastin fibers in the extended state. Calcium is also deposited near the elastin fibers and contributes to the increased thickness of the arterial wall.

The effects of atherosclerosis on the mechanical properties of the arterial wall are complex and difficult to distinguish from those caused by aging. In the early stages, arterial distensibility can actually increase as elastin fibers are disrupted; however, as the disease progresses, fibrosis and calcification tend to make the arterial wall less distensible.

Endarterectomy. During an endarterectomy the atherosclerotic plaque is removed, along with the intima and a portion of the media, leaving behind a tube consisting of the outer media and adventitia. This reduces the wall thickness to approximately one third of its original value

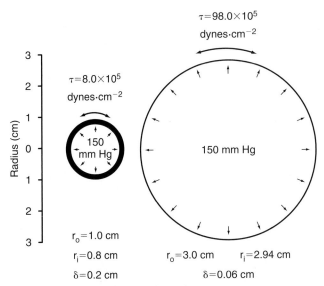

FIGURE 13-10 ■ End-on view of a cylinder, 2 cm in diameter, that is expanded to 6 cm in diameter while the wall area remains constant. δ, Wall thickness; r_i, inside radius; r_o, outside radius; t, wall stress. (From Sumner DS: The hemodynamics and pathophysiology of arterial disease. In Rutherford RB, editor: Vascular surgery, Philadelphia, 1977, WB Saunders.)

and should result in an increase in tangential stress, according to Equation 15. As would be expected, endarterectomy decreases the stiffness of an artery to circumferential expansion.[18] Still, the endarterectomized artery remains stiffer and less distensible than a normal artery; this indicates that the components responsible for strength and stiffness are concentrated in the outer layers of the arterial wall. It is because of this anatomic arrangement that endarterectomy is possible.

Aneurysms. When the structural components of the arterial wall are weakened, aneurysms can form. Rupture occurs when the tangential stress within the arterial wall becomes greater than the tensile strength. Figure 13-10 shows a tube with an outside diameter of 2 cm and a wall thickness of 0.2 cm, dimensions similar to those of atherosclerotic aortas.[1] If the internal pressure is 150 mm Hg, the tangential wall stress is 8.0×10^5 dynes/cm^2. Expansion of the tube to form an aneurysm with a diameter of 6 cm results in a decrease in wall thickness to 0.06 cm. The increased radius and decreased wall thickness increase the wall stress to 98.0×10^5 dynes/cm^2, assuming that the pressure remains constant. In this example, the diameter has been enlarged by a factor of 3, and the wall stress has increased by a factor of 12.

Although the tensile strength of collagen is extremely high, it constitutes only approximately 15% of the aneurysm wall.[19] Furthermore, the collagen fibers in an aneurysm are sparsely distributed and subject to fragmentation. The tendency of larger aneurysms to rupture is readily explained by the effect of increased radius on tangential stress (see Equation 15) and the degenerative changes in the arterial wall. The relationship between tangential stress and blood pressure accounts for the contribution of hypertension to the risk of rupture.

The diverging and converging geometry of aneurysms can result in complex flow patterns that include areas of

boundary layer separation and flow reversal.[20] These patterns explain the frequent accumulation of thrombus in aneurysms, which confines the flow stream to an area not much larger than the native artery. Because this thrombus increases the effective thickness of the vessel wall, it may reduce tangential stress and provide some protection against rupture. However, the tensile strength of thrombus and arterial wall are different, and the contribution of thrombus to the integrity of an aneurysm is impossible to predict.[3] Furthermore, the thrombus within an aneurysm is often not circumferential. In this situation, Equation 15 can be applied to the wall segment without thrombus, and the tangential stress at that site depends on the maximum internal radius.

Another factor to consider is that in approximately 55% of ruptured abdominal aortic aneurysms, the site of rupture is in the posterolateral aspect of the aneurysm wall.[21] The posterior wall of the aorta is relatively fixed against the spine, and repeated flexion of the wall in that area could result in structural fatigue. This fatigue would produce a localized area of weakness that might predispose to rupture.

HEMODYNAMICS OF ARTERIAL STENOSIS

Energy Losses

According to Poiseuille's law (see Equation 8), the radius of a stenotic segment has a much greater effect on viscous energy losses than does its length. Inertial energy losses, which occur at the entrance (contraction effects) and exit (expansion effects) of a stenosis, are proportional to the square of blood velocity (see Equation 9). Energy losses are also influenced by the geometry of a stenosis; a gradual tapering results in less energy loss than an irregular or abrupt change in lumen size. A converging vessel geometry tends to stabilize laminar flow and flatten the velocity profile, whereas a diverging vessel produces an elongated velocity profile and a less stable flow pattern. The energy lost at the exit of a stenosis can be significant because of the sudden expansion of the flow stream and dissipation of kinetic energy in a zone of turbulence.

The energy lost in expansion (ΔP) can be expressed in terms of the flow velocity distal to the stenosis (v) and the radii of the stenotic lumen (r_s) and the normal distal lumen (r):

$$\Delta P = k \frac{\rho}{2} v^2 \left[\left(\frac{r}{r_s} \right)^2 - 1 \right]^2 \qquad [17]$$

Figure 13-11 illustrates the energy losses related to a 1-cm-long stenosis. The viscous losses are relatively small and occur within the stenotic segment. Inertial losses resulting from contraction and expansion are much greater. Because most of the energy loss in this example results from inertial effects, the length of the stenosis is relatively unimportant.[1]

Bruits and Poststenotic Dilatation

The presence of an audible sound or bruit over an artery is usually regarded as a clinical sign of arterial disease. Stenoses or irregularities of the vessel lumen produce

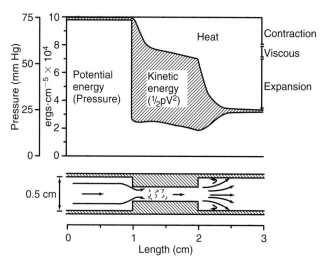

FIGURE 13-11 ■ Energy losses resulting when blood flows steadily through a 1-cm–long stenosis. Inertial losses (contraction and expansion) are more significant than viscous losses. (From Sumner DS: The hemodynamics and pathophysiology of arterial disease. In Rutherford RB, editor: Vascular surgery, Philadelphia, 1977, WB Saunders.)

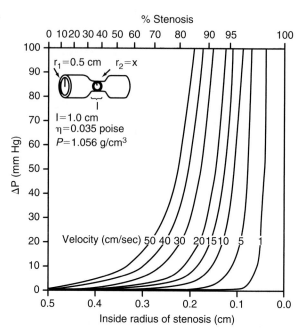

FIGURE 13-12 ■ Relationship of pressure drop across a stenosis (ΔP) to the radius of the stenotic segment (or % stenosis) for various flow velocities. (From Strandness DE, Sumner DS: Hemodynamics for surgeons, New York, 1975, Grune and Stratton.)

turbulent flow patterns that set up vibrations in the arterial wall. These vibrations generate displacement waves that radiate through the surrounding tissues and can be detected as audible sounds. Such vibrations are probably the main source of sound in the arterial system.[3]

Generally, a soft, midsystolic bruit is associated with a relatively minor lesion that does not significantly reduce flow or pressure. A bruit with a loud diastolic component suggests a stenosis severe enough to reduce flow and produce a pressure drop. Thus, the intensity and duration of a bruit serve as a rough guide to the severity of an arterial stenosis. A bruit may be absent when an artery is nearly occluded or when the flow rate is extremely low.

A dilated area distal to a stenosis is a common clinical finding. Poststenotic dilatation has been observed in the thoracic aorta below coarctations, distal to arterial stenoses at the thoracic outlet, and distal to atherosclerotic lesions. The most likely explanation for this phenomenon is that arterial wall vibrations result in structural fatigue of elastin fibers. In a series of animal model studies, poststenotic dilatations did not develop unless a bruit was present distal to the stenosis.[22] It appears that vibrations in the audible range may weaken elastin fibers and break down links between collagen fibers. When this occurs, the arterial wall distal to the stenosis becomes more distensible and subject to localized dilatation.

Critical Arterial Stenosis

The degree of arterial narrowing required to produce a significant reduction in blood pressure or flow is called a critical stenosis. Because the energy losses associated with a stenosis are inversely proportional to the fourth power of the radius at that site (see Equations 8 and 17), there is an exponential relationship between energy loss (pressure drop) and reduction in lumen size. When this relationship is illustrated graphically, the curves have a single sharp bend (Figure 13-12; also see Figure 13-5). These

observations provide theoretical support for the concept of critical stenosis.[23,24]

As previously noted, blood flow velocity is a major determinant of fluid energy losses (see Equations 8, 9, and 17). Thus, the pressure drop across a stenosis varies with the flow rate. Because flow velocity depends on the distal hemodynamic resistance, the critical stenosis value also varies with the resistance of the runoff bed. In Figure 13-12, a system with a high flow velocity (low resistance) shows a reduction in pressure with less narrowing than a system with low flow velocity (high resistance). The higher flow velocities produce curves that are less sharply bent, making the point of critical stenosis less distinct.

Another observation related to critical stenosis is that the decrease in flow is linearly related to the increase in pressure gradient, as long as the peripheral resistance remains constant[24] (Figure 13-13). In this situation, the curves for pressure drop and flow reduction are mirror images of each other, and the critical stenosis value is the same for both. Many vascular beds are able to maintain a constant level of blood flow over a wide range of perfusion pressures by the mechanism of autoregulation. This is achieved by constriction of resistance vessels in response to an increase in blood pressure and dilatation of resistance vessels when blood pressure decreases. For example, autoregulation permits the brain to maintain normal flow rates down to perfusion pressures in the range of 50 to 60 mm Hg.[25]

In general, significant changes in pressure and flow begin to occur when the arterial lumen has been reduced by approximately 50% of its diameter or 75% of its cross-sectional area; however, the concept of critical stenosis is strictly valid only when the flow conditions are specified.

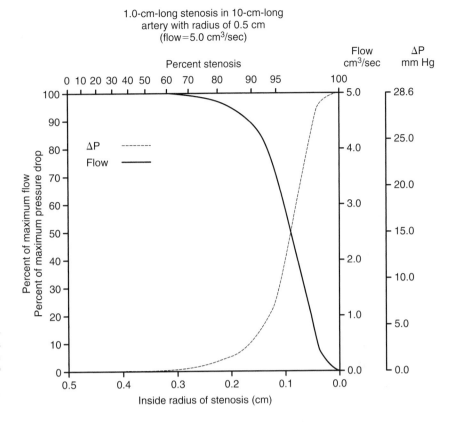

1.0-cm-long stenosis in 10-cm-long
artery with radius of 0.5 cm
(flow=5.0 cm³/sec)

FIGURE 13-13 ■ Effect of increasing stenosis on blood flow and pressure drop across the stenotic segment. Collateral and peripheral resistances are considered to be fixed. (From Strandness DE, Sumner DS: Hemodynamics for surgeons, New York, 1975, Grune and Stratton.)

Consequently, a stenosis that is not significant at resting flow rates can become critical when flow rates are increased by reactive hyperemia or exercise. For example, iliac stenoses that do not appear severe by arteriography may be associated with significant pressure gradients during exercise.[26] Because of the complex geometry of atherosclerotic lesions and the wide variation in arterial flow rates, it is often difficult to predict the hemodynamic significance of a lesion based on the apparent reduction in lumen size. Therefore physiologic testing by blood pressure measurement must be used to document the clinical severity of arterial lesions.[27,28]

Effect of Stenosis Length and Multiple Stenoses

Poiseuille's law predicts that the radius of a stenosis will have a much greater effect on viscous energy losses than will its length (see Equation 8). If the length of a stenosis is doubled, the viscous energy losses are also doubled; however, reducing the radius by half increases energy losses by a factor of 16. Furthermore, inertial energy losses are independent of stenosis length and are especially prominent at the exit of a stenosis (see Figure 13-11 and Equation 17). Because energy losses are primarily due to entrance and exit effects, separate short stenoses tend to be more significant than a single longer stenosis. It has been shown experimentally that when stenoses that are not significant individually are arranged in series, large reductions in pressure and flow can occur.[29] Thus,

multiple subcritical stenoses may have the same effect as a single critical stenosis.

Based on the preceding discussion, several points can be made about stenoses in series. When two stenoses are of similar diameter, removal of one provides only a modest increase in blood flow. If the stenoses have different diameters, removal of the least severe has little effect, whereas removal of the most severe improves blood flow significantly.

These principles apply only to unbranched arterial segments, such as the internal carotid. In the presence of a severe stenosis in the carotid siphon, removal of a less severe lesion in the proximal internal carotid artery is not likely to result in significant hemodynamic improvement. In contrast, when the proximal lesion involves an artery that supplies a collateral bed that parallels a distal lesion, removal of the proximal lesion can be beneficial. For example, when there is an iliac stenosis and a superficial femoral occlusion, removal of the iliac lesion usually improves perfusion of the lower leg by increasing flow through the profunda-geniculate collateral system.

ARTERIAL FLOW PATTERNS IN HUMAN LIMBS

Collateral Circulation

When arterial obstruction occurs, blood must pass through a network of collateral vessels to bypass the diseased segment. The functional capacity of the collateral circulation varies according to the level and extent of occlusive lesions. As mentioned in the preceding example, the profunda-geniculate system can compensate to a large degree for an isolated superficial femoral artery occlusion; however, the addition of an iliac lesion severely limits collateral flow.

A typical hemodynamic circuit includes the diseased major artery, a parallel system of collateral vessels, and the peripheral runoff bed (Figure 13-14). The collateral system consists of stem arteries, which are large distributing branches; a midzone of smaller intramuscular channels; and reentry vessels that join the major artery distal to the point of obstruction.[30] These vessels are preexisting pathways that enlarge when flow through the parallel major artery is reduced. The main stimuli for collateral development are an abnormal pressure gradient across the collateral system and increased velocity of flow through the midzone vessels.[31] This mechanism is consistent with the gradual improvement in collateral circulation that results from a regular exercise program in patients with lower extremity arterial occlusive disease.[32]

Collateral vessels are smaller, longer, and more numerous than the major arteries they replace. Although considerable enlargement can occur in the midzone vessels, collateral resistance is always greater than that of the original unobstructed artery. In addition, the acute changes in collateral resistance during exercise are minimal.[33] Therefore, the resistance of a collateral system is, for practical purposes, fixed.

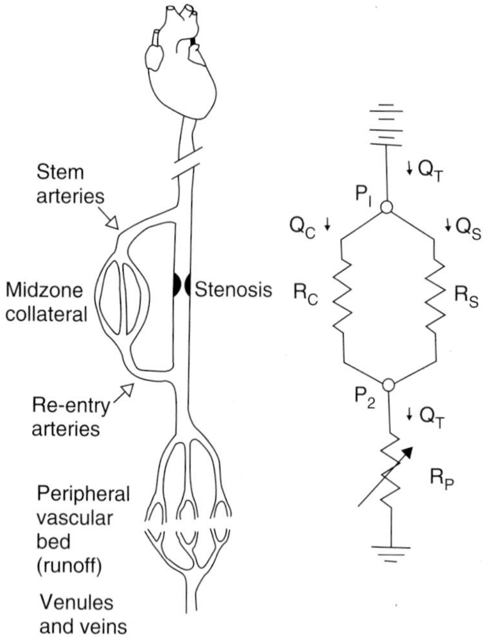

FIGURE 13-14 ■ Major components of a hemodynamic circuit containing a stenotic artery. The analogous electrical circuit is shown on the right, with the heart represented as a battery and the central veins as a ground. Flows are represented by Q_T (total), Q_C (collateral), and Q_S (stenosis). Resistances are represented by R_C (collateral), R_S (stenosis), and R_P (peripheral runoff); R_C and R_S are fixed, and R_P is variable. (From Sumner DS: The hemodynamics and pathophysiology of arterial disease. In Rutherford RB, editor: Vascular surgery, Philadelphia, 1977, WB Saunders.)

Distribution of Vascular Resistance and Blood Flow

Unlike collateral resistance, the resistance of a peripheral runoff bed is highly variable. The muscular arterioles are primarily responsible for regulating peripheral resistance and controlling the distribution of blood flow to various capillary beds. Arteriolar tone is mainly determined by the sympathetic nervous system, but it is also subject to the influence of locally produced metabolites.

When discussing blood flow in the lower limb, it is useful to separate vascular resistance into segmental and peripheral components. Segmental resistance consists of the relatively fixed parallel resistances of the major normal or diseased artery and the bypassing collateral vessels, such as the superficial femoral artery and the profunda-geniculate system. Peripheral resistance includes the highly variable resistances of the distal calf muscle arterioles and cutaneous circulation. The total vascular resistance of the limb can be estimated by adding the segmental and peripheral resistances (see Equations 12 and 13).

Normally, the resting segmental resistance is low and the peripheral resistance is relatively high; therefore the pressure drop across the femoropopliteal segment is minimal. With exercise, the peripheral resistance falls, and flow through the segmental arteries increases by a factor of up to 10, with little or no pressure drop.

With moderate arterial disease, such as an isolated superficial femoral artery occlusion, the segmental resistance is increased as a result of collateral flow, and an abnormal pressure drop is present across the thigh. Because of a compensatory decrease in peripheral resistance, the total resistance of the limb and the resting blood flow often remain in the normal range.[34] During exercise, the segmental resistance remains high and fixed, whereas the peripheral resistance decreases further. However, the capacity of the peripheral circulation to compensate for a high segmental resistance is limited, and exercise flow is less than normal. In this situation, exercise is associated with a still larger pressure drop across the diseased arterial segment. The clinical result is calf muscle ischemia and claudication.

When arterial disease becomes severe, as in combined iliofemoral and tibioperoneal occlusive disease, the compensatory decrease in peripheral resistance may be unable to provide normal blood flow at rest. In this case, there is a marked pressure drop across the involved arterial segments and little or no increase in blood flow with exercise. Claudication is severe, and ischemic rest pain or ulceration may develop.

These changes in the distribution of vascular resistance in the lower limb explain the alterations in blood pressure and flow observed in patients with arterial occlusive disease.

Arterial Pulses and Waveforms

The heart generates a complex pressure pulse that is modified by arterial wall properties and changes in vascular resistance as it progresses distally. Normally, the peak systolic pressure is amplified as it passes down the lower limb[3]; this is due to a progressive decrease in arterial compliance and reflections originating from the relatively high peripheral resistance. Consequently, the systolic pressure at the ankle is higher than that in the upper arm, and the ankle-brachial pressure ratio is greater than 1. However, the diastolic and mean pressures gradually decrease as the blood moves distally.

When blood flows through an arterial stenosis or a high-resistance collateral bed, the distal pulse pressure is reduced to a greater extent than the mean pressure.[35] This indicates that the systolic pressure beyond a lesion is a more sensitive indicator of hemodynamic significance than is the mean pressure. It is well known that palpable pedal pulses in patients with superficial femoral artery stenosis can disappear after leg exercise. This occurs when increased flow through high-resistance vessels causes a reduction in pulse pressure. The contour of the pressure pulse also reflects the presence of proximal arterial disease. These changes can be demonstrated plethysmographically and include a delayed upslope, rounded peak, and bowing of the downslope away from the baseline.[36]

Changes in the flow pulse are also useful to characterize the state of the arterial system. Although the peak pressure increases, the peak of the flow pulse decreases as the periphery is approached.[3] The flow pattern in the major arteries of the leg is normally triphasic (Figure 13-15). An initial large, forward-velocity phase resulting from cardiac systole is followed by a brief phase of flow reversal in early diastole and a third smaller phase of forward flow in late diastole. This triphasic pattern is modified by a variety of factors, including proximal arterial disease and changes in peripheral resistance. For example, body heating, which causes vasodilatation and

decreased resistance, abolishes the second phase of flow reversal; on exposure to cold, resistance increases and the reverse-flow phase becomes more prominent. Because a stenotic lesion is accompanied by a compensatory decrease in peripheral resistance, one of the earliest changes noted distal to a stenosis is the disappearance of the reverse-flow phase (see Figure 13-15). As a stenosis becomes more severe, the distal flow pattern becomes monophasic, with a slow rise, a rounded peak, and a gradual decline toward the baseline in diastole. The character of the flow pulse proximal to an arterial obstruction is variable and depends on the capacity of the collateral circulation. These flow patterns can be studied noninvasively using a Doppler velocity detector.

Pressure and Flow in Normal Limbs

As the pressure pulse moves distally, the systolic pressure rises, the diastolic pressure falls, and the pulse pressure becomes wider. The fall in mean arterial pressure between the heart and ankle is normally less than 10 mm Hg. In normal individuals at rest, the ratio of ankle systolic pressure to brachial systolic pressure (ankle-brachial index) has a mean value of 1.11 ± 0.10.[37] Moderate exercise in normal extremities produces little or no drop in ankle systolic pressure. Strenuous effort may be associated with a drop of several millimeters of mercury; however, pressures return rapidly to resting levels after cessation of exercise.

The average blood flow in the normal human leg is in the range of 300 to 500 mL/min under resting conditions.[3] Blood flow to the muscles of the lower leg is approximately 2.0 mL per 100 g per minute. With moderate exercise, total leg blood flow increases by a factor of 5 to 10, and muscle blood flow rises to approximately 30 mL per 100 g per minute. During strenuous exercise, muscle blood flow can reach 70 mL per 100 g per minute. After cessation of exercise, blood flow decreases rapidly and returns to resting values within 1 to 5 minutes.

Pressure and Flow in Limbs with Arterial Obstruction

If an arterial lesion is hemodynamically significant at rest, there is a measurable reduction in distal blood pressure. Generally, limbs with a lesion at one anatomic level have an ankle-brachial index between 0.9 and 0.5, whereas limbs with occlusions at multiple anatomic levels have an index less than 0.5.[28] The ankle-brachial index also correlates with the clinical severity of disease: in limbs with intermittent claudication, the index has a mean value of 0.59 ± 0.15; in limbs with ischemic rest pain, 0.26 ± 0.13; and in limbs with impending gangrene, 0.05 ± 0.08.[37]

Because of the increased segmental vascular resistance in limbs with arterial occlusive disease, the ankle systolic blood pressure falls dramatically during leg exercise. As indicated in Figures 13-16 to 13-18, the extent and duration of the pressure drop are proportional to the severity

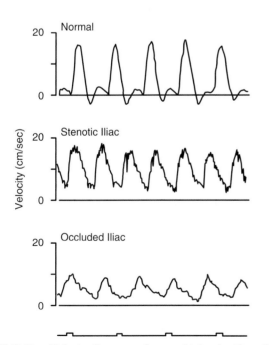

FIGURE 13-15 ■ Velocity flow waveforms obtained with a directional Doppler velocity detector from the femoral artery of a normal subject, a patient with external iliac stenosis, and a patient with common iliac occlusion. (From Strandness DE, Sumner DS: Hemodynamics for surgeons, New York, 1975, Grune and Stratton.)

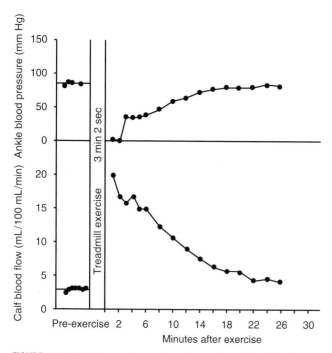

FIGURE 13-16 ■ Pre-exercise and postexercise ankle blood pressure and calf blood flow in a patient with severe stenosis of the superficial femoral artery. (From Sumner DS, Strandness DE: The relationship between calf blood flow and ankle blood pressure in patients with intermittent claudication, Surgery 65:763–771, 1969.)

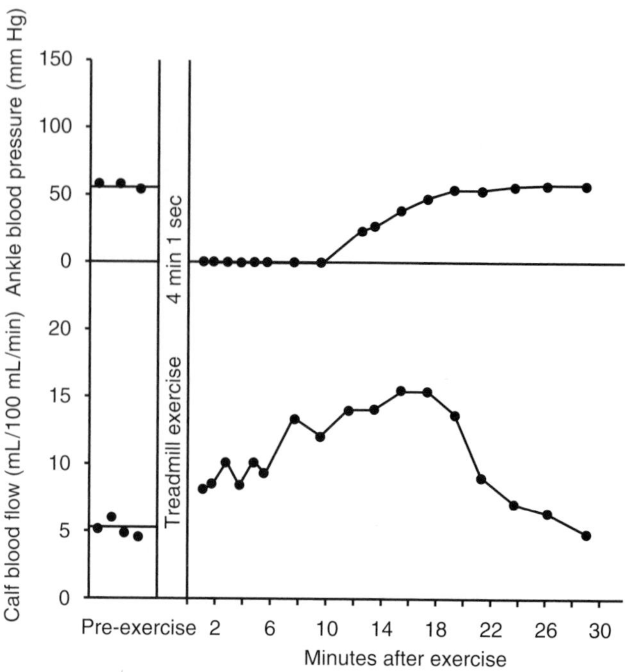

FIGURE 13-17 ■ Pre-exercise and postexercise ankle blood pressure and calf blood flow in a patient with iliac stenosis and superficial femoral artery occlusion. (From Sumner DS, Strandness DE: The relationship between calf blood flow and ankle blood pressure in patients with intermittent claudication, Surgery 65:763–771, 1969.)

of the arterial lesions. Recovery of pressure to resting levels may require up to 30 minutes.[28]

Resting leg or calf blood flow in patients with intermittent claudication is often not significantly different from values obtained in normal individuals. However, the capacity to increase limb blood flow during exercise is quite limited, and pain occurs in the muscles that have been rendered ischemic. The pain of claudication is presumably due to the accumulation of metabolic products that are removed under normal flow conditions. As the occlusive process becomes more severe, the decrease in peripheral vascular resistance can no longer compensate, and resting flow may be less than normal. When this occurs, ischemic rest pain or ulceration may appear. As shown in Figures 13-16 to 13-18, the capacity to increase calf blood flow with exercise depends on the severity of arterial occlusive disease. With increasing degrees of disease, the hyperemia that follows exercise becomes more prolonged, and the peak calf blood flow is both decreased and delayed. In some cases, flow may fall below resting levels.[28] The ankle blood pressure returns to normal after peak flows have started to decline.

The changes in blood pressure and flow in lower limbs with arterial occlusive disease provide the basis for noninvasive diagnostic tests. By monitoring the ankle systolic pressure before and after treadmill exercise or reactive hyperemia, two components of the physiologic response can be evaluated: (1) the magnitude of the immediate pressure drop, and (2) the time for recovery to resting pressure. The changes in both of these parameters are proportional to the severity of arterial disease.[38]

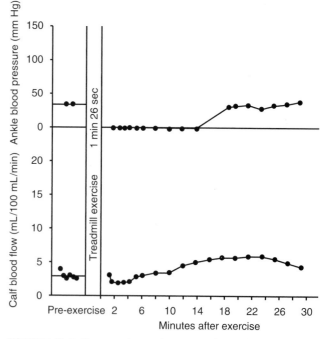

FIGURE 13-18 ■ Pre-exercise and postexercise ankle blood pressure and calf blood flow in a patient with occlusion of the iliac, common femoral, and superficial femoral arteries. This patient had moderate rest pain and severe claudication. (From Sumner DS, Strandness DE: The relationship between calf blood flow and ankle blood pressure in patients with intermittent claudication, Surgery 65:763–771, 1969.)

Vascular Steal

Hemodynamic arrangements in which one vascular bed draws blood away or "steals" from another can occur in a variety of situations. A vascular steal can arise when two runoff beds with different resistances must be supplied by a limited source of inflow.

Multiple-Level Occlusive Disease

One example of the steal phenomenon involves a limb with lesions in both the iliac and superficial femoral arteries.[1] The orifice of the profunda femoris artery, which supplies the variable resistance of the thigh, is between the fixed resistances of these two arterial lesions. The resistance of the distal calf runoff bed is also variable. Under resting conditions, normal leg blood flow can be maintained by a nearly maximal decrease in calf resistance and a moderate decrease in thigh resistance. In this situation the ankle systolic pressure will be abnormally decreased. With the increased metabolic demands of exercise, the thigh resistance can decrease further, but the calf resistance has already reached its lower limit; this results in a further pressure drop across the proximal iliac lesion, which reduces the pressure perfusing the calf. Blood flow to the calf is decreased until the thigh resistance rises and thigh blood flow begins to fall. In this situation, the effect of exercise is to increase thigh blood flow, decrease calf blood flow, and decrease distal blood pressure. The thigh steals blood from the calf because the proximal iliac lesion restricts inflow to both runoff beds.

Subclavian Steal Syndrome

In the subclavian steal syndrome, reversal of flow in the vertebral artery is associated with subclavian artery occlusion and symptoms of brainstem ischemia.[39] When occlusion is present in the proximal subclavian artery on the left or the innominate artery on the right, the pressure at the origin of the ipsilateral vertebral artery is reduced. This can result in reversal of flow in the vertebral artery, which then serves as a source of collateral circulation to the arm. The increased demands of arm exercise tend to augment the reversed flow, and the patient may experience ischemia of the brainstem. The hemodynamic effect is more severe with innominate artery occlusion than with isolated subclavian occlusion. With innominate occlusion, the origin of the right common carotid is also subject to reduced pressure, and the patterns of collateral circulation to the arm and brain become quite complicated. Blood passing down the vertebral artery on the side of the occlusion may be recovered, in part, by the right common carotid artery; however, during arm exercise, flow in the right common carotid may be reduced.

It is important to distinguish between symptomatic and asymptomatic subclavian steal. The presence of reversed vertebral artery flow, as demonstrated by arteriography, may be a normal variant without clinical significance.[40] In true subclavian steal syndrome, there is often a definite relationship between arm exercise and symptoms of brainstem ischemia. There will also be objective evidence of decreased blood flow to the involved arm, such as a diminished radial pulse and lowered brachial blood pressure relative to the contralateral arm.[41]

Extraanatomic Bypass Grafts

When an extraanatomic bypass is performed, a single donor artery must supply several vascular beds. In the case of a femorofemoral crossover graft, one iliac is the donor artery, the leg ipsilateral to the donor artery is the donor limb, and the contralateral leg is the recipient limb. Studies of crossover grafts in animal models have shown that the immediate effect of the graft is to double the flow in the donor artery.[42,43] When an arteriovenous fistula is created in the recipient limb, graft flows may increase by a factor of 10 without any evidence of a steal from the donor limb.

These experimental observations are consistent with hemodynamic data from patients with femorofemoral grafts.[44] Improvement in the ankle-brachial index on the recipient side can be achieved, even in the presence of significant occlusive disease in both the donor and recipient limbs. Although the ankle-brachial index may decrease slightly on the donor side, a symptomatic steal is extremely uncommon. The most important factor contributing to vascular steal with a femorofemoral graft is stenosis of the donor iliac artery. With iliac stenosis, a steal is most likely to occur during exercise when flow rates are increased. A mildly stenotic iliac can be used as a donor artery when high flow rates are not needed, such as in the treatment of ischemic rest pain. However, when increased flow rates are required to improve the walking distance of a patient with claudication, stenosis of the donor iliac may result in a steal from the donor limb. Occlusive disease in the arteries of the donor limb distal to the origin of the graft does not result in a steal, provided that the donor iliac artery is normal.

These principles also apply to other types of extraanatomic bypass grafts, including axillary-axillary, carotid-subclavian, and axillofemoral grafts.[42,45]

HEMODYNAMIC PRINCIPLES AND THE TREATMENT OF ARTERIAL DISEASE

It should be apparent from the preceding discussion that the high fixed segmental resistance of the diseased major arteries and collaterals is responsible for decreased peripheral blood flow. Therefore, to be most effective in improving peripheral blood flow and relieving ischemic symptoms, therapy must be directed toward lowering this abnormally high segmental resistance. Because the peripheral resistance has already been lowered to compensate for the increased segmental resistance, attempts to further reduce the peripheral resistance are seldom beneficial.[46]

Although exercise therapy has been shown to improve collateral function, the degree of clinical improvement is usually modest.[32] In general, exercise therapy is best suited for patients with mild, stable claudication who are not candidates for direct intervention. Another method for improving peripheral blood flow in limbs with arterial disease is medically induced hypertension.[46] The administration of mineralocorticoid and sodium chloride raises systemic blood pressure and increases the head of pressure perfusing the diseased arterial segment. Although this technique has not been applied widely, it has been used successfully in patients with severe distal ischemia and ulceration.

Direct Arterial Intervention

The most satisfactory approach to reducing the fixed segmental resistance is direct intervention by open surgical or catheter-based techniques. Depending on the nature of the lesions, endarterectomy, embolectomy, interposition grafting, or bypass grafting may be indicated. Percutaneous transluminal angioplasty, stenting, or stent-grafting may also be appropriate in selected cases.[47] In patients with occlusive disease involving a single anatomic level, a successful procedure should return all hemodynamic parameters to normal or near normal. This should be evident as an increase in the ankle-brachial index and an improvement in the ankle pressure response to leg exercise.[48] However, because it is seldom possible to perform a perfect arterial reconstruction, it is common to detect a minor degree of residual hemodynamic impairment. When occlusions involve multiple levels, the treatment of one level should result in significant improvement, and the persisting hemodynamic abnormality should then reflect the remaining untreated disease. In such cases, the improvement is usually sufficient to increase claudication distance or relieve ischemic rest pain. The relative severity of lesions at different levels is often difficult to determine clinically; however, the basic principle is to initially treat the most proximal level of hemodynamically significant occlusive disease.

The factors required for optimal function of arterial grafts can be analyzed in terms of basic hemodynamic principles. As noted previously, vessel diameter is the main determinant of hemodynamic resistance, so that the diameter of a graft is considerably more important than its length. All prosthetic grafts develop a pseudointimal layer of variable thickness that further reduces the effective diameter.[3] Therefore, whenever the situation permits, a graft with a relatively large diameter should be used. Graft diameter is often limited by arterial size. To minimize energy losses associated with entrance and exit effects, the diameter of a graft should approximate that of the adjacent artery. When arteries of unequal size must be joined, a gradual transition is preferable. Thus, the graft should be slightly smaller than the proximal artery and slightly larger than the distal artery.

Theoretically, end-to-end anastomoses are preferable to those done end to side, because the end-to-end configuration eliminates energy losses resulting from curvature and angulation. However, these losses appear to be minimal under physiologic conditions, and in most clinical situations the anastomotic angle is determined by technical factors. For example, reversed angulation has been used successfully in the construction of aortorenal and femorofemoral bypass grafts. Nevertheless,

as a general rule, the smallest anastomotic angle that is technically feasible should be used. The width of an end-to-side anastomosis should be approximately equal to the diameter of the graft; the length of an anastomosis is less important but does serve as the main determinant of anastomotic angle. A carefully everted suture line also helps to minimize energy losses at anastomoses.

Bifurcation grafts, such as those used for aortofemoral bypass, are subject to the same general hemodynamic considerations as arterial bifurcations and branches. Most commercially available grafts have secondary limbs with diameters that are half that of the primary tube, resulting in an area ratio of 0.5. In this configuration, each of the secondary limbs has 16 times the resistance of the primary tube, and in parallel they offer 8 times the primary tube resistance. The flow velocity in the secondary limbs is doubled, and almost 50% of the incident pulsatile energy is reflected at the graft bifurcation.[3] As discussed previously, the area ratio determines the hemodynamic characteristics of a bifurcation in regard to pressure gradient, flow velocity, and transmission of pulsatile energy. However, the optimal area ratio for grafts has not been established, and the geometry of bifurcation grafts has received relatively little attention. Instead, the development of prosthetic grafts has emphasized features such as graft material, porosity, and surface characteristics. Despite theoretical disadvantages, commercially available grafts have functioned extremely well in a variety of clinical applications.

Vasodilators

The rationale for the use of vasodilators is that they lower peripheral vascular resistance and improve limb blood flow. Although this may occur in normal limbs, it is unlikely to be beneficial in limbs in which peripheral resistance is already decreased as a result of arterial disease. There is even a theoretical possibility that dilating vessels in relatively normal areas could divert blood away from the areas of ischemia. Most clinical studies of vasodilator therapy have failed to show a significant effect.[49,50] There is no conclusive evidence that vasodilators can increase flow in either collateral vessels or severely ischemic tissues. Consequently, there is no theoretical or clinical support for vasodilator therapy.

Sympathectomy

Because the purpose of sympathectomy is to reduce peripheral resistance by release of vasomotor tone, it is subject to the same general criticisms as vasodilator therapy. Because sympathectomy has little, if any, influence on collateral resistance, there is no rational basis for its use in the treatment of intermittent claudication.[51] Furthermore, exercise-induced muscle ischemia alone is a potent stimulus for peripheral vasodilatation.

The use of sympathectomy for cutaneous ischemia has some physiologic basis, because the predominant effect is dilatation of cutaneous arterioles. However, clinical improvement can occur only if the ischemic tissues are capable of further vasodilatation, as demonstrated by reactive hyperemia testing.[36] Beneficial results have been obtained in patients with mild rest pain and superficial ischemic ulcers; patients with severe rest pain and extensive tissue loss are not likely to respond.[51] Although sympathectomy has been recommended as an adjunct to arterial operations, there is little objective evidence that it improves either the early or the late results of arterial reconstructive surgery.[52]

Rheologic Agents

According to Poiseuille's law, hemodynamic resistance is directly proportional to blood viscosity (see Equations 8 and 11). If the pressure remains constant and viscosity is reduced, flow increases in proportion to the fall in viscosity. Procedures for lowering blood viscosity are most often used in the immediate postoperative period to increase flow through a reconstructed arterial segment.

Low-molecular-weight dextran (molecular weight 40,000) is the most commonly used agent for reducing blood viscosity. The increased peripheral blood flow observed after intravenous administration of low-molecular-weight dextran is the result of both peripheral vasodilatation secondary to blood volume expansion and changes in viscosity due to hemodilution.[3] Dextran solutions also influence red blood cell aggregation and platelet function.[53]

An orally administered rheologic agent, pentoxifylline, has been evaluated in a multicenter clinical trial for the treatment of patients with intermittent claudication.[54] Pentoxifylline reduces blood viscosity by improving the membrane flexibility of red blood cells. The drug also has an inhibitory effect on platelet aggregation. During the clinical trial, the distance walked before the onset of claudication increased in both the pentoxifylline and the placebo groups; however, the degree of improvement was significantly greater in those receiving pentoxifylline. It was concluded that pentoxifylline is a safe and effective drug for use in patients with intermittent claudication. Although this agent may provide a modest degree of functional improvement in some patients, its effect on the progression of arterial disease is unknown.

HEMODYNAMICS OF THE VENOUS SYSTEM

The structure of the vein wall is considerably different from that of the companion arteries. Some of these major differences are as follows: (1) the vein wall is much thinner, being anywhere from one third to one tenth as thick as that of the systemic arteries; (2) there is little elastic tissue in the wall of the vein; (3) the venous media is almost exclusively a muscular layer; (4) venules have no media and no smooth muscle; and (5) a major part of the walls of the larger veins is composed of adventitia. An important characteristic of the veins is the presence of valves, which are essential for proper function. The distribution and number of valves correspond well to regions in which the effects of gravity are greatest; they have a bicuspid structure with a fine connective tissue skeleton covered by endothelium on both surfaces. The major function of venous valves is to ensure antegrade flow and prevent reflux from the deep to the superficial veins.

From a clinical standpoint, the area of greatest interest in the lower extremity venous system is below the knee. This is the most common site for the development of venous thrombosis, and it is also the region of the leg where the complications of post-thrombotic syndrome are evident. The veins of the soleus muscle are often termed the *soleal sinuses* because of their capacious size and lack of venous valves. These sinuses are the most common site for the development of venous thrombosis.

The perforating veins that normally carry blood from the superficial to the deep veins are key elements in venous function. These short channels have the following features: (1) they penetrate the deep fascia; (2) they contain valves; (3) they are found predominantly below the knee; (4) the majority are small and inconstant in location; and (5) they vary in number from 90 to 200.[55] Although not commonly thought of as such, the great and small saphenous veins have all the characteristics of perforating veins. One relatively constant large perforator can be found on the medial aspect of the distal thigh, and this is one of the few that establishes a direct communication between the great saphenous vein and the deep venous system. A common misconception is that the perforating veins along the medial aspect of the lower leg communicate directly with the great saphenous vein. In fact, they communicate most commonly with its major tributary, the posterior arch vein. Normally, there are four relatively constant perforators that join the posterior arch vein, and when these are diseased, they contribute to the pathogenesis of the post-thrombotic syndrome. The region in the vicinity of the lowest two perforating veins is often referred to as the *gaiter area*.[55] As discussed later in this chapter, the function of the venous wall and its associated valves becomes evident when the effects of gravity and the calf muscle pump are considered.

Normal Pressure and Flow Relationships

A major factor in venous physiology that explains the capacitance function of these vessels is that they can undergo large changes in volume with very little change in transmural pressure. This is due not to the elastic properties of the walls, but to the fact that they tend to collapse under the influence of a low transmural pressure. Veins are actually stiffer than arteries when compared at the same distending pressure. This results from the paucity of elastic tissue and the prominent adventitia, which consists largely of collagen.

One of the remarkable features of the venous system is the wide range of flow rates that can be found—from high flows to nearly complete stasis. Flow rates depend on a variety of complex interactive factors such as body position, level of activity, vascular fluid volume, and ambient temperature. Because it is virtually impossible to measure instantaneous venous flow in either the superficial or the deep veins, it is necessary to look at measurements of venous pressure and relate these to specific conditions or disease states.

Resting Venous Pressure

The pressures that exist in the absence of pulsatile flow are shown in Figure 13-19, which shows the hydrostatic model of a 6-foot-tall "dead man." If the case of an open rigid tube is considered, pressure at the top would be zero (atmospheric). In the body, the arteries and veins can be represented as a series of parallel tubes, with the veins being collapsible and the arteries rigid. When the system is filled with fluid, but not enough to entirely distend the collapsible tube (venous), the pressure in the collapsed portion of the tube is atmospheric. Pressures in the rigid tube (arterial) must be equal to those in the collapsible tube up to the zero point. Above the zero pressure point, the pressures in the rigid tube are negative, because the collapsed tube representing the veins prevents free communication between the two segments.

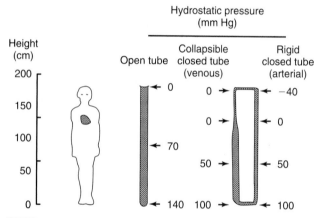

FIGURE 13-19 ■ Hydrostatic pressures measured in the upright "dead man." The pressures in the open tube are those expected in a rigid tube of equal height. The pressures in the closed tubes are those expected in a system of closed, connected parallel tubes. (From Strandness DE, Sumner DS: Hemodynamics for surgeons, New York, 1975, Grune and Stratton.)

When we examine the pressure relationships in a living man, supine and erect, some important facts can be noted[56] (Figure 13-20). There is a point just below the diaphragm where the pressures in the arteries and veins remain constant regardless of position. This has been termed the *hydrostatic indifferent point* (HIP). This point changes only when the subject is placed head down, and then it is located at the level of the right atrium. The zero pressure level is in the region of the right atrium, usually at the level of the fourth intercostal space. The effect of gravity is the same throughout the vascular system in a supine subject. Raising an arm above the head in the erect position produces some dramatic changes. The arteriovenous pressure gradient in the foot remains the same (83 mm Hg), but in the hand it falls to a level of 31 mm Hg.[57]

Although there is no difference in the pressure gradient across the capillaries in the feet between the supine and the standing positions, some important changes do occur. On assuming the standing position, there is a translocation of blood into the veins of the legs (approximately 500 mL).[58] There is also a marked increase in the transmural venous pressure at the foot as a result of the effect of gravity. With this increase in pressure, fluid is forced out of the capillaries into the tissues. Although some of this fluid may be picked up by the lymphatics, other factors must come into play if edema is to be prevented. The single most important element in preventing the continued accumulation of interstitial fluid is the calf muscle pump. This can dramatically lower the pressure in the veins and capillaries, thus promoting the return of interstitial fluid to the circulation.

Pressure Changes during Exercise

Features that distinguish normal subjects from patients with venous disease are best understood by examining the pressure changes that occur with leg exercise. Although patients with chronic arterial disease can usually be distinguished from normal subjects under resting conditions

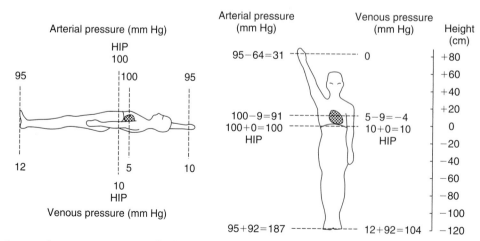

FIGURE 13-20 ■ Intravascular pressures present in the normal supine and erect human. The hydrostatic indifferent point (HIP) is located just below the diaphragm. (From Strandness DE, Sumner DS: Hemodynamics for surgeons, New York, 1975, Grune and Stratton.)

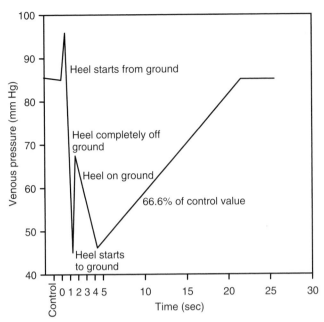

FIGURE 13-21 ■ Changes in the mean saphenous vein pressure measured at the level of the ankle that occur with a single step. (Redrawn from Pollack AA, Wood EH: Human venous pressure in the saphenous vein at the ankle during exercise and changes in posture, J Appl Physiol 1:649–662, 1949.)

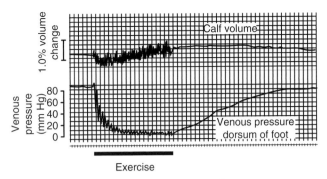

FIGURE 13-22 ■ Normal calf volume and venous pressure response to calf muscle exercise. Pressure changes were measured in a dorsal foot vein. Venous pressure falls rapidly, remains low throughout the period of exercise, and returns slowly to the baseline after calf muscle contraction ceases. (From Strandness DE, Sumner DS: Hemodynamics for surgeons, New York, 1975, Grune and Stratton.)

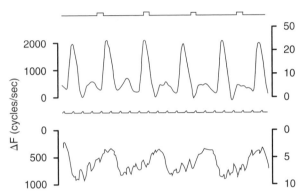

FIGURE 13-23 ■ Comparison of the flow velocity patterns in the common femoral artery *(top)* and common femoral vein *(bottom)* in the supine position with normal respiration. The venous velocity patterns are dominated by the pressure changes that occur with respiration. ΔF, Doppler shift frequency, which is proportional to velocity. (From Strandness DE, Sumner DS: Hemodynamics for surgeons, New York, 1975, Grune and Stratton.)

by measurement of distal arterial blood pressure, this is not the case with venous disease. For patients with venous problems, it is only when the muscle pump is activated that the abnormality is apparent. The calf muscle pump produces important changes in venous volume, flow rate, and flow direction. The muscle pump fulfills three useful functions: (1) it lowers the venous pressure in the dependent limb; (2) it reduces venous volume in the exercising limb; and (3) it increases venous return.

With quiet standing, the venous pressure at the level of the foot remains constant, but this is dramatically altered with even a single step (Figure 13-21). As noted in Figure 13-21, at the completion of a single step, the venous pressure is low and requires several seconds to return to the prestep level.[59] When a normal subject walks, the venous pressure remains at a low and steady level throughout the period of exercise. Calf volume initially falls but gradually increases during exercise as the arterial inflow rises (Figure 13-22). It should be emphasized that the observed pressure changes at the level of the foot are entirely dependent on intact and functioning venous valves in the distal limb. The calf muscle pump essentially empties the local venous system during contraction. With relaxation, the veins are nearly empty, and the venous pressure is very low. These changes are vital to maintaining normal venous return and protecting the limb from edema. As shown later in this chapter, destruction of the valves dramatically alters these changes.

Venous Flow Patterns

Flow on the venous side of the circulation is influenced by a variety of factors, including respiration, the filling

pressure of the right heart, body position, the activity of the calf muscle pump, and the amount of arterial inflow. The patterns of blood flow in the femoral artery and vein are shown in Figure 13-23. Flow velocity in the normal femoral vein is lowest at peak inspiration, when the intraabdominal pressure resulting from descent of the diaphragm is at its maximum. In theory, the changes in velocity of venous flow in the subclavian vein should be opposite to those in the femoral vein—that is, highest at peak inspiration, when intrathoracic pressure is at its minimum.

As noted earlier, the presence of competent valves prevents reflux of blood and an increase in venous pressure. This can be shown when the pressure is suddenly increased above a competent iliofemoral valve (Figure 13-24). A cough and a Valsalva maneuver result in a sharp increase in pressure above the valve but not below it. There is no reflux of blood flow through the valve during either of these maneuvers.

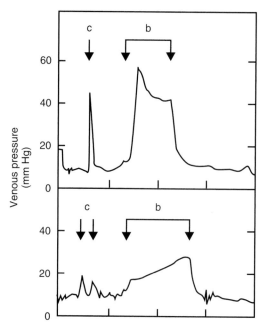

FIGURE 13-24 ■ Effect of a cough *(c)* and a Valsalva maneuver *(b)* on the venous pressure in a patient with a competent valve at the iliofemoral level. *Upper panel,* Pressure changes above the valve. *Lower panel,* Pressure changes below the valve. (From Ludbrook J, Beale G: Femoral venous valves in relation to varicose veins, Lancet 1:79–81, 1962.)

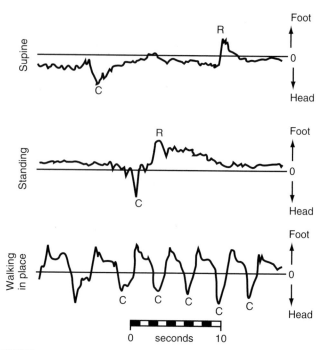

FIGURE 13-25 ■ Venous velocity changes recorded from an incompetent great saphenous vein in a patient with primary varicose veins. The effects of muscular contraction *(C)* and relaxation *(R)* are indicated for the supine and standing positions. The bidirectional flow that occurs with walking is also shown. (From Strandness DE, Sumner DS: Hemodynamics for surgeons, New York, 1975, Grune and Stratton.)

Abnormal Pressure and Flow Relationships

The most common manifestations of abnormal venous function are primary varicose veins and the postthrombotic syndrome. Current evidence suggests that primary varicose veins are often familial. The initial abnormality in this condition appears to be incompetence of the terminal valves of the great and small saphenous veins, which permits reflux of blood. With the passage of time, progressive incompetence of the other valves occurs. Dodd and Cockett[60] also include patients with idiopathic perforator vein incompetence in the primary varicose vein group. Although this may be valid, it is likely that many of these incompetent perforators occur secondary to episodes of calf vein thrombosis that result in destruction of the valves.

The flow abnormality produced by loss of valvular competence at any level of the venous system is easily demonstrated with a Doppler velocity detector. The flow patterns shown in Figure 13-25 are from the great saphenous vein of a patient with primary varicose veins. In the supine position, flow with calf contraction is antegrade, with a slight and transient period of reflux during relaxation; however, with standing, the opposite is noted, with flow being toward the foot. Walking in place clearly illustrates the rapid changes in direction that occur with each step as a result of loss of valvular competence. When the pressure in the veins on the dorsum of the foot is measured during exercise in a patient with primary varicose veins, the deviations from normal are evident (Figure 13-26). The pressure does not fall to normally low levels, and it returns to the pre-exercise level much faster when

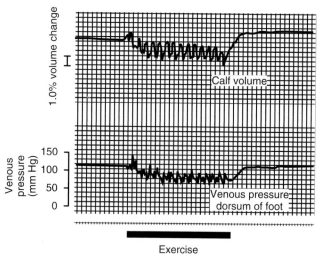

FIGURE 13-26 ■ Calf volume and venous pressure changes recorded from a dorsal foot vein of a patient with primary varicose veins. The pressure does not fall to the low levels seen in normal subjects (see Figure 13-22), and it returns to the baseline much faster. (From Strandness DE, Sumner DS: Hemodynamics for surgeons, New York, 1975, Grune and Stratton.)

walking is stopped. If a tourniquet is placed around the upper calf, this pattern is normalized as long as the valves in the deep system are competent.

With the development of acute deep vein thrombosis, two major factors determine the long-term outcome: (1) the location and extent of the residual venous

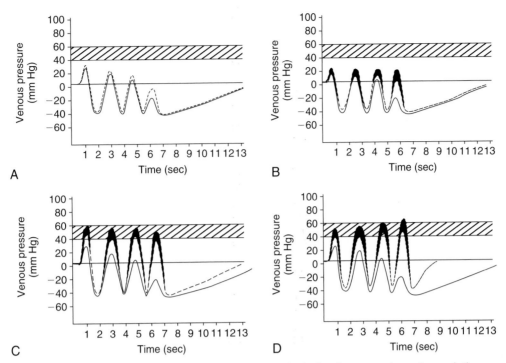

FIGURE 13-27 ■ Pressure changes in the great saphenous vein at the ankle during four steps. In each panel, the normal response is noted by the solid line. **A,** Primary varicose veins and no leg ulcers. **B,** Varicose veins, incompetent ankle perforators, normal deep veins, and no leg ulcers. **C,** Varicose veins, incompetent ankle perforators, normal deep veins, and leg ulcers present. **D,** Varicose veins, incompetent ankle perforators, abnormal deep veins, and leg ulcers present. (From Arnoldi CC, Linderholm H: On the pathogenesis of the venous leg ulcer, Acta Chir Scand 134:427–440, 1968.)

obstruction and (2) the condition of the valves below the knee in the area of the calf muscle pump.[61-64] Because these vary greatly from one patient to another, it is not surprising that the pressure responses also show a wide variation. Four examples of the types of patterns that can be observed are shown in Figure 13-27. It is clear that even with primary varicose veins, the pressure changes at the level of the foot are abnormal with exercise (see Figures 13-26 and 13-27). However, patients with this very common condition generally complain of minimal edema and rarely develop ulceration. The factors that appear to be responsible for the development of post-thrombotic syndrome relate primarily to the status of the deep veins below the knee and the perforating veins. The most abnormal venous pressures and flows occur in the area where ulceration develops and are due to valvular incompetence in both the distal deep veins and their connections with the superficial venous system. With this combination, the high pressures that can be generated by activation of the calf muscle pump result in ambulatory venous hypertension in the lower leg.

In 1978, Browse and Burnand[65] offered a reassessment of the factors responsible for the development of post-thrombotic syndrome. They recognized that the clinical condition could occur only with damage to the deep venous system and postulated that the abnormally high venous pressures would lead to the development of multiple new capillaries in the dermis, with large pores in the venular side. As a result, there would be extravasation of large molecules such as fibrinogen and coagulation factors. These factors, in conjunction with tissue factors, would lead to the conversion of fibrinogen to fibrin. If this were combined with inadequate fibrinolysis, fibrin would accumulate in the tissues and produce a barrier to the diffusion of both oxygen and nutrients. The end result would be tissue anoxia and death of the skin in the affected region.

HEMODYNAMIC PRINCIPLES AND THE TREATMENT OF VENOUS DISEASE

In contrast to the arterial side of the circulation, there are few direct therapeutic approaches that can correct the underlying hemodynamic abnormalities of venous disease. Although obstruction of inflow to a limb is the most commonly treated arterial abnormality, mechanical interference with venous outflow is a rare cause of chronic venous insufficiency.

One exception to this observation is the patient with venous claudication. This entity is uncommon and may not be recognized. It occurs in the specific clinical setting of chronic iliofemoral venous occlusion. In most cases, the major deep veins distal to the groin are patent and competent. With vigorous exercise, the patient is unable to adequately decompress the deep venous system, and the thigh becomes tense and very painful. After the patient stops exercising, it often requires 15 to 30 minutes for the pain and tightness to disappear. It is important to recognize that this syndrome rarely occurs with ordinary exercise and thus tends to be seen in relatively young patients who indulge in vigorous activities such as jogging, skiing, or tennis. The underlying mechanism of venous claudication involves the collateral veins that bypass the obstructed segment and have a relatively high, fixed resistance.[66] This high outflow resistance results in a marked increase in venous volume during exercise. In some circumstances, it may be feasible to provide therapeutic relief with a crossover saphenous vein graft using the proximal saphenous vein from the opposite limb. This is rarely done, however, because the symptoms in most patients produce only minimal disability.

Other surgical procedures designed to treat chronic venous insufficiency do so by either removing the offending vein or interrupting it at some point in its course. This procedure is done to eliminate sites of reflux and restore the pressure-flow relationship to normal. The value of this particular approach is limited because the most common site of the abnormality responsible for chronic venous insufficiency is the distal deep veins, an area that is not amenable to direct surgical intervention.

There has been some interest in promoting valvular competence in the proximal femoral vein in the thigh. This has been done by a direct surgical approach through a longitudinal venotomy or by transposition of a competent venous valve.[67,68] The validity of these techniques is questionable, however, because there is no evidence to support the concept of the so-called critical valve; the alterations of pressure and flow are nearly always secondary to deep venous abnormalities in the distal limb, and proof of the effectiveness of such an approach is currently lacking.

The most common form of therapy for chronic venous insufficiency is the use of support stockings that provide external compression and thus minimize the amount of edema that occurs during ambulation.[69] The exact mechanism of compression therapy remains poorly understood.[70] In theory, the stocking should reduce the transmural venous pressure gradient in a graduated fashion, with the highest compression pressures in the ankle area and diminishing pressures proximally up the limb. The amount of pressure exerted by a stocking depends on the elastic tension in the garment and the radius of the limb. Compression pressure should be in the range of 80 to 90 mm Hg while standing, 50 to 60 mm Hg while sitting, and 0 mm Hg in the recumbent position. This is obviously not possible with any single stocking; therefore a compromise must be accepted.

Elevation of the legs above the level of the heart is also a standard method for relieving the symptoms of chronic venous insufficiency. The physiologic basis for the use of elevation depends on three major effects: (1) it reduces venous pressure by decreasing the hydrostatic component related to gravity; (2) it promotes the reabsorption of edema fluid; and (3) it prevents ambulatory venous hypertension. Periodic elevation and external compression therapy are essential for the treatment of chronic venous insufficiency. When strictly adhered to, a regimen of elevation and compression minimizes edema, improves skin nutrition, and avoids ulceration in the majority of patients.

CONCLUSION

The fundamental principles of hemodynamics often seem remote from the routine clinical problems faced by vascular surgeons. The purpose of this chapter has been to show how these mathematical and physical concepts provide the basis for a rational approach to the pathophysiology, diagnosis, and treatment of vascular disease. These principles are also important for understanding the noninvasive diagnostic techniques that are discussed elsewhere in this book. The use of objective hemodynamic data is an essential step in the clinical evaluation and follow-up of patients. This increased reliance on physiologic testing should encourage vascular surgeons to consider patients with vascular disease in terms of basic hemodynamic principles.

BIBLIOGRAPHY

Berguer R, Hwang NHC: Critical arterial stenosis—a theoretical and experimental solution. Ann Surg 180:39–50, 1974.
Carter SA: Response of ankle systolic pressure to leg exercise in mild or questionable arterial disease. N Engl J Med 287:578–582, 1972.
Flanigan DP, Tullis JP, Streeter VL, et al: Multiple subcritical arterial stenosis: effect on poststenotic pressure and flow. Ann Surg 186:663–668, 1977.
Johnson BF, Manzo RA, Bergelin RO, et al: Relationship between changes in the deep venous system and the development of the postthrombotic syndrome after an acute episode of lower limb deep vein thrombosis: a one- to six-year follow-up. J Vasc Surg 21:307–313, 1995.
Kfu DN, Giddens DP, Phillips DJ, et al: Hemodynamics of the normal human carotid bifurcation—in vitro and in vivo studies. Ultrasound Med Biol 1:13–26, 1985.
Killewich LA, Martin R, Cramer M, et al: Pathophysiology of venous claudication. J Vasc Surg 1:507–511, 1984.
May AG, Van de Berg L, DeWeese JA, et al: Critical arterial stenosis. Surgery 54:250–259, 1963.
Phillips DJ, Greene FM, Jr, Langlois Y, et al: Flow velocity patterns in the carotid bifurcations of young, presumed normal subjects. Ultrasound Med Biol 1:39–49, 1983.
Sumner DS, Strandness DE, Jr: The relationship between calf blood flow and ankle blood pressure in patients with intermittent claudication. Surgery 65:763–771, 1969.
Sumner DS, Strandness DE, Jr: The hemodynamics of the femorofemoral shunt. Surg Gynecol Obstet 134:629–636, 1972.

References available online at expertconsult.com.

QUESTIONS

1. Viscous energy losses in flowing blood result from which of the following?
   a. Changes in the velocity and direction of flow
   b. Friction between adjacent layers of moving blood
   c. Turbulent flow in areas of stenosis
   d. Disturbed flow at points of branching
   e. Areas of boundary layer separation

2. Poiseuille's law states that pressure gradients in an idealized flow model are inversely proportional to which of the following?
   a. Mean flow velocity
   b. Tube or stenosis length
   c. Blood viscosity
   d. Tube or stenosis radius
   e. Volume flow rate

3. Inertial energy losses in blood flow are related primarily to which of the following?
   a. Changes in the velocity and direction of flow
   b. Blood viscosity
   c. Specific gravity of blood
   d. Friction between adjacent layers of moving blood
   e. Mean blood pressure

4. The critical stenosis value for a particular artery depends on which of the following?
   a. Length of the arterial segment
   b. Tangential wall stress
   c. Blood viscosity
   d. Compliance of the arterial wall
   e. Flow rate and peripheral vascular resistance

5. Which of the following statements about the collateral circulation is false?
   a. Collateral vessels are preexisting pathways that enlarge when the parallel major artery is occluded.
   b. The vascular resistance of the collateral bed is relatively fixed.
   c. Collateral artery resistance is usually less than that of the original unobstructed parallel artery.
   d. An abnormal pressure gradient across the collateral bed may stimulate the further development of collateral pathways.
   e. The midzone of the collateral bed consists of small, intramuscular vessels.

6. Which of the following is not related to tangential stress and rupture of arterial aneurysms?
   a. Volume flow rate through the aneurysm
   b. Arterial blood pressure
   c. Internal radius of the aneurysm
   d. Tensile strength of collagen
   e. Thickness of the aneurysm wall

7. With an extraanatomic bypass, such as a femoro-femoral crossover graft, a vascular steal from the donor limb is most likely to occur in which of the following circumstances?
   a. There is occlusive disease in both the donor and the recipient limbs.
   b. There is an occlusive lesion in the donor artery.
   c. Severe occlusive disease is present in the donor limb.
   d. The recipient limb has only mild occlusive disease.
   e. The donor limb is hemodynamically normal.

8. Venous claudication is characterized by all of the following except
   a. Chronic iliofemoral venous occlusion
   b. Thigh pain with vigorous exercise
   c. High-resistance venous collaterals
   d. Minimal disability with ordinary activities
   e. Valvular incompetence in the tibial veins

9. Which of the following is not a function of the calf muscle pump?
   a. It lowers venous pressure in the dependent limb.
   b. It reduces venous volume in the exercising limb.
   c. It improves arterial blood flow to the exercising muscle.
   d. It increases venous return to the right heart.
   e. It minimizes the accumulation of interstitial fluid in the distal limb.

10. All of the following contribute to the pathogenesis of the post-thrombotic syndrome except
    a. Deep vein thrombosis with chronic obstruction of the deep veins
    b. Extravasation of blood components into the sub-cutaneous tissues
    c. Incompetence of the venous valves in the deep veins below the knee
    d. The presence of primary varicose veins
    e. Ambulatory venous hypertension

ANSWERS

1. **b**
2. **d**
3. **a**
4. **e**
5. **c**
6. **a**
7. **b**
8. **e**
9. **c**
10. **d**

The Noninvasive Vascular Laboratory

J. Dennis Baker

In the early days of vascular surgery, patient assessment was based on a careful history and physical examination. Although a few clinicians used the Collins oscillometer to estimate the pulse pressure in an extremity, there was little help available in terms of quantitative assessment of arterial or venous disease. Angiography provided the only objective determination of pathologic changes. Early experience with arteriography and phlebography highlighted some of the limitations of these techniques, especially the problem of underestimating the severity of stenotic lesions on single-plane studies. In addition, the cost, patient discomfort, and risk of complications associated with contrast studies precluded their routine use for screening evaluations and follow-up.

The growing interest in more accurate differential diagnosis, localization of disease, determination of its severity, and documentation of progression stimulated the development of objective measurement techniques. In the 1960s, investigators started working with different plethysmographic techniques to quantitate arterial occlusive disease in the leg. Modification of ultrasound equipment to measure blood flow by the Doppler shift principle represented an important step forward in instrumentation and led to the rapid development of noninvasive studies. Additional techniques were designed to evaluate carotid artery disease as well as deep venous occlusion and insufficiency. This chapter describes the main diagnostic techniques used in the noninvasive laboratory and discusses their clinical application for patients with vascular disease. With an understanding of the merits and limitations of each method, clinicians can make the best use of these tests.

INSTRUMENTATION

Doppler Velocity Measurement Techniques

High-frequency sound waves (2 to 10 MHz) penetrate soft tissues and are reflected by the different interfaces encountered. Reflection from a moving interface results in the reflected frequency being increased if the motion is toward the point of observation and decreased if the motion is away from it. The magnitude of the shift is determined by the following equation:

$$f_s = \frac{2Vf_0 \cos \phi}{C} \qquad [1]$$

where f_s is the frequency shift, V the velocity, f_0 is the transmitted frequency, ϕ is the angle between the ultrasound beam and the velocity vector, and C is the speed of sound in tissue (1540 m/s). For a given velocity, a greater frequency shift is obtained with a higher transmitting frequency. In contrast, tissue penetration varies inversely with probe frequency, so the selection of a frequency for a given application is a balance between depth and velocity requirements.

Continuous-wave detectors are the simplest systems. The probe has two separate crystals, one transmitting and one receiving continuously. This system detects all velocities within the intersecting paths of the sound beams. If this zone includes more than one vessel (e.g., an artery and a vein), the resulting signal represents a combination of both velocities. Pulsed Doppler systems use a single crystal that repeatedly transmits a short burst of sound followed by a waiting period, during which the crystal functions in a receiving mode. By selecting the time and duration of the listening phase, one can define a sample volume, or the portion of the vessel from which velocity is to be measured. Modern duplex scanners use complex scan probes made up of many elements in an array, but the principle of focal sampling is the same.

The shifted frequency obtained from a vessel is within the audible range, so the data can be presented to the examiner as an audio signal. Although qualitative interpretation is helpful in some patient examinations, quantitative measurements provide objective testing. Spectral analyzers are used to determine the main frequency components obtained from a given vessel. This information is usually displayed on a sonogram, which shows the frequency content in time (Figure 14-1).

In some applications, it is more useful to have a measure of velocity rather than the raw frequency data. If the probe angle relative to the direction of flow can be measured, the velocity is estimated using the Doppler equation. The accuracy of the estimate depends greatly on the accuracy of the angle measurement. Errors are greatest when the probe is at a right angle to flow and least when it is at a low angle. Whenever possible, velocities should be measured with an angle less than 60 degrees.

Duplex Scan

During the 1960s, B-mode ultrasound imaging was used for visualization of soft tissue structures. Although early

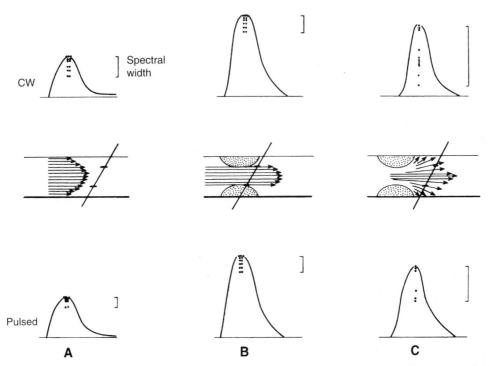

FIGURE 14-1 ■ Comparison of sonograms from continuous-wave (CW) and pulsed Doppler systems. Sonograms display the different frequency contents detected at each point in time. The CW system detects all velocities across the vessel, whereas the pulsed system detects only those velocity vectors within the sample volume, indicated by the marks on the ultrasound beam. **A,** Normal arterial signals. CW has more low-frequency content, because it detects flow near the walls as well as in the center stream. **B,** Within stenosis, there is increased peak frequency, and the frequency distributions of both types of Doppler systems are similar, because the sample volume encompasses the entire flow stream. **C,** Beyond stenosis, peak frequency is elevated, with increased frequency distribution resulting from turbulent flow. Spectral width is greater with CW systems.

devices had only crude resolution, equipment has improved to the point that clear, detailed images of vessels can be produced in real time (Figure 14-2). In general, experience shows that when high-quality imaging is obtained, the diagnostic accuracy is very high; however, in patients with advanced atherosclerosis, it is difficult to obtain optimal studies, and diagnostic accuracy is lower. A common problem is incomplete imaging of the vessel wall as a result of calcification, which is present in varying degrees in up to half of patients studied. The extent of interference may be limited, but in some vessels there is no visualization of substantial portions of the artery. Although calcified plaques stand out sharply in the ultrasound image, some atheromas are visualized poorly or not at all. A major source of error is that recent thrombus may have the same echo density as flowing blood, so that an occluded vessel may look normal on the ultrasound image.

To overcome the limitations of ultrasound imaging, the research team at the University of Washington developed the duplex scanner, combining a real-time B-mode ultrasound image system with a pulsed Doppler detector.[1] The ultrasound image shows not only the vessel under study but also the location of the sample volume of the Doppler beam so that the examiner can position it to study velocity patterns at specific locations in the vessel. The device can study calcified vessels by analyzing the Doppler velocity signal distal to the areas of calcification. The evaluation of the Doppler signal from the common carotid artery and its branches is performed using spectral analysis (Figure 14-3). Based on the peak systolic velocity, end-diastolic velocity, velocity ratios, and degree of spectral broadening, a category of stenosis is assigned to the vessel segment.

In the past 20 years, there has been extensive improvement of duplex scanners in terms of both image resolution and Doppler signal processing. The early devices were limited to the study of superficial vessels; however, the availability of low-frequency probes (2.0 to 3.5 MHz) permits the evaluation of abdominal vessels, including the aorta, vena cava, and main visceral branches. Study of intracranial artery branches is also possible.

An important subsequent development is the color-coded Doppler system. A linear array transducer composed of many separate elements is used to produce a grid of sample volumes encompassing the area covered by the B-mode image (Figure 14-4). A portion of the grid is selected for color coding of velocity information. Each of the sample volumes within the area is examined. If the returning ultrasound signal has no change in phase or frequency, the amplitude information is used to create the gray-scale image at that point in the matrix. If there is a change in phase or frequency, the information is analyzed in terms of velocity. A color is assigned to represent an approximate mean velocity occurring at that point in the field. Red and blue show flow toward and away from the transducer, respectively. The magnitude of the velocity is represented by the hue of the color: a dark shade indicates

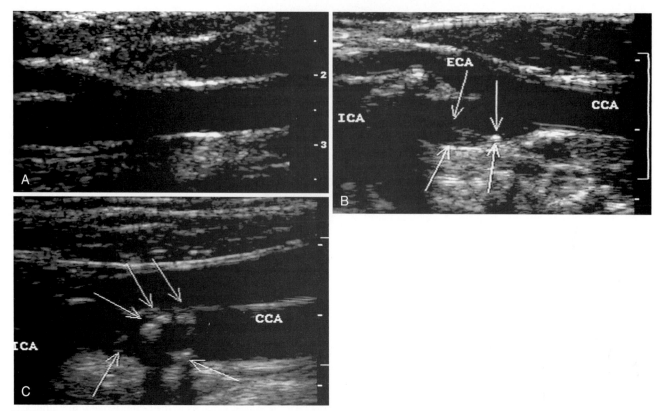

FIGURE 14-2 ■ B-mode images from carotid duplex scan. **A,** Normal bifurcation. **B,** Moderate heterogeneous plaque with varying echogenicity. **C,** Calcified lesion with high echogenicity and shadowing below the plaque. *CCA,* Common carotid artery; *ECA,* external carotid artery; *ICA,* internal carotid artery.

slow flow, and a lighter shade or white indicates high flow. The aggregate of the color representation from the sample volumes detecting motion produces a real-time representation of the flow patterns within the vessels superimposed on the gray-scale image of the stationary tissue. Figure 14-5 (see color plate) illustrates examples of the advantages of color duplex scans. A more recent development is color coding of the Doppler power (as opposed to velocity) detected. Power is proportional to the square of the velocity; therefore this measurement provides more sensitive detection of very slow flow or flow in small vessels. A good example of the benefit of power imaging is the detection of an internal carotid string sign. Squaring the velocity eliminates the positive or negative value, so that power values have no directional representation. Power is represented in a single color, usually orange.

CAROTID ARTERY STUDIES

The internal carotid artery (ICA) poses a unique challenge to physical examination, because it is impossible to palpate a distal pulse. It is not uncommon to find a patient whose carotid pulse in the neck is normal to palpation but who has occlusion of the internal carotid branch. This limitation stimulated the development of physiologic tests to assess the status of the ICA. Most of the early tests provided indirect measurement by detecting

distal changes in blood flow characteristics produced by advanced stenosis. Common features of the indirect methods are that they detect only lesions that are sufficiently advanced to reduce mean blood flow, and they cannot separate a tight stenosis from an occlusion because the physiologic changes in the distal bed may be indistinguishable. These methods achieved a variable degree of clinical use in the 1970s and 1980s, but were ultimately replaced by duplex scanning.

Duplex Scan

The routine examination covers as much of the common carotid artery (CCA) and its branches as can be visualized with the configuration of the transducer used. In some patients, the origins of the CCAs can be visualized. Figures 14-2*A* and 14-5*A* (see color plate) show normal carotid bifurcations. The color image demonstrates the reverse velocity detected in the carotid bulb as a result of the complex flow pattern at the bifurcation. Many older patients have tortuosity that precludes the CCA, the bulb, and the branches from being visualized in a single plane; in such cases, careful scanning is required to obtain satisfactory imaging. Figure 14-5*B* (see color plate) shows an example of tortuosity in an elderly patient. Although such arteries can be studied with a conventional scanner, the color-coded unit simplifies the examination. The scan usually identifies the pathologic regions, but with advanced atherosclerosis, it is often difficult to get an

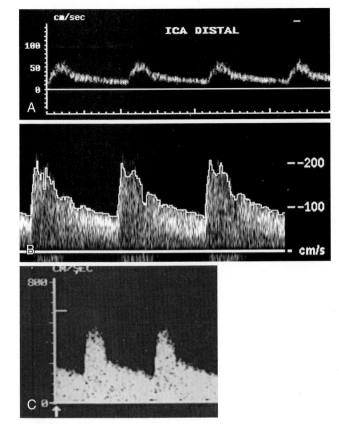

FIGURE 14-3 ■ Doppler sonograms from carotid duplex scans. **A,** Normal study with normal spectral width. **B,** Moderate stenosis with spectral broadening but no increase in peak frequency. (Note that frequency scales are different in the three records.) **C,** Severe stenosis with high peak velocity and extensive spectral broadening.

adequate image to accurately estimate the degree of stenosis. Much of the classification of stenosis is based on interpretation of the Doppler signal. The two branches are distinguished by the image and the velocity signals. The ICA has a low peripheral resistance at all times, resulting in forward flow throughout diastole, whereas the high resistance in the external carotid artery results in a diastolic flow of zero. Stenoses produce an increased velocity at the site of the lesion and turbulence beyond it (see Figure 14-1). The turbulence is identified as spectral broadening on the sonogram (see Figure 14-3). Mild stenoses may not produce a significant increase in peak systolic velocity, but are identified by a moderate degree of spectral broadening.

Based on the peak systolic velocity and the degree of spectral broadening, the ICA is placed into one of six diagnostic categories. There are two sets of criteria that have been used for many years, and although some laboratories have made modifications or adjustments, the basic principles continue to be applied. The criteria developed at the University of Washington use primarily ICA velocity parameters (Table 14-1).[2] Further improvements in accuracy can be obtained using ratios of ICA velocities to CCA velocities in normal portions of the artery (Table 14-2).[3] The diagnosis of ICA occlusion must be based on image and Doppler information, because the low flow found with some "string signs" is below the velocity detection threshold of many scanners. Newer color duplex devices have improved our ability to find small residual flow channels, especially using power flow mapping. Both the stippled appearance of chronic thrombus and a small diameter of the ICA indicate occlusion. Overall, low-grade plaques are best assessed with the image, whereas advanced lesions are best evaluated with the Doppler information.

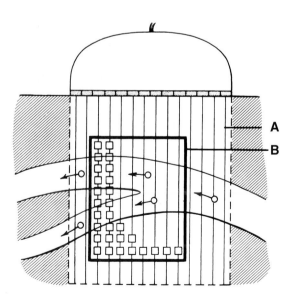

FIGURE 14-4 ■ Color-coded duplex system. A linear array transducer is used to create a matrix of sample volumes. A gray-scale image is created within area *A*. Most examinations are performed with color coding of velocities limited to a portion of the image (area *B*). Within this portion of the matrix, ultrasound signals from sample volumes with a change in phase or frequency are interpreted as velocity data. Otherwise, the data are coded as part of the gray-scale image.

TABLE 14-1	Categories of Internal Carotid Artery Stenosis: University of Washington Criteria	
ICA Stenosis	**ICA Velocity**	**Spectrum**
Normal vessel	Peak systolic velocity <125 cm/s	No broadening
1%-15%	Peak systolic velocity <125 cm/s	Limited broadening in late systole
16%-49%	Peak systolic velocity <125 cm/s	Broadening throughout systole
50%-79%	Peak systolic velocity >140 cm/s; end-diastolic velocity <140 cm/s	Broadening throughout systole
80%-99%	End-diastolic velocity >140 cm/s (severe stenosis may have very low velocity)	Broadening throughout systole
Occlusion	No ICA Doppler signal; flow to zero in common carotid artery	

ICA, Internal carotid artery.

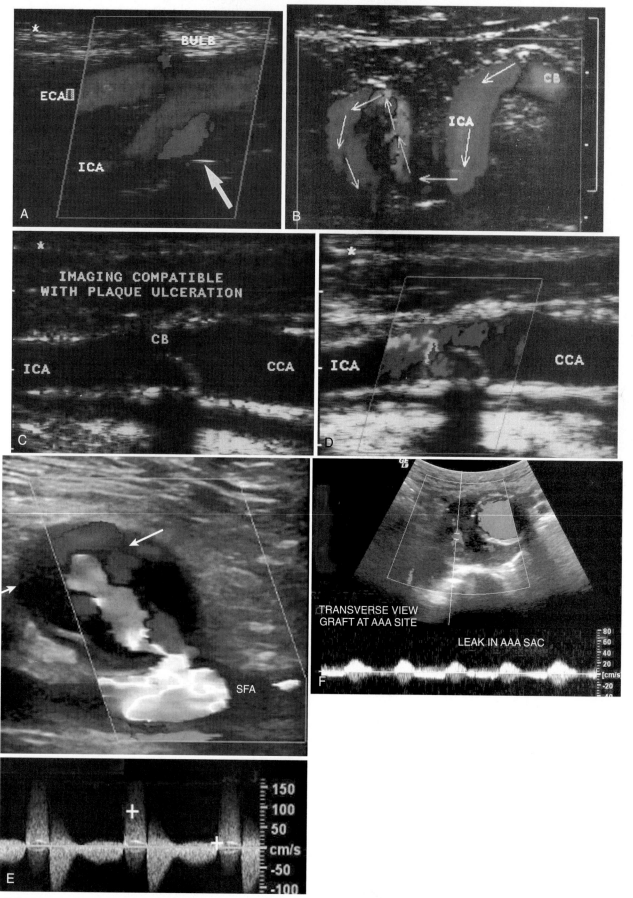

FIGURE 14-5 ■ **A,** Advantages of using color duplex scanning. Normal carotid bifurcation, illustrating the reverse flow occuring in the bulb during peak systole *(arrow)*. **B,** Marked tortuosity of internal carotid artery *(ICA)* is easily demonstrated with color scan. **C,** Conventional gray-scale image does not provide clear identification of large ulcer. **D,** Blood flow within plaque confirms the ulcer. **E,** Pseudoaneurysm originating from the superficial femoral artery *(SFA)* resulting from catheterization. Note the bidirectional flow recorded in the neck. **F,** Type 2 endoleak with flow detected in the aneurysm sac outside of prosthesis.

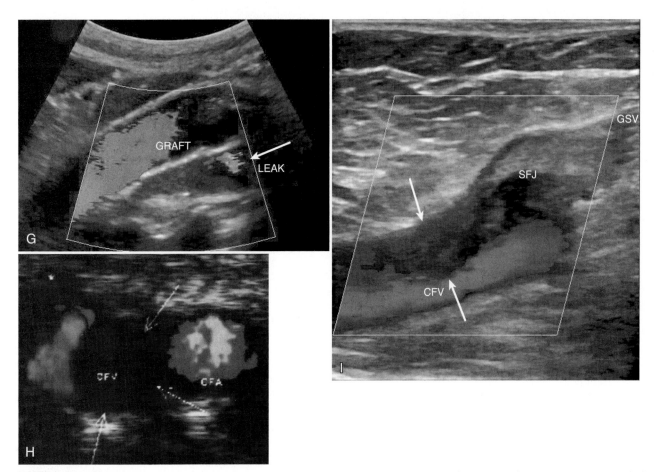

FIGURE 14-5, cont'd ■ **G,** Longitudinal view of same aorta showing leak is posterior to graft. **H,** Blood flow around partial occluding thrombus. **I,** Thrombus extending into common femoral vein, seen 2 days after endovascular ablation of great saphenous vein. See Color Plate 14-5.

TABLE 14-2 Categories of Internal Carotid Artery Stenosis: Bluth Criteria

ICA Stenosis	Peak Systolic Velocity (cm/s)	Diastolic Velocity (cm/s)	ICA/CCA Velocity
Normal vessel	<110	<40	<1.8
1%-39%	<115	<40	<1.8
40%-59%	<130	>40	<1.8
60%-79%	>130	>40	>1.8
80%-99%	>250 (severe stenosis may have very low velocity)	>100	>3.7
Occlusion	No ICA Doppler signal	No ICA Doppler signal	No ICA Doppler signal

ICA, Internal carotid artery; *CCA,* common carotid artery.

There has been a rapid growth in the use of duplex scanning for carotid diagnosis. Different investigators have demonstrated that the technique can be highly accurate. Studies have shown rates of 92% to 96% accuracy in the identification of severe stenosis.[4-6] When these studies are analyzed in terms of correct category of stenosis, exact agreement is found in 77% to 87%, with poor agreement in only 1% to 2%. Of particular importance is the fact that experienced laboratories make few errors in separating severe stenosis from occlusion. Mansour and coauthors[7] reported a 98% positive predictive value and 99% negative predictive value in the correct determination of ICA occlusion.

In addition to estimating the severity of a stenosis, scanners are now being used to study the plaque itself. Most investigators merely distinguish between homogeneous- and heterogeneous-appearing plaques and describe the surface as either smooth or irregular. More elaborate approaches to the description of morphology are being evaluated, but no single approach has been widely adopted.

Although the majority of attention has been focused on the carotid circulation, laboratories routinely investigate the status of the vertebral arteries as well. The examination seeks two types of problems: stenosis in the vertebral artery itself and the abnormal flow produced by subclavian steal. In the majority of cases of significant vertebral stenosis, the lesion is located at the origin of the vessel. In some cases of severe occlusive disease, there is sufficient asymmetry in the waveforms of the two vertebral arteries to point to the problem side. However, a more complete assessment is obtained by examining the origins. Because of its deeper location, the left vertebral

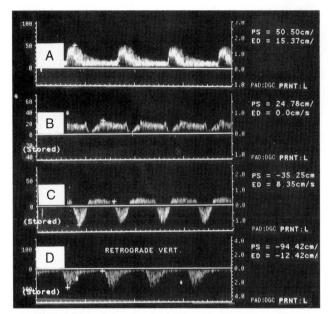

FIGURE 14-6 ■ Vertebral artery Doppler waveforms. **A** is normal. **B** to **D** are signals recorded on the side of severe subclavian stenosis. **B,** Attenuated systolic flow. **C,** Reversed flow in systole, with forward flow in diastole. **D,** Complete flow reversal.

artery is more difficult to study than the right. Ackerstaff and associates[8] found that the status of the ostium could be studied satisfactorily in about 80% of patients. When adequate evaluation of the prevertebral portion was possible, a sensitivity of 80% and a specificity of 97% were achieved in the detection of reductions greater than 50% in diameter. Most clinical cases of subclavian steal are demonstrated by a reverse flow in the vertebral artery on the affected side. Von Reutern and Pourcelot[9] demonstrated that in some cases of subclavian stenosis there is distortion of the waveform rather than complete reversal of flow. The abnormal waveforms may have attenuation of the systolic component or an alternating pattern with reverse flow in systole and forward flow in diastole (Figure 14-6). Such cases can be assessed more fully by recording the Doppler signal after arm exercise or the induction of reactive hyperemia. In the presence of advanced subclavian stenosis, this stress test produces full reversal of flow.

Applications

Symptomatic Patients

A large number of transient ischemic attacks and strokes are caused by thromboembolization from plaques in the carotid bifurcation. In most situations, a duplex scan is the initial workup, identifying the location and severity of lesions in the carotid system. Many centers use the ultrasound study as the definitive test on which to base the decision to treat. Having an experienced vascular laboratory with a validated record of high accuracy in carotid scanning is the critical element in using duplex scanning as the definitive test. In other settings, additional confirmation is obtained with magnetic resonance or computed tomography angiography.

Asymptomatic Carotid Stenosis

Increasing numbers of asymptomatic patients are being referred to vascular laboratories for the evaluation of cervical bruits. Although some of these patients have bruits radiating from the heart or the great vessels, in a considerable number the sound originates from the carotid bifurcation. Duplex scanning can provide accurate separation according to category of stenosis (see Tables 14-1 and 14-2). Patients with severe stenosis are considered at increased risk of stroke and are evaluated for prophylactic carotid endarterectomy. Lesions that fall in the moderate category should have follow-up testing to detect those that progress into the high-risk group. Most people with normal vessels or early disease do not require routine follow-up.

Another indication is the screening of patients with advanced atherosclerotic disease in the coronary or peripheral vessels. Owing to the diffuse nature of atherosclerosis, some of these patients have occult carotid bifurcation lesions, with a resulting increased risk of stroke. Screening is performed most often in patients who are being considered for cardiac or major peripheral arterial operations to detect carotid lesions that may substantially increase the risk of perioperative stroke. Although screening may be appropriate for patients with multiple risk factors or severe occlusive disease in other arteries, routine testing of large populations results in a low yield of stenoses in the 80% to 99% category and is not cost-effective.

Intraoperative Assessment

Over the years, there has been increasing use of completion studies to evaluate the status of the operated artery before closing the neck. Contrast angiography is the most common technique used, usually with a single injection into the CCA below the level of the endarterectomy. Another approach is to examine the repair using a simple continuous-wave Doppler unit with subjective evaluation of the signals. This method detects severe residual stenoses but is not sensitive to other problems. Increasingly, completion duplex scanning is now being used to detect residual defects requiring correction, and studies have shown satisfactory results.[10-12] Bandyk and colleagues[13] used a peak systolic velocity greater than 180 cm/s or a velocity ratio greater than 2.4 as the criterion to perform a confirmatory angiogram or to proceed directly to reopening the artery.[13]

Postoperative Follow-Up

Recurrent stenosis after carotid endarterectomy remains a clinical problem. Early studies reported as much as 5% symptomatic restenosis and 8% asymptomatic restenosis (as identified by noninvasive testing).[14,15] More recent studies applying life-table analysis have found restenosis rates of 20% to 32% with greater than 50% diameter reduction.[16,17] It has been shown that a substantial proportion of restenoses occurs early in the postoperative period. A common practice is to obtain an early postoperative study that can be used as a baseline. Follow-up evaluations are done 6 and 12 months after surgery. If the study remains normal, noninvasive studies are repeated yearly. More recent studies show that in the presence of a normal completion angiogram or duplex scan, follow-up need not be performed until 1 year after operation.[18,19]

LOWER EXTREMITY ARTERIAL STUDIES

Segmental Extremity Pressure Measurement

Indirect measurement of extremity pressures has been performed since the beginning of the 20th century using a sphygmomanometer and auscultation of the Korotkoff sounds with a stethoscope. Although this technique is universally used to measure pressures in the brachial artery, its application in the lower extremity is less practical because of the difficulty of listening for Korotkoff sounds in the popliteal space. The technique is certainly not applicable in the distal portions of the extremity because of the small size of the vessels involved. Investigators overcame this limitation by using a variety of plethysmographic devices. In 1959, Winsor[20] first described the clinical measurement of arterial gradients using a plethysmograph. Systolic pressures in the lower extremity are normally higher than those in the upper extremity. He described the blood pressure index (blood pressure of arm/blood pressure of leg), which in normal persons is less than 1.0. A value greater than 1.0 indicates clinically significant occlusive disease proximal to the point of measurement. (Note that the ratio winsor described is the inverse of the currently used ankle-brachial index.) Likewise, a gradient between two sampling sites localizes the occlusive disease in the intervening segment. The main limitation of this method is that it detects only occlusive lesions that are sufficiently advanced to reduce the systolic pressure, so that it is not possible to detect early disease. Introduction of the Doppler velocity detector greatly simplified the indirect measurement of extremity pressures. For this application, the Doppler device is used merely to detect the presence or absence of the movement of blood in the artery. Measurements made by this method are reproducible, but do not provide diastolic pressure. Plethysmographic techniques are cumbersome and are not used routinely.

In clinical practice, simple screening can be performed by measuring the pressure at the brachial arteries and at the dorsal pedal and posterior tibial arteries on each side. The ankle-brachial index (ABI) is determined by dividing the ankle pressure on each side by the higher of the two brachial pressures. The resulting value reflects the severity of the occlusive disease for the entire extremity. Normally, the ABI should be greater than 1.0, and values less than 0.95 are abnormal. Figure 14-7 summarizes the general relation between ABI values and clinical status.

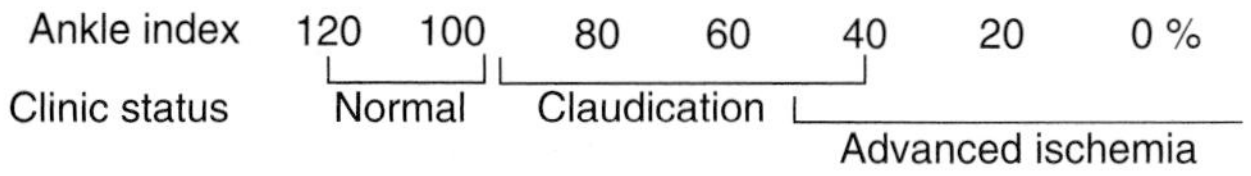

It must be emphasized that this is only a rough correlation and that patients with similar values may have substantial differences in exercise tolerance. Likewise, the index at which rest pain appears varies considerably from patient to patient, ranging from 0.30 to 0.50.

An important limitation of the indirect measurement of extremity pressure is seen in patients with abnormal stiffening of the vessel wall, most often due to heavy calcification. Such conditions occur with diabetes mellitus but can also be found with other disorders. In these cases, the systolic pressure measured reflects the cuff pressure required to collapse the vessel wall in addition to the pressure required to overcome the intraluminal pressure. In a few patients, it is not possible to stop the flow of blood at all. Error due to wall stiffness should be suspected whenever the ABI is greater than 1.3 or its value is out of proportion to the patient's clinical status. In general, a leg with a normal ABI should have an easily palpable ankle pulse. In some patients with stiff arteries, it may be possible to obtain an accurate evaluation by measuring the toe pressure. In a healthy person, there is a gradient of 20 to 30 mm Hg between the ankle and the toe; therefore a correction must be made when toe pressures are being used.

Localization of occlusive disease can be obtained by measuring the pressures at different levels of the leg. Segmental pressure measurements are usually performed by applying cuffs at the thigh, the upper calf, and immediately above the ankle. A standard adult-sized cuff (12 cm wide) is satisfactory for calf and ankle determinations, but a thigh cuff (18 cm) should be used above the knee. (Using a narrower cuff above the knee results in artificially high pressure measurements as a result of the size discrepancy between the cuff and the diameter of the thigh. Thigh measurements with an arm cuff usually result in determinations that are 20 to 30 mm Hg higher than those obtained with the wider cuff.) A thigh pressure lower than the brachial pressure indicates obstruction proximal to the location of the thigh cuff. Gradients of more than 20 mm Hg between measuring sites are diagnostic of occlusive disease in the intervening segment, and higher gradients are usually associated with more severe lesions.

An important limitation of the use of the wide cuff for thigh measurement is that it is possible to make only a single thigh measurement. As a result, it is not possible to distinguish occlusive disease above the ligament from that in the proximal portion of the superficial femoral artery, because both conditions can result in the same thigh pressure measurement. To overcome this problem, some investigators have recommended using 12-cm–wide cuffs to obtain two separate thigh measurements. When this is done, it is necessary to take into account the 20- to 30-mm Hg artifact in the results. In a study comparing the wide cuff with the two narrow-cuff techniques in the same group of patients, Heintz and coworkers[21] reported an increased accuracy in the localization of disease using the two-cuff technique. Both methods of thigh pressure measurement are still being used, so it is important to know which method is being reported when reviewing the results of patient studies. Although segmental pressures have been used extensively to detect proximal

Ankle index	120	100	80	60	40	20	0 %
Clinic status		Normal	Claudication				
				Advanced ischemia			

FIGURE 14-7 ■ Relation of ankle-brachial index to patient symptoms.

disease, diagnostic errors may occur in 25% of patients. Other techniques should be used when an accurate determination of the segmental localization is needed.

Stress Testing

Most patients with advanced arterial insufficiency are adequately evaluated by measurements at rest; however, less severe lesions may not produce a sufficient disturbance at resting flow rates to be detected by the usual methods. An example of this problem is a patient with typical symptoms of claudication who has normal or borderline leg pressures. A more complete evaluation can be obtained by increasing the flow to accentuate the hemodynamic effect of the stenosis. The simplest and most normal way to increase blood flow is to have the patient walk. Exercise produces a decrease in vascular resistance in the leg, with a resulting increase in flow to the leg. With moderate levels of exercise, there is no change in distal pressures in a normal extremity, but increasing the flow through a moderate stenosis causes an increased resistance at the lesion. The resulting energy loss can be detected by noninvasive tests such as a pressure gradient or the attenuation of the pulse waveform.

The stress test is performed by having the patient walk on a treadmill for 5 minutes or until symptoms force the patient to stop. Most protocols use a low level of exercise (2 mph with a 10% to 12% grade). This level of stress is sufficient to yield an abnormal result in most claudication patients, without undue cardiac stress. Baseline arm and ankle pressures are measured with the Doppler detector. As soon as walking is completed, the patient lies down on the examining table for repeated pressure measurements, made at 30-second intervals during the first 2 minutes and at 60-second intervals for the remainder of the examination, usually 5 to 10 minutes. The examiner always asks the patient why he or she stopped walking, because in some cases, the limiting factor is angina or shortness of breath rather than claudication. Identification of these limitations is an important benefit of the stress test, because it may uncover or emphasize the significance of these other conditions.

One objective measurement of the severity of occlusive disease is exercise tolerance (i.e., the time the patient walks at the standardized rate). Further assessment is based on the changes in extremity pressures. Figure 14-8 shows the time-pressure relations seen in control subjects and in different categories of occlusive disease. Healthy people have no significant change in ankle pressures with the modest level of exercise used for the stress test. In contrast, patients with flow-limiting stenoses have a drop in distal pressures as a result of vasodilatation in the muscles. The magnitude of the drop in both ABI and recovery time are increased with more severe occlusive disease. Multiple lesions produce more marked depression of the recovery curve than do single lesions.

There are some situations in which treadmill exercise is not practical or does not offer the best evaluation. In such cases, reactive hyperemia can be used to increase blood flow in the extremities. A thigh cuff inflated above systolic pressure produces local circulatory arrest, resulting in hypoxia and local vasodilatation. When the cuff is

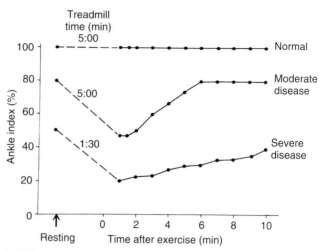

FIGURE 14-8 ■ Changes in ankle-brachial index with exercise. The severity of the arterial stenosis is related to the exercise tolerance and the magnitude of the drop in ankle pressure and recovery time.

released, there is a transient increase in flow, the duration of which is related to the period of ischemia and to the total blood flow to the leg. The magnitude of the pressure drop is comparable to that seen after walking, but the recovery is always more rapid with reactive hyperemia. In contrast to exercise, reactive hyperemia does produce a transient pressure drop (with a rapid recovery) in normal subjects. Criteria for a normal result are lowest ABI greater than 0.80 and return of the index to 90% of the baseline value within 1 minute.[22] The technique provides a useful test method for patients who cannot walk on the treadmill because of disabilities or those who are unwilling to perform adequately on the treadmill, and for the full evaluation of the less-involved limb in patients with marked asymmetry of their occlusive disease.

In general, stress testing is not routinely needed in a majority of patients seen in the vascular laboratory. Those with significant abnormalities at rest always have abnormal responses to exercise. This additional evaluation can be reserved for patients with typical symptoms of arterial insufficiency but normal or near-normal resting studies and those with confusing symptoms in whom one wants to exclude arterial insufficiency as a cause. The stress examination is also useful for research studies in which more sensitivity for the detection of improvement or deterioration is needed.

Doppler Waveform Evaluation

Most commercial Doppler detectors provide an analog signal that is proportional to the velocity of the blood in the vessel studied. This signal can be displayed on a screen or recorded. The overall shape of the waveform reflects the status of the vessel proximal to the point studied (Figure 14-9). In the lower extremity, the normal velocity wave is triphasic, with reverse flow in early diastole. Proximal stenosis first eliminates the reverse flow; with more severe lesions, there is blunting of the systolic upstroke and increasing flow during diastole. The

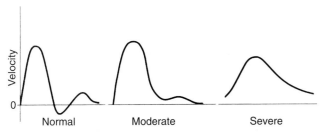

FIGURE 14-9 ■ Doppler velocity tracings in the leg. Increasing stenosis results in elimination of reverse flow, decrease in systolic peak, and increase in flow during diastole.

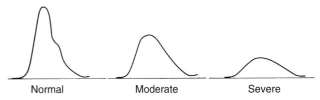

FIGURE 14-10 ■ Pulse-volume recorder tracings in the leg. Increasing stenosis results in loss of the dicrotic notch and flattening of the curve.

simplest analysis of Doppler waveforms is a qualitative interpretation of the curves, allowing the identification of broad categories of disease. One specific application has been the assessment of the aortoiliac segment. However, the method suffers from a high false-positive rate resulting from the fact that an attenuated wave can be caused by proximal disease, distal disease, or a combination of the two.

A variety of techniques for quantitative analysis of the Doppler waveform have been described over the years. These investigations have largely focused on separating significant inflow occlusive disease from that below the inguinal ligament. Although each method evaluated offers some additional diagnostic benefit, none has achieved wide application. Burnham and colleagues[23] proposed the measurement of common femoral artery acceleration time (onset of systole to peak systole) to identify significant aortoiliac disease. An acceleration time greater than 133 msec is found with proximal stenosis.

Segmental Plethysmography

During systole, the blood entering a limb normally causes an increase in the total volume of the extremity, with a return to resting volume during diastole. This phenomenon is responsible for the pulse pressure oscillations seen with the sphygmomanometer while taking blood pressure. The total volume change is small and can be detected only with the aid of sensitive devices. A variety of plethysmographic recorders have been devised using a mercury strain gauge, water displacement, capacitance, and impedance systems, but the majority of these systems have proved to be impractical for routine clinical application. In the early 1970s, the pulse-volume recorder was designed specifically for peripheral arterial diagnosis. The system uses a calibrated recording air plethysmograph with standard blood pressure cuffs applied at the thigh, calf, and ankle levels. The cuffs are inflated to 65 mm Hg to ensure optimal contact of the cuff around the extremity. A sensitive transducer detects the small increase in pressure within the cuff resulting from the volume increase of the extremity during systole. The recorder provides a hard-copy tracing of the pulse wave, which has been demonstrated to be similar to arterial pressure waves measured directly.

The primary diagnosis is based on a qualitative evaluation of the pulse-volume waveform.[24] The tracing from each level is categorized as normal, mildly abnormal, moderately abnormal, or severely abnormal. The normal tracing has a brisk, sharp rise to the systolic peak and usually displays a prominent dicrotic notch (Figure 14-10). Early disease is characterized by the absence of a dicrotic notch and a more gradual, prolonged downslope. Moderate disease is characterized by a rounded systolic peak. Severe occlusive disease produces a flattened wave with a slow upstroke and downstroke. The absolute amplitude measurements are of limited value from patient to patient, because substantial changes result from variations in cardiac output and vasomotor tone. Comparison of amplitudes from each side in the same patient can be of value in assessing unilateral disease. In the presence of bilateral disease, it can be helpful to standardize the amplitude measurements in the lower extremities by comparing them with arm tracings, because most patients do not have major upper extremity occlusive disease. Serial pulse-volume measurements have been shown to be reproducible in patients with stable disease, so that amplitude changes indicate progression of disease.

The pulse-volume recorder has received extensive application. In most situations, the plethysmographic studies are used in combination with segmental Doppler pressure measurements. Vascular laboratories using the device report that it is a useful adjunct to routine pressure measurements. One particular advantage is the ability to accurately assess the presence or absence of occlusive disease in patients with rigid arteries. In addition, the pulse-volume recorder has improved the detection of aortoiliac stenosis. Kempczinski[25] reported the correct identification of advanced inflow disease in 95% of extremities.

Duplex Scan

In recent years, the duplex scan has been used more frequently to evaluate peripheral arteries. With appropriate scan heads, Doppler signals can be obtained from the aorta down to the tibial branches. Screening for occlusive disease can be done by comparing signals from the distal aorta and more distal sites. A more complete assessment is obtained by examining the full length of the segment in question, looking for the increased velocity and spectral broadening produced by a stenosis. The color-coded Doppler scan makes tracking of the vessels and localizing of significant stenoses considerably easier than with conventional scanners. The most common practice is to use the ratio of the peak systolic velocity recorded at the tightest part of the stenosis to the peak systolic velocity recorded in a normal portion of the same artery. A ratio greater than 2 defines a greater than 50% diameter reduction of the lumen.[26,27] Some groups have established additional criteria to distinguish stenosis greater than 75%. Cossman and colleagues[28] consider the stenosis to be greater than 75% if the velocity ratio is greater than 4 or the peak velocity in the lesion is greater than 400 cm/s.[28] Gonsalves and Bandyk[29] identify a severe lesion by a velocity ratio greater than 4, a peak velocity greater than 300 cm/s, or an end-diastolic velocity greater than 100 cm/s.

Scanning is also used for visceral vessels, including the arteries of normal and transplanted kidneys. The anterior approach to visceral branches can be difficult owing to the presence of bowel gas. Flank approaches and examination of a fasting patient increase the rate of successful studies. Most renal artery stenoses occur at the origins, so it is necessary to obtain recordings from the proximal part of the vessel. As with peripheral lesions, the focus has been on identifying hemodynamically significant stenoses. A peak systolic velocity greater than 180 cm/s identifies an abnormal vessel, and a ratio of the peak velocity in the stenosis to the peak velocity in the aorta at the level of the renal arteries greater than 3.5 predicts a stenosis with a greater than 60% lumen diameter reduction.[30-32] Another approach has been to use the waveform recorded in the renal hilum.[33] Although recording hilar signals is usually easier than examining the main renal arteries, this approach does not seem to be as accurate in the diagnosis of significant stenoses.[32] An important limitation of the duplex scan in the evaluation of renal disease is that accessory branches are often missed.

Duplex scanning has also been used to study the mesenteric branches. The celiac trunk and the proximal superior mesenteric artery can be located easily. In contrast, the inferior mesenteric artery is often not found unless it provides significant collateral flow because of occlusions in other branches. Unlike the situation with the kidneys, the perfusion to the gut is highly variable, depending on physiologic responses to feeding. Therefore it is important to obtain baseline studies of patients in a fasting state. There has not been as much investigation of quantitative criteria to define severe mesenteric disease as there has been of other duplex scan applications. Severe stenosis is identified by a significant focal increase in velocity combined with poststenotic turbulence and reduced velocity beyond the stenosis. Moneta and colleagues[34] found that peak systolic velocities greater than 200 cm/s in the celiac artery and 275 cm/s in the superior mesenterica indicate stenosis greater than 70%.[34]

Applications

Severity and Location of Arterial Lesions

The primary use of noninvasive tests in patients with lower extremity problems is to obtain objective determinations to supplement the physical examination. Such measurements permit reproducibility between different examiners as well as from one time to another. In addition, the tests are valuable in measuring the progression of arterial disease and assessing arterial reconstructions. Extremity pressures and pulse plethysmographic recordings are valuable to assess disease severity; however, duplex scanning must be used for an accurate determination of the level and extent of lesions. Kohler and associates[26] found a sensitivity of 89% and a specificity of 90% in the identification of iliac stenosis greater than 50%. Legemate and coworkers[35] used a velocity increase of 150% and found a sensitivity of 92% and specificity of 98%. It is possible to estimate common femoral artery blood flow with duplex scan measurements, but the high variability in repeat measurements in individual patients limits the clinical usefulness of this approach.[36] Although further refinement of quantitative criteria is required, it is clear that duplex scanning can play an increasing role in the evaluation of peripheral arterial insufficiency.

Following the lead of those performing carotid endarterectomy without preoperative angiography, investigators have reported the feasibility of planning arterial operations with only the ultrasound scan.[28,37-40] Wain and coauthors[40] reported that duplex mapping is accurate down to the popliteal level, but in their experience, the technique is not as good at defining an appropriate target vessel at the crural level.[40] More recent studies have shown improved results with mapping of the entire lower leg in order to plan the appropriate bypass operation, including selection of the site of distal anastomosis.[41,42] Adequate visualization of the peroneal artery in the lower calf remains one of the challenges for the examiner.

With the increasing frequency of percutaneous interventional procedures, a need has developed for evaluation of extremity complications. The duplex scan provides a simple tool to assess the appearance of a mass adjacent to an arterial puncture site. The primary question is whether the mass is simply a hematoma or whether there is an early pseudoaneurysm, possibly complicated by an arteriovenous fistula. Figure 14-5E shows a pseudoaneurysm originating from the superficial femoral artery. There is a small diameter neck off the artery with flow into the adjacent space. The Doppler waveform from the neck shows a bidirectional pattern typical of a pseudoaneurysm. In the case of a hematoma, there is a homogeneous mass (with no blood flow) adjacent to the vessels which would appear normal on scan.

Intraoperative Assessment

As with carotid surgery, duplex scanning provides an excellent tool for completion assessment after certain other arterial operations. In many operating rooms, scanning can be done more quickly and provide a more complete examination than can a conventional contrast angiogram. Often, short focal defects such as a retained valve are easily seen on a scan but may not be well demonstrated angiographically, especially with a single film study. Bandyk and associates[43] reported on scanning after infrainguinal bypass grafts. The examination involves scanning the full length of the graft, including both anastomoses. A peak systolic velocity greater than 180 cm/s or a velocity ratio greater than 2.4 indicates a problem for which revision must be considered. Bandyk and associates[43] reported intraoperative revision rates of 14% to 16%. Fifty-two percent of the legs with significant duplex findings that were not repaired at the time of the original operation underwent subsequent revision.

Intraoperative duplex scanning has also been advocated for renal artery repairs to reduce the risk of early occlusion and possible loss of the kidney. Studies from both Bowman Gray and the Mayo Clinic reported an 11% incidence of the detection of defects requiring repair at the time of the original procedure.[44,45] A focal high-velocity jet with a peak systolic velocity greater than 200 cm/s combined with distal turbulence identifies a tight stenosis, whereas lack of flow in the vessel indicates acute thrombosis.[44] Both these findings mandate immediate revision.

Graft Surveillance

Because of the poor secondary patency of vein grafts that thrombose, careful attention has been given to follow-up. As early as 1972, some surgeons advocated postoperative noninvasive testing to identify hemodynamic changes. For many years, graft status was monitored with pressure measurements; however, this technique is limited for patients with stiff arteries or with small-caliber distal bypasses. In 1985, Bandyk and associates[46] reported good results with graft surveillance using the duplex scanner to measure the peak systolic velocity. In this study, a peak velocity of less than 40 cm/s was associated with early graft thrombosis. In later years, the surveillance protocol was expanded to include a sampling of the graft velocity and a scan of the entire graft.[47,48] Such mapping permits the identification of the specific site of stenosis. A peak systolic velocity of 180 to 200 cm/s indicates a problem. Bandyk and Johnson[48] recommended intervention for any lesion with a peak systolic velocity greater than 300 cm/s or a velocity ratio greater than 3.5. A large proportion of stenoses are found within the first postoperative year; therefore a program of close surveillance is advocated by many authors.[49-51] The fact that significant problems can appear later is a reason to continue surveillance beyond the first year, albeit at a reduced frequency.

In the past decade there has been an explosion in the use of endograft placement for treating aortic aneurysms. Unlike open repair, the endovascular procedure was found to have a substantial incidence of postprocedure complications, primarily endoleaks (see Chapter 39). From the early days of the procedure, surgeons used computed tomographic angiography (CTA) to evaluate postoperative results. The common practice was to obtain studies at 6 months, 1 year, and annually after that. Increasing concern over the radiation exposure and the repeated administration of nephrotoxic contrast led some investigators to evaluate the use of ultrasound for the endograft surveillance.[52] Arko and

associates compared findings on postoperative CTA and duplex scan.[53]

There was a close correlation of aneurysm diameters and duplex scan had a 90% negative predictive value. (Most of the endoleaks missed were caused by small lumbar arteries.) Improved skills with scanning techniques and improved equipment have resulted in increasing use of ultrasound surveillance of endografts. Many surgeons obtain an initial postoperative CTA, and if it is normal then limit routine follow-up to a duplex examination.[54] Figures 14-5F and 14-5G (color plate) show a typical type 2 endoleak.

VENOUS DISEASE

The correct diagnosis of venous abnormalities can be challenging. In contrast to arterial occlusive disease, venous disease may be difficult to distinguish from other problems on the basis of the physical examination. In the past, diagnosis depended on phlebography, which, in addition to being painful, can precipitate thrombosis in a normal venous system. In the 1960s, Strandness and coworkers[55] and Sigel and colleagues[56] used the simple continuous-wave Doppler velocity detector to identify normal and abnormal flow patterns in the veins of the leg. With the subsequent development of noninvasive techniques for the arterial system, there was a parallel growth in the methods of venous diagnosis. The 1970s and 1980s saw extensive use of physiologic methods such as impedance phlebography, but these tests have been replaced by duplex scanning.

Doppler Venous Examination

The flow in the extremity veins can be evaluated qualitatively with a continuous-wave Doppler detector. The patient is examined in the supine position with the head slightly elevated. The deep veins are found adjacent to the accompanying arteries. A normal vein has spontaneous flow with a phasic variation with respiration. Breath-holding or a Valsalva maneuver decreases or abolishes flow; with release, there is a transient augmentation of the signal. A quick compression of the extremity distal to the probe produces a brisk augmentation, often followed by a transient decrease on release. Proximal compression decreases or abolishes the flow signal, with augmentation coming on release. Examination of a thrombosed segment of vein shows no flow, and adjacent collateral veins have a high-pitched signal. The patent portion of the vein distal to an obstruction has a continuous flow with no respiratory variation, and the Valsalva maneuver produces no change. Limb compression can produce limited augmentation, but clearly less than that in the normal vein. The vein segment proximal to an occlusion may have phasic flow similar to normal, but distal compression produces little change. The Doppler examination is sensitive to alterations in venous flow patterns, and different forms of extrinsic compression can produce similar changes. Abnormal studies can result from large hematomas, massive edema, or ruptured popliteal cysts. A false-positive test can also occur with advanced pregnancy, ascites, morbid obesity, or abdominal masses compressing the inferior vena cava.

The Doppler venous examination can also detect venous valvular insufficiency. Normally, there should be no flow produced by compression proximal to the probe, because the valves prevent flow toward the probe. With incompetent valves, proximal compression (or a Valsalva maneuver) produces augmentation as a result of the retrograde flow. Demonstration of significant reverse flow is clear evidence of postthrombotic syndrome.

The venous examination with a continuous wave device was once an important test for acute deep venous thrombosis (DVT) in the leg, but it has been supplanted by quantitative and imaging techniques. Because of the simplicity of the Doppler examination, it is still used, primarily as an extension of the physical examination. An abnormal flow pattern in a patient with borderline physical findings can trigger more complete evaluation by the vascular laboratory. Simple Doppler examination is also helpful in detecting deep venous reflux in a patient with varicose veins.

Duplex Scan

The high resolution available with duplex scanners makes it possible to visualize venous thrombosis. In this application, the emphasis is on imaging. Thrombus is seen within the vein lumen with varying degrees of echogenicity (Figure 14-11). On occasion, fresh thrombus may look no different from flowing blood; in these instances, additional assessment is obtained by compressing the vein with the probe. Normally, gentle pressure flattens the vein completely (Figure 14-12). A partially or totally occluding thrombus prevents collapse in response to external pressure. Compression is performed in the transverse mode to ensure accurate evaluation with the maneuver. When examining in the longitudinal orientation, it is possible to move the ultrasound beam off the center of the vein so that the

vein appears to collapse when it does not. Occluded segments can also be identified by the lack of flow on Doppler examination, and determination of flow characteristics should be part of every study. Abnormalities in Doppler velocity signals either at rest or in response to augmentation maneuvers indicate lesions that might not be evident with imaging. Color-coded Doppler is especially helpful in detecting partial occluding thrombi (see Figure 14-5H, see color plate). The color scanner has also improved the examination of the calf veins.

Most centers perform a detailed examination from the inguinal ligament to the calf veins. In addition to the deep system, superficial veins can be imaged. The greatest difficulty in many examinations is following the vein through the adductor canal. The common and superficial femoral veins are examined in the supine position with moderate leg dependency. (The deep femoral vein is usually not

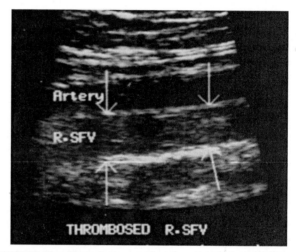

FIGURE 14-11 ■ B-mode scan of venous thrombus. Note the appearance of the vein lumen compared with the normal flow in the adjacent artery. *R-SFV,* Right superficial femoral vein.

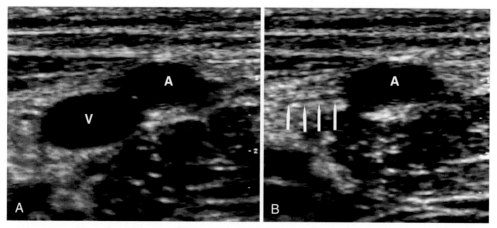

FIGURE 14-12 ■ Transverse duplex scans. **A,** Normal appearance of vein. **B,** Complete collapse of vein in response to external compression with the probe. *V,* Vein; *A,* artery.

followed beyond its origin.) The popliteal vein is best imaged with the patient in the lateral or prone position. Infrapopliteal branches can be difficult to evaluate fully; however, special attention should be given to these whenever the patient has focal calf symptoms. The other problem area is detecting thrombus in the common or external iliac veins. It is difficult to image these veins; therefore one must often rely on indirect evidence given by the flow signal from the common femoral vein. Proximal occlusion causes a loss of phasic variation with respiration and limited or no change with the Valsalva maneuver. Vogel and coworkers described using the change in common femoral vein diameter during the Valsalva maneuver: an increase of less than 10% indicates iliofemoral thrombosis.[57]

Duplex scanning of the deep leg veins for thrombus is technically difficult and requires considerable experience for an accurate diagnosis. Experienced investigators have reported sensitivities and specificities of approximately 95% for the diagnosis of thrombus.[57-60] Although most studies have focused on acute thrombosis, Rollins and associates demonstrated the same high accuracy in the identification of chronic disease.[59] In addition, they reported 89% accuracy in the evaluation of calf veins, compared with 93% for the proximal veins. When thrombus is identified, the clinician usually wants to know the duration of the process. Currently there is no specific method for determining this parameter. Generally an acute thrombus has a hypoechoic, homogeneous appearance on gray scale imaging. The vein lumen is distended, and a "floating tail" may be found at the upper end of the thrombus. In the chronic phase, the lesion is more echoic and typically has a heterogeneous appearance. The vein diameter is smaller than normal and venous collaterals may be found.

Ultrasound is also used to evaluate reflux in specific venous segments. Many laboratories perform this evaluation in a casual fashion, examining patients in the recumbent position. Van Bemmelen and associates[61] emphasized the need to examine the patient in the standing position to re-create the maximum stimulus for reflux.[61] In addition, they pointed out the importance of adequate compression. A reverse velocity of 30 cm/s is necessary for consistent valvular closure.[62] Inadequate compression may result in incomplete closure. In such a case, slow reverse flow can occur through a normal valve, leading to the interpretation of an abnormal segment.

Applications

Acute Deep Venous Thrombosis

Clinicians are aware of the fallibility of physical findings in the diagnosis of acute DVT of the leg; therefore most of the effort toward the noninvasive diagnosis of venous disease has focused on acute occlusion. Duplex scanning became the primary modality used to diagnose acute DVT. Many institutions perform alternative imaging studies only in patients with nondiagnostic scans or when the scan cannot be obtained. This practice has been justified by the high accuracy achieved by different investigators.[57-60] A major advantage of scanning is the ability to identify the specific location of disease, especially when there are thrombi at multiple levels. Another important advantage is the detection of partially occluding thrombi, a key limitation of the physiologic techniques used in the past. In addition to confirming the initial diagnosis, scanning can be used to document change during therapy.

Recurrent Deep Venous Thrombosis

The diagnosis of recurrent DVT in patients with post-thrombotic syndrome presents a great challenge to clinicians. Exacerbation of symptoms can mimic the symptoms of the original thrombosis, and in many cases, patients are given anticoagulants without objective evidence of recurrence. Noninvasive testing can be used to obtain an objective diagnosis. Duplex scanning can identify residual chronic thrombus by its high echogenicity. Other characteristics include thickened vein walls, fibrosed segments of occluded veins, and valvular insufficiency with reverse flow on Doppler examination. These features allow the examiner to use a duplex scan to distinguish recent from chronic clot; this contrasts with the phlebogram, which shows all lesions as filling defects.

Venous Insufficiency

The complications of chronic stasis are usually obvious, but it may be difficult to assess the relative contributions of outflow obstruction and reflux. Although the initial conservative management is similar, further surgical treatment must be directed to the specific cause. Doppler examination can determine the presence of venous reflux. Measurement of reverse blood velocities or flows provides a quantitative assessment that is not available with the simpler tests.[61,63] This information can help in the selection of specific interventions.

Preoperative Vein Mapping

With the extensive use of the greater saphenous vein for in situ bypass grafts, knowledge of the patient's specific anatomy has become more important. Using contrast phlebograms, Shah and associates[64] demonstrated that only 65% of thighs and 45% of calves had a single saphenous trunk. The rest had variants of double systems and cross-connections. Because many surgeons are concerned about the possibility of contrast phlebography inducing acute thrombosis, duplex scanning is now the standard method of mapping the superficial veins in both the arms and the legs.[65,66] The high resolution of the images available on contemporary machines permits a satisfactory demonstration of size, course, double segments, and varicosities. These findings correlate closely with anatomy demonstrated at operation.

Follow-Up of Endovenous Ablation

Endovenous closure has become the leading treatment for major reflux of the great saphenous vein. Early experience with the techniques showed a high incidence of vein closure; however, there was concern about possible extension of the thrombosis into the deep system and chance of subsequent pulmonary embolization (see Chapter 51). Most practitioners obtain a duplex scan in the first week following the procedure looking for proximal extension. Figure 14-5*I* (see color panel) shows thrombus extending from saphenofemoral junction, adherent to the anterior wall of the common femoral vein without occlusion of this vein. Lawrence and colleagues[67] have proposed a classification for levels of thrombosis with ablation procedures.

CONCLUSIONS

Extensive development of noninvasive vascular laboratory techniques has increased the amount of objective data that can be accumulated about a patient. As is the case with other diagnostic modalities, it is critical to remember that the different tests should always supplement, not replace, the information gained from a careful history and physical examination. It is increasingly common to find medical students or young house staff presenting patients in terms of the results of vascular laboratory tests rather than describing presenting symptoms and physical findings. Another area of concern is the common practice of sending patients to the noninvasive laboratory for "diagnosis of vascular condition" without their having been examined. This practice results in too many inappropriate tests (with the corresponding unnecessary costs).

Optimal use of noninvasive test results requires an understanding of the limitations and errors of the specific examinations. The choice of tests must be based on the questions to be answered. There are some questions that cannot be answered by any of these techniques; for example, they cannot detect small ulcers in the carotid arteries. In addition, it must be remembered that errors, both false-positives and false-negatives, occur with all diagnostic methods; therefore it is important to be aware of the accuracy of the tests being used. Published studies often represent the best that can be expected, and newly established laboratories often do not achieve optimal results. Therefore, to apply noninvasive results appropriately, it is important to know the accuracy obtained by the laboratory performing the test.

BIBLIOGRAPHY

AbuRhama A, Bergan J, editors: Noninvasive Vascular Diagnosis, ed 2, New York, 2007, Springer-Verlag.
Mansour MA, Labropoulos N, editors: Vascular Diagnosis, Philadelphia, 2005, Elsevier.
Polak J: Peripheral Vascular Sonography, A Practical Guide, ed 2, Philadelphia, 2004, Lippincott, Williams & Wilkins.
Zierler RE, editor: Strandness's Duplex Scanning in Vascular Disorders, ed 4, Philadelphia, 2010, Lippincott, Williams & Wilkins.
Zwiebel WJ, Pellerito JS, editors: Introduction to Vascular Ultrasonography, ed 5, Philadelphia, 2005, Elsevier.

References available online at expertconsult.com.

QUESTIONS

1. Measuring thigh pressure with a regular arm blood pressure cuff affects the determination in what way?
   a. It is higher than the actual pressure.
   b. It is equal to the actual pressure.
   c. It is lower than the actual pressure.

2. The right ankle index is calculated by dividing the higher ankle pressure by which of the following?
   a. Right brachial pressure
   b. Left brachial pressure
   c. Higher brachial pressure
   d. Lower brachial pressure

3. An ankle-brachial index of 1.60 indicates which of the following?
   a. Normal arterial system
   b. Significant arterial insufficiency
   c. Pathologic vessel wall stiffness
   d. Arteriovenous fistula in the extremity
   e. None of the above

4. When evaluating a patient with an exercise stress test, the severity of occlusive disease is evaluated by what means?
   a. Walking time
   b. Magnitude of drop in ankle-brachial index
   c. Recovery time
   d. All of the above
   e. None of the above

5. Noninvasive cerebrovascular techniques are accurate for all of the following except:
   a. Detecting advanced stenosis of the internal carotid artery
   b. Detecting internal carotid occlusion
   c. Detecting arterial ulceration
   d. Detecting abnormal turbulence in the internal carotid artery

6. For a given arterial velocity, the magnitude of the Doppler frequency shift is related to which of the following?
   a. Distance from the probe
   b. Frequency of the probe
   c. Type of system (pulse or continuous wave)
   d. All of the above
   e. None of the above

7. Which of the following statements is true about spectral broadening of a Doppler signal?
   a. It is greatest proximal to a stenosis.
   b. It is greatest in the stenosis.
   c. It is greatest just beyond a stenosis.
   d. It is the same at all the above sites.

8. When using duplex scanning, very low velocities are best detected by which modality?
   a. Power Doppler imaging
   b. Color Doppler imaging
   c. Sonogram of pulsed Doppler signal

9. Which of these findings is not associated with an acute deep vein thrombosis?
   a. Presence of venous collateral
   b. Enlarge venous diameter
   c. Echolucent mass in vein
   d. "Floating tail" of the thrombus

10. Suitability of a superficial femoral artery for treatment with balloon dilatation can be determined by which of the following?
    a. Segmental pressures
    b. Volume plethysmography
    c. Duplex scan
    d. All of the above
    e. None of the above

ANSWERS

1. **a**
2. **c**
3. **c**
4. **d**
5. **c**
6. **b**
7. **c**
8. **a**
9. **a**
10. **c**

CHAPTER 15

Principles of Imaging in Vascular Disease

Antoinette S. Gomes

Currently there are several imaging techniques used to image the vascular system. These techniques include catheter based conventional digital subtraction angiography, Doppler ultrasound, magnetic resonance angiography (MRA), and computed tomography angiography (CTA).

Conventional digital subtraction angiography (DSA) has long been the gold standard for arteriography because of its high resolution and rapid image acquisition. In digital radiography, the x-ray signal is electronically detected, digitized, and processed before display. Using subtraction techniques, DSA allows rapid visualization of both the arterial and venous phases and enhancement of the parenchymal phase. Small vessels are well seen. Because image acquisition is rapid, and repeated injections can be made, DSA is invaluable in the performance and assessment of the results of endovascular interventional techniques that are performed at the same time as the diagnostic arteriogram.

Limitations of conventional angiography are its invasive nature, with the requirement for catheter placement; the need for conscious sedation; the length of the study; and radiation exposure. The need for patient monitoring both before and after the procedure and the need for patient recovery time add significantly to the cost of the procedure.

Another limitation is that usually images are acquired in only one plane per contrast injection. Newer developments have helped to overcome this limitation. Newer equipment allows rotational angiography that permits acquisition of an image volume as the image intensifier and x-ray tube rotate around patient. The image volume acquired can be reconstructed to obtain three-dimensional volume-rendered images. This technique is helpful in analyzing complex vasculature such as that in aneurysms. The technique is particularly useful in the cerebral circulation. Positioning and timing are more complex in the abdomen. Research in this area is exploring use of this technology for measurement of blood velocity and flow profiles.

Two newer imaging techniques now available for performing angiography are MRA and multislice CTA. These techniques, although representing distinctly different technologies, provide images of the vascular system that are competitive with those obtained from conventional catheter-based angiography. Although the image resolution of these two techniques is less than that of conventional angiography, the image quality is such that

these methods have the potential to supplant, and in many instances already do supplant, conventional diagnostic angiography.

MAGNETIC RESONANCE ANGIOGRAPHY

Magnetic resonance imaging (MRI) uses radiofrequency waves and magnetic field gradients to generate images. It is characterized by high contrast between soft tissue and flowing blood. The different pulse sequences used during MRI permit the enhancement or reduction of signal from different tissues based on their hydrogen density and their response to varying magnetic field gradients. MRI can be used to obtain static images of the body and images of the vascular system.

A variety of pulse sequences have been used to perform MRA. These sequences include two-dimensional time-of-flight, phase-contrast, and, more recently, three-dimensional time-of-flight gadolinium-enhanced MRA. With MRA, conventional MRI images are usually acquired before and after any contrast administration as part of a complete MR examination.

Time-of-Flight Angiography

Time-of-flight angiography is performed using a flow-compensated gradient refocused sequence. Data are typically acquired as a stack of two-dimensional slices or as a single three-dimensional volume. In this technique, stationary tissues in the slice or volume of interest are saturated from repeated radiofrequency pulses and have low signal intensity.[1-3] Blood flowing into the imaging has not been subjected to these radiofrequency pulses and is therefore fully magnetized (unsaturated). When it flows into the volume, it is bright compared with the stationary background tissues. This inflow technique works well in relatively normal arteries and veins, such as carotid arteries, the cerebral vasculature, vessels of the feet, the inferior vena cava, and iliac veins. Selective saturation pulses can be applied, allowing selective saturation of blood entering the imaging volume, such that either the arterial or the venous signal can be suppressed. With this technique, separate images of the arterial and venous system can be acquired.

A limitation of this technique is in-plane saturation, which results in signal dropout when the long axis of the vessel coincides with the scan plane or in the presence of

256

slowly flowing blood in tortuous arteries. Another limitation is turbulence-induced signal loss in and distal to a stenosis.[4,5] In addition, the relatively long echo times required for gradient moment nulling make time-of-flight imaging sensitive to susceptibility artifacts from bowel gas, implanted metallic objects (e.g., clips), or other air-tissue interfaces. These artifacts are a primary reason for the inaccuracy of time-of-flight MRA. In addition, imaging times are lengthy because vessels need to be imaged perpendicular to the long axis of the vessel and a stack of slices must be acquired. Long acquisition times can lead to artifacts caused by slice misregistration or patient motion.

Phase-Contrast Angiography

Phase-contrast angiography uses velocity-induced phase shifts, which occur as blood flows through a magnetic field in the presence of flow-encoding gradients.[1,6,7] Two images created with opposite bipolar flow-encoding gradients are subtracted from each other; in the phase difference image, the residual phase is proportional to velocity. Stationary tissues do not undergo a velocity-induced phase shift in either image; they are suppressed and therefore subtract completely. The flow-encoding gradients can be in any direction or in multiple directions, depending on the selected flow sensitivity. Phase-contrast angiography can be performed as a two- or three-dimensional gradient refocused sequence and is improved after contrast administration.[8] It has been used in the evaluation of the renal arteries, carotid arteries, and portal veins. It is also used to measure flow velocity. When used with cardiac gating, a time-resolved velocity profile can be generated, providing quantitative measurement of the flow rate.

There are limitations to the technique. The amplitude of the preselected bipolar gradient determines the degree of velocity encoding (VENC). Phase-contrast sequences encode only a specified range of velocities.[9] In occlusive disease, turbulence causes a wide spectrum of rapidly changing velocities, which produce intravoxel phase dispersion and signal loss. Artifactual signal loss at sites of vessel stenosis is common. The sequence is also susceptible to measurement degradation from cardiac, respiratory, and translational motion. Background subtraction can be problematic. Currently, because faster MR angiographic techniques are available, phase contrast techniques are used primarily for the measurement of flow velocity.

Three-Dimensional Contrast-Enhanced Magnetic Resonance Angiography

Three-dimensional time-of-flight gadolinium-enhanced MRA is the most widely used and useful of the MRA techniques. It does not rely on motion of blood to create flow signal. A contrast agent, typically gadolinium chelate, is given to shorten the T1 (spin-lattice) relaxation time of blood so that it is significantly shorter than that of surrounding tissues. Blood is imaged directly using a T1-weighted sequence. Blood is bright relative to background tissues during the arterial phase of three-dimensional contrast-enhanced MRA, because contrast transiently reduces the arterial blood T1 to less than that of the brightest background tissue (fat). This technique reduces the sensitivity to turbulence, and in-plane saturation effects are eliminated.[4,5] With this technique, a number of slices are oriented in the plane of the target vessels, permitting rapid imaging of a large field of view covering a large region of the vascular system. Contrast-enhanced MRA is fast and affords high-quality breath-hold and non–breath-hold angiograms. Dynamic contrast-enhanced MRA exploits the transient shortening in blood T1 after the intravenous administration of a contrast agent using a fast, three-dimensional spoiled gradient echo sequence. This is a first-pass technique, because the contrast agents currently used are extracellular agents and the gadolinium chelate rapidly leaks into the extravascular space. However, repeated slice volumes over the region of interest can be acquired during passage of the contrast allowing images in both the arterial and venous phases. Typical repetition times for contrast-enhanced MRA are less than 5 msec, with echo times of 1 to 2 msec and total scan times of 10 to 30 seconds. The sequences that use T1-weighted gradient echo, T1 fast field echo, or fast low-angle shot have high spatial resolution and a high signal-to-noise ratio. The images can be acquired in a breath-hold fashion and reformatted in any plane.[10-14] Because intravascular signal is dependent on T1 relaxation rather than inflow or phase accumulation, in-plane saturation and signal loss owing to turbulence are not significant.[4]

During the first-pass arterial phase, imaging is done before vascular contrast equilibration. Using a first-pass technique, steady-state background signal is nearly eliminated. Once the contrast is injected and dynamic imaging is done, however, a second bolus injection of contrast material must be given to repeat the process over, for example, a second region of interest. When the second dose is given, residual soft tissue enhancement can obscure vascular detail.[15] Subtraction techniques, using a precontrast mask, are typically used to remove background tissues. When the second or third dose of contrast is used, subtraction is mandatory. Timing is important in contrast-enhanced MRA. Unlike CT, MRA does not map spatial data linearly over time.[16] With three-dimensional MRI, all the three-dimensional Fourier or K-space data (the information from which the image is constructed) are collected before individual slices are reconstructed. K-space maps spatial frequencies rather than spatial data. Consequently, K-space data do not correspond to image space directly. Different portions of K-space determine the features of the image. The center of K-space, which records low spatial frequencies, affects contrast, whereas the periphery of K-space records high spatial frequencies, which contribute to the fine details, such as edges.[16,17]

Intravascular T1 signal intensity is determined by the gadolinium concentration at the time the center of K-space is collected.[17] The timing is synchronized so that the midportion of the bolus arrives at the desired site as the center of K-space is being collected. Perfect timing produces maximal arterial signal with minimal venous signal. If central K-space data are acquired too early, while arterial gadolinium is increasing rapidly, ringing or banding artifacts may be generated. Acquiring central K-space data too late leads to reduced arterial signal intensity and enhancement of venous structures. Several methods have been used to obtain proper bolus timing, including simple estimates of the travel time of the bolus from the site of injection to the region of interest. For example, in a healthy patient, the travel time from the antecubital vein to the aorta is approximately 15 seconds; in a patient with cardiac disease or an aneurysm, it is 25 to 35 seconds. To estimate contrast travel time more precisely, a test bolus can be used. In this technique, 1 to 2 mL of contrast followed by a 10- to 15-mL saline flush is injected at the same rate as the planned injection. Multiple single-slice fast gradient echo images of the appropriate vascular regions are then obtained as rapidly as possible—typically, every 1 to 2 seconds for a given period—and the time to peak enhancement (contrast travel time) is determined in the region of interest. A limitation of this technique is the setup time; also, the redistribution of the test bolus to the interstitial space may add to the background signal. Other timing techniques used include MR fluoroscopy.[18] In this technique, two two-dimensional sagittal gradient refocused images are obtained rapidly (<1 second per image) throughout the region of interest. Images are generated in near real time and updated at a rate greater than one image every second. The bolus time is watched, and when it arrives, the operator switches over to the three-dimensional MRA sequence. This technique may be helpful in cases of asymmetrical flow owing to asymmetrical stenoses.

Another technique is a temporally resolved method in which multiple three-dimensional data sets are rapidly acquired (over 2 to 8 seconds) without any predetermined timing; injection and scanning are begun simultaneously.[19-23] The operator then selects the desired image set. Other techniques used to facilitate MRA involve simply scanning faster using parallel imaging techniques and using alternative K-space acquisition techniques.

Respiratory motion causes image blurring, ghosting, and signal loss. In three-dimensional imaging, blurring occurs in the direction of motion, whereas ghosting is more pronounced in the phase-encoding direction.[24] Before the availability of fast imaging systems, MRA techniques were too long to permit breath holding. Breath holding results in improved images in abdominal and thoracic MRA and facilitates the visualization of small vessels, such as the renal arteries.[25] It does not appear to be as critical in the evaluation of the carotids. Most ambulatory patients can hold their breath 20 to 30 seconds, and imaging is usually done on inspiration.

Another MRA technique that is now widely used is a time-resolved three-dimensional MRA technique with very high subsecond temporal resolution and submillimeter spatial resolution, which allows capture of multiple arterial, mixed and venous phase images during the passage of contrast agent through the vascular anatomy (e.g., TWIST sequence). No test bolus or bolus timing is required with this technique. Imaging is so fast that venous contamination is eliminated. The technique is helpful for monitoring flow through vascular beds. It is helpful in determining flow patterns through cerebral and peripheral malformations and in delineation of shunt characteristics.

There is also renewed interest in non–contrast-enhanced MRA techniques using inflow inversion recovery techniques, and these sequences are an area of research interest, particularly for assessment of the renal arteries.

Patient Preparation

Patient cooperation is required for optimal contrast-enhanced MRA, because motion and improper breath holding can render the MRA study nondiagnostic. Valuable scanner time is often squandered during attempts to image an uncooperative patient. Patients should be relaxed, and the procedure should be explained to them beforehand. For patients who are particularly anxious, premedication with a sedative such as diazepam or fentanyl may be helpful. The intravenous (IV) catheter should be placed before the imaging is started and before the patient is in the magnet. A 22-gauge IV catheter or larger is placed in the antecubital fossa or below if the arms are to be extended above the head.

Gadolinium-Based Contrast Agents

Currently, almost all contrast-enhanced MRA studies are performed using gadolinium-based contrast agents. Gadolinium is a paramagnetic metal ion. Paramagnetic atoms or molecules possess unpaired electrons that, when placed in a magnetic field, undergo magnetization (attain magnetic susceptibility). The electrons set up circulating currents in response to the externally applied field. These currents induce an internal magnetization that augments or opposes the external field. When the direction of internal magnetization is the same as that of the external field, the effective field within the object is enhanced. This magnetic field enhancement is known as *paramagnetism.*

Gadolinium decreases both spin-lattice (T1) and spin-spin (T2) relaxation times. Because gadolinium is toxic in its natural form, it is chelated with ligands, such as gadopentetate dimeglumine, gadoteridol, or gadodiamide, to form MR contrast agents.[26] These agents are extracellular and pass from the intravascular compartment into the interstitial space in a matter of minutes.[4,5] Measurements of T1 shortening at different cardiac outputs have shown that injection rates greater than approximately 2 mL/s do not increase T1 shortening. Signal intensity increases asymptotically as the injection rate increases, with negligible increases seen beyond a rate of 4 to 5 mL/s.[27,28]

Most contrast-enhanced MR studies are performed with 0.1 mmol/kg of gadolinium or a double dose of 0.2 mmol/kg, or with a set volume of 15 or 30 mL with an injection rate of 1.5 to 2.5 mL/s. Contrast can be injected manually or, preferably, with a power injector. Either technique is followed rapidly by a 15- to 20-mL saline flush.

With contrast-enhanced MRA, once arterial data are collected, the sequence is repeated to capture the venous and equilibrium phases. With longer scanning times, the patient may take a short breath before repeating the sequences.

From their introduction, these agents were found to have a high safety margin and a low rate of adverse effects. It has been estimated that approximately 6 million doses of gadolinium containing contrast agents are administered annually.[29,30] However, in the late 1990s a new disease was described, and in 2006 was shown to be associated with the use of gadolinium containing contrast agents.[31] This disease, nephrogenic systemic fibrosis, has a low incidence; there are only several hundred cases reported in the literature.[32,33] It is characterized by fibrosis of the skin, connective tissue, and internal organs, eye changes, and flexion and extension contractures. There is currently no consistently successful treatment, and it is potentially fatal. The majority of cases have occurred in patients with end-stage renal disease, chronic kidney disease, acute kidney injury, and acute renal insufficiency of any severity owing to hepatorenal syndrome, and in patients requiring dialysis or those in the perioperative liver transplantation period. These patients and patients with glomerular filtration rate (GFR) of 30 mL/min per 1.73 m² or less are at high risk. It is recommended that gadolinium-based contrast agents be avoided in these high-risk patients and alternative imaging methods be used unless the information cannot be obtained with non-contrast MRI or other methods. It is also recommended that all patients undergo screening for renal insufficiency before receiving gadolinium-based contrast agents and package insert doses not be exceeded.[34] The risk in patients with normal renal function is unknown, and to date there have been no reported cases in patients with normal renal function.

Postprocessing Techniques

Three-dimensional contrast-enhanced MRA produces a contiguous volume of data. In most body MRA studies, the volume is asymmetrical (e.g., 400 × 300 × 64). The slice is typically viewed interactively using a computer workstation. Thin multiplanar reformatting (MPR) can be performed,[1,28] and 1- to 2-mm slices can be viewed in multiple planes (axial, sagittal, and oblique).[35,36]

Because the thin sections do not display the entire vessel, the maximum-intensity projection (MIP) processing technique is often used.[37,38] With this algorithm, the user first selects the volume or portion of the volume to be evaluated. The algorithm then generates rays perpendicular to the viewing plane, records the maximum intensity of any voxel encountered along that ray, and assigns that maximum value to the corresponding pixel in the output image. This process results in images similar in appearance to conventional angiograms.

The MIP algorithm has some limitations. A major problem occurs when stationary tissue or structures within stationary tissue have a higher signal intensity than the vessels of interest. This can occur in the presence of crossing vessels, hemorrhage, fat, metallic susceptibility artifacts, or motion artifacts. This results in mapping of these extra signals into the projection image, producing a discontinuity in vessel signal that mimics vessel stenosis.[1] Reducing the thickness of the MIP subvolume to

exclude as much extraneous tissue as possible can mitigate this limitation. Underestimation of vessel diameter is another limitation of the technique.

Subtraction techniques are also used to improve vessel visibility. These techniques are performed by a complex subtraction of precontrast and postcontrast raw data sets[39,40] and are routinely used in contrast-enhanced MRA of the extremities.

Three-dimensional volume rendering is another postprocessing technique that allows separation of overlapping structures. In many instances, this rendering is preferred over standard MIP images.

Clinical Applications

Extracranial Carotid Arteries

The carotid arteries can be well seen with contrast-enhanced MRA (Figure 15-1). The short circulation time of the carotid circulation (4 to 6 seconds) makes timing critical; otherwise, venous overlap of the images results. Both long and short imaging times have been used to overcome this problem.

High-resolution imaging with short echo time is recommended. A major problem that impedes accurate stenosis assessment is the occurrence of high-speed turbulent jets at the site of stenosis. Specialized coils are recommended. The origins of the vessels from the

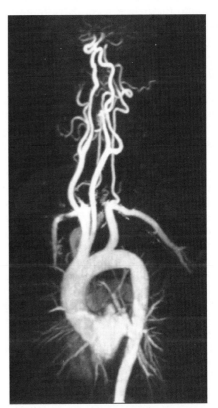

FIGURE 15-1 ■ Contrast-enhanced magnetic resonance angiography of normal carotid arteries. Sagittal oblique maximum-intensity projection of the thoracic aorta shows normal carotid arteries.

aorta should be included in the imaging plane. Numerous studies have shown a high degree of correlation between stenosis measurement with contrast-enhanced MRA and digital subtraction angiography.[41-46] MRI has also been used to evaluate atherosclerotic plaque in the carotid arteries.[47,48]

Thoracic Aorta

Contrast-enhanced MRA is used routinely to evaluate the thoracic aorta. It is the standard of practice for following the status of dissections and monitoring aneurysm enlargement (Figure 15-2). Imaging is usually performed in the oblique sagittal plane or coronal plane. In aortic dissection, the origins of the brachiocephalic vessels should be included. A phased array body coil is recommended when the aneurysm is confined to the thoracic aorta. The ascending, descending, and abdominal aortas are evaluated. A full evaluation of the aorta should include multiplanar cardiac-gated black blood imaging of the aortic wall to detect intramural hematoma.

Abdominal Aorta and Pelvic Vessels

Contrast-enhanced MRA is most often performed in this region to evaluate for aortic dissection or abdominal aortic aneurysm or as part of an evaluation for peripheral artery disease. The images are acquired in the coronal plane using a phased array body coil. A localizer image is obtained first in the sagittal plane, preferably with breath-holding, to determine that the entire volume of the aneurysm will be in the field of view. It is important to note that vessel calcifications are typically not seen with MRA (see Figure 15-2A).

Renal Arteries

Renal contrast-enhanced MRA is performed similarly to an abdominal aortic study, although a thinner coronal slab can be used, allowing decreased slice thickness or acquisition time. High-resolution imaging is preferred. A true slice thickness of less than 2.4 mm is recommended, and breath holding is critical. Otherwise, distal renal artery branches and accessory renal arteries may be difficult to visualize. Typically, renal arteries can be seen out to the interlobar branches. Review of the raw data is critical for full assessment (Figure 15-3).

Small intrarenal branches are not seen well with current techniques. If resolution is not adequate or if motion occurs, fibromuscular dysplasia might not be detected. Examination of the source images can provide information regarding renal size and cortical thickness. A transit time can be calculated for each kidney. Renal transplant arteries can also be seen with contrast-enhanced MRA. Newer techniques that shorten acquisition time and reduce motion artifacts should result in improved visualization of the renal arteries. Although there are multiple studies describing the value of renal artery MRA, it is used largely as a screening tool in patients with acceptable GFR. In hypertensive patients, conventional arteriography is usually deferred if the renal arteries are normal. If an abnormality is detected, conventional arteriography is usually performed, at which time angioplasty or stent placement can be done (Figure 15-4). Using conventional angiography as a reference standard, the reported sensitivity and specificity of contrast-enhanced MRA for diagnosing renal artery stenosis are 88% to 100% and 70% to 100%, respectively.[49]

Mesenteric Vessels

The proximal portions of the mesenteric arteries are usually well seen on renal or abdominal MRA. Contrast-enhanced MRA is used often to evaluate for mesenteric ischemia caused by proximal vessel stenosis or occlusion. Evaluation of the source images and MPR are useful.[50-53] Distal small vessels are usually not visualized well enough to exclude distal small vessel disease. Thin slices are recommended.

Portal Venous System

Contrast-enhanced MRA provides high-quality images of the portal system and hepatic veins. Following arterial phase images, delayed acquisitions are obtained that routinely show the portal and hepatic veins.[53,54] Portal vein thrombosis and collaterals are also seen (Figure 15-5). Again, a review of the source data thin MIP subvolume and often three-dimensional volume rendering are necessary.

Peripheral Vessels

Initially, contrast-enhanced MRA of the runoff vessels of the lower extremities was limited by the restricted field of view of MR scanners.[55] The field of view of most scanners, typically 400 to 500 mm, required repeated injections to cover the entire lower extremity. This imaging was typically performed by first imaging the smaller vessels of the calf, followed by repeated injections while imaging over the knee and thigh. A complete abdominal aorta and peripheral runoff study could not be performed in one setting because of soft tissue enhancement from extracellular gadolinium contrast agent. Newer scanners are equipped with a moving table, which allows image acquisition similar to that of conventional arteriography, whereby a single bolus of contrast can be followed and imaged multiple times as it travels from the aorta to the feet (Figures 15-6 to 15-8). Newer scanners also permit whole-body MRA (Figure 15-9).

It is important to note that optimal visualization of peripheral vessels requires that they be imaged before venous enhancement occurs and obscures arterial vessels. In addition, because they are smaller than pelvic vessels, calf vessels must be imaged with parameters that afford higher resolution. Typically, with bolus-chase techniques, MRI is performed faster and with lower resolution in the pelvis and thigh, and the infusion rate is low to ensure a long bolus. Injection rates of 0.3 to 2.0 mL/s for 30 to 45 seconds can be used. Subtraction improves image quality. The issue of venous enhancement is related not only to imaging delay and contrast injection, but to the underlying disease process. In general, patients with

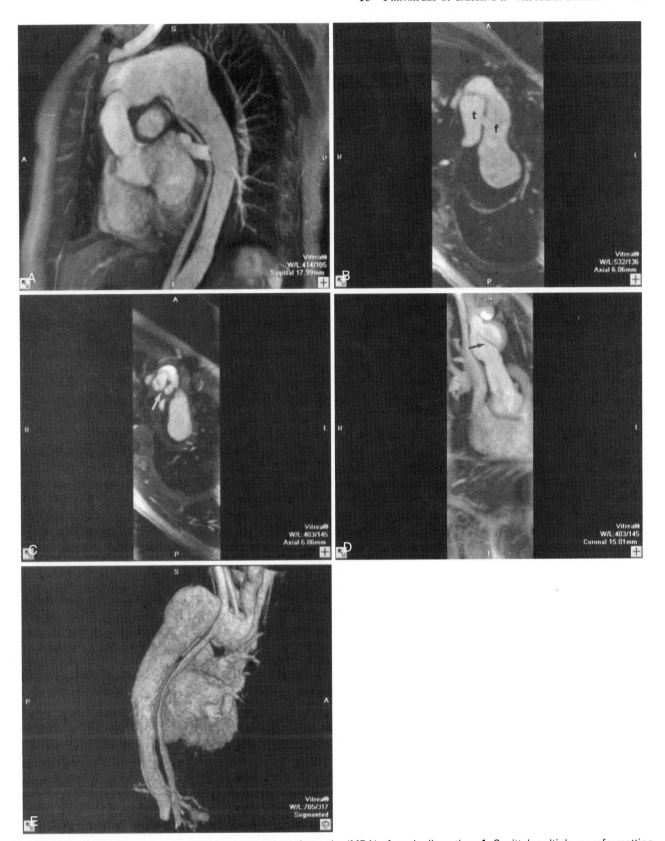

FIGURE 15-2 ■ Contrast-enhanced magnetic resonance angiography (MRA) of aortic dissection. **A,** Sagittal multiplanar reformatting (MPR) in a patient after repair of a type A aortic dissection with valved homograft in the ascending aorta. There is dilatation of the transverse arch. The residual intimal flap is seen as a dark stripe in the descending thoracic aorta. **B,** Axial MPR at the level of the transverse aorta shows the intimal flap with a communication between the large false lumen *(f)* and the true lumen *(t).* **C,** Axial MPR at a higher level shows the intimal flap involving the innominate and left common carotid arteries *(arrow).* **D,** Coronal MPR shows that the intimal flap starts just above the homograft *(arrow).* **E,** Three-dimensional volume-rendered MRA of the thoracic aorta shows the compressed true lumen and the dilated false lumen.

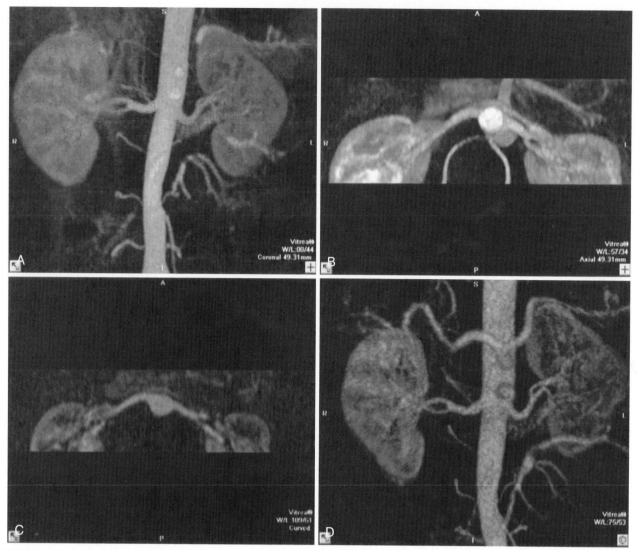

FIGURE 15-3 ■ Contrast-enhanced magnetic resonance angiography of normal renal arteries. **A,** Maximum-intensity projection (MIP) of renal arteries shows normal right and left renal arteries. A plaque is seen in the descending aorta. **B,** Thick-slab MIP in the axial plane shows the origins of the right and left renal arteries. **C,** Curved multiplanar reformatting (MPR) allows visualization of the interlobar arteries. **D,** Three-dimensional volume-rendered image affords visualization of the right and left renal arteries and the proximal interlobar branches.

claudication usually do not exhibit venous enhancement until very late, whereas patients with inflammatory processes, such as cellulitis or venous ulcers, tend to have early venous enhancement. The examination must therefore be tailored to the patient. This need has prompted many imagers to perform two injections; the first injection targets the lower station, and the second injection evaluates the upper and middle stations. This technique has proved to be advantageous.[56,57] In patients with peripheral artery disease (PAD), MRA allows development of an adequate treatment plan.[58]

Magnetic Resonance Venography

MR venography of the pelvis and extremities can also be obtained during the late phase of a contrast-enhanced MR angiogram. Axial two-dimensional time-of-flight

imaging has been used to evaluate venous structures in the upper extremities and venous thrombus in the lower extremities. However, with these studies, vessels parallel to the imaging plane undergo "in-plane saturation," resulting in signal dropout; this can be problematic when evaluating the great veins of the chest because the subclavian and axillary veins are in-plane during an axial acquisition performed to evaluate the superior vena cava. Two-dimensional time-of-flight imaging can also be degraded by patient motion, magnetic field inhomogeneity, and susceptibility artifacts. Despite these limitations, in some circumstances it may be useful to evaluate the pelvic veins and inferior vena cava.[59,60]

Contrast-enhanced MRA overcomes many of the limitations of two-dimensional time-of-flight imaging and is preferred for evaluating the veins of the upper extremity, superior vena cava, jugular veins, inferior vena cava, and

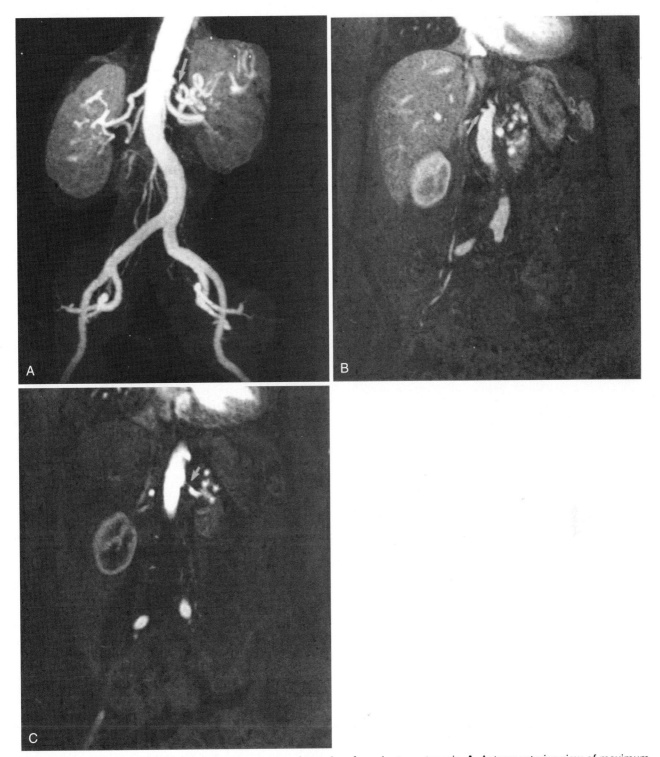

FIGURE 15-4 ■ Contrast-enhanced magnetic resonance angiography of renal artery stenosis. **A,** Anteroposterior view of maximum-intensity projection shows mild irregularity in the right renal artery with high-grade stenosis at the origin of the left renal artery. **B,** Review of raw data shows the origin of the right renal artery *(arrow).* **C,** Adjacent slice of raw data shows high-grade stenosis at the origin of the left renal artery *(arrow).* Inspection of raw data slices from the slab volume is often necessary for accurate diagnosis.

renal veins. These structures can be imaged by obtaining delayed acquisition images on a standard contrast-enhanced MRA study (Figures 15-10 and 15-11). The initial acquisition is timed for the first pass through the arterial system, and multiple acquisitions are obtained following the arterial phase. These late images usually have both arterial and venous enhancement. A selective venous study can be obtained by subtracting the arterial phase study from a mixed venous-arterial phase study.[61,62] Direct venography of upper extremity veins can also be

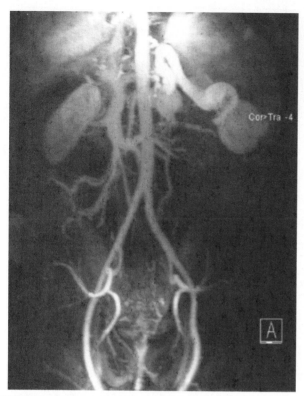

FIGURE 15-5 ■ Venous phase of abdominal contrast-enhanced magnetic resonance angiography. The superior mesenteric vein and portal vein are seen. Large dilated varices are seen in the splenic bed draining into the left renal vein, producing a spontaneous splenorenal shunt.

performed by direct injection of a diluted or full-strength gadolinium contrast agent.[63,64]

Newer techniques, such as true fast imaging with steady state precession (FISP), a steady-state gradient echo sequence, have also been used with some success to evaluate the arterial and venous systems. A rapidly acquired stack of true FISP images provides thin-section viewing of arteries and veins, which are seen as bright blood.

Source data and postprocessing techniques are important in the assessment of venous thrombus, because low–signal-intensity thrombus might not be seen with MIP. The differentiation of acute and chronic thrombus can be difficult with two-dimensional time-of-flight images. With acute thrombus, contrast-enhanced images may show dense periadventitial enhancement.[65] This enhancement is usually not seen with chronic clots and vessel size reductions. Venous mapping using contrast-enhanced MRA is routine at some centers, and it is also useful for quantifying clot burden and determining the presence and size of collaterals. This information is helpful in assessing alternative access sites in patients with venous obstruction from long-term central venous catheters. Contrast-enhanced MRA can also differentiate bland thrombus from tumor thrombus in patients with neoplasms that extend into the venous system. Tumor thrombus enhancement distinguishes it from bland thrombus that does not enhance. MR venography is routinely used to evaluate the patency of upper extremity veins, jugular veins, and the superior vena cava.

Future Directions: New Contrast Agents

New gadolinium chelate agents formulated at 1.0 M (e.g., gadobutrol), rather than the current 0.5 M, and agents with higher relaxivity owing to weak protein interactions (e.g., gadobenate dimeglumine) demonstrate greater intravascular signal than do conventional agents.[66-68] These agents provide better visualization of both large and small vessels. Intravascular blood pool agents are under development, and two main types are currently being evaluated. One type (e.g., MS-325) has a strong affinity for serum albumin,[69-71] and the other type (e.g., gadomer-17) is a macromolecular agent whose size precludes rapid extravasation.[72] Full exploitation of these intravascular agents will necessitate sophisticated subtraction techniques to separate the arteries from the veins.

MULTIDETECTOR ROW COMPUTED TOMOGRAPHY ANGIOGRAPHY

The use of CT for imaging the vascular system has been made possible by the development of multidetector row helical computed tomography (MDCT) scanners. In helical CT, there is continuous CT gantry rotation coupled with continuous table movement through the scanner.[73] This technique permits the rapid acquisition of data and increased data collection with each rotation. Initial spiral scanners were single-row scanners, but the development of multidetector row arrays, faster gantry rotation times, stronger x-ray tubes, and improved reconstruction algorithms has resulted in shorter image acquisition times and improved volume coverage. The three fundamental improvements—speed, volume coverage, and section thickness—are important for CTA. The rapid acquisition speed is such that the contrast bolus can be imaged as it traverses the arterial system. The evolution of 4-, 8-, 16-, 32-, and 64-slice MDCT scanners has resulted in incremental increases in volume coverage and spatial and temporal resolution and reductions in scan time. MDCT scanners with 320 detector rows are now available. With a four-row scanner, the entire thoracoabdominal aorta and iliac arteries can be imaged in 15 to 30 seconds using a 2.5-mm section thickness throughout the entire scan volume. With a 16-row CT scanner, the same anatomic territory can be imaged in 8 to 10 seconds using a 1.25-mm section thickness. CTA is used to image large vessels, such as the thoracic and abdominal aortas, and the major visceral branches of the abdominal aorta, the carotids, and the pulmonary arteries. With faster scans, MDCT permits the entire abdominal aorta and lower extremity runoff to be imaged in a single, high-spatial-resolution scan. Using a 1.25-mm collimation and a table speed of 27.5 seconds (1.6-mm effective section thickness), a distance of 1300 mm can be covered in less than 30 seconds. Sixteen-slice MDCT permits 100 cm to be covered in 21.4 seconds; with the 64-slice scanner, 153 cm can be covered in approximately 15.6 seconds. Although vascular imaging can be performed on four-row scanners, it is generally accepted that 16-row scanners result in more scans being diagnostic, particularly when

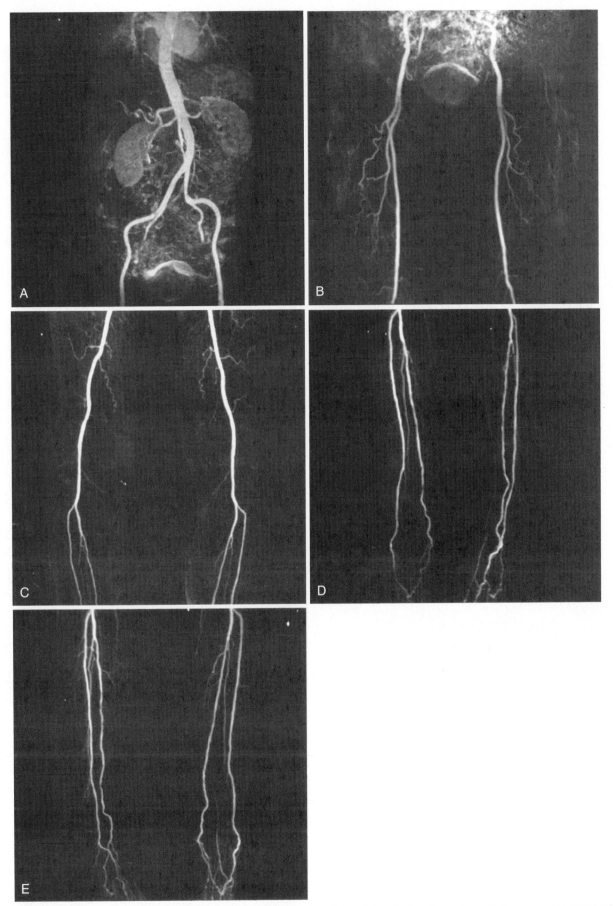

FIGURE 15-6 ■ Contrast-enhanced magnetic resonance angiography of the abdominal aorta and runoff. Images were acquired on 1.5-T system with a moving table. **A,** Abdominal aorta station. There is moderate plaquing in the right and left renal arteries. The pelvic vessels are normal. **B,** Thigh station shows normal common femoral arteries, superficial femoral arteries, and deep femoral arteries. **C,** Knee station shows normal popliteal arteries, anterior tibial arteries, and tibioperoneal trunk. The proximal posterior tibial arteries and peroneal arteries are seen. **D,** Calf station. Anteroposterior projection shows three-vessel runoff bilaterally, including views of the plantar arch. **E,** Calf station oblique view allows separation of the runoff vessels.

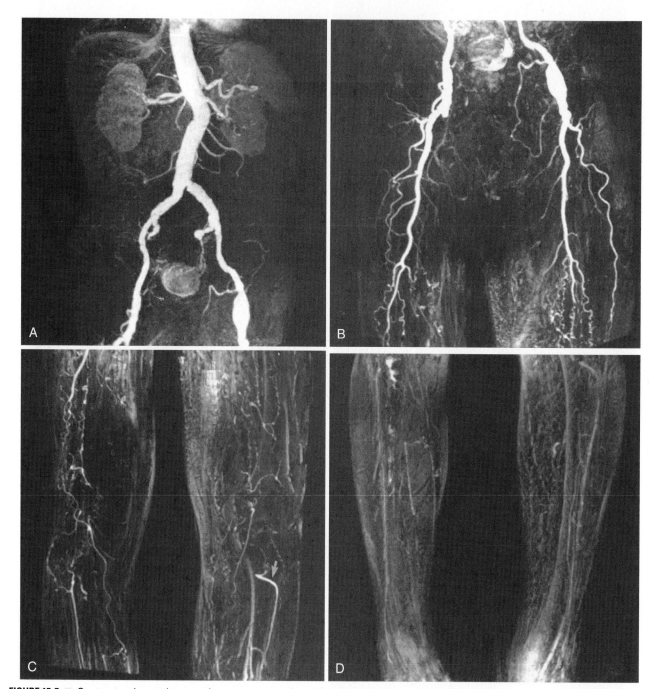

FIGURE 15-7 ■ Contrast-enhanced magnetic resonance angiography abdominal aortogram and runoff in a patient with severe peripheral vascular disease. **A,** Abdominal station shows atherosclerotic changes in the common iliac vessels. An aneurysm is seen in the left common iliac artery. **B,** Thigh station shows occlusion of the right and left superficial femoral arteries, with bilateral enlarged deep femoral collaterals. **C,** Knee station shows severe occlusive disease. There is no filling of either popliteal artery. On the right, collaterals reconstitute a segment of the anterior tibial artery *(arrow)* and a segment of the posterior tibial artery. On the left, a segment of the proximal anterior tibial artery is reconstituted by collaterals. **D,** Calf station. On the right, a diffusely diseased anterior tibial artery is faintly seen. An isolated segment of the posterior tibial artery is identified. On the left, a portion of the anterior tibial artery is faintly seen, and a small portion of the peroneal artery is identified.

large anatomic coverage or small vessel detail is required. Sixty-four–row scanners are now widely used. New scanners with a larger number of detector arrays are under evaluation.

The speed of multislice CT shortens breath-hold examination times and reduces the amount of contrast medium needed to achieve consistent high-quality vascular enhancement.[74-77] The speed of MDCT allows large-volume coverage in a short time. This image acquisition speed can also be used to increase spatial resolution with the acquisition of thinner slices in order to increase the flexibility of a data set. High-resolution imaging requires that thin-slice collimation data be reconstructed to produce a near-isotropic data set of thin, overlapping, transverse images. The 16-row scanner permits the acquisition of 0.625- to 0.75-mm nominal

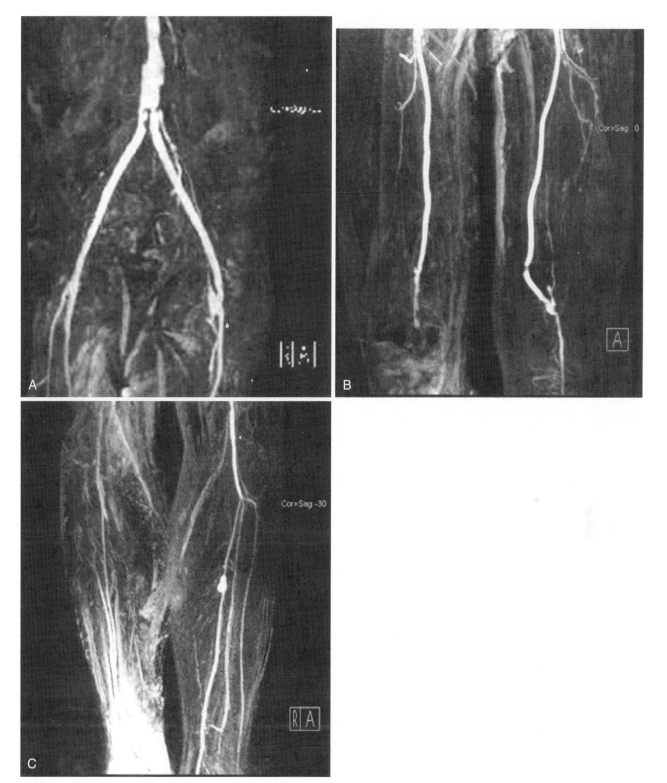

FIGURE 15-8 ■ Contrast-enhanced magnetic resonance angiography in a patient with peripheral grafts. **A,** Aortogram station shows irregularity of the distal abdominal aorta and a patent aortobifemoral graft. A filling defect is seen at the origin of the right limb of the graft. **B,** Thigh station shows bilateral superficial femoral artery grafts. The left graft has a tight stenosis proximal to the distal anastomosis. The right graft is occluded distally. **C,** Calf station on the right shows poor filling of a portion of the anterior tibial artery. On the left, the popliteal artery is patent, with three-vessel runoff. A small aneurysm is seen in the posterior tibial artery.

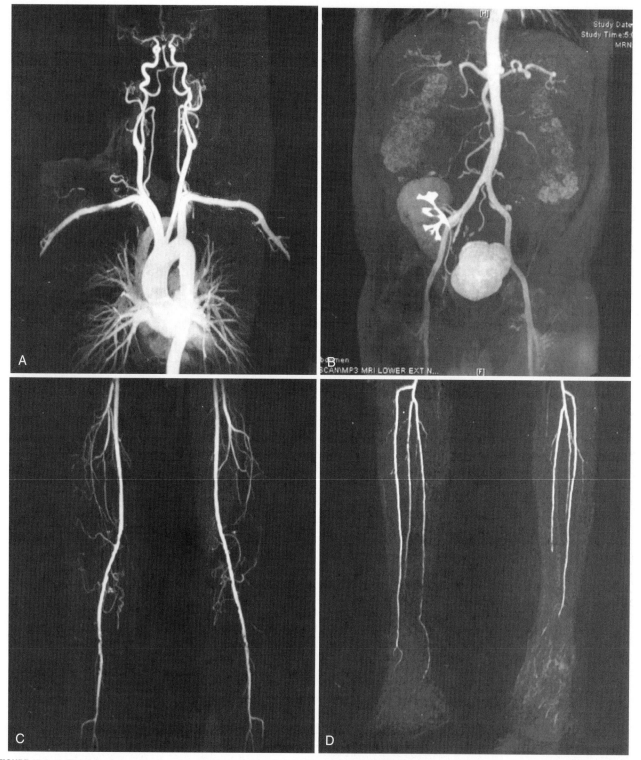

FIGURE 15-9 ■ Total-body magnetic resonance angiography. **A,** The thoracic aorta is normal. **B,** Abdominal aorta and pelvis station show right renal transplant. **C,** Thigh and knee station show mild atherosclerotic plaquing in the superficial femoral arteries. **D,** Calf station. Timing is too early on the left, with poor filling of the left calf vessels.

slice thicknesses with nearly isotropic voxels with almost equal in-plane and through-plane resolution. With the 64-slice MDCT, pitch-independent visualization of 0.4-mm isotropic voxels is possible. Although slice thickness of this degree is not necessary for all CT studies, it enhances visualization of small vessels in the central nervous system, coronary and mesenteric vessels, and vessels of the calf.

Acquisition of extensive volumes with submillimeter resolution generates nearly isotropic data that can be arranged in arbitrary imaging planes with the same high spatial resolution as the original axial section. The

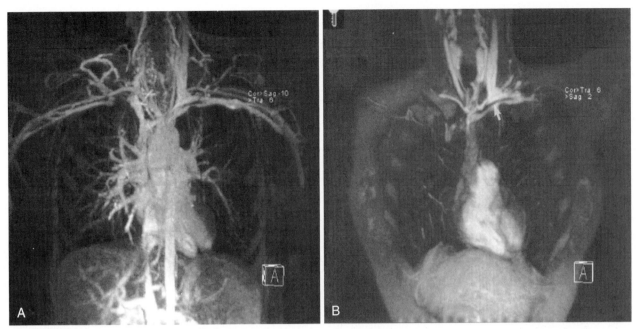

FIGURE 15-10 ■ Contrast-enhanced magnetic resonance angiography venogram of the upper extremities. **A,** Venous phase maximal-intensity projection (MIP) shows occlusion of the right internal jugular vein with multiple collaterals. There is localized occlusion of the right subclavian vein. A dark linear structure is seen in the left subclavian vein and superior vena cava; this represents a catheter. **B,** Thin MIP shows the catheter to better advantage *(arrow).*

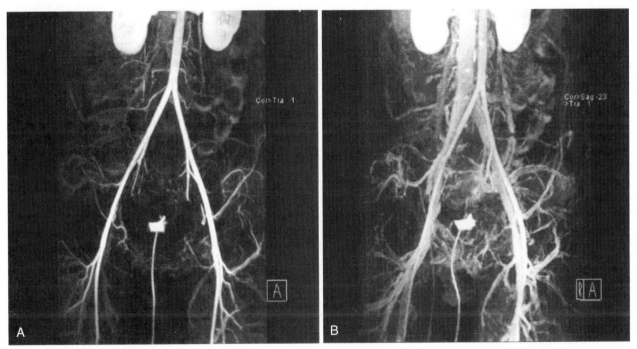

FIGURE 15-11 ■ Contrast-enhanced magnetic resonance angiography pelvic venogram. **A,** Arterial phase shows normal arterial vessels. **B,** Delayed phase shows good filling of pelvic veins and inferior vena cava.

acquisition of high-resolution data enhances the image quality of two-dimensional displays and three-dimensional volume rendering.[78-83]

The rapid acquisition time of MDCT scans allows image acquisition during a breath hold. Image noise is an important consideration, particularly when images are to be reviewed with three-dimensional volume rendering.

The visibility of a structure in the body is dependent on the ratio of that structure and its immediate background to the noise (contrast-to-noise ratio). During CTA, this ratio is affected by the amount of arterial opacification and the noise in the scan. As section thickness is halved, image noise increases by approximately 40%. The goal of decreasing section thickness to visualize small blood vessels and to obtain better detail in large vessels must be balanced with the goal of reducing image noise. Fortunately, image noise is influenced by other factors that do not affect spatial resolution. These include x-ray current and potential and the reconstruction algorithm or kernel used. Depending on the scanner, the pitch can influence scan noise indirectly. According to International Electrotechnical Commission specifications, pitch (*p*) equals the table feed per rotation divided by the total width of the collimated beam. It shows whether data acquisition occurs with gaps (p > 1) or with overlap in the transverse direction (p < 1). Greater tube current is required to compensate for reconstruction strategies that avoid an increase in the effective section thickness as the pitch is increased. For many acquisitions, an increase in pitch will not affect noise. If the maximum tube current is selected for a scan with a given pitch value, and the pitch value is increased, no more current can be supplied to compensate, and the noise will increase.

With MDCT, slice thickness is a reconstruction parameter rather than an acquisition parameter. The narrowest section thickness that can be reconstructed is dependent on the width of the detector groups. Images can be reconstructed at thicker intervals. When images are acquired with thin sections, as long as the raw data are saved, thicker sections can be reconstructed, and the data set that provides the best diagnostic information can be used.

Contrast Medium Administration

Iodinated contrast material is used for CTA. This is the same contrast material used for conventional arteriography and therefore presents the same risks of idiosyncratic allergic reaction and nephrotoxicity. Optimized vessel opacification is an important aspect of CTA because with each new scanner generation, acquisition time decreases and correct synchronization of CT acquisition relative to arterial enhancement becomes more critical.[84] Care must be taken to match the table speed and helical pitch with the first circulation of contrast material through the anatomic region of interest so that data are acquired during peak enhancement and not before or after the contrast bolus has arrived. Image acquisition techniques are modified depending on the number of detector rows in the scanner. With 16-slice MDCT, the entire chest, abdomen, and pelvis can be imaged in less than 15 seconds. With the 16-slice scanner or higher row scanners, care must be taken not to outrun the contrast bolus when imaging the peripheral vessels. With MDCT, the scanning delay following an injection of contrast needs to be timed relative to the patient's contrast transit time (from intravenous injection site to the arterial region of interest). This transit time can be obtained with the injection of a small test bolus. Many scanners have this bolus tracking capability built into the system. When contrast is injected, a series of low-dose scans is acquired while the attenuation in the region of interest is monitored. The transit time equals the time when a predetermined enhancement threshold is reached (e.g., 100 Hounsfield units). The minimum trigger delay to start the CT acquisition after the threshold is reached depends on the scanner (range,

2 to 8 seconds) and on the longitudinal distance between the monitoring series and the starting position of the CT series.[85] Automatic triggering is used, coupled with a dual-head contrast injector that permits a saline flush. The saline flush reduces the total contrast used by eliminating contrast left in the tubing; it also reduces perivenous streak artifacts by removing dense contrast material from the brachiocephalic veins and superior vena cava in thoracic and cardiac CT scans. In routine clinical practice, the injection duration should match the acquisition time. Faster acquisitions require less contrast material volume. Long acquisition times benefit from biphasic injections, with an initially high injection rate followed by a lower one, because they lead to a more uniform enhancement plateau. To ensure adequate vessel opacification with fast MDCT acquisitions, the iodine administration needs to be increased. This is done by increasing the injection flow rate or using contrast material with a higher iodine concentration (e.g., 370 mg/mL of iodine).

Radiation Dose

A variety of measurements have been used to measure or describe CTA dose. Studies using four-slice CTA have shown increased effective collective doses compared with multislice CT. With 16- and 64-row scanners, radiation dose is reduced using dose modulation techniques. In dose-optimized protocols using tube current modulation, the dose is delivered according to the attenuation of the tissues scanned, and the dose is reduced over thinner areas. Depending on scan volume, the dose may be reduced by 10% to 30%.[86] At least two studies have shown an average reduction in dose using the 16-row scanner compared with four-row multislice CT.[86] Nonetheless, the radiation dose from CTA is lower than that of conventional angiography.

Image Reconstruction

The large data sets obtained with multislice CT require three-dimensional workstation viewing. The large number of images prohibits "film" viewing. Typically, comprehensive image analysis is performed, consisting of rapidly scrolling all axial images on a dedicated workstation and performing three-dimensional reconstructions using a variety of algorithms. Postprocessing techniques consist of MPR, MIP, volume rendering, and shaded surface displays. In vascular imaging, heavy calcifications and intravascular stents can impede luminal visualization, but review of the axial transverse images and longitudinal or curved MPR usually permits the evaluation of the vessel lumen.

Applications

MDCT angiography (CTA) is used for imaging most major vessels and even some smaller vessels in the body.

Carotid Arteries

CTA provides high-quality images of the carotid arteries and permits visualization of carotid plaque. CTA with

MPR provides views of the plaque and vessel lumen, making it a useful technique for assessing carotid artery stenosis.[87-90]

Quantification of plaque is feasible. The combined use of noncontrast cranial CT with CT perfusion imaging and CTA of the cerebral vessels is safe and feasible,[91] and such a protocol can facilitate the triage of patients with suspected carotid disease.

Coronary Arteries

Coronary artery CTA differs from CTA in other parts of the body in that electrocardiograph (ECG) gating is needed to freeze cardiac motion. Scanners of 64 rows or greater are preferred. Gating may be retrospective or prospective. With retrospective gating, image reconstruction uses only the data acquired during a short segment of the cardiac cycle. The data are then postprocessed to correlate with the ECG and assign cardiac phase to each segment of the reconstructed data. Prospective ECG gating has been implemented in an effort to lower the radiation dose compared with retrospective gating. With prospective gating, information from prior heart beats is used to estimate the correct time to turn the x-rays off and on during the R-R intervals. The x-rays are turned off completely except during the acquisition phases in diastole when heart motion is less. The scanner acquires one slab during one heart beat, repositions the patient during the next heartbeat, and acquires another slab in the next heart beat. This process requires several heartbeats with 64-row detectors[92] or can be accomplished in a single heartbeat with wider area detector CT scanners.[93] With CTA, artifacts such as calcium blooming and beam hardening can be problematic in interpreting stenoses in heavily calcified coronary arteries. A newer technique is dual-energy CT, in which two x-ray tubes operating at different kilovoltage (kV) acquire data 90 degrees apart; it is based on the energy-dependent tissue attenuation differences.[94] The technique is under evaluation for discrimination of calcified and noncalcified plaque in atherosclerotic vessels.[95]

Pulmonary Arteries

CTA is used routinely as the first-line imaging technique to assess for pulmonary artery embolism. It has largely replaced conventional invasive arteriography for diagnosis. A main advantage of CTA is that in addition to having a high positive and negative predictive value, it reliably demonstrates alternative or additional disease causing the patient's symptoms. In the past, the major limitation of CTA was inadequate visualization of the peripheral lung bed.[96] Newer MDCT scanners, such as the 16-row scanner, cover the entire thorax with submillimeter slices in one short breath hold (10 seconds), with near-isotropic voxels allowing visualization of the proximal and distal vessels.[86] Scans can be acquired with high resolution (thin 0.5- and 1-mm collimation) or in severely dyspneic patients; a faster protocol with wider collimation (2.5 and 1.5 mm) can be acquired. The optimal protocol depends on the equipment used.[86,97-99] MDCT CTA has been used for the combined study of the pulmonary arteries and the

deep veins of the legs using the same injected bolus of contrast.[100] Because of the high positive and negative predictive value of CTA of the pulmonary arteries and the added radiation dose required to study the legs, the current recommendation is that if pulmonary embolism is present, the deep venous system should be evaluated with ultrasonography, except in carefully selected patients such as those with suspected involvement of the inferior vena cava.[101,102]

CTA is useful for assessing the presence of other vascular anomalies of the pulmonary arteries, such as pulmonary artery arteriovenous malformations. It is also used for mapping and evaluating abnormalities of the pulmonary veins.

Thoracic Aorta

CT has long been used to evaluate the thoracic aorta. With current scanners, the entire thoracic and abdominal aorta can be imaged with near-isotropic resolution (Figure 15-12). The traditional helical CT indications for imaging the thoracic aorta have been reemphasized and strengthened with the introduction of MDCT.[103] The availability, speed, and ease of modern MDCT make it the imaging technique of choice for the diagnosis of acute aortic pathology such as aortic trauma, dissection, intramural hematoma, and aneurysm (Figure 15-13; see color plate).[104]

MDCTA is faster, more readily available, and less operator dependent than echocardiography, and it provides more complete organ visualization. MDCT CTA is faster than both MRA and conventional arteriography. It is more suitable than MRA for patients in unstable condition, and it is less invasive than conventional arteriography. The ability to perform multiplanar reformatting and the ability to see both the lumen of the aorta and the wall are distinct advantages over conventional arteriography. Imaging of the thoracic aorta typically is done with noncontrast images of the thorax to identify regions of hyperdensity within the aortic wall suggesting intramural hematoma. This imaging can be performed with wider collimation and slice thicknesses of 2.5 to 5 mm. Narrow-slice collimation is necessary for CTA and requires thin slices of 1 to 2.5 mm to provide adequate spatial resolution and image quality for postprocessing.[86] In cases of aortic root pathology, ECG synchronization of the scan acquisition using either prospective or, more commonly, retrospective ECG gating removes cardiac motion artifact, allowing evaluation of this region.

Abdominal Aorta and Iliac Arteries

The volume coverage capabilities of MDCT have had a major effect on imaging of the abdominal aorta. With current MDCT scanners, the entire abdominal aorta and iliac vessels can be covered with near-isotropic resolution (Figure 15-14; see color plate for Figure 15-14C). The high scan speed allows the use of less contrast material.[105]

In the abdomen, traditional indications for CTA include diagnosis and surveillance of aneurysms, preoperative evaluation of endograft placement and

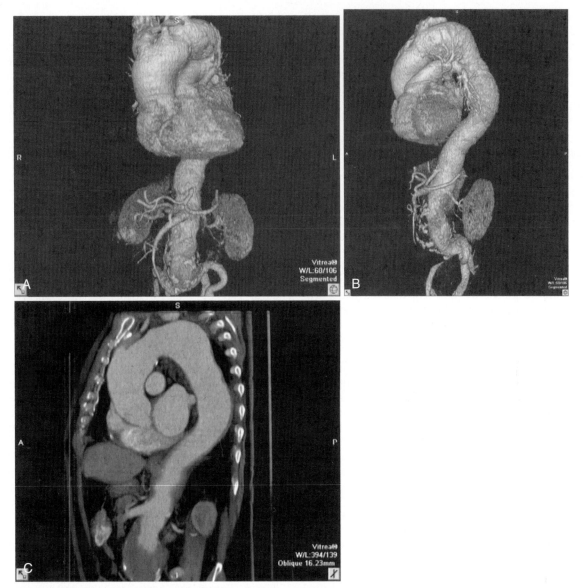

FIGURE 15-12 ■ Multidetector row helical computed tomography angiography of thoracoabdominal aortic aneurysm. **A,** Frontal view shows ascending aorta and abdominal aorta with visceral vessel origins. Calcifications in the aneurysm are seen. **B,** Oblique view. **C,** Curved multiplanar reformatting.

postplacement monitoring, and tumor diagnosis and staging (Figure 15-15). Other routine uses include evaluation of abnormalities of the mesenteric vessels,[106-108] renal artery stenosis, and portal venous system abnormalities. MDCT CTA is routinely used in the evaluation of potential renal donors[109] and liver donors[110-112] (Figure 15-16). It is also used in the assessment of patients undergoing liver lesion embolization. The use of thin collimation reduces volume averaging that impedes small vessel visualization; the improved z-axis resolution allows clear assessment of small mesenteric vessels and the degree of renal artery stenosis. Using a 0.5-second MDCT scanner, Willmann and colleagues[106] obtained high-quality CT angiograms with 92% sensitivity and 99% specificity for the detection of aortoiliac and renal artery stenosis (Figure 15-17). The decision to use MRA or CTA to evaluate the abdominal aorta is determined largely by the patient's ability to cooperate, the status of the patient's

renal function, and the degree of resolution required for diagnosis.

Peripheral Arteries

Imaging of the peripheral arteries is one of the new and exciting applications of CTA. With multislice CTA, noninvasive imaging of the entire abdominal aorta and runoff vessels can be accomplished with high resolution, providing angiogram-like images of the runoff vessels (Figure 15-18; see color plate for Figure 15-18B). Using four-slice MDCT, a high correlation has been found between MDCT results and digital subtraction angiography in the evaluation of lower extremity atherosclerotic vascular disease.[113-115] The ability to see the relationship of vessel calcifications and the ability to perform multiplanar reformatting are advantages that are not available with

Text continued on p. 278.

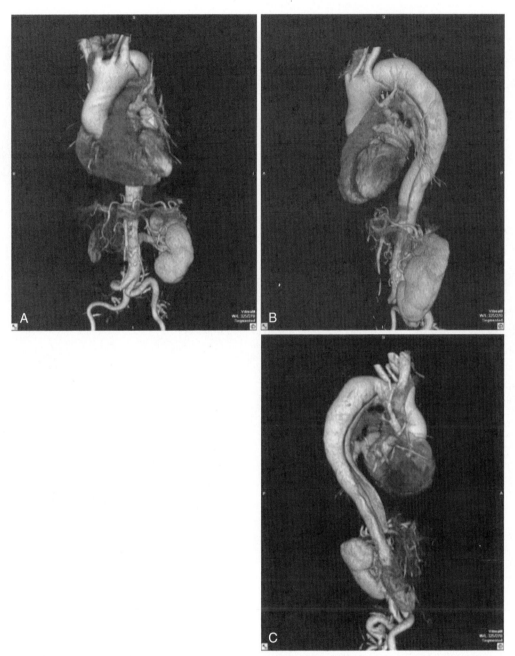

FIGURE 15-13 ■ Multidetector row helical computed tomography angiography of acute aortic dissection on 16-row multislice computed tomography CT scanner. Three dimensional volume rendered images of type B aortic dissection showing the intimal flap and the true and false lumens. Note the clear delineation of the origins of the major branch vessels. See Color Plate 15-13.

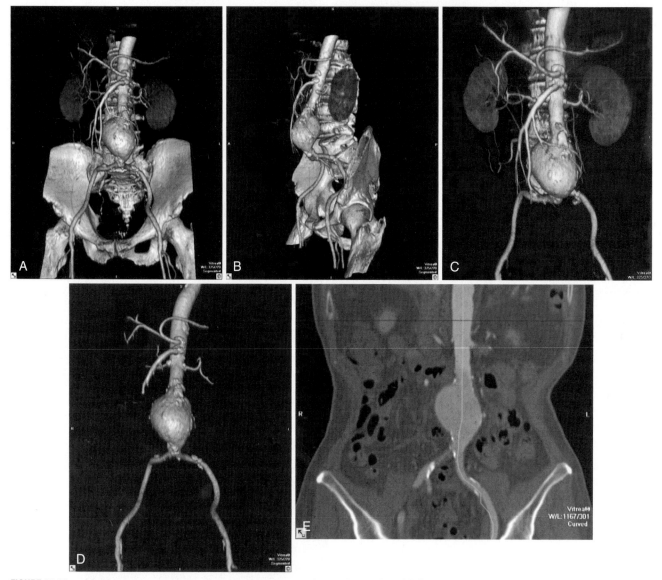

FIGURE 15-14 ■ Multidetector row helical computed tomography angiography of infrarenal abdominal aortic aneurysm. **A,** Three-dimensional volume-rendered image of the abdominal aorta and branch vessels. The celiac artery and superior mesenteric arteries are seen. The infrarenal saccular aneurysm extends to just above the aortic bifurcation. **B,** Oblique view of the aorta. **C,** Partial removal of bone shows the renal arteries and superior mesenteric artery branches. See color plate. **D,** Images with full bone and soft tissue removal show the aneurysm. Note that vessel calcifications are well seen on the computed tomographic angiography images. **E,** Curved multiplanar reformatting allows measurement of vessel diameter. See Color Plate 15-14.

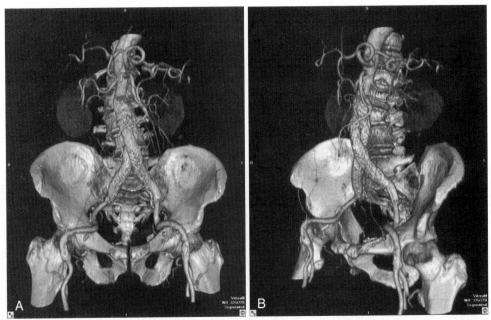

FIGURE 15-15 ■ Multidetector row helical computed tomography angiography of aortic endograft. **A,** Abdominal study shows a bifurcated endograft in the aorta. **B,** Oblique view shows that the limbs of the endograft are crossed; no obstruction is seen.

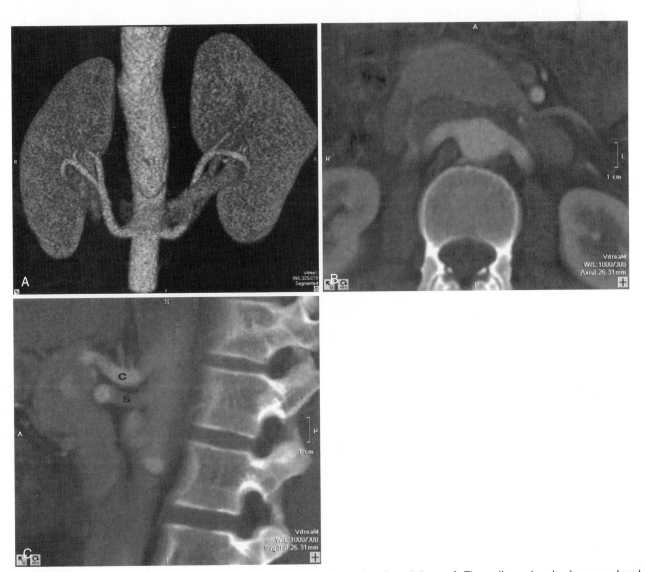

FIGURE 15-16 ■ Multidetector row helical computed tomography angiography of renal donor. **A,** Three-dimensional volume-rendered images of the renal arteries. **B,** Multiplanar reformatting (MPR) of the origin of the renal arteries. **C,** Note that the origins of the celiac *(c)* and superior mesenteric *(s)* arteries are well seen on sagittal MPR.

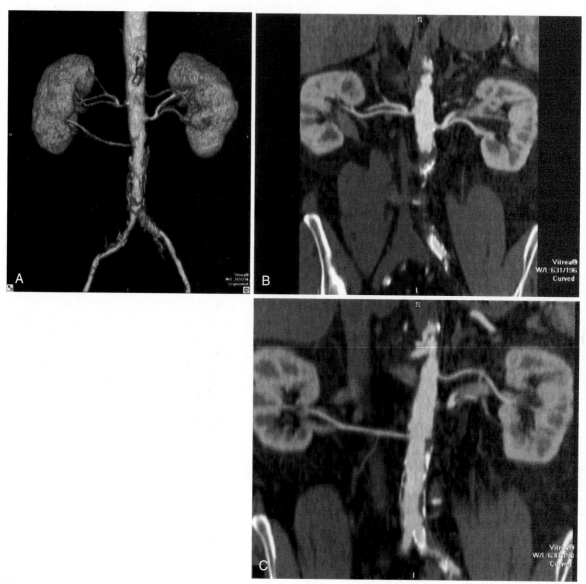

FIGURE 15-17 ■ Multidetector row helical computed tomography angiography of renal artery stenosis. **A,** Three-dimensional volume-rendered image shows high-grade stenosis at the origin of the right renal artery. The left renal artery is normal. An inferior accessory artery is seen on the right, and a superior accessory artery is seen on the left. Note the calcifications in the infrarenal aorta. **B,** Curved multiplanar reformatting (MPR) shows the origins of the right and left renal arteries. **C,** Curved MPR shows the origins and course of the accessory renal arteries.

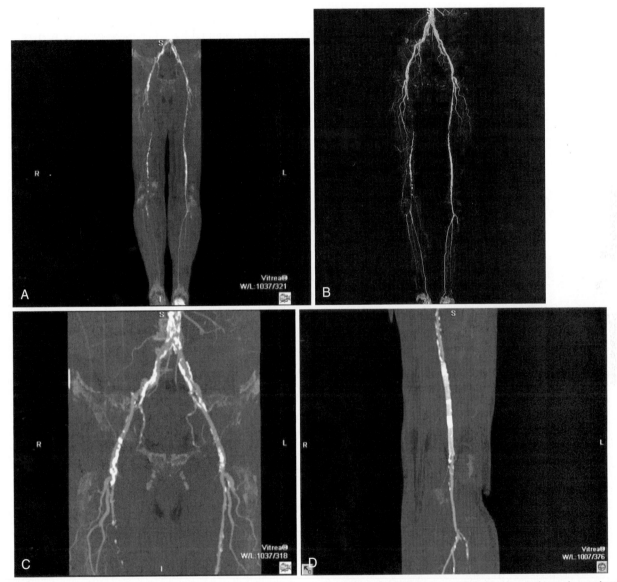

FIGURE 15-18 ■ Multidetector row helical computed tomography angiography of peripheral runoff. **A,** Maximum-intensity projection (MIP) of peripheral runoff study done on a 16-row scanner. Note full coverage of extremities. **B,** Three-dimensional volume rendering may also be performed. See color plate. **C,** Zoomed images of pelvis station show the dense calcifications in the aorta and pelvic vessels. Occlusion of the right superficial femoral artery (SFA) is seen. **D,** Zoomed MIP images of the left distal SFA show the vascular stents. See Color Plate 15-18.

conventional arteriography. Although disadvantages such as the use of ionizing radiation, the need for iodinated contrast material, and the demanding postprocessing requirements need to be considered, there are circumstances when MDCT CTA is preferred. Calcifications can be seen and provide useful pretreatment information about whether to use angioplasty alone or stents. Patients who have had prior stent placement are better evaluated with CTA, which allows the vessel lumen to be visualized. In some situations, such as preoperative endograft planning, CTA is sufficient and angiography is unnecessary. Careful bolus timing is required. With four-row scanners, imaging delay can result in venous opacification, obscuring the arteries of the feet. With 16- and 64-row scanners, care must be taken not to outstrip the bolus and acquire images too early, before vessels are filled.

MAGNETIC RESONANCE ANGIOGRAPHY VERSUS COMPUTED TOMOGRAPHY ANGIOGRAPHY

The determination to use CTA versus MRA is dependent on the nature of the vascular bed to be studied, the information to be obtained, and the status of the patient. MDCT CTA is faster, requires less patient cooperation, and affords higher resolution than MRA, but it involves exposure to ionizing radiation and the use of potentially nephrotoxic iodinated contrast material. MRA has lower resolution, takes longer, and requires more patient cooperation, but it does not involve the use of ionizing radiation. Patients with metallic stents and implants are better evaluated with MDCT CTA because of artifacts that occur with MRA. Patients with pacemakers are not routinely studied with MRA unless the information needed cannot be obtained by other means or the patient has a new MRI-compatible pacemaker.

Both techniques permit the acquisition of volume data, which can be manipulated with postprocessing techniques. Both techniques provide large data sets that require workstation viewing. Subtraction techniques currently available with MRA make postprocessing faster than with CTA, which requires time-consuming background and bone removal (Figure 15-19; see color plate). Both these techniques, however, are noninvasive and are likely to supplant conventional angiography in the diagnosis of vascular disease. As technology improves, other applications of CTA and MRA are anticipated, and improved small vessel visualization is expected.

BIBLIOGRAPHY

Binkert C, Baker P, Petersen B, et al: Peripheral vascular disease: blinded study of dedicated calf MR angiography versus standard bolus-chase MR angiography and film hard-copy angiography. Radiology 232:860–866, 2004.

Fleischmann D: High concentration contrast media in MDCT angiography: principles and rationale. Eur Radiol 13(Suppl 3):N39–N43, 2003.

Foley WD, Karcaaltincaba M: Computed tomography angiography: principles and clinical applications. J Comput Assist Tomogr 27(Suppl 1):S23–S30, 2003.

Gotway MB, Dawn SK: Thoracic aorta imaging with multislice CT. Radiol Clin North Am 41:521–543, 2003.

Hartmann IJC, Wittenberg R: Schaefer-Prokop imaging of acute pulmonary embolism using multidetector CT angiography: an update on imaging technique and interpretation. Euro J Radiol 74:40–49, 2010.

Idee JM, Port M, Dencausse A, et al: Involvement of gadolinium chelates in the mechanism of nephrogenic systemic fibrosis: an update. Radiol Clin North Am 47:855–869, 2009.

Napoli V, Fleischmann D, Chan FP, et al: Computed tomography angiography: state-of-the-art imaging using multidetector-row technology. J Comput Assist Tomogr 28(Suppl 1):S32–S45, 2004.

Prince M: Body MR angiography with gadolinium contrast agents. Magn Reson Imaging Clin N Am 4:11–24, 1996.

Prokop M, Shin HO, Schanz A, et al: Use of maximum intensity projection in CT angiography: a basic review. Radiographics 17:433–451, 1997.

Shoepf UJ, Becker CR, Hofmann LK, et al: Multislice CT angiography. Eur Radiol 13:629–636, 2003.

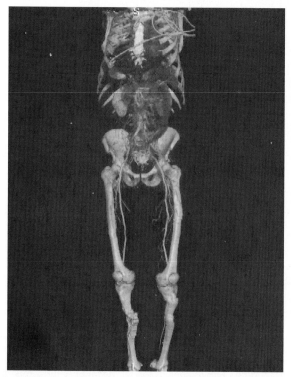

FIGURE 15-19 ■ Total-body magnetic resonance angiography. Imaging of the entire body is possible using 16- or 64-row MDCT scanners. Extensive postprocessing is required to remove bone and soft tissue. See Color Plate 15-19.

References available online at expertconsult.com.

QUESTIONS

1. True or false: MRA and CTA provide similar images because they are based on the same technology and use ionizing radiation.

2. Which of the following statements regarding MRA is correct?
   a. Two-dimensional time-of-flight techniques are best for visualizing tortuous vessels with slow flow.
   b. Contrast-enhanced MRA techniques use conventional iodinated contrast material.
   c. Gadolinium-containing contrast material is recommended in patients with GFR ≤30 mL/min per 1.73 m^2.
   d. Subtraction techniques are used to remove background tissue in both digital subtraction angiography and MRA.

3. Which of the following techniques have been used for MRA?
   a. Two-dimensional time of flight
   b. Three-dimensional time-of-flight contrast-enhanced MRA
   c. Phase-contrast techniques
   d. All of the above

4. Contrast-enhanced MRA is useful for evaluating which of the following vascular beds?
   a. Arch vessels
   b. Abdominal aorta
   c. Runoff vessels
   d. Deep veins of the upper and lower extremities
   e. Tertiary branches of the mesenteric artery

5. Which of the following statements regarding MDCT CTA is true?
   a. It has lower resolution than contrast-enhanced MRA.
   b. Image acquisition time is shorter than for contrast-enhanced MRA.
   c. Postprocessing of images to remove bone and soft tissue is easier with MDCT CTA.

6. Which of the following statements regarding MDCT CTA are true?
   a. It is frequently used for the diagnosis of acute aortic dissection.
   b. It is preferred over contrast-enhanced MRA for follow-up studies in patients with chronic aortic dissection.
   c. It is better than contrast-enhanced MRA in patients with limited ability to cooperate.

7. True or false: Accuracy of stenosis assessment is equal with MDCT CTA and contrast-enhanced MRA.

8. True or false: Peripheral runoff studies can be performed with both MDCT CTA and contrast-enhanced MRA.

9. Which of the following statements regarding MDCT CTA is correct?
   a. Scanners with four detector rows have larger volume coverage than scanners with 16 detector rows.
   b. Slice thickness is a reconstruction parameter with MDCT.
   c. MDCT has higher accuracy than contrast-enhanced MRA for evaluating accessory renal arteries in renal donors.
   d. All of the above

10. Postprocessing techniques used for MDCT CTA and contrast-enhanced MRA include which of the following?
    a. MIP
    b. Three-dimensional volume rendering
    c. MPR
    d. All of the above

ANSWERS

1. **False**
2. **d**
3. **d**
4. **a, b, c, d**
5. **b**
6. **a, c**
7. **False**
8. **True**
9. **d**
10. **d**

ARTERIAL OCCLUSIVE DISEASE

CHAPTER 16

Vascular Grafts: Characteristics and Rational Selection

Luke P. Brewster • Howard P. Greisler

Alexis Carrel, the father of vascular surgery, was the first to describe the utility and shortfalls of autogenous and synthetic grafts. The main limitation identified by him was the lack of durability for small-diameter synthetic grafts.[1,2] Kunlin first used the saphenous vein for arterial bypass,[3] but it took time to implement the use of vein as a preferred conduit for arterial grafting.[4] The first clinical successes of synthetic vascular grafts were reported in the 1950s when Voorhees and colleagues developed the first fabric graft from Vinyon N, a material commonly used in parachutes[5]; several ethylene-based synthetic grafts followed. To date, large vessel grafts have demonstrated excellent results, whereas small-diameter grafts have performed poorly.

Cardiovascular disease has become more prevalent, and it is the leading cause of death in the world and the second leading cause of death for all Americans. Despite improvements in the medical therapy of cardiovascular disease, the number of vascular interventions (combining bypass grafting and angioplasty ± stenting) has at least doubled in recent years.[6] Coupling this finding with an increasing lifespan, the population that will benefit from vascular surgery is expected to continue to increase. With more than 1.4 million bypass operations annually in the United States, finding suitable autogenous veins and arteries for conduit in patients with a lifespan of more than 2 years is critical to optimal therapy in preventing limb loss and delaying mortality.[7] When suitable autogenous conduits are not available, synthetic grafts are useful, particularly for bypassing proximal disease.

This chapter will discuss the normal artery; arterial, venous, and synthetic conduits; the challenges of maintaining bypass patency; and current inroads with cardiovascular conduit engineering.

NORMAL AND PATHOLOGIC COMPOSITION OF THE VESSEL WALL

The arterial intima (tunica intima) is composed of a relatively quiescent endothelial cell (EC) monolayer and its surrounding basement membrane proteins (e.g., type IV collagen, perlecan). Together with the underlying internal elastic lamina, the intima maintains smooth muscle cells (SMCs) in their contractile state and inhibits pathologic SMC activity. Deep to the intima and separated by the internal elastic lamina is the medial layer (tunica media). It is the thickest arterial layer and in

non-pathologic states it is composed of SMCs and many extracellular matrix (ECM) proteins (e.g., elastin and the fibrillar collagens such as type I collagen). Medial SMCs here respond to intimal cues to dilate or contract the vessel. The medial layer in veins is difficult to define because it lacks the internal elastic lamina, but after exposure to arterial flow via vein graft bypass, they develop a defined media over time that has similarities to that of native artery.[8] The external elastic lamina defines the abluminal edge of the media The vaso vasorum, which supplies most of the outer two thirds of the vessel wall's metabolic needs, is prominent in the outer adventitial vessel layer (tunica adventitia). The adventitia is composed of loosely arranged connective tissue and fibroblasts, and it could have an important role in the progression of restenosis and late interventional failure after angioplasty owing to vessel remodeling, because adventitial delivery of therapeutic treatments has reduced these complications.[9]

In the absence of disease or injury, native blood vessels possess an endothelial lining that constantly secretes bioactive substances that inhibit thrombosis, promote fibrinolysis, and inhibit SMC switching from a contractile to synthetic phenotype. Throughout the cardiac cycle, the cells of the vessel wall communicate in a transmural and longitudinal fashion to accommodate systolic flow, provide resistance during early diastole, and then propel blood distally during late diastole. This latter phase is the only part of arterial flow dependent on the artery rather than the heart and is critical to maintaining adequate demand tissue perfusion, which may be a factor contributing to the benefit of autogenous conduits over synthetic grafts for arterial bypass.

CURRENT STATUS OF VASCULAR CONDUITS

The Artery

Few autogenous arteries are available for use as a conduit because of the lack of redundant arterial perfusion and available lengths of medium-sized arteries. However the patency rates of inferior mammary artery conduits in coronary artery bypass grafting is outstanding compared with vein grafts.[10] The benefit is less clear when arterial harvesting is required, such as radial artery grafting.[11] There is also some support for this benefit in patients with challenging distal bypasses.[12] The theoretic advantage is that arteries do not need to adapt to arterial flow, and thus are relatively protected from negative remodeling. However, all bypass targets are not identical, and graft remodeling is also determined in part by the perfusion bed (myocardium versus skeletal muscle).

The Vein

Superficial and deep veins can be used as conduits for arterial bypass. Their benefit over synthetic grafts for small diameter graft bypasses is well accepted.[13] The greater saphenous vein is the most commonly used conduit for coronary and infrainguinal bypass grafting. It is duplicated in approximately 8% of persons,[14] and its course has been well described.[15] The lesser saphenous vein is not easily accessible in the supine position, but it can be useful as a conduit when working posteriorly or through a separate harvest incision.[16-18] More commonly in our practice, bilateral cephalic veins, which are approximately 50 cm, can be sewn together as a composite conduit for distal bypasses.[19,20]

Once implanted, veins undergo arterialization in which they develop a muscular media and elastic lamina. Adaption can be both positive and negative; therefore it is not surprising that a number of vein grafts fail or require adjunctive procedures to maintain patency (Table 16-1). The modes of failure include myointimal hyperplasia (frequently at anastomotic or valve sites or at sites of intraluminal manipulation) and progression of atherosclerosis in the inflow or outflow arteries, or both, or in the vein graft itself. Limiting trauma at time of vein harvest,[21] proper perioperative medication (antiplatelet agents[22] and a statin[23,24]), proper ultrasound surveillance protocols[25] are critical to optimizing patency and clinical benefit of vein grafts. The patency benefit of anticoagulation of vein grafts is modest,[26,27] and the risks of bleeding are generally thought to outweigh these small benefits to vein graft patency.[24]

Cryopreserved Vessels

Cryopreserved allografts provide an alternative to either femoral vein harvest or to antibiotic-soaked Dacron with omental flap coverage for infected aortoiliac reconstruction.[32] However, their poor primary patency rates for infrainguinal bypass,[33-35] even with immunosuppressive therapy,[36] limit this application to patients with infection and without leg or arm vein.

TABLE 16-1 Proper Handling of Vein Grafts

Limiting Injury	Surveillance and Secondary Patency
"No touch" technique	Recommended surveillance protocol
Heparinized blood versus crystalloid solutions[21]	
Limiting time from harvest to implantation	Proper medical management
In situ versus reversed[28-29]	Antiplatelet therapy
Endoscopic versus open harvest[30-31]	Role of anticoagulation

SYNTHETIC GRAFTS

The idea of a nonreactive vascular conduit as an ideal graft is no longer accepted and is likely impossible to create; therefore current initiatives emphasize incorporation into the surrounding tissues. These approaches include the development of nonautologous biologics, synthetic grafts that promote or support tissue ingrowth, and tissue engineered vascular grafts that attempt to mimic certain functional properties of the blood vessel, such as compliance and desirable cell phenotypic characteristics. Readily available large-diameter grafts, such as those used for aortic reconstruction, have superb 5-year patency rates.[37] Conversely, when synthetic grafts are used in the infrapopliteal region, the results are poor, with 1- and 3-year patency rates of 43% and 30%, respectively.[13]

Conduit Patency and Failure

The benefits of vein grafts versus synthetic grafts is well established,[13,38] but recently the PREVENT III and IV trials have demonstrated that even vein grafts have durability limitations for both infrainguinal and coronary revascularizations.[39,40] As described, primary patency rates are strikingly similar to those reported more than 30 years ago.[13] However, secondary patency rates are better, emphasizing the importance of vein graft surveillance and prophylactic reinterventions.

A variety of mechanisms can lead to vascular graft occlusion, and they occur in a defined temporal sequence. Immediate graft failure is usually the result of technical error during the operation or the patient having a hypercoagulable status. Failure in the first month following graft placement is most likely the result of thrombosis secondary to distal flow resistance or, less commonly, restricted inflow into the graft. Small-diameter grafts are prone to early thrombosis because of their lower flow rates and higher resistance in their outflow vessels. Therefore graft thrombogenicity is of primary concern early after graft placement.

Pseudointimal hyperplasia is the most common reason for graft failure from 6 months to 3 years after graft insertion, occurring primarily in the perianastomotic region in the case of synthetic conduits and both there and the sites of valves or mechanical injuries in the case of vein grafts. Later graft failure is frequently due to the progression of distal atherosclerotic disease. Small-diameter grafts are particularly susceptible to anastomotic pseudointimal hyperplasia (IH), which is a false intima composed of smooth muscle cells, inflammatory cells, and activated endothelial cells, forms on the graft material. This is distinguished from neointimal hyperplasia, in which a new intima with confluent endothelium is generated, frequently with an increased diameter compared to the true intima. More generically, the term *myointimal hyperplasia* is used. Its definition encompasses both phenomena and includes the abnormal multiplication or increase in the number of normal cells, often with excessive accumulation of the extracellular matrix, in the innermost part of the blood vessel.

Pathophysiologically, denuded intima of a vein graft or exposed luminal area of a synthetic graft may lead to thrombosis via platelet deposition and activation of the coagulation cascade, which over time promotes pathologic SMC migration, proliferation, and ECM deposition, leading to IH. IH in turn narrows the vessel lumen (restenosis), decreasing blood flow to the point that it can promote local thrombosis or lead to symptomatic ischemia in the relevant distal end organs, such as the brain (cardiovascular accidents), heart (myocardial infarctions), and extremities (critical limb ischemia; Figure 16-1).

Thrombosis and intimal hyperplasia represent the most common causes of graft failure and are both largely mediated at the luminal interface of the vessel or graft; therefore the inner lining of grafts has been the subject of much investigation. This is discussed below in two parts: the body's response to grafts and the design of desirable blood-biomaterial interfaces.

Cellular and Molecular Mediators of Graft Outcome

A confluent quiescent endothelial lining of injured vessels and synthetic grafts is desirable for clinical applications.[41] Re-endothelialization of injured vessels or endothelialization of synthetic grafts can occur through transanastomotic endothelial cell migration (usually limited in

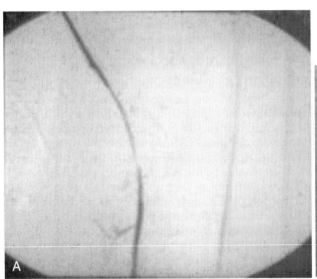
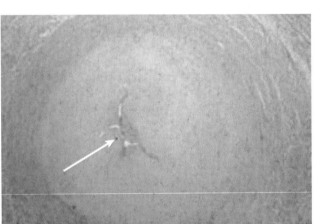

Wave	SMC activity	Growth factor mediators	Time frame after injury	ECM production +<++
1	Proliferation	FGF-2	24–72 hours	+
2	Migration	PDGF, FGF-2, TGF-β	1–7 days	++
3	Proliferation	PDGF, TGF-β	7–14 days	++++
4	ECM production	FGF-2, PDGF, TGF-β, Ang II	> 2 weeks	++++

B

FIGURE 16-1 ■ **Myointimal hyperplasia: arteriographic and histologic findings. A,** Arteriogram showing a focal vein graft stenosis after a femoropopliteal bypass *(left),* and histology of this segment of vein graft *(right).* The *arrow* encompasses the diameter of myointimal hyperplasia. Deep to the *arrow,* a well-organized muscular vessel media is identified. **B,** Summary of the waves of myointimal hyperplasia in experimental models. Of note, the first wave occurs in the media. The second wave occurs in the media to myointimal region, and the third and fourth waves occur in the myointima. Strategies to limit this problem must understand cellular and bioactive proteins in a temporal and transmural fashion. (Reprinted with permission from Elsevier. Brewster LP, Brey EM, Greisler HG et al: Advanced Drug Delivery Reviews, 58 (9) 604–629, 2006.)

humans to 1 to 2 cm), transmural tissue ingrowth accompanied by microvessels from the perigraft tissue, and from deposition of circulating endothelial cells, endothelial progenitor cells (EPCs), or stem cells. Homing can be promoted through affixation of EC attractant antibodies to the grafts in a fashion similar to that used in coronary artery stents.[42]

However, ECs growing on prosthetic graft surfaces are not necessarily the same as their normal quiescent counterparts in uninjured vessels. These ECs are often "activated," secreting bioactive substances (e.g., platelet-derived growth factor [PDGF]) that actually promote thrombogenesis and changes in SMCs to a synthetic phenotype. This has been seen in the perianastomotic region, which is the most frequent site of interventional failure after operation.[43] SMCs found within the myointima of prosthetic grafts are also functionally altered. They produce significantly higher amounts of PDGF, as well as various extracellular matrix proteins, than those of the adjacent vessel, which contribute to the development of intimal hyperplasia along with the body's inflammatory reactions to prosthetic material.[44]

The inflammatory response to vascular interventions is complex. Both inflammatory cells and proteins mediate it in a cooperative manner. Potent chemoattractants like complement 5a (C5a) and leukotriene B_4 recruit neutrophils to the graft surface, where they localize in the fibrin coagulum of the graft's inner and outer capsule via $\beta2$ integrins. In addition, immunoglobulin G binds to the neutrophils' Fcγ receptors activating the neutrophils' proinflammatory response while inhibiting normal clearance of bacteria. Neutrophils also interact with various other deposited proteins including C3bi and factor X, and they adhere to the endothelial cells in the perianastomotic region through selectin- and integrin-mediated mechanisms. L-selectin is thought to modulate neutrophil and endothelial cell interactions by presenting neutrophil ligands to the both E- and P-selectin on the vascular endothelium. In addition, selectin-carbohydrate bonds are important for the initial cellular contact, whereas the integrin-peptide bonds are responsible for strengthening of this adhesion as well as the transmigration of neutrophils. Both intercellular adhesion molecular 1 (ICAM1) and vascular cell adhesion molecule 1 (VCAM1) on the EC surface bind these integrins as well, and ECs upregulate ICAM1 expression and express VCAM1 when stimulated by inflammatory agonists such as interleukin (IL)-1, tumor necrosis factor (TNF)-α, lipopolysaccharide, and thrombin. Furthermore, activated neutrophils release oxygen-free radicals and various proteases, which result in matrix degradation that may inhibit both endothelialization and tissue incorporation of the vascular graft.

Circulating monocytes and macrophages are also attracted to areas of injured or regenerating endothelium, especially in response to IL-1 and TNF-α. There are many plasma monocyte recruitment and activating factors, including LTB$_4$, platelet factor 4, and PDGF. This process is propagated in the presence of these plasma activating factors driving monocytes to differentiate into macrophages that direct the host's chronic inflammatory response via the release of proteases and oxygen-free radicals.

A variety of cytokines are released from inflammatory cells activated by vascular grafts. Cultured monocytes and macrophages incubated with Dacron and expanded polytetrafluoroethylene (ePTFE) have been demonstrated to produce different amounts of IL-1β, IL-6, and TNF-α that are biomaterial specific.[45] Because the inflammatory reaction elicits a cascade of growth processes, it has been proposed that approaches attenuating the initial inflammatory reaction may improve long-term graft patency. Alternatively, directing the inflammatory response to promote favorable cellular and protein responses may promote intimal generation and tissue incorporation.

Creation of a More Hospitable Blood Biomaterial Interface

The long-term patency of vascular grafts depends upon the intrinsic properties of the graft itself and the hemodynamic environment in which the graft is placed, as well as patient variables (e.g., diabetes, renal failure, nutritional status), and may or may not be improved by prior or concomitant interventions such as proximal or distal angioplasty. It is now clear that tissue incorporation is important for graft function; therefore grafts that have this ability are considered desirable for medium- and small-caliber vessel replacement. The compliance mismatch between arteries and grafts causes flow disruption in vivo, which could contribute to anastomotic pseudointimal hyperplasia.[46] For this reason, a number of surgeons have suggested interposing a segment of vein between the synthetic graft and artery, creating a composite graft at the distal anastomosis. This has also led some investigators to design more compliant grafts using more flexible materials or changing the parameters of graft construction to improve graft compliance. Although animal experiments have suggested concept validity, the clinical benefit of this approach remains controversial. Many factors may contribute to this confusion, including longitudinal variability in the diameter and compliance of the arterial tree and the effect of activated endothelium on intimal hyperplasia. Furthermore, there is a robust fibrotic response after implantation that leads compliant grafts to become more noncompliant after implantation; therefore, even if a compliance match were attained initially, this benefit would unlikely persist. Synthesis of a conduit designed to match the compliance of the arterial wall is simplistic, as the compliance of the diseased arteries to which the grafts would be anastomosed is widely variable. Furthermore, in the para-anastomotic region there are dynamic changes in compliance that vary over time. First a para-anastomotic hypercompliant zone exhibits a 50% gain in compliance, then later its compliance is lessened 60% from baseline.[47] It is likely that this bimodal adaptation limits the practical value of graft designs focused on initial mismatch. Addressing later mismatch may be more valuable, but synthetic grafts are intrinsically limited in this ability to adapt over time.

Anticoagulant Affixation

Early platelet deposition on vascular grafts is mediated by von Willebrand factor and platelet membrane glycoproteins. After adherence to a graft, platelets degranulate, releasing many bioactive substances, including serotonin, epinephrine, ADP, and thromboxane A2; these substances in turn activate additional platelets and promote a prothrombogenic reaction. Activated platelets also release growth factors, such as PDGF, epidermal growth factor (EGF), and transforming growth factor-β, which promote SMC migration and proliferation as well as ECM degradation and ECM protein synthesis. In addition, platelets release monocyte chemoattractants such as platelet factor 4 and β-thromboglobulin, which mediate the recruitment of macrophages to the graft. Platelet deposition and activation continues chronically after graft implantation as evidenced by increased thromboxane levels and decreased systemic platelet counts 1 year after Dacron graft implantation in a canine model,[48] and human studies have confirmed platelet adhesion to grafts up to 1 year after implantation.

The deposition and activation of platelets elicit various pathologic cascades; therefore the thrombogenic nature of the synthetic graft surface can lead to both early and late graft failure. A myriad of approaches have been studied to attenuate platelet deposition, aggregation, and degranulation. Antiplatelet agents directly targeting platelet or graft-binding molecules such as platelet surface GPIIb/IIIa and different functional domains of thrombin have been shown to at least transiently decrease the accumulation of platelets on Dacron grafts.[49] The surface thrombogenicity of grafts can be altered experimentally through disruption of the blood system's coagulation cascade on thrombogenic surfaces. We have reported improved patency, thromboresistance, and the absence of intraluminal graft thrombus in heparin-analog–coated ePTFE grafts using a canine bilateral aortoiliac artery model.[50] Similarly, combined data tables of clinical data showed a decrease in subacute thrombosis with heparin-coated coronary artery stents.[51] Genetic approaches to increase thromboresistance have been used by multiple groups through the overexpression of thrombotic inhibitors, but because quiescent ECs themselves are antithrombotic, there may be limited benefit of this approach compared with a functioning endothelium.

A heparin-bonded Dacron graft from Maquet (Wayne, NJ) is currently available on the market. The heparin is bound primarily through Van der Waals bonds to the polyester fiber pretreated with a cationic agent, tridodecilmethyl-ammonium chloride. The external third of the graft wall is coated with collagen to prevent blood extravasation.[52] In a comparative clinical trial involving 209 patients undergoing femoropopliteal bypass grafts, the heparin-bonded Dacron graft exhibited a slightly better but significant ($p = 0.04$) patency with 1, 2, and 3 years of 70%, 63%, and 55%, compared to untreated ePTFE graft of 56%, 46%, and 42%, respectively.[53]

A heparin-bonded ePTFE graft developed by W.L. Gore is currently available worldwide. Heparin binding is through covalent end-point attachment of the heparin to the pretreated bioactive surface of the graft. An animal study showed improved patency of the graft compared with the standard ePTFE graft using a canine carotid interposition model up to 6 months.[54] The surface heparin activity measured by antithrombin III uptake per unit area was 24.7 ± 7.9 pmol/cm^2 at 2 weeks and remained at 15.3 ± 3.7 pmol/cm^2 by 12 weeks after implantation. Clinical data to date suggests decent early results[55] and 5-year results.[56]

Whether the anticoagulation works through continuous release of heparin from the material establishing an effective concentration at the interface between blood and the graft surface or through nonconsumptive mechanisms of active function of the heparin immobilized on the material surface is unclear. A major concern with heparinization of the graft surface is the duration of heparin function. Premature release or disturbance of functional heparin or the presence of a physical barrier owing to adherent blood components implies a theoretical inefficacy of the approach. Although theoretically probable,[57] there have been discordant case reports on whether these grafts cause heparin-induced thrombocytopenia.[58,59]

Prevalent Grafts

Polyethylene terephthalate (PET or Dacron) and ePTFE are the predominant materials currently used in prosthetic vascular grafts, but both Dacron and ePTFE react with blood components and perigraft tissues in both clinically desirable and undesirable manners. All grafts, regardless of their composition and structure, evoke complex but predictable host responses that begin immediately upon restoration of perfusion, and this improved understanding of the cellular and molecular components of biomaterial and tissue interactions has led to more intelligent designs of grafts that maximize beneficial ingrowth while minimizing the chronic inflammatory changes that lead to graft dilation or occlusion. These approaches include protein adsorptive grafts (e.g., growth factors, anticoagulants, antibiotics) and improved graft skeletal construction via synthetic polymers or biologically derived structural proteins that can be bonded to various bioactive cytokines and growth factors to induce a more favorable host response.

Dacron

PET was first introduced in 1939. DuPont (Wilmington, DE) made further developments and patented its well-known Dacron fiber in 1950.[60] Vascular grafts made from Dacron were first implanted by Julian in 1956[61] and DeBakey in 1958.[62]

Clinically available Dacron grafts are fabricated in either woven or knitted forms. In woven grafts, the multifilament Dacron threads are fabricated in an over-and-under pattern in both lengthwise (warp) and circumferential (weft) directions. This structure results in limited porosity and the best dimensional stability of the finished grafts. Accordingly, woven grafts have less bleeding through interstices and less likelihood of structural deformation after implantation. The disadvantages of such grafts are less desirable handling features, reduced compliance, and a tendency to fray at cut edges.

Knitted grafts use a textile technique in which the Dacron threads are looped to form a continuous interlocking chain. Most knitted grafts are manufactured with the threads predominantly oriented in a longitudinal direction (warp knitting) as opposed to a circumferential direction (weft knitting), which has been proved to be structurally unstable. Warp knits have good handling characteristics and reasonable dimensional stability. The loop structure creates greater porosity and radial distension. The velour technique that extends the loops of yarn on the surfaces of the fabrics has been used in the attempt to increase tissue incorporation. An external velour surface permits more extensive and firmer incorporation of the graft into surrounding tissue, but the function of an internal velour structure remains controversial, with the suggestion that it may enhance firm anchorage of the fibrin–platelet pseudointima.[63,64]

Crimping technique is used to increase flexibility, distension, and kink resistance of textile grafts. It is recognized, however, that much of the initial elasticity is lost with the stretching during implantation and with later tissue incorporation. Crimping also reduces the effective internal diameter of the graft and creates an uneven luminal surface. The latter can potentially interfere with laminar blood flow that leads to increased thrombogenicity of the graft. Although such considerations may not be critical in large-diameter grafts, they are important in small-diameter situations. As a result, prosthetic rings or coils are often applied to the graft external surface of grafts to provide external support to resist kinking and mechanical compression.

The high porosity of the knitted graft necessitates preclotting to prevent transmural blood extravasation. Gelatin (Vascutek, U.K.) and collagen (Maquet, Wayne, N.J.) are predominantly used to seal knitted Dacron graft pores. The gelatin and collagen in the Vascutek and Maquet grafts are cross-linked by low concentrations of formaldehyde, a method resulting in a weak linkage that allows the gelatin or collagen to be degraded in the body in less than 2 weeks.[65,66]

Dacron grafts, especially knitted grafts, have been demonstrated to be prone to dilate when implanted into the arterial environment. A 10% to 20% increase in graft diameter size after 1 year following restoration of blood flow is in the expected range. A follow-up study in 95 patients from 2 weeks to 138 months postoperatively (mean, 33 months) demonstrated a mean increase of 17.6% (0% to 84%) compared with initial graft size.[67] Woven grafts are structurally more stable. A direct relationship between uncomplicated graft dilatation and structural failure has not been established. Consequently, there is no recommendation on a specific degree of dilation that constitutes a significant hazard and warrants graft replacement.

Structural failure has been reported sporadically in the literature despite advances in the design and manufacturing of grafts (Figure 16-2).

In 1997, an inquiry to the U.S. Food and Drug Administration by Wilson et al.[68] revealed 68 cases of Dacron graft failure owing to structure defect, with an average time to failure of 7.4 years (range, 4 to 18 years). The true incidence of structure failure is difficult to estimate because most patients with grafts are not followed-up for long periods or are not being evaluated periodically for graft integrity. A number of factors may contribute to the graft degradation including the design of the textile structure, manufacturing process, surgical handling or application of clamps during implantation, mechanical fatiguing due to cyclic stresses of pulsatile blood flow, and chemical or physical alterations associated with biodegradation. The first generation of double-velour knitted Dacron grafts introduced in the mid 1970s, such as the Microvel and Cooley Double Velour grafts (Boston Scientific Meadox, Oakland, N.J.), showed excessive dilation and rupture after implantation.[68,69] It is believed that structural failure of these grafts was related to the fabrication techniques such as the use of trilobal filaments, insufficient strength of guideline yarns, and the weakness of connecting lines where two knitted bands join together to form a tube.[67,70] The trilobal filaments were replaced with more durable cylindrical filaments more than 30 years ago.

After implantation, a coagulum containing fibrin, platelets, and blood cells builds up during the first few hours to days and stabilizes over a period of 6 to 18 months, forming a compacted layer. The histologic characteristics observed within Dacron grafts is a compact fibrin layer on the blood contacting surface and densely packed foreign body giant cells between the outer layer of graft wall and surrounding connective tissue capsule. The fibrin layer within the midgraft region beyond 1 to 2 cm from either anastomosis remains acellular regardless of whether the grafts are woven or knitted. Protein impregnation changes the surface properties of Dacron grafts and may induce more inflammatory reaction, but does not change the clinical patency rates of these grafts.[65,71,72]

ePTFE

PTFE was patented by DuPont in 1937 as Teflon. In the 1960s, ePTFE was developed and is the material used in vascular grafts. The expanded polymer is manufactured by heating, stretching, and extruding processes producing a microporous material that is more supportive of firm tissue adhesion.

The PTFE molecule is biostable, and the graft made from it does not undergo biological deterioration within the body. The surface of the graft is electronegative, which minimizes its reaction with blood components. ePTFE grafts are manufactured by stretching a melt-extruded solid polymer tube that then cracks into a nontextile porous tube. The characteristic structure of ePTFE is a node-fibril structure in which solid nodes connect through fine fibrils with an average internodal distance in the range of 30 μm for standard grafts.

The initial host response to ePTFE grafts is similar to that of Dacron grafts.[63,64] A fibrin coagulum or amorphous platelet-rich material develops over a time sequence similar in both materials. Lack of luminal surface cellular coverage can be found at the midgraft region for years following human implants.[73-75] In outer wrap–reinforced

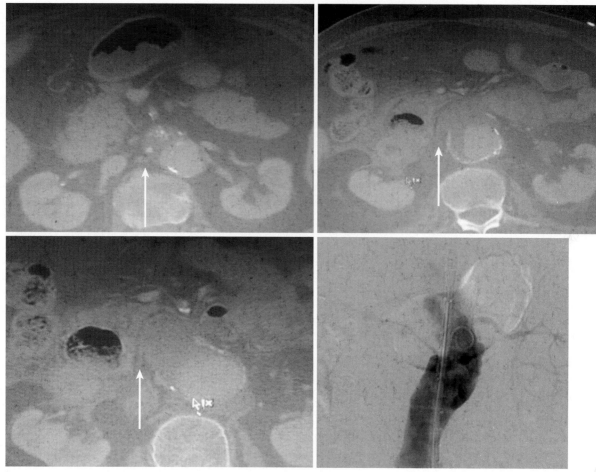

FIGURE 16-2 ■ **Contained rupture of prior aortic aneurysm repair.** Computed tomographic scan images demonstrate rupture of the Dacron graft likely near the proximal anastomosis. Arteriogram at time of reoperation *(bottom right)* demonstrates the dilation of the graft compared to native aorta.

grafts, the wrap delays the infiltration of the cells from perigraft tissue.[64]

In addition to the standard ePTFE graft, a number of modified grafts have been developed to offer specific properties for various applications. Thin-wall grafts, which have a wall thickness of 0.2 to 0.3 mm versus 0.4 to 0.6 mm for the standard grafts, possess better handling characteristics and improved compliance. The grafts failed to show a better patency for hemodialysis arteriovenous access compared with the standard graft[76] and are prone to more postpuncture blood loss. Extended stretch ePTFE graft has longitudinal extensibility that is achieved by a microcrimping of the fibrils. When the stretch graft is extended, the fibrils are extended to their full length, and the microstructure of the graft is then identical to that of the standard ePTFE graft. Stretch ePTFE grafts have somewhat better patency rates when used for atrioventricular access. Unfortunately, no data support such an advantage when used for peripheral reconstructions. Rings or coils are often applied to the abluminal surface of the grafts to provide external support in order to increase the graft resistance to external compression and to reduce kinking.

Still, the rate and extent of tissue ingrowth can be improved by optimizing graft permeability. Clowes et al.[77] have demonstrated enhanced tissue ingrowth and complete reendothelialization of 60 μm or 90 μm internodal distance ePTFE grafts in a baboon model.[77] Transinterstitial capillary ingrowth was not seen with the more commonly used 30-μm internodal distance ePTFE. Human trials using ePTFE with these expanded internodal distances failed to show any advantage in platelet deposition (considered an indicator of endothelial coverage) compared with standard 30-μm internodal distance ePTFE grafts.[78]

The delivery of potent angiogens or genes that promote EC-specific mitogenesis or chemotaxis upon injured vessels or prosthetic surfaces may be used to regenerate a rapid and complete endothelium after vascular intervention. We have demonstrated the feasibility of this approach in endarterectomized canine carotid arteries (Figure 16-3).

Prosthetic devices could store these genes or proteins and provide a controlled expression or release of these genes or proteins locally to circulating or surrounding ECs in a cell-demanded fashion. Ideally, this kind of

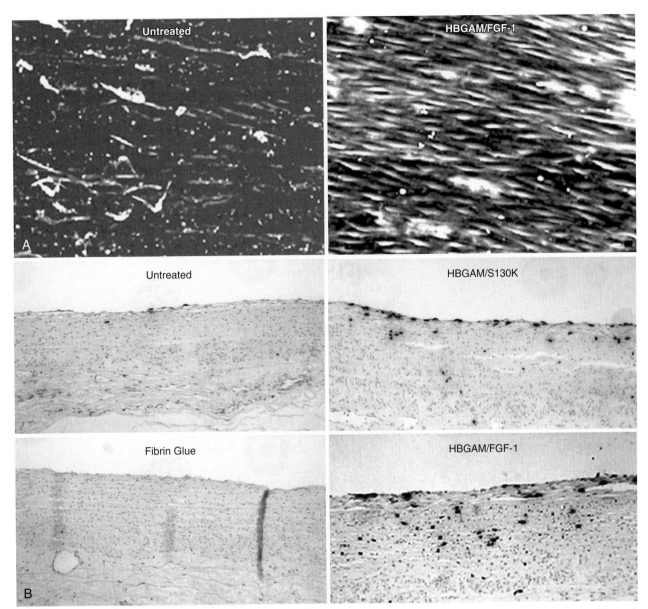

FIGURE 16-3 ■ **Endothelial healing with localized delivery of FGF-1 in fibrin glue. A,** Scanning electron micrograph (×400) illustrating the differences in re-endothelialization between normal saline untreated arteries and treatment arteries at 30 days after balloon angioplasty injury. The *top* micrograph is an untreated artery, and the *bottom* micrograph is an HBGAM/FGF-1 treated artery. **B,** Light microscopy micrograph (×10) comparing mitotic indices of treatment groups to untreated and fibrin glue treated control arteries at 30 days after injury as measured by bromodeoxyuridine (BrdU) incorporation *(brown staining)*. The control arteries have significantly less BrdU incorporation than the treatment arteries (*p* < 0.017). (From Brewster L, Brey EM, Addis M, et al: Improving endothelial healing with novel chimeric mitogens. Am J Surg 192:589–593, 2006.)

prosthetic could then be available as an off-the-shelf alternative to autogenous vein.

Carbon coating (Carboflo; Bard Peripheral Vascular, Tempe, Ariz.) has been used to increase the surface electronegativity so as to diminish thrombus formation. A prospective multicenter clinical study, consisting of 81 carbon-impregnated ePTFE and 79 standard ePTFE grafts for below-knee popliteal and distal bypasses, showed no difference in patency rates between the two groups up to 2 years after implantation.[79] However, a recent report on a multicenter trial in Europe involving 128 carbon-coated ePTFE and 126 standard ePTFE grafts for infrainguinal bypasses demonstrated significantly greater 1- and 2-year patency rates of the carbon-coated versus the standard grafts by life-table analysis.[80]

Applying the concept of the vein cuff, a precuffed graft was developed to improve the hemodynamics at the distal anastomosis.[81] The ePTFE in the cuff is thinner, which results in improved handling. The graft has been tested for both the hemodialysis angioaccess[82] and the infrapopliteal applications.[83,84] The 2-year patency rates for angioaccess were significantly higher with the precuffed graft versus the stretch ePTFE graft.[82] In a nonrandomized study from the United Kingdom, 50 precuffed grafts

(Distaflo, Bard Peripheral Vascular) were inserted into 46 patients with critical limb ischemia. The patency, limb salvage, and survival rates were similar to historical control bypass staffs with a Miller cuff.[83] A North American prospective, randomized, multicenter trial comparing the Distaflo to a standard ePTFE graft with vein modification at the distal anastomosis is currently underway. The midterm results, with a mean follow-up of 12.7 months, showed the primary patency rates of 54.35% (25/46) for the Distaflo graft compared to 55.81% (24/43) for the vein cuff ePTFE graft.[84]

Polyurethane

The compliance of both ePTFE and Dacron grafts do not correlate well with autogenous vessels. The superior elastic and compliant properties and acceptable biocompatibility of polyurethane (PU) make it an appealing material for vascular grafts. Developing PU-based small-diameter vascular grafts has attracted great interest from industry.

The unique mechanical properties of PU come from the molecular structure of the polymer. Segmented PUs are copolymers comprising three different monomers, a hard domain derived from a diisocyanate, a chain extender, and a soft domain most commonly polyol. The soft domain is mainly responsible for flexibility, while the hard domain imparts strength. The selection of the three monomers can produce materials with different mechanical characteristics, which makes PU an attractive biomaterial. Lycra is a trade name of segmented polyether polyurethane, which was commercialized in 1962 by DuPont.

As a biomaterial, PU was first used in manufacturing implantable roller pumps and left ventricular assist devices and as a coating for early artificial hearts.[85] The first generation of PU vascular grafts used polyester polyurethanes such as the Vascugraft by B. Braun Melsungen (Melsungen, Germany). Although an initial report demonstrated good biocompatibility,[86] the graft underwent surface chemical modification and deterioration in vivo.[87,88] A clinical trial using Vascugraft for below-knee bypass was aborted after 8 of 15 grafts had occluded in the first year.[88] It has been reported that PUs with polyester polyols as soft segments are hydrolytically unstable.[89]

Polyether-based PUs were then used, such as the Pulse-Tec (Newtec Vascular Products of North Wales, Deeside, U.K.) vascular access graft. Polyetherurethane is relatively insensitive to hydrolysis but susceptible to oxidative degradation.[89] The Pulse-Tec graft suffered from in vivo biodegradation and died in the product pipeline. Vectra (Thoratec Laboratories Corporation, Pleasanton, Calif.) is another vascular access graft made with polyetherurethaneurea. The graft is manufactured with an average pore size of 15 μm and a nonporous layer under the luminal surface, which makes it impervious to liquids.[90] In a multicenter trial involving 142 patients receiving either Vectra or ePTFE vascular access grafts with a follow-up time up to 12 months, no difference was found in terms of the patency rate or complications between the two grafts but the Vectra grafts allowed earlier access.[91]

However, it was noted that the PU graft elongated over time after implantation and the incidence of pseudointimal formation near the anastomosis was higher compared to ePTFE grafts.[91,92] The Vectra graft received clearance from the U.S. Food and Drug Administration in 2000, and it is currently a part of the Bard product line.

Tissue reactions to PU grafts are discrepant in the literature because factors such as different compositions of polymers, graft fabrication, porosity, and surface modifications all affect the results.[93-95] After so many iterations and years, it is doubtful that PU grafts will be functionally superior to ePTFE or Dacron.

Antibiotic Coated Grafts

Vascular graft infection is rare, but it is catastrophic when it occurs as demonstrated by an amputation rate of approximately 50% and a reported mortality rate that ranges from 25% to 75%. In an attempt to limit this dreaded complication, penicillin and cephalosporins have been successfully bound to Dacron and ePTFE grafts and have been found to limit *Staphylococcus aureus* infection in animal models. Rifampin-bonded gelatin-sealed Dacron grafts have also been shown in vitro to lessen bacterial colonization.[96] Intuitively, tissue ingrowth itself may also provide resistance to infection. Although a number of products are available on the market, the low incidence and delayed manifestation of graft infection (along with the avoidance of synthetic grafts in contaminated fields) limit the benefit of these efforts.

Endovascular Grafts

There are three basic types of stents: balloon-expandable stents, which need balloon inflation to expand the stent into the arterial wall; self-expanding stents, allowing delivery in a collapsed form with the stent expanding to its predetermined size after release from the delivery device; and thermal expanding stents, made by shape memory metal alloys that exist in an easily manipulated form and that restore their memorized shape at a certain transition temperature. All these stents have been used successfully in iliac arteries with a 2-year patency of approximately 84%. Improved endothelialization has also been reported using VEGF gene application to a modified metal stent.[97] Although stenting itself has quickly become an important member of the endovascular armamentarium, the development of biodegradable stents has progressed slowly, mostly because of difficulties in replicating the properties of stainless steel stents.[98] Still, the promise of cell-demanded sustained drug delivery in biodegradable stents has led to a renewed interest in this approach.[99] Preliminary evidence supports the short-term stability of these stents and the ability of these stents to deliver bioactive agents to the vessel lumen, providing proof of concept for this approach.

Stent grafts are a collapsible hybrid product composed of either Dacron or ePTFE with stents providing for radial support. These stent grafts maintain flow through their lumen and are commonly used to exclude flow into aneurysmal portions of arteries. Theoretically, the graft creates a barrier to exclude diseased arterial wall and provides a smooth flow conduit, while the stent support affixes the graft and may enhance luminal patency by resisting external compression. Stent grafts are delivered endovascularly, and since endovascular intervention reduces early operative morbidity and mortality, they have considerable consumer interest. However, the benefits of this approach over traditional operations is not clear, and it appears that outcomes are similar to that of the more traditional operative approach 2 years after intervention or operation. Furthermore, in a large study the subgroup of nonoperative candidates failed to demonstrate a survival benefit from endovascular repair compared to watchful waiting.[100]

The rapid improvements in stent grafts will likely lead to improved durability and decreased frequency of reintervention. Therefore they will likely have a defined role in the treatment of patients with cardiovascular disease. For this reason it is important to define the known differences in healing between stent grafts and traditional bypass grafts.

Compliance changes among stent, unsupported graft, and artery interfaces yield remarkable hemodynamic disturbances. In addition, delivery procedures, such as balloon dilatation, may alter both graft intrinsic characteristics such as porosity and wall thickness, as well as create mechanical injury to the surrounding artery. In addition, unlike conventional bypass, the endovascular graft is placed within the lumen of arteries with perigraft exposure to diseased arterial intima or to thrombus. All these factors change the healing characteristics of stent grafts compared to synthetic grafts. An inflammatory reaction and progressive thickening of neointima have been observed in both ePTFE- and Dacron-based stent grafts. When comparing endovascular grafts to conventional bypass grafting using a canine iliac artery model, endovascular stent grafts composed of ePTFE grafts and balloon-expandable stents resulted in both a greater rate of endothelialization and an approximately fivefold thicker neointima in the midportion of the graft and a higher percentage of stenosis at the distal anastomosis when compared to conventional ePTFE grafts.[101] Pathologic remodeling has also been reported after anchoring to the arterial wall, and it has been reported that stent placement may cause a variety of flow disturbances. The stent components themselves also stimulate a nonspecific inflammatory reaction and induce neointimal formation. Tissue engineering approaches, including cell seeding with genetically modified cells, may limit these complications.[102,103] The accumulation of experience, optimization of devices, and a better understanding of resultant pathologic processes will likely allow the easy transfer of the recent advances in tissue-engineered grafts and vessels to stent grafts. This transfer is probably critical to enhancing their durability over time.

Novel Conduits

Because autogenous tissue is desirable for healing, there has been a sincere effort recently to develop bioresorbable grafts. Unfortunately, aneurysmal dilatation of bioresorbable grafts can be expected to occur after sufficient degradation of the graft material if there is not adequate cell and matrix ingrowth. The first published report of a fully bioresorbable graft was by Bowald and colleagues[104] and described the use of a rolled sheet of Vicryl (a copolymer of polyglycolide and polylactide). We have reported that 10% of PGA (polyglycolic acid) grafts interposed into rabbit aortas have aneurysmal dilation within the first 3 months after implantation, and that this does not increase over the next 9 months, suggesting that the critical time for the development of aneurysms is during prosthetic resorption before the ingrowth of tissue with a sufficient strength to resist hemodynamic pressures. These studies also demonstrated the ability of bioresorbable grafts to support sufficient cellular ingrowth. Four weeks after implantation, these 24 × 4-mm grafts contained an inner capsule with a confluent layer of endothelial cells and myofibroblasts within dense collagen fibers.[105,106] Similarly constructed and implanted Dacron grafts demonstrated an inner capsule containing solely of fibrin coagulum with minimal cellularity. Macrophage infiltration and phagocytosis paralleled the resorption of PGA, which was totally resorbed at 3 months.

In order to limit graft rupture, several approaches have been developed. One is to combine the bioresorbable material with a nonresorbable material to retain a mechanical strut. A second solution involves the combination of two or more bioresorbable materials with different resorption rates so that the more rapidly degraded material evokes a rapid tissue ingrowth while the second material provides temporary structural integrity to the graft. Third, growth factors, chemoattractants, or cells can be applied to the graft to enhance tissue ingrowth, structure, and organization. To date such approaches have not yielded clinical products.

Tissue engineered vascular grafts (TEVGs) are another approach toward creating a conduit more biodynamic than strictly synthetic grafts. The potential benefits of the TEVG include the creation of a responsive and self-renewing tissue graft with functional intimal, medial, and adventitial layers (including both cellular and ECM components) that can be remodeled by the body according to its needs.

Weinberg and Bell[107] were the first to develop a TEVG in vitro. Using collagen and cultured bovine vascular cells, they demonstrated the feasibility of creating a TEVG, but their graft had prohibitively low burst pressures requiring external Dacron for support. In the following decade, L'Heureux and colleagues[60] constructed a human blood vessel with an acceptable burst strength and a thromboresistant endothelium in vitro using cultured umbilical cord-derived human cells,[60] but because of the immunogenic effects of the heterogeneic ECs in vivo, this graft devoid of ECs had only a 50% patency rate at 8 weeks in a canine model. Using a clinically relevant aged fibroblast-derived media, L'Heureux and colleagues[62] demonstrated a TEVG that has suitable bursting strengths at insertion, has a functional endothelium, and demonstrates mechanical stability in a variety of animal models out to 8 months.

A hybrid approach involves seeding autologous endothelial cells onto synthetic grafts. In 1978, Herring and colleagues[63] first reported that endothelial cell seeding onto a graft surface enhanced graft survival. Since then, this subject has been intensively investigated. Zilla and colleagues demonstrated increased patency and decreased platelet deposition in clinically implanted endothelial cell seeded ePTFE femoropopliteal bypass grafts over 3 years compared with unseeded grafts, and this group more recently reported an overall 7-year primary patency rate of 62.8% for 153 endothelialized femoropopliteal ePTFE grafts[64]; this is comparable to the patency rate of saphenous vein grafts in this region. However, the seeded grafts have not yet been reproducibly shown to significantly reduce anastomotic pseudointimal hyperplasia.

In fact, the potential for IH is a major concern with EC-seeded grafts, and this has been described in case reports. In one case, bilateral above-knee grafts seeded with cephalic vein ECs developed stenosis and had to be replaced 41 months after implantation. The central part of this graft was explanted and investigated. The graft had a confluent endothelial lining on a collagen IV–positive basement membrane with subintimal tissue of 1.21 ± 0.19 mm thickness.[65] The unusually thick subendothelial layer was also found in another case in which a microvascular EC-seeded Dacron graft was placed as a mesoatrial bypass and had to be resected because of external mechanical stricture 9 months after implantation.[66]

Besides technical challenges, concern exists as to the ultimate function of those endothelial cells seeded on the graft surface. Unlike their uninjured counterparts, injured endothelial cells produce a variety of procoagulants like von Willebrand Factor, plasminogen activator inhibitor, thrombospondin, and collagen. Higher levels of PDGF and FGF-2 have also been measured in EC-seeded grafts; this is particularly concerning given their potential role in stimulating the migration and proliferation of SMCs, which can lead to IH. There is much discussion about the proper cells to use for cell seeding ex vivo or cell homing in vivo. The EC is the most fastidious vascular cell to grow, and heterogenous ECs are highly immunogenic. Therefore in the absence of immunosuppression, autogenous ECs are currently a requirement for TEVG. Using vascular smooth muscle cells or fibroblasts with or without exogenous matrix scaffolding can create the TEVG media and adventitia. These cells can be harvested from the patient in need, but because these patients are typically older with significant comorbidities, their cells (particularly VSMCs and ECs) might not retain sufficient doubling capacity necessary to generate these TEVGs; this is possibly the result, in part, of the loss of telomere length that occurs with aging.

To counteract this biological limitation, Niklason and colleagues have demonstrated an increase in the population doublings of adult VSMCs through retroviral infection with the human telomerase reverse transcriptase (hTERT) subunit without evidence of inducing cellular transformation.[108] However, these arteries have unacceptably low bursting strengths, and this is probably because hTERT infection did not remediate the stunted production of essential ECM proteins (e.g., collagen) that confer vessel strength in these transformed aged cells. These functional characteristics of TEVG provide proof of concept of this approach to improving conduit choice.

Clinical success has been seen when using TEVGs for vessel replacement in the venous system, which is less challenging hemodynamically. These TEVGs have been implanted in 42 pediatric patients with congenital heart defects. To date these grafts have been resistant to aneurysmal dilatation and had superb patency.[67]

Decellularized tissue scaffolds are appealing because they are already composed of native vascular extracellular matrix proteins that exhibit reasonable structural characteristics as well as providing instructive cues for cellular ingrowth. Using bone marrow-derived cells incubated on decellularized canine carotid arteries, Byung-Soo Kim and colleagues demonstrated cellular incorporation into the scaffold and subsequent differentiation of these cells into endothelial and vascular smooth muscle cells and subsequently into three distinct vessel layers.[68] Others have used a more focused approach and induced or applied endothelial progenitor cells (EPCs) into similar scaffolds with promising results. The benefit of EPCs include a robust replication potential ideal for TEVG engineering, and these cells acquire mature endothelial cell markers and function upon seeding into TEVGs[69]; these attributes may be further augmented by protein and gene therapy.[70]

Using biological gels, such as those composed of type I collagen or fibrin, one can promote tissue ingrowth and direct remodeling in a bioreactor, thereby promoting favorable characteristics such as improved mechanical strength or vessel reactivity over time[71]; such approaches are easily modified by the addition of growth factors with refined delivery systems in order to enhance and sustain cellular ingrowth.[72] Further refinement of these scaffolds can mimic the differential mechanical properties of the intimal and medial arterial layers (Figure 16-4).

Because autogenous cells cannot spontaneously populate a scaffold by migration or proliferation alone, they may also be recruited internally via circulating ECs or EPCs or externally from the surrounding tissue or exogenous source through angiogenic ingrowth during tissue incorporation of the graft. In addition to the benefit provided by the localization of cells, transmural capillary ingrowth also provides for cellular perfusion and nutrient supply that extends beyond the distance supplied by simple diffusion (100 μm). Currently, a group is designing three-dimensional capillary constructs (Figure 16-5) that could provide grafts with the cellular and metabolic infrastructure requisite for the creation of a living TEVG through the induction of a vaso vasorum, which can be incorporated into preexisting capillary networks (inosculation).[73] Proof of concept of this approach has been demonstrated in cardiac sheet grafts.[74] This induction can be supplemented by the delivery of angiogenic proteins or genes to these constructs. With further research, a small diameter, totally resorbable vascular graft may be able to improve the current dismal long-term patency rates of synthetic small caliber grafts.

Endovascular stents were conceptualized before the introduction of angioplasty in 1969, and they have enjoyed increasing popularity in recent years. With more than 1.5 million percutaneous coronary interventions occurring each year and a prevalence of in-stent stenosis ranging from 15% to 60% of patients, there is little wonder that much interest has been paid to the drug-eluting stent (DES). Currently used DESs release broadly suppressive drugs to the surrounding tissue to limit neointimal stenosis, and they likely retard myointimal

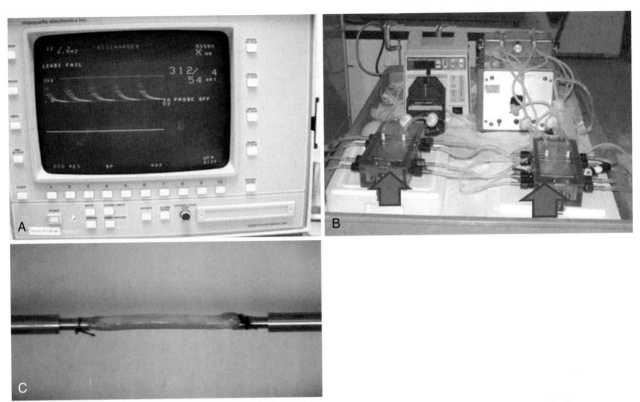

FIGURE 16-4 ■ **Bioreactor utilization of tissue engineered blood vessel. A,** Pulsatile flow through the bioreactor. **B,** Bioreactor apparatus setup. The vessels are inside the boxes *(large arrows).* **C,** The vessel loaded onto the inflow and outflow of the bioreactor.

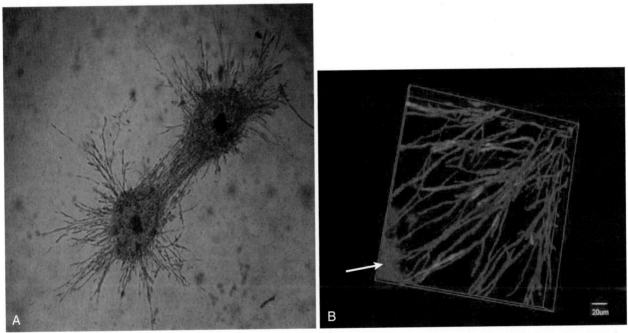

FIGURE 16-5 ■ **Creating a vasa vasorum in vitro. A,** Light microscopy demonstrating inosculation of endothelial cell sprouts from two separate endothelial cell pellets. **B,** Three-dimensional reconstruction of endothelial cell tubule inosculation. The *arrow* designates the closest cell pellet.

thickening rather than facilitate healing. This may be sufficient for short-term benefit, but may compromise the long-term durability of these vascular interventions. Long-term durability is likely to become more critical in the coming years because of the improved mortality rates in patients with cardiovascular disease. Therefore it is critical to avoid complacency in clinical thinking, because what comprises a good result today depends on mortality rates that might not be applicable to today's patients. We firmly believe that promoting healing and not limiting the adverse effects of healing will provide for durable results.

GRAFT SELECTION

Aortic Reconstruction

A variety of prosthetic grafts function adequately in the large-diameter, high-flow positions. For procedures on the thoracic aorta and for extensive thoracoabdominal aortic reconstructions and for emergency repairs of ruptured abdominal aortic aneurysms, tightly woven Dacron grafts are an appropriate choice. Their long-term patency and dimensional stability have been satisfactory, and blood loss through the interstices is minimal.

For elective infrarenal aortoiliac replacement or bypass, both woven and knitted Dacron grafts have excellent, well-documented long-term results.[75] Many surgeons prefer knitted grafts because of their better handling and healing characteristics. Such features are thought to be particularly important for aortofemoral grafts done for occlusive disease that must cross the inguinal ligament, often with anastomoses made to a diseased femoral artery or profunda femoris branch alone.[76] Although Dacron grafts have long been a conventional choice, a randomized multicenter trial comparing stretch ePTFE versus knitted Dacron (collagen- or gelatin-coated) grafts showed no difference in 5-year patency rates among all three grafts when used for aortic bifurcation reconstructions.[109]

In general, all currently available prosthetic grafts perform well for aortic reconstructions. Issues of cost and convenience will probably be the discriminating factors for graft selection.

Infrainguinal Reconstruction

It is well established that autogenous saphenous vein is the preferred choice for infrainguinal bypass, which has a primary patency rate near 70% for above-knee femoral popliteal bypass at 5 years.[13,79,110]

Controversy exists, nevertheless, regarding whether prosthetic grafts should be the graft of choice initially when bypass to the above-knee popliteal level is feasible. A number of well-designed clinical trials have demonstrated no significant differences in patency or limb salvage rates between vein and prosthetic grafts within 2 years; however, the 4- to 5-year patency with vein grafts is higher than with ePTFE grafts (61% to 76% versus 38% to 68%).[80-82] The rationale for the preferential use of prosthetic grafts is that the compromised long-term survival of many of these patients may reduce the importance of long-term graft patency. It is reasoned that even if patency rates with prosthetic conduits are slightly lower, the saphenous vein will still be available for use in reoperation if this is required.[83] The patency rates of reoperations are much higher with autogenous veins than prosthetic grafts.[84-87] The advantages of initial use of prosthetic grafts are the shorter operative time and the need for less dissection that may be advantageous in the high-risk patient population. Yet no study has confirmed the corresponding reduction in mortality and morbidity rates of using prosthetic grafts. Many have shown that prosthetic graft failure is associated with a significantly higher incidence of limb-threatening ischemia,[88] and

more second operations are required with the initial use of prosthetic grafts. The morbidity rate and the risks of associated complications such as graft infection, which are clearly higher with reoperations, must also be considered.[89]

Most surgeons currently agree that, when it is available, saphenous vein should be the first choice, especially for limb salvage situations. Prosthetic grafts may be used preferentially in selected patients, particularly older patients undergoing operation for noncritical ischemia with fairly good runoff.

For infrapopliteal bypasses, every effort should be made to use autogenous vein, as the long-term function of prosthetic grafts in this position is far less than satisfactory. The patency rates for ePTFE grafts are 20% to 58% at 1 year and 18% to 41% at 3 years.[20,90-92]

Adjunctive techniques are often used to improve the results of infrapopliteal bypass with prosthetic grafts, such as the interposition of a venous cuff, patch, or boot at the anastomosis of the prosthetic conduit to the distal artery,[111-115] the creation of prosthetic-vein composite graft,[93] and the addition of a remote distal arteriovenous fistula.[94] Improved patency rates have been demonstrated with these adjunctive procedures, particularly for the below-knee bypass grafts.

The interposition of venous tissue at the distal anastomosis between the artery and prosthetic graft has appealing theoretical advantages deriving from both biological and mechanical factors. Animal experiments have demonstrated a decreased neointimal thickness by the presence of vein at the perianastomotic area.[95,116,117] Venous endothelium may also confer a beneficial effect through fibrinolytic and antiplatelet activity, although these effects remain unproved. Mechanically, vein interposed between a stiff prosthetic graft and a more pliable artery would buffer the compliance mismatch. It is also possible that venous tissue simply enlarges the distal anastomosis so that the formation of hyperplasia must encroach on a wider lumen before becoming clinically significant.

A variety of prosthetic grafts are currently available for lower extremity revascularization procedures, including standard and modified (thin wall, stretch, 60/20 thrupore, carbon-coated, heparin-bond) ePTFE grafts, and biological protein–coated knitted Dacron grafts. ePTFE grafts are more widely used mainly because of their better handling properties. Despite the efforts of manufacturers, the clinical benefits of these adaptations have been limited.[118-121] Solutions for small-diameter vascular reconstructions prove to be a continuous challenge. Applying anticoagulant agents such as heparin to prosthetic grafts may provide some benefit when autologous vein is not available.[55]

Extraanatomic Grafts

The extraanatomic reconstructions, such as axillofemoral, femorofemoral, or axilloaxillary bypasses, often involve remote subcutaneously implanted grafts. Graft compression or kinking is therefore a major concern. The use of externally supported grafts is a common practice, and most recommend a 10-mm graft.

Both the ePTFE and the Dacron grafts have been demonstrated to have equivalently good long-term patency.[122-125] The externally supported ePTFE grafts for axillobifemoral bypass have a 5-year primary patency of 71%,[122] and the externally supported, knitted Dacron grafts used for axillofemoral bypass have a primary patency rate of 78% at 5 years and 73% at 7 years.[123] The 5-year primary patency of femorofemoral crossover grafts in patients with disabling claudication is reportedly 72% with no difference between the Dacron and the PTFE grafts.[124] For carotid-subclavian grafts, some authors have documented higher long-term patency rates with ePTFE or Dacron grafts than with vein grafts.[126-128]

Venous Reconstruction

Ring-reinforced ePTFE grafts are commonly used for large-caliber venous replacements in unusual circumstances, such as the replacement or bypass of the inferior or superior vena cava,[129-132] iliofemoral, jugular,[133] and portal vein[134] or the construction of portosystemic shunts for portal hypertension.[135,136]

The ring-reinforcement in theory resists respiratory compression better, and thus prevents graft collapse that may be a factor in promotion of thrombosis. However, no comparative study with nonringed grafts has been done and is not feasible given the small numbers of patients in even the largest reports with these procedures. A temporary arterial fistula can be added to these venous reconstructions to improve their patency.[137]

Hemodialysis Vascular Access

Typically, long-term access to the vascular system is provided by an arteriovenous fistula or a bridge graft. The prosthetic bridge graft accounts for approximately half of all hemodialysis access procedures performed in patients with end-stage renal disease in the United States. However, only 26% of them remain patent without complication 2 years after placement.[138] The secondary 3-year patency is better at 42% to 60%.[139-141] The failure of prosthetic angioaccess grafts is often associated with stenosis at the venous anastomosis, which leads to subsequent thrombosis.

Standard wall thickness ePTFE grafts are usually the prosthetic choice for angioaccess when a primary arteriovenous fistula for hemodialysis cannot be performed or has failed. Dacron grafts often have patency, bleeding, and wall integrity difficulties. Various modified grafts have been studied for many years in an attempt to improve the performance of the prosthetic grafts for the angioaccess application. The modifications to prosthetic material have included changing the wall structure, adding luminal or extramural coatings, and incorporating relatively impermeable layers.

Tordior and colleagues showed that the evolution of ePTFE to a "stretch" configuration is superior to the standard, nonstretch configurations.[141a] They hypothesized that this advantage was caused by less intimal hyperplasia from poor compliance match problems. Thin-wall ePTFE grafts are also commonly used because of their improved handling characteristics and flexibility, but results from others do not support this advantage.[142]

The tapered ePTFE graft was designed to improve the hemodynamics by changing the geometric configuration, but a randomized multicenter trial showed no difference between tapered and thin-wall stretch PTFE grafts.[143]

A common limitation for angioaccess grafts is that they require a period of time after implantation before being used. Autogenous arteriovenous fistulas typically require a maturation period of 6 weeks to 6 months before first cannulation, whereas prosthetic grafts are not accessed for 2 to 4 weeks to permit tissue incorporation. The Vectra PU graft reportedly allows early access. The time required to reach hemostasis following puncture is significantly shorter with this graft than with ePTFE[144] but long-term graft survival data is needed to prove its advantage. Technical complications manifested by graft kinking (likely owing to rigidity of the PU at the anastomosis to native vessels) were noted by several groups.[145]

Other Locations

Visceral and renal arterial reconstructions can be performed with prosthetic grafts with good results, and in these reconstructions many surgeons prefer prosthetic grafts. Paty and colleagues[146] reported a patency of 97% at 7 years in a series of 489 renal revascularizations with ePTFE grafts. Another study by Cormier and colleagues[147] achieved an 85% patency at 5 years. These good patency rates are likely due in part to their generally short length with high blood flow and not being subjected to mechanical stresses around body joints.

Autogenous veins are usually recommended for distal renal artery grafts in young patients with fibromuscular disease, or visceral or renal procedures that involve bypass to diseased vessels with compromised distal arterial beds. For children, aortorenal vein grafts have a prohibitive incidence of aneurysmal dilatation; therefore direct reimplantation of renal artery or reconstruction using the internal iliac artery are favored.

CONCLUSION

There seems to be a plateau in clinical improvement in recent years. However, current bench research on improving venous conduits and creating tissue engineered vessels holds promise for the future. The unique clinical training of vascular surgeons provides a pioneering opportunity for those involved on this front. As more patients live with cardiovascular disease than die from it, there is little doubt that approaches that maximize autologous tissue use and promote rather than retard graft healing will be the ultimate winners in future graft inroads and development. Still, for patients who are unlikely to live long enough to realize that benefit, temporary inhibition and retardation strategies may be adequate. Both approaches with their respective clinical products will likely coexist for the near future.

References available online at expertconsult.com.

QUESTIONS

1. Saphenous vein grafts for arterial bypass:
   a. Must be of good quality (>3mm and not ectatic) to enjoy superior patency rates over synthetic graft
   b. Can be utilized with synthetic grafts as a composite bypass and exhibit patency rates similar to that of saphenous vein alone
   c. Have patency rates that rival that of the internal mammary artery to left anterior descending artery
   d. Should be reserved for coronary revascularization because synthetic grafts cannot be used for the heart.
   e. Have similar one year patency rates for lower extremity and coronary bypass

2. Heparin-bonded vascular grafts for infrainguinal reconstruction:
   a. Has improved patency rates over saphenous vein grafts
   b. Is superior to cryopreserved artery or vein as bypass conduit
   c. Is very likely to cause heparin-induced thrombosis in patients
   d. Is likely to maintain heparin function for sustained periods of time
   e. Only affects platelet aggregation as heparin is not otherwise bioactive

3. Which of the following is true when comparing Dacron to ePTFE grafts?
   a. Dacron is more resistant to infection than ePTFE
   b. Dacron binds gentamycin better than ePTFE
   c. ePTFE expands more in vivo
   d. ePTFE has greater radial than axial compliance
   e. There is a patency advantage to heparin-affixation on Dacron grafts

4. What is the advantage of using synthetic graft over saphenous vein for above knee bypass?
   a. Quicker operation
   b. Better patency rates
   c. Less susceptible to infection
   d. They spontaneously endothelialize over time
   e. All of the above

5. The initial pseudointima formation:
   a. On Dacron is related to the weave of the graft
   b. On ePTFE assists in the endothelialization of the graft
   c. Is preventable with proper graft sizing
   d. Is initiated by passive protein accumulation
   e. Is an antibody specific mechanism, followed by passive binding of serum proteins.

6. Polyurethane grafts:
   a. exhibit better elasticity and compliance than ePTFE and Dacron
   b. have higher degenerative and pseudoaneurysm complications
   c. are first-line grafts for vascular access
   d. a and b
   e. all of the above

7. Treatment of infected aorto-femoral grafts include all of the following except:
   a. Rifampin-soaking Dacron graft as replacement conduit without systemic antibiotics or omental wrapping
   b. Resecting graft, oversewing aorta, and axillary-bipopliteal ePTFE grafts
   c. Utilizing deep vein for new bypass
   d. Temporizing anastomic leaks with endovascular grafts
   e. Utilizing cryovessels for in situ reconstruction.

8. Endovascular stent grafts are:
   a. Composed of the same materials as open vascular grafts
   b. Should not be expected to suffer consequences of material fatigue
   c. Unlikely to remodel the aorta
   d. Do not accumulate pseudointima over time
   e. Unlikely to fail compared to open bypass grafts

9. Biologic grafts:
   a. Are currently superior in patency to autogenous vein
   b. Can be composed quickly from tissue from the host patient
   c. Are remodeled in part by macrophage activity
   d. Are not expected to develop aneurysmal degeneration
   e. All of the above

10. Regarding graft selection:
    a. Dacron outperforms ePTFE for aortic grafting
    b. Vein grafts outperform prosthetic graft in the above knee bypass over time
    c. Autogenous vein has superior patency over synthetic grafts for carotid-subclavian bypass
    d. Synthetic grafts without external support are most commonly utilized for femoral-femoral bypass
    e. All of the above

ANSWERS

1. **e**
2. **b**
3. **e**
4. **a**
5. **d**
6. **d**
7. **a**
8. **a**
9. **c**
10. **b**

CHAPTER 17

Arterial Access; Guidewires, Catheters, and Sheaths; and Balloon Angioplasty Catheters and Stents

Charlie C. Cheng • Peter A. Schneider • Michael B. Silva, Jr.

The last 2 decades have seen a dramatic shift in the management of vascular diseases, with increasing reliance on percutaneous techniques and a decrease in the use of open surgical alternatives. There has been a democratization of interventional skills throughout the specialty of vascular surgery and great interest in these techniques among parallel subspecialties involved in the care of vascular patients. By devising training and educational programs for dissemination of endovascular skills for both new trainees and practicing surgeons, this remarkable and rapid evolution has been achieved. Although there is much to be sorted regarding the best therapeutic endovascular or open surgical alternative for any given vascular problem, there is now a broad consensus that excellence in performing angiography, catheter manipulations, and endovascular device delivery is just as important in the development of a mature vascular surgical practice as excellence in open surgical technique has always been. The basis, therefore, for an advanced contemporary vascular surgical practice must include a deep working knowledge of endovascular devices and the best manner for their implementation.

The acquisition of endovascular skills is a layering process. One begins with the knowledge and familiarity of the most basic tools such as needles, guidewires, catheters, and sheaths. To this is added experience with using these devices safely and efficiently, understanding the sequence of how they are used together, and the interactions between the tools and vascular lesions. The interventionist must understand imaging. Knowing how to safely perform and expertly interpret the angiographic image is paramount in deciding when and how to intervene. Once these skills are mastered, advanced interventional procedures such as angioplasty and stenting are added to the mix. The contemporary vascular surgeon, with advanced endovascular skills and strong open surgical expertise, is then ideally positioned to participate in the advancement of the field by developing and investigating new procedures and new devices. This chapter begins with the introduction to vascular access, and is followed by description of various wires, sheaths, catheters, balloons, and stents needed for endovascular procedures.

VASCULAR ACCESS

The Access Site

Endovascular intervention begins with vascular access. Appropriate vascular access requires the site to provide a secure, direct, and uninterrupted pathway to the vascular bed of interest or target lesion. The commonly used arterial access sites are the common femoral arteries in the groins and the brachial arteries at the antecubital fossae (Figure 17-1). The femoral approach from the right groin is usually the first choice for angiography and most interventions (Figure 17-2). Its superficial location allows for ease of access, and its relatively large caliber provides blood flow around the sheath to maintain perfusion to the distal lower extremity. In addition, the common femoral artery lies anterior to the femoral head, providing support for pressure to achieve hemostasis should the need arise. This access can be directed in a retrograde fashion toward the pelvis or antegrade toward the thigh. The retrograde femoral puncture provides access to the entire thoracoabdominal aorta and its branches. The contralateral iliofemoral arteries and lower extremity circulation can be easily catheterized from this approach. Alternatively, using an antegrade femoral puncture, distal arteries such as the infrapopliteal and inframalleolar circulation can be visualized in detail and treated most directly.

Arterial puncture in the upper extremity also provides access to thoracoabdominal aorta and its branches. The use of upper extremity access is usually limited to instances in which the common femoral arteries are not available because of occlusive disease in the aortoiliac segment or recent bypass. The left brachial artery is preferably used because the left subclavian artery is a separate branch from the left common carotid artery off the aortic arch. A sheath from the right brachial artery can also be used. It has a potential disadvantage in that it crosses the origin of the right common carotid artery (and also the left common carotid artery in bovine arch) as it enters the aortic arch. This can increase the risk of embolization to the brain from atherosclerotic plaque in the diseased innominate artery during sheath and

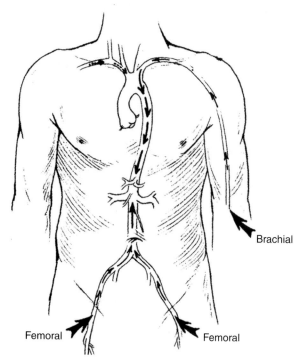

FIGURE 17-1 ■ Sites for arterial access. (From Moore WS, Ahn SS, editors: Endovascular surgery, ed 4, Philadelphia, 2011, Saunders, p 50.)

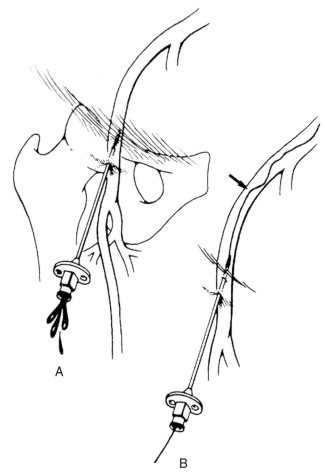

FIGURE 17-2 ■ Common femoral artery puncture. **A,** Entry into common femoral artery. **B,** Maintenance of access with passage of guidewire. (From Moore WS, Ahn SS, editors: Endovascular surgery, ed 4, Philadelphia, 2011, Saunders, p 50.)

catheter manipulations or device delivery. The axillary artery is contained in a neurovascular sheath, and even minimal bleeding in the sheath has the potential to cause nerve compression with resultant upper extremity paralysis. Therefore the axillary artery is not routinely used as an arterial access. The radial artery is frequently used for cardiac interventions; devices deliverable through a 6-French sheath can be used through specially designed radial sheaths, but access at the wrist necessitates very long catheters and devices for imaging or intervening in the infrainguinal vasculature. The advantages and disadvantages of the various access sites are listed in Table 17-1.

For venous interventions, common access sites are the femoral veins in the groins, brachial veins at the antecubital fossa, and popliteal veins behind the knee. In the treatment of deep venous thrombosis with thrombolytic therapy or endovascular mechanical thrombectomy, the contralateral femoral vein is recommended. Although venous valves are a potential impediment for catheter advancement from an up and over approach, it is not difficult to overcome this impediment with guidewire and guide catheter advancement techniques. Using this approach, a removable inferior vena cava (IVC) filter can be placed before catheterization and treatment of the diseased vein in the lower extremity. Simultaneous access of the popliteal vein may also be used to cross the venous lesion. With the leg externally rotated at the hip, ultrasound guidance can be used to locate and access the popliteal vein behind the knee with the patient in the supine position.

In diagnostic venograms, the superficial veins of the upper and lower extremities can be used. In the upper extremities, the cephalic or the basilic veins are used. In the lower extremities, superficial veins on the dorsum of the foot are cannulated and venous tourniquets are used to direct contrast into the deep system.

Vascular Cannulation

Vascular cannulation is a standardized procedure that is applied regardless of the vein or artery selected. There are two methods to obtain vascular access (Figure 17-3): the through-and-through puncture and the single-wall puncture. In the through-and-through (double-wall) method, both the anterior and posterior walls are completely crossed with the needle. The needle is then withdrawn back into the lumen. This is sometimes used for venous entry, but is not recommended routinely for arterial access. The posterior wall puncture can lead to bleeding complications such as retroperitoneal hematoma at the groin or nerve compression in the surrounding perivascular spaces. The posterior wall puncture can also lead to arteriovenous fistula. For arterial access, the single-wall puncture is preferred. A steady pressure is applied to slowly advance the needle. Pulsatile flow after puncture

TABLE 17-1 Comparison of Sites for Arterial Access

Site	Advantages	Disadvantages	Comments
Femoral	Easily accessed Large vessel	Possible tortuosity Long pathway for catheter manipulations to remote targets	First choice among sites Obesity may complicate puncture
	SPR set up for right-handed access	Left side accessed from the patient's right	Predictable complications
	Most devices designed for femoral access Right or left artery available Permits brachiocephalic and aortic runoff access Easily compressed Puncture complication easily managed	May be compromised by ASO	
Brachial	Usually patent and disease free Either side accessible	Prone to thrombosis Patient comfort compromised by arm board	Second-choice site Micropuncture set is a useful adjunctive device
	Most target lesions are accessible	Long, tortuous route for catheter manipulations	Brachial site best for angiography and some simple interventions
Axillary	Large vessel	Major complication, "short hematoma"	Small catheters are best used by experienced operators
	Short working distance to the aorta	Brachial plexopathy	Use is best limited to angiography
	Access from the left avoids crossing the cerebrovascular orifices	Uncomfortable patient position	
Subclavian	Large vessel	Potential for pneumothorax	Useful for angiography, PTA and stenting, thrombolysis
	Very short working distance to the aorta	Prolonged bimanual compression	
	Accessible bilaterally; left side preferred	Increased risk of hematoma with larger catheters	Angle of approach desirable for renal angioplasty
	Access to arch, thoracic aorta, and entire runoff		Sheath removed when PTT returns to normal
	Each leg may be accessed antegradely		Most difficult access; requires experience
Radial	Ease of access and compression for early patient discharge	Very long working distance	A novelty
	Radial artery may be expandable	Radial artery may thrombose; later unusable for bypass graft Hand ischemia potential Nerve damage potential	

From Moore WS, Ahn SS, editors: Endovascular surgery, ed 3, Philadelphia, 2001, WB Saunders, p 39.
ASO, Arteriosclerosis obliterans; *PTA,* percutaneous transluminal angioplasty; *PTT,* partial thromboplastin time; *SPR,* special procedures room.

of only the anterior wall indicates entry into the arterial lumen.

The Seldinger technique is the fundamental method of vascular access that was first described in 1953 (Figure 17-4). A wire, needle, and a sheath are required. In this technique:

1. Angulated entry into the vascular wall is obtained with the needle beveled anteriorly (see Figure 17-4A). The single-wall puncture should be used. Intraluminal position of the needle is indicated by pulsatile flow from the needle hub during arterial puncture or steady blood return into the syringe with negative pressure during venous puncture. A small injection of intravenous contrast under fluoroscopy can also be used to confirm intraluminal needle position.
2. A guide wire is then passed through the needle into the vascular lumen until the stiff portion is well

inside the artery or vein (see Figure 17-4B). The wire should be inserted gently and advance easily without resistance. If there is resistance, fluoroscopy should be used for wire advancement.
3. The needle is removed and exchanged for the appropriate sheath over the guide wire (see Figure 17-4C). There may be instances when the artery is hard from calcified plaque or the surrounding tissue is fibrotic from previous access or surgery. Dilators of increasing size can be used over the guide wire for sequential dilation of the track and arteriotomy until the sheath can be inserted.

For safe vascular access, especially the small arteries such as the brachial artery at the antecubital fossa, a modified Seldinger technique using the micropuncture set is recommended (Figure 17-5). A small, 21-gauge needle is used to obtain vascular entry. A 0.018-inch guidewire is inserted to secure access, followed by

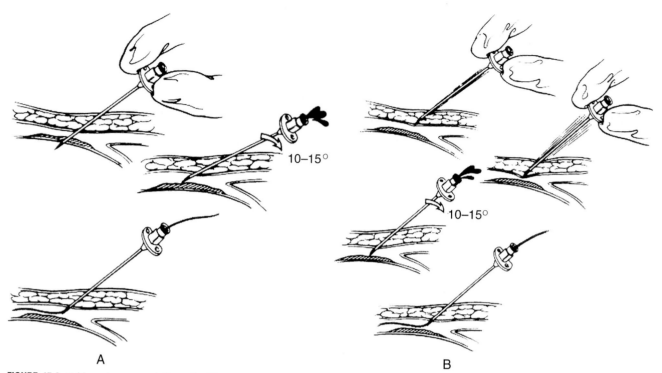

10–15°

10–15°

A

B

FIGURE 17-3 ■ Vascular cannulation. **A,** Through-and-through (double-wall) puncture. **B,** Anterior (single-wall) puncture. (From Moore WS, Ahn SS, editors: Endovascular surgery, ed 4, Philadelphia, 2011, Saunders, p 52.)

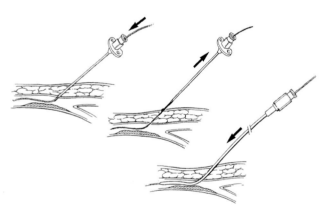

FIGURE 17-4 ■ The Seldinger technique. **A,** Angulated entry into the vascular wall. **B,** Guide wire is then passed through the needle into the vascular lumen. **C,** The needle is removed and exchanged for the appropriate sheath over the guide wire. (From Moore WS, Ahn SS, editors: Endovascular surgery, ed 4, Philadelphia, 2011, Saunders, p 52.)

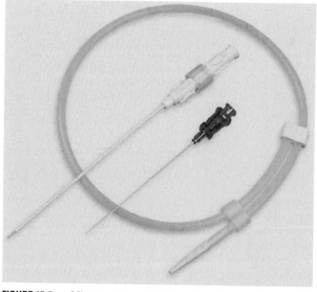

FIGURE 17-5 ■ Micropuncture kit. (From Bard Access System, Salt Lake City, Utah.)

exchange of the needle for a paired coaxial catheter. The small inner catheter accepts the small guidewire and functions as a dilator for the larger outer catheter. The small guidewire and catheter are both removed, and a 0.035-inch guidewire is inserted into the outer catheter. This catheter is then removed for the appropriate sheath. It is common to use ultrasound guidance for real-time vascular wall imaging, in addition to routine reliance on micropuncture technique.

TECHNIQUES FOR ARTERIAL ACCESS

In this section, anatomic landmarks and techniques used for a specific arterial site are described.

Retrograde Femoral Puncture

The common femoral artery can be located using the osseous anatomic landmarks at the groin (Figure 17-6).

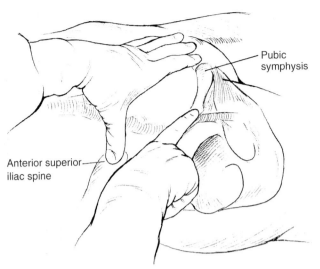

FIGURE 17-7 ■ Antegrade femoral puncture. Localization of the anterior superior iliac spine pubic symphysis. The needle is inserted just distal to the inguinal ligament. (From Moore WS, Ahn SS, editors: Endovascular surgery, ed 4, Philadelphia, 2011, Saunders, p 54.)

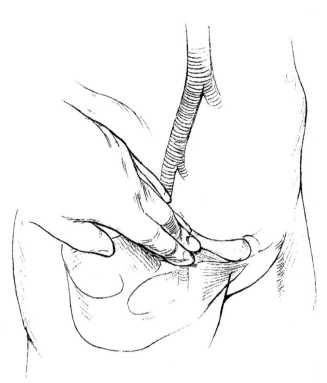

FIGURE 17-6 ■ Retrograde femoral puncture. Localization of the common femoral artery using the osseous anatomic landmarks at the groin. (From Moore WS, Ahn SS, editors: Endovascular surgery, ed 4, Philadelphia, 2011, Saunders, p 53.)

In general, there is approximately 3 to 5 cm of common femoral artery located anterior to the junction of the medial third and middle third of the femoral head. This artery begins proximally at the inguinal ligament and is two fingerbreadths lateral to the pubic symphysis on a line joining the symphysis with the anterior iliac spine. This relationship varies little with the patient's body habitus and age; however, the location of the inguinal ligament and the common femoral artery can be misleading in obese patients. The abdominal panniculus may falsely lead the interventionalist to initiate access more distally, resulting in puncture of the superficial femoral or profunda femoris arteries. Before entry with the needle, the femoral head should first be identified with the fluoroscopy. Inadvertent access of these arteries increases the risk of postoperative hematoma, pseudoaneurysm, or arteriovenous fistula. Using ultrasound to identify the common femoral artery and the profunda femoris and superficial femoral artery origins, at the time of microneedle insertion, reduces these types of complications.

To access the common femoral artery, the surgeon needs to locate the inguinal ligament and be familiar with the relation between skin puncture site, angle of needle entry, and the femoral head. Once there is pulsatile blood return at the needle hub, the guidewire is passed to secure the intraluminal location. Fluoroscopy can be used to verify the location of the needle tip. If the tip is below the femoral head, puff contrast arteriography is performed with the image intensifier in an ipsilateral oblique position to confirm access of the common femoral artery.

This view allows for visualization of the common femoral bifurcation and the proximal superficial femoral or profunda femoris arteries. If the arterial puncture is satisfactory, the guidewire is advanced under fluoroscopic guidance.

Antegrade Femoral Puncture

The antegrade femoral puncture is a useful arterial access for intervention of distal, ipsilateral arterial lesions. This is especially true for tall patients with distal tibial arterial lesions, where there may not be enough catheter length for the angioplasty balloon or stent to reach the target from a contralateral, retrograde femoral puncture. In this technique, the needle is inserted just distal to the anterior iliac spine in an antegrade fashion to access the common femoral artery (Figure 17-7). Similar to retrograde femoral puncture, the location of the inguinal ligament can be misleading in obese patients, resulting in puncture of the superficial femoral or the profunda femoris arteries. In these patients, the abdominal panniculus is retracted in a cephalad direction to allow for appropriate location and angle of needle entry at the skin. The location of the femoral head should be identified with fluoroscopy before skin puncture. Less commonly, the needle may access the external iliac artery; this results in difficulty with guidewire advancement and postoperative bleeding complications (Figure 17-8). Ultrasound guidance should be used routinely.

With antegrade femoral puncture, the guidewire is frequently advanced into the profunda femoris artery. Under fluoroscopic guidance, the needle tip may be moved either medially or laterally to redirect it into the superficial femoral artery. However, this may not be possible if the needle access is too close to the femoral bifurcation. For antegrade punctures, the needle should enter the proximal common femoral artery as close to the femoral head and the inguinal ligament as possible. As mentioned previously, the use of the micropuncture kit is recommended. If the wire is advanced into the profunda femoris artery, the needle is exchanged over wire with the outer sheath in this artery. Contrast is injected through the sheath as it is pulled back until the tip is in the common femoral artery under fluoroscopy. An angled guidewire is then advanced into the superficial femoral artery (Figure 17-9).

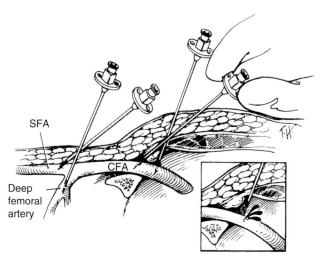

FIGURE 17-8 ■ External iliac artery access during antegrade puncture. Potential difficulty with guide wire advancement and postoperative bleeding complications. (From Moore WS, Ahn SS, editors: Endovascular surgery, ed 4, Philadelphia, 2011, Saunders, p 54.)

Another technique is to sequentially exchange the micropuncture needle over wire to a 6-French sheath. With a 0.014-inch wire in the profunda femoris artery to maintain arterial access, the sheath is pulled back while contrast is injected until the tip is in the common femoral artery. A second, angled guidewire is passed through the sheath and advanced into the superficial femoral artery. The 0.014-inch wire is removed from the profunda femoris artery, and the sheath is advanced over the dilator and guidewire.

Ultrasound Guided Access

A small and portable ultrasound unit such as the Sonosite (General Electric, Bothell, Wash.) can be used to identify and characterize the artery or vein to be accessed (Figure 17-10). The common femoral artery or vein can be located at the groin, the brachial artery or vein at the antecubital fossa, and the superficial veins in the upper or lower extremities. The ultrasound is especially useful when the vascular structure cannot be palpated because of occlusive disease or patient obesity. Under ultrasound imaging, the echogenic tip of the micropuncture needle can be seen as it passes deep into the soft tissue and enters the anterior wall of the artery or vein. In addition, a soft spot in a diseased arterial wall can be identified and entered with needlepoint accuracy.

For access of the common femoral artery, the artery is first identified at the groin. The ultrasound probe is moved in a cephalad direction to image the artery until it dives deep to become the distal external iliac artery at

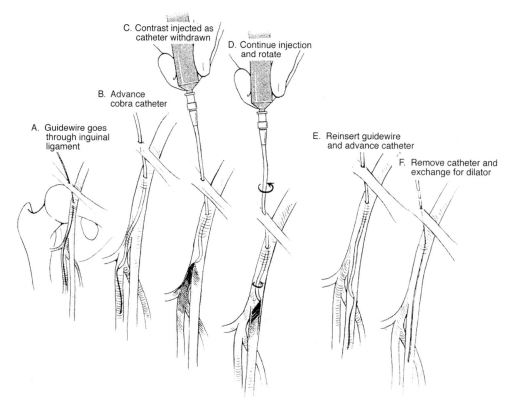

FIGURE 17-9 ■ Redirecting the wire and catheter from the profunda femoris to the superficial femoral artery. (From Moore WS, Ahn SS, editors: Endovascular surgery, ed 4, Philadelphia, 2011, Saunders, p 55.)

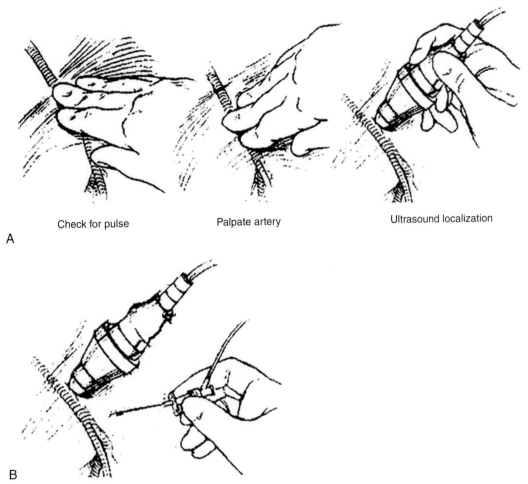

Check for pulse   Palpate artery   Ultrasound localization

A

B

FIGURE 17-10 ■ Ultrasound guided vascular access. **A,** Localization of artery with ultrasound. **B,** Ultrasound guided access using real-time imaging. (From Moore WS, Ahn SS, editors: Endovascular surgery, ed 4, Philadelphia, 2011, Saunders, p 56.)

the inguinal ligament. This is the anatomic landmark for the beginning of the proximal common femoral artery. The probe is then moved in a caudal direction to locate the origin of the superficial femoral and profunda femoris arteries. This is the landmark for the distal common femoral artery at the bifurcation. While the entire common femoral artery is being imaged, attention is given to any potential plaque on the posterior wall or calcification on the anterior wall. These lesions are avoided, and the arterial entry site should be made proximal to these lesions if possible. Once a spot on the anterior arterial wall is selected, skin entry of the needle is made approximately 1 or 2 cm away from the probe to provide a gentle angle of access into the artery. There is a learning curve to this technique, and the surgeon needs to keep in mind the relationship between the skin puncture sites, angle of needle access, and the depth of the artery as imaged. This technique is used for both antegrade and retrograde femoral punctures.

For access of the brachial artery, the artery is first identified at the antecubital fossa. The artery is imaged in a proximal and distal direction to select the location where it is most superficial, and to note the location of the brachial bifurcation. The probe is then lightly placed on the skin, and the artery is imaged again to visualize any potential crossing basilic or antecubital veins overlying the artery. Puncture of the vein and artery is avoided to prevent iatrogenic arteriovenous fistula. The median nerve may also be identified and avoided.

With mastery of this technique, a surgeon will be able to access vascular structures that might not otherwise be safely or easily cannulated. Access complications can be limited by verifying position, avoiding focal plaque, and directing the needle to a healthier arterial segment. The micropuncture technique and ultrasound-guided access can be used for all vascular cannulations. Other than the slight increase in procedure time required during the learning phase, there are no credible arguments against routine use of this technique.

ACCESS SITE COMPLCATIONS

New innovative technologies and techniques in endovascular surgery are rapidly emerging. With increasing use of catheter-based endovascular interventions, it is conceivable that there will be a rise in complications from these procedures. There are unique complications specific to endovascular therapies that are different from conventional open surgeries. It is therefore important that vascular surgeons performing these procedures are knowledgeable in the recognition and management of these complications. Studies have shown that overall complications following endovascular surgery can range from 1.5% to 9%.[1-3] The most frequently encountered complications in endovascular surgery are related to access site problems. Following cardiac catheterization, the incidence of groin complications is 0.05% to 0.7%.[4,5] However, the incidence is much higher following percutaneous transluminal angioplasty, at 0.7% to 9.0%.[5,6] Peripheral vascular complications, in descending order of frequency, include pseudoaneurysm, groin hematoma, and arteriovenous fistula. In the following sections, complications related to vascular puncture will be presented. Complications associated with endovascular procedures will be presented later in the chapter.

Hematoma

Groin hematoma remains one of the most common complications following endovascular procedures. Predisposing factors include the use of anticoagulants during procedure, periprocedural antiplatelet medications, size of access device, surgeon's experience, and type of procedure being performed. Blood from a femoral artery usually collects in the external genitalia, flank, or thigh, and ecchymosis is typically minimal immediately after the procedure but may become significant in the hours following completion. In patients taking anticoagulation and antiplatelet medications, ecchymosis may be more extensive with discoloration extending upward onto the lower abdomen or below onto the thigh and flank as the patient ambulates. Bleeding from the brachial artery may have ecchymosis involving much of the arm.

Symptoms of a hematoma can vary from mild discomfort to severe pain with attendant swelling. Small hematomas rarely lead to severe complications, but large hematomas can result in significant blood loss with hypotension and significant physiologic derangement. Pressure and tension from the mass effect can cause skin necrosis with compression and irreversible nerve injury. The extent of a hematoma can be elucidated with computed tomography; this entails additional radiation and contrast exposure and is not routinely employed, but it may be useful in identifying retroperitoneal hemorrhage associated with the access that is otherwise not externally visible.

When a hematoma is suspected, manual pressure should be applied to prevent further bleeding. Urgent surgical evacuation with repair of the vessel may be necessary to prevent shock and life-threatening complications if direct pressure is inadequate to achieve hemostasis. Other surgical indications include severe pain, nerve compression, venous obstruction, and skin necrosis. After the skin incision is made over the hematoma, dissection is made through the fascial planes to the artery. Usually, one or two interrupted sutures are all that is needed to repair the vessel.

Several factors can assist in the prevention of hematomas. During access, it has been found that needle access 1 cm lateral to the most medial cortex of the femoral head and proper maintenance of a 30- to 45-degree puncture angle can reduce the likelihood of groin hematoma formation.[7] At the time of sheath removal, hypertension control and coagulation status of the patient should be known. The use of commercially available closure devices is recommended to assist in arterial closure and to reduce the time of immobility. If a device is not used, manual pressure at the access site on the artery, not the skin puncture site, is held at 15 to 30 minutes, and longer if necessary. This pressure is followed by limited mobility for 6 to 8 hours. Sandbags or other compression devices have been used; however, they can become dislodged easily and fail to apply pressure directly over the site of arterial puncture and allow for continued hemorrhage. These devices obscure the access site, impede visual inspection, and provide a false sense of security; therefore their use is not recommended.

Pseudoaneurysm

Pseudoaneurysms result from failure of the closure in the arterial puncture site, leading to contained bleeding in the soft tissue adjacent to the site of vascular entry. The wall of a pseudoaneurysm is composed of organized thrombus and adjacent soft tissue rather than the vessel wall, as in true aneurysms. Pseudoaneurysms are most commonly seen in the femoral artery (incidence is 0.05% to 0.4%), likely because it is the site most frequently used for access.[8,9] However, it can be seen in any arterial entry including brachial,[9,10] axillary, radial, and popliteal arteries (as high as 2.9%).[11]

Predisposing factors to pseudoaneurysm formation include anticoagulation, antiplatelet agents, hypertension, and the location of vascular entry.[8] There is a higher rate of pseudoaneurysm formation if the arterial access is below the femoral head in either the superficial femoral or profunda femoris artery, or at the femoral bifurcation.[4,10,12,13] Difficulty in compressing these arteries and the greater ratio of sheath size to artery diameter may be contributing factors.

Pseudoaneurysms typically develop within 24-48 hours after the intervention, but may not be apparent until several days later. They are associated with pain, and ecchymosis may be present. Similar to a hematoma, pressure created from the mass effect can cause irreversible nerve injury, necrosis of overlying skin, and compression of the veins.[9] Rarely, pseudoaneurysms can rupture and cause life-threatening hemorrhage.

At the access site, diagnosis is suggested by the presence of a pulsatile mass that is tender to palpation and has a bruit. Diagnosis is confirmed by duplex ultrasound with visualization of the cavity, neck, and bidirectional flow. The examination should note the size and the character of the neck of the pseudoaneurysm. The neck may be wide or long and narrow. Some pseudoaneurysms are complex with multiple lobes.

There are many treatment options, and management of pseudoaneurysms should be based on size and the presence of complications mentioned previously, such as nerve compression. Many small pseudoaneurysms thrombose spontaneously[8] and may be observed without therapy. Thrombosis usually occurs within 2 to 4 weeks, but possibly later if there is concurrent anticoagulation or antiplatelet therapy. Repeated ultrasound examination for confirmation of closure is recommended.

Surgical repair has been the mainstay of therapy for larger pseudoaneurysms, but it is now seldom used. When needed for enlarging aneurysms or complications, the hematoma is evacuated and the artery is dissected and exposed. The puncture site is then oversewn with suture. It is important not to misidentify a hole in the fascia as the arterial defect. Suture placement in the fascia will lead to recurrent pseudoaneurysm or persistent bleeding.

There are less invasive approaches that are available. Ultrasound-directed compression was first described in the 1990s and uses ultrasound to identify the neck of the pseudoaneurysm. The neck is seen as a high-velocity jet, and direct compression is applied with the transducer. This is associated with significant pain, and is labor intensive. Ultrasound-guided thrombin injection has become the treatment of choice.[9,10] It is preferred over direct ultrasound compression because it produces less patient discomfort and has a higher success rate. Studies have shown it to be successful in 94% of patients, despite 30% of patients being anticoagulated and receiving antiplatelet therapy.[9] The procedure is performed with ultrasound guidance, with the introduction of needle into the cavity as far away from the neck as possible; 500 to 1000 units of bovine thrombin is injected, and ultrasound imaging is used to see clotting and cessation of blood flow into the pseudoaneurysm cavity. Long, narrow necks are ideal, whereas wide necks are contraindicated. Wide necks with direction communication between the pseudoaneurysm and the artery have higher risks of clot embolization and thrombin injection into the artery.

Arteriovenous Fistula

Arteriovenous fistula is a postprocedural direct communication between access artery and vein, caused by inadvertent puncture of the artery and vein. This complication can occur at any vessel access site. Because most access is obtained at the groin, arteriovenous fistulas are most commonly seen between the femoral artery and vein. A prospective study of patients undergoing coronary angioplasty using duplex ultrasound found an incidence of 2.8%.[8] In contrast, an incidence of 0.3% was detected when using audible bruit as an indication for duplex study, likely an underestimation of the true incidence.[14] Predisposing factors include periprocedural anticoagulation, hypertension, female gender, left femoral puncture, and popliteal artery access. The increased incidence associated with left femoral access may be due to alteration of the entry angle while standing on the right side. In popliteal artery puncture, the vein is posterior to the artery and this overlap makes the occurrence of fistula more likely.

Most patients with arteriovenous fistula are asymptomatic. Small fistulae may appear with only a thrill or continuous bruit on auscultation. Larger fistulae may have vessel enlargement, leading to aneurysmal dilatation with time. Steal syndrome can develop with flow from the involved artery into the adjacent vein, leading to limb ischemia. A physiologic shunt can be produced, significant enough to elevate right sided filling pressures

leading to exacerbation of congestive heart failure in at risk patients.

Once an arteriovenous fistula is suggested by the identification of a thrill or bruit, the diagnosis is confirmed with duplex ultrasound. The examination shows the characteristic systolic-diastolic flow pattern with arterialization of the venous signal.

Many arteriovenous fistulae close spontaneously and may be observed without specific treatment.[15] Symptomatic fistulae should be treated. Surgical repaired is performed by dissecting the artery and exposing the defect. Arterial control is obtained either by clamping or digital pressure. Venous control is obtained by direct pressure. The arterial defect is repaired first, using horizontal mattress Prolene sutures. Usually, only one or two interrupted sutures are needed for the repair.

Less invasive approaches have been described. Successful use of ultrasound-guided compression has been attempted.[4] Recently there have been several studies describing the use of endovascular repair with stent grafts.[16,17] Arteriography of the groin shows rapid filling of the venous system. A short, covered stent is used to cover the arteriovenous communication.

Retroperitoneal Hematoma

Retroperitoneal hematoma is perhaps the most feared complication of groin access following femoral arterial puncture. It is rare with an incidence of 0.15%, but can be fatal.[18] Following puncture, the blood tracks into the retroperitoneal cavity, and it may not be visible or palpable at the groin. An iliopsoas hematoma can form if the bleeding is contained in the iliopsoas muscle. If there is bleeding into the retroperitoneum, a large amount of blood can accumulate in this large potential space, leading to compression of the ipsilateral kidney and life-threatening complications associated with the hemodynamic derangement of significant blood loss.

Predisposing factors for significant retroperitoneal hematoma formation include periprocedural anticoagulation, double arterial wall puncture, and arterial entry above the inguinal ligament.[18,19] With through-and-through arterial wall puncture, there may be bleeding into the retroperitoneal space from the arteriotomy on the posterior wall. In arterial access above the inguinal ligament, hemostasis is difficult because compression is not against the femoral head.

Symptoms of retroperitoneal hematoma commonly include lower abdominal and back pain. There is usually no ecchymosis initially, but the pain is more severe than the typical periprocedural pain. As the hematoma enlarges, compression of the lumbar plexus in the psoas muscle can cause thigh pain, numbness, or weakness in the quadriceps. The pressure created from the mass effect can also cause venus obstruction with or without thrombosis[20] or result in the urge to urinate or defecate. Finally, patients with severe blood loss may have life-threatening hypotension and shock. Conversely, patients may also exhibit normal hemodynamics and few external physical findings.

It is important to maintain a high index of suspicion in patients with lower abdominal, back, and flank pain after groin punctures. Patients with symptoms and any of the physical findings described previously should prompt a computed tomographic scan of the abdomen and pelvis. Initial managements of the retroperitoneal hematoma include stopping and reversing anticoagulation and antiplatelet therapy. Patients need to be stabilized with fluids and blood as needed. Most retroperitoneal bleeds are self limited. Indications for surgery include urgent decompression of the hematoma for patients with compression neuropathy and surgical repair of the arterial defect for persistent bleeding and hematoma progression.

Access Site Occlusion

Occlusion of the artery at the access site can result from thrombosis, dissection, and vasospasm. Predisposing factors include peripheral vascular disease, advanced age, female gender, atherosclerosis, prolonged occlusion by manual pressure or compression device, poor distal runoff, and a hypercoagulable state. Atherosclerosis results in luminal area reduction and increases the risk for plaque disruption, facilitating vessel thrombosis.

Patients with acute occlusion at the arterial access site exhibit signs and symptoms typical of acute limb ischemia. The presence of pulses at the groin may come from the distal external iliac artery, even though the common femoral artery is occluded. Occlusion of the radial artery may be asymptomatic because of adequate flow to the palm supplied by the ulnar artery.

Acute limb ischemia requires immediate intervention with heparinization and thrombectomy. Arteriography can be used for confirmation of the diagnosis and identification of the site of obstruction. Endovascular intervention is not typically used for these complications. Open surgical exploration with thrombectomy, arterial repair, and confirmation of successful restoration of distal perfusion is the treatment of choice.

Groin Infection

Soft tissue infections at the vascular access site after catheterization are rare, but can be potentially severe. They are most commonly caused by gram-positive organisms from the skin flora, especially the *Staphylococcus* species.[21,22] Predisposing factors include hematoma at the access site, immunodeficiency, obesity, diabetes, and use of closure devices.[23-25] The foreign materials used by these devices can serve as a nidus for infection and cause more access site infections compared with direct compression.[26]

Patients with access site infections exhibit erythema, induration, and tenderness. There may be purulent drainage associated with an abscess formation or fever and chills from bacteremia. Infections from cellulitis that are mild and superficial respond to antibiotics. More extensive infections may require surgical drainage and debridement in addition to antibiotics. The foreign material from closure devices may need to be removed with repair of any arterial defects.

Several factors may assist in the prevention of soft tissue infection. Percutaneous access should be avoided in areas of soft tissue infection. Repeat access following other recent endovascular intervention should be via a different site if possible. Closure devices should be used only in areas of sterility. Sheaths and catheters should be removed as soon as possible.

GUIDEWIRES, CATHETERS, AND SHEATHS

Most interventionists acquire their knowledge of guidewires, catheters, and sheaths through actual handling of the devices, with little thought given to the complex scientific and engineering processes that led to their development. Suppliers of these products are eager to offer a variety of devices that are tailored to specific needs and may have subtly different handling characteristics, making the task of selecting and stocking an inventory difficult for the practitioner.

The maturation of an endovascular practice goes through predictable phases in the buildup and use of this fundamental inventory. Initially, only a few variants are available, and the interventionist makes do with what is on hand. With growing experience, more difficult anatomic challenges, and a wider offering of therapeutic endovascular alternatives, the perceived need for additional wire, catheter, and sheath options increases substantially. In this second phase, a number of competing products are tested, and inventory increases markedly. Ultimately, the interventionist becomes facile with a wider selection of devices and is able to adapt their different shapes and handling characteristics to a greater number of anatomic conditions. In this mature phase, inventory stabilizes, with new products being introduced as new technologies are developed or significant improvements are made.

This chapter does not promote any particular brand or list of products necessary for the successful conduct of an endovascular practice; rather, it offers background and definitions that may be useful in assisting the practitioner in sorting through the many options presented for consideration. The number and variety of products needed are directly related to the number and variety of procedures performed and the previously mentioned phase of maturation of the particular endovascular practice.

Guidewires

Design Characteristics

Guidewires are designed to have the characteristics of "pushability" and flexibility. Most guidewires have a single steel core, called a *mandrel*, surrounded by a coiled wire and coated with a substance to make the guidewire slippery. The tip of the guidewire, always more flexible than the rigid body, is frequently made of a smaller wire that is bonded to the distal tip of the mandrel. These design characteristics—slipperiness and maximal flexibility—allow the tip of the guidewire to be manipulated past tortuous lesions or tight stenoses while limiting the risk of dissection or perforation. (This is why turning the wire around and using the rigid back end is not recommended.)

Guidewire tips are available in three shapes: straight, angled, or J-shaped. The type of tip chosen imparts variable degrees of steerability under fluoroscopic guidance. *Steerability* refers to the ability to direct the intravascular tip of the guidewire through manipulation of the extraanatomic portion by twisting, pulling, and pushing.

Guidewires are sized by their maximal transverse diameter (in hundredths of inches) and by their length (in centimeters). The guidewires most commonly used in peripheral vascular procedures come in three diameters: 0.035, 0.018, and 0.014 inch. For most angiographic procedures and most aortoiliac interventions, a 0.035-inch guidewire is used. *Trackability* of a wire refers to the ability of a catheter or an endovascular device such as a balloon catheter or stent to pass over the wire through tortuous anatomic configurations. Generally, a larger-diameter wire that is stiffer provides better trackability than one that is smaller and more flexible.

For infrageniculate lesions or tight renal and carotid stenoses, a 0.014- or 0.018-inch wire can be used. These smaller wires allow the operator to advance a lower-profile balloon across a tight lesion in a smaller artery. A balloon with a lower profile has a smaller transverse diameter in its folded or uninflated state, which allows it to traverse a tighter stenosis than one with a higher profile.

Occasionally, a 0.038-inch wire is needed for passage of a large-diameter sheath or delivery of an endograft through a tortuous iliac artery. Passage of these large devices may be facilitated by the additional trackability of a stiffer wire with a greater diameter.

Guidewires come in a variety of lengths. The most commonly used lengths for general-purpose guidewires are 145 and 150 cm. Exchange wires, which allow the exchange of catheters or interventional devices without losing access across a remote lesion, are usually 180, 260, or 300 cm long. Longer wires are more difficult to handle and increase the chance of contamination. When performing any intervention, one should try to maintain the wire across the lesion until the completion angiogram has been obtained and is satisfactory. This allows additional interventional procedures, such as stent placement, to be performed after suboptimal intermediate interventions through a constant channel. A good formula for selecting wire length is as follows:

Total length of wire needed =
    Length of wire from insertion site to lesion +
    Length of catheter or interventional device + 10 cm

With a shorter wire, it may not be possible to remove the catheter while maintaining fixation of the wire across the lesion. Docking devices are available in some wire systems that allow extension of the length of the wire in place by adding a second wire to the end of the first via an attachable dock. These docking systems are of sufficiently low profile that they allow for subsequent passage of catheters and interventional devices over the added wire, over the docking system, and onto the initial wire.

Guidewire tip shapes and coatings facilitate function. Non–hydrophilic-coated J-tip catheters are useful for initial catheter introduction via the Seldinger technique. Although dissection can occur with any type of wire, these wires have characteristics that can reduce the frequency of this complication compared with hydrophilic wires with angled or straight tips. J-tip wires are also useful for passage of a wire through a stent when the use of an angled or straight wire might lead to inadvertent passage through a fenestration in the stent. Angled- or shapeable-tip guidewires are steerable and are therefore useful in manipulating the catheter across a tight stenosis or into a specific branch vessel. The use of straight wires should be limited to catheter exchanges.

Most guidewires have a hydrophilic coating of either polytetrafluoroethylene or silicone, which decreases the coefficient of friction during catheter exchange or while traversing a stenosis. The interventionist should be aware of the tactile differences noted with different wires as they are advanced into an artery. For example, the passage of a highly hydrophilic wire or a reduced-diameter wire in the subintimal plane may offer so little resistance that the technician is unaware that dissection has occurred. In contrast, attempted passage of a standard J-tip wire through an introducer needle and into an artery in an extraluminal plane may offer enough resistance that the operator feels the need to confirm the location with a hand-held injection of contrast agent. This starting wire is recommended for the beginning interventionist. A good practice is to wipe the guidewire with a sponge soaked in heparin and saline solution frequently and routinely between each catheter manipulation. This minimizes the amount of thrombotic debris that accumulates on the wire and decreases friction during subsequent catheter or wire exchanges. Care must be taken when wiping a wire not to inadvertently remove any length of the wire from its intended position. The practice of wiping toward the body reduces this possibility.

Selection

As one gains experience with catheter-based therapy, the number of guidewires and catheters needed to complete an intervention successfully may become fewer. The recommendations in this chapter should serve as a reference for the reader, but are by no means comprehensive (Table 17-2). For initial entry into the artery, a J-tip wire is recommended; it is associated with the lowest risk of dissection. J-tip wires come in a wide variety; some have a movable core that can convert the distal end of the wire from a flexible state to a rigid one. For initial introduction, a nonhydrophilic guidewire with medium rigidity should be chosen. The Bentson wire has a floppy tip, is of medium to firm rigidity and, although straight in its packaged state, forms a large, functional J-tip when being advanced through an artery or vein.

Glidewires (Terumo, Tokyo, Japan) can be either straight or angled and are hydrophilic. Angled Glidewires are steerable and can be manipulated with torque at the skin level, with or without an external torquing device. The use of straight Glidewires is not recommended during initial access because they are associated with the greatest chance of dissection. If dissection is suspected but not confirmed, a few simple tests can be performed. If a J-tip wire is used, one can attempt to spin the wire under fluoroscopy. The curved J-tip will not move freely

TABLE 17-2 Types of Guidewires and Catheters

Guidewire	Diameter (0.001 × in)	Length (cm)	Features	Function
General				
J-tp (Cook, Bloomington, Ind.)	18, 21, 25, 28, 32, 35, 38	80, 100, 125, 145	Variable tip curve 1.5, 3, 7.5, 15 TFE coated	Catheter introduction Passage through stents or tortuous vessels
Bentson (Cook, Bloomington, Ind.)	18, 21, 25, 28, 32, 35, 38	145, 180	15-cm flexible tip with distal 5 cm soft	Atraumatic negotiation of tortuous or strictured vessel
Glidewire (Boston Scientific, Quincy, Mass.)	18, 25, 32, 35	120, 150, 180, 260	Hydrophilic; angled or shapeable tip	Crossing difficult lesions
Exchange				
Amplatz Super Stiff (Cook, Bloomington, Ind.)	35, 38	80, 145, 180, 260	Stiff mandrel with flexible tip	Catheter exchange, good trackability Straightens acute aortoiliac bifurcation
Rosen (Boston Scientific, Quincy, Mass.)	35	150, 180, 260	1.5-mm J-tip	Good trackability Supports advancing catheter
Wholey (Mallinckrodt, St. Louis, Mo.)	35	145, 190, 300	17-cm floppy tip	Steerable tip, stiff core catheterization
Lunderquist-Ring (Cook, Bloomington, Ind.)	38	125	Very stiff	Used through a catheter, flossing, straightening tortuous iliac arteries for endograft delivery
Renal				
TAD (Mallinckrodt, St. Louis, Mo.)	35 tapers to 18 tip	145, 200	36-cm tapered tip Guidewire extension available	Good for crossing a stenosis with little trauma Good trackability with little trauma
TAD II Spartacore (Guidant, Santa Clara, Calif.)	Same as TAD 14	145, 180	20-cm tapered tip Atraumatic tip, 1:1 torquing	Short renal arteries Rigid support Low-profile 14 system

From Moore WS, Ahn SS, editors: Endovascular surgery, ed 3, Philadelphia, 2001, WB Saunders, p 50.
TFE, Tetrafluoroethyl.

in a subintimal plane. One can also perform hand-held contrast agent injection.

Smaller-diameter wires include 0.018- and 0.014-inch wires. These may be useful in renal, carotid, or infrageniculate manipulations. Use of these wires requires use of appropriately sized catheters, balloon angioplasty catheters, and stents. This may necessitate an expanded inventory and some redundancy, however (e.g., 4-mm balloon angioplasty catheters with a 0.018-inch system and different 4-mm balloon catheters with a 0.035-inch system). Small wires are preferable in many instances when the introduction of the lowest-profile balloon catheter is needed. Recent advances in the design of 0.014-inch wires have made their bodies more rigid, allowing for improved trackability. The 0.014-inch system is currently the preferred system for angioplasty and stenting of renal arteries.

Infusion wires have been designed for use during thrombolytic infusion therapy. These wires have a proximal infusion port and a lumen that allows infusion through the distal aspect of the wire. Typically these wires are passed through a multiside hole infusion catheter, such as a Mewissen Infusion Catheter (Boston Scientific, Quincy, Mass.). Using a coaxial system and a Tuohy-Borst adapter (Cook, Bloomington, Ind.), thrombolytic agents can be infused directly into the clot through

the infusion catheter while simultaneously infusing either additional thrombolytic agent or heparin into the distal circulation via the infusion wire.

Catheters

Design

Catheters are made from polyurethane, polyethylene, polypropylene, Teflon, or nylon, with polyurethane catheters having the highest coefficient of friction and Teflon having the lowest. Catheters are sized according to their outer diameter (in French) and their length (in centimeters). Although catheters that have smaller internal diameters are available, most catheters used in angiography will accommodate a 0.035-inch guidewire. The 5-French catheter is most common, but 4- and 6-French catheters are used occasionally. These are matched with appropriately sized sheaths. The most commonly used catheter lengths are 65 and 100 cm.

Functionally, catheters can be either selective or nonselective. Nonselective or flush catheters, which have multiple side and end holes that allow a large cloud of contrast agent to be infused over a short period, are used for large-vessel opacification and in high-flow systems (Figure 17-11). These nonselective catheters can be

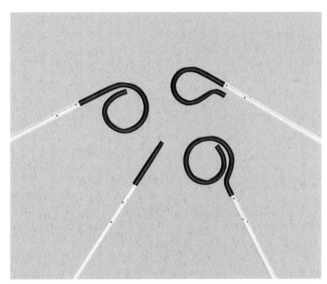

FIGURE 17-11 ■ A variety of nonselective flush catheters. (From Moore WS, Ahn SS, editors: Endovascular surgery, ed 4, Philadelphia, 2011, Saunders, p 65.)

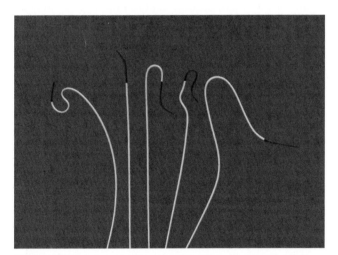

FIGURE 17-12 ■ A variety of selective shaped catheters. (From Moore WS, Ahn SS, editors: Endovascular surgery, ed 4, Philadelphia, 2011, Saunders, p 65.)

TABLE 17-3 Catheter Maximal Flow Rate

Size (French)	Length (cm)	Rate of Contrast Agent (mL/s)
5	65	15
5	100	11
6	65	21
6	100	17

From Moore WS, Ahn SS, editors: Endovascular surgery, ed 3, Philadelphia, 2001, WB Saunders, p 51.

Catheter information, such as maximal flow rate, bursting pressure, inner diameter, outer diameter, and length, is detailed on the package label. The catheter package should be reviewed before being opened; this can reaffirm the catheter's compatibility with the wire and the introducer sheath while visually assessing the shape of the tip relative to the anatomic angles being navigated.

Flow rate (Q) through a catheter varies with its internal radius and is inversely proportional to catheter length. Poiseuille's equation can be used to describe the factors associated with flow through a catheter:

$$Q = \frac{P\pi R^4}{8\eta L}$$

where Q is flow (mL/min), P is the pressure drop (mm Hg) over the length of the catheter, R is the internal radius (mm), η is the viscosity of the fluid, and L is the length of the catheter (mm). Table 17-3 shows the effect of altering radius and length on flow rates for several commonly used catheters.

Selection

Prevention of thrombus formation is desired in any vascular cannulation. There is an increasing likelihood of thrombus formation as catheter size increases with respect to the internal diameter of the vessel lumen. This risk can be minimized by selecting the smallest catheter that will achieve the intended purpose and by removing the catheter as early as possible. Thrombus may also form within a catheter while it is in the lumen of the vessel. Regular aspiration of blood from catheters is recommended before planned injection and flushing with heparinized saline solution once the catheter is found to be free of clot.

The head shape of a catheter determines its function. All catheters, regardless of shape, should be advanced over a wire to limit the potential for intimal injury during advancement and positioning. Nonselective catheters, such as the pigtail catheter, are designed to be used in larger-diameter vessels, such as the aorta. Once the wire has been withdrawn and the curl of the pigtail has been formed in the aorta, the leading edge of the catheter curl offers a relatively blunt profile. As such, these catheters can be carefully advanced or repositioned distally without reinserting the wire. A wire should be reinserted before removing any shaped catheter through the iliac or brachial artery into which it is introduced. This practice

straight or have shaped ends (e.g., Tennis Racquet or pigtail catheters). There are numerous, interchangeable variations of the curled pigtail shape, with subtle modifications of the tightness of the curls.

Selective catheters have only a single hole at the tip and are used to intubate vascular families (branches off the aorta) before advancement of the wire (Figure 17-12). With angiography that includes selective catheterization, smaller amounts of contrast material are used at lower injection rates to obtain adequate arterial opacification. When using selective catheters, care must be taken to avoid intimal injury or dissection of the artery from either direct catheter tip advancement or the forceful injection of contrast material. In addition, a "jet effect" can occur when forceful injection of contrast material pushes the catheter out of the vessel of interest and back into the aorta. Lengthening the "rise of rate" of injection on the power injector control panel can limit these negative effects.

limits the potential for the catheter tip to score and injure the intima as it is removed.

To cannulate the contralateral iliac artery for selective iliac injection, the nonselective flush catheter used for the initial aortogram can often be used. The wire is reinserted and advanced to the tip of the catheter orifice to open the angle of the curl. The catheter is withdrawn to the bifurcation so that the tip engages the orifice of the contralateral iliac artery. The wire is then advanced distally, and the catheter is advanced over the wire. To minimize arterial injury, care should be taken not to advance or withdraw the unfurled pigtail catheter without reintroducing the wire.

For selective cannulation of branches of the aorta, choose a catheter with a head shape that corresponds to the anatomic angle of the branch to be entered. In selective catheterization, the catheter tip itself is manipulated into the orifice of the branch vessel. Injections at lower pressures may be performed after this step; however, for higher-pressure injections, the catheter must be advanced farther into the branch to prevent losing access as a result of catheter whip and recoil. This is accomplished by passing the wire more distally and advancing the catheter over it and into the target vessel.

For arch vessels, start with a vertebral catheter. This catheter has perhaps the most minimally selective design, with a 1-cm tip angled at approximately 30 degrees to the straight access. With practice, however, it is possible to use this catheter for each of the thoracic arch vessels. Alternatively, a number of elaborately designed catheters have been developed to facilitate cannulation of arch vessels. The Headhunter (Balton, Warszawa, Poland) or the Simmons (Terumo, Tokyo, Japan or Balton, Warszawa, Poland) may be appropriate for this task; if these are unsuccessful, the Mani (Merit Medical, Murry, Utah), the Vitek (Cook Medical, Vandergrift, Penn), or the HN4 (Cook Medical, Vandergrift, Penn) can be used.

Most of the more elaborately shaped selective catheters are designed to be reformed in the aortic arch or the abdominal aorta proximal to the vessel that one is attempting to intubate. Once the catheter is reformed into its planned shape, the operator withdraws and rotates the catheter under fluoroscopic guidance until it engages the orifice of the desired branch vessel.

For renal and visceral arteries, a cobra catheter or a Shepherd hook are recommended. The catheter should be advanced above the intended artery and rotated as it is gently pulled inferiorly. This manipulation will result in intubation of the renal or the visceral orifice; its position can be confirmed with a puff of contrast material. Once the orifice of the intended artery has been intubated, a guidewire with a floppy tip is advanced into it distally so that the catheter can then be advanced over the stiffer portion of the wire.

In arteries of the lower extremity, a simple selective straight catheter over a guidewire can be used for selective arteriography. Occasionally, when a guidewire cannot be manipulated across a tight stenosis, the catheter can be advanced to the area of stenosis to support the wire as an additional attempt to cross the lesion is made.

A number of catheters have been designed for specific functions or unusual situations. Catheters with a

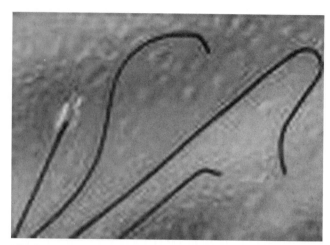

FIGURE 17-13 ■ Terumo Glide catheters. The bottom catheter with the slightly angled head is routinely used to intubate most arch branches. (From Moore WS, Ahn SS, editors: Endovascular surgery, ed 4, Philadelphia, 2011, Saunders, p 66.)

hydrophilic coating, called Glidecaths (Terumo, Tokyo, Japan) or Slip-Caths (Cook, Bloomington, Ind.), may be helpful in crossing tight stenosis (Figure 17-13). For thrombolytic therapy, the Mewissen Infusion Catheter is used in conjunction with Cragg or Katzen wires (Boston Scientific, Quincy, Mass.). When assessing a patient with an aneurysm for the potential use of an aortic endograft, aortography is performed with a 5-French pigtail catheter that is marked with radiopaque markers at 1-cm increments. This allows for the measurement of aortic and iliac segments and aids in the selection of appropriately tailored limbs for the endoprosthesis. In addition, a catheter with radiopaque markings spaced 2.8 cm apart is available. This catheter is useful in obtaining an inferior venacavogram before vena cava filter placement. The 2.8-cm measurement can then be used to determine the transverse diameter of the vena cava and identify those vessels that are too large for standard filter placement.

With the proliferation of accurate noninvasive imaging techniques and the growing acceptance of the appropriateness of endovascular intervention for the treatment of atherosclerotic disease, purely diagnostic angiography is performed infrequently. More commonly, patients undergoing catheterization are candidates for potential intervention in addition to angiographic inspection. As such, catheterizations are performed routinely through introducer sheaths with hemostatic valves. This facilitates the introduction of various endovascular devices while minimizing blood loss and trauma to the artery at the insertion site.

Sheaths

Introducer Sheaths

Once percutaneous access has been obtained and wire access to the blood vessel has been established, the track is dilated gradually with progressively enlarging dilators. Dilators, like catheters, are sized according to their outer diameter (in French). Sheaths, in contradistinction, are sized according to their inner diameter (also in French).

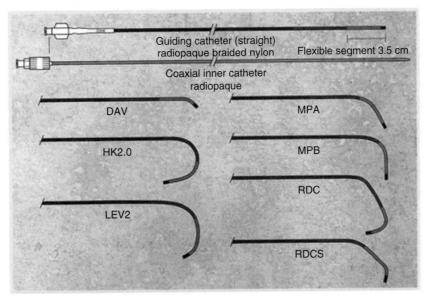

FIGURE 17-14 ■ Guide catheters. Some come with an obturator, sized by outer diameter in French units and length in centimeters do not have a side infusion port. (From Moore WS, Ahn SS, editors: Endovascular surgery, ed 4, Philadelphia, 2011, Saunders, p 67.)

Consequently, if planning to use a 5-French sheath, then sequentially pass 4-, 5-, and 6-French dilators. The final size of the hole in the artery is determined by the outer size of the 5-French sheath, which is just over 6 French. Progressive dilatation causes fewer traumas to the common femoral artery and reduces the potential for iatrogenic injury.

Introducer sheaths all have hemostatic valves and side infusion ports. The side port may be used to monitor pressure or, in some cases, to inject contrast agent and eliminate the need for a catheter. Sheaths come in multiple lengths (measured in centimeters); 15- or 25-cm lengths are most common. A shorter 6-cm sheath is ideally suited for working on arteriovenous grafts or fistulas. These shorter sheaths are adapted for high-volume infusion and may be left in the graft for dialysis after the procedure if the patient requires same-day dialysis. Occasionally, a long 5-French sheath is used to assist with passage of a catheter through a tortuous iliac artery. When planning to perform angioplasty or stenting, the initial 5-French sheath placed for diagnostic angiography is exchanged for a larger-diameter sheath, usually 7 French, through which the interventional devices can be passed. The smallest size sheath required for the planned intervention is recommended.

Guiding Catheters and Guiding Sheaths

Both guiding catheters and guiding sheaths are used to facilitate passage of a smaller catheter or an endovascular device through a tortuous area to a desired treatment location. The larger size of the guiding catheter or the guiding sheath may allow contrast agent injection around the smaller endovascular treatment device while it is in place. For visceral, renal, and carotid artery angioplasty and stenting, use of a guiding catheter or a guiding sheath is preferred. In addition to facilitating passage of the endovascular device, they promote precise positioning by

allowing contrast agent injections around the device, with concomitant maintenance of wire access across the lesion.

Although the terms *guiding catheter* and *guiding sheath* are sometimes used interchangeably, there are differences between them. Guiding catheters are designed with a stronger external reinforcement material, which aids in supporting balloon or catheter passage through long distances in the aorta to branch vessels (Figure 17-14). Unlike guiding sheaths, guiding catheters have no hemostatic valve and require the use of a Tuohy-Borst side-arm adapter. Another important distinction between sheaths and catheters is that guiding sheaths are sized according to their internal diameter, whereas guiding catheters are sized according to their outer diameter (both in French).

Sheaths are packaged with a tapered internal obturator for introduction and advancement into an artery (Figure 17-15). Not all guiding catheters come with internal obturators. The size discrepancy between the internal diameter of the guiding catheter and the wire is usually significant. Advancement of a guiding catheter that is much larger than its wire can be associated with injury to the intima of the artery and an unintentional endarterectomy. To reduce the size mismatch, one can advance a selective catheter over the wire to just beyond the tip of the guiding catheter and then advance both as a unit. It is preferable, however, to use only guiding sheaths and guiding catheters supplied with internal obturators. Both sheaths and catheters are available with radiopaque tips. These are preferred because they allow for accurate identification of the end of the guide in relation to the endovascular device and the lesion being treated.

Guides are available with preformed distal shapes for use in many anatomic scenarios. Use of a hockey stick–shaped catheter that forms a 90-degree angle is useful in the deployment of a renal artery stent. When using a guide to facilitate delivery of a balloon-expandable stent, attempt to advance the guide past the lesion to be stented. If successful, this allows delivery of the stent

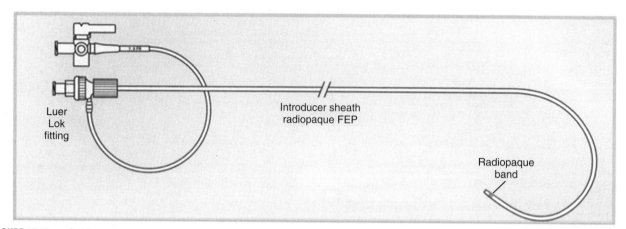

FIGURE 17-15 ■ Guide sheaths. All come with an obturator, sized by inner diameter in French and length in centimeters. Sheaths have an integrated side infusion port. (From Moore WS, Ahn SS, editors: Endovascular surgery, ed 4, Philadelphia, 2011, Saunders, p 68.)

through a protected sleeve, limiting the potential for dislodging the stent from its delivery balloon as it traverses the atherosclerotic lesion. The guide is then withdrawn to the orifice of the involved artery, and contrast material is injected for accurate positioning just before deployment.

The authors have used an externally supported long-shuttle catheter with a straight but malleable tip for angioplasty and stenting of the brachiocephalic vessels. Newer guide sheaths with a variety of tips shaped specifically for accessing the arch vessels and those with hemostatic valves, radiopaque tips, and obturators are currently being developed, which will make carotid angioplasty and stenting less complex.

Guiding sheaths are particularly useful when performing interventions in the contralateral iliac system. In addition to facilitating passage of stents up and over the bifurcation, they protect the ipsilateral iliac artery from the repetitive passage of balloon catheters, diagnostic catheters, and stents. Most important, they allow for intermediate assessment of the results of preliminary angioplasty with pericatheter puff angiography while maintaining wire access across the lesion. If angioplasty of a contralateral iliac artery is performed without a guide sheath, assessment of the results requires removing the balloon catheter and advancing a diagnostic catheter over the wire. The wire must then be removed, and the catheter must be pulled back above the lesion undergoing angioplasty to perform angiography. If it is determined that a stent is required because of suboptimal angioplasty results, it becomes necessary to recross the freshly treated lesion. If the wire does not pass through the center of the lumen but rather tracks through a portion of the fractured plaque, subsequent stenting may prove catastrophic. The use of a guiding sheath is recommended for contralateral iliac endovascular interventions.

When using guiding catheters or guiding sheaths, the operator should note that their diameters are much larger than those of devices used in simple angiographic procedures. The larger the diameter of the introducer, the higher the rate of complications in the iliac and femoral systems. In a smaller patient, the catheter may be of sufficient size to occlude the artery or significantly diminish

flow distal to the insertion site, subjecting the ipsilateral extremity to some degree of ischemia and predisposing to thrombosis. Anticoagulants are administered once these large-diameter devices are in place. Use of these catheters should be limited, and their removal from a vessel should be prompt. With devices of 8 French or larger, percutaneous closure devices may be of benefit.

Summary

There are three rules of endovascular surgery:
1. Once across a lesion with a wire, do not remove it until the case is finished. Unfortunately, wires still get pulled out inadvertently.
2. Read the package. As described in this chapter, sizing methodology for wires, catheters, and sheaths was clearly an afterthought. Wire diameters are in hundredths of an inch, and their lengths are in centimeters; dilators and catheters are described in French by their outer diameters; and sheaths are described in French by their inner diameters with their lengths in centimeters. For guiding sheaths, the inner diameter is in French; for guiding catheters, the outer diameter is in French. Balloon catheters and stents are described by their outer diameter in French in the undeployed state and in millimeters once they are inflated or deployed. The challenge is putting together pieces that fit. Mercifully, all the information needed is on the front of the package for each of these devices. The corollary to this rule is that the package will be found in the trash can.
3. Everything falls on the floor. This is both self-explanatory and prophetic. Be prepared with at least two of everything.

BALLOON ANGIOPLASTY CATHETERS

Role of Balloon Angioplasty in Endovascular Intervention

Endoluminal blood vessel manipulation by means of balloon angioplasty has become a cornerstone of contemporary vascular therapy. The usefulness of balloon angioplasty has increased steadily since 1980, and at present, balloon angioplasty contributes significantly to the management of occlusive disease in most vascular beds. Improvements in technology and catheter-based techniques have broadened the spectrum of lesions that are amenable to percutaneous transluminal angioplasty (PTA). The development of vascular stents has further increased the number of applications for balloon angioplasty.

PTA (with stent placement, as needed) is an essential option in the management of aortoiliac, femoropopliteal, and renovascular occlusive disease.[27] Subclavian, common carotid, and innominate lesions, although less common, have been managed with PTA, with reasonable initial results.[28,29] The results of PTA of the intracranial vasculature and the tibial and pedal vessels are less clear, but there is substantial interest in pursuing these applications.[20,30-32] Balloon angioplasty may be used to treat some lesions within bypass grafts and dialysis grafts. PTA shows promise in the central venous system and represents a potentially significant advance in venous reconstruction. This section presents the concepts, equipment, and techniques that make balloon angioplasty an integral part of contemporary vascular practice.

Structure of Balloon Angioplasty Catheters

Balloon angioplasty is performed using a disposable coaxial catheter selected from among many sizes and types to meet the demands of the particular lesion being treated. The function of a balloon angioplasty catheter is to exert a dilating force on the endoluminal surface of a blood vessel at a desired location. Although a balloon angioplasty catheter is a relatively simple tool, there are multiple variables that must be considered when choosing a catheter for a given situation. These features include balloon diameter and length, catheter size and length, balloon type, and catheter profile (Figure 17-16).

The angioplasty catheter has two lumens: one that permits the catheter to pass over a guidewire during placement, and one to inflate the balloon once it is appropriately placed. Balloon diameters range from 1.5 to 24 mm and are selected with the intent to slightly over-dilate the artery being treated (Table 17-4). Balloon lengths range from 1.5 to 20 cm and should be sufficient to dilate the lesion, with a slight overhang into the adjacent normal arterial segment. Radiopaque markers on the catheter at each end of the balloon permit the operator to place the catheter precisely. The shoulder is the tapered balloon end that extends beyond the radiopaque marker. Because the body of the balloon is always cylindrical, the taper of the shoulder helps define the balloon's overall

TABLE 17-4 Structure and Function of Balloon Angioplasty Catheters

Structure	Function
Balloon diameter	Exert dilating pressure to appropriate diameter on endoluminal surface of blood vessel
Balloon length	Dilate entire length of lesion with slight overhang of balloon onto adjacent artery
Catheter size	Deliver appropriate balloon to lesion on smallest possible catheter
Catheter length	Reach lesion through chosen access site without excessive catheter length
Balloon type based on various materials	Promote use for high-pressure inflation, low-profile catheter passage, stent placement, or scratch resistance
Catheter profile	Determine size of access sheath required
Shoulder	Taper balloon to the catheter shaft and determine inflated shape of balloon
Balloon port	Provide lumen along catheter shaft and into balloon used for inflation
Guidewire port	Provide guidewire lumen for delivery of catheter to its intended site
Radiopaque markers	Mark end of balloon for correct placement

From Moore WS, Ahn SS, editors: Endovascular surgery, ed 3, Philadelphia, 2001, WB Saunders, p 56.

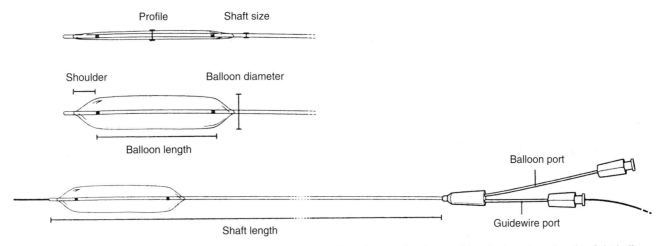

FIGURE 17-16 ■ The balloon angioplasty catheter. The various variables that need to be considered when choosing the right balloon catheter. (From Schneider PA: Endovascular skills, ed 2, New York, 2003, Marcel Dekker, 2003; and Moore WS, Ahn SS, editors: Endovascular surgery, ed 4, Philadelphia, 2001, Saunders, p 72.)

shape when it is fully inflated. A short shoulder is desirable when angioplasty is performed adjacent to an area where dilatation is contraindicated, such as a smaller-diameter branch vessel or an ulcerated or aneurysmal segment. The tip of the catheter, which is the segment that extends beyond the end of the balloon, also varies in length.

The shaft length varies from 40 to 150 cm. The shaft must be long enough to reach from the remote access site to the lesion. In general, the shortest catheter that is able to reach the target site is desirable, because it is less cumbersome and more responsive to manipulation, requires shorter guidewires, and makes exchanges simpler. Angioplasty catheters that pass over a 0.035-inch guidewire are available over a broad range of balloon sizes (3 to 18 mm). Catheter shaft sizes range from 3 to 7 French and are determined by the balloon type and diameter. Standard angioplasty in its most common working range (diameters from 3 to 8 mm) can be performed using 5-French catheters. Larger-diameter balloons or heavy-duty (high-pressure) balloons require larger catheter shafts (5.8 to 7 French). Smaller-diameter balloons (2 to 4 mm) are available on 3.8-French shafts, which pass over 0.014- or 0.018-inch guidewires.

Function of Balloon Angioplasty Catheters

The type of balloon is determined by its material. Standard balloons are constructed of polyethylene, polyethylene terephthalate, or other low-compliance plastic polymers. Burst pressures range from 8 to 12 atmospheres. At higher pressures, low-compliance balloons will exert force without an increase in diameter or the risk of vessel rupture. Thinner-walled balloons are available, which permit a lower profile (discussed later). These are more easily passed through a preocclusive or tortuous lesion, but they are less puncture resistant and are not useful for heavily calcified lesions or stent placement. Reinforced high-pressure polymer balloons, such as the Blue Max (Boston Scientific, Quincy, Mass.), have burst pressures that exceed 17 atm and may be pressurized to more than 20 atm. These balloons have larger shafts (usually by approximately 1 French) than do standard balloons. These thick-walled balloons are useful for treating heavily calcified or sharp lesions and recalcitrant lesions, such as those caused by intimal hyperplasia.

The performance of the catheter can be enhanced by a hydrophilic coating applied by the manufacturer to the balloon surface to permit the balloon to track and cross easily. There are multiple potential applications of this concept of modifying the balloon surface (e.g., antithrombotic therapy and brachytherapy).

The profile of the catheter is the overall diameter of the catheter shaft with the balloon wrapped around it. After a balloon has been inflated, its profile increases in size because the balloon no longer wraps as neatly around the catheter. The used balloon material forms wings, which may be manually rewrapped around the catheter if necessary. The profile of the balloon affects its ability to pass through a lesion. In general, preinflation of the balloon is not performed, because this can make it more difficult to pass the balloon across the lesion. Catheter

profile is the main factor limiting the size of the percutaneous access site and is an important consideration in every angioplasty.

Mechanism of Revascularization with Balloon Angioplasty

Balloon angioplasty causes desquamation of endothelial cells and histologic damage proportional to the diameter of the balloon and the duration of inflation. Longitudinal fracture of the atherosclerotic plaque and stretching of the media and adventitia increase the cross-sectional area of the diseased vessel.[33,34] Plaque compression does not add appreciably to the newly restored luminal diameter.[35] Postangioplasty arteriography almost always reveals areas of dissection and plaque separation caused by PTA. Areas of dissection are seen more frequently with dilatation of calcified lesions. The plaque may become partially separated from the artery wall at the angioplasty site and may remain attached to the proximal and distal arterial walls. Medial dissection occurs at plaque edges or at plaque rupture sites and tends to be somewhat unpredictable.[33,35] The media opposite the plaque becomes thinner. Because most fractures in the plaque are oriented in the direction of flow, there is a relatively low incidence of acute occlusion at the angioplasty site (owing to dissection) or distally (owing to atheroembolization).[27,33] Platelets and fibrin cover the damaged surface, and some endothelialization and surface remodeling soon follow. Follow-up angiography shows that most dissection planes have healed within 1 month.[36]

Mechanism of Balloon Dilatation

The dilating force generated by the balloon is proportional to the balloon diameter, the balloon pressure, and the surface over which the balloon material is applied.[37,38] The dilating force is a result of the hydrostatic pressure within the balloon, the wall tension generated by balloon expansion, and the force vector that results from deformation of the balloon by the lesion.

Hydrostatic pressure is proportional to both the inflation pressure and the endoluminal surface area of the lesion that is dilated by the balloon. At any established level of hydrostatic pressure, wall tension is dependent on Laplace's law and is therefore proportional to the radius of the balloon. This explains why larger balloons are more likely to rupture at a given pressure: the larger radius results in increased wall tension.

Most atherosclerotic lesions require 8 atm of pressure or less for dilatation. When the balloon is inflated, the proximal and distal ends fill first, and the middle section or the body of the balloon, which is usually located at the segment of most severe stenosis, forms a waist (Figure 17-17). This waistlike shape also contributes to the dilating force of the balloon. As the balloon waist is expanded by increasing wall tension, a radial vector force is generated, which is greatest when the waist is tightest. Once the balloon is fully inflated, further inflation to treat a small area of residual stenosis will not contribute to the dilating force, but will increase the likelihood of balloon rupture. For a given stenosis for which there is a choice

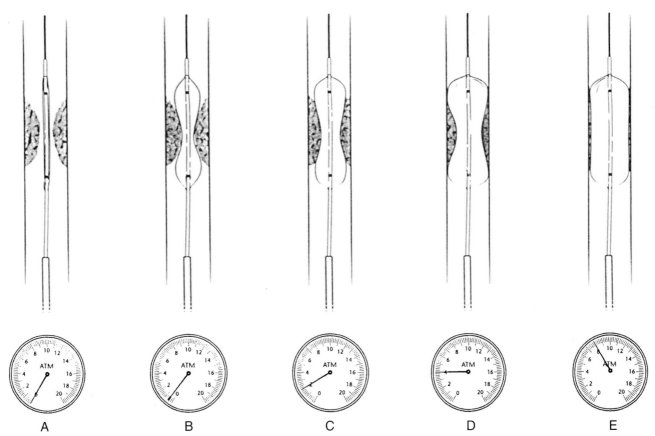

FIGURE 17-17 ■ Dilatation of the atherosclerotic waist. **A,** The balloon catheter is advanced through the lesion. **B,** The proximal and distal ends of the balloon begin to fill at very low pressure. **C,** At 2 atm of pressure, a waist develops where the stenosis caused by the plaque is most severe. **D,** Stenosis remains at 4 atm of pressure as the waist persists. **E,** The waist has been fully dilated. (From Schneider PA: Endovascular skills, ed 2, New York, 2003, Marcel Dekker; and Moore WS, Ahn SS, editors: Endovascular surgery, ed 4, Philadelphia, 2001, Saunders, p 74.)

of possible balloon diameters, a larger balloon will generate a much higher dilating force. The larger diameter increases the wall tension, and the larger balloon size results in a tighter waist at the point of maximal stenosis and a higher radial force vector.

The Perfect Angioplasty Catheter

Balloon angioplasty catheters, like all other catheters, must be pushable and trackable. The balloon material must be durable and resistant to rupture and must permit high pressures (20 atm or more). The compliance of the balloon should be low; once the balloon has reached its intended diameter, further increases in pressure should not be followed by an increase in diameter. The balloon must be scratch resistant, puncture resistant, and reusable and must collapse to the lowest possible profile. The lumen filling the balloon must be large enough to inflate and deflate the balloon in a short time. The catheter must be small enough in caliber to be used safely via standard percutaneous approaches.[18,19]

Present technology does not permit the optimization of all these factors in a single catheter; however, most balloon angioplasty catheters are designed to feature one or more of these strengths. Basic categories of balloons are as follows:

1. A wide variety of lesions that require pressures of 2 to 10 atm and intended diameters of 4 to 10 mm may be treated using standard polyethylene balloons through 5- or 6-French sheaths placed over 0.035-inch guidewires.

2. Small-caliber balloons (1.5 to 4 mm in diameter) are available that can be placed through 4-French sheaths over 0.018-inch guidewires. These catheters confer advantages in specific situations that require small-caliber balloons. Trackability and pushability are poor, however, especially from a very remote puncture site.

3. High-pressure balloons are made of more durable polymer material and may be inflated to pressures in excess of 20 atmospheres. The shaft size is larger (5.8 French or more), and the profile of the thicker balloon material is higher because the wings of the previously expanded balloon material are not completely collapsible. This requires use of a 6-French or larger sheath.

4. Larger-diameter balloons (>10 mm) are available for aortic or central venous angioplasty. Balloons up to 18 mm in diameter are available on 5.8-French shafts; however, the profile of these balloons is high, they require more time to inflate and deflate, and they are often more compliant than is desired.

5. Scratch-resistant balloons have been designed and are being marketed for stent placement. Sharp stent edges can cause balloon rupture. When this occurs during stent placement, it can cause stem embolization or migration.

Current Practice of Balloon Angioplasty

Indications for balloon angioplasty vary significantly from one vascular bed to another.[21,39] Balloon angioplasty plays a role, however, in the management of most vascular occlusive problems. In general, the best candidates for balloon angioplasty are those with less extensive disease or those with medical comorbidities that contraindicate open surgery.[21,39] The lesions that are most amenable to balloon angioplasty are focal stenoses located in large vessels with good runoff.[19,39] Stents have had a significant influence on the feasibility of balloon angioplasty, making it possible to treat more extensive lesions.[22,23]

The advantage of balloon angioplasty is that it permits mechanical intervention with less morbidity than that associated with most open surgical options; however, its use is limited by several factors. Many patients present with disease that is too extensive to be treated with angioplasty. Balloon angioplasty offers limited long-term success in many settings; the patency and durability are less than with surgery. Applications of angioplasty and short- and long-term success are limited in smaller-diameter arteries, especially those less than 5 mm in diameter. The required administration of iodinated contrast agents cannot be tolerated by many patients with renal insufficiency.

Technique of Balloon Angioplasty

Equipment

A wide selection of balloon angioplasty catheters should be readily available to the operator. A facility with trained support staff, an inventory of other endovascular supplies, and satisfactory radiographic imaging capabilities are essential. Supplies that should be opened and placed on the sterile field are listed in Box 17-1.[24-26]

Approach to the Lesion

Before balloon angioplasty, the approach must be planned, based on the location of the lesion, its suitability for angioplasty, and the timing of PTA performance. If the lesion's location and appearance are known as a result of a prior imaging study (e.g., duplex mapping, magnetic resonance angiography, standard arteriography) and it is deemed suitable for angioplasty, the puncture site for vascular access may be chosen accordingly. When arteriography is performed initially and PTA is added to the same procedure, the access site chosen for arteriography may be converted to use for the therapeutic procedure, or a new access site may be selected. The shortest distance that provides adequate working room is usually best. The operator should work forehand for best catheter control (Figure 17-18).

BOX 17-1	Supplies for Balloon Angioplasty

ENDOVASCULAR INVENTORY

- Balloon angioplasty catheters
- Stents
- Access sheaths
- Guidewires
- Angiographic catheters

SUPPLIES for STERILE FIELD

- 4- × 4-inch gauze
- Entry needle
- No. 11 scalpel
- Mosquito clamp
- Iodinated contrast agent
- Lidocaine (local anesthetic agent)
- 10-mL syringe
- 20-mL syringe or larger
- 25-gauge needle
- Inflation device
- Gown
- Gloves, drapes

From Moore WS, Ahn SS, editors: Endovascular surgery, ed 3, Philadelphia, 2001, WB Saunders, p 58.

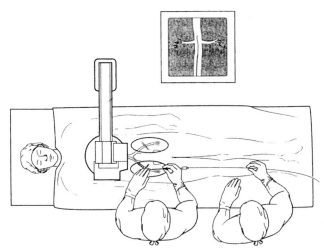

FIGURE 17-18 ■ Working forehand. In this case, the right-handed operator works forehand to manipulate catheters and guidewires. The assistant stands to the side. The fluoroscopic image is observed on the monitor placed on the opposite side of the table. (From Schneider PA: Endovascular skills, ed 2, New York, 2003, Marcel Dekker; and Moore WS, Ahn SS, editors: Endovascular surgery, ed 4, Philadelphia, 2001, Saunders, p 76.)

After the lesion has been identified, it is marked with external markers placed on the field by the observation of bony landmarks or by road-mapping. Arteriography does not usually require a hemostatic access sheath. When an arteriographic procedure is converted to an angioplasty procedure, a sheath is placed to minimize injury to the access vessel. The smallest sheath adequate for the intended balloon catheter is best, because complications increase with increasing French size. Midprocedure sheath changes are cumbersome and inconvenient;

therefore the operator should attempt to place the correct sheath when the decision is made to proceed with PTA. Guidelines for sheath sizing are presented in Table 17-5. The required sheath is selected based on the desired type and diameter of the balloon, the size of the catheter, and the need for a stent.

TABLE 17-5 Sheath Sizing Guidelines for Balloon Angioplasty

Sheath (French)	Balloon Diameter (mm)	Balloon Shaft (French)	Anticipated Procedure
4	2-4	3.8	Small-vessel PTA (0.018-inch guidewire)
5	3-6	5	Infrainguinal, renal, or dialysis graft PTA without stent (0.035-inch guidewire)
6	Up to 8	5	Standard PTA—aortoiliac, infrainguinal, renal, or subclavian
	Up to 7	5	Placement of medium Palmaz stent with low-profile balloon
	Up to 6	5.8	PTA with high-pressure balloon
7	Up to 12	5.8	Aortic PTA
	Up to 8	5.8	PTA with high-pressure balloon
	Up to 9	5	Placement of medium Palmaz stent (4-9 mm) Placement of Wallstent (≤10 mm)
9	Up to 18	5.8	Aortic PTA
	6-8	5	Placement of 8 French guiding catheter for renal, subclavian, or carotid PTA-stent
	8-12	5.8	Placement of large Palmaz stent (up to 12 mm) Placement of large Wallstent (≥12 mm)

From Moore WS, Ahn SS, editors: Endovascular surgery, ed 3, Philadelphia, 2001, WB Saunders, p 59.
PTA, Percutaneous transluminal angioplasty.

The patient is given anticoagulants and if a stent placement is anticipated, antibiotics are administered. The lesion should be crossed with an appropriate guidewire before opening angioplasty catheters or other intervention devices. If the guidewire does not pass easily, the operator may decide on subintimal approach or the use of various catheters to facilitate crossing the lesion with the wire. If there are multiple lesions and the proximal lesion is preocclusive, the operator may need to proceed first with PTA for this lesion.

Balloon Catheter Selection

A slight overdilatation at the angioplasty site is generally recommended. The ranges of balloon sizes available for specific PTA sites are listed in Table 17-6. The diameter of the normal vessel just distal to the lesion is measured to help assess the required balloon diameter (Figure 17-19). Cut film provides a 10% to 20% magnification of the artery, and the diameter of the artery may be taken directly from the radiographic film measurement. Digital subtraction filming requires the use of software measuring packages or the use of catheters with graduated measurement markers for size comparisons. In general, if there is uncertainty about the final desired diameter, it is best to begin with a smaller-diameter balloon and to upsize as needed to avoid overdilatation.

The balloon should be long enough so that there is a short overhang into the adjacent nondiseased arterial segment. If the lesion is lengthy or is juxtaposed to an area where dilatation is contraindicated, it is best to choose a shorter balloon and to dilate the lesion with several sequential balloon inflations. The length of the catheter shaft must be adequate to cover the distance from the access site to the lesion.

Balloon Catheter Placement

The selected balloon catheter is wiped and flushed with heparinized saline solution but is not preinflated. After placement of the correctly sized sheath, the angioplasty catheter is passed over the guidewire, through the sheath,

TABLE 17-6 Selection of Balloon Angioplasty Catheters

Lesion Site	Balloon Diameter (mm)	Balloon Length (cm)	Shaft Length (cm) Femoral Access	Shaft Length (cm) Axillary Access
Common carotid artery	6-8	2 or 4	120	—
Subclavian artery	6-8	2 or 4	120	75
Axillary artery	5-7	2 or 4	120	30
Renal artery	5-7	2 or 4	75	75
Aorta	8-18	4	75	—
Common iliac artery	6-10	2, 4, or 6	75*	120
External iliac artery	6-8	2, 4, or 6	75*	120
Superficial femoral artery	4-7	2, 4, 6, or 10	75†	120
Popliteal artery	3-6	2, 4, or 6	75†	120‡
Infrageniculate artery	2-4	2 or 4	75†	120‡

From Moore WS, Ahn SS, editors: Endovascular surgery, ed 3, Philadelphia, 2001, WB Saunders, p 60.
*Approaching these lesions via a contralateral femoral access site usually requires a 75-cm catheter.
†Approaching these lesions via a contralateral femoral access site usually requires a 120-cm catheter and occasionally may require a 150-cm catheter.
‡May occasionally require a 150-cm catheter.

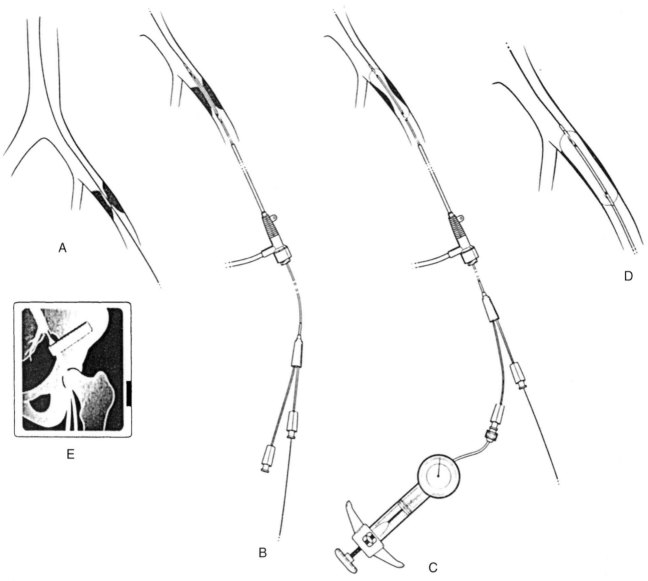

FIGURE 17-19 ■ Balloon angioplasty. **A,** The left external iliac artery stenosis is to be treated. A guidewire is placed across the lesion. **B,** The diameter of the balloon is selected. The diameter may be determined by measuring the diameter of the adjacent uninvolved artery, either by measuring cut film images directly or, if using digital subtraction imaging, by comparing with a known standard such as a catheter with graduated markers. **C,** The angioplasty catheter is passed over the guidewire, through the access sheath, and across the stenosis. **D,** The balloon is inflated by using the inflation device. **E,** The fully dilated shape of the balloon is confirmed by using fluoroscopy. (From Schneider PA: Endovascular skills, ed 2, New York, 2003, Marcel Dekker; and Moore WS, Ahn SS, editors: Endovascular surgery, ed 4, Philadelphia, 2001, Saunders, p 77.)

and into the lesion. The catheter should pass easily through the sheath because the balloon has not yet been inflated. The balloon catheter should track along the guidewire and advance across the lesion using predetermined markers of the lesion's location. The balloon is centered so that its body dilates the portion of the lesion with the most critical stenosis. This is where the force vector will contribute substantially to the dilating force.

The balloon material may break by snagging on a protruding calcific lesion or a previously placed stent. If this is a concern, a longer sheath can be used to deliver the balloon to the lesion. If the balloon catheter will not track along the guidewire, this may be due

to distance, lack of shaft strength, tortuosity, or even subintimal guidewire positioning. If this occurs, consider a stiffer guidewire or a longer sheath.

Occasionally, the lesion itself may be so tight that the balloon catheter cannot be advanced across it. If the balloon will cross the lesion only partially, do not start angioplasty. Withdraw the PTA catheter, and confirm guidewire positioning. Consider (1) adequate anticoagulation, (2) "Dottering" the lesion by advancing a van Andel graduated-tip catheter or a straight 5-French angiographic catheter across the lesion, (3) predilatation with a smaller-diameter (lower profile) balloon, or (4) a balloon with a hydrophilic coating.

Balloon Inflation

After catheter placement, the balloon is inflated without delay to avoid thrombus formation. The balloon is inflated using a 50% contrast agent solution so that the outline of the balloon is visible under fluoroscopy. This permits the operator to observe the location and severity of the atherosclerotic waist as it is being dilated. Solution is forced into the balloon using an inflation device, which also measures the pressure required to dilate the lesion.

The balloon is usually inflated for 30 to 60 seconds, deflated, and then reinflated for another 30 to 60 seconds. A spot film of the inflated balloon is often obtained to document its full expansion. After complete deflation of the balloon, but before moving the catheter, fluoroscopy is used to visualize the balloon and ensure that it is fully deflated. Partially flared balloon wings can disrupt fractured atherosclerotic plaque or damage the tip of the access sheath on withdrawal. During removal of the balloon catheter, the guidewire must be maintained in place across the lesion.

Completion Arteriography

After the balloon catheter is removed, completion arteriography is performed to evaluate the results of PTA. This is usually done through the same access site used for balloon angioplasty. The guidewire may be exchanged for an angiographic catheter, which is placed upstream from the lesion. If the tip of the sheath is in proximity to the lesion, contrast material may be injected through the side arm of the sheath to obtain an arteriogram. Occasionally, it is necessary to perform a second puncture to obtain access for completion arteriography.

When completion arteriography shows a widely patent PTA site without residual stenosis or significant dissection, the procedure is complete. When residual stenosis or dissection are present, its significance may be evaluated using adjunctive means of assessment (Table 17-7). Inadequate angioplasty results can be treated with stent placement.[22,23]

Complications of Balloon Angioplasty

The balloon angioplasty procedure is less likely to result in complications when the catheters are handled with excellent technique. Advice about the use of balloon catheters is presented in Box 17-2.

The tremendous advantage of PTA is that the incidence and severity of complications are generally low. Because the durability is not as good as with surgical reconstruction, PTA is useful only when complication rates are acceptable. Patients with extensive disease (category 3 or 4 lesions) are poor candidates for endovascular intervention and have a high chance of experiencing complications if it is attempted.[39] Complications can occur at the access site, at the PTA site, in the runoff, or systemically. Systemic complications and some access site complications may occur with arteriography alone. The total complication rate should be less than 10%, and the rate of serious complications (or those

TABLE 17-7	Assessing the Results of Balloon Angioplasty
Method	**Comments**
Completion arteriography	Only method required in most cases; usually performed in projection used for PTA (anteroposterior)
Oblique views	Useful in assessing posterior wall residual stenosis or postangioplasty dissection
Magnified views	Evaluation for dissection flaps or contrast trapping in arterial wall
Pressure measurement in small-diameter artery	Only quantitative hemodynamic assessment available; time-consuming; results variable; catheter placement across lesion may affect
Vasodilator use	Adjunct to pressure measurement when there is no gradient despite the appearance of substantial lesion
Intravascular ultrasonography	Expensive; particularly effective in finding and measuring diameter of residual stenosis

From Moore WS, Ahn SS, editors: Endovascular surgery, ed 3, Philadelphia, 2001, WB Saunders, p 61.
PTA, Percutaneous transluminal angioplasty.

requiring operative intervention) should be less than 5% (Table 17-8).[19,21,39]

STENTS

Stents were developed to buttress open a vascular lumen, and to overcome limitations of elastic recoil and dissection after angioplasty. Today, various stents have been developed and approved for the treatment of different vascular beds. These vascular beds include the thoracoabdominal aorta, carotid, renal, iliac, and the superficial femoral arteries. Early stents were made of various metals with different mechanical properties. With innovative technology and development, currently available stents include covered stents, covered stents with heparin-bonding on the luminal surface, and stents with thermal memory. New stents that will be available soon in the United States for use in the treatment of peripheral vascular disease include the drug-eluting and biodegradable stents. In the following sections, various types of stents along with their approved uses will be described.

Mechanical Properties

Stents are made of various metals that include stainless steel, nitinol, platinum, and various metal alloys. Various construction methods include etched, laser-cut, coiled, woven, or knitted. The combination of different metals and construction methods allow for various stents to have different radial strength, hoop strength, flexibility, trackability, pushability, and radiopacity. The radial strength is the ability of a stent to obliterate the luminal stenosis or occlusion of a diseased arterial or venous segment. The hoop strength is the ability of a stent to resist radial

TABLE 17-8 **Complications of Balloon Angioplasty**

Systemic	Puncture Site	PTA Site	Runoff
Renal failure	Hemorrhage	Dissection	Embolization
Fluid overload	AV fistula	Residual stenosis	Thrombosis
Contrast agent allergy	Hematoma	Thrombosis	Spasm
	Ecchymosis	Rupture	
	Pseudoaneurysm		
	Thrombosis		

From Moore WS, Ahn SS, editors: Endovascular surgery, ed 3, Philadelphia, 2001, WB Saunders, p 62.
PTA, Percutaneous transluminal angioplasty; *AV*, arteriovenous.

BOX 17-2 | **Handling Balloon Catheters**

- Pick catheters before the case to save time and ensure that you have what you need.
- Flush and wipe catheter with heparinized saline solution to decrease thrombogenicity.
- Keep profile of catheter low by avoiding preinflation.
- Check catheter size before placement to avoid unintended overdilatation.
- When correct catheter shaft length is unclear, measure outside the body with angiographic catheter of known length for a quick estimation.
- When best arterial diameter is unclear, underestimate to avoid overdilatation.
- Be sure the guidewire is intraluminal before advancing and inflating balloon catheter.
- Push catheter from the tip when entering the hub of the access sheath to avoid kinking the guidewire and catheter.
- Have some options when the catheter will not advance along the guidewire (see text discussion).
- Be ready to inflate as soon as the balloon crosses the lesion.
- Magnify field of view at the PTA site if necessary to ensure correct balloon position.
- Know what to do next when catheter will not advance through lesion (see text discussion).
- Deflate balloon by aspirating with a large syringe before withdrawal of catheter.
- Rotate catheter to fold its wings before pulling it into the sheath.
- Use fluoroscopy during inflation to confirm the location and severity of the lesion.
- Take a spot film of expanded balloon after complete inflation for documentation and size comparisons.
- Maintain guidewire across the lesion until completion study is satisfactory.
- If balloon bursts, inflate rapidly until it will no longer hold pressure, then exchange it for a new balloon.
- If there is evidence of arterial rupture, reinflate balloon at same location to tamponade.

From Moore WS, Ahn SS, editors: Endovascular surgery, ed 3, Philadelphia, 2001, WB Saunders, p 62.
PTA, Percutaneous transluminal angioplasty.

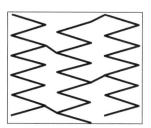
Periodic peak-peak, non-flex connectors e.g., Cordis – Precise

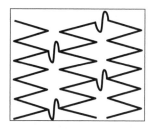
Periodic peak-peak, flex connectors e.g., Optimed – Sinus 5F

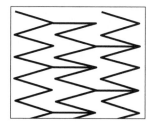
Periodic peak-valley non-flex connectors e.g., Cook – Zilver

FIGURE 17-20 ■ Open cell design. (From Houdart, Cirse 2005 September 10-14, 2005, Nicer, Acropolis.)

compression by external forces. If the external force is excessive, the stent may become crushed or kinked. Flexibility of a stent is the force required to bend it, and a flexible stent is able to reach a distal target lesion after navigating through tortuous proximal vessels. Trackability is the ability of a stent to track over a wire with its delivery system, whereas pushability is the force required to push the delivery system containing the stent over the wire through a vascular system. Radiopacity is the visibility of a stent and depends on the amount of aluminum to make it invisible on fluoroscopy.

The characteristics of stents also differ in terms of thickness, durability, resistance to corrosion, and the amount of open-area–to-metal surface ratio. The *open-area–to-metal surface ratio* refers to the area between the metal rings of the stent that is not covered by the stent itself. In stents with open cell design, the rings of the stents are connected by bridges (Figure 17-20). The surface area between the rings is larger, ranging from approximately 5.8 to 11.5 mm^2. In closed cell stents, the

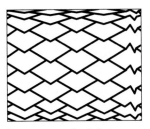
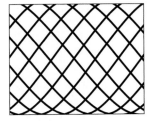

One-to-one cell relation
e.g., Abbott – Xact
Boston Scientific – NexStent

One-to-one cell relation
e.g., Boston Scientific – Wallstent

FIGURE 17-21 ■ Closed cell design. (From Houdart, Cirse 2005.)

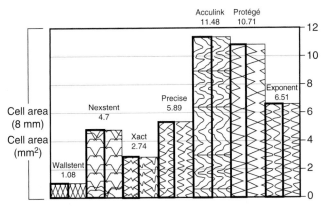

FIGURE 17-22 ■ Comparison of free cell area. (From Houdart, Cirse 2005.)

Comparison of free cell area

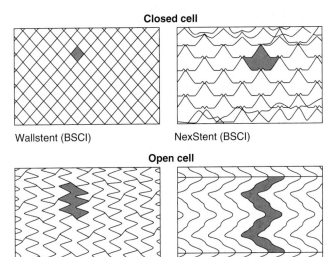

FIGURE 17-23 ■ Treatment with closed cell stent to minimize embolization from the vascular lesion. (From Houdart, Cirse 2005.)

rings are braided or the laser cut (Figure 17-21). The area between the ring is decreased, ranging from 1.1 to 4.7 mm^2 (Figure 17-22). For lesions in which the risk of embolization needs to be minimized, stents with closed cell design should be used (Figure 17-23).

These various properties and characteristics affect the result and biocompatibility of stents in the arterial or venous systems. The ideal stent has high radial and hoop strength to resist recoil, is flexible to navigate tortuosity, is trackable and pushable to easily reach the target lesion, and has high radiopacity for visualization. This stent also has low profile and high expansion ratio, easy deployment system, and minimal foreshortening for accurate placement. After placement, the stent is crush resistant, stimulates minimal intimal hyperplasia or in-stent restenosis for durability, is compatible with magnetic resonance, and has low cost.

Classification

Stents are classified into two main groups: the balloon-expanded stents and self-expanded stents. In balloon-expanded stents, the stents are premounted on a balloon catheter and deployed with inflation of the balloon. The prototypical example is the Palmaz stent (Cordis Endovascular, Warren, N.J.). In self-expanded stents, the stents spring open when they are uncovered by a sheath, the prototypical of which is the Wallstent (Boston Scientific Vascular, Natick, Mass.). Most of

these stents are made of nickel-titanium alloys that take advantage of their thermal memory to expand to their predetermined size and shape when warmed to body temperature.

Balloon-Expanded Stents

The balloon-expanded stents are premounted on a balloon catheter prior to insertion. Using this angioplasty catheter, the stent is delivered to the target lesion and expanded with inflation of the balloon. If needed, balloon-expanded stents can be oversized by reinflation with a larger balloon; this differs from the self-expanded stents, which can open only to its predetermined diameter based on the thermal memory of the nitinol characteristics. Compared to the self-expanded stents, balloon-expanded stents have a higher radial and hoop strength, but less flexibility. It has the theoretical advantage of better results in the treatment of heavily calcified lesions that can recoil.

The prototypical Palmaz Stent (Cordis Endovascular) is a rigid stent configured with staggered rows of rectangular slots circumferentially etched out of its wall (Figure 17-24). It is laser cut from a single tube of malleable stainless steel. These stents can be expanded to a larger diameter, but will foreshorten to a certain degree. These stents have been approved by the U.S. Food and Drug Administration (FDA) for the treatment of iliac and renal arterial diseases. The large Palmaz stents have diameters ranging from 8 to 12 mm with lengths as long as 30 mm. They have the flexibility to go up and over the aortic bifurcation to treat contralateral iliac arterial lesions. The medium Palmaz stents have diameters ranging from 4 to 9 mm with lengths as long as 39 mm. These stents are ideal for treatment of renal ostial lesions in the calcified aortic wall.

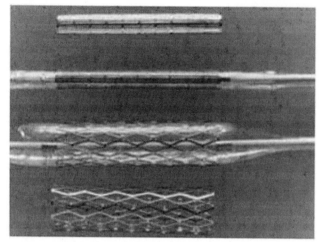

FIGURE 17-24 ■ Palmaz stent (Cordis Endovascular, Warren, N.J.).

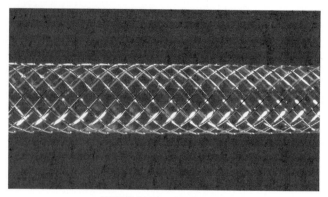

FIGURE 17-25 ■ Wallstent.

Other balloon-expanded stents available in the market include; the Omnilink Stent, RX Herculink Elite Stent, and RX Herculink Plus Stent by Abbott Vascular (Abbot Park, Ill.); Omniflex Stent (AngioDynamics, Queensbury, N.Y.); Valeo Stents (Bard Peripheral Vascular, Tempe, Ariz.); Express LD Stent and Liberte Stent (Boston Scientific Vascular); Formula 418 Stent (Cook Medical, Bloomington, Ind.); Visi-Pro Stent and ParaMount Stent (ev3 Endovascular, Plymouth, Minn.); and Bridge Assurant Stent, Driver Stent, and Racer Stent (Medtronic, Santa Rosa, Calif.). Materials for these stents include stainless steel, platinum, and cobalt-chromium alloy. The balloon catheters use either the over-wire or rapid exchange (monorail) system. These balloon catheters also have different series that are compatible with 0.035-, 0.018-, or 0.014-inch wires.

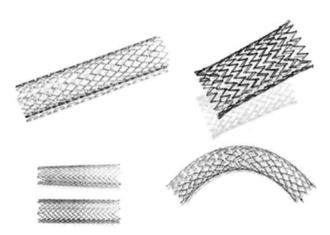

FIGURE 17-26 ■ Nitinol stents with thermal memory.

Self-Expanded Stents

The self-expanded stents are made of stainless steel and compressed within a delivery catheter covered by a sheath. The stent is delivered to the vascular lesion using this catheter, which also holds the stent in position as the outer sheath is withdrawn. As the stent is uncovered, it springs open and expands to its predetermined diameter. These stents are highly flexible, but have less hoop strength compared with balloon-expanded stents.

The prototypical Wallstent (Boston Scientific) is a flexible tubular stent with woven mesh design. The separate wires are able to move freely at their interconnections (Figure 17-25). This flexibility allows the stent to navigate across the aortic bifurcation and be placed in tortuous vessels. The wires are made of thin Elgiloy stainless steel combining cobalt, chromium, nickel, and other metals. The platinum core in the struts allows for radiopacity and visibility, and the low iron content makes the stent compatible with magnetic resonance imaging. The Wallstent is approved for treatment of iliac arterial disease. It has a diameter ranging from 5 to 24 mm and a length of 18 to 94 mm. During stenting, the size of the stent is chosen based on the diameter of the vessel and the length of the lesion. The stent diameter should be oversized by approximately 1 mm relative to the vessel. Shortening of the stent needs to be considered when selecting the length. To deploy the stent, the outer sheath is withdrawn while the stent is held in position with the deliver catheter. During deployment, the stent can be pulled back if it is too distal to the lesion. However, the stent cannot be advanced because the diverging struts will catch and injure the vessel wall.

A subgroup of self-expanded stents is a variety of stents with thermal memory (Figure 17-26). These stents are made of nitinol, a nickel-titanium alloy containing 50% to 55% nickel and 45% to 50% titanium. At approximately 1000°F (538°C, the alloy forms and sets the memory of the stent shape. There is a transition temperature at which the stent will recover its memory and return to its predetermined shape. This temperature is usually 90°F for nitinol stents. Below this temperature, the stent is more pliable. After deployment across the vascular lesion, the stent warms up and returns to its predetermined shape.

A variety of nitinol stents have been approved for intravascular use in the United States and include: Xceed Stent, Absolute Sent, and Xpert Stent (Abbott Vascular); Luminexx Stent and LifeStent Flexstar Stent

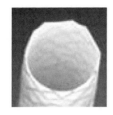

Film-Cast Encapsulation

iCast struts are completely embedded in Advanta™ PTFE during and after deployment.

FIGURE 17-27 ■ iCast Covered Stent (Atrium Medical, Hudson, N.H.).

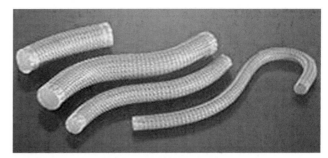

FIGURE 17-28 ■ Viabahn-covered stent (W.L. Gore and Associates, Flagstaff, Ariz.).

(Bard Peripheral Vascular); Sentinol Stent (Boston Scientific Vascular); Zilver Stent (Cook Medical); SMART Stent (Cordis Endovascular); and Complete SE Stent (Medtronic). The delivery system is compatible with 0.035- or 0.018-inch wire.

A subgroup of nitinol stents are designed for the treatment of carotid stents. These self-expanded stents are straight or tapered in shape. The stents are small in profile and use a small delivery system over 0.014-in wire. Most stents have closed-cell design to minimize embolization risk after stent placement. The high coverage of lesion by the stent traps the atherosclerotic plaque outside, minimizing protrusion of plaque between the rings and embolization to the brain. Most stents use the rapid exchange delivery system.

Covered Stent

Balloon-Expanded Stent Grafts

The iCast Covered Stent (Atrium Medical, Hudson, N.H.) is a laser-cut, stainless-steel stent with an encapsulated cover of expanded polytetrafluoroethylene (ePTFE; Figure 17-27). It has a 6/7-French profile on a delivery system that is compatible with 0.035-in wire. The stent has high deployment accuracy with a low foreshortening design. This stent is currently approved by the FDA for the treatment of tracheobronchial stricture caused by malignant neoplasms.

Self-Expanding Stent Grafts

The Viabahn Endoprosthesis (W.L. Gore and Associates, Flagstaff, Ariz.) is a self-expanding, stent graft made of an ePTFE lining with an external nitinol stent (exoskeleton; Figure 17-28). This exoskeleton is made from a single strand of nitinol wire formed into a sinusoidal shape and wound in helical fashion around the polytetrafluoroethylene (PTFE) tube. The luminal surface of the PTFE is covalently bonded to bioactive heparin. The 5- to 13-mm stent grafts are approved for use in the iliac arteries, and the 5 to 8 mm stents are approved for use in the superficial femoral arteries. The length of the stents ranges from 25 to 150 mm. The introducer sheath sizes range from 6 to 12 French, and is compatible with 0.018- or 0.035-inch wires. For treatment of occlusive lesions, the lesion should be predilated. The stent should

be 5% to 20% larger than the healthy native vessel diameter and overlap the proximal and distal margins of the lesion by 1 cm. If more than one stent is needed, there should be at least 1 cm of overlap between the stents. If different diameter stents are needed, the size should not differ by 2 mm, with the larger stent placed after and within the smaller stent. Post-stenting angioplasty is performed to the size of native vessels.

The Flair Endovascular Stent Graft (Bard Peripheral Vascular) is a flexible, self-expanding endoprosthesis composed of a nitinol framework encapsulated within two layers of ePTFE. The inner, luminal layer is carbon impregnated. It is approved for treatment of stenosis at the venous anastomosis of ePTFE or other synthetic arteriovenous graft used for dialysis. It is available in diameters ranging from 6 to 9 mm. It uses a 9-French sheath over a 0.035-in wire. It is a stent graft that can be used in the management of failing dialysis access grafts for management of pseudoaneurysms and venous outflow stenoses.

The Future

Drug-Eluting

In-stent restenosis caused by intimal hyperplasia can limit the efficacy and patency of endovascular angioplasty and stenting. Sirolimus (a natural macrocyclic lactone) and paclitaxel (a cytotoxic agent) are immunosuppressive and antiproliferative that can limit neointimal growth by the vascular smooth muscle cells. Stents can be sprayed or impregnated with these drugs to prevent restenosis.[40] Many multicenter randomized trials have shown that drug-eluting stents are safe and effective after coronary intervention in preventing restenosis.[41,42] However, the efficacy of these stents in the treatment of peripheral vascular disease is still under investigation. For the treatment of SFA diseases, the SIROCCO I and II (Sirolimus-Coated Cordis Self-Expandable Stent) studies randomized patients to either the Smart nitinol bare stent (Cordis) or Sirolimus-coated Smart stent. At 2 years, SIROCCO II did not show any significant difference in in-stent restenosis rate between the two stents. However, the results were better for the paclitaxel-coated Zilver PTX stent (Cook) compared with bare Zilver PTX stents in both the randomized prospective trial and the registry.

The Cypher stent (Cordis) is the only drug-eluting stent with below the knee indication such as the tibial arteries. Experience with this stent using sirolimus is still limited.[43] However, several single-center cohort studies seem to show better results in terms of short to midterm patency and clinical outcome. Currently, there are several ongoing randomized, multicenter studies comparing either sirolimus or paclitaxel-eluting stents with bare stents in the infrapopliteal lesions. Only time will tell if there is any advantage in using these drug-eluting stents in the treatment of peripheral arterial disease.

Biodegradable Stents

Drug-eluting stents have been shown to be effective in limiting in-stent restenosis by intimal hyperplasia after percutaneous coronary intervention. However, there is delayed healing of the stented arterial segment with the presence of the permanent metal stents. Biodegradable stents were developed to enhance vascular wall healing and the return of vascular function.[44] Drug-eluting stents made with biodegradable polymer offer the advantage of controlled elution of the active drug.[45] When the function of the drug is over, the stent polymer degrades to inert organic monomers, eliminating any potential long-term adverse effect on the vascular wall by the permanent metal stents (Figure 17-29, see color plate). Drugs used include sirolimus, next generation everolimus, and paclitaxel. Current ongoing trials are limited to coronary interventions.[45] Recent results at 2 and 3 years did not show any difference between drug-eluting biodegradable polymers and drug-eluting metal stents.[46,47] More research is needed to find the best possible combination of drug and biodegradable polymer to provide the optimal clinical outcome.

Procedural Complications

Dissection

Dissection is arterial wall injury caused by inadvertent vessel wall entry by the wires, needles, or catheter during passage through blood vessels. There are two types of dissections determined by the site of wall entry. The first type occurs at the arterial access site and is caused by incomplete entry of the needle into the arterial lumen. Placement of a guidewire leads to passage of the wire in the intramural layer with resulting subintimal dissection. This can be suspected when there is resistance during passage of the wire or catheter. Dissection can be confirmed with hand injection of 3 to 5 mL of contrast that remains in the arterial wall and does not washout. If identified early, this type of dissection is often self limiting and can be addressed by removing the needle, wire, or sheath and changing the access site.

The second type is caused by iatrogenic subintimal dissection during passage of wire or catheter at sites remote from the access site. The iliac or superficial femoral arteries may be diseased from atherosclerosis, and wire may dissect into a subintimal plan. Similar to the first type of dissection, suspicion is raised when there is resistance during passage of guidewires followed by

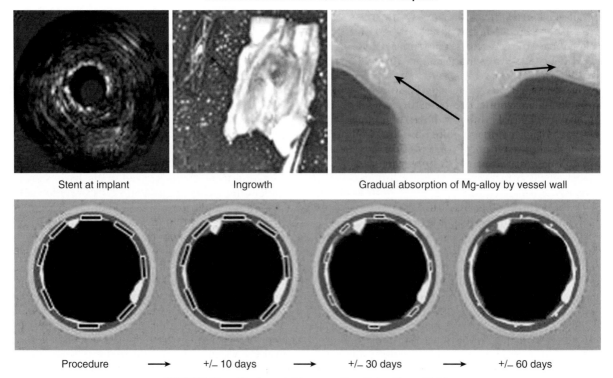

Quick Endotheliazation and Gradual Absorption

Stent at implant   Ingrowth   Gradual absorption of Mg-alloy by vessel wall

Procedure   →   +/− 10 days   →   +/− 30 days   →   +/− 60 days

FIGURE 17-29 ■ Biodegradable stent. See Color Plate 17-29.

lack of blood return through the catheter. Diagnosis is again confirmed by contrast injection. This is treated by pulling back the guidewire and catheter, and the lesion is crossed in the true lumen.

Short retrograde dissections are usually benign without serious consequences. The antegrade direction of the blood flow pushes the flap against the vessel wall without the need for further therapy. Antegrade dissections are potentially more difficult to resolve. The direction of blood flow may cause exacerbate the dissection and compromise the lumen. Occlusions or distal vascular compromise may require endovascular stent placement from the contralateral side or immediate surgical thrombectomy.

Arterial Perforation

Perforation or rupture of an artery during endovascular therapy is an uncommon but known risk. This can occur at the access site or remotely and may be associated with passage of a wire or catheter tip beyond the target or through a smaller side branch. Visualization while advancing wires, catheters, and devices is important to minimize this complication. Overdilation with poorly sized balloons can also result in focal perforations.

With the development of endografts for the treatment of thoracic and abdominal aortic diseases, the catheters are larger to accommodate for the size of the endograft. This can cause perforation or rupture of the smaller, calcified, and tortuous femoral or iliac arteries during passage of these catheters. This complication is usually not apparent while the catheter is in place. When the catheter is removed, the tamponade effect is lost and the bleeding becomes evident.

Arterial perforation is suspected when there is persistent bleeding around the vascular sheath or when there is acute pain during manipulation of guidewire or catheter. Most arterial perforations from guidewires resolve spontaneously without significant blood loss. Small arterial injuries may be repaired endovascularly with prolonged balloon inflation, stent grafting, or embolization. Endovascular intervention might not be possible in larger arterial injury with severe bleeding, leading to hypotension, shock, and life-threatening complications. Bleeding can be controlled by inflating a balloon to tamponade the vessel proximal to the injury. Open surgical exploration with immediate repair is then performed using primary closure, patches, or grafts as appropriate.

Endovascular devices should always be advanced without significant resistance. Wires, catheters, and devices should be advanced only under direct fluoroscopic visualization. Adherence to these tenants will limit the risk of perforation or arterial injury.

Embolization

With endovascular device manipulation against an occluded or severe atherosclerotic segment, distal embolization may occur from dislodged arterial mural thrombus or plaque. Thrombus may also form on these devices or within the sheath and be dislodged with flushing. It is possible that many small embolic events go unnoticed

and do not result in adverse clinical events. However, it has been documented that stroke is a complication of catheter manipulation in an atheromatous aortic arch and wire passage across an internal carotid plaque. Manipulation with endovascular devices should, therefore, be minimized in any vascular bed to prevent embolic complications. Acute vascular compromise requires immediate intervention with catheter-directed thrombolysis or surgical embolectomy.

A rare but serious complication is cholesterol embolization from manipulation of devices against a heavily diseased aortic wall. These cholesterol plaques enter the visceral and peripheral arterial circulation and can result in visceral ischemia, renal failure, and cutaneous necrosis. Symptoms and signs usually present later and are not immediately obvious at the conclusion of the procedure. Patients may have abdominal pain and develop the characteristic livedo reticularis rash. Treatment is mainly supportive with heparinization and fluid resuscitation. Outcomes range from mild to severe.[48,49]

Postprocedure Complications

Device Infection

Infection of endovascular devices is rare, ranging from 0.4% to 0.6%.[50-52] Similar to vascular grafts, most common causes of stent infections are *Staphylococcus aureus* and coagulase-negative staphylococci.[51-53] Infection by *S. aureus* is usually more acute than coagulase-negative staphylococci, and can be as high as 54.5% of cases.[52,53] Device infection probably occurs by either infection at the time of implantation or hematogenous spread by bacteremia.

The diagnosis of graft infection can be difficult because signs and symptoms may be nonspecific. There may be swelling, erythema, pain, and vascular compromise of the ipsilateral limb. Patients with aortic graft infection usually have abdominal discomfort. Infections at the groin can result in sinus tracts, bleeding, or distal embolism. Severe infection can result in multisystem organ failure with sepsis, renal insufficiency, and adult respiratory distress syndrome.

Detection of device infection can be made with various diagnostic modalities that are available. In a study for aortic graft infection, a comparison of these modalities showed an accuracy of 93% for isotopic study with labeled white blood cells, 75% for computed tomography, 50% for endoscopic investigation of aorto-enteric fistulae, and 35.5% for ultrasonography.[54] Presence of perigraft fluid beyond 3 months after surgery is suggestive of infection.[53] Blood cultures should also be obtained.

Individualized treatment is needed for device infections. Aggressive antimicrobial therapy is initiated, but surgery is usually required. Surgical treatment involves stent graft removal and distal revascularization with either in situ or extraanatomic bypass. Infection of bare metal stents has also been reported. Stent infection can result in septic arteritis within the wall of the artery and can lead to pseudoaneurysm formation and vessel rupture.[55,56]

Restenosis and Occlusion

Immediate compromise of the arterial lumen of the vessels intended for treatment or nearby vessels can result from thrombosis, dissection, or poor stent location. For example, arterial occlusion during renal stenting can result from dissection. Similarly, stroke can result from dissection during carotid stenting. In endovascular aneurysm repair of aortic aneurysms, graft placement can result in paralysis by placing the stent graft across arteries providing important direct or collateral flow to the spinal cord. In stenting of abdominal aortas, coverage of renal arteries by proximal stent graft leads to renal failure. Distally, coverage of the inferior mesenteric artery or hypogastric arteries may cause ischemia of the colon.

Restenosis by intimal hyperplasia at the lesion is a late complication after endovascular interventions, and can lead to adverse clinical problems in vascular beds such as the coronary and renal arteries. In renal artery interventions, the rate of restenosis can be as high as 20%.[57,58] After peripheral vascular interventions, there is arterial modeling and induced systemic inflammatory response, as measured by a significantly increased postprocedure level of C-reactive protein.[59] This response may be responsible for early restenosis and was shown to be an independent predictor of 6-month restenosis.[60] The inflammatory response induced can be different in various vascular beds. There was more extensive response in muscular femoropopliteal artery than in elastic iliac and carotid arteries and was independent of lesion morphology and interventional factors.[61] The role of adhesion molecules such as vascular adhesion molecule-1 (VCAM-1), and P-selectin has also been implicated in restenosis.[61,62]

The treatment of restenosis must be individualized. Some restenosis is amendable to repeated endovascular interventions such as angioplasty, atherectomy, and stent placement. Otherwise, surgery with vascular bypass may be needed to reestablish blood flow.

Graft Migration

Graft migration is generally rare, but is a time-dependent phenomenon that increases with time. With the expanded use of endografts in the repair of abdominal aortic aneurysms, migration can range from 10% to 15% over a 30 month follow-up.[63,64] Factors to consider include proximal and distal fixation, device oversizing, length of neck, and neck overlapping. In proximal fixation, predictors of endograft migration were length of proximal fixation and the distance between the renal artery and the stent graft. Factors that were not predictors included preimplantation aortic neck length, neck diameter, degree of device oversizing, device type, placement of proximal extender cuffs, and postprocedure endoleak.[65] Similarly, distal fixation has been shown to be important in the prevention of migration. Patients with greater iliac fixation lengths and shorter distance to the iliac bifurcation had less migration. Good iliac fixation did not result in stent migration, even in the presence of suboptimal proximal aortic fixation.[63] The benefit of device oversizing is controversial and is associated with aortic neck dilation and aortic expansion. Avoidance of greater than 30% in device oversizing is recommended.[66] Given that device migration is frequent after endograft repair of abdominal aortic aneurysms, careful surveillance of the endograft is an important part of postoperative follow-up.

BIBLIOGRAPHY

Abele JE: Balloon catheters and transluminal dilatation: technical considerations. AJR Am J Roentgenol 135:901, 1980.

Block PC, Baughman KL, Pasternak RC, et al: Transluminal angioplasty: correlation of morphologic and angiographic findings in an experimental model. Circulation 61:778, 1980.

Johnston KW: Iliac arteries: reanalyses of results of balloon angioplasty. Radiology 186:207, 1993.

Pentecost MJ, Criqui MH, Dorros G, et al: Guidelines for peripheral percutaneous transluminal angioplasty of the abdominal aorta and lower extremity arteries. Circulation 89:511, 1994.

Roubin GS, Yadav S, Iyer SS, et al: Carotid stem-supported angioplasty: a neurovascular intervention to prevent stroke. Am J Cardiol 78:8, 1996.

Sapoval MR, Chatellier G, Long AR, et al: Self-expandable stems for the treatment of iliac artery obstructive lesions: long-term success and prognostic factors. AJR Am J Roentgenol 166:1173, 1996.

Schneider PA, Rutherford RB: Endovascular interventions in the management of chronic lower extremity ischemia. In Rutherford RB, editor: Vascular surgery, ed 5, Philadelphia, 2000, WB Saunders, p 1035.

Zarins CK, Lu CT, Gewertz BL, et al: Arterial disruption and remodeling following balloon dilatation. Surgery 92:1086, 1982.

References available online at expertconsult.com.

QUESTIONS

1. Which of the following artery is not recommended for vascular access?
   a. Brachial artery
   b. Axillary artery
   c. Common femoral artery
   d. None of the above

2. Ultrasound guided access is recommended because:
   a. Of direct visualization of the vessel to be accessed
   b. Of decreased risk of vascular access complications such as arteriovenous fistula
   c. It is useful for access of pulseless arteries
   d. All of the above

3. Compared to the self-expanded stents, the balloon-expanded stents:
   a. Have more radial strength
   b. Are less flexible
   c. Have more hoop strength
   d. All of the above

4. The diameters of the commonly used guidewires are:
   a. 0.014 inch
   b. 0.018 inch
   c. 0.035 inch
   d. All of the above

5. Which of the following is not a mechanism of balloon angioplasty?
   a. Desquamation of endothelial cells
   b. Plaque compression allows for restoration of luminal diameter.
   c. Stretching of the media and adventitia
   d. Longitudinal fracture of the atherosclerotic plaque

6. Which of the following regarding arterial access is false?
   a. Antegrade femoral access allows for intervention of distal lesions in the infrapopliteal arterial system.
   b. Right brachial artery is preferred over left brachial artery.
   c. Retrograde femoral access allows for proximal aortogram and distal intervention of the contralateral lower extremity.
   d. Brachial access is commonly used in patients with aortoiliac disease.

7. Stents with thermal memory:
   a. Are made of nitinol
   b. Are able to expand to a predetermined shape when warmed
   c. Are a subgroup of self-expanded stents
   d. All of the above

8. Which of the following regarding catheter is not true?
   a. Selective catheters have a single hole at the tip.
   b. Flush catheters have multiple side and end holes.
   c. Catheters do not cause intimal injury or dissection.
   d. Flow rate through a catheter varies with its internal radius.

9. Complications at the vascular access site include all of the following except:
   a. Pseudoaneurysms
   b. Arteriovenous fistulas
   c. Intimal hyperplasia
   d. Hematoma

10. The ideal balloon angioplasty catheter has which of the following characteristics?
   a. Pushability and trackability
   b. Easy to rupture to prevent perforation of the artery
   c. High profile when collapsed
   d. Small filling lumen for inflation and deflation of the balloon

ANSWERS

1. **b**
2. **d**
3. **d**
4. **d**
5. **a**
6. **b**
7. **d**
8. **c**
9. **c**
10. **a**

CHAPTER 18

EXTRACRANIAL CEREBROVASCULAR DISEASE: THE CAROTID ARTERY

Wesley S. Moore

HISTORICAL REVIEW

The development of surgery on the extracranial cerebrovascular circulation was dependent on three principal factors: (1) recognition of the pathologic relationship between extracranial cerebrovascular disease and subsequent cerebral infarction, (2) the introduction of cerebral angiography to identify lesions before the patient's death, and (3) the development of vascular surgical techniques that could be applied to the extracranial vessels once the anatomic patterns of disease were understood and described.

The earliest report linking cervical carotid artery disease to stroke is credited to Savory,[1] who in 1856 described a young woman with left monocular symptoms in combination with a right hemiplegia and dysesthesia. Postmortem examination demonstrated an occlusion of the cervical portion of the left internal carotid artery, along with bilateral subclavian artery occlusions. In 1875, Gowers reported a similar case,[2] and subsequent reports of individual cases were made by Chiari in 1905,[3] Guthrie and Mayou in 1908,[4] and Cadwater in 1912.[5] By 1914, Hunt,[6] in an important publication, emphasized the relationship between extracranial carotid artery disease and stroke. He also described the phenomenon of intermittent cerebral symptoms associated with partial occlusion and used the term cerebral intermittent claudication as a characterizing analogy. Hunt also pointed out that the clinicopathologic observations in patients with stroke were hampered by the fact that routine autopsies did not include examination of the cervical carotid arteries (as is often the case today because of the desire to maintain access to the external carotid artery for the mortician). He emphasized that no examination of cerebral infarction can be considered complete without examination of the neck vessels.[6]

The next major step in the evolution of the management of extracranial cerebrovascular disease came with the development of carotid angiography by Moniz in 1927.[7] By 1937, Moniz and colleagues had described four cases of internal carotid occlusion diagnosed by angiography.[8] In 1938, Chao and colleagues added two more cases,[9] and by 1951, Johnson and Walker had collected from the world literature a total of 101 cases of occlusion of the cervical carotid artery diagnosed by angiography.[10] Despite these early observations, the medical world was still slow to appreciate the relationship between extracranial cerebrovascular disease and cerebral symptoms, as emphasized by the fact that when cerebral angiography came into common use for neurologic diagnosis in the 1950s and 1960s, only the intracranial vessels were included on radiographs films. The area of the carotid bifurcation was seldom examined. By the late 1950s, patients with hemiplegia were still commonly receiving diagnoses of a middle cerebral artery thrombosis, without consideration of the carotid bifurcation as a source of the problem.

The next major steps in the evolution of understanding came from reports by Fisher in 1951 and 1954.[11,12] Fisher reemphasized the relationship between extracranial arterial occlusive disease and cerebral symptoms. He also pointed out that the lesion could be either total occlusion or stenosis. His most important observation, however, was that the disease was often localized to a short segment of the carotid artery, and he predicted that surgical correction might be possible if patients could be identified in the early stages of the clinical syndrome. Fisher stated, "It is even conceivable that some day vascular surgery will find a way to bypass the occluded portion of the artery during the period of ominous fleeting symptoms. Anastomosis of the external carotid artery or one of its branches with the internal carotid artery above the area of narrowing should be feasible."

The surgical phase of understanding and managing extracranial cerebrovascular disease probably began in 1951, but it was not reported in the literature until 1955. This early report by Carrea and colleagues[13] from Buenos Aires described their experience with the management of a patient with carotid artery stenosis. They resected the diseased internal carotid artery and performed an anastomosis between the external carotid artery and the distal internal carotid, as predicted earlier by Fisher.[11] In 1953, Strully and coworkers[14] attempted a thromboendarterectomy of a totally thrombosed internal carotid artery. This attempt was unsuccessful, but the authors suggested that thromboendarterectomy should be technically feasible before thrombosis occurred, as long as the internal carotid artery is patent distally. The first carotid endarterectomy was probably performed by DeBakey and colleagues in an operation done on August 7, 1953, but it was not actually written up until 1959 and then reviewed in 1975.[15,16] The report that was most important in calling the world's attention to the feasibility of carotid artery reconstruction came from Eastcott and associates.[17] Their operation was performed on May 19, 1954, on a patient who was having hemispheric transient ischemic attacks (TIAs) with demonstrable disease at the carotid bifurcation; they used direct, end-to-end anastomosis between the common carotid artery and the internal carotid artery distal to the atherosclerotic lesion.

Although operations on the carotid artery were in the early phase of development, surgical attack was also considered feasible on occlusive lesions of the major arch vessels. In 1956, Davis and colleagues[18] reported their experience with endarterectomy of the innominate artery performed on a patient on March 20, 1954. In 1957, Warren and Triedman reported the second case.[19]

By this time, the stage was set for the explosive development of an aggressive surgical approach to managing extracranial cerebrovascular disease as a means of preventing or treating cerebral infarction.

Thompson,[20] in his 1996 Willis lecture, related in great detail the history of surgery to prevent stroke. Those interested in the definitive history will be rewarded by reading this excellent paper.

NATURAL HISTORY OF EXTRACRANIAL ARTERIAL OCCLUSIVE DISEASE

Therapy aimed at the prevention of cerebral infarction must be compared with the natural history of the disease process. The prognosis for a patient with extracranial arterial occlusive disease differs, depending on the presence or absence of symptoms. When a permanent neurologic deficit is present, the outlook worsens, thus underscoring the importance of prevention. A thorough understanding of the natural history of the disease is essential to formulating a rational and effective therapeutic program. The physician needs to be familiar with the expected results of each available option. This implies that no single alternative is applicable to all situations and that individualization is the key to effective prevention.

In the United States, approximately 600,000 people suffer a first stroke each year. In 200,000 of these cases, death follows, but at any one time approximately 1 million stroke victims are alive and disabled. In 1976, the annual direct and indirect cost of stroke was estimated at $7,363,784,000.[21] Nearly 30 years later, with inflation and the accelerating cost of medical care, this cost has probably quadrupled. The incalculable morbidity of the affected individual adds further to the magnitude of this problem. Prevention remains the most plausible alternative.

The initial mortality of an ischemic stroke ranges from 15% to 33%.[22-24] Survivors remain at an inordinately high risk of subsequent stroke, estimated between 4.8% and 20% per year.[25,26] This implies that half of patients will experience a second event within 5 years.[23,27,28] The average recurrent stroke rate reported in the literature is between 6% and 12% each year. The most common

cause of death in patients with extracranial arterial occlusive disease is myocardial infarction (MI). In an analysis of 535 stroke victims, however, the leading cause of death was recurrent stroke, as opposed to the expected myocardial mortality.[26]

Since 1973, public health statistics have documented an accelerating decline in stroke mortality.[29] Stroke used to be considered the third leading cause of death in the United States. The American Heart and Stroke Association recently reported that stroke has now dropped to the fourth leading cause of death. The reasons for this are multifactorial but include successful efforts at primary prevention including surgical intervention and treatment of carotid bifurcation lesions, improved medical management, and better care of the patient with acute stroke, often in specialized centers. This reduction in stroke mortality has led to the erroneous assumption that a decline has also occurred in stroke incidence, which is not the case.

In 1989, Wolf and colleagues[30] reported the epidemiologic data from the Framingham Study to the 14th International Joint Conference on Stroke and Cerebral Circulation. They reviewed the experience from three successive decades, beginning in 1953. A decline in stroke fatality in both men and women was observed. However, the 10-year prevalence of stroke actually rose, and the incidence of stroke in men rose from 5.7% to 7.6% to 7.9%, without any apparent change in women. The authors postulated that falling case fatality rates might have resulted from changes in diagnostic criteria, a lessening in stroke severity, or improved care of stroke patients.

Harmsen and colleagues[31] reviewed the stroke incidence and fatality in Gothenburg, Sweden, between 1971 and 1987. They noted that the stroke incidence remained the same during that interval, but the stroke fatality rate declined in both sexes. This was more marked for intracerebral hemorrhage and subarachnoid hemorrhage than for infarction. They concluded that the decline in stroke fatality rates might have been related to a decrease in smoking or better management of blood pressure. They could not explain why no corresponding decline in stroke incidence occurred.

Finally, Moden and Wagener[32] examined the epidemiologic aspects of stroke based on death certificate information available from the National Center for Health Statistics' compressed mortality file for all 50 states and the District of Columbia for the period 1968 to 1988. They noted a decline in stroke mortality that continued through the 1970s and 1980s, whereas morbidity remained constant and possibly even increased. They noted similar morbidity and mortality rates in both sexes. They concluded that the observed decrease in stroke mortality rates resulted from improved survival rather than a decline in incidence.[32]

A variety of reasons for the decline in stroke mortality have been postulated, including the more aggressive treatment of hypertension. No one has suggested that the decline of stroke mortality might be related to the increasing use of carotid endarterectomy, as illustrated in Figure 18-1. Although this is not proof of a relationship, a possible relationship cannot be discounted.

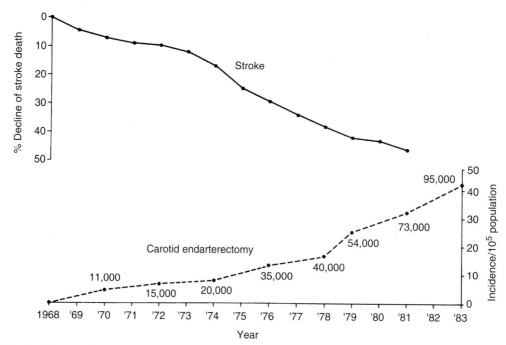

FIGURE 18-1 ■ The declining incidence of stroke-related death from 1968 to 1981 is compared with the accelerated frequency with which carotid endarterectomy was performed during the same period.

Two clinical syndromes deserve special emphasis because of their dismal natural history. Stroke in evolution is also known as *progressing stroke* or *incomplete stroke;* it is an acute neurologic deficit of modest degree that within hours or days progresses to a major cerebral infarct. This can happen in a sequential series of acute exacerbations or in a pattern of waxing and waning signs and symptoms over hours or days, with incomplete recovery eventually leading to a major fixed neurologic deficit. Crescendo transient ischemic attacks is the pattern that allows complete recovery between ischemic events, suggesting repeated frequent embolization from a point arterial source in the affected territory.

In a review of the literature, Mentzer and colleagues[33] identified 263 reported cases of stroke in evolution managed conservatively. Twenty-three percent had complete resolution or mild neurologic deficit on follow-up. Sixty-two percent had a moderate to severe deficit in the early recovery phase. The overall mortality was 14.5%. In their own series, 26 patients with stroke in evolution were treated conservatively. Mortality was 15%, but, more importantly, 66% suffered moderate to severe permanent neurologic deficits, with only five patients recovering completely or experiencing only mild neurologic dysfunction. These results are compared with a series of 17 patients operated on emergently for stroke in evolution. None of these patients had worsening of the preoperative neurologic deficit, four (24%) remained unchanged, and 12 (70%) had complete recovery.[33]

In 1972, Millikan reviewed the natural history of patients with progressing stroke.[34] Of 204 patients, 12% were normal at 14 days, 7% had developed moderate to severe neurologic deficits, and 14% had died. Thus, stroke in evolution treated conservatively carries a poor

prognosis. More than half of patients develop a severe permanent neurologic deficit within a few days of the onset, and approximately 15% die as a result. Only 10% to 20% recover full or partial neurologic function.[34]

Patients who experience TIAs are also at a higher risk of developing a stroke. In the Mayo Clinic population study,[35] 118 patients with TIAs were monitored as a control group without therapy. The stroke rates at 1, 3, and 5 years were 23%, 37%, and 45%, respectively. Most permanent deficits occurred during the first year. This represents a sixteenfold increased risk of stroke compared with an age- and sex-adjusted population. The Oxfordshire project reported an actuarial risk of stroke during the first year after the onset of TIAs to be 11% to 16%.[36] For each subsequent year, the rate was 5% to 9% per year. Some series have reported lower figures,[37,38] but the average reported in the literature is on the order of 30% to 35% at 5 years, or 10% the first year and 6% each year thereafter.

Finally, Toole[39] noted that cerebral infarction in TIA patients goes unrecognized by either patient or physician surprisingly often. These lesions are now identified by better neuroimaging techniques, and there is now evidence to suggest that TIAs are actually small strokes.[39] If a TIA is actually a small stroke, the implied benignity of TIAs must be reexamined, and it may be equally important to prevent TIAs. This consideration is further strengthened by the observations of Grigg and colleagues,[40] who correlated cerebral infarction and atrophy as a function of TIAs and percentage of stenosis. They graded carotid stenosis in symptomatic patients from A (no stenosis) to E (occlusion). In patients with amaurosis fugax, the incidence of cerebral infarction rose from 2% in patients with stenosis grades A, B, and C to 40% in grade D and 58% in grade E. The incidence of atrophy increased in parallel, from 10% in grade A to 30% in grade E.

The natural history of asymptomatic patients with significant extracranial or arterial occlusive disease is difficult to predict accurately. Most studies that have addressed this problem used the presence of a cervical bruit as the sole criterion for inclusion. This inevitably includes patients without significant occlusive disease and omits others without cervical bruit but with high-risk lesions in the extracranial circulation.

As noninvasive studies developed, detection of hemodynamically significant lesions in the carotid system improved. Kartchner and McRae monitored 1130 patients who either were asymptomatic or had nonhemispheric symptoms.[41] The mean interval was 24 months. Of 303 patients with hemodynamically significant lesions, 11.9% had strokes at 2 years. The group with negative noninvasive studies had a much lower stroke rate, on the order of 3% over the same follow-up period. Busuttil and colleagues[42] noted an unfavorable trend toward higher stroke rates in asymptomatic patients with hemodynamically significant lesions in the carotid bifurcation.

In a report by Roederer and colleagues,[43] 167 asymptomatic patients with cervical bruits were monitored with serial duplex scanning regardless of the degree of stenosis at the time of presentation. During follow-up, 10 patients became symptomatic. The development of symptoms was accompanied by disease progression in 80% of patients. By life-table analysis, the annual rate of symptom occurrence was 4%; however, the presence of progression graded at 80% stenosis was highly correlated with the development of either total occlusion of the internal carotid artery or new symptoms. Thus, 89% of the symptoms were preceded by progression of the lesion to greater than 80% stenosis. Progression of a lesion to more than 80% stenosis was an important warning sign, because it carried a 35% risk of ischemic symptoms or internal carotid occlusion within 6 months and a 46% risk at 12 months. Conversely, only 1.5% of the lesions that remained at less than 80% stenosis developed such a complication. These data suggest that careful follow-up with repeated noninvasive evaluation is of great assistance in determining the appropriate management of asymptomatic carotid lesions.[43]

In an analysis of 294 asymptomatic and nonhemispheric patients submitted to cerebrovascular testing, Moore and colleagues[44] found a 15% stroke incidence during the first 2 years in patients with greater than 50% stenosis. In contrast, there was a 3% stroke incidence at 2 years in patients with 1% to 49% stenosis. The difference was found to be statistically significant ($p < 0.05$). The 5-year cumulative stroke incidence was 21% with greater than 50% stenosis, 14% with 1% to 49% stenosis, and 9% in patients with no noninvasive evidence of carotid artery disease.

Chambers and Norris[45] monitored a group of 500 asymptomatic patients with noninvasive studies and clinical evaluation. They identified two high-risk groups: those with stenosis greater than 75%, and those who showed disease progression between studies. For patients with greater than 75% stenosis, the 1-year neurologic event rate (TIA and stroke) was 22%. The 1-year stroke rate alone was 5%. In a later publication,[46] the authors continued to note that neurologic events correlated with an increasing percentage of stenosis as well as disease progression between test intervals. In the study viewed over 5 years, the annual average neurologic event rate was 10% to 15%, with the highest event rate occurring within the first year of diagnosis. Finally, the incidence of silent cerebral infarction as documented by computed tomography (CT) was studied in the same patient population. The authors noted a 10% incidence of cerebral infarction among patients with mild (35% to 50%) stenosis, 17% with moderate (50% to 75%) stenosis, and 30% in patients with severe (>75%) stenosis. The authors concluded that silent cerebral infarction might be an indication for carotid endarterectomy in asymptomatic patients.[47]

Although the natural history of asymptomatic carotid stenosis remains controversial, studies using serial noninvasive cerebrovascular testing have concluded that an increased risk of stroke exists ipsilateral to a 50% or greater carotid artery stenosis. These lesions appear to carry a risk of subsequent stroke on the order of 4% per year. In addition, progression of the disease carries an even higher risk of stroke, with lesions causing greater than 80% stenosis carrying a 35% risk of subsequent symptoms or carotid occlusion at 2 years.

Other studies have suggested that the composition of the plaque influences the stroke risk of carotid artery lesions. In one analysis, 297 patients with carotid stenosis greater than 75% at the time of initial study were at higher risk than peers without significant narrowing or development of symptoms ipsilateral to the lesion.[48] Even those patients with less than 75% stenosis were at greater risk if the associated plaque was less organized (i.e., soft). This was determined by B-mode ultrasonography, which was used to classify plaques as dense, calcified, or soft. A definite trend toward higher risk was seen in plaques of lower density. Only 10% of those patients with calcified plaque in significantly stenotic vessels developed symptoms, whereas 92% of patients with soft plaques and tight stenosis developed symptoms within the first 3 years of follow-up.[48] The morphology of the atherosclerotic plaque, as documented by B-mode ultrasonography, is emerging as one of the more important factors associated with embolic potential and stroke risk. Two studies have concluded that a heterogeneous plaque carries an increased risk of stroke and is a variable independent from carotid stenosis alone.[49,50]

More recently, attempts have been made to better characterize the asymptomatic patient who is at higher risk for a cerebral ischemic event in order to identify subgroups of patients who would benefit from carotid endarterectomy compared to patients with carotid stenosis who are at low risk for an ischemic event. In addition to percent stenosis and plaque composition, two factors have been identified as being associated with increased stroke risk in the asymptomatic patient. These factors include the presence of silent brain infarction as seen on a screening CT scan and silent brain embolic signals as documented using transcranial Doppler. Kakkos and colleagues[51] studied 821 patients with CT scans. In patients with 60% to 99% stenosis and without silent brain infarction on CT, the annual rate of TIA and stroke was 1.3%. In patients with silent brain infarction, the annual event rate was 4.4%, suggesting that this subgroup of patients might benefit from carotid endarterectomy, leaving the low-risk group free from an unnecessary intervention.[51] Markus and colleagues[52] evaluated 467 asymptomatic patients with high-grade carotid stenosis in a multicenter study. Transcranial Doppler identified 77 patients with embolic signals. The annual risk of TIA and stroke was 7.13% in patients with embolic signals compared to 3.04% in patients without embolic signals. For ipsilateral stroke alone, the hazard ratio was 6.37. These findings suggest that screening for silent brain emboli is another method for identifying a high-risk group who are more likely to benefit from intervention.[52]

The embolic potential of ulcerated carotid lesions has been well documented.[53-55] Patients who experience symptoms from these lesions probably have the same prognosis as patients with occlusive lesions. Whether the former patient group responds more favorably to platelet antiaggregants remains to be determined. Moore and coworkers[56] first pointed out that asymptomatic patients with significant ulceration in a carotid plaque in the absence of stenosis appear to be at higher risk of stroke.[56] In a subsequent report, they expanded their series to 153 patients with asymptomatic, nonstenotic ulcerative lesions in the carotid bifurcation. Patients with deep (grade B) or complex (grade C) ulcerations received follow-up and were found to have a stroke rate of 4.5% and 7.5% each year, respectively.[57] Other reports have suggested a similar stroke risk for complex ulcerations in the carotid bulb. However, a much lower stroke risk was reported for deep (grade B) ulcerations, with no significant added risk of stroke observed in these patients. Controversy still exists about deep ulcerations without complex morphology. However, agreement exists that complex ulcerations in the carotid bulb increase the risk of stroke in asymptomatic patients.[58]

The presence of an asymptomatic hemodynamically significant stenosis may increase the risk of stroke during major surgery. Kartchner and McRae reported their experience with 234 patients, 41 of whom had evidence of significant carotid artery stenosis by oculoplethysmography.[59] Seven postoperative strokes developed in the group with positive criteria (17%), whereas postoperative cerebral infarction developed in 2 of 192 patients (1%) with negative noninvasive studies. The mechanisms of stroke and the territory involved were not specifically reported. This high incidence of permanent neurologic deficits led the authors to conclude that prophylactic carotid endarterectomy should be considered in patients with hemodynamically significant carotid stenosis who are undergoing a major cardiovascular procedure.[60]

Other series have reported results to the contrary.[60-63] Using noninvasive vascular evaluation and, in one series, angiography, patients with 50% or greater stenosis in the carotid bifurcation were compared with patients who had lesser degrees of stenosis undergoing cardiovascular surgery. No increased incidence of perioperative strokes was found in patients with positive criteria. Most of these investigators, however, excluded preocclusive stenosis in their considerations. Lesions causing 90% or greater stenosis were excluded from these series and were subjected to prophylactic endarterectomy before cardiovascular operation.

Cardiac surgeons have long been concerned about the presence of carotid stenosis in patients who will be undergoing cardiopulmonary bypass. Their concern is that during bypass there will be a decrease in pump perfusion pressure and a corresponding and unacceptable drop in cerebral blood flow. In fact, the opposite occurs. Von Reutern and colleagues[64] used transcranial Doppler ultrasonography to study middle cerebral artery blood flow before and during cardiopulmonary bypass in patients with and without carotid artery disease. Surprisingly, middle cerebral artery blood flow actually increased during cardiopulmonary bypass. Although the increase was not as great in patients with carotid artery disease, it was clearly an increase over baseline. This observation should dispel concern about the potential drop in cerebral blood flow in patients with carotid stenosis while using the pump.

Patients with a combination of severe carotid stenosis and symptomatic coronary artery disease represent a cohort that is at high risk of death, MI, and stroke. Brener and colleagues[65] performed an extensive literature review that examined complications associated with different treatment strategies. Patients who underwent staging with carotid endarterectomy first had a high cardiac morbidity and mortality. Patients who had coronary bypass first had a higher stroke morbidity. The data suggested that combined or simultaneous coronary artery bypass grafting and carotid endarterectomy might reduce overall morbidity and mortality. However, evidence from retrospective reviews was not sufficiently compelling to make a definitive recommendation.[65] Consensus exists that this is an appropriate topic for a prospective, randomized trial.

The natural history of extracranial arterial occlusive disease cannot be complete without a consideration of the natural history of frequently associated conditions such as coronary artery disease, hypertension, and diabetes. MI remains the most frequent cause of death in these patients. Including these variables in the equation when one is formulating a treatment plan for a particular patient is therefore important. The goal of therapy should be the prevention of a permanent neurologic deficit. When deciding on the most effective way to achieve this, one must consider the life expectancy of the patient and the inherent risk of each particular form of therapy.

PATHOLOGY OF EXTRACRANIAL ARTERIAL OCCLUSIVE DISEASE

The pathology of cerebrovascular disease of extracranial origin can be divided into flow-restrictive lesions and lesions with embolic potential. Each of these can be further subdivided into occlusive and aneurysmal lesions. All entities that have been described as etiologic in extracranial disease fall within these categories.

Atherosclerosis

By far the most common lesion found in patients with extracranial cerebrovascular disease is an atherosclerotic plaque in the carotid bifurcation. This can produce symptoms by reducing blood flow to the hemisphere supplied or, more commonly, by releasing embolic material. Emboli can be composed of clot, platelet aggregates, or cholesterol debris.

The carotid bifurcation appears to be susceptible to the development of atherosclerotic plaques.[66] Frequently, severe changes at the carotid bifurcation occur with minimal or no changes present in the common or internal carotid artery.[67] Several investigators have proposed conflicting theories based on hemodynamic observations in various models. High shear stress and fluctuations in shear stress,[68] disordered or turbulent flow, flow separation, and high and low flow velocity have all been implicated.[69-72] Which of these mechanisms is responsible for plaque formation is not known. Zarins and colleagues[73] used a model of the human carotid bifurcation under steady flow and compared its hemodynamics with those of cadaver specimens. They concluded that carotid lesions localize in regions of low flow velocity and flow separation rather than in regions of high velocity and increased shear stress. They used their model to explain the propensity of the outer wall of the carotid sinus opposite the flow divider to develop atherosclerotic plaques (Figure 18-2). This may have further clinical implications, in that an enlarged carotid bulb after endarterectomy may create a region of reduced flow velocity and increased boundary layer separation, which may favor recurrent plaque deposition.

Once the initial intimal injury is produced by these forces, platelet deposition, smooth muscle cell proliferation, and the slow accumulation of lipoproteins are involved in the reparative process (Figure 18-3). These eventually lead to plaque formation, which further alters the hemodynamics of the system and favors further injury.

The contribution of platelets to atheroma development can take several forms.[74] Platelets may adhere to one another, to the diseased vessel, or both; this can lead to thrombus formation. This process may narrow the vessel lumen, or the thrombus may dislodge, resulting in distal embolization. Vasoactive substances stored in granules within the platelet may be released, causing vasospasm and further contributing to compromise of the arterial lumen. The platelets' interaction with collagen, exposed in an injured intima, may include elaboration of a smooth muscle growth factor that can lead to intimal thickening. The activation of enzymes in platelets, by their contact with collagen, initiates the production of highly active prostaglandins. The production of thromboxane A_2 represents the final common pathway of platelet response to diverse stimuli.[75] This substance is a potent stimulant of platelet aggregation and a powerful vasoconstrictor and is believed to be important in the pathophysiology of plaque formation or the development of symptoms from an already established atheroma.

Hemorrhage into a plaque may also play a significant role in the development of symptoms from an atherosclerotic lesion. Imbalances in wall tension secondary to asymmetrical deposition of plaques can lead to sudden plaque fracture and intraplaque hemorrhage.[76] These can lead to sudden expansion of the atheroma, with acute restriction of flow or breakdown of the intimal surface and concomitant embolization. An alternative mechanism for sudden intraplaque hemorrhage may be related to an increase in neovascularity within the plaque substance. Hypertension may be responsible for precipitating rupture of neovascular vessels, leading to intraplaque hemorrhage and expansion.[77] This process may be responsible for a large number of symptomatic lesions.

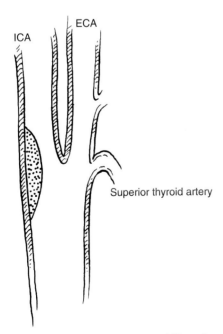

FIGURE 18-2 ■ The common carotid artery bifurcation, the most common site for atherosclerotic plaque deposition, is located on the wall opposite the divider. *ECA,* External carotid artery; *ICA,* internal carotid artery.

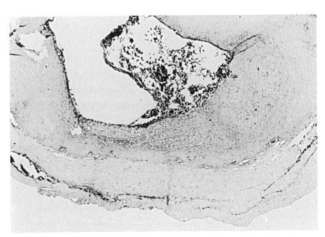

FIGURE 18-3 ■ Microscopic section of an atherosclerotic plaque removed from the carotid bifurcation. Notice the fibrointimal proliferation with cholesterol cleft formation. Thrombotic material is adherent to the luminal surface of the plaque.

In a prospective evaluation of 79 atheromatous plaques removed from 69 patients undergoing carotid endarterectomy, 49 of 53 (92.5%) symptomatic patients had evidence of intramural hemorrhage.[78] In contrast, only 7 of 26 (27%) asymptomatic patients showed recent or acute intraplaque hemorrhage. Rupture of an atherosclerotic plaque with intraluminal release of atheromatous debris has also been correlated with acute stroke and internal carotid occlusion in an autopsy study.[79]

Fibromuscular Dysplasia

Fibromuscular dysplasia is a nonatherosclerotic process that affects medium-size arteries. It was first described in the carotid artery in 1964,[80] and since then it has been recognized as a cause of cerebrovascular symptoms.[81] It may also affect the intracranial arteries, and approximately 30% of patients with cervical involvement have associated intracranial aneurysms.[82] Up to 65% of patients have bilateral disease,[82] and 25% have associated atherosclerotic changes.[83]

Four histologic types of fibromuscular dysplasia have been described[84]:

1. Intimal fibroplasia accounts for about 5% of cases and affects both sexes equally. It usually appears as long tubular stenoses in young patients and as focal stenoses in older patients. It results from an accumulation of irregularly arranged subendothelial mesenchymal cells with a loose matrix of connective tissue. Medial and adventitial structures are always normal.

2. Medial hyperplasia is a rare form of the disease that produces focal stenoses. The intima and adventitia remain normal, whereas the media shows excess smooth muscle.

3. Medial fibroplasia is the most common pattern of fibromuscular dysplasia, accounting for most, if not all, internal carotid artery involvement. It may appear as a focal stenosis or multiple lesions with intervening aneurysmal outpouchings. Histologically, the disease is limited to the media, with replacement of smooth muscle by compact fibrous connective tissue. The inner media may show an accumulation of collagen and ground substance separating disorganized smooth muscle cells. Gradation of these changes correlates with the severity of the lesion. Mural dilatations and microaneurysms are common.

4. Perimedial dysplasia is characterized by the accumulation of elastic tissue between the media and adventitia. It affects renal arteries and is associated with macroaneurysms.

Fibromuscular dysplasia preferentially affects long arteries with few primary branches. Hormonal effects on medial tissue, mechanical stresses on the vessel wall, and unusual distribution of the vasa vasorum in these arteries seem to play a causative role.[84] Some experimental evidence[85] and the fact that women are most commonly affected (92% of cases)[83] support a possible role of hormones in this process. In the appropriate hormonal environment, the normal paucity of vasa vasorum in long, nonbranching arterial segments such as the extracranial carotid artery and the renal artery may predispose to mural ischemia and initiation of the fibroplastic process. Experimental evidence supports this concept.[86]

The exact cause of symptoms is controversial. Thromboembolism from clot, platelets, or both; decreased flow owing to a critical stenosis or a series of noncritical narrowing; intracranial involvement, with or without aneurysm formation; and hypertension have been implicated.[83]

Coils and Kinks

Coils and kinks of the extracranial system on occasion have been associated with fibromuscular dysplasia.[83] More commonly, these are due to embryologic events and changes that occur in the aging process. Neurologic manifestations from these anomalies have been reported in children[87] and in adults.[88-90] Embryologically, the internal carotid artery is derived from the third aortic arch and the dorsal aortic root. In the early stages of development, a normally occurring kink is straightened as the heart and great vessels descend in the mediastinum. Failure of this process may account for the occurrence of coils and loops in children and for its bilaterality in approximately 50% of cases.[90]

In adults, kinking of the extracranial vessels is almost always associated with atherosclerosis. In the aging process, loss of elasticity of the vessel wall occurs, which, in combination with lateral stresses, causes elongation between fixed points—the skull and the thoracic inlet. This produces bowing, with the eventual formation of coils and kinks. Between 5% and 16% of patients submitted for angiographic evaluation have coiling or kinking of one of the extracranial vessels.[88,90] Kinking of the artery is more likely to produce symptoms because of either flow reduction or concomitant plaque formation with distal embolization. Kinking is considered to be an angle of less than 90 degrees between arterial segments (Figure 18-4). Flow restriction is unlikely to exist in the absence of this configuration. This acute angulation is more likely to occur when the head is turned to the ipsilateral side.[87] In other cases, contralateral rotation, neck flexion, and extension may exaggerate the abnormality, leading to markedly reduced flow. A history of TIAs associated with head motion should lead the clinician to suspect the presence of a kink. Abnormal pulsations in the neck, sometimes suggesting an aneurysmal dilatation, may be present on physical examination. Secondary arteriosclerotic changes can occur because of abnormal flow patterns that predispose to plaque formation and ulceration, accounting for the development of neurologic symptoms. Rarely is the vertebral circulation affected by a kink.[88]

Aneurysms

Aneurysms of the carotid artery can cause neurologic symptoms by several mechanisms. Thrombosis and rupture are rare, but embolization is a frequent event.[91] Pressure on cranial nerves can be seen when expansion is rapid, but more frequently this is associated with acute dissection.

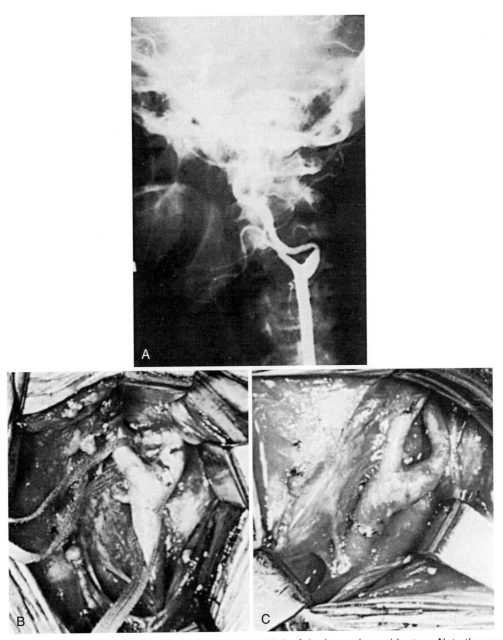

FIGURE 18-4 ■ **A,** Selective left carotid arteriogram demonstrating a kink of the internal carotid artery. Note the angulation of less than 90 degrees and the paucity of contrast material beyond the kink. **B,** Operative appearance of the internal carotid artery kink. **C,** Operative appearance of the internal carotid artery after connection of the kink by mobilization and segmental resection of the common carotid artery. The carotid bifurcation is pulled down, and an end-to-end anastomosis is constructed.

Most extracranial aneurysms are secondary to atherosclerosis. Internal elastic lamina disruption and medial thinning are frequent histologic findings.[92] Two types of aneurysms are recognized: fusiform and saccular. Fusiform aneurysms are more common; they are frequently bilateral and are associated with other arterial aneurysms. Saccular aneurysms are often unilateral and tend to involve the common or internal carotid arteries more often. They may also have a congenital, degenerative, or traumatic origin.[93] Atherosclerotic aneurysms of the extracranial circulation are almost always associated with hypertension.[92]

Trauma is a frequent cause of carotid aneurysms. These are usually saccular and most commonly result from blunt rather than penetrating injury. Hyperextension and rotation of the neck cause compression of the internal carotid artery on the transverse process of the atlas.[94] An intimal injury is produced that frequently leads to thrombosis, but it can also produce aneurysmal dilatation.[92]

Mycotic aneurysms are rare. Syphilis and peritonsillar abscess were once common causes of these aneurysms.[95] *Staphylococcus aureus* is currently the predominant responsible organism.

False aneurysms of the carotid artery may form after penetrating injury, but the most frequent cause is previous carotid surgery. These aneurysms are more common after patch closure of the artery than after primary closure.[91] Disruption of the suture line by infection, suture failure, and technical error are believed to be responsible for their formation. False aneurysms can expand, thrombose, rupture, or lead to distal embolization. The diagnosis of false aneurysm is an indication for surgical repair.

Acute dissection of the carotid artery with or without aneurysm formation is another cause of neurologic events resulting from abnormalities in the extracranial circulation. It can occur secondary to atherosclerosis, fibromuscular dysplasia, or cystic medial necrosis.[96] A history of trauma may or may not be present. On gross inspection, a sharply demarcated transition between the normal color and size of the carotid artery and the dark blue, cylindrical dilatation in the dissected segment is noted.[97] More commonly, the internal carotid artery is affected, and frequently the end of the dissection is not surgically accessible. A double lumen is usually present, with the dissection occurring in the outer layers of the media. Smooth muscle cells are widely separated, and degeneration and fragmentation of the internal elastic membrane occur.[97] The most frequent presentation is a sudden onset of temporal headache or cervical pain associated with a neurologic or visual deficit or Horner syndrome. Acute expansion may cause compression of cranial nerves IX, X, XI, or XII, with concomitant dysfunction.[96] Horner syndrome is thought to be secondary to disruption of periadventitial sympathetic fibers. The carotid artery is far more frequently affected than the vertebral artery. Only a few cases of the latter have been reported, with involvement of the segment between C1 and C2 noted consistently.[96]

Takayasu Arteritis

In 1908, Takayasu described ocular changes in a 21-year-old woman with nonspecific arteritis.[98] These changes consisted of a peculiar capillary flush, with rustlike arteriovenous anastomoses around the papilla and blindness owing to cataracts. Similar cases were later described with the absence of pulses in the arm. Since then, Takayasu arteritis has been recognized as a cause of neurologic symptoms secondary to a nonspecific inflammatory process of unknown cause segmentally affecting the aorta and its main branches. The end result of this process is constriction or occlusion of, and occasional aneurysm formation in, the affected vessels secondary to marked fibrosis and thickening of the arterial wall.[99] Originally thought to be rare in the Western hemisphere, many cases of atypical coarctations of the aorta and other unusual lesions of its main branches are now well recognized as Takayasu arteritis. This explains the many eponyms given to this syndrome.[100]

Four varieties of the disease are recognized.[101] In type 1, involvement is localized to the aortic arch and its branches. Type 2 does not have arch involvement; the lesions are confined to the descending and abdominal aorta. Type 3 has features of both, and type 4 describes any of the first three types plus involvement of the pulmonary artery. In a retrospective study of 107 patients, 84% were female, and 80% were aged 11 to 30 years.[101]

Two phases of the disease are recognized. In the acute or prepulseless stage, systemic symptoms of a nonspecific nature are present. Skin rash, fever, myalgia, arthralgia, pleuritis, generalized weakness, and other nonspecific symptoms develop, making the diagnosis difficult. These symptoms may resolve and go unrecognized by the patient or physician until months or years later, when the second, or occlusive, stage evolves. Next, symptoms of obstruction of the main aortic branches develop. These lesions are not easily managed by endarterectomy, which makes bypass surgery the treatment of choice.

Other forms of arteritis, specifically giant cell arteritis, can cause neurologic symptoms because of extracranial or intracranial involvement. These patients are older than those with Takayasu arteritis, and both sexes appear to be equally affected.[100] Systemic symptoms are usually present. Tenderness over the carotid artery or other affected areas may occur.[102] The histologic picture is characteristic, with changes confined to the media, where a large number of giant cells interspersed with lymphocytes are seen. Early diagnosis is important, because corticosteroid therapy may abort the latter stages of the process.[102]

Radiation Therapy Injury

External cervical radiation therapy is recognized as a cause of accelerated atherosclerotic changes in the extracranial circulation. Experimentally, atherosclerotic lesions similar to the naturally occurring ones can be produced in the abdominal aorta in dogs by x-ray and electron beam radiation.[103] Injury to the endothelial cell, ground substance, elastic lamina, and smooth muscle appears to alter the vessel wall, increasing its permeability to circulating lipids and impairing its ability to repair elastic tissue, leading to the formation of a plaque characterized by fibrosis, fatty infiltration, and intimal destruction.[104] These changes can occur months to years after completion of therapy. Lesions occur in locations unusual for atherosclerosis (Figure 18-5). Blowout of the affected carotid artery may occur, but this is more frequent when surgery is combined with radiation in treating cervical malignancies. Hyperlipidemia and hypercholesterolemia appear to predispose patients receiving radiation therapy to the development of these accelerated changes.[105] Endarterectomy of the affected segments is difficult but can be performed safely.[104,106]

Moritz and colleagues[107] reported their experience with 53 patients who had undergone radiation therapy to the neck an average of 28 months earlier and compared them with a control group of 38 patients who had not had radiation.[107] Thirty percent of the radiated group had moderate to severe lesions of the carotid bifurcation, as detected by duplex scanning, in contrast to only 6% of the control group. Five patients in the radiated group were symptomatic. The authors concluded that patients who receive carotid radiation should undergo periodic follow-up duplex scanning of the carotid arteries.

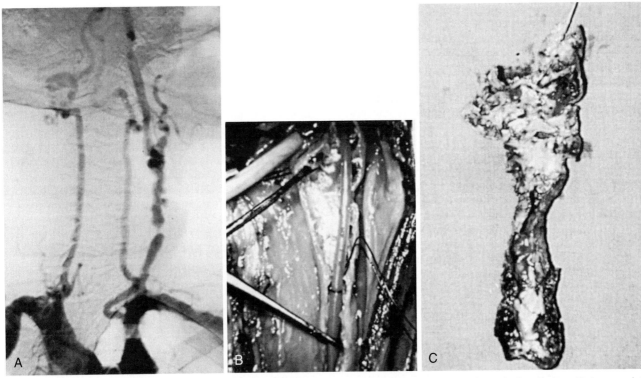

FIGURE 18-5 ■ **A,** Arch angiogram demonstrating carotid artery disease secondary to external cervical radiation. Note complete occlusion of the right common carotid artery. Multiple stenoses are in the left common carotid artery, an unusual site for primary atherosclerosis. **B,** Operative appearance of the lesion secondary to external radiation. **C,** Intimectomy specimen of the lesion produced by external cervical radiation.

Recurrent Carotid Stenosis

Recurrent carotid stenosis has been reported to occur in 1% to 21% of cases[108-113] and may yield an incidence of hemodynamically significant stenosis as high as 32% after 7 years.[108] This can lead to neurologic symptoms by producing emboli or restricting flow. The most common lesion developing within the first 2 years after surgery is myointimal hyperplasia. Histologically, a concentric lesion occurs, with no calcium or lipid deposits. A dense accumulation of collagen and mucopolysaccharides surrounds cellular elements. These substances are produced by the myointimal cell in the normal healing process. Their accelerated production seems to be responsible for the development of the fibroplastic lesion leading to luminal stenosis. An endarterectomy plane is almost impossible to develop.

The morphologic characteristics of the early (<2 years) restenosis suggest a lower risk of stroke compared with arteriosclerotic lesions of a similar degree.[114] In addition, regression of stenosis documented by noninvasive tests has been reported. Thus, controversy exists over the management of early recurrent stenosis after carotid endarterectomy.[115] In the asymptomatic stage, a restenosis documented by successive noninvasive testing should lead the surgeon to consider surgical intervention if progression to greater than 80% of the diameter occurs. Recurrent symptoms are certainly an indication for reoperation unless a different cause is suspected. Interestingly, Bernstein and colleagues[116] showed an inverse correlation

between greater than 50% recurrent stenosis and late stroke and death. Their data suggested that patients with early recurrent stenosis had a better long-term prognosis than those who did not develop recurrent stenosis.

When a stenotic lesion develops more than 2 years after carotid endarterectomy, atherosclerosis is usually the cause. Injury to the vessel by vascular clamps may play a role. Elevated serum cholesterol has a statistically significant association with recurrent carotid stenosis.[109]

These lesions probably carry the same stroke risk as primary arteriosclerotic lesions in the carotid bifurcation. Recommendation for reoperation is thus based on the known risk factors of similar primary arteriosclerotic lesions.

Some investigators have suggested that patch closure at the time of the initial carotid endarterectomy may prevent recurrent stenosis. Several prospective, randomized studies, either completed or in progress, suggest a lower incidence of restenosis with the use of patch angioplasty.[110,117-120] The most compelling argument in favor of patch closure comes from a prospective study by Abu Rahma and colleagues.[121] The authors identified 74 patients with bilateral carotid stenoses in need of bilateral operation. One side was closed primarily, and the opposite side was closed with patch angioplasty. In this manner, demographic and patient characteristics were controlled. The incidence of ipsilateral stroke for primary closure was 4%, versus 0% for patch closure. In the primary closure group, there was a 22% incidence of recurrent stenosis, versus 1% in the patch group ($p < 0.003$). There was an 8% incidence of internal carotid artery occlusion with primary closure, versus 0% with patch closure. Restenosis requiring reoperation occurred in 14% of the primary closure group and in 1% of the patch group. In a life-table analysis, the 24-month freedom from recurrence was 75% in the primary closure group, versus 98% in the patch group.[121] A significant benefit of patch angioplasty appears to be a reduction in technical end point problems. Therefore, patching may be equally important in preventing occurrence and recurrence. The same objective can be achieved by preventing or correcting technical errors at the time of operation when they are identified by completion angiography. Data obtained from experimental hemodynamic studies suggest that an enlarged bulb following patch closure of an endarterectomy site may predispose to areas of low shear stress and therefore recurrent disease. For this reason, it is important not to overenlarge the bulb when using a patch. Overenlargement may be responsible for a higher incidence of recurrence after vein patch angioplasty (9%) versus prosthetic patch angioplasty (2%). However, both were superior to primary closure (34%) in a randomized study.[122]

The benefit of patch closure was also seen in a retrospective analysis of other data from the Asymptomatic Carotid Atherosclerosis Study (ACAS). The study examined the incidence of recurrence for three time intervals: within 3 months of operation (residual disease), 3 to 18 months (myointimal hyperplasia), and 18 to 60 months (recurrent atherosclerosis). The use of patch angioplasty reduced the overall risk of restenosis from 21.2% to 7.1%.[123] Factors associated with early recurrence include an incomplete intimectomy, the use of distal tacking sutures, female sex, continued cigarette smoking, and primary closure of an anatomically small internal carotid artery.[124-126]

Many clinicians routinely prescribe aspirin preoperatively as well as postoperatively, in the hope that embolic events from platelet aggregates can be reduced or eliminated. The rationale is that aspirin will reduce the incidence of myointimal hyperplasia by reducing platelet adhesion or aggregation and interfering with the platelet release reaction. Unfortunately, the carotid artery, like other areas subjected to arterial reconstruction, has not been shown to benefit. A prospective, randomized, placebo-controlled trial failed to show any benefit of aspirin in preventing early carotid restenosis.[127]

Carotid Body Tumors

Vascular surgeons are frequently called on to remove carotid body tumors because of their intimate adherence to the carotid bifurcation and the possible need to clamp, resect, graft, or otherwise repair the carotid artery during the course of resecting the tumor from the neck.

The carotid body is composed of chemoreceptor cells surrounded by a vascular stroma. Carotid body tumors are true neoplasms that arise from chemoreceptor cells. The tumors have an extremely rich blood supply, which makes their surgical removal both difficult and hazardous. Biopsy of a carotid body tumor is absolutely contraindicated because of the risk of uncontrollable

hemorrhage. Immunohistochemical studies suggest that the tumor cells are capable of synthesizing several different neural endocrine substances, yet these tumors seldom have a pathologic endocrine function.

Most carotid body tumors are benign and usually cause problems because of enlargement and compression of adjacent neural or vascular structures. The cranial nerves that can be involved include IX, X, XI, and XII, with associated dysfunction related to the distribution of those nerves. Carotid body tumors, on occasion, can exhibit malignant behavior. Malignancy can be determined only when there is evidence of lymph node or distant metastases. It is not possible to differentiate a benign from a malignant tumor based on histologic examination alone.

PATHOGENETIC MECHANISMS OF TRANSIENT ISCHEMIC ATTACKS AND CEREBRAL INFARCTION

In reviewing the mechanisms for TIA and cerebral infarction, emphasis is placed on those events related to disease in the extracranial vessels. Hemorrhagic stroke is excluded. Cerebral ischemic events related to hypertension and cardiac emboli are briefly reviewed because of their importance in the differential diagnosis and workup of symptomatic patients. Finally, from a pathogenetic standpoint, the difference between TIA and fixed deficit is a matter of degree, duration, and extent of actual infarction. The mechanisms of occurrence are essentially the same. Therefore, for purposes of discussion, we use the general inclusive term ischemic event.

Arterial Thrombosis

When an atherosclerotic plaque expands to produce a critical reduction in blood flow, the vessel ultimately undergoes thrombosis. In the case of the internal carotid artery, if this column of thrombus stops at the ophthalmic artery and remains stable, and if collateral circulation is sufficient via the circle of Willis, the thrombotic event may be entirely asymptomatic (Figure 18-6). If the thrombus propagates beyond the ophthalmic artery to occlude the middle cerebral artery (Figure 18-7), or if small thrombi rather than a thrombotic column form and are subsequently carried to the intracranial vessels by continuous blood flow (Figure 18-8), the patient experiences cerebral symptoms that can vary from transient ocular or hemispheric events to a profound hemiplegia, depending on the extent of propagated thrombus or embolus. In addition, if the collateral circulation to the circle of Willis is poor, the sudden loss of flow through a diseased internal carotid artery may incite a precipitous drop in flow to the hemisphere, resulting in ischemic infarction as a consequence of inadequate proximal blood flow.

Flow-Related Ischemic Events

Although flow-related ischemia used to be considered the most common cause of transient ischemic events, it is

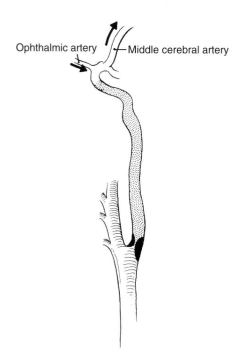

FIGURE 18-6 ■ Thrombus occurring distal to an occlusive lesion of the internal carotid artery. Note that the column of thrombus stops short of the ophthalmic artery, and patency of the middle cerebral artery is maintained.

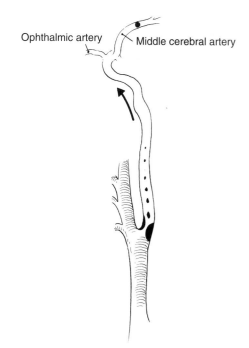

FIGURE 18-8 ■ Emboli released from a plaque strategically placed at the origin of the internal carotid artery can pass into the middle cerebral artery and lodge in the terminal branch. This results in either a temporary or a permanent neurologic deficit in the distribution appropriate to the arterial occlusion.

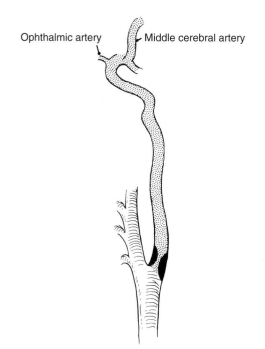

FIGURE 18-7 ■ Thrombus secondary to an occlusive atherosclerotic lesion of the internal carotid artery progresses beyond the ophthalmic artery to involve the middle cerebral artery.

actually a rather rare occurrence. Transient drops in hemispheric blood flow or the development of a chronic low-flow state can be responsible for nonspecific symptoms of lightheadedness, presyncope, or intellectual deterioration.[1,128] It must also be recognized that other, nonvascular causes of these symptoms exist and are probably more frequent.

The collateral blood flow to the brain, via the circle of Willis, is an extremely efficient system. Multiple patients have been described who had bilateral internal carotid artery occlusion, perhaps combined with occlusion of the vertebral artery, but were totally asymptomatic from a central neurologic point of view. Experience obtained performing carotid endarterectomy under local anesthesia has shown that approximately 10% of patients experience neurologic symptoms when the carotid artery is clamped.[55] This 10% may have symptoms on the basis of compromised blood flow when the stenosis progresses or goes on to complete occlusion. Another circumstance that can produce symptoms of global ischemia is simultaneous stenosis or occlusion in more than one extracranial vessel—for example, a carotid occlusion on one side combined with a high-grade stenosis in the contralateral carotid artery. Under these circumstances, transient drops in blood pressure, perhaps posturally related, can produce either global or focal ischemic symptoms. Rarely, patients with unilateral carotid occlusion may have a downstream vascular bed that is marginally perfused. Postural changes under these circumstances can also produce focal ischemia and result in a flow-related TIA. Under these conditions, a patient would be a good candidate for extracranial-to-intracranial bypass grafting.

Flow-restricting lesions in the vertebral arteries or in major vessels proximal to the vertebral origin, such as the innominate or subclavian artery, can produce symptoms related to hypoperfusion in the posterior circulation. One of the most dramatic anatomic observations is the so-called subclavian steal syndrome. If a stenosis or occlusion of the subclavian artery is present proximal to the

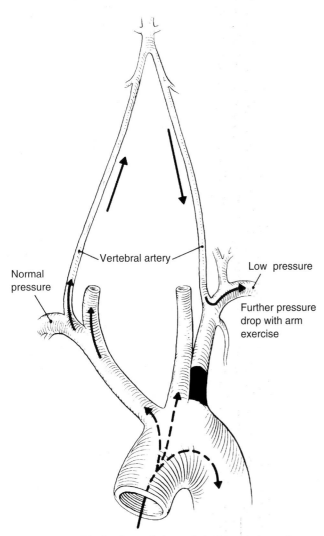

FIGURE 18-9 ■ Mechanism of the subclavian steal syndrome. Note the occlusion in the origin of the left subclavian artery. This produces a pressure gradient with reversal of blood flow in the left vertebral artery, producing a siphoning or steal from the basilar artery.

vertebral artery takeoff, the pressure drop distal to the obstruction causes its branches to serve as sources of collateral blood flow by reversing the normal flow direction. The branches now contribute to the flow of the main trunk rather than receiving flow from the proximally affected artery. The vessels that contribute to collateral blood flow of the distal subclavian artery by reversing flow include the vertebral artery. Under these circumstances, the vertebral artery not only is deprived of the usual antegrade flow but also actually siphons off blood flow from the basilar artery circulation because of flow reversal. This siphoning of blood may be entirely without symptoms if abundant sources of inflow from the other vertebral artery or from the anterior circulation exist. Conversely, if the opposite vertebral artery is small or occluded, a deficiency in basilar artery flow may be present that results in symptoms of basilar artery insufficiency. These symptoms may first appear or become exaggerated if the demand for flow in the affected subclavian artery increases, such as results from active exercise of the arm (Figure 18-9).

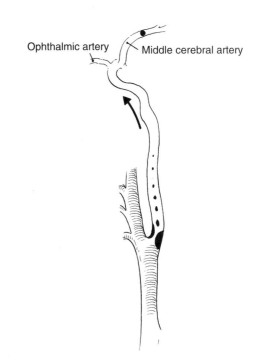

FIGURE 18-10 ■ Embolic fragment in the middle cerebral artery. If this persists, it will lead to focal infarction. If the fragment breaks up and distributes itself through the microcirculation, the ischemic event will be transient.

Cerebral Emboli

The most common causes of cerebral ischemic events are embolic phenomena, primarily arterial in origin and secondarily from cardiac sources. The emboli of arterial origin occur as a consequence of morphologic change present on the luminal surface of a critical artery.[54,55,129,130] These changes most often are associated with atheromatous plaques but can also occur with other lesions such as fibromuscular dysplasia. When an irregular surface produces turbulence, a stimulus for platelet aggregation is present. If the platelet aggregates become large enough and embolize to an important vessel in the brain, symptoms occur. If the platelet aggregates break up quickly from mechanical forces or from the effect of arterial prostacyclin, the symptoms are transient. If the embolic fragment persists, however, it can lead to focal infarction (Figure 18-10).

An atherosclerotic plaque may undergo central degeneration or softening. When this occurs, bleeding into the plaque substance can also occur, leading to sudden plaque expansion with intraluminal rupture,[49,77,112,131] or the plaque may spontaneously rupture into the lumen, discharging its contents into the arterial stream. The plaque contents consist of degenerative atheromatous debris, including various mixtures of cholesterol crystals, calcific material, or thrombotic remnants. If the atherosclerotic plaque is located at a critical point, such as the origin of the internal carotid artery, considerable likelihood exists that embolic atheromatous fragments will be carried to important vascular beds of the brain, producing either transient or permanent neurologic events (Figure 18-11). These events are considered primary embolic events of atherosclerotic plaque origin.

After the plaque has ruptured, a defect is left behind that is called an *ulcer* (Figure 18-12). Further primary emboli can continue to escape from the raw ulcerated surface, or the ulcer itself may serve as a focal point for thrombus or platelet aggregate material to form. These platelet or thrombotic aggregates may secondarily dislodge, owing to blood flow turbulence, and embolize to the brain (Figure 18-13). Thus, the embolic material from an atherosclerotic plaque can consist of atheromatous debris, platelet aggregates, or blood clot. The emboli of arterial origin can be primary, occurring with plaque rupture or on thrombogenic arterial plaque surfaces,[130,132] or secondary, having developed within ulcerative lesions from previous plaque rupture.[133]

Embolic events may produce dramatic focal neurologic events that are immediately appreciated by the patient, or the embolic fragments may travel to more silent areas of the brain, in which case the results are more subtle and appreciated on a chronic basis, such as cerebral atrophy or multiple-infarct dementia.[134,135] The use of transcranial Doppler ultrasonography has provided more objective evidence of emboli from carotid plaques by discerning discrete noise as an embolic particle passes a point of Doppler insonation.[136] Finally, the occurrence of TIAs in a hemisphere distal to a carotid occlusion raises the question of the importance of decreased flow to arterial border zones. Experimental data have demonstrated that emboli originating from a contralateral carotid artery can cross through the circle of Willis and produce focal infarcts in the hemisphere distal to a carotid occlusion.[137] Thus, the contralateral patent carotid artery

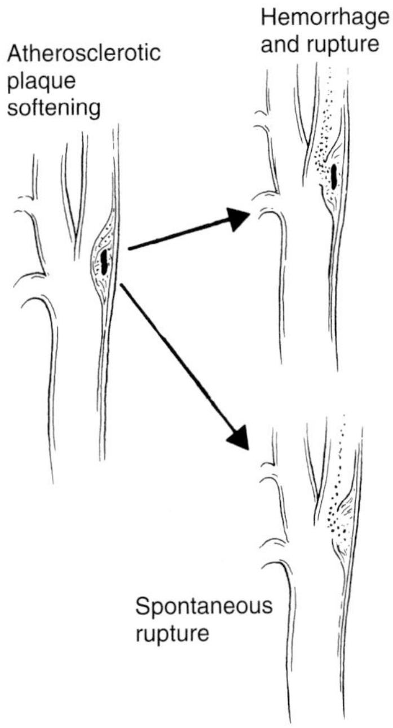

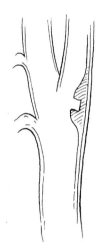

FIGURE 18-11 ■ Atherosclerotic plaque undergoing central softening. Spontaneous hemorrhage may occur into the center of the plaque, producing rupture and discharge of embolic fragments, or the plaque may spontaneously rupture as a result of hydrostatic forces, releasing necrotic embolic debris.

FIGURE 18-12 ■ Following evacuation of an atherosclerotic plaque, a defect or ulcer is left behind.

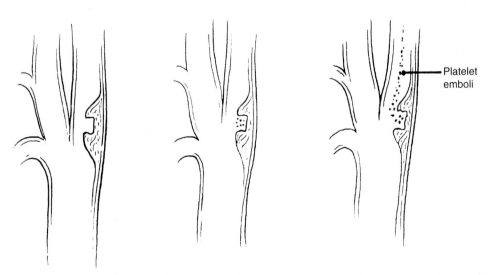

FIGURE 18-13 ■ The ulcerated lesion within an atheromatous plaque can serve as a nidus for platelet aggregation or thrombotic material. These aggregates can secondarily embolize from the ulcer crypt.

should always be considered a possible source of emboli when a patient with a carotid occlusion begins to experience symptoms in the hemisphere distal to the occlusion.

Emboli can also occur from cardiac sources, which include aortic valvular disease, mitral valve prolapse, cardiac arrhythmias, and mural thrombus after MI. Venous thromboembolism passing thru a patent foramen ovale, so-called paradoxical embolism, can also go to the brain. More recently, atherosclerotic plaques of the ascending aorta, as seen with transesophageal echocardiography, have been identified as another source of cerebral embolization.[138-140]

Lacunar Infarction

Focal areas of cerebral necrosis occurring in the basal ganglia, internal capsule, or pons have been described as a consequence of end-vessel occlusive disease involving the lenticulostriate or thalamoperforating arteries. The underlying cause is related to uncontrolled hypertension, and the resulting neurologic deficit is often clinically identified as a pure motor or pure sensory stroke.[141] Although descriptions of this phenomenon date back to the early 1900s, its current understanding is based on the efforts and writings of Fisher.[142]

The clinical picture may often be confused with arterial-arterial emboli, in that antecedent TIAs may have occurred. The differential diagnosis is best made by the very focal neurologic deficit seen clinically and the typical anatomic location seen on the CT scan of the brain. Evidence shows that the so-called lacunae may also be the consequence of emboli of arterial origin.[143-146] Thus, symptoms and imaging of a deep white matter infarct do not rule out atheromatous plaque from the carotid bifurcation as a cause of the event.

CLINICAL SYNDROMES OF EXTRACRANIAL ARTERIAL OCCLUSIVE DISEASE

Extracranial arterial occlusive disease can result in varying symptoms or be completely asymptomatic. A thorough history must be obtained, because this alone can provide clues to the specific nature of the event. Often, one discovers the existence of symptoms that the patient has been ignoring. A complete review of symptoms is mandatory, because this may alter the therapeutic alternatives available. Risk factors for atherosclerosis should be specifically recorded.

Patients can be classified into three categories: asymptomatic patients, patients with TIAs, and patients with cerebral infarction. In asymptomatic patients, a hemodynamically significant lesion or a nonocclusive ulcerated arteriosclerotic plaque in the extracranial circulation may be discovered in the absence of transient or permanent neurologic symptoms. The presence or absence of a bruit in the cervical area should not be a criterion for inclusion in this category. It should be recorded as a general marker of a patient at high risk for atherosclerosis.[147]

In an analysis of 1287 patients with cervical bruits, less than one third of the carotid lesions with bruits proved

to be hemodynamically significant by noninvasive criteria.[41] The fact that significant lesions can occur in the absence of a bruit and vice versa is important. The available data on the natural history of asymptomatic bruits cannot be applied to patients with these lesions. This group of patients is usually discovered by angiography while studying other conditions or by noninvasive studies carried out because of the presence of a bruit or for screening before major surgical procedures. Because of what is known about the natural history of these lesions, as discussed later, therapeutic intervention in the asymptomatic stage may be beneficial. The two categories of symptomatic patients with extracranial arterial occlusive disease are discussed separately.

Transient Ischemic Attacks

General Considerations

TIAs are defined as temporary focal neurologic deficits lasting no more than 24 hours, with complete recovery. The event is caused by ischemia in the territory of the brain supplied by a particular artery or branch. Because of its territorial nature, symptoms tend to be stereotyped. Clinically, symptoms are of sudden onset and without aura, and resolution is often quick. Disappearance of symptoms ordinarily takes only a few minutes.[148] When symptoms last longer than 6 hours, a permanent abnormality is more likely, although it may not be clinically detectable.[149] The frequency of attacks is variable. The patient may experience only one episode or multiple attacks, with variable symptom-free intervals. The most common cause of these transient territorial deficits is extracranial arterial occlusive lesions. The pathology of these lesions has already been discussed. Other important causes in the differential diagnosis include heart disease; hematologic disorders such as systemic lupus erythematosus, hyperglobulinemia, polycythemia, and sickle cell disease; disseminated intravascular coagulation; subacute bacterial endocarditis; paroxysmal embolism; and several rare connective tissue disorders such as pseudoxanthoma elasticum and Ehlers-Danlos syndrome.[149] Migraine, especially when associated with transient neurologic deficit, can be confused with a TIA. A history of migraine in the family, the throbbing quality of the headache, and its occurrence on recovery from the neurologic deficit can be helpful in the differential diagnosis.

An important concept when evaluating patients with symptoms suggestive of TIA is that the symptoms secondary to emboli from a point source such as the extracranial circulation are often the same with every attack. In contrast, patients whose emboli are from the heart tend to have variable symptoms.

Because only about 9% of patients with TIAs are seen by a physician during an attack,[150] the history remains the main factor in establishing the diagnosis. In this regard, family members may be extremely helpful.

Two important syndromes deserve mention. Occasionally, a patient experiences frequent repeated attacks of a specific neurologic deficit with no interval allowing time for complete recovery. If the deficit is the same with each attack and no deterioration in function is seen, this is known as a *crescendo TIA*. If progressive deterioration is seen with each successive attack, a stroke in evolution may be present. In any case, evaluation must proceed on an emergency basis. If a surgically correctable lesion is present and the neurologic deficit is not dense (no loss of consciousness or dense hemiparesis), serious consideration should be given to proceeding with emergency operation.

Carotid Artery Transient Ischemic Attacks

Manifestations of a transient ischemic episode in the territory of the carotid artery include deficits in areas supplied by the anterior and middle cerebral arteries. In older individuals, both anterior and posterior cerebral arteries may be supplied by one carotid artery.[149]

Ischemia in a cerebral hemisphere often produces contralateral symptoms. Motor dysfunction can include weakness, paralysis, or clumsiness of one or both limbs contralateral to the affected hemisphere. Sensory alterations include numbness, loss of sensation, or paresthesia in the opposite side of the face or in one or both limbs. When a patient is examined during an attack, this sensory loss might not be objectively demonstrable.[150]

Ninety-five percent of patients have a dominant left hemisphere. Both receptive aphasia and motor aphasia can occur. When the former is present, the patient or family may interpret it as confusion. Dysarthria can occur as a function of TIA in the nondominant hemisphere, but when it is the sole symptom, vertebrobasilar TIA is more likely. Other functional deficits of the nondominant side include inattention to the patient's own person and environment on the contralateral side.[149] Loss of function of these areas may also be interpreted as confusion.

Transient visual loss (amaurosis fugax) or blurring of vision in the ipsilateral eye is one of the most reliable symptoms of carotid artery TIAs.[151] This may be described as a curtain coming down (altitudinal) or as quadrant field defects. Conjugate eye deviation, as occurs in seizures or completed strokes, is not seen. Homonymous hemianopsia in combination with any of the above-mentioned symptoms suggests carotid TIAs. This is the result of ischemia in the area of the optic radiation emanating from the optic chiasm, which produces loss of vision in the ipsilateral temporal visual field and the contralateral nasal visual field. When TIAs occur secondary to carotid artery disease, these visual field defects are usually limited to a quadrant corresponding to the distribution of the optic radiation. When hemianopsia is complete, it cannot be distinguished from a vertebrobasilar TIA.[149]

Ischemic optic neuropathy is characterized by blindness and is associated with giant cell arteritis in about 10% of cases. In the other 90% of cases, it has been labeled idiopathic. Berguer[152] found a significant correlation between extracranial occlusive disease and idiopathic optic neuropathy. In fact, of 20 symptomatic eyes examined, significant extracranial arterial occlusive disease was found in 12 (60%). An embolic mechanism was suggested as the cause of the optic nerve infarct. A more severe form is seen in patients with very severe extracranial disease, usually occlusion on one side and a high degree of stenosis on the other. These patients develop an ischemic

ophthalmopathy characterized by neovascularization of the iris. The term *rubeosis* has been used to characterize this entity. This suggests that patients with idiopathic optic neuropathy that is not secondary to giant cell arteritis should undergo extracranial vascular evaluation.[152]

Convulsions can occur but are more suggestive of a completed or hemorrhagic stroke. When sensory or motor symptoms are present, they all appear at once, without a march suggestive of focal seizure activity.[149] A combination of symptoms may have more diagnostic reliability than a single symptom alone. In right carotid artery TIA, the combination of ipsilateral visual loss and any contralateral arm symptoms has an increased relationship. In left carotid TIA, diagnostic reliability is increased when language disturbance is combined with right face or extremity weakness or sensory loss.[151]

Altered consciousness or syncope can occur, but it is rarely the only symptom and is more often associated with other disorders, such as cardiac arrhythmias.[149] Other symptoms that make the initial evaluation difficult are dizziness, amnesia, or confusion and impaired vision with alteration in consciousness. These symptoms, without other more specific symptoms, cannot be considered manifestations of TIAs, because they occur most often with other illnesses.

Vertebrobasilar System Transient Ischemic Attacks

Transient ischemia of the area of the brain supplied by the vertebrobasilar system can occur due to flow restriction or emboli from lesions in the vertebral or basilar arteries. Emboli from other sources may also affect this system.

An occlusive lesion at the origin of the subclavian artery can cause vertebrobasilar symptoms as the affected arm is exercised and reversal of flow occurs in the vertebral circulation. This subclavian steal is often accompanied by exertional pain in the arm of the affected side.[149]

Alternating hemiparesis, hemisensory symptoms in repetitive attacks, and bilateral circumoral sensory symptoms associated with unilateral arm or leg weakness or ataxia are highly suggestive of vertebrobasilar TIAs. Symptoms may change from one side to the other with different attacks and may involve all four limbs at one time. Drop attacks, or falling precipitously to the ground without premonitory symptoms, occur in less than 4% of patients.[151] In this syndrome, loss of consciousness is absent or so brief that the patient remembers striking the ground, a feature not present in syncope or seizure.[149]

Equilibratory gait or postural disturbance not associated with vertigo can occur. Complete or partial loss of vision in both homonymous fields or homonymous hemianopsia alone is highly suggestive. Vertigo alone, when not associated with other specific symptoms, should not be considered indicative of TIA. When it occurs in clear relationship to focal weakness of the face, arm, or leg or to ataxia or persistent diplopia, the existence of TIA is likely. Tinnitus is not a feature of vertebrobasilar TIA and is suggestive of labyrinthine vertigo. Single occurrences of bilateral visual blurring, dysarthria, hoarseness, diplopia, dysphasia, confusion, hiccups, vomiting, loss of consciousness, and vital sign alteration may be manifestations of vertebrobasilar TIAs. These symptoms have so many other causes, however, that the diagnosis is uncertain unless they occur in combination or with additional signs of focal brainstem or posterior hemisphere dysfunction.

Cerebral Infarction

A completed cerebral infarction with or without a clinically apparent neurologic deficit can be another manifestation of extracranial arterial occlusive disease. The specific deficits that are clinically detectable are the same as those discussed earlier as manifestations of TIAs.

Accurately estimating the percentage of strokes that are secondary to lesions in the extracranial circulation is difficult. Available studies differ in terms of population, criteria for diagnosis, and therapeutic approach; thus the estimates range from 15% to 52%.[153,154] Extracranial vascular lesions play a major role in the occurrence of cerebral infarction. Approximately 50% of these events are preceded by TIAs, thus providing a clue to diagnosis.[155]

Lacunar infarcts, emboli from a cardiac source, intracerebral or intracranial bleeding, and some hematologic disorders should be included in the differential diagnosis of the cause of stroke. Cerebrospinal fluid examination, electroencephalography (EEG), echocardiography, Holter monitoring, and brain CT are helpful adjuncts. Angiography should be considered, because noninvasive studies do not exclude ulcerative lesions in the extracranial circulation that may be responsible for the embolic infarction. Identification of a cause of the stroke is essential, because these patients remain at high risk of developing a subsequent cerebral infarction.

ROLE OF THE VASCULAR LABORATORY

The role of the vascular laboratory in the evaluation of patients with suspected cerebrovascular disease has been disputed by some and perhaps misused by others. However, it has an increasingly important role, and this section reviews its current application. The vascular laboratory is covered in detail in Chapter 14.

Asymptomatic Patients

Patients without symptoms may come to our attention as possible candidates for extracranial cerebrovascular disease because of the presence of one or more associated risk factors (cigarette smoking, hypertension, diabetes mellitus, coronary artery disease, hyperlipidemia, and peripheral vascular disease) or by the presence of a bruit heard over the carotid artery bifurcation. In the past, the occurrence of a preocclusive carotid stenosis could be ascertained only by carotid angiography, but the incidence of finding a significant lesion by angiographic screening was only 20% to 30%. That means that 70% of the suspect population was subjected to costly and needless hospitalization, plus the risk and discomfort of angiography. Currently, the presence or absence of a hemodynamically significant lesion can be ascertained by carotid duplex scanning. This is an inexpensive, noninvasive test with an accuracy of greater than 95% in qualified vascular laboratories.

Symptomatic Patients

Patients may show territorial neurologic events typical of carotid artery or vertebrobasilar disease, or they may have symptoms that are entirely nonspecific or atypical. In the case of a patient with nonspecific symptoms, such as "dizzy spells," these symptoms may be related to global ischemic events as a consequence of decreased blood flow associated with multiple extracranial occlusive lesions, or they may be due to a myriad of disorders unrelated to cerebrovascular disease. The vascular laboratory serves as an effective screen for these patients, avoiding many negative and hence useless angiograms.

Angiography used to be considered mandatory for the workup of symptomatic patients. This is no longer true. Duplex scanning in a qualified laboratory can provide definitive information necessary for both medical and surgical management. For this reason, a carefully performed duplex scan has become a critical part of the evaluation of symptomatic patients. Contrast angiography is now reserved for patients whose symptoms are not explained by findings on duplex scans or other noninvasive imaging tests such as magnetic resonance angiography (MRA) and CT angiography.

In addition, the preoperative baseline data from the vascular laboratory are extremely helpful in following patients immediately after operation as well as in the late follow-up period. A conversion from a positive to a negative test after operation is expected. If this does not occur, a technical problem is suggested that may require investigation and management. Also, an abnormal study 6 months or a year after surgery in a patient who had a normal study after operation alerts the surgeon to the possibility of recurrent stenosis, often before the onset of symptoms. Finally, the importance of obtaining baseline data on the opposite, asymptomatic carotid artery should not be overlooked. Late strokes that occur in patients who have undergone successful carotid endarterectomy are most often related to the side not operated on. Early identification of progression on the contralateral side permits earlier intervention to prevent contralateral stroke.

BRAIN SCANS AND ANGIOGRAPHY

The advent of CT and magnetic resonance imaging (MRI) has been a benefit in the evaluation of patients with cerebrovascular disease and has virtually eliminated the use of radionuclide scanning. Intracranial space-occupying lesions such as neoplasms, vascular malformations, or subdural hematomas enter into the differential diagnosis of patients with even the most convincing symptoms of transient cerebral ischemia. CT and MRI are quick, noninvasive means of ruling out other abnormalities during the patient workup.

A patient with a TIA may have actually suffered a small cerebral infarction. CT or MRI can identify an unsuspected cerebral infarction and establish a baseline status before operation. The advance knowledge that a small infarction exists is helpful with respect to intraoperative and postoperative management.

Although head scanning may not be a routine part of the preoperative workup, it should become a standard part of the evaluation of symptomatic patients. MRI is replacing CT in some centers. It does not require ionizing radiation or contrast material. It can identify acute cerebral infarction sooner than CT and can image smaller infarcts than CT. Finally, new acquisition programs have enabled the use of magnetic resonance techniques to reconstruct cervical and intracranial arterial anatomy, so-called MRA.

Patients with a clinically overt cerebral infarction should have CT or MRI to document the infarct size and to differentiate between ischemic and hemorrhagic infarction. A hemorrhagic infarction is promptly visible on the CT scan, whereas an ischemic infarction may take several days of evolution before its low-density character is visualized. CT scan data are necessary to determine the proper timing of operation after acute stroke in patients who have had a good neurologic recovery. In fact, of 245 patients with persistent neurologic deficits seen by Dosick and colleagues,[156] 171 were found to have negative CT scan results. Appropriate carotid lesions were found in 110 (64%) of this group. All 110 patients underwent carotid endarterectomy within 14 days of the initial onset of their neurologic deficits. The perioperative morbidity was 0.9%. These investigators concluded that angiography and carotid endarterectomy can be safely performed when indicated in patients with negative CT scan results within the first 2 weeks after a prolonged neurologic deficit.

EEG has generally not been considered helpful in the workup of patients with cerebrovascular disease, with the exception of ruling out seizure disorder in the differential diagnosis. However, a new application of cerebral electrical activity, so-called computerized brain mapping, is of value. This modality uses 32 electrodes (rather than the 16 used with EEG) arranged over both hemispheres. The data are digitized and color coded. The information is analyzed by computer, and hard-copy integrated data are generated. In a report comparing brain mapping, CT, and MRI, brain mapping was more sensitive in identifying small areas of cortical dysfunction.[157]

Aortocranial angiography was once the cornerstone of diagnosis in the workup of patients with suspected cerebrovascular disease. Today, however, the angiogram is no longer a mandatory preoperative study. Current noninvasive studies are sophisticated enough for diagnosis.

Although aortocranial angiography used to be the gold standard for identifying both extracranial and intracranial cerebrovascular disease, most institutions around the world have elected to forgo angiography, provided that noninvasive preoperative testing is of diagnostic quality and correlates with the patient's clinical presentation. Noninvasive testing, primarily carotid duplex scanning, perhaps supplemented with information from MRA or CT angiography, can clearly identify patients with carotid bifurcation disease. MRA or CT may be more accurate in defining the percentage of stenosis than data from

contrast angiography; the contrast angiogram almost inevitably underestimates the percentage of stenosis. Noninvasive testing cannot accurately define carotid ulceration independent of carotid stenosis, but even with angiography, the definition of carotid ulceration is limited. The correlation between the preoperative angiogram and inspection of the plaque at the time of operation was analyzed in the first 540 patients entered into the North American Symptomatic Carotid Endarterectomy Trial (NASCET).[158] The sensitivity and specificity for detecting ulcerated plaques was 45.9% and 74.1%, respectively. The positive predictive value for identifying an ulcer was 71.8%. Thus, even the gold standard of angiography is imperfect in diagnosing ulceration. One possible explanation is that the ulceration may be filled with thrombus when the angiogram is obtained.

The routine preoperative use of angiography has been questioned in the literature. This remains a controversial issue, but the practice has clearly increased in those centers that have validated, certified vascular laboratories.[159]

The benefit of performing carotid endarterectomy without angiography is that angiography carries a significant risk in patients with extracranial arterial occlusive disease. In the ACAS,[160,161] the neurologic morbidity and mortality was 1.2% for angiography alone. This is almost equal to the risk of operation. Although some express the opinion that this complication rate was abnormally high, all patients had been prescreened with ultrasonography and had documented hemodynamically significant lesions. Therefore this represents a select, high-risk group of patients for angiography. With improved techniques of imaging the carotid bifurcation, there has been increasing acceptance of noninvasive imaging as a substitute for preoperative angiography in patients scheduled for carotid endarterectomy. This change in opinion began with the use of improved-quality duplex scanning, and it continues with the use of MRA and CT angiography. Finally, recognizing the limitations of both of these techniques, some suggest combining duplex scanning and MRA for preoperative assessment. When there is clear agreement between the two techniques, this appears to be a safe substitute for contrast angiography; however, when conflicting information is obtained, when the noninvasive study is unsatisfactory, or when the clinical picture is unexplained by noninvasive imaging, the selective use of contrast angiography is clearly indicated.[159,162-172]

SURGICAL CONSIDERATIONS AND TECHNIQUE

Anesthesia and Hemodynamic Monitoring

Patients about to undergo cerebrovascular surgery are probably best managed with general anesthesia. Although some surgeons still prefer to perform carotid endarterectomy using local or cervical block anesthesia,[173] a recent Cochrane analysis of randomized trials failed to show any benefit of regional over general anesthesia.[174] General anesthesia has the advantage of reducing the cerebral metabolic demand of the brain and increasing cerebral blood flow. General anesthesia also provides good airway control, reduced patient anxiety, and a quiet surgical field.

Intraoperative blood pressure control and oxygenation are particularly critical during periods of arterial clamping. These parameters are best monitored with an arterial line, usually placed in the radial artery. The judicious use of nitroprusside or vasopressors by the anesthesiologist to maintain blood pressure in the patient's optimal physiologic range is of paramount importance.

Two primary options are available to monitor cerebral perfusion, which might be required during trial clamping of the carotid artery before a decision to use an internal shunt. These options are the measurement of internal carotid artery back-pressure[175,176] and the intraoperative use of EEG.[173] Although controversy exists as to which is more effective, excellent results have been reported with both techniques. EEG with CT brain mapping is a sensitive and accurate means of identifying patients who require shunting.[157,177] Another technique, that of somatosensory evoked potentials, has been investigated and does not appear to be as sensitive as EEG.[178] Finally, proponents of no monitoring exist; some advocate the routine use of an intraluminal shunt,[179] and others advocate routine operation without a shunt but done in an expeditious manner.[180,181] The literature currently supports either selective shunting based on clinical and monitoring criteria or routine shunting. The consensus is that either of these techniques provides a safe operation with the best outcome.[182,183]

The argument in favor of selective shunting is as follows: because only 10% to 15% of patients actually require an intraluminal shunt, as judged by observations during operations carried out under local anesthesia, why expose the other 85% to 90% of patients to the risks of an internal shunt, which include (1) possible air or atheroma embolism, (2) scuffing or dissection of distal intima, (3) difficulty with end-point visualization, and (4) risk of leaving an intimal flap that may lead to thromboembolic complications? The arguments in favor of the routine use of an intraluminal shunt are that, with routine use, operator facility with the technique is increased and there is less likelihood of complications, and the intraluminal shunt acts as a stent, which can aid in the closure of the internal carotid portion of the arteriotomy.

The criteria for mandatory shunting based on back-pressure measurement, as originally described by Moore and colleagues,[174,175] include a prior cerebral infarction on the side of operation (regardless of back-pressure value) or no prior cerebral infarction but a back-pressure of 25 mm Hg or less in a patient who is otherwise neurologically intact. The EEG criteria for shunt use include a loss of amplitude or slowing of rhythm during trial clamping of the carotid artery.

Carotid Bifurcation Endarterectomy

Indications

The indications for carotid endarterectomy have undergone considerable review and analysis. Data based on retrospective reviews, results of prospective, randomized trials, and committee discussions based on expert opinion have been brought together to define the current indications for carotid endarterectomy.[184-186]

More recently, the Stroke Council of the American Heart Association convened a consensus conference on the indications for carotid endarterectomy. These two reports constitute the most up-to-date agreement concerning indications.[187,188] The ad hoc committee recognized four categories:

1. Proven—the strongest indication, usually supported by results of prospective, randomized trials
2. Acceptable but not proven—a good indication for operation supported by promising but not scientifically certain data
3. Uncertain—data insufficient to define the risk-benefit ratio
4. Proven inappropriate—current data adequate to show that the risk of surgery outweighs any benefit

The recommendations are further stratified by the symptomatic or asymptomatic status of the patient. Finally, the risk of operation based on the comorbid condition of the patient and the individual surgeon's track record is taken into account. Based on this classification, the general indications for carotid endarterectomy can be classified as follows, for symptomatic good-risk patients with a surgeon whose surgical morbidity and mortality rate is less than 6%:

A. Proven indications
   1. One or more TIAs in the last 6 months and carotid stenosis greater than or equal to 70%
   2. Mild stroke with carotid stenosis greater than or equal to 70%
B. Acceptable but not proven indications
   1. TIAs in the past 6 months and stenosis of 50% to 69%
   2. Progressive stroke and stenosis greater than or equal to 70%
   3. Mild or moderate stroke in the past 6 months and stenosis of 50% to 69%
   4. Carotid endarterectomy ipsilateral to TIAs and stenosis greater than or equal to 70%, combined with required coronary bypass grafting
C. Uncertain indications
   1. TIAs with stenosis less than or equal to 50%
   2. Mild stroke with stenosis less than or equal to 50%
   3. Symptomatic acute carotid thrombosis
D. Proven inappropriate indications
   1. Moderate stroke with stenosis less than or equal to 50%, not receiving aspirin
   2. Single TIA, stenosis less than or equal to 50%, not receiving aspirin
   3. High-risk patient with multiple TIAs, stenosis less than or equal to 50%, not receiving aspirin
   4. High-risk patient, mild or moderate stroke, stenosis less than or equal to 50%, not receiving aspirin
   5. Global ischemic symptoms with stenosis less than or equal to 50%
   6. Acute internal carotid dissection, asymptomatic, receiving heparin

For asymptomatic, good-risk patients treated by a surgeon whose surgical morbidity-mortality rate is less than 3%, the indications for carotid endarterectomy are as follows:

A. Proven indications: stenosis greater than or equal to 60% (following ACAS publication)
B. Acceptable but not proven indications: none defined
C. Uncertain indications: high-risk patient or surgeon with a morbidity-mortality rate greater than 3%, combined carotid-coronary operations, or nonstenotic ulcerative lesions
D. Proven inappropriate indications: operations with a combined stroke morbidity-mortality rate greater than or equal to 5%

The Stroke Council of the American Heart Association has updated this report and reaffirmed the indications.[189]

Technique

After the induction of satisfactory anesthesia and the placement of appropriate access and monitoring lines, the patient is positioned supine on the operating table with the head turned away from the side of operation. The neck is moderately extended on the shoulders. The head of the table is flexed approximately 10 degrees to reduce venous pressure, which minimizes bleeding.

This author prefers a longitudinal incision placed along the anterior border of the sternocleidomastoid muscle and centered over the carotid bifurcation. This incision can be extended proximally to the sternal notch for more proximal exposure of the common carotid artery and distally to the mastoid process for extensive exposure of the internal carotid artery, when needed. The use of preoperative ultrasound to identify the location of the carotid bifurcation is helpful in placing the incision accurately and minimizing the incision length. The dissection plane is maintained along the anterior border of the sternocleidomastoid muscle, which permits anterior mobilization of the tail of the parotid gland rather than the bloody division of its substance, with risk of a salivary fistula. The sternocleidomastoid muscle is mobilized off the carotid sheath, and self-retaining retractors are placed. The jugular vein is visualized through the carotid sheath, and the sheath is opened along the anterior border of the vein. The vein is mobilized until the common facial vein is identified. The common facial vein, when present, is a relatively constant landmark for the carotid bifurcation. The common facial vein is divided between ligatures. In the case of a high carotid bifurcation, particular care must be taken to make sure that the hypoglossal nerve is not lurking behind the common facial vein, because this may lead to its inadvertent injury. Once the common facial vein is divided, the jugular vein can be mobilized laterally off the carotid bifurcation, providing excellent exposure. The vagus nerve usually lies in the posterior portion of the carotid sheath, but on occasion it may spiral anteriorly. Particular care must be taken to watch for this anomalous course to avoid nerve injury. Another anomaly is the occasional presence of a nonrecurrent laryngeal nerve that comes directly off the

vagus on the way to innervate the vocal cord. This nerve can cross anterior to the carotid artery and may be mistaken for part of the ansa hypoglossi, resulting in mistaken division and cord paralysis. This anomaly most often occurs on the right side of the neck, but it has also been seen on the left side.

The common carotid artery is mobilized for a sufficient length to get proximal to the atheromatous lesion, as well as to provide sufficient length in case an internal shunt is required. When the dissection approaches the area of the carotid bifurcation, it may be necessary to inject a local anesthetic in the area to block the nerve to the carotid body to prevent or reverse reflex bradycardia. The external and internal carotid arteries are then mobilized for a sufficient length to get completely beyond the atheromatous plaque to a point where the vessels are completely normal circumferentially. When mobilizing the internal carotid artery, particular care must be taken to avoid injury to the hypoglossal nerve (Figure 18-14).

In the case of a high bifurcation or an extensive lesion, mobilizing the internal carotid artery for its maximum extracranial length may be necessary. Several maneuvers are available to gain additional length. The first and most important maneuver is to extend the skin incision all the way up to the mastoid process, with complete mobilization of the sternocleidomastoid muscle toward its

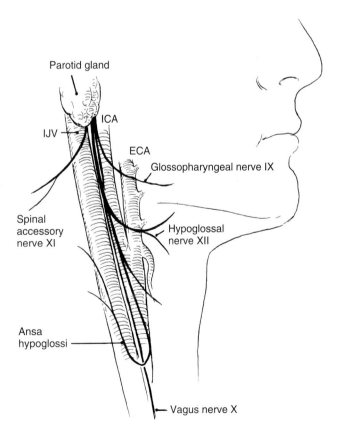

FIGURE 18-14 ■ Anatomic relationship between the carotid bifurcation and the cranial nerves in the neck. Note the intimate relationship between the hypoglossal nerve and the upper portion of the internal carotid artery (ICA). *ECA*, External carotid artery; *IJV*, internal jugular vein.

tendinous insertion on the mastoid process. Care must be taken to avoid injury to the spinal accessory nerve (cranial nerve XI), which enters the substance of the sternocleidomastoid muscle at that level. The posterior belly of the digastric muscle comes into view. This muscle can be mobilized anteriorly or, if necessary, divided with impunity, giving additional exposure of the internal carotid artery. If further exposure is needed, the limiting structures are the styloid process and the ramus of the mandible. The styloid process, after suitable preparation, can be divided with bone rongeurs, and the mandible can be displaced anteriorly. Techniques have also been described for dividing the ramus of the mandible to gain additional exposure, but I have not found this maneuver necessary. Once the carotid artery has been sufficiently mobilized, 5000 units of heparin are administered systemically.

The decision whether to shunt the patient can be made using EEG or back-pressure criteria. If back-pressure is selected, a 22-gauge needle is connected to rigid pressure tubing and hooked up to an arterial pressure transducer. The tubing is flushed with saline, and a 0 pressure level is obtained adjacent to the carotid bifurcation. The needle is carefully bent at a 45-degree angle and inserted into the common carotid artery so that the axis of the distal needle is parallel to the axis of the artery and lies freely within the lumen. The free carotid artery pressure is measured and compared with the radial artery pressure to ensure an accurate reading. When the patient's blood pressure is stable and at the optimal level, the common carotid artery is clamped proximal to the needle, and the external carotid artery is also clamped, thus permitting the reading of the internal carotid artery back-pressure (Figure 18-15). If the back-pressure is greater than 25 mm Hg, the internal carotid artery is clamped and the needle is withdrawn. If the pressure is less than 25 mm Hg, the clamps on the common and external carotid arteries are temporarily removed, the needle is withdrawn, and preparations are made for the use of an internal shunt.

With the common, external, and internal carotid arteries clamped, an arteriotomy is made on the lateral portion of the common carotid artery with a No. 11 blade and is extended toward the plaque and up the internal carotid artery with Potts scissors. The arteriotomy is extended as far as necessary up the internal carotid artery to get beyond the plaque and to expose relatively normal artery. An intimectomy plane is then established between the diseased intima and the internal elastic lamina, attempting to leave the circular medial fibers attached to the arterial adventitia. This facilitates getting a clean distal end point. The proximal end point is obtained by sharply dividing the intima. The intimectomy surface is copiously irrigated with heparinized saline solution to allow the visualization of all bits of debris and facilitate their removal.

The arteriotomy can be closed primarily, but overwhelming evidence indicates better results with patch angioplasty closure. Evidence suggests that female patients, patients with small internal carotid arteries, and patients who continue to smoke are at increased risk of recurrent carotid stenosis.[124,125] The use of patch

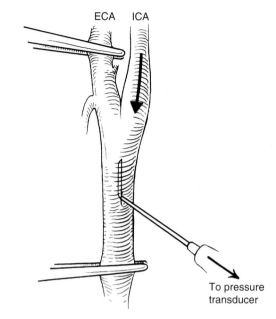

FIGURE 18-15 ■ Technique of measuring the internal carotid artery (ICA) back-pressure. Note the needle placement and needle angulation to maintain the tip of the needle in an axial plane with the common carotid artery. A disease-free portion of the common carotid artery is chosen for arterial puncture. *ECA,* External carotid artery.

angioplasty in these patients may reduce the risk of recurrent stenosis. Trial results indicate that routine use of a prosthetic patch results in the lowest rates of peripheral complications and recurrent stenosis.[121-123] Patch angioplasty should be used routinely when the indication for operation is recurrent stenosis.

Flow is established first to the external and then to the internal carotid artery. I recommend the use of routine completion angiography. There is a 5% to 8% incidence of unsuspected technical errors associated with carotid endarterectomy, and these are best documented with completion angiography.[190,191] Completion angiography is used primarily to identify technical errors involving the internal carotid artery; however, intimal flaps in the external carotid artery occur more commonly and are erroneously considered to be of no consequence. We reported three cases of postoperative stroke secondary to intimal flaps in the external carotid artery: clot formed in the proximal external carotid artery, propagated in a retrograde direction, and then embolized up the internal carotid artery.[192] For this reason, the correction of intimal flaps of the external as well as the internal carotid artery is recommended.

An alternative to completion angiography is the use of intraoperative duplex scanning. Lipski and colleagues[193] reported that the incidence of residual disease and perioperative neurologic complications was statistically significantly reduced in patients who had completion duplex scanning compared with a control group who did not undergo completion imaging.[193] Furthermore, the use of completion duplex scanning identified technical problems and led to their prompt correction in 9 of 39 patients.

Internal Carotid Artery Dilatation

Indications

Internal carotid artery dilatation is uniquely applicable to fibromuscular dysplasia of the carotid artery. It is a major technical advance in simplifying the surgical correction of this lesion.

Technique

The carotid bifurcation is exposed in the usual manner. The internal carotid artery is exposed for its maximal length so that dilatation can be performed under visual and palpable control. Heparin is administered systemically, and the artery is clamped. A vertical arteriotomy, approximately 1 cm long, is made in the carotid bulb, adjacent to the internal carotid artery. Coronary artery dilators are introduced and gently passed toward the base of the skull. I usually start with a 2-mm dilator and progress at 0.5-mm increments to a 4-mm dilator. The surgeon has a sensation of intraluminal septal "popping" as the dilator is passed to the base of the skull. Back-bleeding is allowed to occur after each passage to allow tissue fragments to be washed out and prevent embolization (Figure 18-16). On completion, the arteriotomy is closed, blood flow is restored, and a completion angiogram is obtained to ensure adequate dilatation.

Alternatively, intraoperative balloon angioplasty of the affected segment of the internal carotid artery can be performed. This technique is probably safer because traction injury to the intima is avoided. The intraoperative use of balloon angioplasty, through an open arteriotomy, avoids the possibility of forward embolization from the angioplasty site. After the balloon angioplasty is completed, vigorous back-bleeding of the vessel is allowed, to retrieve any debris loosened by the dilatation. As with progressive dilatation of the vessel, completion angiography is highly recommended to ensure an adequate technical result.

On occasion, the surgeon might not be sure that the dilator has been advanced fully to the base of the skull. Under these circumstances, obtaining a plain radiograph with the dilator in place and comparing that film with the preoperative angiogram to ensure that the dilator has been passed sufficiently far distally is helpful.

Correction of Kinking of the Internal Carotid Artery

Indications

This procedure is indicated for symptomatic kinking of the internal carotid artery and excessive redundancy of the internal carotid artery after mobilization of that vessel for endarterectomy.

Technique

Redundancy of the internal carotid artery can be corrected in a variety of ways, including (1) resection of the redundant internal carotid artery with an end-to-end anastomosis, (2) division of the internal carotid artery with reimplantation onto the proximal common carotid artery, and (3) resection of a segment of the common carotid artery, thus permitting the redundant internal carotid artery to straighten when the carotid bifurcation is brought down for an end-to-end anastomosis (Figure 18-17).

In my experience, the easiest repair is resection of a segment of the common carotid artery, because the anastomosis is the easiest to perform. This requires mobilization of the external carotid artery to move the entire bifurcation proximally.

External Carotid Endarterectomy

Indications

External carotid endarterectomy is indicated in the case of TIAs from embolization or flow reduction and for the correction of significant stenosis or ulceration before extracranial-to-intracranial bypass grafting. In addition, if the internal carotid artery is chronically occluded, there is often a proximal stump left behind that can serve as a nidus for clot or platelet aggregate to reside. The potential exists for this material to embolize via the external carotid artery through collaterals to the brain. Removal of the stump as a part of external carotid endarterectomy will correct this problem.

Technique

The carotid bifurcation is dissected out in the usual manner. The internal carotid artery distal to the

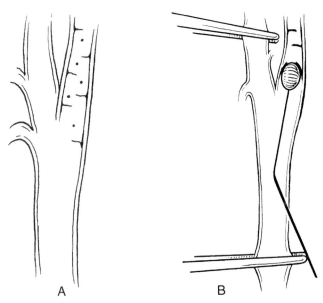

FIGURE 18-16 ■ **A,** Septated lesion of fibromuscular dysplasia. This kind of irregularity leads to symptoms from platelet aggregation and embolization. **B,** A coronary dilator is introduced through a small arteriotomy and advanced up the internal carotid artery. The olive tip of the dilator disrupts the small septa of the fibromuscular dysplastic segment. With an open arteriotomy, back-bleeding flushes any residual intimal segments or platelet aggregates.

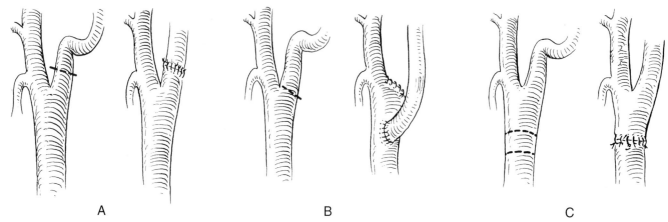

A   B   C

FIGURE 18-17 ■ **A,** A kink of the internal carotid artery can be repaired by segmental resection of the redundant portion of the artery and direct end-to-end anastomosis. **B,** The redundant internal carotid artery can be straightened by dividing it at its origin and moving it proximally to the common carotid artery for end-to-side anastomosis. **C,** The kinked internal carotid artery can be straightened by mobilization of the carotid bifurcation, resection of a segment of the common carotid artery, and direct end-to-end anastomosis, resulting in straightening of the kinked vessel.

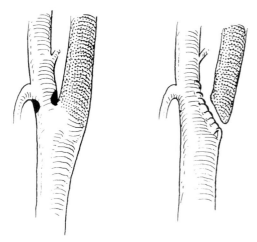

FIGURE 18-18 ■ External carotid endarterectomy can be performed by removing the occluded internal carotid artery and continuing the arteriotomy past the stenotic lesion. This permits endarterectomy under direct vision and primary closure, leaving a smooth taper between the common and external carotid arteries.

obstructed plaque is carefully examined because, on occasion, the vessel may still be patent, thus permitting a standard endarterectomy to be performed, with restoration of blood flow to the internal carotid artery. If the internal carotid artery is confirmed to be occluded, it is divided flush with the carotid bifurcation. An arteriotomy is positioned on the posterolateral aspect of the common carotid artery so that its distal extension passes through the divided orifice of the internal carotid artery and onto the external carotid artery, beyond the atherosclerotic plaque in that vessel. An endarterectomy is then performed. The arteriotomy can be closed primarily, leaving a smooth, tapered transition from the common carotid to the external carotid artery (Figure 18-18). However, the use of a patch is probably preferable. The patch may be of prosthetic material, a vein, or a segment of the occluded internal carotid artery that has been resected and opened. This serves nicely as an autogenous arterial patch.

Resection of Carotid Body Tumor

Vascular surgeons are frequently consulted regarding the surgical management of carotid body tumors. They are familiar with the regional anatomy, and on occasion the tumor may invade the vessel and necessitate segmental resection and arterial reconstruction. The initial approach for exposing a carotid body tumor is the same as that for exposing the carotid bifurcation for endarterectomy. Once the sternomastoid muscle is fully mobilized and the carotid sheath is exposed, the initial maneuver is the circumferential mobilization of the common carotid artery proximal to the tumor mass. When mobilizing the common carotid artery, the vagus nerve should also be identified. After the artery is circumferentially mobilized, the dissection is carried cephalad, with careful separation of the vagus nerve from the artery. As the dissection approaches the area of the carotid bifurcation, the dissection plane, in the periadventitial tissue, continues on the lateral aspect of the bifurcation, on the outer aspect of the internal carotid artery. Once the common facial vein is identified, it can be circumferentially mobilized, clamped, divided, and ligated. This permits the jugular vein to be separated from the carotid bifurcation and the tumor mass. The dissection continues on the lateral aspect of the internal carotid artery. Once the internal carotid artery can be safely and circumferentially mobilized above the tumor mass, this maneuver is completed. Care is taken to identify, protect, and mobilize the twelfth cranial nerve. Dissection is now carried down on the medial aspect of the internal carotid artery, separating the tumor mass from that vessel until the area of the carotid bifurcation is encountered. At this point, the external carotid artery can be carefully mobilized for proximal control. The rich blood supply to the tumor mass is derived from branches of the external carotid artery. In the case of a relatively small tumor, 1 cm or less, it may be possible to separate the tumor mass from the trunk of the external carotid artery by dividing the individual branches that come off the artery and feed the tumor. This can be done until the tumor mass is fully mobilized and excised. More commonly, however, it will be necessary to excise the tumor mass with the entire external carotid artery. Once the external carotid artery is fully mobilized, it can be clamped, divided, and ligated. This will help to control the blood supply inflow to the tumor mass. The outer margins of the tumor are then carefully circumferentially mobilized around the pseudocapsule of the tumor mass. Branches of the external carotid artery are divided as they exit the tumor mass. Once the tumor mass is fully circumferentially mobilized, it can be removed.

In the case of a very large tumor, the mass may, on occasion, encircle and intimately adhere to the internal carotid artery. In this rare instance, the carotid bifurcation may have to be resected with the tumor, and a graft must be placed between the common and internal carotid arteries to restore blood flow. It is common practice to always anticipate this possibility and have the patient monitored with EEG, placed before the operation, to determine whether a shunt will be required or temporary clamping can be used before sewing in an interposition graft. Although a vein graft can be used for this purpose, it is the author's experience that a thin-walled polytetrafluoroethylene graft offers better long-term patency.

POSTOPERATIVE CARE

The first 12 hours are the most critical in managing a patient after cerebrovascular reconstruction. In addition to the usual care required for a patient recovering from general anesthesia, the most important factors are observation of the patient's neurologic status, blood pressure control (either hypotension or hypertension must be appropriately treated), and close wound observation. An expanding hematoma should be identified early, and the patient should be returned promptly to the operating room for identification of the bleeding source and evacuation of the hematoma.

Although intensive care monitoring used to be routine, now only a small percentage of patients actually require an intensive care unit. The majority of patients can be sent to a regular room if they are neurologically intact and hemodynamically stable in the recovery room. Most patients can be discharged safely the next morning. This method of case management has reduced hospital costs.[194-196]

Common practice is to resume antiplatelet drugs. One adult aspirin per day is recommended. If this is not tolerated, Aggrenox or clopidogrel (Plavix) can be used. The rationale for the continued use of antiplatelet drugs is to prevent platelet aggregation and embolization from the new intimectomy site, as well as to serve as prophylaxis in the case of residual, unoperated atherosclerotic plaques in other critical cerebral vessels.

COMPLICATIONS AFTER CAROTID ENDARTERECTOMY

Few vascular operations are as well tolerated as a properly performed carotid endarterectomy. The operative trauma, blood loss, and recovery period are minimal after a successful reconstruction. Unfortunately, the benefits of the procedure, especially in asymptomatic patients, can be negated by a high complication rate. The justification for surgical repair requires that the morbidity of the procedure be kept to a minimum. Possible intraoperative and postoperative complications, their prevention, and their management are discussed.

Intraoperative Complications

One of the most important steps in the prevention of intraoperative problems is adequate preoperative preparation of the patient. Hypertensive patients should have their blood pressure well controlled before the procedure. Patients must be well hydrated, especially if an angiographic procedure has been done within 24 to 48 hours or if they have been receiving continued diuretic therapy. Their myocardial status must be ascertained by careful history, electrocardiography, and other studies such as stress testing as indicated. The use of nitrates during the procedure should be considered in patients with coronary artery disease.

Intraoperative monitoring includes electrocardiographic and continuous blood pressure readings. An intraarterial line can be used to obtain continuous readouts and promptly recognize fluctuations in the patient's blood pressure. The use of Swan-Ganz catheters may be considered in selected patients.

Hypertension and Hypotension

Hypertension and hypotension are frequent during and immediately after carotid endarterectomy. Bove and colleagues[197] found significant hypertension in 19% and hypotension in 28% of 100 consecutive patients undergoing carotid endarterectomy and reported a 9% incidence of neurologic deficits in this group, as opposed to no neurologic morbidity in normotensive patients. This fact, plus the deleterious effects on myocardial function, underscores the importance of early recognition and immediate treatment of extremes of blood pressure. Taking into account the minimal trauma and blood loss that occur during carotid endarterectomy, other factors must have a role in the development of this fluctuation. Some investigators have found a significant increase in the incidence of this problem in chronically hypertensive patients not well controlled preoperatively.[198] The interference with the baroreceptor mechanisms at the carotid sinus may contribute to postoperative blood pressure fluctuations. The postendarterectomy bulb, which is now distensible, might also have a role.[199] Increased cerebral renin production during carotid cross-clamping has been implicated in the development of postendarterectomy hypertension.[200] In a retrospective study of 100 patients, we found a correlation between the use of halogenated fluorocarbon general anesthesia and the development of postendarterectomy hypertension.[201] In a subsequent study, we demonstrated a correlation between cranial norepinephrine levels in jugular venous blood, but not renin, and the development of postoperative hypertension.[202]

Bradycardia during carotid manipulation usually responds to the local injection of 0.5% lidocaine (Xylocaine) in the soft tissues around the nerve to the carotid sinus. Failure of this maneuver to restore a normal heart rate and blood pressure should be followed by immediate investigation and correction of other possible causes. Ranson and colleagues[203] suggested that an uncorrected preoperative deficit in intravascular volume is a critical factor in the development of hypotension and bradycardia. Blocking the reflex arc by the administration of atropine sulfate while volume deficits are corrected frequently returns the blood pressure to within normal limits. If no response is seen after this, the use of vasoconstrictor agents should be considered, and they should be routinely available for immediate administration. Use of these drugs can be deleterious to myocardial function in the presence of hypovolemia.[149,204] The use of dopamine hydrochloride titrated by an infusion pump is preferred by this author.

Hypertension during or after endarterectomy also should be treated promptly. It is preferable to use a short-acting β-blocker initially and sodium nitroprusside by infusion pump, if the hypertension recurs. It is usually started when the systolic blood pressure is greater than 160 mm Hg in normotensive patients and greater than 180 mm Hg in chronically hypertensive patients. It is titrated to keep the systolic levels between 140 and 160 mm Hg. In any case, diastolic pressure is kept at less than 100 mm Hg. The need for intravenous antihypertensive therapy usually lasts less than 24 hours and patients must be monitored in an intensive care unit during that time. In patients with essential hypertension, oral medications are restarted within that period.

Technical Complications

Technical problems during the procedure can be avoided by careful dissection and adherence to a proven established routine. The occurrence of intimal flaps at the distal end point of the endarterectomized segment usually results from incomplete removal of the plaque or too deep a plane of dissection in the media. Several steps must be taken to ensure that no distal intimal flap develops. Following mobilization of the carotid bifurcation, gentle palpation of the internal carotid artery reveal the distal end of the plaque. The arteriotomy should be carried beyond visualization of the distal endpoint. If a shunt is to be inserted, this becomes critical.[205] Only in this manner can the lesion be completely removed under direct vision. As the endarterectomy is carried distally in the internal carotid artery, the most superficial plane in the media that allows complete removal of the plaque should be chosen. In this manner, a tapered endpoint is almost always encountered. Tacking sutures should virtually never be required. The use of intraoperative completion angiograms is encouraged so that distal end-point

defects can be recognized and corrected before completion of the procedure.

Emboli during or after carotid endarterectomy are probably the most frequent cause of neurologic deficits after the procedure. Intraoperatively, these can occur during artery mobilization or shunt insertion or after arteriotomy closure. Care should be taken during the distal insertion of the shunt so that it is done beyond the end of the lesion, as previously mentioned. Failure to do this results in fragmentation of the plaque, with embolization or elevation and wrinkling of the intima. Allowing the shunt to back-bleed freely ensures adequate position and removal of all air. Some clinicians prefer proximal insertion with the shunt fully clamped so that slow, careful release allows immediate reclamping if any air or debris are seen flowing through the shunt.

After the endarterectomy is completed, the area should be free of any loose fragments. Careful irrigation with heparinized saline ensures this. Before completion of the arteriotomy closure, the internal, external, and common carotid arteries should be allowed to bleed freely. Flow should be established to the external carotid artery first to ensure that any debris present goes to this system.

Emboli in the immediate postoperative interval, in the absence of an intimal flap or other technical error, are likely to be from fibrin or platelet aggregates formed in the endarterectomized segment. The use of preoperative antiplatelet agents may prevent such occurrences.

Occasionally, once the procedure is completed, a kink is present in the endarterectomized portion of the internal carotid artery. If the angle between the segments is less than 90 degrees, flow restriction can occur, and disturbances that promote recurrent stenosis are likely. Many times, this can be anticipated when an elongated or coiled artery is present before the endarterectomy. When this situation develops in severe cases, it is preferable to correct the problem by an angioplastic procedure, usually with resection of a segment of the common carotid artery with pull-down and primary anastomosis (see Figure 18-17C). Ligation and division of the external carotid artery are rarely required, because dissection of the trunk and main branches allows sufficient mobility to correct the kink. Ligation and division of the nerve of Hering and surrounding bifurcation tissues are always necessary.

A carotid–cavernous sinus fistula is a feared complication when treating acute carotid thrombosis with balloon catheters placed in the internal carotid artery. On the rare occasion when it is necessary, several maneuvers should be attempted before the use of balloon catheters. The clot should be carefully separated from the intima and gently pulled down. The internal carotid back-pressure is sometimes helpful in this process, and shunting the external circulation can make a difference, allowing extraction of the clot. If the use of balloon catheters is necessary, they should never be inserted beyond the proximal intracranial portion of the artery, and the use of traction force is condemned. Although perforating the carotid artery intracranially with the balloon catheter is possible, the most common mechanism of injury that creates a carotid–cavernous sinus fistula is that of traction with the balloon catheter. This shearing force creates a transverse tear in the portion of the intracranial carotid that is intimately adherent to the cavernous sinus and fixed to the petrous portion of the skull. Therefore traction on the inflated balloon catheter should be gentle. Fluoroscopic guidance may be helpful. Failure of these maneuvers makes abandonment of the procedure mandatory and requires consideration of an extracranial-to-intracranial bypass.

Cranial Nerve Injury

Peripheral cranial nerve injury is another source of morbidity after carotid endarterectomy. In a prospective analysis, Hertzer and colleagues[206] found a 16% incidence of cranial nerve dysfunction after this procedure. Only 60% of injuries were symptomatic. The rest would have gone unnoticed by the patient or physician had further detailed examination been omitted. A similar overall incidence was found by Evans and colleagues[207] on clinical grounds, but when speech pathologists were added as part of the evaluation team, the incidence increased to 39%, mostly related to superior laryngeal and recurrent laryngeal nerve dysfunction. The majority of these deficits were temporary, and when evaluation was repeated in 6 weeks, the incidence was between 1% and 4%. These injuries can be avoided with careful dissection, the principle being to stay in the periadventitial plane of the artery and to be familiar with the anatomy of the area, including well-recognized anomalies (Figure 18-19).

The hypoglossal nerve is frequently visualized during carotid endarterectomy. It can be seen descending along the course of the internal carotid, then crossing the external carotid in a more superficial plane. Mobilization of this nerve may be necessary when a high bifurcation is present or when the lesion extends high in the internal carotid artery. This is accomplished by careful division of small veins that tent the nerve downward. A branch of the external carotid to the sternocleidomastoid muscle is frequently present and requires division. The ansa hypoglossi can frequently be retracted medially, but on occasion it requires division as it comes off the hypoglossal nerve. Traction or retractor injury to the hypoglossal nerve should be avoided. Clinically, the deficit is manifested by deviation of the tongue to the ipsilateral side. Speech, deglutition, and mastication problems have been reported.[206]

The spinal accessory nerve is rarely seen during this dissection, but on high dissections it may be seen entering the sternocleidomastoid muscle superiorly. It can be left attached and retracted with the muscle, but care should be taken not to compress it with the retractor.

The vagus nerve is always seen, usually posterolateral to the carotid artery, between the latter and the jugular vein. On occasion, it lies anteromedial to the artery. Keeping the dissection close to the artery prevents injury to this nerve. The recurrent laryngeal nerve usually lies within the trunk of the vagus at this level, but a nonrecurrent laryngeal nerve on occasion traverses the common carotid artery. Injury to these structures can be asymptomatic or manifested by hoarseness, but hoarseness in the postoperative period is due to vocal cord paresis in approximately half of patients.[206] This underscores the

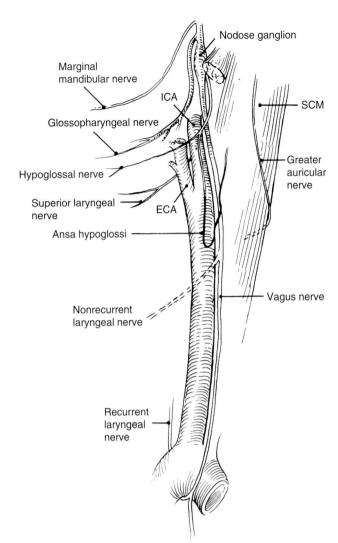

FIGURE 18-19 ■ Surgical anatomy and relationship of structures encountered during exposure of the carotid bifurcation. *ECA*, External carotid artery; *ICA*, internal carotid artery; *SCM*, sternocleidomastoid muscle.

importance of laryngoscopic examination in reaching a specific diagnosis. The asymptomatic injury gains significance when bilateral staged reconstructions are planned, in which case routine laryngoscopic visualization of the vocal cords is highly recommended. Detection of a paralyzed vocal cord mandates delaying the procedure until recovery is complete. If vocal cord paralysis is permanent, appropriate precautions should be taken to avoid bilateral injury, and perioperative airway management should be given special consideration.

The superior laryngeal nerve leaves the inferior ganglion of the vagus (nodose ganglion) and courses behind the internal carotid artery, bifurcating into an internal and an external branch. The internal branch is sensitive to the larynx, and the external innervates the inferior constrictor and cricothyroid muscles. The latter is responsible for the quality of voice, specifically the higher pitches. Injury to the external laryngeal nerve can be avoided by keeping the dissection close to the arterial wall, specifically when controlling the superior thyroid artery.

The glossopharyngeal nerve is usually not seen in the dissection but can be injured when dissections are carried high, especially those requiring division of the digastric muscles.[208,209] This nerve courses posterior to the high portion of the internal carotid artery and can be injured with the application of a vascular clamp that includes tissues other than the artery itself. Again, dissection close to the arterial wall is the key to prevention. Clinically, the dysfunction is evident when tasks requiring oral pharyngeal muscle activity, mostly deglutition, are examined. Horner syndrome may be produced by injury to the ascending sympathetic fibers in the area of the glossopharyngeal nerve.

The cervical branch of the facial nerve lies beneath the platysma, inferior to the angle of the jaw. In some patients, this nerve sends branches to the mandibular branch, and its injury produces sagging of the ipsilateral corner of the lower lip. The marginal mandibular branch can itself be injured when the incision is carried too close to the jaw. Both of these injuries can be prevented by curving the upper portion of the incision toward the mastoid process.[205] Self-retaining retractors should be carefully placed in this area.

The greater auricular nerve courses deep to the platysma over the sternocleidomastoid muscle at an angle toward the ear in the upper portion of the dissection. Its division should be avoided, but is frequently necessary in high dissections. Numbness of the earlobe is the usual consequence, although surprisingly some patients have no complaints after its deliberate division.

The parotid gland lies in the superior portion of the incision anterior to the sternocleidomastoid muscle. Again, curving the incision toward the mastoid process prevents injury in high dissections. Troublesome bleeding and the risk of a parotid fistula can be prevented by this maneuver.

Postoperative Complications

On completion of an operation performed with general anesthesia, the patient is awakened in the operating room. A gross neurologic examination is performed. If no deficit is found, the patient is transferred to the recovery room, where a more detailed examination is performed.

Stroke is the most feared complication of carotid endarterectomy. In experienced hands, it occurs in between 1% and 3% of patients, depending on the indication for the procedure.[210] Most of the low rates of stroke have been reported from specialized centers. Early results from pooled data community surveys showed rates of combined stroke morbidity and mortality ranging from 6.5% to 21%.[211-213] Because carotid endarterectomy is a prophylactic operation used to prevent stroke, these higher complication rates erase most benefits and are clearly unacceptable. A committee of the Stroke Council of the American Heart Association reviewed this problem and set standards for upper acceptable limits of stroke and death as a function of indication for operation. Thus, for patients undergoing carotid endarterectomy for asymptomatic carotid stenosis, the combined operative stroke morbidity and mortality should not exceed 3%; for TIA as an indication, 5%; for prior stroke as an

indication, 7%; and for recurrent carotid stenosis, 10%.[214] A mechanism for individual surgeon audit was described and recommended. Fortunately, more recent results from individual series, prospective randomized trials, and national databases have shown a marked reduction in stroke morbidity and mortality following carotid endarterectomy. These reports will be discussed under results.

TIAs in the first postoperative week have been reported with a frequency as high as 8%. When a neurologic deficit is found on awakening the patient, the main question to be resolved is the patency of the internal carotid artery. If a completion angiogram was performed and no abnormalities were seen, the event is likely to be embolic, and immediate reoperation would likely be of no benefit. If no completion imaging was performed, immediate patency of the vessel should be assessed. This can be done by noninvasive means,[215] but the most expeditious approach is to return the patient to the operating room for exploration. Immediate reoperation and correction of defect including thrombectomy may reverse the deficit.[216] If the vessel appears patent by noninvasive tests, the surgeon needs to determine whether the emboli occurred during the operation or whether a source is present in the operated segment. This is also the case in a patient who is neurologically intact and develops an event in the ipsilateral hemisphere hours or days after surgery. Once patency is evidenced by exploration or noninvasive means, immediate angiography is indicated. Reoperation is necessary if a significant defect or any clot is present. Otherwise, conservative therapy with anticoagulation, antiplatelet agents, or both is warranted. Other factors inevitably influence the decision to reoperate or observe the patient. The difficulty of the initial reconstruction, the patient's general status, and the availability and reliability of ancillary facilities affect this difficult decision (Figure 18-20).

Mortality after carotid endarterectomy has declined significantly as the incidence of postoperative stroke has diminished. Pulmonary problems, renal insufficiency, and sepsis are extremely unusual complications owing to the nature of this procedure. MI remains the most frequent cause of death in the early postoperative period, more so in patients with suspected coronary artery disease.[217] Because of this, preoperative assessment is of paramount importance. Postoperatively, electrocardiographic monitoring for the first 24 hours and a 12-lead electrocardiographic tracing should be obtained. Any suspicion of a myocardial event should be investigated and treated aggressively.

Wound infections after carotid endarterectomy are extremely rare. Routine use of prophylactic antibiotics for 24 hours during the perioperative interval is recommended.

Taking into account that the procedure is performed with full heparinization and that many patients have received platelet antiaggregates preoperatively, the incidence of wound bleeding is low. In Thompson's personal series,[210] reoperation for this problem was required in 7/1022 (0.7%) patients.

Large cervical hematomas may form, and reoperation and drainage should be strongly considered in an otherwise stable patient. The routine use of a Silastic drain has

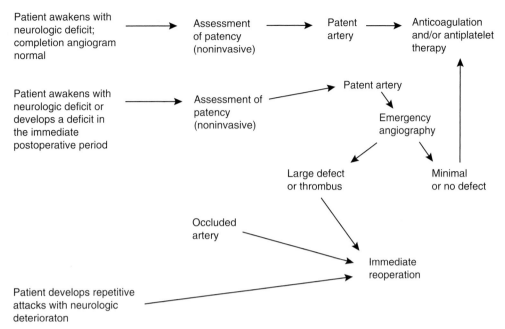

FIGURE 18-20 ■ Algorithm that can be applied to the management of a patient who awakens with a postoperative neurologic deficit after carotid endarterectomy.

not been shown to reduce the incidence of this complication. Bleeding occurs from the suture line rarely. More often, a diffuse ooze is present, requiring reversal of anticoagulation. In any case, drainage of the hematoma and correction of its cause prevent chronic draining wounds, infection, and the rare occurrence of pseudoaneurysm formation. The last is more frequent when closure is performed with a patch.[210]

Headache after carotid endarterectomy is not unusual. It may be associated with a neurologic deficit, in which case a CT scan should be performed. In the majority of cases, however, it runs a self-limited course and is probably related to altered autoregulatory dysfunction of the cerebral circulation. The use of a β-blocker has been effective in treating troublesome headache. Poorly controlled hypertension can result in encephalopathy. The mildest form is headache, which can progress to seizure, and the most severe form is intracerebral hemorrhage, which is often fatal. The risk of this complication mandates careful preoperative and perioperative management of hypertension.

Complications after carotid endarterectomy can be prevented by careful patient preparation, meticulous technique, and adherence to a rational, well-established routine. An uneventful operation is the best way to effectively change the natural history of extracranial arterial occlusive disease.

RESULTS OF SURGICAL TREATMENT FOR EXTRACRANIAL ARTERIAL OCCLUSIVE DISEASE

The most frequently performed operation for extracranial arterial occlusive disease is endarterectomy of the carotid bifurcation. As experience is gained with this procedure, results have improved, and in experienced hands it can be done with morbidity and mortality rates well below the Stroke Council guidelines. When recommending this procedure, the results of the particular surgeon or institution should be considered, because a higher morbidity and mortality may negate any beneficial effects of surgery.

The first multi-institutional study that compared surgical and medical treatment in a prospectively randomized fashion came from the joint study on extracranial arterial occlusion,[218] in which 1225 symptomatic patients with extracranial arterial occlusive disease were randomly allocated to receive either medical or surgical therapy. Long-term survival of as long as 42 months was better in surgically treated patients with unilateral carotid stenosis who were experiencing TIAs or cerebral infarction with minimal residual deficit. The neurologic morbidity in 316 patients who were identified as having hemispheric TIAs as an indication for inclusion in the study was evaluated. The incidence of cerebral infarction at 42 months was reduced in the surgical group. Recurrent TIAs or cerebral infarction usually affected the side not operated on in the surgical patients, in contrast to the medically treated group, in whom neurologic events occurred chiefly in the distribution of the symptomatic artery at the time of randomization. The differences were statistically significant. The combined postoperative morbidity and mortality in the surgically treated group was approximately 8%, which is considered high by today's standards. This may have affected the results of this study in favor of medical therapy.

The preoperative neurologic status of the patient affects the immediate postoperative results. Asymptomatic patients fare better than patients with TIAs, and the latter have lower morbidity than patients with completed strokes. Rothwell and colleagues[219] reviewed 25 studies and performed a metaanalysis. The combined perioperative risk of death and stroke was 3% to 3.5% in asymptomatic patients, compared with 5.18% for symptomatic patients. These differences were consistent across all studies and indicate that operation on asymptomatic patients is safest. In fact, late results may be similarly affected. Bernstein and colleagues[220] reported a series of 456 carotid endarterectomies monitored for 1 to 11 years, with an average follow-up of 45.3 months.[220] Asymptomatic patients who were operated on had a 1.6% incidence of TIAs and a 3.2% incidence of stroke on late follow-up. Those operated on because of TIAs had a 19.5% and 5.2% incidence of recurrent TIAs and stroke, respectively. Patients with a permanent neurologic deficit preoperatively had a 7.9% incidence of TIAs, and 11% developed a stroke on late follow-up.

Similar results were reported by Hertzer and Arison[221] in 329 patients monitored for a minimum of 10 years after carotid endarterectomy. The cumulative incidence of stroke by the life-table method was 24% at 10 years after operation. Only 10% of patients sustained strokes that clearly involved the ipsilateral cerebral hemisphere. Hypertension, preoperative stroke as an indication, and patients with recognized contralateral carotid stenosis had a much higher incidence of stroke on long-term follow-up. Contralateral hemispheric strokes occurred in 36% of patients with uncorrected contralateral lesions, compared with 8% of those who had elective bilateral reconstruction. This difference was statistically significant. Patients undergoing elective myocardial revascularization had a significant increase in long-term survival when compared with patients with uncorrected coronary artery disease. These results suggest that the annual incidence of late stroke, specifically involving the cerebral hemisphere ipsilateral to the previous carotid repair, is 1.1%, a figure within the expected range for the normal population. Stroke in the subset of patients with bilateral carotid arterial disease was fivefold more common in the contralateral than in the ipsilateral cerebral hemisphere. Therefore staged contralateral endarterectomy should be seriously considered in patients with documented but otherwise asymptomatic advanced contralateral carotid stenosis.[221]

Analysis of the available surgical series with long-term follow-up reveals that a successfully performed carotid endarterectomy places the patient at a significantly lower risk of stroke. The results of the various surgical series are summarized in Table 18-1, according to the indications for operation.[222-231] Asymptomatic patients have a 1.2% per year stroke risk, including perioperative morbidity and mortality. Patients with TIA as an indication for endarterectomy have an initial perioperative morbidity and mortality of approximately 3%, with a long-term risk of stroke of 2% per year. Patients whose indication for operation is cerebral infarction have a higher perioperative morbidity, averaging approximately 5%. Long-term results suggest that these patients have an annual stroke rate of approximately 4% per year. The average recurrence of TIAs is on the order of 8% to 10% at 5 years for all indications. These results represent a clear improvement over the natural history of the disease, including the use of antiplatelet drugs; however, they underscore the importance of maintaining the operative stroke rate at acceptable levels for the various indications. A higher figure negates the early and late beneficial results of surgical therapy.

The results of carotid endarterectomy for nonhemispheric symptoms are less predictable. In a series of 107 patients subjected to carotid endarterectomy, the initial perioperative morbidity and mortality were similar to those in patients with specific indications for operation. Carotid endarterectomy was successful in ameliorating symptoms in patients with nonhemispheric symptoms who had greater than 60% diameter reduction of the carotid artery and classic symptoms of vertebrobasilar insufficiency.[232] The same series of 61 patients was updated by Ricotta and colleagues.[233] They compared the results of their cohort of patients with nonhemispheric symptoms to the remainder of their series. Follow-up lasted a mean of 42.3 months. The perioperative stroke rate was 4.9%. Survival was 85.3% at 3 years and 64.9% at 5 years. Stroke-free survival was 77.1% at 3 years and 63.4% at 5 years. During follow-up, 11 patients (18%) developed recurrent nonhemispheric symptoms. These results were not different from the cohort of 553 patients. The authors concluded that carotid endarterectomy provided long-term benefit in this group of patients.

The use of cerebral angiography can also be helpful in selecting patients. The presence of a posterior communicating artery suggests that the anterior circulation may be a major contributor to the vertebrobasilar system. Its presence suggests that removal of a hemodynamically significant lesion in the carotid territory would be beneficial in alleviating posterior circulation systems.

In the absence of significant extracranial carotid artery disease, direct vertebral artery reconstruction is the procedure of choice for patients with vertebrobasilar system lesions secondary to extracranial occlusive disease. The results of direct vertebral artery reconstruction have been good, although the experience is not as extensive as that with carotid artery surgery. In a series of 109 vertebral artery operations, Imparato[234] reported an operative mortality of 3%. Other complications included temporary hemidiaphragm paralysis and Horner syndrome. Two thromboses of the reconstruction occurred; there were no perioperative strokes. Long-term follow-up revealed a stroke incidence of 1.5% per year of follow-up. No controlled series on the natural history of these patients is available for comparison.

The experience with external carotid revascularization is limited; therefore long-term results are not available. In a series of 42 external carotid artery reconstructions, O'Hara and colleagues[235] reported no early morbidity or mortality when the operation was limited to external carotid endarterectomy and patch angioplasty. When the procedure was combined with bypass to the external carotid artery or with an extracranial-to-intracranial bypass, a 33% incidence of stroke was observed. No neurologic symptoms occurred in 25 patients (60%) during follow-up ranging from 1 to 72 months (mean, 27 months). These authors concluded that external carotid endarterectomy can be performed with acceptable risks

TABLE 18-1 **Results of Carotid Endarterectomy According to the Indication for Operation**

Indication	Author	No. of Patients	Follow-up	Operative Morbidity (%)	Operative Mortality (%)	Recurrent TIAs, Ipsilateral (%)	Stroke Ipsilateral (%)	Stroke Contralateral (%)
Asymptomatic	Thompson et al.[179]	132	55.1 mo	0	1.2	0.75	4.7[a]	NS
	Sergeant et al.[222]	43	6.48 mo	2.3	2.3	0	0	0
	Moore et al.[223]	72	6-180 mo	0	0	2.7	5.6[b]	2.7
	Bernstein et al.[224]	87[c]	43 mo	NS[d]	0	NS	6.3[e]	NS
	Hertzer and Arison[221]	126	10-14 yr	NS	NS	NS	9[f]	7[f]
	Lord[225]	226	30-144 mo	2.6	1.1	NS	0.4	1.1
TIA	Bernstein et al.[224]	370[g]	12-132 mo	NS	0	19.5[h]	5.2	NS
	DeWeese et al.[226]	103	60-mo minimum	6.0	0.97	18.4[i]	7.7[i]	10.6
	Thompson et al.[227]	293	Up to 156 mo	2.7	1.4	16.3	4.7	0.6
	Takolander et al.[228]	142	5-yr actuarial	4.9	1.8	14.7	6.5	4.0
	Hertzer and Arison[221]	123	10-14 yr	NS	NS	NS	6[f]	9[f]
Stroke	Thompson et al.[227]	217	Up to 156 mo	5.0	7.4		8.2	NS
	Eriksson et al.[229]	55	21-mo average	3.7	3.7		3.8	NS
	Bardin et al.[230]	127	56-mo average	3.9	3.1		20	NS
	Takolander et al.[228]	60	5-yr actuarial	4.9	5.9	11.6[e]	10	NS
	McCullough et al.[231]	50	41-mo average	3.4	1.7		3.3	NS
	Hertzer and Arison[221]	80	10-14 yr	NS	NS	NS	6[f]	13

TIA, Transient ischemic attack; *NS,* not specified.
[a]Side of stroke not specified; three strokes were fatal.
[b]Two patients suffered transient postoperative deficits with complete recovery.
[c]Number of procedures; exact number of patients not specified.
[d]Perioperative stroke rate of 3% in the entire series of 370 patients.
[e]Side of neurologic event not specified; risk of stroke at 5 years by life-table analysis.
[f]Does not include perioperative strokes.
[g]Total number of patients in series, including TIA patients.
[h]Territory affected not specified.
[i]Includes patients with nonterritorial symptoms.
[j]Includes operative morbidity.

and long-term effectiveness. When the reconstruction involves bypass to the external carotid artery or extracranial-to-intracranial bypass, a higher operative risk can be expected. A similar note of caution was expressed by Halstuk and colleagues,[236] describing 49 external carotid revascularization procedures performed in 36 patients. Indications included ipsilateral TIAs, amaurosis fugax, and a preparatory procedure in anticipation of extracranial-to-intracranial bypass. Twenty patients had preoperative strokes. Twenty-nine patients underwent unilateral external carotid endarterectomy, with the remaining patients undergoing other procedures in addition to the external revascularization. The incidence of postoperative stroke within 8 days of external

carotid revascularization was 13.8%. One operative death occurred, for a mortality rate of 2.7%. Long-term follow-up ranging from 1 to 75 months (mean, 29 months) revealed a 14.2% incidence of late neurologic ischemic events. Three of these were TIAs, one was a reversible ischemic neurologic deficit, and one patient had a stroke 50 months after his initial operation. These results suggest caution in recommending external carotid artery surgery, especially when the revascularization will involve more than just endarterectomy with patch closure.

The perioperative use of aspirin in patients undergoing carotid endarterectomy reduces the risk of stroke and death up to 6 months. Lindblad and associates[237] performed a prospective, randomized trial comparing carotid

TABLE 18-2 Effect of Perioperative Use of Aspirin

Time after Operation	Complication	CEA with ASA, No. of Patients (%)	CEA without ASA, No. of Patients (%)
1 wk	Stroke	0	7 (6)
30 days	Stroke	2 (1.7)	11 (9.6)
6 mo	Stroke	2 (1.7)	11 (9.6)
30 days	Mortality	0.8	4.3
6 mo	Mortality	3-4	6

CEA, Carotid endarterectomy; ASA, acetylsalicylic acid.

endarterectomy in patients with and without aspirin. The results are summarized in Table 18-2. Although the results of individual series are of interest, level 1 data regarding risk and benefit come from prospective randomized trials or population-based analyses.

PROSPECTIVE, RANDOMIZED TRIALS

Despite retrospective data analysis clearly demonstrating the superiority of carotid endarterectomy over medical management in regard to stroke prevention, a number of well-meaning critics point out that retrospective data analysis can be misleading. Retrospective studies compare surgical results with available natural history data. The natural history of a particular disease process can change, often for the better, making the basis of comparison invalid. Likewise, retrospective reviews are often performed in centers of excellence, where surgical complication rates may be lower than the actual risk of operation in the community. For this reason, several prospective, randomized trials were initiated in North America and Europe. The objective of these trials was to scientifically evaluate the efficacy (or lack thereof) of carotid endarterectomy in preventing stroke for a variety of indications when compared with a true, contemporary control group. The trials can generally be categorized into two major classifications: asymptomatic and symptomatic carotid artery disease.

Three asymptomatic trials have completed their data acquisition and reported results: the Veterans Administration Asymptomatic Carotid Stenosis Study, ACAS, and the European Asymptomatic Carotid Surgery Trial. Three symptomatic trials have been completed: NASCET, the Medical Research Council European Carotid Surgery Trial (ECST), and the Veterans Administration Symptomatic Trial.

Asymptomatic Trials

Veterans Administration Asymptomatic Carotid Stenosis Study

Ten Veterans Administration (VA) medical centers entered into a prospective, randomized trial designed to test the hypothesis that carotid endarterectomy plus best medical management (aspirin and risk factor control)

would result in fewer TIAs than treatment with the best medical management alone. The design of the study was published in 1986.[238] Angiography was performed in 713 patients, 3 of whom (0.4%) sustained a neurologic deficit.[239]

A total of 444 patients were randomized over a 54-month interval. In the surgical group, 211 carotid endarterectomies were performed; these patients also received aspirin therapy. In the medical group, 233 patients were treated with aspirin alone. The study spanned a total of 8 years. The 30-day mortality rate for the surgery group was 1.9%, and the incidence of stroke was 2.4%. The combined stroke and mortality rate was 4.3%.[240]

The data analysis demonstrated that all neurologic events (stroke, TIA, amaurosis fugax) in any distribution (including the study artery), combined with deaths, totaled 30 in the carotid endarterectomy group, which represented 14.2% of that population. For the patients treated medically, a total of 55 events occurred, for an event rate of 23.6%. This difference was statistically significant ($p < 0.006$). When the data were analyzed for deaths plus ipsilateral events only, a total of 21 events occurred in the carotid endarterectomy group, for an incidence of 10%; in contrast, there were 46 events in the medically treated group, for an incidence of 19.7%. Once again, this difference was statistically significant ($p < 0.002$). Although the study was not designed to look at stroke alone, this was done retrospectively. A total of 10 strokes occurred in the carotid endarterectomy group ipsilateral to the study artery, for an incidence of 4.7%. A total of 20 strokes occurred in the study artery distribution in the medically treated group, for an incidence of 8.6%. This difference fell just short of statistical significance ($p = 0.056$), probably because of the small sample size. There was no difference in survival rate between the surgically and medically treated groups. This is not surprising, because the major cause of death in this patient group is MI, and prevention of stroke is unlikely to have a beneficial effect on reducing fatal MI. This lack of difference in survival between the surgically and medically treated groups should not be considered a negative factor when interpreting data results, because the objective of operation is to maintain the patient stroke free during his or her remaining lifetime.[241]

Asymptomatic Carotid Atherosclerosis Study

The ACAS, sponsored by the National Institutes of Health (NIH), was the largest multicenter (34 centers), North American, prospective, randomized trial of surgery for asymptomatic carotid stenosis. It tested the hypothesis that carotid endarterectomy plus aspirin and risk factor control would result in fewer TIAs, strokes, and deaths than would aspirin and risk factor control alone.

The design of the study was published in 1989.[242] Initially, 1500 patients were to be randomized, with TIA included as an end point. After criticism of the VA study, the protocol was amended to have stroke and death as the end points. The Data Safety and Monitoring Committee of the NIH gave permission to increase the sample size from 1500 to 1800 patients.

In December 1994, the committee called a halt to the study and informed the investigators, and subsequently the public, that an end point had been reached in favor of carotid endarterectomy,[243] and a full report was published.[160] A total of 1662 patients with diameter-reducing lesions of 60% or greater (as measured by angiography using the North American method; see later) were randomly allocated to receive carotid endarterectomy plus best medical management, including aspirin; the control group received best medical management alone. After a mean follow-up of 2.7 years (4657 patient-years of observation), the aggregate risk over 5 years for ipsilateral stroke, any perioperative stroke, and death was 5.1% for surgical patients and 11% for patients treated medically. The results of surgery, including perioperative morbidity and mortality, reduced the risk of death and stroke by 5.9% absolutely and yielded a 53% risk reduction. This difference was highly significant.

The beneficial effect of surgery in asymptomatic patients was due in large part to the low 30-day perioperative stroke morbidity and mortality. Before the study began, the surgical management committee for ACAS established criteria to audit surgeons who wished to participate in the study.[244] Validation of the audit method was possible on conclusion of the study. Among 825 patients randomized to surgery, the stroke morbidity and mortality rate within 30 days of randomization was 2.3%. However, this included a stroke morbidity and mortality of 1.2% for preoperative angiography. Because of the intent-to-treat design, the angiographic complications were charged to surgery. Of the 724 patients who actually had carotid endarterectomy, mortality was 0.14%, and the stroke rate was 1.38%. Thus, the true 30-day stroke morbidity and mortality rate was 1.52%.[161]

Asymptomatic Carotid Surgery Trial

A group of European investigators, headed by a team from the United Kingdom, embarked on yet another trial. However, included in their trial were methods designed to try to identify a higher-risk group of patients.[245] The investigators reported their results in 2004.[246] A total of 3128 asymptomatic patients with carotid artery stenoses of 70% or greater, as measured by ultrasonography, were entered into the trial from 1993 through 2003. The patients were equally randomized between immediate carotid endarterectomy and indefinite deferral of operation.

The 30-day risk of stroke or death in the surgical group was 3.1%. When analyzing the 5-year results of the two groups, the stroke risk, excluding perioperative events, was 3.8% in the surgical group, versus 11% in the nonsurgical group ($p < 0.0001$). Half the stroke events were disabling or fatal. If perioperative events were included, the 5-year stroke rate in the two groups was 6.4% versus 11.8% ($p < 0.0001$). Comparing fatal or disabling strokes, the event rate was 3.5% in the surgical group versus 6.1% in the nonsurgical group. The investigators found that the results were significant for both men and women when analyzed separately. The authors concluded that, in asymptomatic patients 75 years of age or younger with a diameter-reducing stenosis of 70% or greater as measured by ultrasonography, immediate carotid endarterectomy reduced the net stroke risk by half, from about 12% in the control group to 6% (including a 3% perioperative hazard) in the surgical group. Furthermore, half of the 5-year benefit involved the prevention of disabling or fatal strokes.[246]

Symptomatic Trials

North American Symptomatic Carotid Endarterectomy Trial

The NASCET was a large prospective trial designed to test the hypothesis that symptomatic patients (those with TIA or prior mild stroke) with ipsilateral carotid stenosis (30% to 99%) have fewer fatal and nonfatal strokes after carotid endarterectomy than do patients treated with medical management alone, including aspirin. Investigators anticipated that approximately 3000 patients would be randomly allocated to receive either medical or surgical management and monitored for a minimum of 5 years. The NASCET was also stratified to study two subsets of patients as a function of the degree of carotid occlusive disease: those with 70% to 99% stenosis and those with more moderate lesions ranging from 30% to 69% stenosis.[247] Included in the design of the trial and required by the granting institution (the NIH) was the establishment of an oversight committee that was responsible for reviewing the results of the data from time to time and calling a halt to the study if a clear difference was observed between the two groups.

On February 25, 1991, a clinical alert was issued by the oversight committee, which reported that a clear difference had developed between the two groups, indicating that carotid endarterectomy was superior to medical management in the high-grade stenosis category (70% to 99%). No clear difference had yet occurred in the moderate stenosis group (30% to 69%), and the latter continued to enter patients for randomization.

In the high-grade stenosis category, 295 patients received medical management and 300 patients received surgical management. Sixteen of the medically treated patients (5.4%) actually crossed over to surgery, but because of the "intent-to-treat" design, these patients continued to be analyzed as if they were managed medically, despite their operations. Crossovers become important if the group that patients are leaving is in fact a disadvantaged group, as is the case in this study.

The 30-day operative morbidity and stroke mortality rate for patients managed surgically was 5%. The analysis at the end of 18 months of follow-up, which led the oversight committee to halt this arm of the study. In the surgical group, a 7% incidence of fatal and nonfatal strokes occurred (including perioperative morbidity and mortality). In the medical group, a 24% incidence of fatal and nonfatal strokes occurred. The difference was highly statistically significant ($p < 0.001$). This represents an absolute risk reduction of 17% in favor of surgical management and a relative risk reduction of 71% with surgical management versus medical management at the end of 18 months.

A surprising finding occurred when the mortality rates were analyzed. To date, no study had shown that carotid endarterectomy patients enjoy greater longevity than those treated medically. However, at the end of 18 months, the mortality rate among the medically treated group was 12%, in contrast to 5% for the surgically treated group. Once again, this difference was statistically significant ($p < 0.01$). This indicates a relative mortality risk reduction of 58% in favor of carotid endarterectomy. Further analysis demonstrated that for every 10% increase in stenosis between 70% and 99%, a progressive increase occurred in morbidity and mortality in the control group.[232,248]

The NASCET investigators reported their results in the moderate stenosis group (30% to 69%) in 1998.[249] They demonstrated a beneficial effect of surgery in the 50% to 69% stenosis group but not in those patients with less than 50% stenosis. The 30-day mortality and disabling stroke rate was 2.7%, and the nondisabling stroke rate was 4%, for a total of 6.7%. The 5-year rate for ipsilateral stroke in the surgical group was 15.7%, compared with 22% for patients treated medically. Thus, 15 patients would need to undergo carotid endarterectomy to prevent one stroke over a 5-year interval.

Medical Research Council European Carotid Surgery Trial

The ECST was a large multicenter trial of symptomatic patients with carotid artery disease that was carried out over a 10-year period and reported at approximately the same time as the NASCET. It confirmed the NASCET results reported to date. A total of 2518 patients were randomized over 10 years, providing a mean follow-up of 3 years. This trial stratified the data into three groups: mild stenosis (10% to 29%), moderate stenosis (30% to 69%), and severe stenosis (70% to 99%). In the mild stenosis category, no apparent benefit was evident for carotid endarterectomy compared with the risk of operation. However, in the severe stenosis category, a highly significant benefit in favor of operation was evident. Carotid endarterectomy, despite a 7.5% risk of death and stroke in the perioperative interval, resulted in a sixfold reduction in subsequent strokes over a 3-year interval. This difference was highly statistically significant ($p < 0.0001$).[250]

One interesting and important difference has come to light between NASCET and ECST: they have different methods of measuring carotid stenosis. In the European method,

$$\% \text{ Stenosis} = (1 - R/B) \infty 100$$

where R is minimal residual lumen diameter through the stenosis, and B is the projected diameter of the carotid bulb. This cannot actually be visualized because it is occupied by plaque; therefore an imaginary line is drawn to outline what is believed to be the bulb.

NASCET uses a method common in North America and was previously described in the VA asymptomatic trial. In this method,

TABLE 18-3 Comparison of Carotid Stenosis Estimated by European and North American Methods

Percent Stenosis, European	Percent Stenosis, North American
60	18
70	40
80	61
90	80

Data from Eliasziw M, Smith RF, Singh N, et al: Further comments on the measurements of carotid stenosis from angiograms. Stroke 25:2445–2449, 1994.

$$\% \text{ Stenosis} = (1 - R/D) \infty 100$$

where D is the diameter of the normal internal carotid artery where the walls become parallel.

The result of this difference is most apparent for moderate stenosis, for which the European method appears to greatly overestimate the percentage of stenosis. Eliasziw and colleagues[251] compared the same angiograms using the European and North American methods. Their findings are partly summarized in Table 18-3.

The ECST found significant benefit of carotid endarterectomy in patients with stenosis of 60% to 90%, which corroborated the results in the NASCET moderate stenosis group. The ECST reported no benefit of surgery in the 30% to 69% group as measured by the European method. This is not surprising, because a 69% ECST stenosis is only a 40% stenosis as measured by the North American method.[252]

Veterans Administration Symptomatic Trial

The VA symptomatic trial was a prospective, randomized trial designed to test the hypothesis that patients with greater than 50% ipsilateral internal carotid artery stenosis who were experiencing symptoms (including transient cerebral ischemia and mild stroke) would have fewer neurologic events (including cerebral infarction and crescendo TIAs) in the vascular distribution of the study artery after carotid endarterectomy plus best medical management than those receiving best medical management alone. This study was just getting under way when the results of the ECST and NASCET were reported, which led to its being halted earlier than anticipated. Nonetheless, 189 patients with symptomatic carotid stenoses were randomly allocated to receive either medical or surgical management. When the results were analyzed with a mean follow-up of 11.9 months, 7.7% of the patients randomized to surgical care had experienced stroke or crescendo TIAs during the perioperative or follow-up interval. In contrast, those patients randomized to medical management alone experienced a 19.4% incidence of stroke or crescendo TIAs. This difference was statistically significant ($p = 0.01$). The benefit of operation became apparent within 2 months of randomization.[253]

ALTERNATIVES TO SURGICAL THERAPY

The pathophysiology involved in the development of a stroke from an extracranial lesion has been discussed. The rationale for current medical therapy evolved from an attempt to alter the factors responsible for the development of symptoms secondary to extracranial arterial occlusion. At present, two forms of therapy are considered mainstays in the medical management of this disease: antiplatelet agents and anticoagulation.

Any form of therapy aimed at stroke prevention must also include the control of commonly associated conditions such as hypertension, diabetes, arrhythmias, and coronary artery disease. Cigarette smoking is also a major independent risk factor for the development of carotid bifurcation disease and stroke.[254-256] Any medical approach to stroke risk reduction must begin by advising the patient to stop smoking.

Anticoagulation, mainly with warfarin sodium (Coumadin), has been evaluated in several reports in an attempt to determine whether its use significantly alters the natural history of extracranial arterial lesions. Baker and associates reported a randomized, prospective study in patients with TIAs who were treated with Coumadin.[257] On follow-up, those treated with anticoagulation had a significant reduction in the number of TIAs when compared with control patients. A favorable trend for fewer strokes was noted in the treated group, although the difference in the incidence of cerebral infarction between treated and control patients was not statistically significant.

A reduction in stroke rate was observed in a retrospective study in the community of Rochester, Minnesota, regarding the use of anticoagulants to treat cerebral ischemia.[35] In this study, the net probability of having a stroke within 5 years was approximately for patients treated with anticoagulants. Although this compares favorably with the probability in untreated controls (40%), it represents a significant risk when compared with other available therapies.

Two reports from Sweden also showed a reduction in the development of TIAs and strokes in patients treated with anticoagulants. The first study showed a higher incidence of stroke when anticoagulants were discontinued; therefore long-term therapy was recommended.[258] In the second study, patients treated with anticoagulants showed an increased mortality rate, and serious bleeding complications were seen in this group.[259] Finally, a metaanalysis of 16 randomized studies of anticoagulation failed to show any benefit in patients suffering from TIA or ischemic stroke compared with untreated control groups. However, evidence suggests that patients with thrombosis in evolution may benefit from anticoagulation.[260]

The available evidence indicates that although the incidence of stroke and recurrent TIAs is reduced in patients treated with anticoagulants, it remains high compared with other available therapies. The need for long-term administration, with the concomitant increased risk of complications, makes anticoagulant therapy less desirable.

Antiplatelet agents, mainly aspirin, have been advocated for use in patients with extracranial arterial occlusive disease. The rationale for this therapy is based on evidence that platelets play a major role in the pathophysiology of this disease. Seven double-blind, randomized, prospective studies have compared the use of platelet antiaggregants with placebo in treating patients with cerebral ischemia secondary to extracranial atherosclerosis. In the Canadian Cooperative Study Group,[261] 585 patients who evidenced cerebral ischemia of extracranial origin were prospectively randomized into four treatment regimens. Each regimen was taken four times daily and consisted of a 200-mg capsule of sulfinpyrazone plus placebo, a placebo tablet plus 325 mg of aspirin, both active drugs, or both placebos. Follow-up from 12 to 57 months revealed no statistically significant reduction in TIAs, stroke, or death among patients on sulfinpyrazone. Aspirin reduced the risk for continuing ischemic episodes, stroke, or death by 19%. When analysis was restricted to stroke or death alone, the risk reduction increased to 31%, and when male patients were analyzed separately, the reduction was even higher. No statistically significant differences in stroke or death rate were found among female patients taking any of the four regimens. Based on this observation, the probability of stroke in men taking aspirin was in excess of 5% each year, and in women it was higher than 8% each year.[262] Platelet antiaggregants reduce the incidence of stroke in patients with extracranial lesions. The question still remains whether this reduction equals that achieved by other therapies.

In 1972, a double-blind, randomized, prospective trial of aspirin versus placebo was started in several American centers and continued for 37 months.[263] Sixty percent of these patients had operable lesions in the extracranial territory. The treatment group received 625 mg of aspirin twice daily. At 6 months' follow-up, a statistically significant difference in favor of aspirin was seen when death, cerebral or retinal infarction, and TIAs were grouped together. When each group was considered separately, the difference did not achieve statistical significance. Patients for whom a decision was made to proceed with endarterectomy were also assigned to a randomized, double-blind trial of aspirin during the postoperative period. The results of this trial constitute a separate report.[264] Life-table analyses of these end points at 24 months did not reveal a statistically significant difference in favor of aspirin. When non–stroke-related deaths were eliminated, a significant difference in favor of aspirin emerged. A favorable trend was also noted when the occurrence of TIAs within the first 6 months of follow-up was taken into consideration. In the placebo group, eight brain infarcts occurred among eight patients, reaching an end point in the first 24 months. Eight patients also reached an end point in the aspirin group; however, only two of these suffered a neurologic event.

These two studies showed a favorable trend toward a reduction in the stroke rate among patients receiving aspirin as treatment for symptomatic lesions in the extracranial circulation. In the first, aspirin was used as the principal form of therapy, whereas in the second, aspirin was an adjunct to surgical therapy. The absolute level of cases with an unfavorable outcome in the surgically treated group was about one fifth the percentage of unfavorable outcomes among those treated medically (2% in the surgically treated group, versus 11.3% in the medically treated group). This difference may reflect the independent favorable effect of surgery.

Two other studies have evaluated the use of aspirin in a randomized, controlled, prospective fashion. In a study from France,[265] 604 patients with arteriothrombotic cerebral ischemic events referable to the carotid or vertebrobasilar circulation were entered in a double-blind, randomized clinical trial comparing aspirin 1 g/day, aspirin 1 g/day plus dipyridamole 225 mg/day, and placebo. A comparison of the placebo and aspirin groups showed a significant reduction ($p < 0.05$) of cerebral infarction in the aspirin group. Overall, 66 patients in the entire group suffered cerebral infarction during the trial; this corresponds to a cumulative stroke rate for the placebo group of 18% and a rate of 10.5% for each of the aspirin groups. No significant difference in the aspirin plus dipyridamole group was found. Thus, the incidence of stroke per year was on the order of 6% for placebo versus 3% for the treatment groups. This represents, again, a 50% reduction in stroke risk. In the dipyridamole-aspirin trial in cerebral ischemia, the American-Canadian Cooperative Study Group found no difference in the stroke risk in patients receiving aspirin or aspirin plus dipyridamole for the prevention of stroke during long-term follow-up.[266] Interestingly, the stroke rate in patients treated with either aspirin or aspirin plus dipyridamole was approximately 20% at 5 years. This yields a 4% per year stroke risk, which is not dissimilar to the lower rates reported in natural history studies.

In 1983, a Danish cooperative study comparing the outcomes of patients with extracranial occlusive disease treated with aspirin or placebo was reported.[267] No favorable influence of aspirin in the prevention of ischemic attacks could be determined. Unfortunately, only 203 patients were monitored, which is probably an insufficient number to achieve any statistically valid data. This study has been criticized and probably suffers from type II statistical error.[268]

The objective of any treatment regimen for carotid artery disease should be the reduction of stroke risk. Although each of the prospective, randomized trials of antiplatelet agents showed a trend toward stroke risk reduction, none achieved statistical significance in regard to that parameter. Only when the end points of TIA, stroke, and nonfatal and fatal MI were lumped together did a statistically significant benefit in favor of aspirin emerge. Individual studies lacked sufficient numbers of patients to show a reduction of stroke risk in favor of aspirin; however, in a metaanalysis combining the patients from the various series, the best that could be shown was a 15% stroke risk reduction in favor of aspirin, and this still failed to achieve statistical significance.[269]

The antiplatelet drug ticlopidine hydrochloride was compared with aspirin in a multicenter, prospective, randomized trial of 3069 patients with recent transient or mild persistent focal cerebral or retinal ischemia.[270] The 3-year event rate for nonfatal stroke or death from any cause was 17% for ticlopidine and 19% for aspirin. The rates of fatal and nonfatal stroke at 3 years were 10% for

ticlopidine and 13% for aspirin. The authors concluded that ticlopidine was somewhat more effective than aspirin in preventing stroke in their study population but that the risks of side effects were greater. One of the disadvantages of ticlopidine is a small but finite incidence of thrombotic thrombocytopenic purpura (TTP). This necessitates frequent blood testing while the patient is taking the drug. Clopidagril (Plavix) has emerged as a safer substitute. Although there have been no specific studies comparing aspirin and Plavix for cerebrovascular disease, Plavix has been shown to be efficacious in reducing morbid events in patients with peripheral vascular disease and coronary disease with a much lower incidence of TTP. Earlier studies using the combination of aspirin and dipyridamole failed to show any benefit over aspirin alone. However, newer studies using the combination in a sustained release form (Aggrenox) have shown a benefit over aspirin alone.[271]

Failures of antiplatelet therapy in the treatment of symptomatic carotid artery disease have been reported.[272] Caution should be used in patients who receive platelet antiaggregants as primary therapy for this disease. Partial disappearance of their symptoms should be considered a failure, and alternative forms of treatment should be considered. Patients who experience complete relief of symptoms should be monitored carefully with annual noninvasive studies. Progression of the lesion may be obscured because of suppression of symptoms by the therapy. In a review of 27 aspirin failures requiring urgent operation,[272] 12 of the surgical specimens showed fresh hemorrhage in the atherosclerotic plaque. Whether this was induced or aggravated by aspirin could not be concluded. This incidence of fresh hemorrhage in an endarterectomy specimen appears to be high compared with the findings in elective cases. Finally, good evidence suggests that aspirin is of no benefit to asymptomatic patients with respect to subsequent neurologic events. Cote and colleagues[273] performed a prospective, randomized trial in asymptomatic patients with carotid stenosis of at least 50%.[273] One hundred patients received aspirin, and 184 patients received placebo. The median follow-up was 2.3 years. The annual rates for vascular events were 11% in the placebo group and 10.7% in the aspirin group.

A 1995 report described the use of lovastatin in an attempt to modify carotid plaques.[274] In patients who were in the 60th to 90th percentiles of low-density lipoprotein cholesterol levels, lovastatin appeared to slow the rate of plaque progression. No evidence existed of plaque regression. More recently, clinical trials have shown a clear benefit in reducing stroke risk with the use of statins.[275,276]

In conclusion, the available forms of medical management produce a reduction in the stroke rate in patients with significant atherosclerotic lesions of the extracranial circulation. This reduction does not appear to be as significant as that achieved by successful carotid endarterectomy. Medical treatment for symptomatic extracranial arterial disease should thus be reserved for patients with limited life expectancy or unidentified or surgically inaccessible lesions or for those who are poor surgical candidates.

CONTROVERSIAL TOPICS IN CEREBROVASCULAR DISEASE MANAGEMENT

Carotid Endarterectomy for Acute Stroke

Emergent operation after acute stroke was used early in the history of endarterectomy. Because of several reports indicating a risk of converting an ischemic cerebral infarction into a hemorrhagic one, this procedure was abandoned. In reviewing these reports, it is possible to identify several types of patients who experienced such complications, including those with massive cerebral infarctions and in obtunded states, those in whom an attempt was made to open an occluded internal carotid artery several days to weeks after thrombosis, and those with severe, inadequately controlled hypertension.[277]

Later evidence has suggested improved results if carotid artery surgery is delayed for at least 5 weeks after the acute event. Of 49 carotid endarterectomies performed for acute cerebral infarction, 27 were performed within 5 weeks and 22 were done between 5 and 20 weeks after the acute neurologic event. The latter group showed no morbidity or mortality, whereas patients undergoing early operation had an 18.5% incidence of new postoperative neurologic deficits. The authors concluded that an unstable situation during the early phase of stroke contraindicated endarterectomy. No details about the degree of preoperative neurologic deficit or later recovery were available.[278] Following these guidelines, Dosick and colleagues[156] noted a 21% incidence of recurrent stroke during the 4- to 6-week observation interval. This finding led the authors to select their patients on the basis of CT scans, proceeding with surgery if the scan results were negative. In their series, 110 patients underwent early endarterectomy after a persistent neurologic deficit with negative CT scan results. No patient suffered a neurologic deficit in the territory of the operated artery, and no patient died. Whittemore and colleagues[279] reported a similar experience in 28 patients with small, fixed neurologic deficits undergoing endarterectomy an average of 11 days after the onset of symptoms. There was one postoperative death in this small group of patients and no new perioperative neurologic deficits. The authors recommended proceeding with endarterectomy early in this select group of patients with small cerebral infarcts.

In general, surgical intervention during the acute phase of a stroke is contraindicated. If the patient has a dense neurologic deficit, loss of consciousness, or cardiovascular instability, clearly surgery is not indicated. However, if the patient has a mild to moderate deficit and is fully conscious and otherwise stable, carotid endarterectomy of the responsible lesion can be undertaken soon after the patient has reached a plateau in recovery. This may be days or weeks after the onset of the event. In the small group of patients in whom a clinically unstable lesion exists, manifested by crescendo TIAs or stroke in evolution, emergent endarterectomy should be strongly considered.

Crescendo Transient Ischemic Attacks and Stroke in Evolution

Crescendo TIAs and stroke in evolution used to be considered contraindications to operation. Goldstone and Moore[280] reported experience with a select group of patients with stroke in evolution or crescendo TIAs who were acutely studied with angiography. If an unstable condition such as a free-floating thrombus or a propagating thrombus in the presence of a distally patent internal carotid artery was identified, the patient was taken promptly to the operating room. The net result in a series of approximately 25 patients was no deaths and a return to essentially normal neurologic status, in contrast to the natural history of stroke in evolution, which has an approximately 80% expected mortality.[280]

A similar experience was reported by Mentzer and colleagues[33] with 17 patients operated on emergently for stroke in evolution.[33] None had worsening of the preoperative neurologic deficit, 4 (24%) remained unchanged, and 12 (70%) had complete recovery. One death occurred, for a 6% operative mortality. This compared favorably with a parallel nonrandomized group of 26 patients with stroke in evolution treated conservatively. The medical group had 15% mortality, but more important, 17 patients (66%) suffered moderate to severe permanent neurologic deficits. This report also presented the collated operative results from 90 cases in the literature. After successful endarterectomy, 55% were improved, 25% had no change, and 10% were worse. A 10% mortality for the collated experience was reported. Thus, surgical intervention in the presence of stroke in evolution carries a significantly increased risk of both perioperative stroke and death. However, the results of surgical therapy are considerably better than the natural history of the untreated condition. A specific goal for surgical intervention must be identified by preoperative angiography. Indications for emergent endarterectomy include the presence of an unstable condition such as a free-floating thrombus or propagating thrombus in the presence of a distally patent internal carotid artery. It is highly recommended that CT be used to exclude other associated conditions that could appear to be stroke in evolution. More recently, a derivative report from the VA symptomatic trial identified crescendo TIAs as a surgical imperative.[281]

Possible Deleterious Effect of Antiplatelet Drugs

In patients with asymptomatic carotid bifurcation plaques or with minimal plaques and TIAs who are treated with antiplatelet drugs, there have been reports of progression—more rapid than expected—of the atheromatous lesion to near-total occlusion. Operation at that time indicated a high degree of intraplaque hemorrhage. Thus, antiplatelet drugs may precipitate intraplaque hemorrhage and a rapid progression of the lesion.[272] A subsequent report compared plaque histopathology with the preoperative use of antiplatelet drugs. Patients taking antiplatelet drugs had an 80.1% incidence of multiple intraplaque hemorrhages, in contrast to a 19.7%

incidence of intraplaque hemorrhage in patients not receiving antiplatelet drugs.[282]

Carotid Balloon Angioplasty and Stenting

Carotid balloon angioplasty with stenting is being used with increasing frequency in many centers worldwide. Initially, anecdotal reports provided conflicting data for safety and efficacy. The first large series was reported by Dietrich and colleagues.[283] Between April 1993 and September 1995, 110 nonconsecutive patients underwent treatment using balloon angioplasty and stenting in accord with an approved protocol in a single institution. It is important to note that 72% of the patients in this series were asymptomatic and, therefore, represented the lowest risk group. There were seven periprocedural (in-hospital) strokes, for an incidence of 6.4%, and there were two in-hospital deaths, for an incidence of 1.8%; thus, the combined in-hospital stroke morbidity and mortality was 8.2%. Two patients undergoing stented angioplasty went on to occlusion within 30 days. The same year, Roubin and colleagues[284] reported their experience with 74 patients undergoing placement of 210 stents in 152 vessels. They had one death and nine in-hospital strokes, for a periprocedural stroke morbidity and mortality of 14%.

These and several other anecdotal reports prompted a multidisciplinary group of physicians to write an editorial expressing concern about the proliferation of this procedure without proof of its safety or efficacy. They recommended that a prospective trial comparing stented balloon angioplasty with carotid endarterectomy be performed.[285] Several retrospective comparative studies of carotid endarterectomy and carotid angioplasty with stenting have also been reported. Jordan and colleagues[286] compared percutaneous transluminal angioplasty (PTA) with stenting in 107 patients in their institution with 166 carotid endarterectomies done concurrently.[286] The 30-day combined stroke morbidity and mortality for PTA and stenting was 9.3%, versus 3.6% for carotid endarterectomy. In evaluating the late results (>30 days), including such items as amaurosis, recurrent stenosis, TIA, minor stroke, major stroke, and death, the combined adverse event rate for PTA with stenting was 18.7%, versus 6.6% for carotid endarterectomy. These same authors also did a cost comparison and found that the total cost for carotid endarterectomy was $21,670 per patient, whereas carotid angioplasty with stenting cost $30,140.

Several prospective, randomized trials have also reported their results. The earliest trial, largely from centers in the United Kingdom, noted that the 30-day results were a combined stroke and death rate of 9.9% for carotid angioplasty (CAS) and 9.8% for carotid endarterectomy (CEA).[287] Because this trial was early in the experience, it has largely been discounted because of the unacceptably high complication rates for both CEA and CAS. Nehler and colleagues attempted to do a single-institution prospective, randomized trial,[288] but the trial was stopped after only 17 patients were entered into the study. Ten carotid endarterectomies were performed without death or stroke; however, five strokes occurred during the course of seven angioplasties.

There were also several industry-sponsored trials. The first of these was the Schneider Wallstent trial, whose results were presented at the 26th International Stroke Conference in February 2001.[289] The 2-day periprocedural stroke and death rate was 7.5% in the stent group and 1.8% in the carotid endarterectomy group; the 30-day stroke and death rate was 12.1% in the stent group and 4.5% in the carotid endarterectomy group; and the primary adverse event rate at the end of 1 year was 12.1% in the stent group and 3.6% in the carotid endarterectomy group. The authors concluded that carotid angioplasty and stenting are not equivalent to carotid endarterectomy.

The trials up to this point had been done without cerebral antiembolism devices. Several devices have since been introduced, and most contemporary trials are now being done in conjunction with their use. The most influential industry-sponsored trial to date has been the SAPPHIRE study, sponsored by Johnson and Johnson and Cordis.[290] Both 30-day and 1-year data have been reported, and based on these reports, the U.S. Food and Drug Administration has given conditional approval for the Johnson and Johnson stent and antiembolism device for use in high-risk patients. The trial randomized 159 patients to stent–balloon angioplasty with cerebral protection versus 151 carotid endarterectomies. All these procedures were performed in what was defined as a high-risk patient group. The authors compared a number of parameters, including death and stroke in the postprocedure interval. They also added nonfatal MI, which included both Q-wave and non–Q-wave MI. Interestingly, there was no difference in the death and stroke rate with angioplasty and stenting versus carotid endarterectomy. However, there was a major, statistically significant difference in the incidence of MI in the two groups. The MI rate in the carotid endarterectomy group was 7.9%, whereas in the angioplasty and stenting group it was 2.5%. When comparing all patients, both symptomatic and asymptomatic, the combined death, stroke, and MI rate was 5.8% in the stent group and 12.6% in the carotid endarterectomy group. This difference reached statistical significance in favor of angioplasty and stenting for high-risk patients. The difference held at the end of 1 year, when the major adverse event rate was 11.9% in the stent group and 19.9% in the carotid endarterectomy group ($p = 0.048$). However, after a follow-up interval of 3 years, there was no longer a difference between carotid endarterectomy and carotid angioplasty in this high-risk group.[291] Since this report, several prospective, randomized trials in average risk patients have reported their results. The first report was from France in a trial called EVA-3S. This was a multicenter prospective randomized trial of average risk symptomatic patients. The trial was stopped early by the safety committee because there was a statistically significant difference in favor of CEA over CAS. The 30-day incidence of any stroke and death after CEA was 3.9% versus 9.6% after CAS. These patients have been followed long term, and the 4-year data has now been reported. At 4 years the cumulative death and stroke rate for CEA was 6.2% versus 11.1% for CAS ($p = 0.03$).[292] The next European trial to report was performed in Germany, Austria, and Switzerland (i.e., the

SPACE trial). It was also a multicenter, prospective, randomized trial of average risk, symptomatic patients with severe carotid stenosis. The hypothesis that was being tested was that CAS was not inferior to CEA. After 1200 patients were randomized, the trial was stopped because a futility analysis revealed that the primary hypothesis could not be proved. At the time the trial was stopped, the combined death and stroke rate for CAS was 7.7% versus 6.5% for CEA. Of particular interest was the fact that the incidence of high grade recurrent stenosis was 10.7% for CAS versus 4.6% for CEA.[293] In 2010, the international carotid stenting study investigators reported their interim results from a multicenter, international trial that involved academic medical centers around the world in a study of symptomatic patients with severe carotid stenosis. Seventeen hundred and thirteen patients were enrolled, making it the largest prospective randomized trial of symptomatic patients to date. The incidence of death, stroke, and periprocedural myocardial infarction was 8.5% in the CAS group compared with 5.2% in the CEA group ($p = 0.006$).[294] This trial is of particular interest in that they also studied a subset of 231 patients with preprocedure and postprocedure MRIs looking for new areas of cerebral infarction. In the CAS patients, 50% had at least one new area of infarction compared with 17% of patients undergoing CEA ($p < 0.0001$).[295]

The Carotid Revascularization Endarterectomy versus Stent (CREST) trial is a prospective, randomized trial of both symptomatic and asymptomatic patients. It includes 108 centers in the United States and Canada. It is the only trial to date that has included an asymptomatic arm; with those additional patients, the combined study group of 2502 patients is the largest trial to date. The trial has several unique features. One of the most important is a lead-in phase to qualify those wishing to participate as interventionists performing stent/angioplasty. To be eligible, a potential participant first had to submit their prior experience and results for review by the angioplasty management committee. If their data were satisfactory, they then underwent training in the use of the Acunet/Aculink system and had to submit up to 20 lead-in cases done prospectively. If the results of this second or lead-in phase were satisfactory, they were then allowed to join the study and participate in the randomized trial. Four hundred and twenty seven interventionists applied, but only 227 (52%) were approved, making this a highly selected group of interventionists and assuring the highest level of competence. The primary endpoints of the trial were death, stroke in any distribution, myocardial infarction within 30 days of the procedure, and stroke within the distribution of the study artery afterward. The preliminary results were reported after the last patient entered was followed for 1 year. Because the recruitment spanned 10 years, there was also the opportunity to evaluate cumulative follow-up data, with a mean follow-up of 2.5 years. During the lead-in phase of the trial, the data associated with carotid angioplasty and stenting among the participating centers were reported.[296] Among symptomatic patients, the 30-day morbidity and mortality rate was 5.5%; for asymptomatic patients, it was 2.8%. These results compared well with the surgical series in the NASCET and ACAS. However, it should be recognized

that NASCET and ACAS data are 15 to 20 years old and there is current evidence to indicate that the results of CEA have improved over time. When CREST was unblinded, it was found that the 30 day cumulative results of death, stroke, and MI were 4.5% for CEA and 5.2% for CAS. These differences were not statistically significant. However, when the event rates of death and stroke were analyzed, the combined results for CEA was 2.3% versus 4.4% for CAS ($p = 0.005$). The longer-term analysis also demonstrated that patients older than 70 years did better with CEA than CAS. Finally, a quality-of-life analysis compared patients with and without an adverse endpoint. One year following an adverse event, major stroke followed by minor stroke were identified by patients as having the worst effect on their quality of life. MI, after 1 year, did not affect quality of life compared with patients who did not experience the complication. Finally, since it is known that an MI has an adverse effect on long-term survival, it was a surprise to find that despite there being more MIs in the CEA group, long-term survival was the same as CAS. The reason for this was the fact that stroke, even "minor stroke," also resulted in a shortened life expectancy. Therefore it can be concluded that within the CREST trial, CEA continues to hold an edge over CAS regarding lower rate of stroke and death. When metaanalyses are performed using all level 1 trial data, CEA continues to fare better than CAS.[297]

Asymptomatic Carotid Ulceration

Not uncommonly, a large, nonstenotic, ulcerative lesion in a contralateral carotid artery is discovered incidentally when the ipsilateral symptomatic carotid artery is being studied by angiography. Whether to operate on this ulcerative lesion is a common question. My colleagues and I carried out two retrospective reviews of patients with identified nonstenotic ulcerative lesions that were monitored without treatment. We observed that medium and large ulcerative lesions carried a significant stroke risk, usually not preceded by warning TIAs.[56] In the most recent study, the risk of stroke in patients with large ulcerative lesions being monitored expectantly was approximately 7.5% each year of follow-up after initial identification.[57] While there are good data to suggest that medium grade B and large grade C ulcers, when identified, should undergo prophylactic repair. Unfortunately, contrast angiography is seldom used at present, and there are no valid studies to suggest that less invasive imaging is accurate in identifying ulceration.

Tandem Lesions

Occasionally there is a stenosis of the origin of the internal carotid artery in conjunction with a significant lesion of the carotid siphon. The question often raised is whether operating on the extracranial carotid artery alone is justified if the siphon lesion is larger than the proximal lesion. Several reports indicate that although tandem lesions exist, the embolic potential of the atherosclerotic plaque at the carotid bifurcation greatly outweighs the thrombotic or embolic risk of the lesion in the carotid siphon.[298] This author's practice is to operate on the carotid bifurcation lesion in symptomatic patients in spite of the presence of a siphon lesion.[299] A retrospective review compared the perioperative morbidity, mortality, and late results in patients undergoing carotid endarterectomy with and without angiographically documented intracranial arterial occlusive disease. There was no difference between the two groups. The perioperative stroke rate was 1.9% versus 1.8%; mortality was 0.5% versus 0.7%; and the 3-, 5-, and 10-year stroke rates were 93% versus 92%, 87% versus 90%, and 79% versus 85%, respectively.[300]

Combined Carotid and Coronary Occlusive Disease

The carotid-coronary area is particularly controversial, and treatment depends on whether symptoms exist in either vascular bed. In patients with symptomatic coronary artery disease in whom an asymptomatic carotid stenosis is found, it is difficult to know whether the carotid artery should be fixed first, followed by coronary artery bypass; whether both lesions should be fixed simultaneously; or whether surgery for the carotid artery lesion should be put off until after coronary artery bypass. The literature is controversial on this subject, and I continue to individualize treatment, depending on which lesion appears to be more critical. For example, if a patient has triple coronary artery disease with unstable angina and an asymptomatic carotid stenosis, I usually recommend that the coronary artery surgery be performed first and that the carotid lesion be evaluated after recovery. Conversely, if a patient has relatively stable angina and symptomatic carotid artery disease or a preocclusive (<90%) stenosis, operating on the carotid artery first and then managing the coronary artery lesions a few days later may be wise. Finally, if a patient has both symptomatic carotid artery disease and unstable angina, a simultaneous, combined approach would be justified. The alternative approach would be the use of carotid angioplasty before coronary bypass. The problem with this approach is that CAS must be done in the presence of dual antiplatelet therapy (aspirin and Plavix). Dual antiplatelet therapy would preclude the use of coronary bypass because of perioperative bleeding problems. Another approach might be to perform CAS, then go immediately to the operating room for coronary bypass. Currently there are no scientific data to support these alternatives.

Intellectual Testing and Improvement with Carotid Endarterectomy

After carotid endarterectomy, patients and their families often report that the patient appears intellectually brighter and is able to carry out tasks that have been alien for quite some time. Numerous attempts have been made to quantitate this intellectual improvement, usually without success. We must be careful not to regard intellectually impaired patients as routine candidates for carotid endarterectomy, because the majority of these patients are suffering from organic brain disease rather than compromised blood flow. Although multiple embolization to presume silent areas of the brain has been shown to compromise intellectual function, so called multiple-infarct dementia.

Extracranial-to-Intracranial Bypass Grafting

The technical ability to connect an extracranial arterial branch such as the temporal artery to a cortical branch of the middle cerebral artery has been developed over the past 15 years. To determine whether extracranial-to-intracranial (EC-IC) bypass surgery would benefit patients with symptomatic atherosclerotic disease of the internal carotid artery, an international randomized trial began in 1977 and completed in 1982.[301] In that study, 1377 patients with recent hemispheric strokes, retinal infarction, or TIAs who had narrowing or occlusion of the ipsilateral carotid artery or middle cerebral artery were randomized: 714 were assigned to best medical care, and 663 were assigned to surgery. In the latter group, an EC-IC arterial bypass was performed, with a patency rate on long-term follow-up of 96%. The 30-day surgical mortality was 6.6%, with a stroke morbidity of 2.5%. Nonfatal and fatal strokes on long-term follow-up occurred both more frequently and earlier in patients treated with EC-IC bypass. Survival analysis comparing the two groups demonstrated a similar lack of benefit from surgery. Reduction in the number of TIAs was noted in 77% of the surgical patients. An almost equal number (80%) of the medical patients also showed a reduction or disappearance of TIAs. In all parameters studied, EC-IC bypass failed to improve the results of medical therapy. The large number of patients with long-term follow-up, the uniformity of the disease process in the population studied, the randomization method (which produced a balanced treatment group), the presence of complete and accurate records of all entry and event dates, and the achievement of effective anastomosis with acceptably low morbidity and mortality suggest that this conclusion is not only statistically powerful but also clinically significant.

Magnetic Resonance Angiography

In the continuing quest to find a substitute for invasive contrast angiography, the use of MRA of the vascular system has been developed: so-called MRA. Various computer programs for postprocessing of magnetic resonance images to delineate the vascular system are under active development. To date, excellent imaging of the cervical and intracranial vessels has been achievable. However, several limitations of MRA have been identified. In several instances, the image suggested total occlusion, whereas contrast angiograms showed a patent vessel with a string sign. MRA also tends to overestimate the percentage stenosis, making minimal lesions look like hemodynamically significant lesions. Finally, MRA cannot delineate surface irregularity or ulceration.[302-304]

KEY REFERENCES

Abu Rahma AF, Robinson PA, Saiedy S, et al: Prospective randomized trial of bilateral carotid endarterectomies: primary closure versus patching. Stroke 30:1185–1189, 1999.

Chervu A, Moore WS: Carotid endarterectomy without angiography: personal series and review of the literature. Ann Vasc Surg 8:296–302, 1994.

Dixon S, Pais SO, Raviola C, et al: Natural history of nonstenotic, asymptomatic ulcerative lesions of the carotid artery: a further analysis. Arch Surg 117:1493, 1982.

Eastcott HHG, Pickering GW, Rob C: Reconstruction of internal carotid artery in a patient with intermittent attacks of hemiplegia. Lancet 2:994–996, 1954.

Executive Committee for the Asymptomatic Carotid Atherosclerosis Study: Endarterectomy for asymptomatic carotid artery stenosis. JAMA 273:1421–1428, 1995.

Halliday A, Mansfield A, Marro J, et al: Prevention of disabling and fatal strokes by successful carotid endarterectomy in patients without recent neurological symptoms: randomized control trial. Lancet 363:1491–1502, 2004.

Moore WS, Barnett HJ, Beebe ME, et al: Guidelines for carotid endarterectomy: a multidisciplinary consensus statement from the ad hoc committee, American Heart Association. Stroke 26:188–201, 1995.

Moore WS, Hall AD: Importance of emboli from carotid bifurcation in pathogenesis in cerebral ischemia attacks. Arch Surg 101:708, 1970.

Moore WS, Kempczinski RF, Nelson JJ, et al: Recurrent carotid stenosis: results of this asymptomatic carotid atherosclerosis study. Stroke 29:2018–2025, 1998.

North American Symptomatic Carotid Endarterectomy Trial collaborators: beneficial effect of carotid endarterectomy in symptomatic patients with high-grade carotid stenosis. N Engl J Med 325:445–453, 1991.

Thompson JE: The evolution of surgery for the treatment and prevention of stroke: the Willis lecture. Stroke 27:1427–1434, 1996.

References available online at expertconsult.com.

QUESTIONS

1. What is the most common cause of perioperative neurologic deficit after carotid endarterectomy?
   a. Thrombosis of the repair
   b. Lack of cerebral perfusion
   c. Tandem lesions in the carotid system
   d. Low cardiac output
   e. None of the above

2. Carotid endarterectomy for asymptomatic disease (1) is a proven indication for stenosis of 60% or greater, as documented by angiography; (2) carries the lowest perioperative morbidity and mortality; (3) should be considered when progression to 80% stenosis is documented; (4) may prevent stroke, which is the most common initial manifestation of asymptomatic carotid disease. Which of the preceding statements are true?
   a. 1, 2, 3
   b. 1, 3
   c. 2, 4
   d. 4
   e. 1, 2, 3, 4

3. Which of the following statements about tandem lesions in the intracranial carotid system is true?
   a. They carry a similar stroke risk compared with a carotid bifurcation lesion.
   b. They carry a lower stroke risk than a similar extracranial bulb lesion.
   c. They carry a higher stroke risk than a similar extracranial bulb lesion.
   d. They should deter the surgeon from recommending bifurcation endarterectomy.
   e. They are more frequently the source of symptoms when combined intracranial and extracranial disease is present.

4. In regard to fibromuscular dysplasia: (1) it is best described as an atherosclerotic process affecting medium-size arteries; (2) 30% of patients with cervical involvement may have intracranial aneurysms; (3) medial hyperplasia is the most common type affecting the carotid system; (4) it most commonly affects women, suggesting a hormonal factor. Which of the preceding statements are true?
   a. 1, 2, 3
   b. 1, 3
   c. 2, 4
   d. 4
   e. None

5. Which of the following statements about kinks of the carotid artery is true?
   a. They are frequently the cause of cerebrovascular symptoms.
   b. They may be congenital.
   c. They never cause symptoms.
   d. They frequently require excision and grafting for repair.
   e. They are rarely associated with atherosclerosis.

6. Transient ischemic attacks (1) carry a 40% risk of stroke over 5 years when secondary to extracranial arterial occlusive disease; (2) are always secondary to platelet emboli; (3) may be a manifestation of lacunar infarction; (4) as a manifestation of cardiac emboli, are usually stereotyped, with similar symptoms with each occurrence. Which of the preceding statements are true?
   a. 1, 2, 3
   b. 1, 3
   c. 2, 4
   d. 4
   e. 1, 2, 3, 4

7. Which of the following statements about the use of an internal shunt during carotid endarterectomy is true?
   a. It is necessary in approximately 50% of patients.
   b. It can be predicted based on angiographic findings.
   c. It carries no added risk.
   d. All of the above
   e. None of the above

8. Which of the following statements about external carotid endarterectomy is true?
   a. It carries significant risks when combined with extracranial-intracranial bypass.
   b. It rarely requires patch closure.
   c. It frequently relieves amaurosis but rarely relieves hemispheric TIAs.
   d. All of the above
   e. None of the above

9. Stroke in evolution (1) may be a manifestation of lacunar infarction; (2) suggests an unstable process requiring urgent evaluation and therapy; (3) has a 10% mortality with surgical therapy; (4) should be treated with prompt medical therapy in view of the increased risk of surgery. Which of the preceding statements are true?
   a. 1, 2, 3
   b. 1, 3
   c. 2, 4
   d. 4
   e. None

10. In regard to carotid endarterectomy for acute stroke: (1) the risks of surgical intervention during the acute phase of a stroke are high, so surgery is never indicated; (2) if a CT scan done within 12 hours of the event is negative, endarterectomy can be safely performed; (3) level of consciousness, hypertension, and severity of the deficit should not influence the timing of surgical intervention; (4) if the patient shows continual recovery without deterioration, endarterectomy can be safely performed once a plateau has been reached. Which of the preceding statements is (are) true?
    a. 1, 2, 3
    b. 1, 3
    c. 2, 4
    d. 4
    e. None

ANSWERS

1. e
2. e
3. b
4. c
5. b
6. b
7. e
8. a
9. a
10. d

CHAPTER 19

SURGICAL RECONSTRUCTION OF THE SUPRA-AORTIC TRUNKS AND VERTEBRAL ARTERIES

Ramon Berguer

The supra-aortic trunks (SATs) are the branches of the aortic arch that ascend through the mediastinum and terminate short of the carotid bifurcation and the origin of the vertebral arteries. These trunks carry the entire blood supply to the head and upper extremities. The vertebrobasilar system is composed of the two vertebral arteries, the basilar artery, and their branches to the brainstem, spinal cord, cerebellum, and occipital lobes.

The three most common variants in the anatomy of the SATs have implications in terms of the technique chosen for their reconstruction. These variants are a shared ostium (16%) or a common origin (8%) for the innominate and left common carotid arteries, a left vertebral artery with a separate origin from the aortic arch (6%), and a right retroesophageal subclavian artery (0.5%). A separate origin of the left vertebral artery is associated with an abnormally high (C4 or C5) entry of this artery into the transverse foramina of the cervical spine. A retroesophageal right subclavian artery is associated with a thoracic duct that empties on the right jugulosubclavian confluent, a nonrecurrent right inferior laryngeal nerve, and, in approximately half these patients, a common carotid trunk giving origin to both common carotid arteries.

Through the mechanisms of low flow or atheroembolization, occlusive disease of the SATs can cause symptoms in any of the territories supplied: the hemispheric (carotid) territory, the posterior (vertebrobasilar) territory, and, in the case of proximal subclavian disease, the upper extremity. Vertebral artery occlusive disease may restrict inflow into the basilar artery, resulting in vertebrobasilar ischemia. This is more likely if compensatory flow from the carotid system is not available because of an internal carotid occlusion or a minute or absent posterior communicating arteries.

The SATs are involved by atherosclerosis in the fifth or sixth decade of life. This results in the development of plaques that can obstruct flow or embolize (atheroembolism). Aneurysmal atherosclerotic disease of the SATs is rare. In some locations, the SATs are a common site for Takayasu arteritis, usually in younger individuals.

Traumatic and mycotic aneurysms of the SATs are uncommon but life-threatening conditions.

The incidence of atherosclerotic disease is lower in the SATs than in the internal carotid and vertebral arteries. Nevertheless, the extensive study of extracranial arterial disease reported in 1968 by Hass and colleagues[1] showed that one third of patients undergoing arteriography had a severe lesion involving one or more of the SATs. The morphology of atherosclerotic lesions of the SATs is not defined as well as that of the plaques found in the internal carotid artery, partly because for several years the SATs were not routinely visualized during arteriography of the cerebral vessels. In addition, the SATs are difficult to image with ultrasound techniques, which provides valuable morphologic information in the carotid bifurcation. Because there is limited knowledge of the natural history of these lesions, surgical indications are based partly on inferences. In addition, SAT lesions are often found in individuals who already have concomitant disease of the carotid or vertebral arteries—a situation that confuses the identification of the offending lesion. Stenosing lesions of the SATs usually appear at their origin from the aortic arch and often involve more than one artery. Plaques located in the ostia of the SATs are usually continuous with atheroma that extends over the dome of the aortic arch.

Outlining SAT lesions by arteriography requires an arch injection, preferably in two oblique projections (right and left posterior oblique). If circumstances permit, the arteriographic study should also include selective injections of both common carotid and subclavian arteries (four-vessel arteriogram). The high incidence of concomitant carotid and vertebral artery lesions makes it mandatory to outline the extracranial and intracranial cerebrovascular supply when evaluating a patient for cerebrovascular symptoms.

Vertebrobasilar ischemia can be caused by poor inflow through the carotid and vertebral arteries, reversal of blood flow in a vertebral artery caused by a proximal subclavian artery occlusion (subclavian steal), reversal of right carotid and vertebral artery flow from an innominate artery occlusion, and embolization from the proximal subclavian or vertebral arteries.

SYMPTOMS OF OCCLUSIVE DISEASE OF THE SUPRA-AORTIC TRUNKS

Patients with occlusive disease of the SATs may show symptoms of carotid, vertebrobasilar, and upper extremity arterial ischemia. Although there is no pathologic evidence to support this view, it has traditionally been taught that in patients with disease of the SATs, cerebral symptoms are due to low flow rather than atheroembolization. This concept runs contrary to clinical evidence suggesting that the mechanisms of cerebral ischemia from disease of the SATs are similar to those from atheroma of the carotid bifurcation.

Obliteration of the SATs is suggested by absent pulses in the neck (subclavian, carotid) or arm (axillary, brachial) on one or both sides and by the recording of unequal or abnormally low pressures in the upper extremities. Waveforms recorded by Doppler tracings are dampened in arteries whose origins are stenosed or occluded. Bruits may be present. In patients with subclavian steal, a pulse lag may be felt between the radial arteries of the two arms or, more precisely, a pulse wave delay of greater than 30 msec can be measured by simultaneously recording both brachial artery waveforms.[2] Claudication of the arm and digital artery embolization may be present in subclavian artery disease. A computed tomographic scan of the brain is an essential part of the workup for patients with disease of the SATs. The scan may reveal clinically silent cerebral infarctions.[3]

In symptomatic vertebral (or basilar) artery occlusive disease, the patient may have any combination of the following symptoms: dizziness, vertigo, diplopia, perioral numbness, blurred vision, tinnitus, ataxia, bilateral sensory deficits, and drop attacks. The mechanism that triggers the symptom (e.g., standing up, rotating the neck) must be sought when evaluating these patients. Patients with orthostatic hypotension have vertebrobasilar symptoms when they stand abruptly after sitting or lying down. Blood pressure measurements taken immediately after they stand up and experience symptoms shows a drop in systolic pressure greater than 20 mm Hg. This mechanism is particularly common in diabetic patients with sympathetic paralysis leading to loss of venomotor tone because a substantial amount of blood is pooled in their legs on standing.

The presence of vertebrobasilar ischemia related to turning of the neck suggests osteophytic compression on the vertebral arteries or inner ear disease. In general, in patients with labyrinthine disorders, symptoms appear with brief, head-shaking motions. Patients who develop symptoms by extrinsic compression of the vertebral arteries usually require a few seconds with the neck rotated maximally in a particular direction to develop symptoms. In addition to orthostatism and osteophytic compression, other conditions are capable of causing vertebrobasilar ischemia and must be ruled out. Dissection of a vertebral artery is accompanied by neck pain. In these patients, the symptoms of brain ischemia may be due to critical compromise of the true lumen of the vertebral artery by an intramural dissecting hematoma or thromboembolization from the distal reentry point of the dissection. A number of medical conditions also present with symptoms of vertebrobasilar ischemia; among the most common are inappropriate antihypertensive medication, cardiac arrhythmia, anemia, brain tumor, and subclavian steal.

INDICATIONS FOR SURGERY

No morphologic database exists for atherosclerotic lesions of the SATs comparable to that available for internal carotid artery disease. It is known from arteriograms and postmortem studies that the SATs are less frequently involved by atherosclerotic disease than is the carotid bifurcation. In general, clinicians do not have the ability to use ultrasonography to study the composition of SAT plaques, and the specimens obtained at operation are few because the interventions to reconstruct the SATs are bypasses rather than endarterectomies. The few specimens available for pathologic study show degenerative features similar to those seen in carotid plaques: surface thrombus, ulceration, and intraplaque hemorrhage. One may reasonably infer that the same pathologic mechanisms operate in both carotid artery plaques and SAT lesions. Until more precise information becomes available, it seems sensible to use criteria similar to those applicable to carotid disease to determine treatment guidelines. These criteria, however, must be tempered by the fact that the risk of surgical reconstruction of the SATs is higher than that of carotid endarterectomy.

Indications for surgical repair of SAT lesions are (1) lesions encroaching on more than 70% of a SAT diameter, or plaques with ulceration or surface irregularities in patients with appropriate symptoms (ipsilateral carotid or vertebrobasilar); (2) the same lesions plus ipsilateral internal carotid disease for which an endarterectomy is indicated (the operation should correct both); (3) the same lesions plus a nonacute ipsilateral hemispheric infarction (overt or silent); and (4) preocclusive lesions (>90% cross-sectional area loss) in asymptomatic patients who are good surgical risks and have more than 5 years of life expectancy. This last indication is arbitrary albeit reasonable.

The primary indication for reconstructing a vertebral artery is to treat vertebrobasilar ischemia. Severe occlusive disease of the vertebral artery may be found in individuals who have no symptoms of vertebrobasilar ischemia and do not require surgical treatment. Conversely, many systemic causes of vertebrobasilar ischemia are not related to vertebral artery disease. Therefore the decision to reconstruct a vertebral artery must be based on a strong anatomic and clinical presumption that the symptom (vertebrobasilar ischemia) is secondary to the anatomic lesion (occlusive disease of the vertebral arteries).

Vertebrobasilar ischemia may be due to stenosis or occlusion of the vertebral or basilar arteries, restricting flow in the territory supplied by these arteries. This is the so-called low-flow (or hemodynamic) mechanism. These patients often have repetitive transient ischemic attacks triggered by positional or postural mechanisms. Although their risk for stroke is lower than that in patients with carotid disease, they may suffer serious traumatic injuries because of loss of balance (such as syncopal attack while driving). In patients with low-flow symptoms of ischemia in the vertebrobasilar territory, the surgical indication rests on the assumption that the basilar artery is not receiving adequate inflow from the vertebral arteries. Ischemia of the vertebrobasilar territory may also be due to microembolization (atheroemboli). Contrary to prevalent views in the neurologic literature, approximately one third of vertebrobasilar ischemic episodes are caused by atheroembolization from plaques or mural lesions of the vertebral arteries.[4] Patients with embolic symptoms are at high risk for infarctions of the brainstem, cerebellum, and occipital lobes. The mechanism here is microembolization from the irregular surface or from the core of a plaque in the proximal subclavian or vertebral arteries or from a lesion in the wall of the vertebral artery secondary to repetitive trauma from an osteophyte or from intramural dissection.

In patients with low-flow symptoms, and because two vertebral arteries usually supply the basilar artery, the presence of a normal vertebral artery contraindicates an operation on the opposite artery, regardless of its anatomic condition. A vertebral artery of normal caliber emptying into a basilar artery is enough to supply the basilar territory. This means that for a lesion in the vertebral arteries to be considered significant, it must be severe (>75% stenosis) and the opposite vertebral artery must be equally diseased, hypoplastic, or absent.

My approach to a patient with low-flow vertebrobasilar ischemia is first to determine whether any other clinical condition (e.g., orthostatism, arrhythmia) capable of producing these symptoms is present. If so, it should be corrected. If symptoms persist after treatment, an arteriogram is indicated. If the arteriogram shows a lesion that fulfills the anatomic criteria listed previously and the operation appears to be technically feasible, a reconstruction of the vertebral artery is indicated.

In patients with vertebrobasilar ischemic symptoms secondary to embolization, the indication for surgery rests on demonstration of the emboligenic lesion, regardless of the condition of the opposite vertebral artery. The criteria of bilateralism and degree of severity that apply to low-flow lesions are irrelevant when considering treatment for atheroembolic disease.

RECONSTRUCTION OF THE SUPRA-AORTIC TRUNKS

The main decision involved in reconstruction of the SATs is whether to do the repair through the chest or through the neck. Cervical repairs are traditionally done by means of a bypass from a suitable donor vessel to the diseased one. Most of these bypasses run transversely either between vessels on the same side of the neck (carotid and subclavian) or across the neck (remote bypasses). Bypass procedures between the ipsilateral carotid and subclavian arteries are largely being superseded by transposition procedures that provide the advantage of a single arterial anastomosis without the need for a saphenous vein graft or a prosthetic tube. Transthoracic or axial repairs require

a partial or total sternotomy for a direct approach to these vessels. The lesions are corrected with a bypass from the ascending aorta.

The choice between transthoracic (axial) and cervical (transverse) repairs can be made using the following general guidelines. Axial repairs are preferred in younger patients who have innominate artery lesions or multiple lesions (usually innominate and left common carotid). They are also the natural choice for patients in whom a simultaneous coronary bypass operation is indicated. In patients with atherosclerotic disease of the SATs and coronary arteries, repairing concomitant severe lesions of the first segment of the left subclavian artery is advisable even if this stenosis is asymptomatic. This repair permits a later myocardial revascularization using the left internal mammary artery.

Cervical repairs are preferred in older patients, in those who are at high risk of thoracotomy, and in those who have had previous transsternal procedures. Cervical repair is the choice for all single arterial lesions (other than those of the innominate artery).

Cervical Repairs

In the early 1970s, techniques for revascularization of the SATs consisted of a transverse bypass between a donor and a recipient (diseased) artery. The insertion of a bypass between the carotid and subclavian arteries, although described in 1957,[5] did not become popular until the 1970s. These bypasses were between the midsegment of the carotid artery and the second (retroscalene) segment of the subclavian artery. In some cases, the carotid artery acted as the donor vessel, and the bypass corrected a blockage of the first portion of the subclavian artery. In others, the subclavian artery was the donor vessel to bypass a proximal common carotid artery lesion. In subclavian-carotid bypasses, when the anastomosis to the carotid artery is of the end-to-side type, there is always the possibility of a source of proximal embolization (from the diseased proximal common carotid artery) or of extension of the proximal thrombus across the end-to-side anastomosis. As a result, an end-to-end anastomosis (see later) into the common carotid artery is recommended.

Carotid-subclavian bypasses became the standard operation for the correction of subclavian steal syndrome in the 1970s. When use of the carotid as the donor vessel was not advisable (because it was the only patent carotid artery or because of disease in the proximal common carotid artery), correction of subclavian steal was achieved with bypasses between both subclavian arteries or both axillary arteries. These remote bypasses became known as extraanatomic operations. Although they offer the advantages of avoiding a thoracotomy and carrying a lower operative mortality, they have lower long-term patency rates than those achieved by axial or shorter reconstructions. These remote bypasses are constructed with the graft crossing the neck in front of the sternum, giving a poor cosmetic result and subjecting them to external compression. Most significantly, bypasses in this anterior, low-neck location may interfere with an eventual tracheostomy and certainly with a midsternotomy that might be required for coronary revascularization later on.

Many of the cervical bypasses done in the 1970s used saphenous vein as the preferred graft material. There was fear of embolization from the "neointima" of prosthetic tubes and doubts about their long-term patency. However, saphenous veins also presented specific problems. They were not always available, and gross mismatches in caliber often occurred between the vein and the recipient arteries. In addition, the length required for remote bypasses led to the possibility of axial rotation or compression or kinking of the vein graft with rotation of the neck. Because of these difficulties, surgeons explored the use of prosthetic substitutes for arterial bypass in the neck. The reported results indicate that polytetrafluoroethylene (PTFE) grafts are preferable to saphenous vein for bypasses in the neck; they provide a good-caliber match, and their patency rates are excellent,[5] probably as a result of the high flow rates usually measured in these arteries.

Anatomic Indications

Innominate Artery Occlusion or Stenosis. A variety of cervical techniques are available to correct flow deficits caused by innominate artery stenosis or occlusion. Subclavian-subclavian and axilloaxillary bypasses can supply the right carotid artery through retrograde flow into the proximal right subclavian or axillary arteries. Carotid-carotid bypasses are technically feasible, but for the correction of severe innominate artery disease, they represent an unnecessary risk because both carotid systems will likely be severely hypotensive during the proximal anastomosis of the bypass to the donor left common carotid artery, unless shunted.

If the innominate artery lesion is suspected to be embolizing—or if it exhibits a grossly irregular surface or large ulcerations—the distal innominate artery should be ligated (excluded) at the completion of the remote bypass procedure. This may not be possible using a supraclavicular approach. A complex solution is an end-to-end anastomosis between the proximal subclavian artery and the proximal right common carotid artery, with ligation of the proximal carotid stump and then revascularization of the middle or distal third of the right subclavian through a remote bypass from the other side of the neck. Axial reconstructions (see later) are preferable for innominate artery lesions.

Common Carotid Artery Occlusion or Stenosis. The common carotid artery can be revascularized by means of a subclavian-carotid bypass from the ipsilateral subclavian artery, with the distal anastomosis being performed end to end to avoid embolization from the diseased proximal common carotid artery. When the entire carotid system on one side is not visualized on the arteriogram, one must consider the possibility that the carotid bifurcation is patent, with retrograde flow from the external carotid artery perfusing the internal carotid artery antegradely. Delayed subtraction films may show this late opacification, but duplex imaging is the best way to show patency of the carotid bifurcation and this peculiar

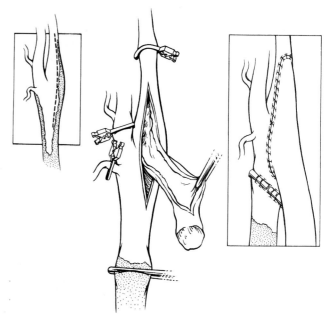

FIGURE 19-1 ■ Traditional method of anastomosing the distal limb of a graft to the carotid bifurcation following endarterectomy of the latter. Occlusion of the common carotid artery immediately below the anastomosis transforms it into a functional end-to-end junction *(inset, right)*.

combination of retrograde (external carotid) and antegrade (internal carotid) flow. In these patients, atheromatous plaque is usually found at the origin of the internal carotid artery, necessitating endarterectomy before performing the distal anastomosis. The traditional means of constructing a distal anastomosis for a graft at the level of the carotid bifurcation is with an end-to-side junction (an onlay patch), with or without a concomitant endarterectomy of the carotid bulb (Figure 19-1). This end-to-side anastomosis is functionally transformed into an end-to-end junction by ligation of the common carotid artery below the anastomosis, in the soft segment created by endarterectomy of the distal portion of the common carotid artery. A preferable technique for the distal anastomosis is (Figure 19-2): to amputate of the distal common carotid artery, the carotid bulb is then everted for endarterectomy (type 2 eversion). The round cross section of the carotid bifurcation allows a simple end-to-end anastomosis to the bypass arising from the subclavian artery.

If the stenosing lesion of the common carotid artery is located at its origin and its distal two thirds are free of disease, transposing the midportion of the common carotid artery to the subclavian artery is a better solution than a subclavian-carotid bypass. It requires only one anastomosis and no prosthesis. At times, a thrombosed common carotid artery with a patent bifurcation can be thrombectomized after dividing it low in the neck and doing an eversion endarterectomy up to the bifurcation. The distal portion of the endarterectomy is terminated under direct vision through the standard arteriotomy used for a conventional carotid endarterectomy. After endarterectomy, the common carotid artery is reimplanted into the second portion of the subclavian

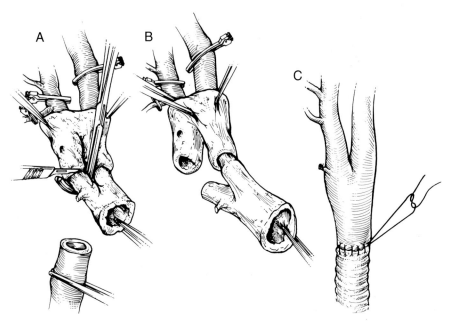

FIGURE 19-2 ■ My preference for anastomosing the graft to the carotid bifurcation is an eversion endarterectomy followed by an end-to-end anastomosis. **A,** Eversion of the external carotid after exposing the flow divider in the plaque. **B,** Eversion of the internal carotid component of the plaque. **C,** Anastomosis of the graft to everted bifurcation.

artery. Subclavian-carotid bypass and transposition of the carotid into the subclavian are easier on the right side, where the subclavian artery is more accessible.

In cases in which the ipsilateral subclavian artery is not a suitable donor vessel, a common carotid artery lesion can be corrected by means of a carotid-carotid bypass. This operation is traditionally done by placing a bypass between both carotids in front of the airway. Instead, I prefer the shorter retropharyngeal route (see later in this chapter).

Subclavian Artery Occlusion. Reconstruction of the proximal subclavian artery is done (1) to correct a symptomatic subclavian steal, (2) to correct an emboligenic lesion of the proximal subclavian, (3) to revascularize the subclavian before an internal mammary transposition to the coronary arteries, or (4) to transpose the left subclavian to the left common carotid artery before extending a thoracic stent-graft across its origin. Carotid-subclavian bypass is a proven operation to revascularize the subclavian artery. If the subclavian lesion has been the source of embolization, the prevertebral subclavian artery must be ligated at the time of the bypass. It has been the author's preference for the last 15 years to use a direct transposition of the subclavian artery (prevertebral portion) to the common carotid artery. Although this operation is slightly more complex than the bypass, it involves only one anastomosis, excludes the diseased proximal subclavian artery, and does not require a graft.

Techniques

Carotid-Subclavian or Subclavian-Carotid Bypass and Carotid (or Subclavian) Transposition. The

approach is through a supraclavicular incision dividing the clavicular head of the sternocleidomastoid muscle. The dissection is first lateral to the jugular vein, which is retracted medially. The prescalene fat pad is entered, and the anterior scalene muscle is exposed. The subclavian artery is isolated beneath the anterior scalene (second portion) or lateral to it (third portion) if a bypass is planned. In the first case, the phrenic nerve is isolated from the surface of the anterior scalene, and the subclavian artery is exposed after division of this muscle. The site chosen for anastomosis of the bypass is usually lateral to the thyrocervical trunk. Alternatively, the subclavian artery can be exposed in the third segment, between the brachial plexus and the anterior scalene muscle, with partial division of the latter.

The dissection is then moved medial to the jugular vein, and the common carotid artery is exposed. A suitable site is selected for the anastomosis of the graft to the carotid artery. In the case of a carotid-subclavian bypass for subclavian steal, the vein graft or prosthetic tube is anastomosed to the side wall of the carotid artery and then passed under the jugular vein into proximity with the subclavian artery (Figure 19-3). Both anastomoses are end to side.

If the bypass is intended to revascularize the common carotid artery, the subclavian artery anastomosis is done first; the graft is then tunneled under the jugular vein and anastomosed end to end to the common carotid artery or to its bifurcation (Figure 19-4), ligating the proximal carotid stump. Another alternative is to do an end-to-side anastomosis to the common carotid artery and ligate the common carotid artery immediately proximal to the anastomosis, which makes it functionally an end-to-end junction. The proximal exclusion is necessary to avoid embolization from the proximal common carotid artery

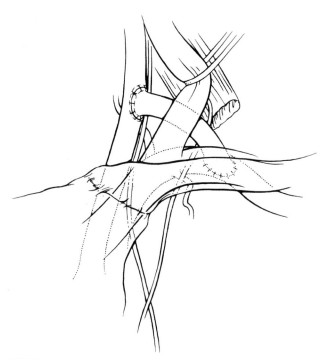

FIGURE 19-3 ■ Carotid-subclavian bypass graft tunneled under the jugular vein.

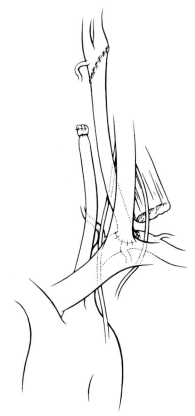

FIGURE 19-4 ■ Bypass from the left subclavian artery to the left carotid bifurcation.

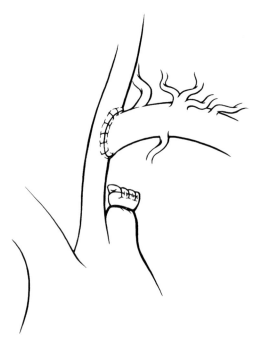

FIGURE 19-5 ■ Transposition of the left subclavian artery to the left common carotid artery.

or extension of the thrombus into the distal common carotid artery.

The bypass technique between the carotid and subclavian arteries is used, in cases of common carotid artery occlusion and in patients with a left internal mammary artery–coronary anastomosis. Transposing one of these arteries into the other is a more elegant surgical solution (Figure 19-5), in that only one artery-to-artery anastomosis is required. The long-term patency rates for carotid-subclavian transposition are superb. The drawbacks are the greater technical difficulty and the possibility of mediastinal bleeding from improper handling of the stump of the left subclavian artery. The transposition operation is particularly easy when the common carotid artery is the one being transposed; once freed, the common carotid, which has no branches, moves about the neck with ease. Translocation of the subclavian artery into the common carotid artery may be difficult on the left side, where the subclavian artery may have a deep location or the vertebral artery may have a low origin. When this low origin interferes with good proximal control of the much shorter first portion of the subclavian, the vertebral artery is divided at its origin and the subclavian artery low in the neck, but distal to the stump of the vertebral artery. The subclavian artery is transposed to the common carotid artery and, separately, the vertebral artery is transposed into either of the two vessels.

When transposing the subclavian artery to the common carotid artery, care must be taken to ensure proper position of the vertebral artery when the subclavian is brought into apposition to the common carotid before the anastomosis. Excessive length of the vertebral artery, once the subclavian artery is freed and moved upward, may cause kinking of this vessel and thrombosis. Although some authors have written that division of the left internal mammary artery facilitates the transposition, this is not so; it is an unwise maneuver that negates the possibility of a later myocardial revascularization using the internal mammary artery.

Subclavian-Subclavian Bypass. There is hardly any indication for subclavian-subclavian bypass. The incision is supraclavicular on both sides, and the second or third portions of the subclavian are approached in the manner described earlier. The tunnel connecting the two subclavian arteries is made behind the sternocleidomastoid muscle, staying as low as possible to protect the graft behind the upper edge of the manubrium. Care is taken to avoid any axial rotation of the graft when tunneling across the neck.

Axilloaxillary Bypass. Axilloaxillary bypass is rarely, if ever, indicated. Axillary arteries are exposed between the sternal and clavicular heads of the pectoralis major. Removal of part or all of the pectoralis minor from the coracoid process improves exposure of the axillary artery. The graft is tunneled under the sternal part of the pectoralis major and through presternal subcutaneous tissue into the opposite axillary artery. Both anastomoses are end to side.

Carotid-Carotid Bypass. Carotid-carotid bypass is used to revascularize a common carotid artery whose origin in the mediastinum is involved by disease. One carotid acts as the donor vessel to the other. Because exposure of the common carotid arteries is a reasonably simple procedure, carotid-carotid bypass is a good technique to revascularize one common carotid trunk when the other one is healthy and the ipsilateral subclavian artery is not a suitable donor vessel. The bypass between both common carotid arteries lies low in the midline, partially hidden by the upper edge of the manubrium. Although these grafts make a rather lengthy loop and take off from the donor site at an oblique angle, their patency rate is excellent, provided the donor vessel is free of disease. These bypasses are sometimes cosmetically poor and, as mentioned previously, the grafts run a lengthy trajectory to link two vessels that, anatomically, are only four fingerbreadths apart. It is preferable to tunnel the bypass across the neck through the retropharyngeal space (Figure 19-6), which is a shorter and straighter path. The tunnel for the bypass is behind the pharynx and in front of the prevertebral lamina. This space is loose and easily admits an 8-mm prosthesis without any pharyngeal compression.[6]

The distance between both carotids in the retropharyngeal space (approximately 5 cm) is short enough that it permits the direct reimplantation of one carotid into the other without a graft (Figure 19-7). This procedure has the disadvantage of requiring clamping of both common carotid arteries simultaneously; because of this, it is one of the few instances in which the protection of a shunt may be required to perfuse a clamped (donor) common carotid artery.

Axial Repairs

Endarterectomy was the first technique reported for reconstruction of the innominate artery,[7] and it was later formally described and perfected by Carlson and colleagues.[8] Innominate endarterectomy is no longer used because of safety concerns. Its main drawback is the

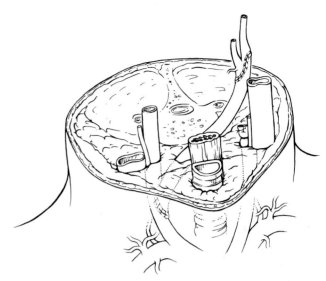

FIGURE 19-6 ■ Cross section of the neck showing the trajectory of a carotid-carotid bypass through the retropharyngeal space.

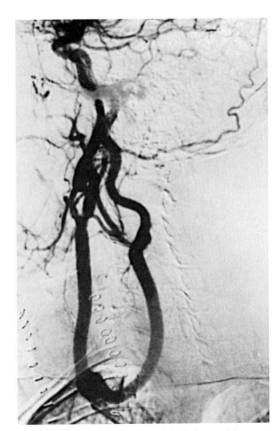

FIGURE 19-7 ■ Direct transposition of the left carotid artery to the right common carotid artery using the retropharyngeal route. (From Berguer R: The short retropharyngeal route for arterial bypasses across the neck. Ann Vasc Surg 1:127–129, 1986.)

difficulty of clamping the origin of the innominate artery without occluding the left common carotid artery or damaging the plaque that may be present about the ostium of either. A common origin of the innominate and left common carotid arteries is found in 17% of individuals. The left common carotid is a branch of the innominate in another 8% of individuals. In either case, a clamp placed to exclude the origin of the innominate artery would result in bilateral hemispheric ischemia. When an innominate endarterectomy is done in a patient who has a common ostium for the innominate and left common carotid arteries, a temporary shunt from the ascending aorta to the left common carotid artery is mandatory. With innominate endarterectomy, it is also difficult to achieve a satisfactory proximal termination of the endarterectomy in the aortic arch wall, where tacking sutures are often required. Finally, approximately half the patients with symptomatic innominate artery stenosis have severe lesions of either the left common carotid or left subclavian artery. These concomitant lesions are not suited for endarterectomy using the transsternal approach.

Rather than endarterectomy, a bypass from the ascending aorta is preferred to correct innominate artery and other associated lesions that may be present. The technique of bypass from the ascending aorta was introduced by DeBakey and associates.[9]

Technique

Midsternotomy. Traditionally the anterior mediastinal arteries (innominate and right common carotid) were approached through a midsternotomy (Figure 19-8). The sternotomy is prolonged through a short incision that

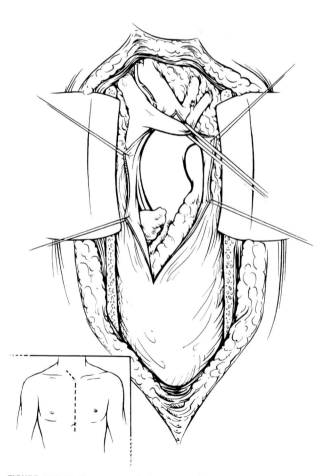

FIGURE 19-8 ■ Exposure of the ascending aorta and anterior supra-aortic trunks through the traditional full sternotomy (*inset* shows the skin incision).

follows the right anterior edge of the sternocleidomastoid muscle to expose and obtain control of the proximal right common carotid and right subclavian arteries. After dividing the sternum, the innominate vein is dissected, and the thymic veins are ligated. The thymus is separated through its midline and preserved, to be used as tissue interposed between the graft and the sternum at the time of closure. The ascending aorta is approached below the innominate vein after opening the pericardial sac. The dissection continues over the origin of the innominate artery and onto its bifurcation. During dissection of the innominate bifurcation, care is taken not to injure the recurrent nerve near the origin of the right subclavian artery.

Partial Midsternotomy. In 1991, after being confronted with a poorly executed midsternotomy, it became apparent that approaching the ascending aorta and the anterior trunks did not require complete splitting of the sternum. Since then, my preferred technique has been to approach the anterior SATs with a partial sternotomy, splitting only the upper three sternal segments (Figure 19-9). The manubrium is sewn down to the third intercostal space, where a small notch is made laterally with the oscillating saw. This notch facilitates a subperiosteal fracture at this site when the sternal spreader is used. Dissection of the brachiocephalic vein and thymus and exposure of the ascending aorta follow the same steps described for the full sternotomy. The advantages of this partial midsternotomy are that the chest cage remains intact and stable in its lower half, postoperative pain is noticeably reduced, and the chance of sternal instability is minimal.

Bypass from the Ascending Aorta. If the intent is to replace the innominate artery with a bypass (Figure 19-10), the first inch of the right subclavian and right common carotid arteries are exposed. More often, however, one and sometimes both carotid bifurcations need to be exposed to be revascularized. The carotid bifurcation in this case is exposed through the standard neck incision used for carotid endarterectomy. After isolating the proximal right subclavian and common carotid arteries, an appropriate prosthetic tube is selected for the bypass. An 8- to 10-mm PTFE or Dacron fabric tube matches the caliber of the innominate artery, requires only a moderate amount of aortic wall to be excluded, and does not occupy much space in the anterior mediastinum.

The proximal end of the prosthesis is beveled. Safe exclusion clamping of the ascending aorta requires the use of a nitroglycerin drip to reduce the systolic pressure to 110 mm Hg. The exclusion clamp is placed on the proximal aorta (Figure 19-11). With the clamp secured, the aorta is opened, and the beveled end of the graft is anastomosed to the ascending aortotomy with continuous 4-0 polypropylene sutures. Before unclamping and to avoid air embolization, the patient is momentarily placed in 15 degrees of Trendelenburg position, and the proximal anastomosis is vented and tested. If it is found to be satisfactory, a clamp is placed on the graft immediately above the anastomosis, and the table is returned to the horizontal position.

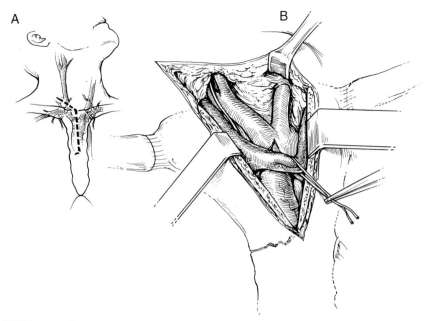

FIGURE 19-9 ■ Skin incision (A) and exposure (B) obtained through a partial sternotomy.

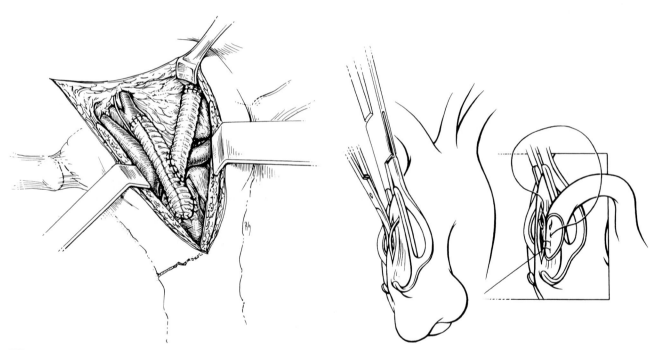

FIGURE 19-10 ■ Ascending aorta–to–innominate and left common carotid artery bypass completed through a partial sternotomy.

FIGURE 19-11 ■ Exclusion clamping of the ascending aorta and anastomosis of the main prosthesis to the aortotomy.

The patient is then systemically heparinized. Occluding clamps are placed first in the proximal right carotid and subclavian arteries and in the proximal portion of the innominate artery. The innominate artery is divided proximal to its bifurcation and prepared for anastomosis. The bypass graft, which is placed over the brachiocephalic vein, is cut to appropriate length and anastomosed to the innominate artery with continuous 5-0 polypropylene sutures. The graft and the distal vessels are bled before completing the anastomosis, and flow is reestablished first into the right subclavian artery and then into the right common carotid artery. The proximal stump of

the innominate artery is closed with a continuous double running suture.

In cases in which additional arteries need to be revascularized (usually the left common carotid), an additional 8-mm PTFE or Dacron side branch is anastomosed at an appropriate angle to the 10-mm main prosthesis after the proximal suture line is completed (Figure 19-12). Any anticipated side branches are added before the distal anastomosis is done to avoid having to reclamp the innominate portion of the bypass after establishing flow through it. With the side branch anastomosed and excluded, one can perfuse the right carotid and vertebral

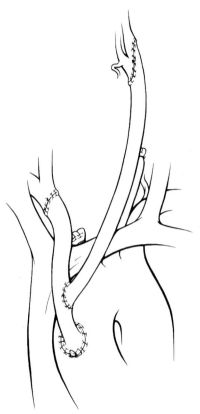

FIGURE 19-12 ■ Common pattern for revascularization of the anterior supra-aortic trunk: the main prosthesis (10 mm) replaces the innominate artery, and an 8-mm side branch supplies the left carotid system.

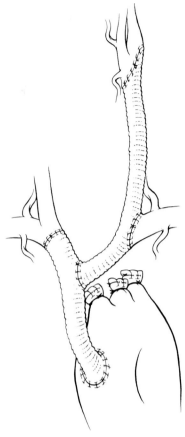

FIGURE 19-13 ■ Revascularization of all three supra-aortic trunks completed by transposing the left subclavian artery to the prosthesis that replaces the left carotid system.

arteries while constructing the left carotid anastomosis. In multiple replacements of the SATs (Figure 19-13), the main bypass is the one supplying the right-sided trunk (innominate, right carotid, right subclavian). From this trunk emerge the branches supplying the left carotid or left subclavian artery or both.

Results and Complications of Reconstruction of the Supra-Aortic Trunks

Transthoracic reconstructions are generally done in younger patients with multiple-vessel involvement. Cervical repairs are done in older patients who are less likely to tolerate a thoracotomy and in patients with single-vessel disease of the common carotid or proximal subclavian arteries.

Any comparison of the results of the thoracic and cervical approaches must be done with reticence because of the differences between the two groups of patients. In addition to age and anatomic extent of disease, other considerations affect the choice of the approach, such as pulmonary function, previous coronary artery bypass surgery, and life expectancy.

A review of my experience with SAT reconstruction from 1982 to 1998 encompassed 282 cases—182 cervical repairs and 100 transthoracic repairs (Table 19-1). The most frequent indication for cervical repair in my practice is single-trunk disease (carotid or subclavian artery) or a history of myocardial revascularization. All innominate artery lesions are operated on through the chest.

TABLE 19-1	**Morbidity and Mortality of Repair of the Supra-Aortic Trunks**		
Approach	**No. of Patients**	**TIA or Stroke (%)**	**Deaths (%)**
Cervical	182	3.8	0.5
Thoracic	100	8.0	8.0

TIA, Transient ischemic attack.

Reported operative mortality for transthoracic repair ranges from 3% to 19%,[10,11] with most authors reporting series of 20 to 40 patients; some smaller series reported no mortality.[11] Increasing experience, refinement in anesthesia and perioperative care, and better patient selection have reduced the mortality of transthoracic repair from 10% to 5% in reports from the Baylor group[11,12] and from 10% to 3.8% between the first and second halves of my experience.[13]

Reported mortality for cervical repairs is lower than that for thoracic repairs, between 0% and 4%. In the series by Berguer and colleagues,[14] the morbidity from stroke and transient ischemic attack in patients undergoing cervical repair was 3.8%. Patients undergoing cervical repair are some of the highest-risk patients among those with cerebrovascular disease; many have had previous myocardial revascularization procedures or are limited by restrictive pulmonary disease.

Over the last 14 years, a change in operative techniques has led to a reduction in operative complications and an increase in patency rates. Whereas 15 years ago, the author performed subclavian-carotid and carotid-subclavian grafts for single-vessel disease, today most of these reconstructions are direct transpositions of one vessel to the other. The patency rate for cervical transposition procedures in Berguer and colleagues[14] was 100% after 5 years.

Likewise, the techniques for transthoracic reconstruction have been refined and extended. Partial sternotomy has been a standard approach for 20 years. Endarterectomy of the innominate artery is no longer performed. The goal is to extend the revascularization of the SATs to the left subclavian artery in patients who are likely candidates for future myocardial revascularization. With these refinements and changes in patient selection criteria in the latter half of the author's experience (1988 to 1998), the combined mortality and morbidity has been the same (3.8%) for cervical and transthoracic repairs. Table 19-1 shows the incidence of stroke and death following cervical and transthoracic repair in the entire series.

The most frequent and serious complication reported after either cervical or transthoracic repair of the SATs is myocardial infarction.[15,16] The second most frequent complication is stroke, which can develop during the operation or 3 to 4 days afterward. A delayed stroke may be hemorrhagic and is likely related to hyperperfusion and regional hypertension. In the author's experience, stroke has been a more frequent complication than myocardial infarction. Perioperative strokes are more common in patients with multiple intracranial and extracranial involvement.[11] Some postoperative strokes may be due to technical flaws resulting in distal embolization or to prolonged clamp ischemia times. The latter can be managed with the usual cerebral protection methods. Intravenous dexamethasone is used routinely before clamping, controlled heparin activity (activated clotting time), and—in patients with extensive and multiple disease—mild superficial hypothermia. Shunts for SAT repair are not recommended, with the rare exception noted under the description of carotid-carotid bypass.

Technical problems may cause perioperative or postoperative bleeding, which can be severe and life threatening. Suture line bleeding, aortic wall tears from clamp or suture injury, and bleeding from an innominate artery stump can result in serious perioperative bleeding and severe tension hemothorax. Postoperative graft thrombosis and infections are rare.

The long-term outcome of these patients is largely determined by the progress of their coronary atherosclerotic disease. For patients undergoing cervical and transthoracic repairs, the 10-year survival is 50%.[16-18] Myocardial infarction is the most common cause of death (80%).

The long-term patency of these reconstructions is excellent.[17] Cumulative primary patency rates at 10 years are 82% and 88% for cervical and thoracic repairs, respectively.[13,14] Transpositions have the best patency rate (100% at 5 years) of all cervical repairs. Saphenous veins fare worse than synthetics when used for SAT

reconstruction; axial rotation, caliber mismatches, kinking, and intimal hyperplasia probably account for this.

In conclusion, cervical reconstruction is indicated in patients who have had previous myocardial revascularization and in those with single lesions of the common carotid or subclavian arteries. In this last group, it is preferable to use transposition techniques between the carotid and the subclavian and, if the midline needs to be crossed, a retropharyngeal bypass. Reconstructive techniques using short (retropharyngeal) bypasses or no bypasses at all (transpositions) have outstanding patency rates, in contrast to the poor patency rates reported for conventional extraanatomic bypasses. The transthoracic approach is favored for patients with multiple-vessel disease. SAT reconstruction may be done in conjunction with coronary artery bypass grafts. This approach should be confined to centers with experience in these techniques, where the operative mortality is similar to that obtained in cervical repairs.[17]

RECONSTRUCTION OF THE VERTEBROBASILAR SYSTEM

The indications for vertebral artery reconstruction were discussed earlier. The vertebral artery is generally reconstructed at two levels: in its proximal segment for stenosing disease of its ostium, and in its distal segment (above C2) for compression or thrombosis or a source of embolization from the intraspinal segment of this artery.

Reconstruction of the Proximal Vertebral Artery

Although the first reconstructions of the vertebral arteries were endarterectomies,[19-22] this technique is seldom used today. Vertebral artery bypass was advocated in the 1970s.[23] Today, most proximal vertebral artery lesions are dealt with by transposition of the artery into the neighboring common carotid artery[24-26] (Figure 19-14). The appeal of this operation is that it consists of one artery-to-artery anastomosis and does not require a vein graft (needed for bypass) or extensive dissection of the subclavian artery (needed for endarterectomy).

The operation is done through a supraclavicular incision. The approach is between the bellies of the sternocleidomastoid muscles. The vertebral artery is isolated below the vertebral vein, dissected from its origin up to the point where it disappears under the longus colli, and freed from the overlying sympathetic ganglion or crossing sympathetic fibers. After clearing the adventitia of the chosen transposition site in the posterolateral wall of the common carotid artery, the patient is heparinized and the vertebral artery is divided above the stenotic area, suture-ligating its proximal stump. The distal segment of the artery is swung into the common carotid artery (Figure 19-15). Using an aortic punch, a small arteriostomy is made in the common carotid wall to which the vertebral artery is anastomosed in end-to-side fashion using 7-0 polypropylene sutures and an open-type anastomosis.

In a few cases, this technique is not possible. The most frequent reason is a contralateral common or internal

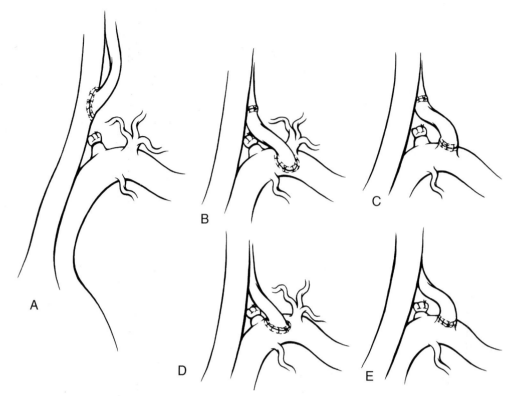

FIGURE 19-14 ■ Common techniques for reconstruction of the proximal vertebral artery. **A,** Transposition of the proximal vertebral artery to the common carotid artery. **B,** Bypass from the subclavian to the proximal vertebral artery. **C,** Subclavian-vertebral bypass originating in the amputated stump of the thyrocervical trunk. **D,** Transposition of the vertebral artery to another subclavian site. **E,** Transposition of the vertebral artery to the stump of the thyrocervical trunk.

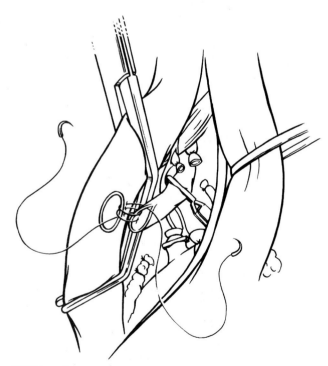

FIGURE 19-15 ■ Technique for transposition of the left vertebral artery to the left common carotid artery. The thoracic duct has been double ligated. The proximal vertebral artery stump has been clipped and suture-ligated. The sympathetic chain, left intact, is now seen behind the vertebral artery as the latter is brought close to the common carotid artery for anastomosis.

carotid artery occlusion or an abnormally short first segment of the vertebral artery entering the cervical spine through the transverse process of C7 rather than C6. If the opposite common or internal carotid artery is occluded, clamping the remaining ipsilateral common carotid artery to transpose the vertebral artery to it carries severe risk of brain ischemia. In this situation, a subclavian-to-vertebral artery bypass is preferred. If the vertebral artery is too short to be brought easily to the common carotid artery wall, it can also be bypassed from the subclavian artery using a saphenous vein graft.[22,23] The bypass originates from the subclavian artery lateral to the thyrocervical trunk and is anastomosed end to end to the vertebral artery below the longus colli muscle. This procedure does not require any type of shunting. The most frequent complications from proximal vertebral artery dissection and transposition are partial Horner syndrome from manipulation (or injury) of the intermediate sympathetic ganglion overlying the vertebral artery and an occasional lymphocele from injury to, or failed ligature of, the main or accessory thoracic ducts.

Reconstruction of the Distal Vertebral Artery

Regardless of the level between C6 and C2 where the external compression or occlusive process occurs, the distal vertebral artery is reconstructed at the space between the C1 and C2 transverse processes (Figure 19-16). This is the widest gap between transverse processes in the neck and is also the segment where the

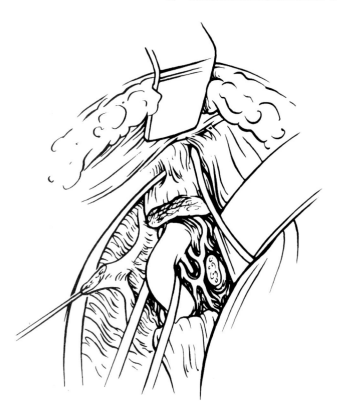

FIGURE 19-16 ■ Exposure of the vertebral artery between the transverse processes of C1 and C2. The anterior ramus of the C2 nerve has been divided, and its anterior end is retracted with a stay suture. The artery has been dissected away from the surrounding vertebral plexus, which is now seen behind it.

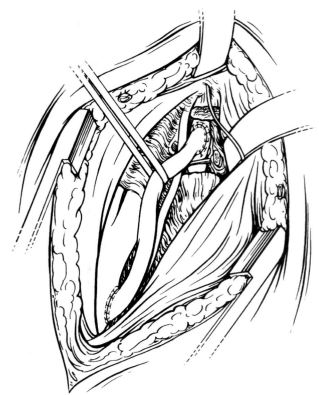

FIGURE 19-17 ■ Completed common carotid–to–distal vertebral artery bypass graft. A metal clip occludes the distal vertebral artery immediately below the anastomosis, making it function as an end-to-end junction.

vertebral artery is often maintained patent by collaterals from the occipital artery when the proximal segment of the artery is occluded.[24-26]

The operation is done through an incision similar to that used for carotid endarterectomy. Exposure of the vertebral artery at this level requires dissecting posterior to the jugular vein and identifying the spinal accessory nerve and the levator scapulae muscle. The levator is cut, exposing the transverse course of the anterior ramus of the C2 nerve. The artery lies below the ramus and is perpendicular to it. The ramus is cut, and the artery is exposed. Dissection of the vertebral artery may be made difficult by the plexus of veins that surrounds it.

Once the artery is isolated, it can be reconstructed in several ways. The most common reconstruction is a bypass from the common carotid artery to the distal vertebral artery immediately below the transverse process of C1 using autogenous vein (Figure 19-17). This requires dissection of the common carotid below the bifurcation and the availability of a saphenous vein with a caliber approximating that of the vertebral artery. Once the end-to-side anastomosis of the vein graft to the vertebral artery is completed, the latter is ligated immediately below the anastomosis to avoid embolization from its proximal segment.

Another alternative is to use the external carotid artery (or, in rare cases, the occipital artery) to revascularize the distal vertebral artery (Figure 19-18). The external carotid is skeletonized and transposed below the jugular

vein, anastomosing it end to end to the distal vertebral artery. The appeal of this procedure is that it does not require clamping of the internal carotid supply and that the caliber match between the distal external carotid artery and the vertebral artery is usually good. This choice obviously requires that the external carotid artery and the carotid bifurcation be free of atherosclerotic disease. I use this type of operation most often in individuals who have external compression or occlusion of the vertebral artery by osteophytes during neck rotation. These patients are generally younger and free of disease of the carotid bifurcation.

A third solution is transposing the distal segment of the vertebral artery to the neighboring internal carotid artery by means of an end-to-side anastomosis. This, again, has the appeal of a limited dissection and no need for a vein graft. The shortcoming is that one needs to clamp the internal carotid artery for the end-to-side anastomosis. This technique should not be used in patients in whom the opposite internal carotid artery is severely diseased or occluded.

A few patients have extrinsic compression or disease of the vertebral artery above the level of C1. In these patients, the reconstruction is done in the distalmost segment of the extracranial vertebral artery before it penetrates the dura mater as it courses over the lamina of the atlas (the pars atlantica). The approach is posterior through a racquet-shaped incision (Figure 19-19) with the patient in the park-bench position. The semispinalis,

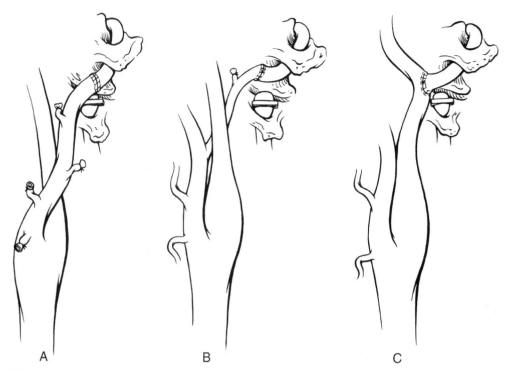

FIGURE 19-18 ■ Alternative methods for reconstruction of the distal vertebral artery. **A,** External carotid transposition to the distal vertebral artery. **B,** Occipital artery transposition to the distal vertebral artery. **C,** Transposition of the distal vertebral artery to the distal internal carotid artery.

splenius, and longus capitis muscles are cut, and the sternomastoid is de-inserted from the mastoid process. The transverse process of C1 is identified, and the obliquus capitis superior muscle is cut. The artery rests on the posterior lamina of the atlas, covered by a dense plexus of veins and tethered by one or two muscular branches, which are divided. The vein bypass is anastomosed end to side. The distal cervical internal carotid artery can be isolated after dissecting away the vagus and hypoglossal nerve trunks, which, in this posterior approach, overlie the internal carotid artery. The bypass is anastomosed end to side to the distal cervical internal carotid artery (Figure 19-20). In some patients, the vertebral artery pathology is extrinsic bony compression of the artery between the occipital ridge and the posterior lamina of C1. In this situation, once the vertebral artery is dissected (using the suboccipital approach described here), laminectomy of C1 eliminates the lower element of compression. Unless there is demonstrable damage to the wall of the vertebral artery by the bony impingement, a bypass is not needed.

The risks and patency rates of vertebral artery operations are different for proximal and distal repairs.[26] Proximal reconstructions are technically easier. Distal reconstructions are more demanding and lengthier procedures. Berguer and colleagues[26] reported on 252 proximal vertebral artery reconstructions with a combined mortality and morbidity of 0.9%. No stroke or death occurred in 159 patients undergoing only a proximal vertebral artery reconstruction. The only morbidity and mortality occurred in patients undergoing simultaneous carotid and vertebral artery reconstruction. The cumulative secondary patency rate for proximal reconstructions was 92% at 10 years.

In 117 distal vertebral reconstructions, the combined mortality and morbidity was 3.4%, fourfold greater than that for proximal repairs. Kieffer and colleagues reported 2.4% mortality.[27] Refinements in patient selection and surgical safeguards in the last 12 years have reduced the combined morbidity and mortality rates for proximal (0%) and distal (1.3%) vertebral reconstructions.

Postoperative thrombosis of a proximal reconstruction is rare, seen in 3 of 252 cases (1.2%) in the author's experience. In all three cases, a short vertebral artery (entering at C7) could not be repaired by a standard vertebral-to-carotid transposition, and a subclavian-vertebral or carotid-vertebral bypass was performed. In one case, tension at the anastomotic line, and in two others, a kink of the interposition vein graft, resulted in postoperative thrombosis. All patients underwent reoperation and thrombectomy, and the technical flaw was corrected. These three reoperations were recorded as patent at 3, 5, and 7 years postoperatively. Other complications of proximal reconstruction are an occasional lymphocele and a partial Horner's syndrome from manipulation of or injury to the lower cervical sympathetics. In one case of distal reconstruction, the spinal accessory nerve was damaged.

Postoperative thrombosis is more frequent following operations on the distal vertebral artery. The author has seen it in 4 of 117 distal reconstructions (3.4%). The causes were faulty anastomoses or inadequate vein grafts. Thrombectomy and replacement with a new graft reestablished patency in two of the four failures.

Presenting symptoms of vertebrobasilar ischemia were relieved in 83% of patients.[22,25] Among survivors, the 5-year rate of protection from stroke was 97%.

References available online at expertconsult.com.

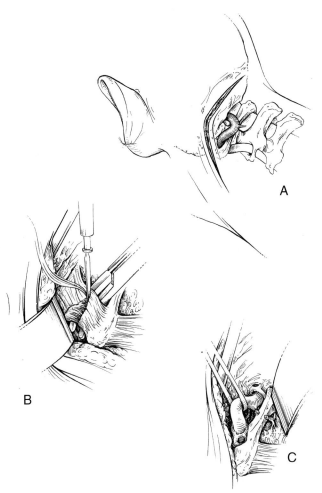

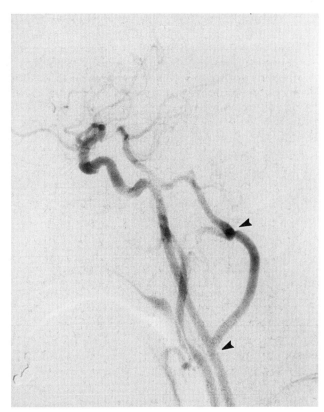

FIGURE 19-20 ■ Postoperative arteriogram showing a bypass from the cervical internal carotid artery to the suboccipital vertebral artery *(arrowheads)* before its entry into the foramen magnum.

FIGURE 19-19 ■ **A,** Incision to approach the suboccipital segment of the vertebral artery. **B,** Division of the obliquus capitis superior. **C,** The looped vertebral artery is lifted from the underlying lamina of C1. A descending muscular branch has been ligated and divided. (From Berguer R: Revascularization of the vertebral arteries. In Nyhus LM, Baker RJ, Fischer JE, editors: Mastery of Surgery, Boston, 1996, Little Brown.)

QUESTIONS

1. In a patient with a retroesophageal right subclavian artery, which of the following associated anomalies are expected or likely to occur: (1) nonrecurrent right inferior laryngeal nerve; (2) thoracic duct emptying on the right side; (3) common trunk as the origin of both common carotid arteries; (4) right vertebral artery arising from the right common carotid artery; or (5) left vertebral artery arising from the left common carotid artery?
   a. 1, 3, 4, 5
   b. 2, 3, 4, 5
   c. 1, 2, 3, 4
   d. 1, 2, 3, 4, 5

2. What is the most efficient operation to correct a severe stenosis of the origin of a vertebral artery?
   a. Subclavian–to–vertebral artery autogenous vein bypass
   b. Transposition of the vertebral artery to the common carotid artery
   c. Endarterectomy and patch of the origin of the vertebral artery
   d. Balloon angioplasty of the stenotic origin

3. Vertebrobasilar ischemia may be the result of which of the following: (1) a hemodynamically significant lesion of the vertebral artery; (2) a hemodynamically significant lesion of the basilar artery; (3) microembolization from a vertebral artery lesion; (4) microembolization from a subclavian artery plaque; or (5) microembolization from a dissected vertebral artery?
   a. 1, 3, 4, 5
   b. 1, 3, 5
   c. 1, 2, 5
   d. 1, 2, 3, 4, 5

ANSWERS

1. **c**
2. **b**
3. **d**

CHAPTER 20

ENDOVASCULAR REPAIR OF EXTRACRANIAL CEREBROVASCULAR LESIONS

W. Austin Blevins, Jr. • Peter A. Schneider

Each year in the United States, nearly 800,000 individuals experience a new or recurrent stroke, accounting for direct and indirect costs of more than $40 billion and untold damage to patients and their families. Stroke is responsible for 1 out of every 18 deaths in the United States, making it the number three cause of death after heart disease and cancer.[1] Carotid bifurcation stenosis and resultant ischemia producing emboli is a major cause of preventable stroke. Efforts to address this major health issue have focused on risk factor management, including medical therapy and surgical or endovascular intervention.

Treatment of carotid disease has evolved considerably over the past 60 years with the introduction of the carotid endarterectomy (CEA) in the 1950s and carotid angioplasty in the late 1970s. During the 1990s several landmark, randomized controlled trials (RCTs) in North America and Europe were published that demonstrated the superiority of CEA plus medical management over medical management alone, affirming CEA as the gold standard for patients with carotid bifurcation stenosis.[2-9] Carotid stenting was introduced in the mid 1990s and has evolved with advances in technique, equipment, operator experience, and the routine use of cerebral protection devices. Carotid angioplasty and stenting (CAS) is a viable minimally invasive alternative to CEA for select patient populations and is continuing to develop as an option for treating carotid bifurcation stenosis. The purpose of this chapter is to describe the technique of CAS, provide an overview of current results, and offer perspective as to the value of this treatment in the management of extracranial cerebrovascular disease.

TECHNIQUE

Patient Selection for Carotid Angioplasty and Stenting

Part of the motivation in the development of CAS was to address the needs of patients at high risk for CEA in an attempt to improve results of carotid revascularization. In the United States, the Centers for Medicare and Medicaid Services (CMS) has established criteria for patient eligibility for endovascular carotid interventions on the basis of being high risk for CEA, identifying both physiologic and anatomic factors making the patient a high-risk candidate for an open surgical procedure (Box 20-1).

The use of CAS for patients at high risk for CEA is now an established practice. The rate of perioperative myocardial infarction in the CREST Trial (detailed later in this chapter) was about twice as high after CEA than after CAS. It may be that going forward, patients with any significant history of coronary artery disease are considered to be at increased risk for CEA and may be better served with CAS.

However, there are also factors that make patients high risk for CAS; these are primarily anatomic. Examples of poor anatomy for CAS include: severe tortuosity of the aortic arch, great vessels or carotid bifurcation, heavy calcification of these vessels, or access problems. Marked angulation, kinks, and coils of the internal carotid artery might not allow adequate room for appropriate deployment of cerebral protection devices (CPDs) with adequate wall apposition.[10] If these areas are straightened by stents, the angulation is usually displaced distally and may be more exaggerated. Difficult arch anatomy or severe calcification of the aortic arch and proximal branch vessels may preclude a safe carotid intervention. Carotid bifurcation lesions that are recently symptomatic or are composed of soft plaque should also be avoided, if possible. These lesions can also be treated using proximal protection, so that the cerebral circulation is protected from emboli before crossing the lesion. Carotid bifurcation lesions that are too long to treat with a single stent also tend to add risk to the CAS procedure. Poor early results of CAS in older patients have prompted a high level of caution in octogenarians. Extra evaluation for high-risk anatomy, preexisting brain lesions, evidence of cognitive problems, or other factors that may make repair more risky or limit its long-term value should be performed. In the early phases of CAS, these high-risk factors for performing CAS were not yet established. It is now well recognized that CAS in its current form and with existing technology is not a direct replacement product for CEA. The results of CAS have improved steadily over the past 15 years. One of the reasons for this is improved patient selection based on a better understanding of which patients are at high risk for CAS.

The patient must be neurologically intact and able to follow commands to permit safe carotid stenting. Patients who cannot lie flat on the fluoroscopy table because of shortness of breath from cardiac or pulmonary problems will not tolerate intervention. Morbid obesity makes femoral access more challenging, as well as control of access site after of the procedure. Patients who cannot be treated safely with antiplatelet agents before and after the procedure, or who are at high risk for hemorrhagic complications, should not undergo endovascular carotid interventions.

Preprocedure Evaluation

Thorough evaluation and preparation of the patient before the procedure is essential for safe carotid intervention. The brachiocephalic anatomy is studied before the procedure to assess candidacy for the percutaneous approach. A thorough understanding of the arch, carotid, and cerebral arterial anatomy can be obtained with catheter-based arteriogram, computed tomographic (CT) angiogram, or magnetic resonance angiography. Several anatomic factors can be considered relative contraindications to CAS as mentioned previously. A National Institutes of Health (NIH) stroke scale or other objective evaluation is completed before to CAS. A CT or magnetic resonance image (MRI) of the brain is obtained in symptomatic patients and in those 80 years of age or older to evaluate for preprocedure cerebral pathology. Octogenarians have a higher risk of stroke with CAS; therefore it should be performed with caution.[11] Antiplatelet therapy is administered; aspirin daily and clopidogrel (Plavix) 75 mg/day for 5 days before the procedure. In all cases, patients should have received clopidogrel (total dose of 300 mg) before the intervention. Antihypertensive medication is held or decreased on the day of the procedure. If antihypertensive is required during the procedure, it is best to use a short-acting agent. Postoperative hypotension or bradycardia can occur after CAS as a result of baroreceptor stimulation. Patients with aortic stenosis may have cardiovascular collapse in this setting, and external pacing pads or a temporary internal pacemaker should be placed. In patients with absent

femoral pulses owing to aortoiliac occlusion, a transbrachial approach may be considered.

The CAS procedure is performed using local anesthesia with minimal or no sedation to facilitate patient cooperation and continuous neurologic monitoring. Continuous arterial pressure monitoring is required. Techniques such as squeezing a rubber toy aid in simple and effective neurologic monitoring during the procedure.

Approved carotid stenting systems are limited to use in patients with symptomatic ≥50% stenosis, or asymptomatic ≥80% stenosis. CAS in standard risk patients and those at high risk for CEA, but who are asymptomatic, are not currently approved for reimbursement under Medicare guidelines, unless it is performed as part of an approved clinical research protocol. Reconsideration of the extent of coverage of CAS by the CMS is likely to take place as a result of data accumulated through the CREST Trial.

Access

The overwhelming majority of CAS cases are performed through femoral artery access. The right common femoral approach is the most convenient for catheter manipulations by the right handed surgeon, but the left is acceptable as well if the right side is hostile. A micropuncture set (21-gauge needle) can be used for the initial femoral access; this has significantly reduced the number of femoral access complications. The use of ultrasound during puncture has become routine, and it has enhanced the ability to use closure devices at the conclusion of the procedure. Following guidewire access, an introducer sheath is placed in the common femoral artery that is the same size as that intended for the carotid stent placement (typically 6 or 7 French). If the right common femoral approach offers unfavorable anatomy, the contralateral groin or the upper extremities can be used. If a brachial approach is planned, access to the common carotid artery is usually best obtained from the contralateral brachial artery. Direct percutaneous or open carotid access through a short transverse skin incision has also been described in patients with complex arch anatomy.

Arch Evaluation

Arch manipulation carries a risk of neurologic events. In several studies of CAS, up to 1% of patients sustained a stroke in the contralateral hemisphere, suggesting that carotid access is a contributor to morbidity.[12,13] Administer systemic heparin before aortic arch manipulation. An ACT of 250 seconds or greater is desired.

Following systemic anticoagulation, an arch aortogram is performed using a multi-sidehole flush catheter (e.g., pigtail catheter) with the image intensifier in a left anterior oblique (LAO) position. The goal is to obtain an en face view of the aortic arch as it traverses posterior and laterally to the left along the spine. An angle of 30 to 45 degrees LAO usually provides an optimal view of the origins of the arch vessels. The pigtail catheter is subsequently withdrawn over a 260-cm angled guidewire. The guidewire and pigtail catheter should be pulled back together into the descending aorta where the pigtail can

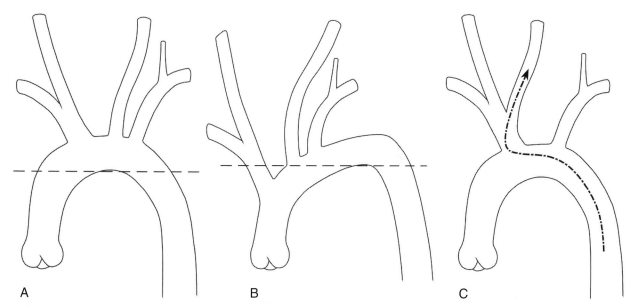

FIGURE 20-1 ■ Evaluation of the aortic arch. The arch of the aorta can be assessed rapidly for anticipated challenge in selective catheterization of the arch branches. Draw a horizontal line across the upper, inner crest of the aortic arch. **A,** When arch branches originate from the top of the arch, they are usually straightforward to selectively catheterize. **B,** When arch branches originate from the upslope of the ascending aorta, the upper, inner aspect or crest of the arch serves as a fulcrum over which the cerebral catheter must work to achieve selective access. This is the situation in which a reversed curve catheter is particularly helpful. This can be assessed easily by drawing a horizontal line across the upper inner aspect of the arch of the aorta. **C,** The bovine arch configuration can be a challenge when treating the left carotid artery. The origin of the artery is displaced toward the patient's right and the vessel path courses to the patient's left, creating a sharp turn from the arch into the left common carotid artery (see *dotted line*).

then be removed and the guidewire can be advanced into the ascending aorta. As few manipulations as possible are performed in the aortic arch and great vessels to lower the risk of an iatrogenic embolic event.

Hypertension and advanced age are associated with increased tortuosity of the access pathway to the carotid bifurcation. This makes no difference in the performance of CEA, but directly influences the challenges posed for CAS. Negotiating the tortuous arch requires more manipulation for catheterization, a more embedded position of the exchange guidewire, and more maneuvers to achieve sheath placement. The tortuosity of the arch can be assessed rapidly by drawing a horizontal line across the apex of the inner curvature of the arch.[14] Vessels that originate below the horizontal line at the apex of the aortic arch (e.g., branches that arise from the ascending aorta) are more difficult to selectively cannulate (Figure 20-1). The authors caution against carotid stenting in the setting of a "difficult arch" until the operator has become expert with selective cannulation of the common carotid arteries in this situation. Even then, the tortuous arch likely poses a slight increase in the overall risk of CAS. Training and credentialing documents suggest varying numbers of carotid arteriograms as a prerequisite to initiating CAS training.[15,16]

SELECTIVE COMMON CAROTID CANNULATION

Selective cannulation can be accomplished using one of two preshaped catheters; a simple curve catheter such as

a vertebral catheter or a complex curve catheter such as the reversed-angle Vitek catheter (VTK). The image intensifier is maintained in its fixed position (i.e., LAO) and landmarks or roadmapping can be used to guide vessel cannulation. The first choice catheter in most cases is a simple curve, such as a vertebral catheter. The angle formed by the vertebral catheter along with the tip angle on an angled guidewire is adequate to cannulate the common carotid artery. The simple curve catheter is passed into the ascending aorta. The guidewire is retracted into the shaft of the catheter to permit the catheter tip to function properly. The catheter is withdrawn slowly into the arch, and its tip is rotated superiorly. When the catheter tip engages the arch branch, the catheter is rocked gently side to side to allow it to "seed" itself into the common carotid artery. The guidewire is advanced, slowly at first to ensure that it does not catch on the wall and kick the catheter tip out of the artery. Once the guidewire has accessed the common carotid artery, the vertebral catheter is advanced over the guidewire into the midcommon carotid artery for selective angiograms of the carotid artery and its bifurcation. Be careful to avoid inadvertently passing the guidewire into the carotid artery bifurcation. As the cerebral catheter rounds the turn from the arch into the common carotid artery, it tends to straighten the wire out and may prompt it to jump forward. Meticulous adherence to fundamentals of wire and catheter handling is essential to avoid unintentional movement of devices in the carotid or introduction of air bubbles.

Complex curve or reversed-angle catheters such as the Vitek or VTK are usually required when the aortic arch

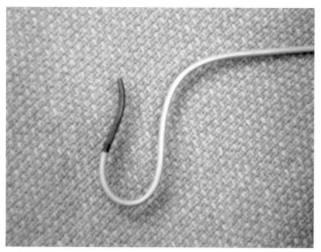

FIGURE 20-2 ■ Complex-curve or reversed-curve cerebral catheters, such as the Vitek, can be used to catheterize branches arising from a tortuous arch. A severely retroflexed common carotid artery or a bovine arch configuration may also be approached with the Vitek catheter. There is a first bend near the tip of the catheter and a second more acute bend to approximately 180 degrees (an elbow shape), which allows the tip of the catheter to point in a direction that is reversed from the direction of the catheter shaft.

is tortuous, the common carotid arteries are retroflexed toward the patient's left, or there is a bovine arch configuration (Figure 20-2). Complex curve catheters are best reformed in the proximal descending aorta and then pushed proximally into the arch. The catheter is advanced with the tip angled anteriorly and then the tip is angled superiorly as the branch of choice for catheterization is approached. After the tip is engaged into the common carotid artery of choice, the catheter is adjusted slightly, usually with a gentle pull, to allow the elbow of the catheter (located at the second curve of a reversed curve or complex cure catheter) to reach its optimal intended configuration and seed itself in the artery origin. Arteriography can be performed from this position, and the catheter is unlikely to slip out. However, reversed-angle catheters cannot be as easily advanced into the branch vessels after cannulation of the origin. They are used mainly to access the origin of the branch vessels for a selective angiogram of the carotid arteries. Advancing the reverse curve catheter into the external carotid artery requires as much wire as possible be placed beyond the catheter tip. Because of the reverse angle, a forward push on the catheter shaft when it does not have a reasonably robust rail of wire to pass along will advance the catheter further proximally into the aortic arch and actually drag the tip out of the common carotid artery.

After selective cannulation of the common carotid artery, angiograms are performed with half-strength contrast. The carotid bifurcation is best visualized in the ipsilateral oblique or lateral position. Multiple views may be needed to best open the carotid bifurcation, as the next step usually involves selective cannulation of the external carotid artery. If an arteriogram or CT angiogram was performed before the CAS procedure, optimal angles for viewing the open carotid bifurcation can usually be

derived from these studies. If a lateral view of the carotid bifurcation is required to open the carotid bifurcation and cannulate the external carotid artery, after the exchange guidewire is anchored in place, the sheath is best advanced using an LAO view.

Lateral and craniocaudal anteroposterior intracranial images are obtained if cerebral artery imaging has not already been done before CAS to identify any intracranial pathology and to document the intracranial circulation before CAS. Contrast is administered at 3 or 4 mL/s for 2 seconds with a rate of rise of 0.5 seconds.

CAROTID SHEATH ACCESS

Carotid sheath access requires placement of an adequate length of exchange guidewire into the common carotid artery. When the arch is straightforward and there is no tortuosity and the common carotid artery is of adequate length, this can be accomplished by placing the tip of the exchange guidewire in the distal common carotid artery. However, usually to place an adequate length of exchange guidewire, the external carotid artery must be catheterized and used to anchor the stiff guidewire (Figure 20-3). Selective external carotid cannulation can be accomplished with a 260-cm angled guidewire and the vertebral catheter. An attempt should be made to reach as distal as possible in the external carotid artery. This allows adequate guidewire length for the subsequent placement of the carotid sheath. Passage of the stiff exchange guidewire into the small external carotid artery branches must be done with caution to avoid injury or perforation to these branches. CAS can usually be accomplished with a 6- or 7-French sheath. The guidewire is then withdrawn from the vertebral catheter, and a 260-cm Amplatz Super Stiff or other exchange guidewire is passed into the external carotid artery. Caution should be used during wire exchanges. Removing the wire too quickly can create a vacuum, resulting in introduction of air emboli. It is sometimes helpful to administer contrast into the catheter to confirm external carotid placement. Contrast injections into the carotid system should not be done unless free backflow of blood is present at the hub of the diagnostic catheter. Otherwise there is a risk of pushing microbubbles into the system. In the external carotid artery, back bleeding can at times be diminished by the tight fit of the catheter in the small external carotid artery branches. In this event, the cerebral catheter is slowly withdrawn until adequate backflow is noted.

The vertebral catheter is withdrawn, leaving the Amplatz guidewire in the external carotid artery. The groin access sheath is removed. A 90-cm long sheath (Destination by Terumo [Somerset, NJ] or Shuttle Sheath by Cook [Bloomington, IN]) is advanced over the Amplatz guidewire into the common carotid artery. Image the tip of the Amplatz guidewire in the external carotid artery and the last turn from the arch into the common carotid artery during sheath passage. If the tip of the advancing sheath hangs at the turn into the common carotid artery or the tip of the guidewire moves back, it indicates that the sheath is not advancing appropriately over the guidewire. Reassess the curvature in the system and ensure that

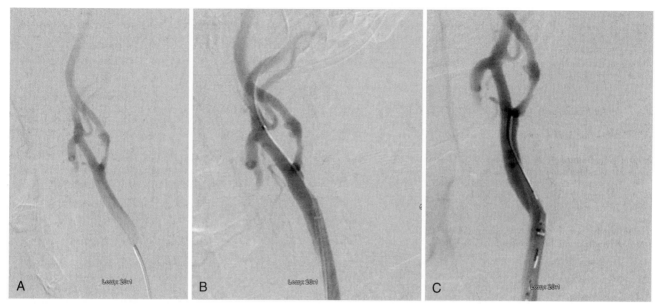

FIGURE 20-3 ■ Carotid sheath placement. The external carotid artery is usually catheterized and a stiff exchange guidewire is placed. The cerebral catheter is withdrawn and the exchange guidewire is used as a rail over which to place a 6- or 7-French, 90-cm–long carotid access sheath. During sheath advancement, the image intensifier is placed in the LAO position, and the tip of the exchange guidewire is observed. The progress of the sheath tip is monitored as it makes the turn from the aortic arch into the common carotid artery. If the tip of the guidewire begins to back up, sheath advancement should be stopped because this is a sign that the rail is not adequate for sheath passage. A landmark is selected from the carotid angiogram performed before sheath placement, and this is used to help decide where to place the tip of the sheath and to stop sheath advancement.

an adequate length of stiff exchange guidewire is present. The dilator tip for the 90-cm carotid sheath is long and not well visualized during fluoroscopy. Identify the optimal length for the dilator to protrude from the sheath and lock the Y-adaptor on the back end of the dilator in this position. After the dilator and sheath are advanced fully into the common carotid artery, and if a position closer to the bifurcation is needed, the dilator is held steady while the sheath is advanced over it. The stiff exchange guidewire and the dilator are withdrawn, and the carotid angiogram is repeated through the carotid sheath with a road map of the carotid bifurcation stenosis in preparation for filter placement.

CEREBRAL PROTECTION

There are no large randomized trials comparing CAS with and without cerebral protection devices, although their use has become standard of practice after early data suggested a decrease in embolic complications.[10] The CMS also mandates CPD use for endovascular carotid interventions. There are numerous commercially available CPDs (Box 20-2) that are categorized as follows: distal filter, distal occlusion balloon, and proximal occlusion with or without reversal of flow.

Distal filter placement is by far the most commonly used CPD. The filter is placed distal to the lesion before stent placement, typically on a 0.014-inch guidewire system. These devices vary in shape and deployment, but once in place, they permit continuous antegrade flow into the intracranial internal carotid artery while serving as a barrier to embolic debris. Distal filters generally capture

---

BOX 20-2 | Commercially Available Cerebral Protection Devices by Category

DISTAL FILTER
- Angioguard XP
- Emboshield
- FilterWire EX, EZ
- AccuNet
- SPIDER
- Interceptor
- Rubicon Filter
- Fibernet

DISTAL OCCLUSION
- PercuSurge Guardwire
- Tri-Active
- Guardian

PROXIMAL OCCLUSION
- PAES
- Mo.Ma
- Cordis
- Abbott
- Boston Scientific
- Abbott
- EV3
- Medtronic
- Rubicon Medical
- Lumen
- Medtronic
- Kensy Nash
- Rubicon-Abbott
- Gore
- Invatec

| BOX 20-3 | Advantages and Disadvantages of Distal Filter |

ADVANTAGES

- Preservation of flow
- Less spasm than distal occlusion devices
- Angiographic evaluation of lesion during procedure

DISADVANTAGES

- Larger crossing profile
- Importance of exact diameter sizing
- Potential thrombosis or occlusion of filter
- Prolonged procedure time
- Unprotected during passage of filter
- Must pass retrieval catheter through stent

| BOX 20-4 | Advantages and Disadvantages of Distal Occlusion |

ADVANTAGES

- Complete protection of distal ICA
- Low crossing profile
- High flexibility
- No sizing issues

DISADVANTAGES

- Interruption of blood flow during protection
- Potential dissection/spasm in distal ICA
- Potential embolization via ECA
- No angiographic evaluation of lesion during procedure
- Prolonged procedure time
- Unprotected during passage of balloon

ICA, Internal carotid artery; *ECA*, external carotid artery.

| BOX 20-5 | Advantages and Disadvantages of Proximal Occlusion |

ADVANTAGES

- Complete protection prior to lesion manipulation
- Not limited by tight or tortuous lesions
- No guidewire restrictions
- Angiographic evaluation of lesion during procedure

DISADVANTAGES

- Larger introducer size
- Interruption of flow during procedure
- Potential dissection/spasm in common carotid artery or ECA

ECA, external carotid artery.

---

particles greater than 100 μm in size. Filters may be fixed to the wire or separate from the initial guidewire. The fixed-guidewire systems are simpler and require fewer steps. However, in the fixed-guidewire system, any guidewire movement after the filter is deployed results in movement of the filter itself. In addition, the attachment of the filter to the guidewire limits the handling of the guidewire during lesion traversal. The free-guidewire systems permit a choice of guidewires. When there is substantial tortuosity, a complex lesion, or other challenges, the free-guidewire systems have an advantage. The advantage of filters is that they allow continued cerebral perfusion, particularly in patients who have inadequate collateral circulation to permit temporary carotid occlusion (Box 20-3).

Distal balloon occlusion devices prevent antegrade flow in the internal carotid artery during the period of angioplasty and stenting (Box 20-4). The balloon can be inflated from 3 to 6 mm and is a component of the 0.014-inch guidewire. This system has a lower crossing profile than distal filters. Angioplasty balloons, catheters, and stents can then be loaded onto the wire and removed while the balloon occludes the internal carotid artery. At the completion of the procedure, the static column of blood in the internal carotid artery is aspirated to remove any embolic particles that may have accumulated. None of the distal occlusion balloon systems are commonly used in the United States for CAS, but they are common in some countries.

Proximal balloon occlusion devices do not require crossing the lesion before establishing embolic protection (Box 20-5). Such devices provide protection by occluding the common and external carotid arteries, after which collateral flow through the circle of Willis creates a back-pressure that prevents antegrade flow into the internal carotid artery (ICA). Reversal of flow in the ICA can also be augmented by connecting the common carotid artery catheter to an external filter and then to the femoral vein, creating an arteriovenous fistula. This technique requires the use of a larger access sheath (8 French) and occlusion of the external carotid artery, but it also offers the advantage of performing carotid interventions with the potential for less microembolization. Intolerance to reversed flow is a major concern, but is present in less than 5% of cases. There is a high likelihood that reversed flow will be a major addition to CAS and will permit stenting of more dangerous bifurcation lesions.

TECHNIQUE FOR USE OF DISTAL FILTERS

The filter should be placed only after the sheath is in a stable position in the common carotid artery. Any movement of the sheath after filter placement could also move the filter. If the sheath should flip back into the arch during the procedure while the filter is deployed, the filter may be withdrawn into the lesion or tangle with the stent. The supporting guidewire for the filter is not sturdy enough to support a repeated advancement of the sheath. After placement of the common carotid artery sheath, the appropriate guidewire for the selected filter is used to cross the target lesion. The tip of the leading guidewire is hand shaped with a curve to provide directionality for crossing the lesion. Most lesions that are isolated to the proximal internal carotid artery are posterior wall plaques. In passing the guidewire tip to cross the lesion, the best pathway is usually anterior in the proximal internal carotid artery, just behind the flow divider. Bifurcation lesions that involve the distal common carotid artery are usually more complex and less predictable. The key is to lead with the guidewire tip; do not make a loop, and be gentle in probing the lesion. Once

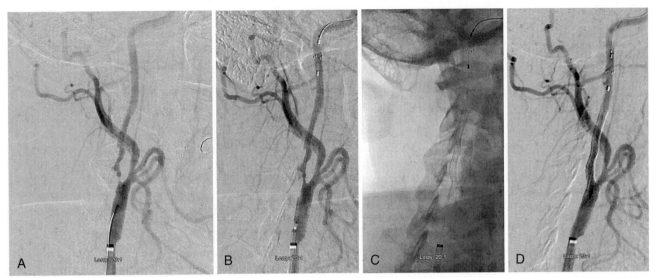

FIGURE 20-4 ■ Stent placement. **A,** The filter is placed distal to the carotid lesion. **B,** Predilation is performed. **C,** The carotid stent is placed across the lesion, from nondiseased internal carotid artery distal to the lesion to the common carotid artery. **D,** After poststent dilation, there is excellent prograde flow across the internal carotid artery and a widely patent stent.

the lesion is crossed with the guidewire tip, the filter device is advanced across the target lesion into a straight, normal segment of the distal extracranial internal carotid artery distal to the lesion by a few centimeters and deployed. Placing the device into a tortuous segment may be difficult and could impede filter function. The landing zone for the filter is assessed in advance; it must be reachable with the proposed filter and be long enough and straight enough to accommodate the filter. An activated clotting time (ACT) of 250 seconds or higher is required before placing filter devices.

The crossing profile of the filter is often larger than the residual lumen in a tight stenosis. Occasionally it may be difficult to cross extremely stenotic, tortuous, or calcified lesions. A "buddy wire" may be helpful in providing extra support during filter placement. A slightly larger sheath is needed to accommodate a buddy wire, such as a 7-French sheath. If tortuosity is the issue, sometimes it can be improved by placing a stiff but low-profile guidewire into the external carotid artery. Tortuosity may also be improved by having the patient change the neck position, capitalizing on the natural mobility of the carotid artery. When a tight lesion cannot be crossed with a filter, occasionally a balloon predilatation with a 2.0- or 2.5-mm–diameter angioplasty balloon is required. When critically stenotic carotid lesions or highly tortuous carotid bifurcations are involved, the use of a "free-wire" filter system (e.g., Emboshield [Abbott Vascular, Santa Clara, CA], Spider [Covidien, Minneapolis, MN]) has advantages over a fixed-wire system (e.g., Accunet [Abbott Vascular, Santa Clara, CA], Filterwire [Boston Scientific, Natick, MA]).

After each step of the intervention, flow of contrast through the CPD must be observed. The image intensifier is positioned such that the tip of the sheath is visible on the inferior aspect of the monitor screen and the filter is visible on the superior aspect. If the device becomes filled with debris, it must be aspirated. When removing a full device following completion angiogram, it is important not to recapture it completely, because debris may be extruded from it and embolize distally. If there is evidence of a filling defect within the filter, or some indication that it may contain debris, catheter aspiration is performed. The usual tendency during the procedure is for any tension on the guidewire to result in partial withdrawal of the filter; this can induce spasm or spill any debris that the filter holds. Another potential problem is for the filter to tangle with the stent. If this occurs, it might not be possible to fix it without open surgery.

STENT PLACEMENT

Predilation is performed selectively before stent placement with a 3-mm rapid exchange balloon, usually 4 cm in length to avoid "watermelon seeding" of the balloon upon inflation (Figure 20-4). Some operators routinely administer small doses of atropine (0.25 to 0.5 mg) before balloon dilatation, except in patients with a recurrent stenosis, because the carotid bulb is already denervated in these patients. The pressure used for predilatation is nominal for the balloon used. Use higher pressure (14 to 16 atm) in heavily calcified stenoses. The duration of the predilatation depends on the appearance and behavior of the balloon. If the balloon immediately attains its full shape, the predilatation time is shorter. Observe the monitor for bradycardia if a prolonged inflation is required. If there is significant bradycardia with predilation, there is a high likelihood that bradycardia will occur after stent placement and dilation.

A variety of self-expanding stents are available for use with the respective CPDs. Self-expanding stents are classified as open cell or closed cell. The open cell stents have larger cells, in general, and there is suggestion that this may invite more late-stage emboli through the tines of the stent. However, post-CAS neurologic events are multifactorial, which is a difficult variable to isolate. The open cell stents are also more easily contoured than the closed cell stents and can handle tortuosity better. Closed cell stents have smaller cells, more outward radial force in general and are less flexible. Closed cell stents are also easier to cross with the filter retrieval catheter. The self-expanding stent is deployed using landmarks, such as a bifurcation roadmap or the nearby vertebral bodies. The stent is placed from normal artery distal to the lesion to normal artery proximal to the lesion. The self-expanding stent is usually postdilated with a 5-mm balloon; rarely is a 6-mm PTA required after stent deployment. Following stent deployment, shorter (2-cm) balloons are used to dilate the narrow portion of the stent where the residual stenosis is visible using fluoroscopy. Avoid overdilation, even though this is how lesions in multiple other vascular beds are treated. The difference in the carotid is that the stent is used as scaffolding, the stent provides continuous expansile energy after the procedure, and there is a desire to avoid disrupting the lesion more than necessary. The patient may again be pretreated with a small dose of atropine to blunt the carotid sinus response to stretching. A residual stenosis may be accepted. The balloon used for PTA after stenting is always maintained within the stent to avoid dissection. Nominal pressure is used to fully expand the balloon and the stent. Some operators avoid postdilation whenever possible under the idea that this maneuver generates the most microemboli during transcranial Doppler monitoring. In the majority of the cases, the stent is placed across the bifurcation into the common carotid artery, crossing the origin of the external carotid artery. Deployment of the stent across the external carotid artery has not resulted in adverse events; follow-up arteriograms and duplex studies have demonstrated that the external carotid artery remains patent in most patients.

Kinks and bends in the ICA may pose a problem with stent implants. Deploy stents across significant bends only if they are isolated. Avoid placing the distal end of the stent into kinks and tortuous segments of the ICA, especially if more than a single bend is noted. Tortuosity cannot be eliminated, is displaced distally, and can become more exaggerated when a stent is placed and results in stiffening of a segment of artery. A highly tortuous internal carotid artery should be considered a relative contraindication for CAS, as acute occlusions are more common following stent placement in these tortuous vessels. In addition, there may be difficulty in advancing the stent delivery catheter into place in this situation.

FILTER REMOVAL, COMPLETION ANGIOGRAM, AND ACCESS SITE MANAGMENT

The filter is maintained in place until the carotid reconstruction is evaluated and continued flow through the filter is documented. Following stent placement, completion angiograms are acquired in the projection that had demonstrated the maximum stenosis. Attention is paid to the ICA immediately distal to the stent. Spasm in this segment may be encountered, especially where the filter is located (Figure 20-5). If significant spasm is encountered, a small dose of intraarterial nitroglycerine (50 to

100 μg) is administered directly into the internal carotid artery. Distal dissections are unusual and when present can be remedied with an additional stent of appropriate size. Reasonable prograde flow through the stented segment and the filter should be present. If there is slow flow or there is a filling defect within the filter, an aspiration catheter is used before filter removal. The filter retrieval catheter is passed carefully through the stent to capture the filter. Open cell stent designs have excellent contour ability, but also have diamond-shaped points in the lumen that can snag the retrieval catheter. If the retrieval catheter catches on the stent, do not push the catheter forward, because this will tend to withdraw the filter down toward the stent. Have the patient rotate or extend the neck to permit a straight shot of the retrieval catheter along the wire through the stented portion.

After filter retrieval, intracranial angiograms are obtained after CAS by most operators as a routine, and these may be compared with preoperative studies. If there is any concern about the potential for kinks of the ICA distal to the stent, the carotid arteriogram is repeated without the guidewire and filter in place. The neurologic status of the patient is monitored during the procedure and is assessed at its conclusion.

In suitable patients, access site hemostasis is achieved at the end of the procedure using one of several approved closure devices. A femoral arteriogram is performed in the oblique projection. If a calcified vessel is encountered during needle puncture, closure devices are not used. In this situation, the long sheath is exchanged for a short sheath of the same caliber that is removed when the ACT is less than 180 seconds, and manual pressure is held for the appropriate time period.

POSTOPERATIVE CARE AND FOLLOW-UP

Patients are monitored in the hospital overnight. It is not uncommon for patients to respond to carotid sinus distension with bradycardia and hypotension. Occasionally, 24 to 48 hours of inotropic support is required before the carotid sinus adapts to the radial force of the self-expanding stents. Avoidance of extreme oversizing of the stents helps to decrease the incidence of bradycardia and hypotension following CAS. The presence of significant hypotension in the absence of bradycardia is unusual in the immediate postprocedure period, and other causes (e.g., retroperitoneal bleed related to access site problems) should also be considered. Other potential perioperative complications include stroke, myocardial infarction, and access site complications. A predischarge evaluation and an NIH stroke scale are completed. Medications include aspirin (ASA) (325 mg per day indefinitely) and clopidogrel (75 mg per day for 1 month). Follow-up includes 1-month, 6-month, and yearly clinical evaluation and duplex examination.

RESULTS OF CAROTID STENTING

Early interest in carotid interventions during the 1980s and early 1990s was limited because of a lack of outcome

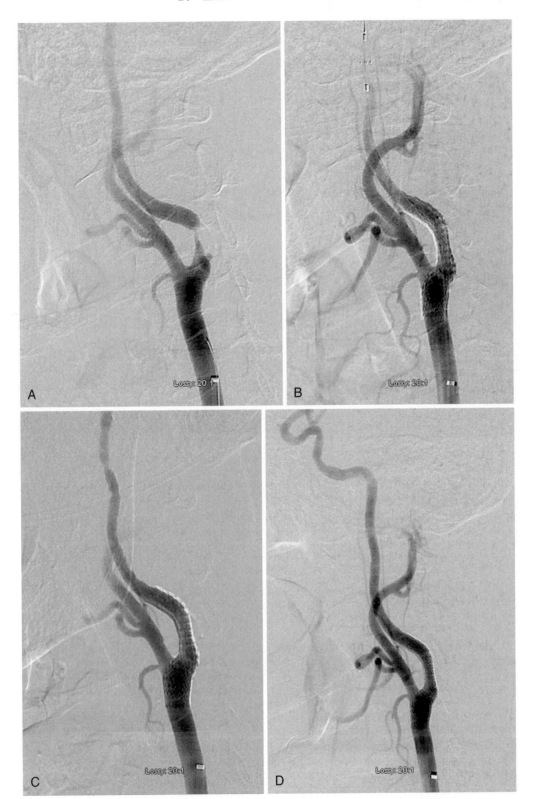

FIGURE 20-5 ■ Spasm of the distal internal carotid artery. This may be induced by the filter. The key is to finish the case and retrieve the filter in an expedition manner. However, if spasm occurs in the middle of the procedure, it may be helpful to administer small doses of nitroglycerine while completing the stent procedure.

data and fear of cerebral embolism. In 1994, Marks and colleagues[17] reported the first use of carotid angioplasty supported by stents. Soon thereafter, balloon angioplasty was replaced by stent-supported angioplasty of the carotid artery. Interest in the procedure grew rapidly with

improvement in stents as well as the introduction of cerebral protection devices, whose use was first described by Theron and colleagues in 1996.[18]

Numerous observational studies and registry trials were performed to evaluate the safety and efficacy of

TABLE 20-1 Summary of Published Results of Observational Studies of Carotid Angioplasty and Stenting

Study	Year of Publication	No. of Lesions	Cerebral Protection (%)	30-Day Outcome	
				Death (%)	Stroke (%)
Wholey et al.[20]	1997	114	0	1.8	3.5
Yadav et al.[21]	1997	126	0	0.8	7.1
Henry et al.[21a]	1998	174	18	0	2.9
Mathias et al.[31]	1999	799	NG	—	2.1
Shawl et al.[34]	2000	192	0	0	2.6
Wholey et al.[36]	2000	5210	Very low	1.9	3.9
d'Audiffret et al.[25]	2001	83	18	—	4.4
Reimers et al.[32]	2001	88	100	—	1.1
Roubin et al.[33]	2001	604	0	1.6	5.8
Al Mubarak et al.[22]	2002	164	100	1.2	1.2
Criado et al.[24]	2002	135	0	0	2.2
Guimaraens et al.[26]	2002	194	100	1.9	1.0
Henry et al.[27]	2002	184	100	0.5	2.2
Koch et al.[29]	2002	167	0	—	7.5
Macdonald et al.[29a]	2002	150	50	1.3	6.0
Whitlow et al.[35]	2002	75	100	0	0
Cremonesi et al.[23]	2003	442	100	—	2.0
Hobson et al.[28]	2003	114	0	1.8	0.9

TABLE 20-2 High-Risk Prospective Registry Data

Name	Company	No. of Patients	Stent	Embolic Device	MAE (%)	Stroke (%)	Year Presented
ARCHER 1	Guidant	158	Acculink	None	7.6	4.4	2003
ARCHER 2	Guidant	278	Acculink	Accunet	8.6	6.8	2003
ARCHER 3	Guidant	145	Acculink	Accunet	8.3	7.6	2003
BEACH	BSC	480	Wallstent	Filterwire	5.8	4.4	2005
CABERNET	BSC	454	Nexstent	Filterwire	3.9	3.4	2005
CREATE	EV3	160	Acculink	SPIDERX	5.6	4.4	2005
SECuRITY	Abbott	305	Xactstent	Emboshield	7.5	6.2	2003
MAVErIC	Medtronic	399	Exponent	PercuSurge	5	3	2004

ARCHER, The Acculink for Revascularization of Carotids in High-Risk Patients; *BEACH,* Boston Scientific EPI: a carotid stenting trial for high risk surgical patients; *CABERNET,* Carotid Artery Revascularization Using the Boston Scientific Filterwire EX system and the EndoTex NextStent Carotid Stent; *CREATE,* Carotid Revascularization with the EV3 Arterial Technology Evolution; *SECuRITY,* Registry Study to Evaluate the Neuroshield Bare Wire Cerebral protection System and X-act Stent in Patients at High Risk for Carotid Enadrterectomy; *MAVErIC,* Evaluation of the Medtronic Self-Expanding Carotid Stent with Distal Protection of Carotid Artery Stenosis.

CAS. A summary of the largest observational studies is shown in Table 20-1.[19-36] These studies not only demonstrated the feasibility of CAS, but they also provided a significantly better understanding of the clinical issues associated with CAS and distal protection devices. Using the data from Table 20-1, weighted averages of stroke rates from studies published in 1996 to 1998, 1999 to 2001, and 2002 to 2003 were 4.7%, 3.8%, and 2.6%, respectively. Technical success, defined as residual angiographic stenosis of less than 30%, was achieved in greater than 95% of the cases in all of the studies. Although the results of these observational studies were encouraging, the majority were notable for their poor documentation and lack of long-term follow-up.

A number of industry-sponsored clinical registries have also provided a great deal of clinical information (Table 20-2). These nonrandomized studies differed from earlier observational studies by having predefined inclusion and exclusion criteria, independent neurologic assessments, and standardized use of equipment and cerebral protection. Technical success rates mirrored earlier studies though stroke rates and major adverse event (MAE) rates were higher, failing to meet the benchmarks for perioperative stroke and death established in ACAS and NASCET (3% for asymptomatic, 6% for symptomatic).[2-9] The risk of contralateral events is persistent through several trials, reinforcing the importance of safe arch access.[12,13] Although distal embolic protection is widely accepted, the efficacy of these devices in preventing perioperative events has been difficult to prove.[37,38] When CAS was implemented by those with catheter skills, adequate proficiency was obtained in performing CAS with approximately 25 cases.[38] Octogenarians were found to have worse than expected outcomes than younger patients, with higher rates of stroke after CAS.[11,38]

TABLE 20-3 Randomized Controlled Trials

Trial	Year	No. of Patients	CPD (%)	Asymptomatic (%)	F/U (Months)	Completed
CAS vs. CEA	1998	23	0	0	1	No (harm)
Wallstent	2001	219	0	0	12	No (futility)
Brooks	2001	104	0	0	48	Yes
CAVATAS	2001	504	0	3	36	Yes
Brooks	2004	85	0	100	48	Yes
SAPPHIRE	2004	334	96	71	36	No (slow enrollment)
EVA-3S	2004	527	92	0	6	No (futility/harm)
SPACE	2006	1200	—	0	1	No (funding)
TESCAS-C	2006	166	100	—	6	Yes
BACASS	2006	20	—	0	45	Yes
Steinbauer	2008	87	0	0	64-66	Yes
CREST	2010	2502	96	47	30	Yes
ICSS	2010	1703	72	0	3	Yes

Modified from Brott TG, Hobson RW 2nd, Howard G, et al; CREST Investigators: Stenting versus endarterectomy for treatment of carotid-artery stenosis, N Engl J Med 363:11–23, 2010.

CPD, Cerebral protection device; *F/U,* follow-up; *CAS,* carotid angioplasty and stenting; *CEA,* carotid endarterectomy; *CAVATAS,* Carotid and Vertebral Artery Transluminal Angioplasty Study; *SAPPHIRE,* Stenting and Angioplasty with Protection in Patients at High Risk for Endarterectomy; *TESCAS-C,* trial of endarterectomy versus stenting for the treatment of carotid artery atherosclerosis in China; *BACASS,* carotid artery stenting versus carotid endarterectomy. A prospective, randomised trial with long term follow-up. *EVA-3S,* Endarterectomy Versus Stenting in Patients with Symptomatic Severe Carotid Stenosis; *SPACE,* Stent-Protected Angioplasty versus Carotid Endarterectomy; *CREST,* Carotid Revascularization Endarterectomy versus Stent Trial; *ICSS,* International Carotid Stenting Study.

RANDOMIZED CONTROLLED TRIALS

Landmark RCTs comparing CEA (with best medical therapy) to best medical therapy alone were published in the early 1990s and provided level I evidence for the use of CEA as the standard for treatment of carotid occlusive disease.[2-9] To date, 13 RCTs comparing CAS to CEA have been conducted with mixed results (Table 20-3). Of these, eight have been completed, with the two largest studies being published in 2010.

The first RCT comparing CAS and CEA was a small, single-center trial conducted by Naylor and colleagues[39] in the United Kingdom. This study was stopped after the first 17 patients were randomized because of high complication rates in the CAS arm. Five of seven patients in the CAS arm suffered periprocedure strokes, with three remaining disabling at 30 days. There were no complications in the CEA arm. The second RCT, the Wallstent trial, was also stopped early because of significant adverse outcomes in the CAS arm.[40] This multicenter study randomized 219 symptomatic patients with greater than 60% stenosis to CAS with the Wallstent versus CEA. Interim analysis revealed combined risk of stroke or death, or both, at 30 days of 12.1% in the CAS group versus 4.5% in the CEA group. Notably, cerebral protection was not used and this was thought to contribute in part to the high risk associated with CAS in this study. A subgroup analysis of this trial also demonstrated worse CAS results in centers with limited carotid stenting experience.

The first completed randomized trial comparing endovascular and surgical treatments for carotid artery stenosis (the Carotid and Vertebral Artery Transluminal Angioplasty Study) was designed to compare balloon angioplasty alone without embolic protection to CEA in symptomatic patients.[41] Stents were incorporated once they became available, but were used in only 26% of patients in the endovascular arm. For the 504 patients enrolled, there was no significant difference found in the composite stroke or death rate at 30 days (10.0% endovascular group vs. 9.9% CEA group) or at 3 years (14.3% endovascular group vs. 14.2% CEA group).[41] However, this study was criticized for a number of reasons. The lack of embolic protection and 26% stent usage are in contrast to current standard practice, and the substantially higher stroke rate of 9.9% in the CEA arm makes comparison with other CEA trials difficult.

More encouraging were the results of the trials conducted by Brooks and colleagues,[42,43] the first of which was published in 2001 and involved symptomatic patients, and the second of which was published in 2004 and involved asymptomatic patients. Extremely low complication rates were observed in both arms and the results of both trials suggested equivalence of CAS to CEA. However, enthusiasm was appropriately guarded because these were small, single-institution studies performed by a highly select, experienced team.

The Stenting and Angioplasty with Protection in Patients at High Risk for Endarterectomy (SAPPHIRE) trial demonstrated promise for CAS and was the first randomized trial to evaluate patients who were at high risk for CEA.[12] SAPPHIRE was also the first randomized trial of CAS to use mandatory distal embolic protection. The majority of patients (more than 70%) were asymptomatic. The 30-day combined periprocedural adverse event rate was 4.8% for CAS patients and 9.8% for CEA patients ($p = 0.09$). At 1 year, the combined major adverse event rate was 12.2% for CAS patients and 20.1% for CEA patients ($p = 0.004$ for noninferiority analysis; $p = 0.05$ for intention-to-treat analysis).[44] These data showed noninferiority of CAS for patients at high risk for CEA. A significant difference in event rates between CAS and CEA was due to the greater association of CEA with non–Q-wave myocardial infarction. Excluding myocardial infarction, there was no significant difference found between CAS (5.5%) and CEA (8.4%) patients. The long-term follow-up data at 3 years revealed a substantial cumulative incidence in death from cardiac and nonneurologic causes (18.6% CAS vs. 21.0% CEA).[45] Nevertheless, SAPPHIRE was viewed as the trial that proved the noninferiority of CAS in high-risk patients. CAS continues to be a mainstay in treatment in most U.S. centers for patients with compelling indications for carotid repair, but who are at high risk for conventional repair with CEA.

Two European RCTs, Stent-Protected Angioplasty versus Carotid Endarterectomy (SPACE) and Endarterectomy Versus Stenting in Patients with Symptomatic Severe Carotid Stenosis (EVA-3S) sought to establish noninferiority in standard-risk, symptomatic patients.[46,47] In the SPACE trial, the primary endpoint was ipsilateral stroke or death, or both, at 30 days. A variety of different stents were used, and embolic protection was not mandated. The initial aim of the study was to enroll 950 patients per group to achieve a power of 80%. The interim analysis in the SPACE trial comprised 1183 patients and reported a primary event rate of 6.84% in the CAS group versus 6.34% in the CEA group ($p = 0.09$ for noninferiority analysis).[46] Although SPACE CAS patients were treated variably with embolic protection, there was no significant difference in results between those who were treated with and without CPD. Furthermore, in most endpoints there was a favorable trend toward the surgical arm, although none were statistically significant. After this interim analysis, the steering committee decided to terminate the study on the basis of both futility and financial constraints because it was revealed that 2500 patients would be needed to adequately power the study to achieve trial endpoints. Thus, the SPACE trial failed to prove noninferiority of CAS compared with CEA, despite the similar perioperative stroke and death rates for the two procedures. The authors concluded that CEA should remain the preferred treatment for patients with symptomatic stenosis, because evidence was lacking to support equivalent endovascular treatment. Subsequent subgroup analysis from the SPACE trial revealed that there was an excess risk in stenting in men than in women ($p = 0.03$) and in patients older than 70 years ($p = 0.08$).[48]

Similarly, the EVA-3S trial failed to demonstrate noninferiority of CAS in symptomatic patients. The primary endpoint was defined as a composite of any stroke or death occurring within 30 days after treatment. The goal was to enroll 872 patients per group to achieve a power of 80%. A variety of different stents was used at different centers, and cerebral protection was initially not required until the safety committee instituted a protocol change as a result of a 25% 30-day rate of stroke or death in patients treated without EPDs.[49] The study randomized 527 patients and was subsequently ended prematurely for safety reasons after interim analysis revealed significantly higher 30-day event rate in the CAS group (9.6%) compared with the CEA group (3.9%; $p = 0.01$). These results persisted at 6 months, with an event rate of 11.7% in the CAS arm versus 6.1% in the CEA group ($p = 0.02$).[47] The EVA-3S results have been criticized for the significantly

higher 30-day stroke rate observed in the CAS arm of the study as compared with other published results. The trial also did not compare groups of physicians with equal experience. Whereas the surgeons performing CEA had performed at least 25 endarterectomies within 1 year before trial entry, interventionists were certified after performing less than half that number of CAS and were allowed to enroll study participants while completing their training and certification, a factor that could also increase stroke risk in the CAS arm. Despite these claims, however, subgroup analysis failed to show any statistically significant difference between operators based on level of experience.[47] The conclusion from the EVA-3S authors supported the notion that CEA remains an excellent option for symptomatic carotid stenosis with low complication rates that were not matched by CAS.

The International Carotid Stenting Study (ICSS) enrolled 1713 symptomatic patients with at least 50% internal carotid artery stenosis to compare efficacy of CEA and CAS.[50] Surgeons were required to have performed at least 50 CEA operations and interventionists were required to have performed at least 50 stenting procedures with at least 10 in the internal carotid artery. Evaluated endpoints were stroke, myocardial infarction (MI), and death. Interim analysis of data at 120 days demonstrates that the incidence of stroke, MI, or death in the CAS group was significantly higher than in the CEA group (8.5 vs. 5.2, respectively; $p = 0.006$).[50] The ICSS study has been criticized for bias toward the surgical arm because of the poor experience level of those performing CAS. A subgroup of the ICSS patient cohort underwent diffusion-weighted MRI brain imaging after treatment, and patients who underwent stent placement had a significantly higher incidence of asymptomatic lesions on cerebral imaging. Further research will be required to understand what these represent and whether they are of long-term clinical significance.

The Carotid Revascularization Endarterectomy versus Stent Trial (CREST) is an NIH-sponsored, prospective, randomized, multicenter trial comparing the efficacy of CEA and CAS in both symptomatic and asymptomatic patients.[51] The primary endpoints include 30-day periprocedural composite of stroke, MI, and death, or any ipsilateral stroke during the 4 years following randomization. A total of 2502 symptomatic and asymptomatic patients from 117 centers in Canada and the United States were enrolled. To address concerns from previous trials, CREST required rigorous credentialing for surgeons and interventionists. Surgeons had to document that they had performed at least 12 CEAs in the previous year with rates of complications and deaths less than 3% and 5% for asymptomatic and symptomatic patients, respectively. Interventionist were certified after satisfactory evaluation of their endovascular experience, CAS results, participation in hands-on training, and participation in a lead-in phase of up to twenty cases.[11,51]

CREST investigators reported no significant difference between the CAS and CEA arms in regard to the combined end points of stroke, MI, and death (Table 20-4).[51] Analysis of each endpoint individually showed a higher rate of stroke after CAS at 30 days (4.1% vs. 2.3%; $p = 0.01$) and a higher rate of myocardial infarction

TABLE 20-4	CREST Trial Results: Endpoints According to Treatment with CAS or CEA		
Endpoint	CAS (n = 1262)	CEA (n = 1240)	p Value
Any periprocedure stroke or postprocedure ipsilateral stroke (%)	4.1 ± 0.6	2.3 ± 0.4	0.01
Major stroke (%)	0.9 ± 0.3	0.6 ± 0.2	0.52
Minor stroke (%)	3.2 ± 0.5	1.7 ± 0.4	0.01
Myocardial infarction (%)	1.1 ± 0.3	2.3 ± 0.4	0.01
Death (%)	0.7 ± 0.2	0.3 ± 0.2	0.18
Primary study endpoint* perioperative (%)	5.2 ± 0.6	4.5 ± 0.6	0.38
Primary endpoint* to 4 years (%)	7.2 ± 0.8	6.8 ± 0.8	0.51
Cranial nerve palsy	0	5%	—

From Berkefeld J, Chaturvedi S: The International Carotid Stenting Study and the North American Carotid Revascularization Endarterectomy Versus Stenting Trial: Fueling the Debate About Carotid Artery Stenting. Stroke 41:2714–2715, 2010.
CREST, Carotid Revascularization Endarterectomy versus Stent Trial; *CAS*, carotid angioplasty and stenting; *CEA*, carotid endarterectomy.
*Primary study endpoint was any periprocedural stroke or myocardial infarction or death or postprocedural ipsilateral stroke.

TABLE 20-5	CREST Results: Asymptomatic and Symptomatic Patients		
Endpoint	CAS	CEA	p value
Any Periprocedural Stroke or Postprocedural Ipsilateral Stroke (%)			
Asymptomatic	2.5 ± 0.6	1.4 ± 0.5	0.07
Symptomatic	5.5 ± 0.9	3.2 ± 0.7	0.25
Primary Study Endpoint* (%)			
Asymptomatic	3.5 ± 0.8	3.6 ± 0.8	0.56
Symptomatic	6.7 ± 1.0	5.4 ± 0.9	0.69

From Berkefeld J, Chaturvedi S: The International Carotid Stenting Study and the North American Carotid Revascularization Endarterectomy Versus Stenting Trial: Fueling the Debate About Carotid Artery Stenting. Stroke 41:2714–2715, 2010.
CREST, Carotid Revascularization Endarterectomy versus Stent Trial; *CAS*, carotid angioplasty and stenting; *CEA*, carotid endarterectomy.
*Primary study endpoint was any periprocedural stroke or myocardial infarction or death or postprocedural ipsilateral stroke.

after CEA (2.3% vs. 1.1%; $p = 0.03$). The estimated 4-year rates of combined primary endpoints was 7.2% versus 6.8% for CAS and CEA, respectively ($p = 0.51$). Cranial nerve injury occurred in 5% of CEA patients and none after CAS. Both CEA and CAS outcomes were within the AHA guidelines for periprocedural stroke and death for carotid repair (≤3% for asymptomatic patients and ≤6% for symptomatic patients; Table 20-5). A sub-analysis of CREST data is awaited to elucidate findings in octogenarians, gender differences, and any changes in results with CAS over time. The carotid stenting systems used during the CREST, the Accunet filter and Acculink stent, were established at the initiation of the trial and used for the course of the study. Over the ensuing decade, other carotid stenting systems became available and other methods of cerebral protection were developed but were not included in the trial. During the CREST enrollment period (2000 to 2008), concurrent registry studies demonstrated a steady decrease in the risk of adverse outcomes with CAS. This may reflect better patient selection based on an improved understanding of which patients are at high risk for CAS (e.g., tortuous or heavily calcified arch, great vessels or carotid bifurcation). Because the equipment used in CREST was held static for the study, any improvement in results over time may be due to better technique, more experience, and especially improved patient selection for CAS.

CREST was a huge, lengthy, and largely successful undertaking, the results of which will significantly influence the practice of CAS. CREST showed excellent results for both CAS and CEA. This was also the first major randomized trial to use rigorous credentialing standards for study operators. Some potential disadvantages of the study design: the CAS systems used were rigidly established so that other options for cerebral protection and stenting were not included, and there is concern about the potential lack of generalizability to the community. Additional arguments suggest that the two study arms are not in fact equivalent because the effect of stroke and MI on the patient are probably not interchangeable.[52] More subgroup analysis will be released that will specifically address the effect of age, perioperative myocardial infarction, and other factors to fully understand the results of CREST.

CONCLUSION

CEA has a long track record of success in carotid revascularization, whereas CAS has improved significantly and is competitive with CEA. CAS is established therapy for patients at high risk for CEA, especially those with a hostile neck. According to the National Center for Health Statistics, CAS is a routinely performed procedure in both academic and community settings. Whether CAS will be expanded to standard-risk populations awaits further evaluation and further analysis of CREST data. As this and long-term data reflecting the durability of CAS continues to accumulate, greater operator experience is acquired, and new stenting technology develops, the application of CAS will continue to mature and likely expand.

References available online at expertconsult.com.

QUESTIONS

1. Carotid stenting is approved for use in the U.S. for patients with characteristics that make the patient high risk for carotid endarterectomy. These factors include which of the following:
   a. Patient chooses to have carotid stent
   b. Patient has an extensive history of GI bleeding
   c. Patient is a non-responder to clopidogrel
   d. Patient has a tracheal stoma
   e. Patient has an asymptomatic moderate stenosis

2. Anatomic factors that increase the periprocedural risk of carotid stenting include all of these, except:
   a. tortuous arch
   b. highly calcified arch
   c. recently symptomatic critical carotid stenosis
   d. restenosis after previous carotid endarterectomy
   e. Fresh thrombus at the site of the bifurcation lesion

3. Periprocedural medications for use in the carotid stent procedure includes all of these, except:
   a. aspirin
   b. papavarine
   c. clopidogrel
   d. nitroglycerine
   e. atropine

4. A common method of establishing carotid sheath access is:
   a. Place a stiff exchange guidewire in the external carotid artery and advance the carotid sheath over the exchange guidewire.
   b. Advance the carotid sheath over the soft guidewire used for selective catheterization of the common carotid artery.
   c. Place the stiff guidewire into the internal carotid artery beyond the lesion and advance the carotid sheath over the exchange guidewire.
   d. Advance the sheath into the arch and then cannulate the common carotid artery using a stiff exchange guidewire.

5. Which of the following is true about the use of cerebral protection devices?
   a. Only one filter is approved for use with CAS
   b. CMS mandates the use of cerebral protection devices during CAS
   c. Filters have been shown in large randomized trials to provide a lower risk of periprocedural stroke than when no filter is used.
   d. The dwell time for a filter has no correlation with periprocedural risk of stroke.
   e. Filters are just as simple to place when the artery distal to the bifurcation is extremely tortuous.

6. In the first few hours after carotid stent placement, an average patient's vital signs are more likely to trend toward:
   a. Bradycardia and hypotension
   b. Hypertension and tachycardia
   c. Hypertension and bradycardia
   d. No significant change from prior to stent placement

7. Randomized, controlled trials of carotid stenting and carotid endarterectomy include all of these, except:
   a. NASCET
   b. CREST
   c. SAPPHIRE
   d. ICSS
   e. SPACE

8. The primary endpoint for the CREST Trial was:
   a. Stroke and death at 30 days
   b. Stroke, death, myocardial infarction, and cranial nerve injury at 30 days
   c. Stroke, death, and myocardial infarction at 4 years
   d. Stroke, death and myocardial infarction at 30 days and post-procedural ipsilateral stroke at long-term follow-up
   e. Stroke, death and myocardial infarction, cranial nerve injury and positive diffusion-weighted MRI at 30 days

9. The CREST results showed that:
   a. The risk of periprocedural myocardial infarction was higher with stenting than with endarterectomy
   b. The risk of minor stroke was higher with endarterectomy than with stenting
   c. The risk of persistent cranial nerve injury beyond 6 months after carotid endarterectomy was 0%.
   d. There was no significant difference in the risk of major stroke or death between carotid stenting and carotid endarterectomy

10. Name some of the advantages of the use of embolic protection during carotid stenting.
    a. Distal filters permit preservation of prograde flow to the brain during the CAS procedure.
    b. Proximal occlusion can be performed with a smaller caliber carotid sheath than other types of protection.
    c. When using proximal protection, it is simple to avoid patients who are at high risk for intolerance of reversed flow by evaluating cerebral collaterals based on pre-procedure MRI scanning.
    d. Distal filters permit the use of any guidewire the operator would like to use for passage of the balloon and stent into the carotid artery.

ANSWERS

1. **d**
2. **d**
3. **b**
4. **a**
5. **b**
6. **a**
7. **a**
8. **d**
9. **d**
10. **a**

CHAPTER 21

SURGICAL MANAGEMENT OF AORTOILIAC OCCLUSIVE DISEASE

Michael Belkin • Christopher D. Owens

Arteriosclerotic occlusive disease of the abdominal aorta and iliac arteries is a common cause of ischemic symptoms in the lower extremities of middle-aged and elderly patients in the Western world. Although not as common as occlusive disease of the femoropopliteal arterial system, with which it may be combined, aortoiliac occlusive disease may be more disabling because of the greater number of muscle groups subjected to diminished perfusion. The initial manifestation of occlusive disease of the distal aorta or iliac arteries is intermittent claudication with symptoms involving muscles of the thigh, hip, buttock, and calf. Because the calf muscles are usually the only muscle groups affected by intermittent claudication caused by superficial femoral artery occlusion, the involvement of more proximal muscles in the symptom complex may help to distinguish aortoiliac occlusive disease from femoropopliteal occlusive disease. Unfortunately, a sizable minority of patients with aortoiliac disease complain only of calf claudication. In addition to claudication, male patients with aortoiliac occlusive disease may complain of difficulty in achieving and maintaining an erection because of inadequate perfusion of the internal pudendal arteries. The Leriche syndrome in males consists of the manifestations of aortoiliac occlusive disease and includes claudication of the muscles of the thigh, hip, and buttock; atrophy of the leg muscles; impotence; and diminished femoral pulses.[1]

Aortoiliac occlusive disease per se is rarely the cause of ischemia at rest or ischemic tissue loss, except by embolization. The collateral circulation that develops around the occlusive process in the aorta and iliac arteries is usually rich and sufficient to supply the lower extremities with adequate quantities of arterial blood to ensure good resting tissue perfusion. However, arteriosclerotic plaques in the aorta and iliac arteries may cause the so-called blue toe syndrome (i.e., microembolization of arteriosclerotic debris to the terminal vessels in the foot).[2-5] Such symptoms can occur in a patient who otherwise appears to have adequate distal arterial supply, including palpable pedal pulses in some instances. Under these circumstances, a search must be made by angiography for a proximal source of microembolization.

When aortoiliac occlusive disease is combined with femoropopliteal occlusive disease—a finding more common in elderly patients—resting ischemia may result.[6] As in any arterial system, tandem lesions in the

arteries supplying the extremities are more significant than single lesions.

The risk factors for aortoiliac occlusive disease are those for atherosclerosis in general and include cigarette smoking, hypertension, elevated serum cholesterol, and diabetes.[7-18] In our experience, patients reporting symptoms of claudication caused by aortoiliac occlusive disease are on average nearly a decade younger than those complaining of claudication from superficial femoral artery occlusion. However, patients with ischemia at rest from the combination of aortoiliac and femoropopliteal occlusive disease are generally in the seventh decade of life and are not notably younger than those who develop ischemic rest pain from femoropopliteal disease.

The initial lesions of aortoiliac occlusive disease usually begin at the terminal aorta and the proximal portions of the common iliac arteries or at the bifurcations of the common iliac arteries (Figure 21-1). The lesions then progress proximally and distally. Approximately 33% of the patients treated by authors for symptomatic aortoiliac disease have had disease at the origin of the deep femoral arteries in the groin, and more than 40% have had superficial femoral artery occlusions. The natural history of aortoiliac occlusive disease is one of slow progression.[19,20] The ultimate anatomic result of aortoiliac atherosclerosis is variable, but can lead to occlusion of the distal abdominal aorta, with progression of the thrombus up to the level of the renal arteries (Figure 21-2). Although occlusion of the terminal aorta, once it occurs, may remain stable for years, it does not always have a benign course, as reported by Starrett and Stoney.[21] They observed that more than one third of patients with aortic occlusion went on to show thrombosis of the renal arteries over a period of 5 to 10 years (Figure 21-3). However, Reilly and colleagues[22] later suggested that the renal arteries remain patent; no instances of thrombosis occurred in 21 patients followed up with arteriography after a mean of 27.7 months.

Variants in the pattern of aortoiliac occlusive disease occur, including relatively circumscribed occlusive lesions of the midabdominal aorta described in early middle-aged women who are heavy cigarette smokers (Figure 21-4). Although the upper abdominal aorta is ordinarily spared in patients with aortoiliac occlusive disease, a minority of these patients have marked involvement of this aortic segment, with occlusive disease at the

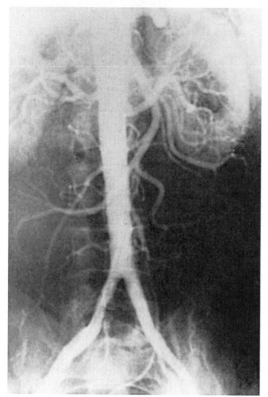

FIGURE 21-1 ■ The earliest manifestations of aortoiliac occlusive disease are evident in the terminal aorta and proximal common iliac vessels.

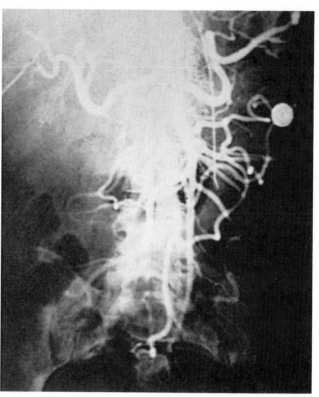

FIGURE 21-3 ■ The end result of aortoiliac occlusive disease consists of total aortic thrombosis, which may include the origins of the renal arteries.

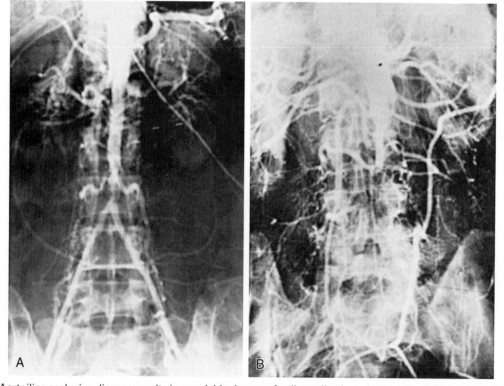

FIGURE 21-2 ■ Aortoiliac occlusive disease results in a variable degree of collateralization, shown as a discrete channel from a lumbar to the deep iliac circumflex artery **(A)** and as a multiplicity of small vessels that supply the hemorrhoidal and gluteal arteries that reconstitute the femoral vessels via iliac and femoral circumflex arteries **(B)**.

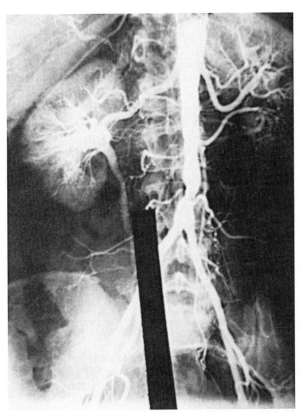

FIGURE 21-4 ■ Aortoiliac occlusive disease may consist of a short-segment circumferential lesion, especially common in younger women. Such a lesion may be amenable to localized endarterectomy.

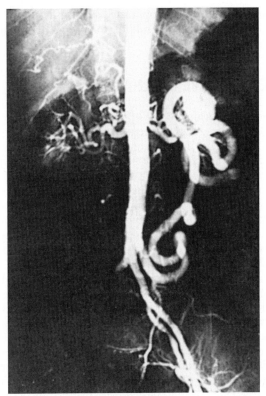

FIGURE 21-5 ■ A large meandering mesenteric artery associated with total superior mesenteric artery celiac occlusion, renal artery stenosis, complete occlusion of the right common iliac artery, and distal left external iliac stenoses with a single patent hypogastric artery. End-to-side proximal anastomosis may best preserve both mesenteric and pelvic circulation.

origins of the major visceral vessels and renal arteries (Figure 21-5).

DIAGNOSIS

The diagnosis of aortoiliac occlusive disease is ordinarily and easily made on the basis of the patient's symptoms. Complaints of high claudication, with or without accompanying sexual dysfunction in males, certainly suggest this disease process. Claudication symptoms, however, must be distinguished from symptoms of nerve root irritation caused by spinal stenosis or intervertebral disk herniation, which may be associated with activity and relieved by sitting or lying down in some individuals.[23] These patients can ordinarily be distinguished easily from patients with true claudication by the fact that their symptoms are produced as much by standing still as by walking and by the typical sciatic distribution of the pain.

A patient with intermittent claudication owing to aortoiliac disease ordinarily has lower extremities that appear healthy and well perfused at rest, although the muscles may be somewhat atrophic from disuse. Diminished or even absent femoral pulses are often a principal clue to the level of the occlusive process. Bruits heard in the groins can also call attention to proximal occlusive lesions. However, stenotic lesions at the origins of the superficial or deep femoral arteries can also cause femoral bruits.

Easily palpable pedal pulses at rest may be found in patients with severe claudication from aortoiliac occlusive disease, even when the femoral pulses are barely discernible. This reflects the rich collateral circulation that is ordinarily present in such patients.

Segmental Doppler pressures at all levels in the lower extremity are ordinarily lower than the brachial pressure. If no accompanying superficial femoral occlusive disease exists, no impressive gradient occurs between the high thigh pressure and the ankle pressure; however, disabling symptoms can occur in patients with aortoiliac disease who have resting ankle pressures in the near-normal range and a normal ankle-brachial pressure index. Thus, in evaluating these patients, repeating the pressure measurements after a period of graded exercise is often wise.[24] A marked fall in ankle pressure immediately after exercise occurs if the patient's symptoms are caused by significant aortoiliac occlusive disease. More sophisticated Doppler waveform analysis or the use of a pulse-volume recorder may reveal patterns suggestive of proximal occlusive lesions.[25-27] We have found, however, that resting and postexercise Doppler pressure measurements are satisfactory for the evaluation of the majority of patients.

The indications for surgery in symptomatic aortoiliac occlusive disease are disabling claudication and ischemia at rest manifested by rest pain in the foot, ischemic ulceration, or pregangrenous skin changes. Patients with aortoiliac disease and ischemia at rest ordinarily have accompanying femoropopliteal disease unless the ischemic lesions are the result of microemboli, as noted earlier.

PREOPERATIVE EVALUATION

Preoperative evaluation of a patient with aortoiliac occlusive disease includes a careful evaluation of any accompanying cardiac and pulmonary disease. In the authors' experience, approximately 40% of patients with symptomatic aortoiliac occlusive disease have clear clinical and electrocardiographic evidence of coronary artery disease. Symptomatic unstable coronary artery disease in such individuals clearly demands investigation, including cardiac catheterization and coronary angiography in many cases. If coronary artery reconstruction is indicated, this procedure should be done first and the aortoiliac occlusive disease repaired as a second procedure. Patients with mild or stable coronary artery disease can ordinarily undergo aortoiliac reconstruction without great risk. Older patients with severe cardiopulmonary disease who are not good candidates for coronary artery reconstruction are probably best managed by extraanatomic bypass procedures of lesser magnitude than formal aortoiliac or aortofemoral reconstruction. Patients with severe restrictive pulmonary disease may require a period of preoperative preparation that includes bronchodilators, broad-spectrum antibiotics, and abstinence from cigarette smoking.

Angiography has historically played a major role in the preoperative evaluation of patients with symptomatic aortoiliac disease and can generally be performed by the retrograde Seldinger technique using the femoral approach.[28] When angiography is not possible, magnetic resonance angiography (MRA) is particularly well suited for evaluating the aorta and renal and iliac arteries. New and faster acquisition techniques and high-quality, three-dimensional postprocessing capabilities make MRA an attractive, noninvasive, and accurate alternative. In some institutions, computed tomography angiography is favored over MRA as a more clinically useful, noninvasive alternative to standard angiography. Regardless of the modality, the goal of the radiographic examination is to provide views of the entire abdominal aorta in two planes to demonstrate unexpected lesions of the celiac axis or superior mesenteric artery origins, to provide anteroposterior and oblique views of the pelvis to define any iliac artery lesions in more than one plane, and to demonstrate possible lesions at the origins of the deep femoral arteries. Views should also be obtained of the vessels in the thighs, at the knees, and in the calves to demonstrate associated femoropopliteal occlusive disease and the quality of the runoff. At the time of angiography, obtaining pull-back pressures across iliac artery lesions of doubtful significance is a useful technique because it can demonstrate whether such lesions are likely to interfere with flow. Measurements should be taken at rest and after papaverine injection or during a period of reactive hyperemia after tourniquet ischemia to mimic the hemodynamic situation that occurs during exercise.[29] Intraarterial digital subtraction angiography has become quite

useful for evaluation of the aortoiliac arterial segment. The advantages of this technique include the use of small amounts of contrast medium and good resolution of the vessels studied.

Percutaneous balloon therapy with or without stenting has supplanted surgical reconstruction as the most common therapy for aortoiliac occlusive disease. The recent TransAtlantic Intersociety Consensus (TASC II) document delineated which patients are best served by percutanous versus surgical therapy.[32] It is generally believed that TASC types A and B lesions (focal, short-segment lesions [≤3 to 10 cm], unilateral or bilateral) are best treated with endovascular techniques. Conversely, TASC type D lesions (long-segment occlusions and diffuse, severe long-segment disease, particularly bilateral) are best treated with open surgery. Intermediate TASC type C lesions can be treated appropriately with either technique, but are increasingly being treated initially with percutaneous approaches.

AORTOFEMORAL BYPASS GRAFT

Over the past 2 decades, the aortofemoral bypass graft has remained the gold standard for the treatment of severe symptomatic aortoiliac occlusive disease. This procedure's 30-day operative mortality rate of 5% to 8% in the early 1970s has been reduced in our own experience to less than 2% over the past 15 years, a level consistent with reports from other surgeons and similar to that observed in patients undergoing elective abdominal aortic aneurysm repair.[33-39] Arterial insufficiency of the lower extremities is a manifestation of a systemic process that results in clinically evident coronary artery disease in approximately 50% of these patients.[40-42] Reduced operative mortality has been observed and is associated with a concomitant reduction in the number of early cardiac deaths. The improved perioperative management of patients with diseased hearts has resulted from a number of factors, including selective employment of preliminary cardiac surgery for certain individuals, sophisticated pharmacologic management of the damaged myocardium, and more precise perioperative fluid management tailored to the individual patient's myocardial reserve.[39]

Surgical Technique

The femoral vessels are typically exposed first through bilateral longitudinal incisions to reduce insensible fluid loss through the exposed abdomen. The aorta is exposed through a transabdmonial approach with typically a longitudinal incision though some prefer a transverse incision. Some surgeons expose the infrarenal aorta through a retroperitoneal exposure, which is an attractive alternative for patients with multiple prior intraabdominal procedures. Once all vessels are exposed, systemic anticoagulation is instituted. The aorta should be palpated for an appropriate place to apply a cross clamp. It may be necessary to apply the clamp in an anterior-posterior configuration in the event of severe posterior calcification to prevent traumatic clamp injury.

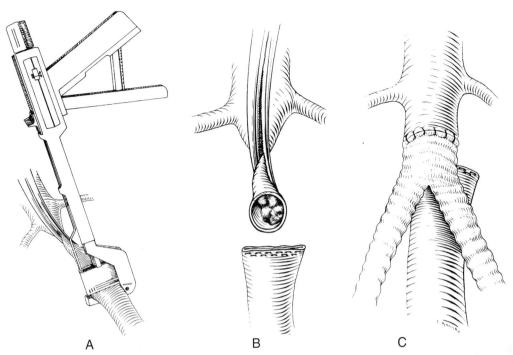

FIGURE 21-6 ■ End-to-end proximal anastomosis for aortofemoral reconstruction can be initiated with the infrarenal aortic cross-clamp placed in an anteroposterior direction, with minimal dissection as close to the origin of the renal arteries as possible. The aorta is then stapled or occluded with a second clamp just proximal to the origin of the inferior mesenteric artery (**A**). After transection of the infrarenal aorta and complete thromboendarterectomy of the proximal infrarenal aortic cuff (**B**), end-to-end anastomosis is completed with continuous 3-0 polypropylene sutures (**C**).

The knitted Dacron prosthesis is the standard graft material used by most surgeons with experience in aortoiliac reconstruction. This material, usually impregnated with collagen or gelatin, may provide a more stable pseudointima than woven prostheses do.[43,44] An important factor contributing to improved results has undoubtedly been recognition of the critical role of the deep femoral artery in providing sustained patency of the aortofemoral graft limb.[33,36,45,46] The current practice of extending the distal anastomosis down over the origin of the deep femoral artery to ensure an adequate outflow tract has been widely accepted and is important in patients with tandem superficial femoral occlusions and in patients with stenosis of the deep femoral origin. We have found, however, that if extensive profundaplasty or endarterectomy is necessary, this vessel is better closed with an autogenous tissue patch of saphenous vein, bovine pericardial patch, or endarterectomized superficial femoral artery than attempting to make a long deep femoral patch with the distal end of an aortofemoral prosthesis.[45]

The incidence of graft infection has been minimized with preoperative and intraoperative antibiotics.[33,47-49] Aortoenteric fistulas can be prevented by closure of retroperitoneal tissue and the posterior parietal peritoneum over the graft and proximal suture line to prevent erosion of the graft into the duodenum.[33,50,51] The abandonment of silk sutures in favor of permanent prosthetic suture material has undoubtedly helped to reduce the incidence of false aneurysm formation.

A good deal of controversy remains over the proper method of performing the proximal anastomosis of an aortobifemoral graft.[33,52,53] Most surgeons favor the end-to-end technique of proximal anastomosis, with transection of the aorta between clamps approximately 1 to 2 inches below the renal arteries and oversewing or stapling of the distal end (Figure 21-6). This permits an endarterectomy or thrombectomy of the proximal aortic stump under direct vision before constructing the anastomosis. It also has the advantage of not requiring flow to be reestablished in the more distal aorta, where arteriosclerotic plaque and mural thrombus may have been loosened by application of the distal clamp. This may avoid intraoperative emboli to the lower extremities.

Some authors claim that the end-to-end technique reduces the incidence of aortoduodenal fistulas because the end-to-end anastomosis does not project anteriorly, as does an end-to-side aortofemoral reconstruction. Unfortunately, the controlled studies that are available do not substantiate that the results of the end-to-end technique are significantly superior to those of the end-to-side technique. Therefore the end-to-end technique is probably more appropriate for patients who will not suffer any hemodynamic disadvantage from interruption of forward flow in the abdominal aorta. This technique also appears to be desirable for patients who have already suffered complete aortic occlusion. The end-to-side technique (Figure 21-7) is reserved for individuals who would lose perfusion of an important hypogastric or inferior mesenteric artery if forward flow in the aorta were sacrificed at the time of surgery.[52] Arteriographic studies in patients with indications for an end-to-side anastomosis are shown in Figures 21-5 and 21-8.

Although aortofemoral reconstruction has the potential to restore potency to males with sexual dysfunction

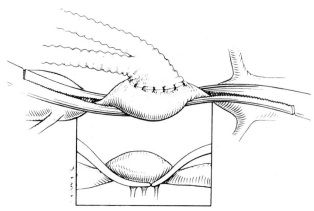

FIGURE 21-7 ■ End-to-side proximal anastomosis for aortofemoral reconstruction is required to preserve antegrade pelvic perfusion when retrograde perfusion from distal femoral anastomoses is doubtful. The infrarenal aorta is occluded proximal to the origin of the inferior mesenteric artery and just distal to the origin of the renal arteries. After longitudinal arteriotomy and thorough thromboendarterectomy, if required, the anastomosis is constructed using continuous polypropylene sutures.

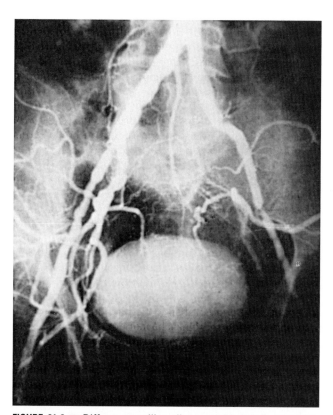

FIGURE 21-8 ■ Diffuse aortoiliac disease with left hypogastric occlusion and minimal left pelvic collateralization may warrant end-to-side proximal anastomosis to preserve the right hypogastric system.

because of inadequate hypogastric artery perfusion,[52,53] surgical dissection in the area of the terminal aorta and proximal left common iliac artery can also cause difficulty with both erection and ejaculation by interfering with the autonomic nervous plexus, which sweeps over these vessels.[54] When performing aortofemoral bypass grafting, confine the dissection of the aorta to the area

between the renal arteries and the inferior mesenteric artery. The aorta is exposed anteriorly and laterally, without distorting the vessel, to avoid embolization of arteriosclerotic debris. After systemic heparinization, the distal clamp is placed proximal to the inferior mesenteric artery; then the aorta is cross-clamped below the renal arteries, where the aortic wall is likely to be considerably less diseased. The aorta is divided transversely, and the distal end is beveled and oversewn.

In the case of an end-to-side anastomosis, the longitudinal aortotomy is placed high, up near the renals in the more normal aorta, and great care is taken to remove all loose debris and mural thrombus from the lumen in the excluded aortic segment. At completion of an end-to-side anastomosis, attention is also given to adequate backflushing of all loosened debris and clot from the distal aorta before forward flow is reestablished. In performing either type of proximal anastomosis, a short stem of a graft is sutured to the aorta with a running suture of 3-0 polypropylene. Knitted Dacron prostheses are invariably used; the size is selected so that the limb diameter corresponds to the diameter of the patient's common femoral arteries. The average prosthesis size used for males is 16 × 8 mm or, in larger individuals, 18 × 9 mm. For females, the most commonly used sizes are 12 × 6 mm and 14 × 7 mm. After completion of the proximal anastomosis, the limbs are tunneled retroperitoneally into the groins. On the left, the tunnel ordinarily passes beneath the sigmoid mesentery and ureter and into the groin in a rather lateral channel that avoids trauma to the nerve plexuses at the terminal aorta. On the right, the tunnel is made along the course of the right common iliac artery beneath the ureter. In the groin, end-to-side anastomoses are fashioned in the distal common femoral artery with 5-0 polypropylene. The anastomoses are carried down into the deep femoral arteries for a short distance if there is any evidence of incipient stenosis of the origins of these vessels or if the superficial femorals are occluded. The end of the graft thus acts as a patch, widening the orifice of the deep femoral artery.

Despite significant advances in laparoscopic general surgery, applications of this new technique to vascular surgery have been few. However, several authors have applied laparoscopic techniques to aortofemoral reconstruction. Whether performed completely via the laparoscopic approach or through limited incisions with laparoscopy-assisted dissection, the procedure has proved to be time-consuming and technically challenging.[55,56] As the technology evolves and intracorporeal anastomotic techniques are refined, however, the role of laparoscopic aortofemoral bypass will expand and become clearer.

In patients with well-localized aortoiliac lesions, aortoiliac endarterectomy may be a suitable option. This operation, even in the hands of enthusiasts, is confined to patients whose disease ends distally near the bifurcation of the common iliac arteries (Figure 21-9; see also Figure 21-4).[33] Endarterectomy of the external iliac artery is tedious and unrewarding for most surgeons. There is little evidence to suggest that endarterectomy is superior to a properly performed aortofemoral bypass graft in terms of early or late results. In our practice, aortoiliac endarterectomy is confined to a minority of individuals

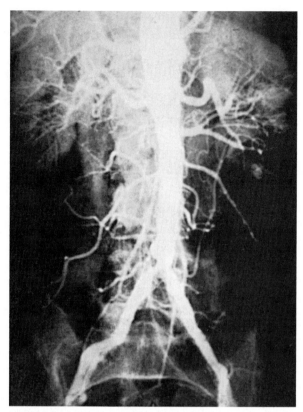

FIGURE 21-9 ■ Aortoiliac occlusive disease with significant lesion confined to the origin of the right common iliac artery, amenable to either local endarterectomy or percutaneous transluminal angioplasty.

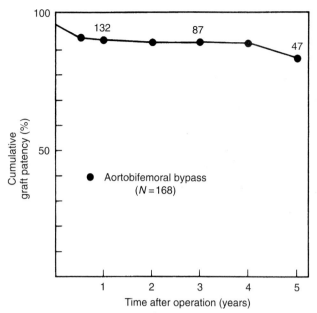

FIGURE 21-10 ■ For 168 aortobifemoral graft limbs inserted in 84 consecutive patients, the 5-year cumulative patency was 86%.

who appear to have principally aortic disease with little involvement of the iliac arteries. This group of patients characteristically consists of early middle-aged women with occlusive disease of the midabdominal aorta that ends at the aortic bifurcation or in the proximal portions of the common iliac arteries. We avoid aortoiliac endarterectomy in males because of concerns about interfering with the autonomic nerves at the terminal aorta and proximal left common iliac artery. Currently, most patients who would be considered candidates for aortoiliac endarterectomy from an anatomic standpoint are treated with percutaneous balloon angioplasty with or without stenting.

Results

Initial aortobifemoral graft limb patency rates approach 100%, and the 5-year patency is greater than 80% in a number of reports.[33,34,36,57,58] Long-term patency has also improved to an anticipated 75% at 10 years.[33] A number of refinements of operative technique may be responsible for the low incidence of graft limb thrombosis in recent years. The more prevalent use of the aortobifemoral graft as opposed to aortoiliac bypass or extended aortoiliofemoral endarterectomy has negated the effect of unsuspected or progressive atherosclerosis in the external iliac vessels. Meticulous avoidance of graft limb redundancy and an awareness of the desirability of compatibility

between the diameter of the graft limb and that of the vessel into which it is implanted have also probably helped to maintain long-term patency.

Our results with aortofemoral bypass grafting are illustrated in Figure 21-10. The 5-year cumulative patency of 86% is comparable with that reported in a number of other studies.[33,34,36,57] Thirty-day operative mortality was slightly less than 1%. This low mortality rate undoubtedly reflects careful patient selection as well as improved operative management and anesthetic technique. However, because aortoiliac occlusive disease is rarely life threatening (although it may be limb threatening), it is preferable to treat high-risk patients with procedures of lesser magnitude.

Although most authors have reported excellent patency rates after aortofemoral bypass, several subgroups with inferior results have been identified. Younger patients and those with small aortas are more vulnerable to late graft failure. A study of aortofemoral reconstructions in 73 patients younger than 50 years documented a 50% primary patency rate 5 years after bypass.[53] In that study, patients with aortas less than 1.8 cm wide had significantly lower patency rates (6-year patency of 20%) than did those with aortas larger than 1.8 cm (6-year patency of 60%). Similarly, we have documented lower patency rates in younger patients: 5-year patency rates were only 66% in patients younger than 50 years, compared with 87% for 50- to 60-year-olds and 96% for those older than 60 years.[59] Younger patients also had significantly smaller aortas, corroborating the influence of aortic size on long-term outcomes. There were no significant differences in patency rates for patients operated on for limb salvage versus claudication, and no significant differences between the genders.

Although the excellent graft patency rates for aortofemoral bypass grafts do not necessarily reflect functional results, approximately 95% of patients are initially rendered asymptomatic or improved; after 5 years, about 80% remain in this category.[36,57] A study from the United Kingdom indicated that among patients fully employed before aortobifemoral bypass, 85% returned to full employment an average of 4 months after surgery, and more than 50% of those not previously employed returned to work after bypass.[60] Other studies have documented a more sobering functional outcome after successful aortofemoral arterial reconstruction. One study, employing the SF-20 questionnaire, found that after aortobifemoral bypass, patients had decrements in physical and role function and general health perception similar to those of patients with congestive heart failure or recent myocardial infarction.[61] Clearly, more functional outcome analysis is necessary after the treatment of aortoiliac occlusive disease.

The 5-year cumulative survival rate for patients undergoing aortofemoral bypass grafting remains some 14% lower than that anticipated for a normal age-corrected population. However, nearly 80% survive 5 years, whereas less than 50% survive 10 years.[41]

Concomitant Distal Reconstruction

When patients have threatened limb loss from a combination of aortoiliac and femoropopliteal occlusive disease, repair of the proximal or inflow lesions is necessary to salvage the extremity. However, it is not always clear whether concomitant distal reconstruction, such as femoropopliteal bypass, should be performed at the time of the initial operation. Results reported in the literature suggest that in the majority of patients with ischemia at rest caused by combined aortoiliac and femoropopliteal disease, repair of the aortoiliac occlusive disease and restoration of normal perfusion to the deep femoral arteries achieve limb salvage in the vast majority (probably 80%) of patients.[46,62] However, in patients who have extensive tissue necrosis of the skin of the forefoot or heel, particularly individuals with diabetes, restoration of pulsatile flow in the foot may be necessary to achieve healing. Under these circumstances, we believe that a combination of both proximal and distal reconstructive procedures may be necessary at the initial operation. The combined procedure has the disadvantage of increasing the operating time and surgical trauma in a group of patients who are likely to be elderly with a high incidence of coronary artery disease; however, with modern anesthetic management and a two-team operative approach, this combined reconstruction can be performed safely and within a reasonable time.

ALTERNATIVES FOR HIGH-RISK PATIENTS

Although transabdominal arterial reconstruction for aortoiliac occlusive disease can be performed successfully with low morbidity and mortality in many patients, less extensive procedures may be preferable in patients who are high risks for major surgery under general anesthesia. In such patients, distal aortic and proximal iliac occlusions can be treated by axillofemoral bypass grafts, which

are discussed later.[63-67] If the occlusive disease is limited to one common, or external, iliac artery, then alternatives to axillofemoral bypass are warranted in poor-risk individuals. The use of the patent iliac system as the origin for a bypass permits a shorter graft segment and affords better long-term patency. The femorofemoral bypass is an example of such a procedure.[68] An anatomically similar procedure, the iliofemoral graft, has received little attention in the literature.

Ilioiliac and Iliofemoral Bypass Grafts

The authors have reviewed their experience with 94 patients undergoing ilioiliac or iliofemoral bypass grafting from 1982 to 1992. Poor-risk patients, particularly those with severe cardiopulmonary impairment, who had no important occlusive disease in the aorta or in the proximal segment of at least one common iliac artery were considered for reconstruction using a patent common or external iliac artery for the proximal anastomosis (see Figure 21-5). The iliac site for anastomosis has several technical advantages, including exposure through an oblique, suprainguinal, renal transplant incision, which is technically simple, even in obese patients. The graft is more deeply placed and therefore more cushioned than in the femorofemoral position. Ilioilial grafts are shorter than femorofemoral grafts, and no disturbance of inguinal lymph nodes or lymphatics occurs. The femoral artery on the donor side is left undisturbed for later use as the origin for a distal bypass, if indicated.

The mean age of the 94 patients undergoing ilioiliac or iliofemoral bypass was 60 years, and 26% had diabetes mellitus. Forty-one percent had clear clinical and electrocardiographic evidence of coronary artery disease, and 43% had significant hypertension. Fifty-eight percent of the patients were operated on for claudication, and 42% for limb salvage. Twenty-three patients had ilioilial grafts, and 91 patients had iliofemoral grafts. Fifty-seven iliounifemoral grafts and 14 iliobifemoral grafts were performed.

In patients subjected to iliac artery reconstruction, the patent iliac segment was exposed extraperitoneally through a curvilinear incision parallel to and above the inguinal ligament, identical to the approach for renal transplantation. Limited iliac endarterectomy was necessary in a few instances. Separate vertical groin incisions were made to expose the common femoral arteries. For ilioiliac bypass, symmetrical incisions were made to expose the iliac vessels, and the graft was positioned in the retroperitoneum (Figure 21-11A). The grafts to the femoral arteries were placed under the inguinal ligament (see Figures 21-11B, 21-11C). For patients undergoing bilateral iliofemoral reconstruction, the crossover limb was placed from the iliofemoral graft retroperitoneally in the iliac fossa or, in a few cases, subcutaneously to the contralateral femoral artery (see Figure 21-11C).

The 30-day operative mortality for these procedures was zero. The 4-year cumulative patency for the ilioiliac grafts (23 limbs) was 96%, and that for the iliofemoral grafts (91 limbs) was 72%. The 4-year patency for iliobifemoral grafts (28 limbs) was 72%, and that for iliounifemoral grafts (63 limbs) was 71% (Figure 21-12). When

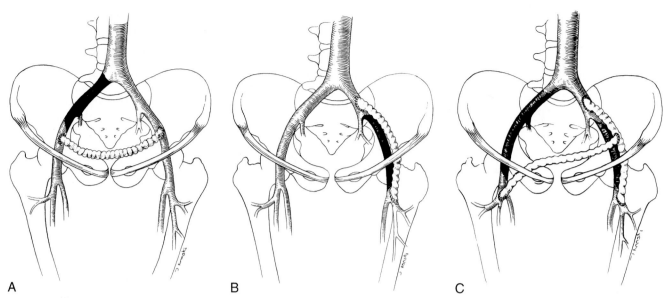

A   B   C

FIGURE 21-11 ■ A patent common or external iliac artery may be used as a donor vessel for ilioiliac **(A)**, iliofemoral **(B)**, or iliobifemoral **(C)** bypasses in appropriate patients who would otherwise require axillofemoral reconstruction.

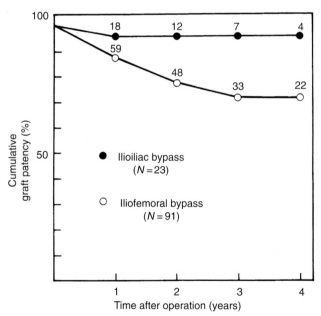

FIGURE 21-12 ■ Using a patent iliac vessel as the donor artery, the 4-year cumulative graft patency for 23 ilioiliac grafts was 96%, whereas the patency for 91 iliofemoral graft limbs was 72%.

both the superficial and deep femoral arteries were patent, the cumulative patency rate for iliofemoral grafts was higher (85%) at 4 years than when only the deep femoral artery was patent (62%). Demonstration of a statistically significant difference in late patency between aortofemoral grafts and iliofemoral grafts was not possible, although the aortofemoral grafts had numerically superior 4- and 5-year patencies. We thus believe that the iliofemoral bypass is an adequate substitute for aortofemoral bypass in certain elderly and poor-risk individuals who have proximal occlusive disease confined largely to the external iliac arteries or to one iliac system.

Femorofemoral Bypass Graft

In patients whose occlusive disease is confined to one iliac artery and whose aorta and contralateral iliac system are free of hemodynamically significant lesions, the femorofemoral bypass is often used. The femorofemoral bypass depends on one iliac artery to supply adequate blood flow to support both lower extremities. One of the most common current indications for femorofemoral bypass is for patients undergoing endovascular aortounifemoral repair of aortic aneurysms necessitating contralateral revascularization or in patients having a previous endoprosthesis re-lined and converted to an aorto-uni-iliac device. Maini and Mannick,[66] Vetto,[68] Brief and coworkers,[69] and Plecha and Pories,[70] demonstrated that these operations yield quite satisfactory long-term results (60% to 80% 5-year patency). Failure of these grafts because of progressive worsening of proximal atherosclerosis has been uncommon. Such worsening may be retarded by increased flow through the donor iliac system, which is required to supply both of the lower extremities with blood. Berguer and coworkers[71] reported experimental support for this hypothesis by demonstrating in animals that intimal hyperplasia correlates inversely with blood flow and shear stress. However, experimental results yielding the opposite conclusion have also been reported.[72]

The femorofemoral graft is particularly applicable to high-risk patients because it can be performed easily under epidural or spinal anesthesia. The two common femoral arteries are exposed through short vertical groin incisions. The groin incisions are connected by a subcutaneous suprapubic tunnel created by blunt dissection on the deep fascia. It is preferable to have the graft form a C configuration, with the anastomoses placed in the distal common femoral arteries and the graft traveling proximally up through the suprapubic tunnel and down to the opposite common femoral artery (Figure 21-13). In our experience with femorofemoral bypass, 60% of patients

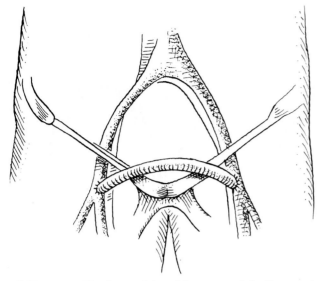

FIGURE 21-13 ■ The femorofemoral bypass graft is illustrated, with the preferred C configuration of the subcutaneous tunnel constructed well above the pubis.

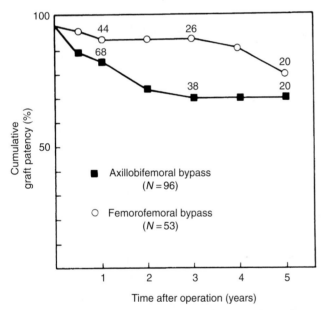

FIGURE 21-14 ■ The 4-year cumulative graft patency for 53 femorofemoral grafts was 80%, and the patency for 48 axillobifemoral grafts (96 limbs) was 70%.

were operated on for limb salvage and 40% for disabling claudication. The average age of these patients was 61 years. Forty-one percent had clinical evidence of coronary artery disease, 33% were diabetic, and 44% had significant hypertension. The 5-year cumulative graft patency was 80% (Figure 21-14). Although the difference in late patency rates for femorofemoral and aortofemoral bypass is not statistically significant, femorofemoral bypass is slightly inferior numerically. In select patients with focal common iliac artery stenosis, donor limb angioplasty and stenting followed by a femorofemoral bypass has been reported to be safe and efficacious.[73] This practice could expand the patient population who are

eligible for femorofemoral bypass. The reasonably good long-term results, the ease of performance, and the low morbidity associated with femorofemoral bypass suggest that it might logically be used in good- and poor-risk patients who have proximal occlusive disease confined to one iliac arterial segment. Although it is difficult to argue against this point of view, the fact that the groins have been operated on and the common femoral arteries dissected during the performance of a femorofemoral graft makes an aortobifemoral reconstruction in such individuals technically more difficult if progression of proximal disease causes a return of symptoms or late failure of the femorofemoral bypass. Therefore, in good-risk patients with evidence of arteriosclerotic disease in the aorta or in the patent iliac system, the recommendation is aortobifemoral bypass at the outset in an attempt to avoid possible future reoperation.

Axillofemoral Bypass Graft

In very elderly and high-risk patients who are in danger of limb loss from a combination of aortoiliac and femoropopliteal occlusive disease and whose proximal occlusive lesions involve the aorta and proximal iliac arteries, the axillofemoral bypass graft is a logical alternative to aortoiliac reconstruction or primary amputation. Extraanatomic reconstruction may also prove useful for patients with multiple prior abdominal procedures, multiple adhesions, or previous pelvic irradiation. Intraabdominal sepsis, sometimes resulting from an infected aortic graft, is another common indication. If an axillofemoral graft is chosen for such individuals, a bifemoral graft is preferred to a unifemoral one, because several reports, beginning with that of LoGerfo and colleagues,[65] showed that the axillobifemoral graft has a decidedly better 5-year cumulative patency.[67] The probable reason for this finding is that the axillobifemoral graft has approximately doubled the flow rate in its axillary limb as the axillounifemoral graft.

In constructing an axillobifemoral graft, the first portion of the axillary artery is exposed by an incision placed beneath the clavicle on the side selected for the proximal anastomosis (Figure 21-15). It is common to split the pectoralis major and divide the pectoralis minor muscle to provide better operative exposure and more space for the graft as it emerges from the axilla into the subcutaneous plane. The common femoral arteries are exposed through bilateral short groin incisions.

A DeBakey tunneling instrument can then be passed from the infraclavicular incision laterally to a subcutaneous plane in the midaxillary line. The curve in the tunneler is used to direct the tunnel anteriorly above the iliac crest and then in front of the inguinal ligament into the ipsilateral groin incision. An externally supported Dacron or polytetrafluoroethylene prosthesis, usually 8 mm in diameter, is attached to the tunneling instrument and drawn back through the tunnel into the axillary incision for anastomosis with the first portion of the axillary artery. A side limb is attached to the graft in the ipsilateral groin incision just proximal to the anastomosis with the common femoral artery. The side limb is then passed through a subcutaneous suprapubic tunnel into the

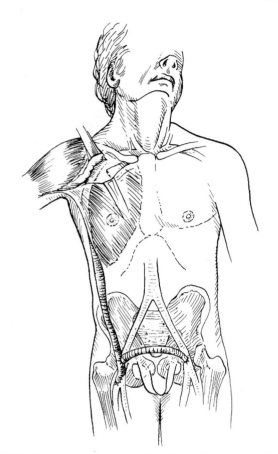

FIGURE 21-15 ■ Subcutaneous axillobifemoral bypass graft completed with proximal anastomosis to the right axillary artery, right distal anastomosis to the common and deep femoral arteries, and extension of the prosthesis with a side limb to the left common femoral artery.

opposite groin in a manner similar to that used for a femorofemoral graft.

Because neither the thoracic nor the abdominal cavity is entered when an axillofemoral graft is performed, this procedure usually does not interfere with the patient's ability to breathe, cough, or take oral feedings. On the first postoperative day, most patients are ambulatory and on a regular diet. From 1982 to 1992, we performed axillobifemoral grafts electively in 48 poor-risk patients for symptomatic aortoiliac occlusive disease. All but two of these patients were operated on for limb salvage necessitated by a combination of far-advanced aortoiliac and femoropopliteal disease. The 5-year cumulative graft patency in this group of patients was 70% (see Figure 21-14). Although this figure is not completely discouraging, it is statistically significantly inferior to the results achieved with aortofemoral bypass grafting during the same period. Therefore axillofemoral grafts should be offered only to poor-risk individuals in danger of limb loss and should not be used for the treatment of symptoms of claudication alone.

When axillofemoral grafts fail, they can frequently be reopened by thrombectomy using local anesthesia if the patient presents promptly after graft thrombosis has occurred. Approximately 25% of grafts thrombectomized

in this fashion go on to long-term patency.[65] Thus the functional results achieved with axillobifemoral grafting may be somewhat better than the 70% graft patency figure indicates.

Patency rates associated with axillofemoral reconstruction range from a low of 30% to a high of 85%.[74-76] The reasons for this extraordinary variability can be explained in large part by patient selection, indication, and status of the outflow vessels. Extraanatomic reconstruction for nonocclusive disease, such as in patients with intraabdominal sepsis or an infected aneurysm repair, achieves better patency rates than does operation primarily for occlusive disease. Patients with claudication fare better than those requiring limb salvage because of inherent outflow restriction in the latter group. In similar fashion, patients who undergo simultaneous distal femoropopliteal reconstruction show better results than those whose infrainguinal disease is not addressed. Finally, in some series, axillobifemoral grafts sustain a significantly better 5-year patency rate than do unilateral reconstructions. Flow through the descending axillary limb in bilateral reconstructions is twice that of axillounilateral grafts, perhaps explaining the improvement in some series. Other investigators have found no significant difference between bilateral and unilateral reconstructions, again probably reflecting patient selection and status of outflow.

Some of the most favorable results were reported by Harris and colleagues in 1990.[75] They achieved an 85% patency rate after 4 years in a group of 76 patients, 26% of whom were operated on for nonocclusive disease, 20% of whom underwent simultaneous outflow reconstruction, and all of whom had axillobifemoral grafts. This series was also performed in a single institution using a technique that had been standardized for many years. Similar excellent 5-year patency and limb salvage rates of 74% and 89%, respectively, were reported by Passman and colleagues.[77] These authors believe that more liberal application of the axillobifemoral bypass is warranted. In contrast, a less favorable patency rate (29%) was reported by Donaldson and colleagues[74] for 72 patients managed in several institutions by a group of 30 surgeons operating on patients with predominantly occlusive disease. Finally, many authors have reported secondary patency rates, either exclusively or in addition to primary rates, which further confuses the statistics. These series clearly show that the secondary patency rate is significantly better than the primary, attesting to the fact that up to 25% of axillobifemoral grafts require subsequent thrombectomy to maintain patency.

Descending Thoracic Aorta–To–Femoral Artery Bypass

The descending thoracic aorta can be used as an inflow source for bypass to the femoral arteries.[78,79] Although seldom indicated as a primary procedure, this bypass offers a durable alternative after aortic failure, aortic graft infection, or other problems that necessitate avoidance of the abdominal aorta. We generally expose the thoracic aorta through a sixth or seventh interspace incision. A 10-mm synthetic graft is tunneled through the diaphragm at the posterior pleural reflection and down through the retroperitoneal space to the left groin. We usually make a small lateral flank incision to facilitate safe tunneling through the retroperitoneum. The descending thoracic aorta is generally of good quality and is usually clampable with a partially occluding clamp. The procedure is completed with a femorofemoral bypass. Relatively few reports focusing on this procedure are available in the literature. McCarthy and colleagues[78] achieved a 100% 4-year patency rate with 21 thoracic aorta–to–femoral artery bypasses, whereas Criado and Keagy[79] reported an 83% 6- to 8-year secondary graft patency rate.

Percutaneous Transluminal Angioplasty

Percutaneous catheter dilatation of atheromatous vascular stenoses was introduced by Dotter and Judkins in 1963.[80] However, this technique did not become widely applied until Gruntzig designed and developed the double-lumen balloon catheter for percutaneous transluminal angioplasty in the early 1970s. In the Gruntzig technique, the balloon catheter is inserted into a stenotic arterial region with the Seldinger technique and expanded to a fixed diameter. In one of Gruntzig's original reports in 1977,[81] percutaneous dilatation was attempted in 41 patients with isolated iliac artery stenosis and proved to be initially successful in 90%.

Early success is not necessarily sustained, as evidenced by the lower 50% to 60% 5-year success rate reported by Johnston and coworkers[82] among 684 iliac angioplasties performed in Toronto between 1978 and 1986. If initial technical failures are excluded, however, success rates improve by 10% to 15%, as confirmed in a randomized, prospective, multicenter trial reported by Wilson and coworkers.[83] This study demonstrated that successful results were sustained for 3 years in 73% of dilated iliac lesions, which is not significantly different from the 82% success rate observed with conventional surgery. Success rates for percutaneous transluminal angioplasty are maximal when the procedure is performed for claudication resulting from common iliac stenosis with excellent runoff (75%); they are minimal when it is performed for critical ischemia caused by external iliac occlusion with poor runoff (19%). This technique has been useful in the initial management of patients with symptomatic short-segment iliac stenoses (see Figure 21-9). High-risk patients with appropriate lesions can be palliated effectively without the need for anesthesia and major surgery. Even in good-risk patients, percutaneous transluminal angioplasty has an advantage as an initial therapy for symptomatic lesions, in that it does not jeopardize a future surgical approach to the aorta or iliac arteries if the angioplasty ultimately fails.

The application of intraluminal stents has increased the number of iliac lesions amenable to balloon angioplasty. Whether used secondarily to correct a technically inadequate angioplasty (e.g., a dissection, residual stenosis, or residual arterial pressure gradient) or primarily to open a long-segment occlusion, stents have increased the technical success rates of percutaneous angioplasty. The Dutch Iliac Stent Trial demonstrated that selective stent placement had better improvement in symptoms than did patients treated with primary stent placement.[84] A review of 230 iliac Palmaz stent placements in 184 patients followed up with angiography at 6 months confirmed an 86% 4-year primary patency rate.[85] Most restenotic lesions were successfully treated with follow-up angioplasty.

The cost-effectiveness of a successful procedure is unquestionable, because patients may be discharged from the hospital on the day of or the day after dilatation. Despite the increasing enthusiasm for percutaneous therapy, it has not been shown to offer superior long-term benefit when compared with aggressive risk factor modification and exercise. Selection for intervention is best individualized, based on the degree of patient disability, risk of intervention, and pathologic anatomy.

References available online at expertconsult.com.

QUESTIONS

1. Symptoms of the Leriche syndrome include all of the following except:
   a. Claudication of the thigh and buttock
   b. Rest pain of the feet
   c. Impotence
   d. Diminished femoral pulses

2. Blue toe syndrome is usually characterized by which of the following?
   a. Severe claudication symptoms
   b. Absence of distal palpable pulses
   c. Palpable pedal pulses
   d. Severe tibial artery occlusive disease

3. Which of the following statements is true of patients with isolated aortoiliac occlusive disease?
   a. They generally do not suffer from ischemic rest pain.
   b. They often have relatively normal ankle-brachial indices at rest.
   c. They frequently have palpable pedal pulses.
   d. All of the above
   e. None of the above

4. Advantages of the end-to-end technique for proximal anastomosis of an aortobifemoral bypass graft include all of the following except:
   a. Decreased incidence of aortoduodenal fistula
   b. More complete endarterectomy of the proximal aortic stump
   c. More complete preservation of pelvic blood flow
   d. Decreased incidence of distal atheroemboli

5. The end-to-side technique for aortobifemoral bypass grafts is preferred in patients with which of the following?
   a. Extremely calcified infrarenal aortas
   b. Occluded inferior mesenteric arteries
   c. Common iliac artery occlusions
   d. External iliac artery occlusions

6. Reported results of aortobifemoral bypass surgery suggest which of the following?
   a. 5-year cumulative patency rates greater than 80%
   b. Poor patency rates for patients with small (<1.8 cm) aortas
   c. Significant decrements in physical and social role function despite successful bypass
   d. All of the above

7. Reported results of aortobifemoral bypass surgery suggest which of the following?
   a. Younger patients enjoy superior long-term results.
   b. Aorta size is not a major predictor of long-term outcome.
   c. Results are relatively equal between the genders.
   d. Superficial femoral artery outflow is an important predictor of long-term patency.

8. Success rates for percutaneous transluminal angioplasty of the iliac arteries are better for which of the following?
   a. Common iliac rather than external iliac lesions
   b. Patients with claudication rather than rest pain
   c. Stenotic rather than occlusive lesions
   d. All of the above

9. Which of the following statements about the use of intraluminal stents for iliac angioplasty is true?
   a. It should be performed as an adjunct for all iliac angioplasty.
   b. It should be reserved for only technical failures of primary balloon angioplasty.
   c. It has increased the number of iliac lesions amenable to balloon angioplasty.
   d. It has had no significant impact on the primary patency of iliac angioplasty.

10. Concomitant inflow and infrainguinal revascularization is indicated in which of the following situations?
    a. In all patients with complete superficial femoral artery occlusion
    b. For patients with severe rest pain
    c. For patients with extensive tissue necrosis
    d. For diabetics

ANSWERS

1. **b**
2. **c**
3. **d**
4. **c**
5. **d**
6. **d**
7. **c**
8. **d**
9. **c**
10. **c**

CHAPTER 22

Angioplasty and Stenting for Aortoiliac Disease: Technique and Results

Carlos A. Rueda • Ruth L. Bush

HISTORY OF ENDOLUMINAL TREATMENT

The concept of endovascular therapy of atherosclerotic occlusive disease was introduced in the 1960s when Dotter performed the first transluminal angioplasty in a patient with ischemic extremities.[1] His novel technique, however, could not reliably maintain luminal patency and did not receive wide acceptance as a treatment of vascular occlusive lesions. Subsequent device modifications led to the development of an angioplasty balloon composed of latex material. The clinical success of this new construct was limited, in part because of its improved compliance, and could not fully dilate a calcified lesion. The introduction of an angioplasty balloon made of polyvinyl chloride in 1976 by Gruntzig and Hopff,[2] followed by rigid balloons composed of polyethylene and polyethylene terephthalate, marked a significant advance in endovascular therapy. The latter angioplasty balloons displayed a low compliance and high radial force in a fully inflated condition. As the technology and techniques of endovascular therapy continued to improve as well as become more widely accepted as outcomes data became available, transluminal balloon angioplasty evolved to an important modality in the treatment of peripheral vascular disease.

Despite numerous studies demonstrating the short-term clinical success of transluminal angioplasty, it has several limitations, in part because of the architectural variation of atherosclerotic lesions. Early restenosis or occlusion following angioplasty can occur because of either elastic recoil of the arterial wall or intimal dissection.[3,4] Vessels that are heavily calcified, completely occluded, or that contain ulcerated plaques might not be amenable to balloon angioplasty. Moreover, residual luminal irregularities following angioplasty occasionally trigger mural thrombus formation, leading to thrombotic occlusion.[5,6] Late restenosis following angioplasty can occur as a result of intimal hyperplasia or atherosclerotic progression.[7-9]

In an effort to deal with these limitations of transluminal angioplasty, researchers proposed the concept of intravascular stents as a means of maintaining vessel patency against the restenotic process, as well as improving the clinical outcome of balloon angioplasty. Since

Dotter first reported his successful deployment of intravascular stents in canine femoral and popliteal arteries in 1969,[10] a variety of stent devices composed of various materials have been introduced.[11-14] Intravascular stenting is recognized as a potentially effective modality in overcoming elastic recoil of the arterial wall, stabilizing intimal dissection at the site of angioplasty, and maintaining the luminal patency of arteries with calcified and eccentric atherosclerotic plaques.

CLASSIFICATION OF AORTOILIAC OCCLUSSIVE DISEASE

The 2007 Trans-Atlantic Inter-Society Consensus (TASC II) guidelines were developed to assist physicians in the prevention and management of peripheral arterial disease.[15] The classification of inflow of aortoiliac lesions was updated in 2007 to reflect the advances in endovascular technology. General guidelines included in the TASC II document state that lesions classified as TASC A (Table 22-1) should be treated preferentially with endovascular techniques, whereas lesions classified as TASC D should be treated preferentially with open surgery. Lesions classified as TASC B or C have less clear recommendations. Good surgical judgment including surgical experience, available technology, and patient overall health needs to be considered when deciding on the appropriate initial treatment plan.

GENERAL PRINCIPLES OF ENDOLUMINAL STENTS

The desired characteristics of an intravascular stent depend on the anatomic placement and lesion characteristic for which it will be used. In general, the optimal stent needs to be encased in a low-profile device to cross high-grade lesions, and the stent should be deployed easily and accurately. Flexibility and durability are important characteristics that need to be combined with a low thrombogenic nature and high radial force. Moreover, the stent should have noticeable radiographic opacity to facilitate visualization. Finally, the ideal stent would be

TABLE 22-1 TransAtlantic Inter-Society Consensus II: Morphologic Stratification of Iliac Lesions

Type	Definition	Treatment Choice
A	Unilateral or bilateral stenoses of CIA Unilateral or bilateral single short (<3 cm) stenosis of EIA	Endovascular
B	Short (≤3 cm) stenosis of infrarenal aorta Unilateral CIA occlusion Single or multiple stenosis totaling 3-10 cm involving the EIA not extending into the CFA Unilateral EIA occlusion not involving the origins of internal iliac or CFA	Endovascular preferred
C	Bilateral CIA occlusions Bilateral EIA stenoses 3-10 cm long, not extending into CFA for good-risk patients Unilateral EIA stenosis extending into the CFA Unilateral EIA occlusion that involves the origins of the internal iliac and/or CFA Heavily calcified unilateral EIA occlusion with or without involvement of origins if internal iliac and/or CFA	Open surgery preferred
D	Infrarenal aortoiliac occlusion Diffuse disease involving the aorta and both iliac arteries requiring treatment Diffuse multiple stenoses involving the unilateral CIA, EIA, and CFA Unilateral occlusions of both CIA and EIA Bilateral occlusions of EIA Iliac stenosis in patients with AAA requiring treatment and not amendable to endograft placement or other lesions requiring open aorta or iliac surgery	Open surgery

CIA, Common iliac artery; *EIA,* external iliac artery; *CFA,* common femoral artery; *AAA,* abdominal aortic aneurysm.

TABLE 22-2 Characteristics of Stents

Self-Expanding	Balloon-Expandable	Covered Stent
Flexible	Rigid	Flexible
Low radial force	High radial force	Low radial force
Longer lengths	More effective at short lengths	Longest lengths available
Covering sheath in delivery system	Premounted on a balloon	Sheath or balloon premounted
Shortening is variable	Some shortening	Minimal shortening
Nitinol frame	Steel frame	Nitinol or steel frame
Radiopacity is low	Radiopacity is moderate	Radiopacity is moderate
Less accurate placement	Accurate placement	Variable accuracy

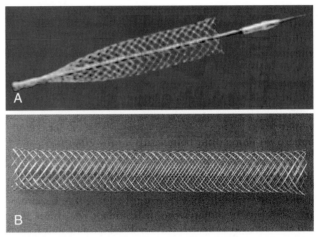

FIGURE 22-1 ■ A, Deployment of the Wallstent is achieved by withdrawing the constraining sheath. **B,** The fully deployed Wallstent.

biocompatible, to promote endothelialization without causing intimal hyperplasia.

Intravascular stents can be separated into three distinct types: self-expanding stents, balloon-expandable stents, and covered stents (Table 22-2). Within each of these categories, there are numerous stents with different structural materials, deployment devices, and biocompatible characteristics.[11,12,16-19] In addition, there are many stents undergoing clinical trials. However, the Wallstent (Schneider, Minneapolis, Minn.), the Palmaz stent (Cordis, Warren, N.J.), the Medtronic Vascular Complete SE Vascular Stent System (Medtronic Vascular, Santa Rosa, Calif.), the Express LD Iliac Premounted Stent System (Boston Scientific Corp, Natick, Mass.), the E-LUMINEXX Vascular Stent (Bard Peripheral Vascular, Tempe, Ariz.), the Zilver Vascular Stent (Cook,

Bloomington, Ind.), the S.M.A.R.T. Nitinol Stent System (Cordis, Miami Lakes, Fla.), the Viabahn endoprosthesis (W.L. Gore, Flagstaff, Ariz.) have been approved by the U.S. Food and Drug Administration (FDA) specifically for iliac artery placement.

Self-Expanding Stents

Self-expanding stents are generally manufactured so that the stents are constrained within a delivery sheath. The prosthesis is placed intravascularly through an introducer sheath that is advanced over a guidewire for deployment. Deployment is achieved by withdrawing the constraining sheath while keeping the stent in position, thus permitting the stent to self-expand and anchor to the vessel lumen (Figure 22-1). Stents in this category are generally noted for their ease of deployment and high degree of flexibility meandering around the curves typically found in an iliac artery. These characteristics are advantageous because they tend to be more forgiving if they are not placed exactly accurately. Compared with balloon-expandable stents, however, they may have lower hoop strength or radial force, which is the resistance to radial compression. These stents require oversizing by 2 to 3 mm to maintain outward radial force after deployment. Most delivery systems of self-expanding stents have a smaller diameter compared with those of balloon-expandable stents. Besides, the Wallstent and the Gianturco-Z stent (Cook, Bloomington, Ind.) are available.

Another type of self-expanding stent is the nitinol stent, which was first introduced by Dotter and colleagues in 1983.[20] Nitinol is a nickel-titanium alloy that has a unique temperature-associated memory property. The nitinol wires can be shaped into a coil spring configuration to serve as a stent when heated to 500°C. As it cools down to 0°C, the nitinol coil straightens into a linear alignment that can be constrained into a delivery catheter for stent deployment. The exposure to warm body temperature after deployment causes the nitinol stent to resume its original coil spring shape. Several clinical studies have evaluated the application of these stents in vascular occlusive lesions.[20-23] Common examples of nitinol stents include the Symphony stent (Boston Scientific Vascular, Watertown, Mass.), Cragg stent (Mintech, France, Elsenfeld, Germany), S.M.A.R.T. stent (Cordis, Miami, Fla.), and Memotherm stent (Bard/Angiomed, Karlsruhe, Germany).

Balloon-Expandable Stents

The balloon-expandable stent is first mounted and compressed onto an angioplasty balloon. The original stents were all operator mounted; newer stents are premounted by the manufacturer. Once the stent is positioned intraluminally, it is deployed by inflating the balloon to expand the stent (Figure 22-2). Unlike a self-expanding stent, the balloon-expandable stent can be expanded further by a larger angioplasty balloon catheter beyond its predetermined diameter. Most balloon-expandable stents are characterized by excellent hoop strength owing to intrinsic stent rigidity once deployed, which can be advantageous in treating stenotic vessels containing calcified plaques. The rigid property of such a stent, however, can create a technical dilemma when treating lesions in tortuous vessels. Moreover, it makes a contralateral approach for iliac artery stenting a challenge, although newer stents are more trackable and flexible. Commonly used examples of balloon-expandable stents include the Palmaz stent (Johnson and Johnson Interventional

Systems, Warren, N.J.), Strecker stent (Boston Scientific Vascular, Watertown, Mass.), Gianturco-Roubin stent (Cook, Bloomington, Ind.), Ave stent (Arterial Vascular Engineering, Santa Rosa, Calif.), Absolute Stent (Medtronic, San Diego, Calif.), and Intrastent (Intratherapeutics, Minneapolis, Minn).

Covered Stents

The first covered stent approved by the FDA for the use in the iliac system is the Gore Viabahn (Gore, Flagstaf, Ariz.). It is a flexible Nitinol stent lined with expanded polytetrafluoroethylene. The Nitinol flexibility, as in self-expanding stents, allows it to conform to the vessel shape closely. In addition, it has a heparin-bioactive surface providing a thromboresistent surface. It is important to conduct predeployment percutaneous transluminal angioplasty (PTA) of the affected area with subsequent coverage of the entire PTA-treated area with the covered stent. This stent is deployed by untwisting the screw-connector at the base of the deployment knob and slowly pulling the knob away from the adapter. In the Gore Viabahn Endoprosthesis Feasibility Study, 45 limbs in 42 subjects were treated for iliac artery occlusive disease.[24] This was the first-generation endoprosthesis without the heparin bioactive surface. There was a 12-month primary patency of 86% and a procedural success rate of 93%.

The Advanta V12 (Atrium, Australia/Pacific, Ulfimo, New South Whales, Australia) balloon-expandable polytetrafluoroethylene-covered stent is mounted in a stainless steel frame and comes in diameters suitable for the treatment in iliac arteries. It is not approved by the FDA, but is widely used in other countries to treat iliac occlusive disease. The United States version of the Advanta is the iCast stent (Atrium, Hudson, N.H.), which is currently approved for tracheobronchial lesions and is presently being evaluated for use in the treatment of iliac artery occlusive disease.

The main argument for the use of a covered stent rather than an uncovered stent is that the layer material will provide a direct barrier to tissue ingrowth from neo-intima hyperplasia.[25] However, restenosis can develop at the edges not coverd by graft material where intima injury may have occurred.[26,27]

Interim results from the Covered versus Balloon Expandable Stent Trial conducted in Australia have provided excellent results for challenging aortoiliac occlusive disease.[28] Patients with classification of TASC B, C, or D in the iliac level were randomized to the Advanta V12 group versus a bare metal stent group. They were followed with duplex ultrasound at various intervals and freedom from stent occlusion was assessed. The covered stent group had significantly lower restenosis rate and greater freedom from stent occlusion than the bare metal stent group. The covered stent also showed superiority when treating TASC C and D lesions.

INDICATIONS FOR STENT PLACEMENT

Indications approved by the FDA for iliac stent placement include stenotic or occlusive atherosclerotic lesions

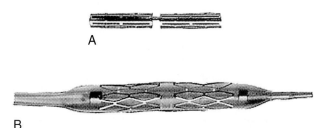

FIGURE 22-2 ■ **A,** The Palmaz stent is crushed to a small caliber and mounted on an angioplasty balloon. Sizes most commonly used for iliac interventions are already premounted by the manufacturer. **B,** The Palmaz stent is deployed by inflating the angioplasty balloon.

BOX 22-1	Indications to Intravascular Stent Placement

- Residual stenosis of 30% or greater
- Unstable intimal flaps
- Dissection
- Transstenotic pressure gradient of 10 mm Hg or greater
- Early restenosis following percutaneous transluminal angioplasty
- Nearly or totally occluded iliac arteries
- Ulcerative plaques
- When combined with an infrainguinal bypass operation

BOX 22-2	Contraindications to Intravascular Stent Placement

- Arterial perforation with contrast extravasation in the target vessel (covered stent may treat this complication)
- Severely calcified vessels
- Marked vessel tortuosity (not a contraindication for Wallstent placement)
- Target lesions cross areas of flexion, such as the inguinal ligament, knee, or shoulder
- Coexistent aneurysmal disease requiring surgical intervention
- Successful balloon angioplasty
- Presence of hypercoagulable disorder
- Long-standing arterial occlusion
- Target vessels that may serve as the proximal or distal site of a bypass grafting procedure

---

or failed or inadequate balloon angioplasty in the iliac artery (Box 22-1). The latter condition can be assessed by angiography, intravascular ultrasound (IVUS), or hemodynamic means. Angiographic or IVUS detection of residual stenosis of 30% or greater, unstable intimal flaps, and dissection along the subintimal or medial layers are all considered inadequate angioplasty results that warrant intraluminal stent placement. Furthermore, a transstenotic pressure gradient of 10 mm Hg or greater following angioplasty is considered an indication for iliac stent placement. Provocative testing using pharmacologic agents that stimulate vasodilatation may be necessary to identify a hemodynamically significant lesion. Up to 75% of patients without a translesion pressure gradient will have a significant gradient following injection of a vasodilator. Either 100 to 200 μg/mL of nitroglycerin or 30 to 60 mg of papaverine can be injected directly into the vessel in question. Immediate arterial dilatation is induced, thus mimicking exercise. A pressure drop of 10 mm Hg or more is considered indicative of a hemodynamically significant stenosis.

In addition to the FDA-approved indications for iliac artery stenting, certain other arterial conditions may be considered for stent placement. In the case of early restenosis following balloon angioplasty, stent placement is appropriate rather than repeated angioplasty alone. The 2-year patency rate of the iliac artery following angioplasty is between 65% and 81% and is affected by numerous factors, such as the degree of stenosis, the length of narrowing, and the distal vessel patency.[3,29,30] Restenosis of the iliac artery frequently occurs at the original angioplasty site,[7,9,11,31] which can be caused by neointimal hyperplasia or rapid atherosclerotic progression. Iliac artery stenting in such a condition can delay the restenotic process.

Primary stent placement, as opposed to stenting following inadequate angioplasty, has been used more frequently in the treatment of difficult iliac lesions. Nearly or totally occluded iliac arteries may be appropriate for primary stenting because angioplasty alone in these situations generally yields poor long-term patency rates.[14,32-36] Stenotic iliac vessels with ulcerative plaques can cause distal embolization when treated with balloon angioplasty.[6,37] It is appropriate to perform primary stent placement in such a condition to prevent plaque

dislodgment. Moreover, primary stenting can be used as an adjunct procedure to improve iliac inflow when combined with a planned infrainguinal bypass operation.[38-40] A randomized controlled trial comparing primary stent placement versus primary angioplasty followed by selective stent placement found similar cumulative patency at 2 years (71% vs. 70%, respectively; $p = 0.6$).[41] The authors concluded that because angioplasty followed by selective stent placement is less expensive than primary stent placement, the former seems to be the treatment of choice for intermittent claudication owing to iliac artery occlusive disease.

CONTRAINDICATIONS TO STENT PLACEMENT

Box 22-2 summarizes the contraindications for intravascular stent placement. Arterial perforation as a result of balloon angioplasty, as evidenced by contrast extravasation, is considered a contraindication for intraarterial stent placement. Stent placement in such a condition can lead to severe hemorrhagic complications or pseudoaneurysm formation. In these challenging situations, placement of a covered stent may be more appropriate.[42,43] Stent placement should also be avoided in aneurysmal arteries, because persistent blood flow around the stent can lead to further aneurysm expansion unless a covered stent is used. Because balloon-expandable stents, such as the Palmaz stent, are relatively rigid, they are less than ideal in tortuous vessels. Self-expanding stents, such as the Wallstent, have greater flexibility and are more appropriate in vessels with marked tortuosity. Severely calcified arteries often are not amenable to balloon angioplasty; similarly, stent placement should not be expected to restore the normal vessel lumen, because stent deployment requires the same basic techniques as balloon angioplasty. Long-standing arterial occlusion is considered a relative contraindication to stent placement. In this setting, the risk of plaque embolization resulting from stent expansion may outweigh the potential benefit of arterial recanalization. Finally, stent deployment

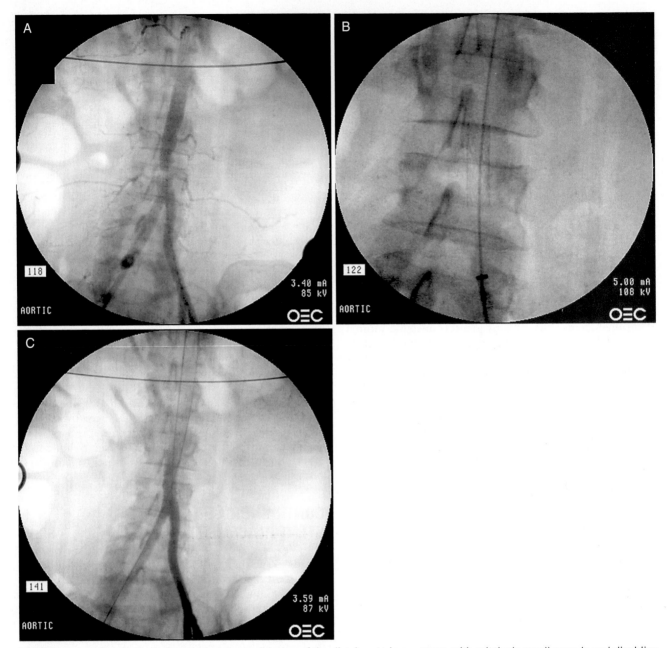

FIGURE 22-3 ■ **A,** Focal atherosclerotic "apple core" lesion of the distal aorta in a woman with relatively small vessels and disabling claudication. A pressure gradient of 50 mm Hg existed across the lesion. **B,** Unilateral femoral access was gained, and a balloon-expandable stent was placed across the lesion. **C,** Follow-up imaging demonstrates no residual stenosis, with no further pressure gradient measures.

should be avoided in arteries that might serve as either the proximal or distal site of a bypass grafting procedure. In a stented artery, application of vascular clamps might not only cause significant damage to the arterial wall, but also crush the stent so that reexpansion is impossible. If vascular control is needed in a stented artery, intraluminal occlusion balloon catheter should be used rather than vascular clamps.

AORTOILIAC OCCLUSIVE DISEASE

In the infrarenal aorta, short segment stenoses can occur that are unrelated to the bifurcation. Atherosclerotic occlusive disease is the cause in the vast majority of cases. Primary stent implantation for the endovascular treatment of such focal atherosclerotic stenoses has demonstrated in small studies to be technically feasible, relatively easy to perform, and with satisfactory midterm results (Figure 22-3).[44-46] These patients usually exhibit disabling claudication and are between 30 and 70 years of age. The disease may be a focal infrarenal stenosis or, more commonly, involve the origins of the common iliac arteries.

The spectrum of symptoms is commonly referred to as the *Leriche syndrome*, a combination of diminished or absent femoral pulses, thigh and buttock claudication, and erectile dysfunction in men. Women may exhibit these types of lesions because of the intrinsically small caliber of their vessels. Female patients tend to be younger, be heavy smokers, and have elevated lipid levels. Alternatively, distal embolization presenting as blue toe syndrome may be the first manifestation of disease.

In patients deemed appropriate for intervention, non-invasive studies to determine the physiologic nature of the obstruction and angiography (conventional, MRA, or computed tomographic angiography) are valuable in analyzing the extent of the lesion and planning appropriate treatment. The type of lesion, patient characteristics, concomitant comorbidities, and acuteness of symptoms are all factors to consider in choosing percutaneous therapy versus surgical modalities. Percutaneous techniques are a viable alternative to major surgical reconstruction, with lower costs, morbidity, and mortality. Evaluation of aortic lesions with IVUS and subsequent evaluation after stent deployment has improved long-term clinical outcome of balloon angioplasty and stented aortic lesions.[47]

AORTIC STENOSIS

Techniques used for angioplasty, with or without stenting, of the aorta and iliac segments are similar. Although PTA has demonstrated excellent results in focal stenoses of the abdominal aorta and iliacs, primary stenting may reduce the degree of restenosis with PTA alone and decrease distal embolization, especially if there is significant irregularity on the vessel surface and a substantial amount of plaque.[32,35,43,46,48-50] Focal aortic stenoses are treated by mounting a balloon-expandable stent on a larger-caliber angioplasty balloon or using a large self-expanding stent. When using a balloon-expandable stent, the operator should consider passing a sheath and dilator through the lesion to avoid dislodgement of the stent off the balloon by the lesion. Often the stent is initially mounted on a smaller balloon and then serially dilated until the angiographic result or hemodynamic gradient is improved. In addition, a heavily calcified lesion has a high risk of rupture if it is aggressively dilated, and a self-expanding stent may be the safer option. Self-expanding stents have a large diameter relative to the size of the sheath; therefore a larger self-expanding stent than a balloon-expandable stent will fit through the same sheath. As a result, the length of the lesion to be covered needs to be carefully measured, and the operator must be familiar with the behavior of these stents. The role of covered stents, such as cuffs made for endoluminal abdominal aortic aneurysm repair, needs more rigorous study.

The aortic diameter should be sized with a calibrated catheter, with IVUS, or by preintervention computed tomographic scanning to avoid undersizing. Balloon size usually ranges between 12 and 18 mm. A single stent is generally required in most cases, with no special technical requirements. Large Palmaz-type stents (Palmaz XXL) have been used successfully and can be inflated up to 25 mm in diameter. Concentric aortic stenosis may encroach on the inferior mesenteric artery; coverage of this vessel may be unavoidable. Furthermore, only midabdominal aortic lesions should be treated in this fashion. Different techniques (described later) are used when the lesion involves the aortic bifurcation. For focal aortic stenoses, the technical success, safety, and adequate patency rates have been reported with primary stent placement.[35,45,46,51,52] Durability appears satisfactory in properly selected patients.

ILIAC STENOSIS OR OCCLUSION

Patients with iliac lesions exhibit a wide spectrum of symptoms, depending on the amount of involvement of the iliac arteries, whether the lesions are focal or multisegmental, and the degree of infrainguinal disease. Indications for intervention are severe disabling claudication, rest pain, tissue loss, or blue toe syndrome. Individual risk factors and possible adverse outcomes associated with each procedure must also be taken into consideration when deciding on the best treatment option. Initially, iliac artery angioplasty with subsequent stent placement was used for only focal lesions; however, with technologic advances, more complex multisegmental lesions are now approached endoluminally with varied results.

RESULTS OF ILIAC ANGIOPLASTY AND STENTING

Multiple studies have documented excellent results following both focal and complex iliac artery stenting procedures, with most reporting superior results over angioplasty alone (Figures 22-4 and 22-5).* In a large, representative systematic review by Bosch and Hunink,[61] technical success with angioplasty alone was 91%; with stent placement, it was 96%. This report of more than 2100 patients compared the PTA cohort (n = 1300) with the stent cohort (n = 816) and demonstrated similar complication rates between the two groups; however, the patients with stents had improved long-term patency rates. When performed for claudication, 4-year primary patency rates were 65% for stenosis and 54% for occlusion after angioplasty, versus 77% for stenosis and 61% for occlusion after stenting. The rate differential was similar, although the overall percentages were lower, when procedures were performed for critical limb ischemia. Statistical analysis showed a 39% reduction in long-term failure after stent placement compared with PTA.

As seen in Table 22-2, there is currently no consensus about the best treatment for moderately severe iliac artery lesions (TASC type B and C lesions). In a review of their experience with percutaneous and surgical treatment of these complex iliac lesions, Timaran and colleagues[29] evaluated the primary outcome of patency and also analyzed potential variables that may preclude successful revascularization.[29] At all time points (1, 3, and 5 years), patients with surgical reconstruction (n = 52) had higher patency rates than patients with stents (n = 136). Poor runoff was the only independent predictor of

---

*References 13, 14, 22, 29, 32, 39, and 53-62.

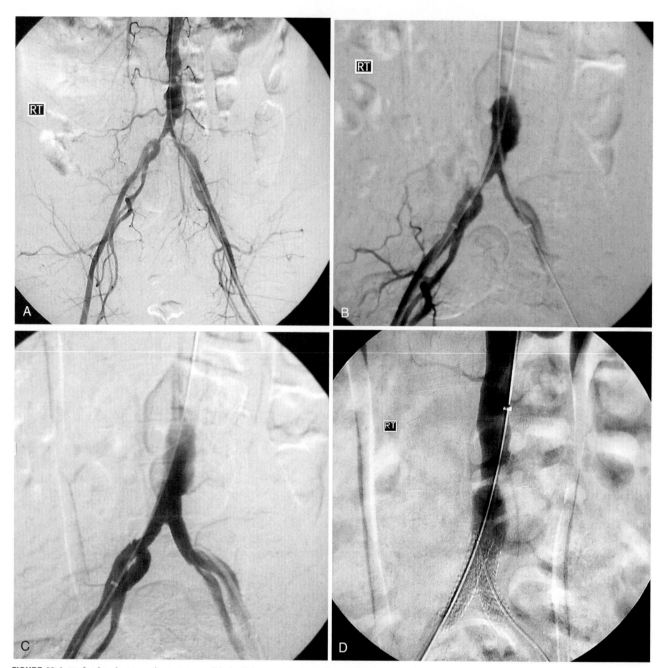

FIGURE 22-4 ■ **A,** Angiogram in a man with Leriche syndrome demonstrates focal atherosclerotic disease at the distal aorta and proximal common iliac arteries. **B,** Bilateral percutaneous femoral access was obtained with placement of 6-French sheaths. **C,** Initial improved result after angioplasty of the common iliac arteries. **D,** Completion angiogram after deployment of bilateral "kissing" balloon-expandable stents.

primary failure in either cohort. Furthermore, in patients with poor runoff, iliac stenting was associated with inferior outcomes compared with surgical reconstruction. This finding has been supported by other studies of either surgical or endovascular interventions.[55,63,64] In a review of the treatment of TASC type D lesions, the most severe type, Ballard and colleagues[64] found that ipsilateral superficial femoral artery obstruction was also an independent predictor of both stent and bypass graft failure.

The endovascular management of complex iliac artery occlusions targeting TASC C and D lesions was evaluated by Leville and colleagues.[62] They reported on 89

patients with symptomtic iliac occlusions classified as TASC B, C, or D. Twenty-four percent of the patients in the TASC C and D groups required hybrid procedures with femoral artery endarterectomy and patch angioplasty and half required multiple access sites. However, the 3-year primary patency was 76%, and secondary patency was 90% with a 97% limb salvage rate. The authors concluded that complex iliac occlusions can be treated safely with endovascular means with results comparable to open reconstruction.

In most gender-based comparisons, women have inferior results following iliac stent placement compared with

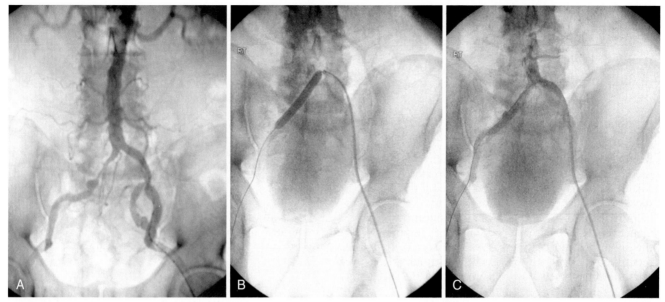

FIGURE 22-5 ■ **A,** High-grade lesion of the right common iliac artery. **B,** Access from the contralateral femoral artery was used for initial angioplasty. **C,** Results after balloon angioplasty, with no apparent residual stenosis. The patient went on to have a self-expanding stent placed across the lesion (not shown).

their male counterparts.[64-66] Conversely, in a retrospective study of 44 women having iliac angioplasty compared with men matched for comorbidities, female gender was not a negative predictor of outcome. Although women in this series had smaller vessels and a higher incidence of pretreatment total occlusion, no statistically significant difference existed in 2-year primary patency, percutaneous primary-assisted patency, or limb salvage rates. However, stent placement was not performed in these patients. Perhaps the use of stents in smaller vessels in women should be limited. Full critical evaluation awaits future randomized prospective trials or larger retrospective series or registries.

CHRONIC TOTAL OCCLUSION OF THE ILIAC ARTERY

The use of endovascular techniques to treat stenotic common and external iliac arteries is well established.* However, endovascular techniques for chronic total occlusions of these arteries continue to be described. Recanalization of the common and external iliac arteries has many challenges, but likely the most important is crossing the lesion safely, particularly in the area of the aortic bifurcation. This is often achieved through subintimal recanalization. In recent years, this specific technique has been shown to be achieved with the new so-called reentry devices such as the Pioneer catheter (Medtronics, Minneapolis, Minn.) or the Outback catheter (Cordis, Miami, Fla.).

APPROACHES TO COMMON AND EXTERNAL ILIAC ARTERY OCCLUSIONS

Approaches for complete occlusions of the iliac artery include using the contralateral or ipsilateral iliac artery in a retrograde manner or the transbrachial artery technique. When using the contralateral retrograde crossover approach, a curved catheter can be used to approach the occlusion by engaging the stump of the common iliac artery. At this point, a stiff hydrophilic 0.035-inch wire can be used to cross the occlusion followed by percutaneous balloon angioplasty and stenting. This approach has the disadvantage that there is minimal support from the catheter; therefore there might not be enough support to successfully cross the lesion. In addition, this approach may not adequately align the balloon and stent with the aortic bifurcation leaving suboptimal results. Finally, it may also impede the use of any reentry devices because of the angulation.

The transbrachial approach, usually from the left brachial artery, has several advantages including improved support, pushability, and a straight approach to the involved iliac artery. Disadvantages include the need to use longer sheaths (at least 90 cm) to reach the aortic bifurcation, the risk of cerebral embolization, and limited sheath size (maximum recommended size of 6 French). However, as technology continues to improve, more devices, catheters, balloons, and stents become available at lower profiles.

The ipsilateral retrograde iliac artery approach may be a difficult access site because it is distal to the occlusion in a pulseless femoral artery. Ultrasound as well as fluoroscopy combined with road-mapping may be necessary to cannulate the pulseless femoral artery. In addition, subintimal recanalization may be taken too far into the aorta and a retrograde dissection may be created with serious consequences. Therefore this approach may be the least desirable to recanalize the occluded iliac artery. Of course, confirmation or entry back into the true arterial lumen should be performed either with contrast visualization or IVUS.

REENTRY DEVICES

Reentry devices such as the Pioneer catheter (Medtronics, Minneapolis, Minn.) or the Outback catheter (Cordis, Miami, Fla.) may occasionally be needed if there is not a successful reentry into nondiseased artery. These devices help by saving time and avoiding complications if other maneuvers have been unsuccessful. More importantly, if the subintimal space is excessively dissected, then the reentry device will not work as well or at all. Therefore the subintimal space must remain tight for the successful use of a reentry device.

The Outback catheter has an external marker to help orient the needle into the lumen using fluoroscopy. The Pioneer catheter uses IVUS technology to guide the reentry needle toward the true lumen. Once the needle is in the true lumen, a 0.014-inch wire may be advanced, and the reentry catheter is removed and angioplasty and stenting can be conducted as planned.

Multiple small series report success and rapid reentry times (routinely less than 3 minutes) with both catheters.[67,68] In addition, they report no patients requiring conversion to open surgery. And most authors believe that this technology has opened the endovascular world to TASC C and D lesions, which otherwise would require management with open surgical approaches. However, the utility and success of these devices involves a learning curve and they should be considered as adjuncts not primary procedures.

COMPLICATIONS OF INTRALUMINAL STENT PLACEMENT

The complication profile is similar for either aortic or iliac interventions (Box 22-3). Because the deployment of a balloon-expandable stent requires the physical mounting of the stent on a balloon catheter, accidental dislodgment of the stent from the catheter delivery system may occur. Similar complications occur that are nonspecific for percutaneous procedures, including those related to puncture sites, arterial dissection, and vessel rupture. Unlike with self-expanding stents, which constantly exert an outward radial force, external compression on balloon-expandable stents owing to vascular clamping injury can result in permanent stent deformity. Although short-term failure is mainly due to thrombosis in the stented vessel, long-term patency can be adversely affected by restenosis induced by intimal hyperplasia. Factors associated with stented artery thrombosis are iliac artery occlusion, multiple stent deployment, and hypercoagulable disorders. Stent placement in an occluded iliac artery is particularly prone to restenosis, in part because of the lack of an endothelial lining in the occluded vessel. Stent

| BOX 22-3 | Complications Associated with Intravascular Stent Placement |

- Local complications
- Hematoma
- Pseudoaneurysm
- Arteriovenous fistula
- Plaque distal embolization
- Stent dislodgment in delivery system
- Stent migration and embolization
- Stent misplacement
- Contrast allergic reaction
- Vessel perforation
- Side branch occlusion
- Accelerated intimal hyperplasia
- Extrinsic compression of stent
- Stent infection

deployment may further denude the intimal lining, thereby reducing the protective antithrombotic function of endothelium. In addition, the incidence of distal embolization following the stent placement is 2.4% to 7.8%.[37] As with all radiographic interventions, transient contrast-induced nephropathy can occur after an interventional procedure.

CONCLUSIONS

Intravascular stent placement has proved to be an invaluable tool in both the primary treatment of aortoiliac occlusive disease and the management of complications of balloon angioplasty. Clinical application of iliac stents has also extended to the treatment of patients with total iliac occlusion and restenosis. Although balloon angioplasty has met with limited success in treating totally occluded iliac arteries, the use of intravascular stents has improved the success rate to approximately 80% at 3 years, with a late occlusion rate similar to that of stenotic lesions. The benefit of primary stenting of the iliac artery has been demonstrated in several series, with a favorable 5-year patency rate of greater than 90%, which is comparable to conventional surgical reconstruction. The primary weakness of intravascular stenting is the induction of intimal hyperplasia leading to restenosis. The incidence of restenosis within 1 year of stent placement has been shown to be greater than 20%. There are many areas for future research to focus on in an attempt to solve this dilemma including covered stent technology. Promising techniques, including the use of drug-eluting stents, vascular brachytherapy, cutting balloons, and aggressive antiplatelet regimens, are being tested to improve clinical outcomes.[69-75]

BIBLIOGRAPHY

Ballard JL, Bergan JJ, Singh P, et al: Aortoiliac stent deployment versus surgical reconstruction: analysis of outcome and cost. J Vasc Surg 28:94–101, 1998.
Brewster DC: Current controversies in the management of aortoiliac occlusive disease. J Vasc Surg 25:365–379, 1997.

Dotter CT, Judkins MP: Transluminal treatment of arteriosclerotic obstruction: description of a new technique and a preliminary report of its application. Circulation 30:654–670, 1964.

Greiner A, Dessl A, Klein-Weigel P, et al: Kissing stents for treatment of complex aortoiliac disease. Eur J Vasc Endovasc Surg 26:161–165, 2003.

Harnek J, Zoucas E, Stenram U, et al: Insertion of self-expandable nitinol stents without previous balloon angioplasty reduces restenosis compared with PTA prior to stenting. Cardiovasc Intervent Radiol 25:430–436, 2002.

Martin D, Katz SG: Axillofemoral bypass for aortoiliac occlusive disease. Am J Surg 180:100–103, 2000.

Mohamed F, Sarkar B, Timmons G, et al: Outcome of "kissing stents" for aortoiliac atherosclerotic disease, including the effect on the non-diseased contralateral iliac limb. Cardiovasc Intervent Radiol 25:472–475, 2002.

Murphy TP, Ariaratnam NS, Carney WI, Jr, et al: Aortoiliac insufficiency: long-term experience with stent placement for treatment. Radiology 231:243–249, 2004.

Norgren L, Hiatt WR, Dormandy JA, Nehler MR, et al: Inter-society consensus for the management of peripheral arterial disease (TASCII). J Vasc Surg 45(Suppl S):S5–67, 2007.

Schneider JR, Besso SR, Walsh DB, et al: Femorofemoral versus aortobifemoral bypass: outcome and hemodynamic results. J Vasc Surg 19:43–55, 1994.

Stoeckelhuber BM, Meissner O, Stoeckelhuber M, et al: Primary endovascular stent placement for focal infrarenal aortic stenosis: initial and midterm results. J Vasc Interv Radiol 14:1443–1447, 2003.

Tetteroo E, van der Graaf Y, Bosch JL, et al: Randomised comparison of primary stent placement versus primary angioplasty followed by selective stent placement in patients with iliac-artery occlusive disease. Dutch Iliac Stent Trial Study Group. Lancet 351:1153–1159, 1998.

Timaran CH, Prault TL, Stevens SL, et al: Iliac artery stenting versus surgical reconstruction for TASC (TransAtlantic Inter-Society Consensus) type B and type C iliac lesions. J Vasc Surg 38:272–278, 2003.

Timaran CH, Stevens SL, Freeman MB, et al: Infrainguinal arterial reconstructions in patients with aortoiliac occlusive disease: the influence of iliac stenting. J Vasc Surg 34:971–978, 2001.

Treiman GS, Schneider PA, Lawrence PF, et al: Does stent placement improve the results of ineffective or complicated iliac artery angioplasty? J Vasc Surg 28:104–112, 1998.

Waksman R: Vascular brachytherapy vs drug-eluting stents for the treatment of in-stent restenosis: the jury's still out. Catheter Cardiovasc Interv 62:290–291, 2004.

References available online at expertconsult.com.

QUESTIONS

1. All of the following are indications for stent placement except:
   a. Intimal dissection
   b. Residual stenosis greater than 15%
   c. Recurrent stenosis following angioplasty alone
   d. Symptomatic atherosclerotic iliac lesions

2. Which of the following statements about pharmacologic agents in angiography are true?
   a. They may induce peripheral vasodilatation that unmasks significant stenosis.
   b. Either papaverine or nitroglycerin may be used.
   c. They are injected directly into the intraarterial catheter or sheath in the vessel under investigation.
   d. They cause significant vasospasm.

3. Covered stents may be used in the iliac arteries in all of the following conditions except:
   a. Arteriovenous fistulas
   b. Vessel ruptures
   c. Aneurysms
   d. Mycotic aneurysms
   e. Atherosclerotic occlusive lesions

4. Complications of iliac stent placement include which of the following?
   a. Distal embolization
   b. Thrombosis
   c. Stent malposition
   d. Vessel rupture
   e. All of the above

5. The classic definition of Leriche syndrome consists of all of the following except:
   a. Decreased femoral pulses
   b. Blue toe syndrome
   c. Buttock claudication
   d. Impotence

6. Iliac stenting has been recommended as the primary treatment for which of the following lesions?
   a. TASC type A
   b. TASC type B
   c. TASC type C
   d. TASC type D

7. The outcome after stenting of which vessel most closely approximates surgical results?
   a. Common iliac artery
   b. External iliac artery
   c. Common femoral artery

8. Long-term patency of intravascular stents is limited by which of the following?
   a. Vessel size
   b. Neointimal hyperplasia
   c. Progression of atherosclerosis
   d. Stent durability

9. Complications common to percutaneous procedures include which of the following?
   a. Contrast-induced nephropathy
   b. Puncture site hematoma
   c. Vascular injury
   d. Nerve damage

10. All of the following are (relative) contraindications for intravascular stent placement except:
    a. Target area across from an area of flexion, such as the knee joint
    b. Arterial perforation with contrast extravasation
    c. Residual stenosis of 40% following balloon angioplasty
    d. Multisegmental iliac disease

ANSWERS

1. **b**
2. **a, b, c**
3. **d**
4. **e**
5. **b**
6. **a**
7. **a**
8. **b, c**
9. **a, b, c**
10. **c**

DIAGNOSIS AND SURGICAL MANAGEMENT OF THE VISCERAL ISCHEMIC SYNDROMES

Lewis B. Schwartz • Tina T. Ng • James F. McKinsey • Brian Funaki • Bruce L. Gewertz

Although the causal relationship between acute mesenteric vascular occlusion and intestinal gangrene had been known for centuries, it was not until 1895 that the first successful case of preoperative recognition and treatment by intestinal resection was reported by Elliot.[1] Recognition of the chronic form soon followed, with the term angina abdominis applied by Goodman to illustrate the similarities to the newly described angina pectoris.[2] Indisputable evidence was provided in 1936 by Dunphy,[3] a surgical resident at the Peter Bent Brigham Hospital in Boston who described the clinical course of a 47-year-old man with weight loss and periumbilical pain out of proportion to the findings on physical examination. The patient died suddenly in the hospital, and postmortem examination revealed chronic mesenteric disease with fresh thrombus completely occluding the celiac trunk. Dunphy reviewed 12 other deaths from mesenteric vascular occlusion and found an antecedent history of chronic recurrent abdominal pain in 7.

The first successful reports of mesenteric revascularization appeared in 1958.[4] In that year, Shaw and Maynard[4] from the Massachusetts General Hospital reported two cases of superior mesenteric artery (SMA) thrombosis superimposed on atherosclerotic occlusive disease. Both patients were treated with SMA thromboendarterectomy and survived. The surgeons made the astute observation that although the responsible atherosclerotic lesions involved all three mesenteric arteries, they were confined to the proximal segments, such that vascular reconstruction was technically feasible.

Since that time, intestinal ischemic disorders have been recognized as uncommon but clinically important causes of abdominal pain. Although their incidence is estimated at only a few cases per 100,000 population, their lethal nature requires vigilance and a high index of clinical suspicion to avoid catastrophe. This chapter reviews the pathophysiology, clinical presentation, and treatment of intestinal ischemic disorders.

VASCULAR ANATOMY

The mesenteric circulation consists primarily of three branches of the abdominal aorta (Figure 23-1): the celiac axis, the SMA, and the inferior mesenteric artery (IMA).

Their multiple branch points and interconnections form such a rich anastomotic network that compromise of two of the three major arteries is usually required for the development of chronic ischemic symptoms. Knowledge of the normal and variant anatomy is essential for surgical diagnosis and revascularization.

Celiac Axis

The celiac axis supplies the stomach, liver, spleen, portions of the pancreas, and the proximal duodenum. It originates from the ventral portion of the abdominal aorta, near the level of T12 to L1, between the diaphragmatic crura. Its origin is encased in the median arcuate ligament, a dense, fibrous portion of the central posterior diaphragm draped across the aortic hiatus. In most patients, the celiac axis branches soon after its origin into the common hepatic, splenic, and left gastric arteries. In 1% of cases, the SMA arises from the celiac axis as well, forming a common celiomesenteric trunk.

The hepatic artery is usually the first branch of the celiac axis. It may also arise from the SMA (the so-called replaced right hepatic artery) in approximately 12% of cases. Additional variants include the replaced common hepatic artery (approximately 2.5%) and direct origin of the common hepatic artery from the aorta (approximately 2%). The common hepatic artery gives rise to the right gastric artery and the gastroduodenal artery, which further divides into the right gastroepiploic and superior pancreaticoduodenal arteries. The remaining proper hepatic artery gives rise to the cystic, right hepatic, and left hepatic arteries, which serve the gallbladder, the right and caudate hepatic lobes, and the middle and left hepatic lobes, respectively.

The second branch of the celiac axis is the splenic artery. Its first named branch is the dorsal pancreatic artery, supplying the posterior body and tail of the pancreas. Just before entering the splenic hilum, the splenic artery gives rise to the left gastroepiploic artery and multiple short gastric arteries, providing blood flow to the gastric fundus.

The final branch of the celiac axis is the left gastric artery. It courses cephalad and to the left to supply the gastric cardia and fundus along the lesser curvature of the stomach, joining centrally with the right gastric artery from the hepatic artery. In approximately 12% of the

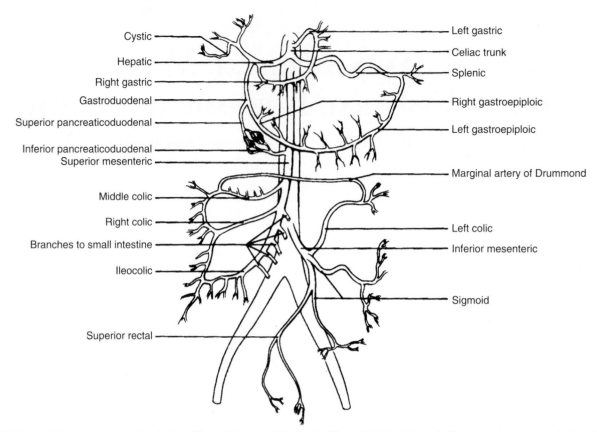

Cystic —
Hepatic —
Right gastric —
Gastroduodenal —
Superior pancreaticoduodenal —

Inferior pancreaticoduodenal —
Superior mesenteric —

Middle colic —
Right colic —
Branches to small intestine —
Ileocolic —

Superior rectal —

— Left gastric
— Celiac trunk
— Splenic

— Right gastroepiploic

— Left gastroepiploic

— Marginal artery of Drummond

— Left colic
— Inferior mesenteric

— Sigmoid

FIGURE 23-1 ■ The mesenteric circulation. (From Schwartz LB, Davis RD Jr, Heinle JS, et al: The vascular system. In Lyerly HK, Gaynor JW Jr, editors: The handbook of surgical intensive care, ed 3, St Louis, 1992, Mosby Year Book, p 287.)

population, the left hepatic artery originates from the left gastric artery.

Superior Mesenteric Artery

The SMA arises from the aorta just distal to the celiac axis at the level of L1 to L2. It passes behind the neck of the pancreas, in front of the uncinate process, and over the third portion of the duodenum. Its first branch, the inferior pancreaticoduodenal artery, courses superiorly to join the superior pancreaticoduodenal artery (from the gastroduodenal) and forms the most proximal collateral pathway with the celiac axis. The central branches of the SMA supply the midgut from the ligament of Treitz to the midtransverse colon. These include the middle colic (serving the proximal two thirds of the transverse colon), right colic (mid-ascending and distal ascending colon), and ileocolic (distal ileum, cecum, appendix, and proximal ascending colon).

Inferior Mesenteric Artery

The IMA arises from the left side of the aorta 8 to 10 cm distal to the SMA at the level of L3. It travels caudad and to the left before dividing into the left colic and sigmoid arteries. The IMA supplies the distal third of the transverse colon, the descending and sigmoid colons, and the proximal rectum. It has anastomotic communications with the left branch of the middle colic from the SMA

and with portions of the middle and inferior rectal arteries from the internal iliac.

Collateral Circulation

The mesenteric circulation has a redundant collateral network that serves to maintain perfusion even with compromise of the proximal main channels. The celiac axis and SMA communicate primarily via the superior and inferior pancreaticoduodenal arteries (via the gastroduodenal artery). The SMA and IMA communicate via the centrally located arch of Riolan (often referred to as the *meandering mesenteric artery*), as well as by the multiple communications at the periphery of the colon called the *marginal arteries of Drummond*. In addition to these collateral pathways, muscular branches of the aorta may contribute to intestinal perfusion, including the lumbar intercostal arteries, internal mammary arteries (via the deep epigastric arteries), middle sacral artery, and internal iliac arteries (via collaterals between the inferior and superior rectal arteries). Because of this plentiful collateral network, it is understandable that in most instances of gradual occlusion, at least two of the three major mesenteric orifices must be blocked to produce the clinical syndromes of chronic intestinal ischemia. In contrast, sudden occlusion of one widely patent vessel can cause acute ischemia because collaterals may be underdeveloped.

ACUTE ISCHEMIA

Pathophysiology

There are four primary causes of acute mesenteric ischemia (AMI): embolization to the SMA (approximately 50% of all cases), thrombosis of a preexisting atherosclerotic lesion at the origin of the vessel (20%), nonocclusive mesenteric ischemia (20%), and mesenteric venous thrombosis (10%).[5,6] In earlier series, the phenomenon of nonocclusive mesenteric ischemia was not well appreciated and was frequently misdiagnosed as acute venous occlusion. For example, Cokkinis[7] reported in 1935 that acute mesenteric venous thrombosis accounted for the majority of cases of AMI.

Other unusual arteriopathies, such as Takayasus arteritis, fibromuscular dysplasia, and polyarteritis nodosa, may first present with intestinal ischemia. Isolated dissections of the SMA also have been reported,[8] although the more common mechanism is extension of dissections of the descending thoracic aorta into the SMA and celiac axis.[9,10]

If untreated, intestinal ischemia commonly leads to intestinal infarction. Tissue loss may result from both hypoxia during flow interruption and reperfusion injury once intestinal arterial blood flow is restored. Reperfusion injury is principally mediated by activation of the enzyme xanthine oxidase and the recruitment and activation of circulating polymorphonuclear neutrophils (PMNs).[11,12] In the presence of oxygen and hypoxanthine (a by-product of adenosine triphosphate metabolism), xanthine oxidase produces oxygen-derived free radicals that cause severe local tissue injury through lipid peroxidation, membrane disruption, and increased microvascular permeability.[13] PMNs are attracted to reperfused tissue by the local secretion of cytokines (tumor necrosis factor-α, interleukin-1, platelet-derived growth factor) by ischemic endothelium.[14-16] Subsequent rolling, adherence, and activation of the PMNs in the microcirculation result in the secretion of myeloperoxidase, collagenases, and elastases that can further injure the already ischemic and vulnerable tissue.[17-19] Activation of the inflammatory cascade may also have systemic effects, with cardiac, pulmonary, and other organ system dysfunction.[20]

Acute Mesenteric Arterial Embolism

Most mesenteric arterial emboli originate from left atrial or ventricular mural thrombi or cardiac valvular lesions. These thrombi are usually associated with cardiac dysrhythmias such as atrial fibrillation or hypokinetic regions from previous myocardial infarctions. The majority of mesenteric emboli lodge in the SMA because of its high basal flow and nearly parallel course to the abdominal aorta. Only 15% of SMA emboli remain impacted at the origin of the vessel. The majority of emboli progress distally 3 to 10 cm to the tapered segment of the SMA just past the origin of the middle colic artery (Figure 23-2). A substantial fraction (10% to 15%) of mesenteric emboli are associated with concurrent emboli to another arterial bed.[21] Intestinal ischemia owing to embolic arterial occlusion can be compounded by reactive mesenteric

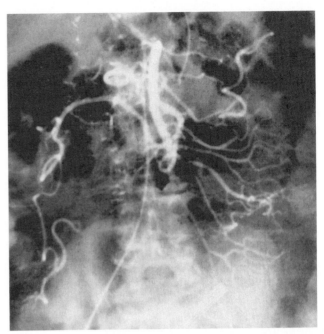

FIGURE 23-2 ■ Anteroposterior view of the aorta revealing embolic occlusion of the proximal superior mesenteric artery (SMA). Note the normal-appearing proximal jejunal arterial branches and then an abrupt cutoff of the SMA. (From McKinsey JF, Gewertz BL: Acute mesenteric ischemia. Surg Clin North Am 77:307–318, 1997.)

vasoconstriction, which further reduces collateral flow and aggravates the ischemic insult.

Acute Mesenteric Arterial Thrombosis

Thrombosis of the SMA or the celiac axis is usually associated with preexisting arterial lesions. When carefully questioned, many of these patients have histories consistent with chronic mesenteric ischemia (CMI), including postprandial pain, weight loss, "food fear," bloating, and early satiety. By far, the most common underlying lesion is an atherosclerotic plaque that slowly progresses to a critical stenosis over years, until the residual lumen suddenly thromboses during a period of low flow. Unlike embolic occlusions, thrombosis of the SMA generally occurs flush with the aortic origin of the vessel.

As noted previously, an unusual cause of AMI is aortic dissection involving the origins of the visceral vessels. The intimal flap of the dissection can exclude, compress, or extend into the visceral vessels, resulting in acute thrombosis. The symptoms of bowel ischemia may be masked by the pain associated with the aortic dissection, leading to a delay in diagnosis and treatment. AMI following coronary artery bypass grafts is rare but highly lethal, with mortality rates as high as 70%. As would be expected, ischemia occurs in patients with severely stenotic mesenteric vessels that occlude during the nonpulsatile perfusion of extracorporeal bypass.[22,23]

Nonocclusive Mesenteric Ischemia

Mesenteric ischemia unassociated with anatomic arterial or venous obstruction can occur during periods of low cardiac output. Such low-flow states can result from cardiac failure, sepsis, or administration of α-adrenergic agents or digitalis compounds. Although less common, mesenteric vasospasm can also follow elective revascularization procedures for chronic SMA occlusion, in which case vasoconstriction of small- and medium-size vessels is precipitated by early enteral feeding.[24] The older mean age of the population has produced a group of people with severe medical problems at risk for this type of mesenteric ischemia. The diagnosis is made at the time of angiography. Radiographic criteria suggesting the diagnosis include (1) narrowing of the origins of multiple branches of the SMA; (2) alternate dilatation and narrowing of the intestinal branches (the "string-of-sausages" sign); (3) spasm of the mesenteric arcades; and (4) impaired filling of the intramural vessels.[25] The mortality of this specific subset of patients is relatively high regardless of treatment, owing to the serious underlying medical conditions and the frequent delay in diagnosis.[26]

Mesenteric Venous Thrombosis

Mesenteric venous thrombosis (MVT) is thrombosis of the veins draining the intestine (inferior mesenteric, superior mesenteric, splenic, and portal veins). The obstruction in venous return leads to edema, distension, and eventual infarction of affected segments. Primary MVT is idiopathic, although given the improved understanding of predisposing conditions, the number of patients in this category is diminishing. Patients in whom a causative factor is identified are said to have secondary MVT. These factors include myriad clinical syndromes, including trauma, surgery, cancer, cirrhosis, pancreatitis, dehydration, and increasingly recognized hypercoagulable syndromes such as polycythemia vera, thrombocytosis, protein C and S deficiency, antithrombin III deficiency, antiphospholipid antibody syndrome, and factor V Leiden mutation (activated protein C resistance).[27]

Patients with MVT have a somewhat different presentation from those who have ischemia caused by arterial obstruction; the onset of symptoms may be insidious and the findings more subtle. Pain out of proportion to the physical examination is still an essential feature. The test of choice to confirm the diagnosis is contrast-enhanced computed tomography (CT), although duplex scanning and magnetic resonance imaging (MRI) are gaining popularity. Thrombus is located in the superior mesenteric vein in 70% of patients, with portal and inferior mesenteric vein thrombus found in about 30%.[28]

Symptomatic acute MVT is a lethal disease, with a 30-day mortality of about 25% and a 3-year survival of 35%.[28] Patients with evidence of chronic thrombosis fare somewhat better, because collateral venous channels form to augment intestinal venous drainage.

Clinical Presentation and Diagnosis

AMI can appear precipitously with decompensation over hours or insidiously with progression over days. Classic symptoms of AMI include sudden abdominal pain out of proportion to the physical examination, with gut emptying at the onset of pain. The subacute pattern of mesenteric ischemia is characterized by a more gradual development of vague abdominal signs and symptoms. These include less intense and nonspecific abdominal pains with nausea, vomiting, and changes in bowel habits. The abdomen may become distended but still have active bowel sounds.

Predictably, physical signs intensify as the syndrome progresses. In the early phases, signs of peritoneal irritation such as abdominal guarding and rebound are absent. As the bowel becomes more ischemic, necrosis progresses from the mucosal layers to the seromuscular layers. After full-thickness bowel infarction, the abdomen is often grossly distended, with absent bowel sounds and exquisite tenderness to palpation. Bowel infarction can impart a feculent odor to the breath.

Ancillary laboratory evaluations often reveal an increase in hemoglobin and hematocrit, consistent with hemoconcentration. There is a marked leukocytosis with a predominance of immature white blood cells (left shift). Although no specific laboratory findings are diagnostic, serum levels of amylase, lactic dehydrogenase, creatine phosphokinase, and alkaline phosphatase, singly or severally, are often elevated, along with a metabolic acidosis with a persistent base deficit.[29] Unfortunately, most of these abnormalities do not develop until after bowel necrosis has occurred.

Plain abdominal radiographs are used to exclude other potential causes of abdominal pain rather than confirm the diagnosis of AMI. In fact, completely normal plain abdominal films are seen in more than 25% of patients with mesenteric ischemia.[30] Subtle signs of AMI on plain abdominal films include a dynamic ileus and distended air-filled loops of bowel. Bowel wall thickening from submucosal edema or hemorrhage can be prominent, especially in cases of acute MVT. In advanced stages, pneumatosis of the bowel wall and portal vein gas portend an extremely poor prognosis.

Barium contrast evaluations of the upper and lower gastrointestinal tracts are contraindicated because residual intraluminal contrast material can limit visualization of the mesenteric vasculature during diagnostic angiography. On the rare occasion when barium studies are performed in a patient with the gradual development of abdominal pain, the submucosal edema and hemorrhage of intestinal ischemia are manifest by thickening of the bowel wall, strictures, or ulcerations.

Duplex ultrasonography may be of some benefit in visualizing flow in the SMA and celiac axis. With expert technical assistance, these tests can document proximal stenoses in the SMA or celiac axis or complete occlusion of these vessels.[31] In newer series, color Doppler ultrasonography has been shown to be a valuable screening tool for AMI; it is far more specific than clinical evaluation alone.[32,33] Unfortunately, a significant percentage of patients at risk for mesenteric ischemia have dilated air-filled loops of bowel that make ultrasonography difficult if not impossible.

CT of the abdomen and pelvis can delineate subtle changes consistent with subacute bowel ischemia such as focal or segmental bowel wall thickening.[34] Thrombus within the mesenteric veins or the lack of opacification of the veins after intravenous contrast administration is often seen in MVT.[35] Nonenhancement of the arterial vasculature with timed intravenous contrast injections can be noted in acute mesenteric arterial thrombosis or embolization. CT scans can also vividly demonstrate pneumatosis or portal vein gas.

Advances in contrast-enhanced and cine phase magnetic resonance angiography have allowed better visualization of the visceral vasculature and have a more important role in the diagnosis of AMI.[36] Specifically, when MRI is coupled with magnetic resonance oximetry, both anatomic and physiologic information regarding the mesenteric circulation can be obtained.[37]

Despite these aforementioned developments, the definitive diagnostic study remains mesenteric angiography via either CT angiography or catheter-based studies if the former is not available. Image manipulation (three-dimensional reconstruction) or multiple views are often needed for adequate assessment of the vessels at risk. The origins of the celiac axis and the SMA can be visualized only by lateral views, whereas the more distal celiac axis and SMA distributions are best viewed through anteroposterior projections. On occasion, selective cannulation of the origins of the celiac axis and SMA is often required to completely define the anatomy and pathophysiology. Thorough aortography is also needed to evaluate potential inflow and outflow sites for bypass grafts, as well as to clarify the extent and location of other atherosclerotic lesions in the iliac artery and the IMA.

In patients with nonocclusive ischemia, angiography usually reveals multiple areas of narrowing and irregularity in major branches. The small- and medium-size arterial branches may be decreased or absent, and the vasculature is diffusely pruned, with an absent submucosal "blush." In MVT, selective angiograms may demonstrate reflux of contrast material back into the aorta owing to extremely slow flow and heightened outflow resistance. A prolonged arterial phase with accumulation of contrast and thickened bowel walls is also characteristic. In extreme cases, angiographic contrast may extravasate into the bowel lumen, which is indicative of active bleeding. The definitive diagnosis of MVT is made during the venous phase; either a filling defect is noted within the portal vein or, in more severe cases, the entire venous phase is absent.

Treatment Options

Initial treatment of AMI includes volume resuscitation, correction of acidosis, and administration of appropriate antibiotics. Heparin anticoagulation should be started immediately to prevent further propagation of thrombus. A urinary catheter, as well as a peripheral arterial catheter, should be placed for monitoring intravascular volumes and hemodynamic status. A nasogastric tube should be placed to decrease the chance of aspiration.

Contrast-enhanced imaging studies, such as CT angiography, should be performed immediately. Although mesenteric angiography remains a definitive diagnostic tool, it is increasingly used in association with planned endovascular treatment. In select patients with an early diagnosis of SMA embolus unassociated with bowel

necrosis, a trial of thrombolytic therapy and angioplasty may be appropriate.[38,39] Such treatments are usually limited to patients with abdominal pain for less than 8 hours' duration without signs of peritoneal irritation. If lysis is not evident within 4 hours of commencing high-dose thrombolytic therapy, or if peritoneal signs develop, the infusion should be discontinued and immediate surgical exploration should be performed.

An increasing number of case reports and series have detailed the use of percutaneous angioplasty to dilate significant atherosclerotic plaques of the SMA that are unmasked by thrombolytic therapy.[40-42] Owing to the variable angle of the origin of the SMA from the aorta, placement and removal of the angioplasty catheter and stent placement may be more difficult than for lower extremity angioplasties.[10] Restenosis rates range from 25% to 50% in earlier series,[40,41] but the largest single-center retrospective review to date demonstrated more promising results. In a 9-year series of 70 patients with AMI, the Cleveland Clinic vascular group achieved an 87% success rate in endovascular treatment of AMI. Patients in the endovascular group were slightly older (65 ± 12 vs. 60 ± 13 years), were weighted with more thrombotic occlusion cases (72% vs. 64%), and had longer duration of symptoms (median, 62 vs. 26 hours). The primary mode of endovascular treatment was thrombolysis infusion; additional therapy included vasodilator (papaverine or nitroglycerin) therapy (51%), mechanical thrombectomy (12%), and PTA plus stent (33%). Successful endovascular therapy resulted in fewer laparotomies (69% vs. 100% in traditional therapy), lower rates of acute renal failure (27% vs. 50%) and pulmonary failure (27% vs. 64%), and lower mortality rates (36% vs. 50%).[43] Those who failed endovascular treatment had the same high 50% mortality rate as the open surgical group. Still, while endovascular therapy is increasingly used for AMI at major center, open surgical revascularization remains the predominant treatment across the United States.[44]

When an aortic dissection involves the origin of one or more of the visceral vessels, endovascular repairs have been attempted through stent placement[45,46] and balloon fenestration of the dissection septum.[47] Although such minimally invasive treatments are highly attractive, they are currently limited by the frequently rapid onset of ischemic symptoms, inability to gain access to the dissection channel, or the need for surgical repair of an associated aortic aneurysm.

Regardless of the cause, most patients with acute arterial occlusion require early surgical exploration and reestablishment of mesenteric flow to prevent or minimize bowel infarction. A generous midline incision should be made, and the extent of mesenteric ischemia and necrosis should be assessed. If the entire small bowel is frankly gangrenous, enterectomy with lifelong hyperalimentation is the only option. In many instances, patient preferences and family consultation may argue for simple abdominal closure with terminal pain relief as a more appropriate choice. If bowel infarction is not profound, surgical revascularization should be performed.

To achieve adequate exposure, the transverse colon is retracted superiorly, and the fourth portion of the

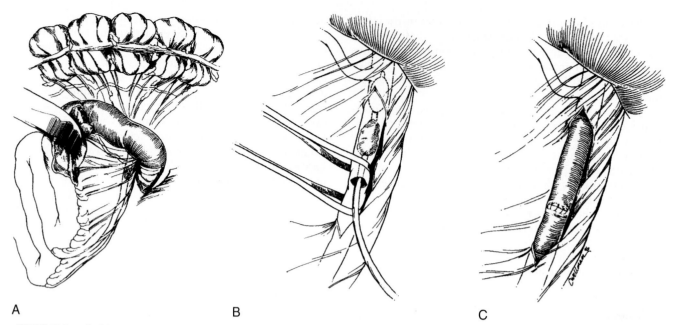

A B C

FIGURE 23-3 ■ **A,** Mobilization of the transverse colon and duodenum to expose the superior mesenteric artery. **B,** Balloon-tipped catheter extraction of a mesenteric embolus through a transverse arteriotomy. **C,** Primary closure of the arteriotomy without stricture. (From McKinsey JF, Gewertz BL: Acute mesenteric ischemia. Surg Clin North Am 77:307–318, 1997.)

duodenum is mobilized to the ligament of Treitz. The SMA is identified by palpation of the root of the mesentery. If the cause of mesenteric ischemia is an embolus, a more proximal SMA pulse is often noted. The SMA is encircled at or just distal to the level of obstruction (Figure 23-3A), and a transverse arteriotomy is made. Balloon-tipped embolectomy catheters are inserted retrograde, and the embolus is extracted (see Figure 23-3B). Embolectomy catheters should also be passed distally to ensure that no fragmentation of the clot or discontinuous thrombosis has occurred. Transverse arteriotomies are closed primarily with interrupted fine monofilament sutures to ensure that the vessel is not stenosed (see Figure 23-3C). If a longitudinal arteriotomy is required, closure is best accomplished with a vein patch. Appropriately selected longitudinal arteriotomies can also be used for distal anastomoses of bypass grafts if thrombectomies are unsuccessful in obtaining arterial inflow.

When flow is restored, the bowel is reinspected for persistent regions of ischemia. Segments that previously demonstrated equivocal viability may improve with revascularization, and resection may be avoided; lengths of bowel that are obviously nonviable must be removed. Bowel continuity can be restored primarily, or stomas may be exteriorized if the patient is unstable. In most instances, a second-look operation should be performed at 24 to 36 hours to assess the cumulative effects of reperfusion. Planning for this reexploration allows the surgeon to minimize the amount of bowel resected primarily and to ensure that the final bowel anastomoses are performed with viable bowel.

The management of SMA thrombosis caused by underlying atherosclerotic lesions is more challenging because simple surgical thrombectomy is unlikely to be durable.[48] The proximal SMA should be opened through a longitudinal arteriotomy. If thrombectomy is temporarily successful, an intraarterial shunt is placed while the exposures needed for definitive revascularization are performed. The longitudinal arteriotomy in the SMA can serve as the distal anastomotic site for both antegrade bypasses originating in the supraceliac aorta and retrograde bypasses from the infrarenal aorta or iliac vessels. If there is a high likelihood of bowel resection, an autologous conduit should be used for the bypass.

In syndromes of nonocclusive ischemia, the primary therapy is selective arterial administration of vasodilating agents such as papaverine. Such treatment must be coupled with the cessation of α agonists or other vasoconstrictors. Heparin should also be administered to prevent thrombosis in the cannulated vessel, but the drug must be infused through a peripheral intravenous catheter to avoid precipitation when mixed with papaverine. If a patient demonstrates signs of continued bowel ischemia or necrosis, as evidenced by rebound tenderness or guarding, surgical exploration is required. All necrotic bowel should be resected while arterial infusions of vasodilators continue. The room temperature should be elevated, and the bowel should be kept in moist laparotomy pads to minimize vasoconstriction during exploration. Most patients should undergo a second-look operation in 24 to 48 hours to reassess bowel viability.

The surgical treatment of MVT is restricted to fluid resuscitation, correction of any underlying coagulopathy, and resection of nonviable bowel. Unfortunately, venous thrombectomy is of limited durability and has not proved effective in most instances. The extent of bowel resection should be generous, and repeated exploratory laparotomy is often required to ensure that adequate bowel resection has been performed. Because many patients succumb despite these measures, a more aggressive stance toward early surgical thrombectomy or fibrinolysis has been advocated by some.[49,50] The risks of these maneuvers are considerable, however, and intervention should be reserved for patients who do not improve with conventional therapy.

Although the detection of frankly necrotic bowel is not difficult, the determination of viability in marginally perfused bowel is more challenging. Simple indicators of viability include visible peristalsis as well as a pink and normal color of the serosa. Along with palpation of the distribution of the SMA for arterial pulsations, Doppler ultrasonography can be used to further evaluate arterial signals within the vascular arcades. If any question remains, the bowel should be reassessed at a minimum of 30 minutes after revascularization. Administration of intravenous fluorescein followed by illumination with a Wood ultraviolet light will confirm perfusion of the bowel. The primary limitation of fluorescein is that it is eventually absorbed in fat; therefore it can be administered only once before it diffuses throughout all tissue and loses its specificity. Unfortunately, no combination of tactics is sufficiently sensitive or specific for error-free evaluation of bowel viability.[51]

Long-term patient outcomes after acute intestinal ischemia are strongly dependent on the timeliness of diagnosis, the underlying lesion, and the associated cardiovascular status. In a comprehensive report by Klempnauer and colleagues[52] of 90 patients suffering from intestinal ischemia, 31 patients survived and were discharged from the hospital. Cumulative 5-year survival was approximately 50% (16 of 31). Mortality was greatest during the first year after the incident. The worst survival (20% at 5 years) was seen in patients who suffered mesenteric arterial thrombosis, and the best survival was seen in patients with emboli or nonocclusive ischemia (about 70%). Only one patient who survived the first episode of arterial thrombosis died because of recurrent bowel ischemia. Remarkably, 8 of the 15 surviving patients returned to work.

CHRONIC MESENTERIC ISCHEMIA

In contrast to the varied causes of AMI, CMI is a result of end-stage atherosclerosis in more than 90% of cases. Risk factors parallel those of atherosclerosis in general, including a positive family history, smoking, hypertension, and hypercholesterolemia. Interestingly, in most series, there is a slight female preponderance, and nearly 50% of patients have a history of prior cardiovascular surgery.[53] Nonatherosclerotic causes of CMI include thrombosis associated with thoracoabdominal aneurysm, aortic coarctation, aortic dissection, mesenteric arteritis, fibromuscular dysplasia, neurofibromatosis, middle aortic syndrome, Buerger disease, and extrinsic celiac artery compression by the median arcuate ligament.

Clinical Presentation

The sine qua non of CMI is postprandial abdominal pain. The pain is characteristically dull and crampy, occurring primarily in the epigastrium or midabdomen. The discomfort results from activation of visceral afferent nerves that respond to distension and ischemia but that poorly localize pain. The pain occurs 15 to 45 minutes after eating, with increasing severity according to the size and nature of the meal. The temporal relationship between pain and food ingestion often leads to "food fear," another classic but not invariable complaint.

Weight loss is the second classic symptom of CMI. Although malabsorption can contribute to malnutrition in severe cases, most weight loss is simply due to the patient's fear of eating. Many patients become so emaciated that they undergo extensive evaluations for occult neoplasms.

Other less common symptoms of CMI include diarrhea, nausea and vomiting, and constipation. The variability in signs and symptoms is due in part to the region of the gut affected. Foregut ischemia (celiac axis distribution) is usually accompanied by nausea, vomiting, and bloating, whereas midgut ischemia (SMA) causes classic postprandial abdominal pain and weight loss. The infrequent findings of constipation, occult blood in the stool, and ischemic colitis on colonoscopic biopsy may signify hindgut (IMA) involvement. The lack of specificity of the signs and symptoms of this syndrome often leads to a delay in diagnosis, and it is common for affected patients to have undergone myriad interventions, including antacid or antireflux therapy, cholecystectomy, hysterectomy, and adhesiolysis.

The findings on physical examination are also nonspecific, but the astute clinician can recognize several clues indirectly suggesting the diagnosis. Unexplained weight loss and emaciation alone should arouse suspicion of the syndrome. Manifestations of atherosclerosis in other vascular beds are common, including a cervical or peripheral bruit, decreased peripheral pulses, and signs of chronic lower extremity ischemia. An abdominal bruit can be heard in up to 70% of affected patients.

Diagnosis

Routine laboratory evaluation is rarely helpful, although malnutrition may be accompanied by hemoconcentration, immunoincompetence, hypoalbuminemia, hypoproteinemia, or hypocholesterolemia. Tests for panmalabsorption, such as stool fat content, D-xylose tolerance, or vitamin B_{12} absorption, may be positive but are nonspecific. Plain abdominal films may reveal aortic or arterial calcification, suggesting mesenteric atherosclerosis. Additional imaging studies, such as endoscopy, gastrointestinal contrast examination, and CT, rarely establish the diagnosis but are useful in excluding more common clinical syndromes.

Ultrasonography has added a new dimension to the diagnostic evaluation of patients with suspected CMI. The ability to screen patients with chronic abdominal pain without incurring the risk of contrast arteriography has been a significant advance in the identification of affected patients. Predictive values in excess of 80% have been documented using peak systolic velocity criteria of greater than 275 cm/s for the SMA and greater than 200 cm/s for the celiac axis.[54,55] The test is highly operator dependent, however, and independent confirmation of accuracy is necessary for each noninvasive vascular test laboratory using this technique.

For positive or equivocal ultrasound examinations, diagnostic arteriography is required for more exact lesion localization and for planning revascularization. A complete examination consists of anteroposterior and lateral aortic views, as well as selective injections of the celiac axis, SMA, and IMA (Figure 23-4). Occlusion of two or three of the main trunks is generally required for development of the CMI syndrome (Figure 23-5). Significant mesenteric occlusive disease combined with the development of large collateral vessels is essentially pathognomonic (Figure 23-6). Celiac axis occlusion by the median arcuate ligament is also readily demonstrated by contrast arteriography and may be responsible for CMI in younger patients[56] (Figure 23-7).

More recent developments in CT and image processing have allowed such detailed reconstructions of the visceral aortic branches that catheter-based arteriography may become unnecessary in many cases. As demonstrated in Figures 23-8 and 23-9, identification of a highly calcified plaque at the SMA origin prompted contrast-enhanced CT reconstruction. Significant orificial lesions with poststenotic dilatation of both the celiac axis and the SMA were demonstrated in this patient with symptoms of CMI and a large abdominal aortic aneurysm.

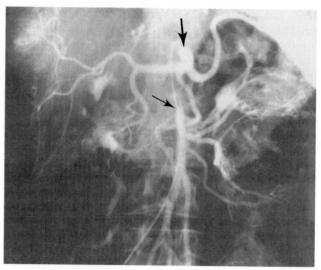

FIGURE 23-4 ■ Chronic mesenteric ischemia in a 67-year-old woman who had undergone antrectomy, vagotomy, and cholecystectomy and who presented with nausea, vomiting, and a 40-pound weight loss. Anteroposterior arteriogram with direct celiac injection shows critical stenosis of the celiac axis *(thick arrow)* and distal reconstitution of an occluded superior mesenteric artery *(thin arrow)*. (From Schwartz LB, Gewertz BL: Chronic mesenteric arterial occlusive disease: clinical presentation and diagnostic evaluation. In Perler BA, Becker GL, editors: Vascular intervention: a clinical approach, New York, 1998, Thieme Medical, p 522.)

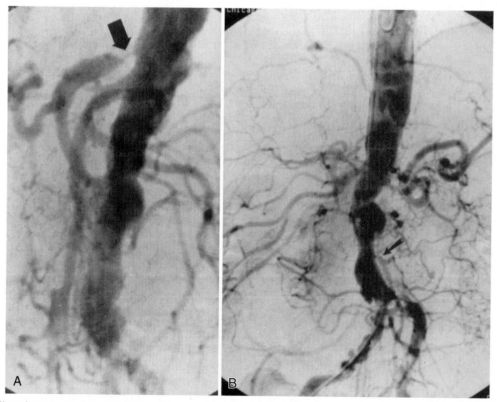

FIGURE 23-5 ■ Chronic mesenteric ischemia in a 78-year-old woman who had undergone coronary artery bypass and carotid endarterectomy and who presented with claudication, a 30-pound weight loss, and postprandial pain. **A,** Lateral aortogram shows critical celiac axis stenosis *(arrow)*. **B,** Anteroposterior aortogram shows severe infrarenal aortic disease and critical inferior mesenteric artery stenosis *(arrow)*. (From Schwartz LB, Gewertz BL: Intestinal ischemic disorders. In Yao JST, Pearce WH, editors: Modern trends in vascular surgery, Stamford, Conn, 1999, Appleton and Lange, pp 347–367.)

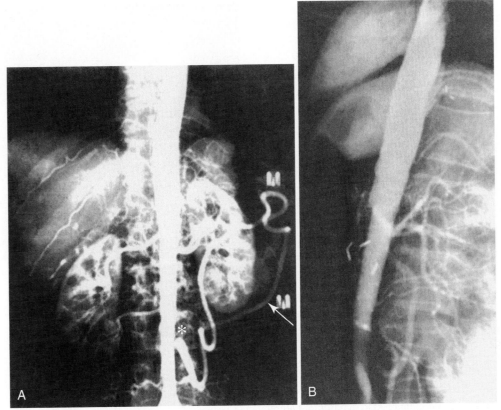

FIGURE 23-6 ■ Chronic mesenteric ischemia in a 67-year-old woman with postprandial abdominal pain and a 30-pound weight loss. **A,** Anteroposterior aortogram (early phase) shows occlusion of the celiac axis and superior mesenteric artery (SMA), along with critical stenosis of the inferior mesenteric artery (IMA) origin *(asterisk).* Note the presence of a meandering mesenteric artery *(arrow).* **B,** Lateral aortogram demonstrating occlusion of both the celiac and superior mesenteric arteries at the orgin. (From Schwartz LB, Gewertz BL: Chronic mesenteric arterial occlusive disease: clinical presentation and diagnostic evaluation. In Perler BA, Becker GL, editors: Vascular intervention: a clinical approach, New York, 1998, Thieme Medical, p 521.)

Treatment Options

Because there is no effective medical therapy for CMI, its treatment is focused on the mechanical relief of occlusive lesions and restoration of blood flow. Open mesenteric bypass has been the gold standard of treatment in the past; however, endovascular therapy, consisting of percutaneous transluminal angioplasty and stenting (PTA/stent), has emerged recently as the most favored treatment modality for CMI[57] (Figure 23-10). The Nationwide Inpatient Sample from 1988 to 2006 demonstrated that whereas there were 6342 cases of endovascular intervention and 16,071 open surgical repairs for all causes of mestenteric ischemia (both acute and chronic), patients with CMI were more frequently treated endovascularly than with open bypass (62% vs. 38%). Reasons for this trend were attributed to lower cardiac and pulmonary morbidity and mortality rates,[44] although some major academic centers have demonstrated comparable outcomes for both open and endovascular repairs.[58-60]

In 2009, the Mayo Clinic group published their analysis of risk-stratified outcomes in their retrospective review of 229 open or endovascular treated CMI patients. Patients who underwent percutaneous intervention were signficantly older and of higher risk. Interestingly, the mortality rate was not statistically different, although

open surgical patients had higher cardiac and pulmonary complication rates (36% vs. 18%) and longer hospital stays (12 ± 8 vs. 3 ± 5 days).[60]

Despite these documented advantages of percutaneous therapy, open surgical repair has shown to have superior durability; therefore the choice of therapy should be tailored to the patient's comorbidities and disease process. In general, endovascular therapy is associated with fewer complications, but it does demonstrate lower primary patency rates and a greater need for earlier reintervention.[58-60] One of the largest series with intermediate-term (3 years) follow-up describes 49 patients treated endovascularly for symptomatic CMI. Primary patency was 63.9% ± 8.5% and approximately 30% of patients required reintervention with mean time to first reintervention of 15.5 ± 4.3 months.[61] The extensive plaque burden from aortic atherosclerosis has been proposed as the principle mechanism for the high restenosis rate.

Surgical revascularization remains the most durable treatment for CMI. Early reports emphasized single-vessel reconstruction using autologous vein and a retrograde approach with bypass grafts originating from the infrarenal aorta.[62,63] Although this procedure avoids supraceliac aortic dissection and clamping, the geometry of a retrograde bypass is theoretically unfavorable, with

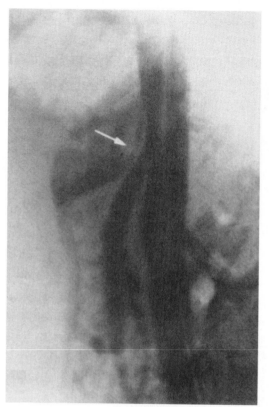

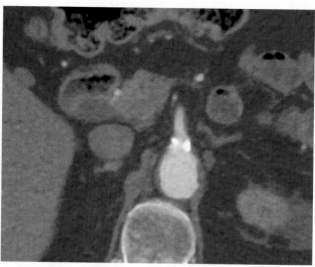

FIGURE 23-8 ■ Calcified plaque is noted at the origin of the superior mesenteric artery.

FIGURE 23-7 ■ Median arcuate compression syndrome. Lateral aortogram in a 27-year-old woman with postprandial abdominal cramping, bloating, and occasional nausea and vomiting. Note the compression of the celiac axis and superior mesenteric artery *(arrow)*. Her twin sister had similar complaints and arteriographic findings. (From Bech F, Loesberg A, Rosenblum J, et al: Median arcuate ligament compression syndrome in monozygotic twins. J Vasc Surg 19:935, 1994.)

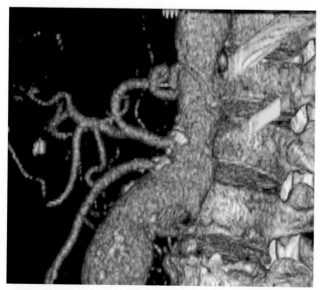

FIGURE 23-9 ■ Contrast-enhanced reconstruction of computed tomography scan confirms the hemodynamic significance of orificial lesions of the celiac axis and superior mesenteric artery. Note the detail of the distal vessels on the image, allowing operative planning.

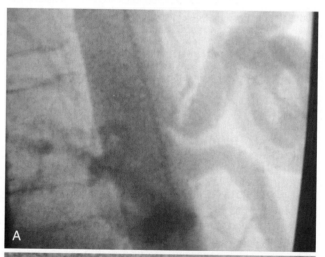

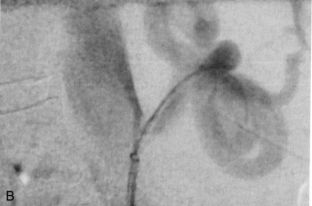

FIGURE 23-10 ■ **A,** Severe stenosis of the celiac axis in a patient with foregut ischemic symptoms. **B,** Successful angioplasty with stent placement despite angulation of the artery origin.

the potential for compression by the overlying abdominal viscera. In the modern era, antegrade bypass using grafts originating in the supraceliac aorta has become the preferred surgical technique.[64]

Regardless of the method of revascularization, proper patient selection is critical to optimize results. Other common gastrointestinal disorders should be excluded, and the diagnosis of CMI should be ascertained. Concurrent extracranial carotid and coronary artery disease should be detected and treated appropriately. Medical or percutaneous treatment for myocardial ischemia is preferred, because patients with CMI are at increased risk for intestinal infarction during and after coronary artery revascularization.

Although hypoproteinemia with serum albumin of less than 3 mg/dL frequently accompanies CMI, postponement of operative therapy to nourish the patient is rarely helpful. The risk of intestinal infarction during the preoperative period is significant and is often associated with catastrophic results. In patients with life-threatening malnutrition, consideration should be given to endovascular therapy as a temporizing measure before surgical reconstruction.

Antegrade Bypass

Aortic-celiac-mesenteric bypass is best performed through a transperitoneal approach. After a thorough exploration of the abdomen, attention is directed toward exposure of the distal thoracic aortic inflow source. This portion of the aorta is usually spared from atherosclerosis. The triangular ligament of the left lobe of the liver is divided, and moist laparotomy packs are inserted to protect the liver parenchyma. Although exposure is greatly facilitated by the use of self-retaining retractor systems, care should be taken to avoid excessive force. The lesser sac is entered by division of the gastrohepatic ligament. The esophagus is retracted to the left, and final aortic exposure is achieved by division of the diaphragmatic crura and median arcuate ligament. This allows isolation of 8 to 10 cm of the distal thoracic aorta without division of the diaphragm.

The mesenteric arterial branches are identified next. The origin of the celiac axis is already substantially exposed during the aortic dissection. Dissection along its length is continued until a soft patent distal target is appreciated (usually within the distal celiac axis before its branching). Following this, the operative field is temporarily shifted to the midabdomen by lifting and superiorly displacing the transverse colon. The small bowel and the fourth portion of the duodenum are retracted to the right. The SMA is palpated in the small bowel mesentery as the vessel courses from the retroperitoneum at the inferior margin of the pancreas. The peritoneal membrane is incised, and a suitable segment is isolated. Blunt dissection is used to develop a tunnel behind the pancreas on the left side of the aorta.

Intravenous heparin (100 units/kg) and mannitol (25 g) are administered. A longitudinal incision is made in the aorta, and additional arterial wall is removed as needed. A bifurcated Dacron or polytetrafluoroethylene graft (typically 14 × 7 mm) is delivered to the field.

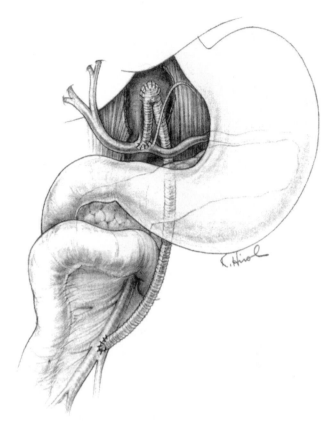

FIGURE 23-11 ■ Aorta–carotid artery–superior mesenteric artery bypass using a bifurcated Dacron graft. (From Zarins CK, Gewertz BL: Atlas of vascular surgery, New York, 1989, Churchill Livingstone, p 109.)

Proximal aortic followed by distal celiac axis anastomosis is performed, and the viscera are reperfused. SMA anastomosis is performed last, after the second limb of the graft is tunneled beneath the pancreas (Figure 23-11). An alternative but equally effective technique involves sequential bypass using a single 8-mm Dacron graft[64-66] (Figure 23-12).

Retrograde Bypass

Mesenteric bypass grafts originating from the infrarenal aorta or iliac arteries (retrograde bypass) were the first techniques used in surgical correction of mesenteric arterial lesions.[6] This approach offers the advantages of limited dissection and avoidance of supraceliac aortic occlusion. Despite these features, retrograde bypass has been used less frequently in recent years. Results from a number of clinical series suggest (but do not prove) that retrograde bypass is less durable than its antegrade counterpart.[67,68] This is presumed to be due to the tendency for SMA grafts to kink or twist when the viscera are returned to their normal anatomic positions. Although the use of stiffer prosthetic conduits and meticulous technique can improve the orientation of these reconstructions, retrograde bypass should be considered a third option to be used only if antegrade bypass and aortomesenteric endarterectomy are not feasible. Specific

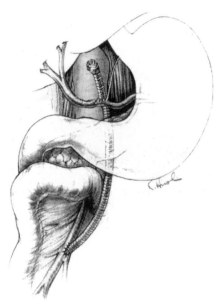

FIGURE 23-12 ■ Sequential aorta–celiac axis–superior mesenteric artery bypass using an 8-mm Dacron graft configured in sequential fashion. (Modified from Zarins CK, Gewertz BL: Atlas of vascular surgery, New York, 1989, Churchill Livingstone, p 109.)

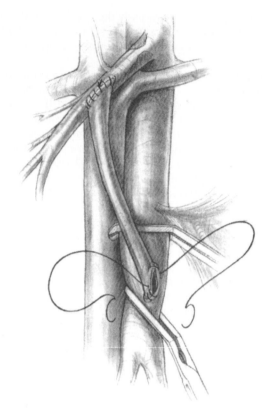

FIGURE 23-13 ■ Retrograde infrarenal aorta–superior mesenteric artery bypass using autologous vein. (From Zarins CK, Gewertz BL: Atlas of vascular surgery, New York, 1989, Churchill Livingstone, p 107.)

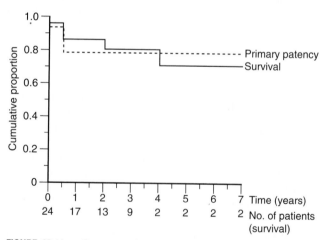

FIGURE 23-14 ■ Symptom-free survival (n = 24) and primary patency (n = 19) in patients undergoing surgical revascularization for chronic mesenteric ischemia. Calculation was done using the life-table method. Number of patients per interval is shown at the bottom. (Modified from Moawad J, McKinsey JF, Wyble CW, et al: Current results of surgical therapy for chronic mesenteric ischemia. Arch Surg 132:616, 1997.)

indications for retrograde bypass currently include (1) emergency revascularization in patients undergoing laparotomy for AMI, (2) inaccessible supraceliac aorta due to previous surgery or subphrenic inflammation, (3) severe cardiac disease with contraindications to supraceliac aortic occlusion, and (4) the need for simultaneous infrarenal aortic and mesenteric revascularization.

Retrograde mesenteric bypass begins with exposure of the most proximal suitable segment of the SMA as it exits from beneath the pancreas. The more proximal the anastomosis in the SMA, the less likely it is that kinking will occur, because the graft will lie geometrically parallel to the aorta. The mesentery is then returned to its normal position as the graft is pulled taut to lie adjacent to the aorta. A soft portion of the aorta or iliac artery is located, and the proximal anastomosis is performed; a fair amount of tension must be maintained on the graft to avoid laxity and kinking when the abdomen is closed (Figure 23-13).

Access to the celiac axis is problematic with this approach; therefore celiac revascularization is usually performed via anastomosis to the common hepatic artery or, less commonly, the splenic artery. The common hepatic anastomosis (distal anastomosis) is performed in an end-to-side fashion at 90 degrees. After the Kocher maneuver, the graft can be tunneled behind the duodenum and head of the pancreas, en route to the infrarenal aorta. In this position, torsion and kinking are minimized. When the less robust splenic artery is used, grafts are tunneled behind the tail of the pancreas and anterior to the left renal vein.

Outcomes of Surgical Treatment

A review of collected series of the surgical treatment of CMI during the 1980s and 1990s reveals an overall operative mortality rate of 6%, with 20% of patients sustaining major complications.[69] Although documentation of nearly 500 cases appears in the literature, most of these represent small case series, and the rarity of the syndrome implies that few institutions have extensive experience. Most clinicians agree that recurrence is less likely if more than one vessel is revascularized. This concept was first championed by Robin and colleagues,[50] who noted differential recurrence rates corresponding to the number of vessels treated. Subsequent reports confirmed this finding,[70,71] making complete revascularization the standard.

Although many clinicians report excellent symptomatic relief after surgical revascularization for CMI, only a few have rigorously examined graft patency.[64,72,73] McMillan and coworkers[72] used duplex scans and arteriography to document graft patency in 25 patients undergoing mesenteric bypass. Their series included 16 patients treated for CMI and 9 treated for AMI, in whom the perioperative morbidity was predictably higher. Considering the 22 patients who survived for more than 1 month, graft patency after a mean of 35 months was 89%. The success rates of retrograde and antegrade grafts were indistinguishable, as were the outcomes of prosthetic and autogenous vein reconstructions. It was noted that two of the three patients experiencing occluded grafts were asymptomatic, emphasizing that patency cannot be inferred from clinical criteria alone.

Expected results in the modern era are typified by the University of Chicago experience with 24 consecutive patients undergoing mesenteric revascularization over a 10-year period.[64] All patients had significant SMA involvement, and 21 also had lesions of the celiac axis. Seventeen antegrade and seven retrograde bypasses were performed. Calculated 5-year primary patency was 78%, documented by duplex scans, arteriography, or both; 5-year patient survival by life-table analysis was 71% (Figure 23-14).

References available online at expertconsult.com.

QUESTIONS

1. What is the incidence of a "replaced right hepatic artery" arising from the SMA rather than the celiac axis?
   a. 2%
   b. 5%
   c. 12%
   d. 20%
   e. 40%

2. What is the most common site of origin of a mesenteric embolus?
   a. Midthoracic aorta
   b. Left ventricle
   c. Aortic valve
   d. Supraceliac aorta
   e. Pelvic veins (paradoxical embolus)

3. Nonocclusive mesenteric ischemia is associated with all of the following except:
   a. Digitalis toxicity
   b. Low cardiac output
   c. Administration of α-adrenergic agents
   d. Sepsis
   e. Inotropic administration

4. What is the most common cause of mesenteric venous thrombosis?
   a. Leukemia
   b. Hypercoaguable states
   c. Intra-abdominal abscess
   d. Primary portal hypertension
   e. Pancreatic cancer

5. What is the most common location for a clinically significant acute embolic obstruction of the mesenteric circulation?
   a. Origin of the celiac axis
   b. Origin of the SMA
   c. Origin of the IMA
   d. Mid-SMA just distal to the origin of the middle colic artery
   e. None of the above

6. What is the most common location for a clinically significant chronic obstruction of the mesenteric circulation?
   a. Origin of the celiac axis
   b. Origin of the SMA
   c. Origin of the IMA
   d. Mid-SMA just distal to the origin of the middle colic artery
   e. None of the above

7. What is the best clinical indicator of the presence of acute intestinal ischemia?
   a. Severe leukocytosis
   b. Severe abdominal pain without rebound tenderness
   c. Acidosis
   d. Atrial fibrillation
   e. Hyperamylasemia

8. All of the following statements about angioplasty for mesenteric vascular disease are true except:
   a. The immediate failure rate is less than 5%.
   b. The periprocedural mortality is lower than that for operative therapy.
   c. Percutaneous transluminal angioplasty is useful in ischemia related to aortic dissection.
   d. Durability (defined as relief of symptoms) is less than that with operative repair.
   e. Stenting has improved patency.

9. What is the principal advantage of antegrade mesenteric bypass versus retrograde bypass for chronic mesenteric ischemia?
   a. Lower operative mortality
   b. Higher blood flow in grafts
   c. Allows use of autogenous conduits
   d. Avoids potential kinking of grafts
   e. Lower cardiac stress

10. What is the most reliable sign or symptom when making the clinical diagnosis of chronic mesenteric ischemia?
    a. Postprandial pain
    b. Weight loss
    c. Melena
    d. Postprandial vomiting
    e. Hypoalbuminemia

ANSWERS

1. **c**
2. **b**
3. **c**
4. **b**
5. **d**
6. **b**
7. **b**
8. **b**
9. **d**
10. **a**

CHAPTER 24

MANAGEMENT OF RENOVASCULAR DISEASE

William B. Newton III • Racheed J. Ghanami • Kimberley J. Hansen

HISTORICAL BACKGROUND

Renovascular Hypertension

Goldblatt defined a causal relationship between renovascular disease and hypertension through his innovative work published in 1934,[1] but Bright of Guy's Hospital, London, first called attention to a potential association between hypertension and renal disease 100 years earlier.[2] Bright observed that patients with "dropsy" and albuminuria during life had shrunken kidneys and an enlarged heart (cardiac hypertrophy) at autopsy. He suggested that the altered quality of the blood so affected the small circulation as to render greater action necessary to force the blood through the terminal divisions of the vascular system.

Although Bright failed to recognize the relationship between increased blood pressure and cardiac hypertrophy, his observations stimulated many theories. Among them was Traube's speculation that elevated blood pressure led to increased myocardial work and subsequent hypertrophy.[3] Based on Bright's observations and subsequent hypotheses, several investigators described experimental models intended to re-create the clinical lesions observed in the kidney and heart. In 1879, Growitz and Israel[4] produced acute occlusion of one renal artery and performed contralateral nephrectomy to decrease functioning renal mass. Although these investigators created what they thought was cardiac hypertrophy in some animals, elevated blood pressures occurred in none.

Lewinski might have predated Goldblatt's observations had his experiments included blood pressure measurements.[5] In 1880, he reported that 6 of 25 dogs developed cardiac hypertrophy after partial constriction of the renal arteries. In 1905, Katzenstein[6] created hypertension in dogs by producing partial occlusion of the renal arteries, although complete occlusion after torsion of the renal pedicle did not produce elevated blood pressures. Katzenstein demonstrated that the elevated pressures returned to normal when constricting rubber bands were removed. However, he mistakenly concluded that the blood pressure changes were not related to a chemically mediated mechanism. In 1898, Tigerstedt and Bergman published the landmark description of a renal pressor substance in rabbits, a crude extract they termed *renin*.[7] Although their work was confirmed in 1911 by Senator,[8] these and other investigators did not consider renin central to the pathogenesis of hypertension.

In 1934, Goldblatt[1] demonstrated that constriction of the renal artery produced atrophy of the kidney and hypertension in the dog. As a clinical pathologist, Goldblatt noticed that extensive vascular disease was often present at autopsy in patients with hypertension and was frequently severe in the renal arteries. In his own words: "Contrary, therefore, to what I had been taught, I began to suspect that the vascular disease comes first and, when it involves the kidneys, the resultant impairment of the renal circulation probably, in some way, causes elevation of the blood pressure."[1] Goldblatt's elegant experiments introduced a new era by demonstrating that renal artery stenosis could produce a form of hypertension corrected by nephrectomy.

In 1938, Leadbetter and Burkland[9] described the first successful treatment of this correctable form of hypertension. They cured a 5-year-old child with severe hypertension by removal of an ischemic ectopic kidney. The photomicrographs published from that renal artery specimen were the first documentation of a renovascular origin of hypertension. In subsequent years, numerous patients were treated by nephrectomy, based on the findings of hypertension and a small kidney on intravenous pyelogram. Smith reviewed 575 such cases in 1956 and found that only 26% of patients were cured of hypertension by nephrectomy.[10] This led him to suggest that nephrectomy should be limited to strictly urologic indications.

In 1954, Freeman performed an aortic and bilateral renal artery thromboendarterectomy in a hypertensive patient, which resulted in resolution of the hypertension.[11] This first cure of hypertension by renal revascularization, in combination with the widespread use of aortography, was followed by enthusiastic reports describing blood pressure benefit after renal revascularization.[12-15] Nevertheless, by 1960 it became apparent that renal revascularization in hypertensive patients with renal artery stenosis was associated with a beneficial blood pressure response in fewer than half of individuals. These clinical results fostered general pessimism regarding the value of operative renal artery reconstruction for the treatment of hypertension.

Contemporary operative management of renovascular hypertension began with the introduction of tests of functional significance. Split renal function by Howard and Connor,[16] Stamey and associates,[17] Page and Helmes,[18] and others[19-21] identified the role of the renin-angiotensin system in blood pressure control, thus describing the pathophysiology of renovascular hypertension. After accurate assays for plasma renin activity became available, physicians could accurately predict which renal artery lesion was producing renovascular hypertension.

Renovascular Renal Insufficiency

Until the current era, the pathophysiology and management of renovascular disease focused solely on hypertension; however, contemporary reports have emphasized the relationship between renovascular disease and renal insufficiency.[22-30]

The term *ischemic nephropathy* has been adopted to recognize this relationship. By definition, ischemic nephropathy describes the presence of severe occlusive disease of the extraparenchymal renal artery in combination with excretory renal insufficiency. In 1962, Morris and associates reported on eight azotemic patients with global renal ischemia who experienced improved blood pressure and renal function after renal revascularization.[31] Novick, Libertino, and Dean and their groups found a similar beneficial functional response when bilateral renal lesions were corrected in azotemic patients.[24,25,27,28] These early reports and the reports that followed suggested that ischemic nephropathy could mediate renal insufficiency that was rapidly progressive, contributing to end-stage renal disease. In this chapter, diagnostic studies and methods of management for renovascular disease (RVD), renovascular hypertension (RVH), and ischemic nephropathy are reviewed.

PATHOLOGY

Occlusive lesions of the renal artery can be divided into two main categories: atherosclerosis and fibromuscular dysplasia. Atherosclerosis of the renal artery is not unique. The pathogenesis parallels atherosclerotic lesions elsewhere, with cholesterol-rich lipid deposition and intimal thickening. Later, this atheroma may undergo central degeneration and even calcification. Atheromas typically occur at or near the renal artery ostium (Figure 24-1). This ostial lesion reflects aortic atheroma that spills over into the renal artery orifice. Most commonly, these lesions are found on the left and account for approximately 70% of patients with RVH. Like atherosclerosis elsewhere, angiographic findings that are pathognomonic for a hemodynamically significant lesion include poststenotic dilatation and the presence of collateral vessels. Often there is simultaneous angiographic involvement of the abdominal aorta and its bifurcation. Most commonly, the renal artery lesion is only one manifestation of generalized atherosclerosis.

Fibromuscular dysplasia of the renal artery encompasses a variety of hyperplastic and fibrosing lesions of the intima, media, or adventitia. They are most frequently seen in young women. This is of no predictive value, however, because fibrodysplastic lesions can be found at any age and in either sex. Medial fibroplasia is the most common lesion, accounting for 85% of dysplastic lesions. The right renal artery is more commonly affected than the left, but bilateral involvement is present in the vast

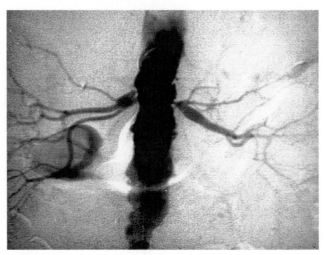

FIGURE 24-1 ■ Arteriogram showing typical appearance of ostial atherosclerotic renal artery stenosis. Aortic atheroma spills over into the renal artery to create stenosis.

majority of patients. The basic cause of medial fibroplasia remains unknown, but its frequent occurrence in multiple arteries suggests a systemic arteriopathy. It often involves long segments of the renal artery and its branches, producing a characteristic "string-of-beads" appearance angiographically. Embryologic variations, hormonal influences, autoimmune mechanisms, and even recurrent trauma during youth have been suggested as possible causative factors. None of these explanations is adequate, however, and the supporting evidence remains mostly conjectural.

Based on the angiographic appearance of fibromuscular disease, several methods of categorization have been suggested. To establish a uniform terminology, Harrison and McCormack[32] combined their experience and developed a classification of these lesions correlating the histologic and angiographic appearance. Depending on the layer predominantly involved, lesions may be categorized as intimal, medial, or adventitial (Figure 24-2). Clinically, however, it may be difficult to segregate individual lesions into one of these categories. The most common variety of fibromuscular dysplasia is medial fibroplasia (85%) with mural microaneurysms (Figure 24-3). Less commonly, the dysplastic lesions may appear as a single mural stenosis (see Figure 24-2), which is consistent with intimal fibroplasia (5%). Perimedial dysplasia (10%) demonstrates the same gender predilection and arterial septa as medial fibroplasia; however, mural microaneurysms are absent.

PATHOPHYSIOLOGY

The kidney, because of its influence on circulating plasma volume and on the modulation of vasomotor tone, is a dominant site of blood pressure regulation. To examine the pathophysiology of RVH, a review of the normal homeostatic activities of the kidney in blood pressure regulation is appropriate.

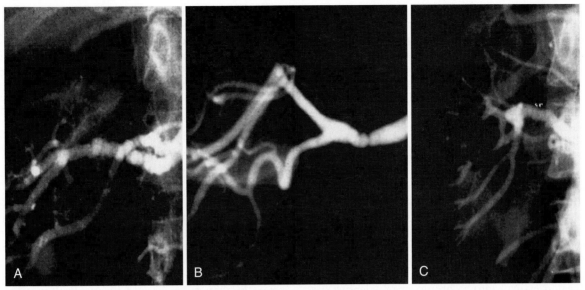

FIGURE 24-2 ■ Angiographic appearance of fibromuscular dysplasia: alternating septa and mural microaneurysms of medial fibroplasia **(A)**, focal stenosis of intimal fibroplasia **(B)**, and fine septa without microaneurysms characteristic of perimedial dysplasia **(C)**.

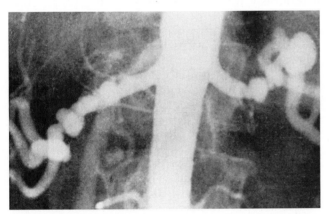

FIGURE 24-3 ■ Arteriogram demonstrating typical "string-of-beads" appearance of medial fibroplasia with fine septa and microaneurysm.

Renin-Angiotensin-Aldosterone System

The renin-angiotensin-aldosterone system is a complex feedback mechanism that normally acts to maintain a stable blood pressure and blood volume under varying conditions. Richly innervated modified smooth muscle cells located along the afferent arterioles in juxtaposition to the renal glomerulus (juxtaglomerular apparatus) are sensitive monitors of perfusion pressure. Diminished perfusion pressure stimulates these cells to release renin, a proteolytic enzyme. Renin interacts with angiotensinogen, an α-globulin manufactured in the liver, to produce angiotensin I. Angiotensin I, an inactive and labile decapeptide, is converted to the potent vasoconstrictor angiotensin II by angiotensin-converting enzyme, which is abundant in the lungs and other tissues. In addition to its potent vasoconstrictor properties, angiotensin II, through its conversion to angiotensin III, also increases blood pressure by stimulating aldosterone release from the zona glomerulosa of the adrenal cortex. This, in turn, increases plasma volume by increasing sodium and water resorption in the renal tubules. Through these actions of angiotensin II and III, blood pressure, plasma volume, and plasma sodium content are increased. In addition, the adjacent cells of the distal convoluted tubule (macula densa) may play a role by acting as sensors of sodium concentration in the distal tubules and exerting a positive feedback mechanism on renin release. As these mechanisms increase perfusion pressure in the juxtaglomerular cells, further renin production and release are suppressed, and blood pressure is modulated within a narrow range.

Potentially, two forms of hypertension may be produced by hemodynamically significant RVD: renin-dependent hypertension and volume-dependent hypertension. Through the mechanisms just described, decreased perfusion activates the renin-angiotensin-aldosterone axis of vasoconstriction and volume expansion. Current information regarding the nature of RVH suggests that a functionally significant unilateral renal artery stenosis activates the angiotensin II–mediated increase in peripheral resistance and blood pressure as well as the aldosterone-mediated volume expansion. When the contralateral renal artery and kidney are normal, the feedback mechanisms in the normal kidney produce a natriuresis and compensatory reduction in circulating plasma volume. In this scheme, an angiotensin II–vasoconstrictive source of hypertension is created.

In contrast, when the contralateral renal artery or kidney is also diseased, this compensatory diuresis is lost and volume expansion occurs, producing an angiotensin-aldosterone–mediated, volume-dependent hypertension. Modification of renal perfusion by renal revascularization can effectively diminish or abolish the underlying mechanism producing either of these varieties of RVH.

It would be simplistic to think that these factors provide a complete description of all the mechanisms activated by the onset of renal hypoperfusion. In the clinical context, however, the pathophysiology of renal hypertension can be characterized by a sustained elevation in peripheral vascular resistance that is mediated by the activation of both the renin-angiotensin and the sympathetic nervous systems and their concomitant contribution to vascular endothelial dysfunction. Although the contribution of increased renin secretion and angiotensin II production is a sustaining stimulus for the hemodynamic and hormonal response, the actions of angiotensin II on the vascular endothelium may play the biggest role in sustained blood pressure elevation. Both the renin-angiotensin and the sympathetic nervous systems appear to act in concert to regulate the integrated hormonal response that operates to regulate sodium and potassium balance and arterial pressure.

It is well accepted that RVH is caused by increased activity of the renin-angiotensin system produced initially by hypersecretion of renin from the juxtaglomerular apparatus of the ischemic kidney. However, as hypertension evolves into a chronic stage, adaptive cardiovascular changes may become an essential mechanism for the maintenance of elevated blood pressure and peripheral vascular resistance. The effect of hypertension on precapillary resistant vessels triggers a myogenic response that is evidenced by the combination of hypertrophy and hyperplasia of the vascular smooth muscle.[33,34] This augments vascular reactivity to pressor agents. There is also evidence that renin may be trapped in structural elements of the vascular wall.[35] Local production of angiotensin II by tissue renin-angiotensin systems may contribute to the remodeling of resistance vessels.[36] Angiotensin-converting enzyme exists in the plasma membrane of vascular endothelial and smooth muscle cells. Thus, the necessary components for the production of angiotensin II may be found in both vascular and cardiac tissue. In the chronic phases of the hypertension process, hypersecretion of renin from the ischemic kidney may be less important than increased production of vascular angiotensin II as the mechanism that sustains the elevation in arterial pressure.

The pathophysiology of renovascular renal insufficiency (i.e., ischemic nephropathy) is incompletely understood.[37] The earliest clinical reports suggested a "glomerular filtration failure" based on hypoperfusion of the kidney,[38] but the molecular basis for ischemic nephropathy is poorly characterized. Like RVH, the renin-angiotensin system likely contributes to ischemic nephropathy through its paracrine effects—intrarenal angiotensin peptides increase efferent arteriolar tone.[39] In the presence of a pressure-reducing renal artery lesion, this paracrine effect increases glomerular capillary pressure to support glomerular filtration. In contrast to these positive effects, angiotensin peptides have also been shown to promote tubulointerstitial injury in the presence of a renal artery lesion.[40] This observation is supported by the induction of transforming growth factor-β and interstitial platelet-derived growth factor-β, which are associated with increased extracellular matrix and interstitial fibrosis.[41-44] Disruption of the tubular cell cytoskeleton and the loss of tubular membrane polarity have also been suggested. Besides these potentially reversible contributors to excretory renal insufficiency, an

atherosclerotic renovascular lesion can also be a source of atheroemboli.[45] The inability to distinguish potentially reversible ischemic nephropathy from irreversible renal parenchymal disease has enormous clinical importance. Recovery of renal function after renovascular intervention has proved to be the strongest predictor of dialysis-free survival.[23,26]

PREVALENCE OF RENOVASCULAR HYPERTENSION AND ISCHEMIC NEPHROPATHY

RVH is generally thought to account for 5% to 10% of the hypertensive population. Tucker suggested an even lower prevalence.[46] Likewise, Shapiro and colleagues[47] suggested that the identification and successful operative treatment of RVH in patients older than 50 years are so unlikely that diagnostic investigation for a correctable cause in that group should be undertaken only when hypertension is severe and uncontrollable. Estimates of the prevalence of hypertension in the United States from all causes range from 60 to 80 million people, and hypertension may be present in 25% to 30% of the adult population.

The actual contribution of RVD to hypertension or renal insufficiency has been uncertain because the population-based prevalence of RVD was unknown. Past prevalence estimates of RVD were extrapolated from case series, autopsy examinations, or angiography obtained to evaluate diseases of the aorta or peripheral circulation.[31,48-54]

Recently, the population-based prevalence of RVD has been estimated for participants in the Cardiovascular Health Study (CHS) sponsored by the National Heart, Lung, and Blood Institute. The CHS is a longitudinal, prospective, population-based study of coronary heart disease and stroke in elderly men and women. This study showed that hemodynamically significant RVD was present in 6.8% of this elderly, free-living cohort.[55] Multivariate analysis demonstrated that increasing participant age ($p = 0.028$; odds ratio [OR], 1.44; 95% confidence interval [CI], 1.03 to 1.73) and increasing systolic blood pressure at baseline ($p = 0.007$; OR, 1.44; 95% CI, 1.10-1.87) were significantly and independently associated with the presence of RVD. Moreover, renal insufficiency was associated with RVD, but only when renal artery disease coexisted with significant hypertension. Contrary to historical assumptions, RVD demonstrated no significant relationships with gender or ethnicity.[55]

Like in the general population, the incidence of RVH is undoubtedly low when all patients with hypertension are considered. Because RVH tends to produce relatively severe hypertension, its prevalence in the large population of mildly hypertensive patients (diastolic blood pressure <105 mm Hg) is probably negligible. In contrast, however, it is a frequent cause of hypertension in the smaller group of patients with severe hypertension. In our experience, the presence of severe hypertension at the two extremes of life carries the highest probability of its being RVH. Our review of the causes of hypertension in 74 children admitted for diagnostic evaluation over a

TABLE 24-1 **Classification of Hypertension in 74 Children by Age**

	0-5 Yr	6-10 Yr	11-15 Yr	16-20 Yr
Total no. of children	9	9	29	27
Essential hypertension	1	5	24	21
Correctable hypertension	8 (89%)	4 (44%)	5 (17%)	6 (22%)

From Lawson JD, Boerth RK, Foster JH, et al: Diagnosis and management of renovascular hypertension in children. Arch Surg 112:1307, 1977.

TABLE 24-2 **Results of Renal Duplex Sonography in 629 New Hypertensive Adults**

Renal Vascular Disease	No. Present (%)	Absent (%)	Total (%)
All patients	154 (24)	475 (76)	629 (100)
<60 yr + DBP ≥ 110 mm Hg	98 (52)	91 (48)	189 (30)
DBP ≥ 110 mm Hg + SCr ≥ 2.0 mg/dL	53 (71)	22 (29)	75 (12)

From Deitch JS, Hansen KJ, Craven TE, et al: Renal artery repair in African-Americans. J Vasc Surg 26:465–473, 1997.
DBP, Diastolic blood pressure; SCr, serum creatinine.

5-year period showed that 78% of the children younger than 5 years had a correctable renin-dependent cause (Table 24-1).[56] In 1996, our center screened 629 hypertensive adults older than 50 years for RVD (Table 24-2). Overall, 25% of subjects demonstrated significant renal artery disease. However, 52% of those older than 60 years whose diastolic pressure was greater than 110 mm Hg had significant renal artery stenosis or occlusion. When serum creatinine was elevated in conjunction with this age and blood pressure, 71% of subjects demonstrated hemodynamically significant RVD.

Based on these data, the probability of finding RVH correlates with patient age, the severity of hypertension, and the presence of associated renal insufficiency. Accordingly, the search for RVD should be directed toward the subset of patients at the extremes of age who have severe hypertension, especially when it is associated with renal insufficiency. The reader should keep in mind, however, that the severity of hypertension is based on its level without medication and does not refer to the difficulty of medical control.

CHARACTERISTICS OF RENOVASCULAR HYPERTENSION

Because of the small proportion of RVH among the entire hypertensive population, many reports have focused on the value of demographic factors, physical findings, and screening tests to discriminate between essential hypertension and RVH. Most frequently cited

as discriminate factors suggesting the presence of RVH and a need for further study are recent onset of hypertension, young age, lack of family history of hypertension, and presence of an abdominal bruit. The most complete study comparing the clinical characteristics of patients with RVH to those with essential hypertension was the Cooperative Study of Renovascular Hypertension.[57] In that study, the prevalence of certain clinical characteristics in 339 patients with essential hypertension was compared with their prevalence in 175 patients with RVH secondary to atherosclerotic lesions (91 patients) and fibromuscular dysplasia (84 patients). Although the prevalence of several characteristics was significantly different in RVH compared with essential hypertension, none of the characteristics had sufficient discriminant value to be used to exclude patients from further diagnostic investigation for RVH. Certainly, the finding of an epigastric bruit in a young white female with malignant hypertension is strongly suggestive of a renovascular origin of the hypertension. The absence of such criteria, however, does not exclude the presence of RVH, and such criteria should not be used to eliminate patients from further diagnostic study.

In a review of the first 200 patients with RVH treated in our center, 64% had family histories of hypertension, 46% had no audible abdominal bruit, and ages ranged from 5 to 80 years (mean, 56 years).[58] Because RVH can be secondary to any of several diseases affecting the renal artery, and because each of these diseases has its own clinical characteristics, the use of demographic or physical findings such as age, abdominal bruit, and duration of hypertension to exclude patients from study inappropriately excludes some patients with RVH from further evaluation. Therefore, the decision to undertake diagnostic study should be based on the severity of hypertension. Mild hypertension has a minimal chance of being renovascular in origin. In contrast, the more severe the hypertension, the higher the probability that it is from a correctable cause. With this in mind, we evaluate all adult patients with diastolic blood pressures greater than 105 mm Hg who would be considered for intervention to evaluate for a renovascular lesion as a correctable origin of hypertension. Children are evaluated when their blood pressure exceeds the 95th percentile for height and age.[59]

NATURAL HISTORY OF ATHEROSCLEROTIC RENOVASCULAR DISEASE

The rationale provided for renal artery intervention frequently cites the presumed natural history of the atherosclerotic renal artery lesion. Much of the information regarding atherosclerotic renovascular disease and its natural history has been extrapolated from angiographic case series and ultrasound examinations from retrospective reviews or from prospective studies in select hypertensive patients. Although the quality of these studies and their interpretation vary widely, most commonly, anatomic progression of atherosclerotic renovascular disease has been considered a certainty, one that is associated with inevitable decline in kidney size and kidney

TABLE 24-3   **Prospective Angiographic Natural History Studies of Atherosclerotic Renal Artery Stenosis**

	Year	Patients (n)	Renal Arteries (n)	Mean Follow-Up (mo)	Anatomic Progression (% Patients)	Progression to Occlusion (% Arteries)	Blood Pressure Change	Decrease in Renal Length (% Patients)	Serum Creatinine Increase (% Patients)	GFR Decline (% of Patients)
Dean and colleagues[97]	1981	41	—	44	17	12	—	37	46	3*
Plouin and colleagues[132]	1998	26	—	6	—	—	−24/+12	—	NS	NS
Webster and colleagues[133]	1998	30	—	—	13†	0†	−28/−16‡	—	NS	—
van Jaarsveld and colleagues[134]	2000	50	100	12	20	5	−17/−7	–	NS	NS
Pillay and colleagues[62]	2002	85	159	30	–	–	NS	NS	—§	—

Modified from Pearce JD, Craven BL, Craven TE, et al: Progression of atherosclerotic renovascular disease: a prospective population-based study. J Vasc Surg 44:955–963, 2006.)
GFR, Glomerular filtration rate; *NS,* not significant.
*Greater than 50% increase, data for 30 patients.
†Of eight patients with serial angiography.
‡From referral to last follow-up.
§Unilateral group had significant increase; bilateral group did not.

function. This "natural history" of atherosclerotic renovascular disease has been cited to support intervention for disease when encountered.[60]

Prospective angiographic clinical studies of atherosclerotic renovascular disease are summarized in Table 24-3. Forty years ago, Dean[61] reported on patients with renovascular hypertension randomized to medical management or open surgical repair. Forty-one patients were randomized to medical management with high grade, atherosclerotic renal artery stenosis, hypertension, and positive renal vein renin assay or split renal function studies. Over an average of 44 months, 17 patients crossed over to the surgical arm. Each of these patients had controlled hypertension, but 15 demonstrated declining renal function as demonstrated by 10% loss in renal length, a 100% increase serum creatinine level, or 50% reduction in measured glomerular filtration rate. Among medically treated patients, 54% demonstrated a 50% decline in glomerular filtration rate; however, 13% demonstrated improved renal function when measured serially. Overall, the decline in renal function was variable with 97% of patients experiencing less than 50% decline in glomerular filtration.

A recent prospective study by Pillay and colleagues[62] described the change in blood pressure and serum creatinine among patients with atherosclerotic renovascular disease. Ninety-eight patients in this multicenter, nonrandomized observational study were noted to have greater than 50% renal artery stenosis during aortography to evaluate peripheral vascular disease. On a minimum duration of 2 years of follow-up, 64 patients with unilateral renal stenosis and 21 patients with bilateral disease were managed medically. Twelve patients with bilateral disease underwent percutaneous intervention or open operative repair. The overall 2-year estimated mortality was 32%. Mortality was equivalent for patients treated with renal artery intervention and for those treated

medically. There was no change in median blood pressure, number of anti-hypertensives, or change in renal size in follow-up among survivors. A small but statistically significant increase in serum creatinine was observed in patients who underwent renal artery intervention. Patients with bilateral renovascular disease treated medically had stable serum creatinine over 2 year follow-up. This study lacked a specific measure of glomerular filtration; however, it demonstrated stable length and stable serum creatinine with controlled hypertension in medically managed patients who had anatomic disease but no clinical indication for renovascular hypertension.

Prospective duplex ultrasound studies are summarized in Table 24-4. A series of consecutive reports described prospective duplex studies performed at the University of Washington. These authors first reported on serial duplex examinations performed on 80 patients with hypertension. Renal arteries were classified according to four categories: normal, stenosis less than 60%, stenosis greater than 60%, or renal artery occlusion. The rate of progression to greater than 60% stenosis during 3 years of follow-up was 8% for renal arteries that were initially classified as normal and 43% initially classified as having less than 60% diameter reducing stenosis. Incident renal artery occlusions were observed only in arteries previously categorized as having 60% diameter reducing stenosis. The 3-year risk for occlusion among the entire group was 7%. Lesion progression was associated with increasing patient age, increasing systolic blood pressure, smoking, female sex, and poorly controlled hypertension.

A most informative prospective study of atherosclerotic renovascular disease among hypertensive patients utilizing renal duplex was provided by Capps and colleagues,[63] who described 5-year follow-up for 170 patients with 295 kidneys. Disease progression was defined by 100 centimeter per second increase in renal artery peak

TABLE 24-4 **Prospective Duplex Sonography Natural History Studies of Atherosclerotic Renal Artery Stenosis**

Reference	Year	Patients (n)	Kidneys (n)	Mean Follow-Up (mo)	Anatomic Progression (% Patients)	Progression to Occlusion (% Arteries)	Blood Pressure Change	Decrease in Renal Length> 1 cm (% Arteries)	Serum Creatinine Increase (% Patients)	GFR Decline (% Patients)
Zierler and colleagues[135]	1994	80	134	13	8	3	—	8	—	3
Zierler and colleagues[136]	1996	76	132	32	20	7	—	—	—	NS
Caps and colleagues[63]	1998	177	295	33	31	3	—	—	—	—
Caps and colleagues[137]	1998	122	204	33	—	2	—	16	—[†]	NS

Modified from Pearce JD, Craven BL, Craven TE, et al: Progression of atherosclerotic renovascular disease: a prospective population-based study. J Vasc Surg 44:955–963, 2006.)
GFR, Glomerular filtration rate.
[†]Seven subjects with bilateral atrophy increased 0.33 mg/dL/year; remainder were not significant.

systolic velocity or progression to renal artery occlusion. By these criteria, disease progression was detected in 31% of renal arteries; 3% of arteries progressed to occlusion and all of these were considered to be diseased at baseline. A model to predict the 2-year calculated risk of progression included diabetes and systolic blood pressure greater than 160 mm Hg.

The data reviewed in the reports above are frequently cited as rationale for intervention for atherosclerotic renovascular disease discovered incidentally during assessment for cardiac or other vascular diseases. However, more recent prospective duplex studies suggest otherwise, at least in patients without severe associated hypertension. Davis and colleagues[64] reported on 119 participants in the Cardiovascular Health Study with 235 kidneys followed over an 8-year period. None of these subjects demonstrated severe hypertension. Controlling for within subject correlation, the overall estimated change in renovascular disease among all 235 kidneys was 14% (95% CI, 9.2%-21.4%) with hemodynamically significant renovascular disease in 4% (95% CI, 1.9%-8.2%).[64] No hemodynamically significant stenosis at baseline progressed to renal artery occlusion on follow-up. Increased blood pressure and decrease in renal length were not associated with renovascular disease at baseline examination. These findings cast doubt on the value of renal artery intervention in the absence of renovascular hypertension or renal insufficiency.

DIAGNOSTIC EVALUATION

The selection and appropriate sequence of diagnostic studies in patients with suspected RVD are still ill defined. The general evaluation of all hypertensive patients should include a careful medical history, physical examination, serum electrolyte and creatinine determination, and electrocardiography. Electrocardiography is important to gauge the extent of secondary myocardial hypertrophy or associated ischemic heart disease. Serum electrolyte and serial serum potassium determinations can effectively

exclude patients with primary aldosteronism if potassium levels are greater than 3.0 mg/dL. One must remember, however, that hypokalemia is often due to salt-depleting diets and previous diuretic therapy. Finally, estimation of renal function is mandatory. Preexisting renal disease may reduce renal function and cause hypertension. Conversely, renal dysfunction may reflect ischemic nephropathy.

Screening Studies

Identification of a noninvasive screening test that accurately identifies all patients with RVD that may warrant interventional management remains an elusive goal. Prior methods such as peripheral plasma renin activity, rapid-sequence intravenous pyelography, and saralasin infusion have been abandoned. Screening studies are basically of two types: functional studies or anatomic studies. Of the functional type, isotope renography continues to be proposed as a valuable screening test, but the methods used are continually modified with the hope of improving its sensitivity and specificity. The newest versions of isotope renography consist of renal scans performed before and after the administration of an inhibitor to angiotensin I–converting enzyme. Of these, only captopril renal scanning has gained widespread use and acceptance as a screening tool. Anatomic screening studies include renal duplex sonography and arteriography.

Captopril Renal Scanning

To understand the basis of captopril renal scanning, one must consider some of the features of renal physiology and the importance of the renin-angiotensin system in the maintenance of homeostasis. Glomerular filtration is governed partially by the relative tone of the afferent and efferent arterioles. During periods of reduced blood pressure recognized by the juxtaglomerular apparatus (e.g., proximal renal artery stenosis), increased renin is released, which ultimately leads to an increase in the level

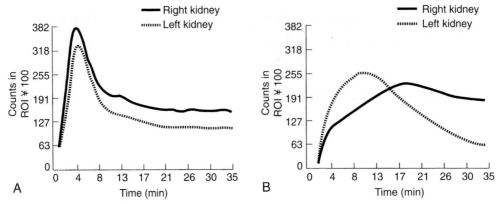

FIGURE 24-4 ■ Captopril renal scintigraphy before **(A)** and after **(B)** captopril administration demonstrates the positive finding of a time delay in reaching peak radioactivity after captopril. *ROI,* Region of interest.

of intrarenal angiotensin II. Angiotensin II acts predominantly to constrict the efferent arteriole to maintain renal glomerular perfusion pressure and filtration. When an angiotensin I–converting enzyme inhibitor such as captopril is given in this circumstance, an acute reduction in the amount of angiotensin II occurs. This leads to a reduction in constriction of the efferent arteriole and a decrease in the glomerular filtration rate (GFR). Captopril renal scanning is composed of a baseline renogram and a repeat renogram obtained after a dose of captopril. A test is considered positive when a normal baseline scan becomes abnormal after captopril administration—that is, when the time to peak activity increases to more than 11 minutes or when a normal glomerular filtration ratio between the two sides increases to greater than 1.5:1 (Figure 24-4). In experienced hands, this study is reported to be highly reliable.[65] Unfortunately, it is less reliable when significant parenchymal disease is present. For that reason, we do not rely on its results to eliminate RVD in azotemic patients.

Renal Duplex Sonography

Through continued improvements in probe design and duplex sonographic technology, imaging and Doppler shift interrogation of deep abdominal vasculature have been introduced as screening methods to identify and quantify visceral and renal artery occlusive disease. We have evaluated the role of duplex sonography as an initial surface screening test, as an intraoperative study to confirm the technical success of reconstructive procedures, and as a postoperative surveillance method to follow progression of disease and stability of reconstructions.[59,66-69]

Technically successful studies, defined as a complete main renal artery interrogation from aortic origin to renal hilum, can be obtained in almost 95% of cases. These results are ensured by proper patient preparation and method of examination. Details of the conduct of the procedure are covered elsewhere.[66]

The criteria for identifying renal artery stenosis by renal duplex sonography are given in Table 24-5. Assuming that renal artery peak systolic velocity (PSV) varies with the degree of renal artery stenosis and aortic PSV

TABLE 24-5 Doppler Velocity Criteria for Significant Stenosis and Occlusion

Defect	Criteria
<60% diameter-reducing RA defect	RA-PSV from entire RA < 1.8 m/s
≥60% diameter-reducing RA defect	Focal RA-PSV ≥ 1.8 m/s and distal turbulent velocity waveform
Occlusion	Doppler-shifted signal from RA B-scan image
Inadequate study for interpratation	Failure to obtain Doppler samples interpretation from entire main RA

From Hansen KJ, Tribble RW, Reaves SW, et al: Renal duplex sonography: evaluation of clinical utility. J Vasc Surg 12:227–236, 1990; and Motew SJ, Cherr GS, Craven TE, et al: Renal duplex sonography: main renal artery versus hilar analysis. J Vasc Surg 32:462–471, 2000.
RA, Renal artery; *RA-PSV,* renal artery peak systolic velocity.

(i.e., inflow), most authors have advocated using the ratio of renal artery PSV to aortic PSV (the renal-to-aortic ratio) to define critical renal artery stenosis.[70-73] In contrast, we have found no relationship between renal artery PSV and aortic PSV in the presence or absence of disease (Figure 24-5). Focal renal artery PSV of 1.8 m/s or more in combination with distal post-stenotic turbulence correlates highly with the angiographic presence of diameter-reducing renal artery stenosis of 60% or greater.[66] In 122 kidneys with single renal arteries and renal angiography for comparison, renal duplex sonography correctly identified 67 of 68 kidneys with normal arteries or less than 60% renal artery stenosis, and 35 of 39 kidneys with 60% to 99% renal artery stenosis. All 15 renal artery occlusions were correctly identified by failure to obtain a Doppler-shifted signal from an imaged renal artery. Using this method and these criteria for interpretation, renal duplex sonography was 93% sensitive and 98% specific.

Renal Angiography

Controversy continues over the use of aortography and renal angiography in the routine screening of

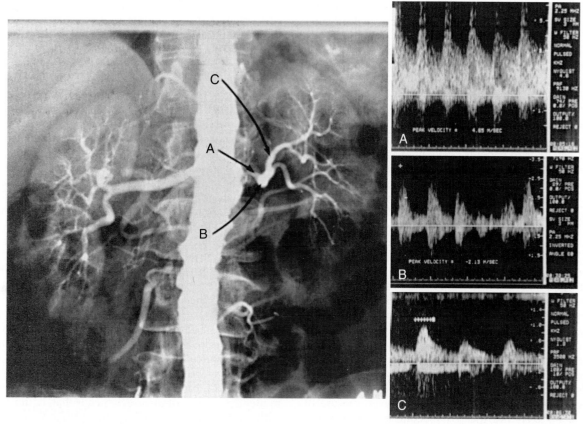

FIGURE 24-5 ■ Radiographic cut-film angiogram demonstrating high-grade left renal artery stenosis. **A,** Doppler spectral analysis at the site of stenosis demonstrating focal increase in renal artery peak systolic velocity (RA-PSV; 4.6 m/s). **B,** Distal spectral analysis demonstrating turbulent waveform and decreased RA-PSV with irregular spectral envelope and spontaneous bidirectional signals. **C,** Spectral analysis several vessel diameters distal to stenosis demonstrating return of nearly normal waveform.

hypertensive individuals. Some believe that these methods should be reserved for select groups of patients. We do not share this view and proceed with angiography in the circumstances summarized earlier.

Details of performing angiography to evaluate aortic and branch disease are addressed elsewhere. Currently, intraarterial digital subtraction angiography is used to evaluate the majority of patients. The fact that angiography in patients with severe renal insufficiency, especially those with concomitant diabetes mellitus, can aggravate renal failure is widely recognized. Nevertheless, we believe that this risk is justified in patients with severe or accelerated hypertension and in those with positive renal duplex sonography results. In these circumstances, the potential benefit derived from the identification and correction of a functionally significant renovascular lesion exceeds the risk of contrast exposure. In addition, the use of carbon dioxide and gadolinium as alternatives may reduce the risk of nephrotoxicity.[74,75] However, gadolinium should be used with caution in patients with chronic renal insufficiency due to its association with nephrogenic systemic fibrosis.

Because the mortality and the morbidity of contrast nephropathy leading to dialysis dependence are high, measures to protect renal function during angiography should be taken. Conventional contrast agents have iodine incorporated into their structure to absorb x-ray

photons, thereby achieving visualization of the vasculature. The nephrotoxicity of such iodinated contrast agents has been recognized for many years. The principal site of contrast-induced nephrotoxicity is the renal tubule from transient regional renal ischemia, whereas the effect on glomerular function appears to be mild.[76,77] It was thought that the ionization and high osmolarity of early contrast agents may have contributed to their nephrotoxicity. Nonionic contrast agents (e.g., iohexol) are available that provide comparable absorption of x-ray photons, but are significantly less charged than traditional agents. It was hoped that the reduced ionic nature would decrease their nephrotoxicity, but the occurrence of severe adverse renal events did not differ between ionic and nonionic contrast media in a large randomized clinical trial.[78]

Renal nephrotoxicity after exposure to ionic agents occurs most commonly in patients with preexisting renal insufficiency (3.3 relative risk) alone or in combination with diabetes mellitus, especially juvenile-onset diabetes.[78] Other risk factors such as dehydration, volume of contrast used, and simultaneous exposure to other nephrotoxins contribute to the likelihood of acute contrast nephrotoxicity.[79] Other risk factors include multiple myeloma and heavy proteinuria. Overall, the incidence of acute renal dysfunction following contrast angiography varies from 0% to 10%, although these estimates are skewed by several studies that included only juvenile diabetics. In one study, hospital-acquired nephropathy occurred in 12% of patients.[80] In patients with normal renal function, however, the incidence of contrast nephropathy is only 1% to 2%.[81] The effect of diabetes on the risk of acute renal failure following angiography appears to be dependent on the type of diabetes and the magnitude of secondary diabetic nephropathy.

Patients with type 1 diabetes appear to be more susceptible to contrast-induced acute renal failure than do those with type 2 diabetics. Harkonen and Kjellstrand[82,83] found that 20 of 26 patients (76%) with a prestudy serum creatinine level greater than 2 mg/dL who underwent excretory urography also developed acute renal failure.[83] Weinrauch and associates[84] reported that acute renal failure following coronary angiography developed in 12 of 13 patients (92%) with juvenile-onset diabetes and severe diabetic nephropathy. In addition, the cause of chronic renal insufficiency appears to affect recovery from contrast-induced acute renal failure. Whereas both diabetic and nondiabetic patients with renal insufficiency are at increased risk for contrast-induced acute renal failure, diabetics appear to recover less often and are at greater risk of permanent dependence on dialysis as a consequence of contrast-induced acute renal failure.[82-84]

Specific measures to minimize the risk of contrast-induced acute renal failure remain controversial, and the results from controlled studies are largely inconclusive. Nevertheless, the basic relationship between the use of contrast material and the risk of contrast nephropathy appears to be related to the amount of time the kidney is exposed to the contrast material. For this reason, maximizing urine flow rate during and immediately after angiography and limiting the quantity of contrast agent used are important considerations. Maximal urine flow rate should be achieved by preliminary intravenous hydration of the patient. Studies that examined the optimal preparation of patients with renal insufficiency indicated that hydration with 0.45% saline provides better protection against acute decline in renal function associated with radiocontrast agents than does hydration with 0.45% saline plus mannitol or furosemide.[85] Recent evidence suggests that administration of sodium bicarbonate before contrast exposure may significantly reduce renal dysfunction.[86]

By scavenging reactive oxygen species, acetylcysteine may protect against contrast-induced nephrotoxicity. Tepel and colleagues[87] studied patients with chronic renal dysfunction who required nonionic contrast for computed tomography. They documented a significant reduction in serum creatinine with the use of oral acetylcysteine and hydration compared with placebo and hydration.

Although further study is needed to better define the role of acetylcysteine during aortography, we administer two oral doses of acetylcysteine (600 mg) before and after these studies in patients at high risk for contrast nephropathy.[68] We routinely admit any patient at risk for contrast nephropathy 12 hours before angiography for intravenous hydration at 1.5 mL/kg per hour. The patient receives two 600-mg oral doses of acetylcysteine immediately before angiography and a bolus of intravenous fluid (3 to 5 mL/kg) with or without sodium bicarbonate. Finally, intravenous hydration is continued for 4 to 6

hours, and two additional doses of acetylcysteine are administered after completion of the study.

Although attempts to calculate a safe upper limit of contrast material have met with some success, no definitive limit currently exists. Even small doses (30 to 60 mL) may induce renal failure in patients with extreme renal insufficiency (GFR ≤ 15 mL/min). Conversely, more than 300 mL of contrast material can be administered safely to other patients with no risk factors for acute renal failure.[83] The authors' practice is to limit the quantity of non-ionized contrast agent to less than 50 to 75 mL in patients with a significant reduction in GFR (<20 to 30 mL/min).[88] If additional contrast material is required to complete the vascular evaluation, we postpone further study and approach the total evaluation in a sequential manner. In almost all instances, digital subtraction techniques have been useful in limiting the quantity of contrast material required. A single midstream aortic injection, using 10 to 20 mL of low-osmolar, nonionic contrast material and digital subtraction, provides images approaching the quality of prior conventional cut-film studies.

Adjuncts or alternatives to angiography are appropriate in many instances. In addition to the use of digital subtraction techniques, carbon dioxide gas can be used for angiography with minimal renal risk.[89] Because it offers limited detail, carbon dioxide angiography is often used to identify the site of disease, which is then better defined with conventional contrast agents. Other alternatives to conventional angiography that reduce or eliminate the risk of nephrotoxicity include the use of gadolinium as a contrast agent for angiography,[74,75] magnetic resonance angiography,[90] and abdominal ultrasonography with visceral or renal artery duplex sonography.

Finally, high-dose loop diuretics, angiotensin-converting enzyme inhibitors, and angiotensin II receptor antagonists are held for at least 72 hours before aortic reconstruction or exposure to arterial contrast agents. Selective β-blockers and calcium channel blockers are substituted when necessary.[91]

Both aortography and selective renal angiography using multiple projections may be necessary to adequately examine the entire renal artery. The proximal third of the left renal artery usually courses anteriorly, the middle third transversely, and the distal third posteriorly, whereas the right renal artery arises from the anterior aorta and then pursues a more consistent posterior course. Lesions in the renal artery that are coursing anteriorly or posteriorly are frequently not seen or may appear insignificant in an anteroposterior aortogram. Oblique aortography or oblique selective renal angiography projects these portions of the vessels in profile and reveals the stenosis. Figure 24-6 illustrates how the delicate septal lesions of fibromuscular dysplasia may be unrecognizable or appear insignificant in the anteroposterior projection, whereas the true severity is demonstrated in the oblique projection.

Functional Studies

Two tests—renal vein renin assays and split renal function studies—have proved valuable in confirming the

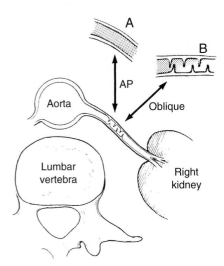

FIGURE 24-6 ■ Graphic illustration of how the septa of medial fibroplasia can be missed. *A*, When the vessel is viewed with an anteroposterior (AP) arteriogram, the septa are masked by the overlying dye column. *B*, In the oblique projection, the septa are demonstrated because they are parallel to the direction of the x-ray.

functional significance of renal artery stenosis. Neither has great value, however, when severe bilateral disease or disease in the renal artery supplying a single kidney is present. In these circumstances, the decision for operation is based on the severity of hypertension and the degree of renal insufficiency. Furthermore, urologically performed split renal function studies are no longer done in any center studying patients with RVH. The reader is referred to earlier texts describing their use.[92,93]

Renal Vein Renin Assays

When a unilateral obstructive renal artery lesion is found by renal angiography, its functional significance should be evaluated. Most centers rely solely on renal vein renin assays (RVRAs) to establish the diagnosis of RVH. The unfortunate consequence of this trend is that one must presume that all patients with RVH have lateralizing RVRAs. Results of the evaluation of this study in our center underscore the fallacy of this presumption. Many factors can affect the RVRA; if these are not properly managed, erroneous results may occur.

The effect of antihypertensive medications and unrestricted sodium intake on renin release, and thereby the RVRA, is widely recognized. Many antihypertensive medications, especially those that function through β-adrenergic blockade, suppress renin output and can lead to false nonlateralization of the RVRA. Before presuming that no drug is interfering with the release of renin, all such medications must be withheld for at least 5 days—preferably 2 weeks—before the RVRA. Similar effects on renin levels are seen when sodium intake is not restricted. For this reason, the patient must be on no more than a 2-g sodium diet for at least 2 weeks before the study. The preparation of patients for RVRA is summarized in Box 24-1.

BOX 24-1   **Patient Preparation for Renal Vein Renin Assay**

1. Chronic salt restriction (2-g sodium diet daily)
2. Discontinuance of all antihypertensive drugs except diuretics and calcium channel for at least 5 days before the study
3. Oral furosemide (40 mg) diuresis the night before the study
4. Nothing by mouth for 8 hours before the study
5. Strictly flat bed rest for 4 hours before and during the study
6. Prestudy sedation with intramuscular diazepam (5 mg)

The technical aspects of performing the RVRA cannot be overemphasized. The left renal vein contains not only renal venous effluent but also adrenal, gonadal, and lumbar venous effluent. Misplacement of the venous catheter into the origin of one of the nonrenal branches or sampling in the proximal renal vein, where a mixture from these other sources is present, may dilute the renin activity coming from the kidney. This leads to erroneously low measurements of renin activity and produces a false interpretation of the RVRA.

The time of sampling the two renal veins for renin activity is also a potential source of error in the RVRA. In studies performed with a single catheter, several minutes may elapse between sampling the two renal veins as the catheter is switched from one side to the other. Furthermore, catheter manipulation and patient discomfort can affect renin release. Not surprisingly, when a single catheter is used, both false-positive and false-negative renal vein renin ratios are common.

Several methods of stimulating renin release have been suggested. These methods include tilting the patient to the upright posture during the study, stimulation with intravenous hydralazine hydrochloride, and nitroprusside stimulation. Although all these methods increase renin release, they also increase false-positive determinations and reduce the reliability of the RVRA to unacceptable levels.

Vaughan and colleagues[94] stressed the importance of expressing the RVRA in relation to the systemic renin activity rather than simply evaluating the ratio of renin activity between the two renal veins. In patients with RVH secondary to unilateral renal artery stenosis, one should find hypersecretion of renin from the ischemic kidney and suppression of renin secretion from the normal kidney. Through application of this hypothesis, Stanley and Fry[95] showed a statistically significant difference in the renal-systemic renin indices in patients who were cured of RVH by operation compared with those who were only improved. Although this method has appeal as a predictor of the extent of benefit, its value in patients with bilateral renal artery lesions is limited. Because both lesions may be producing RVH, both this method and renal vein renin ratios have less validity as predictors of response to operation. If one bases the decision for operative management solely on whether absolute cure is expected, many patients with severe

TABLE 24-6   Frequency of Severe Deterioration in Parameters of Renal Function during Drug Therapy

Parameter	No. of Patients Monitored	Mean Follow-Up (mo)	Failure Event	Number Affected	Percentage Affected
Renal length	38	33	≥10% decrease	14	37
Serum creatinine	41	25	≥100% increase	2	5
Glomerular filtration rate or creatinine clearance	30	19	≥50% decrease	1	3

From Dean RH, Kieffer RW, Smith BM, et al: Renovascular hypertension. Arch Surg 116:1408, 1981.

hypertension who would benefit from its reduction to a mild, easily controlled level would be excluded from consideration as operative candidates. Therefore, this method of RVRA interpretation should be considered only as an additional predictive tool and not as an alternative to the evaluation of renal vein renin ratios.

RVRAs also may be inaccurate in patients with accessory or segmental renal artery stenosis if renal venous sampling is limited to the main renal vein. Because recognition of renin hypersecretion depends on sampling the ischemic areas of the kidneys, selective segmental venous sampling must be done in these patients. When segmental sampling is required, the renin activity from the segment sampled is compared with the simultaneously collected contralateral main renal vein sample to calculate the renal vein renin ratio.

MANAGEMENT OPTIONS

The question of what constitutes the best method of management for patients with RVH or ischemic nephropathy is unanswerable. There are no prospective, randomized trials that compare all available treatment options. In the absence of level I data, advocates of medical management, percutaneous transluminal angioplasty (PTA), or operative intervention cite selective clinical data to support their particular views.

A majority of the medical community evaluates patients for RVH only when medications are not tolerated or hypertension remains severe and poorly controlled. The study by Hunt and Strong[96] remains the most informative study available to assess the comparative value of medical therapy and operation. In this nonrandomized study, the results of operative treatment in 100 patients were compared with the results of drug therapy in 114 similar patients. After 7 to 14 years of follow-up, 84% of the operated group was alive, compared with 66% of the drug therapy group. Of the 84 patients alive in the operated group, 93% were cured or significantly improved, compared with only 21% of the surviving patients in the drug therapy group. Death during follow-up was twice as common in the medically treated group as in the operated group, resulting in differences that were statistically significant in patients with either atherosclerosis or fibromuscular dysplasia of the renal artery.

Additional prospective data regarding medical therapy for RVH suggest that a decrease in kidney size and renal function may occur despite satisfactory blood pressure control. Dean and colleagues[97] reported the results of serial renal function studies performed on 41 patients with RVH (i.e., hypertension and positive functional studies) secondary to atherosclerotic renal artery disease who were randomly selected for nonoperative management (Table 24-6). In 19 patients, serum creatinine levels increased between 25% and 120%. GFRs dropped between 25% and 50% in 12 patients, and 14 patients lost more than 10% of renal length. In four patients, a significant stenosis progressed to total occlusion. Overall, 17 patients (41%) had deterioration of renal function or loss of renal size that led to operation, and one patient required removal of a previously reconstructible kidney. Of the 17 patients in whom renal function deteriorated, 15 had acceptable control of blood pressure during the period of nonoperative observation. This experience suggests that progressive decline of renal function in medically treated patients with atherosclerotic RVD, and RVH occurs despite medical blood pressure control.

The detrimental changes that can occur during medical therapy alone are often cited as supporting evidence for intervention for all renovascular lesions. It should be emphasized, however, that the only prospective angiographic data were obtained from patients with proven RVH (i.e., high-grade renal artery stenosis with severe hypertension and positive physiologic studies).[97] Accordingly, these data should not be applied to asymptomatic patients. Indications for interventional management include all patients with severe, difficult-to-control hypertension[60,63]; this includes patients with complicating factors such as branch lesions and extrarenal atherosclerotic disease, including those with associated cardiovascular disease that would be improved by blood pressure reduction. Moreover, young patients whose hypertension is moderate, who have no associated end-organ disease, and who have easily correctable atherosclerotic or dysplastic main renal artery lesions are also candidates for operative intervention. The chance of curing moderate hypertension is good in such patients, and it remains to be proved that medical blood pressure control is equivalent to the cure of hypertension. Finally, no evidence exists that age, type of renovascular lesion (whether atherosclerotic or dysplastic), duration of hypertension, or presence of bilateral lesions accurately estimate the likelihood of successful surgical management. Consequently, the presence or absence of these factors should not be used as determinants of intervention.

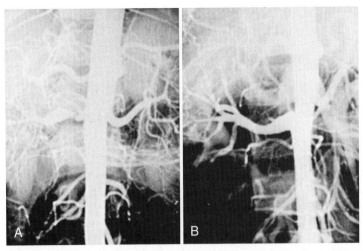

FIGURE 24-7 ■ Preoperative **(A)** and postoperative **(B)** arteriograms in a 5-year-old child who underwent right renal artery reimplantation.

OPERATIVE TECHNIQUES

A variety of operative techniques have been used to correct renal artery stenoses. From a practical standpoint, three basic operations are most frequently used: aortorenal bypass, thromboendarterectomy, and reimplantation. Bypass is most versatile. Endarterectomy has particular application to artificial atherosclerosis, especially when renal-type arteries are involved. When the renal artery is sufficiently redundant, reimplantation is technically easiest and has particular application in children (Figure 24-7).

Antihypertensive medications are reduced during the preoperative period to the minimum necessary for blood pressure control. Frequently, patients requiring large doses of multiple medications for control have significantly reduced requirements while hospitalized and on bed rest. If continued therapy is required, vasodilators (e.g., nifedipine) in combination with selective β-adrenergic blockers (e.g., atenolol) are the drugs of choice. There is little effect on hemodynamics when these agents are combined with anesthesia. If the patient's diastolic blood pressure exceeds 120 mm Hg, the pressure must be brought under control, and operative treatment must be postponed until this is accomplished. If blood pressure is difficult to control, the patient may be transferred to the intensive care unit, where intravenous nitroprusside therapy with continuous intraarterial monitoring of blood pressure is instituted for 24 hours before operation. Similarly, if the patient has a significant history of heart disease, then pulmonary artery wedge pressure and cardiac performance are monitored to maintain optimal cardiac hemodynamics and recognize and correct adverse changes before they become clinically significant.

Certain measures and maneuvers are applicable to almost all renal artery operations. Mannitol (12.5 g) is administered intravenously early in the operation. Just before renal artery cross-clamping, heparin (100 units/kg) is given intravenously, and systemic anticoagulation is verified by activated clotting time. Protamine is rarely required for the reversal of heparin at the end of the reconstruction.

Mobilization and Dissection

Through a midline xiphoid-to-pubis incision, the posterior peritoneum overlying the aorta is incised longitudinally, and the duodenum is reflected to the patient's right to expose the left renal artery (Figure 24-8). By extending the posterior peritoneal incision to the left along the inferior border of the pancreas, an avascular plane behind the pancreas can be entered to expose the entire renal hilum on the left (Figure 24-9).

This exposure is of special significance when distal lesions must also be managed. The left renal artery lies behind the left renal vein. In some cases, the vein can be retracted cephalad to expose the artery; in other cases, caudal retraction of the vein provides better access. Usually the gonadal and adrenal veins, which enter the left renal vein, must be ligated and divided to facilitate exposure of the artery. Frequently, a lumbar vein enters the posterior wall of the left renal vein, and it can be avulsed easily unless special care is taken while mobilizing the renal vein. The proximal portion of the right renal artery can be exposed through the base of the mesentery by ligating two or more pairs of lumbar veins and retracting the left renal vein cephalad and the vena cava to the patient's right. However, the distal portion of the right renal artery is best exposed by mobilizing the duodenum and right colon medially (Figure 24-10). Next, the right renal vein is mobilized and usually retracted cephalad to expose the artery.

When bilateral renal artery lesions are to be corrected, and when correction of a right renal artery lesion or bilateral lesions is combined with aortic reconstruction, we modify these exposure techniques. First, we extend the base of the mesentery exposure to allow complete evisceration of the entire small bowel and the right and transverse portions of the colon; in this exposure,

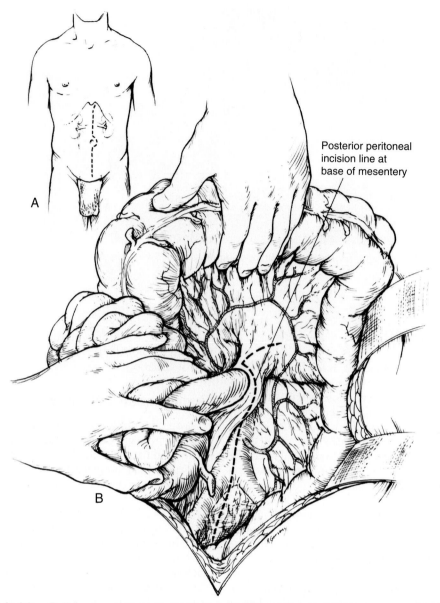

Posterior peritoneal
incision line at
base of mesentery

FIGURE 24-8 ■ **A,** Skin incision. **B,** Exposure of the aorta and left renal hilum through the base of the mesentery. Extension of the posterior peritoneal incision to the left, along the inferior border of the pancreas, provides entry to an avascular plane behind the pancreas. This allows excellent exposure of the entire left renal hilum as well as the proximal right renal artery. (From Benjamin ME, Dean RH: Techniques in renal artery reconstruction: part I. Ann Vasc Surg 10:306–314, 1996.)

the posterior peritoneal incision begins with division of the ligament of Treitz and proceeds along the base of the mesentery to the cecum and then up the lateral gutter to the foramen of Winslow (Figure 24-11). Second, we extend the incision to the left along the inferior border of the pancreas to enter a retropancreatic plane, thereby exposing the aorta to a point above the superior mesenteric artery. Through this modified exposure, simultaneous bilateral renal endarterectomies, aortorenal grafting, or renal artery attachment to the aortic graft can be performed with wide visualization of the entire area.

Another technique is to partially divide both diaphragmatic crura as they pass behind the renal arteries to their paravertebral attachment. By partially dividing the crura, the aorta above the superior mesenteric artery is easily visualized and can be mobilized for suprarenal cross-clamping.

Aortorenal Bypass

Three types of graft are usually available for aortorenal bypass: autologous saphenous vein, autologous hypogastric artery, and synthetic prosthesis. The decision of which graft to use depends on a number of factors; the saphenous vein is preferred by some. However, if it is small (<4 mm in diameter) or sclerotic, the hypogastric artery or a synthetic prosthesis may be preferable. A thin-walled, 6-mm polytetrafluoroethylene graft is satisfactory when the distal renal artery is of large caliber.

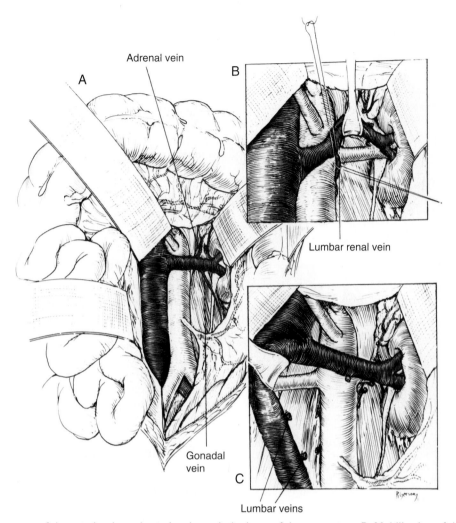

Adrenal vein

A

B

Lumbar renal vein

Gonadal
vein

C

Lumbar veins

FIGURE 24-9 ■ **A,** Exposure of the proximal renal arteries through the base of the mesentery. **B,** Mobilization of the left renal vein by ligation and division of the adrenal, gonadal, and lumbar renal veins allows exposure of the entire left renal artery to the hilum. **C,** Two pairs of lumbar vessels have been ligated and divided to allow retraction of the vena cava to the right, providing adequate exposure of proximal renal artery disease. (From Benjamin ME, Dean RH: Techniques in renal artery reconstruction: part I. Ann Vasc Surg 10:306–314, 1996.)

When an end-to-side renal artery bypass is used, the anastomosis between the renal artery and the graft is done first. Silastic slings can be used to occlude the renal artery distally. This method of vessel occlusion is especially applicable to this procedure. In contrast to vascular clamps, these slings are essentially atraumatic to the delicate renal artery. The absence of clamps in the operative field is also advantageous. Furthermore, when tension is applied to the slings, they lift the vessel out of the retroperitoneal soft tissue for more accurate visualization.

The length of the arteriotomy should be at least three times the diameter of the renal artery to guard against late suture line stenosis. A 6-0 or 7-0 monofilament polypropylene suture material is employed with loop magnification.

After the renal artery anastomosis is completed, the occluding clamps and slings are removed from the artery, and a small bulldog clamp is placed across the vein graft adjacent to the anastomosis. The aortic anastomosis is then done. First, an ellipse of the anterolateral aortic wall is removed, and then the anastomosis is performed. If the

graft is too long, kinking of the vein and subsequent thrombosis may result. If any element of kinking or twisting of the graft occurs after both anastomoses are completed, the aortic anastomosis should be taken down and redone after appropriate shortening or reorientation of the graft. In most instances, an end-to-end anastomosis between the graft and the renal artery provides a better reconstruction. This is especially true for combined aortorenal reconstruction. In this circumstance, the renal artery graft is attached to the Dacron aortic graft before its insertion. After the aortic graft is attached and flow is restored to the distal extremities, the renal artery can be transected and attached to the end of the saphenous vein graft without interrupting aortic flow.

Thromboendarterectomy

Thromboendarterectomy is used only for atherosclerotic renal artery stenosis. It is not applicable in fibromuscular disease. Transaortic endarterectomy of bilateral main renal artery lesions has been strongly advocated by Wylie

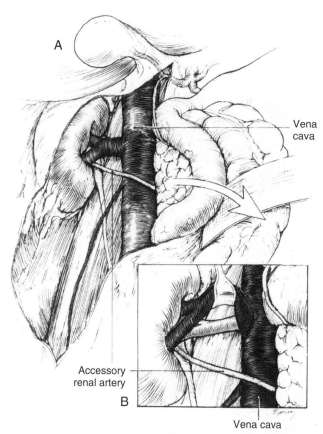

FIGURE 24-10 ■ **A,** Not uncommonly, an accessory right renal artery arises from the anterior aorta and crosses anterior to the vena cava. **B,** The right renal vein is typically mobilized superiorly for exposure of the distal right renal artery. (From Benjamin ME, Dean RH: Techniques in renal artery reconstruction: part I. Ann Vasc Surg 10:306–314, 1996.)

and colleagues[98] (Figure 24-12). In this procedure, the proximal aortic clamp must usually be placed above the superior mesenteric artery. If it is placed below this artery, it seriously compromises the exposure of the orifices of the renal arteries. Visualization of the distal end of the renal artery endarterectomy is facilitated by inversion of the renal artery into the aorta. Alternatively, a transrenal endarterectomy uses a transverse aortotomy, carrying the incision across the stenoses and into each renal artery. By this method, the entire endarterectomy can be performed under direct vision with Dacron patch closure.

Extraanatomic Bypass

Extraanatomic procedures have become increasingly popular as an alternative method of renal revascularization for high-risk patients.[99] We do not believe that these procedures are equivalent to direct reconstructions, but they are useful in a highly select subgroup of high-risk patients.

Hepatorenal Bypass

A right subcostal incision is usually used to perform the hepatorenal bypass. The hepatoduodenal ligament is incised, and the common hepatic artery both proximal and distal to the gastroduodenal artery origin is encircled. Next, the descending duodenum is mobilized with the Kocher maneuver, the inferior vena cava is identified, the right renal vein is identified, and the right renal artery is encircled where it is found, either immediately cephalad or caudad to the renal vein (Figure 24-13).

A greater saphenous vein graft is usually used to construct the bypass. The hepatic artery anastomosis of the vein graft can be placed at the site of the amputated stump of the gastroduodenal artery or proximal to this branch when it must be saved as a collateral for gut perfusion. After completion of this anastomosis, the renal artery is transected and brought anterior to the vena cava for anastomosis end to end to the graft.

Splenorenal Bypass

Splenorenal bypass can be performed through a midline or a left subcostal incision. The posterior pancreas is mobilized by reflecting the inferior border cephalad. When the retropancreatic plane has been entered, the splenic artery can be mobilized from the left gastroepiploic artery to the level of its branches. The left renal artery is exposed as described earlier. After the splenic artery has been completely mobilized, it is divided distally, spatulated, and anastomosed end to end to the transected renal artery (Figure 24-14).

Ex Vivo Reconstruction

Ex vivo management is necessary in patients with fibromuscular dysplasia and aneurysms or stenoses involving renal artery branches; patients with fibromuscular dysplasia, renal artery dissection, and branch occlusion; patients with congenital arteriovenous fistulas of renal artery branches requiring partial resection; and patients with degeneration of previously placed grafts to the distal renal artery. Several methods of ex vivo hypothermic perfusion and reconstruction are available. A midline xiphoid-to-pubic incision is used for most renovascular procedures and is preferred when autotransplantation of the reconstructed kidney or combined aortic reconstructions are to be performed. An extended flank incision made parallel to the lower rib margin and carried to the posterior axillary line is used for complex branch renal artery repairs and is the preferred approach for ex vivo reconstructions without autotransplantation. The ureter is always mobilized but left intact, and an elastic sling or noncrushing clamp is placed around it to prevent collateral perfusion, inadvertent rewarming, or continued blood loss through the ureteric collaterals.[100]

After the kidney is mobilized and the vessels divided, the kidney is placed on the abdominal wall and perfused with a renal preservative solution. Continuous perfusion during the period of total renal ischemia is possible with complex perfusion pump systems and may be superior for prolonged renal preservation during storage periods. However, simple intermittent flushing with a chilled preservative solution provides equal protection during the shorter periods (2 to 3 hours) required for ex vivo dissection and complex renal artery reconstructions. For

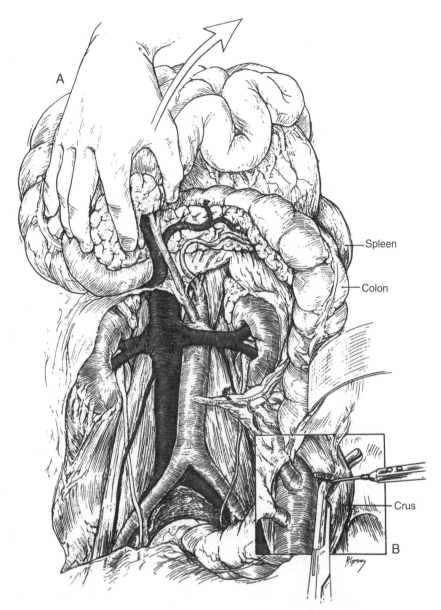

FIGURE 24-11 ■ **A,** For bilateral renal artery reconstruction combined with aortic repair, extended exposure can be obtained with mobilization of the cecum and ascending colon. The entire small bowel and right colon are then mobilized to the right upper quadrant and placed onto the chest wall. **B,** Division of the diaphragmatic crura exposures the origin of the mesenteric vessels. (From Benjamin ME, Dean RH: Techniques in renal artery reconstruction: part I. Ann Vasc Surg 10:306–314, 1996.)

intermittent flushing, refrigerate the preservative over-night, add the additional components (Table 24-7) immediately before use to make up 1 L of solution, and hang the chilled (5°C to 10°C) solution on an intrave-nous stand to provide gravitational perfusion pressure of at least 2 m. Five hundred milliliters of solution is flushed through the kidney immediately after its removal from the renal fossa. If arterial exposure is adequate, the vein may be left intact, controlled with an atraumatic clamp and a small venotomy made for the egress of perfusate. Regardless of whether the vein is divided or left intact, as each anastomosis is completed, an addi-tional 150 to 200 mL of solution is flushed through the kidney, a procedure that also shows any leaks at the suture line.

Surface hypothermia is used to maintain constant hypothermia during ex vivo renal artery reconstruction. One method of surface hypothermia consists of the fol-lowing steps.

- Place two 1-L bottles of normal saline solution in ice slush overnight.
- After removing the kidney, place it in a watertight plastic sheet from which excess saline solution can be suctioned away and place laparotomy pads over the kidney.
- Keeping it cool and moist by a constant drip of the chilled saline solution.

With this technique, it is possible to maintain renal core temperatures of 10°C to 15°C throughout the period of ischemia.

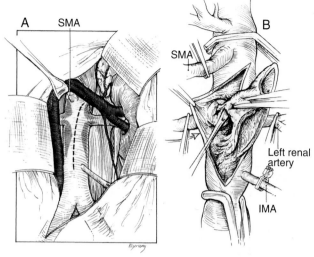

FIGURE 24-12 ■ Exposure for a longitudinal transaortic endarterectomy is through the standard transperitoneal approach. The duodenum is mobilized from the aorta laterally in standard fashion or, for more complete exposure, the ascending colon and small bowel are mobilized. **A,** The dotted line shows the location of the aortotomy. **B,** The plaque is transected proximally and distally, and with eversion of the renal arteries, the atherosclerotic plaque is removed from each renal ostium. The aortotomy is typically closed with a running 4-0 or 5-0 polypropylene suture. *IMA,* Inferior mesenteric artery; *SMA,* superior mesenteric artery. (From Benjamin ME, Dean RH: Techniques in renal artery reconstruction: part I. Ann Vasc Surg 10:306–314, 1996.)

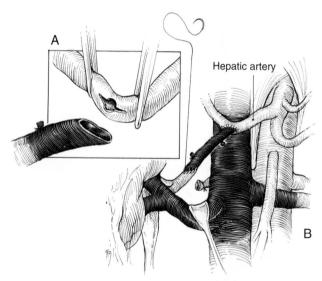

FIGURE 24-13 ■ The reconstruction is completed using a saphenous vein interposition graft between the side of the hepatic artery **(A)** and the distal end of the transected right renal artery **(B).** (From Benjamin ME, Dean RH: Techniques in renal artery reconstruction: part II. Ann Vasc Surg 10:409–414, 1996.)

When both the renal artery and renal vein have been divided, autotransplantation to the iliac fossa is not necessary for most ex vivo reconstructions, even though it is an accepted method for reattachment of the ex vivo reconstructed renal artery. Autotransplantation of the reconstructed kidney to the iliac fossa was adapted from renal transplant surgeons, with no thought given to the

significant difference between the two patient populations. Reduction in the magnitude of the operative exposure, manual palpation of the transplanted kidney, potential use of irradiation for episodes of rejection, and ease of removal when treatment of rejection has failed are all historical and practical reasons for placing the transplanted kidney into the recipient's iliac fossa, but none of these advantages apply to patients requiring ex vivo reconstruction.

Rather, the factors most important in this patient population are related to improving the predictability of permanent patency after revascularization. Because many ex vivo procedures are performed in relatively young patients, the durability of the operation should be measured in terms of decades. For this reason, attaching the kidney to the iliac arterial system within or below sites that are highly susceptible to significant atherosclerotic occlusive disease subjects the repaired vessels to disease that may, in time, threaten their patency. Furthermore, subsequent management of peripheral vascular disease can be complicated by the presence of the autotransplanted kidney. Finally, if the kidney is replaced in the renal fossa and the renal artery graft is properly attached to the aorta at a proximal infrarenal site, the result should mimic that of the standard aortorenal bypass and thus carry a high probability of technical success and long-term durability.

For replacement of the kidney in its original site, the Gerota capsule must be opened during mobilization. Before transection of the renal vein begins, a large vascular clamp is placed to partially occlude the vena cava where it is entered by the renal vein. An ellipse of vena cava containing the entrance site of the renal vein is then excised, and the kidney is removed for ex vivo perfusion and reconstruction (Figure 24-15). When the distal renal artery–graft anastomoses are completed and the kidney is replaced in its bed, the ellipse of vena cava is reattached. This technique protects against stenosis of the renal vein anastomosis as a result of technical error. The renal artery graft is then attached to the aorta in the standard manner.

Nephrectomy

Nephrectomy is a procedure that should be limited to a subgroup of patients with RVH in whom the kidney responsible for the hypertension has nonreconstructible vessels and negligible residual excretory function. In these circumstances, nephrectomy can be of benefit because it controls hypertension without diminishing overall excretory function. In all other circumstances in which significant residual excretory function is present, the price of nephrectomy (loss of functioning renal mass) is greater than the potential benefit. This extreme conservatism regarding nephrectomy is based on the knowledge that more than 35% of patients with atherosclerotic lesions develop severe contralateral lesions during follow-up. Such lesions place the patient at risk for clinically severe renal failure and recurrent hypertension. This risk is even more important in children, because 50% of those who initially show a unilateral lesion subsequently develop contralateral disease.

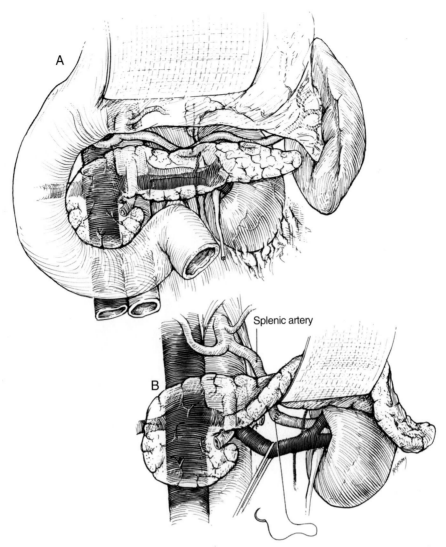

FIGURE 24-14 ■ **A,** Exposure of the left renal hilum in preparation for splenorenal bypass. The pancreas has been mobilized along its inferior margin and retracted superiorly. **B,** The transected splenic artery is anastomosed end to end to the transected left renal artery. A splenectomy is not routinely performed. (From Benjamin ME, Dean RH: Techniques in renal artery reconstruction: part II. Ann Vasc Surg 10:409–414, 1996.)

TABLE 24-7 Electrolyte Solutions* for Ex Vivo Repair

Composition		Ionic Concentration		Additives to 930 mL of Solution at Time of Use
Component	**Amount (g/L)**	**Electrolyte**	**Concentration (mEq/L)**	
K_2HPO_4	7.4	Potassium	115	50% dextrose: 70 mL
KH_2PO_4	2.04	Sodium	10	Sodium heparin: 2000 units
KCl	1.12	Phosphate (HPO_4^{2-})	85	
$NaHCO_3$	0.84	Phosphate ($H_2PO_4^-$)	15	
		Chloride	15	
		Bicarbonate	10	

*Electrolyte solution for kidney preservation supplied by Travenol Labs, Deerfield, Ill.

EFFECT OF OPERATION ON HYPERTENSION

Most of the controversy surrounding the role of open surgical treatment of RVH relates to the morbidity and mortality associated with operation, the frequency of technical failure, and the low rate of a favorable blood pressure response to operation. Certainly, the literature documents the fact that poorly performed operations in poorly selected patients seldom result in a blood pressure benefit. Current results of operative intervention in centers experienced with the management of RVD, however, underscore the high rate of long-term patency

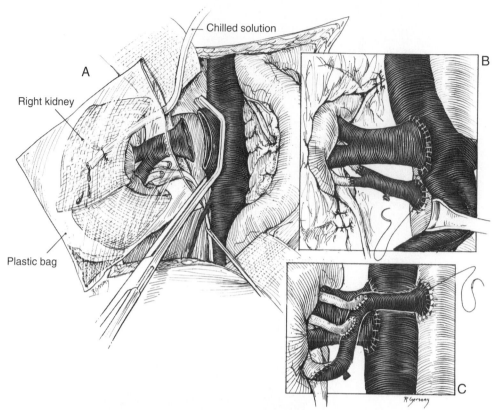

FIGURE 24-15 ■ Renal reconstruction requiring longer than 40 to 45 minutes of warm renal ischemia is facilitated by cold perfusion techniques. **A,** An ellipse of the vena cava containing the renal vein origin is excised by placement of a large, partially occluding clamp. After ex vivo branch repair, the renal vein can be reattached without risk of anastomotic stricture. **B,** The kidney is repositioned in its native bed after ex vivo repair. The Gerota fascia is reattached to provide stability to the replaced kidney. Arterial reconstruction can be accomplished via end-to-end anastomoses (as in **B**). **C,** Alternatively, reconstruction is occasionally performed with a combination of end-to-end and end-to-side anastomoses. If exposure is adequate, the renal vein can be controlled but left intact with a small venotomy for egress of perfusate. (From Benjamin ME, Dean RH: Techniques in renal artery reconstruction: part II. Ann Vasc Surg 10:409–414, 1996.)

and benefit to both blood pressure and renal function. Although our cumulative experience spans more than 40 years and includes the operative management of more than 1500 patients, a review of the results of a recent series of 500 consecutive atherosclerotic patients exemplifies current experience.[23]

Among patients with nonatherosclerotic RVD, 92% had a beneficial hypertension response, but only 43% were considered cured—a lower cure rate than that reported in the earlier surgical series.[30,101] This difference may be explained by the number of older patients, the number of patients with uncorrected contralateral lesions, and the duration of hypertension in many of these patients with nonatherosclerotic RVD. In contrast to the blood pressure results obtained in the entire group, patients younger than 45 years who had all anatomic renal artery lesions corrected and who had been hypertensive for less than 5 years had a cure rate of 68% and an improvement rate of 32%. This response rate is comparable with results from earlier reports.

Although operation was accomplished in the nonatherosclerotic RVD group without death, the operative mortality of 4.7% among 1076 patients with atherosclerotic RVD was high.[23,26,138-141] Blood pressure benefit (i.e., cured and improved) was observed in 88% of

patients, of which 49% were cured and 39% improved. Unfortunately, 13% of the patients failed to see a benefit (Table 24-8).

EFFECT OF RENAL REVASCULARIZATION ON RENAL FUNCTION

Little information is available regarding the incidence, prevalence, or natural history of ischemic nephropathy. Nevertheless, circumstantial evidence suggests that it may be a more common cause of progressive renal failure in the atherosclerotic age group (55 years or older) than previously recognized. In a 1988 report, 73% of patients with end-stage renal disease were in the atherosclerotic age group.[102] In a report by Mailloux and colleagues,[103] a presumed renovascular cause of end-stage renal disease increased in frequency from 6.7% for the period 1978 to 1981 to 16.5% for the period 1982 to 1985. The median age at onset of end-stage renal disease for that group was the oldest of all groups, falling in the seventh decade of life.

In 1076 patients (see Table 24-8), 44% experienced improved renal function with a range of 23%-58% among the individual studies. In addition, 44% experienced no

Table 24-8 Surgical Renal Artery Revascularization*

Reference	Year	Patients	Bilateral Repair (%)	Preoperative Renal Dysfunction (%)	Renal Function Response (%)			Hypertension Response (%)			Perioperative Mortality (%)	Perioperative Morbidity (%)
					Improved	Unchanged	Worsened	Cured	Improved	Failed		
Fergany and colleagues[139†]	1995	175	2.3	92.3	35	47	18	46	54	0	2.9	NR
Geroulakos and colleagues[138†]	1997	38	NR	47	45	37	18	3	53	44	2.6	23.6
Hansen and colleagues[26]	2000	232	64	100	58	35	7	11	76	13	7.3	30
Cherr and colleagues[23]	2002	500	59	48.8	43	47	10	73	12	15	4.6	16
Marone and colleagues[140]	2004	96	27	100	42	41	16	NR	NR	NR	4.1	NR
Grigoryants and colleagues[141†]	2007	35	57	46	23	60	17	9	79	12	2.8	NR
Mean %[‡]					44	44	12	49	39	13	4.7	20.6

*Renal function and hypertension responses expressed percentage of patients surviving operation.
†Weighted mean based on number of patients with reported data categorized according to column.
‡References in which data were not reported or categoric response categories were combined are not included in calculation.
NR, Not reported.

change in their renal function after open repair. Renal function worsened in 12% of the patients.

To improve understanding of ischemic nephropathy, Dean and colleagues[104] undertook a retrospective review of data collected during a 42-month period from 58 consecutive patients with ischemic nephropathy who were admitted for operative management. They examined the rate of decline in their renal function during the period before intervention and the effect of operation on their outcome. Their ages ranged from 22 to 79 years (mean, 69 years). Based on serum creatinine values, immediate preoperative estimated GFR ranged from 0 to 46 mL/min (mean, 23.85 ± 9.76 mL/min). Patients with at least three sequential measurements for the calculation of estimated GFR changes during the 6 months before operation (n = 50) and the first 12 months after operation (n = 32) were used to describe the preoperative rate of decline in estimated GFR and the effect of operation on this decrease in the operative survivors. In addition, comparative analyses of data from patients with unilateral versus bilateral lesions and patients classified as having improvement in estimated GFR versus no improvement after operation were performed. Comparison of the immediate preoperative and immediate postoperative estimated GFRs for the entire group showed significant improvement in response to operation (Figure 24-16). Likewise, the rate of deterioration in estimated GFR for the total group was improved after operation (Figure 24-17). A similar improvement in the rate of deterioration in estimated GFR was seen in the subgroup of patients who had an immediate improvement in response to operation (Figure 24-18).

From this review, it was found that the site of disease (unilateral or bilateral), the anatomic status of the distal renal artery, and the rate of deterioration in renal function were significant predictors of a beneficial effect on renal function. Conversely, unilateral disease, absence of severe hypertension, and diffuse branch vessel occlusive disease were negative predictors of such benefit.

The data presented in this retrospective review argue that ischemic nephropathy is a rapidly progressive form of renal insufficiency. The effect of renal revascularization on renal function, however, was heterogeneous. Nevertheless, the frequency of both retrieval of renal function and slowing the rate of its deterioration during follow-up was gratifying and encourages continued study of the role of operation in properly selected patients.

Recently, we reviewed the functional response to operation in more than 200 consecutive hypertensive patients treated for ischemic nephropathy.[26] Overall, two thirds of patients had early improvement in excretory renal function (i.e., ≥20% increase in estimated GFR), and three quarters of dialysis-dependent patients were permanently removed from dialysis after operation (Table 24-9). When estimated survival was stratified to renal function response, only patients who were improved demonstrated increased dialysis-free survival. Patients who were unchanged or worse had nearly identical rates of follow-up death or eventual dialysis dependence (Figure 24-19). Hypertension response in this subgroup with ischemic nephropathy had no apparent effect on survival (Figure 24-20).

Experience suggests a potential benefit of operation on both GFR and its rate of deterioration in a subset of patients. Nevertheless, the risk associated with operation is not inconsequential. This risk and the rate of survival must be placed in context with the probability of survival without operation. In a study of the duration of survival after the institution of dialysis, Mailloux and coworkers[103] found that end-stage renal disease caused by uncorrected RVD was associated with the most rapid rate of death during follow-up. In their study, patients with RVD had a median survival after the initiation of dialysis of only 27 months and a 5-year survival rate of only 12%. In patients who progress to dialysis dependence, median survival has been 16.5 months.[26] These findings equate with a death rate in excess of 20% per year. In a group of 20 patients who were dialysis

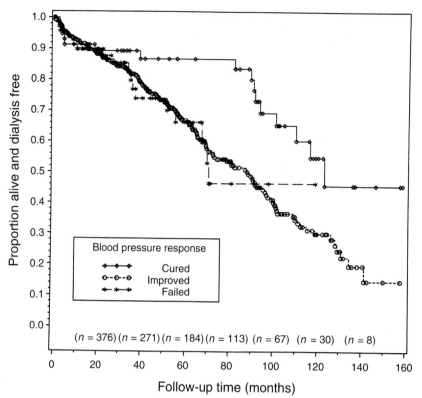

FIGURE 24-16 ■ Product limit estimates of time to death or dialysis according to blood pressure response to operation for athero-sclerotic renovascular disease (n = 472). (From Cherr GS, Hansen KJ, Craven TE, et al: Surgical management of atherosclerotic renovascular disease. J Vasc Surg 35:236–245, 2002.)

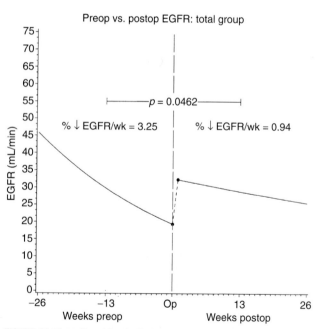

FIGURE 24-17 ■ Graphic depiction of the percentage deterioration of estimated glomerular filtration rate (EGFR) per week for the entire group during the 6 months before (n = 50) and after (n = 32) operation (Op). The immediate effect of operation on the EGFR is also depicted. The *p* values for differences are determined using the *t* test for unpaired data. Note the improvement in the slope of decline in EGFR after operation. (From Dean RH, Tribble RW, Hansen KJ, et al: Evolution of renal insufficiency in ischemic nephropathy. Ann Surg 213:446–455, 1991.)

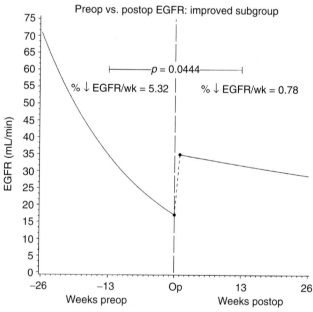

FIGURE 24-18 ■ Graphic depiction of the percentage deterioration of estimated glomerular filtration rate (EGFR) per week during the 6 months before (n = 23) and after (n = 25) operation (Op) in the improved group of patients (i.e., those who had at least a 20% improvement in EGFR following operation). The immediate effect of operation on EGFR in this improved group is also depicted. The *p* values for differences are determined using the *t* test for unpaired data. Note the improvement in the slope of decline in EGFR after operation in this group. (From Dean RH, Tribble RW, Hansen KJ, et al: Evolution of renal insufficiency in ischemic nephropathy. Ann Surg 213:446–455, 1991.)

TABLE 24-9 Renal Function Response versus Preoperative Serum Creatinine

Renal Function Response	Preoperative SCR 1.8-2.9 mg/dL	Preoperative SCR ≥ 3.0 mg/dL	Dialysis Dependent	Total
Improved (%)	52	59	75	58
No change (%)	39	33	25	35
Worse (%)	9	8	—	7

From Hansen KJ, Cherr GS, Craven TE, et al: Management of ischemic nephropathy: dialysis-free survival after surgical repair. J Vasc Surg 32:472–482, 2000.
SCR, Serum creatinine.

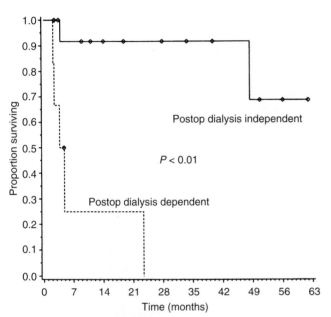

FIGURE 24-19 ■ Product limit estimate of patient survival according to dialysis status after operation for dialysis-dependent ischemic nephropathy (n = 20). (From Hansen KJ, Thomason RB, Craven TE, et al: Surgical management of dialysis-dependent ischemic nephropathy. J Vasc Surg 21:197–211, 1995.)

dependent at the time of operation, no operative deaths occurred, and 16 (80%) were rendered free of dialysis postoperatively.[105] Their life-table estimate of survival is shown in Figure 24-19. Survival in those rendered dialysis independent was excellent. Those not freed from dialysis by operation had a death rate during follow-up similar to those in Mailloux's group[103] who were not submitted to operation.

This experience underscores two important points. In the contemporary patient population with ischemic nephropathy, severe hypertension is the clinical characteristic favoring a correctable renovascular cause for renal insufficiency. However, renal function response after operation is the key determinant of dialysis-free survival. Only patients with an incremental increase in function are spared eventual dialysis. Although patients whose renal function is unchanged are frequently considered "preserved," these data suggest that such patients progress to death or dialysis dependence at a pace equivalent to that of patients who are worse after surgery. Most important, the results argue that a carefully controlled, prospective, randomized trial comparing operation with balloon angioplasty and medical therapy is

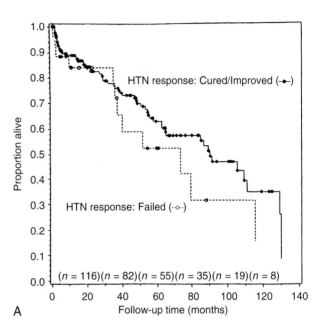

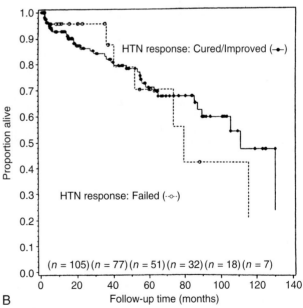

FIGURE 24-20 ■ **A,** Product limit estimates of all-cause mortality for patients with ischemic nephropathy as a function of hypertension (HTN) response to operation. **B,** Product limit estimates of cardiovascular or renal mortality for patients with ischemic nephropathy as a function of hypertension response to operation. Hypertension response did not affect the rate of death or cardiovascular death. (From Hansen KJ, Cherr GS, Craven TE, et al: Management of ischemic nephropathy: dialysis-free survival after surgical repair. J Vasc Surg 32:472–482, 2000.)

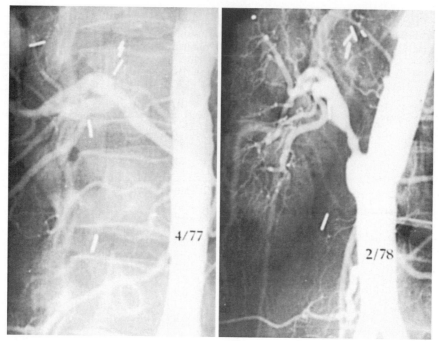

FIGURE 24-21 ■ Postoperative arteriograms showing fibrous narrowing of the saphenous vein graft secondary to subendothelial fibroblastic proliferation.

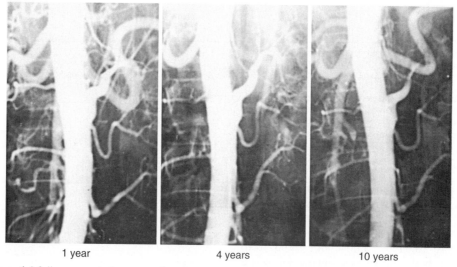

1 year   4 years   10 years

FIGURE 24-22 ■ Sequential follow-up arteriograms of a 10-year-old child who underwent a hypogastric autograft to the left renal artery and an iliac vein autograft to the superior mesenteric artery. Ultimately, both grafts required replacement.

necessary to confirm the value of operation in patients with controlled hypertension. Only through this method can we accurately clarify the role of intervention in dialysis-free survival among patients with ischemic nephropathy.

LATE FOLLOW-UP RECONSTRUCTIONS

From our experience with the operative management of RVH, 1- to 23-year follow-up sequential angiography of 198 reconstructions is available for evaluation.[106] Ten grafts developed suture line or midgraft stenoses requiring revision from 1 to 8 years after the initial operation (Figure 24-21). Four patients had graft occlusions during follow-up and probably represent missed graft stenoses that progressed to occlusion. Three grafts required correction of aortic anastomotic false aneurysms in Dacron prostheses in two patients at 8 and 20 years postoperatively. The remaining grafts (88%) had no untoward changes and continued patency during follow-up.

Five saphenous vein grafts and two hypogastric autografts underwent aneurysmal dilatation. Only one of these, a hypogastric autograft, required replacement (Figure 24-22). The remaining six stabilized, and the patients remained cured of hypertension. Aneurysmal dilatation of autogenous grafts (vein or artery) has occurred only in young children in our experience. This suggests that the saphenous vein in young patients is particularly susceptible to this phenomenon. For this reason, we prefer the normal hypogastric artery as the conduit of choice for this group. In the two instances of autogenous arterial graft aneurysmal degeneration, fibromuscular dysplasia of the donor hypogastric artery was identified in retrospective microscopic evaluation.[106]

Follow-up angiography and renal duplex sonography showed progression of mild to moderate contralateral RVD in 38% of patients. This is most important in children, as 7 of 15 with fibromuscular dysplasia had bilateral involvement.[56] In only three of these seven children was the contralateral disease evident at the time of initial evaluation and operation; in the remaining four, the development and progression of contralateral disease were documented subsequently. This occurrence of contralateral stenosis has led us to perform nephrectomy in children only if blood pressure is uncontrollable and revascularization is impossible. Because the longest follow-up was only 10 years, the true incidence of subsequent contralateral disease in children is unknown.

Although the failure of operative repairs is infrequent, the dialysis-free survival of patients with failed repairs is decreased.[107] Figure 24-23 compares patients requiring secondary intervention with patients having only primary renovascular repair. Patients requiring secondary intervention demonstrated a significant and independent

increased risk of eventual dialysis dependence (relative risk [RR], 12.6; 95% CI, 4.5-34.9; $p < 0.001$) and decreased dialysis-free survival (RR, 2.4; 95% CI, 1.1-5.4; $p = 0.035$). It is not known whether failed balloon angioplasty with or without stenting demonstrates similar associations with eventual dialysis dependence.

EFFECT OF BLOOD PRESSURE RESPONSE ON LONG-TERM SURVIVAL

The rationale for the management of hypertension of any cause is to decrease long-term cardiovascular morbidity and improve event-free survival. Consequently, we reviewed the outcome of 71 patients who underwent operative management of RVH 15 to 23 years previously.[106] Complete follow-up was available in 66 of the 68 patients who survived operation. Comparison of the initial blood pressure response after operation (1 to 6 months postoperatively) with the blood pressure status at the time of death or current date (up to 23 years later) showed that the effect of operative treatment is maintained over long-term follow-up (Figure 24-24). In patients who required repeated renovascular operation for recurrent RVH during follow-up, the majority of the operations were performed for the management of contralateral lesions that had progressed to functional significance (i.e., produced RVH).

Assessment of the effect of blood pressure response on late survival produced results that are not surprising.

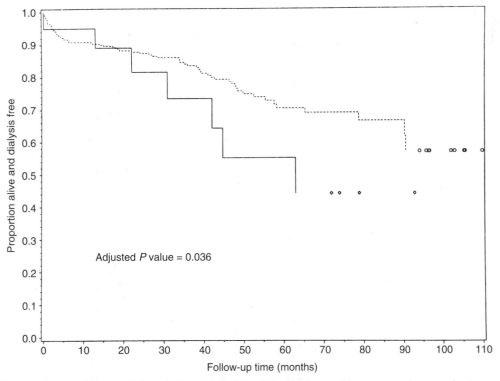

FIGURE 24-23 ■ Product limit estimates of dialysis-free survival for 20 patients requiring a secondary renal artery operation (solid line) and 514 patients having primary renal artery repair only *(broken line)* with adjusted *p* values. Operative failure was associated with a significant and independent decrease in dialysis-free survival. (From Hansen KJ, Deitch JS, Oskin TC, et al: Renal artery repair: consequences of operative failures. Ann Surg 227:678–690, 1998.)

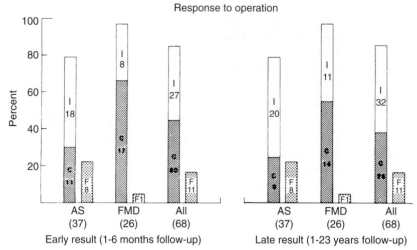

FIGURE 24-24 ■ Comparison of initial benefit and late blood pressure response in the different types of lesions treated in the 1960s. *AS,* Arteriosclerotic lesion; *FMD,* fibromuscular dysplasia.

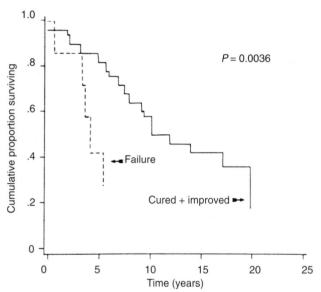

FIGURE 24-25 ■ Kaplan-Meier life-table analysis for patients treated in the 1960s, showing survival by response to operation in 37 arteriosclerotic patients (deaths from cardiovascular causes). These observations differ significantly from those in the contemporary population with atherosclerotic renovascular disease (see Figure 24-16). (From Dean RH, Tribble RW, Hansen KJ, et al: Evolution of renal insufficiency in ischemic nephropathy. Ann Surg 213:446–455, 1991.)

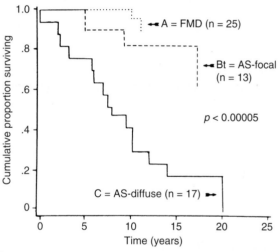

FIGURE 24-26 ■ Kaplan-Meier life-table analysis of survival of patients who benefited from operation by type and stage of disease, with 55 patients cured or improved from the 1960s (deaths from cardiovascular causes). *AS-diffuse,* Diffuse atherosclerosis; *AS-focal,* focal atherosclerosis; *FMD,* fibromuscular dysplasia. (From Dean RH, Tribble RW, Hansen KJ, et al: Evolution of renal insufficiency in ischemic nephropathy. Ann Surg 213:446–455, 1991.)

Although the subgroup of nonresponders was small, they experienced a significantly more rapid death rate during follow-up than did patients who had a positive blood pressure response to operation (Figure 24-25). This finding confirms the validity of the premise that inadequate management of RVH leaves the patient at higher risk of early death from cardiovascular events. The presence of angiographically diffuse atherosclerosis at the time of evaluation and operation was predictive of a more rapid rate of death during follow-up (Figure 24-26).[104]

This difference in subsequent death rate was present even though a comparison between patients with diffuse atherosclerotic disease and those with focal atherosclerotic disease was undertaken only in patients experiencing a significant blood pressure response. In view of the suggestion by some physicians that the presence of diffuse disease precludes a high rate of blood pressure response to operation, it is important to note that no significant difference occurred in the frequency of response between the focal (80%) and diffuse (77%) groups in this study. In addition, although the presence of diffuse disease was associated with a more rapid death rate, it does not preclude the probability of a longer survival in this subgroup compared with a similar group of patients who either did

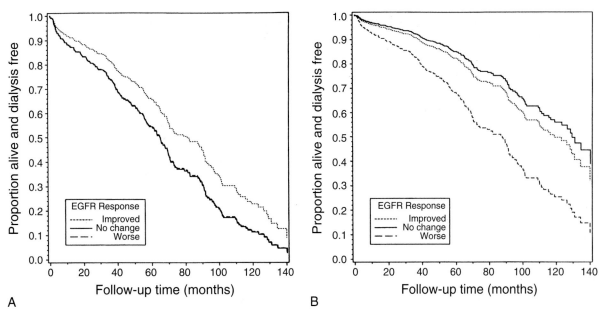

FIGURE 24-27 ■ Predicted dialysis-free survival according to postoperative renal function response for patients with a preoperative estimated glomerular filtration rate (EGFR) of 25 mL/min/m² (25th percentile) or 39 mL/min/m² (median value). The interaction between preoperative EGFR and renal function response for dialysis-free survival was significant and independent. (From Cherr GS, Hansen KJ, Craven TE, et al: Surgical management of atherosclerotic renovascular disease. J Vasc Surg 35:236–245, 2002.)

not undergo operation or received no blood pressure benefit from such intervention. Furthermore, if one considers that diffuse disease is only a later stage of focal disease, it is not surprising that the end point of clinically significant disease—namely, death from cardiovascular events—arrives sooner when one begins follow-up or removes a risk factor that causes its acceleration later in its natural history.

In contrast, a contemporary group of 500 atherosclerotic patients did not demonstrate improved event-free survival in association with beneficial blood pressure response to operation (Figure 24-27).[23] As noted earlier, only atherosclerotic patients who are cured (i.e., normotensive without medications) have demonstrated increased survival. Although there are a number of possible explanations for this observed difference, renal function response among contemporary patients demonstrated a significant and independent association with follow-up survival. Global renal disease treated with complete renal artery repair after rapid decline in renal function provided the best opportunity for improved glomerular filtration. Patients whose renal function was unimproved or worse remained at increased risk for eventual dialysis dependence. In the contemporary population, progression to dialysis dependence was the single strongest risk factor for death.

PERCUTANEOUS TRANSLUMINAL ANGIOPLASTY

The introduction of PTA as an alternative interventional modality by Gruntzig and colleagues[108] in 1978 led to a new era in the management of patients with renal artery stenosis. This technique uses the principle of coaxial dilatation of the vessel by inflation of a balloon-tipped catheter introduced across the stenotic renal artery lesion. The stenotic lesion is disrupted and, by stretching the vessel wall itself, portions of the media are disrupted, leaving the vessel diameter greater than it was before dilatation. The increased luminal diameter is created primarily by disruption of the intima and the atherosclerotic or fibrodysplastic lesion and by dilatation of the less diseased arterial wall. Early reports of the results of this technique showed that stenotic renal arteries could often be dilated successfully, with immediate improvement in hypertension in patients with RVH.

By reviewing the reported experience with PTA and observations from the operative management of unsuccessful PTA, one can formulate indications for the preferential use of each procedure in the treatment of RVH.[109-128] Reported experience with PTA of medial fibroplasia shows early results similar to those of open surgical repair. Beneficial blood pressure responses have been reported to be as high as 100% after PTA in properly selected patients, and although vessel perforation, hemorrhage, and branch occlusions have been reported, their incidence is less than 5%.[109] One would anticipate that such complications would be most likely in patients with diffuse fibromuscular dysplasia affecting both the distal main renal artery and its branches. When the procedure is performed by an experienced interventionist, the cure rate after PTA of fibromuscular dysplasia ranges from 37% to 51%.[110] Fibromuscular dysplasia involving the branch level is best managed primarily by an open operative approach, and PTA should be reserved for the

TABLE 24-10   Renal Artery Revascularization with Angioplasty and Stenting*

Reference	Year	Patients	Bilateral Treatment (%)	Preprocedure Renal Dysfunction (%)	Renal Function Response (%)			Hypertension Response (%)			Periprocedure Mortality (%)	Periprocedure Morbidity (%)
					Improved	Unchanged	Worsened	Cured	Improved	Failed		
Burket and colleagues[142]	2000	126	NR	29	43	24	56	8	NR	NR	2	4
Lederman and colleagues[120]	2001	265	41	37	7.5	78	14	NR	70	30	<1	2
Bush and colleagues[143]	2001	73	16	68	23	51	26	6	89	5	1.4	9
Rocha-Singh and colleagues[144]	2002	51	55	100	77	18	5	NR	91	9	0	14
Gill and Fowler[145]	2003	100	26	75	31	38	31	4	79	17	2	18
Zeller and colleagues[146]	2004	456	NR	52	34	39	27	NR	46	54	<1	NR
Nolan and colleagues[147]	2005	82	NR	59	23	53	24	0	81	0	0	7
Kayshap and colleagues[148]	2007	125	36	100	42	23	25	0	0	0	1.6	6
Corriere and colleagues[149]	2008	99	11	75	28	65	7	1	21	78	0	5.5
Mean%[†]			31	55	28	38	31	4	54	29	1	6.6

NR, Not reported.

*Series selected based on publication in 2000 or later, use of angioplasty and stenting, and inclusion of more than 50 patients, and categorical reporting of renal function or hypertension responses, or both.

[†]Weighted mean based on number of patients with reported data categorized according to column; references where data was not reported or categoric response categories were combined were not included in calculation.

subgroup of patients with medial fibroplasia limited to the main renal artery.

Stenotic lesions occurring in children are usually discrete narrowings and therefore appear to be ideal for PTA. However, the stenotic area is commonly a congenital hypoplasia of the entire vessel wall and is composed predominantly of elastic tissue. When such a hypoplastic vessel is subjected to PTA, the original diameter returns after dilatation or, if the vessel has been overdistended, rupture of the vessel wall is likely. Therefore PTA is an inappropriate method of intervention in children with renal artery stenosis, and lifelong success is best achieved by operative correction.

Finally, a review of series reporting results with PTA for atherosclerotic lesions illustrates the frequency of failure with this lesion as well. An early report by Miller and colleagues[111] in 1985 noted that only 45% of ostial and mixed lesions were improved after 6 months; Sos and colleagues reported only a 14% benefit rate when bilateral ostial lesions were treated.[105] These results show that PTA alone has little value in the treatment of this type of lesion; one must accept the risks of cholesterol embolization, vessel thrombosis, and loss of renal function for only a minimal chance of prolonged benefit.

Endoluminal stenting of the renal artery as an adjunct to PTA was first introduced in the United States in 1988 as part of a multicenter trial.[112] During this same period, the Palmaz stent and Wallstent were being used in Europe. Currently, the most common indications for the use of stents are: (1) elastic recoil of the vessel immediately after angioplasty, (2) renal artery dissection after angioplasty, (3) restenosis after angioplasty, and

(4) primary application in ostial atherosclerosis. With 263 patients entered, results from the multicenter trial demonstrated cure or improvement of hypertension in 61% of patients at 1 year. At follow-up of less than 1 year, angiographic restenosis occurred in 32.7% of patients.

Recognizing the poor immediate success of PTA alone for ostial atherosclerosis, some have advised the primary placement of endoluminal stents for these lesions.[113] Table 24-10 summarizes single-center reports on renal function and angiographic follow-up after treatment of ostial atherosclerosis by PTA in combination with endoluminal stents in 1377 patients since 2000.[120,142-148] These studies differ in regard to criteria for ostial lesions, evaluation of the clinical response to intervention, and parameters for significant restenosis. Despite these differences, these cumulative results provide the best available estimates of early hypertension response, change in renal function, and primary patency. The overall hypertension cure rate was 4%, with a range of 0% to 8%; 54% of the patients had improved blood pressure control, with a range of 0% to 91%. With improvement defined as a 20% or greater decrease in serum creatinine concentration, response rates ranging from 7.5% to 77% were observed (mean, 28%). A number of authorities also make use of the concept of "stabilized" renal function, defined as a less than 20% change in serum creatinine concentration. By this definition,[120,142-149] renal function was stabilized in the majority of patients included in the studies published between 2000 and 2008 (range, 18% to 78%; mean response rate, 38%; see Table 24-10). Again, these results are similar to those reported in the meta-analysis from 2000 (range, 0% to 64%; mean response rate, 38%).[55,149] A significant percentage of treated patients (range, 0% to 56%; mean, 31%) also experienced post-PTAS worsening of renal function. However, it is also important to note that the periprocedural morbidity was 6.6% and periprocedural mortality was 1% for these patients. To date, only one prospective, randomized, controlled study has compared endovascular treatment with surgical revascularization for the treatment of renovascular hypertension.[128] In this report, 58 patients with renovascular hypertension were randomly assigned to either surgical revascularization or angioplasty. In both groups, hypertension was cured or improved in approximately 90% of patients. However, more than half of the patients in whom angioplasty failed were switched to the surgical arm for revascularization. On the basis of these results, the authors recommended angioplasty as the treatment of choice for selected renovascular lesions contributing to renovascular hypertension, with aggressive follow-up and repeat intervention (endovascular and surgical) carried out as needed. Other investigators have reported that the beneficial blood pressure response seen after open surgical repair for failed angioplasty may be less than that seen in patients who undergo primary surgical repair without previous endovascular treatment.[129] Moreover, a previous endovascular procedure may make open surgical repair technically more demanding, especially if an endoluminal stent is present.

The Angioplasty and Stenting for Renal Artery Lesions (the ASTRAL trial) commenced patient recruitment in September 2000.[130] The trial randomized patients with significant anatomic atherosclerotic renovascular disease to either PTRA-S with best medical management (e.g., statins, antiplatelet, antihypertensive therapy) or to optimal medical management alone. The primary end point was the rate of change in renal function over time. Secondary end points included blood pressure control, adverse heart and vascular events, and mortality. Fifty-seven centers recruited patients into ASTRAL, 53 of these were from the United Kingdom and 4 were from Australia.

The first published report of ASTRAL trial results is available.[130] A total of 806 patients (403 randomized to each group) were enrolled into the ASTRAL trial. The trial included a mean follow-up of 33.6 months, with all surviving patients having completed a minimum of 12 months follow-up. At base line, trial group demographics were virtually identical for the two groups. The average degree of stenosis for the most severe renal artery lesion was 76% diameter reducing; 60% of patients had renal artery stenosis exceeding 70%. Mean blood pressures were reported as 149/46 and 152/76 mm Hg in the PTRA-S and medically managed groups respectively. Patients averaged 2.8 antihypertensive medications in both groups.

The ASTRAL trial demonstrated no difference in blood pressure, renal function, adverse renal events, vascular events, or mortality between the two groups; 6.8% of subjects in the PTRA-S group suffered significant complications, including renal artery perforation, thrombosis, embolization, and significant renal insufficiency. Ignoring complications requiring admission, another 20% of PTRA-S patients experience less serious complications consisting primarily of groin hematoma and mild renal insufficiency. Although the ASTRAL trial represents the largest published prospective randomized clinical trial to examine the role of PTRA-S, the trial has received substantial criticism. Patients were excluded from randomization if their physician believed that they would benefit from PTRA-S. As a consequence, it can be argued that patients who would likely benefit from PTRA-S were systematically omitted. In addition, 403 patients randomized to PTRA-S 40% had stenosis between 50% and 70% diameter reducing. Moreover, pressure gradients across the stenosis were not measured either before or after therapy. Finally, only 359 of 403 patients randomized to PTRA-S underwent the procedure, whereas 24 of 403 patients assigned to medical management underwent intervention. However, when the trial results are examined on a per protocol basis there was no apparent benefit for PTRA-S.

Currently there are no level I data demonstrating any association between improved hypertension control after renal artery PTAS and either increased survival or reduced morbidity and mortality from adverse cardiovascular events. There are at least three more large ongoing prospective randomized clinical trials which compare PTAS with best medical management.[150-151] Of these, the Cardiovascular Outcomes in Renal Atherosclerotic Lesions (CORAL) trial is the most eagerly awaited trail to report.

In summary, experience with the liberal use of PTA has helped to clarify its role as one of the therapeutic options in the treatment of RVH, but the data argue for its selective application. In this regard, PTA of nonorificial atherosclerotic lesions and medial fibroplasia limited to the main renal artery yields results comparable with those of operation if performed by persons experienced in the technique. In contrast, the use of PTA for the treatment of congenital stenotic lesions, fibrodysplastic lesions involving renal artery branches, and ostial atherosclerotic lesions in association with ischemic nephropathy is associated with inferior results and with increased risk of complications. Operation remains the initial treatment of choice for patients in these groups, although the type of interventional therapy for RVD must always be individualized.

References available online at expertconsult.com.

QUESTIONS

1. Which test is most sensitive for the identification of all hypertensive patients who might have renovascular hypertension?
   a. Isotope renography
   b. Rapid-sequence intravenous pyelography
   c. Arteriography
   d. Peripheral plasma renin activity

2. Which finding is most accurate in confirming the presence of renovascular hypertension?
   a. Demonstration of collaterals by renal arteriography
   b. Lateralization (1.5 : 1) of renal venous renin assays
   c. Absence of function on rapid-sequence intravenous pyelography
   d. Elevation of peripheral plasma renin activity
   e. Presence of severe renal artery stenosis in a patient with hypertension

3. What endogenous pressor substance causes elevation of blood pressure in patients with renovascular hypertension?
   a. Angiotensinogen
   b. Renin
   c. Angiotensin I
   d. Prostaglandin E2
   e. Atrial natriuretic factor

4. Which of the following factors is most predictive of renal function retrieval by renal revascularization?
   a. Low volume with hypoconcentration of creatinine in urine from the affected kidney
   b. Normal intrarenal vessels on arteriography
   c. Hyperconcentration of nonreabsorbable solutes in the urine of the affected kidney
   d. Normal glomeruli and tubules on microscopic evaluation of renal biopsy
   e. None of the above

5. Which operative technique is never an acceptable method for treatment of an orificial renal artery occlusion?
   a. Thromboendarterectomy
   b. Saphenous vein aortorenal bypass
   c. Synthetic graft aortorenal bypass
   d. Renal artery reimplantation
   e. None of the above

6. In terms of long-term durability, which material is best for renal revascularization in children?
   a. Normal saphenous vein
   b. Expanded polytetrafluoroethylene
   c. Normal hypogastric artery
   d. Polyester
   e. None of the above

7. What is the apparent incidence of progressive loss of renal function in kidneys of patients treated medically for renovascular hypertension secondary to atherosclerotic renal artery stenosis?
   a. Less than 10%
   b. 10% to 20%
   c. Greater than 30%
   d. Greater than 60%
   e. Greater than 80%

8. What technical success rate is acceptable when performing renal revascularization?
   a. Less than 50%
   b. 50% to 70%
   c. 70% to 80%
   d. 80% to 90%
   e. Greater than 95%

9. Which factor most frequently determines the likelihood of long-term maintenance of initially successful blood pressure reduction by operative management of renovascular hypertension?
   a. Graft material used for aortorenal bypass
   b. Progression of contralateral disease
   c. Development of stenosis of graft anastomosis
   d. Development of new lesions beyond the bypass in the kidney operated on
   e. None of the above

10. What is the most important determinant of dialysis-free survival following operative treatment for ischemic nephropathy?
    a. Blood pressure response
    b. Renal function response
    c. Number of functioning kidneys
    d. Failure of operative renal artery repair
    e. b and d

ANSWERS

1. c
2. b
3. e
4. c
5. e
6. c
7. c
8. e
9. b
10. e

CHAPTER 25

Endovascular Treatment of Renovascular Disease

Douglas B. Hood • Kim J. Hodgson

Although surgical revascularization of renal artery occlusive disease has long been known to benefit patients with renovascular hypertension, as well as selected patients with renal insufficiency, the associated morbidity and mortality of these procedures discouraged their use in all but the most severe cases. Endovascular renal revascularization offers the opportunity to gain the therapeutic benefits of surgery with reduced periprocedural risk and recovery time, albeit with potentially less durability. Development of endovascular techniques led to an explosion in renal artery interventions, often with poorly defined indications. Nonetheless, all endovascular practitioners should know the indications for and the technique of percutaneous renal revascularization, because many patients seen in the average vascular practice will benefit from this procedure.

Renal artery stenosis (RAS) is the most common cause of secondary hypertension, with an estimated incidence of 5% in the hypertensive population. Congenital anomalies, arteritis, trauma, arterial dissection, fibromuscular dysplasia, and atherosclerosis are all recognized causes of RAS. Among these, atherosclerosis is by far the most common, accounting for 60% to 80% of all cases of clinically significant renal artery disease. This chapter summarizes the current status of endovascular management of atherosclerotic RAS, with a focus on recently reported technical and clinical results. The indications for renal artery angioplasty and stenting continue to be investigated in light of improvements in the medical therapy of renovascular disease, particularly hypertension.

NATURAL HISTORY

Atherosclerosis affecting the renal arteries is a progressive disease that often results from encroachment of aortic plaque into or across the renal artery orifice. Because of this characteristic pattern, most clinically relevant atherosclerotic renal artery lesions are ostial in location, occurring within the most proximal 5 mm of the vessel. Once RAS becomes hemodynamically significant (>60%), progression to renal artery occlusion is a real possibility. Using sequential angiograms, Tollefson and Ernst[1] found that RAS progressed at approximately 5% per year, irrespective of the level of stenosis, and that occlusion was associated with greater degrees of stenosis. Caps and associates[2] showed that 49% of patients

with RAS greater than 60% measured by duplex ultrasonography showed disease progression over a 3-year period.[2] Zierler and colleagues[3] reported that in renal arteries with stenosis greater than 60%, progression to occlusion was 5% at 1 year and 11% at 2 years. Renal artery occlusion is associated with loss of nephrons and atrophy of the kidney parenchyma, with a mean decrease in kidney length of 1.8 cm in Zierler's report. Renal atrophy can also occur in association with stenotic but nonoccluded renal arteries.

DIAGNOSIS

Patients with atherosclerotic RAS are more often male and older than 60 years, and they have the typical atherosclerotic risk factors of diabetes, hyperlipidemia, tobacco use, and hypertension. The diagnosis of renovascular hypertension is suggested by unstable or accelerated hypertension that can occur in combination with progressive deterioration of renal function (ischemic nephropathy). Development of malignant hypertension in a patient with a prior history of easily controlled essential hypertension is particularly suggestive of RAS. A less common clinical scenario is rapidly progressive renal insufficiency associated with mild hypertension. Flash pulmonary edema in the setting of accelerated hypertension may also indicate the existence of significant RAS. The physical finding of an abdominal or flank bruit supports the diagnosis, but is present in only 25% of patients. Laboratory findings consistent with RAS include refractory hypokalemia and an elevated peripheral renin assay, but each is found in only an occasional patient. Any of these clinical findings, alone or in combination, raises the index of suspicion and should prompt diagnostic imaging of the renal arteries.

IMAGING STUDIES

In the past, renal artery imaging required invasive angiographic procedures. The need for angiography and its associated morbidity dissuaded many practitioners from aggressively pursuing the diagnosis of RAS in patients who were medically compromised. The development of less invasive imaging techniques that provide a thorough investigation of renal artery anatomy has increased the recognition of RAS.

Renal duplex ultrasonography has emerged as an excellent test to screen patients for RAS. Although it requires significant technical expertise, it is a safe and relatively inexpensive modality that can provide information concerning kidney size, cortical thickness, renal artery hemodynamics, and velocity profiles, as well as nonvascular anatomic renal abnormalities such as cysts. Several authors have documented the accuracy of using renal artery peak systolic velocities to detect RAS. A peak systolic velocity greater than 180 cm/s, along with a renal-to-aortic velocity ratio of 3.5 or greater, is used in many vascular laboratories to identify significant RAS. In the author's experience, a peak systolic velocity greater than 220 cm/s identified RAS with 91% sensitivity and 85% specificity.[4] Importantly, the negative predictive value of 95% of this threshold value in our laboratories essentially eliminated the possibility of RAS, making duplex ultrasonography a highly useful screening test. Limitations of ultrasound imaging of the renal arteries include large body habitus and overlying bowel gas obscuring identification of the renal arteries.

Renal duplex ultrasonography to measure renal arterial resistance may also offer a method to predict outcomes following therapy for RAS.[5,6] In a study by Radermacher and colleagues,[5] duplex ultrasonography was used to measure the renal resistance index in 138 patients who had unilateral or bilateral renal artery stenosis of more than 50% and underwent renal angioplasty or surgery. The procedure was technically successful in 95% of patients. Creatinine clearance and 24-hour ambulatory blood pressure were measured before renal artery stenosis was corrected and at intervals of 3, 6, and 12 months and yearly thereafter. Mean follow-up was 32 months. Patients with an elevated renal resistance index (27% of the cohort) failed to realize an improvement in blood pressure, whereas those with a normal index experienced a statistically significant improvement in mean arterial pressure at 3-year follow-up. Creatinine clearance declined in 80% of patients with an elevated renal resistance index despite technically successful revascularization. Forty-six percent of patients with an elevated renal resistance index became dependent on dialysis during follow-up, and 29% died. Patients with a normal resistance index experienced a significant increase in creatinine clearance, followed for 60 months.

Magnetic resonance angiography (MRA) using gadolinium is also a useful tool for evaluating renal artery anatomy. It has a sensitivity of 90% to 100% and a specificity of 76% to 94% when compared with conventional arteriography.[7,8] As a screening modality, MRA is more expensive and less patient friendly than duplex scanning, but it has become a valuable diagnostic tool and is often the first-line screening test in institutions without reliable duplex scanning results.

Contemporary computed tomographic (CT) imaging, including multislice CT angiography, provides very accurate reconstructions of abdominal vascular anatomy and pathology. The major limitations to widespread use of this modality for RAS screening are the need for iodinated contrast, exposure to ionizing radiation, and significant cost. These factors also limit the use of this modality for serial surveillance of known subcritical stenoses.

Using any of these modalities, the diagnosis of RAS can be reliably excluded, but conventional angiography is usually required for confirmation of positive results and to guide endovascular interventions. In the presence of renal insufficiency, carbon dioxide or gadolinium have been used instead of iodinated contrast agents.[9-11] Although carbon dioxide and gadolinium have limitations, and the image quality is inferior to that obtained using conventional iodinated contrast agents, renal artery imaging is possible and reproducible using either of these alternatives. These agents are particularly valuable for patients with ischemic nephropathy, in whom even small amounts of iodinated contrast may be injurious. Recent concern regarding the use of gadolinium in patients with renal dysfunction and its association with nephrogenic systemic fibrosis has limited its use.[12]

When considering intervention for RAS, the clinician must recognize that the presence of anatomic RAS does not necessarily establish it as the pathophysiologic cause of hypertension or renal dysfunction. Unfortunately, physiologic tests such as peripheral or renal vein renin sampling and nuclear scanning have not been proved sufficiently reliable to be of value in selecting patients for treatment. Consequently, the decision to intervene is ultimately a clinical judgment and can never be made with absolute certainty of benefit. In general, intervention is considered when unilateral or bilateral RAS of greater than 60% is documented and any of the following clinical parameters is present: poorly controlled blood pressure despite aggressive medical management, hypertension complicated by congestive heart failure or flash pulmonary edema, or progressive renal insufficiency.

ENDOVASCULAR MANAGEMENT

Following is a description of one technique that has been used successfully for the endovascular management of renal artery lesions. It should be noted, however, that there are many variations of this technique, and an operator may find different combinations of sheaths, guidewires, and other instruments equally efficacious.

Groin access via the femoral artery is used most commonly, although a brachial artery approach should be considered for renal arteries with significant caudal angulation or in patients with significant aortoiliac occlusive disease (Figure 25-1). For unilateral RAS, it is preferable to access the contralateral femoral artery, which can provide more secure access to the target vessel. Following percutaneous arterial access and placement of a 5-French sheath, a multi–side-hole catheter is placed in the abdominal aorta and positioned at the level of the L1 to L2 vertebral interspace for flush aortography. Complete visualization of the renal artery origins usually requires anteroposterior and oblique views. Catheterization of one or both renal arteries may be required for definitive angiographic detail. Translesion pressure measurements may be performed for lesions of questionable hemodynamic significance. Documentation of significant RAS is followed by upsizing to a 6- or 7-French sheath. Several sheaths are available with preformed curves at their tips that are designed for

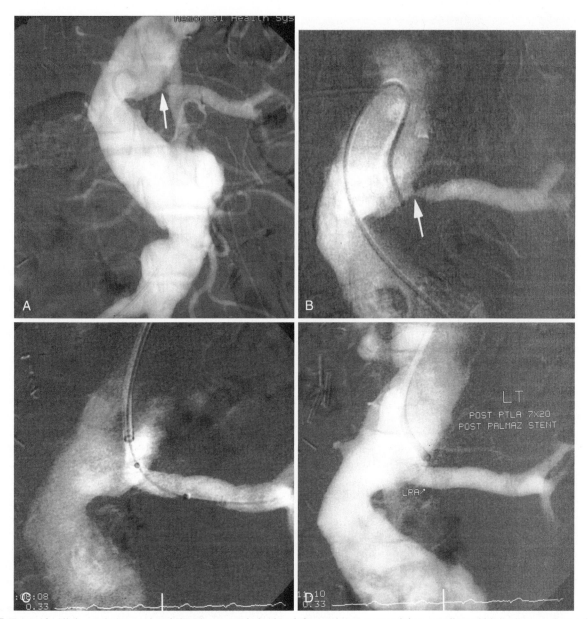

FIGURE 25-1 ■ **A,** High-grade stenosis of the downward-sloping left renal artery supplying a solitary kidney in a patient with an abdominal aortic aneurysm and aortoiliac tortuosity. **B,** Difficult selective catheterization from the femoral approach. **C,** Simplified access from the left brachial approach. **D,** Completion arteriogram after angioplasty and stenting.

placement into the aortic branches. Alternatively, the operator may choose to place a shaped guiding catheter through the femoral sheath and into the renal artery. The shaped sheath or guiding catheter provides support against the opposite aortic wall that helps to stabilize access to the renal artery.

Placement of the sheath or guiding catheter at the renal orifice allows small amounts of contrast to be injected to guide the precise placement of angioplasty balloons and stents (Figure 25-2). In addition, the sheath or guiding catheter provides external support for the subsequent passage of guidewires, balloons, and stent delivery systems. This arrangement also allows complete imaging without the loss of the guidewire crossing the lesion.

After systemic heparinization, the renal artery lesion is traversed with a guidewire. Most contemporary systems for renal artery intervention are based on 0.014-inch guidewire platforms. The wire tip is placed into a proximal segmental renal branch. Caution must be exercised with the passage of any wire, because renal artery or parenchymal perforation is possible, particularly with the hydrophilic wires. Atherosclerotic lesions in the midportion of the main renal artery may be well treated with balloon angioplasty alone, but the more common ostial lesions generally require stent placement. Premounted, balloon-expandable stents are preferred; several type are available commercially. These systems are more flexible and have lower crossing profiles than the 0.035-inch systems of the past. Predilatation is generally not required

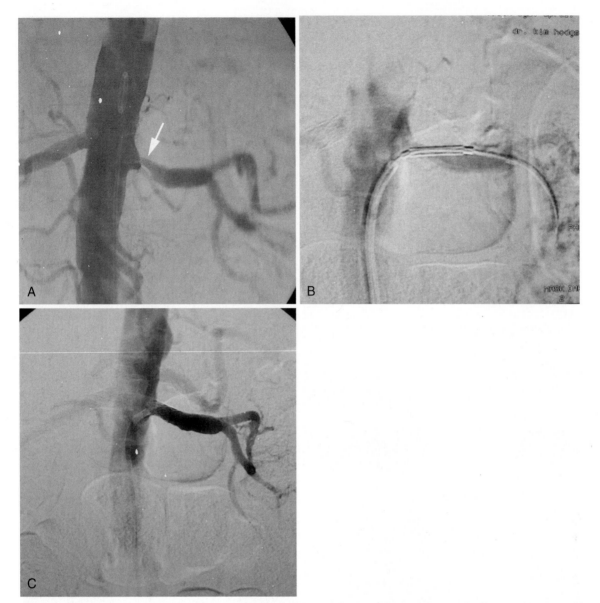

FIGURE 25-2 ■ **A,** Selective catheterization of the renal artery orifice with a guiding catheter to facilitate guidewire crossing of the lesion. **B,** Predeployment angiogram to confirm proper stent positioning. **C,** Completion angiogram after angioplasty and stenting.

and may be associated with microembolization of plaque fragments to the renal parenchyma. Most cases require a stent 20 mm long or less mounted on a 5- or 6-mm balloon. The stent is positioned across the lesion, with 2 to 3 mm of stent projecting into the aorta for ostial lesions. Once the stent is deployed, the balloon is deflated and withdrawn, being careful to maintain wire access across the lesion.

Completion angiography is performed with contrast injected through the side arm of the sheath or guiding catheter. The completion study should be critically assessed for technical success (<30% residual stenosis) and for the complications of renal artery dissection, thrombosis, emboli, or perforation of the renal parenchyma. Having confirmed a successful result, a closure device is used to seal the femoral puncture site after the sheath is removed.

RESULTS

Prospective trials comparing endovascular intervention with medical management or open surgical repair of RAS are few, but a substantial body of nonrandomized descriptive literature is available. In general, published reports describe the results of endovascular treatment according to technical success, blood pressure response, renal function, and survival criteria.

Initial Technical Success and Procedural Complications

A number of series have analyzed the initial technical results of endovascular intervention. Interpretation of technical results in the various studies is sometimes challenging because of the varying definitions of success and

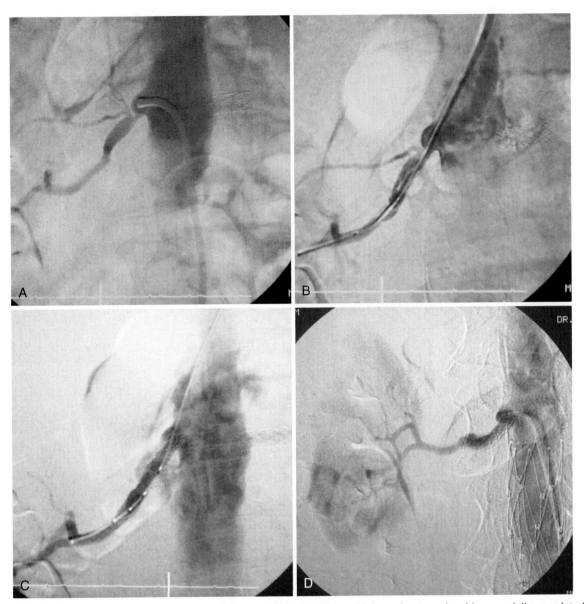

FIGURE 25-3 ■ **A,** Scout angiogram of the right renal artery demonstrating a high-grade stenosis with a caudally angulated renal artery. **B,** Guidewire-induced dissection of the right renal artery approached from a femoral access site, now crossed with a guidewire from the brachial approach. **C,** Successful stenting of the dissection. **D,** Follow-up angiogram 6 months later.

the inconsistent use of postprocedural imaging and pre-angioplasty and postangioplasty pressure measurements. Technical success is most commonly defined as a residual stenosis of less than 30%, with no evidence of flow-limiting dissection (Figure 25-3), perforation, or branch vessel compromise. An inability to traverse the lesion with a guidewire is the most common cause of technical failure and occurs in 2% to 5% of cases.[13]

The use of stents has resulted in increased technical success and patency rates when compared with balloon angioplasty alone. In series published during the 1990s, technical success rates varied between 24% and 91% using primary angioplasty alone, with stenting reserved only for rescue indications.[13] In an effort to clarify the role of primary stenting in the treatment of atherosclerotic ostial stenosis, van de Ven and coworkers[14] performed a randomized, prospective study that included 84

hypertensive patients. All patients had ostial RAS, defined as a 50% or greater reduction in luminal diameter within the first 10 mm of the aortic lumen. Immediate technical success was significantly better in the stent group than in the angioplasty group (88% vs. 57%), with equivalent complication rates. Analyzed on an intent-to-treat basis, the rate of primary patency (free of restenosis) at 6 months was only 29% in the angioplasty group and 75% in the stent group; secondary patency (including treatment of restenosis) at 6 months was 51% and 80%, respectively (Figure 25-4). Clinical results at 6 months showed no difference between the groups in terms of blood pressure or serum creatinine levels. In all, 12 patients in the angioplasty group received stents during follow-up, either for an unsuccessful initial result (5) or for recurrent stenosis (7). These authors concluded that by following a policy of selective stenting, with stent

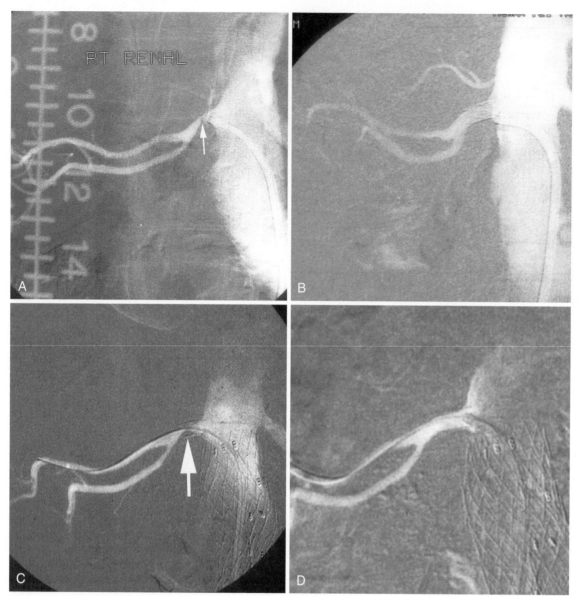

FIGURE 25-4 ■ **A,** Scout angiogram of a high-grade right renal artery stenosis. **B,** Completion arteriogram after angioplasty and stenting. **C,** In-stent recurrent stenosis at 6 months. **D,** Result after simple repeat balloon angioplasty of in-stent restenosis.

placement used only for technical failures and recurrent stenoses, stents could be avoided in approximately 40% of patients. However, because of the need for repeated interventions in patients treated initially with angioplasty alone, primary stenting is probably more efficacious for patients with atherosclerotic ostial RAS. A metaanalysis of primary renal artery stenting by Isles and associates[15] documented a technical success rate of 96% to 100%. Restenosis rates following primary stenting were 9% and 39% at 6 and 12 months, respectively. A more recent publication by Sivamurthy and colleagues[16] reported primary patency of 82% and primary assisted patency of 100% at 5 years.

The rate of procedural complications has also been evaluated. Alhadad and coworkers[17] found a 30-day mortality rate of 2% for renal artery interventions. Beutler and coauthors[18] reported initial technical success in 61 of 63 patients (97%), with a 6% renovascular complication rate. More importantly, in Beutler's series, 8% of patients showed clinical signs of cholesterol emboli, and at least 20% of patients experienced a decrease in renal function. Martin and associates[19] reviewed complication rates from two large series and two metaanalyses that included 2994 revascularizations. Periprocedural complication rates ranged from 12% to 36%. The most common complications were groin hematoma and puncture site trauma, both occurring in approximately 5% of patients. The incidence of symptomatic renal artery embolization varied from 1% to 8%, with renal artery occlusion rates between 0.8% and 2.5%.

Blood Pressure Response

Three randomized trials have compared the blood pressure response to endovascular intervention and pharmacologic therapy. Webster and coworkers[20] published the first randomized trial of angioplasty versus medical therapy in 1998, including 55 patients with hypertension and RAS in excess of 50%. Both medical and angioplasty groups demonstrated a significant reduction in blood pressure, with no significant difference between groups. Subgroup analysis, however, showed that patients with bilateral ras had an improved blood pressure response with angioplasty. Plouin and associates[21] randomized 49 patients to either angioplasty alone or medical therapy. There was no significant difference in mean blood pressure between the two groups at 6 months, but significantly more patients were rendered free of pharmacologic treatment in the endovascular group. Van Jaarsveld and colleagues[22] also prospectively compared the results of medical therapy versus angioplasty and failed to show a compelling difference in blood pressure control between groups.[22] Nevertheless, the number of antihypertensive medications prescribed was significantly lower in the angioplasty group. Of note, 44% of patients in the medical arm ultimately underwent angioplasty after 3 months owing to poor blood pressure control.

These prospective, randomized trials compared renal artery angioplasty with or without selective stent placement to medical therapy. The benefit of routine primary stenting compared with medical therapy has not been evaluated. However, given the improved technical outcome with primary stenting compared with selective stenting, it would be reasonable to conclude that primary stenting may provide better blood pressure benefit than was demonstrated in these early series. A more recent retrospective study of 100 patients with RAS by Pizzolo and associates[23] supports this assumption. In this study, primary stenting was performed in the majority of patients (67%) undergoing endovascular therapy. A significant improvement in blood pressure control was observed when compared with patients treated medically. Almost twice as many patients manifested an improvement in blood pressure control with endovascular intervention (57% vs. 29%). No patient in either group was cured.

A summary analysis of these cited studies suggests that the endovascular management of RAS results in a better blood pressure response than that achieved with medical therapy, requiring fewer antihypertensive agents for control. Furthermore, it appears that this response can be enhanced by the use of stents.

Renal Function

The results of endovascular intervention for ischemic nephropathy have been less compelling. The randomized trials already cited also examined the renal response to intervention, and all failed to show consistent improvement in renal function compared with preintervention status. In the reports by Plouin and colleagues[21] and van Jaarsveld and colleagues,[22] mean serum creatinine levels and creatinine clearance at 6 and 12 months were unchanged from pretreatment values. Webster and colleagues[20] documented no change in serum creatinine levels; creatinine clearance was not evaluated.[20]

In a retrospective study of patients with rapidly declining renal function, Beutler and colleagues[18] found that stent placement resulted in stabilization of renal function in 87% of patients.[18] No effect on renal function was evident when patients with stable renal function were treated. Consistent with Beutler's findings is a report by Ramos and coworkers[24] in which patients with lower glomerular filtration rates (GFRs) had larger improvements in GFR after endovascular intervention than did patients with higher preprocedure GFRs. In addition, when considering all patients as a group, a significant increase in renal function was evident. Burket and colleagues[25] reported that 43% of patients with baseline renal insufficiency showed significant improvement in renal function after intervention. A retrospective review by Gruneiro and colleagues of 79 patients who had undergone renal artery stenting revealed that 25% experienced an increase in serum creatinine of 20% or more over the average follow-up period of 24 months, despite maintenance of anatomic patency (<50% restenosis) in 88%.[26] Of note, dialysis was ultimately required in 44% of patients with baseline preprocedure creatinine levels of 2 mg/dL or greater, but in only 3.4% of patients with preprocedure creatinine levels of less than 2 mg%, suggesting that early intervention, before the development of renal excretory dysfunction, may be important for overall preservation of renal function.

There are two primary explanations of why endovascular intervention has had a less beneficial effect on renal function than expected, despite excellent technical results. First, iodinated contrast agents may cause injury from which the compromised kidney cannot recover. The use of less nephrotoxic contrast agents, such as carbon dioxide, in patients with compromised renal function (serum creatinine >1.8 mg/dL) may lessen the effects of this toxin. Satisfactory renal artery imaging using carbon dioxide with digital imaging can guide endovascular revascularization. At the least, the use of carbon dioxide drastically reduces the amount of iodinated contrast required for renal interventions and thereby limits contrast-induced parenchymal injury.

The second explanation for the less than expected response is cholesterol embolization. This has led to the recent use of distal protection devices originally designed for coronary and carotid interventions. Holden and Hill[27] described their results using a distal protection device in 37 patients, 14 of whom exhibited improved renal function at 1-year follow-up. In contrast, in 20 patients who underwent stenting without the use of a protection device, none had improvement in renal function at 1 year. Subsequently, Holden and colleagues[28] reported a prospective series of renal stenting in patients with baseline renal dysfunction. Interventions were performed in 83 arteries, all with embolic protection. Follow-up at 6 months showed that 97% of patients had stable or improved renal function. Cooper and colleagues[29] reported a series of 100 patients who were randomized to renal stenting with and without embolic protection and abciximab. Decline in renal function was seen in patients who received neither intervention or either alone. In comparison, patients who received both embolic protection and abciximab showed no decline in renal function at 1 month.

Two recently published randomized trials have addressed renal artery stent placement and renal dysfunction. The STAR trial randomized 140 patients with impaired renal function and 50% or greater atherosclerotic RAS by noninvasive imaging.[30] Subjects were assigned to stent placement with medical treatment or medical treatment alone. Medical treatment included antihypertensive treatment, a statin, and aspirin. The investigators concluded that there is no advantage to stenting in terms of progressive renal functional impairment, but this study has been criticized for a number of potential confounding flaws. For example, 18 of 64 patients in the stent group did not receive the assigned treatment, most because the stenosis was less than 50% by angiography.

The ASTRAL trial was a larger trial including 806 patients that also investigated changes in renal function in patients randomized to medical therapy alone or in combination with renal artery stenting, and this trial also concluded that there is no worthwhile clinical benefit to revascularization.[31] Unfortunately, this trial also suffered from significant methodologic flaws that may have introduced significant selection bias.

Surgical revascularization remains the one other option available for the treatment of ischemic nephropathy owing to RAS. Reports by Marone, Hansen, and Hallett and their respective coauthors have all documented that surgical revascularization provides substantial improvement in renal function, particularly if the RAS is bilateral or affects a solitary kidney.[32-35] In addition, the more severe the renal insufficiency, the greater the benefit seen. A randomized series of 50 patients comparing open surgical reconstruction and stenting for RAS showed longer durability and, perhaps surprisingly, lower morbidity of the open reconstructions.[36]

Survival

The expectation that improvement in blood pressure control and renal function following endovascular intervention will result in enhanced survival has yet to be conclusively documented. Only two studies have addressed this issue. Pillay and coworkers[37] found an overall mortality of 30% at 2 years in patients with either unilateral or bilateral RAS. No significant difference in survival was evident between patients who underwent endovascular treatment versus patients receiving optimal medical management.[10] However, patients in the endovascular group had a significantly higher baseline serum creatinine level. In contrast, Pizzolo and colleagues[23] found that 87% of patients treated with stent placement were alive at a median follow-up of 28 months, compared with 67% of patients treated medically. Subsequent regression analysis, used in an effort to explain the observed benefit, found endovascular treatment to be the sole independent predictor of improved survival.

SUMMARY

The technical success of primary stenting, along with the low incidence of morbidity and mortality, has made endovascular management the primary therapy for atherosclerotic RAS in many institutions. Surgical revascularization of atherosclerotic RAS is largely limited to patients with renal artery occlusions, multiple renal arteries, hilar or segmental renal artery lesions, or dissections or those who fail endovascular management.

References available online at expertconsult.com.

QUESTIONS

1. What is the most common cause of secondary hypertension?
   a. Pheochromocytoma
   b. Renal artery stenosis
   c. Hyperthyroidism
   d. Coarctation of the aorta

2. What is the most likely cause of renal artery occlusive disease?
   a. Takayasu arteritis
   b. Fibromuscular dysplasia
   c. Posttraumatic dissection
   d. Atherosclerosis

3. In patients with hemodynamically significant renal artery stenosis, progression to vessel occlusion occurs in what percentage at 1 year?
   a. 1%
   b. 5%
   c. 25%
   d. 40%

4. Abdominal or flank bruits are audible in up to what percentage of patients with renal artery stenosis?
   a. 5%
   b. 15%
   c. 25%
   d. 50%

5. Noninvasive methods of renal artery imaging include all of the following except:
   a. Duplex scanning
   b. Magnetic resonance angiography
   c. Computed tomography–angiography
   d. Renal scintigraphy

6. Alternatives to iodinated contrast agents that may be used for angiography in patients with renal insufficiency include which of the following?
   a. Iopamidol
   b. Carbon dioxide
   c. Oxygen
   d. Gadolinium

7. What is the most common cause of technical failure of renal artery interventions?
   a. Inability to traverse the lesion with a guidewire
   b. Residual stenosis greater than 30%
   c. Vessel perforation
   d. Branch vessel compromise

8. True of false: In the treatment of renal artery ostial stenosis caused by atherosclerosis, primary stenting produces an inferior result compared with angioplasty alone.

9. True or false: Compared with medical therapy, endovascular management of renal artery stenosis provides at least an equivalent blood pressure response, with fewer antihypertensive agents required.

10. Endovascular intervention may have little beneficial effect on renal function, despite adequate technical results, owing to which of the following?

a. Intrinsic renal parenchymal disease
b. Use of nephrotoxic contrast agents
c. Intraprocedural microembolization
d. All of the above

ANSWERS

1. **b**
2. **d**
3. **b**
4. **c**
5. **d**
6. **b, d**
7. **a**
8. **False**
9. **True**
10. **d**

Surgical Management of Femoral, Popliteal, and Tibial Arterial Occlusive Disease

Frank J. Veith • Neal S. Cayne • Nicholas J. Gargiulo • Evan C. Lipsitz • Enrico Ascher

This chapter discusses open surgical options for femoral, popliteal, and tibial arterial occlusive disease. Although some of these procedures may be performed occasionally for disabling intermittent claudication, the vast majority should only be performed for critical lower limb ischemia. This can be defined as sufficiently poor arterial blood supply to pose a threat to the viability of the lower extremity. Manifestations of critical ischemia are rest pain, ulceration, and gangrene. These manifestations typically occur because of arteriosclerotic occlusive disease of large, medium-sized, or small arteries, although other etiologies can produce or contribute to these ischemic conditions. For example, many nonvascular causes result in limb pain at rest; infection may cause or contribute to gangrene; and trauma and decreased sensation may produce ulceration. Although thromboembolism and other etiologies can produce acute critical limb ischemia, this chapter will address only chronic lower extremity ischemia owing to obliterative arteriosclerosis. Over the last 3 decades, it has become increasingly apparent that limbs that are threatened by this process almost always have multilevel occlusive disease, which often includes occlusions of arteries in the thigh, leg, and foot.[1]

Surgical options for chronic critical lower limb ischemia include local amputations of toes and other portions of the foot, a variety of debriding procedures including open amputations of portions of the foot to control infection, and a variety of traditional surgical revascularization procedures, primarily vein and prosthetic arterial bypasses above or below the inguinal ligament. Occasionally these may be supplemented with localized endarterectomies with or without patch angioplasties. Except for an occasional patient with common femoral artery (CFA) or deep femoral artery (DFA) lesions, these operations are rarely required and are rarely sufficient to save a severely ischemic limb.

TOE AND FOOT AMPUTATIONS, DEBRIDEMENTS, AND CONSERVATIVE TREATMENT

Although a detailed description of these procedures is beyond the scope of this chapter, certain principles should be emphasized. Gangrenous and infected toes can be successfully amputated by closed or open techniques in patients with good circulation as manifest by pedal pulses. Extensive debriding and partial foot amputations will also usually heal in such patients if all infected and necrotic tissue is excised. Such procedures will result in patients regaining an effective walking status. Amputation of one or more gangrenous or ulcerated toes or limited debriding may also sometimes result in a healed foot in patients without distal pulses and substantial arterial occlusive disease (e.g., an occluded superficial femoral artery). Determination of moderately good collateral circulation by ankle-brachial indices or pulse volume recordings may be helpful in predicting such healing. However, sometimes in patients with borderline circulation, a trial at such local procedures is warranted before proceeding with a major effort at revascularization. If prompt healing does not result, revascularization is justified and should be performed without delay.

In addition, some patients with critical ischemia as manifest by mild ischemic rest pain or limited gangrene or ulceration can be treated conservatively with good foot care, antibiotics, analgesics, and limited ambulation.[2] Conservative treatment is indicated in patients who might not tolerate revascularization procedures because of major comorbidities. Long periods of palliation and occasional healing of small ulcerations or gangrenous patches may occur in a few patients with critical ischemia.[2]

HISTORY OF AGGRESSIVE APPROACH TO LIMB SALVAGE IN PATIENTS WITH CRITICAL ISCHEMIA DUE TO INFRAINGUINAL ARTERIOSCLEROSIS AND EVOLUTION OF THE RELATIONSHIP BETWEEN OPEN BYPASS SURGERY AND ANGIOGRAPHIC TECHNIQUES AND ENDOVASCULAR TREATMENTS

In the 1960s and 1970s, major below-knee or above-knee amputation was regarded as the safest and best treatment for gangrene and ulceration from arteriosclerotic

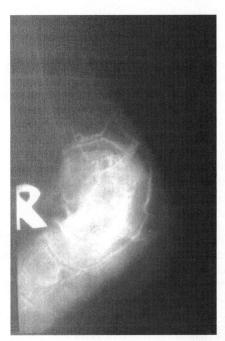

FIGURE 26-1 ■ This 83-year old patient with diabetes had a gangrenous great toe. A vein bypass to the posterior tibial artery in 1971 resulted in limb salvage for 10 years after the limb-threatening event. (From Veith FJ, Cayne NS, Gargiulo NJ III, et al: Surgical options for critical limb ischemia. In Bosiers M, Schneider P, editors: Critical limb ischemia, New York, 2009, Informa Healthcare, pp 195–208.)

occlusive disease below the inguinal ligament,[3] despite the effectiveness of reconstructive arterial surgery (bypass and endarterectomy) for aortoiliac occlusive disease and despite some occasional positive results from femoropopliteal and even femorotibial bypasses. Because we had access to unusually good arteriography that visualized all the arteries in the leg and foot (Figure 26-1), we developed and promoted an aggressive approach to salvage threatened limbs, including those with extensive gangrene.[4] More than 96% of patients with threatened limbs were subjected to an effort to save the limb. Only 4%, those with severe dementia or gangrene extending beyond the midfoot, were excluded. Only 6% of all patients with threatened limbs, when examined by this extensive arteriography, had no patent artery in the leg or foot that could serve as an outflow site for a bypass.[4] With improvements in technique, this proportion of patients with arteries unsuitable for a bypass fell to 1% to 2%.[1,5-11] Successful foot salvage was achieved in 81% to 95% of patients in whom bypasses were performed for the period that they lived up to 5 years.[1,4] However, 52% of these limb salvage patients had many medical comorbidities and died, usually from cardiac causes, within the first 5 years after their initial bypass.[4] More than two-thirds of the patients who lived beyond 5 years retained a useable limb and were able to ambulate beyond the 5-year time point.[4] However, to maintain limb salvage many of these patients required some form of reoperation or reintervention, because they developed a failed (thrombosed) or failing (threatened but patent) graft from a lesion in their graft or its inflow or outflow tract.[1,4,5] These worthwhile

limb salvage results were in part achieved because of a myriad of improvements in the surgical techniques,[1,4-11] development of methods to facilitate the many reoperations these patients required,[12-14] and importantly because of improved anesthetic and intensive care management of these limb-salvage patients who often had advanced cardiorespiratory disease, poor kidney function, and diabetes. Collectively, these improvements made it possible to attempt limb salvage in almost every patient with a threatened limb and intact brain functions.[1,4,9] In addition, many vascular centers throughout the world adopted these policies and were able to achieve equally good results.

EARLY USE OF ENDOVASCULAR TECHNIQUES (ANGIOPLASTY AND STENTING) WITH BYPASS SURGERY

In the mid 1970s, some centers embraced the use of percutaneous transluminal angioplasty (PTA) to treat these old, sick patients with threatened lower limbs.[4] Initially, PTA was used to correct hemodynamically significant iliac artery stenosis. In most instances, it was combined with some form of infrainguinal bypass. However, as PTA techniques improved, balloon angioplasty was used to treat short iliac occlusions and some superficial femoral artery (SFA) lesions. Approximately 19% of patients with a threatened limb could be treated with PTA alone without an adjunctive bypass, whereas another 14% required some form of open surgical revascularization along with their PTA.[1] These percentages increased and results improved with the introduction of iliac stents. As technical improvements in endovascular technology were developed, it became possible to use popliteal, infrapopliteal, and tibial PTA to facilitate the treatment of these limb salvage patients, to manage them less invasively, and to avoid some of the systemic and local complications of the lengthy and sometimes difficult distal operations in these old, sick patients.[15,16,17] When possible, these endovascular techniques could be used to help in the treatment of patients with failed or failing bypasses, because reoperative procedures were often more difficult than primary bypass operations.[1,4,18,19] Sometimes (in approximately 20% of patients) PTA eliminated the need for a secondary bypass: more often it made the secondary bypass simpler. In addition, we developed a number of unusual approaches to lower extremity arteries to facilitate reoperations by eliminating the need to redissect previously dissected arteries.[12-14,20]

CURRENT AND FUTURE RELATIONSHIP BETWEEN ENDOVASCULAR TREATMENTS AND OPEN BYPASS SURGERY

Recent improvements in catheter, guidewire, stent, and stent-graft technology have transformed the treatment of lower limb ischemia from a primarily open surgical (bypass) modality supplemented by some catheter-based treatments to a primarily endovascular modality. Most who treat critical ischemia regard endovascular treatments as the first option to treat chronic obstructive arteriosclerosis at all levels, including disease in the leg and foot. Indeed, there are some endovascular enthusiasts who mistakenly believe they have originated the limb salvage concept, and some maintain that if a limb cannot be salvaged by endovascular treatment, the next option should be a major amputation.

Although endovascular treatment should be the first therapeutic option to revascularize a critically ischemic limb in most patients, some patients whose leg and foot cannot be saved by some form of endovascular treatment can undergo an open surgical bypass procedure or a partially open removal of a resistant clot with a successful salvage of the foot.

Although almost all experts will agree that there are still some indications for open surgical bypasses for limb threatening ischemia, there is wide variation in opinions about the proportion of patients with critical ischemia that will require an open bypass at some point in their disease process. At least 20% to 35% of patients with critical ischemia will require open surgery at some point in the course of their disease, although endovascular techniques continue to improve so that this proportion may decrease in the future. We also believe that such procedures will usually be indicated after failures of one, or usually more, endovascular treatments, although there are some patients with extensive foot gangrene, long occlusions, limited target outflow arteries, and a good greater saphenous vein in whom a bypass should be considered as the best initial treatment option.[21,22] To some extent, such an option will depend on many factors, such as the age and health of the patient, the pattern of disease, and the skills of the involved interventionalist and surgeon. One real concern is that, as fewer bypasses will be required, fewer surgeons will be skilled in these demanding bypass techniques, particularly in the difficult circumstances in which they will be needed. Perhaps referral centers for bypasses should be established for the same reasons that such centers have been recommended for patients who require open thoracoabdominal aneurysm repair.

It has been recognized for many years that repetitive or redo procedures are an important component of care for patients with critical ischemia[1,4,5]; this will continue. Endovascular procedures may be used to salvage limbs after failed or failing open surgical bypasses.[1,18,19] This tendency will increase as technology improves. Similarly, bypass operations or partially open thrombectomy will be required after early or late failure of endovascular treatment or prior bypasses in patients in whom no further endovascular options are available. Most of the 20% to 35% of critical ischemia patients who will require an open surgical bypass or thrombectomy will require it in such a setting.

There are certain principles and precautions that should be followed by those performing endovascular interventions for limb ischemia. These interventions should be used in a way that preserves at least one good target outflow artery, thereby leaving the option of an open surgical rescue if the intervention fails. In addition, care must be taken not to render initially patent arterial segments unusable, thereby necessitating a more distal

bypass than would have been required before the endovascular procedure. Moreover, key collateral vessels should be preserved so that the patient will not be worse than he originally was if the intervention fails. This is particularly important to avoid the need for some reinterventions if ulcerated or gangrenous lesions have healed.

SPECIFIC OPEN SURGICAL REVASCULARIZATION PROCEDURES

Open surgical revascularization procedures fall under two major headings: bypass procedures and thrombectomy and revision of failed (thrombosed) prior bypasses that cannot be rescued by endovascular means. The latter circumstance is usually associated with an organized fibrinous plug that cannot be lysed, dilated, or removed at either the proximal or distal anastomosis of a prosthetic bypass.

SUPERFICIAL FEMORAL ARTERY AND ABOVE-KNEE POPLITEAL OCCLUSIVE DISEASE

With the introduction of improved techniques for crossing total occlusions, subintimal or intraluminal PTA can be used to treat most occlusions of the SFA and above-knee popliteal artery. Nitinol self-expanding stents and stent-grafts (Viabahn, W. L. Gore, Flagstaff, AZ) can be used as adjuncts to these procedures.[23-25] When performing these procedures, care must be taken not to violate the principles and precautions outlined previously and to preserve important collateral vessels, such as the DFA. In the unusual instance when these endovascular interventions fail and cannot be restored to patency or when technical difficulty is encountered, a femoropopliteal bypass can be performed to the below-knee popliteal artery or tibioperoneal trunk via standard medial approaches.[26] This bypass is best performed with a reversed greater saphenous vein harvested via skip incisions, although endoscopic vein harvest has been described[27]; however, this technique requires special equipment and technical expertise. In situ vein bypass offers no advantage in the femoropopliteal position. If the groin is heavily scarred or infected, the distal two-thirds of the deep femoral artery can be accessed directly in the thigh and used for bypass inflow (or outflow if a bypass ends in the groin).[13] In circumstances in which the medial approaches to the popliteal artery are rendered difficult or impossible because of scarring or infection, both the above-knee and the below-knee popliteal arteries can be accessed via lateral approaches and used for bypass outflow.[14] If this is done, the graft can be tunneled laterally in a subcutaneous plane. If patients do not have a saphenous vein or arm vein or if their veins are too small (<3.5 mm in distended diameter) or involved with preexisting disease[28] and they require a femoropopliteal bypass, a 6-mm polytetrafluoroethylene (PTFE) conduit may be used.[29] If this is done or if a vein is used, duplex surveillance is warranted and reintervention is justified for a failing (threatened) graft. However, if the graft has failed (thrombosed), reintervention is indicated only if the failure results in critical ischemia, which occurs in approximately 65% of cases in whom the original bypass was performed for critical ischemia.[12]

TIBIAL AND PERONEAL ARTERY BYPASSES

Tibial and peroneal artery bypasses may be indicated after multiple failures of endovascular treatments. Some also believe that these bypasses also indicated when long segments of all three crural vessels and the below knee popliteal or tibioperoneal trunk are occluded, especially if extensive foot necrosis is present. However, even in this circumstance some believe long-segment tibial subintimal PTA is effective.[30] However, no one has been able to duplicate Bolia's tibial artery results despite enthusiasm for subintimal PTA for shorter lesions and in the SFA and popliteal arteries.[31]

For tibial and peroneal bypasses, autologous vein is the graft of choice if it is disease free.[28] The source of the superficial vein can be from any limb or site, and the vein can be used in either the reversed or in situ configuration. A randomized comparison of reversed and in situ vein grafts to crural arteries demonstrated no significant patency or limb salvage differences, except for veins less than 3 mm in distended diameter.[32] In this circumstance, in situ grafts performed better, but the difference was not statistically significant. To facilitate the use of vein as the conduit, the grafts should be as short as possible. In addition, the SFA, the popliteal artery, and even tibial arteries have proved to be effective sites of origin for these distal bypasses when there is no important proximal disease (Figures 26-2 to 26-4).[6-8,10] If proximal disease is present, it can often be treated with PTA enabling a distal short vein graft without compromising patency.[33] Moreover, if there is a patent popliteal blind or isolated segment (without tibial or peroneal outflow) and limited lengths of autologous vein, a composite sequential bypass may be performed with the distal component being a vein graft

from the isolated popliteal to a patent tibial artery and the proximal component being a PTFE graft from a femoral artery to the proximal end of the vein graft.[34] If a patient with critical ischemia is faced with an imminent amputation and is totally without satisfactory autologous vein, a PTFE tibial bypass is in an acceptable option, and good secondary patency and limb salvage results have been demonstrated (43% 5-year secondary patency and 66% 5-year limb salvage) in this setting (Figures 26-5 and 26-6).[29,35] Although some advocate the use of a distal vein

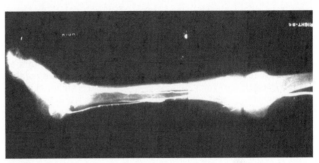

FIGURE 26-3 ■ This tibiotibial bypass performed with a reversed vein graft was patent after 12 years. (From Veith FJ, Ascer E, Gupta SK, et al: Tibiotibial vein bypass grafts: a new operation for limb salvage, J Vasc Surg 2:552–557, 1985.)

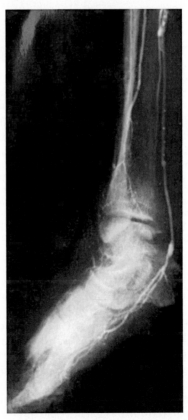

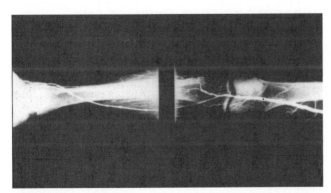

FIGURE 26-2 ■ This arteriogram was obtained 10 years after a reversed vein bypass from the below-knee popliteal artery to the distal anterior tibial artery. (From Veith FJ, Cayne NS, Garbiulo NJ III, et al: Surgical options for critical limb ischemia. In Bosiers M, Schneider P, editors: Critical limb ischemia, New York, 2009, Informa Healthcare, pp 195–208.)

FIGURE 26-4 ■ A magnified arteriographic view of the foot of the patient shown in Figure 26-3. Twelve-year limb salvage was achieved despite an incomplete plantar arch. (From Veith FJ, Ascer E, Gupta SK, et al: Tibiotibial vein bypass grafts: a new operation for limb salvage, J Vasc Surg 2:552–557, 1985.)

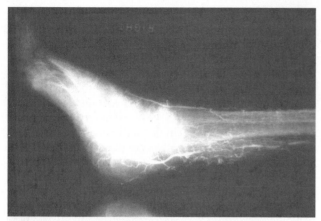

FIGURE 26-5 ■ This arteriogram is from a patient with great toe gangrene. There is only an isolated posterior tibial artery segment. No other patent arterial segments were available as targets for revascularization, and no autologous vein available for a bypass. (From Veith FJ, Cayne NS, Gargiulo NJ III, et al: Surgical options for critical limb ischemia. In Bosiers M, Schneider P, editors: Critical limb ischemia, New York, 2009, Informa Healthcare, pp 195–208.)

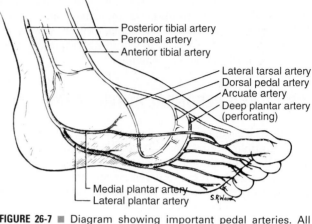

FIGURE 26-7 ■ Diagram showing important pedal arteries. All these named arteries can be used for limb salvage revascularizations. (From Ascer E, Veith FJ, Gupta SK: Bypasses to plantar arteries and other tibial branches: an extended approach to limb salvage, J Vasc Surg 8:434–441, 1988.)

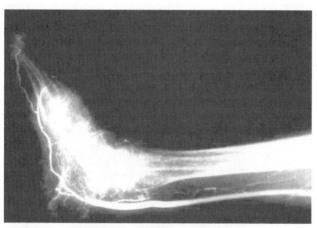

FIGURE 26-6 ■ A prosthetic bypass with a PTFE graft was performed to the isolated segment shown in Figure 26-5. This arteriogram was obtained 4 years after the original operation. Patency was maintained until the patient's death 6 years after the operation. (From Veith FJ, Cayne NS, Gargiulo NJ III, et al: Surgical options for critical limb ischemia. In Bosiers M, Schneider P, editors: Critical limb ischemia, New York, 2009, Informa Healthcare, pp 195–208.)

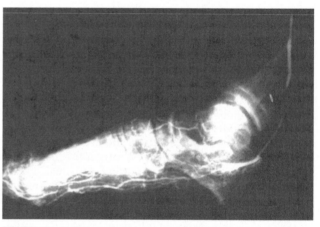

FIGURE 26-8 ■ This arteriogram was obtained 4 years after a reversed vein graft to the lateral plantar artery. (From Veith FJ, Cayne NS, Gargiulo NJ III, et al: Surgical options for critical limb ischemia. In Bosiers M, Schneider P, editors: Critical limb ischemia, New York, 2009, Informa Healthcare, pp 195–208.)

BYPASSES TO FOOT ARTERIES AND THEIR BRANCHES

patch or cuff to improve patency,[36] others have not been convinced that any of these adjunctive procedures improve patency results more than a carefully constructed distal PTFE graft anastomosis. In the authors' recent experience with PTFE bypasses to leg arteries, they have a role in achieving and maintaining limb salvage when other options are not available.[37] The graft must, however, be implanted into a leg artery that has luminal continuity to its normal terminal branches and preferably richly supplies the foot, and the surgeon must be willing to do a secondary or redo prosthetic tibial bypass if the original graft fails.[37] Many groups have not been able to duplicate these results, although others have.[38,39]

In the late 1970s and early 1980s, it was realized that many patients who were thought to have patterns of arteriosclerosis totally unsuited for revascularization actually had patent named arteries in their foot that could be used as outflow sites for distal bypasses;[1,4,7,10] (Figure 26-7). By performing bypasses to these vessels, it was possible to substantially increase the number of critical ischemia patients that could have their threatened limb saved (Figures 26-8 and 26-9).[1,7,10] Many other groups subsequently confirmed these initial results.

These very distal grafts can be performed only with vein as a conduit. However, many of these grafts can originate from the below-knee popliteal artery or even from patent proximal tibial arteries (see Figures 26-2 to

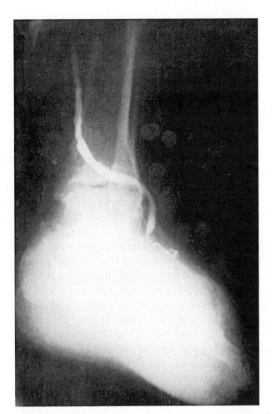

FIGURE 26-9 ■ This arteriogram was obtained 12 years after a reversed vein bypass to the lateral tarsal artery. Note the forefoot amputation required to obtain healing. Despite this, the patient walked normally. (From Ascer E, Veith FJ, Gupta SK: Bypasses to plantar arteries and other tibial branches: an extended approach to limb salvage, J Vasc Surg 8:434–441, 1988.)

26-4).[1,6,7,10] As with all infrainguinal bypass grafts, and especially those to crural arteries, the procedures must be performed with care and technical perfection. Any technical error in graft preparation, tunneling, or anastomotic construction will result in failure. Good lighting (headlight), a dry field, and patience are essential. Magnification and microsurgical instruments are often required, and care must be taken to treat outflow arteries atraumatically and to preserve all outflow branches, even the small ones that are unnamed. Completion arteriography (cinefluoroscopy) is also essential, as with all infrapopliteal bypasses to assure good anastomotic configuration and bypass flow rates. If spasm or decreased flow is noted, vasodilators (nitroglycerin, papaverine) may be helpful.[40] Additional technical details and illustrations are provided in a recent textbook chapter that goes beyond the scope of this chapter.[26]

Although these foot artery procedures were developed before endovascular approaches existed to revascularize these very distal arteries, these foot artery bypasses still have a role. Coronary balloons, 0.14 in guidewire-based systems, and stents are now being used to revascularize patent arteries in the lower leg and foot. Although these techniques can work well in the short term, long-term results are unclear, and it remains to be determined how these results will compare with those of bypass operations.

NEWER TECHNIQUES FOR REDO PROCEDURES AFTER FAILED BYPASSES: THROMBECTOMY AND TOTAL OR PARTIAL RESCUE OF A FAILED POLYTETRAFLUOROETHYLENE BYPASS OR TOTALLY NEW BYPASSES

It is well known that infrainguinal revascularization procedures, both endovascular and open surgical, are associated with a progressively increasing failure rate, with a diminished luminal caliber followed by thrombosis. This is due to both intimal hyperplasia, which is largely a reaction to vascular injury, and progression of the arteriosclerotic process. When bypasses or PTAs that have been performed for critical ischemia fail after a patency interval of 6 months or longer, the originally threatened limb is only threatened again in approximately 65% of patients. This may be due to healing of the original gangrenous or ulcerated lesion and the fact that greater blood flow is required to achieve healing than to maintain it. Alternatively, the maintenance of a healed foot after a revascularization failure may be due to improved collateral blood flow or absence of the trauma or infection that contributed to the gangrene or ulceration in the first place.

Whatever the reason, management strategies for patients with failed revascularization procedures should be influenced by the fact that critical ischemia might not recur. Only then should a secondary intervention be undertaken, because such secondary procedures are generally more difficult and have worse results than primary procedures. Thus, redo procedures are not indicated to prevent critical ischemia from developing. The one exception is when a primary procedure is determined by physical examination, symptoms, or noninvasive testing to be in the failing state (i.e., threatened by the development of a new or recurrent lesion that reduces flow but without thrombosis of the revascularization).

A full description of all possible redo procedures that are indicated when a primary bypass (with vein or prosthetic) fails is beyond the scope of this chapter and is available elsewhere.[12] Nevertheless some principles deserve emphasis, in addition to those already mentioned. First, endovascular interventions should always be considered the first option in patients requiring a redo procedure even if the original revascularization was a bypass. Improved technology that was previously unavailable may be effective and may provide sufficient increased blood flow to maintain foot viability.

Second, redissection of previously dissected arteries, particularly in the groin, should be avoided because they are difficult and prone to a fivefold increased risk of infection. If a totally new bypass is required, as is usually the case when a failed vein graft cannot be freed of clot, alternate or new approaches to patent arteries should be used and these have been well described.[12-14,20]

Third, complete preprocedure arteriography should precede any reoperative attempt. Planning can be optimized only when the surgeon or interventionist is fully aware of the location and extent of all occlusive and stenotic arterial disease throughout the iliac system and the entire lower extremity.

Fourth, if the failed bypass is a prosthetic conduit, an effort should be made to restore patency percutaneously using mechanical thrombectomy devices and lytic agents. This is often facilitated if the proximal anastomotic hood of the original graft can be seen angiographically to facilitate guidewire passage. Only if interventional procedures fail should reoperation be undertaken; this is generally required when the proximal or distal organized thrombotic plug cannot be lysed or removed by percutaneous means. In this circumstance the PTFE graft is approached at its most accessible midportion, usually in a subcutaneous position and remote from any anastomosis. The graft is opened longitudinally, and the liquefied clot is removed gently with balloon catheters. Next, using fluoroscopic guidance, guidewires and catheters are gently used to traverse the anastomosis. Fluoroscopy with contrast injections is used to identify any inflow or anastomotic lesions and similarly any outflow lesions. A double-lumen balloon catheter is then passed over the guidewire across the anastomosis, the balloon is inflated with dilute contrast, and under fluoroscopic control the balloon is withdrawn gently to remove free clot. By observing the distortion of the balloon, hyperplastic and arteriosclerotic lesions can be observed and corrected by PTA without or with stent placement.[41,42] Balloon distortion within the proximal graft indicates the presence of an organized gelatinous or fibrinous plug that usually cannot be removed with a balloon catheter.[42] In that case and because loose clot has been removed, there may often be some flow in the opened graft, presenting a problem with hemostasis. If so, a 9-French hemostatic sheath is placed into the graft, and bleeding around the sheath is controlled with doubled vessel loops. The sheath and its dilator are passed over the wire across the anastomosis. The dilator is removed and an adherent clot removal catheter (Edwards Laboratory) is passed within the sheath under fluoroscopic control. The sheath is retracted and the wires of the clot removal catheter are deployed only within the graft under fluoroscopic control to engage the adherent plug and remove it without injuring the adjacent artery.[42] Angiography is used to demonstrate the absence of residual luminal defects. A similar procedure is then performed distally. If unobstructed distal flow cannot be obtained after PTA and stent placement, the proximal graft (now with unobstructed inflow) is transected and used as the origin for a partially new bypass to another patent distal artery accessed via a virginal approach.[12,14,20] Completion contrast fluoroscopy should be used to confirm an adequate lumen without defects and unimpeded flow through the graft and into the outflow tract.

MULTIPLE REDO PROCEDURES

Some patients are subject to repetitive failure of lower extremity revascularization procedures including bypasses. Some believe that patients who have failure of two or more bypasses in the same lower extremity should, if they redevelop critical ischemia, undergo a major amputation. Lipsitz and colleagues[43] do not agree with this concept and have recently demonstrated the value of repetitive redo bypasses, usually performed over several years (up to 15), in preserving the limb and life style of these patients. They observed the duration of patency following more than three bypasses was substantial and resulted in more than 3 years of extended limb salvage in more than 50% of the patients who would otherwise have required an amputation.[43] These beneficial results were obtained only when the repetitive bypasses were performed according to the principles already outlined. Moreover, these repetitive bypasses should be performed only when the patient would otherwise require an immediate major amputation.

CONCLUSIONS

The bottom line of all these treatment efforts for critical ischemia is that everything possible should be done to salvage the threatened foot in these elderly, sick patients who do not walk well after one major amputation and certainly do not do so after bilateral amputations, which 25% of this population may otherwise require at some point in their course. Although the methods needed to save limbs initially and maintain this salvage may be time consuming and technically demanding, and although they require continuing commitment on the part of the vascular surgeon or vascular specialist, they are gratifying to those who perform them effectively and are rewarding in maintaining an acceptable life style in this group of patients with advanced atherosclerosis.

References available online at expertconsult.com.

QUESTIONS

1. True or false: Multiple reinterventions and redo bypasses are often indicated and worthwhile after a failed primary vein bypass.

2. Bypasses to arteries below the popliteal artery should be performed for limb salvage with PTFE grafts in which of the following circumstances?
   a. When no acceptable autologous vein is present in the involved lower extremity
   b. Only when no autologous vein is available in any of the patient's four extremities
   c. In no circumstances
   d. Only to the posterior tibial artery
   e. None of the above

3. True or false: Heavily calcified, incompressible tibial arteries are unsuitable for use in limb salvage arterial bypasses.

4. True or false: Studies have clearly shown that in situ vein bypasses are uniformly superior to reversed vein bypasses.

5. True or false: The standard arteriogram for femoropopliteal occlusive disease should visualize all arteries from the renal arteries to the forefoot.

6. True or false: Vein and PTFE bypasses to isolated popliteal artery segments have a poor chance of being successful in treating critical limb ischemia and should be avoided if possible.

7. When is bypass to a tibial artery at the ankle level or in the foot indicated for disabling intermittent claudication?
   a. Always
   b. Almost never
   c. Almost always
   d. Frequently
   e. Never

8. True or false: Toe amputation or foot debridement should never be combined with arterial revascularization.

9. True or false: The presence of pedal pulses is evidence of sufficiently good circulation in the foot that a toe amputation for infection is likely to heal.

10. True or false: In patients with a failed infrainguinal bypass and a rethreatened limb, there is a poor chance of saving the foot by performing a secondary revascularization.

ANSWERS

1. **True**
2. **b**
3. **False**
4. **False**
5. **True**
6. **False**
7. **b**
8. **False**
9. **True**
10. **False**

CHAPTER 27

ENDOSCOPIC HARVESTING OF THE SAPHENOUS VEIN

Juan Carlos Jimenez • Christian Eisenring

Open vein harvest for coronary artery bypass grafting and infrainguinal bypass procedures is associated with increased patient morbidity and postoperative wound complications.[1] In the limb salvage population, patients exhibit severe peripheral arterial occlusive disease, marginal distal perfusion, poor nutrition, and infected wounds. These factors make it difficult to heal lower-extremity skin incisions required to harvest long, continuous segments of saphenous vein required for optimal bypass patency. Over the past decade, endoscopic harvest of the saphenous vein and the radial artery has been increasingly used by cardiac surgeons for coronary artery bypass grafting and has become the standard of care within this specialty.

More recently, these techniques have been used increasingly for minimally invasive harvest of autogenous conduits in conjunction with peripheral vascular surgery. Because longer, continuous segments of conduit are required for infrainguinal revascularization, especially infrapopliteal bypass, certain technical modifications have been required to facilitate use for lower extremity limb salvage procedures.[2]

RESULTS

Endoscopic Vein Harvesting: Coronary Artery Bypass Grafting

Several prospective, randomized trials have compared endoscopic vein harvest (EVH) with traditional open saphenous harvest during coronary artery bypass grafting and have demonstrated superior outcomes for EVH. Advantages include lower wound complication rates, decreased postoperative pain, increased patient satisfaction, improved cosmesis, and equivalent graft patency rates.[3-8] Griffith and colleagues[9] performed a histologic analysis of veins harvested by open techniques and EVH. There was no difference in endothelial, smooth muscle, and elastic lamina continuity between the two groups. Medial and adventitial connective tissue uniformity was also not significantly altered.

Despite multiple supportive studies validating EVH for coronary artery bypass grafting (CABG), a recent study by Lopes and colleagues[10] questioned the superiority of this technique. They reviewed the outcomes of 1753 patients who underwent EVH for CABG and compared them to 1247 patients in the open harvest group.

They demonstrated a higher rate of vein-graft failure at 12 to 18 months in the EVH group compared with the open cohort (46.7% vs. 38%, respectively). At 3 years, endoscopic vein harvest was also associated with higher rates of death, myocardial infarction, and repeated revascularization. Critics of this study highlighted the elevated vein-graft failure and death rates in both open and EVH groups compared with similar published series. Additional criticisms included an overall lower use of internal mammary artery conduits, which are associated with superior patency compared with vein grafts, and that 20% of the procedures in this patient cohort were performed off-pump.

A recent study performed by the Northern New England Cardiovascular Disease Study Group demonstrated a decreased risk of leg wound infections with EVH, but an increased adjusted risk of bleeding requiring a return to the operating room.[11] Endoscopic harvest was also associated with a significant reduction in long-term mortality in these patients. The results also demonstrated that between 2001 and 2004, the use of EVH increased from 34% to 75% in patients requiring CABG.

Endoscopic Vein Harvesting: Infrainguinal Revascularization

Several studies have demonstrated similar favorable results for EVH during distal arterial bypass for limb salvage, although no randomized controlled trials have been conducted (Table 27-1).[12-15] Jordan and colleagues[12] performed 164 saphenous vein EVHs for lower extremity arterial reconstructive procedures over a 6-year period.[12] A review of patency rates using Kaplan-Meier analysis at 1, 3, and 5 years demonstrated vein graft patencies of 85%, 74%, and 68%, respectively. Fourteen patients (8.5%) developed wound infections during the 30-day postoperative period, and two patients developed harvest site hematomas. None of these wound complications led to either graft failure or limb loss. The limb salvage rate was 89%.

A review by Erdoes and Milner[14] examined the outcomes following EVH for infrainguinal arterial bypass in 214 limbs over a 6-year period. The indication for bypass was limb salvage in 88.3%, claudication in 9.3%, and trauma and aneurysm in 2.4%. Assisted primary patency at 18 months was 77.2% by Kaplan-Meier analysis. Wound complication rates were 7.5%, with 2.5% of

TABLE 27-1 **Results of Endoscopic Vein Harvest Used in Conjunction with Peripheral Arterial Bypass**

Study	Year	Mean Operative Time (Min)	Primary Patency (%)	Overall Limb Salvage (%)	Overall Wound Complication Rate (%)
Jordan and colleagues[12]	2001	NA	69 (12 mo)	89	0.9
Suggs and colleagues[13]	2001	295	93 (12 mo)	92	4
Illig and colleagues[13a]	2003	NA	60 (12 mo)	98	20.4
Erdoes and Milner[14]	2005	248	71.5 (18 mo)	91	7.5
Gazoni and colleagues[15]	2006	241.5	92.8 (21 mo)	96.5	13.8
Pulatt and colleagues[15a]	2006	NA	30 (12 mo)	85	6
Jimenez and colleagues[2]	2007	410.4	78.5 (12 mo)	100	14
Hinesand colleagues[15b]	2010	NA	73.2 (72 mo)	63	37
Juilliard and colleagues[16]	2011	NA	42.2 (36 mo)	81	20.2

NA, Not available.

patients requiring readmission to the hospital. Only one patient early in the series required conversion to an open harvest.

Gazoni and colleagues[15] reported results for patients who underwent femoral to below-knee arterial bypass grafting over a 27-month period.[15] Fifty-nine patients underwent traditional open saphenectomy, and 29 had EVH. There was a trend toward improved patency rates in the EVH group compared with open harvest, although no statistically significant difference was noted (92.8% vs. 80.6%). No significant differences were found between the two groups in postoperative complications, operative time, length of hospital stay, patency rates, limb salvage, and death. The incidence of wound complications was 3.4% in the EVH group and 15.3% in the open harvest group, although this difference also was not statistically significant. Similarly, Hines and colleagues examined outcomes over a 5-year period for 27 patients who underwent femoral-popliteal bypass with EVH in patients with Trans-Atlantic Inter-Society Consensus (TASC) D disease of the superficial femoral artery.[15b] Kaplan-Meier primary and primary assisted patency rates were 73.2% and 80.8% at 1 year, respectively, and these rates were maintained for 70 months. Only one patient developed a superficial wound infection.

Following formal systematic training by vascular surgeons and implementation of technical modifications specific to limb salvage procedures at our institution, we noted 30-day primary and primary-assisted patency rates of 85.7% and 92.9%, respectively.[2] Kaplan-Meier primary assisted patency was 63.6%. No patients required primary amputation at 19 months. One graft occlusion occurred within 30 days as a result of a tunnel hematoma in a patient who sustained a postoperative myocardial infarction and required therapeutic anticoagulation. One late hematoma was noted, and one patient demonstrated skin necrosis at the level of the ankle requiring prolonged hospitalization. Complete wound healing was achieved in 75% of patients with preoperative tissue loss owing to critical limb ischemia.

Recently, the long-term durability of EVH for lower-extremity bypass has been questioned following a study by Julliard and colleagues.[16] Over a period of 8.5 years, 363 patients underwent infrainguinal bypass; 170 patients underwent EVH, and 193 underwent traditional open saphenous vein harvest. No differences in indication for surgery were noted between groups. Primary patency rates were significantly lower in the EVH group compared with the open group at 6, 12, and 36 months. There were no differences in length of stay or wound complication rates. Limb salvage and survival were also identical between groups. The differences were not significant in patients with claudication and in those without diabetes.

TECHNIQUES

Endoscopic Harvest of the Greater Saphenous Vein

Although several endoscopic vein-harvesting systems are currently available, at the University of California–Los Angeles (UCLA), the Vasoview Hemopro II Harvesting system is used (Maquet, Wayne, NJ). Preoperative color duplex mapping is performed to assess vein diameters, caliber, patency, and location of branches. In addition, intraoperative ultrasound is performed to mark the course of the vein under sterile conditions before EVH to maximize incision placement accuracy.

An incision is made three fingerbreadths posterior to the medial femoral or tibial condyles depending on whether harvest will be performed above or below the knee. A longitudinal 2 cm incision is made and the GSV is identified. A Silastic vessel loop is placed around the GSV for mobilization (Figure 27-1). At this time, several more centimeters of vein are bluntly dissected and mobilized from the surrounding subcutaneous tissue to ease placement of the blunt tip trocar (BTT) in the direction of intended vein harvest. The BTT is placed into the subcutaneous space overlying the GSV, and sufficient air is inflated into the port balloon to ensure a good seal with the adjacent skin. Leakage of CO_2 outside the harvest tunnel can lead to suboptimal visibility and bleeding during vein mobilization. A CO_2 cannula is then attached to a port on the BTT and continued at a flow rate of 3 to 5 L/min up to a maximum pressure of 10 to 15 mm Hg. Carbon dioxide insufflation should not exceed central venous pressure to avoid embolism. Insufflation of the vein harvest tunnel facilitates placement of the 5-mm camera through the main port of the BTT and enhances visualization of the GSV within the subcutaneous space.

A conical tip is placed on the tip of the camera, and the vein is dissected bluntly along its anterior and posterior surfaces (Figure 27-2). Branches are skeletonized from surrounding soft tissue and exposed to maximal length before division with the bipolar dissector. The main goal before division of branches is to suspend the entire length of the vein by its branches in the center of the harvest tunnel and allow maximal CO_2 insufflation for good visibility (Figure 27-3). Care must be taken at this time to avoid avulsion of large branches. Generally the disruption of minor venous branches is not problematic, because the insufflation tends to control bleeding from these tributaries without the need for additional cauterization.

Following complete blunt dissection, the BTT is replaced with the vein-harvesting cannula, which serves to retract, cauterize, and divide all branches. The Vasoview system provides a retractable C-ring that is used in conjunction with the harmonic scalpel dissector to mobilize the main vein and provide counter-tension at each

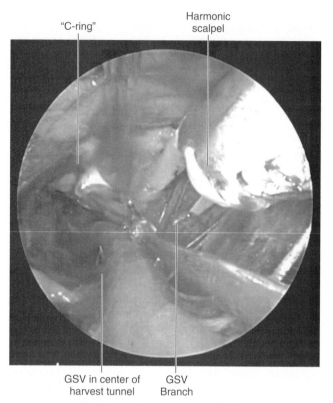

FIGURE 27-3 ■ Branch ligation in the insufflated endoscopic harvest tunnel following circumferential vein dissection.

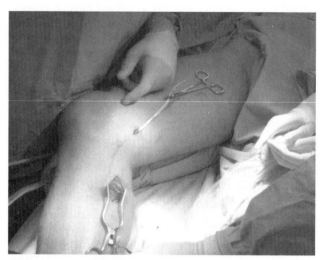

FIGURE 27-1 ■ A 3-cm longitudinal incision is made either above or below the knee for initial mobilization of the greater saphenous vein and placement of the blunt tip trocar.

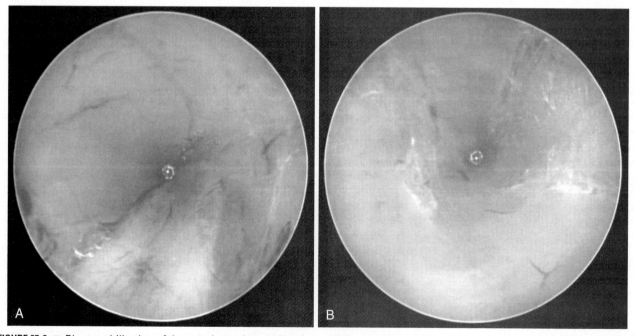

FIGURE 27-2 ■ Blunt mobilization of the anterior and posterior planes of the greater saphenous vein using the conical tip of the 5-mm camera.

individual branch site. A retractable harmonic dissector is then used to cauterize and divide all branches, while avoiding direct or collateral thermal injury to the vein wall. Care must be taken to avoid overly aggressive retraction at this time, which can result in branch avulsion and bleeding within the tunnel. Once all branches are cauterized and divided, the vessel cradle (the C-ring) is then run along the entire length of harvested vein to ensure that no branches remain. The vein can then be removed through a proximal and distal stab incision made directly at opposite ends of the harvest tunnel. All cauterized side branches should be reinforced before limb salvage bypass with individual silk and Prolene sutures. Injured segments of vein must be repaired directly with Prolene suture and, if luminal compromise is present, the affected segment of vein must be excised and venovenostomy is performed. The vein is then prepared and flushed in usual fashion.

Endoscopic Harvest of the Lesser Saphenous Vein

EVH of the lesser saphenous vein is performed in the prone position. Preoperative vein mapping can be useful to determine length, diameter, and caliber of this vessel for use in lower extremity limb salvage procedures. The LSV usually has more large branches than the GSV, and it lies deeper within the subfascial plane. Care must be taken to avoid injury to the sural nerve, which lies adjacent to the LSV in the leg. A 2-cm transverse incision is made in the upper leg below the knee joint distal to where the LSV dives deep and joins the popliteal vein. The vein is harvested and removed in similar fashion. A stab incision can then be made in the distal calf to remove the vein in its entirety (Figure 27-4). Minimally invasive popliteal to posterior tibial artery bypass can also be performed in this position with placement of the vein through the harvest tunnel in either reversed or nonreversed fashion (following treatment with a semiclosed valvulotome.)

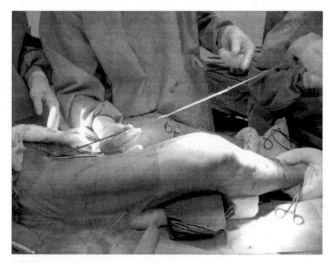

FIGURE 27-4 ■ Long, continuous saphenous vein segments required for infrainguinal revascularization can be obtained using endoscopic vein harvest.

Technical Modifications in the Limb Salvage Population

Although the techniques of harvest are similar for both cardiac surgeons and those performing limb salvage procedures, certain technical adjustments have been applied to infrainguinal bypass for limb salvage. At UCLA, vascular surgeons and fellows underwent formal training on operative simulators before implementation in the operating room. This training included familiarization with the different components of the device during formal sessions with industry representatives and the review of video and other interactive materials during didactic sessions.

Certain technical modifications have been implemented during EVH by vascular surgeons; these modifications facilitate use during lower-extremity limb salvage procedures. Longitudinal vein harvest incisions are preferred over the traditional transverse incisions, performed during cardiac surgery procedures, because they can be extended proximally or distally, or both, and used to expose arterial targets for bypass simultaneously. A medial EVH incision just above the knee at the level of the femoral condyle can be used subsequently to expose the above-knee popliteal artery after the GSV has been removed. A harvest incision just below the knee at the level of the tibial condyles can also be used for exposure of the below knee popliteal artery, the tibioperoneal trunk, and the proximal peroneal and posterior tibial arteries. A longitudinal incision just proximal to the medial malleolus can be extended to expose the distal posterior tibial artery.

When ipsilateral GSV harvest is performed for limb salvage procedures, the harvest tunnel is frequently used for subcutaneous placement of the vein. It can either be reversed or left in situ with subsequent valve lysis with the use of a semiclosed valvulotome. Meticulous hemostasis must be ensured within the harvest tunnel because bleeding and hematoma formation can jeopardize graft patency. Compression bandages should be avoided when ipsilateral harvest is performed for limb salvage procedures, whereas this technique is frequently used following EVH for coronary artery bypass grafting. Patients are instructed to discontinue oral clopidogrel (Plavix) 7 days before the operation to minimize bleeding risk. Immediate postoperative therapeutic heparin drips or subcutaneous low molecular weight heparin should be avoided. Platelet antiaggregation therapy with aspirin or clopidogrel can usually be reinstated safely 24 to 48 hours after the operation.

COMPLICATIONS OF ENDOSCOPIC VEIN HARVEST

All wound complications associated with open saphenous vein harvest can occur with minimally invasive techniques. These complications include infection, dehiscence, hematoma, lymphocele, and limb swelling. A metaanalysis of randomized trials conducted by Athanasiou and colleagues[17] compared minimally invasive versus conventional vein harvesting and found that

EVH techniques were associated with an overall reduced risk of wound infections. However, infections occurring within the harvest tunnel following EVH usually require drainage of fluid collections contained in a closed space. Allen and colleagues[18] identified three closed-space tunnel infections out of 1259 patients who underwent EVH. These three patients also had early postoperative hematomas and wound cultures that were positive for *Staphylococcus aureus*. Two patients were treated by unroofing the tunnel with an incision over its entire length. One patient was managed successfully using closed-space irrigation with a Blake drain irrigated every 8 hours and gradually withdrawn over a 10-day period.

Carbon dioxide insufflation during EVH can result in hypercarbia,[19] pneumoperitoneum,[20] and CO_2 embolus, especially when the insufflation pressure exceeds central venous pressure.[21] Chiu and colleagues[21] randomly assigned 498 patients to high (15 mm Hg) and low (12 mm Hg) CO_2 insufflation groups for EVH during CABG. Transesophageal echocardiography with transgastric inferior vena cava views was used to monitor for the appearance of CO_2 bubbles. The incidence of CO_2 embolus was significantly elevated in the high-pressure insufflations group (13.3% vs. 6.5 %; $p < 0.05$). Two patients in the high-pressure group required immediate cessation of insufflation. Although no patient exhibited hemodynamic alterations in either group in this study, massive CO_2 embolus with circulatory collapse has been noted in separate reports. All patients with visible CO_2 bubbles on TEE were converted to open harvest and these patients all exhibited subclinical injury to the vein wall.

When EVH is performed on the ipsilateral GSV during minimally invasive distal arterial bypass, care must be taken to avoid postoperative tunnel hematomas because the compressive effects may compromise vein graft patency. Because the vein graft is usually placed within the EVH tunnel, meticulous hemostasis in the subcutaneous tissue and reinforcement of all ligated branches must be ensured. Extension of existing incisions should be used in selected instances when significant bleeding is noted. Immediate postoperative anticoagulation should be avoided, as well as compression wraps when the ipsilateral GSV is used for graft tunneling because of possible compression of the vein within its subcutaneous position.

Although rare, skin necrosis has been reported following EVH, especially in the lower leg at the level of the ankle where minimal subcutaneous fat exists. Conversion to open harvest at this level should be performed if excessive resistance is noted during blunt dissection. At UCLA, one patient exhibited full thickness skin necrosis requiring flap coverage and ultimately leading to late graft failure. Early recognition and flap coverage is crucial, especially when the harvest tunnel is used for graft placement.

References available online at expertconsult.com.

QUESTIONS

1. A 2011 study by the Northern New England Cardiovascular Disease Study Group demonstrated which of the following results?
   a. A significant reduction in long-term mortality
   b. A decreased risk of leg wound infections
   c. An increased adjusted risk of bleeding
   d. An increase in the use of EVH between 2001 and 2004
   e. All of the above

2. A 2009 study published in the New England Journal of Medicine by Lopes and colleagues demonstrated which of the following results?
   a. Equivalent outcomes following both EVH and open harvest
   b. Higher rates of vein graft failure with open harvest
   c. Higher rates of vein graft failure following EVH
   d. Lower rates of death with EVH
   e. Lower rates of myocardial infarction with EVH

3. Complications following EVH include the following:
   a. Tunnel hematoma
   b. Skin necrosis
   c. Hypercarbia
   d. Lymphocele
   e. All of the above

4. Specific technical modifications to EVH which facilitate use in limb salvage procedures include the following:
   a. Longitudinal harvest incisions
   b. Avoidance of the harvest tunnel for placement of the vein graft
   c. Routine use of compression Ace bandages following bypass
   d. Transverse harvest incisions
   e. Routine therapeutic heparinization following bypass

5. When harvesting the small saphenous vein, the following is true:
   a. Branches are encountered less frequently than EVH of the great saphenous vein
   b. Care must be taken to avoid injury to the sural nerve
   c. Care must be taken to avoid injury to the epigastric vein
   d. Dissection is performed deep to the muscular fascia
   e. The small saphenous vein connects directly with the femoral vein in most patients

6. Closed space wound infections following EVH should be treated with:
   a. Warm compresses
   b. Warm compresses and aspirin
   c. Warm compresses and ibuprofen
   d. Unroofing of the harvest tunnel and drainage
   e. All of the above

7. Technical details of EVH for limb salvage procedures should include the following considerations:
   a. A medial EVH incision can be used for exposure of the above or below knee popliteal artery
   b. A longitudinal EVH incision at the medial ankle can be used for both vein harvest and exposure of the anterior tibial artery
   c. The GSV should never be harvested through the femoral incision
   d. Only reversed GSV bypasses can be performed following EVH
   e. Reinforcement of cauterized vein branches is not usually necessary for hemostasis prior to bypass

8. Technical differences between EVH for coronary artery bypass surgery and limb salvage procedures include the following:
   a. The preferred use of longitudinal incisions in limb salvage procedures
   b. Longer lengths of vein are usually required for limb salvage procedures
   c. Harvest of the great and small saphenous veins can be performed for both
   d. Overall decreased risk of wound infections has been demonstrated for both
   e. All of the above

9. Carbon dioxide insufflation during EVH has been known to cause the following:
   a. Hypercarbia
   b. Pneumoperitoneum
   c. CO2 embolus
   d. Circulatory collapse
   e. All of the above

10. The following statements are true regarding EVH:
    a. Randomized, controlled trials have demonstrated superior outcomes for EVH compared with open vein harvest following limb salvage procedures
    b. No histologic studies have been performed following both types of harvest
    c. Endoscopically harvest GSV has superior patency compared with the internal mammary artery
    d. Lower extremity skin incisions in the limb salvage population are difficult to heal due to poor nutrition, infected wounds, and atherosclerotic disease
    e. All of the above

ANSWERS

1. **e**
2. **c**
3. **e**
4. **a**
5. **b**
6. **d**
7. **a**
8. **e**
9. **e**
10. **d**

CHAPTER 28

Infrainguinal Endovascular Reconstruction: Technique and Results

Brian G. DeRubertis • Peter A. Schneider

Management of infrainguinal arterial occlusive disease continues to move away from open surgery and toward percutaneous procedures, and the number of percutaneous options is growing rapidly. This chapter focuses on standard techniques for arterial access, diagnostic imaging, lesion crossing, and options for treating occlusions and stenoses of the femoropopliteal and tibial circulation.

PATIENT SELECTION AND PREOPERATIVE IMAGING

Infrainguinal occlusive disease can usually be diagnosed by history and physical examination. Confirmatory studies are usually performed—either duplex mapping or magnetic resonance angiography—in order to plan the therapeutic approach and limit the amount of contrast required for arteriography. Diagnostic arteriography does not currently exist in many practices, because most patients do not undergo arterial access unless there is an intention to treat. Occasionally, what initially appeared to be a lesion appropriate for angioplasty based on duplex scanning or magnetic resonance angiography turns out to be more complex, and only an arteriogram is obtained.

Infrainguinal occlusive disease can be classified by its morphology, which assists in determining which patients are best managed with endovascular intervention and which ones require surgery. The TransAtlantic Inter-Society Consensus (TASC) classification (Box 28-1) and others have defined disease morphology in an effort to clarify the issue of lesion severity.[1] The general concept is that endovascular techniques are preferred in patients with less severe forms of disease and among those with shorter life expectancies or greater periprocedural risk factors. Conversely, open surgical approaches have a better risk-benefit profile in patients with fewer medical comorbidities or more severe forms of disease, such as long-segment occlusions, in which endovascular procedures are less durable. The recommendation from the TASC group is that type A lesions be treated with endovascular intervention, type D lesions be treated with surgery, and types B and C lesions be treated with either, depending on the patient's comorbidities, general medical condition, expected longevity, and availability of conduit for bypass.

Over the past decade, many practices have seen a steady movement toward the use of endovascular techniques for infrainguinal arterial occlusive disease, to the point that some approach all patients with an "endovascular first" strategy with open surgical bypass reserved for failures of endovascular therapy. However, some lesions or disease patterns continue to be best treated with open surgery, such as common femoral disease or long-segment femoropopliteal occlusions with distal tibial reconstitution, although even these difficult disease patterns can be treated with some of the newer percutaneous modalities, such as laser or excisional atherectomy.

Approaches

Percutaneous intervention for infrainguinal occlusive disease is usually performed through the contralateral femoral artery using an up-and-over approach or through the ipsilateral femoral artery using an antegrade approach (Table 28-1). Infrainguinal interventions can also be performed through the brachial artery, but this approach is rarely required and may be more challenging because of the longer distances involved and the higher likelihood of access-related complications. The primary advantages of the up-and-over approach, which is most commonly used, are the following: an aortogram with runoff can be easily converted to endovascular therapy; it permits evaluation of the inflow aortoiliac arteries before treatment of infrainguinal lesions; only a simple retrograde femoral puncture is required; and it facilitates selective catheterization of the superficial femoral artery (SFA) orifice and treatment of proximal SFA lesions, which can be difficult via the ipsilateral antegrade approach. Furthermore, puncture site management is contralateral to the intervention site rather than proximal to it. The antegrade approach may be used for better guidewire and catheter control in infrapopliteal intervention and also in patients who have contraindications to the up-and-over approach. The likely approach is determined before the procedure in order to facilitate room setup and the availability of supplies, but both groins are always prepared in case an alternative approach is required during the procedure.

TransAtlantic Inter-Society Consensus Classification of Femoropopliteal Lesions

TYPE A LESIONS

- Single stenosis <3 cm

TYPE B LESIONS

- Single stenosis 3 to 10 cm long, not involving the distal popliteal artery
- Heavily calcified stenosis up to 3 cm
- Multiple lesions, each <3 cm (stenosis or occlusion)
- Single or multiple lesions in the absence of tibial runoff to improve inflow for distal surgical bypass

TYPE C LESIONS

- Single stenosis or occlusion >5 cm long
- Multiple stenoses or occlusions, each 3 to 5 cm

TYPE D LESIONS

- Occlusion of the common femoral artery, popliteal artery, proximal trifurcation arteries
- Occlusion of the superficial femoral artery >10 cm long

From Schneider PA, Nelken N, Caps MT: Angioplasty and stenting for infrainguinal lesions. In Yao JST, Pearse WH, Matsumura JS, editors: Trends in vascular surgery, Chicago, 2003, Parmentier Publishing, p 292.

TABLE 28-1 **Comparison of Approaches to Infrainguinal Interventions: Up-and-Over versus Antegrade**

	Up-and-Over Approach	Antegrade Approach
Puncture	Simple retrograde femoral	More challenging, less working room
Catheterization	Challenging with tortuous arteries, narrow or diseased aortic bifurcation; easier to catheterize SFA when going up and over femoral	Entering SFA from antegrade approach requires proximal puncture and selective catheter
Guidewire and catheter control	Fair	Excellent
Catheter inventory	More supplies needed	Minimal, shorter catheters
Specialty items	Up-and-over sheath, long balloon catheters	None
Indications	Proximal SFA disease, CFA disease ipsilateral to infrainguinal lesion, obesity	Infrapopliteal disease, patients with contraindication to up-and-over approach

From Schneider PA: The infrainguinal arteries—advice about balloon angioplasty and stent placement. In Endovascular skills, ed 2, New York, 2003, Marcel Dekker, p 316.
CFA, Common femoral artery; *SFA,* superior femoral artery.

Platforms

Percutaneous intervention in the infrainguinal circulation can be achieved with either 0.035-inch or 0.014-inch platforms, using sheath sizes ranging from 4 to 7 French. Most diagnostic angiograms and interventions are begun with a standard 0.035-inch platform. This platform has several advantages: the guidewires and catheters are easy to handle, the inventory is usually readily available, the fluoroscopic visualization of these larger-caliber devices is simpler, and the larger guidewires and catheters are often more helpful than the smaller diameter devices when crossing chronic or heavily calcified occlusions. However, there are also some significant disadvantages of 0.035-inch systems: the larger-caliber guidewires and catheters may not easily cross critically diseased segments and may be more prone to cause arterial damage; at longer distances, these catheters lose their "pushability" because of high friction; and in small arteries such as tibial vessels, the standard platform devices may be too big. In addition to their smaller crossing profiles, the smaller 0.018- and 0.014-inch platforms tend to be more trackable in small, tortuous vessels at distant locations from the access site, especially when using monorail (rapid-exchange) systems with longer guiding sheaths or catheters. Most of the coronary devices are on a 0.014-inch or 0.018-inch platform, as are current atherectomy systems; therefore the array of available balloon catheters and stents is much broader with this system. Monorail balloon catheters permit better pushability because the friction of the guidewire on the balloon catheter lumen occurs over a much shorter distance than with coaxial balloon catheters. Monorail systems have the additional advantages of greater ease of use (especially with a single operator), shorter required guidewire lengths, and less guidewire movement during catheter exchanges.

Sheaths

For initial diagnostic angiography, a 5-French sheath is generally used in conjunction with 5-French diagnostic catheters (Omni-Flush [AngioDynamics, Queensbury, N.Y.] or VCF [Cook Medical, Bloomington, Ind.] catheter for aortography with runoff; Kumpe or Angled Glide [Cook Medical] catheter for selective angiograms). Although angioplasty alone can be performed through 4- or 5-French sheaths, especially when using balloons designed for 0.014- or 0.018-inch platforms, most stents and atherectomy devices require larger sheaths. As a result, most interventionists will change to a larger sheath for intervention once diagnostic angiograms have been performed and the operator has decided to proceed with intervention. It is important to note that with the advent of better percutaneous closure devices, sheath size has become a less important consideration because the larger puncture holes can be closed safely and easily in a percutaneous fashion in most patients, without the need for manual compression.

TABLE 28-2 Supplies for Up-and-Over Approach to Infrainguinal Intervention

Category	Type	Function	Diameter	Length	Other Features
Guidewires	Bentson	Starting	0.035 inch	145 cm	
	Glidewire	Selective, therapy	0.035, 0.018 inch	150, 260 cm	Steerable
	Rosen	Exchange	0.035 inch	180 cm	Sheath placement
	Amplatz	Exchange	0.035 inch	180 cm	Sheath placement
	Ironman	Therapy	0.014 inch	190, 300 cm	
Catheters	Omni-flush	Flush, selective	4 French	65 cm	
	Straight	Flush, exchange	5 French	90 cm	Multi–side hole
Glidecath	Selective, exchange, 4, 5 French	100 cm	Angled tip		
Sheaths	Destination	Guide sheath	5, 6 French	45 cm	Straight
	Rabbe	Guide sheath	6 French	45, 70 cm	Straight
Balloons	Multiple	PTA infrainguinal	0.035, 0.018, 0.014 inch	75, 90, 110 cm OTW	Balloon diameters, 2-6 mm
				Rapid exchange	Balloon lengths, 2, 4, 5, 10 cm
Stents	SMART	Stent SFA, popliteal Self-expanding	0.035 inch	80, 120 cm OTW	Stent diameters, 7-8 mm Stent lengths, 4, 6, 10 cm
	Precise	Stent SFA, popliteal	0.018 inch	120 cm	OTW, Stent diameters, 7-8 mm
		Self-expanding		Rapid exchange	Stent length, 4 cm
	Multiple	Stent tibials	0.014 inch	150 cm	Stent diameters, 2.5-4 mm
		Balloon-expandable		Rapid exchange	Stent length, 2 cm

OTW, Over the wire; *PTA*, percutaneous transluminal angioplasty; *SFA*, superficial femoral artery.

Technique

Up-and-Over Approach

Supplies required for an up-and-over approach are listed in Table 28-2. This approach requires longer guidewires, catheters, and sheaths than the antegrade approach. A standard retrograde common femoral artery puncture is performed contralateral to the symptomatic side. A floppy-tipped guidewire is passed into the aorta. A hook-shaped, multi–side-hole flush catheter, such as a 65-cm Omni-flush (AngioDynamics), is passed into the aorta, and an aortoiliac arteriogram is obtained. If bilateral runoff is required, it can be performed at that time with the catheter head placed in the infrarenal aorta. When only unilateral runoff on the symptomatic side is indicated, the catheter is passed over the aortic bifurcation, and lower extremity arteriography is performed. After evaluating the infrainguinal lesions, determining that the aortic bifurcation can accommodate an access sheath, and deciding that the up-and-over approach is best, an up-and-over sheath is placed (Figure 28-1).

The aortic flush catheter is withdrawn to the aortic bifurcation, and its tip is rotated toward the contralateral side to direct the guidewire into the contralateral iliac artery. The advancing guidewire, usually a steerable, angled-tip Glidewire (Terumo Medical, Tokyo, Japan), must be steered into the external iliac artery and then into the infrainguinal arteries. From this approach, the guidewire usually tends to select the contralateral internal iliac artery if there is tortuosity of the iliac system. The guidewire also tends to select the SFA rather than the deep femoral artery. Either of these destinations for the guidewire is satisfactory from the standpoint of sheath placement, as long as the guidewire is well anchored distal to the groin. The catheter is advanced over the bifurcation, and a stiffer exchange-length (260 cm) guidewire (Stiff

Angled Glidewire [Terumo Medical], Supra-Core Wire [Abbott Vascular, Abbott Park, Ill.] or Rosen Wire [Cook Medical]) is placed. The tip of the exchange guidewire should be distal to the groin as far as it will easily travel. If there is a proximal SFA lesion that is planned for treatment, the guidewire is usually directed into the deep profunda femoris artery. If there is excessive iliac tortuosity, an Amplatz Superstiff guidewire (Cook Medical) may be required.

Dilators are used to enlarge the arteriotomy. Because dilators are sized by their outside diameter and sheaths are sized by their inside diameter, if a 6-French sheath is planned for placement, the tract should be dilated using a 7-French dilator. The guide sheath is placed on the guidewire; when a curved sheath is used, it is oriented such that its curved end is pointing toward the contralateral side and the side arm of the sheath is on the side of the operator. The sheath is advanced over the guidewire using fluoroscopy. Passage over a narrow or diseased aortic bifurcation is performed with care and patience. The sheath is advanced to its hub, if possible. It is important to remember that the tip of the dilator extends beyond the radiopaque marker on the end of the sheath tip for a short distance, and injury to the arteries can occur if this dilator advances beyond the end of the guidewire. The tip of the sheath will generally terminate somewhere between the mid external iliac artery and the very proximal SFA, depending on the height of the patient. Heparin is usually administered (100 U/kg) as the sheath is placed, and an activated clotting time (ACT) is checked (goal ACT > 250 seconds).

Figure 28-2 demonstrates the steps required for infrainguinal intervention using an up-and-over approach. The exchange guidewire is replaced with a steerable 260-cm Glidewire (Terumo Medical). The diseased infrainguinal segment is road-mapped through the side

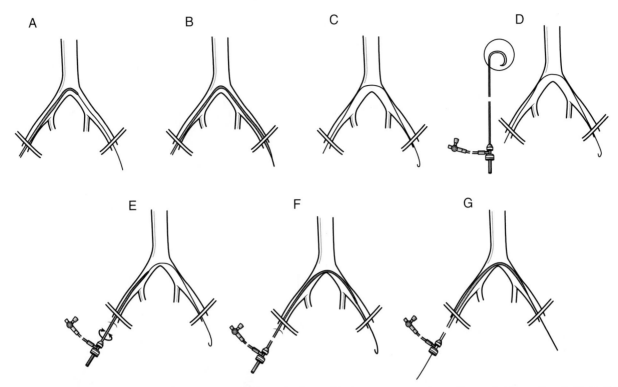

FIGURE 28-1 ■ Placement of an up-and-over sheath. **A,** A guidewire and catheter are passed over the aortic bifurcation. **B,** The catheter is advanced to the contralateral femoral artery. **C,** An exchange guidewire is placed, and the catheter is removed. **D,** The sheath is oriented with its tip pointing toward the contralateral side. **E,** The sheath is advanced over the guidewire. This is visualized using fluoroscopy. **F,** The sheath is advanced to its hub. There must be enough guidewire ahead of the sheath tip to permit a smooth advance. **G,** The dilator is removed, and the sheath is ready to use. (From Schneider PA: The infrainguinal arteries—advice about balloon angioplasty and stent placement. In Endovascular skills, ed 2, New York, 2003, Marcel Dekker, p 195.)

arm of the sheath, and the Glidewire is used to cross the lesion to be treated. Lesion crossing is facilitated by supporting the Glidewire with a hydrophilic catheter, such as a 5-French Angled Glidecath (Cook Medical) or Quick Cross catheter (AngioDynamics). If treatment of tibial lesions is planned, a 5-French, 100-cm-long catheter is advanced into the distal popliteal artery, and road mapping is performed through this catheter. A low-profile guidewire, usually an 0.014-inch hydrophilic wire such as an Asahi Grandslam (Abbott Vascular) is used to cross the tibial lesions, and the 5-French diagnostic catheter is exchanged for a 135-cm–long, 0.014-inch Quick Cross catheter (AngioDynamics) to support the wire. Interval arteriography may be performed through the side arm of the sheath or through the selective catheter using a Tuohy-Borst adapter during attempts at lesion crossing. Once the lesion has been crossed, the supporting catheter is advanced down to the level of the reconstituted artery, the wire is removed to assess for blood return from the catheter lumen, and confirmatory angiography is performed to demonstrate the intraluminal position of the catheter.

Antegrade Approach

Supplies required for an antegrade approach are listed in Table 28-3. An antegrade common femoral artery puncture is performed ipsilateral to the symptomatic side. This approach is well suited to patients who have normal aortoiliac inflow, especially if tibial angioplasty is required or if there is a need to limit the use of contrast material. The puncture should be performed as proximally as possible along the common femoral artery to leave some working room between the puncture and the origin of the SFA. A steerable guidewire, such as the Wholey guidewire (Mallinckrodt, Hazelwood, Md.), is used; the shaft of this guidewire is more supportive for catheter and sheath passage than a Glidewire. The Wholey guidewire can often be steered anteromedially into the SFA. If not, the guidewire is advanced into the deep femoral artery, and an angled-tip catheter is placed over it (Figure 28-3). The image intensifier is placed in the ipsilateral anterior oblique position to open the femoral bifurcation, and the catheter is withdrawn enough to perform road mapping by refluxing contrast material into the SFA. The catheter is used to steer the guidewire into the SFA.

If the lesion is in the proximal to mid SFA, the artery is road mapped using the catheter, and the guidewire is advanced across the lesion (Figure 28-4). The same guidewire can be used for sheath placement. If the lesion is more distal in the artery, the guidewire is advanced without crossing the lesion, and the sheath is placed. The sheath size required may be 4, 5, or 6 French, depending on the platform used and treatment modality desired. An appropriately sized dilator is used to enlarge the arteriotomy before sheath placement.

After the sheath is placed, femoral arteriography is performed through its side arm. Heparin is administered

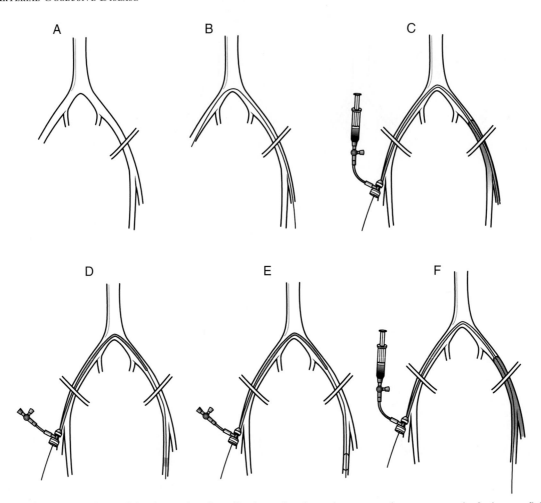

FIGURE 28-2 ■ Balloon angioplasty of the femoral and popliteal arteries through an up-and-over approach. **A,** A superficial femoral artery lesion is identified. **B,** A guidewire is introduced through the contralateral femoral artery and passed over the aortic bifurcation. **C,** An up-and-over sheath is placed, and arteriography is performed. **D,** The guidewire crosses the lesion. **E,** Balloon angioplasty is performed. **F,** Completion arteriography is performed through the sheath. (From Schneider PA: The infrainguinal arteries—advice about balloon angioplasty and stent placement. In Endovascular skills, ed 2, New York, 2003, Marcel Dekker, p 323.)

TABLE 28-3 Supplies for Antegrade Approach to Infrainguinal Intervention

Category	Type	Function	Diameter	Length	Other Features
Guidewires	Wholey	Starting, selective	0.035 inch	145 cm	Steerable
	Glidewire	Selective, therapy	0.035 inch	150, 180 cm	Steerable
	Rosen	Exchange	0.035 inch	180 cm	Sheath placement
	Ironman	Therapy	0.014 inch	190 cm	
Catheters	Kumpe	Selective, exchange	5 French	40 cm	Short, angled tip
Glidecath	Selective, exchange	4, 5 French	70 cm	Angled tip	
	Straight	Flush, exchange	5 French	70 cm	Multi–side hole
Sheaths	Standard	Access, guide	5, 6 French	12-20 cm	Straight
Balloons	Multiple	PTA infrainguinal	0.035, 0.018, 0.014 inch	75, 90 cm	Balloon diameters, 2-6 mm; balloon lengths, 2, 4, 6 cm
Stents	SMART	Stent SFA, popliteal Self-expanding	0.035 inch	80 cm OTW	Stent diameters, 7-8 mm Stent lengths, 4, 6, 10 cm
	Precise	Stent SFA, popliteal Self-expanding	0.018 inch	80 cm OTW Rapid exchange	Stent diameters, 7-8 mm Stent length, 4 cm
	Multiple	Stent tibials Balloon-expandable	0.014 inch	100 cm Rapid exchange	Stent diameters, 2.5-4 mm Stent length, 2 cm

OTW, Over the wire; *PTA,* percutaneous transluminal angioplasty; *SFA,* superficial femoral artery.

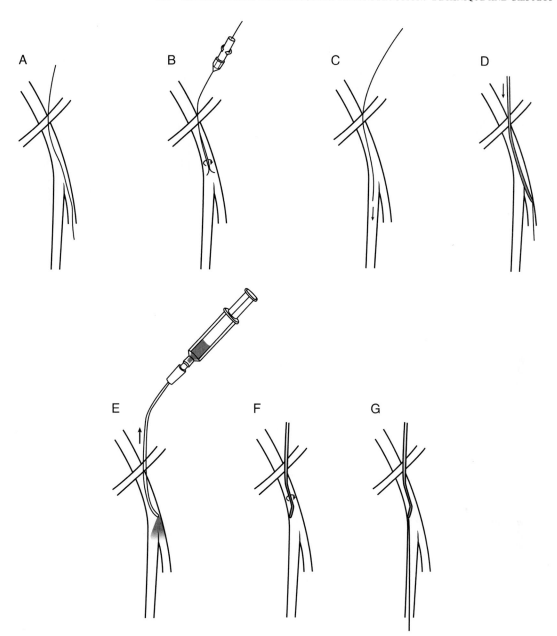

FIGURE 28-3 ■ Catheterization of the superficial femoral artery (SFA) through an ipsilateral antegrade approach. **A,** After antegrade femoral puncture, the guidewire tends to advance into the profunda (deep) femoral artery (PFA). **B,** A Wholey guidewire can be used with a torque device to direct the guidewire into the SFA. **C,** The guidewire tip is rotated anteriorly and medially to enter the SFA. **D,** Another option is to pass an angled-tip catheter into the PFA. **E,** The guidewire is removed, and the catheter is slowly withdrawn while puffing contrast material to demonstrate the femoral bifurcation. **F,** The catheter tip is rotated toward the SFA. **G,** The guidewire is advanced through the catheter into the SFA. (From Schneider PA: The infrainguinal arteries—advice about balloon angioplasty and stent placement. In Endovascular skills, ed 2, New York, 2003, Marcel Dekker, p 109.)

(100 mg/kg) and the ACT is assessed. Standard-length, 180-cm, 0.035-inch guidewires may be used for lesions above the knee. Longer 260-cm, 0.014- or 0.018-inch guidewires are used for infrageniculate intervention, especially in tall patients. As with the contralateral approach, the lesion is then evaluated angiographically, and a steerable guidewire and supportive hydrophilic catheter is used to cross the lesion. Arteriography is repeated after the guidewire is across the lesion to be certain that the guidewire is in the distal artery and not in a perigenicular collateral. The lesion is then treated

with the operator's preferred treatment modality, and the completion arteriography is performed through the sheath while maintaining guidewire control until the results are assessed.

TREATMENT MODALITIES

Approach, sheath placement, and lesion crossing are performed similarly regardless of the ultimate treatment modality that is chosen. Once the lesion has been crossed

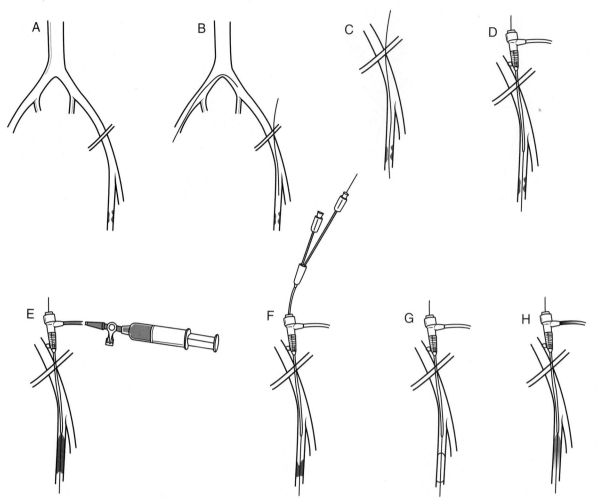

FIGURE 28-4 ■ Balloon angioplasty of the superficial femoral artery (SFA) and popliteal artery through an antegrade approach. **A,** Stenosis of the SFA is suitable for balloon angioplasty. **B,** The lesion may be approached from either the contralateral or the ipsilateral femoral artery. **C,** The guidewire is placed across the stenosis through an antegrade approach. **D,** An access sheath is placed into the proximal SFA. **E,** Arteriography is performed through the side arm of the sheath to evaluate the lesion and confirm guidewire position. **F,** The balloon angioplasty catheter is passed over the guidewire and advanced into the lesion. **G,** Balloon angioplasty is performed. **H,** Completion arteriography is performed. Guidewire position is maintained until the results are assessed. (From Schneider PA: The infrainguinal arteries—advice about balloon angioplasty and stent placement. In Endovascular skills, ed 2, New York, 2003, Marcel Dekker, p 318.)

and confirmation of true-luminal reentry has been ascertained, the operator can choose from an increasing number of percutaneous treatment modalities. Although much of this decision is based on operator preference and comfort level, certain modalities are better suited for specific disease patterns.

Balloon Angioplasty

Balloon angioplasty has been used since the 1980s and has the advantage of being technically simple and quick to perform, thus minimizing contrast usage and radiation exposure. Most superficial femoral and popliteal artery lesions are treated with balloons ranging from 4 to 6 mm in diameter, and a number of vendors provide balloons in lengths up to 200 mm. Tibial arteries range from 1 to 4 mm in diameter, but most are treated with balloons ranging from 2 to 3.5 mm in diameter and up

to 150 mm in length. Increased balloon lengths allow long-segment lesions to be treated faster by minimizing the number of inflations and reducing the number of times a recently treated area is subjected to stagnation of blood flow because of a balloon inflation proximal or distal to it. Most modern angioplasty balloon catheters are relatively noncompliant in nature, thus ensuring that the balloon diameter varies little, even at high-pressure inflations.

Catheter length must be anticipated before selecting the balloon. Most of the standard 0.035-, 0.014-, or 0.018-inch platform balloons are on shafts that are either 75 to 80 cm long or 120 to 150 cm long. A 75-cm balloon catheter shaft passed up and over the bifurcation will reach anywhere from the common femoral artery to the distal SFA, depending on the patient's height. An estimation of the distance to the lesion can be obtained by using a 75-cm–long straight exchange catheter for guidewire exchanges. The up-and-over sheath also provides clues because its length is known.

When performing angioplasty of an infrainguinal lesion, the balloon catheter is passed over the guidewire and into the lesion. The location of the lesion may be marked using road mapping or an external marker. The balloon is then inflated until the waist on the balloon profile is resolved, which generally requires inflations up to 6 to 10 atm. The duration of balloon inflation is anywhere from a few seconds to several minutes. If the waist caused by a lesion fails to resolve even at high inflation pressures, this can sometimes be remedied by exchanging a long balloon for a short (2 cm long) balloon which is then centered directly at the waist and inflated to the balloon's rated burst pressure. Following treatment, the completion arteriogram is obtained through the side arm of the sheath. Balloon angioplasty of the superficial femoral and popliteal arteries almost always produces some evidence of dissection on completion arteriography. In this setting, deciding which patients require a stent may be challenging, though stents are generally used in patients with flow-limiting dissections, large spiral dissections, or residual stenoses or dissections resulting in greater than 30% reduction in flow lumen diameter.

Stent Implantation

Early reports of stent use in the infrainguinal circulation were plagued with poor patency outcomes, mostly because of a high number of stent fractures and subsequent occlusions owing to the use of balloon-expandable stainless steel stents. Most contemporary series of femoropopliteal stent implantation demonstrate improved patency results, likely owing to the use of self-expanding nitinol stents that have increase flexibility and resistance to stent fractures; however, most continue to carry only biliary or tracheobronchial indications and are used in the arterial circulation in an off-label fashion. These stents are highly flexible and can be oversized between 1 and 3 mm larger than the intended artery segment. Self-expanding nitinol stents are available for 0.035-inch platforms ranging in diameter from 4 to 7 mm and lengths of 2 to 150 cm for the femoropopliteal circulation. These stents generally require a 6-French delivery sheath, although lower profile systems using a 0.018-inch platform that can be delivered through a 4-French sheath are increasingly available. The newer nitinol stents foreshorten only minimally and have markers on the ends for better visualization. Stent delivery catheters are either 80 or 120 cm long, based on the length of the balloon catheter required. Self-expanding stents deploy by unfurling from the tip end of the catheter, back toward the hub end. Most stents are deployed with the same mechanism: the pushing rod is held steady while the stent delivery catheter hub is pulled back. This action withdraws the membrane covering the stent, and it deploys (Figure 28-5). The stent is visualized with fluoroscopy. The constrained stent is passed slightly beyond the lesion and pulled back slightly with a fine-tuning adjustment as its tip end begins to open. After the stent is deployed, balloon angioplasty is repeated.

Stents can be used either as a primary modality or selectively following angioplasty as described previously for flow-limiting dissections (with or without contrast trapping in the wall of the artery), spiral dissections, or residual stenosis of the artery lumen greater than 30%. Primary stent placement has been shown in a single randomized trial to result in improved patency rates relative to angioplasty alone, although many continue to use selective stenting preferentially. Primary stent implantation is also used in most cases following recanalization of long-segment occlusions where the likelihood of early rethrombosis is thought to be increased.

Atherectomy

Atherectomy, whether performed by excisional, orbital, or laser atherectomy devices, has the advantage of allowing for plaque debulking with the potential for improved results over angioplasty alone without leaving behind a stent. This advantage has particular importance in specific areas, such as the popliteal or tibial circulation, where stents do not perform particularly well. In addition, atherectomy systems have the ability to treat vessels without changing the options for subsequent open surgical revascularization. The most commonly used atherectomy systems currently available include the SilverHawk and TurboHawk excisional atherectomy systems (eV3, Plymouth, Mass.), the Diamondback 360 orbital atherectomy system (Cardiovascular Systems, St. Paul, Minn.), and the TurboElite excimer laser catheter (Spectranetics, Colorado Springs, Colo.).

The SilverHawk excisional atherectomy system received U.S. Food and Drug Administration (FDA) approval in 2003. This single-use, battery-powered atherectomy catheter allows for directional atherectomy in which the plaque is excised by a rotational cutter and packed into the nose cone of the device. It is compatible with 6- to 7-French sheaths and is used with a 0.014-inch platform in a monorail fashion. Although the original SilverHawk catheters offer treatment ranges from 1.5 7 mm vessel diameter, the newest iterations of the device (the TurboHawk SX-C and LS-M devices) offer improved cutter efficiency and wider vessel diameter treatment ranges, allowing a single catheter to treat vessel diameters of 2 to 4 mm and 3.5 to 7 mm, respectively.

The Diamondback 360 atherectomy catheter received FDA approval in 2007 for the treatment of arterial lesions in the peripheral vasculature. This device consists of a diamond-tipped burr or crown that is positioned eccentrically on a flexible drive shaft of the catheter that runs over a 0.018-inch platform. The drive shaft generates an orbital speed of 80,000 to 200,000 rpm, which allows the crown to sand down plaque into debris that is small enough (2 to 6 µm) to pass through the capillary circulation. This mechanism of action makes this device well suited for tough fibrous lesions or heavily calcified lesions; therefore it has been applied most frequently to infragenicuate lesions.

The TurboElite laser atherectomy system is composed of the catheter and separate generator that creates a xenon laser in the ultraviolet wavelength that vaporizes plaque. Tissue penetration is 10 µm, thus resulting in

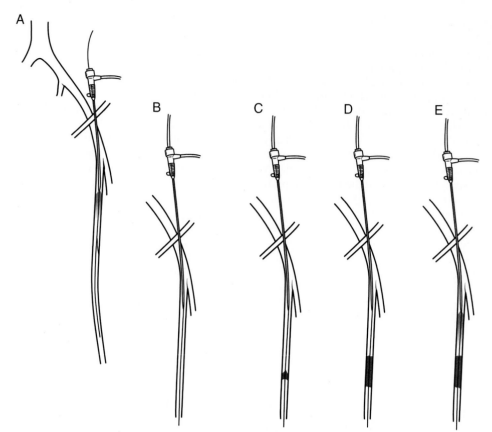

FIGURE 28-5 ■ Stent placement in the superficial femoral artery. **A,** Dissection is present after balloon angioplasty. **B,** A self-expanding stent delivery catheter is placed over the guidewire and advanced into the segment of dissection. **C,** The stent is deployed from the tip end to the hub end of the catheter. **D,** Post-stent balloon angioplasty is performed to bring the stent to its appropriate profile. **E,** Completion arteriography is performed. (From Schneider PA: The infrainguinal arteries—advice about balloon angioplasty and stent placement. In Endovascular skills, ed 2, New York, 2003, Marcel Dekker, p 321.)

minimal temperature change to neighboring tissue. The catheters range in diameters from 0.9 to 2.5 mm, but can be used in conjunction with the TurboBooster catheter, which allows directional orientation of the laser catheter to create a significantly larger lumen than the catheter alone. As a result, lumen diameters can range from 1.5 to 6 mm. The catheters require 0.014- or 0.018-inch platforms and are compatible with 6- to 8-French sheaths, depending on whether the TurboBooster catheter is used.

The steps required for atherectomy in the infrainguinal circulation begin in a similar fashion as for angioplasty and stenting. An appropriately sized up-and-over sheath for the device of choice is placed following diagnostic angiography. Next, the patient is given 100 units/kg of IV heparin for systemic anticoagulation, and the lesion must be crossed. Although the stenosis or occlusion can be crossed with any size guidewire, 0.035-inch wires must then be exchanged for a 0.014- or 0.018-inch wire depending on the system chosen. Atherectomy is then performed, generally with slow and deliberate advances of the catheter to avoid distal embolization. Some clinicians prefer to use distal embolic protection devices during atherectomy, but most systems do not require this and rates of clinically relevant embolization are low in most series. After several passes of the atherectomy catheter, generally in different orientations when using directional catheters, the device is removed and

angiography is repeated. Areas of residual luminal irregularity owing to dissections or residual plaque can be post-dilated with low-pressure balloon angioplasty. Rarely, stent implantation may be necessary after plaque debulking if residual flow-limiting lesions exist. In general, all atherectomy systems are more complex and require somewhat longer procedure times relative to balloon angioplasty and stenting. In addition, increased contrast usage is typical because of the multiple passes required and the repeated angiography needed to assess treatment response. However, benefits of atherectomy include minimization of the barotrauma associated with angioplasty and avoidance of stent implantation in most cases.

Covered-Stent Grafting

The most common mode of failure following percutaneous interventions for the infrainguinal circulation results from restenosis owing to intimal hyperplasia. To combat this process, some clinicians have adopted the placement of covered stent grafts in the superficial femoral artery. This technique prevents ingrowth of intimal hyperplasia and excludes other thrombogenic material on the surface of the treated artery from the arterial lumen. Currently available stents include expanded polytetrafluoroethylene–covered nitinol self-expanding stents (Viabahn [W.L. Gore, Flagstaff, Calif.]

and Fluency [Bard, Murray Hill, N.J.]) and balloon-expandable stainless steel stents (iCast [Atrium Medical Group, Hudson, N.H.] and Jostent [Abbott Vascular]). Of these, the Viabahn endoprosthesis is used most frequently and is available in a range of diameters and lengths appropriate for the superficial femoral artery. Increasingly smaller delivery catheters are available, allowing treatment of most patients with sheaths as small as 6 French. The technique for placement of these stents is similar to that of nitinol stents, although there are additional issues that should be considered to ensure that the risk of stent graft thrombosis and resultant ischemia is minimized. First, as with any surgical bypass, it is important that the patient has adequate inflow and distal tibial runoff. Second, debulking with atherectomy or predilatation with balloon angioplasty, as well as postimplantation angioplasty is important to allow full expansion of the stent graft. In addition, oversizing should be avoided to prevent infolding and kinking of the graft. Finally, while all diseased segments of the artery should be covered, care should be taken to avoid unnecessary coverage of significant collaterals if at all possible, because the coverage of such collaterals can result in acute limb-threatening ischemia if the graft occludes. Antiplatet therapy with aspirin and clopidegrel is important in all percutaneous interventions, but it should be considered mandatory in patients undergoing stent-grafting of the superficial femoral artery.

RESULTS OF PERCUTANEOUS INFRAINGUINAL INTERVENTION

Balloon Angioplasty for Femoropopliteal Lesions

The patency of percutaneous transluminal angioplasty (PTA) of a short femoropopliteal lesion under favorable circumstances is 70% to 80% at 1 year and 50% to 60% at 5 years.[2-12] This type of lesion is ideally suited to PTA. Endovascular intervention is cost effective compared with surgery in this setting and is the treatment of choice.[13] Unfortunately, most situations in which femoropopliteal balloon angioplasty is considered are more

complex and factors are not as favorable. The technique of subintimal angioplasty for long-segment occlusions of the femoropopliteal arteries, which involves the intentional entry into a subintimal dissection plane followed by reentry into the true lumen after the occlusion is crossed, was first described in the late 1980s. Technical success rates with this procedure range from approximately 70% to 90%.[14-18] The major obstacle to technical success is the difficulty in reentering the true lumen distal to the occlusion. Preliminary results using two commercially available systems designed for true lumen reentry are promising and may improve technical success rates.[19,20] In one of the largest studies of long-segment femoropopliteal lesions treated with subintimal recanalization with long-term follow-up, patency rates following technically successful procedures were 71% at 1 year and 58% at 3 years.[17]

Data accumulated over 20 years provide a deeper understanding of femoropopliteal balloon angioplasty across a variety of patient and lesion characteristics. In a summary of studies covering 1241 patients, the results (weighted averages) for femoropopliteal balloon angioplasty were as follows: 90% technical success rate, 4.3% complication rate, 1-year patency of 61%, and 5-year patency of 48%.[1] In a review of several large studies published in the early to mid 1990s, before the broad availability and use of stents, patency rates ranged from 47% to 63% at 1 year and 26% to 48% at 5 years.[2] Multiple factors affect the results of femoropopliteal PTA, including lesion length, clinical stage (claudication vs. limb salvage), runoff, lesion type (stenosis vs. occlusion), proximal location, and lack of residual stenosis after PTA (Tables 28-4 and 28-5).[3-5] Metaanalyses have demonstrated the effect of lesion type and clinical stage (see Table 28-4).[6,7] Lesion length is not addressed in as many studies, and length classifications have not been standardized; however, it appears that length also has a significant effect on results (see Table 28-5).[8-11]

Stent Implantation for Femoropopliteal Lesions

Over the past 5 years, stent placement has become integrated into infrainguinal intervention. This evolution has

---

TABLE 28-4 **Metaanalyses of Femoropopliteal Balloon Angioplasty: Effect of Lesion Type and Clinical Stage**

Reference	No. of Limbs	Lesion Type	Clinical Stage	Primary Patency (%)		
				1 Year	3 Years	5 Years
Hunink and colleagues[6]	4800	Stenosis	Claudication	79	74	68
		Stenosis	Limb threat	62	54	47
		Occlusion	Claudication	52	43	35
		Occlusion	Limb threat	26	18	12
Muradin and colleagues[7]	923	Stenosis	Claudication		61	
		Stenosis	Limb threat		43	
		Occlusion	Claudication		48	
		Occlusion	Limb threat		30	

From Schneider PA, Nelken N, Caps MT: Angioplasty and stenting for infrainguinal lesions. In Yao JST, Pearse WH, Matsumura JS, editors: Trends in vascular surgery, Chicago, 2003, Parmentier Publishing, p 293.

TABLE 28-5 Effect of Lesion Length on Results of Femoropopliteal Balloon Angioplasty

Reference	Lesion Length (cm)	Patency (%)	Follow-Up
Murray and colleagues[8]	<7	81	6 mo
	>7	23	6 mo
Currie and colleagues[9]	<5	59	6 mo
	>5	4	6 mo
Jeans and colleagues[10]	<1	76	5 yr
	>1	50	5 yr
Krepel and colleagues[11]	<2	77	5 yr
	>2	54	5 yr

From Schneider PA, Nelken N, Caps MT: Angioplasty and stenting for infrainguinal lesions. In Yao JST, Pearse WH, Matsumura JS, editors: Trends in vascular surgery, Chicago, 2003, Parmentier Publishing, p 293.

TABLE 28-6 Results of Randomized Trials Comparing Primary versus Selective Stent Placement for Femoropopliteal Occlusive Disease

Author	Year	Patency After Stent Placement (%)		Follow-Up (Yr)
		Primary	Selective	
Vroegindeweij and colleagues[21]	1997	74	85	1
Cejna and colleagues[22]	2001	65	65	2
Grimm and colleagues[23]	2001	62	68	3
Becquemin and colleagues[24]	2003	44	57	4
Schillinger and colleagues[28]	2006	63	37	1

Modified from Schneider PA, Nelken N, Caps MT: Angioplasty and stenting for infrainguinal lesions. In Yao JST, Pearse WH, Matsumura JS, editors: Trends in vascular surgery, Chicago, 2003, Parmentier Publishing, p 293.

been prompted by the development of a variety of simple, low-profile, user-friendly, self-expanding stents that can be easily placed when needed or when the immediate results of PTA are not satisfactory. Earlier studies have shown no patency benefit to primary stent implantation over selective stenting, but these studies focused on the use of rigid stainless steel balloon-expandable stents, which are not well suited for the femoropopliteal circulation (Table 28-6).[21-24] More recent data suggest that modern self-expanding nitinol stents may significantly improve patency results over balloon-expandable stents, as nonrandomized studies have shown 70% to 80% primary patency at 3 years.[25-27] In addition, a randomized trial comparing primary stenting of the superficial femoral artery with self-expanding nitinol stents to selective stenting for residual stenoses or dissections suggested

that primary stenting of all lesions is associated with decreased rates of restenosis and increased ankle-brachial indices compared to selective stenting.[28] In this study of 104 patients with severe claudication or limb-threatening ischemia owing to lesions in the superficial femoral artery, the rate of restenosis on angiography at 6 months was 24% in the stent group and 43% in the angioplasty group ($p = 0.05$); at 12 months the rates on duplex ultrasonography were 37% and 63%, respectively ($p = 0.01$).

Although the merits of primary stent placement continue to be debated, it is clear that selective stent placement has an important role in successful percutaneous intervention. The immediate success of intervention is higher with the availability of stents. Approximately 15% of patients undergoing PTA alone require selective stent placement or experience immediate failure.[22,24] The least favorable results of PTA come from the treatment of long lesions, occlusions, residual stenoses, and limb-threatening ischemia. Stents are an essential tool if endovascular intervention is to be an option in treating these complex lesions and unfavorable clinical situations. A metaanalysis of 423 stent implantations for femoropopliteal occlusive disease demonstrated 66% patency at 3 years, which was not dependent on clinical indication or lesion type.[7] Stents have also yielded promising results with long, chronic occlusions.[29]

Just as self-expanding nitinol stents appear to provide additional benefit over stainless steel stents, advances in stent technology contine to offer promise of improved results. Additional examples of this emerging technology include several spiral-shaped stents that have been developed (aSpire Stent [LeMaitre Vascular, Burlington, Mass.] and IntraCoil Stent [ev3/Covidien, Plymouth, Mass.]) and have high radial strength and flexibility; the ability to accommodate bending, shortening, and elongation; and the capability to preserve potentially important collaterals, which may also have an important role in endovascular infrainguinal revascularization. Despite these potential advantages and the fact that the IntraCoil stent had been the only stent that carried an FDA indication for the superficial femoral artery until recently, these designs did not gain wide clinical use nor support in the medical literature because patency rates with these stents have been similar to balloon angioplasty alone, and ultimately each of these devices have been removed from production by their manufacturers.[30,31] Another new stent design is demonstrated in the Supera Veritas stent (IDEV Technologies, Webster, Tex.), which is composed of six pairs of nitinol wires interwoven in a helical fashion with a closed cell geometry that is delivered through a 7-French sheath (6 French in Europe) over a 0.014- or 0.018-inch platform, with diameters from 4 to 8 mm and lengths up to 120 mm. The interwoven nitinol helix provides the stent with fourfold the radial force and more than threefold the crush resistance of standard self-expanding nitinol stents, and early European data suggest that the stent may perform well in long lesions. Recently presented data on 159 patients who underwent stenting of femoropopliteal arteries and 23 patients who underwent isolated popliteal stenting demonstrated a 74% and 83% 12-month patency rate (by duplex), respectively. Moreover, the average lesion length in the femoropopliteal group was 240 mm, with 40% TASC D classification and 57% total occlusions, suggesting that these patients had long complex lesion anatomy. Finally, subgroup analysis showed no stent fractures at 24 months.[32]

Drug-Eluting Stent Implantation for Femoropopliteal Lesions

Drug-eluting stents have been used extensively in the coronary circulation in recent years and have been shown to result in reduced restenosis after intervention. Currently available balloon-expandable drug-eluting coronary stents include the Taxus stent (Boston Scientific, Natick, Mass.), which is a paclitaxil-coated stent in diameters of 2.25 to 4 mm and lengths of 8 to 38 mm, and the Cypher stent (Cordis; Johnson and Johnson, Miami Lakes, Fla.), which is a sirolimus-coated stent in diameters of 2.25 to 3.5 mm and lengths of 8 to 33 mm. Despite the prolific use of these stents in coronary arteries, the concept of drug-eluting stents in the periphery remains a relatively new area of research and clinical practice. Currently, there are no commercially available drug-eluting stents for the peripheral circulation in the United States, although several clinical trials have evaluated the safety and efficacy of self-expanding drug-eluting stents in the United States and abroad. The first such stent studied in the periphery was a sirolimus-coated SMART stent (Cordis; Johnson and Johnson) which was implanted for superficial femoral artery lesions in claudicants and patients with limb-threatening ischemia in the SIROCCO I and SIROCCO II Trials.[33,34] These randomized trials did not show a statistically significant benefit for the sirolimus-coated stents relative to bare metal stents at 6 months, and at 24 months the restenosis rates were nearly identical. More recently, two studies are underway with drug-eluting stent platforms designed more specifically for use in the femoropopliteal circulation. These studies include the STRIDES registry, a European study of the everlimus-coated DYNALINK-E stent (Abbott Vascular, Brussels, Belgium), and the Zilver PTX Trial, which evaluates the paclitaxel-eluting Zilver (Cook Medical) self-expanding nitonol stent in the superficial femoral artery.[35,36] This latter trial was a multicenter randomized trial in which 479 patients were treated with primary Zilver PTX stent placement, angioplasty alone, or provisional bare metal or Zilver PTX stent placement after failed angioplasty. Two-year follow-up data for 278 patients demonstrated a 50% reduction in restenosis in patients treated with the drug-eluting stent. In the provisional group, 81.2% of the arteries treated with the drug-eluting stents remained patent compared with 62.7% of those treated with bare metal stents alone.[36]

Covered Stent-Grafting of the Femoropopliteal Arteries

Several groups have reported outcomes following the use of these covered stent-grafts in the superficial femoral artery with follow-up periods of up to 4 years.[37-40] The only published data from a randomized trial using covered stent grafts for the treatment of infrainguinal occlusive disease compared percutaneous placement of the Viabahn stent graft (W.L. Gore) with surgical femoral-popliteal (above-knee) bypass with expanded polytetrafluoroethylene and found favorable results for the use of covered stents in this setting.[40] This study randomized 100 limbs (86 patients) to treatment with either Viabahn stents or bypass and followed the patients postoperatively with ankle brachial index and arterial duplex up to a median of 18 months. The two groups had equivalent primary and secondary patency rates at 12 months (74% and 84%, respectively, for the stent graft group and 74% and 84%, respectively, for the bypass group). A continued concern in using covered stent grafts in the femoropopliteal circulation is the risk of acute limb ischemia following occlusion of these grafts. While this problem does occur, the rates of acute ischemia remain relatively low in published studies.

Balloon Angioplasty and Stent Placement for Infrapopliteal Lesions

The patency of infrapopliteal balloon angioplasty is not as well established as that for more proximal lesions. Most of these patients have limb-threatening ischemia, multilevel disease, and multiple or diffuse tibial lesions that require treatment. Results have been assessed most often by evaluating limb salvage rather than patency. A metaanalysis of 1282 treated limbs demonstrated a technical success rate of 93% and a 2-year limb salvage rate of 74%.[41] Stent placement is technically feasible using low-profile, balloon-expandable coronary stents on a 0.014-inch platform. Although this approach may help to salvage an unsuccessful tibial balloon angioplasty, there are insufficient data to determine whether stents are of any significant value in the infrapopliteal arteries.

Balloon Angioplasty for Infrainguinal Bypass Graft Stenosis

The results of balloon angioplasty for failing infrainguinal bypass grafts have been mixed,[42,43] in part because of the nature of lesions caused by myointimal hyperplasia. These lesions are smooth and fibrous and are often not sufficiently remodeled by standard balloon angioplasty; there is a relatively high probability of elastic recoil. Preliminary studies on the use of cutting balloons for infrainguinal bypass graft stenoses have demonstrated promising results.[44,45] Cutting balloons (Flextome Cutting Balloon; Boston Scientific) are available on a 0.014-inch platform and contain three or four longitudinally placed atherotomes designed to create a controlled series of incisions in the lesion, thereby promoting more effective remodeling. Currently, cutting balloon diameters range from 2 to 4 mm and are available in lengths of 6, 10, and 15 mm. Cutting balloon angioplasty is frequently followed by larger standard balloon angioplasty to improve luminal diameter.

Atherectomy for Femoropopliteal and Tibial Lesions

Like most data concerning percutaneous intervention in the infrainguinal circulation, much of the efficacy data available on atherectomy come from nonrandomized registries or retrospective studies. For the SivlerHawk atherectomy system, the multicenter TALON registry provides one of the biggest data sets and examined 6- and 12-month target lesion revascularization rates in 748 limbs in 601 patients.[46] In these cases, atherectomy was the sole modality used in 73%, and stents were used in only 6.3% of lesions, with an overall technical success (less than 50% residual stenosis after atherectomy) rate of 95%. Target lesion revascularization–free survival was 90% and 80% at 6 and 12 months, respectively. Among the largest studies of the use of the SilverHawk system in both femoropopliteal and infrageniculate disease is a recent prospective single-center series that evaluated 579 lesions in 275 patients.[47] Sixty-three percent of patients were treated for critical limb ischemia; lesion distribution included femoropopliteal disease in 53.4%, tibia disease in 37.6%, and multilevel disease in 9.0%. At a mean follow-up of 12.5 months, 18-month primary and secondary patency was 58% and 83%, respectively, for claudicants, and 49% and 70%, respectively, for patients with critical limb ischemia. Limb-salvage at 18-months in patients with critical limb ischemia 92.4%.

Among the most widely cited studies regarding outcome following laser atherectomy with the Spectranetics excimer laser is the Laser Angioplasty for Critical Limb Ischemia trial.[48] This international multicenter trial evaluated the excimer laser in patients who were deemed poor open surgical bypass candidates because of poor bypass targets, lack of available conduit, or presence of severe comorbid illness putting the patient at high-risk for surgical complications. One hundred fifty-five limbs were treated in 145 patients with limb-threatening ischemia. Popliteal or infrageniculate vessels were treated

in more than 50% of the limbs, and mean treatment length per limb was greater than 150 mm. The 6-month limb-salvage rate in this group of patients was 93%, despite their severe degree of disease. In addition to the use of this laser atherectomy device in patients with critical limb ischemia, some have used the Spectranetics laser in claudicants. In the Peripheral Excimer Laser Angioplasty trial, 251 patients with claudication were randomized to either excimer laser–assisted angioplasty or balloon dilation alone. The 12-month patency rates and functional status were found to be similar in both groups.[49]

CONCLUSIONS

Although the results of endovascular intervention for occlusive disease of the iliac arteries are excellent, whether this success can be extrapolated to the infrainguinal arteries remains controversial. It is clear, however, that the lower periprocedural morbidity and rapid recovery associated with endovascular approaches make them attractive to physicians and patients, while also establishing them as an important tool in the vascular surgeon's arsenal in combatting lower extremity arterial occlusive disease. A full-service vascular surgery practice must include a broad variety of both endovascular and surgical options for treating infrainguinal arterial occlusive disease. Infrainguinal endovascular intervention and its growing cadre of associated options have a high likelihood of improving the care of patients with vascular disease in the years to come.

References available online at expertconsult.com.

QUESTIONS

1. Which of the following is an advantage of endovascular intervention over open surgery for infrainguinal arterial occlusive disease?
   a. Less morbidity
   b. Improved patency
   c. Superior durability
   d. All of the above

2. The ipsilateral antegrade femoral approach for infrainguinal intervention is preferred over the contralateral up-and-over approach in which of the following circumstances?
   a. Preprocedural imaging demonstrates absence of iliac inflow disease.
   b. Chronic renal insufficiency
   c. Planned infrapopliteal intervention
   d. All of the above

3. Which of the following is an advantage of the smaller (0.014- or 0.018-inch) platforms over standard (0.035-inch) systems in infrainguinal endovascular intervention?
   a. Smaller crossing profiles
   b. Better fluoroscopic visualization
   c. Improved ability to cross chronic occlusions
   d. All of the above

4. When using smaller platforms, why are monorail (rapid-exchange) catheters preferred over coaxial catheters?
   a. Less friction and improved trackability
   b. Reduced guidewire movement during catheter exchanges
   c. Shorter required guidewire lengths
   d. All of the above

5. Which of the following statements regarding sheath selection for infrainguinal endovascular intervention is true?
   a. Balloon angioplasty requires a sheath sized 6 French or larger.
   b. Stent placement requires a sheath sized 6 French or smaller.
   c. Sheaths are sized according to their outer diameter.
   d. All of the above

6. Which of the following factors is associated with improved outcome in patients undergoing femoropopliteal balloon angioplasty?
   a. Long lesions
   b. Absence of residual stenosis after angioplasty
   c. Poor outflow
   d. All of the above

7. Which of the following statements regarding the use of stents for femoropopliteal disease is true?
   a. All stenotic lesions should be stented primarily.
   b. Balloon-expandable stents are more effective than self-expanding stents.
   c. Postangioplasty dissection with contrast trapping should be stented.
   d. All of the above

8. Major obstacles to technical success with infrainguinal subintimal angioplasty include which of the following?
   a. Entering the subintimal plane from the true lumen above the occlusion
   b. Reentering the true lumen below the occlusion
   c. Perforation
   d. All of the above

9. Endovascular intervention for infrainguinal bypass graft stenoses differs from de novo atherosclerotic lesions in which of the following respects?
   a. Increased incidence of elastic recoil
   b. Increased incidence of dissection
   c. Increased need for stents
   d. All of the above

10. Which of the following statements regarding infrapopliteal balloon angioplasty is true?
    a. Patency rates are well established.
    b. Unsuccessful PTA can be salvaged with balloon-expandable coronary stents.
    c. Contralateral up-and-over approach is preferred over ipsilateral antegrade approach.
    d. All of the above

ANSWERS

1. **a**
2. **d**
3. **a**
4. **d**
5. **b**
6. **b**
7. **c**
8. **b**
9. **a**
10. **b**

CHAPTER 29

ENDOVASCULAR THERAPY FOR INFRAPOPLITEAL ARTERIAL OCCLUSIVE DISEASE

Matthew L. White • Joseph L. Mills, Sr.

Endovascular therapy (EVT) has increasingly become the initial clinical option for treating both claudication and critical limb ischemia (CLI).[1] Similar to the evolution of open bypass surgery, EVT began above the knee and has been progressively extended to the infrapopliteal segment, now even including the pedal and arch vessels. Enthusiasm for infrapopliteal EVT was tempered by poor initial results,[2] but advances in technique, equipment, and patient selection have led to improved outcomes and more widespread EVT application. This chapter discusses standard techniques for infrapopliteal EVT and reviews the contemporary results of tibial angioplasty, stenting, and atherectomy.

PATIENT SELECTION

The revised TransAtlantic Inter-Society Consensus (TASC II) guidelines provide the current consensus recommendations for EVT.[3] TASC II guidelines do not delineate specific anatomic criteria for infrapopliteal disease and do not formally recommend infrapopliteal EVT, whereas previous TASC guidelines included anatomic criteria for infrapopliteal lesions (Table 29-1).[4] TASC II guidelines mention growing evidence to support EVT for infrapopliteal occlusions in patients with comorbidities in whom in-line flow to the foot can be reestablished. In addition, the guidelines also point out that failed angioplasty does not usually preclude subsequent bypass. Graziani and colleagues[5] also proposed a classification system for patients with CLI secondary to multilevel infrainguinal disease (Figure 29-1).[5] Arterial lesions were graded class 1 to class 7, indicating progressive disease severity with decreasing transcutaneous oxygen tension ($TcPO_2$).

The decision to proceed with infrapopliteal EVT is based on many factors gathered from a complete history, physical examination, laboratory studies, noninvasive imaging, and frequently diagnostic angiography. A surgeon must carefully consider the indication (claudication vs. CLI), disease severity, functional status, age and medical comorbidities, availability and quality of an autologous vein conduit, and prior extremity interventions. EVT is preferred in patients with less severe disease, more comorbidities, shorter life expectancy, and absent suitable autologous vein. Open bypass surgery is more strongly considered for younger, healthier patients, especially when a good autologous vein conduit is available.

TECHNIQUE

Infrapopliteal EVT is best performed through the ipsilateral common femoral artery (CFA) using an antegrade approach. The proximal CFA should be accessed to allow working room between the puncture site and superficial femoral artery (SFA). Accessing the contralateral CFA for an up-and-over approach is also possible, but is probably better reserved for treating lesions above the knee. The antegrade approach has distinct advantages: better wire and catheter control and "pushability" using shorter devices, no routine use of a long sheath, and no requisite crossing of the aortoiliac vessels. Both groins should always be prepared in case an alternative approach is required.

Once the ipsilateral CFA has been accessed, a guidewire is manipulated anteromedially to cannulate the SFA. If this is not possible, the wire can be advanced down the profunda femoris artery, and a short, angled-tip catheter is advanced over the wire. Lateral anterior oblique positioning of the image intensifier helps to open the femoral bifurcation. The catheter is withdrawn slowly while puffing contrast until the femoral bifurcation is clearly demonstrated. The catheter tip is steered medially and anteriorly toward the SFA, and the guidewire is advanced into the SFA (see Figure 28-3). The access sheath diameter is typically 5 French, although tibial angioplasty with 0.014- and 0.018-inch platforms can be performed through a 4-French sheath. If an up-and-over approach is used, a long sheath with its tip in the popliteal artery facilitates tibial interventions.

After sheath placement, a diagnostic angiogram is performed through its side port. Lesions above the knee are well delineated in this manner. A short 0.035-inch guidewire is maneuvered into the popliteal artery below the knee, and a 4- or 5-French Glidecath (Medi-Tech, Watertown, Mass.) is advanced to the end of the wire.

Digital subtraction angiography is then used to identify lesions in the trifurcation and distal runoff vessels into the foot. Lateral views of the foot are routinely obtained.

Both transluminal and subintimal approaches can be used for infrapopliteal angioplasty. When choosing a wire for crossing infrapopliteal lesions, several characteristics must be considered, including size (0.035, 0.018, or 0.014 inches), length (180 to 300 cm), coating (bare or hydrophilic), base metal construction (stainless steel, nitinol), stiffness, weight and tip construction (stiffness, length, coating, shape). Smaller caliber wires (0.014 or 0.018 inches) with a hydrophilic coating and floppy tip are often used to cross tibial lesions. The preferred wires are 0.014-inch, nonhydrophilic, medium-weight with short floppy tips for crossing tibial stenoses. Occlusions, particularly when calcified and long, are more difficult to cross. The

V18 wire (Boston Scientific, Natick, Mass.) is particularly useful for crossing tibial occlusions.

If difficulty arises when attempting to cross stenotic lesions or occlusions with a particular wire, several additional maneuvers are available to facilitate success. Particularly hard or calcified plaque can cause 0.014- and 0.018-inch wires to coil, especially if they have floppy tips. Upsizing to a 0.035-inch wire may give the additional support needed to navigate across the difficult lesion. Another option is the use of a catheter, such as the hydrophilic Glidecath, which can be advanced to the end of the wire and lend additional support. Crossing catheters, such as the Quick-Cross (Spectranetics, Colorado Springs, Colo.), feature a firmer, tapered tip, which facilitates lesion crossing. Predilation with a small, 2- to 2.5-mm–diameter coronary balloon may fracture a particularly difficult lesion and subsequently allow passage of a wire or low-profile crossing catheter. Guidewires with dilatable tips are also available for this technique. Devices specifically designed for crossing a chronic total occlusion (CTO) are a more recent development. These devices use different strategies to facilitate lesion crossing, including plaque microdissection (Frontrunner XP CTO Catheter; Cordis, Bridgewater, N.J.), fast and bidirectional catheter spinning (Cross-Boss CTO Catheter; BridgePoint Medical, Plymouth, Minn.), and catheter tip deflection capability with spiral wedges to facilitate advancement (Wildcat Catheter; Avinger, Redwood City, Calif.).

Subintimal angioplasty is a useful technique first described by Bolia and coworkers[6] in 1989 for the treatment of long-segment femoropopliteal occlusions.[6] This technique may also be successfully applied to infrapopliteal lesions as well (Figure 29-2, see color insert). A wire is used to intentionally create a subintimal dissection plane just proximal to an occlusion. The wire is typically formed into a short J shape and is advanced in the subintimal plane until the occlusion has been passed. If reentry into the true lumen is difficult, it may be facilitated by a special reentry device, such as the Outback

Classification	Lesions Characteristics
TASC A	Single stenosis <1 cm long in tibial or peroneal vessels
TASC B	Multiple focal stenoses of tibial or peroneal vessels <1 cm long
	One or two stenoses <1 cm long involving the trifurcation
	Short tibial or peroneal stenosis with femoropopliteal PTA
TASC C	Stenoses 1 to 4 cm long in tibial or peroneal vessels
	Occlusions 1 to 2 cm long in tibial or peroneal vessels
	Extensive stenosis of the trifurcation
TASC D	Occlusion >2 cm long in tibial or peroneal vessels
	Diffusely diseased tibial or peroneal vessels

TABLE 29-1 TASC I Classification of Infrapopliteal Lesions

PTA, Percutaneous transluminal angioplasty.

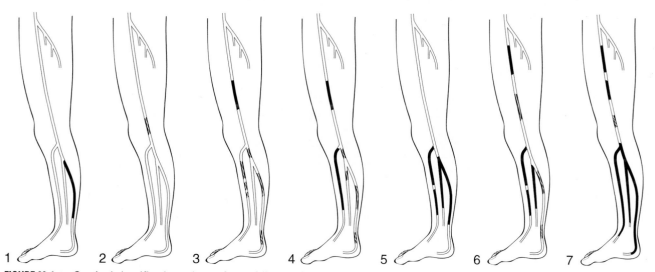

FIGURE 29-1 ■ Graziani classification scheme for multilevel infrainguinal disease. (From Graziani L, Silvestro A, Bertone V, et al: Vascular involvement in diabetic subjects with ischemic foot ulcer: a new morphologic categorization of disease severity. Eur J Vasc Endovasc Surg 33:453–460, 2007.)

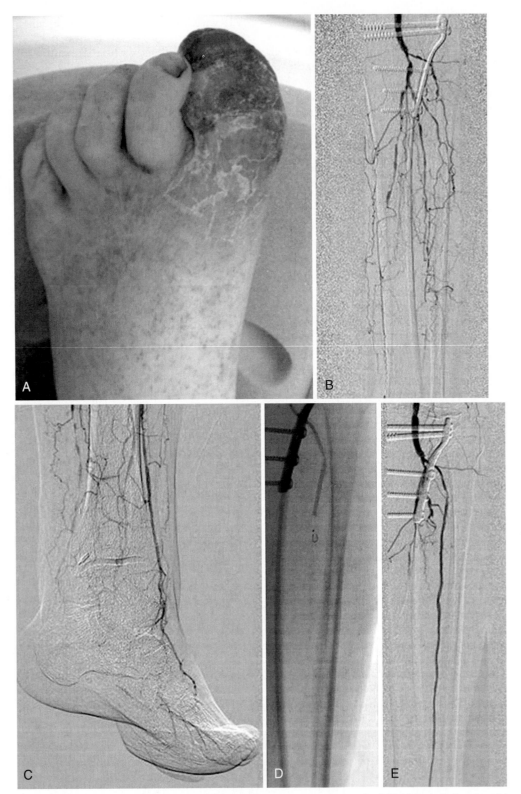

FIGURE 29-2 ■ A 77-year-old high-risk patient with diabetes and great toe gangrene. **A,** Critical limb ischemia with ankle-brachial index (ABI) of 0.39. **B,** Three-vessel long-segment (>25 cm) tibial artery occlusions, with **(C)** distal anterior tibial artery reconstitution. **D,** Subintimal angioplasty of long-segment occlusion. **E,** Anterior tibial artery after long-segment subintimal angioplasty with ABI improved to 0.81. Toe amputation healed and the vessel remains patent 6 months after intervention. See Color Plate 29-2.

LTD catheter (Cordis) or Pioneer catheter (Medtronic, Minneapolis, Minn.).

Once a stenosis or occlusion has been crossed successfully, balloon angioplasty is possible (Figure 29-3, see color insert). Balloon angioplasty stretches the arterial wall causing plaque fracture and sometimes local dissection, which is usually not flow limiting. Treating long-segment tibial lesions with longer balloons is a useful technique, but some short, focal lesions require a shorter balloon with more directed dilation force. A cutting balloon (Boston Scientific), which features three to four microsurgical blades fixed longitudinally along the outer surface of a noncompliant balloon, is particularly useful for the intimal hyperplasia near graft anastomoses. Creating controlled cuts in the intima theoretically allows less vessel wall disruption, less neutrophil activation, and more controlled balloon dilation.[7] Drug-coated balloons are another emerging technology.[8]

Stenting in the infrapopliteal segment has traditionally been reserved for obviating emergency surgery because of poor angioplasty results, such as a flow-limiting dissection. More recently, drug-eluting stents have been used for the treatment of infrapopliteal disease, with encouraging results.[9] Other infrapopliteal maneuvers, such as atherectomy and cryotherapy, may add more cost than real benefit compared to angioplasty alone.[10]

RESULTS

The outcome of infrapopliteal EVT depends on many factors, including indication for the procedure, lesion characteristics, runoff status, comorbidities, and technical factors, such as dissection or persistent stenosis (Table 29-2). Poorer outcomes appear to be predicted by the following factors: CLI versus claudication,[11] longer lesion length,[12-14] poor runoff status,[11,12,15] comorbidities of diabetes[16,17] and renal failure,[11,18] smoking,[17] and untreated intraprocedure flow-limiting dissection and persistent stenosis greater than 30%.

Angioplasty

Giles and associates[12] retrospectively reviewed 163 consecutive patients (176 limbs) who underwent infrapopliteal EVT for CLI; 102 patients (58%) also had concomitant femoropopliteal angioplasty or stenting, or both[12]; and 97 lesions (55%) were TASC C or D. Subintimal angioplasty was performed only for complete occlusions that could not be crossed transluminally. The technical success rate was 93%, and 1- and 2-year primary patency rates were 53% and 51%, respectively. The 3-year limb salvage was 84%. On multivariate analysis, predictors of restenosis were TASC D lesions and lack of a bypass target, whereas multilevel intervention was protective. Sadek and colleagues[19] retrospectively reviewed 85 patients (89 limbs) who underwent either single-level tibial (29 limbs) or multilevel (60 limbs) interventions. Overall, 77% of patients had CLI. The technical success rate was 91%, and 12- and 18-month primary patency rates were 34% and 27%, respectively, in the single-level interventions and 58% and 48%, respectively, in the

multilevel interventions. The 12- and 18-month limb salvage rates were 75% and 67%, respectively, in the single-level interventions and 84% and 63%, respectively, in the multilevel interventions. The difference of primary patency and limb salvage between the two groups did not reach statistical significance. Peregrin and associates[15] retrospectively reviewed 1268 patients (1445 limbs) who underwent infrapopliteal angioplasty for CLI. Almost all lesions were classified as TASC D. The technical success rate was 89%, and the primary and secondary limb salvage rates at 1 year were 76% and 84%, respectively. Interestingly, the number of patent infrapopliteal arteries at the end of angioplasty significantly correlated with 1-year limb salvage rates. As the number of patent crural arteries increased from 0 to 3, the 1-year limb salvage rate increased from 56% to 83%. Conrad and colleagues[11] retrospectively reviewed 144 patients (155 limbs) who underwent infrapopliteal angioplasty; 133 limbs (86%) were treated for CLI, and 116 limbs (75%) had TASC C or D lesions. The technical success rate was 95%, and the 24- and 40-month primary patency rates were 71% and 62%, respectively. Multivariate analysis showed poor runoff, CLI, and dialysis as negative predictors of patency. The 40-month limb salvage rate was 86%; negative predictors of limb salvage included dialysis and failure to improve runoff.

Data are also available regarding angioplasty for long-segment infrapopliteal disease. Schmidt and coworkers[20] studied 58 patients (62 limbs) with CLI who underwent infrapopliteal angioplasty for lesions 8 cm or greater in length.[20] The technical success rate, defined by restoration of flow in at least one infrapopliteal vessel, was 95%. At short-term follow-up of 3 months, angiography demonstrated restenosis less than 50% in 31% of treated arteries, restenosis greater than 50% in 31%, and occlusion in 38%. Clinical improvement (wound healing or improvement of rest pain) was present in 76% of treated limbs. All arteries with restenosis greater than 50% or occlusion were retreated. At 15 months, 77% of limbs showed further clinical improvement, and the limb salvage rate was 100% without bypass.

Subintimal Angioplasty

Groups have also published specifically regarding subintimal angioplasty. Tartari and colleagues[21] reported on 117 subintimal angioplasty procedures for complete occlusions, 82 (15 TASC C and 67 TASC D) of which were infrapopliteal. Technical success, defined as recanalization of at least one tibial vessel with adequate flow to the foot, was possible in 83% of cases. At a mean follow-up of 13.5 months, 12.5% of this cohort underwent major amputation and 11.3% underwent surgical bypass. Vraux and coworkers[13] reviewed 46 patients (50 limbs) with CLI and tibial occlusions. Technical success was possible in 82% of cases. Primary patency was 46% at 12 months and 42% at 24 months. Limb salvage was 87% at 12 and 24 months. Longer lesion length and the need to extend treatment to the popliteal artery were associated with lower clinical patency rates. Ingle and colleagues[22] retrospectively reviewed 67 consecutive patients (70 limbs) who underwent infrapopliteal angioplasty for occlusive

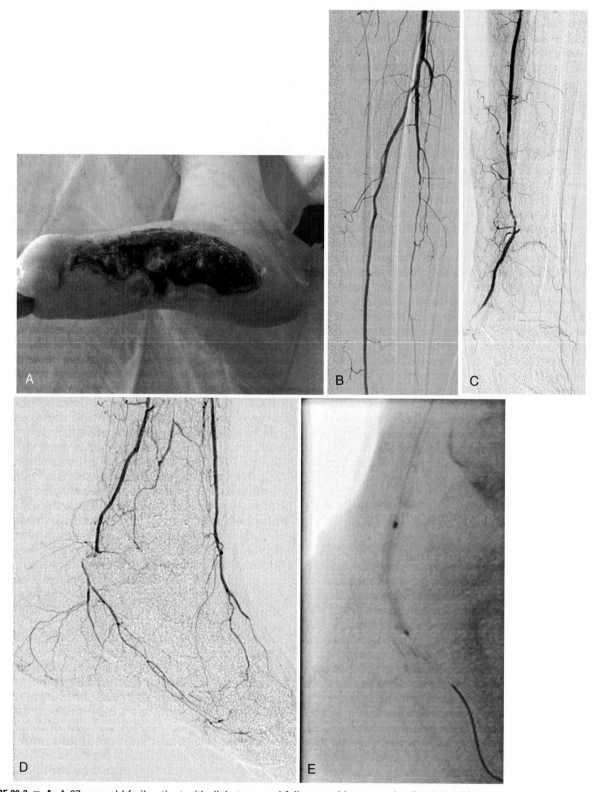

FIGURE 29-3 ■ **A,** A 67-year-old frail patient with diabetes; renal failure; and large, nonhealing lateral foot wound and ankle-brachial index (ABI) of 0.71 after angioplasty of the superficial femoral artery owing to long-segment tibial disease. **B,** Angiogram with catheter placed in popliteal artery shows patent posterior tibial artery proximally. **C,** Multiple distal posterior tibial artery stenoses. **D,** Calcified, total inframalleolar posterior tibial artery occlusion and severe angulation. **E,** 2 mm × 2 cm balloon angioplasty of tibial occlusion.

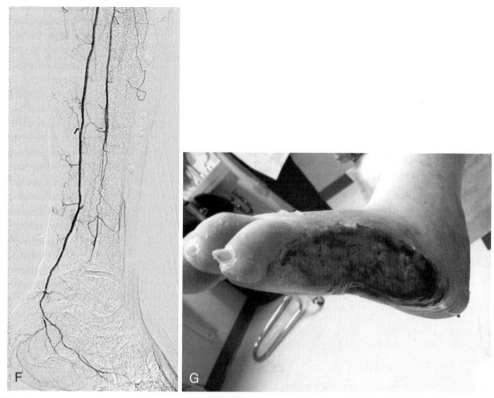

FIGURE 29-3, cont'd ■ **F,** Posterior tibial artery with continuous flow into the foot after 2.5 mm angioplasty of the distal posterior tibial artery and 2 mm angioplasty of the inframalleolar posterior tibial occlusion. **G,** ABI improved to 1.01 with good wound granulation after repeated debridement. See Color Plate 29-3.

lesions; 61 patients (91%) had CLI. The technical success rate was 86% and the limb salvage rate at 3 years by Kaplan-Meier life-table analysis was 94%.

Cutting Balloon Angioplasty

Data from cutting balloon angioplasty are also available. Vikram and associates[23] compared conventional and cutting balloon angioplasty in 36 patients with failing infrainguinal vein grafts. Short-term primary patency seemed to be better in the cutting balloon cohort; however, primary patency for angioplasty at 1 year was not significantly different between the two groups. Engelke and colleagues[24] treated 16 anastomotic stenoses after infrainguinal bypass. Cutting balloon angioplasty was successful in 15 lesions (94%), including 6 lesions that were resistant to conventional angioplasty; there were no perforations. The primary lesion patency at 12 months was 76%. Ansel and coworkers[25] reviewed their treatment of 73 patients (93 vessels) with cutting balloon angioplasty, 52 (71%) of whom had CLI. Most vessels treated (71%) were infrapopliteal. Technical success was possible in 81%, with all failures being successfully stented. There were no perforations. At 1-year follow-up, the limb salvage rate was 89%.

Drug-Coated Balloon Angioplasty

Although infrapopliteal data are lacking on drug-coated balloons, Tepe and colleagues[8] compared conventional and paclitaxel-coated balloon angioplasty of the femoropopliteal segment in 102 patients. There was a significantly decreased restenosis rate at 6 months in lesions treated with the paclitaxel-coated balloons (17% vs. 44%).[8] In addition, target lesion revascularization at 2 years was significantly reduced in the paclitaxel-coated balloon cohort (15% vs. 52%). These results provide encouragement for extension of this technology to the infrapopliteal segment.

Stenting

Bosiers and colleagues[26] prospectively collected data on 443 patients (681 lesions) who underwent infrapopliteal EVT for CLI. Patients were allocated to PTA plus stenting (300 patients), PTA alone (79 patients), or excimer laser atherectomy (64 patients). Mean lesion length was not specifically reported, but 21% of treated lesions were occlusive. Laser atherectomy was generally used for single, long lesions. At 1-year follow-up, primary patency rates for PTA, PTA plus stenting, and laser atherectomy were 68.6%, 75.5%, and 75.4%, respectively. Limb salvage rates at 1 year for PTA, PTA plus stenting, and laser atherectomy were 96.7%, 98.6%, and 87.9%, respectively. Randon and colleagues[27] enrolled 35 patients (38 limbs) with CLI for randomization to angioplasty (22 limbs) or primary stenting (16 limbs); 64% of treated lesions were occlusive, with most occlusions greater than 2 cm in length. At 1-year follow-up, there was no difference between angioplasty and stenting in regard to

TABLE 29-2	**Results of Infrapopliteal Angioplasty, Stenting, and Atherectomy**						
Author	**Year**	**Number Treated**	**CLI**	**Mean Lesion Length**	**Technical Failures**	**Primary Patency**	**Limb Salvage Rate**
Angioplasty							
Giles and colleagues[12]	2008	176	100%	NR	7%	53%, 1 yr 51%, 2 yr	84%, 3 yr
Conrad and colleagues[11]	2009	155	86%	NR	5%	71%, 2 yr 62%, 3.3 yr	86%, 3.3 yr
Sadek and colleagues[19] (Single vs. multilevel PTA)	2009	89	77%	NR	9%	34%, 1 yr Single level 58%, 1 yr Multilevel	67%, 1.5 yr Single level 63%, 1.5 yr Multilevel
Peregrin and colleagues[15]	2010	1445	100%	NR	11%	NR	76%, 1 yr
Schmidt and colleagues[20]	2010	62	100%	18.3 cm	5%	50%, 3 mo	100%, 15 mo
Subintimal Angioplasty							
Ingle and colleagues[22]	2002	70	91%	NR	14%	NR	94%, 3 yr
Vraux and Bertoncello[13]	2006	50	100%	78% >10 cm	18%	46%, 1 yr 42%, 2 yr	87%, 1 yr 87%, 2 yr
Tartari and colleagues[21] (SFA only in 27 limbs)	2007	109	100%	59% ≥10 cm	17%	NR	87%, 1 yr 85%, 2 yr
Cutting-Balloon Angioplasty							
Engelke and colleagues[24]	2002	16	31%	NR	6%	67%, 1 yr	93%, 10 mo
Ansel and colleagues[25]	2004	73	71%	2.7 cm	0%	NR	89%, 1 yr
Vikram and colleagues[23]	2007	11	NR	NR	18%	50%, 1 yr	NR
Drug-Coated Balloon*							
Tepe and colleagues[8]	2008	48	15%	7.5 cm	2% All cases	80%, 6 mo	96%, 6 mo
Stenting							
Feiring and colleagues[28]	2004	92	68%	NR	7%	NR	87%, 1 yr
Bosiers and colleagues[26]	2006	300	100%	NR	NR	76%, 1 yr	99%, 1 yr
Donas and colleagues[29]	2009	34	100%	6.5 cm stenosis; 7.5 cm occlusion	3%	91%, 10 mo	100%, 10 mo
Randon and colleagues[27]	2010	16	100%	38% ≥10 cm	13%	56%, 1 yr	92%, 1 yr
Drug-Eluting Stent							
Scheinert and colleagues[9]	2006	30	63%	NR	0%	100%, 6 mo	100%, 9 mo
Feiring and colleagues[32]	2010	130	100%	NR	9%	NR	88%, 3 yr
Karnabatidis and colleagues[17]	2011	51	100%	7.7 cm	0%	30%, 3 yr	NR
Rastan and colleagues[30]	2011	82	51%	3.0 cm	0%	81%, 1 yr	98%, 1 yr
Atherectomy							
Zeller and colleagues[14]	2007	36	53%	4.6 cm	2%	67%, 1 yr 60%, 2 yr	100%, 2 yr
Safian and colleagues[33]	2009	124	32%	3.0 cm	2.5%	NR	100%, 6 mo

CLI, Critical limb ischemia; *NR*, not reported; *PTA*, percutaneous transluminal angioplasty.
*Femoropopliteal.

primary patency (66% vs. 56%), limb salvage (90% vs. 92%), or survival (69% vs. 74%). The only significant difference between the cohorts was an increased need for redo angioplasty in the PTA group after 6 months (3 vs. 0 in the stenting group). Feiring and colleagues[28] reviewed their experience treating 82 patients with infrapopliteal lesions; six occlusions were not able to be crossed, leaving 76 patients (86 limbs) treated with infrapopliteal stents. CLI was the indication for stenting in 68% of patients. A total of 197 stents were deployed in the study, which were an assortment of balloon expandable and self-expanding coronary stents. At 1-month follow-up, CLI patients had a significantly improved mean ankle-brachial index (ABI;

0.32 to 0.9). Between 6 and 12 months of follow-up, two patients developed in-stent restenosis, which was successfully treated. At 1-year follow-up, the limb-salvage rate for CLI patients was 96%; however, expressed on an intention-to-treat basis, the 1-year limb salvage rate was 87%. Donas and coworkers[29] treated 34 CLI patients with infrapopliteal stenting. Indications for stenting were long-segment stenoses or occlusions, or flow-limiting dissection or elastic recoil after PTA. Immediate (12 to 24 hours) improvement in ABI was realized (0.45 to 0.92), which was partially sustained at 6 months (0.77). The 6-month limb-salvage rate was 100%, and primary patency was 91% at a mean follow-up of 10.4 months.

Drug-Eluting Stents

Scheinert and colleagues[9] studied 60 consecutive patients with infrapopliteal obstructions treated with a bare-metal stent (BMS) or sirolimus-eluting stent (SES).[9] At 6 months follow-up, the SES cohort had a significantly lower mean degree of in-stent restenosis (1.8% vs. 53.0%). Likewise, Rastan and colleagues[30] conducted a randomized, double-blinded, multicenter study of 161 patients with infrapopliteal disease who received either a BMS (79 points) or SES (82 points). The 1-year primary patency rate was significantly higher in the SES cohort (80.6% vs. 55.6%). In addition, the median change in the Rutherford classification[31] was –2 in the DES cohort compared with –1 in the BMS cohort. Karnabatidis and colleagues[17] prospectively studied 81 patients with CLI and long segment (>4.5 cm) infrapopliteal lesions treated with either a BMS (34 points) or everolimus-eluting stent (47 points). At 3-year follow-up, the everolimus-eluting stent cohort had a significantly higher primary patency rate (30% vs. 21%). Regression analysis revealed that smoking and diabetes were significant predictors for increased restenosis and reduced patency. Feiring and colleagues[32] prospectively enrolled 118 patients (130 limbs) with CLI for treatment with at least one infrapopliteal drug-eluting stent (DES). A total of 228 stents were deployed in the study, and 35% of patients received overlapping stents. On an intention-to-treat basis, the 3-year limb salvage rate was 88%.

Atherectomy

Data on infrapopliteal atherectomy are lacking, but Zeller and associates[14] studied infrapopliteal directional atherectomy with the SilverHawk device (FoxHollow Technologies, Redwood City, Calif.) on 36 patients (49 lesions). CLI was the indication for intervention in 19 (53%) patients. The mean lesion length was 46 mm, and the mean percent diameter stenosis was 89%; there were 11 (22%) occlusions. Predilation was performed in 16 (33%) lesions, and following atherectomy, 19 lesions (38%) were treated with additional balloon angioplasty. After atherectomy, there was an immediate increase in mean ABI (0.48 to 0.81), which was partially sustained at 1-year follow-up (0.72). Primary patency was 67% at 1 year and 60% at 2 years. Lesions with a length of 50 mm or greater had a significantly higher restenosis rate (44% vs. 26%). Safian and colleagues[33] studied 124 patients (201 stenoses) in a nonrandomized, prospective fashion. They used the Diamondback 360° Orbital Atherectomy System (Cardiovascular Systems, St. Paul, Minn.) to perform infrapopliteal atherectomy; CLI was the indication to intervene in 40 (32%) patients. The mean lesion length was 30 mm, and the mean percent diameter stenosis was 87%. Following atherectomy, adjunctive angioplasty was performed in 79 (39%) lesions. At 6-month follow-up, there was an increase in mean ABI (0.68 to 0.82), and 78% of patients had improvement in chronic limb ischemia based on the Rutherford-Becker ordinal scale.

POSTPROCEDURAL MANAGEMENT

Following EVT, patients should be maintained on their preprocedure medical regimens for control of hypertension, CHF, angina, and arrhythmia. Diligent fluid management is especially important in patients with CHF, who may become easily volume overloaded. Beta blockade should be continued if there are no contraindications; in this same moderate and high-risk population, targeted heart rate control has been shown to reduce cardiac complications and improve mortality after open vascular operations.[34,35] Metformin, a commonly prescribed antihyperglycemic drug, should be withheld around the time of contrast administration because of the possibility of lactic acidosis with worsening renal function.[36] For patients with normal renal function, metformin should be withheld immediately before contrast administration and for 48 hours after the study. For patients with renal dysfunction, metformin should be withheld 48 hours before and 48 hours after contrast administration. In both cases, metformin should only be restarted in the absence of an acute decline in renal function.

ANTIPLATELET THERAPY

Patients with claudication or CLI are usually already taking aspirin (81 or 325 mg daily). Aspirin has well-established cardiac and cerebral protective effects and may improve patency after PTA and stenting.[37-39] Aspirin has a rapid onset of action, within minutes, with a peak action of less than 30 minutes; it produces approximately 20% platelet inhibition, lasts 5 to 7 days, and is the most cost-effective antiplatelet therapy.[40] Clopidogrel is another antiplatelet option,[41] which can be added to aspirin to provide up to 40% platelet inhibition. It takes 5 days to reach peak activity, which can be reduced to hours with a loading dose of 300 mg.[42] Clopidogrel is significantly more expensive than aspirin and may have an increased risk of complications compared with aspirin alone.

CONCLUSIONS

A growing body of evidence supports the use of infrapopliteal EVT for CLI. Advances in technique, technology, and patient selection have fostered short-term results similar to bypass. Infrapopliteal EVT for CLI maximally benefits older, higher-risk patients with shorter life expectancies who do not require the durability of a bypass, but rather the shorter-term augmentation in blood flow to heal a wound or resolve ischemic rest pain. Newer technologies, such as drug-coated balloons, drug-eluting stents, and atherectomy, have shown promise for infrapopliteal application and may further increase the ability to successfully treat CLI in an endovascular fashion.

References available online at expertconsult.com.

QUESTIONS

1. Which of the following projections of the left common femoral artery usually best delineates the origin of the left deep femoral artery?
   a. Straight AP
   b. LAO
   c. RAO
   d. 30 degree craniocaudal
   e. True lateral

2. Antegrade femoral access would be of greatest utility when performing endovascular therapy for which of the following lesions?
   a. Proximal common femoral to posterior tibial bypass graft stenosis
   b. SFA origin stenosis
   c. PFA stenosis
   d. Aorto-bifemoral graft limb stenosis
   e. Below-knee popliteal artery stenosis

3. Which of the following best describes a TASC (I) C infrapopliteal artery lesion?
   a. Multiple < 1 cm long focal posterior tibial artery stenosis
   b. 1.5 cm long mid peroneal artery occlusion
   c. 4 cm long anterior tibial artery occlusion
   d. Two < 1 cm long stenoses in the tibioperoneal trunk
   e. Solitary tibial stenosis < 1 cm in length

4. Poorer outcomes of infrainguinal angioplasty are associated with all of the following *except:*
   a. Poor runoff
   b. Diabetes mellitus
   c. End stage renal disease
   d. Claudication
   e. Residual stenosis > 30%

5. Which of the following statements about tibial angioplasty is most correct?
   a. Initial technical success rates are less than 80% in most series.
   b. One-year patency rates are generally poor (<50%).
   c. Limb salvage rates in patients with critical limb ischemia are < 75% at one year.
   d. Runoff does not have a major impact on patency.
   e. Cutting balloon angioplasty patency rates are better at one-year compared to angioplasty with standard balloons.

6. All of the following are advantages of the antegrade approach for infrapopliteal angioplasty *except:*
   a. Wire pushability
   b. Avoidance of iliac artery disease and tortuosity
   c. Catheter control
   d. Ease of access in obese patient
   e. Sheath passage

7. Based on most published data, improved results following tibial angioplasty are most strongly suggested for which one of the following therapies or adjuncts?
   a. Cutting balloon angioplasty
   b. Atherectomy
   c. Subintimal angioplasty
   d. Bare metal stents
   e. Drug-eluting stents

ANSWERS

1. **b**
2. **e**
3. **b**
4. **d**
5. **b**
6. **d**
7. **e**

CHAPTER 30

THORACIC AND LUMBAR SYMPATHECTOMY: INDICATIONS, TECHNIQUE, AND RESULTS

Peter Gloviczki

Minimally invasive endoscopic technology has rapidly transformed both thoracic and abdominal surgery and the field of surgical sympathectomies was no exception. For thoracic sympathectomy, the thoracoscopic procedure is used almost exclusively.[1-3] Laparoscopic[4] and retroperitoneoscopic techniques[5,6] have also been developed for ablation of the lumbar sympathetic chain. Because of its relatively less invasive nature, the open technique for lumbar sympathectomy is still performed, but with rapidly decreasing frequency.[7,8] Indications for both thoracic and lumbar sympathectomies have changed during the past decades. Earlier indications such as claudication, uncomplicated primary Raynaud syndrome, or scleroderma are not used.[9] Refractory palmar and plantar hyperhidrosis, chronic pain syndrome, Buerger disease, frostbite, and complicated primary Raynaud syndrome and secondary Raynaud phenomenon with nonhealing digital ulcerations have become the most common indications for endoscopic sympathectomy.[2,8,10]

HISTORICAL BACKGROUND

Although Jabouley suggested sympathetic denervation for vasospastic disorders as early as 1899, periarterial sympathectomy was introduced by Leriche only in 1913 for ischemic lesions caused by vasospasm.[11] The first lumbar sympathectomy was performed by Royle in 1923 to treat a patient with spastic paralysis of the lower limb.[12] The concept of sympathectomy was soon adopted by Adson and Brown,[13] who performed lumbar sympathectomy to relieve vasospasm of the lower extremities. Adson and Brown[14] were the first to perform cervicothoracic sympathectomy in 1929.

Using the single-scope technique, thoracoscopic sympathectomy was popularized by Kux[15] in Austria as early as 1954. With the advent of endoscopic surgery, both thoracoscopic[1-3] and laparoscopic or retroperitoneoscopic procedures[5,6] have been developed for sympathetic denervation.

ANATOMY AND PHYSIOLOGY

The peripheral nervous system includes both somatic and autonomic components. The somatic efferent motor nerves control the voluntary striate muscles, and the afferent nerves transmit somatosensory information to the brain. The autonomic nervous system transmits information from the abdominal viscera and from the smooth and cardiac muscles and the exocrine glands. Autonomic nerves are composed of the sympathetic and parasympathetic nervous systems.

Anatomy

The sympathetic nervous system consists of the central autonomic network, which includes the brainstem, diencephalons, and cortex, and of the peripheral sympathetic pathways. The peripheral sympathetic pathway consists of preganglionic and postganglionic neurons. Information from the brainstem and hypothalamus descends through the lateral funiculus of the spinal cord to the preganglionic sympathetic fibers. The preganglionic sympathetic neurons originate in the anteromedial column of the thoracolumbar cord, between T1 and L2. These myelinated white nerve fibers travel in the ventral root of the spinal cord to the paravertebral sympathetic ganglia, where they synapse onto the postganglionic unmyelinated grey fibers. It is likely that each preganglionic axon innervates about ten postganglionic neurons.[16] The postganglionic axons can leave the parasympathetic ganglia at the level of the synapse or can travel first up or down in the sympathetic chain before exiting the ganglion via grey rami. The regional activity of the sympathetic chain is the product of reflex arcs between somatic afferent fibers and preganglionic efferent fibers. For sympathetic denervation of the upper limbs, the interruption of the sympathetic chain from T2 to T4 is required. Although the stellate ganglion has some innervation to the upper limbs, resection of the stellate ganglion results in Horner syndrome (ptosis, myosis, and enophthalmos). Because of this associated

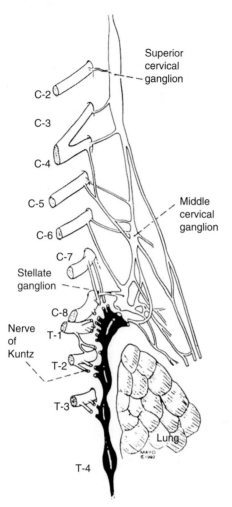

FIGURE 30-1 ■ Lower cervical and upper thoracic sympathetic chain. The nerve of Kuntz, originating at the level of T2 provides direct communicating fibers to the brachial plexus. (From Lowell RC, Gloviczki P, Cherry KJ, Jr, et al: Cervicothoracic sympathectomy for Raynaud's syndrome. Int Angiol 12:168–172, 1993.)

between the T1 (and C8) ganglion and the T2 ganglion to minimize axonal and potential neuron injury that may increase side-effects, particularly compensatory hyperhidrosis after sympathectomy.[2]

In addition to the paravertebral ganglia, there is another subtype of peripheral sympathetic ganglia: the prevertebral ganglia. These include the celiac, aortorenal, and superior and inferior mesenteric ganglia located in the abdominal cavity, on the top and around the aorta. These ganglia send postganglionic fibers to the abdominal and pelvic organs.

Physiology

The sympathetic nervous system modifies basal organ functions and mediates the body's response to stress ("fright, flight and fight response"). The primary function of the peripheral sympathetic nervous system is to prevent heat loss by reducing the blood flow to skin and subcutaneous tissue of the limbs. The increased activity of the postganglionic sympathetic nerves, mediated by norepinephrine, results in decreased blood flow because of stimulation of the vasoconstrictor fibers innervating the blood vessels. There is increased sweating caused by stimulation of the sudomotor fibers innervating the exocrine glands (an activity mediated by acetylcholine, adenosine and other neuropeptides), and there is piloerection mediated through the activity of the pilomotor fibers which innervate the erector pili muscles.[16] The sympathetic system antagonizes the vasodilatory effect of the parasympathetic nerves on arterial resistance vessels, on the cutaneous precapillary sphincters, and on the capacitance venules.

As a result of sympathetic denervation, the blood flow to the skin increases, there is a loss of sweating and piloerection, and the hands after thoracic sympathectomy/sympathotomy and the feet after lumbar sympathectomy become warm, pink, and dry. Sympathectomy also results in decreased pain of the ischemic limb, likely owing to an enhanced tolerance to pain stimuli. The pain tolerance is better because of decreased tissue concentration of norepinephrine and because of a reduced spinal augmentation of pain transmission to cerebral centers.

The maximal effect of the sympathectomy/sympathotomy is immediate, although vasodilation will be less 1 week because of compensatory mechanisms. Blood flow changes recorded at 6 months following sympathectomy are minimal because of incomplete denervation, regeneration of fibers, and a hypersensitivity of the receptors to circulating catecholamines.

Several authors have investigated the effect of sympathectomy on blood flow of the limbs. Cronenwett and colleagues[17] found no increase of nutrient capillary perfusion as a result of sympathectomy. Using intradermal xenon clearance, Moore and Hall[18] observed increased flow to the cutaneous capillary circulation. Rutherford and Valenta[19] failed to confirm increased muscle flow as a result of sympathectomy. Dalessandri and colleagues,[20] however, described increased collateral circulation in patients who underwent sympathectomy.

It is evident that the effect of sympathectomy on cutaneous blood flow is transient, but this period may be

morbidity, the stellate ganglion is not removed surgically. The nerves of Kuntz (Figure 30-1) are important because they provide direct collaterals from the T2 and T3 ganglia to the upper limbs. Resection of T2 and T3 ganglia (sympathectomy) is thought to be essential to achieve good and durable sympathetic denervation of the arms. The preganglionic fibers may bypass the paravertebral ganglia to synapse with more distal intermediate ganglia or may cross over to innervate the contralateral side as well. Therefore, as mentioned previously, a complete sympathectomy includes division of the preganglionic fibers and excision of the relay ganglia T2 and T3 and the intercommunicating fibers (the nerve of Kuntz). Several authors advocate T4 and T5 resection, especially in patients who undergo the operation for axillary hyperhidrosis.[3]

Figure 30-2 depicts the finer anatomy of the nerves and illustrates the difference between T2 sympathectomy and T1-T2 sympathotomy at the level of the second rib. Atkinson and colleagues[2] advocate performing sympathotomy by severing all visualized sympathetic branches

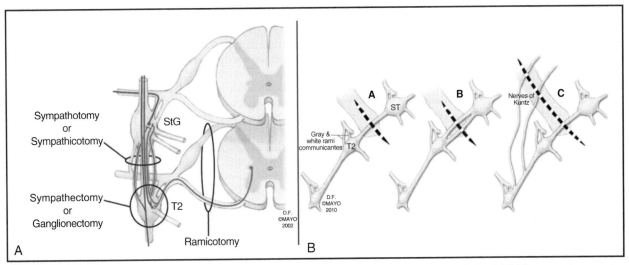

FIGURE 30-2 ■ **A,** Illustration of the two different techniques of interruption of the sympathetic chain, *1,* T1-T2 sympathotomy has a lesser chance of compensatory hyperhidrosis and a lesser chance to injure of axonal injury *(red)* from the neuron in the spinal cord. *2,* Sympathectomy has a higher chance of axon injury that may also cause neuron injury and more chance for compensatory hyperhidrosis. *StG,* Stellate ganglion. **B,** During sympathotomy all nerves are severed, including the nerves of Kuntz that run across the second rib between the StG and the T2 ganglion. *A,* Single sympathetic trunk. *B,* Multiple trunks. *C,* Trunk with lateral nerves of Kuntz (**16 patients**). (With permission from Atkinson JL, Fode-Thomas NC, Fealey RD, et al: Endoscopic transthoracic limited sympathotomy for palmar-plantar hyperhidrosis: outcomes and complications during a 10-year period. Mayo Clinic Proceed 86:721–729, 2011.)

TABLE 30-1 Indications for Sympathectomy

Indication	Thoracic Sympathectomy	Lumbar Sympathectomy
Best	Hyperhidrosis Causalgia Frostbite Buerger disease Raynaud phenomenon caused by stable arterial occlusions (e.g., traumatic subintimal fibrosis, distal emboli, digital gangrene) Facial blushing	Hyperhidrosis Causalgia Frostbite Buerger disease Atheroembolism (blue toe syndrome)
Acceptable	Primary Raynaud syndrome with digital ulcerations or Distal arterial occlusions	Inoperable Buerger or atherosclerotic arterial occlusions with limited tissue loss Rest pain in nondiabetic patient owing to small arterial occlusions (e.g., distal Buerger atherosclerosis, arterial emboli) with or without Raynaud phenomenon
Contraindications	Uncomplicated Raynaud disease	Claudication Diabetes with neuropathy

sufficient to heal superficial ulcerations. The more lasting effects of sympathectomy are on sweating, abnormal vasomotor tone, and pain relief.

THORACIC SYMPATHECTOMY

Indications

In an earlier study from the Mayo Clinic, Lowell and colleagues[9] reviewed indications for cervicothoracic sympathectomy in 68 patients. The most frequent indications were atheroembolism followed by Raynaud syndrome, causalgia, hand ischemia, reflex sympathetic dystrophy, and Buerger disease. The most frequently used indications for thoracic sympathectomy are medically refractory palmar-plantar hyperhidrosis and causalgia.[2,3] Additional indications include distal digital occlusion, vasospastic disorders with digital ulcerations not responding to medical treatment, Buerger disease, and frostbite.[1,10,21-23] There is a beneficial effect of sympathectomy on facial blushing.[10] Uncomplicated Raynaud disease and scleroderma are contraindications to cervical sympathectomy (Table 30-1).

Surgical Technique

Thoracic sympathectomy can be performed using open surgical technique, via transaxillary, transthoracic approach, or cervical approach, or using the thoracoscopic approach. Open techniques are rarely performed, usually only if thoracotomy or cervical incision is needed for another reason, such as vascular reconstruction or cervical or first rib resection.

Open Surgical Techniques

Transaxillary Approach. Patients who undergo transaxillary approach to the thoracic sympathetic chain are placed into a 90-degree lateral decubitus position with the arm elevated by the surgical assistant or with the help of an arm board. The transverse skin incision is performed in the axillary fossa, just distal to the axillary hairline. The dissection is carried down to the third rib, avoiding injury to the long thoracic nerve anteriorly and the subscapular artery and thoracodorsal nerve posteriorly. The pectoralis major muscle is retracted anteriorly, and the latissimus dorsi is retracted posteriorly. A 6-cm–long segment of the third rib is dissected from its periosteum, and it is removed. The pleura is entered, and the lumbar sympathectomy chain is dissected in the paravertebral region posteriorly by incising the posterior pleura (Figure 30-3). The chain is located 2-3 cm centimeters lateral to the azygos vein. The chain between T1 and T5 is sharply dissected, and the sympathetic chain with T2-T3 and usually T4 ganglia is removed. The stellate ganglion should not be removed, and dissection toward the neck should be avoided.

Cervical Approach. The cervical approach is through a supraclavicular skin incision. A 6-cm–long transverse incision is made 2 cm proximal to the clavicle, and the posterior belly of the sternocleidomastoid muscle is divided. The external jugular vein is ligated and divided, and the anterior scalene muscle is divided, carefully retracting the phrenic nerve medially. The subclavian artery is gently retracted caudally, and the stellate ganglion is exposed medial and anterior to the brachial plexus. It usually lies immediately lateral to the vertebral artery (Figure 30-4). The stellate ganglion is preserved, and dissection is carried down into the thoracic cavity, retracting the pleural dome as much as possible. The T1, T2, and T3 ganglions can usually be removed through this approach. On the left side, the dissection is similar, but attention must be paid to avoid injury to the thoracic duct. If injury to the thoracic duct or to one of the larger cervical ducts and leak of chyle is identified, ligation of the duct is warranted to avoid the complications of a chylocutaneous cyst or fistula.

Thoracoscopic Sympathectomy

The technique of thoracoscopic sympathectomy was first described in detail by Kux in 1978 using a single-scope technique.[15] Modern endoscopic instrumentation resulted in significant modification of the original technique, using multiple ports, as reported by Ahn and colleagues[1] (Figure 30-5). There have been many subsequent modifications to this technique, and currently a large number of patients, primarily with hyperhidrosis, undergo thoracoscopic sympathectomy, using one, two, or three endoscopic ports.

An excellent description of the uniportal and the biportal sympathectomy was given by Johnson and Patel[24] (Figure 30-6A, B). The operation is performed under

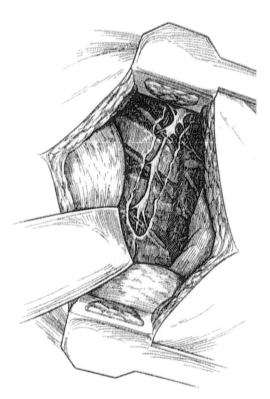

FIGURE 30-3 ■ Transaxillary minithoracotomy through the third intercostal space, performed with resection of a 6-cm-long segment of the third rib. After opening the pleura, the sympathetic chain distal to the stellate ganglion is resected, including the T2 and T3 segments. (With permission from T Rutherford RB: Atlas of Vascular Surgery, Philadelphia, 1993, WB Saunders.)

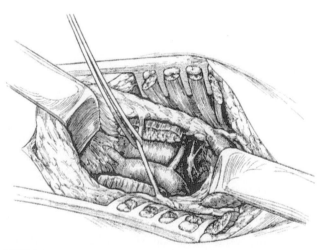

FIGURE 30-4 ■ Right supraclavicular approach for thoracic sympathectomy. The stellate ganglion is just lateral to the vertebral artery, which is exposed after transaction of the anterior scalene muscle. Note the phrenic nerve on a vessel loop. T1 to T3 is resected, gaining further exposure with downward retraction. (With permission from Rutherford RB: Atlas of Vascular Surgery, Philadelphia, 1993, WB Saunders.)

general anesthesia using a double-lumen endotracheal tube for deflation of the ipsilateral lung during the procedure. For bilateral procedures, the patient is positioned supine with the arms abducted bilaterally. For unilateral procedures, the patient is laid on the side.

Standard thoracoscopic instrumentation is used with a 5-mm rigid scope (with 30-degree and right-angle camera), electrocautery, and Harmonic scalpel (Ethicon

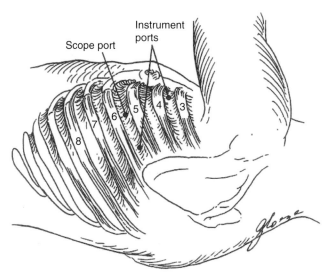

FIGURE 30-5 ■ Thoracoscopic sympathectomy using three endoscopic ports: two instrument ports in anterior and posterior axillary line, and scope port in midaxillary line. (With permission from Ahn SS, Machleder HI, Concepcion B, Moore WS: Thoracoscopic cervicodorsal sympathectomy: preliminary results. J Vasc Surg 20:511–519, 1994.)

Endo-Surgery, Cincinnati, Ohio) for dissection and ablation of the sympathetic ganglia and fibers. The port is placed through the third intercostal space for the uniportal procedure and the third and fifth spaces for the biportal operation, both in the anterior axillary line (see Figure 30-6A, B). Some surgeons use three thoracoscopic ports to help retraction of the lung during sympathectomy.[1] The uniportal procedure is performed with the instruments placed through the port beside the endoscope. The sympathetic chain courses over the rib heads just lateral to the vertebral bodies. The sympathetic chain and ganglia are well visualized through the posterior pleura. The sympathectomy procedure by this and many other groups involves incision of the posterior pleura and cauterization of the T2 and T3 ganglia that provide most sympathetic innervation to the arm and hand via the nerve of Kuntz. Most authors suggest ablating the T4 ganglia as well. On the right side, the azygos vein on the left of the hemiazygos vein can be close to the ganglia, and they should be avoided. Sometimes intercostal veins cross over the sympathetic chain, and injury or cauterization can result in bleeding from these vessels.

A recently introduced technique at Mayo Clinic by Atkinson and colleagues[2] has been gaining popularity because it is aimed at decreasing side effects of sympathectomy, like postsympathectomy neuralgia and reactive hyperhidrosis. The technique of T1-T2 sympathotomy differs in some detail from the previously described procedure.

The operation is performed using general anesthesia, followed by placement of a double-lumen endotracheal tube. Both arms are abducted to 90 degrees and the back elevated to 40 degrees. The chest wall is perforated through a small (<1 cm) transaxillary skin incision or,

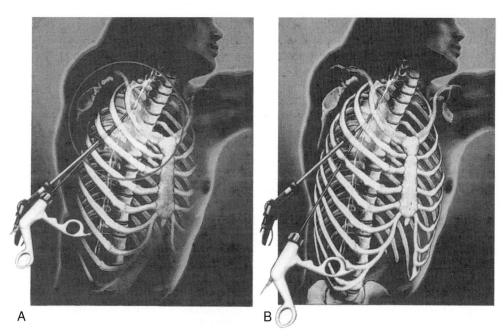

FIGURE 30-6 ■ **A,** Port location and instrument placement for uniportal thoracoscopic sympathectomy. **B,** Port locations and instrument placement for biportal thoracoscopic sympathectomy. (With permission from Johnson JP, Patel NP: Uniportal and biportal endoscopic thoracic sympathectomy. Neurosurgery 51:78–79, 2002.)

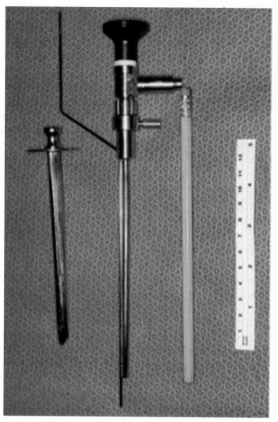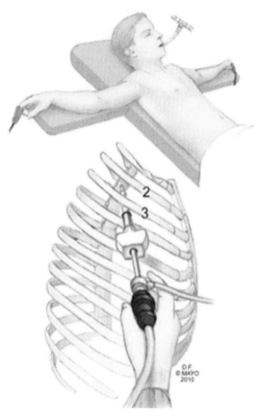

FIGURE 30-7 ■ *Left,* Instruments used for sympathotomy at Mayo Clinic. Hollow trocar with obturator for perforating chest wall allows penetration of the chest wall through a small (<1 cm) incision, removal of the inner obturator, and passage of the endoscope with attached monopolar cautery probe (second object). A pencil and tape measure provide perspectives of size. *Right, upper,* Position of patient at surgery. *Lower,* Single small incision and uniportal access with endoscope and cautery combined. (With permission from Atkinson JL, Fode-Thomas NC, Fealey RD, et al: Endoscopic transthoracic limited sympathotomy for palmar-plantar hyperhidrosis: outcomes and complications during a 10-year period. Mayo Clinic Proceed 86:721–729, 2011.)

occasionally, in the anterior midclavicular area between the second and third ribs, to place a small endoscope and the attached monopolar cautery. There is no gas insufflation with this technique (Figure 30-7). Sympathotomy is performed above the T2 ganglion and below the T1 ganglion (or the stellate ganglion) by transection of all nerve fibers across the second rib using an electrocautery. Once both sides are done, bilateral pediatric feeding tubes are placed and the wounds are closed. The intrapleural air is aspirated through the bilateral pediatric feeding tubes, which are then removed. Most patients are discharged within 23 hours.

The Mayo group also uses a Doppler palmar blood flow device to confirm the elevation of skin blood flow after sympathotomy. This technique provides immediate feedback to the surgeon about the efficacy and completeness of the operation.[2]

Results

Hyperhidrosis

Zacherl and colleagues[25] reported on long-term results of 630 operations performed in 352 patients. Complications included pneumothorax in 1.3%, Horner syndrome in

3.8%, and subcutaneous emphysema in 2.1%. The median follow-up of this study was 16 years; 68% of the patients were fully satisfied; 26% were partially satisfied with the procedure. Permanent cure was obtained in 93% of the patients, although 67% complained of compensatory sweating. Just like other authors, this article also reported lower success rate in axillary hyperhidrosis.[25]

Drott and colleagues[22] published results of 850 thoracic sympathectomies performed for hyperhidrosis of the palms, axillae, and face.[22] For palmar hyperhidrosis, cure is almost 100% after thoracoscopic sympathectomy, and the success rate was dependent on resection or ablation of T2 ganglion.

Compensatory hyperhidrosis appears to be frequent, although according to some authors avoiding resection of T3 and T4 likely decreases the risk of this complication. Overall satisfaction rate of the operation for palmar hyperhidrosis has been reported to be between 87% and 95%. For axillary hyperhidrosis, satisfaction rate is much lower (60%), and some surgeons avoid sympathectomy completely. Resection of T4 and T5 is frequently required to achieve good results.

A recent consensus document of The Society of Thoracic Surgeons' General Thoracic Workforce reviewed 1097 published articles on this topic, including 12 randomized controlled trials and 90 comparative studies. The document concluded that primary hyperhidrosis of the extremities, axillae, or face is best treated by endoscopic thoracic sympathectomy. Interruption of the sympathetic chain can be achieved either by electrocautery or clipping. The literature suggests that the highest success rates occur when interruption is performed at the top of the third rib (R3) or the top of R4 for palmar-only hyperhidrosis. R4 may offer a lower incidence of compensatory hyperhidrosis[26] but moister hands. For palmar and axillary, for palmar, axillary, and pedal, and for axillary-only hyperhidrosis, interruptions at R4 and R5 are recommended. The top of R3 was thought to be best for craniofacial hyperhidrosis.

Wolosker and colleagues[27] prospectively followed 453 patients with hyperhidrosis who underwent endoscopic thoracic sympathectomy to evaluate long-term improvement in quality of life. Quality of life improved immediately after surgery in 91% of the patients, and this improvement was sustained at 5 years after surgery.

Atkinson and colleagues[2] performed a retrospective review of 155 patients who underwent thoracoscopic T1-T2 sympathotomy disconnection surgery for medically refractory palmar-plantar hyperhidrosis. No patient had Horner syndrome, intercostal neuralgia, or pneumothorax. Two patients (1.3%) developed hemothorax. All 155 patients had immediate improvement. At a mean of 40 months after surgery, 97% had successful control of palmar sweating; 69% experienced decreased axillary sweating. Compensatory hyperhidrosis did not occur in 32%; it was mild in 62%, moderate in 5%, and severe in 1%.

Reflex Sympathetic Dystrophy

In patients who have complex regional pain syndrome or reflex sympathetic dystrophy, sympathectomy has been reported to effectively decrease pain. Singh and colleagues[28] analyzed long-term results in 42 patients. Thirty-two underwent thoracoscopic and 10 had open cervicothoracic sympathectomy. Early improvement was reported in all patients. There was no morbidity or major early complications. The hospital stay was shorter in the thoracic sympathectomy group, and these patients had a better outcome. These authors did not find preoperative stellate ganglion blockade predictive of postoperative clinical outcome. Because of the obvious benefit of thoracoscopic sympathectomy, they recommended it as a procedure of choice for patients with complex regional pain syndrome over open surgical sympathectomy.

Raynaud Syndrome

Lowell and colleagues[9] reported on results of open surgical treatment of 20 patients who underwent open cervicothoracic sympathectomies for Raynaud syndrome. No mortality was reported, but Horner syndrome was observed in five patients (transient in three and mild in two). Three patients had postsympathectomy neuralgia, two patients had phrenic nerve palsy, and one patient had pneumothorax. Nineteen of the 20 patients had immediate improvement following surgical treatment. This early

benefit, however, disappeared in all patients at 6 months, and the authors concluded that cervicothoracic sympathectomy in patients with uncomplicated Raynaud syndrome is not recommended.

In a recent systematic review, Coveliers and colleagues[29] analyzed the evidence for a total of 728 thoracic sympathectomies in the management of digital ischemia caused by both primary Raynaud disease (PRD) and secondary Raynaud phenomenon (SRP). Early improvement was reported in 92% of PRD patients and in 89% of SRP patients, but long-term beneficial effect was only 58% for PRD and 89% for SRP. Most benefit in PRD patients was limited to the first 6 months, and no improvement was noted afterward in 42%. Ulcer healing or early improvement was still achieved in 95%, suggesting that thoracic sympathectomy may maximize tissue preservation or prevent amputation, and it remains a useful treatment for both PRD and SRP.

Conclusions

The technique of thoracoscopic sympathectomy is currently the operation of choice for patients who need surgical denervation of the thoracic sympathetic chain. Of the open techniques, if needed in the occasional patient, the best is the transaxillary transthoracic sympathectomy. Resection or thoracoscopic ablation of at least T2-T3 ganglia is reported to achieve good results with this operation. Highly selective T1-T2 sympathotomy for palmar hyperhidrosis offers a high long-term success rate and low complication rate.

The best indications for cervical sympathectomy include refractory palmar hyperhidrosis and causalgia resulting in chronic pain syndrome. Chronic occlusive arterial disease caused by arteritis such as Buerger disease or Raynaud disease with nonhealing superficial ulcerations is also a good indication for sympathectomy. Preoperative stellate block does not always predict outcome, and complications for the operation include compensatory sweating, Horner syndrome, and postoperative neuralgia. Compensatory swelling appears to be less frequent with sympathotomy. Compensatory sweating can be such a disabling condition that techniques of reversal of the thoracic sympathectomy have been recently entertained: reconstructions using nerve grafts and applying clips to the nerves during the first operation with the idea to remove them at a later stage should compensatory sweating develop was recommended.

LUMBAR SYMPATHECTOMY

Indications

Causalgia, plantar hyperhidrosis, frostbite, Buerger disease, pain from atheroembolism (blue toe syndrome), and digital ulcerations are current indications for lumbar sympathectomy. Patients who have critical limb ischemia but an ankle brachial index greater than 0.3 have also been suggested as candidates for lumbar sympathectomy. Patients who have claudication or diabetes with diabetic neuropathy should not undergo lumbar sympathectomy.

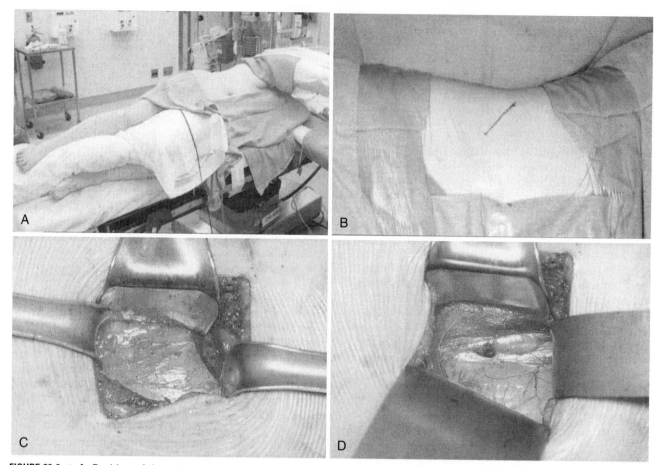

FIGURE 30-8 ■ **A,** Position of the patient on the operating table for right lumbar sympathectomy. **B,** An 8-cm skin incision is made from the tip of the eleventh rig toward half way between the umbilicus and the pubis. **C,** The abdominal muscles are split along their fibers. **D,** Blunt retroperitoneal dissection is made to explore the space between the medial edge of the psoas muscle and the inferior vena cava.

Techniques

Open Surgical Lumbar Sympathectomy

The operation is performed in a semilateral decubitus position (Figure 30-8). An 8-cm oblique flank incision is made from the tip of the eleventh rib either toward the umbilicus or slightly lower halfway toward the umbilicus and the pubis. The dissection is carried down to the abdominal muscles; the muscles are split along their fibers, and the retroperitoneum is entered. On the right side, the peritoneum with the ureter is retracted medially, and the lumbar sympathetic chain is identified between the inferior vena cava and the psoas muscle (see Figure 30-8C, D). On the left side, the sympathetic chain is located between the aorta and the psoas muscle. The genitofemoral nerve that lies over the psoas muscle is identified and carefully preserved (Figure 30-9A, B). Attention is paid to avoid any retractor injury to the aorta that may cause embolization into the lower limbs, not infrequently into the right leg. The sympathetic chain is dissected from the rim of the pelvis all the way up to the level of L1. Usually three ganglia (L2 to L4) are removed with the intervening sympathetic chain. Frequently the chain runs under the lumbar vessels, and dissection has

to be careful to avoid injury to these vessels. To avoid sexual dysfunction, L1 must be preserved in males, and bilateral resection of L1 ganglia should not be performed at all in young males. After excision of the ganglia and the chain, careful hemostasis is performed and the muscles, the subcutaneous tissue, and the skin closed in layers.

Retroperitoneoscopic Lumbar Sympathectomy

This technique was well described by Beglaibter and colleagues[6] and more recently by Rieger and colleagues.[30,31] The procedure is performed with anesthesia and endotracheal intubation, with the patient with hyperextended flank (Figure 30-10). Balloon dissection of the retroperitoneal space is done by inserting the balloon through a small incision in the flank. Two or three ports are used for retraction and dissection. The chain is ablated with excision and electrocautery. To facilitate the localization of the various levels of the lumbar sympathetic trunk, Rieger recommends that the projection of the lumbar vertebral bodies on to the anterior abdominal wall is marked fluoroscopically.

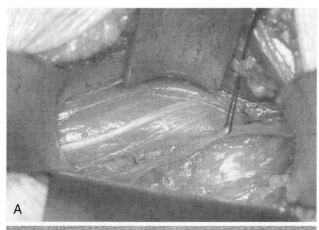

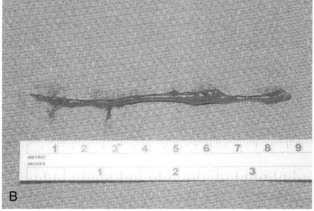

FIGURE 30-9 ■ **A,** The lumbar sympathetic chain is on a black silk. Note the genitofemoral nerve over the psoas muscle. **B,** The resected sympathetic chain with T2, T3, and T4 ganglia.

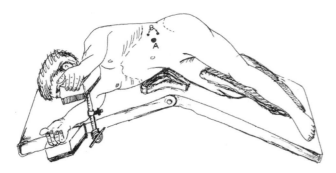

FIGURE 30-10 ■ Position and port placement for retroperitoneoscopic lumbar sympathectomy. (With permission from Beglaibter N, Berlatzky Y, Zamir O, et al: Retroperitoneoscopic lumbar sympathectomy. J Vasc Surg 35:815–817, 2002.)

Results

The most frequent early complication of lumbar sympathectomy is postsympathectomy neuralgia that has been described in 20% to 50% of the patients.[8] Paradoxic gangrene is usually the result of embolization from the aortoiliac vessels, and careful retraction of the tissues during the operation will prevent this complication. As mentioned previously, bilateral resection of L1

sympathetic ganglia may result in disturbance in ejaculation or potency.

Persson and colleagues[32] reported on results of lumbar sympathectomy for ischemic rest pain and ulcers in 37 patients who had inoperable disease. All patients had an ankle-brachial index greater than 0.3. There was no neuropathy, and patients had limited tissue loss; 78% of these patients had long-term pain relief, and only 11% required amputation. On the contrary, Fulton and Blakeley[33] reported no effect of sympathectomy on amputation of patients with severe distal ischemia. Seventeen unselected patients in this series with advanced arteriosclerosis underwent lumbar sympathectomy with a 70% rate of amputation discrediting this operation. This report and others caused significant controversy regarding this operation and decreased the use of lumbar sympathectomy for the indication of critical limb ischemia.

Bandyk and colleagues[8] reported on results of sympathectomy in 73 patients who underwent surgical treatment for reflex sympathetic dystrophy. Forty-seven of these patients underwent thoracic sympathectomy, and 37 had lumbar sympathectomy. The authors found that greater than 50% reduction in pain score for more than 2 days after sympathetic block predicted good response to the operation. No mortality or major morbidity was reported. Transient neuralgia was noted in 20% of the patients after lumbar sympathectomy; 90% of patients reported excellent results at 3 months. At 1 year, 25% still had significant pain relief and 50% had improvement. Overall patient satisfaction was 77%.

Beglaibter and colleagues[6] presented the results of 29 retroperitoneoscopic lumbar sympathectomies performed in 27 patients. Twenty-two had ischemia of the lower limb, five because of Buerger disease, and five patients had severe reflex sympathetic dystrophy. Improvement in symptoms was noted in all patients.

Five patients in the series previously underwent computed tomography–guided chemical sympathectomy. It should be noted that reported complications related to attempts at chemical sympathectomy using phenol or alcohol injections resulted in complications related to the injection itself and to the effects of the chemicals that are injected. Ureteral damage, including stricture and necrosis, retroperitoneal abscess formation, or fibrosis have been reported.[34]

Rieger and colleagues[30] performed 178 endoscopic lumbar sympathectomies at L3 and L4 levels for plantar hyperhidrosis in 90 patients. Post-sympathetic neuralgia occurred in 42%, and compensatory sweating occurred in 42%. Post-sympathetic neuralgia, however, was only minor and temporary, and only one patient had severe compensatory sweating. One patient had temporary loss of ejaculation. At 24 months, 97% of the patients had their hyperhidrosis cured.

Conclusion

Lumbar sympathectomy is effective and durable in patients with plantar hyperhidrosis. Lumbar sympathectomy also has good results in patients who have causalgia, Buerger disease, or frostbite. Patients with reflex sympathetic dystrophy with confirmed sympathetically mediated pain syndrome can have long-term benefit from this operation. With the advent of lower limb revascularizations, indications for critical limb ischemia have decreased significantly. Good results have been reported with Buerger disease and in nondiabetic patients with distal atherosclerosis who have rest pain, limited tissue loss, and an ankle brachial index better than 0.3. The most frequent complication of the operation is postsympathectomy neuralgia that is usually transient and responds well to pain medications. Open lumbar sympathectomy will soon be completely replaced by retroperitoneoscopic procedures.

BIBLIOGRAPHY

Atkinson JL, Fode-Thomas NC, Fealey RD, et al: Endoscopic transthoracic limited sympathotomy for palmar-plantar hyperhidrosis: outcomes and complications during a 10-year period. Mayo Clinic Proceed 86(8):721–729, 2011.

Bandyk DF, Johnson BL, Kirkpatrick AF, et al: Surgical sympathectomy for reflex sympathetic dystrophy syndromes. J Vasc Surg 35:269–277, 2002.
Cerfolio RJ, De Campos JR, Bryant AS, et al: The Society of Thoracic Surgeons expert consensus for the surgical treatment of hyperhidrosis. Ann Thor Surg 91(5):1642–1648, 2011.
Coveliers HM, Hoexum F, Nederhoed JH, et al: Thoracic sympathectomy for digital ischemia: a summary of evidence. J Vasc Surg 54(1):273–277, 2011.
Rieger R, Pedevilla S, Pochlauer S: Endoscopic lumbar sympathectomy for plantar hyperhidrosis. Br J Surg 96(12):1422–1428, 2009.

References available online at expertconsult.com.

QUESTIONS

1. The peripheral nervous system includes all components except
   a. Somatic efferent motor nerves
   b. Somatic afferent motor nerves
   c. Somatic efferent nerves to the exocrine glands
   d. Autonomic nerves to the abdominal viscera
   e. Autonomic sympathetic and parasympathetic nerves

2. Most experts agree that for sympathetic denervation of the upper limb interruption of the sympathetic chain at the following level is required
   a. Stellate ganglion
   b. Stellate ganglion and T1
   c. T2 to T4
   d. T4-T5
   e. T5

3. In patients with axillary hyperhidrosis resection of the following ganglions as extension of a T2-T3 sympathectomy is recommended
   a. T4
   b. T4-T5
   c. T1
   d. C8
   e. C8-T1

4. Indications for thoracoscopic sympathectomy include all of the following except
   a. Hyperhidrosis
   b. Buerger's disease with digital ulcers
   c. Uncomplicated Raynaud's syndrome associated with scleroderma
   d. Frostbite
   e. Causalgia

5. The right sympathetic chain with T2-T5 ganglia is located 2 to 3 cm lateral to the
   a. Phrenic nerve
   b. Azygos vein
   c. Hemiazygos vein
   d. Long thoracic nerve
   e. Right atrium

6. Direct collateral sympathetic fibers to the arm at T2-T3 levels are located in the
   a. Nerve of Herring
   b. Intercostobrachial nerve
   c. Nerve of Kuntz
   d. Paravertebral ganglia
   e. Brachial plexus

7. The right lumbar sympathetic chain is located
   a. Lateral to the psoas muscle
   b. Medial to the inferior vena cava
   c. Lateral to the genitofemoral nerve
   d. Between the psoas muscle and the inferior vena cava
   e. Just lateral to the aorta

8. To avoid sexual dysfunction, lumbar sympathetic ganglia at what level must be preserved in males
   a. L1
   b. L2
   c. L3
   d. L4
   e. L5

9. Which of the following is usually a contraindication to lumbar sympathectomy
   a. Digital gangrene
   b. Causalgia
   c. Frostbite
   d. Diabetic neuropathy
   e. Buerger's disease

10. Sympathectomy results in all of the following changes in a limb except:
    a. Decreased sweating
    b. Increased skin circulation
    c. Decreased pain
    d. Increased circulation to the skeletal muscles
    e. Increased parasympathetic tone

ANSWERS

1. **c**
2. **c**
3. **b**
4. **c**
5. **b**
6. **c**
7. **d**
8. **a**
9. **d**
10. **d**

CHAPTER 31

Thoracic Outlet Syndrome and Vascular Disease of the Upper Extremity

Samuel S. Ahn • Toshifumi Kudo • Justin S. Ahn

THORACIC OUTLET SYNDROME

Thoracic outlet syndrome (TOS) is defined as symptomatic compression of the neurovascular bundle at the thoracic outlet. This syndrome can take three main forms—neurogenic, venous, and arterial—depending on the specific structures compressed. Most patients with TOS have neurologic symptoms, although vascular problems may be present. This chapter reviews the history and the current etiologic, diagnostic, and therapeutic theories concerning TOS and its treatment.

History

TOS is still a controversial subject in regard to its diagnosis, conservative management, and surgical treatment. The concept of the disease and the anatomic structures focused on have changed over the centuries. In 1821, Cooper noted that subclavian artery thrombosis was due to compression by a cervical rib.[1] This compression became known as *cervical rib syndrome*. From 1920 to 1931, the scalene muscles, first rib, and congenital ligaments became the focus to explain neurovascular compression in the thoracic outlet region.[2-4] Next, the term *scalenus anticus syndrome* became popular, and an association with trauma was described.[5,6] The *costoclavicular syndrome*, compression between the clavicle and first rib, was described in 1943.[7] Peet and colleagues introduced the term *thoracic outlet syndrome* in 1956,[8] and Rob and Standeven proposed the term *thoracic outlet compression syndrome* in 1958.[9] More recent studies have emphasized histologic abnormalities indicating scalene muscle fibrosis in TOS patients.[10,11]

Over the years, various surgical approaches have been proposed. Coote performed a cervical rib resection in 1861.[12] Murphy performed a first rib resection in 1908.[13] Because of the high nerve complication rate associated with this procedure, the first scalenectomy was performed by Adson and Coffey in 1927,[14] but it was realized that division of the muscle alone eventually led to reattachment of the muscle fibers and scarring, causing recurrent symptoms. Clagett reintroduced the first rib resection with a posterior approach in 1962.[15] In 1966, Roos described the transaxillary approach for first rib resection,[16] which is less invasive and more cosmetic and has become one of the standard approaches. In the late 1960s, an approach using an infraclavicular incision alone was described[17]; however, this approach produced a large, cosmetically unpleasant scar and, more importantly, provided only limited exposure posteriorly. Sanders and coworkers[18] reintroduced scalenectomy for the treatment of recurrent TOS after first rib resection and posttraumatic TOS in 1979. For the purpose of total decompression, Atasoy introduced a combined approach, a transaxillary first rib resection and transcervical anterior and middle scalenectomy, in 1996.[19]

Incidence and Demographics

The incidence of TOS is reported to be approximately 0.3% to 2% in the general population.[19,20] The most common age range is 25 to 40 years. Patients in their teens as well as octogenarians have also been diagnosed with TOS, although rarely. Women are more commonly affected than men, with a female-to-male ratio of 4:1.

Anatomy

A knowledge of the complex anatomy of the thoracic outlet is crucial to understanding the pathogenesis of TOS and making the diagnosis. The thoracic outlet is defined as the musculoskeletal structures surrounding three important structures: subclavian artery, subclavian vein, and brachial plexus. This triangle is formed by the anterior scalene muscle, middle scalene muscle, and first rib (Figure 31-1). The subclavian artery arises from the upper mediastinum, passes behind the anterior scalene muscle, and arches over the first rib; it therefore courses through the scalene triangle, which is bordered by the anterior and middle scalene muscles and has the first rib as its floor. The nerve roots (C5 to T1) of the brachial plexus, after exiting the intervertebral foramina, unite to form the upper (C5 and C6), middle (C7), and lower (C8 and T1) trunks of the brachial plexus. They lie posterior, lateral, and superior to the subclavian artery and travel through the scalene triangle with the artery, with the lower trunk having a close relationship with the artery. The subclavian vein follows a similar course but, in contrast to the subclavian artery and brachial plexus, does not traverse the scalene triangle. It courses anterior to the

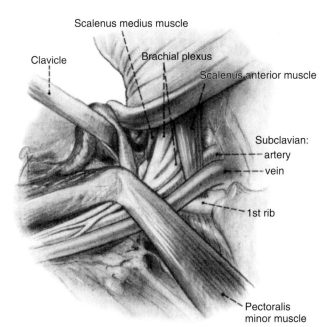

FIGURE 31-1 ■ Anatomic dissection showing the anatomy at the thoracic outlet. The cadaver's head is turned to the left, and the clavicle is reflected laterally. (From Machleder HI, editor: *Vascular disorders of the upper extremity,* ed 3, Mt. Kisco, N.Y., 1998, Futura Publishing.)

insertion of the anterior scalene muscle on the first rib, outside the scalene triangle, and runs inferior and lateral to the subclavius tendon and costocoracoid ligament. All three structures then follow a similar course, passing under the clavicle and subclavius muscle and beneath the pectoralis minor near its insertion into the coracoid process and giving off several branches before entering the upper arm. Throughout their course, the neuromuscular structures are confined by various myofascial coverings.

Three main spaces in the thoracic outlet region are potentially responsible for compression of the neurovascular structures as they travel to the upper extremity: scalene triangle, costoclavicular space, and retropectoralis minor space. The scalene triangle is the most common site of nerve compression. Its contents are the brachial plexus and subclavian artery. The costoclavicular space, bordered by the clavicle and the first rib, is distal to the scalene triangle. It is traversed by all three structures: artery, vein, and nerve. The retro-pectoralis minor space is formed by the coracoid process and the insertion of the pectoralis minor and by the ribs posteriorly. It is outside the thoracic outlet area and is less important in TOS. The brachial plexus may be compressed or tethered around the coracoid process with arm abduction or elevation.

In addition to the brachial plexus, two nerves in this area are surgically important. The phrenic nerve, a motor nerve to the diaphragm, arises primarily from C4 and usually receives branches from C3 and C5. The nerve travels on the anterior surface of the anterior scalene muscle, crossing lateral to medial. Because of this anatomic relationship, the nerve is vulnerable to injury during scalenectomy. Thirteen percent of the population

has a double phrenic nerve.[21] The long thoracic nerve arises primarily from C6 and usually receives branches from C5 and C7. It courses through or just posterior to the middle scalene muscle and then descends over the first rib to reach the serratus anterior muscle. Injury to the nerve results in winging of the scapula. Another surgically important structure is the thoracic duct, which empties into the left subclavian vein and is susceptible to operative injury resulting in troublesome lymphatic leakage.

Cause

The cause of neurogenic TOS is hypothesized to be a combination of osseous changes, soft tissue abnormalities, trauma, and inflammation—in other words, congenital predisposing anatomic structures and acquired extrinsic factors that may produce further compression of the neurovascular structures in the thoracic outlet area. In vascular TOS, the cause of arterial TOS is usually a bony abnormality—a cervical rib or a rudimentary first rib. Primary venous TOS is generally due to the costoclavicular ligament and subclavius muscle compressing the subclavian vein. It is important to consider the interaction between the neurovascular structures and the surrounding bony and muscular framework as a dynamic rather than a static process to understand the pathogenesis of TOS. Tumor can also be the cause of TOS; 1% to 2% of patients with TOS have underlying tumor at the thoracic outlet in our series (unpublished data).

Osseous Changes

Cervical ribs, present since birth, are regarded as predisposing factors. They have an incidence of 0.5% to 1.5% in the general population[22-24]; approximately 50% are bilateral,[25,26] and there is a female-to-male ratio of 2:1. Most are asymptomatic,[27] but they are found with increasing prevalence in patients with TOS, reportedly occurring in 4% to 11% of patients who undergo TOS decompression surgery.[23,28,29] The size of the cervical rib may vary. The ribs often have rudimentary or incomplete ossification, with a fibrous band extending from the tip and inserting on the first rib (Figure 31-2). Complete cervical ribs often insert on the first rib and occasionally are accompanied by an area of hyperostosis or even a fairly well-developed joint structure (Figure 31-3). The brachial plexus is stretched over the cervical rib or accompanying fibrous bands, which produces compression, usually in the lower trunk.[30] Other osseous factors predisposing a patient to symptomatic TOS include a long transverse process of C7, first rib fracture, bifid first rib, and malunion of the clavicle. Poor posture with anterior displacement[31] and saggy or droopy shoulders are also included in this category. It should be noted that the presence of a radiographically observed anatomic anomaly is not always necessary for the diagnosis.

Soft Tissue Abnormalities

Congenital fibromuscular bands and ligaments are observed in a majority of patients with neurogenic TOS.[30]

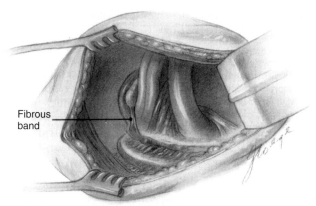

FIGURE 31-2 ■ View of a fibrocartilaginous band from the tip of the right-sided seventh cervical transverse process from the transaxillary surgical approach. This abnormality can compress the brachial plexus and subclavian artery, causing symptoms identical to those resulting from a cervical rib. The fibrocartilaginous band commonly occurs with an elongated C7 transverse process and represents partial formation of a cervical rib. (From Makhoul RG, Machleder HI: Developmental anomalies at the thoracic outlet: an analysis of 200 consecutive cases. J Vasc Surg 16:534–545, 1992.)

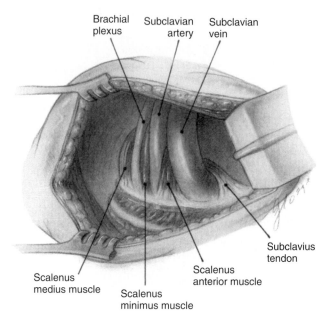

FIGURE 31-4 ■ Appearance of the scalenus minimus abnormality from the transaxillary surgical approach. (From Makhoul RG, Machleder HI: Developmental anomalies at the thoracic outlet: an analysis of 200 consecutive cases. J Vasc Surg 16:534–545, 1992.)

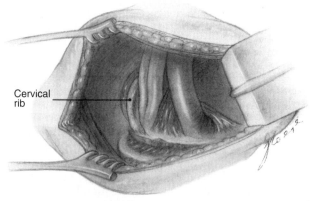

FIGURE 31-3 ■ View of thoracic outlet structures from the transaxillary surgical approach. The brachial plexus and subclavian artery are compressed and displaced by a right-sided cervical rib. This cervical rib articulates in the center of the first thoracic rib. (From Makhoul RG, Machleder HI: Developmental anomalies at the thoracic outlet: an analysis of 200 consecutive cases. J Vasc Surg 16:534–545, 1992.)

Some authors report anomalous bands or ligaments found at the time of surgery in more than 80% of their patients.[32,33] These bands and ligaments have been present since birth and are categorized into nine different types.[30,34]

Scalene muscles are the most important structures that cause upper extremity symptoms. Congenital or acquired scalene muscle changes may be observed. One anatomic variation is the smallest scalene muscle (scalenus minimus) originating from the transverse process of the C7 vertebra, interdigitating between the subclavian artery and the brachial plexus, inserting in conjunction with the anterior scalene muscle on the first rib, and producing further compression (Figure 31-4). The role of the smallest scalene muscle has previously been underappreciated, but our review of 185 patients undergoing TOS surgery

revealed that it was a prevalent (68.1%) and clinically significant marker for contralateral TOS surgery (unpublished data).

Another variation is a narrow scalene triangle, which could have a significant role in the development of TOS symptoms.[35] The anatomic relationship between the scalene angle and the brachial plexus—the nerve roots emerging from the apex of the scalene triangle (a higher anatomic region)—might also contribute to symptoms.[35] A hypertrophied subclavius muscle may be a factor in TOS as well.

Trauma

In addition to anatomic predispositions, trauma has been implicated as a precipitating factor for symptomatic TOS. Typical major trauma includes whiplash injuries of the neck[36] and blows to the shoulders resulting in acute hyperextension injury, often occurring during motor vehicle accidents. Some reports note that approximately 80% of TOS patients have symptoms precipitated by trauma to the neck and shoulder girdle area.[37,38] Stress injury, caused by repetitive motion or specific occupational activities over a prolonged period (e.g., continual abduction of the arms or excessive computer use), can also lead to TOS. Even upper extremity injury can cause TOS. Trauma causes spasm, inflammation, edema, and swelling, followed by scarring and fibrosis; this leads to increased muscle thickness, narrow interscalene spaces, and eventually compression of the neurovascular structures during contraction. The onset of symptoms may be delayed by days to weeks or even months.[35] Significant histologic muscle fiber changes have been demonstrated in the scalene muscles of patients with neurogenic TOS.[10,11]

Pathology

Studies focusing on the histochemical and morphometric analysis of the anterior scalene muscle have opened a new area of investigation into the causes of neurovascular compression at the thoracic outlet.[10,11] This research has been particularly useful in demonstrating the changes that occur in posttraumatic neurogenic TOS and often appear in the absence of obvious structural abnormalities.

Vertebrate skeletal muscle is composed of several distinctive muscle fiber types, each having different morphologic, metabolic, and contractile characteristics that are distinguishable by specific histochemical staining methods. Despite a high degree of specialization, these fibers retain the capacity to accommodate changes in demand and patterns of stimulation, responding with alterations in basic biochemical elements.

Human skeletal muscle usually comprises predominantly type 2, quick-reacting fibers, which have a low oxidative enzyme capacity. A smaller percentage of slow tonic-contracting type 1 fibers, characterized by a greater oxidative capacity, is present. These latter fibers (type 1) are common to postural muscle groups. Anterior scalene muscle demonstrates type 1 fiber predominance, which indicates that this muscle has a uniquely structured fiber composition to sustain protracted periods of tonic contraction.

Striking increases in type 1 fiber composition and selective hypertrophy of the type 1 fiber system occur in patients with posttraumatic TOS. The anterior scalene muscle in these patients demonstrates an extraordinary adaptive transformation and recruitment response in the type 1 fiber system, possibly reflecting chronic increased tone or motor neuron stimulation. It seems likely that in posttraumatic TOS, stretch injury to the muscle initiates a response of muscle contraction or denervation and reinnervation, compromising the scalene triangle (between the anterior and middle scalene muscles) and constricting the brachial plexus, which both accentuates and perpetuates the neurovascular compressive phenomenon.

Clinical Presentation

The signs and symptoms of TOS are representative of the neurovascular structures involved in compression: the brachial plexus and the subclavian artery and vein. Symptoms may develop spontaneously or after trauma of a type that causes chronic muscle spasm in the neck or shoulder region. Presenting symptoms span a broad range of severity, from mild to disabling. Some patients report the onset of symptoms after a cervical injury or motor vehicle accident. More commonly, the onset of neurogenic symptoms is insidious; they may be mild and intermittent at first and are generally ignored by the patient. The symptoms gradually increase in frequency and severity, followed by progression that affects job, sleep, or activities of daily living. Patients may experience upper extremity pain, paresthesia, and numbness. Headache, neck pain, chest pain, and almost any upper extremity complaint may be attributable to TOS. Patients with vascular TOS may have a sudden onset.

Neurologic Symptoms

Neurologic symptoms caused by thoracic outlet compression of the brachial plexus predominate in 94% to 97% patients.[37,39] The symptoms of neurogenic TOS are basically the same as those of nerve compression in other regions of the body: pain, paresthesia, tingling sensation, and weakness for peripheral nerves; and Raynaud's syndrome, temperature change, and color change for autonomic nerves. Typically, two patterns of brachial plexus compression have emerged. Lower plexus (C8 and T1) involvement is regarded as more common than upper plexus (C5 and C6) involvement; however, the picture is often mixed.[40]

Lower brachial plexus thoracic outlet compression usually causes sensory disturbance to the ulnar nerve distribution. Patients complain of pain and paresthesias in the medial (ulnar) aspect of the arm from the axilla, through the brachial area and the forearm, down to the hand (the fourth and fifth fingers). Ulnar-innervated muscles include the hypothenar, interosseous, and deep flexors of the ring and little finger. Pain in the anterior or posterior shoulder region and the side or back of the neck radiating into the occipital or mastoid area of the skull is also characteristic.[41]

Patients with upper plexus TOS usually exhibit symptoms in the forearm and upper arm, rather than the hand. Upper plexus TOS also produces pain in the side of the neck that radiates upward to the ear and may include the mandible, face, temple, and occipital regions, with hemicranial headaches.[40] The pain radiates posteriorly into the rhomboid area, anteriorly across the clavicle into the upper pectoral region, laterally through the trapezius and deltoid muscle areas, and down the outer arm.[41] Compression of the upper trunk may cause evidence of C5 to C7 nerve root involvement or sensory disturbance to the median nerve distribution.[42]

Brachial plexus compression can cause subjective coldness of the hand, even pallor, which may be mistakenly interpreted as arterial insufficiency or complex regional pain syndrome type I (reflex sympathetic dystrophy). In more advanced cases, weakness of the hand and loss of dexterity of the fingers frequently develop.[22] The lateral thenar muscles are most severely affected. In late cases there is muscle atrophy, impaired use of the arm without paralysis, or even a "claw" hand.

TOS can appear with headache as the primary component. Occipital and orbital headaches that radiate forward are common. In contrast, frontal headaches are not due to TOS. Surgical decompression of the thoracic outlet can be effective in treating TOS-related headaches. In a review of 227 TOS patients, the prevalence of headache was 41%, and the primary and secondary success rates of TOS surgery for relieving headache were found to be 52.7% and 75.2%, respectively, at 1 year, using life-table analysis (unpublished data).

Venous Symptoms

Venous TOS is less common than neurogenic TOS and accounts for 2% to 3% of cases.[21,39] Venous obstruction produces swelling, edema, cyanosis, and discomfort of the arm that is aggravated with exercise. Patients may have a sudden onset of symptoms because of subclavian vein thrombosis. The natural clinical course is protracted, with continued disability. Collateral venous circulation develops over time and may be evident as distended superficial veins of the shoulder and chest. Vigorous activity is often difficult in the presence of chronic subclavian vein occlusion.

Arterial Symptoms

Arterial involvement is the least common form of presentation, constituting 1% to 2% of cases.[21,39] These patients exhibit signs of ischemia: pain, pallor, pulselessness, and coolness of the affected side. They often experience fatigue of the arm with exercise and ischemic claudication, particularly with the arm elevated. Ischemic ulcers on the hand or gangrenous fingertips may occur because of thrombosis or embolization; this indicates severe narrowing or aneurysm of the subclavian artery. Retrograde embolization to the brain circulation can occur. In the authors' series, 1.5% of all surgical TOS patients (43% of arterial TOS patients) exhibited vertebrobasilar stroke (unpublished data).

Exacerbating Factors

Symptoms are typically exacerbated with increased arm activity and elevation, particularly overhead, abducted, and externally rotated arm positions. Common activities such as combing the hair, reaching or working with the arms overhead, or even driving a car with the hands on top of the steering wheel can cause symptoms. With prolonged use of the upper extremities, patients may describe feelings of tiredness, weakness, or heaviness and note relief with lowering the arms. The paresthesias are often nocturnal, awakening the patient with a feeling of numbness or, more commonly, pain. Sleep disturbance is common. Heavy work during the day may be followed by misery at night.

Diagnosis

The diagnosis of TOS is still controversial, because objective findings are few. No single clinical or objective test has been accepted as definitively establishing the diagnosis. The overall clinical evaluation is critical, because the diagnosis of TOS is usually based on patient history, subjective complaints, and findings on physical examination. The workup begins with a thorough history, including onset of symptoms, any exacerbating or alleviating factors, history of trauma, and complaints in the head, neck, shoulder, and upper extremity.

Physical Examination

The physical examination should not be limited to testing for TOS. It should focus on all the patient's problems and be geared toward ruling out more common causes of symptoms in the upper extremity, such as cervical stenosis, carpal tunnel syndrome, or cubital tunnel syndrome. After a general examination, attention is turned to the neck, shoulder, and upper extremities, especially to the intrinsic muscles of the hand and the distribution of sensory changes. Both extremities need to be examined, regardless of whether they are symptomatic. Patients with obvious venous or arterial TOS may have a much clearer clinical picture and objective findings than those with neurogenic TOS.

Inspection and Palpation

The initial examination of the upper extremity should begin with inspection and palpation for discoloration, such as blanching, cyanosis, or gangrene; muscle atrophy; abnormal fingernail and hair growth; and temperature, moisture, and pulse. A note should be made of abnormal distension of veins, which could be collateral vessels, particularly around the shoulder. The symmetry and positional change of the vessels should be noted.[43] Muscle atrophy, particularly in the hypothenar, is not common, but not rare, in TOS. The hands should be examined at the same time and compared with each other.

The supraclavicular and infraclavicular areas should be examined by palpation. In patients with TOS, there is often tenderness to compression over the anterior scalene muscle. Reduced sensation to light touch may be present in the involved fingers. Peripheral pulsation and blood pressure should be examined in both arms. A difference in blood pressure between the two arms of more than 20 mm Hg suggests blockage of the arterial circulation. The Allen test is useful for evaluating the integrity of the palmar arch; however, it is generally not helpful in diagnosing TOS.

Auscultation

Auscultation should begin in the supraclavicular fossa bilaterally. It should then be performed with the stethoscope just beneath the middle third of the clavicle beginning with the arm in the neutral position and then gradually bringing it up into the abducted and externally rotated position. This is done while palpating the radial pulse. If obliteration of the radial pulse occurs, the stethoscope should be moved laterally in the infraclavicular area, then medially in the supraclavicular area, to detect bruits and a site of compressive occlusion. Because blood flow may be totally obliterated at the thoracic outlet, the maneuver should be performed slowly so as not to overlook bruits.[43]

Muscle Strength Test

Because muscle weakness can be one of the objective findings of TOS, the strength of all muscle groups of the arm should be tested. Patients may have weakness of the shoulder girdle muscles (deltoid), biceps, and triceps in cases of upper plexus compression (C5 to C7) and weakness of the intrinsic muscles of the hands in lower plexus compression (C8 to T1). Note that most TOS patients (85% to 90%) have combined symptoms of upper and lower plexus compression.[40] The patient is asked to make a ring with the thumb (the thenar muscle innervated by the median nerve) and the little finger (the hypothenar muscle innervated by the ulnar nerve) against resistance. The interosseous muscles are tested using the interdigital card test and spreading the fingers apart against resistance. Grip strength should be measured with dynamometry.

Provocative Clinical Tests

Positional and pressure maneuvers that increase pressure on the nerve may be used to elicit symptoms and make a clinical diagnosis. The patient should complain of reproduction of symptoms in the correct nerve distribution. However, these results should be interpreted carefully. Obliteration of a peripheral pulse or even the production of symptoms during the examination does not necessarily mean pathology; this may occur in normal individuals. These tests should be used to supplement other physical, radiographic, or historical findings that point to the diagnosis. These provocative tests (pressure, position, and Tinel) should also be performed at the common distal sites of nerve compression in the upper extremity to determine any concomitant sites of nerve compression that may be present and contributing to the patient's symptoms.[23]

Tinel's Sign. Tinel's sign (distal tingling on percussion) should be considered positive if the patient complains of a radiating tingling sensation in the arm when tapping over the brachial plexus at the supraclavicular area.

Adson Test. The Adson test is performed by holding the patient's arm down while the head is turned toward the affected side with slight cervical extension.[14] The radial pulse is evaluated when the patient inspires deeply. This maneuver may narrow the scalene triangle, compressing the subclavian artery and brachial plexus. It should be considered positive when the radial pulse is obliterated or diminished or symptoms are reproduced.

Abduction and External Rotation Test and Wright's Hyperabduction Test. The abduction and external rotation test requires abducting the arms to 90 degrees in external rotation, which rotates the clavicle and subclavius muscle posteriorly and inferiorly. Wright's hyperabduction test is performed with the shoulders hyperabducted to 180 degrees and rotated externally while turning the head away from the affected side.[44] Symptoms caused by a narrow interscalene space are aggravated by abduction of the extremity because the nerves are pushed up against the tight, narrow area, increasing pressure on them. Deep inspiration with breath holding may accentuate an ambiguous response. The patient is checked for any change in pulse and any symptoms in the arm. The test should be considered positive when the radial pulse is obliterated or diminished or if symptoms, such as weakness, tiredness, and numbness in the arm and paresthesia in the fingers, are reproduced. The duration of these provocative tests should not exceed 2 minutes and preferably should last only 1 minute. Care must be taken to avoid misdiagnosing an ulnar nerve neuropathy at the elbow.

Elevated Arm Stress Test. The elevated arm stress test (or Roos test) requires the shoulders to be abducted and externally rotated 90 degrees and the elbows flexed 90 degrees with rapid opening and closing of the hands.[30] This test is performed for up to 3 minutes, as long as the patient has no complaint. Reproduction of symptoms, such as fatigue, cramping, pain, or paresthesia, within 3 minutes is considered a positive test.

Laboratory Tests

Electrophysiologic Tests

Because the majority of symptoms of TOS are caused by neural compression, a variety of electrophysiologic tests have been proposed for the objective diagnosis of TOS. However, because compression is positional and intermittent, and electrophysiologic change may occur in late cases,[41] these tests have a low level of sensitivity for TOS diagnosis.[19] A positive electrophysiologic study confirms the clinical diagnosis of TOS, but a negative finding does not exclude its presence. These tests may also be useful in the differential diagnosis of more peripheral nerve lesions, such as median nerve compression at the carpal tunnel or ulnar nerve compression at the cubital tunnel or Guyon canal.

Electromyography. Sensory function is involved in most patients with TOS. Because electromyography evaluates motor nerve function, findings are usually normal.

Nerve Conduction Velocity. The typical findings of nerve conduction studies in patients with TOS are as follows: normal sensory and low-amplitude motor responses in the median nerve region; low-amplitude sensory and relatively low- or normal-amplitude responses in the ulnar nerve region.[19,45]

F-Wave Responses. When a peripheral nerve is stimulated percutaneously and the centrally propagated (antidromic) impulse reaches the motor neuron in the spinal cord, some of the impulses will be reflected back down the axon in an orthodromic direction. This "reflected" potential is called an *F wave*.[46] In some settings, quantitative measurements can enhance the sensitivity of this electrophysiologic response.[47]

Somatosensory Evoked Potentials. Progress has been made in facilitating the objective evaluation of neurogenic TOS by recording somatosensory evoked potentials across the brachial plexus and in the supraclavicular fossa and cervical spinal cord.[48,49] The most characteristic abnormality found in patients with neurogenic TOS is a reduction in the amplitude of the ulnar nerve response at the N9 electrode, or Erb's point, or the brachial plexus recording electrode, whereas the median somatosensory evoked potential is normal. This dampening of the N9 amplitude can be accentuated, or the potential completely ablated, by placing the arm in the abducted and externally rotated position, which is the most symptomatic position for patients with TOS.

Anatomic Studies

Plain Radiography. Plain radiographs of the cervical spine and shoulder should be obtained in all patients being evaluated for TOS to identify bony or other abnormalities that might be the cause of compression, including cervical disk disease, an abnormal first rib, a cervical rib, elongated C7 transverse processes, or shoulder pathology. Cervical ribs and long transverse processes at C7 may be the origin of radiolucent congenital bands to the first thoracic rib.[22,41] Patients with a low-lying shoulder girdle have a narrow costoclavicular space. A chest radiograph should be obtained to rule out the presence of Pancoast tumor at the apex of the lung.

Computed Tomography and Magnetic Resonance Imaging. Computed tomography (CT) scanning is not conclusively diagnostic in TOS patients. Brantigan and Roos claimed that a high-speed multidetector CT study with contrast is a promising technique because spatial resolution is much better than with magnetic resonance imaging (MRI), and the study is faster.[41] Individual muscles can be visualized and peeled back using computer techniques.

MRI has also been proposed for the diagnosis of TOS because of its better visualization of soft tissues; fibrous bands and brachial plexus deviation have been shown.[50] Using special sequences, Collins and others[51] have performed detailed studies of the thoracic outlet with a high degree of accuracy in diagnosing TOS compression. These tests are helpful to confirm compression, but it should be noted that such compression may not necessarily be the cause of the patient's symptoms. MRI is also useful to rule out other causes, such as tumor. Impaired venous flow at the thoracic outlet can be demonstrated by MRI without contrast medium.

Arteriography. Angiography is not indicated in patients with neurologic symptoms alone. Positional arterial obstruction can usually be confirmed by simple physical examination. Arteriography should be reserved for patients in whom arterial involvement is suspected by clinical findings: an infraclavicular or supraclavicular bruit, absent radial pulse, significant blood pressure difference between arms (>20 mm Hg), limb ischemia, suspicion of embolization, or pulsating paraclavicular mass.

In patients with arterial thoracic outlet compression, arteriography and venography in the upper extremities should be performed in the neutral position, with the arm at the patient's side, and in the stress position, with the upper arm at right angles to the chest. The use of digital intravenous angiography, which allows the patient to be radiographed in the sitting position, demonstrates a much higher yield of arterial compression lesions, correlating much more closely with the clinical findings (Figure 31-5). We often perform the positional exposures with the patient's hand behind the head. If this is not done, many of the compressive abnormalities at the thoracic outlet are missed.

Venography. Venography is indicated if venous involvement is suspected. Venograms with the patient's arm

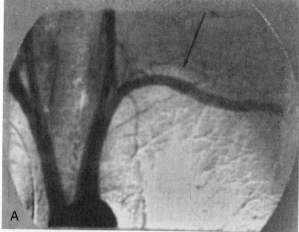
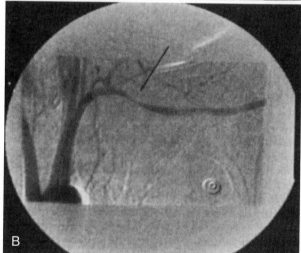

FIGURE 31-5 ■ Digital intravenous axillosubclavian angiogram obtained in the supine **(A)** and sitting **(B)** positions to demonstrate thoracic outlet compressive changes *(arrows)*, which are often seen only in the sitting position.

in various positions can show intermittent occlusion or complete occlusion with collateralization (Figure 31-6). Magnetic resonance angiography is also being used for that purpose.[41] Early venography combined with catheter-directed thrombolysis is indicated in a patient with acute occlusion of the axillosubclavian vein, an acutely swollen upper extremity, or when the possibility of Paget-Schroetter syndrome exists.

Provocative Tests (Scalene Muscle Block)

A newer test with high sensitivity and specificity for the diagnosis of neurogenic TOS is the electromyogram-guided selective scalene block. The method and results have been reported by Jordan and Machleder.[52] Anesthetic blocks of the anterior scalene muscle have been used as a method of diagnosing and confirming TOS and for predicting which patients may benefit from surgical decompression.[28] When a local anesthetic agent is injected into the anterior scalene muscle and paralyzes it temporarily, the patient's symptoms caused by compression are

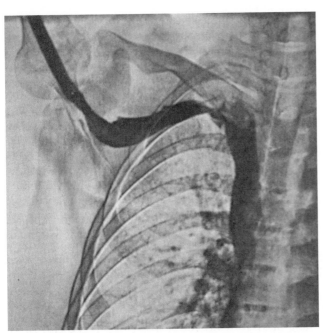

FIGURE 31-6 ■ Typical venographic picture of axillosubclavian compression at the thoracic outlet that eventually leads to thrombosis and an acute clinical presentation. Note that the right upper extremity is hyperabducted.

relieved for a few hours to a few days. However, the standard technique of using surface landmarks often results in inadvertent somatic and sympathetic block because there is no reliable way to verify needle tip localization.[19]

Jordan and Machleder[47,52] reported that electrophysiologic guidance facilitates accurate needle tip placement in the performance of anterior scalene muscle blocks. A Teflon-coated, 25-gauge hypodermic needle, bared at the tip, is advanced through the sternocleidomastoid muscle. Electromyographic activity is monitored as the needle is advanced through the tissue layers; the anterior scalene muscle can be activated with lateral neck bending against resistance and with deep inspiration. In most patients, a twitch of the scalene muscles is visible with electrical stimulation. The patient is asked whether pain is produced and whether insertion at this depth produces pain that is similar in quality and location to the usual pain experienced. After an injection of 2 mL of 2% lidocaine into the anterior scalene muscle, the arm is placed into a stress position and exercised for 1 minute; the patient is then asked to rate the pain. Attempts to activate the anterior scalene muscle are performed again with lateral neck movement and with deep inspiration, but only distant motor action potentials can be identified. Electrical stimulation can no longer produce a visible twitch of the scalene muscles. A positive test occurs if the patient has greater than 50% improvement in the elevated arm stress pain score after anesthetic injection of the anterior scalene muscle compared with a baseline examination. The results of these blocks correlate with surgical outcomes; a positive result predicts a good outcome to surgical decompression. Note that the absence of pain relief does not exclude the presence of TOS, as long as the patient has symptoms and clinical findings.

Differential Diagnosis

Failure to make the correct diagnosis or to appreciate the presence of other problems is a major concern in the treatment of patients with TOS.[53] It is not uncommon for TOS to coexist with other conditions; in particular, lung tumors, cardiac disease, and psychiatric disorders should be considered, as well as cervical spine, neurologic, and musculoskeletal disorders.

Cervical Spine Disorders

Neurovascular compression of the cervical spine can cause intermittent pain and tenderness in the neck and back of the head, often radiating down the arm in the radial nerve distribution. Provocative maneuvers include head turning with tilting back and the Spurling test (pressing the forehead downward), which can reproduce symptoms. MRI of the cervical spine is useful for the diagnosis.

Neurologic Disorders

A double-crush syndrome may be present in TOS patients, which refers to two coexisting entrapment syndromes, commonly carpal tunnel syndrome or cubital tunnel syndrome combined with brachial plexus compression.[54,55] If surgical intervention is necessary, the more peripheral entrapment should be treated first.

Cubital Tunnel Syndrome (Ulnar Nerve Entrapment at the Elbow). The ulnar nerve originates from the C8 to T1 nerve routes and supplies motor branches to the flexor carpi ulnaris and the medial half of the flexor digitorum profundus. It can be entrapped as it courses through the ulnar groove behind the medial condyle of the humerus. Its compression at the elbow produces tingling pain, with paresthesias and numbness in the ulnar distribution (the last two fingers) but few symptoms in the shoulder and neck. The presence of medial forearm numbness can also help to delineate TOS from ulnar neuropathy, because that area is innervated by the medial antebrachial cutaneous nerve (lower cord of brachial plexus; C8 and T1 nerve roots). Electrophysiologic tests are useful for the diagnosis.

Carpal Tunnel Syndrome. Carpal tunnel syndrome is caused by compression of the median nerve by the carpal ligament at the wrist. Because it is a pure median neuropathy, the first three fingers are involved predominantly, delineating it from TOS. Carpal tunnel syndrome typically produces symptoms that originate in the hand and radiate up the arm, in contrast to TOS, which produces pain in the neck and shoulder that moves down to the hand. Tinel sign elicited by tapping the volar wrist crease and the Phalen test (wrist flexion) are helpful in making the diagnosis. Confirmation is achieved with electrodiagnostic studies that show delayed nerve conduction across the wrist.

Musculoskeletal Disorders

Shoulder Pathology. Inflammation or tears of the tendons around the shoulder cause reduced shoulder range of motion and tenderness at the biceps and rotator cuff tendons. MRI is helpful in making the diagnosis.

Complex Regional Pain Syndrome. Complex regional pain syndrome (CRPS) is a neuropathic pain disorder that involves dysfunction of the peripheral and central nervous systems.[56,57] It may develop after trauma. CRPS type I (without a definable nerve lesion) and type II (with a definable nerve lesion) were formerly known as *reflex sympathetic dystrophy* and *causalgia*, respectively. CRPS is clinically characterized by sensory (burning, spontaneous pain, allodynia, hyperalgesia), autonomic (edema, sweating abnormalities, change in skin color or temperature), and motor (muscle weakness, postural or action tremor, decreased range of motion, muscle spasms, dystonia) disturbances. In chronic stages, trophic changes such as abnormal nail growth, increased or decreased hair growth, fibrosis, thin glossy skin, and osteoporosis may be present. Patients with CRPS commonly suffer from psychological dysfunction (depression, anxiety, phobia).

Conservative Management

In general, conservative treatment should be tried initially in every patient with TOS except for those with severe, long-standing symptoms and those with obvious neurologic signs, ischemic symptoms, or venous obstruction.[19] It includes education and instruction, several types of physical therapy modalities, and medication.

Education

Patient education is important to encourage compliance with treatment. The purpose of treatment and its expected benefits should be understood. Even a simple explanation of the syndrome and reassurance may satisfy some patients. A review of factors that exacerbate or relieve symptoms and previous successful or unsuccessful treatment is valuable. In some cases, modification of activities of daily living or work habits can help the patient's symptoms, particularly the avoidance of repetitive activities, overhead work, and weight lifting. A slower work pace with frequent short breaks should be emphasized. Many individuals experience sleep disturbances. These patients should be instructed how to rest and protect the cervical spine at night to avoid irritating positions. Obesity, breast hypertrophy, and general physical condition may contribute to symptoms in some patients.

Posture

Most patients with TOS have subtle or obvious posture deformities. Forward-flexed postures exacerbate TOS symptoms.[23,58] A postural assessment, including the spine, should be performed initially.[59,60] Rebalance and strengthening of the muscular and skeletal system, particularly the cervicoscapular muscles, can correct poor posture, which helps relax the neck muscles and decompress the brachial plexus. Good posture should be maintained when sitting, standing, and walking.[59]

Exercise

The home program is initially directed toward range-of-motion exercises and stretching exercises for scalene muscles and other tight muscles. Then it can gradually strengthen the shoulder girdle muscles, including the trapezius, rhomboids, and levator scapulae muscles.[19,28] Elevating the arms above 90 degrees abduction should be avoided. It may take more than 2 to 3 months for symptomatic improvement to occur.

Medication

Patients can get relief from various medications, including analgesics, muscle relaxants, nonsteroidal antiinflammatory drugs, and antidepressants. Pain clinics and biofeedback can be recommended for pain relief. Edema control with compressive garments, elevation, and retrograde massage is beneficial if swelling is present. Most patients are helped by conservative treatment and can manage their lives and tolerate their discomfort without surgery. If the symptoms have improved enough so that the patient can live with them, conservative therapy should be continued.

Surgical Considerations and Technique

Indications

The goal of surgery is to decompress the neurovascular structure at the thoracic outlet space. If there are vascular complications, direct approaches to the subclavian artery and vein should be considered, as well as decompression. Surgical procedures are directed toward a variety of normal and abnormal structures, including the anterior and middle scalene muscles (two sides of the scalene triangle), the first rib, the cervical rib, fibrous bands, and ligaments. Besides confirming the diagnosis and ruling out more common causes of symptoms in the upper extremity, indications for surgery include (1) failure of conservative management and physical therapy after several months; (2) completion of treatment of all associated conditions; (3) disability in terms of work, recreation, or daily activities; and (4) vascular complications. Kashyap and colleagues[61] reviewed some of the advantages and disadvantages of different surgical approaches.

Transaxillary Rib Resection and Partial Scalenectomy

The transaxillary rib resection and partial scalenectomy was originally described by Roos in 1966 and is arguably the most common approach used for thoracic outlet decompression.[16] First rib resection is recommended mainly for the lower type of TOS with C8 to T1 root symptoms.[19] Supraclavicular scalenectomy is applicable in patients with the upper type of TOS involving C5 to C7 roots[40] or in those with recurrence after first rib resection, thought to be due to scarring of the scalenes.[62] The surgical strategy for neurogenic TOS is (1) transaxillary first rib resection and subtotal lower scalenectomy as a primary procedure and (2) completion scalenectomy with a supraclavicular approach for patients with recurrent symptoms who need surgery.

Technique. The patient is placed in the semisupine lateral position (45 to 60 degrees) with a soft axillary roll placed under the dependent axilla. The ipsilateral arm, neck, chest wall, and axilla are prepared. The arm is covered with a sterile cotton stockinette, wrapped with a gauze bandage, and placed in a sterile arm holder for retraction. Retraction of the arm to the contralateral side and upward provides better visualization of the neurovascular structures in the axillary tunnel. However, it is important to avoid overzealous arm retraction with this approach, and occasional intermittent release of traction prevents arm ischemia or brachial plexus injury.

A transverse incision is made just below the hair-bearing area in the axilla between the pectoralis major

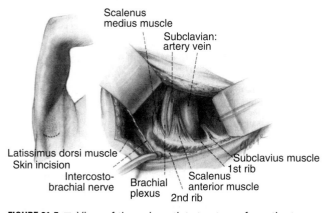

FIGURE 31-7 ■ View of thoracic outlet structures from the transaxillary approach to first rib resection. (From Machleder HI, editor: Vascular disorders of the upper extremity, ed 2, Mt. Kisco, N.Y., 1989, Futura Publishing.)

and latissimus dorsi muscles (Figure 31-7). The incision is deepened in the subcutaneous tissue until the chest wall is reached. The thoracoepigastric vein should be divided for adequate exposure. The brachiointercostal nerve may also have to be sacrificed to gain adequate exposure. A tissue plane deep to the axillary fascia and on top of the serratus anterior is bluntly dissected superiorly and anteriorly through loose areolar tissue. The highest thoracic artery, a branch from the axillary artery penetrating the first intercostal space, should be identified, ligated, and divided to avoid troublesome bleeding. Using further blunt dissection with a sponge-tipped hemostat, the loose tissue is cleared to identify the first rib. The subclavian vein, anterior scalene muscle, subclavian artery, brachial plexus, and middle scalene muscle are carefully dissected (see Figure 31-7). The phrenic nerve anterior to the anterior scalene muscle must be identified and carefully protected. It is necessary to lift the arm carefully to facilitate the exposure. To avoid serious injury, the blade of the retractor must not apply traction to the nerve roots or the brachial plexus.

Once the anterior scalene muscle is dissected and the vessels are free, a right-angled clamp placed under the muscle elevates it away from other structures as the muscle is divided with scissors as far from the first rib as possible. The smallest scalene muscle, if it exists, is divided off the Sibson fascia and the C7 transverse process. The middle scalene muscle is dissected and divided with scissors at the highest level feasible, with a right-angled clamp placed to hook the muscle. The long thoracic nerve posterior to the middle scalene muscle must be identified and carefully protected. The first rib resection is performed in an extraperiosteal fashion, except in areas where the vein or artery may be adherent to the periosteum and prone to tearing, where subperiosteal dissection is required. The intercostal muscle is pushed away by blunt dissection with a periosteal elevator (Figure 31-8*A*). The first rib is then

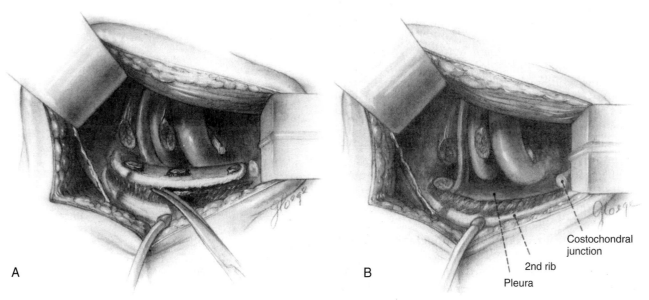

FIGURE 31-8 ■ Steps in transaxillary first rib resection. **A,** Division of subclavius, anterior scalene, and middle scalene tendons, as well as initial incision of the intercostal muscle. **B,** Relationship of structures after removal of the first rib.

freed circumferentially by the periosteal elevator and a blunt-tip right-angled clamp anteriorly and posteriorly. With a Roos nerve protector shielding the C8 and T1 nerve roots, an angled bone-cutting instrument is carefully placed on the posterior neck of the rib and applied to cut the rib posteriorly. The subclavius tendon is divided sharply to the sternal joint space with a scalpel under direct vision, with careful protection of the vein. The rib is then divided anteriorly with a Bethune rib shear. The rib is thus detached and removed from the field (see Figure 31-8*B*). A large-angled bone rongeur is used to trim the anterior remaining end of the rib to the sternal joint. The posterior stump of the first rib is further truncated close to the transverse process using a box-shaped bone cutter. Any sharp bony fragments must be identified with visual inspection or palpation and removed. Any additional soft tissue bands crossing the brachial plexus nerve roots are sought and carefully divided. The remaining anterior and middle scalene muscles are trimmed further until the stumps are above the neurovascular bundle.

A drainage tube connected with closed suction is brought out through a separate stab wound below the incision. After closure of the subcutaneous tissue, the skin is closed using monofilament polypropylene suture with plastic surgery technique.

During the performance of this operation, adequate lighting and visualization need to be maintained because of the configuration and depth of the operative field. Cautery must not be used after reaching the first rib for fear of injuring the neurovascular structures.

Advantages and Limitations. This approach allows rapid exposure of the first rib without much manipulation of the subclavian vessels or brachial plexus. The incision itself is cosmetically appealing and allows for rapid recovery, and most patients leave the hospital on the first postoperative day. Many groups have used this procedure with short- and long-term success.[40,63,64] A cervical rib can be managed through the axillary approach.

The drawbacks of this approach are directly related to the operative view. Visualization is through a long axillary tunnel that must be adequately lighted to prevent injury, which occurs most commonly to the axillary vein or T1 nerve root.[65] A supplementary light source from a headlight is indispensable, and a fiber-optic lighted retractor is paramount for the safe conduct of this operation. Congenital fibromuscular bands are sometimes hidden from view because they are most often medial and superior to the first rib and obscured by the neurovascular bundle.

In patients with arterial complications, an associated upper dorsal sympathectomy can be added easily. However, satisfactory exposure of the subclavian-axillary artery and its reconstruction are technically daunting.

Supraclavicular Scalenectomy with or without Rib Resection

Procedures performed through a supraclavicular approach include anterior and middle scalenectomy alone or combined with first rib resection.

Technique. This anterior approach to the thoracic outlet requires that the patient be placed supine. An incision is made in the supraclavicular area approximately 1 to 2 cm above and parallel to the clavicle between the internal and external jugular veins. Subplatysmal flaps are constructed, and the clavicular head of the sternocleidomastoid must be divided. The internal jugular vein is retracted medially, and if one is operating on the left side, the thoracic duct is carefully identified and may be ligated. The scalene fat pad must be reflected laterally or superiorly to arrive at the anterior scalene muscle. Coursing on the anteromedial surface of the anterior scalene muscle is the phrenic nerve, which must be carefully dissected free of the muscle and protected without undue tension. Next, the muscle is transected at a low point, with care to avoid injuring the underlying subclavian artery. A simple scalenectomy has been advocated by some and requires division of the muscle close to its origin at the cervical transverse processes.[66,67] However, many practitioners advocate completion of the decompression by removing the first rib as well. Rib resection requires mobilization of the brachial plexus and division of the middle scalene muscle (Figures 31-9 and 31-10). The long thoracic nerve exits in the posterolateral aspect of the middle scalene muscle and indicates the lateral margin of muscle division. Even after division of the scalenes, the operative wound should be palpated to identify any remaining fibrous or muscular bands causing compression. If a cervical rib is present, it will be found within the fibers of the middle scalene muscle. An extraperiosteal first rib resection is performed and requires detachment of the intercostal muscles at the inferior aspect of the first rib.[68] A subperiosteal resection of the rib may allow easier separation of the intercostals and less bleeding; however, reossification in the periosteal bed may lead to recurrent symptoms. Division of the first rib posteriorly is done as close to the transverse process as possible and requires gentle retraction of the brachial plexus

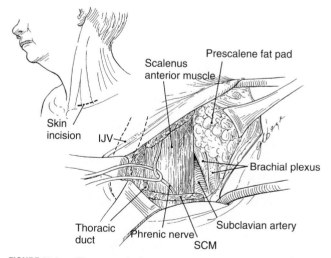

FIGURE 31-9 ■ Transcervical approach to scalenectomy for relief of thoracic outlet compression syndrome. The relationship of major surrounding anatomic structures is depicted. *IJV*, Internal jugular vein; *SCM*, sternocleidomastoid muscle. (From Machleder HI, Moll FL: Surgery for thoracic outlet syndrome. In Trout HH 3rd, DePalma RG, editors: Reoperative vascular surgery, New York, 1987, Marcel Dekker.)

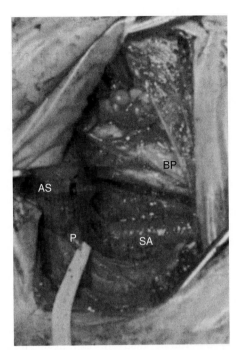

FIGURE 31-10 ■ Operative view of transcervical approach after resection of anterior scalene muscle. *AS,* Anterior scalene muscle stump; *BP,* brachial plexus; *P,* phrenic nerve; *SA,* subclavian artery.

anteromedially. After separation of the pleura and subclavian vessels from the first rib periosteum with blunt dissection, the rib is divided as anteriorly as possible, with retraction and separation of the subclavian vein and artery. The anterior division of the first rib has proved problematic in some patients, and some authors recommend a routine infraclavicular counterincision for rib division close to the costochondral junction, which is usually required for venous TOS.[69]

Advantages and Limitations. The main advantages of the supraclavicular approach are an excellent view of the structures in the thoracic outlet, with wide exposure and the ability to perform arterial reconstruction if necessary. Cervical ribs or prolonged transverse processes are easily removed with this approach.[70] Long-term success in correcting compressive symptoms has been documented.[71,72]

This approach requires the dissection and mobilization of the phrenic nerve, brachial plexus, and long thoracic nerve, which leads to its major disadvantage—the risk of nerve damage caused by traction injury or transection of these structures.[65] This approach is also limited for venous TOS.

Combined Approach

Technique. The combined approach requires the patient to be placed in the lateral decubitus position for the transaxillary approach and then moved to the supine position for the supraclavicular approach. Once the first rib resection is complete, the anterior and middle scalenectomy can be performed easily because most of the distal insertions were already released from the first rib during resection.

Advantages and Limitations. The transaxillary approach allows removal of the first rib in a safe and expeditious manner, and the supraclavicular approach allows complete scalenectomy and arterial reconstruction. The combination of both procedures allows complete decompression of the thoracic outlet and correction of the arterial source of embolization in one setting. This approach can be used in selected patients but is not needed for most patients with TOS.[73,74]

Posterior Approach

Technique. The posterior approach requires a posterior periscapular incision, with division of the trapezius muscle and elevation of the scapula. With superior retraction, the thoracic outlet can be reached and the first rib freed from the surrounding structures. In Clagett's original description,[15] the rib is essentially removed subperiosteally, but then as much periosteum is removed as necessary to prevent bony regeneration.

Advantages and Limitations. Experience with this approach indicates that it might have a role in a few selected patients needing exposure of the proximal brachial plexus roots, particularly at the intraforaminal level.[75] Patients with prior anterior irradiation and tissue fibrosis who require exposure of the thoracic outlet or those requiring reoperations for TOS may also benefit from this approach.

This approach has not been widely accepted because of the relatively high morbidity compared with other surgical options. The incision and posterior dissection lead to considerable postoperative pain and shoulder disability. Furthermore, visualization of the anterior structures is difficult, and arterial reconstruction is impossible with this approach.

Postoperative Care

An upright chest radiograph is performed in the recovery room to detect pneumothorax or phrenic nerve injury. A large pneumothorax may need transthoracic aspiration, but small air collections usually resolve spontaneously. Pain medication should be prescribed. Most patients leave the hospital on the first postoperative day. The closed suction drain is usually removed in the outpatient clinic once the total amount of lymphatic fluid discharge is less than 30 mL per 24 hours. Showering with sutures in place is allowed once drain sites are closed. Patients are encouraged to use the affected side to perform activities of daily living and to begin a home exercise program (arm exercises at least three to four times per day) starting on day 1. These exercises help to prevent a "frozen" shoulder. Heavy lifting (more than 5 lb) should be avoided until 3 to 4 weeks after surgery. Patients are usually seen for a follow-up visit within 2 weeks after surgery. Many patients return to work in 4 to 6 weeks. Sutures with plastic surgery technique should be removed 3 to 4 weeks postoperatively to prevent hypertrophic scars and keloids.

Typically, patients undergoing surgery have had symptoms for a long time, and even after decompression surgery, they often have some residual or intermittent symptoms of dysesthesia, numbness, or other tolerable symptoms that may need ongoing attention.

Surgical Complications

Vascular, nervous, and lymphatic injuries can occur from decompression surgery for TOS.

Pneumothorax

Intraoperative pneumothorax occurs once the pleura is torn during the rib resection. It has been reported in up to one third of cases, being the most common complication of first rib resection.[53] However, the condition usually resolves spontaneously or by transthoracic aspiration without a chest tube. A closed suction drain is used routinely and usually eliminates the need for a chest tube.

Nerve Injuries

Brachial plexus injury, either temporary or permanent, represents one of the most serious complications. This occurs as a result of excessive and prolonged traction of the arm in the transaxillary approach. Occasional intermittent release of arm traction is important during surgery. Another cause is inadvertent nerve traction during exposure of the scalene muscle or the first rib in the supraclavicular approach. Direct operative injury may also occur; the lower plexus (C8 and T1) is more commonly injured because it is in close proximity to the posterior end of the first rib. This injury is major and usually permanent. The motor deficit includes the long flexors of the fingers and the intrinsic muscles of the hand, although the sensory deficit involves only the small finger in the hand and the medial side of the forearm.[53] In large series, the incidence of permanent brachial plexus is less than 1% with each approach.[37,40,66]

The phrenic nerve, based on its relationship with the anterior scalene muscle, is prone to injury during scalenectomy, particularly with supraclavicular approach. The nerve should be carefully defined, using a nerve stimulator if necessary, before anterior scalenectomy. It should then be kept within a vessel loop. Although most injuries are temporary, they may take months to resolve. In patients with bilateral TOS requiring operation on the contralateral side, it is essential to ensure that phrenic nerve paresis has completely resolved before a second operation. If not, it can result in complete diaphragmatic paralysis and severe ventilatory incapacity.[76]

Long thoracic nerve injury can occur during middle scalenectomy. The nerve should be identified before excising the muscle. Traction injury to the long thoracic nerve may result in a winged scapula, although this is usually transient. Division of the nerve results in a permanent winged scapula.

The intercostobrachial nerve usually originates from the second intercostal nerve. It appears under the second rib in the midaxillary line, at the midpoint of the transaxillary wound. Injury to this nerve results in temporary or permanent numbness or paresthesias on the medial aspect of the arm. The nerve is often sacrificed deliberately to allow better exposure of the thoracic outlet structures.

Injury to the Subclavian Artery and Vein

Vascular injury in the transaxillary approach may be difficult to visualize, because the exposure is deep and limited, and the rib or the muscle may hide the injury. If the field becomes bloody, it is prudent to pack the operative field for a few minutes rather than proceeding. Most injuries are small initially. After tamponade of the vessel or removal of the rib, vessel repair can proceed. Another incision may be necessary to control the artery proximally if the bleeding is major.

Lymphatic Leakage

The thoracic duct usually empties into the venous system at the junction of the left subclavian vein and the internal jugular vein. However, the anatomy may be variable; there may be double ducts or significant branches.[77] Injury to the thoracic duct can occur in the supraclavicular approach on the left side, but it is rare through the transaxillary approach or on the right side. The duct should be controlled with a suture or a vascular clip to prevent chylothorax.

Results of Surgical Treatment for Neurogenic Thoracic Outlet Syndrome

Decompression surgery for TOS has few standard objective criteria for evaluation, and most postoperative results are reported with a subjective grading of success that relies on the patient's response to treatment. Functional outcome is an important parameter, as is improvement of symptoms. Thus, the patient's ability to return to the same job provides a good index of operative success. Recent studies reported that the *Disabilities of the Arm, Shoulder, and Hand* questionnaire can be a valid and objective test for evaluating the functional state after TOS surgery.[78,79]

Primary success can be defined as 50% improvement or greater on the ipsilateral side of the operation or the patient's return to preoperative work status without the need for an additional ipsilateral procedure. Secondary success is similarly defined following an additional ipsilateral procedure. Altobelli and colleagues[80] conducted a review of 9 years of experience with 254 primary first rib resections with partial scalenectomy via a transaxillary approach, followed by 80 secondary operations for recurrent symptoms using the supraclavicular scalenectomy in 185 patients.[80] The initial success rate at 2 months was 86.6% for primary procedures. Life-table analysis revealed that the primary success rates were 46.9% at 18 months, 37.6% at 36 months, and 36.0% at 72 months. The secondary success rates were 71.7% at 18 months, 58.9% at 36 months, and 49.1% at 72 months (Figure 31-11). In evaluating these results, length of follow-up is a crucial factor, because recurrent TOS usually occurs within 18 months after the initial surgery; 90% and 65%

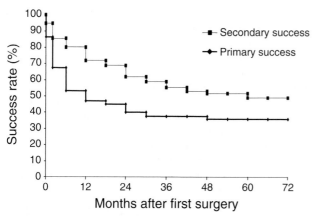

FIGURE 31-11 ■ Life-table analysis for primary and secondary clinical success rates after transaxillary first rib resection with partial scalenectomy followed by supraclavicular scalenectomy. Note that 90% and 65% of failures occur within 18 months of primary and secondary success, respectively. (From Altobelli GG, Kudo T, Haas BT, et al: Thoracic outlet syndrome: pattern of clinical success following surgical decompression. J Vasc Surg 42:111–117, 2005.)

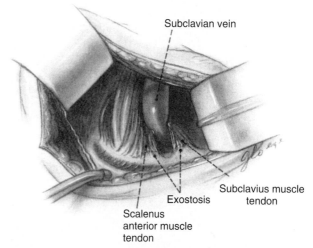

FIGURE 31-12 ■ Typical Paget-Schroetter abnormality. Hypertrophy of the subclavius tendon and associated exostoses are seen at the subclavius and anterior scalene insertions to the first rib (visualized from the transaxillary surgical approach). The vein is compressed in the most medial area of the thoracic outlet. (From Kunkel JM, Machleder HI: Treatment of Paget-Schroetter syndrome: a staged multidisciplinary approach. Arch Surg 124:1153–1158, 1989.)

of failures occurred within 18 months of primary and secondary success, respectively. Therefore reports with short-term follow-up could mask the overall success rate of the procedures performed.

Reported results in the literature were similar. Improvement of neurogenic TOS symptoms may be noticed shortly after surgery, sometimes immediately.[19] The initially high percentage of improvement generally decreases after a few years.[19] When comparing different approaches, Sanders' review of the surgical results for TOS showed some interesting data.[81] Transaxillary, supraclavicular, infraclavicular, posterior, and transpleural first rib resection, as well as scalenectomy and combined rib resection, all had similar success rates. In addition, in Sanders and coworkers' own series,[37,82] which included transaxillary first rib resection, anterior and middle scalenectomy, and combined scalenectomy and rib resection, the 3- to 5-year success rate—with *success* being defined as enough symptomatic improvement for the patient to believe that the surgery was worthwhile—was approximately the same, and the overall improvement was 70% using life-table methods.

One of the main causes of recurrent TOS is scar tissue formation around the brachial plexus and subclavian vessels, which follows nerve decompression operations anywhere in the body during the healing process. To minimize the effect of scar tissue and give early mobility to the brachial plexus and subclavian vessels, patients should be instructed to perform active range-of-motion exercises beginning the day after surgery, as mentioned earlier.

The most significant variable reported is the cause of the TOS. Occupational repetitive stress injuries were reported to be associated with poor outcome following TOS surgery.[28] Other studies have found that preoperative depression[83] and surgeries for some other compression syndrome, such as carpal or cubital tunnel syndrome, were associated with a worse outcome. On the other hand, a recent study reported that compliance with TOS-specific physical therapy, improvement in quality-of-life scores after physical therapy, young age, and competitive athletics were associated with improved surgical outcomes.[84]

In patients with recurrent TOS, symptoms may develop several weeks or months after the primary surgery. After 2 years, symptoms of recurrence occur less frequently.[85] In Sanders and colleagues' series of 134 operations in 97 patients for recurrent TOS using the transaxillary and transcervical approach over 22 years, the 84% initial success rate dropped to 59% at 1 to 2 years, 50% at 3 to 5 years, and 41% at 10 to 20 years.[62]

Vascular Thoracic Outlet Syndrome

Venous Thoracic Outlet Syndrome (Paget-Schroetter Syndrome)

Spontaneous, or effort-related, thrombosis of the axillo-subclavian vein is a disabling disorder of young, otherwise healthy individuals. This type of thrombosis was described independently more than 100 years ago by Paget in England and Von Schroetter in Germany—hence, Paget-Schroetter syndrome.[86] With subsequent investigations, it is now understood that despite the apparent spontaneous nature of the event, there is an underlying chronic venous compressive anomaly at the thoracic outlet plus repetitive trauma (Figures 31-12 and 31-13). The subclavius muscle tendon can be demonstrated to be the site of obstruction in many cases in which intermittent obstruction is present but has not yet led to thrombosis. Physical findings include obvious arm swelling and dilated collateral veins in the shoulder girdle region. Venography confirms the diagnosis. Pulmonary embolism from axillosubclavian vein thrombosis has been well documented,[87,88] and deaths from pulmonary embolism from

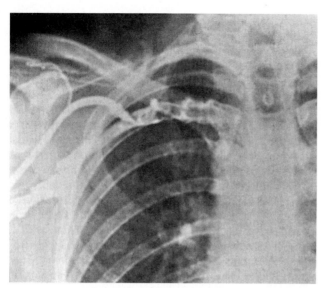

FIGURE 31-13 ■ Axillosubclavian vein thrombosis characteristic of Paget-Schroetter syndrome or the effort thrombosis variant of thoracic outlet compression syndrome. Note the collateral vessels and intraluminal thrombus.

these sources have been recorded in the surgical literature.[88] Furthermore, severe thromboembolic pulmonary hypertension is an infrequent but potentially fatal complication of Paget-Schroetter syndrome.[89] Studies of relatively large groups of patients have shown the value of immediate catheter-directed thrombolytic therapy with urokinase followed by a period of anticoagulation to allow the acute phlebitic process to subside. Patients are then treated with transaxillary first rib resection to relieve the external compression. In patients with long-standing compression of the vein, stricture and fibrosis can result; this can be treated with transvenous balloon angioplasty after the external compressive elements have been removed. With this course of therapy, an excellent functional result can be expected.[90-92] Of note, there is no role for stenting of the subclavian vein in the region of the thoracic outlet before operative decompression and that the persistent mechanical forces in this region likely lead to stent malfunction and failure, thus making the situation worse.[93] Although studies have validated the staged, multidisciplinary approach, there have been reports of successful immediate surgical decompression following thrombolytic therapy; however, these cases are insufficient in number to result in a publication available for general review.[92] Recent studies reported successful outcomes using multidisciplinary approach based on (1) early diagnostic venography and thrombolysis; (2) paraclavicular thoracic outlet decompression with external venolysis and frequent use of subclavian vein reconstruction; and (3) temporary postoperative anticoagulation, with or without an adjunctive arteriovenous fistula.[94,95]

Arterial Thoracic Outlet Syndrome

The earliest lesion of arterial TOS is usually simple stenosis of the vessel lumen, which can spontaneously reverse after thoracic outlet decompression. However,

long-standing, repeated compression of the subclavian artery may eventually result in post-stenotic dilatation and aneurysm formation with chronic inflammation. The most common cause is the presence of bony abnormalities (complete or incomplete cervical rib, elongated C7 transverse process, or malunion following fracture of the clavicle or first rib).[96-98] In addition, isolated congenital bands, hypertrophic anterior scalene muscles, and physiologic drooping of the shoulder girdle can lead to arterial entrapment. The consequences range from relatively minor microembolic events to major vessel thromboembolic complications resulting in potentially limb-threatening ischemia.[99]

Even when TOS has been recognized, the arterial manifestations may be overlooked because of the belief that nerve compression is causing the patient's symptoms.[98,100] As a result, the appropriate diagnosis might not be made until obvious ischemic changes of the upper extremity occur. Factors such as unilateral involvement, a predominant distribution in the hands and digits, and the absence of any underlying vascular disorders suggest artery-to-artery embolization. The diagnosis may be suggested by a pulsatile mass, subclavian artery bruit, atrophic skin changes, gangrene or ulcerations of the fingertips, history of fractured clavicle or ribs, and decreased blood pressure in the affected extremity. Duplex scan imaging of the vascular system at the subclavian artery can be useful. Transfemoral arteriography of the entire upper extremity vascular system, including positional views, should be used in any patient suspected of having arterial thoracic outlet compression.

Options for the surgical treatment of vascular TOS consist of (1) management of ischemia of the extremity, (2) decompression, (3) repair of the arterial lesion, and (4) dorsal sympathectomy. Surgical thrombectomy or catheter-based thrombolysis should be done after diagnostic angiography in the operating room. Usually, decompression surgery, including rib resection and scalenectomy, should be performed later to reduce the risk of hemorrhage. Vessels with aneurysmal changes or post-stenotic dilatation more than 2 cm should be resected and reconstructed with autogenous saphenous vein or synthetic prosthesis using the supraclavicular approach with an infraclavicular incision. An arterial lesion less than 2 cm can be left alone, and only rib resection and scalenectomy should be performed using the transaxillary approach. Dorsal sympathectomy can be performed through the axillary incision or under thoracoscopic guidance.[101,102] Increased cutaneous perfusion and improved pain threshold can be observed. Generally, excellent outcomes can be expected with timely diagnosis and treatment.[96,97]

VASCULAR DISEASE OF THE UPPER EXTREMITY

The upper extremities are subject to a variety of unique intrinsic arterial and venous disorders, as well as the peripheral manifestations of systemic collagen vascular diseases. Patients developing arterial insufficiency of the upper extremities generally demonstrate one of three different clinical patterns: (1) attacks of Raynaud disease symptoms, (2) digital ischemia and gangrene, or (3) crampy pain with exercise, often referred to (with disregard for the word origin) as *claudication*. The initial examination of the upper extremity should begin with inspection, palpation, and auscultation. Noninvasive vascular testing, such as segmental systolic pressure measurement with Doppler flow detector, digital plethysmography, and duplex scan, can be used to further document the disorder.

Afflictions of the Major Vascular Structures

Approximately 50% of cases of acute arterial insufficiency of the upper extremity are secondary to embolization; of the remainder, 25% are the result of primary arterial thrombosis and 25% are iatrogenic in origin, including arterial blood pressure monitoring, sampling of arterial blood gases, and creation of an arteriovenous fistula for dialysis. Brachial artery catheterization is a well-documented cause of upper extremity ischemia.[103] Trauma to the brachial vessels generally carries a poor prognosis secondary to the commonly associated nerve injury (Figure 31-14). When signs of ischemia accompany an upper extremity fracture, fracture reduction should be done as a primary maneuver, and reassessment of arterial integrity should be done promptly. Takayasu arteritis should be considered, particularly in a relatively young female patient.

The vast majority of embolic arterial occlusions in the upper extremity are of cardiac origin, but brachiocephalic aneurysmal disease occasionally results in embolic episodes. The diagnosis of upper extremity ischemia is straightforward. The triad of symptoms—pain, paresthesias, and pallor—is generally accompanied by a loss of radial and ulnar pulse and diminished segmental pressures on noninvasive testing. Diagnostic and therapeutic measures must be prompt in episodes of acute upper extremity embolization. It has been documented that patients treated within 12 hours of the embolic episode have excellent long-term results.[104,105] Two modes of therapy may produce satisfactory results: the immediate administration of continuous intravenous heparin with careful monitoring of the thromboplastin time, and embolectomy with careful observation for the development of compartment syndrome. High-dose local infusion of urokinase (250,000 units of urokinase dissolved in 100 mL of normal saline over 30 minutes) by a transarterial catheter has been effective in the lysis of intra-arterial thrombi.[106] This technique can be used intraoperatively to more effectively remove thrombotic material from the very vasoactive vessels of the upper extremities. If there is any clinical or radiographic evidence of vasospasm, 30 mg of papaverine can be infused via the same catheter.[107] Experience has also been accumulating on the use of recombinant tissue-plasminogen activator.[108]

Small Vessel Occlusion in the Upper Extremity

The collagen vascular diseases manifest themselves by deposition of immune complexes in the intimal and subintimal surfaces of small vessels. In addition, obliterative, proliferative processes characterize diseases such as scleroderma and diabetes. Scleroderma is the most common entity manifesting with digital ischemia. The fact that digital ischemia may precede systemic manifestations of these diseases adds to the difficulty of the initial diagnosis and emphasizes the need for a logical approach, which may have to be repeated during the evolution of the patient's disease.[109,110] The response to cigarette smoking, particularly in men suspected of suffering from Buerger disease, is characteristic in this group of patients. The presence of digital gangrene in a young patient without evidence of atherosclerosis or aneurysmal disease, and particularly in the presence of normal upper extremity segmental pressures, should lead one to suspect a generalized collagen vascular disease. The process of gangrene in the fingers is quite different from that of necrosis, which is a wet suppurative process. Fingertip gangrene is more often a process of desiccation and mummification. Serologic tests are the basis of the diagnostic workup in these patients. Plain radiographs of the hands are also indicated. Evidence of skin atrophy and shiny tenseness or calcinosis of the skin are also valuable diagnostic findings. In cases in which skin biopsy is performed, immunofluorescence staining is extremely helpful. Specific arteriographic findings of collagen vascular diseases have been well documented: bilateral lesions; arterial obstruction without calcification; absence of atherosclerotic changes; smooth narrowing of the arterial lumen; total arterial occlusion or a stringlike appearance; multiple lesions, predominantly in the forearm and hand; less collateral circulation, giving a winding, corkscrew appearance; and small, attenuated terminal digital branches having the appearance of a "tree root."[111] Arteriography is also useful in excluding proximal lesions,

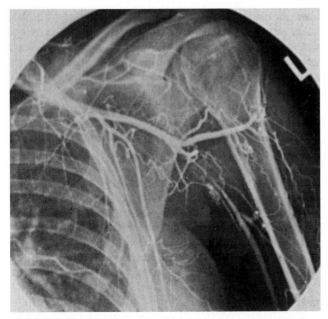

FIGURE 31-14 ■ Intimal dissection and occlusion of the axillobrachial artery at the level of the brachial plexus cords. This lesion is best repaired by reverse vein grafting, with care being taken to avoid entrapment of brachial plexus elements.

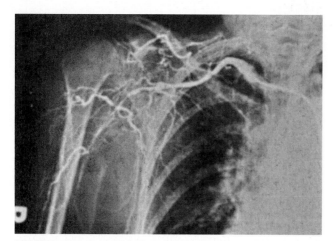

FIGURE 31-15 ■ Typical pattern of axillosubclavian arterial occlusive disease seen in giant cell arteritis.

although it rarely demonstrates specific changes characteristic of certain types of arteritis (Figure 31-15). Medical management includes avoidance of cold exposure, use of gloves, discontinuation of tobacco use, and medication such as nifedipine, which is useful in relieving arterial spasm and associated digital ischemia.

Raynaud disease is a vasospastic condition. Although associated with the collagen diseases, it can also be idiopathic. The chief symptom is a peculiar blanching and cyanosis of the fingertips owing to profound vasoconstriction of the capillary beds caused primarily by exposure to cold and aggravated by the use of tobacco and caffeine. The diagnosis is confirmed by arteriography. Intraarterial injection of 25 mg tolazoline (Priscoline) during arteriography relieves the spasm momentarily and elucidates the spastic process. Initial treatment is with calcium channel blockers, such as nifedipine (30 to 60 mg daily). Surgical treatment is a dorsal sympathectomy, often performed by a thoracoscopic approach.

Arteriography

Arteriography can be useful in the diagnosis and assessment of vascular disorders of the upper extremity. The transfemoral route is preferred, particularly to enable visualization of the proximal aortic vessels and to avoid the need to traverse a potentially diseased axillosubclavian vessel. Proximal aneurysmal dilatation and atherosclerotic occlusive disease, as well as thrombosis and ulcerating plaques, are generally well identified radiographically. Proximal subclavian occlusion with subclavian steal phenomenon and retrograde flow in the vertebral artery is easily demonstrated. This lesion should be suspected whenever there is a pressure discrepancy greater than 20 mm Hg in the contralateral brachial artery pressure.

Magnification views of the hand during arteriography, particularly if augmented by hand cooling or warming, or injection of intraarterial vasodilating drugs, such as papaverine or nitroglycerin, can differentiate between Raynaud phenomenon, which is generally associated with

segmental occlusions, and Raynaud disease, which is generally identifiable only by vasospastic hypersensitivity. The angiographic characteristics of arterial vasospasm are marked delay in flow, a threadlike appearance, and tapered areas of occlusion relieved by the injection of vasodilating drugs or hand warming.

Iatrogenic Venous Insufficiency of the Upper Extremity

Although thoracic outlet compression can lead to axillosubclavian vein thrombosis, the vast majority of venous occlusive processes result from trauma or iatrogenic injury. Long-term intravenous alimentation, upper-extremity intravenous access for therapy, or procedures such as central venous pressure monitoring and Swan-Ganz monitoring can result in axillosubclavian thrombotic episodes. It is important to recognize that chronic axillosubclavian vein thrombosis may be an indolent and relatively silent process and is seldom associated with symptoms in the upper extremity. Whenever this problem has been examined prospectively, however, the incidence of venous thrombosis in the major upper extremity veins approaches 25%. Heparin therapy rarely leads to lysis, but it might prevent extension of thrombosis with removal of cannulas. Thrombolytic therapy with streptokinase or recombinant tissue plasminogen activator may prove efficacious. Reports of successful surgical therapy by either thrombectomy or interposition grafting do not demonstrate any superiority over conservative management, and the failure rate is sufficiently high that enthusiastic recommendation of surgical intervention cannot be supported.

Upper Extremity Deep Venous Thrombosis in Air Travelers

Deep venous thrombosis (DVT) of the lower extremities in extended duration air travel is well known and documented because of a concern for pulmonary embolism; however, case reports suggest an association of air travel with upper extremity thrombosis as well. One case series out of a single center documented five separate cases of upper extremity DVT in association with air travel.[112] All patients were admitted after 5- to 10-hour flights. The five patients had risk factors present before their flight, which included a previous history of shoulder injury with DVT, chronic atrial fibrillation, past clavicle fracture, and Paget-Schroetter syndrome. The timeframe for initial symptom presentation (typically extremity swelling and pain) varied from during flight to 3 days afterward. An additional single case report was documented in a patient following a 15-hour flight.[113] This patient's venous thrombosis started at the insertion site of a pacemaker, which was placed 2 months earlier. A full hypercoagulation workup was unremarkable. Three patients with upper-extremity DVT were observed in the Los Angeles area following air travel, which included a flight attendant (not documented). These patients all responded to standard treatment, which included anticoagulation, catheter-directed thrombolysis, balloon angioplasty, or first-rib resection.

There are numerous theories regarding the etiology of upper DVT in air travelers. Current literature suggests that the airline cabin's arid and hypoxic hypobaric conditions contribute to a prothrombotic state via increased plasma viscosity, decreased fibrinolysis, and induced coagulation.[114-116] Venous stasis and pooling, though more commonly associated with DVT of the lower extremity in air travelers, is also another consideration given the restricted mobility in typical airline seats. Air travelers, particularly frequent fliers that carry heavy bags over their shoulders could also be at risk because of chronic compression of the thoracic outlet. In addition, flight attendants may also be predisposed, secondary to Paget-Schroetter syndrome from frequent and strenuous overhead arm movement. Predisposed air travelers have the potential to develop upper extremity DVT. Patients with upper extremity DVT or pulmonary embolism should be questioned regarding recent air travel. Future studies may further elucidate the true incidence of upper extremety DVT in air travelers, as well as explore upper extremety-specific thrombotic risk factors.

BIBLIOGRAPHY

Altobelli GG, Kudo T, Haas BT, et al: Thoracic outlet syndrome: pattern of clinical success following surgical decompression. J Vasc Surg 42:111–117, 2005.

Atasoy E: Thoracic outlet compression syndrome. Orthop Clin North Am 27:265–303, 1996.

Durham JR, Yao JS, Pearce WH, et al: Arterial injuries in the thoracic outlet syndrome. J Vasc Surg 21:57–70, 1995.

Jordan SE, Machleder HI: Diagnosis of thoracic outlet syndrome using electrophysiologically guided anterior scalene blocks. Ann Vasc Surg 12:260–264, 1998.

Machleder HI: Evaluation of a new treatment strategy for Paget-Schroetter's syndrome. J Vasc Surg 17:305–317, 1993.

Machleder HI, Moll F, Verity MA: The anterior scalene muscle in thoracic outlet compression syndrome: histochemical and morphometric studies. Arch Surg 121:1141–1144, 1986.

Melby SJ, Vedantham S, Narra VR, et al: Comprehensive surgical management of the competitive athlete with effort thrombosis of the subclavian vein (Paget-Schroetter syndrome). J Vasc Surg 47:809–821, 2008.

Novak CB, Mackinnon SE: Thoracic outlet syndrome. Orthop Clin North Am 27:747–762, 1996.

Oates SD, Daley RA: Thoracic outlet syndrome. Hand Clin 12:705–718, 1996.

Sanders RJ, Haug CE, Pearce WH: Recurrent thoracic outlet syndrome. J Vasc Surg 12:390–400, 1990.

Sanders RJ, Pearce WH: The treatment of thoracic outlet syndrome: a comparison of different operations. J Vasc Surg 10:626–634, 1989.

Urschel HC, Jr, Razzuk MA: Neurovascular compression in the thoracic outlet: changing management over 50 years. Ann Surg 228:609–617, 1998.

References available online at expertconsult.com.

QUESTIONS

1. The Allen test is useful in evaluating which of the following?
   a. Thoracic outlet compression
   b. Presence of cervical rib
   c. Integrity of palmar arch
   d. Digital blood flow
   e. Acute effort thrombosis

2. The thoracic outlet is bounded by which of the following structures? (More than one may be correct.)
   a. Medial border of sternum
   b. First thoracic rib
   c. Clavicle
   d. Subclavian artery
   e. Subclavius tendon

3. The thoracic outlet is traversed by which of the following structures? (More than one may be correct.)
   a. Subclavian artery
   b. Brachial plexus
   c. Anterior scalene muscle
   d. Pectoralis major tendon
   e. Middle scalene muscle

4. Digital gangrene is not associated with which of the following?
   a. Buerger disease
   b. Vasculitis
   c. Raynaud disease
   d. Arterial thoracic outlet syndrome
   e. Paget-Schroetter disease

5. Digital plethysmographic tracings are most apt to be misinterpreted secondary to which of the following?
   a. Cuff malfunction
   b. Transducer malfunction
   c. Segmental arterial occlusions
   d. Changes in sympathetic activity
   e. Poor light

6. Which of the following is a common cause of prominent right-sided supraclavicular pulsation?
   a. Common carotid aneurysm
   b. Subclavian aneurysm
   c. Subclavian tortuosity or elongation
   d. Innominate artery aneurysm
   e. Mycotic aneurysm

7. Effort thrombosis of the subclavian vein is often associated with which of the following?
   a. Straining at bowel movement
   b. Hypercoagulation syndrome
   c. Thoracic outlet compression syndrome
   d. Calcinosis cutis, Raynaud phenomenon, sclerodactyly, and telangiectasia (CRST syndrome) or scleroderma
   e. Collagen vascular disease in general

8. What is the correct course when peripheral pulses are absent following fracture-dislocation of the humerus?
   a. Arteriography should be done promptly before reduction.
   b. Arterial exploration should be done at the fracture site as the first step.
   c. Fracture reduction should be followed by arterial re-evaluation.
   d. Sympathetic block should be performed immediately.
   e. Pulses should be rechecked in approximately 1 hour, before fracture manipulation.

9. Diagnosis of thoracic outlet syndrome has to fulfill which of the following criteria?
   a. Symptoms referable to the thoracic outlet neurovascular bundle
   b. Compression of the neurovascular bundle at the thoracic outlet space
   c. Symptoms related to compression
   d. No other explanation for symptoms
   e. All of the above

10. When diagnosing neurogenic thoracic outlet syndrome, the single best test to determine whether symptoms are related to the compression of the neurovascular bundle at the thoracic outlet is which of the following?
    a. Magnetic resonance angiography
    b. Magnetic resonance venography
    c. An electrophysiologic test, such as electromyogram or somatosensory evoked potential test
    d. EMG-guided scalene muscle stimulation and block test
    e. Provocative Adson or abduction and external rotation test

ANSWERS

1. c
2. b, c, e
3. a, b
4. e
5. d
6. c
7. c
8. c
9. e
10. d

CHAPTER 32

Natural History and Nonoperative Treatment of Chronic Lower Extremity Ischemia

Amir F. Azarbal • Erica L. Mitchell • Gregory J. Landry • Gregory L. Moneta

Despite the focus on operative and endovascular interventions in vascular surgery, most patients with peripheral chronic lower extremity ischemia do not require intervention. Nonoperative therapy and risk factor modification are the primary elements of treatment for the majority of patients.

Although only 1% to 2% of people younger than 50 years suffer from symptoms of intermittent claudication, this figure rises to 5% in those aged 50 to 70 years and to 10% in those older than 70.[1-3] It is estimated that 8 to 12 million people in the United States,[4] and 27 million people in North America and Europe,[5] suffer from peripheral arterial disease (PAD), and this number is expected to rise as the population ages.

STRATIFICATION AND EPIDEMIOLOGY

Chronic lower extremity ischemia represents a clinical spectrum. Clinical manifestations range from asymptomatic disease and atypical symptoms to classic intermittent claudication and critical limb ischemia with impending tissue loss. Intermittent claudication is typically reported as the number of blocks a patient can walk on level ground at a normal speed without having to stop; however, patients are frequently poor judges of objective walking distance. Pharmaceutical trials have stratified patients based on walking distances (initial or absolute claudication distances) or claudication times during either fixed or graded load treadmill testing. Recently, tools such as the Walking Impairment Questionnaire have assisted in the stratification of intermittent claudication.[6] Combining the objective measurements of ischemia (ankle-brachial pressure index, toe pressure, pulse-volume recordings) with the clinical situation helps to define the natural history of various patient groups with chronic lower extremity ischemia.

Lower extremity PAD is an independent risk factor for cardiovascular morbidity and mortality. Atherosclerotic cardiovascular disease is a systemic process affecting multiple arterial beds, including the coronary, cerebrovascular, upper and lower extremities, and visceral arteries. There is often significant disease overlap in the various arterial segments.[7,8] A number of large, population-based epidemiologic studies have reported on the incidence and prevalence of PAD. PAD incidence and prevalence is dependent on the definition of PAD used.

Asymptomatic Arterial Insufficiency

Asymptomatic PAD is defined as a decreased ankle-brachial index (ABI) without lower extremity symptoms. Most studies use an ABI of less than 0.9 as a reference standard for PAD.[5] The presence of asymptomatic lower extremity occlusive disease varies, but available data indicate that for every patient with intermittent claudication, there are probably three others with similar disease who do not complain of symptoms or have atypical symptoms.[9] Ratios of symptomatic to asymptomatic patients range from 1:1.8 to 1:5.3.[1,2,10,11]

The prevalence of asymptomatic PAD was 25.5% among 1537 participants in the Systolic Hypertension in the Elderly Program.[12] Data from a nationwide cross-sectional study, based on more than 350 primary care practices, demonstrated that 13% of 6979 patients older than 50 years had abnormal ABIs, with or without symptoms of intermittent claudication.[7] Only 24% of patients with chronic lower extremity ischemia had a previous diagnosis of PAD. Asymptomatic patients accounted for 48% of newly diagnosed PAD.

Incidence of Symptomatic Peripheral Arterial Disease

The majority of epidemiologic studies of PAD have focused on patients with intermittent claudication, defined as leg pain with walking (most often calf pain, but it can involve the thighs and buttocks as well). Pain is induced by exercise and is relieved by rest. The reported incidence of PAD varies between 2.2% of a population aged 33 to 82 years and 17% of a population aged 55 to 70 years.[1,2] In the Framingham Heart Study, the incidence of PAD was based on symptoms of intermittent claudication in subjects 29 to 62 years old. The annual incidence of intermittent claudication per 10,000 subjects at risk rose from 6 in men and 3 in women aged 30 to 44 years to 61 in men and 54 in women aged 65 to 74 years.[13] The average rate of development of intermittent claudication over a 2-year period in subjects older than age 50 was 0.7% in men and 0.4% in women.[13]

In the Edinburgh Artery Study of almost 1600 subjects older than 55 years, the 5-year cumulative incidence of PAD was 9%.[14] Bowlin and coworkers[15] followed 8343 Israeli men over a 21-year period and found a cumulative incidence of 43.1 per 1000 population. In the Quebec Cardiovascular Study of 4570 men followed over 12 years, an incidence of 41 per 10,000 population per year was noted.[16] In the large prospective Physicians' Health Study, 433 incident cases of PAD were reported among 22,071 relatively healthy men.[17]

Prevalence of Symptomatic Peripheral Arterial Disease

Epidemiologic studies have used both questionnaires and noninvasive vascular laboratory screening to estimate the prevalence of PAD in the elderly adult population. Before the development of reliable noninvasive testing, the diagnosis of PAD was based on standardized patient questionnaires. Among questionnaires, the World Health Organization/Rose Questionnaire and the Edinburgh Classification Questionnaire (ECQ) have been the most extensively studied. The ECQ appears to be more robust, with a sensitivity of 91% and a specificity of 99% for the diagnosis of intermittent claudication.[18] Using the ECQ, the prevalence of lower extremity arterial disease was estimated to be 4.6% in the Edinburgh Artery Study in men and women between the ages of 55 and 74 years.[2] Other studies have found the prevalence of intermittent claudication in adults older than age 45 to be approximately 1% to 5% (Table 32-1).

When ABI is used as a reference standard, the detected prevalence of lower extremity arterial occlusive disease is even greater, likely because of the inclusion of patients who are asymptomatic or have atypical symptoms. The overall age-adjusted prevalence of PAD diagnosed on the basis of the ABI is approximately 12%; for intermittent claudication, it is 1% to 2% up to age 50 and 5% to 7% from the seventh decade onward.[19] In the Cardiovascular Health Study, the prevalence of a decreased ABI (<0.9) was 12.4% in adults aged 65 years or older in four U.S. communities.[12] Using the same criteria, investigators in the Rotterdam Study reported a PAD prevalence of 19% in subjects older than 55 years.[10] In the Edinburgh Artery Study, the prevalence of lower extremity arterial occlusive disease diagnosed using ABI was 17% in subjects between the ages of 55 and 74 years.[2] In a Danish study, the prevalence of lower extremity arterial occlusive disease in 60-year-old subjects was 16% for men and 13% for women (Table 32-2).[20] Thus, objective standards of measurement identify a greater number of patients with PAD than does reliance on patient description of symptoms.

Several factors might explain the lack of sensitivity of questionnaires and the increased prevalence of PAD with noninvasive testing.[2,21] First, symptoms might not occur until the disease is advanced. This is particularly relevant in older patients who may rarely walk more than one or two blocks at a time in the performance of their activities of daily living, or who may assume that leg pain while walking is a natural part of the aging process. Second, patients with PAD may have other comorbidities, such as

TABLE 32-1   Prevalence of Intermittent Claudication by History or Questionnaire in Large Population Studies

Study	No. of Patients	Age (Yr)	Intermittent Claudication Prevalence (%)
Schroll and Munck (1981)[11]	360 men	60	5.8
	306 women	60	1.3
Reunanen and colleagues (1982)[251]	5738 men	30-59	2.1
	5224 women	30-59	1.8
Fowkes and colleagues (1991)[2]	1592 men and women	55-74	4.5
Stoffers and colleagues (1991)[252]	3654 men and women	45-54	0.6
		55-64	2.5
		65-74	8.8
Smith and colleagues (1990)[111]	18,388 men	40-64	0.8
Skau and Jonsson (1993)[253]	7254 men and women	50-89	4.1
Newman and colleagues (1993)[12]	5084 men and women	65-85	2.0
Stoffers and colleagues (1996)[19]	1719 men	55-75	1.5
	1935 women	55-75	2.8
Zheng and colleagues (1997)[254]	15,106 men and women	45-64	1.0
Meijer and colleagues (1998)[10]	3052 men	70	2.2
	4663 women	70	1.2

arthritis, cardiac disease, or pulmonary disease, that affect their walking ability to a greater degree than PAD.

RISK FACTORS

Smoking

The specific mechanisms by which tobacco exerts its adverse effects on arteries remain poorly understood; however, a direct relationship between tobacco smoking and peripheral vascular disease has been well established.[22] All epidemiologic studies of lower extremity arterial disease have confirmed cigarette smoking as a strong risk factor for the development of such disease, with relative risk ratios ranging from 1.7 to 7.5.[1,10,12,23-27] A case-control study revealed a sevenfold higher risk of developing PAD in ex-smokers compared with those who had never smoked, and the risk increased to sixteenfold in current smokers compared with those who had never smoked.[28] The diagnosis of lower extremity arterial disease is made up to a decade earlier in smokers compared with nonsmokers. More than 90% of all patients referred to vascular clinics for PAD have a history of smoking.[29]

In addition to the chronic effects of smoking on the development of atherosclerosis, smoking has acute effects

TABLE 32-2 Prevalence of Peripheral Arterial Disease Based on Ankle-Brachial Index Abnormalities in Large Population Studies

Study	No. of Patients	Age (Yr)	Intermittent Claudication Prevalence (%)
Schroll and Munck (1981)[11]	360 men	60	16.0
	306 women	60	13.0
Criqui and colleagues (1985)[1]	613 men and women	38-82	11.7
Hiatt and colleagues (1990)[255]	950 men and women	44-68	11.9
Newman and colleagues (1991)[256]	1592 men and women	55-74	24.6
Coni et al.and colleagues (1992)[21]	265 men and women	>65	9.1
Newman and colleagues (1993)[12]	2214 men	>65	13.9
	2870 women	>65	11.4
Stoffers and colleagues (1991)[252]	1719 men	55-75	11.0
	1935 women	55-75	8.6
Meijer and colleagues (1998)[10]	2589 men	>55	16.9
	3861 women	>55	20.5

on lower extremity function. Smoking two cigarettes within a 10-minute period resulted in an acute lowering of the ABI in chronic smokers from 0.64 ± 0.14 to 0.55 ± 0.11 ($p = 0.008$).[30] In addition to having adverse influences on atherosclerosis, the carbon monoxide in tobacco smoke may directly contribute to claudication. Smoking is associated with acute drops in treadmill walking distances, presumably owing to carbon monoxide.[31] An immediate and significant decrease in the time or distance that patients can walk on the treadmill before they get claudication symptoms has been demonstrated when air containing carbon monoxide is breathed.[31,32] Smokers have an increased risk of peripheral vascular disease progression,[33] myocardial infarction, stroke, and death.[34] Smokers also have an increased risk of major amputation.[35,36]

Diabetes Mellitus

A strong association exists between diabetes mellitus and PAD. Two types of vascular disease are seen in patients with diabetes: microcirculatory dysfunction involving the capillaries and arterioles of the kidneys, retina, and peripheral nerves, and a macroangiopathy involving the peripheral and coronary arterial circulation.[37] The Framingham Study was one of the first major epidemiologic studies to demonstrate the association between diabetes and PAD. Diabetes increased the risk of claudication by a factor of 3.5 in men and 8.6 in women.[38] Numerous subsequent studies have associated impaired glucose tolerance with a twofold to fourfold increase in the risk of developing intermittent claudication.[39-44] In an elderly white population, 20.9% of patients

with diabetes mellitus and 15.1% of patients with an abnormal glucose tolerance test had an ABI less than 0.9.[45] In a Swedish study, 21% of patients with diabetes had signs of PAD.[46] The duration and severity of diabetes mellitus correlate strongly with the incidence and severity of PAD.

Patients with diabetes mellitus often develop symptomatic forms of PAD and have poorer lower extremity function than do those with PAD alone.[47] The prevalence of diabetes in patients undergoing lower extremity revascularization ranges from 25% to 50%, compared with a prevalence of 6% in the general population.[48] The rate of lower extremity amputation is sevenfold to tenfold higher in diabetic patients than in those without diabetes.[23,49-51] In fact, diabetes leads to most of the nontraumatic lower extremity amputations in the United States. In addition to diabetes, insulin resistance and hyperinsulinemia are also risk factors for PAD.[26,52]

Gender

Early epidemiologic studies focused on the prevalence of PAD in men. The popular notion based on the Framingham Study was that symptomatic PAD in women lagged behind men by 10 years[53] and that women were generally not affected by PAD until after menopause. However, more recent epidemiologic studies indicate that PAD prevalence and incidence in men and women are similar. Several studies have demonstrated that the age-adjusted incidence of intermittent claudication is equal in both genders,[20,54] with the frequency of PAD among diabetic women markedly higher than that among diabetic men.[20] Among subjects with a low ABI, coronary artery disease was less prevalent among women. Women also had a lower frequency of cerebrovascular disease.[54] In another study, the prevalence of PAD was almost identical in men and women; however, other cardiovascular disease was twice as prevalent in men.[7] Progression of PAD, as measured by changes in ABI, appears to be the same in men and women.[55] However, women may suffer faster functional decline. A prospective trial of 380 men and women showed that at 4-year follow-up, women were more likely do have a decline in walking distance and more likely to develop mobility related disability than men. These functional differences seem to be attributable to smaller baseline calf muscle area in women.[56] Epidemiologic studies have shown that women may be more susceptible to aortoiliac arterial occlusive disease than men are.[57] Autopsy findings also provide important information about gender differences in the occurrence of atherosclerotic changes in various arterial beds. Compared with men, women have a greater extent of fatty streaks in the abdominal aorta, but not in the coronary arteries.[58]

It is possible that PAD is underdiagnosed in women to a greater degree than in men. Studies have shown that women are less likely than men to have diagnosed PAD on the basis of symptoms, even if clinically significant PAD is present on noninvasive examinations.[59,60] In addition, it has been shown that infrainguinal arterial reconstructions performed on women tend to be for more advanced disease compared with men, and the women tend to be older.[61,62] The reasons for the more advanced presentation in women are unclear. It has been speculated that because women more frequently assume a caretaker role, they are more likely to ignore their own medical care; or perhaps women are more likely to ignore mild to moderate pain, attributing it to a consequence of old age.[63] It is clear that the previous dictum of PAD being primarily a disease of men is changing as more data about its effect on women emerge.

Race

Few studies have assessed differences in PAD prevalence among different ethnic groups. One early study indicated that African American patients with PAD typically had a higher occurrence of infrapopliteal atherosclerosis, which was associated with a greater incidence of limb loss.[64] Certain studies also indicate that PAD may be underreported in the African American population. In the Atherosclerosis Risk in Communities Study, more than 4000 African Americans were screened for PAD. Despite a greater prevalence of hypertension and diabetes, the prevalence of PAD measured by questionnaire was lower among African American men than among white men. However, 3.3% of African Americans had an ABI less than 0.9, compared with only 2.3% of whites.[54] In the Cardiovascular Health Study, the nonwhite population tested had a 3.5-fold increased frequency of an ABI less than 0.8.[12]

Hyperlipidemia

It is estimated that up to 50% of patients with lower extremity arterial disease have hyperlipidemia. In the Framingham Study, a fasting cholesterol level greater than 270 mg/dL was associated with a doubling of the incidence of intermittent claudication.[53] Population studies have demonstrated that the relative risk of PAD is 2.05 in patients with hypercholesterolemia,[65] 1.7 in patients with hypertriglyceridemia,[24] and 2.0 in patients with elevated levels of lipoprotein (a).[66] Other studies have suggested that triglyceride levels are not an independent risk factor for PAD when corrected for other serum lipid variables.[24,67]

Ridker and colleagues[68] evaluated multiple plasma lipid constituents, including total cholesterol, high-density lipoprotein (HDL) and low-density lipoprotein (LDL) cholesterol, lipoprotein (a), and apolipoproteins A-I and B-100, and the risk of developing PAD. Of the lipid markers tested, the ratio of total cholesterol to HDL cholesterol was the strongest predictor of PAD development, and the addition of screening for other lipid abnormalities did not improve predictive values. The addition of screening for two nonlipid variables—C-reactive protein and fibrinogen—did, however, improve the prediction of PAD risk.

Hyperhomocysteinemia

A number of prospective and retrospective studies have suggested an association between elevated levels of plasma homocysteine and premature vascular disease in the coronary, cerebrovascular, and peripheral circulation.[69-72] Early studies suggesting this association, however, were based on small numbers of patients. Darius and colleagues[73] evaluated plasma homocysteine levels as an independent risk factor for PAD in 6880 primary care patients older than 65 years. Although PAD (defined as an ABI < 0.9) was more frequently diagnosed in patients in the highest quintile of homocysteine levels (24.3%) than in the lowest quintile (13.0%; crude odds ratio 2.1), the association was less strong after adjusting for other atherosclerotic risk factors (odds ratio 1.4). Thus, the association between hyperhomocysteinemia and atherosclerosis is likely mild.

Serum Markers

Fibrinogen and C-reactive protein have been implicated in the pathogenesis of PAD in numerous studies.[34,74-79] The role of these factors in the pathogenesis of atherosclerosis is unclear; however, they are thought to be potential markers of endothelial dysfunction.[80] Elevated fibrinogen levels were independent risk factors for the development of PAD in both the Edinburgh and Rotterdam studies.[10,81]

C-reactive protein is an acute phase reactant that is elevated in acute inflammatory conditions. Persistent elevations are observed in chronic inflammatory disorders. The elevation of this factor in patients with atherosclerosis has led to the theory that inflammation contributes to the development of atherosclerosis. Whether C-reactive protein itself causes atherosclerosis is unknown. Other atherogenic risk factors such as age,[82,83] smoking,[84] diabetes,[85] and hyperlipidemia[86] are associated with elevated levels of C-reactive protein in the absence of PAD. Therefore elevated C-reactive protein may be an epiphenomenon associated with, but not causative of, an atherogenic state.

McDermott and colleagues[87] evaluated the association of elevated inflammatory biomarkers and physical performance in patients with PAD. Both elevated C-reactive protein and D-dimer, a marker of ongoing fibrin formation and degradation, were associated with poorer physical functioning in PAD patients. Measurements of walking distance, walking speed, and balance were significantly worse in patients with elevated C-reactive protein and D-dimer.

Infection

Although controversial, there is evidence that atherosclerosis may be associated with an inflammatory process caused by chronic infection with *Chlamydia pneumoniae*.[88,89] Many existing studies have explored the role of *Chlamydia* species infection in coronary artery disease.[90-92] A recent metaanalysis was performed in which the pooled data from 38 studies were examined.[93] The overall odds ratio was 1.6, suggesting only a mild causative role at best. Skeptics argue that *C. pneumoniae* is an innocent bystander in the atherosclerotic process rather than a cause. In support of this argument, the association between atherosclerosis and *C. pneumoniae* infection appears to be higher in retrospective cross-sectional and case-control studies than in prospective case-control studies, and the association is inversely proportional to length of follow-up.[93]

Alcohol Consumption

Mild to moderate alcohol consumption is associated with a reduced risk of cardiovascular disease and reduced cardiac mortality.[94-97] Several epidemiologic studies have suggested an inverse relationship between alcohol consumption and PAD.[17,98-101] In nonsmoking men, researchers from the Rotterdam Study found an odds ratio for PAD of 0.68 with consumption of more than 20 g of alcohol per day, with an odds ratio of 0.41 in a comparable group of women. The beneficial effects of alcohol are thought to be due to its influence on hemostasis,[81] its lipid profile,[102] and the generation of oxygen free radicals.[103]

NATURAL HISTORY

Once the diagnosis has been made, patients and physicians fear both disease progression and limb loss, in addition to the functional limitations caused by intermittent claudication. Multiple longitudinal studies of large groups of claudicants with objective criteria for enrollment provide an accurate database.[104-107]

Vascular Overlap

Because atherosclerosis is a systemic process, significant overlap exists between PAD and other forms of cardiovascular disease—namely, coronary artery disease and cerebrovascular disease. Hertzer and colleagues[108] clearly demonstrated a high incidence of coronary artery disease in vascular surgery patients. Their conclusions were based on a series of 1000 patients undergoing major vascular surgery in whom they performed preoperative coronary angiography, regardless of the history of coronary artery disease or symptoms. More than 90% of patients had clinically significant coronary artery disease, much of which was asymptomatic. The authors also found an increased frequency of severe coronary artery disease with age, from 22% among patients younger than 50 years to 41% among patients 70 years or older. Table 32-3 summarizes the data from this important study.

In the Cardiovascular Health Study, 60% of patients with PAD had a history of other symptomatic cardiovascular disease, such as myocardial infarction, angina, or stroke.[12] Conversely, 40% of patients with coronary artery or significant cerebrovascular disease also had PAD. Similar findings were reported in the large epidemiologic study by Aronow and Ahn,[8] in which 1886 patients older than 62 years were screened for cardiovascular disease. Seventy percent of patients with PAD had associated coronary artery or cerebrovascular disease (34% cerebrovascular, 58% coronary artery). The well-recognized overlap between PAD and other types of cardiovascular disease has been confirmed in numerous large epidemiologic studies and clinical trials (Table 32-4).

Progression of Symptoms

Knowledge of the natural history of PAD is essential when planning therapeutic strategies. When patients

TABLE 32-3 Incidence of Coronary Artery Disease in 1000 Consecutive Patients with Peripheral Vascular Disease Screened by Angiography

Extent of Disease	Unsuspected		Suspected	
	No. of Patients	(%)	No. of Patients	(%)
Normal coronary arteries	64	14	21	4
Mild to moderate CAD	218	49	99	18
Advanced compensated CAD	97	22	192	34
Severe correctable CAD	63	14	188	34
Severe incorrectable CAD	4	1	54	10

Data from Hertzer NR, Beven EG, Young JR, et al: Coronary artery disease in peripheral vascular patients: a classification of 1000 coronary angiograms and results of surgical management, Ann Surg 199:223-233, 1984; table from Taylor LM Jr, Porter JM: Natural history and nonoperative treatment in chronic lower extremity ischemia. In Moore WS, editor: Vascular surgery: a comprehensive review, Philadelphia, 1993, WB Saunders.
CAD, Coronary artery disease.

TABLE 32-4 Concomitant Cerebrovascular and Coronary Artery Disease in Patients with Peripheral Arterial Disease

Study	Cerebrovascular Disease (%)	Coronary Artery Disease (%)
Ogren and colleagues (1993)[257]	33	51
Szilagyi and colleagues (1986)[258]	19	47
Mendelson and colleagues (1998)[259]	35	62
Aronow and Ahn (1994)[8]	34	58
CAPRIE (1996)[123]	19	40
Meijer and colleagues (1998)[10]		
Men	9	39
Women	8	14

CAPRIE, Clopidogrel versus Aspirin in Patients at Risk of Ischemic Events.

with intermittent claudication are followed for 5 years, approximately 50% to 75% have either no change in symptoms or experience improvement. Approximately 25% experience symptom progression, with 5% to 25% requiring therapeutic intervention and only 2% to 4% requiring major amputation.[19,109] Both continued tobacco use[33] and diabetes mellitus[109] are correlated with progressive deterioration. However, the most important consistent predictor is the severity of objectively determined arterial occlusive disease at the first patient encounter.[51]

Life Expectancy

In contrast to the relatively benign lower extremity prognosis in most patients with PAD, the prognosis for morbidity and mortality from other manifestations of

TABLE 32-5	**Relative Risk of Mortality in Patients with Peripheral Arterial Disease Compared with Those Without**		
Study	**No. of Patients**	**Follow-Up (Yr)**	**Relative Risk**
Reunanen and colleagues (1982)[251]	5738 men	5	3.0
McKenna and colleagues (1991)[113]	744 men and women	5	2.4
Criqui and colleagues (1992)[110]	565 men and women	10	3.1
Ogren and colleagues (1993)[257]	477 men	10	2.5
Vogt and colleagues (1993)[114]	1492 women	4	4.0
Kornitzer and colleagues (1995)[115]	1592 men	10	3.3
Leng and colleagues (1996)[14]	1592 men and women	5	1.6

cardiovascular disease is worse. Life expectancy is clearly reduced in patients with PAD, attributable primarily to an increase in cardiovascular disease (Table 32-5).* The relative risk of a patient with intermittent claudication having a fatal or nonfatal myocardial infarction or stroke is twofold to threefold that of a nonclaudicant. All-cause mortality is also twofold to fourfold higher, with 60% of deaths from myocardial infarction and 15% from stroke.[110,112] According to the TransAtlantic Inter-Society Consensus document, the 5-year mortality of the average claudicant is 30%, with the majority of deaths caused by manifestations of cardiovascular disease.[20] An additional 5% to 10% will experience a nonfatal cardiovascular event.[19] The prevalence of asymptomatic carotid artery disease in patients with chronic lower extremity disease has also been examined. Screening carotid duplex scans in patients requiring infrainguinal revascularization have demonstrated a 30% incidence of asymptomatic internal carotid artery stenosis greater than 50% in that population.[116,117] Given the demonstrated prevalence of concomitant coronary and carotid vascular disease, reduced long-term survival in patients with chronic lower extremity ischemia is not surprising.

Multiple risk factors have been defined as important contributors to the increased long-term cardiovascular mortality of patients with lower extremity arterial occlusive disease. These include advanced age, continued tobacco use,[34] diabetes,[118] and dialysis dependence.[119-121] Of these, end-stage renal disease is the most pronounced, predicting 2-year survival rates of 50% to 65%.

Survival is inversely related to the degree of objectively determined chronic lower extremity ischemia at presentation.[122] McDermott and coworkers[122] showed that patients with an ABI less than 0.3 had significantly higher mortality than those with an ABI of 0.3 to 0.9

(relative risk 1.8).[122] In a group of patients followed for 10 years, Criqui and associates[110] demonstrated progressively decreasing survival with increasing PAD disease severity. Among patients with a normal ABI, asymptomatic PAD, moderately symptomatic PAD, and severe symptomatic PAD, 10-year survival rates were approximately 85%, 55%, 40%, and 25%, respectively. In another study, Vogt and coworkers[114] found that patients with multilevel PAD had a relative mortality risk of 7.2 compared with controls. In contrast, patients with PAD confined to the aortoiliac arterial segment had a relative mortality risk of 2.0 compared with controls. Multiple randomized trials in large populations with coronary disease indicate that aggressive risk factor modification reliably reduces near-term cardiac mortality.[123-129]

Critical Limb Ischemia

At the far end of the spectrum of clinical severity are those patients with critical limb ischemia (CLI). CLI is defined as arterial blood flow that is inadequate to accommodate the metabolic needs of resting tissue. Clinically, CLI describes a group of patients with limb-threatening ischemia and includes patients with rest pain, ischemic ulcerations, and gangrene. Objective circulatory measurement of CLI populations provides the best stratification of prognosis. The likelihood of near-term limb loss is related to the severity of ischemia at the time of patient presentation and the presence of tissue loss. Data on the incidence and prevalence of CLI are less definitive than data for intermittent claudication. Using multiple different extrapolation methods, it is estimated that between 500,000 and 1 million new cases occur each year.[130,131] This means that 1 new patient per year develops CLI for every 100 patients with intermittent claudication in the population, mostly in older patients. Few epidemiologic studies of CLI exist, compared with the myriad studies addressing the epidemiology of intermittent claudication. In a 7-year prospective study from the Lombardy region of northern Italy, CLI was estimated by three methods: conversion of intermittent claudication to CLI in prospectively followed patients, hospital admissions for CLI over a 3-month period, and rates of major limb amputations.[130] Surprisingly similar results were obtained with each method, with the incidence of CLI ranging from 450 to 650 cases per 1 million population per year. A national survey of the Vascular Surgical Society of Great Britain and Ireland found a similar incidence of 400 patients per 1 million population per year.[131]

Patients with CLI and those with intermittent claudication share similar risk factors, but most patients with CLI do not have a clear history of intermittent claudication. Major risk factors for advanced limb ischemia include age, smoking, and diabetes. The incidence of major amputation rises markedly with age. A Danish national discharge survey reported that the incidence of major lower extremity amputations increased from 0.3 per 100,000 per year for patients younger than 40 years to 226 per 100,000 per year for those older than 80 years. Patients with diabetes who smoke require amputation earlier in life than do patients without diabetes who do not smoke.[131]

*References 1, 2, 12, 14, 20, 110-115.

TABLE 32-6 **Chronic Lower Extremity Ischemia in Younger Patients**

Study	No. of Patients	Follow-Up (Yr)	Stable/Improved (%)	Worse (%)	Dead (%)	Amputated (%)
McCready and colleagues (1984)[142]	21	4-6	38	52	10	—
Pairolero and colleagues (1984)[141]	50	13.5	64	36	10	30
Evans and colleagues (1987)[140]	153	5.5	—	—	17	16
Valentine and colleagues (1990)[137]	22	2.2	76	24	4.5	0
Levy and colleagues (1994)[260]	109	2.3	—	—	—	27

Not all CLI is truly critical. Clearly, patients with progressive gangrenous changes and constant ischemic pain have an unstable clinical situation requiring prompt therapy. However, abundant clinical experience indicates that patients who have CLI manifested by intermittent rest pain may experience noticeable improvement at times, presumably secondary to improved cardiac hemodynamics. Small ulcerations may heal with protective dressings alone. Several randomized pharmacologic trials have documented ulcer healing in up to 40% of CLI patients randomized to placebo,[132,133] although in most of these trials, fewer than half the control patients were alive without a major amputation after 6 months.[134,135]

Chronic Lower Extremity Ischemia in Younger Patients

Lower extremity ischemia in patients younger than 40 years is infrequent. Peripheral vascular disease in young patients has several unique features that must be considered (Table 32-6).[136-142] These patients are almost universally heavy smokers. One prospective study performed detailed evaluations for hypercoagulable states in younger patients with chronic lower extremity ischemia and demonstrated that 90% had laboratory abnormalities (deficiencies in natural anticoagulants, defective fibrinolytic activity, or the presence of antiphospholipid antibodies).[139] Another study demonstrated significant abnormalities in LDL cholesterol oxidation in younger patients with PAD compared with older PAD patients.[136]

Despite attempts at revascularization, younger patients who manifest limb-threatening symptoms frequently progress rapidly to limb loss. Limited survival of reconstructions and the need for more frequent operative revisions characterizes these patients.[136,143] Although survival is reduced in younger patients with peripheral vascular disease compared with age-matched controls, on balance, coronary atherosclerosis in younger patients with severe PAD does not appear to be as aggressive as the atherosclerosis affecting their lower extremities.[144,145]

Nonoperative management with aggressive risk factor modification (cessation of tobacco use, lipid control) is the initial therapy of choice in younger patients with claudication. However, the greater functional expectations and frequent limitations on gainful employment experienced by younger patients with claudication complicate their ability to tolerate a prolonged course of nonoperative therapy. Despite this complication, revascularization attempts should be made judiciously, with an understanding of the diminished longevity of these

procedures in this age group and the higher amputation rate after failure.

Amputation

The incidence of major lower extremity amputation appears to have reached a plateau or decreased in the last decade, possibly owing to improved methods of revascularization and limb salvage, reduction in smoking, and improved diabetic control.[146-148] As with the larger subgroup of patients with CLI, patients who undergo major amputation often have not experienced a steady disease progression from claudication to rest pain to tissue necrosis to amputation.

In a review of 713 patients who were undergoing below-knee amputations for ischemia, more than half had experienced no ischemic symptoms as recently as 6 months before the amputation.[149]

Overall, the ratio of below-knee amputations to above-knee amputations is equal and has not significantly changed in several decades.[144,150-152] However, the introduction of aggressive limb salvage teams has increased the rate of below-knee amputations at selected centers.[153] Primary healing of below-knee amputations ranges from 30% to 90%.[153,154] Revision to attempt below-knee salvage varies from 4% to 30%.[155-157] Half of all below-knee amputees who fail to achieve primary healing ultimately require above-knee amputation.[158-160]

More below-knee than above-knee amputees achieve ambulation.[151,161,162] Overall, however, only a small number of major amputees for ischemic disease achieve meaningful independent ambulation. Initial rehabilitation can take 9 months or longer. After 2 years, 30% of amputees who had been walking no longer use their prostheses.[151] Advanced age and female gender bode poorly for ambulation.[163] Fifteen percent of amputees require contralateral amputation, and another 20% to 30% die within 2 years.[151,153,164]

NONOPERATIVE TREATMENT

The nonoperative treatment of chronic lower extremity ischemia includes risk factor modification, exercise, and pharmacologic therapy.

Management of Risk Factors

The first step in the management of PAD patients is treatment of risk factors. Multiple randomized trials in

TABLE 32-7	Recommendations for Risk Factor Reduction in Patients with Chronic Lower Extremity Ischemia	
Parameter	Target Goal	Therapy
LDL cholesterol	<100 mg/dL	Diet, statins
HDL cholesterol	Men, ≥35 mg/dL Women, ≥45 mg/ dL fibrates	Diet, exercise, niacin
Triglycerides	<150 mg/dL	Diet, exercise, gemfibrozil, niacin
Blood pressure	Systolic <130	β-Blockers
Diastolic	<85	ACE inhibitors
Antiplatelet therapy	All patients on some form	Aspirin, clopidogrel
Diabetes	HbA₁c < 7%	Insulin, ↑insulin sensitivity
Tobacco cessation	Complete abstinence	Nicotine replacement, antidepressant

LDL, Low-density lipoprotein; *HDL*, high-density lipoprotein; *ACE*, angiotensin-converting enzyme; *Hb A₁c*, glycosylated hemoglobin.

large populations at high risk for coronary disease indicate that aggressive risk factor modification (lipid reduction, antiplatelet therapy, diabetes management, and blood pressure control) reliably reduces near-term cardiac mortality.[123,124,126-129] Table 32-7 describes basic guidelines for risk factor modification based on these trials.

Smoking Cessation

Smoking cessation is by far the most important treatment for patients with PAD. PAD symptoms are unlikely to progress and may even improve once smoking is stopped completely.[165] In patients with intermittent claudication, improvement in walking distance up to 40% has been reported.[165,166] Improved patency of arterial repairs in nonsmokers has been demonstrated for both aortofemoral and femoropopliteal reconstructions,[167-170] and the degree of tobacco use (measured by carboxyhemoglobin levels) bears directly on the incidence of graft occlusion.[171]

Patients with PAD are often unaware of the strong association between smoking and lower extremity disease. In one study, only 37% of smokers with PAD recognized smoking as a risk factor.[172] The initial effort, therefore, on the part of all physicians must be to educate patients about the relationship between tobacco use and PAD and to inform patients unequivocally that smoking is the most important factor responsible for their leg condition. Studies have shown that strong and repeated advice by physicians to quit smoking results in abstinence in more than one third of smokers.[173]

Physicians must be prepared to provide a plan to help the patient achieve the goal of smoking cessation. Reassuring the patient is extremely important. Multiple attempts at quitting are common. For most people who eventually quit, 2 to 5 years and an average of six abstinence-relapse cycles are required.[174] Although half of all smokers make an attempt to discontinue tobacco use each year, as few as 3% to 5% remain abstinent at 1 year.[175] A recent randomized control trial demonstrated that patients enrolled in an intensive smoking cessation program consisting of education, counseling, behavioral therapy, and advice regarding pharmacologic adjuncts were threefold more likely to abstain from smoking at 6 months compared with patients only receiving advice from their physician.[176] Pharmacologic adjuncts for the treatment of smoking addiction may be helpful in facilitating cessation. Current adjuncts include nicotine replacement therapy, partial nicotine receptor agonists, and antidepressant therapy. Most nicotine replacement agents provide up to 30% of a smoker's regular daily nicotine intake and reduce or prevent withdrawal symptoms. Nicotine gum is the oldest form of nicotine replacement and is currently available without a prescription. Drawbacks include the requirement of specific chewing techniques to maximize nicotine release and drug inactivation with pH changes if beverages are consumed during use. Nicotine transdermal patches (dose ranging from 7 to 21 mg/24 hours) are easier to use. Reviews of randomized, double-blinded nicotine replacement trials for smoking cessation therapy in younger patients (30 to 40 years old) document biochemically confirmed 6-month abstinence rates of 20% to 45% in the treatment groups, compared with 5% to 25% in the control groups, depending on the setting (with treatment initiation in a smoking cessation clinic superior to that in a primary care office).[177,178] No benefit was derived from treatment longer than 8 weeks or from the tapering of nicotine. Intermediate-dose (14 mg/24 hour) nicotine patches have been used cautiously in patients with symptomatic coronary artery disease.[179]

Partial nicotine receptor agonists, such as varenicline, have recently gained popularity as adjuncts to smoking cessation. A recent Cochrane database metaanalysis showed that varencicline appears to be superior to placebo and buproprion for smoking cessation, but not significantly better than nicotine replacement therapy.[180] Finally, nicotine and citrate inhalers have been used in several small, randomized trials with or without nicotine patches.[181,182] These devices maintain reinforcement of the ritual and sensory phenomena of smoking. Although short-term abstinence with these devices has been achieved in 20% to 30% of cases, long-term success has been disappointing.

Smoking cessation programs now focus on depression as an important component of the smoker profile and as a major factor in withdrawal symptoms.[183] The antidepressant agents buproprion and fluoxetine have been used in randomized trials, with 12-week biochemically confirmed cessation rates of 30% to 40%.[184] In addition to diminishing withdrawal symptoms (which share many characteristics with chronic depression), these agents appear to attenuate some of the weight gain observed with smoking cessation. These agents have also been used in combination with nicotine replacement (patch or inhaler), with improved results compared with either agent alone.[185]

Treatment of Diabetes

Although diabetes is clearly recognized as a risk factor for PAD, it is not clear how optimizing glycemic control affects the progression of PAD. There is evidence that glycemic control prevents the microvascular complications of diabetes; however, its effect on macrovascular complications is less clear.[186] In the Diabetes Control and Complications Trial, 1440 patients with type 1 diabetes were randomized to intensive versus conventional insulin therapy. Although patients receiving intensive insulin had fewer cardiovascular events, there was no effect on the progression of PAD.[187] Similarly, in the United Kingdom Prospective Diabetes Study, in which 3867 patients with type 2 diabetes were randomized to drug treatment with sulfonylureas or insulin versus dietary control, intensive treatment resulted in fewer deaths from myocardial infarction but no difference in amputations or death from PAD.[188] Thus, recommendations for optimal glycemic control (hemoglobin $A_{1c} < 7\%$) are based primarily on its beneficial effect on cardiac rather than on peripheral arterial end points.

Treatment of Hyperlipidemia

Hyperlipidemia is a risk factor for all manifestations of atherosclerotic arterial occlusive disease, including PAD. A number of studies have evaluated the effects of treatment of hyperlipidemia on the progression of PAD. In general, lipid-lowering therapies are associated with stabilization or regression of PAD, as measured by angiography and severity of symptoms.[186,189] In the Cholesterol Lowering Atherosclerosis Study, 188 men with PAD and coronary artery disease were randomized to treatment with colestipol and niacin versus placebo. Lipid-lowering therapy was associated with stabilization of femoral atherosclerosis.[190] In the Program on Surgical Control of the Hyperlipidemias study, 838 patients with a history of myocardial infarction and hyperlipidemia were randomized to ileal bypass surgery versus placebo and followed for 10 years. A significant reduction in PAD progression was noted in the surgical group, with a 44% risk reduction for the development of an abnormal ABI (i.e., <0.95) and a 30% risk reduction for the development of intermittent claudication.[191] Similar results were found in the Scandinavian Simvastatin Survival Study, in which cholesterol reduction was associated with a 38% reduction in the risk of new or worsening symptoms of intermittent claudication.[192] By consensus agreement, the goals of lipid-lowering therapy are an LDL level less than 100 mg/dL and a triglyceride level less than 150 mg/dL.[193,194] Initial recommended therapy is a 3-hydroxy-3-methylglutaryl-coenzyme A reductase inhibitor (i.e., statin). Niacin can also be an important adjunct in increasing HDL levels and decreasing triglyceride levels.[195]

Treatment of Hypertension

Although hypertension is a risk factor for PAD, there is little evidence that management of hypertension alters disease progression. As a result, the goal of hypertension management in patients with PAD is to reduce the risk of myocardial infarction and stroke. There has been concern that the use of β-blockers might result in a worsening of PAD symptoms; this was based on early reports of reduced blood flow to the lower extremities with β-blocker therapy.[196] However, metaanalyses found no evidence that β-blockers adversely affect mild to moderate claudication.[197]

In the Heart Outcomes Prevention Evaluation Study, the angiotensin-converting enzyme inhibitor ramipril was shown to significantly decrease rates of myocardial infarction, stroke, and cardiovascular death in patients at high risk for these events. Forty-four percent of these patients had a history of PAD.[124] These results could not be explained solely on the basis of lowering blood pressure. Most patients did not have hypertension at the time of study entry, and the mean reduction in systolic blood pressure was only 3 mm Hg.

Treatment of Hyperhomocysteinemia

Hyperhomocysteinemia is a recognized risk factor for PAD and other manifestations of cardiovascular disease. Elevated plasma homocysteine levels can be lowered with vitamin B and folate supplements. There is, however, no evidence that treatment of hyperhomocysteinemia alters the course of PAD.

Antiplatelet Therapy

Although there is no clear evidence of improvement in PAD symptoms with antiplatelet therapy, there is growing evidence that patients with PAD benefit from antiplatelet therapy to reduce the risk of cardiovascular morbidity and mortality. The most frequently used antiplatelet medications include aspirin and the glycoprotein IIa/IIIb inhibitors (clopidogrel, ticlopidine).

Aspirin

The Antiplatelet Trialists' Collaboration reviewed 189 controlled studies involving the prevention of cardiovascular events in more than 100,000 patients with clinical evidence of cardiovascular disease. Overall, there was a 25% relative risk reduction of fatal and nonfatal myocardial infarction, stroke, and cardiovascular death associated with antiplatelet therapy at 3 years of follow-up.[198] However, in a subgroup analysis of 3295 claudicants, the risk reduction in these end points after a mean follow-up of 27 months was not significantly different. The small number of patients in the subgroup analysis may have accounted for this lack of statistical difference. Similar benefit was shown for aspirin doses ranging from 75 to 350 mg/day. Similar benefits of aspirin therapy were noted in the Physicians' Health Study, in which 22,071 male physicians were enrolled. Aspirin at a dose of 325 mg every other day resulted in a 54% risk reduction in the subsequent need for peripheral arterial surgery compared with placebo.[199] Based on these findings, aspirin has been recommended as antiplatelet therapy in patients with PAD by groups such as the American College of Chest Physicians[200] and the TransAtlantic Inter-Society Consensus.[20] The efficacy of aspirin therapy as primary prevention for cardiovascular events in patients with asymptomatic PAD has yet to be demonstrated. In fact, a recent randomized controlled trial of 3350 patients without evidence of cardiovascular disease and an ABI less than 0.95 showed no difference in myocardial infarction and stroke rates or all-cause mortality between the aspirin-treated group and the control group.[201]

Glycoprotein IIb/IIIa Inhibitors

The glycoprotein IIb/IIIa inhibitors inhibit platelet activation by blocking adenosine diphosphate receptors. Drugs in this class include ticlopidine and clopidogrel.

Ticlopidine. Ticlopidine has been shown to significantly lower the risk of ischemic carciovascular events, including stroke and fatal and nonfatal myocardial infarction.[202] Ticlopidine also decreases the need for lower extremity revascularization procedures compared with placebo in patients with PAD.[203] However, ticlopidine is rarely used because of rare but severe hematologic side effects, including thrombotic thrombocytopenic purpura, thrombocytopenia, and neutropenia.[204]

Clopidogrel. The most recently and extensively studied antiplatelet medication is clopidogrel. In the Clopidogrel versus Aspirin in Patients at Risk of Ischemic Events (CAPRIE) trial, 19,185 patients with recent stroke, myocardial infarction, or stable PAD were randomized to receive clopidogrel (75 mg daily) or aspirin (325 mg daily).[123] The study showed a significant relative risk reduction of 8.7% ($p = 0.04$) for subsequent cardiovascular events (myocardial infarction, ischemic stroke, or vascular death) in the patients treated with clopidogrel. In the subgroup of more than 6000 patients with PAD, the relative risk reduction was even greater, at 24%.

The safety profiles of aspirin and clopidogrel were comparable in the CAPRIE study. Clopidogrel and ticlodipine have similar antiplatelet effects, but clopidogrel is associated with fewer hematologic side effects. The risk of thrombotic thrombocytopenic purpura in patients taking clopidogrel is estimated at 4 per 1 million population. Routine hematologic monitoring is not considered necessary.[205]

Exercise Therapy

Patients with intermittent claudication typically reduce their walking in response to the discomfort induced by walking. Severely affected individuals may become housebound. Many patients believe that the pain manifested as claudication indicates injury, and they avoid walking to prevent adverse consequences. Exercise therapy in the management of claudication has been studied for more than 30 years. It is the best documented therapy and is an essential component of the nonoperative treatment of intermittent claudication. Regular walking results in a measurable improvement in walking distance, quality of life, and community-based functional capacity in most patients with intermittent claudication.[206-209] The major limitation of exercise

therapy is the presence of associated medical conditions that limit the ability to exercise. Initial evaluation includes functional assessment followed by exercise to determine pain-free and maximal walking distances. Success is defined as improvement in pain-free and maximal walking distances on a treadmill, improvement in scores on quality-of-life questionnaires, or both.

Exercise programs can increase walking distances from 80% to a 234%.[206,207] A metaanalysis of supervised exercise programs found a mean increase of 179% in patients' initial claudication distance and a mean increase of 122% in maximal walking distance.[208] Although better results have been achieved with supervised exercise programs, some benefit has consistently been measured in simple physician-recommended programs as well. In addition, a recent randomized controlled trial showed that the use of a step activity monitor in an unsupervised setting was as effective in increasing peak walking time and claudication onset time as supervised exercise therapy.[210]

The optimal frequency and duration of exercise as therapy for intermittent claudication are unclear; however, in a recent Cochrane analysis, significant benefits in claudication symptoms were detectable with 30 minutes of exercise 3 days a week.[211] In randomized trials that compared exercise to other treatment modalities, exercise therapy was superior to angioplasty at 6 months. Surgery may be more effective than exercise, but the attendant morbidities and potential mortality must be considered.[211]

The mechanism by which walking exercise improves symptoms of claudication is not completely understood. Neither ankle blood pressure nor calf muscle blood flow are objectively improved in claudicants with improved walking tolerance after an exercise program.[207,212-214] Elevated levels of proangiogenic vascular endothelial growth factor have been detected in exercised muscle.[215] The current belief is that adaptation of the muscle cells, likely by enzyme induction, to the relatively decreased oxygen delivery in an ischemic limb is largely responsible for the improved muscle performance seen with exercise training. Other possible mechanisms include improved hemorheologic blood cell characteristics, changes in gait with more efficient use of muscle groups, better fatty acid metabolism, and an increased ratio of muscle fibers to capillaries after regular exercise.[212,213,216]

Pharmacologic Therapy

Intermittent Claudication

The initial focus of treatment for patients with intermittent claudication is risk factor modification. Pharmacologic therapy should also be considered and is occasionally useful in improving symptoms. A number of drug classes, including vasodilators, hemorheologic agents, prostaglandins, antiplatelet agents, and anticoagulants, have been studied in recent years for the treatment of claudication symptoms. Currently two drugs, pentoxifylline and cilostazol, have been approved by the U.S. Food and Drug Administration for the treatment of patients with intermittent claudication.

Pentoxifylline. Patients with chronic lower extremity ischemia have abnormal hemorheology. Blood from patients with claudication demonstrates reduced flow rates through filters with uniform pore size.[217] Multiple studies have demonstrated decreased erythrocyte and leukocyte deformability, increased platelet aggregation, increased leukocyte and platelet adhesion, and increased blood viscosity in patients with chronic lower extremity ischemia.[218,219] Pentoxifylline is a hemorheologic agent that decreases blood viscosity and platelet aggregation and improves red blood cell flexibility. A modest improvement in claudication symptoms can be anticipated in some patients treated with pentoxifylline.[220,221] Less than 10% of patients demonstrate greater than 100% improved walking distances. Patients with ABIs less than 0.80 and symptoms of less than 1 year's duration appear to experience the most benefit. The most common side effect is gastrointestinal distress.

A metaanalysis of randomized, placebo-controlled clinical trials from 1976 to 1994 demonstrated an absolute increase of 29.4 and 48.4 m in pain-free and maximal walking distances in the pentoxifylline group compared with placebo.

Cilostazol. Cilostazol is a phosphodiesterase inhibitor that has many possible mechanisms of action, including vasodilatation, inhibition of platelet aggregation and smooth muscle proliferation, and improvement of lipid profile. Randomized, multicenter, placebo-controlled trials have demonstrated the superiority of cilostazol over placebo in improving initial and absolute claudication distances in patients with intermittent claudication.[222-225] These trials demonstrated an improvement in initial claudication distance of 35% to 59%, and an improvement in absolute claudication distance of 41% to 51%, after 12 to 24 weeks of treatment with cilostazol versus placebo. Effects seem to disappear after discontinuation of the drug.[226] The usual dose of cilostazol is 100 mg orally twice a day.

One randomized prospective trial comparing pentoxifylline to cilostazol demonstrated significantly greater improvement in walking distance in patients receiving cilostazol compared with pentoxifylline or placebo.[227] In 54 centers, 698 patients were randomized to receive pentoxifylline (n = 232), cilostazol (n = 227), or placebo (n = 239). After 24 weeks of treatment, mean maximal walking distance in patients receiving cilostazol had increased by 107 m, compared with 64 m in patients receiving pentoxifylline and 65 m in those receiving placebo. Quality-of-life assessments using Medical Outcome Study SF-36 questionnaires also demonstrated the efficacy of cilostazol. Side effects include headache, diarrhea, and dizziness.

Other Pharmacologic Agents. A number of additional pharmacologic agents have been investigated in the treatment of intermittent claudication. Although each has exhibited some benefit in limited, small trials, none has proved efficacious in large randomized trials.
Naftidrofuryl. Naftidrofuryl is a vasoactive drug frequently used for intermittent claudication in Europe. It is not available in the United States. Naftidrofuryl is a

serotonin antagonist that improves aerobic metabolism in oxygen-depleted tissues (via stimulation of carbohydrate and fat entry into the tricarboxylic acid cycle). It may also reduce both erythrocyte and platelet aggregation.[228] Systematic reviews of randomized, controlled trials comparing naftidrofuryl with placebo revealed modest but statistically significant increases in both pain-free walking distance and total walking distance. Treatment with naftidrofuryl does not change ABI.[229]
Carnitine. Intermittent claudication is the result of blood flow abnormalities to the lower extremities and metabolic abnormalities in skeletal muscle. Carnitine metabolism has been shown to be abnormal in patients with intermittent claudication; they have an accumulation of acylcarnitines (intermediates of oxidative metabolism) in skeletal muscle, inhibiting transport of free fatty acids into the mitochondria.[230] The amount of acylcarnitine in muscle corresponds to the degree of walking impairment. This has led to the hypothesis that carnitine supplementation can improve muscle performance. The mechanism of action includes promoting pyruvate entry into the citric acid cycle and facilitating transport of free fatty acids into the mitochondria. These actions have been demonstrated in several small phase II trials. In three randomized multicenter trials, treatment of patients with intermittent claudication with carnitine analogs (L-carnitine or propionyl L-carnitine) resulted in significant improvements in treadmill walking and quality of life compared with placebo.[231-233] Carnitine is not approved for use in the United States as a treatment for PAD.
Prostaglandin Analogs. Prostaglandin analogs (synthetic prostaglandin E_1 and prostaglandin I_2, or prostacyclin) are potent vasodilators that inhibit platelet aggregation.[234] Prostaglandins have been evaluated primarily for the treatment of critical limb ischemia, with fewer trials performed in patients with claudication. Intravenous prostaglandin E_1 was evaluated in two randomized controlled trials that demonstrated significant improvements in maximal walking distance (371% increase in absolute claudication distance) and quality of life compared with placebo.[235,236] Side effects include frequent vasoactive flushing and headache.

Because intravenous preparations are not practical for widespread use in patients with intermittent claudication, oral prostaglandin analogs have been developed. Beraprost sodium is an oral prostacyclin analog with vasodilatory and antiplatelet effects. A multicenter randomized European trial suggested that beraprost increased walking distance in claudicants.[237] However, a large, multicenter, randomized, placebo-controlled trial in the United States failed to show any statistical benefit.[238]
Vasodilators. Vasodilator drugs were the first class of drugs used to treat intermittent claudication. Examples include α-blockers, calcium channel blockers, and direct-acting vasodilators such as papaverine. Several controlled trials have shown that vasodilators have no efficacy in treating intermittent claudication.[239] In theory, the reason for this is that ischemic muscle beds are already maximally vasodilated during exercise. Vasodilators therefore do not augment arterial flow in muscle beds distal to stenoses, but they may cause vasodilatation of

noischemic muscle beds, thereby creating a "steal" phenomenon, taking blood away from ischemic tissue.

Anticoagulants. Anticoagulants (heparin, low-molecular-weight heparin, oral anticoagulants) result in no significant improvement in either pain-free or maximal walking distances. An increased risk of bleeding has been noted with these agents. Anticoagulants are not indicated for the treatment of intermittent claudication.[240]

Buflomedil. Buflomedil, a vasoactive, hemorheologic agent, has been used for the treatment of intermittent claudication in Europe for many years. Blufomedil reduces vasoconstriction through both α_1 and α_2 adrenolysis. The use of this medication is based on scant clinical evidence. A recent metaanalysis examining clinical trials of buflomedil found only two small trials that conformed to accepted reporting standards. Although modest improvements in walking distance have been reported, the data are not strong enough to support the recommendation of this medication for treatment of intermittent claudication. It is not available in the United States.[241]

L-Arginine. L-Arginine is an amino acid demonstrated to enhance nitric oxide formation and endothelium-dependent vasodilatation in patients with atherosclerosis. Two small trials demonstrated improvements in initial and absolute claudication distances, but larger trials are needed to define the role of L-arginine in claudication therapy.[242,243]

Critical Limb Ischemia

The mainstay of treatment for chronic CLI is either surgical or endovascular revascularization; however, this is not always required when the only manifestations are intermittent rest pain or shallow ulcers. The natural history of intermittent rest pain is not necessarily one of inevitable progression to gangrene and limb loss. This was clearly shown in randomized controlled trials of prostaglandin treatment in patients with CLI, in which approximately 50% of patients with rest pain or ulcer improved on placebo.[132,244] Situations in which patients refuse surgery or are not surgical candidates (owing to severe comorbidities or lack of target vessels, small ulcers, or rest pain) can improve on occasion without revascularization.

Novel nonoperative therapies for critical limb ischemia have focused on three main areas: intermittent pneumatic compression (IPC) devices, stem cell therapy, and gene-directed therapy. Intermittent pneumatic compression devices aim to increase vascular flow to ischemic limbs by increasing the arteriovenous pressure gradient of the limb. Hemodynamic improvement of limbs with CLI has been demonstrated with the use of intermittent pneumatic compression devices.[245] There have been randomized controlled trials demonstrating improved ABI, claudication distance, and quality of life in stable claudicants randomized to IPC therapy compared with controls[246]; however, there are no randomized trials of IPC therapy for limb salvage in patients with CLI.

Stem cell therapy arose from the discovery that a subset of bone marrow derived mononuclear cells are able to differentiate into endothelium and promote new vessel growth. Currently, progenitor cells can be obtained from bone marrow aspiration or peripheral blood sample aphoresis. These progenitor cells are then delivered to the ischemic limb via intraarterial or intramuscular injection. A metaanalysis of more than 701 patients treated with stem cell therapy showed significant benefit in ABI, transcutaneous partial pressure of oxysen (TCO_2), pain-free walking distance, pain scale, ulcer healing, and amputation rates.[247] Intramuscular administration appears superior to intraarterial administration, but the preference of bone marrow versus peripheral blood derived stem cells is controversial.

Gene-induced angiogenesis introduces angiogenic genes or gene products into an area of ischemia using gene transfer approaches and viral and plasmid vectors. Trials of vascular endothelial gowth factor (VEGF), fibroblast growth factor (FGF), hepatocyte growth factor, and *DEL1* gene have been reported.[248] A recent metaanalysis of trials of gene therapy identified one trial of gene therapy (using basic fibroblast growth factor) that reported clinical benefit. All other trials and the pooled data showed no benefit in patients with claudication or critical limb ischemia when only gene therapy trials were included.[249] A recent clinical trial also showed no benefit in treating patients with unilateral intermittent claudication with vascular endothelial growth factor.[250]

CONCLUSION

Appropriate management of patients with chronic lower extremity ischemia is complex. Understanding of the natural history of this disease is important for patient education and management. Patients with peripheral vascular disease often have concomitant atherosclerotic disease of other vascular beds. Risk factor modification is aimed at preventing both disease progression and adverse cardiovascular events. Intermittent claudication usually confers a low risk of limb loss, and initial treatment is generally non-operative with a trial of exercise and pharmacologic therapy. The risk of limb-loss is greater in patients with critical limb ischemia, and patients with CLI generally require surgical or endovascular revascularization. Newer treatments including gene and progenitor cell derived therapies are emerging, but there is limited evidence for their use.

References available online at expertconsult.com.

QUESTIONS

1. An abnormal ABI is present in approximately what percentage of patients older than 50 years?
   a. 1%
   b. 2%
   c. 15%
   d. 25%
   e. 35%

2. What is the increased risk of developing peripheral arterial disease in current smokers versus those who have never smoked?
   a. Two times
   b. Four times
   c. Six times
   d. Sixteen times
   e. Thirty-two times

3. What disease process leads to the most nontraumatic amputations in the United States?
   a. Diabetes
   b. Buerger disease
   c. Tobacco abuse
   d. Obesity
   e. Connective tissue disorders

4. What is the prevalence of peripheral arterial disease in women versus that in men?
   a. 10% that in men
   b. 50% that in men
   c. 75% that in men
   d. Equal to that in men
   e. 150% that in men

5. The relative risk of a patient with intermittent claudication having a myocardial infarction or stroke compared with a nonclaudicant is increased by what factor?
   a. One to two times
   b. Two to three times
   c. Four to five times
   d. Six to eight times
   e. Ten times

6. What proportion of patients undergoing amputation for ischemia experienced ischemic symptoms 6 months before the amputation?
   a. Less than 50%
   b. 60% to 70%
   c. 70% to 80%
   d. 80% to 90%
   e. 100%

7. The relative risk reduction for myocardial infarction, ischemic stroke, or vascular death in patients with peripheral arterial disease managed with clopidogrel versus aspirin is approximately which of the following?
   a. 5%
   b. 10%
   c. 15%
   d. 20%
   e. 25%

8. The most likely mechanism by which exercise therapy improves walking distance in patients with intermittent claudication is which of the following?
   a. Increase in ankle-brachial index
   b. Muscle cell adaptation to decreased oxygen delivery
   c. Increased collateral formation
   d. Improved cardiac output
   e. Improved blood hemorheology

9. Which of the following is currently the most effective drug available in the United States for improving walking distance in patients with peripheral arterial disease and intermittent claudication?
   a. Cilostazol
   b. Pentoxifylline
   c. Warfarin
   d. Aspirin
   e. Carnitine

10. Which of the following is a contraindication to the use of cilostazol for the treatment of intermittent claudication?
   a. Congestive heart failure
   b. Walking distance less than 100 feet
   c. CYP 3A inhibitors
   d. Warfarin therapy
   e. Use of β-blocker drugs

ANSWERS

1. **d**
2. **d**
3. **a**
4. **d**
5. **b**
6. **a**
7. **e**
8. **b**
9. **a**
10. **a**

CHAPTER 33

THROMBOLYSIS FOR ARTERIAL AND GRAFT OCCLUSIONS: TECHNIQUE AND RESULTS

Vikram S. Kashyap • Niren Angle • William J. Quiñones-Baldrich

Thrombolytic therapy is an important modality in the treatment of patients with peripheral arterial and venous thrombosis. Randomized clinical trials have compared thrombolytic therapy with traditional surgical options, thus providing guidelines for patient selection. As a therapeutic intervention, lytic therapy may be the best alternative in certain clinical situations. In many other cases, it is just one aspect of the overall care of patients with thrombotic complications of peripheral vascular disease.

This chapter provides an overview of the fibrinolytic system and the available agents. This information can be translated into guidelines to help clinicians select patients who may benefit from thrombolytic therapy. Methods, dosages, complications, and promising new areas are also discussed.

HISTORY

The fluidity of blood post mortem is an observation that dates to the Hippocratic school in the fourth century BC.[1] Almost 2000 years later, it was rediscovered by the Italian anatomist Malpighi.[2] In 1761, Morgagni noted that blood does not retain its liquid state after death but frequently forms clots.[3] This is followed by partial or complete reliquefaction.

In 1906, Morawitz observed that postmortem blood destroys fibrinogen and fibrin in normal blood.[4] Thus, the presence of an active fibrinolysin was postulated. The term *fibrinolysis* had been coined by Dastre in 1893 to describe the disappearance of fibrin in unclottable blood obtained from dogs subjected to repeated hemorrhage.[5] From the latter part of the nineteenth century until the present, intense investigation has been undertaken to elucidate the complex and vital functions of the fibrinolytic system. The role of the fibrinolytic system from a homeostatic point of view is fully appreciated. The interplay of components, activators, and inhibitors are becoming more appreciated. The potential to harness the fibrinolytic system for therapeutic means has emerged in the last few decades, and results from prospective clinical trials are now available, providing guidelines to patient selection and therapy. For the vascular specialist, thrombolytic therapy represents one of the most promising therapeutic modalities for arterial and venous thrombosis, but careful dosing and monitoring of thrombolytic therapy are required. In addition, careful attention and observation of the patient and often the limb undergoing treatment is required.

FIBRINOLYTIC SYSTEM

The complex and intricate relationships among all components of the fibrinolytic system are only partially understood. Much progress has been made, however, mostly owing to recognition of the importance of the fibrinolytic system as a homeostatic system. This same process has been harnessed for a therapeutic effect in cases of clinical thrombosis. The concept of dynamic equilibrium was proposed by Astrup in 1958.[6] In a delicate balance, fibrinolysis breaks down fibrin, which is continuously being deposited throughout the cardiovascular system. This is the result of limited activation of the coagulation system. This baseline fibrinolytic activity is probably under local and central control mechanisms. The feedback loop that prevents systemic fibrinolysis involves both inhibitors at the activator level and specific inhibitors of the proteolytic enzyme plasmin.

The final common pathway in the fibrinolytic system is the conversion of the proenzyme plasminogen to the active enzyme plasmin. Plasminogen is a glycoprotein produced by the liver. Full-sized plasminogen can be divided into a heavy N-terminal region that consists of five homologous but distinct triple-disulfide–bonded domains (kringles) fused to a lighter catalytic C-terminal domain. At least four forms occur in plasma, based on variations in the N-terminal and the degree of glycosylation. The two main forms are Glu-plasminogen and Lys-plasminogen.[7] Glu-plasminogen contains glutamic acid and exists in high concentrations in plasma. Lys-plasminogen, containing mostly lysin in the N-terminal, results from limited proteolysis of the Glu form; it has a shorter half-life and is found in higher concentrations in thrombus, most likely secondary to its higher affinity for fibrin.[8] A schematic view of the fibrinolytic system is presented in Figure 33-1.

The kringle portion of plasminogen is a nonprotease, or heavy chain, consisting of five homologous domains. These domains exhibit a high degree of sequence homology with one another and with domains found in prothrombin, tissue plasminogen activator (t-PA), urinary plasminogen activator, and factor XII. Kringle-4 shares homology with apolipoprotein A. The function of these

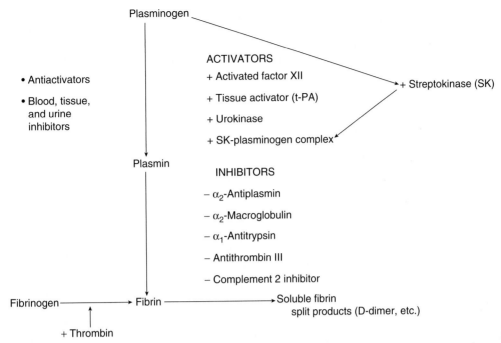

FIGURE 33-1 ■ Simplified scheme of the fibrinolytic system with endogenous and exogenous activators.

kringles is thought to be of paramount importance in the binding of plasminogen and plasmin to fibrin, α_2-antiplasmin, and other macromolecules.[9,10] In addition, the kringle portion of plasminogen has been implicated in mediating neutrophil adherence to endothelial cells.[11] On binding, conformational changes occur that transform a closed structure into an open structure. ε-Aminocaproic acid and tranexamic acid induce this change from the closed structure to the open structure. Because of this change, plasminogen is far more readily cleaved to the active enzyme plasmin by plasminogen activators. The open conformation also binds more readily to exposed lysine residues on fibrin's surface. Concentrations of lysine analogs, such as tranexamic acid and aminocaproic acid, that actually promote the more active, open conformation of Glu-plasminogen also prevent its binding to fibrin and therefore exhibit an antifibrinolytic effect.[12]

The primary substrates for the proteolytic activity of plasmin in circulation are fibrinogen and fibrin. Circulating fibrinogen is composed of three polypeptide chains known as the α, β, and γ chains. These chains are bonded together by disulfide bonds, which are also linked to a second identical chain, thus making fibrinogen a dimer of trimers. Thrombin, the common pathway of the coagulation cascade, removes several amino acid peptides from the end terminal of the α chain, the β chain (fibrinopeptide B), to form fibrin. As new sites are exposed, staggered polymerization is initiated.[7] Through catalysis by factor XIIIa, the domains are brought together and chemically cross-linked. Plasmin catalyzes the hydrolysis of these bonds, producing peptides that can be assayed in circulation. Specifically, those produced after the cleavage of fibrinogen consist of truncated polypeptides collectively known as X *fragments*. X fragments can be

incorporated into both newly forming and existing thrombi, causing them to be more fragile. This has been proposed as a possible explanation of why fibrin-specific fibrinolytic agents such as t-PA do not result in fewer bleeding complications compared with nonspecific agents. Because t-PA is such a potent fibrinolytic activator, the accumulation of these X fragments could make existing thrombi more susceptible to its fibrinolytic action. Several fragments are specifically produced by the action of plasmin on fibrin, as opposed to fibrinogen. Unique fragments such as D-dimers can be assayed, documenting fibrinolysis as opposed to fibrinogenolysis.[13]

Plasmin is a relatively nonspecific protease and thus can hydrolyze many proteins found in plasma and extracellular spaces. Known targets of plasmin are factors V and VIII and von Willebrand factor.[1] Prothrombotic activity can be shown with the initial administration of fibrinolytic agents (specifically t-PA and streptokinase, which may relate to the release of fibrinopeptide A). Plasminogen can also cause the release of kinin from high-molecular-weight kininogen. In addition, it can directly and indirectly activate prekallikrein, again inducing kinin formation.[14,15] Plasmin can also attack protein components of the basement membrane, as well as other active proteases within the matrix, including fibronectin, collagen, and laminin.[7]

Activation of factor XII by various stimuli results in initiation of the coagulation cascade, conversion of prekallikrein to kallikrein and kinin (inflammatory response), and formation of plasmin from plasminogen. This intrinsic mechanism of activation is complemented by a second intrinsic pathway that is not dependent on factor XII. The main pathway for plasminogen activation is known as the extrinsic system. Two activators are recognized in humans: urokinase-type plasminogen activator (u-PA) and t-PA. Their physiologic activity is controlled by inhibitors, mostly plasminogen activator inhibitor (PAI) type 1 (PAI-1) and type PAI-3. These inhibitors control the activity of the activators in plasma and possibly at the cellular level. PAI-1 is synthesized in the liver and vascular endothelial cells and is normally present in trace amounts in plasma. PAI-1 elevation leading to prothrombotic states is becoming increasingly recognized. When pharmacologic doses of these agents are administered, the inhibitor activity is suppressed. It is estimated that one third to half of the initial pharmacologic dose of urokinase, for example, becomes inactivated shortly after administration.[11] Once plasminogen has been converted to plasmin, inhibitors of plasmin come into play. The main physiologic inhibitor of plasmin is α_2-antiplasmin. This protease inhibitor is a single-chain glycoprotein that inhibits plasminogen in two steps: a fast reversible binding step, followed by the formation of a covalent complex involving the active site of plasmin.[7] The half-life of this complex is approximately 12 hours.[16] Other inhibitors of plasmin include α_2-macroglobulin, protease nexin, and aprotinin. Protease nexin is a broad-spectrum inhibitor of serine proteinases and inhibits, among others, trypsin, thrombin, urokinase, plasmin, and one- or two-chain t-PA. Once bound, these proteases are internalized via nexin receptors on the cell surface and rapidly degraded.[17] Aprotinin, also known as *basic pancreatic trypsin inhibitor*, has been isolated and purified and is sold under the name Trasylol (Bayer, West Haven, Conn.). It is also a potent inhibitor of trypsin and kallikrein, in addition to plasmin. The use of bovine aprotinin to reduce postoperative bleeding after major surgery has been reported.[18,19] In animal models, it has been shown to serve as an antidote to bleeding induced by the administration of recombinant t-PA (rt-PA).[20] Because aprotinin inhibits plasmin and not the activator, it should work with other plasminogen activators.

This complex system is capable of maintaining a balanced equilibrium between clotting and lysis, so that blood fluidity is ensured. It is important to recognize that although plasmin is highly selective for fibrin, it also digests fibrinogen and other plasma proteins. Circulating plasmin inhibitors prevent this otherwise disordered lytic action and preclude free circulating plasmin under normal conditions.

A link between lipoprotein metabolism and fibrinolytic function has been suggested by the demonstration of significant homology between the amino acid sequence of apolipoprotein A and the structure of plasminogen. Thus, a prothrombotic function by virtue of interference with the numerous physiologic functions of plasminogen has been suggested in patients with increased levels of apolipoprotein A. Apolipoprotein A has also been found to competitively inhibit the binding of plasminogen to fibrinogen and to the plasminogen receptor on endothelial cells.[26]

Plasma levels of both t-PA and PAI-1 exhibit circadian variations. For example, t-PA activity is lowest in the early morning and highest in the afternoon. Plasma PAI activity peaks in the early morning and passes through a trough in the afternoon. Thus, overall there is decreased fibrinolytic activity in the morning.[27-30] Differences in patterns have been observed between men and women, suggesting a hormonal influence.[31] Furthermore, PAI activity has been noted to vary secondary to diet, with caffeine-containing beverages possibly enhancing fibrinolytic activity. Conversely, cigarette smoking induces an acute increase in t-PA; this increase in t-PA may deplete normal stores and thus paradoxically decrease fibrinolytic capacity.

From the foregoing discussion, it is evident that the fibrinolytic (plasminogen-plasmin) system plays a vital role in biological homeostasis. In addition, it has a pivotal role in certain disease states, ranging from atherosclerosis to carcinogenesis.

From a therapeutic standpoint, drugs capable of converting plasminogen to plasmin achieve their lytic effect to a great extent by overwhelming circulating plasmin inhibitors and generating an abundance of plasmin (exogenous fibrinolysis). Circulating plasmin not only produces the desired fibrinolysis but also proceeds to digest circulating fibrinogen. A more desirable situation results in the activation of thrombus-bound plasminogen (endogenous fibrinolysis) by these agents. Thrombus-bound plasminogen is, to a certain extent, protected from circulating inhibitors and thus proceeds with fibrin digestion much more effectively. Current investigations are concentrated on producing agents with a high affinity for thrombus-bound plasminogen and little activation of the circulating zymogen. Clinical experience to date has failed to demonstrate this theoretical benefit. With better understanding of the complexity of the fibrinolytic system, it is possible that these benefits can be realized.

THROMBOLYTIC AGENTS

The use of thrombolytic agents has clearly resulted in a significant improvement in the outcome of patients with acute cardiac ischemia, myocardial infarction, and cerebral infarction. It has also resulted in a modification in the treatment algorithm for patients with peripheral arterial occlusion. Thrombolytic therapy is an important treatment option for patients with vascular occlusive disease. Table 33-1 summarizes the characteristics of some of the common thrombolytic agents. Several schemes may be used to classify thrombolytic agents. The agents can be grouped by their mechanism of action—those that directly convert plasminogen to plasmin versus those that are inactive zymogens and require transformation to an active form before they can cleave plasminogen. Agents can be classified by their mode of production. In addition, thrombolytic agents can be classified by their pharmacologic actions—those that are fibrin specific (i.e., bind to fibrin but not to fibrinogen) versus those that are nonspecific, and those that have a great degree of fibrin affinity (i.e., bind avidly to fibrin) versus those that do not. Another useful classification of thrombolytic agents is groups based on their origin: the streptokinase compounds, the urokinase compounds, the tissue plasminogen activators, and an additional group consisting of novel agents. In the following sections, we have divided thrombolytic drugs chronologically.

TABLE 33-1 **Thrombolytic Agents**

Characteristics	Streptokinase	Urokinase	Tissue Plasminogen Activator	Reteplase
Source	β-Hemolytic *Streptococcus*	Fetal renal cell culture	Recombinant DNA technology	Plasminogen activator
Metabolism	Liver	Liver	Liver	Liver
Advantages	Low cost	Direct activator; no allergic reaction	Fibrin-selective direct activator	Plasminogen activator in presence of fibrin
Disadvantages	Allergic reactions; complex mechanism of action	High cost	High cost	High cost
Regional infusion dosage	Low dose: 5000-10,000 U/hr High dose: 30,000-60,000 U/hr	30,000-50,000 U/hr 2000-4000 U/min for 1-2 hr, then 1000-2000 U/min	0.05-0.1 U/kg/hr	0.5 U/hr IV; no bolus Rate may be adjusted up to 0.75-1.0 U/hr or down to 0.25 U/hr

IV, Intravenously.

First-Generation Thrombolytic Drugs

First-generation thrombolytic agents—namely, streptokinase and urokinase—are highly effective at thrombolysis, but their potency is limited by the fact that they are not fibrin specific. They also convert circulating plasminogen to plasmin, but because circulating plasminogen and the plasminogen in thrombus are in equilibrium, the plasminogen in thrombus would be depleted, thus limiting the efficacy of the agent. This has been termed *plasminogen steal* and is thought to reduce clot lysis.

Streptokinase

Streptokinase is a single-chain nonenzymatic protein produced by β-hemolytic streptococci. Its discovery by Tillett and Garner[32] in 1933 revived an interest in fibrinolysis that has spanned the past 7 decades. Early clinical experience was complicated by a multitude of pyogenic and allergic reactions. This prompted manufacturers to refine the drug, achieving the currently purified product and a marked reduction in febrile and allergic reactions.

The mechanism of action of streptokinase is complex. It initially forms an equimolar complex with plasminogen to form a plasminogen activator. Thus, it requires plasminogen as a cofactor and a substrate. The initial reaction is species specific, having excellent affinity for human and cat plasminogen, relatively poor affinity for dog and rabbit plasminogen, and no reaction with bovine proenzyme. Once the activator complex is formed, it is an excellent activator of all mammalian plasminogen. Besides converting uncomplexed plasminogen to plasmin, plasminogen within the activator complex is converted to plasmin, and during this conversion, streptokinase undergoes rapid progressive degradation.

The kinetics of these reactions have been studied in vitro. In vivo, a more complicated series of reactions occurs. Infusion of streptokinase is followed initially by neutralization by circulating antistreptococcal antibodies. The remaining drug then combines with circulating plasminogen to form the activator complex. This then converts uncomplexed plasminogen to plasmin, which combines with any excess free streptokinase, is neutralized by circulating antiplasmins, or binds to preformed fibrin. The last produces the desired effect of thrombolysis. However, when activity is measured, two half-lives are detected—16 minutes and 83 minutes—indicating that these complex interactions have a significant effect on the concentration and activity of the drug.

From the foregoing discussion, it is evident that precise control of thrombolysis is not possible because the dose-response relationship of streptokinase varies from patient to patient. Initially, clinical use was guided by titers of antistreptococcal antibodies and measurement of the various components or products of the system. This proved impractical, and current practice relies on standardized dosages that achieve the desired effect in the great majority of cases. A potential drawback of this approach is that excess amounts of drug could use most of the circulating plasminogen to form activator complex; this might leave inadequate amounts of zymogen to convert to plasmin. This problem of exceeding plasminogen availability may be important during regional, rather than systemic, administration. Some investigators have combined streptokinase with plasmin administration, resulting in improvements in measured parameters such as plasminogen level, fibrinogen level, and potential fibrinolytic capacity.[33] Similar results are obtained by intermittent rather than continuous infusion of the drug. Unfortunately, the results of these noncontrolled trials have raised doubts about the effectiveness of such regimens. Streptokinase has largely fallen out of favor, partly because of the immunogenicity of even the refined form, which can result in fever, allergic reactions, and acquired drug resistance. A complex of streptokinase and anisoylated plasminogen streptokinase activator complex (APSAC), or anistreplase, was developed in an attempt to solve some of the problems inherent to streptokinase. It is an acylated complex of SK with human lys-plasminogen. The potency of APSAC has been found to be tenfold that of SK, but it has a longer half-life. Although conceptually sound, clinical trials were unable to demonstrate any increase in efficacy or any decrease in antigenicity with the administration of APSAC.

Streptokinase is the only thrombolytic agent approved by the U.S. Food and Drug Administration (FDA) for use in peripheral arterial and venous thrombolysis, but it is rare to find it being used for that purpose, for the reasons stated earlier. The newer thrombolytic agents have much better safety profiles and better therapeutic efficacy; therefore off-label use of these alternative thrombolytic agents is the norm.

Urokinase

Urokinase is a serine protease with direct activator activity; it is normally present in urine as a product of renal tubular cells. It was originally isolated by MacFarlane and Pilling in 1947.[34] Urokinase is present in varying molecular weights, with variable activity. Original purification was done from urine, yielding small amounts of the enzyme at a considerable cost. Newer production methods use human fetal kidney cell culture.

Urokinase is nonantigenic, and its mechanism of action is much more direct compared with that of streptokinase. Urokinase cleaves plasminogen (its only known protein substrate), by first-order reaction kinetics, to plasmin. It is pH and temperature stable. The lack of circulating neutralizing antibodies and its direct mechanism of action allow for a predictable dose-response relationship. Although allergic reactions are rare, over the last few years a febrile response to drug administration has become more common. It has been suggested that this may be related to interleukins that are still present in recently manufactured drug batches. In the past, when the use of urokinase was less common, aging of the drug actually allowed the interleukins to become inactive. These febrile reactions respond readily to antipyretics. Interestingly, urokinase does not contain any lysine binding sites and therefore does not have any fibrin binding properties.[35] High-affinity receptors for urokinase, however, have been demonstrated in several cell types and have been postulated as a mechanism by which cells can invade the intracellular matrix and play a role in other physiologic and pathologic processes.[36-38]

Urokinase is a serine protease and hydrolyzes synthetic esters containing arginine and lysine. Unlike streptokinase, urokinase directly activates plasminogen by cleaving the Arg560-Val561 activation bond. The activation of plasminogen by urokinase occurs by proteolysis. When administered intravenously, urokinase is rapidly removed from the circulation, mainly via hepatic clearance. It has been estimated that the half-life of urokinase in humans is on the order of 14 minutes. Urokinase also reacts with other proteins, including fibrinogen. Urokinase is much more effective in cleaving the susceptible site in plasminogen when it is in the Lys form than in the Glu form. However, the activation reaction of the latter by urokinase may be enhanced by the presence of fibrin.[39] Administration of exogenous plasminogen may also accelerate thrombolysis by urokinase.

Controversy exists regarding the actual thrombolytic effect of urokinase when administered in vivo. Experimental studies have suggested exogenous fibrinolysis as the main pathway, with limited activation of plasminogen within the thrombus (endogenous fibrinolysis).[40] In clinical practice, the results of urokinase therapy have paralleled those achieved with streptokinase, with a decreased incidence of bleeding complications suggested by several investigators.[42-44] Whereas major bleeding complications are seen in 15% to 20% of patients treated with streptokinase, such complications have been reported in only 5% to 10% of patients treated with urokinase. Thus, the benefits observed in laboratory results and the reduced incidence of significant plasminemia with urokinase seem to translate into a decreased incidence of bleeding complications in clinical practice. Although the cost of urokinase remains high compared with that of streptokinase, when complications are considered, the cost of therapy for streptokinase and urokinase is comparable.[45]

Residual thromboplastic activity was detected in the early urokinase preparations,[46] and this may account for the initial hypercoagulable state reported by Kakkar and Scully.[47] At present, this does not appear to be a clinically significant problem.

Despite the drug's record of safety and efficacy accrued over the years, the U.S. Food and Drug Administration halted the release and use of urokinase, manufactured by Abbott Laboratories, on the grounds of deviations from the FDA's current good manufacturing practices guidelines, developed to prevent the manufacture of unsafe products. The FDA inspection of Abbott's manufacturing facility in North Chicago in 1998 raised concerns about the neonatal kidney cells that were being used as a source of urokinase.[48,49] The cells originated from Cali, Colombia, and were obtained through a separate company. The source population was thought to be at high risk for various diseases, including tropical ones, and although there were no documented cases of infectious transmission resulting from urokinase administration, the FDA stated that any connection between the drug and such cases might have gone unrecognized.

In October 2002, the FDA approved the reintroduction of urokinase to the market after Abbott made significant changes in its quality-control and manufacturing practices. Urokinase was approved for use in the treatment of pulmonary embolism. Although it has not been approved for use in the peripheral arterial and venous systems, many practitioners have experience with off-label use in the periphery. During the time that urokinase was unavailable, increased experience and familiarity were gained with other agents, such as rt-PA and reteplase.[50]

Second-Generation Thrombolytic Drugs

Unlike first-generation thrombolytic drugs, second-generation agents are supposed to be fibrin selective. These agents were developed to avoid systemic depletion of circulating fibrinogen and plasminogen and the consequent systemic thrombolytic state; these agents are represented by t-PA, or alteplase, and single-chain u-PA, or pro-urokinase. There is considerable evidence that the plasminogen activator agents are not appreciably fibrin or thrombus specific and that they activate the complement system and damage the cell membranes of platelets and endothelial cells.

Tissue Plasminogen Activator

Tissue plasminogen activator is a naturally occurring enzyme present in all human tissues. Its concentration is variable, with high levels detected in the uterus and moderate amounts in the heart, skeletal muscles, kidneys, ovaries, lungs, thyroid, pituitary, and lymph nodes. Scant amounts of t-PA are found in the liver, spleen, brain, and testes.[51] It is thought to originate from vascular endothelium, and, with the exception of the liver and spleen, tissue concentration correlates with vascularity.

Isolation and purification of t-PA were initially hampered by inadequate sources and procedures. In 1979, Rijken and associates[52] were successful in obtaining 1 mg of t-PA from 5 kg of human uterine tissue. Recognizing the potential of this drug, investigators have concentrated on other sources.

At present, there are two main sources of t-PA. The Bowes melanoma cell line is uniquely efficient in producing large quantities of t-PA,[53] which was subsequently proved to be identical to uterine t-PA.[54] Another source has emerged from the use of recombinant DNA technology, and efforts in the cloning and expression of the t-PA gene from the melanoma cell line have been successful. Since 1987, when rt-PA was approved for the treatment of acute myocardial infarction, it has been used for peripheral thrombolysis as an alternative to urokinase.

In general, plasminogen activators do not cause clot dissolution directly; they must first find and activate molecules of plasminogen in the vasculature at the site of the clot. t-PA is a direct plasminogen activator. Its main advantage is its high affinity for thrombus-bound fibrin. The agent exhibits significant fibrin specificity. t-PA is a poor enzyme in the absence of fibrin. However, the presence of fibrin strikingly enhances the activation rate of plasminogen by t-PA. Two types of t-PA are recognized, with a commercial preparation being a mixture of both types. A single-chain form is cleaved by plasminogen to yield two-chain t-PA. The one- and two-chain forms of t-PA are comparable in activity, with the one-chain form being quickly converted to the two-chain type as lysis proceeds. Most of the circulating t-PA is in the single-chain form. Its selective action promises to produce fewer systemic effects when compared with streptokinase or urokinase.[55] The half-life of t-PA has been estimated to be between 4 and 7 minutes in vivo.[56] With its presumed nonantigenicity and high affinity for fibrin, t-PA theoretically should produce improved clinical results.

When fibrin-selective agents are used for regional infusion, most of the thrombolytic effect is secondary to fibrin-bound plasminogen. However, the importance of a fresh supply of plasminogen to maintain the fibrin-bound plasminogen pool has been emphasized. Experimental studies have suggested that clot lysis induced by the activation of plasminogen is dependent on clot-associated plasminogen, which in turn depends on the concentration of plasminogen in plasma. Depletion of both contributes to less frequent and less rapid recanalization, which is more noticeable with non–fibrin-selective agents than with fibrin-selective ones, likely the result of the depletion of plasminogen induced by the nonselective agents.[57]

Trials comparing rt-PA with streptokinase in patients with acute coronary thrombosis have failed to establish that this more specific drug is a better thrombolytic agent. Systemic bleeding complications have been similar, despite a milder homeostatic defect by laboratory

evaluation in the rt-PA groups.[58] Questions still exist regarding proper dosage to achieve effective local lysis with minimal systemic effects.

Tissue plasminogen activator may also bind and be activated on platelet surfaces.[59] Owing to this binding to platelet receptors, platelets can direct t-PA action on their surface, leading to rapid cleavage of glycoprotein Ib and the loss of platelet binding to von Willebrand factor. This may explain why concentrations of t-PA achieved early in therapy may inhibit platelet aggregation.

In animal models of thrombolysis, it has been suggested that multiple bolus administrations of t-PA have greater lytic efficacy than equal doses given as a single bolus or a continuous infusion.[60] This may have significant implications for clinical therapy, in which protocols requiring continuous infusion of the agent have shown a greater incidence of bleeding complications than protocols in which the drug is administered in bolus form. This might be explained by the accumulation of partially degraded fibrin (X fragments), which might increase the affinity of t-PA for plasminogen by about 17-fold.[7]

In a study in which 17 patients were infused with rt-PA at a rate of 0.1 mg/kg per hour, all patients demonstrated thrombolysis, with 16 showing clinical improvement.[61] More important, there were no systemic complications, with a mean fibrinogen drop of 42% of baseline. The infusion time was 1 to 6 hours, compared with the usual 48 to 72 hours necessary for streptokinase infusion. One patient died from an intracranial hemorrhage during postinfusion heparin therapy. Experience in randomized trials has suggested that a lower dose is just as effective, with a decreased risk of bleeding. The recommended lower dose is 0.05 mg/kg per hour.[62]

Systemic complications may be more related to dose and method of administration with t-PA than with urokinase or streptokinase. It appears that t-PA is more potent and faster than the older agents, perhaps because of its high fibrin affinity. In this regard, t-PA may be ideally suited for intraarterial administration, because a 4- to 6-hour trial could be followed by timely surgical intervention. In addition, intraoperative use could be a welcome adjunct to surgical embolectomy.

Pro-Urokinase

Saruplase, also known as recombinant single-chain urokinase-type plasminogen activator, or pro-urokinase, is a prodrug produced from a naturally occurring physiologic protease.[62] Pro-urokinase is a single-chain polypeptide of 411 amino acids that is converted by plasmin into an active, low-molecular-weight form of urokinase with 276 amino acids.[63] Pro-urokinase functions as a potent plasminogen activator of fibrin-bound plasminogen without requiring extensive systemic conversion to two-chain urokinase. Thus, the entire thrombolytic process is confined to the fibrin clot itself. Administration of pro-urokinase causes decreases in α_2-antiplasmin and fibrinogen and an increase in fibrinogen degradation products. Pro-urokinase is highly effective in the conversion of Lys-plasminogen to plasmin. In contrast, it has little or no activity in the conversion of Glu-plasminogen to plasmin. Because Lys-plasminogen is present in high concentrations in thrombus, this gives pro-urokinase fibrin-specific properties. In addition, plasminogen that is absorbed in thrombus changes its configuration to a pseudo–Lys-plasminogen, which is also attacked by pro-urokinase, converting it to Lys-plasmin. Circulating pro-urokinase is very stable in plasma because of its resistance to plasma inhibitors and ionized calcium.[64] The fibrin specificities of t-PA and pro-urokinase appear to rely on different mechanisms. Whereas t-PA is fibrin clot binding, the fibrin-selective properties of pro-urokinase are thought to be secondary to its preference for activation of Lys-plasminogen or Lys-like–plasminogen substrate found in thrombus. This effect prolongs half-life, which has been estimated to be several days. Such a prolonged half-life has theoretical advantages in clinical situations in which prolonged activity is desired. However, in peripheral arterial occlusions, if the regional infusion fails to produce the desired result and the patient must go to the operating room shortly after discontinuation of the infusion, this prolonged effect may be undesirable.

A recombinant form of pro-urokinase is Prolyse (Abbott Laboratories, Chicago, IL). This urokinase compound has the advantage of not originating in a human cell source. Many of the clinical trials using this drug have been studies of patients with myocardial infarction, where the notable finding was an increased incidence of intracranial hemorrhage (0.9%).[65] The most recent trial was the Prolyse in Acute Cerebral Thromboembolism II (PROACT II) study, which evaluated intraarterial pro-urokinase for acute ischemic stroke.[66] Early intracranial hemorrhage with neurologic deterioration within 24 hours occurred in 10% of pro-urokinase patients and 2% of control patients. Although pro-urokinase is effective at thrombolysis, the increased bleeding risk has limited its widespread use. A phase II trial evaluating pro-urokinase versus urokinase for thrombolysis of acute peripheral arterial occlusion showed that pro-urokinase had a greater efficacy, but an increased risk of bleeding complications at a dose of 8 mg/hour; with a dose of 2 mg/hour, there was a slightly lower rate of thrombolysis, combined with a lower incidence of bleeding complications and fibrinogenolysis.[67]

Third-Generation Thrombolytic Drugs

The last few years have seen the development of a new generation of thrombolytic drugs, including mutant molecules of single-chain u-PA and t-PA; chimeric plasminogen activators; conjugates of plasminogen activators with monoclonal antibodies against fibrin, platelets, or thrombomodulin; and plasminogen activators of animal and bacterial origin.[50]

Reteplase

Reteplase is a single-chain deletion mutant of alteplase, consisting of just the kringle-2 and protease domains.[68] Reteplase has a fivefold decrease in fibrin binding and a half-life of 14 to 18 minutes because of the aforementioned structural differences. Reteplase has less binding to endothelium and monocytes compared with t-PA, and this reduced binding results in increased circulating levels in the bloodstream.[69] Reteplase catalyzes the cleavage of

endogenous plasminogen to generate plasmin. The activation of plasminogen is stimulated in the presence of fibrin and is mediated by the kringle-2 domain.[10,70] Plasmin then degrades the fibrin matrix of the thrombus, thus exerting its fibrinolytic action.

The fact that plasminogen activators in general activate plasminogen molecules in or near the clot allows efficient lysis in small clot burdens such as the coronary circulation. The absolute dependence on a sufficient amount of available plasminogen limits the dose-related efficacy when the clot burden is large. Long, retracted (i.e., organized) clots, such as those in the peripheral arterial circulation, are often deficient in plasminogen. Despite this deficiency, plasminogen activators such as reteplase and t-PA are efficacious when delivered through a catheter directly into the thrombus rather than systemically.

Reteplase has increasingly been used in the treatment of peripheral vascular occlusion, given the unavailability of urokinase for a few years. Nevertheless, published studies regarding its use in controlled trials are relatively few in number. There are two pilot studies that evaluated the dosing regimen of reteplase in the treatment of myocardial infarction.[71,72] These studies demonstrated that reteplase produced significantly higher TIMI-3 (thromboembolism in myocardial infarction) flow rates at 60 and 90 minutes than did front-loaded alteplase. However, in two subsequent trials—the International Joint Efficacy Comparison of Thrombolytics (INJECT)[73] and Global Use of Strategies to Open Occulated Coronary Arteries (GUSTO III)[74] trials—despite the higher TIMI-3 flow rates, this did not translate into a lower mortality in the reteplase-treated patients (7.5% for reteplase vs. 7.2% for alteplase).[15] Reteplase has lower fibrin affinity and thus appears to penetrate thrombus effectively and activate fibrin-bound plasminogen within the clot, resulting in faster clot lysis. Thrombolytics may also cause platelet activation, and this may have been responsible for some of the previously noted lack of efficacy. The addition of glycoprotein IIb/IIIa inhibitors appears to increase the efficacy of thrombolytic agents, as well as speed the lysis.

Tenecteplase

Tenecteplase (TNK-t-PA) is a t-PA mutant in which a threonine molecule (100Thr) is replaced by Asn, and the sequence Lys-His-Arg-Arg is changed to Ala-Ala-Ala-Ala. This change confers high fibrin selectivity and prolongs the half-life to 15 to 19 minutes. TNK-t-PA is highly effective in arterial, platelet-rich thrombi and is more resistant to plasminogen activator inhibitor. Although most of the published data regarding TNK-t-PA have been related to acute coronary syndromes, there is increasing experience in peripheral arterial thrombolysis. One group published its experience with continuous tenecteplase infusion in conjunction with glycoprotein IIb/IIIa inhibition with tirofiban for peripheral arterial thrombolysis.[75] The dose of TNK-t-PA infusion was 0.25 to 0.50 mg/hr, with a mean infusion time of 7.5 hours. Of 48 patients with iliofemoral arterial thrombosis, complete lysis was achieved in 35 patients (73%). There were no deaths, no intracranial bleeding, and no embolic events. It appears, at least from this study, that lysis time is shorter; however, the longer half-life has implications for surgical intervention, as addressed earlier.

Staphylokinase

Staphylokinase is a plasminogen activator produced by certain strains of *Staphylococcus aureus* and was first described as having fibrinolytic properties in 1948.[76] The gene has been cloned from genomic DNA of a lysogenic strain of *S. aureus*. When exposed to a fibrin clot in human plasma, staphylokinase reacts with plasmin at the clot-plasma interface; this staphylokinase-plasmin complex activates thrombus-bound plasminogen and exerts its fibrinolytic activity. Any plasmin that is liberated from the clot is rapidly inactivated by α_2-antiplasmin. In this manner, plasminogen activation by staphylokinase is confined to the thrombus, and the collateral effects of fibrinogen depletion and serum plasminogen activation are minimized. Patients treated with staphylokinase do, however, develop neutralizing antibodies, the titers of which can remain elevated for several months.[77]

Immunofibrinolysis

In an attempt to develop fibrin-specific agents, monoclonal antifibrin antibodies have been bonded to urokinase or streptokinase, rendering these agents fibrin selective. These monoclonal antibodies do not appear to cross-react with fibrinogen and thus show a marked increase in in vitro fibrinolysis compared with unmodified activator.[78] The clinical applicability of these agents remains to be determined; they may significantly alter the current approach to the management of thrombotic disease. Nevertheless, repeated therapy would require different monoclonal antibodies to prevent adverse immunologic reactions.

Fibrolase is a direct-acting fibrinolytic enzyme. It is a metalloprotease isolated from the venom of the southern copperhead snake, which dissolves fibrin through rapid hydrolysis. There is some data to suggest that fibrolase dissolves thrombi much quicker than the plasminogen activators. An added advantage of fibrolase is the rapid inactivation by α 2-macroglobulin, which is relatively abundant in the systemic circulation. Alfimeprase (Nuvelo, Inc, San Cerlos, CA), a recombinant variant of fibrolase, underwent evaluation in clinical trials of peripheral arterial occlusion with inconclusive results. Also, amediplase (Menarini Group, Florence, Italy) is undergoing evaluation in clinical trials. Amediplase is a chimeric protein that combines part of the t-PA and part of the single-chain urokinase plasminogen activator (sc-UPA). In animal models, amediplase is a more potent and longer-lasting thrombolytic than alteplase.

Summary

Most of the clinical experience to date has been with streptokinase, urokinase, and, most recently, t-PA. The effectiveness and complication rates of each of these agents are discussed later in the specific sections dealing with the various clinical entities. Based on the experience to date, streptokinase seems to be a less desirable agent for use in peripheral vascular thrombosis, probably

because of its complex mechanism of action, which translates into dosage difficulties and clinical complications.

Bleeding associated with thrombolytic therapy, regardless of the agent used, is most frequent at sites used for cardiac catheterization, arterial blood gas studies, intravenous infusion, or venipuncture. At any invaded site, the vascular endothelium is disrupted, resulting in an inflammatory reaction. The major components of an inflammatory reaction are fibrin and two different cell types that form the hemostatic plug. The fibrin in the hemostatic plug is identical to the fibrin in a pathologic thrombus in freshly (recently) formed thrombi and is much more susceptible to lysis. Thus, if a fibrin-specific thrombolytic agent is infused into the circulation, it will interact with molecularly identical fibrin in both the hemostatic plug and the pathologic thrombus; this brings about dissolution of the hemostatic plug, thereby inducing bleeding. This may be the reason why, in all recently completed studies comparing first- and second-generation thrombolytic agents, there is as much if not more bleeding with the newer, second-generation agents as with the older ones.

The degradation products of fibrinogen or fibrin are the absolute index of the degree of activation of the fibrinolytic system. When there are high levels of these fibrin degradation products, they are easily detected and signify an intense activation of the plasminogen-plasmin proteolytic system. There is good evidence that all the newer agents, despite assertions to the contrary, do induce the systemic fibrinolytic system, and this probably explains why the rate of distant hemorrhage is no different from that of older generation agents. Regional administration of agents (vs. systemic), dosage, and duration of therapy could have an important role in realizing the clinical benefits of a fibrin-specific agent.

VENOUS THROMBOLYSIS INCLUDING SYSTEMIC THROMBOLYTIC THERAPY

This section briefly discusses systemic thrombolytic therapy for venous thromboembolism and venous occlusions. Treatment of acute coronary thrombosis and stroke are purposely omitted. Although systemic thrombolytic therapy has been used for peripheral arterial occlusions, results have been disappointing, with bleeding complications outweighing any benefit obtained. Local intra-arterial administration prevents many of the systemic complications and is used for peripheral arterial and graft occlusion. This route allows directed thrombolytic therapy to the site of occlusion, minimizes the dose and duration of thrombolytic agent, and is highly effective. Even venous thrombolysis is most effective when it is catheter directed. Patient selection is probably the most important factor in obtaining good results with either modality.

Patient Selection

During the course of systemic thrombolytic therapy, a systemic lytic state is achieved in which fibrin is lysed wherever it has been deposited in the body. Thus, hemostatic plugs are as vulnerable as the clot or thrombus for

---

BOX 33-1   **Contraindications to Systemic Lytic Therapy**

ABSOLUTE

- Active internal bleeding
- Recent (<2 mo) cerebrovascular accident
- Intracranial pathologic condition

RELATIVE MAJOR

- Recent (<10 days) major surgery, obstetric delivery, or organ biopsy
- Active peptic ulcer or gastrointestinal disorder
- Recent major trauma
- Uncontrolled hypertension

RELATIVE MINOR

- Minor surgery or trauma
- Recent cardiopulmonary resuscitation
- High likelihood of left heart thrombus (e.g., atrial fibrillation with mitral valve disease)
- Bacterial endocarditis
- Hemostatic defects (e.g., renal or liver disease)
- Pregnancy
- Diabetic hemorrhagic retinopathy

---

which therapy was initiated. Selection of patients for systemic lytic therapy is based on the presence of an appropriate documented indication and careful evaluation for the presence of contraindications.

Contraindications to systemic therapy are listed in Box 33-1. Absolute contraindications are active internal bleeding and recent (within 2 months) cerebrovascular accident or other intracranial condition. Relative major contraindications include recent (within 10 days) major surgery, trauma, obstetric delivery, organ biopsy, or puncture of a noncompressible vessel; recent gastrointestinal bleed; and severe hypertension. Relative minor contraindications carry a higher risk of complications, but the benefits of therapy may still outweigh the hazards. Peripheral embolization from a central source is a potential hazard of systemic lytic therapy. Therefore valvular heart disease, atrial fibrillation, and previous history of emboli are relative contraindications to systemic lytic therapy. The presence of a mural thrombus is a relative contraindication to fibrinolytic therapy because of the potential for peripheral embolization due to fragmentation, which could have devastating consequences. In patients with a thrombus in the left side of the heart demonstrable by echocardiography, alternative forms of treatment should be considered. It must be recognized, however, that successful lysis of ventricular thrombi with urokinase has been reported.[79] Severe liver disease affects drug metabolism, making the response unpredictable. During pregnancy, a systemic lytic state may precipitate abruptio placentae or lead to hypofibrinogenemia in the fetus, with an increased risk of bleeding. Streptokinase is specifically contraindicated in patients with known allergy, previous therapy within 6 months, or recent streptococcal infection.

One of the most devastating complications of fibrinolytic therapy is intracranial hemorrhage. The incidence

of this complication is approximately 1% of treated patients in trials for acute myocardial infarction. The median time between the start of thrombolytic therapy and the onset of clinical signs of intracranial hemorrhage ranges from 3 to 36 hours, with a mean of 16 hours. Mortality is high for this complication, with an estimated mortality of 66%. Factors predictive of intracranial hemorrhage by multivariate logistic regression analysis include oral anticoagulation before admission, body weight less than 70 kg, and age older than 65 years. An increased incidence of intracerebral hemorrhage has been observed in patients receiving higher doses of t-PA. In the Thrombosis in Myocardial Infarction (TIMI) trial,[80] 1.3% of patients receiving 150 mg of t-PA suffered an intracerebral hemorrhage, as opposed to 0.4% of patients receiving 100 mg of the drug. Interestingly, in the TIMI-II trial, patients who received immediate β blockade as part of their regimen had no incidence of intracerebral hemorrhage when given 100 mg of t-PA, compared with 0.5% in the group that did not receive β blockade. This was not true, however, for patients treated with 150 mg of t-PA. The mechanism by which β-blockers may protect against intracerebral bleeding has not been established.[81]

In the Surgery versus Thrombolysis for Ischemia of the Lower Extremity (STILE) trial, patients were randomized to thrombolytic therapy with t-PA or urokinase versus surgery for the treatment of lower limb ischemia.[82] When evaluated with an intent-to-treat analysis, the incidence of life-threatening hemorrhage was 5.3% to 5.7%. When analyzed on a per-protocol basis, the incidence of this complication was 7.8% in the thrombolysis group. The incidence was similar in patients treated with t-PA and urokinase; these patients also received aspirin and heparin, which may have added to the risk. However, patients with bleeding complications did not receive more heparin or a higher dose of lytic agent; they appeared to respond differently to the therapy. At the end of the infusion, patients with bleeding complications had a significantly lower fibrinogen level than did patients without hemorrhagic complications (188 vs. 310 mg/dL). Measurement of fibrinogen levels, along with the international normalized ratio and partial thromboplastin time (PTT), may be helpful in guiding dose and duration of therapy.

Indications

Pulmonary Embolism

In 1968, a cooperative, controlled, randomized study to evaluate the use of urokinase in pulmonary embolism was initiated.[83] By 1970, 160 patients were entered and assigned to one of two therapeutic arms. Pulmonary angiography was performed on all patients before and after therapy, with lung scans repeated at 3, 6, and 12 months. The minimal eligibility was occlusion of at least one segmental pulmonary artery on angiography. Excluded from the trial were patients who had recent operations and those with contraindications to heparin or thrombolytic therapy. Seventy-eight patients received anticoagulants alone (heparin 75 units/lb loading dose,

10 units/lb per hour for 12 hours), and 82 received urokinase (2000 units/lb per hour for 12 hours). After the 12-hour infusion, all patients received heparin for a minimum of 5 days to maintain a prolonged bleeding time.

The randomization produced a reasonably good balance between the treatment groups. Urokinase therapy resulted in a significantly accelerated resolution of pulmonary emboli at 24 hours, as shown by pulmonary arteriograms, lung scans, and right-sided pressures. No significant differences in mortality or recurrence rates were observed. Patients receiving urokinase tended to respond better if they were younger than 50 years old, the embolus was less than 48 hours old, or the embolus was large, especially if shock was present.

Bleeding complications were significant in both groups (heparin, 27%; urokinase, 45%). This high complication rate is likely the result of demands in the protocol for multiple, frequent invasive procedures, including cutdowns performed for pulmonary angiography. The study group concluded that further study was needed before specific therapeutic recommendations could be made.

In 1974, the second phase of this cooperative study was reported.[84] This study followed the same guidelines as in phase I, comparing 12 hours of urokinase therapy with 24 hours of urokinase therapy and 24 hours of streptokinase therapy. A group treated with heparin alone was not included because the protocol was almost identical to that in the phase I trial, which showed urokinase to be superior to heparin in clot resolution. Fifty-seven patients were given urokinase (2000 units/lb loading dose, 2000 units/lb per hour for 24 hours), and 61 patients received the same regimen for 12 hours. Fifty-eight patients received streptokinase (250,000 units loading dose, 100,000 units/hr for 24 hours).

As expected, the drop in plasminogen during therapy was steeper for patients receiving streptokinase; otherwise the lytic effect was similar. Patients receiving 12 hours of urokinase infusion had nearly equivalent results to those in the phase I trial receiving urokinase. No benefit was seen from extending the urokinase infusion to 24 hours. In patients with massive embolism, however, the greatest improvement was seen with 24-hour urokinase infusion, although the differences were not statistically significant. Streptokinase and urokinase yielded similar results, with small differences favoring urokinase. The study group concluded that all three regimens were more effective in accelerating the resolution of pulmonary thromboemboli than heparin alone.

One of the major problems with the use of thrombolytic therapy for pulmonary embolism is that these patients usually have major contraindications to thrombolytic therapy. For example, this is the case with pulmonary embolism in a postoperative patient. In 1992, an experience with 13 patients treated for angiographically proven pulmonary embolism within 14 days of surgery was reported.[85] The protocol used urokinase (2200 units/kg body weight) injected directly into the clot through a catheter positioned in the pulmonary artery. A continuous infusion at the same dosage was then maintained for up to 24 hours, with the simultaneous administration of heparin at 500 units/hr. The fibrinogen level was maintained at less than 0.2 g/dL. No deaths or bleeding complications were seen, with complete lysis achieved in all patients. This selective therapy for pulmonary embolism may be appropriate for patients in the early postoperative period who suffer a major life-threatening pulmonary embolus.

The long-term results of patients randomized to the Urokinase Pulmonary Embolism Trial (UPET) suggest the clinical importance of resolution of the obstructive process in the pulmonary circulation. Several patients from this study were reexamined 7 years after the original pulmonary embolus. Those assigned initially to thrombolysis had significantly higher pulmonary capillary blood volumes and preservation of the normal pulmonary vasculature response to exercise at 7 years. In contrast, patients who had been treated with anticoagulants alone demonstrated a lower pulmonary capillary blood volume at 1 year and a markedly abnormal increase in pulmonary artery pressure and pulmonary vascular resistance when undergoing exercise testing during right heart catheterization.[86] These data suggest that initial management with thrombolysis can offer improved quality of life years after the event.

More recently, rt-PA has been evaluated in the treatment of acute massive pulmonary embolism. In a multicenter trial, the intravenous administration of rt-PA was compared with intrapulmonary administration in 34 patients with massive pulmonary emboli.[87] All patients were systemically anticoagulated with heparin. The patients received 50 mg of intravenous or intrapulmonary rt-PA over 2 hours, with 22 patients receiving another 50 mg over the subsequent 5 hours. No difference was noted between the intrapulmonary group and the intravenous group, and 7-hour administration was superior to a single infusion of 50 mg over 2 hours. In all groups, up to 38% resolution of the angiographically determined embolism occurred. A decline in the pulmonary arterial pressure was documented in all groups. Fibrinogen levels dropped significantly, and bleeding complications were limited to puncture or operative sites; only four patients required blood transfusions.

In a separate trial, 36 patients with angiographically documented pulmonary emboli received 50 mg of rt-PA over 2 hours, followed by repeated arteriography and, if necessary, an additional 40 mg of rt-PA over 4 hours.[88] Thirty-four of the 36 patients had angiographic evidence of clot lysis, with marked improvement in 24 of the 36. Two bleeding complications occurred, one related to a pelvic tumor and the other 8 days after coronary artery bypass surgery. Again, significant improvement in the clinical condition of these patients was documented.

A randomized, controlled trial of rt-PA versus urokinase in the treatment of acute pulmonary embolism was reported in 1988.[89] Forty-five patients were randomized to 100 mg of rt-PA over 2 hours versus urokinase at systemic doses. At 2 hours, 82% of the rt-PA patients had complete lysis, as opposed to 48% of patients receiving urokinase. Eight of 23 urokinase patients required premature termination of the infusion because of bleeding complications. There was no difference in plasma fibrinogen level or improvement in lung scans between the two groups.

In 1980, the National Institutes of Health Consensus Development Conference concluded that thrombolytic therapy results in greater improvement and normalization of the hemodynamic responses to pulmonary emboli than that observed with heparin alone.[90] Lytic therapy may prevent permanent damage to the pulmonary vascular bed by lysing emboli and restoring the pulmonary circulation to normal. The conference report also stated that although the incidence of bleeding complications was high, contemporary clinical experience suggested an incidence of approximately 5%, which was certainly within the acceptable range.

The thrombolytic agents currently approved by the FDA for use in the treatment of patients with pulmonary embolism are t-PA, given in a 100-mg dose over 2 hours, and, since 2002, the newly reintroduced urokinase. As stated earlier, there is no evidence of improved survival or outcomes in patients with pulmonary embolism who are hemodynamically stable. Tebbe and colleagues[91] evaluated the efficacy of reteplase, given as two 10-unit boluses 30 minutes apart, compared with t-PA in the 100-mg dose. There was no difference in clinical outcomes, complications, or mortality. The rates of stroke and intracranial hemorrhage were similar. However, reteplase reduced pulmonary vascular resistance more quickly than t-PA did. However, it should be emphasized that there is no level I evidence that thrombolysis for the improvement of pulmonary embolism offers any survival advantage, except in cases of massive embolism with hemodynamic compromise.

In current clinical practice, thrombolytic therapy should be considered in all patients with an established diagnosis of pulmonary embolism, any evidence (clinical or monitoring) of hemodynamic compromise, and no absolute contraindication to systemic lytic therapy. This excludes small pulmonary emboli in a patient who remains clinically stable after the initial episode. In this situation, the benefits of thrombolytic therapy over heparin alone are not clear.

It is important that the diagnosis of pulmonary emboli be well documented. Helical or spiral computed tomography (CT) scans are increasingly being used to detect pulmonary embolism. With current technology, image acquisition can be done in 20 seconds, the equivalent of a single breath-hold. The sensitivity and specificity of helical CT in the diagnosis of acute pulmonary embolism range from 69% to 92% and 86% to 96%, respectively.

Under these guidelines, a patient who has a large pulmonary embolism and evidence of right ventricular dysfunction should be considered for a trial of lytic therapy. Systemic anticoagulation with heparin is critical as soon as the diagnosis is strongly suspected. Pulmonary embolectomy is then reserved for hemodynamically compromised patients who fail lytic therapy or have an absolute contraindication to thrombolytic therapy. Once again, it should be emphasized that thrombolytic therapy has not been shown to affect mortality after pulmonary embolism; its efficacy is reflected in secondary end points, not in survival.

Deep Venous Thrombosis

The goal of therapy for deep venous thrombosis (DVT) is the prevention of pulmonary embolism and of long-term sequelae characterized by the postphlebitic syndrome. Anticoagulation has been highly effective in achieving the former but ineffective in preventing valvular damage and thus avoiding the latter. The incidence of such long-term complications can be as high as 90%.[92]

Several well-controlled, randomized, prospective studies have compared systemic lytic therapy with conventional heparin therapy in the treatment of DVT.[93-97] All concluded that dissolution of DVT with lytic therapy is faster and more complete than that observed with heparin alone. On average, complete lysis was seen in 35% of patients, compared with 4% of those treated with heparin alone. At 3 to 6 months' follow-up, valve function was preserved in 7% of heparin-treated patients, compared with 50% of patients treated with thrombolytic agents. The incidence of pulmonary embolism was similar for both regimens, with no difference in mortality. Bleeding complications averaged 4% and 17% for heparin and lytic therapy, respectively. In one study, phlebography at a mean of 7 months after treatment suggested an improved outcome for patients treated with fibrinolytic agents. Normal venograms were found in 40% of streptokinase-treated patients, compared with 8% of those who had received heparin. Clinical symptoms were related to therapeutic results and previous thrombosis. Longer follow-up was reported by Arnesen and colleagues,[98] who phlebographically evaluated 35 patients at a mean observation period of 6.5 years after they had randomly received streptokinase or heparin. Only seven patients had phlebographically normal veins, and all were in the streptokinase group. On clinical examination, 76% of patients in the streptokinase group had normal legs, compared with 33% of patients in the heparin group. Contrasting results were reported from a small prospective study in which 24 patients with major proximal DVT treated with heparin were compared with 25 patients similarly afflicted and treated with streptokinase.[99] After 2.5 years of follow-up, no major difference in hemodynamic status, as measured by foot volumetry, was seen between the two groups. The authors questioned the validity of treatment with lytic therapy, given its higher complication rate. In all these studies, thrombi older than 3 to 5 days were less likely to respond.

A randomized trial of rt-PA for the treatment of proximal DVT was performed by Turpie and colleagues.[100] Twenty patients with proximal DVT were randomized to intravenous rt-PA (0.5 mg/kg) or placebo over 4 hours, following initiation of a therapeutic dose of intravenous heparin. Patients were randomized to rt-PA (0.5 mg/kg) or saline over 1 hour if repeated venography within 72 hours did not show complete lysis. Five of 10 patients treated with rt-PA under this protocol showed partial or complete lysis, compared with 1 of 10 patients treated with heparin. A systemic lytic effect was demonstrated by a drop in plasma fibrinogen and α_2-antiplasmin concentration, with positive fibrin degradation split products and elevated euglobulin lysis time. Thus, modest effectiveness was demonstrated in this study, similar to that achieved by urokinase or streptokinase. Long-term follow-up data on these patients are not available. Three other randomized trials have yielded similar results.[101-103]

Use of systemic thrombolysis for DVT is hampered by concerns over bleeding risk, but regional thrombolytic therapy for DVT is increasingly popular. The concept of regional thrombolytic therapy for DVT is attractive because it can relieve the obstructive process and aid in the preservation of valvular function. These two features are established predictors of the development of the post-thrombotic syndrome.[104] The early reports of success with thrombolysis for DVT led to the development of a national multicenter registry for the evaluation of catheter-directed thrombolysis for lower extremity DVT.[105] The early results in 473 patients were published in 1999 and demonstrated that the methods used to deliver the lytic agent (in this case, urokinase) affect the anatomic result. Attempts to lyse the thrombus by a pedal infusion were remarkably unsuccessful, with a failure rate of 80%. In contrast, catheter-directed lysis, with the agent laced directly into the clot, achieved substantial lysis in 83% of cases and complete lysis in 33%. This experience provides a strong argument in favor of abandoning systemic infusion for thrombolysis because the rates of lysis are not improved, but the dose of lytic agent administered is higher with systemic infusion. Major bleeding complications occurred in 11% of patients, most at the puncture site, and mortality was less than 1%. Comerota and colleagues[106] published a report evaluating health-related quality-of-life variables in patients with iliofemoral DVT treated with thrombolysis versus those treated with anticoagulation alone. Patients treated with thrombolysis reported better overall physical functioning, less health distress, less stigma, and fewer postthrombotic symptoms ($p < 0.05$ for each outcome measure).

Whether preservation of valve function is achieved by this more aggressive form of therapy is uncertain. Nevertheless, it is difficult to ignore the significant improvement in the obstructive component of DVT with thrombolysis, considering that the combination of obstruction and valvular incompetence likely results in the most severe form of postphlebitic syndrome. In view of this, should lytic therapy be offered to all patients with DVT? Recently, the ATTRACT Trial (Acute Venous Thrombosis: Thrombus Removal with Adjunctive Catheter-Directed Thrombolysis) has been initiated. This study involves randomization of consecutive symptomatic patients with acute proximal DVT to best endovascular therapy plus standard DVT therapy or standard DVT therapy alone. The primary objective is to determine whether catheter-directed thrombolytic therapy reduces the occurrence of postthrombotic syndrome (PTS) compared with anticoagulation alone. This study may answer lingering questions about thrombolytic efficacy in DVT.

Of note, when thrombolytic therapy is started more than 5 days after the onset of symptoms, effectiveness is significantly decreased. The incidence of DVT is highest in postoperative patients, women during pregnancy or after childbirth, trauma victims, and patients suffering cerebrovascular accidents or spinal injuries. Lytic therapy is contraindicated in these instances, as well as in septic thrombophlebitis. Prior episodes of thrombophlebitis are likely to have destroyed delicate vein valves, making the benefits of lytic therapy in recurrent attacks uncertain. If clinical evidence of valve competence is present, an attempt to prevent further damage from a recurrent attack and resolve the obstructive component is a reasonable goal. In addition, lytic therapy seems to offer an advantage in more proximal thrombosis (i.e., popliteal vein or higher); thus, treatment of isolated calf thrombi with lytic therapy is of questionable value.

Phlegmasia cerulea dolens at onset causes massive iliofemoral thrombosis with limb-threatening venous outflow occlusion. Historically, the results of venous thrombectomy have been variable, with a significant incidence of rethrombosis and mortality, although more recent experience has been encouraging.[107,108] A much more compelling argument can be made for the use of thrombolytic therapy in the treatment of phlegmasia cerulea dolens. There is no real consensus on treatment, but the advent of catheter-directed thrombolysis presents an attractive and effective treatment option for this disease, which historically resulted in 20% to 40% mortality and a significant amputation rate in survivors.[109] Patel and colleagues[110] reported on two patients with phlegmasia cerulea dolens who were successfully treated with catheter-directed thrombolytic therapy and stenting, without limb loss. This is one of many case reports that demonstrate the feasibility and efficacy of this approach. Lytic therapy offers an important advantage over surgical thrombectomy, because multiple peripheral thrombi not accessible to the catheter may be dissolved. In addition, a general anesthetic, frequently required for venous thrombectomy, is avoided. Although the experience with thrombolytic therapy in this disease is limited, 13 of 14 reported cases were judged to have achieved excellent results, with no mortality.[93,111-113]

Axillary Vein Thrombosis

Axillary vein thrombosis (effort thrombosis) usually occurs in young individuals, and its sudden clinical manifestations lead the patient to seek early medical attention. As a result, this entity is ideally suited for thrombolytic therapy. Anticoagulation rarely leads to resolution and merely arrests the process, allowing for collateral drainage and amelioration of symptoms. This frequently leads to some degree of disability. Catheter-induced axillary subclavian vein thrombosis usually has a more gradual presentation, with slow, progressive occlusion allowing for collateral venous drainage. The clinical presentation aids in the decision whether to offer lytic therapy to a patient with catheter-induced axillary subclavian vein thrombosis. When symptoms develop rapidly over the course of a few days, there is a good probability that the thrombotic material will be sensitive to lytic agents. A combination of infusion through the catheter and in the ipsilateral peripheral vein is most effective. However, if symptoms develop over weeks or months, they tend to be milder in nature and less responsive to fibrinolytic agents. This is likely a result of organization of the thrombotic material.

Both forms of axillary thrombosis have been successfully managed with lytic therapy (Figure 33-2).[114-116] Either systemic or local low-dose infusion appear to be effective.[114] Local infusion requires that the catheter be lodged in thrombus; otherwise, venous collaterals will decrease its effectiveness. A systemic lytic state is avoided in the majority of patients treated by local infusion.

Once complete resolution of the clot is achieved, repeated venography with the extremity in abduction and external rotation is recommended. If an underlying thoracic outlet compression is identified, surgical correction should be advised. Surgical decompression of the thoracic outlet can be performed at the same admission (i.e., after thrombolysis), because no increase in bleeding complications or rethrombosis rates have been noted. After thoracic decompression, a repeat venogram is obtained at 2 weeks. If a stenosis of the vein is identified, balloon dilatation may be successful in avoiding rethrombosis.[114]

Superior Vena Cava Thrombosis

Superior vena cava thrombosis is frequently the result of neoplastic, traumatic, or infectious processes in the mediastinum. In these instances, external compression or inflammation precludes successful resolution of the process with lytic agents. Thrombosis secondary to an indwelling catheter is usually a slow process, allowing for organization and fibrotic replacement of the clot. It is unlikely that this thrombosis will respond to lytic therapy, and surgical decompression may be an option in these patients. Conversely, patients who develop rapidly progressive symptoms may respond to lytic therapy by means of dissolution of the most recently formed clot, which is likely to be sensitive to lysis.

Thrombosis is idiopathic in approximately 4% of patients. Successful resolution of idiopathic vena cava thrombosis has been reported with systemic thrombolytic therapy.[117]

Complications

Bleeding is the most frequent and important complication of systemic lytic therapy. However, most lytic treatments for peripheral arterial or venous thrombosis are done by catheter-directed techniques rather than by systemic administration of thrombolytics. The major exceptions are thrombolytics for stroke and myocardial infarction, which are administered via a bolus and short-term infusion rather than prolonged infusion. The reported incidence of major bleeding (requiring transfusion or discontinuation of the drug) varies from 7%[118] to as high as 45%.[83] Major bleeding occurs in an average of 15% of cases and correlates with the number and type of invasive procedures during therapy. Duration of therapy also seems to influence the incidence of bleeding.

Two broad categories of bleeding are observed. Superficial bleeding, seen at invasive sites, is frequently controlled with pressure. Avoidance of unnecessary procedures and preservation of an intact vascular system are the best preventive measures. Internal bleeding, usually seen in the gastrointestinal tract or the intracranial space, is frequently the result of poor patient selection. Internal

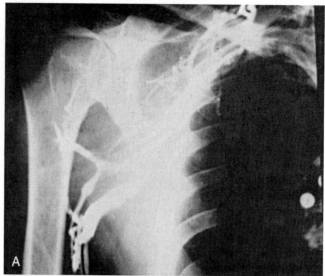

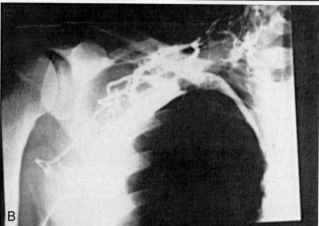

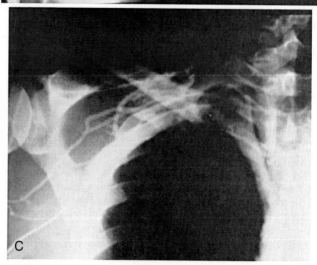

FIGURE 33-2 ■ Venograms of a 28-year-old man with acute onset of pain and swelling in the right upper extremity. **A,** Ascending venogram confirms axillary vein thrombosis. Low-dose streptokinase infusion (10,000 units/hr) was initiated. **B,** Twenty-four hours later, intraluminal thrombus is seen, with patency of the system. **C,** Forty-eight hours later, there is complete resolution of the occlusion.

bleeding should be suspected with unexplained drops in hematocrit. As a rule, any change in the neurologic status of a patient receiving fibrinolytic therapy is considered a complication of therapy until proved otherwise. The infusion is discontinued immediately, and appropriate diagnostic and therapeutic measures are instituted.

Superficial bleeding, which is controlled by local measures, can be tolerated in the final stages of therapy. Its occurrence early in the infusion, or any significant bleeding requiring transfusion, should lead to discontinuation of therapy. The hemostatic defect is corrected by the administration of fresh frozen plasma or cryoprecipitate. These two components are rich in fibrinogen and usually result in resolution of the lytic state. ε-Aminocaproic acid administration (plasmin inhibitor) is rarely recommended and carries a significant risk of aggravating the process for which lytic therapy was instituted. Increasing the dose of streptokinase to decrease its proteolytic effect is scientifically correct but unnecessary. It is interesting to note that bleeding tends to occur in the lag period between termination of lytic therapy and anticoagulant administration.[53,119] Thus, heparin administration should be delayed until the thrombin time or PTT is less than twice normal, and it should be initiated without a loading dose.

Laboratory parameters correlate poorly with the risk of bleeding. However, extremely low fibrinogen levels (<20% of baseline or <100 mg/dL) in the presence of an otherwise minor bleeding complication do increase the chances of continued bleeding, requiring cessation of therapy. An alternative is to temporarily discontinue the drug, administer fresh frozen plasma or cryoprecipitate, and restart the infusion several hours later.

Allergic reactions are not infrequent with streptokinase, although most are minor febrile episodes of no clinical consequence. Serious allergic reactions are extremely rare with the current preparations, and the few reported cases have responded well to conventional therapy.[90]

Pulmonary embolism can occur during treatment for DVT. The incidence appears to be similar to that seen with conventional heparin therapy. In the absence of other complications, continuation of lytic therapy is the treatment of choice. If recurrent emboli are observed, discontinuation of the fibrinolytic agent, heparin administration, and placement of a caval filter may be lifesaving.

REGIONAL INTRAARTERIAL THROMBOLYTIC THERAPY

The management of acute arterial and graft occlusions by the intraarterial local administration of fibrinolytic agents has emerged as an alternative and a frequent adjunct to surgical therapy in a selected group of patients. Recently completed prospective, randomized clinical trials have helped establish the role of lytic therapy in the treatment of patients with peripheral vascular disease. Excellent results with low morbidity and mortality are now possible with modern vascular techniques. It is difficult to estimate the effects of intraarterial lytic therapy based on cases in which surgical management has traditionally been successful.

Emerging from the literature are guidelines that help to define the role of intraarterial lytic therapy. Unquestionably, patient selection is the most important factor in achieving good results with this nonoperative approach. As experience in manipulating the fibrinolytic system increases, improvements in areas where surgical results are poor may follow.

Patient Selection

As a rule, intraarterial fibrinolytic therapy should be considered when the surgical alternative carries a high risk of morbidity or mortality or when the surgical approach has traditionally yielded poor results. In patients with previous multiple vascular reconstructions, lytic therapy may offer an alternative to a difficult and unpredictable surgical intervention. In some cases, it may facilitate such an undertaking, thus serving as a true adjunct to surgical therapy.

In the early experience of intraarterial fibrinolytic therapy, low doses of the agent were administered close to the thrombus to minimize systemic effects. With a low-dose regimen, dissolution of intraarterial thrombi is a slow, gradual process, requiring 12 to 72 hours or longer. If this method is chosen, the viability of the ischemic tissues should be ensured. Otherwise, these patients are better managed surgically, because prompt revascularization can be accomplished. Candidates for intraarterial lytic therapy must be able to tolerate ischemia for the duration of the infusion. With the advent of multiple percutaneous mechanical thrombectomy devices, restoration of some blood flow can be accomplished early after initiation of the endovascular procedure.

Cumulative retrospective and prospective analysis has helped to define guidelines for patient selection. In a prospective study of 80 consecutive patients receiving intraarterial urokinase for acute (<14 days) ischemia, successful lysis was accomplished in 71% (57 patients).[120] Most of these patients required additional adjunctive procedures to maintain patency; only 28% of patients avoided the need for additional interventions. Prosthetic graft and native arterial occlusions responded equally well (78% and 72%, respectively), whereas vein graft occlusions were less likely to respond (53%). Diabetics fared significantly worse compared with nondiabetics. Most important, placement of the catheter within the substance of the thrombus and passage of the guidewire through the occlusive process were the best predictors of success. The location of the occlusion influenced the need for adjunctive procedures. Whereas 88% of aortoiliac and 82% of infrainguinal occlusions required adjunctive procedures, only 17% of upper extremity procedures required additional interventions. The investigators underscored the importance of patient selection, noting that unsuccessful thrombolysis not only delays revascularization but also increases the risk of bleeding complications.[120]

Absolute and relative contraindications to intraarterial fibrinolytic therapy are listed in Box 33-2. Approximately 50% of patients receiving low-dose intraarterial infusion of lytic drugs will develop a systemic lytic state.

BOX 33-2	Contraindications to Intraarterial Fibrinolytic Therapy

ABSOLUTE

- Active internal bleeding
- Cerebrovascular accident within 3 mo
- Intracranial pathologic condition

RELATIVE

- Recent major surgery or trauma
- Minor gastrointestinal bleeding
- Severe hypertension
- Valvular heart disease
- Atrial fibrillation
- Endocarditis
- Coagulation disorder
- Pregnancy
- Minor surgery
- Severe liver disease
- Axillofemoral graft or knitted Dacron graft

Thus, patients with active internal bleeding, recent cerebrovascular accidents (within 2 months), or intracranial lesions are not candidates for any form of fibrinolytic therapy.

Relative contraindications represent risk factors associated with a higher incidence of complications. Recent major surgery or trauma significantly increases the risk of bleeding in the presence of a systemic lytic state. Individual judgment is required, but the presence of relative contraindications should not deter the clinician from using regional lytic therapy if significant benefit is anticipated.

Several cases of embolization to the ipsilateral extremity during intraarterial lytic therapy for occluded axillofemoral grafts have been reported.[120] The length of these grafts makes them less suitable for lytic therapy, so that surgical thrombectomy remains the therapy of choice. Dissolution of the fibrin layer that seals Dacron prostheses can occur with systemic absorption of the drug, leading to oozing through these porous prostheses. Discontinuation of therapy usually results in stabilization of the hematoma by the surrounding capsule.

Indications

Thrombosis after Endovascular Therapy

Percutaneous angioplasty is frequently performed for stenotic arterial lesions in the iliac and femoral systems. Thrombosis after balloon angioplasty is relatively infrequent, but when it occurs, local thrombolytic therapy is highly effective in restoring patency. The onset of occlusion is usually within 24 hours of dilatation; thus, the thrombotic material is fresh and highly sensitive to fibrinolysis. The underlying stenosis has been relieved by the angioplasty, and when thrombosis occurs immediately, it is a simple matter to change catheters so that proximal infusion is promptly initiated.

More than 80% of cases of post–balloon dilatation thrombosis can be treated successfully with intraarterial lytic therapy.[121-123] The duration of therapy is short because the infusion is started early and the thrombotic material is fresh; thus thrombectomy of a friable, recently dilated artery can be avoided. If dilatation of an iliac lesion was performed through an ipsilateral puncture, there is a risk of bleeding and pseudoaneurysm formation (Figure 33-3). If patency was restored by the infusion, repair of the pseudoaneurysm can consist of simple closure of the puncture site without embolectomy.

Native Vessel Occlusion

Acute occlusion of a native artery can be the result of thrombosis secondary to an underlying stenosis or embolization from a central source. In selecting patients for intraarterial lytic therapy, it is important to attempt to delineate the mechanism of occlusion. Lytic therapy appears to be more effective when applied to peripheral embolization.[120] Whereas 50% to 60% of thrombotic occlusions resolve with thrombolytic therapy, approximately 80% of embolic occlusions can be lysed effectively. Conversely, surgical management of proximal lower extremity emboli by transfemoral embolectomy is highly successful, with low morbidity and mortality. In addition, some investigators have noted that emboli secondary to atrial fibrillation may have well-organized components and thus be resistant to fibrinolysis.[124] For these reasons, surgical embolectomy is preferred for proximal (iliac, femoral) emboli secondary to atrial fibrillation. If the embolus is secondary to a recent myocardial infarction (i.e., the surgical risk is increased and the embolus is usually fresh clot), intraarterial fibrinolytic therapy should be considered. It must be kept in mind that the presence of mural thrombus in the ventricle, usually secondary to a recent myocardial infarction, is a relative contraindication to lytic therapy. Although the absence of such findings on echocardiography does not absolutely exclude the possibility, their presence should raise the level of concern about performing lytic therapy.

The management of multiple distal emboli must be individualized, depending on the viability of the extremity and the surgical risk. Intraarterial lytic therapy is a reasonable option in these patients when the extremity is viable and the anticipated surgical reconstruction is difficult. If the ischemia is not well tolerated, proceed with popliteal exploration, thrombectomy, and, on occasion, intraoperative lytic therapy (discussed later).

The use of local fibrinolytic therapy for thrombotic arterial occlusions should be based on the anticipated difficulty, morbidity, and mortality of the surgical alternative. The success rate of fibrinolytic therapy alone in thrombotic occlusion is variable. Of 25 patients with atherosclerotic occlusion, Risius and associates[125] succeeded in treating 13 (52%); of these 13, only 4 required no further therapy, 3 had successful percutaneous transluminal angioplasty, and the remaining 6 required surgery or distal amputations. Of 40 patients with thrombotic occlusions treated by Katzen and colleagues with intraarterial lytic therapy, 32 (80%) achieved successful outcomes.[122] Successful lysis was achieved by Graor and colleagues[121]

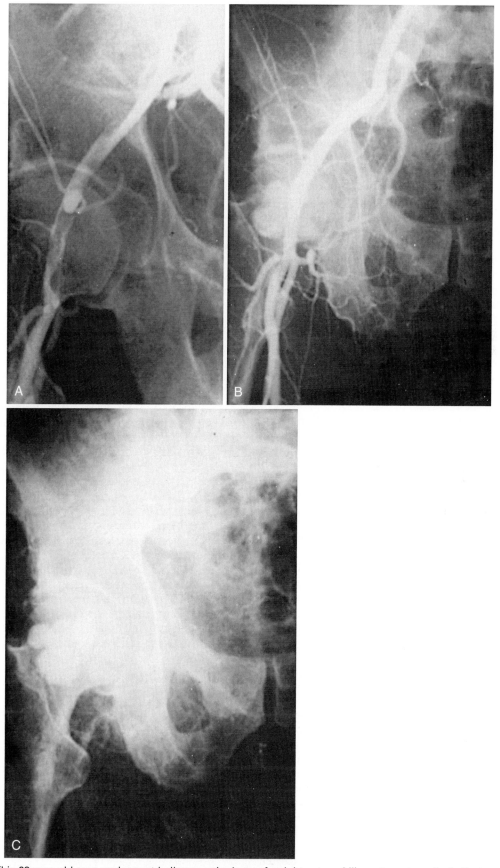

FIGURE 33-3 ■ This 63-year-old man underwent balloon angioplasty of a right external iliac artery stenosis. **A,** Postprocedure angiogram shows thrombosis of the dilated segment. **B,** After 12 hours of intraarterial streptokinase, there is complete resolution of the thrombus. **C,** A pseudoaneurysm is evident on angiography. Repair was limited to suture closure of the perforation, with no need for thrombectomy.

in 25 of 45 patients (56%) with thrombotic arterial occlusions. Eighteen of these 25 patients required secondary procedures. Seventy-eight percent of patients whose thrombi were less than 30 days old were successfully lysed, compared with 37% of patients with older occlusions. This trend has been observed by others and confirmed by recently completed randomized, prospective clinical trials (see later).

Careful analysis of the reported series reveals that although the lytic infusion may reestablish patency, additional procedures are often required. If surgical management becomes necessary, this is often simplified because better preoperative planning is possible. Thus, if the ischemia is well tolerated, the anticipated surgical intervention complex, the occlusion fairly recent (within 2 weeks), and the patient at significantly increased surgical risk, thrombolytic therapy seems justified. Based on the reported experience, long-term results depend mainly on whether a correctable lesion is identified and on the location of the occlusion. Larger vessel occlusions resolved by intraarterial lytic therapy tend to do better, with an expected patency of 60% at 2 years. Similarly treated superficial femoral and popliteal occlusions have a lower long-term patency of about 30% at 2 years.[126] If a correctable lesion is identified and appropriately treated, long-term results are significantly improved. Patencies as low as 20% at 2 years have been reported when no causative lesion was identified.[127]

There are specific instances when surgical intervention has traditionally achieved poor results. Emboli or thrombosis of the popliteal artery with distal clot propagation or multiple tibial emboli carry a risk of amputation of 40%, despite prompt surgical embolectomy.[3,128,129] In patients with a viable extremity at presentation in whom no major runoff vessels are seen on angiography, a trial of local fibrinolytic therapy may improve these results. Surgical correction of the underlying lesion (stenosis or aneurysm) can be performed in a timely fashion. When severe ischemia precludes lytic therapy, it is best to proceed with popliteal exploration and embolectomy. Intraoperative intraarterial infusion of lytic agents in an attempt to lyse clots that are inaccessible to the embolectomy catheter may improve the results of embolectomy alone.

Thrombosis or embolization to the renal arteries is a promising area in which thrombolytic therapy may offer significant advantages over surgical intervention (Figure 33-4). As a complication of myocardial infarction, an embolus to the renal artery carries an inordinate risk with surgical intervention. Capsular collaterals frequently maintain viability of the renal parenchyma to allow sufficient time for success with thrombolytic therapy. The clot material is sensitive to lysis, and the length of the occlusion is short. The reported experience is limited but has been highly successful.[122,130] If a stenosis is uncovered during infusion, percutaneous dilatation or elective surgical repair may be undertaken, as deemed appropriate.

Acute mesenteric artery occlusion has been treated successfully with local intraarterial streptokinase infusion (Figure 33-5).[131] In contrast to the kidneys, the bowel is exquisitely sensitive to ischemia and reperfusion. It is

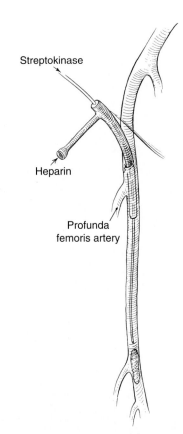

FIGURE 33-4 ■ Preferred delivery method for intraarterial lytic therapy for distal lower extremity occlusions. Low-dose heparin is infused through the coaxial system to avoid upstream thrombus.

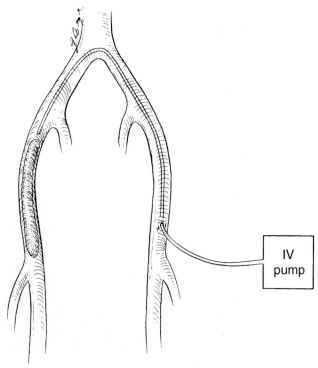

FIGURE 33-5 ■ Preferred method of intraarterial lytic therapy for proximal (iliac, common femoral) occlusions. If possible, the catheter tip should be within the thrombus.

difficult to clinically assess the tolerance to ischemia on presentation and during therapy. If lytic therapy is elected for acute mesenteric ischemia, any deterioration in the overall clinical status, persistent acidosis, or sepsis mandates emergency exploration. Otherwise, frequent angiographic assessment, as often as every 6 hours, is advisable. Failure to show progress during these intervals should trigger early, rather than delayed, exploration.

Acute Graft Occlusion

Acute occlusion of an arterial graft frequently leads to recurrent symptoms and, on occasion, limb-threatening ischemia. Thrombectomy, with or without revision, achieves excellent results in prosthetic grafts and variable results in autogenous vein grafts.[132] Autogenous vein grafts frequently require extensive revision and replacement. Intraarterial thrombolytic therapy, in contrast, has been highly unsuccessful in resolving prosthetic graft occlusions. Of 25 patients with prosthetic graft occlusions treated with local lytic therapy by Sussman and coworkers,[120] the treatment was successful in only 6 patients, 5 of whom required surgical correction of the offending lesion. In the 19 failures, amputation followed in 12 patients. In the experience reported by Van Breda and colleagues,[129] among 19 patients with 20 prosthetic graft occlusions, only 4 patients were managed nonoperatively, 2 of whom required percutaneous transluminal angioplasty. Despite this, lytic therapy was considered beneficial because it allowed elective surgery in 12 patients and improvement in the surgical risk in an additional 2 patients. An adjunctive role for lytic therapy was proposed. Although achieving successful lysis in 7 of 10 polytetrafluoroethylene (PTFE) grafts with thrombolytic therapy, Graor and associates[121] noted that surgical revision was required in most of these patients.[121] In view of the excellent results obtained with surgical thrombectomy, one must seriously question the value of thrombolytic therapy in the management of prosthetic graft occlusions.

The results obtained with lytic therapy in the management of occluded autogenous grafts have been somewhat more gratifying. In the experience of Perler and colleagues,[133] occluded vein grafts were more susceptible to lytic therapy than were PTFE grafts. This experience is shared by others.[134] Graor and coworkers,[121] however, observed a similar response between PTFE and vein grafts, reporting a 75% success rate in vein grafts occluded for less than 14 days. Taking into account the variable results with surgical thrombectomy in the management of occluded autologous grafts, a trial of lytic therapy is an attractive alternative if the event is recent. However, long saphenous vein grafts to tibial vessels in the lower third of the leg or ankle are less responsive to lytic therapy; this may have to do with limited supplies of plasminogen in these very low-flow grafts. Nevertheless, even in unsuccessful attempts, it is not unusual to find liquefied, thickened blood in the graft at operation, thus minimizing the need for mechanical thrombectomy. The operation may actually be limited to removal of the most distal occlusive material and revision of an identified lesion. Retrieving an occluded vein graft in these circumstances is possible with minimal mechanical trauma to the endothelium.

A recent study of acute limb ischemia (ALI) of the lower extremities delineated outcomes in 129 limbs treated in 119 patients.[159] Technical success was achieved in 82% cases. The 30-day mortality rate was 6.0% with all 30-day deaths occurring in females. One (0.76%) central nervous system hemorrhage was noted in this cohort. Primary patency for the entire cohort at 12 and 24 months was 50.1% (95% confidence interval [CI], 39.5 to 60.7) and 37.7% (95% CI, 26.2 to 49.1), respectively, while secondary patency was 74.0% (95% CI, 64.9 to 83.1) and 65.3% (95% CI, 54.5 to 76.2). Multivariable analyses identified patients presenting with femoropopliteal (Hazard Rotio (HR), 2.63) or tibial thrombosis (HR, 2.80); graft thrombosis (vs. native artery thrombosis; HR, 2.57) and long-term dialysis (HR, 3.66; 95% CI, 2.35 to 5.71; $p < 0.001$) were associated with poorer primary patency rates. Cumulative limb salvage at 24 months was 68.8% (95% CI, 59.5 to 78.1) with female gender (HR, 3.34 $p = 0.002$) and thrombolysis for 3 days or greater (HR, 2.35; $p = 0.019$) associated with an increased risk of limb loss. Overall 36-month survival was 84.5% (95% CI, 77.5 to 91.6). Women had decreased survival rates both in the short and mid term (HR, 6.29; 95% CI, 1.78 to 22.28; $p = 0.004$). This study highlighted that endovascular therapy with thrombolysis remains an effective treatment option for patients presenting with lower extremity ALI. However, thrombolysis should be limited to shorter than 3 days. Female gender negatively affected the rates of limb salvage and survival.

It is important to consider several factors when deciding whether to use lytic therapy for an occluded graft. Certainly, surgical risk must be assessed. Infrequently, surgery is avoided altogether. If delaying surgical intervention allows an improvement of the overall risk, lytic therapy should be considered. If little improvement is expected, it is preferable to proceed with thrombectomy in a timely fashion. When dealing with a prosthetic graft occlusion, thrombectomy remains the therapy of choice. In patients in whom multiple previous reconstructions make a surgical approach less desirable, a trial of lytic therapy is a reasonable option; however, one must realize that the chances of success without eventual surgical correction are low. The management of an occluded vein graft differs, in that the results of surgical thrombectomy are less predictable. Thus, if the ischemia is well tolerated, a trial of lytic therapy may help restore patency of the vein graft. Correction of the causative lesion may then be undertaken without the need for thrombectomy of the graft. This can be accomplished percutaneously if the lesion is less than 0.5 cm long; surgery is preferable for longer lesions. Long-term results of this approach tend to correlate with preocclusion history of the bypass. Grafts that fail within the first year after implantation fare worse than those that have been patent for longer periods. Thus, an early failure of a vein bypass graft in which a complex lesion is identified may be best treated with a new reconstruction if autogenous tissue is available. Failure of a vein graft beyond 1 year may be best treated with a trial of lytic therapy and correction of the causative lesion.

Results of Randomized Trials

Lower Extremity Ischemia

Despite a multitude of retrospective reviews of the results of thrombolytic therapy in the management of thrombotic complications of peripheral arterial disease, the precise role of this form of therapy could not be clearly established. For this reason, several investigators embarked on prospective, randomized trials comparing surgery to thrombolysis for ischemia of the lower extremities.

The largest trial to date (STILE) randomized 393 patients with native arterial or bypass graft occlusion to either optimal surgical therapy or intraarterial, catheter-directed thrombolysis with rt-PA or urokinase.[82] Outcomes were analyzed on an intention-to-treat basis to maintain statistical validity. The dosage of rt-PA was 0.05 mg/kg per hour for up to 12 hours; for urokinase, a 250,000-unit bolus injection was followed by 4000 units/min for 4 hours, then 2000 units/min for up to 36 hours. End points measured included death, ongoing or recurrent ischemia, major amputation, and major morbidity. Additional end points included reduction in surgical procedure, clinical outcome classification, length of hospitalization, and outcome by duration of ischemia. The randomization produced equivalent groups in terms of risk factors and comorbid conditions. A monitoring committee terminated the study before its anticipated patient recruitment because a significant primary end point occurred in the first interim analysis. Failure or inability to place the catheter in the thrombolytic group occurred in 28% of patients who were randomized, and these were considered treatment failures. A significant benefit of surgical therapy compared with thrombolysis occurred at 30 days, primarily because of a reduction in ongoing or recurrent ischemia. Clinical outcome classification at 30 days was similar. Stratification by duration of ischemia suggested that patients with ischemia of less than 14 days' duration had lower amputation rates with thrombolysis and shorter hospital stays. Patients with ischemia of longer duration (more than 14 days) who were treated surgically had less ongoing or recurrent ischemia and trends toward lower morbidity. At 6 months, there was an improved amputation-free survival in acutely ischemic patients treated with thrombolysis. However, chronically ischemic patients who were treated surgically had lower major amputation rates. Fifty-five percent of patients treated with thrombolysis had a reduction in the magnitude of their surgical procedure. No difference between rt-PA and urokinase was noted, with fibrinogen depletion being a predictor of hemorrhagic complications. The investigators concluded that surgical revascularization of patients with ischemic symptoms of less than 6 months' duration was more effective and safer than catheter-directed thrombolysis. Crossover to surgical treatment from the thrombolytic group probably accounted for the clinical outcomes being similar in both groups at 30 days. Patients with fewer than 14 days of ischemia who were treated with thrombolysis had an improved amputation-free survival compared with patients who underwent surgical treatment. Of concern was the 28% of patients in the thrombolytic arm who did not receive thrombolytic therapy because of failure to place the catheter within the thrombus. Subsequent analysis revealed that even if these patients were eliminated from the analysis as failures in the thrombolytic arm, the results and conclusions did not change.

Further analysis of those patients in the STILE study who had native, nonembolic arterial thrombosis has been completed.[135] Two hundred thirty-seven patients with lower extremity ischemia owing to iliofemoral or superficial femoropopliteal native artery occlusion, with symptomatic deterioration within 6 months, were randomized to either thrombolytic therapy or surgical revascularization. Before randomization, the optimal surgical procedure was determined for subsequent comparison with eventual outcome. For patients randomized to lytic therapy, the catheter could be properly positioned and the lytic agent delivered in 78% of patients; thus 22% of patients in that group did not receive lytic therapy owing to an inability to position the catheter. A reduction in the subsequent surgical procedure performed occurred in 58% of patients with femoropopliteal occlusions and in 51% of patients with iliofemoral occlusions. Urokinase and rt-PA were equally effective and safe, but lysis time was shorter with rt-PA than with urokinase (8 vs. 24 hours). At 1 year, the incidence of recurrent ischemia was significantly higher in patients treated with thrombolytic therapy than in those treated with surgery (64% vs. 35%). Major amputation rates were also higher in the thrombolytic therapy group, with 10% of patients eventually requiring a major amputation in the thrombolytic arm of the study versus no patients in the surgical arm. Factors associated with poor lytic outcome included femoropopliteal occlusion, diabetes, and presence of critical ischemia. There was no difference in mortality observed at 1 year between the surgical and lytic therapy groups. The investigators concluded that surgical revascularization for lower extremity native arterial occlusions is more effective and durable than thrombolysis. A reduction in the planned surgical procedure occurred for the majority of patients treated with thrombolysis. However, long-term outcome was inferior, particularly in those patients with femoropopliteal occlusions, diabetes, or critical ischemia.

A prospective, randomized comparison of thrombolytic therapy and operative revascularization in the initial management of acute peripheral arterial ischemia was performed in a single institution and published in 1994.[136] In this study, patients with limb-threatening ischemia of less than 7 days' duration were randomly assigned to intraarterial, catheter-directed urokinase therapy or operative intervention. If an anatomic lesion was unmasked by the thrombolytic infusion, this was treated with either balloon angioplasty or surgery. Primary end points included limb salvage and survival. A total of 114 patients were randomized; 57 received thrombolytic therapy, and an equal number had surgery. Thrombolytic therapy resulted in dissolution of occluding thrombus in 70% of patients in the lytic group. Cumulative limb salvage was similar in the two treatment groups, at 12 months (82%). Cumulative survival, however, was significantly improved in patients randomized to thrombolysis

(84% vs. 58% at 12 months). The higher mortality in the surgical arm was primarily due to an increased frequency of in-hospital cardiopulmonary complications. The benefits of thrombolysis appeared to be accomplished without significant differences in the duration of hospitalization and with a modest increase in hospital costs (median, $15,672 vs. $12,253). Intraarterial thrombolytic therapy was associated with a reduction of in-hospital cardiopulmonary complications and therefore improved patient survival.

Based on these results, and to further elucidate the possible effect of thrombolytic therapy on 1-year survival, a multicenter, randomized, prospective trial comparing thrombolysis and peripheral arterial surgery was carried out.[137] Phase I was designed to be a dose-ranging trial to evaluate the safety and efficacy of three doses of recombinant urokinase in comparison with surgery. Two hundred thirteen patients who had acute lower extremity ischemia of less than 14 days' duration were prospectively randomized to one of two groups. The first group received one of three dosages of recombinant urokinase (2000, 4000, or 6000 IU/min for 4 hours, then 2000 IU/min for a maximum of 48 hours). The second group underwent surgical revascularization. Successful thrombolytic therapy was followed by either surgical or endovascular intervention when a lesion responsible for the occlusion was recognized. Follow-up on an intent-to-treat basis was performed for 1 year. The most effective dose of recombinant urokinase was found to be 4000 IU/min. This dose accomplished complete thrombolysis in

35 of the 49 patients (71%) who were randomized to this dose in the lytic therapy group. Mean infusion time was 23 hours. Patients who received 2000 IU/min had a 67% success rate, whereas patients who were randomized to the highest dose (6000 IU/min) had a 60% success rate. Hemorrhagic complications were 2%, 13%, and 16% in the 4000-, 2000-, and 6000-IU/min groups, respectively. When comparing the 4000-IU/min group with the surgical group, the 1-year mortality rate was similar (14% vs. 16%), and amputation-free survival was not statistically different (75% vs. 65%). Again, patients treated with lytic therapy had a decrease in the planned surgical procedure that was statistically significant. The investigators concluded that recombinant urokinase is most effective at 4000 IU/min. Thrombolytic therapy and surgical therapy had similar rates of survival and limb salvage.

From the foregoing results, it is evident that in patients with relatively acute ischemia, thrombolytic therapy is an important and effective treatment, with results that compare favorably with those of surgery. Considerable judgment is required in patient selection, which should account for the duration of the ischemia, the complexity of the anticipated surgical intervention, the presence of contraindications to thrombolytic therapy, and the tolerance of the limb to ischemia (Figure 33-6). Although the number of vein grafts included in these trials was not sufficient to allow specific recommendations, retrospective information suggests that the long-term outcome of thrombolytic therapy in the management of thrombosed vein grafts is best when the vein graft has failed late (more

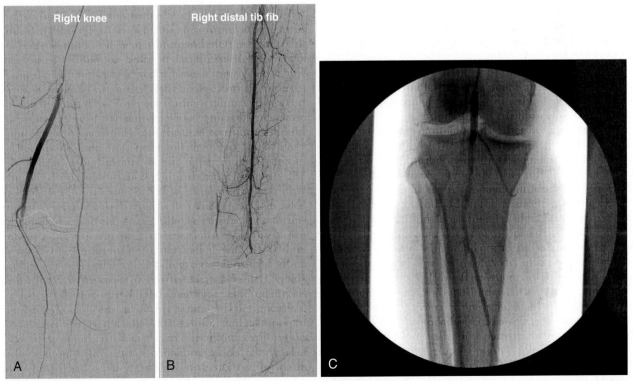

FIGURE 33-6 ■ **A,** Selective angiography of the right leg in a 73-year-old female with acute limb ischemia documents an embolic cutoff in the popliteal artery. **B,** Distal imaging reveals pedal emboli as well with absence of runoff vessels to the foot. **C,** Catheter-directed thrombolytic therapy is initiated, which partially resolves the proximal embolic material but fails to clear the runoff preventing limb salvage.

than 1 year) and when a specific lesion can be identified and corrected after completion of the lytic infusion.

Hemodialysis Access

Thrombosed arteriovenous fistulas can be managed successfully with intragraft administration of fibrinolytic agents. Usually the diagnosis is established early, when the patient notices the absence of a thrill; thus, the thrombotic material is very sensitive to lysis. Administration is by direct puncture because there are no collaterals to dilute the effect of the agent. It is usually best to lace the intragraft thrombus with the lytic agent and then proceed with high-dose intragraft administration. Graor and colleagues[121] were successful in treating 40 of 46 arteriovenous fistulas (87%); PTFE and vein fistulas were equally responsive.[121] Thrombi older than 4 days were less susceptible to lysis (29%). Unfortunately, most patients required surgical revision of the venous anastomosis, and lytic therapy was only a temporizing intervention. In some patients, however, this allowed better preoperative preparation and elective, rather than urgent, operation.

A new method of opening thrombosed grafts is pulse-spray pharmaco-mechanical thrombolysis, followed by balloon maceration. This allows successful lysis of the graft, but more quickly than with intragraft administration and with a smaller dose of lytic agent. The pulse-spray can be done with heparinized saline or with a thrombolytic agent. A relatively underappreciated but well-documented phenomenon resulting from pulse-spray thrombolysis of clotted hemodialysis access grafts is the development of pulmonary embolism. A prospective, randomized, double-blinded study was conducted to evaluate the incidence of pulmonary embolism following the use of this technique with urokinase versus heparinized saline. Although pulmonary embolism occurred in both groups, as documented by lung perfusion scan, the incidence was 18.2% with urokinase and 64.3% with heparinized saline ($p = 0.04$).[138] All the patients, it should be noted, were asymptomatic.

Many studies have attempted to perform cost-benefit analyses of thrombolysis versus surgical thrombectomy. The most common reason for dialysis graft failure is a lesion, usually neointimal hyperplasia, at the venous anastomosis. The interventional techniques allow thrombolysis and identification of the underlying anatomic lesion; this can be treated with balloon angioplasty. Although angioplasty is successful in many cases, surgical revision is usually required at some point in the future.

Acute Stroke

In June 1996, the FDA approved t-PA as a safe and effective treatment for acute stroke, if given within 3 hours of the onset of symptoms.[139] Since then, there has been a proliferation of large clinical trials testing the efficacy of antiplatelet and antithrombotic treatment regimens. The approval of the use of intravenous t-PA was based on the results of the National Institute of Neurological Disorders and Stroke (NINDS) Recombinant Tissue Plasminogen Activator Stroke Study, in which 624 patients with

ischemic stroke were treated with 0.9 mg/kg of t-PA within 3 hours of the onset of symptoms.[140] Of the t-PA group, 31% to 50% had complete or near-complete recovery at 3 months, compared with 20% to 38% of the placebo group. This benefit prevailed for 1 year. However, there was a 6.4% incidence of symptomatic brain hemorrhage in the t-PA group, versus 0.6% in the placebo group. The mortality rates were similar between the groups. The presence of a mass effect or a greater severity of initial neurologic deficit presented an increased risk of hemorrhage. The beneficial effect of t-PA was not observed in three other large trials (the European Cooperative Acute Stroke Study I and II and the Alteplase Thrombolysis for Acute Noninterventional Therapy in Ischemic Stroke [ATLANTIS] trial).[141-143] However, patients in these three trials were treated much later (only 14% treated within 3 hours) than those in the NINDS rt-PA study (622 of 624 enrolled within 3 hours, and 48% treated within 90 minutes).

There have been two large randomized trials evaluating intraarterial thrombolytic therapy for stroke. PROACT II evaluated patients with angiographically documented occlusion of the middle cerebral artery or a first-order branch.[66] By 2 hours, there was partial or complete lysis in 67% of patients in the pro-urokinase group, compared with 18% in the heparin-only group ($p < 0.001$). The primary outcome measure analyzed was the ability to live independently 3 months after the stroke. The percentage of patients able to attain this end point was 40% in the pro-urokinase group and 25% in the heparin group ($p < 0.05$). Intracerebral hemorrhage with neurologic deterioration occurred in 10% of patients in the pro-urokinase group and in 2% in the heparin group ($p = 0.06$). This trial was the first to show a clinical benefit from the use of intraarterial thrombolysis of a middle cerebral artery occlusion. To date, there are no randomized controlled trials comparing the efficacy of intravenous versus intraarterial thrombolytics. It is, however, clear that thrombolytic therapy for acute ischemic stroke can no longer be considered experimental. It has been shown to have clinical benefit as long as patient selection is strictly in accordance with the criteria set forth in the trials and the NINDS guidelines.

Technique

A plethora of strategies for thrombolysis have been used and are described in a recent consensus document.[160] In this comprehensive review, 33 recommendations were made by a panel of experienced surgeons and interventionists from North America and Europe. The areas covered in this publication cover management of patients with lower limb arterial occlusion from presentation to postoperative monitoring. The critical recommendations that deserve emphasis are that thrombolysis for peripheral arterial occlusion should be via a catheter-directed delivery of agent, and that systemic thrombolysis should no longer be used. The likelihood of success with thrombolysis is related to the ability to cross the thrombosed region ("guidewire traversal test"), and placement of an infusion catheter and/or wire embedded into the thrombus. Perhaps, most importantly, identifying and treating the culprit lesion that led to the thrombotic episode is paramount for a long-term successful outcome. Of note, more than 40 dosage schemes were reviewed and described for thrombolytic infusion. These schemes included strategies of continuous versus stepwise infusion, bolusing or lacing the clot, and intraoperative thrombolysis. The most popular strategies included using urokinase 4000 units/min for 4 hours, and then decreasing to 2000 units/min for a maximum of 48 hours, t-PA at a dose of 1 mg/hr and lacing the clot to increase thrombolytic efficiency.

The preferred current technique is described below. First, and of particular importance, thrombolysis should not be attempted in any patient whose ischemia has been of sufficient severity or duration to cause severe motor or sensory impairment or in patients whose ischemia cannot tolerate the anticipated duration of the infusion. Because a systemic lytic state can occur with prolonged regional intravascular thrombolytic therapy, absolute contraindications include active internal bleeding, recent surgery or trauma to the area to be perfused, recent cerebrovascular accident, or documented left heart thrombus. Relative contraindications include gastrointestinal bleeding, severe hypertension, mitral valve disease, endocarditis, hemostatic defects, or pregnancy. After a decision to proceed with thrombolysis, expeditious management in an endovascular suite should ensue.

The chosen approach should maximize access to the occlusion and minimize morbidity. Arterial punctures distal to the presumed occlusion are avoided. Sites where bleeding may cause serious morbidity (e.g., axillary, translumbar) are avoided. When the suspected occlusion is below the superficial femoral artery (strong femoral pulse), an antegrade ipsilateral puncture is preferred (Figure 33-7). When the suspected occlusion is at the femoral level or above, a contralateral puncture with passage of the catheter around the aortic bifurcation is preferred (Figure 33-8). Multiple puncture attempts can

be avoided with the use of Duplex ultrasound in patients with diminished pulses or scarring. Infusions in the upper extremities or aortic branches are carried out through a transfemoral approach. Multi–side-hole catheters are used for infusion, with the infusion length portion of the catheter imbedded in the thrombus. When the infusion is at the popliteal level or below, small (3 French) catheters or infusion wires are used through a coaxial system to prevent upstream clot formation (Figure 33-9). A flush heparin infusion is maintained through the coaxial catheter. If the catheter does not properly penetrate the thrombus, lysis is slowed and inefficient because the lytic agent is "washed out" through collaterals.

Creation of a channel into the thrombus with the angiographic guidewire is of prognostic significance and is technically necessary. Failure to pass the guidewire through the occlusion implies either plaque or a well-organized thrombus, which may be resistant to fibrinolysis. Easy passage of the guidewire through the occlusion not only establishes a channel in which the fibrinolytic agent can concentrate but also implies soft thrombi that can be dissolved. After confirmation of distal arterial patency, the next step is usually power-pulse thrombolysis using a percutaneous mechanical thrombectomy system (i.e., the Possis AngioJet system). This step is performed with a minimal amount of thrombolytic agent (2 mg in 50 mL of saline) that is laced throughout the clotted region with short bursts of the catheter. After 20 minutes, mechanical thrombectomy can be performed without any lytic agent to restore a channel and blood flow into the distal vasculature. The next step is thrombolysis with t-PA. Bleeding complications appear to correlate most closely with duration of therapy rather than with the total dosage of the agent. Therefore it believed that higher-dose, short-term infusions are better tolerated than longer-term, low-dose infusions. A higher dose initially (urokinase 4000 units/min, t-PA 1 mg/hr) appears to be effective with switching to a lower-dose regimen when

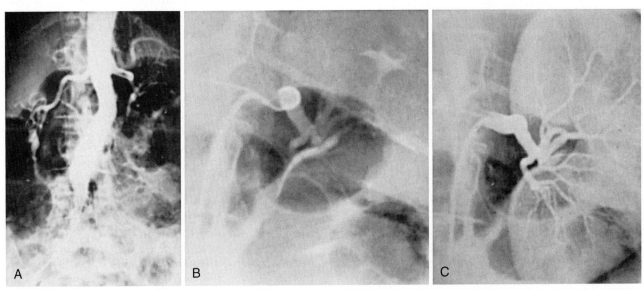

FIGURE 33-7 ■ **A,** Aortogram showing left renal artery embolus. **B,** After 1 hour of high-dose intraarterial urokinase, there is partial clearing and improved perfusion to the left kidney. **C,** Complete clearance of embolus after 3 hours of high-dose intraarterial urokinase.

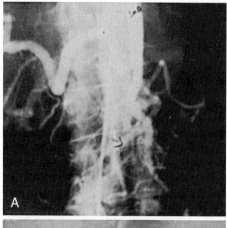
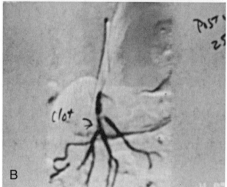
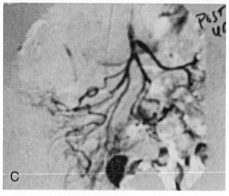

FIGURE 33-8 ■ **A,** Selective superior mesenteric artery angiogram showing occlusion of the distal tree. **B,** Partial clearing of embolus after 250,000 units of intraarterial urokinase administered over 1 hour. **C,** Complete resolution of superior mesenteric artery occlusion after 2 hours (500,000 units) of intraarterial urokinase therapy.

there is remnant thrombus on lytic check angiography (urokinase 1000 to 2000 units/min, t-PA 0.2 to 0.5 mg/hr). Valved infusion catheters and infusion wires are used singly or in combination to achieve the appropriate infusion length for intrathrombus infusion. After dissolution of the thrombus, treatment of the culprit lesion is critical to durable patency of the thrombolytic procedure.

Duration of the infusion is guided by periodic angiographic and clinical monitoring but should rarely exceed 72 hours.[159] The patient is monitored in an intensive care unit, and angiography is repeated daily or more often, depending on the clinical response. Before initiating therapy, baseline fibrinogen, thrombin time, PTT, and fibrin degradation product measurements are obtained. These are repeated 12 hours after commencing the

infusion and then daily. It is expected that the fibrinogen level will drop and fibrin degradation products will become positive. Prolongation of the PTT or thrombin time suggests a systemic lytic state and occurs in approximately 50% of patients. Although specific parameters do not correlate with the risk of bleeding, presence of a systemic lytic state increases the risk. If good progress is being made by the infusion, a low fibrinogen value (<50% of baseline) or evidence of a lytic state in the absence of bleeding complications is tolerated, and therapy is continued. In the absence of a systemic lytic state when little progress is evident, the dosage is increased and the result reassessed. Therapy should be discontinued if there is no improvement in any 24-hour interval, persistent or worsening ischemia, or a major bleeding complication.

The administration of heparin during regional thrombolytic therapy is advocated by most investigators. Clearly, in patients with profound ischemia and very low flow in the extremity, and when pericatheter thrombus formation would be significant (e.g., when 3 to 4 cm of the catheter is in a vessel with low or no flow), concomitant heparin administration should be strongly considered. Heparin administration may also be useful in increasing thrombolysis and minimizing the adverse consequences of a potential episode of distal clot migration or embolization. Heparin therapy, however, may increase the incidence and severity of pericatheter bleeding during lytic therapy and may increase the risk of distant bleeding. For these reasons, it is common to proceed with heparin administration via a continuous infusion to maintain a prolonged PTT at 1.5 to 2.0-fold the control only till thrombolysis is initiated. After lysis begins, a lower dose of heparin is administered; usually 500 units/hr through the sheath side-arm. It is important that the PTT not exceed 60 seconds at the time of catheter and sheath removal. Heparin can then be restarted without a bolus.

When emergency surgery is required, the lytic agent is discontinued and fresh frozen plasma is administered if the fibrinogen level is less than 100 mg/dL. The half-life of these agents is short and is usually not a problem in this setting.

Complications

As with any form of lytic therapy, bleeding is the most feared and frequent complication of low-dose fibrinolytic therapy. The risk of major bleeding (requiring cessation of therapy or blood transfusion) ranges from 5% to 15% when appropriate precautions are observed.[121,144] Bleeding is usually related to systemic effects of the drug, and management was discussed earlier in this chapter.

Considering that high-risk patients may be treated preferentially by this nonsurgical approach, the incidence of bleeding with intraarterial lytic therapy must be considered. The most recent experience indicates that the risk of bleeding correlates more with duration than with total dosage. It is therefore preferable to use higher-dose protocols, especially when a short occlusion is being treated. Although specific coagulation parameters do not correlate with the risk of bleeding, the presence of a systemic lytic state increases this risk. It is important to

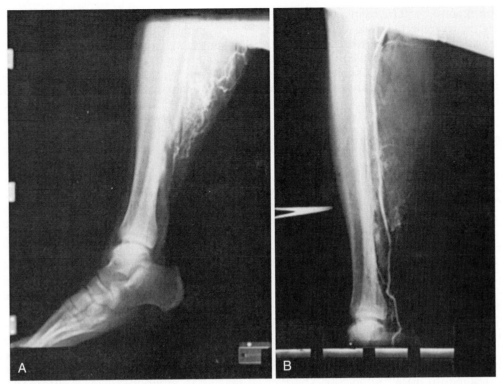

FIGURE 33-9 ■ **A,** Intraoperative completion angiogram after popliteal embolectomy. Note the absence of runoff vessels to the foot. **B,** Repeated angiogram after intraoperative infusion of streptokinase 60,000 units and heparin 1000 units over 30 minutes through the same catheter used for angiography. Note the remarkable improvement in runoff.

document whether systemic effects of the drug are present, because such knowledge helps determine the most appropriate course of action. Systemic effects are heralded by a 50% drop in fibrinogen from baseline, a prolongation of the thrombin time to twofold greater than normal (or higher), or both. If significant progress is being made, continuation of therapy is warranted, despite systemic fibrinolysis. If no significant improvement is noted within the last interval, reassessment should be made, weighing the risks and benefits of the alternatives.

Treatment of hemorrhagic complications depends on their severity and on the progress made during lytic therapy. A small amount of oozing around the catheter entry site, without hematoma formation during the final stages of the infusion, can be controlled locally, keeping the patient under close observation until therapy is completed. The same situation in the early stages of the infusion, when more than 12 to 24 hours of therapy are anticipated, should lead to discontinuation of the drug. Development of a significant hematoma or bleeding at a remote site warrants cessation of therapy. Fibrinogen should be replaced by the administration of fibrinogen-rich components, such as cryoprecipitate or fresh frozen plasma. This usually suffices because the half-life of both urokinase and streptokinase is short.

Distal embolization occurs more frequently than is clinically appreciated. Continuation of therapy is preferable, with perhaps a temporary increase in the hourly dose. When severe ischemia is seen as the result of distal emboli, discontinuation of lytic therapy with prompt surgical embolectomy is indicated.

Several cases of embolization to the ipsilateral extremity have been reported during intraarterial lytic therapy for occlusion of axillofemoral grafts.[121] The length of these grafts makes them unsuitable for lytic therapy; therefore surgical thrombectomy remains the therapy of choice.

Allergic reactions to streptokinase were discussed earlier. Routine administration of 100 mg of intravenous hydrocortisone may prevent some of these reactions and is recommended.

Pseudoaneurysm formation is rare but may occur secondary to bleeding from an arterial puncture site. Surgical repair is recommended.

Intracranial bleeding is a recognized complication of any form of lytic therapy. Any change in the patient's neurologic status during therapy should be viewed as related to the fibrinolytic agent until proved otherwise. Bleeding from an unrecognized intracranial lesion must be ruled out. Lytic therapy should be discontinued while the evaluation is proceeding.

Fatal pulmonary emboli have been reported during intraarterial fibrinolytic therapy.[123] A possible mechanism for this complication is decreased venous circulation in the ischemic extremity, with clot formation, partial lysis, and eventual pulmonary embolization. This is a rare occurrence. Treatment options include cessation of lytic therapy with heparinization or a switch to systemic intravenous lytic therapy. If the latter is chosen, leaving the intraarterial catheter in place may decrease the risk of bleeding through the arterial puncture site.

Conversion of an ischemic myocardial infarction into a hemorrhagic infarct as a complication of fibrinolytic therapy has been reported.[123] The relationship between lytic therapy and the few reported cases is unclear. Deterioration of cardiac function in the presence of an acute myocardial infarction during fibrinolytic therapy should lead the clinician to consider this possibility. Therapy should be discontinued until the cause of the cardiac decompensation is determined.

INTRAOPERATIVE THROMBOLYTIC THERAPY

Approximately 30% of lower extremity embolectomies are incomplete, with residual intravascular defects demonstrable by completion angiography.[145] Experimental studies suggest that the true incidence may be as high as 80%.[146] The idea of removing the bulk of thrombus surgically and lysing any remaining defects is attractive from a therapeutic standpoint. Alternatives include repeated embolectomy with the balloon catheter,[147] irrigation in an attempt to flush the residual clot,[148] passage of Dormia catheters,[149] and distal exploration. These alternatives will further injure the endothelium and thus increase its thrombogenicity. Certain endovascular procedures, such as endoscopy, atherectomy, or dilatation, may also temporarily increase the thrombogenicity of these vessels, leading to early thrombosis. Further mechanical manipulation is likely to result in further injury and thus is unlikely to solve the problem. For these reasons, controlled chemical intraoperative fibrinolysis may be a welcome alternative in the treatment of these complications. When dealing with delayed intervention in the presence of a thrombotic process, propagation of clot into the branches of the arterial tree may be problematic. Once these clots lose their integrity with the parent thrombus, they are difficult to retrieve, and enzymatic dissolution may be the only alternative.

Bleeding complications secondary to intraarterial fibrinolytic therapy are the result of prolonged infusions necessary to lyse extensive thrombus. The potential for intraoperative or perioperative lytic therapy has been suggested by several investigators.[150-152] Common to all these observations was the lack of bleeding complications. There are several advantages to the intraoperative use of lytic agents when compared with the percutaneous method. First, the bulk of the thrombus has been surgically removed, so that less lysis is required. Second, a higher concentration of the agent, with control of inflow (and therefore circulation time), can be accomplished. Finally, infusion within the thrombus or adjacent to it is theoretically unnecessary, and repeated embolectomy with reassessment of the intervention can be done with repeated infusions, as necessary.

In 1985, Quiñones-Baldrich and colleagues[153] reported initial experience with five patients in whom intraoperative infusions of 20,000 to 100,000 units of streptokinase were successful in restoring adequate circulation to limbs still threatened after embolectomy. This experience has been expanded to 23 infusions in 22 patients.[154] In 17 of these patients, both preinfusion and postinfusion arteriograms were available; improvement following lytic therapy was seen in 13 patients (76%). Only one of these reconstructions rethrombosed in the postoperative period. All four patients without angiographic improvement suffered rethrombosis. Thus, it appears that preinfusion and postinfusion arteriography has prognostic significance, implying that failure to improve after intraoperative infusion of the lytic agent suggests a high likelihood of failure; therefore alternative methods of reconstruction need to be considered at the time of surgery.

Bleeding is the most feared complication of intraoperative lytic therapy. Among the 23 patients in whom lytic infusions were performed intraoperatively, 5 had hematomas. All the hematomas occurred in patients who were fully heparinized postoperatively. Among 12 patients who were not heparinized after surgery, there were no bleeding complications. Therefore bleeding after intraoperative lytic therapy is secondary to aggressive antithrombotic and anticoagulation regimens rather than to the lytic therapy itself.

Clinical experience to date is summarized in Table 33-2.[119,153,155-157] Five additional clinical series have been reported since the initial report. Cohen and colleagues[119] performed 13 bolus infusions of 25,000 to 250,000 units of streptokinase. Eight (61%) of the infusions were successful. Five bleeding complications occurred, one of them resulting in death secondary to retroperitoneal bleeding during aortoiliac reconstruction. This result suggests that caution should be exercised when using lytic agents during major abdominal or retroperitoneal surgery. Norem and associates[156] reported their experience with 19 infusions of 50,000 to 200,000 units of streptokinase by bolus injection. They followed the infusion with repeated embolectomy and were able to retrieve additional thrombus in each instance. Two wound hematomas occurred in the postoperative period. Low doses of heparin (200 to 500 units/hr) were maintained postoperatively. With this regimen, bleeding complications were minimized. In a report from Spain, investigators studied 66 femoropopliteal or distal acute arterial occlusions by means of arteriography and Doppler imaging before and after surgery. Patients were prospectively evaluated after either mechanical thromboembolectomy as a single technique (n = 35) or thromboembolectomy plus 250,000 IU of urokinase administered over 30 minutes intraarterially at completion of the operation (n = 31). Intraoperative angiography revealed residual thrombus in 30% of patients and unsuspected arterial lesions in 34%. Recurrence of thrombosis was associated with residual thrombus and amputation. Patients who received the intraoperative thrombolytic infusion had higher ankle-brachial indexes postoperatively than did those who underwent mechanical thromboembolectomy alone. Amputations and the need for distal revascularization were no different between the two groups, although quantitatively, the results were better in the lytic group than in the thromboembolectomy-only group (failure rate, 9.68% vs. 22.86%). There were no bleeding complications with routine intraoperative use of lytic therapy after mechanical thromboembolectomy.

The preferred technique for intraoperative infusion of fibrinolytic agents consists of a drip infusion of the agent without occlusion of the inflow. Experimental evidence suggests that maintenance of blood flow in the system during administration of fibrinolytic agents enhances

TABLE 33-2   Results of Intraoperative Regional Fibrinolytic Therapy

Author	No. of Cases	Drug Dose and Method	Successful (%)	Complications	Remarks
Cohen and colleagues[119]	13	SK: 25,000-250,000 U by bolus	61	Five rethromboses; five bleeding complications; one death after retroperitoneal surgery	Two renal infusions, one partly successful; death related to retroperitoneal bleeding
Norem and colleagues[156]	19	SK: 50,000-200,000 U by bolus	100	Two wound hematomas	All patients underwent repeat embolectomy; postoperative heparin in low doses (200-500 U/hr)
Parent and colleagues[157]	28	SK: 50,000-150,000 U by bolus UK: 35,000-150,000 U by bolus	88	Bleeding 11%; compartment syndrome 21%; two deaths	Deaths not related to lytic therapy; bleeding complications in two patients after retroperitoneal surgery
Comerota and colleagues[155]	38	SK: maximum 50,000 U UK: maximum 150,000 U by bolus in 2 patients; isolated limb, UK 1 million U	74	One wound hematoma; five deaths	Deaths not related to lytic agent
Quiñones-Baldrich and colleagues[153]	23	SK: 60,000-100,000 U UK: 250,000-375,000 U plus heparin 1-4 U/mL; gravity infusion over 30 min	74	Six rethromboses; five wound hematomas	All wound hematomas in patients fully heparinized postoperatively

SK, Streptokinase; *UK,* urokinase.

their effectiveness. This can be accomplished by insertion of a cannula distal to the arteriotomy after repair of the latter. Urokinase, 250,000 units dissolved in 100 mL of saline delivered over 30 minutes, is preferred. On the basis of an original experimental study, the addition of heparin to the infusate at 1 to 4 units/mL is recommended.[146] Preinfusion and postinfusion arteriography is recommended to document the effectiveness of the agent. Failure to show improvement in the postinfusion angiogram suggests a high likelihood of failure and that alternative management should be considered. More recently, the use of isolated limb perfusion with an extracorporeal pump has shown promise in further enhancing the effectiveness of the lytic agent.[158]

Urokinase appears to be a safer agent for intraoperative use. Allergic reactions are not seen. The mechanism of action is direct, and the risk of plasminogen depletion, which may occur with streptokinase, is eliminated. The best method of administration and the appropriate dosage, however, have not been determined. The logistic advantages of bolus infusion are obvious. Nevertheless, a slow infusion has the theoretical advantage of providing a constant amount of the drug while plasminogen is being supplied by the collateral circulation. Bolus infusion, although achieving a high concentration of the agent rapidly, is likely to be washed out, resulting in a short-lived effect. An experimental study was carried performed to further elucidate the best method of infusion. In addition to bolus infusion and slow 30-minute infusion, the study included a group of animals in which the limb was isolated with a proximal tourniquet and the artery and vein connected to an extracorporeal pump. Angiographic results were significantly improved with use of the isolated limb perfusion technique with similar doses of urokinase.[158] In addition, maintenance of inflow during the slow infusion seemed to improve results compared with occluded inflow. However, these differences were not statistically significant, probably because of the number of animals studied. Thus, isolated limb perfusion with extracorporeal pump support of the extremity during revascularization may enhance fibrinolytic activity and improve the efficacy of drug delivery. Clinical experience with this technique is promising but limited.

The high selectivity of t-PA for fibrin and the positive early results with relatively short-term infusion suggest that this agent is promising for intraoperative use. To date, there are no reports of intraoperative use of reteplase.

In summary, one can proceed with an intraoperative fibrinolytic infusion when faced with either residual thrombus inaccessible to the balloon catheter or persistent ischemia after restoration of flow. Although the best method of delivery and most appropriate dosage have not been fully determined, reported clinical experience has allowed guidelines that permit the clinician to obtain the benefits of fibrinolytic infusion in these difficult cases with both safety and efficacy.

References available online at expertconsult.com.

QUESTIONS

1. Streptokinase and urokinase have which of the following similarities: (1) both are bacterial products, (2) both are enzymes, (3) both are highly fibrin specific, or (4) both are direct fibrinolytic agents?
   a. 1, 2, 3
   b. 1, 3
   c. 2, 4
   d. 4
   e. None of the above

2. Which of the following statements about increasing the dose of streptokinase to decrease its lytic effect is true?
   a. It is indicated when bleeding occurs during therapy.
   b. It is a predictable response.
   c. It is scientifically correct but unnecessary.
   d. It increases the risk of bleeding.
   e. None of the above

3. Which of the following statements about tissue plasminogen activator is true?
   a. It is a nonenzymatic protein.
   b. It has fibrinolytic activity in plasminogen-free media.
   c. It is highly antigenic.
   d. It is mainly an exogenous fibrinolytic activator.
   e. None of the above

4. Which of the following statements is true of a patient with deep venous thrombosis of the femoral system: he or she (1) is a candidate for lytic therapy if the thrombosis is recent and it is the first episode, (2) may be treated with low-dose local lytic therapy, (3) has an approximately 50% to 60% chance of failure to clear the clot completely with lytic therapy, or (4) is at higher risk of pulmonary embolism with lytic therapy than with heparin?
   a. 1, 2, 3
   b. 1, 3
   c. 2, 4
   d. 4
   e. None of the above

5. Which of the following statements about intraarterial lytic therapy is true?
   a. It is initiated with a loading dose.
   b. It is highly effective in graft thrombosis.
   c. It is highly effective in postdilatation thrombosis.
   d. It can be safely administered in patients after a stroke.
   e. It usually prevents a systemic lytic state.

6. What is the dose of urokinase?
   a. Guided by plasminogen levels
   b. 2000 units/kg per hour without a loading dose
   c. 2000 units/kg per hour with a loading dose of 2000 units/kg over 10 minutes
   d. 2000 units/lb per hour
   e. None of the above

7. Which of the following statements about pulmonary emboli is true?
   a. They may be a complication of lytic therapy.
   b. They require at least 72 hours of systemic lytic therapy to completely resolve.
   c. They can be effectively treated by streptokinase 2000 units/kg per hour.
   d. They should always be treated with systemic thrombolytic therapy.
   e. None of the above

8. Which of the following statements is true of complications of thrombolytic therapy?
   a. They are caused by the antigenicity of the agent.
   b. They are caused by plasminemia.
   c. They are reduced by the avoidance of invasive procedures.
   d. They are sometimes treated by increasing the dose.
   e. All of the above

9. Which of the following statements is true of intraoperative thrombolytic therapy: it (1) is contraindicated because bleeding results from systemic absorption, (2) may improve the results of incomplete thrombectomy, (3) is done by intravenous administration of the agent, or (4) should include heparin in the infusate?
   a. 1, 2, 3
   b. 1, 3
   c. 2, 4
   d. 4
   e. None of the above

10. Which of the following statements about streptokinase administration is true?
    a. It results in a drop in plasminogen.
    b. It is contraindicated in patients who have received streptokinase any time in the past.
    c. It is more effective than urokinase when given intraarterially.
    d. It results in a predictable lytic response.
    e. None of the above

ANSWERS

1. **d**
2. **c**
3. **e**
4. **b**
5. **c**
6. **d**
7. **a**
8. **e**
9. **c**
10. **a**

ARTERIAL ANEURYSM DISEASE

Descending Thoracic and Thoracoabdominal Aortic Aneurysms: General Principles and Open Surgical Repair

Kristofer M. Charlton-Ouw • Ali Azizzadeh • Anthony L. Estrera • Charles C. Miller III • Hazim J. Safi

Although descending thoracic and thoracoabdominal aortic aneurysms are not as common as infrarenal aortic aneurysms, repair is problematic because of the involvement of visceral arteries and vital lumbar arteries supplying the spinal cord. The classification systems for descending thoracic and thoracoabdominal aortic aneurysms were devised because different aneurysm extents have different levels of risk (Figure 34-1). Since its inception, thoracoabdominal aortic aneurysm repair has been plagued with complications stemming from spinal, mesenteric, and renal ischemia. Adjunctive surgical techniques led to significant reductions in morbidity, especially because of spinal ischemia.

The first reported repairs of descending thoracic aortic aneurysms were published in the early 1950s.[1,2] The first to successfully perform a thoracoabdominal aortic aneurysm repair was Samuel Etheredge and colleagues in 1955 in Oakland, California.[3] One year later, Michael DeBakey and colleagues performed a true thoracoabdominal repair using a homograft. Subsequently, the same group devised an ingenious method of using a Dacron tube graft from the descending thoracic aorta to the infrarenal aorta, and sequentially bypassing the celiac axis, superior mesenteric artery, and both renal arteries. This technique both decreased the load on the heart and the ischemic time to the bowels and the kidneys. Dr. Crawford's repair of thoracoabdominal aortic aneurysm incorporated three principles of vascular surgery: the Matas inclusion technique,[4] whereby the aneurysm sac is opened but not resected; the reattachment of the intercostal arteries to the graft (as described in an animal model by Spencer in 1950[5]); and the reattachment of the small arteries into a large artery attributed to Carrell and Guthrie in 1906. Crawford accrued 28 cases by 1973 and published his results of a large group of aneurysm cases treated for the first time with the same clamp-and-sew technique.[6] This technique depended on expeditious repair with short aortic clamp times because the spine and visceral vessels suffered ischemia during repair. Several adjunctive methods for spinal cord and visceral protection later emerged, including distal aortic perfusion,[7-9] cerebrospinal fluid (CSF) drainage,[10] and systemic or regional profound hypothermia.[11]

By the end of the 1980s, the preferred method of treatment was still the clamp-and-sew technique, but it continued to be associated with high complication rates, predominantly because of spinal neurologic deficits and renal failure. Since 1992, supported by animal models and clinical experience, the clamp-and-sew technique has been largely abandoned in favor of left atriofemoral bypass with the addition of perioperative CSF drainage and moderate passive hypothermia. This chapter provides a review of the authors' experience in descending thoracic and thoracoabdominal aortic aneurysm repair, including its natural history, pathology, diagnosis, open surgical treatment, postoperative complications, and management.

NATURAL HISTORY

The exact prevalence of descending thoracic and thoracoabdominal aortic aneurysms can only be inferred. The incidence of thoracic aneurysms is increasing likely because of better detection with echocardiography and computed tomography. One population-based study from Olmsted County, Minnesota, estimated the incidence of thoracic aneurysms at 10.4 per 100,000 people.[12] The most common thoracic aneurysm occurs in the ascending aorta, but descending thoracic aortic aneurysms account for 45%, whereas thoracoabdominal aortic aneurysms account for approximately 5% of all thoracic aortic aneurysms.[13]

Nearly 13,000 people die annually from thoracic aortic aneurysm, making it the nineteenth leading cause of death in the United States.[14] This rate reflects a dramatic increase to 13.5 and 33.4 per 100,000 in age groups of 65 to 74 and 75 to 84 years.[15] Overall, aortic aneurysm and dissection accounted for 4.3 deaths per 100,000 people in the United States in 2007. Death from thoracic aortic aneurysm is primarily due to rupture. The rate of rupture increases with aneurysm expansion.[16,17] The

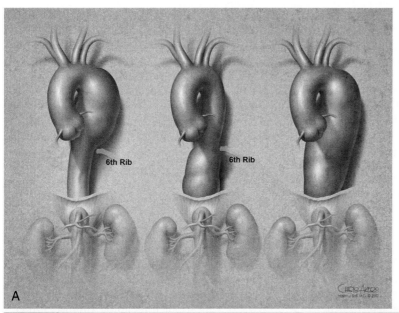

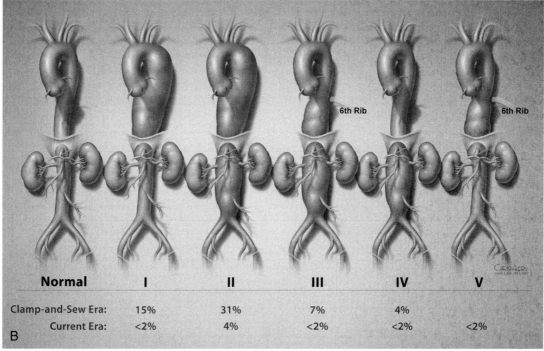

	Normal	I	II	III	IV	V
Clamp-and-Sew Era:		15%	31%	7%	4%	
Current Era:		<2%	4%	<2%	<2%	<2%

FIGURE 34-1 ■ Classifications for thoracic aortic aneurysms. **A,** Descending thoracic aortic aneurysms. **B,** Thoracoabdominal aortic aneurysms with rates of postoperative neurologic deficit in the clamp-and-sew and current eras.

natural history of thoracic aortic aneurysm is expansion at a median 0.1 to 0.3 cm/year.[16,18] After 5 cm, growth and rupture can occur unpredictably. In the Olmsted County study, no ruptures occurred in thoracic aneurysms less than 4 cm. The 5-year rupture risk increased to 16% for aneurysms less than 6 cm and was greater than 30% for aneurysms larger than 6 cm.[12] After rupture, the mortality rate is greater than 90% in the first 24 hours.[19] Most patients die before reaching the emergency room.

Based on the natural history and risk of rupture, descending thoracic and thoracoabdominal aortic aneurysms are considered for repair when maximum diameter reaches 5 to 6 cm. Saccular aneurysms and those with growth of greater than 5 mm in 6 months are also considered for repair, regardless of size. Aneurysms in patients with Turner syndrome, Marfan syndrome, and other connective tissue diseases are repaired at smaller diameters.

PATHOLOGY

An aneurysm is a localized or diffuse dilatation greater than 50% of the reference diameter. Most aneurysms are due to medial degeneration and appear to occur sporadically, but genetic factors are increasingly recognized. Marfan syndrome is an inherited connective tissue disorder caused by a mutation of fibrillin-1 protein that is encoded in the *FBN1* gene. Other syndromes that predispose individuals to abdominal aortic aneurysms include Loeys-Dietz syndrome, variants of Ehlers-Danlos syndrome, and Turner syndrome. Mutations in α-actin, such as *ACTA2*, highlight the importance of vascular smooth muscle function in aortic aneurysm and dissection.[20] In addition, other genes contributing to thoracic aortic disease include *MYH11*, *TGFBR*, and *SMAD3*.[21] The recognition of genetic variants in the development of aortic aneurysm will surely increase because many patients report multiple family members with thoracic aortic disease despite a negative genetic workup.

Like atherosclerosis, aortic aneurysm pathophysiology includes a robust inflammatory component. However, unlike atherosclerosis, which primarily affects the intima and causes occlusive disease, the inflammation in aneurysms occurs in the media and adventitia. Histology of degenerative aortic aneurysms is characterized by thinning of the media with distraction of the smooth muscle and elastic tissue (elastin). There is infiltration of inflammatory cells, including mast cells with neovascularization.[22] There is also activation of proteolytic enzymes and their inhibitors within the aortic wall.[23]

A small percentage of aneurysms are related to infection or so-called mycotic infection, or to trauma, such as pseudoaneurysm. Bacteria or septic emboli may seed the atherosclerotic or ulcerated aortic wall. Infection may also spread from an adjacent empyema or lymph nodes. Organisms associated with aortic infection include *Salmonella* species, *Haemophilus influenzae*, *Staphylococcus* species, *Mycobacterium tuberculosis*, and *Treponema pallidum*. These aneurysms are usually saccular and carry a high risk of rupture. Traumatic injuries of the thoracic aorta are also prone to rupture and should be repaired unless the injury is confined to the intima.[24-27]

CLINICAL MANIFESTATION

Many thoracic and thoracoabdominal aneurysms are discovered incidentally and most often develop without symptoms. Indications for surgical intervention depend on the size of the aneurysm and the presence or absence of symptoms. Symptoms are usually due to sudden expansion of the aneurysm, which can cause a vague pain in the back or sometimes a sharp pain that may denote the presence of rupture or impending rupture. Other symptoms are related to pressure on adjacent structures, such as pressure on the bronchus that can cause respiratory distress or pressure on the recurrent laryngeal nerve causing vocal hoarseness (Figure 34-2). Pressure on the esophagus can cause difficulty swallowing. On rare occasions, paraplegia and paraparesis can be caused by occlusion of critical intercostal arteries. There is also a risk of distal embolization causing "blue toe" syndrome (Figure 34-3).

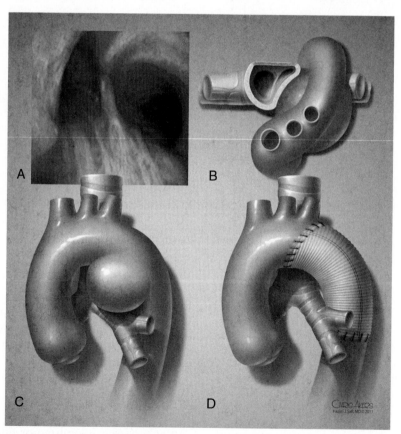

FIGURE 34-2 ■ Saccular descending thoracic aortic aneurysm causing compression of the right main bronchus. **A,** Bronchoscopic view showing right main bronchus compression. **B,** Illustration of aneurysm view in caudal direction before repair. **C,** Coronal illustration of aneurysm before repair. **D,** Illustration after repair.

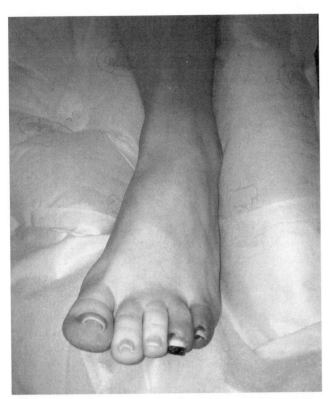

FIGURE 34-3 ■ Example of blue toe syndrome. See Color Plate 34-3.

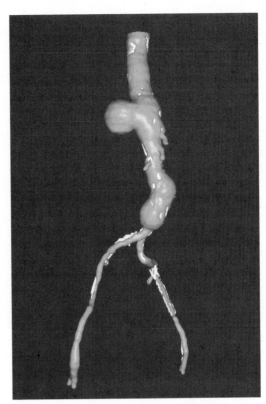

FIGURE 34-4 ■ Three-dimensional reconstruction of saccular thoracoabdominal aortic aneurysm extent V before repair. Note the aneurysm proximity to the celiac artery, the presence of a left iliac stent, and a synchronous infrarenal abdominal aortic aneurysm. See Color Plate 34-4.

Certain manifestations of rupture in 10% to 20% of thoracoabdominal aortic aneurysms include the sudden onset of severe or sharp pain radiating to the back causing a drop in hemoglobin and blood pressure. In a review of more than 100 ruptured descending thoracic and thoracoabdominal aortic aneurysms, the most common site of rupture was the pleural cavity.[28] Other sites of rupture occurred into the lung, esophagus, mediastinum, retroperitoneum, and peritoneal cavity. Thus, in addition to back, chest, or abdominal pain, patients may also exhibit with hemoptysis or hematemesis.

DIAGNOSIS

In the past, the definitive diagnostic tool was the aortogram; however, with the emergence of axial imaging, computed tomography (CT) or magnetic resonance angiography (MRA) are the modalities of choice. CT allows for visualization of the aortic wall, the aneurysm size, the presence or absence of clot formation, intercostal arteries, and effects on the surrounding tissues. The disadvantage of CT is the effect of ionizing radiation and the contrast media, which can exacerbate poor renal function. Three-dimensional reconstruction of axial imaging provides an additional view of thoracoabdominal aortic aneurysms (Figure 34-4). MRA is widely available and has the advantage of not using ionizing radiation, but it takes longer, provokes claustrophobia, and is contraindicated for patients with cerebral aneurysm clips, certain mechanical valves, or other internal metallic hardware. MRA is used less frequently because of these limitations.

Transesophageal echocardiography (TEE) provides excellent views of the ascending and descending aorta as well as heart function. TEE is an important tool in the diagnosis of acute aortic dissection. The limitation of TEE is that it is invasive, requires an expert echocardiographer, and does not provide adequate imaging of the aortic arch or below the level of the diaphragm.

Intravascular ultrasound (IVUS) is emerging as a useful adjunct, especially when there is diagnostic uncertainty such as in traumatic aortic injury (Figure 34-5). This modality allows for high-resolution imaging of the aortic wall and can often distinguish intimal lesions better than axial imaging.[29] The drawback is that it requires invasive intraarterial access, as well as the additional cost of the catheter and computerized ultrasound equipment.

THORACIC ANEURYSM CLASSIFICATION

Descending thoracic aortic aneurysms are divided into three extents (see Figure 34-1A).[30] Extent A designates an aortic aneurysm from the distal origin of the left subclavian artery to the level of the sixth thoracic intercostal space (T6). Extent B is from T6 to the twelfth thoracic intercostal space (T12). Extent C denotes the entire descending thoracic aorta from the left subclavian artery to T12.

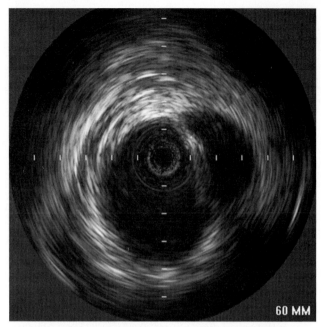

FIGURE 34-5 ■ Intravascular ultrasound of traumatic injury to the descending thoracic aorta causing pseudoaneurysm (grade 3 injury).

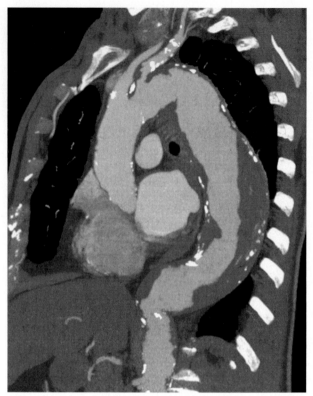

FIGURE 34-6 ■ Parasagittal computed tomographic reconstruction of a thoracic aortic aneurysm with extensive thrombus and atheromatous disease in the aortic wall.

Thoracoabdominal aortic aneurysms are classified in five categories (see Figure 34-1*B*). Extent I is from the left subclavian to above the most proximal renal artery. Extent II is from the left subclavian artery to below the renal arteries. Extent III is from the sixth intercostal space to below the renal arteries. Extent IV is from T12 to below the renal arteries. Extent V, which was introduced in the last 2 decades, is from T6 to just above the renal arteries. The importance of the classification scheme is that it correlated with the incidence of neurologic deficits and mortality especially when using the clamp-and-sew technique.

PREOPERATIVE EVALUATION

Preoperative evaluation of patients for elective thoracoabdominal aortic aneurysm should include a thorough history, physical examination, and determination of the presence of cardiovascular, pulmonary, and renal diseases. Pulmonary function testing is obtained in all patients, especially those with a history of pulmonary disease. However, there is still controversy regaining optimal preoperative cardiac workup for noncardiac vascular disease, despite published practice guidelines.[31,32] Preoperative left ventricular ejection fraction was the strongest cardiac predictor of mortality,[33] and echocardiography is obtained in all patients to assist in stratifying risk and to determine the need for additional cardiac testing. Treatment of coronary artery disease can be treated with medical therapy, coronary artery angioplasty, or coronary artery bypass before thoracoabdominal repair. It is unclear whether preoperative coronary artery or carotid artery revascularization are beneficial.[34,35]

Placement of stents during percutaneous coronary interventions requires antiplatelet medications to prevent in-stent thrombosis.[36] However, administering these can present a problem because newer antiplatelet medications are more potent and can predispose patients to bleeding after major aortic surgery.[37] Cessation of antiplatelet medications with drug-eluting stents is associated with greater than threefold the thrombosis rate compared with bare metal stents. In addition, more than one in four people require noncardiac surgery within 5 years after stent implantation.[38] Current guidelines suggest waiting 2 to 3 months after bare metal coronary stenting and 1 year after drug-eluting stent placement before holding antiplatelet medications for elective surgery.[39] However, the thrombosis risk for drug-eluting stents persists even after 12 months from implantation.[38,40,41]

Renal function should be evaluated with estimation of the glomerular filtration rate (GFR). Normal values are greater than 90 mL/min per 1.73 m^2. GFR is easy to estimate by several methods (e.g., Cockcroft-Gault, Modification of Diet in Renal Disease, or Chronic Kidney Disease Epidemiology Collaboration formulas) and is a better predictor of risk than serum creatinine.[42] Many formulas are available in smart phone applications and can be calculated in seconds.

Axial imaging of the entire chest, abdomen, and pelvis is mandatory to determine the extent of the aneurysm as well as synchronous aneurysms (Figure 34-6). Use of intravenous contrast is helpful in determining the presence of thrombus and atheromatous disease in the

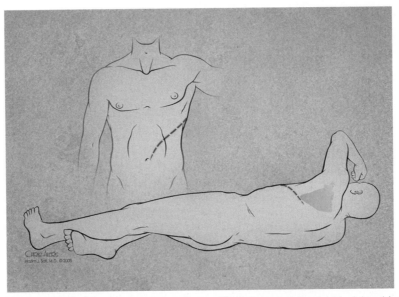

FIGURE 34-7 ■ Right lateral decubitus position for modified thoracoabdominal incision *(dashed line)*.

aortic wall (see Figure 34-6). Echocardiography is also helpful to evaluate for atheromatous disease in the thoracic aorta.

SURGICAL TECHNIQUE

General endotracheal anesthesia is induced with a double-lumen tube for selective single-lung ventilation. A pulmonary artery catheter and neuromonitoring leads for motor-evoked and somatosensory evoked potentials are placed. The patient is positioned in the right lateral decubitus position for placement of the CSF drain. After securing the drain, the hips are tilted slightly posteriorly to gain access to the left femoral artery (Figure 34-7). The shoulders are positioned perpendicular to the table. CSF pressure is kept at 10 mm Hg or less. This pressure is maintained intraoperatively and for 3 days postoperatively.

A thoracoabdominal incision is tailored to fit the extent of the aneurysm. In descending thoracic aortic aneurysm (DTAA) and thoracoabdominal aortic aneurysm (TAAA) extent I and V, a smaller modified thoracoabdominal incision is preferred (see Figure 34-7). The full thoracoabdominal incision begins posterior to the tip of the scapula and proceeds medially along T6. The incision is extended inferiorly at the midline toward the umbilicus. Next, the latissimus dorsi is divided and the serratus anterior muscle is mobilized. After the left lung is deflated, the left chest is entered. The sixth rib is resected or cut posteriorly and left in place, and a self-retaining retractor is used to aid in exposure.

The level of dissection depends on the aneurysm extent. For TAAA extent II, the dissection begins at the pulmonary hilum with opening of the pericardium to expose the left inferior pulmonary vein. The ligamentum arteriosum is divided after identification and preservation of the recurrent laryngeal nerve. The aorta proximal to the aneurysm is circumferentially dissected free. The

lateral muscular portion of the diaphragm may be divided and a retroperitoneal plane can be developed. The abdominal contents are retracted medially to the right of the abdominal aorta, including the left kidney (left visceral medial rotation).

Cannulas are placed for distal aortic perfusion. A purse-string suture is placed in the left inferior pulmonary vein, and the vein is incised. Intravenous heparin is given at 1 mg/kg, and the left inferior pulmonary vein is cannulated with the catheter tip directed toward the left atrium. The catheter is attached to a centrifugal pump with an in-line heat exchanger. The left common femoral artery is exposed and a graft is sewn in an end-to-side fashion to provide inflow. Instead of directly cannulating the femoral artery, a side-arm graft is used to preserve renal function and reduce extremity muscle ischemia.[43,44]

A segmental clamp is applied to the proximal descending thoracic aorta and the mid-thoracic aorta before transecting the aorta. In general, the inclusion technique at the proximal anastomosis is no longer used. The proximal aorta is divided completely and separated from the underlying esophagus to mitigate the risk of graft-esophageal fistula (Figure 34-8). A collagen or gelatin-impregnated woven Dacron graft is sutured end-to-end with 2-0 or 3-0 polypropylene sutures. In cases of acute dissection, 4-0 polypropylene sutures can be used. After completion of the proximal anastomosis, the clamp is moved distally to the celiac axis. The remaining thoracic aorta is opened, and upper intercostal arteries are ligated. Lower thoracic intercostal arteries are temporarily occluded with balloon-tipped catheters.

Patent intercostal arteries from T8 to T12 are reattached, and the graft is passed through the aortic hiatus. The extent and timing of lower intercostal artery reattachment depends on intraoperative neuromonitoring results.[45] An end-to-side loop graft can be used to reattach patent lower intercostal arteries, especially in patients with known connective tissue disease. The distal clamp is moved to the infrarenal abdominal aorta. The upper

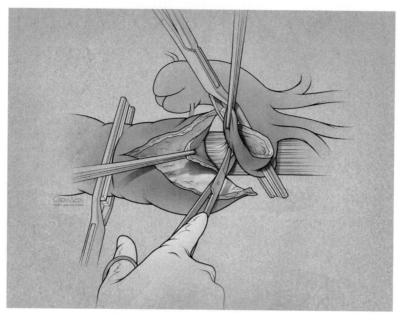

FIGURE 34-8 ■ Separation of the aorta from the underlying esophagus in preparation for the proximal anastomosis.

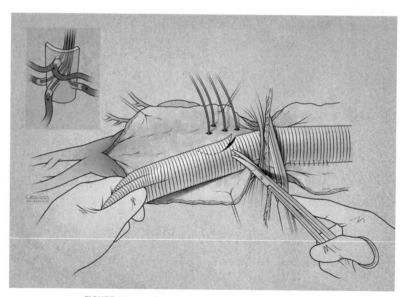

FIGURE 34-9 ■ Graftotomy for the visceral patch.

abdominal aorta is opened and the viscera are perfused via balloon-tipped catheters with cold blood via the centrifugal pump. The kidneys are perfused with cool crystalloid to maintain renal temperature of 15°C. The patient's core temperature can passively drift to 33°C. The viscera are usually attached as a patch (Figure 34-9) unless the patient is young or there is a known connective tissue disorder when the viscera are reattached with a commercially available side-branched thoracoabdominal aortic graft (Figure 34-10).[46] Distal anastomosis can be performed after pulsatile flow is restored to the viscera and renal arteries.

After completion of the distal anastomosis, the graft is de-aired and clamps are released. The anastomoses are checked for hemostasis, and the distal aortic perfusion cannulas are removed once the nasopharyngeal

temperature reaches 36°C. Coagulopathy is corrected with protamine sulfate and blood products as necessary.

The diaphragm is reapproximated with a running no. 1 polypropylene suture. Three large-bore chest tubes are placed. The lung is reinflated and the chest is closed with interrupted no. 2 polyglycolic acid sutures. The remainder of the chest and abdomen are closed in standard fashion. The double-lumen tube is usually exchanged for a single-lumen endotracheal tube before transfer unless there is significant airway edema.

IMMEDIATE NEUROLOGIC DEFICIT

Spinal cord ischemia during thoracic aortic aneurysm repair occurs because of cessation of blood flow to

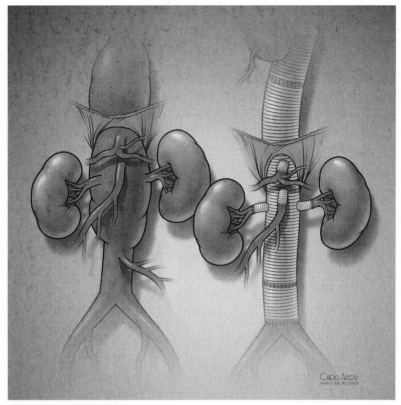

FIGURE 34-10 ■ Side-branched thoracoabdominal aortic graft in cases of young patients, Marfan syndrome, or other known connective tissue disease.

intercostal arteries, inadequate collateral circulation, reperfusion injury, and decreased cerebrospinal perfusion pressure. Several techniques minimize spinal ischemia during aortic clamping and after reconstruction. These techniques include intercostal artery reattachment, distal aortic perfusion, cardiopulmonary bypass, regional[47] or systemic hypothermia,[48] and CSF drainage.

The proposed effect of CSF drainage is to lower spinal fluid pressure and thereby increase blood perfusion pressure.[49] A metaanalysis found that the use of CSF drainage in thoracic aortic aneurysm repair led to an absolute risk reduction in neurologic deficit of 9%.[50] It is possible that the risk reduction is even greater because the meta-analysis included older studies that limited CSF drainage to 50 mL intraoperatively.[51] It is typical to drain 400 to 500 mL over 3 days intraoperatively and postoperatively, with an incidence of subdural hematoma of less than 0.5%.[52] Cases of intracranial bleeding should be rare after instituting a strict postoperative CSF drain protocol.

In addition to CSF drainage, distal aortic perfusion from the left atrium via a cannula placed in the left inferior pulmonary vein can be performed as described previously. Blood flows through a roller pump with an inline heat exchanger into the left femoral artery graft (Figure 34-11). Despite the heat exchanger, the body is allowed to passively cool to 33°C. Other reported methods of distal perfusion include axillofemoral bypass[53] and aortoiliac bypass.[54]

Our spinal protective adjuncts are CSF drainage, mild-moderate passive hypothermia, and left atriofemoral

bypass. With these techniques, recently published data for descending thoracic aortic aneurysm repair showed immediate neurologic deficits in only 0.6%.[55] In the clamp-and-sew area, the rate was more than triple at 5% overall, but increased to 9% in the highest risk extents.[56]

In the clamp-and-sew era, the incidence of neurologic deficits in thoracoabdominal aortic aneurysm extent I was 15%, 31% in extent II, 7% in extent III, and 4% in extent IV (see Figure 34-1B).[57] In addition to aneurysm extent, other predictors of neurologic deficit in the clamp-and-sew era included aortic clamp time and preoperative renal insufficiency. The use of adjuncts has mitigated aortic clamp time as a risk factor for immediate neurologic deficits. In more than 1000 thoracoabdominal aortic aneurysm repairs by the authors, aortic clamp times increased by an average of 34 seconds per year, yet the risk of neurologic deficit significantly decreased in extent II cases, from 1 in 5 to 1 in 30.[58] The strongest risks for postoperative spinal paralysis or paraparesis—collectively termed *neurologic deficits*—were extent II, preoperative renal insufficiency, current smoking, and clamp-and-sew technique.[58] Thus, for the purpose of neurologic risk stratification in the modern era, the groups can be separated into extent II and non–extent II. In a recent series, Safi and colleagues reported postoperative neurologic deficit rates of 4% in extent II and 1.1% in non–extent II cases.[59] Other groups report similar results with neurologic deficits occurring in 6% to 22% of extent II and 2.6% to 8% in non–extent II cases.[60,61]

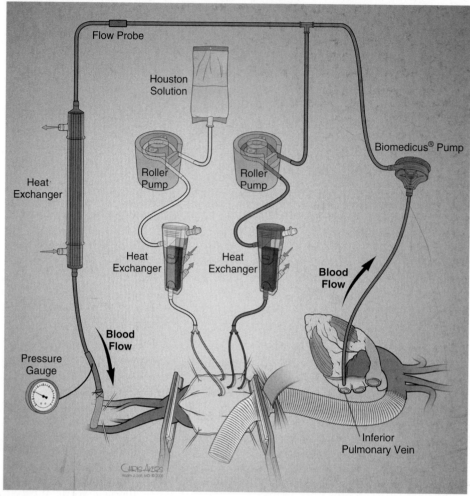

FIGURE 34-11 ■ Left atriofemoral bypass. Inflow is usually from the left inferior pulmonary vein, and roller pumps can provide perfusion via visceral cannulas. Outflow is usually via a graft placed end-to-side on the left common femoral artery. Visceral perfusate is cold blood. Renal perfusate is cold crystalloid solution via a separate roller pump.

DELAYED NEUROLOGIC DEFICIT AND CEREBROSPINAL FLUID DRAINAGE

The patient should be awakened as soon as possible postoperatively to ascertain neurologic status. The goal for mean arterial pressure is greater than 80 mm Hg, and the CSF pressure goal is less than 10 mm Hg. A maximum of 15 mL of CSF fluid is drained each hour to prevent intracranial hypotension and hemorrhage. If blood is noted in the effluent, the drain is capped and any coagulopathy is corrected. The drain is usually removed on the third postoperative day if the patient is neurologically intact. Neurologic function is frequently assessed to detect delayed deficit.

Estrera and colleagues[45] report a current rate of delayed neurologic deficit of 3% (3/105) in cases of descending thoracic and thoracoabdominal aortic aneurysm repair. Neurologic function recovered in two of those three patients before discharge. If delayed neurologic deficit occurs, several maneuvers—identified by the cerebrospinal fluid drain status/oxygen delivery/patient status (the COPS acronym)—are performed with the goal of increasing the spinal oxygenation and perfusion pressure (Figure 34-12).[52] Supplemental oxygen is given, and the patient is kept supine. The mean arterial pressure goal is raised to greater than 90 mm Hg, and the cardiac index is kept at greater than 2.5 L/min. Blood transfusions are given to keep the hemoglobin level greater than 12 g/dL. The CSF drain is opened to keep CSF pressure at less than 5 mm Hg. The drain is kept in place for a total of 7 days in cases of delayed deficit.

Complications of CSF drainage are low but include CSF leak, headache, and intracranial hemorrhage (Table 34-1).[52] The overall complication rate was 1.5% in more than 1100 patients. Serious complications occurred in less than 1%. The most common complication was CSF leak with spinal headache. Most CSF leaks required hydration and blood patch, but resolved without additional invasive management. Meningitis occurred in two patients (0.2%) who developed delayed neurologic deficit with prolonged catheter insertion. The authors have not noted intracranial hemorrhage in recent cases since limiting the CSF drainage to 15 mL/hr in neurologically intact patients.

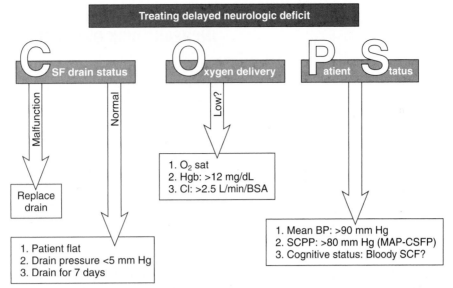

FIGURE 34-12 ■ The COPS protocol for treatment of patients with delayed neurologic deficit: **c**erebrospinal fluid drainage, supplemental **o**xygen, maximizing **p**atient **s**tatus (increasing blood pressure and spinal cord perfusion pressure).

TABLE 34-1	Complications of Cerebrospinal Fluid Drainage

Complication	Frequency (%)
CSF leak without spinal headache	0.1
CSF leak with spinal headache	0.54
Intracranial hemorrhage	0.45
Meningitis	0.2
Spinal headache without CSF leak	0.2
Fractured catheter	0.1

Modified from Estrera AL, Sheinbaum R, Miller CC, et al: Cerebrospinal fluid drainage during thoracic aortic repair: safety and current management. Ann Thorac Surg 88:9–15, 2009.
CSF, Cerebrospinal fluid.

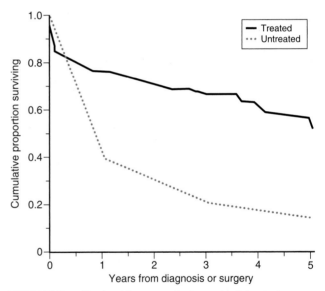

FIGURE 34-13 ■ Kaplan-Meyer survival graph of treated versus untreated thoracic aortic aneurysm from time of diagnosis.

RESULTS

Mortality for descending thoracic and thoracoabdominal aortic aneurysm repair primarily depends on comorbid conditions and aneurysm extent. In 300 cases of open DTAA repair, 30-day mortality was 8% with preoperative renal insufficiency and female sex emerging as risk factors.[30] Other groups reported similar results with rates of 30-day mortality ranging from 2.2% to 14% and spinal neurologic deficit rates between 1% and 7.4%.[61-64]

Published short-term mortality in elective thoracoabdominal aortic aneurysm repair ranges from 4% to 7%.[48,57,60,65,66] Long-term mortality reflects comorbid conditions such as cerebrovascular and coronary disease. Nevertheless, thoracoabdominal aortic aneurysm repair is highly effective in reducing aneurysm-related death. Repair of thoracic aortic aneurysm nearly restores mortality to age-matched controls. In a study comparing untreated historical controls to patients receiving surgical repair, 5-year survival in the untreated group was only 13% compared with 61% in the surgical treatment group (Figure 34-13).[67] Postoperative complications, such as

acute renal failure and manifestations of gastrointestinal ischemia, predict decreased survival.

POSTOPERATIVE RENAL FAILURE

Postoperative renal injury is defined according to the risk, injury, failure, loss, end stage (RIFLE) criteria[68] where there is an increase in creatinine of greater than 1 mg/dL per day over 2 consecutive days or a need for hemodialysis. In a review of the authors' experience in more than 1000 open thoracoabdominal repairs since 1991, the strongest predictor of postoperative renal failure was low preoperative GFR. Other risk factors

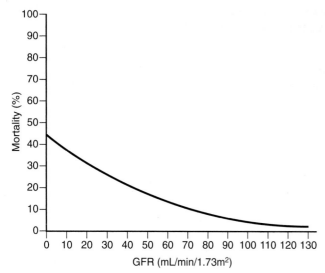

FIGURE 34-14 ■ Graph showing postoperative mortality as a function of preoperative glomerular filtration rate.

include aneurysm extents involving the renal arteries (extent II, III, and IV) and clamp-and-sew technique.[69] The risk of postoperative renal failure was 17% in patients with normal preoperative GFR. In patients with a GFR of 40 or less, the risk of postoperative renal dysfunction was 38%.[43] Preoperative renal function inversely correlates with postoperative mortality (Figure 34-14).

Miller and colleagues[43] showed that using a femoral artery end-to-side graft to provide distal perfusion inflow instead of direct artery cannulation decreased this risk to 30%. They speculated that avoiding occlusion of the femoral artery with the cannula would decrease skeletal muscle ischemia in the extremity (see Figure 34-11), which in turn may decrease release of nephrotoxic factors and rhabdomyolysis.[70] The use of cold perfusate has also been shown to decrease incidence of hospital mortality.[71] However, the dramatic improvements of adjunctive techniques on rates of neurologic deficits have not yet been noted with renal failure.

POSTOPERATIVE GASTROINTESTINAL COMPLICATIONS

Gastrointestinal (GI) complications affect 7% of DTAA and TAAA repairs.[72] Overall mortality increased nearly threefold compared with the entire cohort, and even mild GI complications increased the risk of death. Involvement of the visceral aorta (extent II, III, and IV) and low preoperative GFR were risk factors. The pathophysiology is postulated to be released of atheromatous debris during aortic manipulation and visceral ischemia after aortic clamping. The manifestations include pancreatitis, ileus (>5 postoperative days), GI bleeding, peptic ulcers, liver dysfunction, bowel ischemia, and cholecystitis. The most common GI complication was bowel ischemia (2.5%), which conferred a 62% mortality. Interestingly, acalculous cholecystitis (0.3%) was the highest harbinger of mortality risk at 75%.

CHRONIC AORTIC DISSECTION DOES NOT INCREASE RISK OF REPAIR

There is evidence that rupture occurs at a smaller size in cases of aortic dissection. In a review of ruptured thoracic aortic aneurysms, 40% of ruptures in acute dissection occurred in patients with an aortic diameter less than 6 cm.[28] The median diameter at rupture in chronic dissection cases was 8 cm. Open repair of descending thoracic and thoracoabdominal aortic aneurysms in the setting of chronic dissection has excellent results with the use of adjuncts. No increased risk was noted in nearly 200 elective cases of chronic dissecting descending thoracic and thoracoabdominal aortic aneurysm.[73] However, thoracic aortic operations in cases of acute dissection are fraught with high morbidity and mortality. Medical management for acute type B dissection with strict blood pressure control is the treatment of choice. Surgery is reserved for cases of medical failure, malperfusion syndromes, and rupture. The operative mortality rate in acute type B dissection is 14%, with spinal neurologic deficits in 32%.[74] The higher rate of spinal ischemia is multifactorial. Adjunctive spinal protection techniques, such as distal aortic perfusion and CSF drainage, are often not used because of hemodynamic instability. Critically, intercostal artery reimplantation is contraindicated because of the risk of bleeding. Several ongoing trials are evaluating selective use of stent-grafts in acute, complicated type B dissection.

RUPTURE AND TRAUMATIC AORTIC INJURY

Most patients with a ruptured thoracic aortic aneurysm die before reaching the hospital.[19] Although elective repair of thoracic aneurysms restores actuarial survival to near normal, patients suffer increased morbidity and mortality even after successful repair of a ruptured aneurysm.[75] Thirty-day mortality was 24% in one early series in which more than half the patients suffered cardiac arrest preoperatively.[28] Other reviews showed early mortality ranging from 12% to 54%, with neurologic deficits in 5% to 9%.[76-78]

Blunt traumatic aortic injury (TAI) is a major cause of death due to rupture. Similar to ruptured degenerative aneurysms, open repair of TAI carries a higher risk of early death, neurologic deficits, and pulmonary complications. Data from 255 patients over a 12-year period show improved outcomes with selectively delaying open repair.[25] Patients with left atriofemoral bypass had improved mortality and neurologic outcomes compared to those without (14% vs. 31% and 10% vs. 0%). Improved early results were also noted for endovascular repair.[27,79,80] Since 2005, endovascular repair has become a primary modality for repair of blunt TAI to the descending thoracic aorta. In addition, endovascular repair is being used increasingly in cases of ruptured degenerative descending thoracic aortic aneurysms that meet anatomic criteria. Until commercially available branched or fenestrated stent-grafts become available, endovascular repair for ruptured thoracoabdominal aortic aneurysms remains investigational.

CONCLUSION

Descending thoracic and thoracoabdominal aortic aneurysms are deadly conditions, with the aneurysm size being the currently accepted factor in determining timing of elective repair. Open repair offers durable and proven mortality benefits compared with nonoperative management. Current adjunctive techniques have successfully reduced the risk of spinal ischemia to acceptable levels—even in high-risk patients. Visceral and renal failures continue to be problematic, especially in more extensive thoracoabdominal aneurysms. Aneurysm extent

and preoperative renal function are important risk predictors.

Endovascular repair offers an alternative method of repair. Approved devices for the descending thoracic aorta appear to have a lower short-term mortality, but have higher reintervention rates and similar long-term mortality compared with open repair. Endovascular thoracoabdominal aortic aneurysm repair is a promising alternative to open surgical repair, but there is concern about neurologic deficits, especially in the more extensive aneurysms. Future endovascular techniques will likely have to allow revascularization of the critical lower thoracic intercostal arteries to maintain the improvement in rates of neurologic deficits.

References available online at expertconsult.com.

QUESTIONS

1. Increasing size correlates with risk of thoracic aortic aneurysm rupture. For thoracic aneurysms less than 6 cm, the 5-year risk of rupture is 16%. For thoracic aneurysms greater than 6 cm, the estimated 5-year risk of rupture is:
   a. Less than 15%
   b. Between 15-30%
   c. Between 31-90%
   d. Greater than 90%

2. Signs and symptoms of thoracoabdominal aortic aneurysm rupture can include
   a. Pain
   b. Hypotension
   c. Hemoptysis
   d. Hematemesis
   e. All of the above

3. The risk of spinal paralysis or paraparesis in open repair of extent II thoracoabdominal aortic aneurysm with spinal protective adjuncts is:
   a. Less than 5%
   b. 5%-10%
   c. 11%-15%
   d. >15%
   e. Not dependent on aneurysm extent

4. A 58-year-old woman had an incidental finding on a CT scan of a 4.5-cm extent I thoracoabdominal aortic aneurysm. Your decision to operate is based on the genetic workup showing the presence of a mutation in:
   a. TGF beta receptor type II (TGFBR2)
   b. BRCA1
   c. BCR-ABL
   d. Myosin heavy chain 11 smooth muscle (MYH11)
   e. Tissue inhibitor of matrix metalloproteinase 9 (MMP9)

5. A 65-year old woman had normal neurologic function immediately following open repair of her extent II thoracoabdominal aortic aneurysm. Nursing noted that she stopped moving her lower extremities in the ICU. The next best step in management is:
   a. Steroid administration
   b. MRI of spine
   c. Cerebrospinal fluid (CSF) drainage
   d. Cardioversion
   e. Extubation as soon as possible

6. A 65-year-old man with an extent V thoracoabdominal aortic aneurysm has a serum creatinine of 0.8 mg/dL with an estimated glomerular filtration rate (GFR) of 90 ml/min/1.73m^2. His predicted mortality after open repair is:
   a. 5%
   b. 10%-15%
   c. 15%-20%
   d. >25%

7. The most common complication with CSF drainage is:
   a. Meningitis
   b. Intracranial hemorrhage
   c. CSF leak with headache
   d. Fractured catheter
   e. Spinal paralysis

8. A 40-year-old man with hypertension presents with acute type B aortic dissection. Medical management has begun, but open surgical repair is offered if there is:
   a. Need for greater than 3 oral antihypertensive agents
   b. Visceral malperfusion
   c. Need for greater than 1 intravenous antihypertensive agents
   d. Spinal headache
   e. Estimated GFR >60 mL/min/1.73m^2

9. Patients with chronic thoracic aortic dissection and aneurysm are at no significantly increased risk of death or spinal neurologic deficits after open surgical repair.
   a. True
   b. False

10. Reattachment of intercostal arteries for prevention of spinal neurologic deficit is most important at the level of:
    a. T1-T4
    b. T4-T8
    c. T8-T12
    d. L1-L4

ANSWERS

1. c
2. e
3. a
4. a
5. c
6. a
7. c
8. b
9. a
10. c

CHAPTER 35

ENDOVASCULAR REPAIR OF THORACIC AORTIC ANEURYSM

Eric Hager • Jae S. Cho • Michel S. Makaroun

Thoracic aortic aneurysms (TAAs) are less frequent than abdominal aneurysms but are no less significant. The estimated incidence is 10.4 cases per 100,000 population.[1] With the aging population in the United States coupled with advances in imaging technology, there has been a steady increase in the number of diagnosed TAAs. The natural history of these aneurysms is not well characterized, although it has been shown that approximately 70% of patients who forgo treatment will progress to rupture, with a fatality rate approaching 90%.[2]

Traditionally, repair of TAAs has been limited to open aortic replacement with significant morbidity related to thoracotomy, single lung ventilation, aortic cross clamping, and prolonged visceral or renal ischemia with a prolonged hospital stay and recovery. The reported mortality rates with open repair of TAA at centers of excellence have ranged from 3% to 8%, with paraplegia rates of 3% to 5%.[3,4] The first endovascular exclusion of a thoracic aorta was reported by Dake in 1994.[5] Development of commercial thoracic endografts, however, was slow because of the relatively low prevalence of thoracic aneurysms, the hostile hemodynamic forces of the thoracic aorta and the need for large devices and delivery systems. The U.S. Food and Drug Administration (FDA) approved the first thoracic endograft in March 2005 after a nonrandomized trial showed that thoracic endovascular repair (TEVAR) compared favorably to the standard open procedure. Since then, there has been a paradigm shift in the treatment of descending thoracic aneurysm (DTA), with high-risk patients being offered TEVAR, thus expanding the pool of patients that could undergo treatment. Despite the lack of randomized trial data comparing it with open surgical repair, TEVAR has become the preferred method of treatment for all DTA.

INDICATIONS FOR THORACIC ENDOVASCULAR REPAIR

The decision to intervene on a DTA depends on its size, location, rate of growth, and symptoms and the overall medical condition of the patient. The indications for TEVAR should not differ from those for open repair and typically include aneurysms greater than 6 cm in diameter. Saccular and symptomatic aneurysms are often repaired at a smaller size. It is also suggested that aneurysms with a rapid growth rate (more than 1 cm per year, or 0.5 cm in 6 months) should be considered for early

repair.[6] TEVAR has also been used in other types of thoracic pathology, including acute complicated type B dissection, traumatic thoracic aortic injury, large penetrating aortic ulcers, and intramural hematomas[7] (Box 35-1). The discussion in this chapter will be limited to aneurysmal disease.

PREOPERATIVE PLANNING: IMAGING

The decision to proceed with TEVAR requires detailed imaging for procedural planning. Important anatomic characteristics include landing zones, vessel tortuosity, aneurysm location in relationship to branch vessels, and access size and quality. Computed tomographic angiography (CTA) is the modality of choice for evaluation of aortic pathology and TEVAR planning. Multiplanar reconstructions and three-dimensional modeling provide invaluable information regarding vessel sizes, angulation, length, and anatomic relationships as well as severity of calcification and presence of thrombus. The availability of advanced software such as Vitrea (Vital Images, Minnetonka, Minn.) and Aquarius (TeraRecon, San Mateo, Calif.) has brought the power of workstation analysis to simple desktop computers, allowing operators to perform accurate graft sizing and predeployment planning. For patients who cannot undergo CTA safely, magnetic resonance angiography has also been used successfully, although patients with renal failure are at risk for nephrogenic systemic fibrosis.[8]

ANATOMIC CONSIDERATIONS

Sizing

Accurate measurements of the proximal and distal seal zones and access vessel diameter are of the utmost importance in planning TEVAR. Most endografts require oversizing by 10% to 20% of the seal zone diameter, depending on device parameters. Excessive oversizing can lead to folding, gutter formation, and accelerated aneurysm degeneration. Undersized grafts can lead to migration and endoleaks. Diameter measurements are best obtained in a plane orthogonal to the centerline of flow for accurate sizing of the endograft. Distal landing zone diameters are often smaller than the proximal seal zone, requiring the use of multiple grafts to correct the discrepancy. Use of tapered grafts can alleviate this problem if

- Thoracic aneurysm >5.5 cm
- Aneurysm growth >1 cm per year
- Aneurysm growth >0.5 cm in 6 months
- Traumatic aortic transection
- Complicated type B dissection
- Large penetrating aortic ulcers

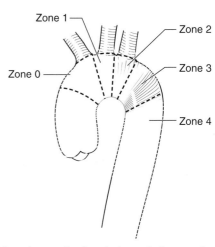

FIGURE 35-1 ■ Anatomic description of the proximal landing zones.

the length of the aneurysm can be properly bridged with one graft. Aortic coverage lengths can be difficult to approximate, however, and are usually underestimated by centerline measurements. The natural tortuosity of the aorta, coupled with the large cavity of an aneurysm and the tendency of the endograft to sit against the greater curvature, usually result in a longer trajectory for graft coverage. These factors should be taken into consideration during graft planning and deployment.

Access

The thoracic aortic diameter is typically larger than the abdominal aorta and requires larger devices and delivery systems. Many devices have a 24-French profile and require at least an 8-mm access channel for safe delivery and deployment. Particular attention should be given to the proximal external iliac artery; this area is prone to atherosclerotic narrowing and calcification, particularly in women. In such a setting, the common iliac artery can be accessed by a small retroperitoneal incision and the use of an iliac conduit. Conduits measuring 10 mm in diameter are preferred and can be used through the retroperitoneal incision or tunneled to the femoral region to avoid angulations in large individuals. Occasionally, this conduit can serve the function of a bypass at the end of the procedure in case of severe external iliac artery disease. On rare occasions, the infrarenal aorta can be accessed directly at the time of exploratory laparotomy. A pure endovascular approach consisting of aligning the iliac system with a graft limb, followed by aggressive balloon dilatation, has been described as a means to obtain satisfactory access. One disadvantage to this approach is the loss of patency of an internal iliac artery.

Landing Zones

The tortuosity and high shear force in the thoracic aorta mandate a longer seal zone than infrarenal aneurysm repair. It is recommended that at least 2 cm of seal zone be used at either end of the graft to prevent migration. These seal zones should be longer in areas of severe angulation, such as the apex of the arch, and may also have to be adjusted upward for thrombus or calcification in the wall. It is also important to recognize that the longer the aortic coverage, the greater the number of excluded intercostal arteries, which affects paraplegia rates.

The proximal seal locations have been classified into five zones (Figure 35-1). Each zone is divided by a tangential line along the distal side of each great vessel; zone 0 involves the origin of the innominate artery, zone 1 the origin of the left common carotid artery (LCCA), zone 2 the origin of the left subclavian artery (LSA), zone 3 the proximal descending thoracic aorta down to the T4 vertebral body, and zone 4 the remainder of descending thoracic aorta. The location of the proximal landing zone depends on the aneurysm morphology; however, the ideal location in terms of anatomic accommodation of the graft is in zones 3 and 4. An important consideration for the proximal seal zone is the angle of the aortic arch. Grafts that are placed within the aortic arch (zones 2 and 3), especially one with an acute angle, may fail to properly appose to the inner curvature of the arch (Figure 35-2). This configuration has occasionally resulted in untoward effects such as migration and collapse, mostly in non-aneurysmal applications. Recent endograft modifications such as the Zenith Pro-Form (Cook, Bloomington, Ind.) and the C-TAG (W.L. Gore, Flagstaff, Ariz.) have been designed to specifically address this problem.

Management of the Left Subclavian Artery

In approximately 20% of cases, adequate coverage of the TAA can be achieved only by extending the graft into zone 2, effectively excluding the LSA from circulation[9] (Figure 35-3). The management strategy of the LSA has evolved since the inception of TEVAR. Prophylactic revascularization of the LSA, either through a carotid subclavian bypass or a transposition, was used routinely in the first study of TEVAR. Intentional coverage without revascularization was later tolerated as a relatively safe practice especially in emergency settings and in the presence of good collateral circulation. Absolute contraindications include an occluded or atretic right vertebral artery or a left internal mammary bypass to the coronary circulation. A review of 22 patients who underwent intentional coverage of the LSA found that almost 70%

of the patients remained asymptomatic, with the remaining 30% suffering only mild left arm claudication symptoms.

The practice of LSA coverage has come under severe scrutiny lately with EUROSTAR data linking it to an increased risk of spinal cord ischemia. Several reports of

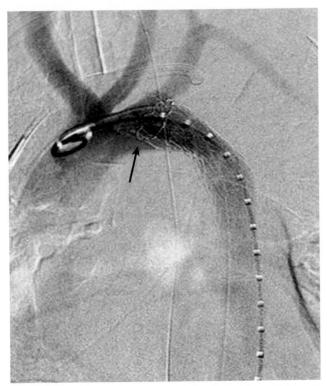

FIGURE 35-2 ■ Angiogram showing "bird beaking" of the proximal endograft.

brain stem strokes and other complications have also surfaced. Peterson and colleagues[11] observed a 63% (5/8) stroke and upper extremity ischemic symptom rate in patients who had LSA coverage without revascularization. A review of a random segment of the literature disclosed a 23% complication rate with LSA coverage compared with a 3% rate when flow to the LSA was maintained.[11,14] The current Society for Vascular Surgery (SVS) guidelines recommend routine preoperative revascularization in elective TEVAR and expectant management in acute settings excluding absolute contraindications.[15]

In order to safely deploy a stent-graft at the level of the left subclavian artery, it is often helpful to gain access to the aortic arch through the left brachial. This allows visualization of the junction between the subclavian and the aorta easier and also allows for salvage stenting in the event of inadvertent coverage.

Management of the Celiac Axis

The ideal distal landing zone places at least 2 cm of graft proximal to the celiac axis. When the aneurysm is more extensive, coverage of the celiac artery is a possibility, allowing for a longer seal zone. Concerns for bowel ischemia and hepatic failure should prompt careful assessment of the collateral network, especially through the gastroduodenal and pancreaticoduodenal arcades. A recent review reported selective coverage of the celiac axis in 31 patients during TEVAR.[16] Of these patients, two (6%) patients had bowel ischemia, and five (16%) had an endoleak that required reintervention. The findings illustrate the fact that celiac coverage is feasible in many cases, but potentially morbid in the absence of adequate collaterals, and should be undertaken with caution.

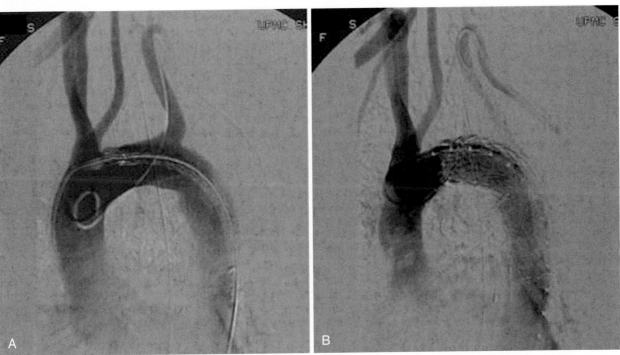

FIGURE 35-3 ■ Predeployment angiogram **(A)**, and postdeployment **(B)**. Note the complete coverage of the left subclavian artery.

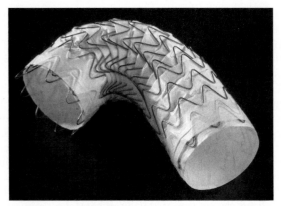

FIGURE 35-4 ■ Gore TAG device. (Courtesy W.L. Gore & Associates.)

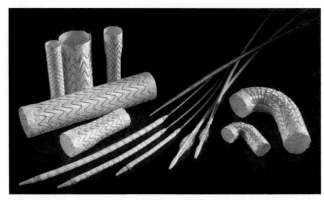

FIGURE 35-5 ■ The conformable Gore TAG thoracic endoprosthesis. (Courtesy W.L. Gore & Associates.)

STENT GRAFT DESCRIPTION

Since the FDA approval of TEVAR in 2005, there has been a rapid increase in the number of stent-grafts available with new modifications and new grafts along the way. Commercial release in the United States typically lags behind the rest of the world because of the regulatory environment.

Gore TAG

The TAG graft (W.L. Gore, Flagstaff, Ariz.) was the first FDA-approved device for the treatment of DTAs (Figure 35-4). As such, it is the most common device implanted for both on- and off-label use in the United States. The graft is an expanded polytetrafluoroethylene (ePTFE) tubular graft reinforced with a layer of fluorinated ethylene propylene (FEP) material and external Nitinol self-expanding stents. The marketed TAG endograft has a lower porosity to help avoid the sac enlargement associated with the earlier version of the device.[17,18] The FEP wrap was also added as a replacement of the longitudinal deployment wire tested with the original device. The stent wire-forms are secured to the graft with a bonding tape made of ePTFE and FEP. Effective proximal and distal seals are achieved by flared edges of the graft as well as an additional ePTFE cuff. The graft has an inlaid gold band that marks the proximal and distal edges, although the flared ends protrude 7 to 9 mm beyond these edges.

The TAG device is constrained in a sleeve of ePTFE/FEP film that is bound by a longitudinal seam running the entire length of the device. This seam is held together by an ePTFE line connected to a deployment knob located at the control end of the delivery catheter. The device is deployed by pulling on the string, which unzips the seam, thereby deploying the stent-graft. The device is available in diameters of 26 to 45 mm and lengths of 10, 15, or 20 cm. It is delivered through a 20- to 24-French sheath. The Gore TAG device is designed to be oversized by 7% to 22%, which is incorporated into the instructions for use (IFU) device sizing guide.

Advantages of the TAG device include a simple deployment mechanism and flexibility that allows easy

accommodation of tortuous thoracic aortas. The endograft deploys from the middle of the graft out toward both ends. This design theoretically avoids the wind sock effect that can occur if the proximal end is released first. Once the graft is deployed, the seal zones are ballooned with a tri-lobed balloon that allows for continuous antegrade blood flow.

The new conformable TAG (C-TAG) device has been modified to increase conformability, especially to the lesser curvature of the arch by changing the wire form strength and pattern (Figure 35-5). The proximal covered scallops have also been replaced by short bare metal stents ranging in length from 3 to 6.5 mm. A 21-mm device has been added to the size range so that patients with smaller aortic diameters can be treated. Two tapered devices (26 to 21 mm and 31 to 26 mm) were also added, providing added flexibility in sizing. Other changes include the addition of a 46-mm device in 2010 and the introduction of a new pressurized hemostatic valve on its sheath to minimize blood loss.

Medtronic Talent

The Talent device (Medtronic, Santa Rosa, Calif.) was approved for commercial use in the United States in June 2008. The device has been available worldwide since 1997 and was widely used outside the United States.

The graft is composed of a nitinol skeleton attached to a woven polyester graft. There is a bare metal component at the proximal end to allow for extended fixation while maintaining flow to the branch vessels. There are a number of tapered and nontapered configurations available as well as different configurations for the last stent (Figure 35-6). The support bar of the device is intended to be aligned along the greater curvature of the aorta, and can be identified by the radiopaque "8" that marks the bar. The Talent is available in a wide range of diameters, from 22 to 46 mm, but was initially limited to 112- to 116-mm lengths, which required many devices to be used to cover a long aortic segment, an average of 2.7 devices in the VALOR trial.[18,19] The device is usually oversized by 10% to 20% over the aortic landing zones and uses a 22- to 25-French delivery catheter.

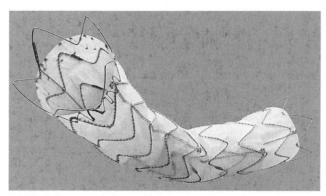

FIGURE 35-6 ■ Medtronic Talent device. (From Moore WS: Endovascular surgery, ed 4, Philadelphia, 2011, Saunders.)

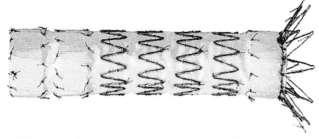

FIGURE 35-7 ■ Cook TX2 device. (From Moore WS: Endovascular surgery, ed 4, Philadelphia, 2011, Saunders.)

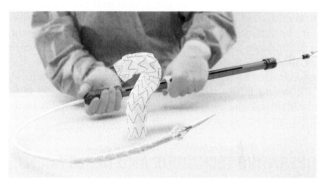

FIGURE 35-8 ■ Bolton Relay device. (From Moore WS: Endovascular surgery, ed 4, Philadelphia, 2011, Saunders.)

The talent device has undergone a series of modifications and improvements, including a much improved delivery catheter and a controlled deployment mechanism. In addition, graft lengths greater than 20 cm are available to overcome one major disadvantage of the earlier system.

The next generation of the device, the Valiant (Medtronic, Fridley, Minn), has finished all regulatory trials in the United States and is awaiting final approval. It uses the Xcelerant (Medtronic, Fridley, Minn) delivery system, which touts greater trackablity for the tortuous aorta because of a hydrophilic outer coating and shorter tip on a braided sheath. Changes to the implant were also introduced to improve flexibility and radial strength of the graft while reducing pressure points in the landing zones by increasing the number of shorter peaks on its uncovered stents from five to eight. The longitudinal support bar was removed, and longer devices were made (up to 227 mm).

Cook TX2

The Cook TX2 stent-graft (Cook Medical, Bloomington, Ind.) was approved by the FDA for commercial use in the United States in 2008. It is a modular device consisting of two components with active fixation. The graft is constructed of a stainless steel skeleton covered in woven Dacron. The entire length of Dacron is supported by an exoskeleton except at the proximal end, where the stents line the inside. This design optimizes the Dacron to aorta apposition at the ends of the graft while maintaining support. The TX2 device uses active fixation on both components in the form of proximal, caudally oriented barbs to prevent distal migration, and distal, cranially oriented barbs to prevent proximal migration. The distal end is a bare stent designed to allow additional coverage of visceral vessels if needed while maintaining patency (Figure 35-7).

There are four gold radiopaque markers near the end of the graft allowing for careful visualization and placement of the graft. The device is available in diameters of 28 to 42 mm in 2-mm increments and in lengths of 120 to 216 mm. There is also a tapered proximal graft that allows for a 4 mm difference between the proximal and distal necks. The delivery system is 20 to 22 French based

on the size of the device. Cook recommends at least a 3-cm overlap at the proximal and distal landing zones.

The TX2 device is deployed in a staged, controlled fashion. The outer sheath is first withdrawn, allowing initial graft release. Once position is confirmed, deployment is completed by releasing the trigger wire. A balloon is then inflated as needed to secure the device in position.

Recent modifications include the introduction of a mechanism (i.e., Pro-Form) that allows the first stent to deploy at an angle to the second stent facilitating apposition to the lesser curve in the arch. A newer, nitinol-based device with lower-profile construction and improved flexibility is still in clinical testing.

Bolton Relay

The Bolton Relay thoracic graft (Bolton Medical, Sunrise, Fla.) has a skeleton of self-expanding nitinol stents covered with a compliant polyester fabric (Figure 35-8). The proximal portion of the device has an exposed bare metal stent that acts to anchor the device in place while maintaining patency of branch vessels. The device is delivered via the transport system, which consists of a primary introduction sheath, a curved flexible secondary delivery sheath, and a thru lumen. The graft is released via the apex release mechanism. There is a double S configuration of the support bar, which is designed to mimic the natural curve of the aorta while providing columnar strength.

A number of platinum and iridium radiopaque markers are embedded in the graft to allow visualization of the device. The device is available in both tapered and non-tapered configurations. The nontapered grafts are available in diameters ranging from 22 to 46 mm, and in lengths of 100 to 250 mm. The delivery system requires a primary introducer sheath of 22 to 26 French, depending on the device size. The tapered grafts are designed to gradually taper in 4-mm increments and the recommended oversizing is 10% to 15%. The graft requires at least a 25-mm proximal and 30-mm distal landing zone. When the coverage zone is long, and multiple grafts are used, the company recommends a minimum of 50 mm of overlap between devices.

Deployment of the relay is achieved by first positioning the primary sheath in the abdominal aorta and then navigating the secondary sheath to the desired location for the device. The release mechanism is much like the TX2 and entails a slow, controlled pull of the outer sheath to allow expansion of the endograft. A separate mechanism is used to expand the proximal bare stents. Typically, ballooning is not required after deployment. The U.S. clinical trial has been completed, and the device is in its final approval stages.

OPERATIVE TECHNIQUE AND DEPLOYMENT

Deployment of these stent grafts differ slightly, but a series of general rules and tips are helpful. Once bilateral access is obtained, a pigtail catheter is placed from the contralateral side to guide deployment while a stiff wire (Lunderquist [Cook Medical, Bloomington, Ind]) is advanced into the ascending aorta from the ipsilateral access. Aortography is performed with the image intensifier rotated to give the best orthogonal view of the desired deployment zone. For proximal images, a left anterior oblique projection of 40 to 60 degrees is usually best, while the projection for distal deployments can be variable. Angiography serves as the last check for device length choice and land marking, but this step can be omitted in patients with compromised renal function.

The chosen stent-graft is then introduced and the deployment steps are followed. Usually the stent-graft is advanced beyond the target region initially and retracted to its desired landing zone, to eliminate any stored forward energy in the graft. During deployment, constant forward pressure is applied on the wire to buttress the graft against the outer curve of the aorta, limiting the tendency for distal migration and poor apposition to the landing zone. Adjunctive techniques have been used successfully to assist in accurate proximal deployment of the endograft, such as pharmacologic reduction of the blood pressure, transient asystole induced by adenosine, and rapid ventricular pacing. These maneuvers help to reduce the shear force on the expanding graft, and can help to prevent the wind sock effect and distal migration. The maneuvers are not universally required, but can be helpful in difficult cases. Proper sizing and deployment technique and newer modified devices can improve lesser curve apposition and improved sealing.

If the extent of the aneurysm requires more than one graft for adequate coverage, the smaller device should be deployed first to allow for an adequate sealing between grafts. The overlap zone should typically be at least 5 cm in length. When the devices are the same size, a longer overlap zone (7 to 10 cm) is typically needed to avoid type 3 endoleaks.

RESULTS

Open repair is a morbid procedure that carries a combined paraplegia and mortality rate of greater than 20% in reports using national and regional databases.[19] Five- and 10-year survival rates following open thoracic aortic aneurysm repair are somewhat limited at 60% and 38%, respectively.[3,4] Results comparing TEVAR to open repair are limited by the lack of prospective randomized trials. Most available information is gleaned from single center reports and registry experience. These data are difficult to interpret because of the inclusion of a multitude of pathologies, different anatomic locations, device types, and patient comorbidities, which makes a direct comparison impossible. Premarket regulatory device trials still provide the best comparative information of TEVAR results to open repair, because relatively similar groups are involved.

Early Results

Technical Success

Technical success in endograft deployment has been reported as high as 98% in all three FDA trials and the Talent thoracic registry.[18,20-22] Most failures were due to access problems preventing the delivery of the device. Interestingly, the EUROSTAR and United Kingdom thoracic registries report a lower deployment success rate, reflecting wider application of the technology in current clinical practice outside of trial guidelines.

Mortality

A significant operative survival benefit is observed with TEVAR when compared with open repair in the U.S. trials (2% vs. 6%). The EUROSTAR registry of TEVAR reports a higher but still favorable mortality rate of 5.3%, likely because 52% of its patients were deemed to be too high risk for open repair and thus represented a sicker cohort.[23] A recent metaanalysis of published literature shows clear survival benefits with TEVAR compared with the open procedure.[24]

Neurologic Complications

Neurologic complications still represent one of the most feared and devastating complications after TAA repairs, whether by endovascular or open means. Advances in endograft technology have not helped much in improving the significant stroke rates associated with TAA repair. Stroke rates for both procedures range from 3% to 5%.[11,18,20,25,26] Strokes are believed to occur with TEVAR primarily because of instrumentation of the aortic arch causing embolization and occasionally coverage of a critical source of blood to the brain.[27] Deployment of stent grafts proximal to the left subclavian artery has been associated with an increased risk of post-operative stroke. In the phase II TAG study, stroke occurred in 14% of patients with endograft deployment proximal to the LSA compared with only 1% when the graft was deployed in zone 3. Similarly, in the VALOR High-Risk trial, the incidence of stroke was 26% when the stent-graft was deployed proximal to zone 3.[10] Interestingly in the STARZ trial, all four strokes occurred with stent-graft deployment distal to the LSA.[20] These strokes may have been related to the recommended deployment sequence of the TX2, starting proximal to the desired deployment zone with a distal readjustment technique used to deploy it.[6] Minimal manipulation and meticulous cleansing of wires, catheters, and delivery system as well as limiting the use of balloon molding to the inside of the graft cannot be overemphasized in minimizing the risk of stroke during TEVAR. Other independent predictors of stroke from the EUROSTAR data include female sex and prolonged procedure time (>2 hours 40 min).[26]

Paraplegia remains a catastrophic complication after TAA repair and is one of the most important predictors of death.[28] Data from the three FDA trials showed a cumulative advantage to TEVAR over open repair (6% vs. 10%). The incidence of paraplegia in the control groups, however, is significantly higher than reported rates from centers of excellence (as low as 3%), but similar to national data from administrative databases.[29,30] Part of the difference involves the inclusion of all spinal cord ischemia events in regulatory trials while mild transient deficits are often overlooked in individual center reports. The moderate protective effects of TEVAR against spinal cord ischemia (SCI) may be due to avoidance of thoracic aortic clamping and reduced local hemodynamic disturbances at the spinal cord level secondary to lack of blood loss from intercostal backbleeding. It should also be noted that SCI is not confined to the perioperative period as delayed and recurrent SCI and paraplegia have also been reported after TEVAR.[31,32]

Several factors have been linked to an increased risk of SCI after TEVAR: concomitant or previous open infrarenal aortic replacement, lack of spinal drainage, extensive thoracic aortic coverage (especially T9 to T12), renal insufficiency, intraoperative hypotension (systolic blood pressure <80 mm Hg), emergency surgery, and coverage of the hypogastric artery, the LSA, or both.[11-13,26,27,33-35] Some of these risk factors are beyond the clinician's control, but coverage of the LSA and hypogastric arteries can be averted by modifying the operative plan. Occlusion of the LSA has been associated with a significant increase in the incidence of paraplegia by the EUROSTAR collaborators, and recent reports suggest that LSA revascularization may be required more frequently than previously recognized for either spinal cord protection or avoidance of left upper extremity ischemic symptoms.[11-14,26] The recent SVS Practice Guidelines recommend revascularization of the LSA in routine elective cases in which the LSA must be sacrificed for effective proximal seal (grade 2, level C evidence).[15] It has also been noted that lumbar and pelvic collaterals account for 25% of spinal cord blood supply,

and a compromised hypogastric blood flow contributed to the development of SCI.[36] Preservation of internal iliac blood flow and a staged repair of synchronous TAA and abdominal aortic aneurism (AAA) to allow development of collaterals has been recommended.[37]

The use of spinal cord protective techniques is typically at the discretion of the practitioner. Most operators use cerebrospinal fluid (CSF) drainage to aid in the protection of the cord. The premise for CSF drainage is based on the principle that spinal perfusion pressure is equal to the mean arterial pressure minus the intrathecal pressure. Reducing the CSF pressure through drainage thus helps to maintain better spinal perfusion. Although drainage is used routinely in few centers, most operators use it selectively based on the estimated risk of paraplegia of individual patients. The drain is inserted preoperatively and maintained for 24 to 48 hours keeping the CSF pressure under 10 cm of water. The efficacy of drainage has also been observed in reversal of delayed onset paraplegia after TEVAR and open procedures. Although the practice can be associated with hemorrhagic complications from catheter placement with a reported incidence of 0% to 3%, CSF drainage should be used when an elevated potential for SCI exists, such as extensive coverage of the thoracic aorta or with associated abdominal aortoiliac pathology.[28]

Vascular Complications

Access site difficulties and other vascular complications are more common after TEVAR than open repair. These complications lead to deployment failures and other significant early morbidity that has been reported to be as high as 14% in some instances.[10] The size discrepancy between small iliac arteries and the large sheaths often required for endograft deployment accounts for most of these complications. This is especially apparent in women, who have smaller native arteries and constitute approximately 40% of patients with TAA. With increased awareness of this complication, its incidence has decreased steadily and was only reported in 6% of procedures in the confirmatory TAG trial.[25]

Endoleaks

The classification of endoleaks is the same as infrarenal endografts. The overall incidence of endoleaks after TEVAR is 9% to 38%. In a recent literature review of 3004 patients, Ricotta[38] reported the overall endoleak rate to be 10.4% at 30 days and 9.5% at 1 year, with the majority being type I or type II. Nearly half of the patients (46%) underwent a secondary procedure with technical success in nearly 86%.[39]

Late Results

Late Survival

Aggregated 1 year data from the three published U.S. trials show a clear aneurysm-related survival benefit for TEVAR over open repair (95% vs. 89%, respectively).[10,18,20] The VALOR trial reported a statistically significant aneurysm related survival advantage over open repair (3.1% vs. 11.6%) at 1 year, whereas the STARZ Trial data noted no differences between groups.

The survival advantage persisted at the 5-year follow-up in the TAG study, which was the first to report long-term data. Although all-cause mortality was not different between groups (68% vs. 67%), aneurysm-related death rates remained significantly less for TEVAR than the open repair cohort, almost entirely because of the perioperative survival benefit.[10] There were a total of four aneurysm-related deaths in the TAG group (2.8%) compared with 11 in the open surgical cohort (11.7%; $p = 0.008$). Major adverse events occurred in 28% of TAG patients and 70% of surgical controls ($p < 0.001$) in the postoperative period; this advantage for the TAG patient persisted at 12 months (42% vs. 77%; $p < 0.001$) and at 5 years (58% vs. 79%; $p = 0.001$).

For high-risk patient populations, studies from Stanford University have shown that late outcomes are poor, with an actuarial survival rate of 31% at 5 years.[39] This observation is akin to the findings of the EVAR-2 trial and of EUROSTAR data for patients with AAA, and raises the question of the efficacy of such treatment in this patient cohort.

Migration

Device migration is a rare occurrence with a reported incidence ranging from 0.7% to 3.9%. Graft migration greater than 10 mm occurred in 2.8% (3/107) of patients at 12 months with TX2, although none resulted in endoleak or reintervention. All were noted to have had implantation of the barbed segment either in an acutely angled segment or within thrombus. With the Talent device, the incidence was 3.9% resulting in one reintervention.

Sac Behavior and Aortic Rupture

Aneurysm sac enlargement has been reported to occur in 7.1% to 14.5% of patients after TEVAR at 1 year.[23,40] The incidence appears similar among all three graft types. In the TAG pivotal trial,[10] aneurysm sac decrease of 5 mm or greater was observed in 50% of patients, while sac growth was noted in 19% of patients. These results, however, reflect data from the original, normal porosity ePTFE grafts and do not reflect long-term performance of currently available devices. Following the introduction of the low porosity material, patients with sac enlargement in the confirmatory TAG trial decreased from 12.9% to 2.9% at 2 years.

Stent-Graft Collapse

Stent-graft collapse and luminal obstruction is a rare complication that has been mostly reported with trauma patients, especially after excessive oversizing of the endograft. This phenomenon has been extremely rare with aneurysmal disease. Poor apposition to the lesser curvature of the arch and high flow rates in the thoracic aorta have been blamed for this potentially fatal complication.[41,42] Fortunately, many of these situations can be treated with further endovascular means. Several reports suggest that the majority of stent-graft collapses can be repaired with either a balloon expandable stent or further stent graft.[43,44]

CONCLUSION

There has been a clear evolution in the treatment of thoracic aortic aneurysms with the introduction of TEVAR, now considered the treatment of choice for most patients. Even patients who were deemed too high risk for conventional open repair may now be treated. TEVAR is a safe and effective therapeutic modality. Safe use of the technology requires a thorough understanding of the different devices available as well as their deployment behavior in a variety of settings. Device modifications introduced over the last 2 years have already improved device handling and performance. Disease-specific engineering, branched offerings, and lower-profile devices are all on the horizon. These are expected to provide a safer, more applicable, and more effective TEVAR in the future. As with all endovascular technology, close long-term follow-up of the patient is imperative.

References available online at expertconsult.com.

QUESTIONS

1. What are the indications for endovascular repair of descending thoracic aortic aneurysms?

2. How much are endografts oversized to achieve seal, and what are the problems with over or undersizing the graft?

3. What are the landing zones of the thoracic aorta?

4. What is the current recommendation for the management of the left subclavian artery?

5. What is the current recommendation for management of the celiac axis?

6. What are the important steps in the deployment of the thoracic endograft?

7. What are the risk factors for paraplegia with TEVAR?

8. What is the risk of stroke with TEVAR and what is the primary cause believed to be?

9. What is the perioperative mortality of TEVAR?

10. What are the 1 and 5 year survival benefits of TEVAR over open repair?

ANSWERS

1. The indications for TEVAR are the same as for open repair and typically include aneurysms greater than 6 cm in diameter, although saccular and symptomatic aneurysms are often repaired at a smaller size. It is also suggested that aneurysms with a rapid growth rate (more than 1 cm per year, or 0.5 cm in 6 months) should be considered for early intervention.

2. 10%-20% is the ideal amount to oversize the aortic diameter at the seal zones, which should be no less than 2-cm long. Grafts that are oversized can lead to folding and gutter formation. Grafts that are undersized tend to migrate and have persistent endoleaks.

3. Each zone is divided by a tangential line along the distal side of each great vessel; zone 0 involves the origin of the innominate artery, zone 1 the origin of the left common carotid artery (LCCA), zone 2 the origin of the left subclavian artery (LSA), zone 3 the proximal descending thoracic aorta down to the T4 vertebral body, and zone 4 the remainder of descending thoracic aorta. The location of the proximal landing zone depends on the aneurysm morphology; however, the ideal location in terms of anatomic accommodation of the graft is in zones 3 and 4.

4. Current SVS guidelines recommend routine preoperative revascularization in elective TEVAR with expectant management in emergency situations. Severely stenotic or occluded right vertebral artery or presence of a cardiac bypass from the left internal mammary are the only absolute contraindications to coverage without subclavian revascularization.

5. After careful interrogation of the gastroduodenal and pancreaticoduodenal arcades and verifying their patency, the celiac access may be covered to assure for a good 2cm distal seal zone.

6. a. Bilateral femoral access is obtained, then a pigtail catheter is placed from the contralateral side to guide deployment.
   b. A stiff wire (curved Lunderquist) is advanced into the ascending aorta from the ipsilateral access.
   c. Aortography is performed with a left anterior oblique projection of 40 to 60 degrees
   d. Angiography serves as the last check for device length choice and land marking, but this step can be omitted in patients with compromised renal function.
   e. The chosen stent-graft is then introduced and the deployment steps are followed.
   f. Usually the stent-graft is advanced beyond the target region initially and retracted to its desired landing zone, to eliminate any stored forward energy in the graft.
   g. During deployment, constant forward pressure is applied on the wire to buttress the graft against the outer curve of the aorta thus limiting the tendency for distal migration.

7. Data from the three FDA trials showed a cumulative advantage over open repair, with a rate of 6% (vs. 10% in open TAA repair). Several factors have been linked to an increased risk of SCI after TEVAR: concomitant or previous open infrarenal aortic replacement, lack of spinal drainage, extensive thoracic aortic coverage (especially T9 to T12), renal insufficiency, intraoperative hypotension (systolic blood pressure < 80 mm Hg), emergency surgery, and coverage of the hypogastric artery, the LSA, or both.

8. The stroke rates associated with TAA range from 3%-5% and are believed to occur primarily because of instrumentation of the aortic arch causing embolization and occasionally coverage of a critical source of blood to the brain.

9. The published data shows the perioperative mortality risk to be 2% (vs. 6% in open repair). The EUROSTAR registry reports a higher but still favorable mortality rate of 5.3%, likely because the patients in the study were deemed not eligible for open repair due to comorbidities and thus represented a sicker cohort.

10. Aggregated data from the three published U.S. trials show a clear aneurysm-related survival benefit for TEVAR over open repair (95% vs. 89%, respectively) at 1 year. The VALOR trial's results mirrored this (3.1% mortality vs. 11.6%). The survival advantage persisted at the 5-year follow-up in the TAG study. Although all-cause mortality was not different between groups (68% vs. 67%), aneurysm-related death rates remained significantly less for TEVAR than the open repair cohort.

CHAPTER 36

Combined Endovascular and Surgical (Hybrid) Approach to Aortic Arch and Thoracoabdominal Aortic Pathology

Wesley Kwan Lew • William J. Quiñones-Baldrich

A combined approach consisting of surgical bypass and aortic endovascular stent graft placement was first used at the University of California–Los Angeles to treat a type IV thoracoabdominal aneurysm in 1999. This procedure was performed to minimize morbidity and mortality of an open repair in a high-risk patient.[1] As this technique has evolved, it is now used to treat more extensive aneurysms of the aortic arch and thoracoabdominal aorta (Figure 36-1, see color plate).

A hybrid repair of thoracoabdominal aneurysms avoids proximal aortic cross clamping and thoracotomy, and it minimizes the visceral ischemia time. For the aortic arch, avoidance of hypothermic circulatory arrest makes a hybrid approach appealing. The use of thoracic stent-grafts in association with open surgical debranching is considered an off-label application of the device.[2]

This chapter will focus on patient selection for hybrid repairs and discuss the techniques of debranching and stent-grafting for both the aortic arch and thoracoabdominal aortic pathology. Additional considerations such as staging the procedures, access, use of spinal protection, and postoperative management will be discussed. The literature and outcomes from case series will be reviewed.

PATIENT SELECTION

Indications

The indications to treat an aortic aneurysm with a hybrid approach are no different than those used for open aneurysm repair. They include aneurysm diameter greater than 6 cm, growth greater then 1.0 cm/yr, unusual aneurysm morphology suggesting a higher risk of rupture (pseudoaneurysm), or symptomatic aneurysm. The hybrid approach should be reserved for patients that are considered high risk because of comorbidities or prior aortic or abdominal surgery.

Anatomy Considerations

Patients are considered for a hybrid repair if an appropriate proximal and distal landing zone is present, or can be created, allowing for exclusion of the aneurysm by a stent graft. Partial or complete debranching of the aortic arch is performed to create additional proximal landing zones. For pathology involving the visceral aorta, critical vessels, such as the celiac artery, superior mesenteric artery (SMA), and renal arteries, can be covered by aortic stent grafts after a surgical bypass has been established. A distal landing zone must be present in the native aorta or a preexisting aortic graft. Open infrarenal aortic replacement may be necessary to create a distal landing zone in patients with an infrarenal aneurysm and a short segment of nonaneurysmal aorta.

Open versus Hybrid Approach

The choice of an open or hybrid approach is dependent on a combination of the patient's history, comorbidities, and overall condition. Patients considered high risk include those who cannot tolerate a thoracotomy given severe chronic obstructive pulmonary disease or previous left chest operations. Patients with severe renal insufficiency with an increased risk of renal failure after open repair are also candidates for a hybrid approach. Patients with significant cardiac conditions, unable to tolerate proximal aortic clamping and increased afterload, should also be considered. Conservative management should be offered to patients with shortened life expectancies or those who are debilitated from coexisting medical conditions.

Open aortic repair has been shown to be a durable procedure with acceptable results and is the treatment of choice in young patients and those with acceptable operative risk. The hybrid repair is currently reserved for high risk patients that are considered poor candidates for an open repair.

Aortic Arch Aneurysm

Open repair of aortic arch aneurysms require a sternotomy, extracorporeal circulatory support often with deep hypothermic circulatory arrest, and hemiarch or total arch replacement.[3] In cases of concomitant descending

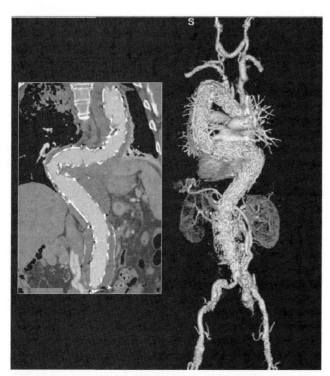

FIGURE 36-1 ■ Type II thoracoabdominal aortic aneurysm with partial aortic arch debranching and visceral debranching. The aortic stent graft spans nearly the entire aorta, from distal to the innominate artery to above the aortic bifurcation. See Color Plate 36-1.

thoracic aorta involvement, an "elephant trunk" technique can be used where a second intervention addresses the descending thoracic aorta component.[4,5] In high-risk patients, a hybrid approach is attractive because it avoids the need for hypothermic arrest, and in cases of descending thoracic involvement the procedure can be done in one stage.

Safi and colleagues[6] published one of the largest case series of open aortic arch aneurysm repair with thoracic or thoracoabdominal aortic involvement in 2004. They replaced the ascending aorta and aortic arch, leaving an elephant trunk in the descending thoracic aorta in 218 patients. Strokes occurred in 2.7%, and 30-day mortality was 8.7%. Of the surviving 199 patients, 2% expired before returning for the second-stage thoracic or thoracoabdominal aortic repair completion. Of those completing the second surgery, 9.7% died within 30 days of the second surgery.[6] Smaller case series of open arch repair in association with ascending or thoracoabdominal aortic aneurysms involve heterogeneous populations and report a wide range of perioperative mortality from 5.3% to 30.8%.[3]

There have been no randomized trials of hybrid versus open repair, but institutions have compared cohorts of open and hybrid repairs. At the University of Florida in Gainesville, they identified 58 patients with aortic arch aneurysms and descending thoracic aortic involvement. An open cohort using a two-staged approach with aortic arch replacement and elephant trunk repair (n = 21) was

compared to a cohort using a hybrid approach (n = 37). Rates of spinal cord ischemia (0% vs. 0%), stroke (10% vs. 11%), 30-day mortality (19% vs. 16%), and survival at 12 months (73% vs. 72%) were similar between the open and hybrid cases. These comparable results were present even though 68% of the hybrid cases still used cardiopulmonary bypass.[7]

In 2010, a more recent, single institution study compared 27 hybrid arch procedures with a contemporary series of 45 cases of open arch repairs. The incidence of permanent cerebral neurologic deficit (4% vs. 9%) and in-hospital mortality (11% vs. 16%) were similar for the hybrid versus open cohort. In the open arch group, it was noted that patients older than 75 years had significantly higher mortality than those younger than 75 years (36% vs. 9%; $p = 0.05$).[8]

Two metaanalyses of hybrid case series have been published. Antoniou and colleagues[9] reviewed 18 studies with a total of 195 patients. Complete arch debranching was performed in 122 patients (63%). The overall technical success rate was 86%. Overall perioperative morbidity and mortality rates were 21% and 9%, respectively. The stroke rate was 7%, and four aneurysm-related deaths were reported during follow-up (2%). No long-term data was reported.[9] A second metaanalysis identified 15 studies with 463 patients in studies published up to May 2008. The overall 30-day mortality was 8.3%, stroke rate was 4.4%, paraplegia rate was 3.9%, and the endoleak rate was 9.2%. Treatment on-pump or off-pump did not affect any of the endpoints.[10]

As increasing data on the hybrid approach emerge, the morbidity and mortality rates are comparable with open repair. Considering that hybrid series most often include higher risk patients, a benefit of the hybrid approach may be implied.

Thoracoabdominal Aneurysm

Open repair of thoracoabdominal aneurysms involve a laparotomy, thoracotomy, proximal aortic cross clamp, and global visceral ischemia. Techniques to optimize open repairs have included left heart bypass and retrograde perfusion of the renal and mesenteric vessels. In high-volume centers, case series of open thoracoabdominal aneurysm repair demonstrate reasonable mortality of 5% to 8.3% with rates of spinal cord ischemia from 3.8 to 16%.[11-14] Late survival at 5, 10, and 15 years were 54% to 67%, 29%, and 21%, respectively.[13,14]

In a contemporary series of open thoracoabdominal aneurysm repair, 305 patients were reviewed.[15] Twenty percent underwent an urgent or emergent repair, and 57% were Crawford extents type I or II. The majority had cerebrospinal fluid drainage (97%) and left heart bypass (89%). Operative mortality was 8%, renal failure necessitating hemodialysis at discharge was 6%, and permanent paraplegia was 3%. Actuarial survival at 2 years was 79%.[15]

Despite these single center outcomes, database outcomes find mortalities to be more dismal. In California, after open repair, patient mortality was 19% at 30 days and 31% at 1 year. An increase in 1-year mortality was noted for patients of increasing age: 18% for patients 50

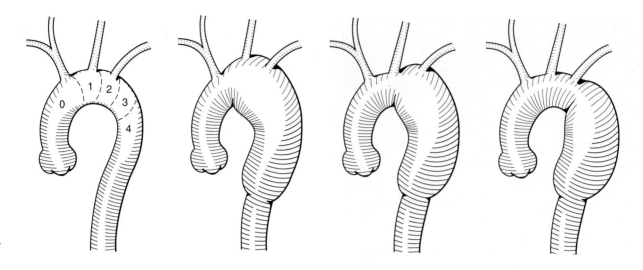

FIGURE 36-2 ■ Thoracic landing zone diagram and aortic arch aneurysm configurations.

to 59 years old, versus 40% for patients 80 to 89 years old.[16] Nationwide, in-hospital mortality was found to be 22.3%. Higher mortality was seen when comparing low- versus high-volume hospitals (27.4% vs. 15.0%; $p < 0.001$) and low- versus high-volume surgeons (25.6% vs. 11.0%; $p < 0.001$).[17]

There have been no randomized comparisons of open versus hybrid thoracoabdominal aneurysm repair. At the Massachusetts General Hospital they compared a contemporary cohort of open (n = 77) versus hybrid (n = 23) thoracoabdominal repairs. Of note, the hybrid patients were not open surgical candidates. Although not significant, the hybrid groups had a higher 30-day mortality (17.4% vs. 7.8%; $p = 0.23$), in-hospital mortality (26.1% vs. 10.4%; $p = 0.27$), and reoperation rates (39.1% vs. 20.8%; $p = 0.03$). However, paraplegia rates (hybrid, 4.3%, vs. open, 3.9%; $p = 0.98$) and 1-year survival (hybrid, 68%, vs. open, 73%) were similar for both groups.[18] Additional series of hybrid repairs are limited to small, heterogeneous patient populations, with varying extents of type II and III thoracoabdominal aneurysms.

Thus far, the outcomes from hybrid thoracoabdominal and aortic arch aneurysm repair have not exceeded that of open surgery. It should be acknowledged that patients in hybrid case series are often high risk and do not qualify as candidates for open surgical repair. As experience and indications with the hybrid technique continue to grow, it may eventually prove to be an acceptable option for more than just high-risk patients.

Contraindications

An absolute contraindication to a hybrid aortic aneurysm repair is the lack of, or inability to create, a proximal and distal seal zone. Relative contraindications include the inability to safely perform debranching at the aortic arch or abdomen. The left carotid and left subclavian arteries require extraanatomic bypass for debranching. In hostile necks from previous surgery or radiation, exposure of

the vessels and tunneling of grafts may not be feasible. The same applies in the abdomen. Exposure of the renal or visceral arteries may be difficult in a reoperative abdomen.

DEBRANCHING THE AORTIC ARCH

The surgical component of a hybrid repair to the aortic arch is used to create a proximal seal zone for an endograft. This is done to treat the proximal extent of thoracic or thoracoabdominal aortic aneurysms or to treat isolated aortic arch aneurysms. The anatomy of the aneurysm will determine which vessels need to be addressed. A classification scheme separates the aortic arch into proximal seal zones and identifies which vessels will be affected[19] (Figure 36-2). Zone 0 involves the origin of the innominate artery, and a stent-graft landing there compromises blood flow to the left subclavian, left common carotid, and innominate arteries. Zone 1 involves the orifice of the left common carotid artery, and a stent-graft landing there compromises the left subclavian and left common carotid circulation. Zone 2 involves the origin of the left subclavian artery, and a stent-graft landing there affects only the left subclavian artery. Zones 3 and 4 are both distal to the left subclavian artery, within the descending thoracic aorta, leaving the arch vessels unaffected.

Left Subclavian Artery

Early in the endovascular treatment of thoracic aneurysms, coverage of the left subclavian artery (zone 2) was routinely done and appeared safe. It was assumed a patent right vertebral artery would provide enough collateral circulation to both the basilar system and the left subclavian artery via retrograde flow from the left vertebral artery.[20,21] More recent data are conflicting. Meta-analysis suggest no neurologic benefit from subclavian

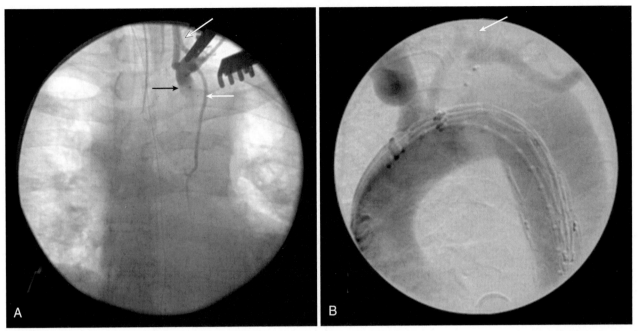

FIGURE 36-3 ■ **A,** Left carotid to subclavian artery bypass completed with Amplatzer plug placed at left subclavian origin *(black arrow).* Left vertebral and internal mammary arteries are preserved *(white arrow).* **B,** Angiogram prior to stent graft deployment in zone 2. Carotid-subclavian bypass can be seen *(white arrow).*

revascularization,[22] but in a registry from Europe, multivariate regression analysis found the risk of spinal cord ischemia to increase with left subclavian artery coverage.[23] Late development of subclavian steal and arm claudication was seen in 15% of patients in one series requiring further intervention.[24] We recommend revascularization of the left subclavian artery in all elective cases. In unstable patients, coverage of the left subclavian artery may be reasonable.

A left supraclavicular incision is used to perform either a left subclavian to carotid artery transposition or left common carotid to subclavian artery bypass. Regardless of the method, left vertebral artery flow should be preserved. In all cases where a bypass is used, ligation or endovascular occlusion of the subclavian proximal to the vertebral origin is recommended to avoid a type II endoleak. Endovascular occlusion can be done using an Amplatzer plug (ADA Medical Corporation, Plymouth, Minn.) or iliac occlusion plug (Zenith Iliac Plug, Cook, Bloomington, IN or Talent Occluder, Medtronic, Minneapolis, MN) deployed in retrograde fashion though the distal anastomosis of the carotid-subclavian artery bypass (Figure 36-3). If an Amplatzer plug is used, it should be done after the aortic stent graft is deployed to prevent developing thrombus from embolizing while there is still antegrade flow through the device and subclavian artery. In cases where a left internal mammary artery has been used for a coronary bypass graft, a transposition cannot be performed. In constructing the carotid-subclavian artery bypass, the subclavian anastomosis should be distal to the origin of the internal mammary artery, thereby maintaining native flow during sewing of the anastomosis. After the anastomosis and bypass are complete, the origin of the left subclavian artery is ligated, and retrograde flow will fill the internal mammary artery.[25]

Partial Arch Debranching

Partial arch debranching involves revascularization of the left common carotid and left subclavian arteries using the right common carotid artery as inflow, in preparation to deploy an endograft just distal to the innominate artery origin (zone 1). This can be done with extraanatomic bypasses, without the need for a sternotomy or thoracotomy (Figure 36-4).

The left subclavian artery revascularization is performed as mentioned previously. This is followed by a right carotid to left carotid artery bypass through bilateral neck incisions made anterior to the sternocleidomastoid muscle to expose the common carotid arteries. A retropharyngeal or subcutaneous tunnel is created between the two common carotid arteries, and a bypass is performed with a Dacron graft. The tunnel is made with a gentle downward curve. If placed subcutaneously, carrying the tunnel behind the manubrium gives the best cosmetic result. Damage to this bypass can occur if a sternotomy is ever needed, and patients should be so informed.[26] The left common carotid artery is ligated proximal to the distal carotid-carotid artery bypass anastomosis. Care is taken to avoid bilateral recurrent laryngeal or vagus nerve injury.

Intraoperative brain monitoring is usually not necessary when clamping is limited to the common carotid artery as external to internal carotid artery collaterals will maintain adequate flow to the affected internal system.

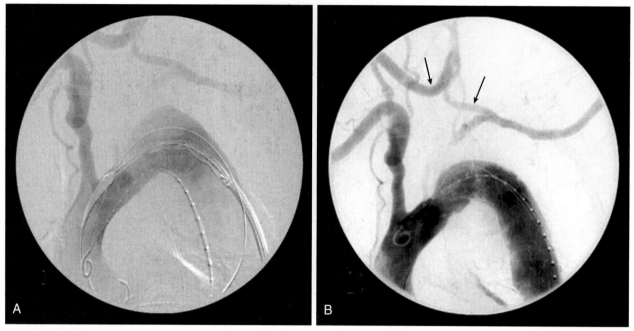

FIGURE 36-4 ■ Angiogram of the aortic arch before **(A)** and after **(B)** a stent-graft is deployed in zone 1 of the aortic arch. Partial arch debranching has been done with a right-to-left carotid artery bypass *(arrow)* and left carotid to left subclavian artery bypass *(arrow)*.

Similarly, common carotid artery shunting has not been necessary.

Complete Arch Debranching

Complete aortic arch debranching involves revascularization of the innominate, left carotid and left subclavian arteries to create a landing zone in the ascending aorta proximal to the innominate artery (zone 0). This is most often done through a median sternotomy[27] and cardiopulmonary bypass is typically not necessary. A side biting clamp is placed on the ascending aorta and either a small bifurcated Dacron graft or a larger tube graft (8 to 12 mm) with a side arm (6 to 8 mm) is fashioned to bypass the right innominate and left common carotid arteries, both in an end to end fashion (Figures 36-5 [see color plate] and 36-6). The latter option is easier to configure and avoids compression or kinking after sternotomy closure.

The left subclavian artery cannot be accessed via a sternotomy and requires a separate left supraclavicular incision. This is best done before the sternotomy as a carotid-subclavian bypass or transposition. During innominate artery clamping, the left subclavian artery will provide collateral flow through the vertebral-basilar pathway to the right subclavian and carotid systems. The origins of any bypassed vessel should be ligated or embolized to prevent a type II endoleak. Before sternotomy, patients should be screened for any cardiac pathology that should be addressed at the same intervention.

The tortuosity and distance from the femoral artery to proximal aortic arch can make tracking an endovascular device difficult. In addition, the endograft delivery system may not be long enough to reach the ascending aorta. The addition of a 10-mm Dacron graft onto the hood of the ascending aortic graft can serve as a conduit for antegrade deployment of the stent graft[28] (see Figures 36-5 and 36-6). It is critical that the location of the conduit to graft anastomosis lead directly into the aorta. Tension at the heel of the ascending aortic graft anastomosis can develop during deployment because of the angle of entry of the deployment catheter; this risks a tear of the aorta and is to be avoided. Tunneling the conduit through an appropriately located stab wound can reduce this risk.[29]

Frozen Elephant Trunk

When aneurysms involve the ascending aorta, there is no proximal landing zone for a stent graft. To reconstruct these aneurysms, the frozen elephant trunk is a one-stage hybrid technique. Hypothermic cardiac arrest is required, hence the term *frozen*. The ascending aorta is replaced with a Dacron graft. A bypass is then taken off this graft to the innominate and left carotid arteries. The arch is then opened, and a modified Dacron graft with a stent attached distally is constrained in a sheath and deployed under fluoroscopy into a distal landing zone, usually the descending thoracic aorta. The proximal end of the modified Dacron graft is then sewn to the ascending aortic graft completing the reconstruction. This technique eliminates the two-stage operation needed with standard aortic arch and elephant trunk operations, but it requires circulatory arrest and for this reason will not be discussed further in this chapter.[30-33]

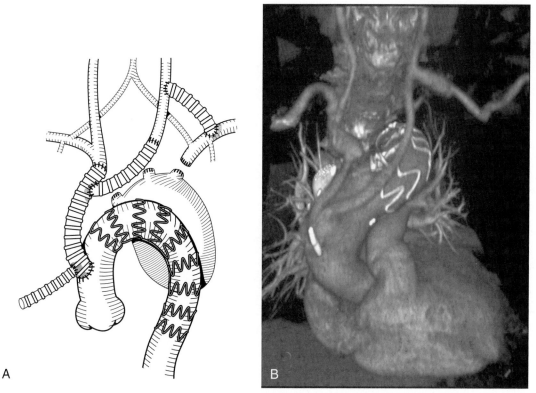

FIGURE 36-5 ■ Schematic **(A)** and three-dimensional **(B)** reconstruction of a complete aortic arch debranching. The bypass graft originates off the ascending aorta to right innominate and left carotid artery. A left carotid to subclavian artery bypass can also be seen. In the schematic there is a conduit off the ascending aortic graft. See Color Plate 36-5.

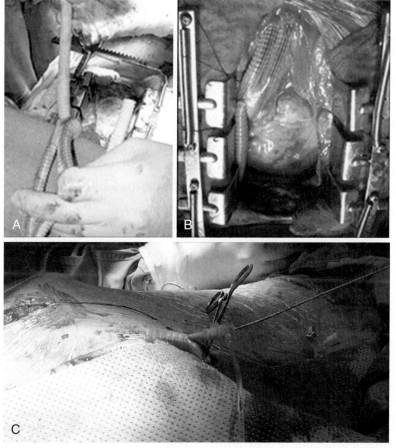

FIGURE 36-6 ■ Operative images of a complete arch debranching. **A,** Bifurcated Dacron graft with additional limb sewn on as conduit. **B,** Bypass graft sewn onto ascending aortic arch. **C,** Conduit tunneled with sheath in place for antegrade stent graft deployment.

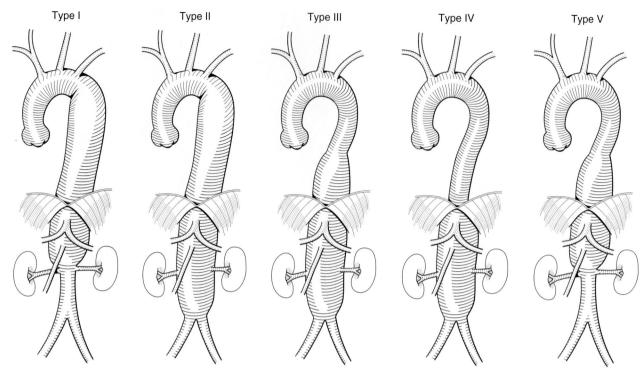

Type I   Type II   Type III   Type IV   Type V

FIGURE 36-7 ■ Diagram of modified Crawford type thoracoabdominal aneurysms.

DEBRANCHING THORACOABDOMINAL ANEURYSMS

Given that the visceral vessels are in close proximity to one another, all four vessels (celiac, SMA, and bilateral renal arteries) will need to be bypassed in most hybrid thoracoabdominal aneurysm repairs. In pararenal aneurysms, debranching one or both kidneys may provide the needed seal zone for a hybrid repair.[34] In patients with preexisting renal failure, on hemodialysis, only the mesenteric arteries require debranching.

Origin of the Visceral Bypass Grafts

Occasionally patients will have had a prior aortic repair, and this preexisting graft can serve as a takeoff for a retrograde visceral graft. If not, the anatomy of the aneurysm will dictate where a bypass graft can originate. The Crawford classification of thoracoabdominal aneurysms can help predict this (Figure 36-7). It is preferable not to use the external iliac arteries given their small size and presence of atherosclerosis, which may not properly support circulation to the entire viscera.

In a type I Crawford thoracoabdominal aneurysm, the native common iliac artery or infrarenal aorta is adequate for use as a graft origin (Figure 36-8, see color plate). In a type II and III Crawford thoracoabdominal aneurysm, aneurysmal involvement of the infrarenal aorta and common iliac arteries makes this a more challenging hybrid repair. If the aneurysm is continuous throughout the iliacs, without a spared segment of nonaneurysmal aorta, a hybrid repair is not feasible and an open repair is the only option (Figure 36-9, see color plate). If there

is a region of nonaneurysmal aorta that can be clamped, a tube or bifurcated aortoiliac graft can be placed for a distal landing zone, and the debranching graft sewn onto the aortic graft (Figure 36-10).

In a type IV thoracoabdominal aneurysm, open surgical repair is still preferred over a hybrid approach. Open repair can be accomplished via a retroperitoneal approach without a thoracotomy. Cross clamping of the supraceliac aorta is better tolerated than control at the proximal thoracic aorta. If a hybrid repair is undertaken, a debranching graft can originate from the descending thoracic aorta, infrarenal aorta, or common iliac artery.

Abdominal Debranching techniques

Patients are placed supine and a midline transabdominal incision is preferred. A retroperitoneal approach can be used, but access to the right renal artery can be difficult. To create a retrograde debranching bypass graft, a trifurcated Dacron prosthesis is preferred. Two limbs are used to bypass the right and left renal arteries with an end-to-end distal anastomosis if feasible. The third limb is used for the SMA in an end-to-side fashion. A jump graft is then taken off the SMA graft, to the celiac artery. The routing of the retrograde bypass grafts will be determined by whether the grafts originate from the right or left aortoiliac systems (Figure 36-11).

To expose the left renal artery, the left renal vein is mobilized by ligation of the inferior mesenteric, gonadal, and adrenal veins; this allows access to the proximal left renal artery. To expose the distal left renal artery, the descending colon is mobilized and rotated medially. The bypass graft is tunneled through the mesentery of

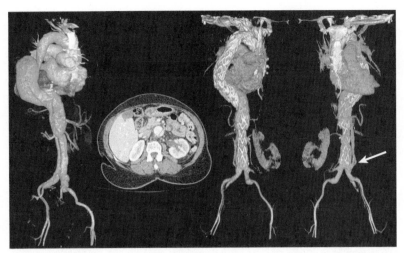

FIGURE 36-8 ■ Aneurysmal degeneration of a type B dissection resulting in a type I thoracoabdominal aortic aneurysm *(left)*. The infrarenal aorta is not aneurysmal *(middle)*, allowing for replacement of the infrarenal aorta with an aortoiliac graft onto which a bypass graft *(arrow)* originates and provides the distal endograft seal zone *(right)*. See Color Plate 36-8.

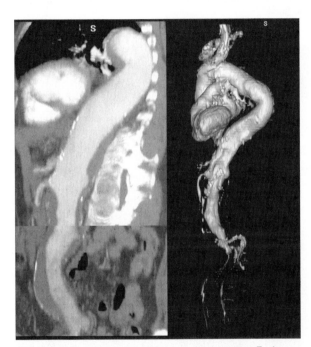

FIGURE 36-9 ■ Type II thoracoabdominal aneurysm. Entire aorta is aneurysmal without a spared segment for a hybrid repair. See Color Plate 36-9.

the descending colon for distal left renal artery bypass, otherwise no tunneling is needed to bypass the proximal left renal artery.

The proximal right renal artery is identified posterior to the vena cava. The distal right renal artery can be accessed by medial mobilization of the right colon, takedown of the hepatorenal ligament, and kocherization of the duodenum. The retrograde bypass grafts is tunneled posteromedial to the vena cava for proximal right renal revascularization, and anterior to the vena cava for more distal right renal artery revascularization. Preoperative planning should identify whether a proximal or distal renal anastomosis will be preformed, and whether multiple renal arteries are present.

The celiac artery is exposed by entering the lesser sac through the gastrohepatic ligament. A nasogastric tube will decompress the stomach and help to identify the esophagogastric junction. Following either the hepatic or the splenic artery, the bifurcation of the celiac artery is identified. To gain access to the main celiac branch, the dense celiac plexus is divided, and the coronary vein is ligated. If more exposure is needed, the left gastric artery can also be ligated. The graft anastomosis is performed in an end-to-side manner to either the hepatic or splenic artery. An anastomosis can be performed at the celiac bifurcation, but exposure is difficult and leaves little room for ligation of the main celiac artery to prevent a type II endoleak.

If the retrograde bypass to the SMA originates in the right common iliac system, the graft is tunneled between the leaves of the mesentery at its base, heading toward the SMA at the base of the transverse mesocolon. Exposure of the SMA is then performed similar to an embolectomy. The mesocolon is elevated, and the middle colic artery identified. Following its course will lead to the SMA. An end-to-side anastomosis is then performed just distal to the middle colic artery, and the SMA is then ligated proximal to the middle colic artery. A jump graft to the celiac artery is then brought through the transverse mesocolon and tunneled anterior to the pancreas.

When the SMA bypass originates from the left iliac system, the graft is routed toward the SMA at its origin with aorta. SMA exposure is accomplished with full mobilization of the left renal vein after dividing the inferior mesenteric, gonadal, and adrenal veins. The third and fourth portions of the duodenum are mobilized to the right, and the SMA is identified posterior to the pancreas and superior to the left renal artery. The jump graft to the celiac artery is then tunneled posterior to the pancreas. Alternatively, the jump graft can be placed in a C-loop configuration to avoid retropancreatic tunneling, but the C-loop is more difficult to isolate from contact with the intestines. In an effort to prevent graft to bowel fistula, all bypass grafts are covered with

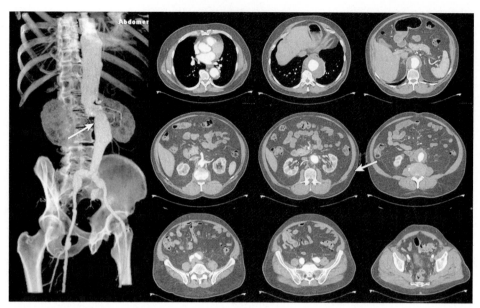

FIGURE 36-10 ■ Type II thoracoabdominal aneurysm with a spared segment of infrarenal aorta *(arrow)*. Open infrarenal aortic repair was performed, and a debranching bypass was based off the aortoiliac graft.

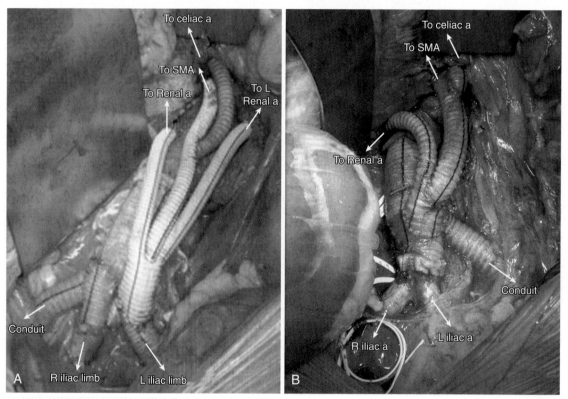

FIGURE 36-11 ■ Different configurations of thoracic aortic aneurysm debranching grafts. In both cases the infrarenal aortic graft allows for an adequate length of distal landing zone. **A,** Debranching graft based off left limb of aortoiliac graft. Conduit can be seen off right iliac limb. **B,** Debranching graft and conduit originating off a tube graft. The left renal bypass arm is behind the SMA limb and cannot be seen in this image.

retroperitoneal tissue whenever possible or omentum if necessary.

It is important to ligate the origins of the debranched visceral vessels to prevent a type II endoleak. Ligation of the origins also prevents competitive flow, which can lead to graft occlusion. Clips can be used, but given the

potential of clip dislodgement,[35] a silk ligature is added. Division of the vessel and oversewing the stump is an alternative.

To minimize contrast during stent-graft placement, the origin of the retrograde bypass graft is marked. Two partially closed clips are sewn to the native aorta or aortic

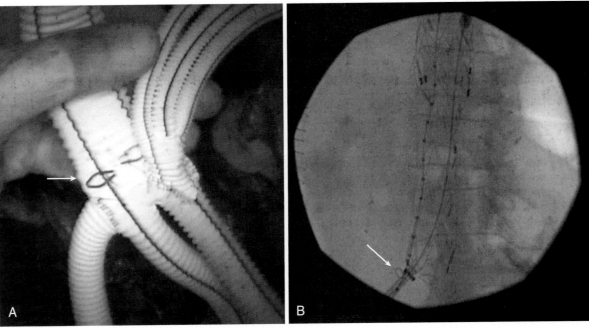

FIGURE 36-12 ■ Partially closed clips sewn onto an aortobifemoral graft creating a "pair of eyes" *(arrow)*, indicating the lowest point the stent graft can be landed to prevent covering the bypass graft.

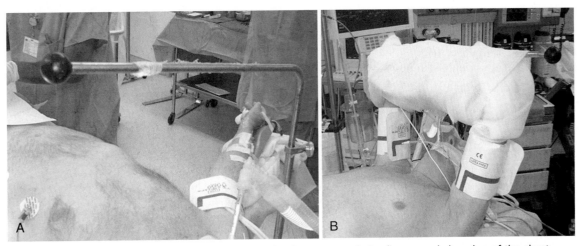

FIGURE 36-13 ■ Ether bar used to suspend the patient's arm to optimize fluoroscopic imaging of the chest.

graft just proximal to the takeoff of the bypass graft, creating "a pair of eyes" (Figure 36-12). This is easily under fluoroscopy and identifies the lowest point where the stent-graft can be landed to prevent covering the visceral bypass graft.

ENDOVASCULAR STENT GRAFT PLACEMENT

Positioning

The patient is placed supine for imaging of the abdominal and descending thoracic aorta. If the aortic arch needs to be visualized, the arms are suspended from an ether bar above the patient's face to image the chest and obtain a steep left anterior oblique view to open the thoracic arch (Figure 36-13).

Access for Endograft Deployment

Arterial access is either through the common femoral artery (open or percutaneous) or from a preplaced conduit. If a percutaneous arterial approach is chosen, two 6F Perclose Proglide (Abbott Vascular, Redwood City, Calif.) devices are deployed before placement of the large sheath to allow for arteriotomy closure at the completion of the case.[36]

The constrained diameters of endovascular grafts vary depending on manufacturer and device, but in general the devices can be quite large. If the femoral or external iliac arteries are less than 8 mm, heavily calcified, or both, the arteries can be injured. In addition, tortuosity in the iliac system can create excess length and issues with pushability. To avoid these concerns, a conduit can be

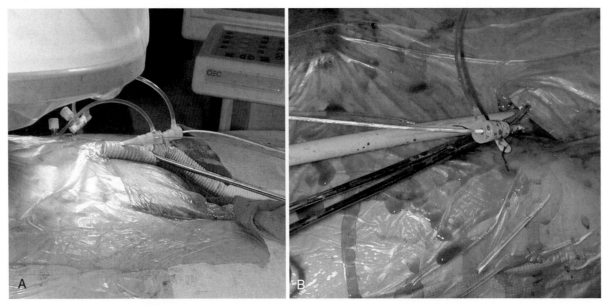

FIGURE 36-14 ■ Conduits used to accommodate multiple sheaths.

created. A 10-mm Dacron graft is used and can accommodate both the large endograft delivery sheath and the smaller (5 French) sheath for the pigtail injection catheter (Figure 36-14).

For complete aortic arch debranching, using a conduit on the ascending aorta bypass graft to deploy the endograft in an antegrade fashion is the preferred approach. If an antegrade approach cannot be used, and there are concerns with the femoral approach, a conduit can be created off the native common iliac artery through a retroperitoneal approach.

In cases of thoracoabdominal aneurysms, a conduit can be added easily when the infrarenal aorta has been replaced with a tube graft or aortobifemoral graft (see Figure 36-11). If the hybrid repair is to be staged, the conduit is marked with clips then left in the subcutaneous tissue. At the second stage, fluoroscopy can be used to identify the clips, and a small cutdown is made to expose the conduit. A thrombectomy is then done to clear the conduit for use (Figure 36-15). After the endovascular procedure is complete, the conduit is ligated as proximally as possible and buried in the subcutaneous tissue. It is important to maintain sterility when handling the conduit, because any infection of the conduit can infect adjacent bypass grafts.

Proximal and Distal Landing Zones

The basic principles of endovascular aneurysm repair involve at least 2 cm of nonaneurysmal native vessel or graft, proximal and distal to the aneurysm, for a proper endograft seal. Preoperative planning is the key to a successful case. Proximal landing is dependent on the anatomy and which vessels have been debranched. In general, landing within an acute angle within the arch is not recommended given the potential for poor apposition of the proximal graft to the inner curve of the aorta (bird beaking).[37] In these situations, debranching of additional

arch vessels is recommended in order to extend the proximal landing beyond the acute angulation. Landing within the arch can be safe when the arch has a wide curvature. Distally, the origin of the retrograde visceral grafts must not be placed within the seal zone.

Stent Graft Placement

In partial arch debranching, there is no antegrade delivery option. To track an endograft into the aortic arch via a retrograde approach, a stiff Lunderquist (Cook, Bloomington, Ind.) with a floppy "Q" tip is used. The tip of the wire can be positioned into the left ventricle to allow more wire support to help the device track. During deployment the wire is pushed to the outer curve of the aortic arch to minimize migration during deployment. Temporary rapid pacing or adenosine during deployment are not used routinely, but both can be an adjuvant to help precise delivery.[38] A flossing technique can also be used to help track devices by straightening tortuosity; this is done with a right brachial artery approach snaring the retrograde wire.

Stent grafts with uncovered struts allow for additional proximal aortic support, which can be helpful in the aortic arch curvature. Oversizing can also lead to bird beaking and should be avoided.[37] With larger diameters in the ascending aorta and arch, care must be taken to assure that the diameter of the aorta at the proximal landing zone can create a seal with the chosen stent graft. Currently the largest FDA-approved thoracic stent graft is 46 mm diameter, which is appropriate to treat a 41- to 42-mm aorta.

In the abdominal aorta, a stiff Amplatzer wire (Cook) can straighten tortuosity and facilitate device tracking. Ideally stent grafts are placed in a distal-to-proximal fashion. To minimize the amount of contrast used, the first device is deployed without contrast. The most distal extent of the landing zone is identified by the "pair of

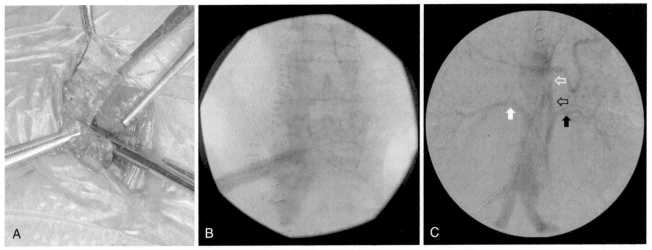

FIGURE 36-15 ■ **A,** Conduit identified in the subcutaneous tissues. **B,** Angiogram of a conduit verifying clearance of thrombus. **C,** Pigtail placed through conduit, debranching graft seen with branches to right kidney *(closed white arrow)*, left kidney *(closed black arrow)*, SMA *(open black arrow)*, and jump graft to celiac artery *(open white arrow)*.

eyes" previously placed just above the origin of the debranching graft. Without additional angiograms the devices are deployed, with the appropriate manufacturer required overlap, until the proximal landing zone is reached. The first aortogram is then performed with a power injector, and the final device is deployed.

A completion angiogram is performed to identify endoleaks. A type I endoleak is treated with balloon inflation, or additional stent-grafts if there is more aorta to cover. With proper planning and technique, bird beaking or inadequate seals should not be encountered, but if present a Palmaz Stent (Johnson and Johnson, Warren, NJ) can help compensate as a last resort.[37] A type III endoleak can be treated with an interposition stent graft component, and a type II endoleak is monitored at follow-up.

Aortic degeneration from dissections is a common cause of aortic aneurysms. Stent-grafts should be placed within the true lumen to seal fenestrations and thrombose the false lumen. In the thoracic aorta, the use of transesophageal echocardiogram can help to identify which lumen the wires traverse. In the abdomen, endovascular ultrasound can be used. When patients have had an interposition graft as the initial treatment for their dissection in the proximal descending thoracic aorta, and the distal landing is in either a normal nondissected segment of aorta, or a surgically placed infrarenal graft, the false lumen can be used for placement of the endovascular graft. In this situation, the false lumen is typically the larger of the two and allows the stent-graft to deploy fully.

STAGING THE HYBRID APPROACH

A single operation is preferred for aortic arch aneurysms without visceral involvement. In a complete arch debranching, the conduit cannot be tunneled for later use; therefore antegrade delivery of the endograft must occur

at the same operation. In the cases of partial arch debranching and left subclavian-carotid bypass or transposition, the operations are all extraanatomic and can be done in a reasonable time with minimal surgical trauma.

Debranching the visceral vessels in a hybrid thoracoabdominal aneurysm repair can be a long operation, with periods of warm ischemia to the kidney and viscera during anastomosis. Before a contrast load, a compromised kidney may need time to recover. For these reasons staging the procedures is preferred, particularly for type II-III thoracoabdominal aortic aneurysms. The second endovascular stage should be performed as soon as the patient has recovered, preferably during the same admission.[27] Interval aneurysm rupture has been noted when patients are discharged from the hospital after debranching, awaiting stent graft placement.[39, 40]

If the thoracoabdominal aneurysm involves the aortic arch, the first stage should be the abdominal debranching, followed by the second stage, which would include arch debranching and stent graft deployment. In any hybrid repair, staging the procedure should be considered if during the operation there is cardiovascular instability, an intraoperative complication, or the procedure becomes exceedingly prolonged.

SPINAL PROTECTION

In open thoracoabdominal aneurysm repair, the use of spinal drainage has been shown to reduce postoperative paraplegia and paraparesis in a randomized trial (13.0% vs. 2.6%; $p = 0.03$).[41] Although the mechanism of paralysis and paraplegia in open and endovascular repair may differ,[42] the use of spinal drainage has been shown to be beneficial and even to reverse cases of postoperative paraplegia in endovascular aortic repairs.[43]

Spinal drainage is recommend when there has been previous aortic surgery, a large coverage of aorta is planned, or collateral circulation from the internal iliac

618 ARTERIAL ANEURYSM DISEASE

and subclavian arteries is compromised.[23,43] When the repair is limited to the aortic arch and proximal descending aorta, spinal drainage is not necessary.

Spinal catheters are placed 1 day before the endovascular portion to avoid delaying the case because of a bloody tap. If this happens, overnight observation usually resolves the issue, thus allowing safe heparinization. During the procedure and in the postoperative period, spinal catheters are allowed to drain continuously at 10 cm of water. To maximize the spinal perfusion pressure, the mean arterial pressure is maintained at greater than 80 mm Hg using a phenylephrine drip if needed. After 48 to 72 hours, if the patient is hemodynamically stable and neurologically intact, the pressure of spinal drainage is increased to 20 cm of water for 6 hours, and then closed to assure no neurologic changes before removal.[42,43]

If the patient develops postoperative paraplegia, the spinal drain is assessed and replaced if malfunctioning. The drainage pressure of the spinal drain can also be decreased to improve spinal perfusion. A magnetic resonance image of the spine is also obtained to rule out reversible causes of paraplegia, such as a spinal cord hematoma.

POSTOPERATIVE MANAGEMENT

After a visceral debranching, patients are given nothing by mouth until bowel function returns. Pancreatitis can occur from pancreas manipulation during graft tunneling. Death from pancreatitis has been reported, and amylase and lipase should be monitored postoperatively.[44,45]

Graft occlusions ranged from 0% to 14% in various case series (see Table 36-2). Although grafts can be occluded without clinical significance,[45] bowel ischemia and death,[44,46,47] as well as permanent renal failure requiring dialysis, have been reported.[39] Renal graft patency is monitored with urine output and laboratories. Worsening renal function should be promptly evaluated with duplex ultrasound or computed tomographic scan to check for patency. Celiac and SMA grafts are monitored clinically and by laboratories. If there is bowel ischemia, the patient will become septic and imaging should be urgently performed. In cases of patent bypass grafts, embolic events during the bypass creation, or during wire and catheter manipulation, can lead to bowel necrosis. If there is suspicion of bowel ischemia, laparotomy should be performed emergently.[47]

Management of an occluded bypass graft will depend largely in part on the patients overall clinical condition. If patients are asymptomatic from the graft occlusion, then reintervention might not be warranted. With worsening renal failure or persistent sepsis, the decision to revise a graft should be considered.

In the aortic arch, transient ischemia attacks or permanent strokes can result from graft failures. Intervening for an occluded graft that has caused a significant stroke can worsen the patient's overall condition. Transient ischemic attacks should be promptly investigated with imaging of the grafts and revision if problems are

identified. Embolic events from wire and catheter manipulation in the arch will manifest immediately after surgery. Management is often supportive.

With any endovascular aneurysm repair, serial imaging is required to assure that the aneurysm sac is decreasing in diameter and there are no endoleaks or problems with the stent grafts. A computed tomographic scan is ordered in the first few weeks after surgery, then at 6 months, and then every year if no issues are identified. If there is renal insufficiency, a magnetic resonance angiogram can be done using minimal gadolinium.

Type II leaks can be monitored if there is no aneurysm sac expansion, but type I and III endoleaks need to be addressed. In case series, up to 17% of patients may required secondary interventions.[18,35]

RESULTS

Aortic Arch Debranching

Case series of hybrid aortic arch aneurysm repair are difficult to interpret given the heterogeneous patient populations and a lack of standardized reporting from individual studies. Table 36-1 summarizes the outcomes from series with more than 10 patients, focusing on aortic repairs with the proximal landing in either zone 0 or zone 1. Patients with descending thoracic aorta aneurysms requiring coverage of the left subclavian artery (zone 2) are not the topic of this discussion. Although a benefit of the hybrid aortic arch repair is the lack of cardiopulmonary bypass, it has been used in a number of patients, thus complicating analysis of outcomes and comparisons.

In one of the earliest case series by Saleh and Inglese[48] from Egypt, 15 high-risk patients had complete arch debranching with zone 0 proximal landing. No cardiopulmonary bypass was used. Success was 100%, with no mortality, paraplegia, or stroke.[48]

These excellent results were not seen in another similar cohort of 26 patients in the series by Weigang and colleagues[29] from the University of Mainz in Germany. All patients were high risk and had complete arch debranching without cardiopulmonary bypass. The 30-day mortality was one of the highest of all case series at 15%. All deaths were from adverse cardiovascular events. There were no episodes of paraplegia or stroke.[29]

In two other series, all patients had complete arch debranching, but cardiopulmonary bypass was used in a subset of cases. In the series by Bavaria and colleagues[49] from the University of Pennsylvania, they included 27 patients, of which 4 were treated with a frozen elephant trunk. These 4 required cardiopulmonary bypass, as well as an additional 15 patients in whom a side-biting clamp could not be applied given that a limited amount of aorta existed between the sinotubular junction and the ascending aorta. Mortality rate was 11%, stroke rate was 11%, and paraplegia rate was 7%.[49]

In the series by Lee and colleagues,[7] they compared patients who underwent open versus hybrid repairs. In the hybrid group of 37 patients, the 30-day mortality was 16%, stroke rate was 11%, and paraplegia rate was 0%. One-year survival was 72%. This series had one of the highest mortality rates, but 68% of the patient required

TABLE 36-1 Summary of Case Series (>10 patients) on the Hybrid Approach to the Aortic Arch

Primary Author	Year	Institute	No. of Patients	High Risk for Open Repair (%)	Emergent Cases (%)	Isolated Arch Aneurysm (%)	CPB/ Circulatory Arrest (%)	Proximal Landing Zone				Mortality (%)	Morbidity (%)	Stroke (%)	Paraplegia (%)	Mean Follow-Up (Mo)	Overall Survival
								Zone 0	Zone 1	Zone 2	Frozen Elephant Trunk						
Saleh[48]	2006	Ain Shams University, Cairo, Egypt	15	100	NA	13	0	15	0	0	0	0	26	0	0	18	93%
Bergeron[27]	2006	St Joseph's Hospital, Marseille, France	25	100	NA	NA	0	15	10	0	0	8	12	8	0	15	88%
Schumacher[51]	2006	Heidelberg, Germany	25	100	32	NA	0	9	16	0	0	20	64	4	0	21	76%
Chan[52]	2008	University of Hong Kong	16	NA	31	NA	6	5	8	3	0	0	67	19	0	14	100%
Gottardi[54]*	2008	University of Vienna, Austria	73	58	NA	NA	0	13	36	24	0	7	NA	1	NA	37	1 yr: 90% 3 yr: 86% 5 yr: 72%
Weigang[29]	2009	University Hospital Mainz, Germany	26	10	NA	NA	0	26	0	0	0	15	13	0	0	NA	NA
Czerny[55]*	2007	University of Vienna, Austria	27	NA	NA	NA	0	10	17	0	0	7	NA	0	0	15	1 yr: 83% 3 yr: 72%
Hughes[50]	2009	Duke University	28	NA	0	NA	43	12	9	0	7	0	21	0	4	14	3 yr: 70%
Chiesa[56]	2010	Vita-Salute, Milan, Italy	51	NA	NA	NA	0	24	27	Not included	0	6	16	6	0	23	NA
Holt[53]	2010	St George, London, U.K.	26	NA	15	NA	0	9	17	Not included	0	6	NA	0	6	NA	NA
Bavaria[49]	2010	University of Pennsylvania	27	NA	NA	NA	74	27	0	0	0	11	NA	11	7	NA	NA
Lee[7]	2011	University of Florida, Gainesville	37	NA	NA	14	68	37	0	0	0	16	32	11	0	NA	1 yr: 72%
Ham[57]	2011	University of Southern California	16	NA	NA	100	0	8	8	0	0	6	50	6	0	13	1 yr: 83% 3 yr: 80%

CPB, Cardiopulmonary bypass; *NA*, not available.
*Patients may be duplicated in these two studies.

cardiopulmonary bypass and 46% required an ascending aortic replacement. The indications for ascending aorta replacement were diameters greater than 36 mm, which would not have sealed a stent graft.[7]

From Duke University, Hughes and colleagues[50] published a series of 28 patients; 43% required cardiopulmonary bypass at the time of hybrid repair. This series included seven patients who had a modified frozen elephant trunk aortic reconstruction, four who required a concomitant cardiac procedure, and one with a pulmonary artery injury that required cardiopulmonary bypass to repair. Despite these challenging patients 30-day in-hospital rates of death, stroke, and permanent paraplegia or paresis were 0%, 0%, and 4%, respectively. Morbidity was limited to 21%, and 3-year survival was 70%.[50]

Series that have treated patients emergently have had varying outcomes. In the series by Schumacher et al[51] out of Heidelberg, Germany, 25 high risk patients were reviewed. Nine patients had complete arch debranching, and 16 had partial debranching. The 30-day mortality and morbidity were quite high at 20% and 63%, respectively, but 32% of the patients were treated emergently for contained ruptures. Another series from the University of Hong Kong treated 31% of the patients emergently. Sixteen patients (five complete debranching, eight partial debranching with carotid-carotid artery bypass, and three with carotid to left subclavian artery bypass) were identified. One patient also required cardiopulmonary bypass (6%), but in contrast to the previous series, there was no 30-day mortality. Of note, the morbidity was high at 67%, with 19% having strokes.[52]

Holt and colleagues[53] also had a series with 26 patients. Complete debranching was done in 9 patients, and partial debranching was done in 17 patients. Mortality was 6%, stroke rate was 0%, and paraplegia rate was 6%. They also treated 15% emergently, and none required cardiopulmonary bypass.[53]

The remaining series were all elective operations without cardiopulmonary bypass being used. These series include a combination of proximal landing in zones 0 or 1. From the University of Vienna, Austria, Gottardi and colleagues[54] had one of the largest case series with 73 patients, but 24 (33%) had landing in zone 2, and 31 (42%) patients had other nonaneurysmal pathologies including acute dissections. The results of the patient were all combined, and in the entire cohort the 30-day mortality was 7% and stroke rate was 1%.[54]

A subgroup of patients in the series from Gottardi and colleagues[54] had been previously published by Czerny and colleagues[55] 1 year earlier. This group consisted of 27 patients, with no zone 2 proximal landing. Ten had complete arch debranching, and 17 had partial arch debranching. In-hospital mortality was 7%, and there was no stroke or paralysis. One-year survival was 83%, and 3-year survival was 72%.[55]

Bergeron and colleagues[27] reported on 25 patients with a 30-day mortality of 8%, stroke rate of 8%, and no paraplegia. Over 10 years, Chiesa and colleagues[56] at the Vita-Salute University in Milan, Italy, identified 52 patients with proximal zone 2 coverage and 51 patients with complete or partial arch debranching. Of the latter 51 patients, 24 required complete arch debranching (proximal zone 0), and 27 required partial arch debranching (proximal zone 1). In these 51 patients, mortality, stroke, and paraplegia rates were 6%, 6%, and 0%, respectively. Thirty-day mortality rates in patients with complete and partial debranching were 13% and 0%, respectively.[56]

A single institution report from the University of Southern California reported the outcomes of hybrid thoracoabdominal and aortic arch repairs. The subset of data from the hybrid approach to the aortic arch identified 16 patients. Eight had zone 0 proximal landing, and eight had zone 1 proximal landing. Mortality was 6%, but morbidity was 50%. Strokes occurred in 6%, and none had paraplegia.[57]

This discussion suggests that complete arch debranching has a higher mortality then partial arch debranching. This may be partially due to the use of cardiopulmonary bypass required in certain patients with complete arch debranching. As one would expect, emergent operations also had worse outcomes compared with elective and urgent cases. Long-term data are limited for hybrid repair. Follow-up in the case series range from 1 to 3 years. One-year overall survival has ranged from 70% to 100% (see Table 36-1).

Hybrid Thoracoabdominal Aneurysms Repair

Case series reporting on the hybrid repair of the thoracoabdominal aorta have been reported worldwide with increasing frequency since first described in 1999.[1] Defining outcomes from these case series can be difficult given the heterogeneous groups of patients in these reports. In Table 36-2, factors such as the extent of aneurysmal involvement based on Crawford classification, emergent, and high-risk patients have been noted and should be kept in mind when examining outcomes. In general, reported mortalities range from 0% to 31%; these are based either on 30-day or in-hospital mortalities. Morbidities range from 17% to 65%, but these values can range depending on how complications have been classified. Permanent paraplegia ranges from 0% to 14%.

One the first series from the University of North Carolina–Chapel Hill published in 2005, reviewed 10 patients. Their outcomes were impressive, with no death or paraplegia, but there were no type I-II thoracoabdominal aortic aneurysms (TAA) in this series. Twenty percent of patients were type IV TAA, 30% were suprarenal abdominal aortic aneurysm (AAA), and 50% were juxtarenal AAA. The patients had an average of 1.3 bypasses per patient, and most did not involve clamping the aorta. Six patients had a single iliorenal bypass, three with a hepatorenal bypass and one with complete visceral revascularization.[34] A recent series (n = 24) from the University of Southern California also had a high proportion of type IV (50%) and pararenal AAA (38%). The remaining 12.5% of patients were either Crawford type I, II, or III TAA. The mortality and paraplegia rates were 4.2%.[57] The patients in both series were considered high risk for surgery.

Van de Mortel and colleagues[46] look at all hybrid procedures done in the Netherlands and identified 16

TABLE 36-2 Summary of Case Series (>10 patients) on the Hybrid Repair of Thoracoabdominal Aortic Aneurysms

Primary Author	Year	Institute	No. of Patients	High Risk for Open Repair (%)	Crawford Classification						Emergent Cases (%)	30-Day Mortality (%)	Paraplegia (%)	Morbidity (%)	Follow-Up (Mo)	Overall Survival	Graft Occlusion Based on No. of Bypasses Created	Late Reintervention (%)
					I	II	III	IV	V	Other								
Fulton[34]	2005	University of North Carolina	10	80	—	—	—	4	3	Juxta, 5	0	0	0	60	Mean, 8.7	100%	0/13 (0%)	10
Resch[58]	2006	Cleveland Clinic	13	100	3	5	2	1	—	Dsxn, 5	15	23	9	NA	Mean, 23	62%	NA	31
Black[35]	2006	St Mary's, London	29	80	3	18	7	1	—	3 Debranching, aborted	10	24	0	62*	Median, 8	NA	2/94 (2%)	17
Zhou[59]	2006	Baylor University	31	100	3	3	8	7	—	10 Arch aneurysms	NA	3	0	19	Mean, 16	90%	2/31 (6.4%)†	0
Lee[40]	2007	University of Florida	17	82	—	2	8	7	—	—	0	24	0	24	Mean, 8	NA	2/56 (3.5%)	6
Böckler[39]	2008	University of Heidelberg, Germany	28	96	2	8	4	1	—	Dsxn, 7 Patch, 1 Plaque, 1 Missing, 4?	22	14	14	59	Mean, 22	3 yrs, 70%	4/28 (14%)†	7
van de Mortel[46]	2008	The Netherlands	16	50	1	1	1	4	6	Juxta, 3	6	31	0	56	Mean, 13	69%	7/58 (13%)	0
Patel[18]	2009	Massachusetts General Hospital	23	100	9	5	9	—	—	—	9	23 in hospital deaths	4	65	Mean, 5.5	1 yr, 68% 2 yr, 34%	7/70 (10%)	17
Quinones[60]	2009	University of California–Los Angeles	20	100	—	3	8	4	1	Pararenal, 1 Arch, 3	0	0	5	30	Mean, 16.6	75%	0/20 (0%)†	5
Chiesa[44]	2009	Milan, Italy	31	100	12	3	6	3	—	Patch, 7	3	19	3	36	Median, 11.9	61%	6/88 (6.8%)	3
Donas[61]	2009	Zurich Hospital, Switzerland	58	100	3	5	9	13	—	Pararenal, 28 VORTEC used for debranching anastomosis	0	9	3	NA	Mean, 22.1	74%	3/113 (3%)	7
Drinkwater[62]	2009	Combined series from Böckler, Wolfe, and Black	107	NA	1	45	32	1	1	Complex, 17	0	15	8	38*	NA	NA	14/107 (13%)	NA
Biasi[63]	2009	St George's Hospital, London	18	NA	2	8	7	—	1	—	11	17	6	17	Median, 23	72%	1/54 (2%)	6
Wolf[45]	2010	Munich, Germany	20	75	1	11	7	—	1	—	10	10	10	45	Median, 5.8	75%	4/70 (5.7%)	10
Muehling[47]	2010	University of Ulm, Germany	16	100	3	3	1	9	—	—	38	31	6	44	Median, 12	81%	2/31 (6.5%)	13
Kabbani[84]	2010	University of Michigan	36	NA	1	10	12	10	—	Pararenal, 3	8	8	0	47	Mean, 6	6 mo, 80%	9/123 (7%)	6
Ham[57]	2011	University of Southern California	24	100	—	3	—	12	—	Pararenal, 9	NA	4	4	39	Mean, 13.3	1 yr, 84% 3 yr, 54%	3/77 (3.9%)	NA

NA, Not available; *VORTEC,* Viabahn open revascularization technique; *Juxta,* juxtaposition; *Dsxn,* dissection.
*Calculated from available data in manuscript.
†Calculated per patients rather than per visceral bypass graft.

patients. In this seemingly uncomplicated group, in which only 50% were deemed unfit for open repair and only 19% were Crawford type I, II, or III TAA, they had one of the highest mortality rates (31%) of any series. They also had a 13% graft occlusion rate (7/58 grafts), accounting for 3 of the deaths. Two patients died from colonic ischemia secondary to an occluded SMA bypass graft, and the third patient died from gallbladder necrosis but also had renal failure requiring hemodialysis from a right renal artery graft occlusion.[46]

Another series of 16 patients, from the University of Ulm in Germany also had a high mortality (31%) in a series of mainly type IV TAA (56%). This high mortality may be explained by the number of emergent operations (38%). All patients were considered high risk. Emergent mortality was 50% (3 of 6) compared to the elective–urgent mortality of 20% (2 of 10). Of the deaths, two were due to graft occlusion with bowel ischemia and subsequent death.[47]

Additional series with high mortalities had more patients with extensive Crawford types I-III TAA. From the Cleveland clinic, 13 consecutive patients, all deemed unfit for conventional thoracoabdominal repair, had aortic dissections with aneurysmal degeneration (n = 5) or TAA aneurysms (n = 8). Mortality was 23%, and six patients required either a proximal or distal aortic repair (two infrarenal reconstructions, three arch elephant trunk grafts, and one ascending aortic repair).[58] St Mary's Hospital in London reported on 29 patients. The TAA distribution was Crawford type I in 3, type II in 18, type III in 7, and type IV in 1. They had no paraplegia in their series, but overall mortality was 24% (7/29). Three patient had debranchings aborted. Two were secondary to intraoperative cardiac instability. These patients survived and were managed conservatively. The third patient had poor inflow for the debranching bypass because of an aortic dissection. This patient died 10 days after the procedure. Of the completed hybrid repairs, the mortality was 23% (6/26). Three patients treated emergently all died. In three elective or urgent patients who died, one was from a pulmonary embolus, another from MI, and the last from emboli to the viscera. Mortality was 100% (3/3) for emergent repairs and 13% (3/23) for urgent and elective patients.[35]

At the University of Florida–Gainesville, 17 patients with TAA (Crawford extent: two type II, eight type III, and seven type IV) were reported. Perioperative mortality was 24%.[40] From the Massachusetts General Hospital, 23 high-risk patients with TAA (Crawford extent: 9 type I, 5 type II, 9 type III) had a 30-day mortality of 17.4%, and in hospital mortality of 23%. This series also had a total of 5/23 (22%) endoleaks during the limited mean follow-up of 5.5 months. Three endoleaks were type I, and two were type II. A total of three patients required endovascular reintervention. Of note, this series also compared the hybrid to a cohort of contemporary open TAA repairs (see earlier discussion).[18]

Of the series with the lowest mortalities, Zhou and colleagues[59] reported on 31 patients with a mortality of 3% (n = 1). This series combined 21 TAAs with 10 cases of aortic arch aneurysms. In those with TAA, Crawford types were type I in three patients, type II in

three patients, type III in eight patients, and type IV in seven patients. Aortic arch reconstructions were performed in 3 patients, supra-aortic trunk debranching in 13 patients, and visceral vessel bypasses in 15 patients. Despite the complex patients the outcomes were encouraging.[59]

From the University of California–Los Angeles, 20 patients were treated using a hybrid approach. Three had aortic arch aneurysm, but the remainder were TAA (Crawford type I, 0; type II, 3; type III, 8; and type IV, 4), symptomatic supravisceral AAA (one), and contained perirenal pseudoaneurysm rupture (one). There was no mortality and only one patient with paraplegia. The latter patient had the entire aorta covered with a stent-graft from the left subclavian to aortic bifurcation treated in a single stage.[60]

In one of the largest series, Donas and colleagues[61] used a novel technique they described as the Viabahn open revascularization technique (VORTEC). The bypass anastomoses were created by using a Viabahn stent graft (Gore, Flagstaff, Ariz.) deployed through one wall of the visceral vessel. The other end was directly sutured end to side with the main feeding bypass graft or fixed into an interposition branch graft off the main bypass. This technique avoided suturing an anastomosis and clamping of the visceral vessels with its associated warm ischemia time. In this series of 58 patients, all were treated electively. Thirty patients had TAA (Crawford types I, 3; type I, 5; type III, 9; type IV, 13; type V, 0), and 28 patients had pararenal AAA. Ninety eight renal and 15 visceral vessels were revascularized using VORTEC. The primary patency of the bypass was 97%, and assisted primary patency rate was 98%, as two occluded Viabahn grafts were reopened by thrombolysis and thrombus aspiration. Thirty-day mortality rate was 8.6%, and permanent paralysis occurred in 3.4%.[61]

In the largest case series report to date (n = 107), Drinkwater and colleagues[62] used data from three major European Vascular Units: St Mary's Hospital, London, University of Heidelberg, Germany, and University of Munich, Germany. Each of these three centers already had individual case series published, but this was a collaborative update on their patients.[35,39,45] There were no emergent cases. Long-term follow-up was not included. The Crawford type TAA distribution was eleven type I, 45 type II, 32 type III, one type IV, one type V, and 17 defined as complex. The 30-day mortality rate was 15%; 12.1% of the patients suffered spinal cord ischemia, and in 8.4% it was complete and permanent; 3.7% of the patients required long-term dialysis, and 2.8% of the patients had bowel resection for an infarcted segment of bowel. The morbidity was not well defined, but was at least 38%. Three patients ruptured their aneurisms before the stenting procedure was undertaken.[62]

From the case series discussed, follow-up is difficult to interpret. A number of series report the outcomes based on median rather then mean months of follow-up, and range from 5.5 to 23 months. From Table 36-2, a rough estimate of survival appears to at least 80% at 1 year. The longest follow-up for any patient is 14 years. This patient was treated in 1999[1] with the first hybrid procedure and continues to do well at the time of this writing, without additional interventions.

SUMMARY

The hybrid approach to aortic arch and thoracoabdominal aortic pathology is a feasible operation. There have been no randomized trials comparing open to hybrid approaches, but based on prospective and retrospective case reports, morbidity and mortality seem comparable. Patient selection is critical, and the success of a hybrid aortic repair is dependent on preoperative planning and execution. A hybrid approach to aortic arch and thoracoabdominal aortic pathology should be included in the armamentarium of vascular surgeons involved in the care of these complex, high-risk patients.

References available online at expertconsult.com.

QUESTIONS

1. In a debranching procedure for a type 3 TAA which artery should not be used as inflow for the bypass graft?
   a. Infrarenal aorta
   b. Common iliac artery
   c. External iliac artery
   d. Descending thoracic aorta

2. In an isolated arch aneurysm, which vessel is not debranched with a complete arch debranching?
   a. Celiac artery
   b. Inominate artery
   c. Left common carotid artery
   d. Left subclavian artery

3. True or false, use of a stent graft for a combined endovascular and surgical (hybrid) approach to treat aortic arch and TAA aneurysms is an **on-label** approved use of the device.
   a. True
   b. False

4. True or false, there have been randomized trials of hybrid versus conventional open repair that suggest a hybrid approach should be favored over open repair for patients with acceptable surgical risks.
   a. True
   b. False

5. Which procedure is not needed in a partial arch debranching where the proximal seal zone is expected to be in zone 1?
   a. Carotid to subclavian artery bypass
   b. Carotid to carotid artery bypass
   c. Sternotomy
   d. Placement of stent graft from the a femoral approach

6. True or false, all hybrid procedures they should be done in two stages.
   a. True
   b. False

7. What is a contraindication to a hybrid repair of a TAA aneurysm?
   a. Replaced right hepatic
   b. Inability to create a proximal or distal landing zone
   c. Previous infrarenal AAA
   d. Aneurysmal degeneration of a aortic dissection

8. Follow-up imaging after a hybrid repair should be:
   a. There is no additional imaging needed
   b. The same as open surgery
   c. The same as any other endovascular aneurysm repair
   d. Done only if there are problems

9. Spinal drainage in not needed in a hybrid repair of the TAA if:
   a. A large amount of aorta is being covered
   b. The bilateral internal iliacs have been previously ligated
   c. Spinal drainage is usually recommended
   d. The patient has had a prior infrarenal AAA

10. If a patient is undergoing complete aortic arch debranching with a sternotomy, which of the following is the least important to assess preoperatively?
    a. Coronary arteries.
    b. Aortic valve
    c. Femoral Arteries
    d. Ascending aorta

ANSWERS

1. **c**
2. **a**
3. **b**
4. **b**
5. **c**
6. **b**
7. **b**
8. **c**
9. **c**
10. **c**

CHAPTER 37

Branched and Fenestrated Grafts for Endovascular Thoracoabdominal Aneurysm Repair

Roy K. Greenberg • Tara M. Mastracci • Matthew J. Eagleton

Thoracoabdominal aortic aneurysms (TAA) can extend from the origin of the left subclavian artery to the aortic bifurcation and are categorized according to the Crawford classification.[1] Since Etheredge described the first open thoracoabdominal repair,[2] perioperative techniques have evolved to limit lower extremity, visceral, and spinal cord ischemia (SCI). Despite the advances, the perioperative mortality risk ranges from 2% to 19%, with the highest risk being derived from statewide Medicare analyses.[3-7] The risk of SCI may be as high as 11%, while worsening renal function is seen in up to a quarter of treated patients.[5,7-9] On the other end, the risk of rupture of untreated large TAA is considerable and is associated with a dismal prognosis when a patient exhibits ruptures. Even in elective conditions, the magnitude of the open surgical procedure relegates otherwise healthy patients to a considerable risk of complications, while patients with significant comorbidities are generally precluded from repair. Consequently, alternative techniques have been developed to address this complex surgical problem. Hybrid repairs involve the surgical creation of extraanatomic bypasses to the visceral and renal branches based off the distal aorta or iliac artery.[10,11] The endovascular portion involves placement of thoracic or bifurcated abdominal graft excluding the involved segment. For less extensive aneurysms that simply abut the visceral or renal arteries, the "snorkel" technique has been described.[12,13] This technique involves placement of stents into the target visceral or renal vessel from above that lay parallel to the aortic component, allowing for antegrade flow into the branch vessel and the aortic graft. However, an endovascular seal must be created above the aneurysm, in the region of the snorkel stents or within the neck immediately below the branches. This is not possible in some circumstances, and the durability of such repairs remains in question. Perhaps the simplest conceptual method of endovascular repair of thoracoabdominal aneurysms is that involving fenestrated and branched devices, as they most closely resemble the principles of open surgical repair (SR). The aorta is basically relined, and whenever there is a critical branch, it is incorporated into that repair. Many improvements to the original designs[14-17] have been implemented, and the technology is used commercially in Europe, Australia, and areas of Asia. However, dissemination of these technologies into clinical practice

has been challenging, similar to the challenges that face the widespread treatment of thoracoabdominal aneurysm in an open surgical manner.

DEVICES

Aortic Components

Fenestrated grafts are currently commercially available within the United States, and these are based on the Zenith platform. Other versions are currently available under clinical investigational trials. Fenestrations and side-arm branches are the two basic models used to make an array of thoracoabdominal devices, each of which has their own merits and limitations (Table 37-1).[18] Fenestrations are circular or elliptical holes created in the graft fabric in a specific location, reinforced with a nitinol ring to provide a stable region against which to expand a balloon-mounted stent-graft (Figure 37-1). The fenestrations may be small (6 mm wide and 6 or 8 mm high, typically used for the renal arteries) or large (8 to 12 mm in diameter, usually used for visceral vessels; e.g., celiac and superior mesenteric artery). Large fenestrations may have a crossing strut or may be strut free depending on whether it is desired to place a mating stent-graft into the target branch vessel. Scallops are U-shaped openings at the ends of a stent-graft that may be used to accommodate branches when such branches are not directly involved in the aneurysm. Side-arm branches are most frequently used in the setting of larger TAAs (types II and III) and may be oriented axially (straight up and down) or angled (simple angle or helical wraps; Figure 37-2). Side-arm branches are most often directed in a caudal direction, but occasionally have been directed cranially. The branches may reside within (internal), exterior (external), or both (internal–external) to the aortic graft. Covered stents are coupled with branch devices to exclude the aneurysm from blood flow. A balloon-expandable stent-graft (Jomed [Abbott Park, Ill] or Atrium [Atrium USA, Hudson NH]) is used to create a seal between the aortic component and the target vessel when fenestrations are used. The proximal (aortic end) of such stents is flared against the nitinol ring attached circumferentially to the aortic fenestration to achieve a seal. In contrast, self-expanding stent-grafts (Fluency [Bard Medical,

TABLE 37-1	Advantages and Limitations of Devices Using Fenestrations and Side-Arm Branches for Excluding Thoracoabdominal Aortic Aneurysms	
	Fenestrations	**Side-Arm Branched**
Advantages	Less aortic coverage, thus minimizing paraplegia risk	Errors or design and deployment are better tolerated
	Can be loaded into a low-profile sheath	Greater overlap between aortic component and mating stent graft
	Can be easily angled in line with the native vessel geometry. side-arm branches impart a downward angle. This can place stress on the target vessel and bridging stent if the target vessel traverses upward and not downward.	Optimal for vessels oriented longitudinal to the aortic axis (such as superior mesenteric artery)
		Flexibility of self-expandable stent grafts reduces target artery distortion and damage
		More proximal aortic coverage required
	Not prone to kinks	Profile is increased because of side arms
Limitations	Errors of design are not well tolerated	Mating stent grafts, transcending through a distance of unsupported aneurysm, may link
	Less sealing zone between the main aortic segment and mating stent graft	Aortic component must be tapered in small aortic lumens, thus decreasing the cross-sectional area and increasing the risk of late migration
	Balloon-expandable stent grafts are more prone to fracture in the arterial environment	
	Challenging to traverse long distances from the fenestration origin to the target branch vessel	

From Qureshi MA, Greenberg RK: Endovascular stent grafting for TAAA. In Franco KL, Thouraui VH, editors: Cardiothoracic surgery review, Philadelphia, 2011, Lippincott Williams Wilkins.

Covington, Ga] or Viabahn [W.L. Gore and Associates Ins, Flogstaff, Az]) are typically used with side-arm branches to better accommodate long distances, tortuosity, and achieve better overlap with the aortic device. Often, hybrid fenestrated or branched devices are used (ones that contain both fenestrations and side-arms) to better accommodate for specific types of anatomy (Figure 37-3).

The devices may be customized to fit patient-specific anatomy or work "off-the-shelf" when a standardized design allows for treatment of a subset of patients with common anatomy akin to branched grafts used to preserve internal iliac patency.[19] The later types of devices rely on the concept that there is some consistency between aneurysm patients in regard to visceral branch morphology. However, the aortic diameter, and extent of the aneurysm vary in most patients, and thus patients considered for standardized devices must be lumped into groups (e.g., juxtarenal aneurysms, type IV thoracoabdominal aneurysm, type II and III thoracoabdominal aneurysms) to assess the proximal and distal extent of the required repair. Evaluation of preoperative images for patients intended for fenestrated stent-grafts demonstrated that several off-the-shelf models would be required to fit the majority of patients[20]; however, with modifications that provide a greater range of target vessels for individual fenestrations, it appears that only one or two visceral segment designs will be necessary to accommodate the majority of patients with juxtarenal and pararenal aneurysms.[18]

Mating Stent-Graft Components

Balloon expandable stent-grafts are constructed with expanded polytetrafluoroethylene (ePTFE) and stainless steel stents. Two designs are frequently used with fenestrated devices and include the Atrium and the Jomed systems. The Atrium stent-graft is provided premounted onto a balloon and consists of two layers of ePTFE sandwiching a stainless steel stent platform. The Jomed stent is provided as either a premounted system or independent from a balloon, allowing for mounting at the time of the procedure. The Jomed device is an ePTFE graft sandwiched by two stainless steel stents. The length of the desired mating balloon-expandable stent-graft is determined at the time of the procedure when a proper assessment of the distance between the fenestration and target vessel can be made. The most commonly used self-expanding stent-grafts are the Fluency and the Viabahn. Both are constructed out of nitinol and ePTFE, but differ considerably in regard to deployment and conformability. The Fluency is a stiffer device that provides more columnar support than the Viabahn, and as a result does not conform as well to tortuous anatomy. Although the Viabahn is more flexible, it must be delivered through a separate sheath placed into the target vessel, and it is often difficult to deploy in the setting of marked tortuosity. When self-expanding stent-grafts are coupled with side-arm branched devices, there is often considerable overlap with the aortic component, the extent of which can vary to a certain degree, providing interventionist with more flexibility in choosing a length of the self-expanding stent-grafts.

Delivery Systems

All branched devices are loaded onto a 16- to 24-French delivery system, depending on the graft diameter and the number of branches. (The larger diameters are reserved for large-diameter [>38 mm] arch branch devices.)

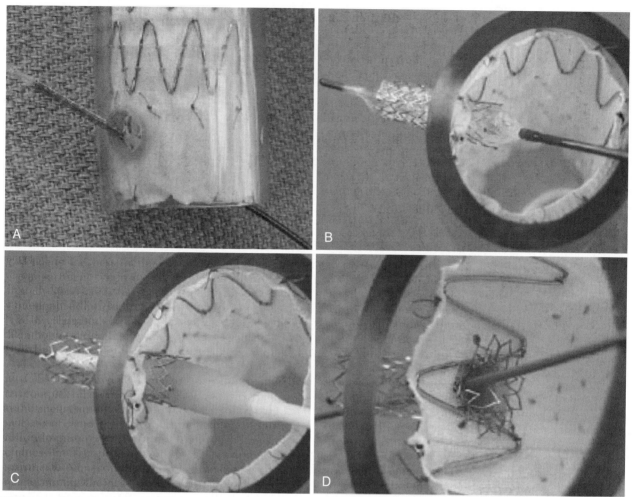

FIGURE 37-1 ■ The aneurysm is excluded using a fenestrated endograft by coupling the aortic component with a balloon expandable stent that is placed through the fenestration. **A,** A stent-graft is placed into the target vessel through the graft fenestration. **B,** The balloon-expandable stent is deployed, leaving a portion of the stent within the main body of the graft. **C,** A larger balloon is placed inside the proximal portion of the deployed stent. **D,** Inflation of this balloon results in flaring of the aortic portion of the stent and creation of the seal. (Reprinted with permission from Greenberg RK: Treating large complex ameurisms: techniques and technologies involving branched or fenestrated devices have emerged to offer ΣVAR options. Endovasc Surg Today 4[3]:43–50, 2005.)

Braided hydrophilic sheaths are used to constrain the graft and enable the devices to be navigated through tortuous and calcified iliacs, allowing for the necessary rotational adjustments that are required to properly align branches. There are two critical delivery system adjuncts that are used with fenestrated grafts. These adjuncts include the fixation of the device to the delivery system such that after sheath withdrawal, longitudinal and rotational adjustments can be made to optimally align the fenestrations, and the use of constraining wires to prevent complete graft expansion following sheath withdrawal, thus providing a space between the fenestrated device and target vessel facilitating cannulation. Side-arm branches do not require placement to be as precise as fenestrated devices, although fixation to the delivery system and graft constraint are used in these devices as well. Frequently, side-arm branches are preloaded with a catheter and wire. When this wire is brought out, an alternative access site (i.e., the branchial artery for the visceral segment, termed *through-and-through access*) provides direct access into the branch from above and confers significant stability for the

delivery of the mating stent-grafts, which is particularly critical in tortuous anatomy. A low-profile version of fenestrated and branched grafts has also been used. The construct uses thinner polyester fabric coupled with nitinol stents and is housed within a 16- to 18-French sheath.

PREOPERATIVE PLANNING AND DEVICE SELECTION

High-resolution computed tomography angiography (CTA) of the chest, abdomen, and pelvis is required with thin (z-plane) reconstructions. This must be accomplished with a contrast injection and a properly timed bolus to allow for opacification of the entire aorta and its branches. These images are then evaluated using a three-dimensional imaging program that allows for the creation of centerline-of-flow (CLF) reconstructions allowing for accurate and reproducible diameter measurements and the assessment of visceral branch

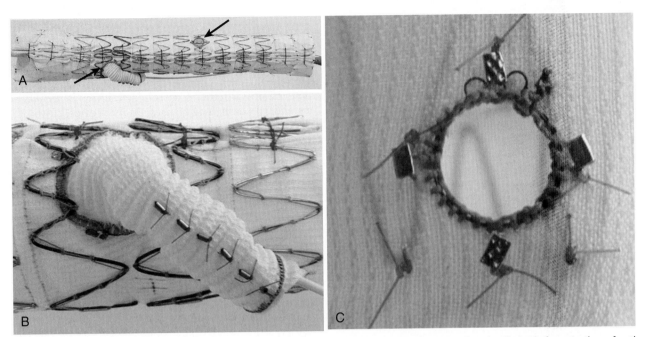

FIGURE 37-2 ■ **A,** Custom-designed main body device tethered to the delivery system demonstrating branch fenestrations for the renal arteries and a helical branch providing antegrade perfusion of the celiac artery. **B,** The helical branch is an 8-mm polyester graft sewn to the aortic prosthesis above the target vessel. These directional branches provide long regions (2 cm) of overlap, allowing mating of a self-expanding stent-graft (Fluency) sized to the visceral vessel. The helical branch construct provides a more secure seal into both the mating vessel and the aortic component given the extensive potential for overlap with both sealing regions, resulting in a reduced tendency to develop endoleaks or component separation. **C,** The fenestrated branch is a nitinol-reinforced opening in the main body device that is sized and aligned with the target vessel ostium. This is mated with a balloon-expandable stent-graft lumen, and the aortic portion is subsequently flared with a compliant balloon to achieve a seal around the fenestration. (From Soltesz EG, Greenberg RK: Endovascular repair of thoracoabdominal aortic aneurysms with fenestrated-branched stent-grafts. Operative Techniques Thorac Cardiovasc Surg 15:86–99, 2010.) See Color Plate 37-2.

relational morphology (Figure 37-4, see color plate). The CLF reconstructions are typically done in a semiautomated fashion, allowing the clinician to ensure the accuracy and modify the computed CLF to ensure accuracy specific to the repair strategy. Some companies offer these services via an internet network (or "cloud network") in an effort to support the planning and sizing of the endovascular grafts. Regardless of the method used to obtain and process the imaging, the following pieces of information are critical to choose and design an appropriate device.

1. The proximal extent of the disease will determine the cranial extent of the repair and which vessels should be incorporated into the repair. All attempts should be made to extend the repair into healthy aorta regardless of the number of visceral vessels that are required to incorporate. One can assume that healthy aorta will be cylindrical, not excessively tortuous, have a length of 2 cm or more, and be generally free of debris; this will provide the stability for the repair in the long term. Aneurysms should be classified in accordance with the Society for Vascular Surgery (SVS) reporting standards classifications system.[21]

2. The proximal aortic diameter orthogonal to the CLF. Devices are then oversized 10% to 20% in comparison to the measured aortic diameter.

3. The geometric relationship between the visceral vessels (the longitudinal and radial location of each

vessel intended to be incorporated into the repair) and the orientation of the visceral vessels to the aortic centerline is required to access eligibility to be treated with a standardized device, or to customize a fenestrated or branched device. This relationship (in conjunction with the luminal diameter around the visceral segment) will help to define whether fenestrations or branches should be used, how the fenestrations should be oriented, and whether branches should be oriented in an upward or downward fashion.

4. The location and morphology of the distal seal (i.e., distal aorta, old surgical graft, or iliac arteries).

5. The tortuosity of the arterial system. This will help to define an overall strategy for the repair, such as when visceral vessels should be accessed from above or below, from which side the main device should be introduced, and the orientation of a contralateral limb (if required).

In addition to these items, certain additional factors also must be considered. Thoracoabdominal aortic aneurysm (TAAA) can be extensive, with diseased aortic lengths in excess of 350 mm. The creation and deployment of such grafts creates many challenges; consequently, nearly all such repairs are modular with the longest graft components rarely longer than 270 mm. In such circumstances, the thoracic component of the aneurysm is repaired with conventional thoracic devices. The visceral segment is repaired with a fenestrated or branched

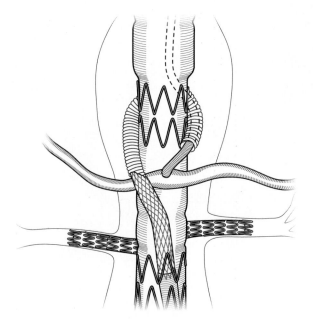

FIGURE 37-3 ■ The main body device is then orientated outside the body, keeping in mind the necessary position for branches and fenestrations. The device is then advanced through the femoral artery to the level of the visceral segment and aligned with the appropriate branch arteries. Multiple low-dose contrast injections may be needed at this step to confirm accurate placement. Gold markers on the fenestrations and helical branches assist in this process. A long hydrophilic wire (St. Jude Medical, Minnetonka, Minn.) is then preloaded into the celiac catheter of the main body device, advanced into the arch, and snared from the left axillary access. This provides through-and-through access to the celiac helical branch. The two top stents are then partially deployed, and the device position is repositioned if necessary by adjusting the longitudinal and rotational planes. The main body device sheath is then completely removed to allow partial expansion of the device; the remaining constraining wire prevents full deployment. The renal fenestrations are cannulated by gaining access into the main body of the device from the contralateral groin. Stents are systematically placed in each branch. (From Soltesz EG, Greenberg RK: Endovascular repair of thoracoabdominal aortic aneurysms with fenestrated-branched stent-grafts. Operative Techniques Thorac Cardiovasc Surg 15:86–99, 2010.)

device that is subsequently mated proximally to the thoracic device and distally to a bifurcated device when necessary. Attention must be directed to the overlap between modular components in regard to sealing and resistance to late separation. In general, when barbs are not used to secure joints between devices, a minimum of four stents of overlap is desired.[22,23] The use of barbs that extend from the inner device to the outer device drops the required overlap length to two stents, provided that the overlap occurs in the straight portion of the aorta. Nearly all fenestrated and most branched devices taper to a distal diameter of 22 to 24 mm, allowing for mating with standard bifurcated components. Most commonly the tapers are created immediately below the lowest renal fenestration, allowing for large graft diameters in the region of the fenestrations to supplement seal and fixation. In the setting of side-arm branches, the tapers usually occur as the side-arms exit from the aortic lumen.

STANDARDIZED VISCERAL SEGMENT DEVICES

Certain anatomic considerations must be evaluated when determining whether a customized device is required or a standard device may be used. In most cases, customized devices will more accurately fit the anatomy for which it was designed, unless the morphology of the patient conforms exactly to the geometry of the intended design. However, the extent to which the target vessels are offset from the design will have implications as to the technical challenges that may be encountered during deployment as well as the long-term integrity of the repair. Discrepancies between target vessel location and the location of aortic fenestrations must be accommodated for by the placement of mating stent-grafts that create a certain amount of stability, forcing the fenestration to align with the vessel and vice versa. Branches provide more leeway in both design and required alignment characteristics than fenestrations, but the mating stent-grafts still must bridge any cranial–caudal discrepancies as well as rotational angulation.[24,25] An assessment of the acceptable mating stent-graft length that travels in an unsupported manner through the aneurysm must be made when considering patients for standardized side-arm branch designs. Most critically, standardized devices have an intended sealing location (i.e., below the kidneys, below the superior mesenteric artery, within the straight portion of the thoracic aorta, or the ascending aorta). It would be inadvisable to treat a patient with disease proximal to the intended sealing location with a standardized device if at all avoidable. Device manufacturers provide a range of morphologies that are acceptable for a standardized design, but at this point, none have published any sizable series, and no long-term results exist. The repercussions of late growth around the sealing and fixation portion of any repair involving aortic branches are considerable, making potential salvage of the endovascular device extremely complicated. Therefore, analogous to the use of infrarenal devices,[26] it would be prudent to exercise caution when straying from the guidelines provided by manufacturers for fenestrated and branched devices.

PROCEDURE

Implantation is typically performed using general endotracheal anesthesia, although regional anesthesia can be used for reasonably short cases. A lumbar drain is placed for drainage of cerebrospinal fluid when extensive coverage of the aorta is anticipated or interruption of contributing blood supply to the artery of Adamkiewicz (T8 to Ll) is coupled with another pathology (e.g., compromised internal iliac arteries or prior abdominal aortic aneurism [AAA] repair). Bilateral femoral arteries are accessed (via cutdown or percutaneously), and selective exposure of brachial or axillary artery access sites is performed (in case of side-arm branches). The primary device is delivered over a stiff wire that is usually placed into the ascending aorta. The device is then oriented appropriately and then unsheathed, with the fenestrations or side

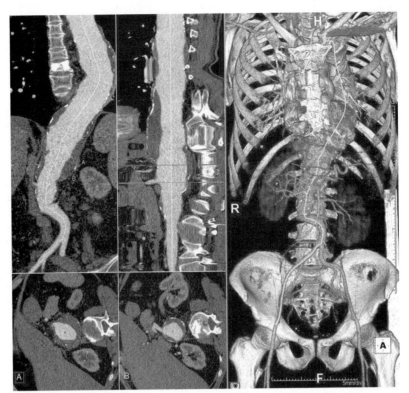

FIGURE 37-4 ■ Accurate planning and construction of the custom-designed branched thoracoabdominal stent-graft require detailed computerized three-dimensional modeling to provide a 360-degree view of the aortoiliac and visceral branch anatomy. Centerline-of-flow analysis allows the surgeon to generate a straightened image of the aorta and assess the precise angle of visceral branches as well as the distance between branches **(A)**. Orthogonal slices through the centerline-of-flow provide measurements that are then used for branched stent-graft construction. These reference points are usually described as a location from the origin as noted on a clock face **(B, C)**. *SMA,* Superior mesenteric artery. (From Soltesz EG, Greenberg RK: Endovascular repair of thoracoabdominal aortic aneurysms with fenestrated-branched stent-grafts. Operative Techniques Thorac Cardiovasc Surg 15:86–99, 2010.) See Color Plate 37-4.

arms corresponding to their respective branch vessels. The sequences of mating the aortic component with the target vessels are detailed as follows. In general, each visceral branch is cannulated from within the aortic prosthesis. After access into each visceral vessel, the aortic component is allowed to completely expand by removing the constraining wires. Balloon expandable stent-grafts (fenestrations) or self-expanding stent-grafts (side-arm branches) are then delivered and deployed. Balloon-expandable stent-grafts are flared proximally. It is common to reinforce the lining of the self-expanding mating stent-grafts in some designs with supplemental stents to ensure the absence of kinking and provide stiffness to the system. The aortic delivery system is removed, and proximal thoracic, distal bifurcated, or internal iliac components are added as required to complete the repair. Repeated angiography is performed at the conclusion of the procedure to ensure effective sac exclusion, preserve essential vessels, and detect any endoleaks. Once sac exclusion is confirmed, the device sheath is removed, and arteriotomies are repaired. Procedural details have been outlined in other publications.[27]

Reinforced fenestrated branches:
1. Access primary aortic graft from contralateral groin.
2. Selectively cannulate the desired fenestration.
3. Establish 6- to 7-French sheath access into the target branch.
4. Deploy balloon-expandable stent-graft mounted on a balloon sized to the target vessel diameter.
5. Flare the aortic portion of the balloon-expandable stent-graft with a 10- to 12-mm balloon. Optionally, larger aortic balloons may be used.
6. Repeat for each reinforced fenestration.

Directional branch:
1. Snare preloaded wire from remote access site (brachial or axillary).
2. Place a sheath (7 to 9 French) over preloaded wire.
3. Deploy primary aortic stent-graft after proper longitudinal and rotational alignment.
4. Advance sheath over preloaded wire into target directional branch.
5. Double puncture brachial–axillary sheath and advance hydrophilic catheter or wire into branch.
6. Cannulate target branch vessel and place stiff wire (Rosen wire).
7. Remove preloaded wire, thus losing all through-and-through access.
8. Advance self-expanding stent-graft into desired location and deploy with a minimum of 2 cm overlap into target vessel and 2 cm overlap into aortic endograft.
9. Selectively used additional stents or stent-grafts to ensure adequate overlap and an absence of kinking.
10. Repeat for each directional branch.

IMAGING ADVANCES

The complexity of the devices and procedures has increased as clinicians have tackled more challenging anatomy. The ability to more accurately visualize the three-dimensional vascular architecture intraoperatively has improved as well. The recent incorporation of flat-panel detectors on virtually all new imaging units has provided the ability to perform intraoperative three-dimensional (3D) imaging using rotational angiography. C-arm cone-beam computed tomography (CBCT) is an advanced imaging capability that uses C-arm flat-panel fluoroscopy systems to acquire and display 3D images. The flat-panel detector functions much like the multiline detectors used in MDCT and provides CT-like images in multiple viewing planes. CBCT systems are commercially available and can be used in fenestrated and branched endografting in two manners. The first would be to perform an intraoperative CBCT with contrast injected from a catheter located immediately proximal to the desired volume to be assessed. The 3D angiogram is then registered with the table and C-arm location. As the interventionist navigates through the vascular system, the image provides a moving roadmap. Alternatively, a non–contrast CBCT can be obtained, and the preoperative high-resolution CT scan is imported into the system. Next, bony landmarks and aortic calcifications are used to fuse the two images (Figure 37-5, see color plate); this is then registered with the C-arm and table position, thus providing a 3D map of the entire vascular system. In either case, the arteries that are displayed can be distorted by respiration or the insertion of catheters, wires, or sheaths. Furthermore, if the patient moves, the scans must be re-registered with the new position. These techniques have been shown to be useful in regard to limiting the required contrast dose,[28] as well as detecting problems with endovascular repairs at the time of the operative repair rather than waiting for a postoperative CT scan.[28-30]

OUTCOMES

Extensive experience with endovascular repair of thoracoabdominal aneurysms has been limited to a few high-volume centers in the United States, Europe, and Australia. The Cleveland Clinic has the largest series, involving more than 750 patients,[31] and other centers have reported successful treatment with similar devices.[32-36] It is important to examine the outcomes of such procedures in the context of the patient's disease. Given that fenestrated and branched devices are used for patients with aneurysms involving the juxtarenal aorta, varying extents of thoracoabdominal aorta as well as arch disease, efforts have focused on segregating results into disease extent for clinical outcomes, because device-related outcomes are generally pooled with all devices of a similar construct. Therefore, mortality, paraplegia, and similar events are reported in the context of the extent of disease, while branch patency, component separation, stent fracture, and other endovascular endpoints include the conglomerate of patients.

SURVIVAL

Survival following any elective procedure provides the fundamental basis of establishing the risk–benefit relationship between intervention versus alternative management options. If the risk of rupture is less than the risk of death or serious complications related to the procedure, then repair is not justified. In that context, survival must be viewed in conjunction with aneurysm size (implying rupture risk) along with the potential effect that the

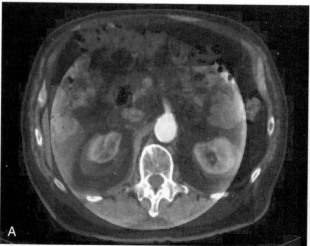
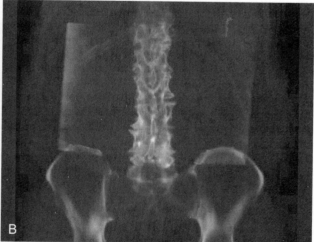

FIGURE 37-5 ■ Images depicting the fusion of the cone-beam computed tomography (CBCT) performed before stent-graft introduction. The colored images represent those of the preoperative multidetector computed tomography (MDCT), and the grayscale images are the ones obtained from the CBCT. The images are aligned in multiple planes including axial **(A)**, anterior **(B)**, and lateral (not shown). Once the scans are registered, or fused, with each other, the images from the MDCT can be overlaid on the live fluoroscopic image. (From Dijkstra ML, Eagleton MJ, Greenberg RK, et al. Intraoperative C-arm cone-beam computed tomography in fenestrated aortic endografting: a preliminary experience. J Vasc Surg 53:583–590, 2011.) See Color Plate 37-5.

TABLE 37-2 **Survival Estimates, Using Life Table Techniques in Accordance with the Extent of Treated Disease**

Extent of Repair	No. of Patients	Perioperative Death, 30 Days (%)	Estimated Survival, 24 Mo (%)	Estimated Survival, 48 Mo (%)
Total	633	3.2		
Juxtarenal	227	1.8	82	65
Type I TAAA	16	12.5	70	NA
Type II or III TAAA	172	5.2	74	59
Type IV TAAA	218	2.3	82	70

Data from Greenberg RK, Eagleton MJ, Mastracci TM: Branched endografts for thoracoabdominal aneurysms. J Thorac Cariovasc Surg 140:S171–S178, 2010.
TAAA, Thoracoabdominal aortic aneurysm, *NA*, not applicable.

effect intervention (or the lack thereof) will have on the patient's quality of life. Survival comparisons intended to contrast treatment options, such as open surgical treatment of TAAA versus endovascular treatment of TAAA that are not randomized, must account for the inherent treatment bias that exists when assessing such patients. Our treatment paradigms include both open and endovascular repair of thoracoabdominal aneurysms. Open repairs are more often performed on younger, healthier patients, whereas endovascular repair is more commonly used in older patients with more significant comorbidities. Survival data reflective of our total experience with a prospective trial of fenestrated and branched devices was published in 2010 (Table 37-2; Figure 37-6, see color plate).[31] The risk of perioperative death for the older and sicker endovascular patient is similar, if not lower, than the risks in younger, healthier, open surgical patients.[7] Long-term survival data from other centers, although retrospective in nature, do not differ markedly (Table 37-3). It is interesting to juxtapose the open and endovascular survival curves of various studies. Despite marked differences in the physiologic status (age and comorbidities) of patients, the curves are closely overlayed (Figure 37-7).

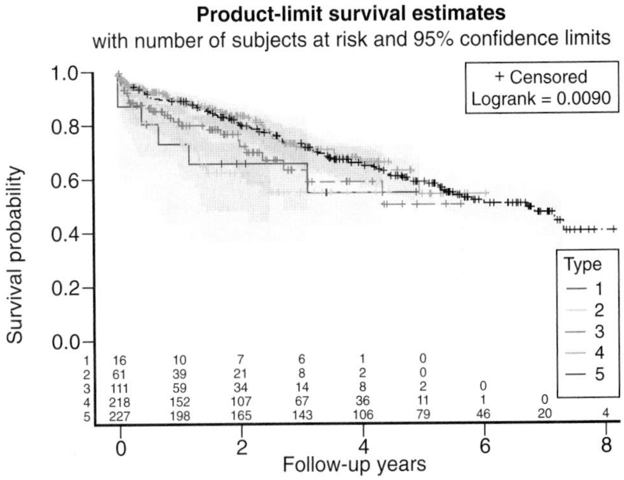

SPINAL CORD ISCHEMIA

Spinal cord ischemia (SCI) is likely the most devastating complication of open or endovascular thoracoabdominal aneurysm repair. It is extremely difficult to determine an individual patient's risk or to council patients and families with respect to their willingness to undergo an elective repair when there is a potential for paraplegia. Patients must understand this risk before any intervention, and clinicians must be attentive to the details of the operative strategy and postoperative management to decrease the potential for a neurologic deficit. Data suggest that the risk of SCI is slightly higher when open SR is performed when compared with endovascular repair (ER; 4.3% ER vs. 7.5% SR; $p = 0.08$); however, when classified in accordance with the extent of the disease, there were no statistical differences between patients undergoing open versus endovascular surgery.[7] The more extensive the repair, the greater the risk of paraplegia for either procedure, which confirms results in other publications.[37-39] In

Product-limit survival estimates
with number of subjects at risk and 95% confidence limits

CCF categories	Baseline	1m	6m	1y	2y	3y	4y	5y	6y
Type 1	16	14	14	10	9	6	1	0	0
Type 2	61	58	50	42	25	13	3	0	0
Type 3	111	109	90	68	50	21	11	4	1
Type 4	218	212	189	164	129	85	51	20	4
Fen repair	227	190	180	166	148	117	88	58	22

FIGURE 37-6 ■ Life table analyses with 95% confidence intervals were constructed for each type of aneurysm treated (type I, II, III, IV, and juxtarenal). *Curve 5* indicates the survival curve for juxtarenal aneurysms. *CCF,* Cleveland Clinic Foundation. (From Greenberg RK, Eatleton MJ, Mastracci TM: Branched endografts for thoracoabdominal aneurysms. J Thorac Cardiovasc Surg 140:S171–S178, 2010.) See Color Plate 37-6.

fact, a prospective contemporary comparative analysis has made it evident that the anatomic extent of the disease drastically overshadowed all other potential factors associated with the risk of paraplegia (Table 37-4). Furthermore, the analysis suggests that endovascular repair may temper the anatomic risk, and that internal iliac pathology had a more detrimental effect on the risk of paraplegia in the setting of endovascular repair (where no intercostals are reimplanted) in contrast to open SR.[7] Concomitant abdominal surgery, long segments of aortic coverage, and occlusion of anterior spinal artery collateral beds were noted to be significant risk factors for

TABLE 37-3 **Summary of Outcomes of Endovascular Repair of Thoracoabdominal Aortic Aneurysms**

Study	No. of Patients	Technical Success (%)	Follow-up (Mo)	Endoleak (%)	Rupture (%)	Bowel Ischemia (%)	Renal Failure Requiring Dialysis (%)	Spinal Cord Ischemia (%)	Branch Vessel Patency (%)	Mortality at 30 Days (%)	Mortality at 12 Months (%)
Greenberg[77]	352	ND*	12	ND	0	ND	ND	4.3	ND	5.7	15.6
Greenberg et al. and Roselli et al[55]	73	93	12	11	0	ND	1.4	2.7	100	5.5	11
Verhoeven[53]	30	93	12	ND	ND	ND	3.3	16.7	>90	6.7	24
Chuter[16]	22	100	12	9.1	ND	ND	0	0	98.75*	9.1	13.6
Ferreira[56]	11	100	8	0	ND	ND	0	27.2	95.3	18.1	NA
Bicknell[57,†]	15	93	12	40	6.6	6.6	13.2	6.6	97	0	6.6
Anderson[15]	4	92.3	12	0	0	ND	0	0	100	25	25

Data from Qureshi MA, Greenberg RK: New results with the Zenith graft in the treatment of aortic aneurysms. J Cardiovasc Surg (Torino) 51:503–514, 2010.
ND, No data; *NA*, not applicable.
*At 1 month.
†The report by Bicknell is a combined report of fenestrated devices (for juxtarenal aneurysms) and branched devices for TAA.

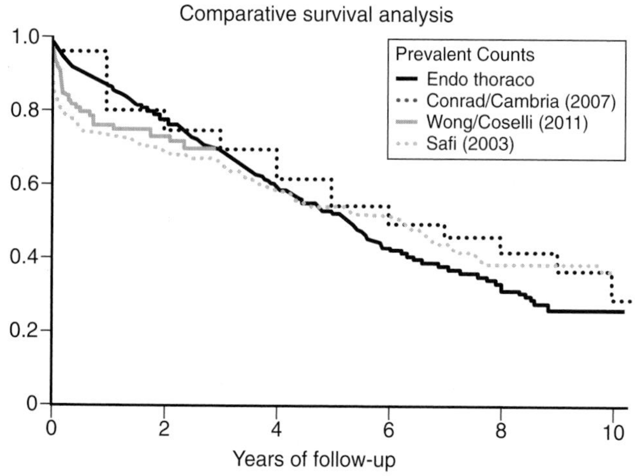

Comparative survival analysis

FIGURE 37-7 ■ Comparative survival analysis of open and endovascular cohorts of thoracoabdominal aortic aneurysm repair in the published literature.

the development of paraplegia in registry data as well (Table 37-5).[39]

There is mounting evidence to suggest that staging an extensive aortic repair may, in fact, decrease the risk of SCI. Experimental evidence of this was published by the Mount Sinai group. They randomized pigs to undergo open lumbar segmental ligation followed by endovascular thoracic repair in either a staged approach (with a 1-week interval) or at a single setting. Paraplegia following the single-stage procedure was 50%, with none of the pigs that underwent a two-stage operation developing neurologic deficits.[40] In fact, staged ERs are commonly performed, and although some clinical evidence exists to support the practice, numbers are small.[41] It is possible that such a strategy minimizes the complexity and overall risk of each procedure, particularly in regard to paralysis. Patients with extensive thoracoabdominal aneurysms that involve the arch or majority of the descending thoracic aorta will often undergo an endovascular arch and descending thoracic repair (even if a complete distal seal is not achievable at the time of thoracic repair), extending

TABLE 37-4 **Multivariable Association of Patient Characteristics and Spinal Cord Ischemia, Stratified by Repair Technique**

Patient Characteristic	SR		ER	
	OR	95% CI	OR	95% CI
Age	1.0	0.5-2.1	1.2	0.3-4.7
Gender (male or female)	1.5	0.6-4.3	1.3	0.3-6.2
African American	0.7	0.1-3.7	0.6	0.03-1.3
Smoking	1.3	0.5-3.3	3.3	0.7-1.7
Diabetes	0.002	—*	1	0.17-6.1
CAD	1.4	0.6-3.6	0.5	0.1-1.7
History of COPD	0.6	0.2-2.1	0.2	0.04-1.2
History of cancer	1.1	0.3-4.1	0.3	0.03-2.6
GFR	1.2	0.7-2.2	0.4	0.2-9.0
Aortic diameter	0.9	0.6-1.5	1.6	0.7-3.2
Extent of aneurysm repair				
I vs. 0	26.5	2.9-242.1	20	2.2-181.3
II vs. 0	38.8	4.8-317.4	14.1	1.1-188.6
III vs. 0	14.3	1.5-133.6	2.6	0.1-54.8
IV vs. 0	1.8	0.1-32.5	2.6	0.2-35.8
Chronic dissections	1.3	0.5-3.7	0.0009	—*
History op. of proximal aorta	0.8	0.3-2.1	1	0.2-5.3
History op. of distal aorta	1.8	0.6-5.6	3	0.8-1.2

Data from Greenberg RK, Lu Q, Roselli E, et al: Contemporary analysis of descending thoracic and thoracoabdominal aneurysm repair: a comparison of endovascular and open techniques. Circulation 118:808–817, 2008.
SR, Surgical repair; *ER*, endovascular repair; *OR*, odds ratio; *CI*, confidence interval; *CAD*, coronary artery disease; *COPD*, chronic obstructive pulmonary disease; *GFR*, glomerular filtration rate *op*, operation.
*Broad and nonsignificant CI.

the coverage down to the celiac artery. Next, at a second setting, often 1 to 2 months later, the visceral, infrarenal, and iliac segments are repaired. There is clearly an interprocedure risk of rupture, but the magnitude of a single-stage operation, particularly regarding SCI, is often too

TABLE 37-5 Multivariate Regression Analysis for Paraplegia

Risk Factor	p Value, Paraplegia (n = 15)	OR (95% CI)
Degenerative aneurysm	0.1406	2.75 (0.72-10.6)
Localization disease at proximal, middle, and descending thoracic aorta	0.4866	0.54 (0.10-3.03)
No. of stent grafts ≥3	0.0428	3.49 (1.04-11.7)
Left subclavian artery covering without transposition/bypass	0.0274	3.94 (1.17-13.3)
Occlusion by device T10	0.2474	2.07 (0.60-7.11)
Renal failure (score ≥1)*	0.0215	3.63 (1.21-10.9)
Concomitant open abdominal surgery	0.0371	5.52 (1.11-27.5)

Data from Buth J, Harris PL, Hobo R, et al: Neurologic complications associated with endovascular repair of thoracic aortic pathology: incidence and risk factors. A study from the European Collaborators on Stent/Graft Techniques for Aortic Aneurysm Repair (EUROSTAR) Registry. J Vasc Surg 46: 1103–1111, 2007.
OR, Odds ratio; *CI*, confidence interval.
*Society for Vascular Surgery/American Association for Vascular Surgery risk classification.

TABLE 37-6 30-Day Mortality, 30-Day Cardiac-Related Mortality and Incidence of Cardiac Events in Patients Undergoing Thoracoabdominal Surgical and Combined Endo and Surgical Approach Repair

	No. of Patients	30-Day Mortality	Cardiac-Related Death	Cardiac Events
Open TAA				
Coselli[58]	2286	150 (6.56%)	NA	181 (7.9%)
Schepens[59]	571	51 (8.9%)	14 (2.5%)	NA
Conrad[5]	455	39 (8.6%)	5 (1%)	67 (14.7%)
CESA				
Quinones-Baldrich[60]	20	0	0	1
Black[61]	17	3 (18%)	1	NA
Resch[11]	13	3	0	NA
Our	266	17 (6.3%)	5 (2%)	45/266 (17%)

Data from Bub GL, Greenberg RK, Mastracci TM, et al. Perioperative cardiac events in endovascular repair of complex aortic aneurysms and association with preoperative studies. J Vasc Surg 53:21–27, 2001.
TAA, Thoracic aortic aneurysm; *NA*, not applicable; *CESA*, combined endovascular and surgical approach.

great for patients with any comorbidities. An alternative strategy that has been suggested to mitigate paraplegia risk is the use of a perfusion branch.[42] This design involves the creation of a side branch that is intentionally left open to the aneurysm sac, creating a large endoleak that is intended to perfuse critical intercostal vessels. The side branch is then closed using embolization techniques at a later time to completely exclude the aneurysm. Few cases have been done with such designs, and studies intended to compare single-stage aneurysm exclusion, staged repair, or the use of concepts akin to perfusion branches are unlikely to be performed in the near future.

Spinal cord drainage and left subclavian revascularization is also used selectively in an attempt to diminish the risk of SCI. Although little prospective data exist regarding the benefits of elective left subclavian revascularization, it is common to follow the SVS practice guidelines.[43] Therefore, in patients with extensive aortic coverage and when coronary vasculature is dependent on an internal thoracic artery, a carotid subclavian bypass is performed. Lumbar spinal drains are used in most patients that undergo extensive aortic coverage, particularly when it involves the mid to distal thoracic aorta or when there is internal iliac compromise. The drains are placed and allowed to drain to 10 cm of water. Should neurologic deficits arise, the drainage can be lowered to 5 or 0 cm of water to encourage spinal cord perfusion. Simultaneously, attention is directed at the maintenance of adequate blood pressure. A mean arterial pressure in excess of 80 mm Hg is targeted throughout the procedure and during the perioperative period. The concern for SCI decreases after 72 hours or when evidence is provided by

CT scanning that the aneurysm sac is completely excluded. At that time, the spinal drainage catheter is removed, and the patient is closely observed for an additional 12 to 24 hours. Treatment options for patients with transient deficits or those with symptoms that are recurrent when cerebrospinal fluid drainage systems are removed include allowing for higher systemic blood pressures (usually achieved by reduction of the antihypertensive regimen) and revascularization of any diseased internal iliac or subclavian arteries.

CARDIAC

The incidence of cardiac events following endovascular thoracoabdominal aneurysm repair has been detailed in a single publication.[44] In this retrospective analysis, 266 patients were assessed for evidence of myocardial infarction and atrial and ventricular arrhythmias. It is difficult to compare these outcomes with other studies, and most of the historical open surgical series did not delineate patients with arrhythmias unless they required intervention (Table 37-6). However, this analysis reviewed only patients who underwent preoperative functional cardiac testing, ultimately concluding preoperative echocardiography to be of limited value in predicting which patients would suffer myocardial infarctions. Only echocardiographic evidence of mitral annular calcification was somewhat associated with postoperative myocardial infarction. That is not to say that such tests are not useful for patient selection or intraoperative management decisions, only that we could not define variables that were predictive in this patient group for myocardial infarctions. In contrast, ventricular arrhythmias were more common in patients with larger left atrial cavities, low ejection fractions, and large left ventricular mass or mass index; however, such events were not linked with death, and thus such patients warrant more intensive monitoring.[44]

The current paradigm for workup of patients before thoracoabdominal aneurysm repair differs depending on whether an endovascular or open surgical approach is planned. All patients undergo transthoracic echocardiography to assess ventricular and valvular function. Stress tests are still obtained for patients who will require extensive aortic repairs, patients with prior coronary artery bypasses or stents, and all patients who are sedentary to the point that they would be unlikely to elicit cardiac symptoms because of a lack of exercise. Catheterization is performed on any patient undergoing an open type II or III thoracoabdominal repair or in a selective manner for endovascular patients when functional studies question the integrity of the coronary circulation. Issues remain regarding how coronary artery disease, when detected, should be managed in the setting of a large, complicated aneurysm. Open surgical revascularization is associated with a considerable delay in aneurysm treatment with the interim risk of rupture; therefore it must be considered carefully on a case-by-case basis. Percutaneous intervention often requires the use of clopidogrel for a minimum of 30 days when conventional stents are used, or for years following placement of drug coated stents. Although endovascular repairs can be done while patients are receiving multiple antiplatelet agents, the placement of spinal drainage catheters may become an issue. The later factor may deter the use of drug-coated stents in patients requiring percutaneous revascularization before procedures that will place patients at risk for paraplegia, or it may deter the use of spinal drainage catheters in patients who will truly benefit from the use of drug-coated stents.

PULMONARY

Patients with thoracoabdominal aneurysm frequently have chronic obstructive pulmonary disease (COPD) as well. In an analysis of 905 patients undergoing abdominal and thoracoabdominal aneurysm repair, 32% had COPD.[45] Pulmonary disease is likely the most common factor that precludes patients from undergoing open SR of thoracoabdominal aneurysms owing to the high risk of pulmonary complications. In this series,[45] COPD patients had a slightly longer hospital and intensive care unit stays, but equivalent perioperative mortality when compared with patients who did not have COPD. Even patients with severe pulmonary disease (GOLD classification III and IV[46]) fared as well as non-COPD patients in the perioperative period. However, during follow-up, COPD patients had shorter life expectancy and a greater risk of late pulmonary death. Akin to the paraplegia analysis, the presence of pulmonary disease as an independent risk factor for perioperative complications was overshadowed by other factors, including the extent of aneurysmal

disease, age, renal failure, and larger aortic diameters. During follow-up, the presence and severity of the COPD were indicative of survival differences for patients with infrarenal[47] or thoracoabdominal aneurysms.[45] In this light, the presence of COPD is not a contraindication for endovascular repair of thoracoabdominal aortic lesions in regard to perioperative risks, but it certainly alters the long-term survival benefit of elective aneurysm repair.

The presence of COPD has a paradoxical benefit when examining specific endovascular outcomes. For some reason, patients with COPD have fewer endoleaks and more favorable sac behavior when compared with non-COPD patients.[45,48,49] Perhaps this relates to the pathophysiology of aneurysm formation in COPD patients or to the effect of smoking (more common in COPD patients) on the small vessels that potentially contribute to type II endoleaks. Despite the fact that multiple authors have noted this observation,[45,48,49] there is no scientific explanation.

RENAL

Renal complications rank second to paraplegia in the factors that may dissuade clinicians from offering treatment options to patients with thoracoabdominal aneurysms. Only 55% of the patients examined by the authors for fenestrated or branched devices had estimated glomerular filtration rate greater than 60 mL/min per 1.73 m². Renal outcomes can be evaluated from the clinical perspective and in the context of endovascular complications. Clinically, the overall incidence of detrimentally effecting renal function (defined by a persistent decrease in estimated glomerular filtration rate (eGFR) more than 30% from baseline or a categorical change from no renal disease to mild, moderate, or severe disease based on the national kidney foundation definitions of renal dysfunction) was 12% to 13%. The bulk of the risk (more than 60% of clinical renal events) occurred during the perioperative period and was often attributed to technical issues with the procedure (renal vessel loss, stent thrombosis, distal renal dissection, or atheroembolic issues).[50] These observations draw attention to the need for careful management of the renal vessels during a repair, limiting the amount of catheter and wire manipulation within the aneurysm sac or the renal artery.

Mating stent-graft device choice may also influence late renal outcomes following fenestrated or branched endograft placement. Initial reports of fenestrated repairs noted a relatively high incidence of renal stenosis or occlusion following successful placement of a fenestrated device.[51] However, subsequent analysis demonstrated that many of these complications can be avoided by the use of covered renal stents rather than uncovered stents, although the latter is not an option for patients with thoracoabdominal aneurysms. Mohabbit's analysis of 518 renal arteries (287 patients) with a mean follow-up of 25 months calculated an estimated freedom from stenosis at 12, 24, and 36 months of 95%.[52] When uncovered renal stents were evaluated separately from covered stents, the freedom from renal artery stenosis at 36 months was 89% versus 95%, respectively ($p = 0.04$).[52] Consequently, it is uncommon to use an uncovered stent in isolation with any fenestrated or branched device.

ENDOVASCULAR

Device durability is the subject of many questions and controversies. There is no question that, as endovascular devices have become more complicated, the risk of endovascular specific complications and device integrity issues has increased. Even data pertaining to infrarenal aneurysms treated with endovascular grafts have been subject to renewed skepticism in regard to long-term aneurysm exclusion.[26] Problems can manifest in many ways, including stent fractures, fabric tears, component separation, device migration, branch thrombosis, type I or III endoleaks, and aneurysm growth. Although the overall incidence of any one of these device-related complications may be low, as a group they drive the need for follow-up vigilance and act as a potential deterrent for younger, healthy patients who might outlive their devices. The identification of these complications is only possible when patients undergo proper follow-up testing, which is then thoroughly reviewed by the clinicians. The resolution of such imaging studies will determine whether stent fractures can be detected.

The literature for branched and fenestrated endografts provides more detail about durability than contemporary reports of open thoracoabdominal repair. The patency of branch vessels, as well as other events that may lead to reintervention, is reported in Table 37-7. The overall

TABLE 37-7 Branch Vessel Patency Following Fenestrated Aortic Endograft

Reference	Vessel Patency (%)	Follow-up (Mo)
Semmens et al.[62]	90.5	17
O'Neill et al.[63]	90.7	19
Muhs et al.[64]	92	46
Ziegler et al.[65]	92.2	72
Scurr et al.[66]	96.6	24
Bicknell et al.[57]	97	12
Kristmundsson et al.[67]	96	25

Data from Semmens JB, Lawrence-Brown MM, Hartley DE, et al: Outcomes of fenestrated endografts in the treatment of abdominal aortic aneurysm in Western Australia (1997-2004). J Endovasc Ther 13:320–329, 2006; O'Neill S, Greenberg RK, Haddad F, et al. A prospective analysis of fenestrated endovascular grafting: intermediate-term outcomes. Eur J Vasc Endovasc Surg 32:115–123, 2006; Muhs BE, Verhoeven EL, Zeebregts CJ, et al: Mid-term results of endovascular aneurysm repair with branched and fenestrated endografts. J Vasc Surg 44:9–15, 2006; Ziegler P, Avgerinos ED, Umscheid T, et al: Fenestrated endografting for aortic aneurysm repair: a 7-year experience. J Endovasc Ther 14:609–618, 2007; Scurr JR, Brennan JA, Gilling-Smith GL, et al: Fenestrated endovascular repair for juxtarenal aortic aneurysms. Br J Surg 95:325–332, 2008; Bicknell CD, Cheshire NJ, Riga CV, et al: Treatment of complex aneurysmal disease with fenestrated and branched stent grafts. Eur J Vasc Endovasc Surg 37:175–181, 2009; and Kristmundsson T, Sonesson B, Malina M, et al: Fenestrated endovascular repair for juxtarenal aortic pathology. J Vasc Surg 49:568–574, 2009.

1-year patency of all branches is approximately 95%. There are no long-term surgical series with radiographic follow-up that define branch patency after open repair. Surrogate endovascular outcomes such as endoleaks, migration, and sac growth remain critical because they contribute to the need for reintervention in an effort to prevent late catastrophic events.

Not many groups have series with long enough follow-up to report branch stent patency for more than 1 year; however, in the study reported in 2010 of 100 patients and a total of 275 implanted branches by Verhoeven and colleagues, the 5 year patency is 93%.[53] Early in the current authors' at the Cleveland clinic, it was possible to perform an analysis of the renal branched and outcomes in the juxtarenal and group IV thoracoabdominal population. These branches were a focus because many of the early grafts involved renal arteries alone. As reported in 2009, the incidence of occlusion was 2.2% in the 231 renal arteries, with a mean follow-up of 15 months.[52] The type of stent was found to be important regarding occlusions, and secondary intervention was required for patients who had covered stents versus uncovered stents. Although contemporary reports of direct comparison between fenestrated and open procedure are not prevalent, Oderich and colleagues[54] reported outcomes in homemade fenestrated devices compared with debranching of aortic aneurysms. In their experience, the patency of primary branch or target vessels at 1 year was 97%, whereas the branch patency for debranching procedures was 98%.[54]

In the experience recently reported at the Cleveland clinic, 633 patients underwent fenestrated or branched endografting over a period of 10 years.[31] There were five late ruptures (0.8%) at a mean of 18 months after treatment. Three of the late ruptures were attributed to component separation and one to a noncontiguous aneurysm rupture. One patient died following failure of an open surgical graft distal to the endovascular repair. These observations, among others, have prompted careful scrutiny of device design plans along with analysis of late radiographic follow-up. Preliminary data suggest that the 30-day freedom from secondary intervention is 98% (95% CI, 96% to 99%), and the 5-year freedom from secondary intervention is 84% (95% CI, 78% to 90%) for all thoracoabdominal aneurysm repairs (Mastracci and Greenberg, personal communication, 2011). The incidence of component separation is 2% to date, and the risk of graft migration is 1%, with a mean event occurrence at 14 months (interquartile range [IQR], 6.1 to 14.9; Mastracci and Greenberg, personal communication, 2011). Mating stent-graft fracture incidence is low (less than 1% for each renal or visceral bed), and aortic stent-graft body stent fractures are exceedingly rare. As experience grows, the modes of failure for branched grafts will be reported in greater detail, and surveillance programs or device design changes will evolve the devices.

CONCLUSIONS

Endovascular repair of thoracoabdominal aneurysms is feasible and often safer than open surgical alternatives.

Although hybrid approaches exist, whereby extraanatomic bypasses are created to critical visceral branches followed by stent-graft placement, the procedure remains invasive and fraught with morbidity and mortality that might not differ significant from conventional surgery at experienced institutions. Fenestrated and branched grafting clearly mitigates the risk of pulmonary complications, the need for extensive dissections, and aortic cross-clamping, thus minimizing the physiologic effect on the patient. However, the procedure remains somewhat complicated, akin to open SR, and is associated with endovascular-specific complications including endoleak, device integrity issues, and migration. Iterative improvements of the devices used to treat such aneurysms continue to occur, and parallel technologies, specifically imaging advances, will facilitate the dissemination of this method of repair. Comparative and longer-term studies are anxiously awaited by clinicians to help determine the optimal management strategies for these complex patients.

References available online at expertconsult.com.

QUESTIONS

1. Fenestrated endografts were developed to:
   a. Achieve more proximal aortic seal when performing an endovascular repair of an abdominal aortic aneurysm (AAA)
   b. Repair concomitant aortic aneurysms and renal artery stenosis
   c. Reduce the incidence of spinal cord ischemia associated with endovascular aneurysm repair.
   d. Maintain perfusion of the false lumen of an aortic dissection

2. Currently commercially available fenestrated endografts:
   a. Are "off-the-shelf" in design, where one size fits most
   b. Must be customized with fenestrations
   c. Can include both fenestrations and true branches
   d. Are not currently commercially available within the United States.

3. Fenestrations are mated with the target vessels using:
   a. Bare metal balloon expandable stents
   b. Bare metal self-expanding stents
   c. Covered self-expanding stents
   d. Covered balloon-expanding stents

4. One of the most important aspects in performing a fenestrated endograft surgery is:
   a. Preoperative sizing and planning
   b. Securing a diverse stock of endovascular tools
   c. Preoperative imaging with aortic angiography
   d. Ensuring that the patient can tolerate a general anesthetic

5. Survival following fenestrated and branched aortic endografting is:
   a. Not significantly different than those undergoing open surgical repair
   b. Dependent on aneurysm extent
   c. Deaths are not typically related to aneurysm-related mortality
   d. All of the above

6. Spinal cord ischemia associated with fenestrated/branched endografting for thoracoabdominal aortic aneurysms is best defined by:
   a. Occurring at a rate similar to that observed in open surgery
   b. Being influenced most by the extent of aortic repair
   c. Concomitant occlusive disease in the hypogastric and/or subclavian arteries may increase in the risk.
   d. All of the above

7. The factor(s) associated with the development of postoperative renal failure include:
   a. The presence of preoperative renal insufficiency
   b. Technical issues with stent deployment in the renal artery
   c. The use of bare metal stents
   d. All of the above

8. One method to possibly reduce the risk of spinal cord ischemia associated with extensive aortic endografting include:
   a. Staged occlusion of the hypogastric arteries
   b. Staged repair with coverage of a portion of the aorta at one surgery, and then completion of the repair at another
   c. Performance of the surgery under controlled hypothermia
   d. Performance of the surgery under regional anesthesia

9. One of the most common co-morbidities that excludes patients from conventional surgical repair is:
   a. A history of carotid artery stenosis
   b. Congestive heart failure
   c. Chronic obstructive pulmonary disease
   d. Renal failure

10. True or False. Unlike conventional endograft repair, fenestrated/branched endografting is void of endoleak development.

ANSWERS

1. **a.** Fenestrated endografts were developed in order to provide a more durable proximal seal when treating AAA with an endograft. It allows the seal zone to be placed in the region of the renal and mesenteric vessels while preserving flow to these important structures.

2. **b.** Currently, fenestrated devices are available within the United States. These provide for customized devices with fenestrations that can be placed to accommodate renal and mesenteric arteries. True branched endografts (with directional branches) are not available in the United States outside of clinical trials, and "off-the-shelf" designs are only available within clinical trials at the time of this publication.

3. **d.** Fenestrations are mated with the target vessels using covered balloon expandable stents. Early data demonstrated that patency rates were significantly higher when covered stents were used compared with bare metal stents. While self-expanding stent designs can be used with directional branches, they are not appropriate for use with fenestrations as they do not provide sufficient radial force at the site of the fenestration to obtain a seal.

4. **a.** Preoperative sizing and planning is the most important aspect of fenestrated endografting. The patient's anatomy must be visualized along the length of aorta, iliac arteries, and femoral arteries. Surgeons must assure the ability to deliver the stent graft system into the aorta, and must design a fenestrated endograft configuration that will sustain target vessel patency and exclude the aneurysm. It is essential that preoperative imaging be obtained with high-resolution computed tomography with the ability to perform reconstructions. While the procedures are typically performed under a general anesthetic, they can be performed under local anesthesia with sedation or regional anesthesia.

5. **d.** All of the above. Despite the fact that patients enrolled in fenestrated/branched endograft trials are typically older, with more co-morbidities, than corresponding patients undergoing open surgical repair – survival differences between these two groups does not differ significantly. Mortality is high in patients that have more extensive aneurysms, as would be expected. Patients that undergo successful fenestrated endograft placement have a very low aneurysm-related mortality.

6. **d.** All of the above. Spinal cord ischemia (SCI) is a devastating complication of aortic surgery, and the use of fenestrated/branched endografts does not ameliorate its occurrence. It occurs more commonly in patients that have extensive aortic aneurysmal disease, such as type II thoracoabdominal aortic aneurysms. Concomitant occlusive disease in vascular beds that can provide collateral flow to the spinal cord (such as the internal iliac arteries and subclavian arteries) can increase the risk of developing this complication.

7. **d.** All of the above. Certainly the presence of preoperative renal insufficiency places patients at increased risk for the development of renal failure. Patients are exposed to iodinated contrast agents, and likely experience some degree of atheroembolization during renal artery manipulation. All of these factors can worsen the already poor renal function and lead to renal failure. Technical problems with stent deployment which can injure the renal artery (i.e., causing occlusion or dissection) significantly contributes to postoperative renal failure. The conversion to the use of covered balloon expandable stents has greatly reduced the incidence of renal branch failure in follow up.

8. **b.** There are a number of adjuncts that have been evaluated to help lower the risk of spinal cord ischemia. These include spinal cord drainage and left subclavian artery revascularization. There is mounting evidence that staging an extensive aortic repair may, in fact, decrease the risk of spinal cord ischemia. Much like the subclavian artery, maintaining patency to the hypogastric arteries likely reduces the risk of developing this complication.

9. **c.** Chronic obstructive pulmonary disease. Pulmonary disease is likely the most common factor that precludes patients from undergoing open surgical repair of thoracoabdominal aortic aneurysms repair. Nearly $\frac{1}{3}$ of patients undergoing fenestrated/branched endografting have severe COPD. These patients, however, did well after endovascular repair and fared as well as the non-COPD patients except for having a longer hospital stay.

10. False. Fenestrated/branched endografting is complicated by the development of endoleaks. Despite the more proximal seal zone, a small rate of type 1 endoleaks is identified. More common than in EVAR and TEVAR, patients undergoing fenestrated endografting have higher rates of type 3 endoleaks, likely due to the increased number of components that must interact with each other. Type 2 endoleaks appear to occur at similar rates.

CHAPTER 38

ACUTE AND CHRONIC AORTIC DISSECTION: MEDICAL MANAGEMENT, SURGICAL MANAGEMENT, ENDOVASCULAR MANAGEMENT, AND RESULTS

Juan Carlos Jimenez

Aortic dissection is one of the most complex clinical conditions encountered by vascular surgeons and is associated with significant morbidity and mortality in patients presenting with this disease. The first descriptions of aortic dissection occurred in the sixteenth century and were described in the autopsy of King George II of England in 1761.[1] First termed *aneurisme dissequant* by Laennec in 1819, arterial dissection occurs when a tear in the intimal layer of the vessel leads to separation of wall layers allowing blood to enter between two distinct channels. The newly formed channel layer is termed the *false lumen* and is separated from the true lumen by a septum composed of the aortic intimal and medial layers. Antegrade blood flow extends into the false lumen distally and may extend to aortic branches (arch, visceral, lower extremity), causing significant end-organ ischemia.

CLASSIFICATION

Acute versus Chronic

An aortic dissection is classified as *acute* if the diagnosis is made within 2 weeks of the initial onset of symptoms. Diagnosis beyond this time period leads to the classification of *chronic* dissection. Treatment varies based on the age of the dissection and the anatomic location of the entry tear; therefore appropriate classification is crucial for institution of proper therapy.

Anatomic Classification

Two distinct classification systems are currently used to classify aortic dissection based on the location of the intimal tear and the degree of distal extension (Figure 38-1). The DeBakey classification, first developed in 1965, classifies aortic dissection into four types:
- Type I: The entry tear originates in the ascending aorta and extends from the aortic arch into the descending or abdominal aorta for varying distances.
- Type II: The dissection originates and is confined to the ascending aorta.

- Type IIIa: The entry tear is just distal to the left subclavian artery, and the extent is limited to the descending thoracic aorta.
- Type IIIb: The dissection originates just distal to the left subclavian artery and extends for a variable distance of the abdominal aorta.

The Stanford classification categorizes the dissection primarily based on the location of the intimal tear. It is the more clinically relevant and referenced system for classification of aortic dissection.
- A Stanford type A dissection originates in the ascending aorta and encompasses DeBakey types I and II.
- A Stanford type B dissection originates in the descending aorta and includes DeBakey types IIIa and IIIb.

The majority of patients with Stanford type A dissections require urgent surgical repair because this disease entity is associated with high rates of mortality if left untreated. Common complications associated with untreated type A dissections include: intrapericardial rupture with cardiac tamponade, extrapericardial rupture, and occlusion of the arch branches resulting in end-organ ischemia. Conversely, patients with Stanford type B dissections do not usually require urgent surgical treatment and are treated with medical therapy. Certain indications for acute surgical treatment exist for these patients, which will be discussed later in this chapter.

INCIDENCE AND SURVIVAL RATES OF AORTIC DISSECTION

The annual age- and sex-adjusted incidence of acute aortic dissection has been estimated at 2.9 to 3.5 per 100,000 persons in modern series.[1,2] It occurs more commonly in men (4:1 male-to-female ratio) and type A dissections are more common than type B dissections.[1] Dissections are seen most frequently in the 40- to 70-year age range; however, patients with collagen vascular disorders (e.g., Ehlers-Danlos syndrome, Marfan syndrome) are usually seen at a much younger age.[3,4]

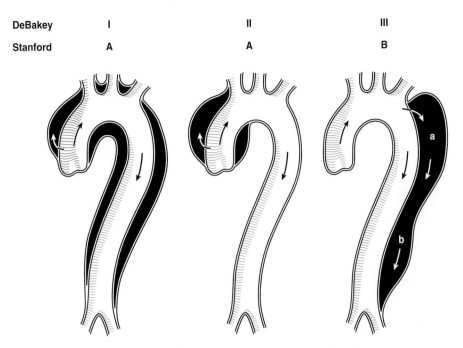

DeBakey   I   II   III

Stanford   A   A   B

FIGURE 38-1 ■ The DeBakey and Stanford classification systems for aortic dissection. (With permission from Erbel R, Alfonso F, Boileau C, et al: Diagnosis and management of aortic dissection. Eur Heart J 22:1642–1681, 2001.)

The mortality associated with acute aortic dissection is high and was estimated at 30% in the first 24 hours, 50% by 48 hours, and 90% at 1 year in a classic study by Hirst and colleagues.[4] Surgical mortality for acute type A dissections has been found to be 25.1% in a recent review of a population-based International Registry of Acute Aortic Dissection (IRAD) registry.[5] Operative mortality in patients with acute, complicated type B dissection approach 25% to 50%.[6] Despite the development of improved medical therapy regimens, early mortality for patients with acute type B aortic dissection ranges from 10% to 12%.[7]

RISK FACTORS

The most common risk factors for aortic dissection include advanced age, hypertension, and structural abnormalities of the aortic wall. More than 70% of patients are hypertensive. In a study by Juvonen and colleagues, older age, chronic obstructive pulmonary disease, and elevated mean blood pressures were unequivocally associated with aortic rupture following type B dissection.[8] Associated structural abnormalities of the aortic wall include: bicuspid aortic valve, aortic coarctation, and chromosomal abnormalities including Turner syndrome and Noonan syndrome. Hereditary conditions associated with collagen vascular disease are also risk factors (e.g., Ehlers-Danlos syndrome, Marfan syndrome). Marfan syndrome is the most common associated disorder in patients younger than 40 years with acute aortic dissection. In patients with Marfan syndrome, a mutation in the fibrillin gene leads to an alteration of the extracellular matrix in connective tissue,

resulting in aortic dilatation and dissection.[9] Pregnancy, especially with accompanying preeclampsia and hypertension, has also been shown to be an independent risk factor for this condition.[10] Cocaine and methamphetamine abuse are also associated with aortic dissection, especially in hypertensive male smokers.[11-13]

Seasonal variation has been observed in the development of aortic dissection with more patients being seen in the winter months.[14] It is also more likely to occur during the hours of 6:00 AM and 12:00 PM.[15] As with acute myocardial infarction or myocardial ischemia, physical and mental activities can also be triggers for acute aortic dissection.[16]

PATHOPHYSIOLOGY OF AORTIC DISSECTION

Aortic dissection is believed to occur when intraluminal wall stress exceeds aortic wall strength.[17] Therefore known risk factors such as hypertension and vessel diameter increase aortic wall stress, and collagen vascular disorders contribute to a reduction of wall strength, both contributing to the pathophysiology of the disease. Acute type A dissections tend to occur at the sinotubular junction, and type B dissections occur distal to the origin of the left subclavian artery. Nathan and colleagues[17] recently demonstrated, in a study using electrocardiogram-gated computed tomography angiography in 47 patients, that peaks of aortic wall stress exist in the sinotubular junction and distal to the left subclavian artery ostium, likely contributing to the development of type A and type B dissections in these locations. They also found that the wall stress proximal to the sinotubular junction exceeded that of the area distal to the left subclavian artery, thus supporting the increased prevalence of type A dissections compared with type B (Figure 38-2).

Once an intimal tear occurs, propagation of the dissection is a dynamic process that can result in both antegrade and retrograde (less common) propagation of blood flow through the false lumen. Fenestrations between the two channels connect the true and false lumen and occur downstream, usually at the origin of branch vessels. The most common location of the false lumen in type B dissections is in the posterolateral aorta (Figure 38-3, see color plate). Although significant variation occurs, the celiac trunk, the superior mesenteric artery, and the right renal artery most commonly arise from the true lumen, and the left renal artery arises from the false lumen.

The aortic wall surrounding the false lumen is significantly weaker than that of the true lumen. In the majority of patients, the false lumen has the larger diameter. A large false lumen diameter relative to the size of the true lumen has been shown to be a strong predictor for secondary dilatation in chronic dissections.[18] Sueyoshi and colleagues[19] followed 62 patients with chronic type B dissections and demonstrated that 83.9% of patients had one or more aortic segments increase in size during the follow-up period (mean, 49.1 months). Patients with blood flow in the false lumen had a significantly higher mean growth rate (3.3 mm/yr) than the group without blood flow (–1.4 mm/yr). The presence of blood flow in the false lumen was also the only significant risk factor for increase in the diameter in the univariate and multivariate analysis.

In a model of chronic type B dissection, Tsai and colleagues[20] demonstrated that diastolic false lumen pressures were highest in the setting of smaller proximal tear size and the lack of a distal tear. Therefore, the lack of an outflow tear may lead to false lumen expansion and dissection-related morbidity and mortality. Significant atherosclerosis is relatively infrequent in patients with acute aortic dissection, and it has been hypothesized that the presence of atheromatous plaque may serve to terminate or limit the extent of the dissection. One potential theory is enhanced fusion of the aortic wall layers secondary to inflammatory aortic wall plaques.

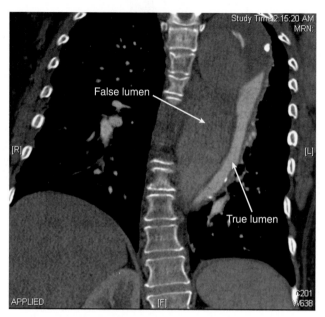

FIGURE 38-2 ■ Enlarged false lumen relative to the true lumen in a chronic type B aortic dissection.

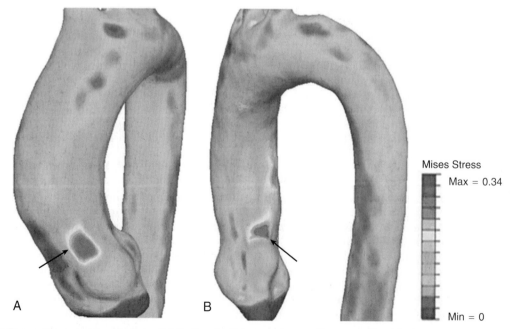

FIGURE 38-3 ■ Three-dimensional wall stress distribution for the normal ascending aorta. The black arrows indicate maxima of stress on the convex (**A**) and concave (**B**) sides of the ascending aorta. (From Nathan DP, Xu C, Gorman III JH, et al: Pathogenesis of acute aortic dissection: a finite element stress analysis. Ann Thorac Surg 91:458–464, 2011.) See Color Plate 38-3.

Weakening of medial collagen and elastin fibers within the aortic wall is a pathologic process referred to as *cystic medial necrosis* and has been implicated in the development of aortic dissection.[21] Patients with hereditary connective tissue disorders such as Marfans or Ehlers-Danlos syndromes universally demonstrate cystic medial necrosis in the aortic wall. Patients without these disorders but with aortic dissection also tend to have a higher degree of cystic medial necrosis than the general population.

CLINICAL PRESENTATION

Pain in the chest, back, and abdomen is the most common symptom of acute aortic dissection. It is usually described as abrupt in onset and typically associated with a "ripping and tearing" substernal chest pain when type A dissection is present. Cardiac tamponade and aortic valve dysfunction can result in syncope, especially in the presence of a type A dissection. Horner syndrome from compression of the adjacent sympathetic ganglia is less common but has been reported. Type B dissection is associated more with back and flank pain that may be migratory in nature. Paresthesias to the lower extremity can occur from lumbar plexopathy, and severe limb pain can occur in the setting of acute arterial ischemia from malperfusion. Pulse deficit with or without extremity ischemia in a patient with severe chest or back pain should raise the suggestion of an acute aortic dissection. Spinal cord ischemia can occur in up to 10% of patients with dissection in the descending thoracic aorta.

Malperfusion Syndrome

Malperfusion following aortic dissection is defined as the loss of adequate blood supply to vital organs owing to aortic branch vessel obstruction resulting in end-organ ischemia. This accompanying clinical process is a significant risk factor for increased morbidity and mortality in patients with aortic dissection.[22] In a study by the IRAD investigators, 15% of all deaths following aortic dissection were related to mesenteric ischemia.[23,24] Approximately one third of patients with type A dissection will also exhibit some manifestation of malperfusion syndrome.[25] Malperfusion can be classified into two distinct categories based on the physiologic mechanism of obstruction: dynamic and static.

Dynamic Malperfusion

Dynamic occlusion of aortic branches occurs when the dissection flap intermittently obstructs the vessel origin, resulting in end-organ malperfusion. This process can occur with both prolapse of the dissection flap into the vessel ostium, compression of the true aortic lumen resulting in inadequate blood flow to affected organs, or both. This type of malperfusion can vary with changes in hemodynamic forces influenced by blood pressure, cardiac output, heart rate, and peripheral vasoconstriction and resistance. The concept of dynamic obstruction is important to understand because patency of a branch on angiography or static imaging may not necessarily ensure vessel patency and adequate end-organ perfusion.

Augmented pressure within the false lumen may also contribute to significant compression of the true lumen and lead to increased dissection related-mortality.[26] Tsai and colleagues demonstrated that partial thrombosis of the false lumen was associated with increased postdischarge mortality in patients with type B acute aortic dissection.[24] The proposed hypothesis for this increased risk is that thrombus within the false lumen occludes distal tears, resulting in restricted outflow with a subsequent increase in false lumen pressure.[18] Medical management primarily through blood pressure reduction may improve the end-organ ischemia in patients with dynamic malperfusion. Patients who demonstrate clinical signs of persistent malperfusion despite optimal medical therapy will likely require endovascular or surgical treatment.

Static Malperfusion

Static malperfusion occurs when the dissection flap extends directly into the vessel orifice resulting in luminal narrowing or complete occlusion. This type of obstruction occurs less frequently than dynamic obstruction. Unlike dynamic malperfusion, this process is rarely improved despite optimal medical therapy or improved flow through the true arterial lumen. Thrombosis of the vessel distal to obstruction may exacerbate the degree of end-organ ischemia. Endovascular or surgical treatment, or both, are usually required for patients with continued malperfusion with static obstruction.

DIAGNOSTIC PITFALLS

The diagnosis of aortic dissection may often be misleading because the common clinical signs and symptoms in these patients are often attributed to various other clinical syndromes. As many as 65% of aortic dissections are misdiagnosed upon initial presentation in the emergency department.[27] Acute chest pain is commonly associated with myocardial infarction and acute coronary syndrome, and delayed or incorrect diagnosis can occur if a high index of suspicion for dissection is not present. In addition, positive electrocardiogram and serologic markers for acute myocardial infarction do not rule out associated aortic dissection. Peripheral neurologic symptoms may also be mistakenly attributed to musculoskeletal pain, neuropathy, or radiculopathy.

The following clinical scenarios should prompt immediate imaging studies to confirm the diagnosis of aortic dissection as well as urgent surgical consultation[28]:

- Chest pain with neurologic symptoms
- Chest pain with radiation to the back
- Chest pain with signs of arterial insufficiency
- Migratory chest pain
- Chest pain with associated severe back or abdominal pain
- Chest pain with widened mediastinum on chest radiograph
- Chest pain with a murmur of aortic insufficiency

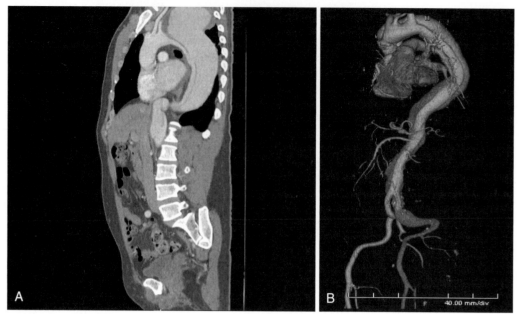

FIGURE 38-4 ■ Three-dimensional reconstruction following computed tomography for aortic dissection delineates the complex anatomy of this disease process. See Color Plate 38-4.

With these scenarios, initiation of intravenous antihypertensive therapy is imperative to prevent propagation of the dissection.

DIAGNOSTIC IMAGING

Chest Radiography

Chest radiography may reveal the presence of a widened mediastinum and aid in the diagnosis of aortic dissection. However, 10% to 20% of patients with aortic dissection have a normal chest radiograph.[29] Although chest radiographs should be obtained in all patients suspected of having this disorder, additional noninvasive imaging is usually required for confirmation of the diagnosis.

Computed Tomography

Computed tomography angiography (CTA) has become the noninvasive imaging study of choice to evaluate aortic pathology. Continued advances in CT scanning in regard to high spatial and temporal resolution have allowed comprehensive analysis of detailed elements for even the most complex dissections (Figure 38-4, see color plate).[30] Several recent studies have demonstrated a sensitivity and specificity for detection of aortic dissection and aortic intramural hematoma to be near 100%.[31-34] Reliable imaging of both the true and false lumens, location of the intimal flap, fenestrations and branch vessel involvement can be achieved with this diagnostic modality. Multidetector CTA with electrocardiograph-gated synchronization improves diagnosis of type A aortic dissections by decreasing motion-related artifacts in the ascending aorta and aortic valve.[35] Three-dimensional reconstructions can be rendered and used for endovascular or surgical planning.

Transthoracic and Transesophageal Echocardiography

Transesophageal echocardiography (TEE) allows high resolution imaging from the aortic root to the descending thoracic aorta. The proximity of the esophagus to the aorta, as well as decreased interference from the chest wall and lung allow high-quality images of the proximal aorta to be obtained. It is superior to transthoracic echocardiography (TTE) for imaging of the intimal tear, true and false lumens, coronary artery involvement, pericardial effusion, aortic valve regurgitation, and flow within the false lumen. Several studies have demonstrated the accuracy of TEE for the diagnosis of aortic dissection with a sensitivity of 86% to 100%, specificity of 90% to 100%, and a negative predictive value of 86% to 100%.[36,37] Sensitivity and specificity for TTE have ranged from 78% to 90% for ascending aortic dissections, but only 31% to 55% for descending aortic dissections. Specificity ranges from 87% to 96% for type A dissections and 60% to 83% for type B dissections.[35] Although TEE is superior for definitive diagnosis of aortic dissection, TTE can be performed rapidly in the emergency room setting and may be used to reliably evaluate the location of the intimal flap in the proximal ascending aorta, pericardial effusion and tamponade, and left ventricular function. It is important to note that a negative TTE result does not rule out aortic dissection, and additional imaging is required if there is a high degree of suspicion despite negative TTE results.

Magnetic Resonance Angiography

Because of long acquisition times, magnetic resonance angiography (MRA) is not as useful for immediate diagnosis of suspected acute aortic dissection. However,

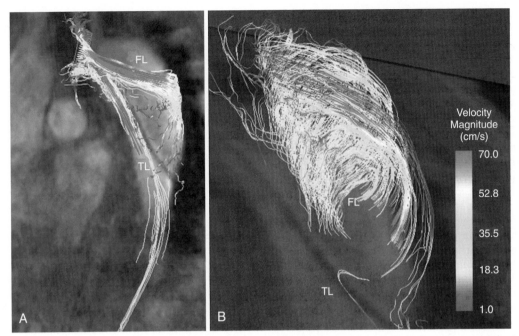

FIGURE 38-5 ■ Streamline visualization shows **(A)** parasagittal view of blood flow in the true and false lumen and **(B)** a double-oblique view of blood flow in the false lumen distal to the primary entry. (From Müller-Eschner M, Rengier F, Partovi S, et al: Tridirectional phase-contrast magnetic resonance velocity mapping depicts severe hemodynamic alterations in a patient with aortic dissection type Stanford B. J Vasc Surg 54:559–562, 2011.) See Color Plate 38-5.

contrast-enhanced three-dimensional MRA has an excellent reported sensitivity and specificity (95% to 100%) for the diagnosis of this disorder.[38] Similar to CTA, MRA can accurately determine the presence or absence of intimal flaps and branch vessel involvement. Information regarding false lumen perfusion can also be readily obtained and may be helpful in the evaluation of visceral ischemia and impaired branch vessel perfusion. Recently newer techniques, such as three-dimensional velocity-encoded cine magnetic resonance imaging, are being used increasingly for superior visualization of pathophysiologic hemodynamics and geometrically triggered changes in blood-flow characteristics within the dissected aortic lumens (true and false; Figure 38-5, see color plate).[39] Limitations of MRA include inability to perform the study in patients with pacemakers or other metallic implants, long examination times, poor tolerance in claustrophobic patients, and the association with nephrogenic systemic fibrosis in patients with advanced chronic kidney disease.

Angiography

The routine use of angiography in patients with aortic dissection is no longer indicated because of its invasiveness and the evolution of the previously described noninvasive imaging modalities for diagnosing aortic dissection. The IRAD investigators reported an overall sensitivity of 87% with aortography for diagnosing aortic dissection.[40] Sensitivities for type A and type B dissections were 87% and 89%, respectively. False negatives may also occur in the presence of intramural hematoma

and a thrombosed false lumen. The main indication for aortography is for endovascular treatment of aortic branches (e.g., angioplasty, stenting), the thoracic or abdominal aorta in association with stent-grafting, or fenestration. These techniques will be discussed later in this chapter.

TREATMENT OF AORTIC DISSECTION

Medical Therapy

Medical therapy is the treatment of choice for uncomplicated type B aortic dissections, with more invasive therapy (endovascular, surgical) reserved for patients with complications such as malperfusion and rupture. Because of high associated mortality if patients are left surgically untreated, medical therapy in patients with type A dissections is reserved for those who are not candidates for surgical therapy. Mortality in this patient group is extremely high. Inpatient admission to an intensive care unit and initiation of intravenous antihypertensive therapy for the purpose of lowering systolic blood pressure and pulse rate is the mainstay of treatment. Central venous access and arterial pressure monitoring should be used as well as Foley catheter measurement of urine output. β-Blockers, calcium-channel blockers, and vasodilators (nitroglycerin, sodium nitroprusside) can be used with the goal of reducing systolic blood pressure to less than 120 mm Hg and keeping the mean arterial pressure less than 80 mm Hg.[41] The patient should remain in the intensive care unit until blood pressure and pain are adequately controlled, and changes in clinical condition should be strictly monitored. Aggressive pulmonary therapy, deep venous thrombosis prophylaxis, nutritional support, and patient mobilization should be undertaken.[39] Indications for endovascular or surgical intervention include: rupture, expansion of the false lumen, retrograde dissection into the proximal aorta, malperfusion, or intractable pain.[39] Follow-up imaging with CTA should be performed just before inpatient discharge and subsequently at 6-month intervals if the dissection remains stable. Chronic dissections that remain unchanged can be followed with yearly CTA or MRA.

Despite optimal medical therapy, in-hospital mortality for uncomplicated type B aortic dissection has been reported at 8.3% in modern series.[39] Estrera and colleagues[7] reviewed the outcomes of 129 consecutive patients with the confirmed diagnosis of acute type B dissection. In-hospital mortality was 19% when vascular intervention was required. Complications included rupture (4.7%), stroke (4.7%), paraplegia (8.5%), acute renal failure (21%), and peripheral ischemia (4.7%). Mean hospital length of stay was 15 days (1 to 88 days), and the mean intensive care unit stay was 8 days (1 to 58 days). One-year and 4-year survival rates were 81.6% and 72.3%, respectively.

The IRAD investigators reported 13% overall in-hospital mortality for 384 patients with acute type B aortic dissections.[20] Most patients were managed medically (73%) with β-blockers used in 79% of nonhypotensive patients. Surgery and endovascular therapy was required in 15% and 12% of patients, respectively. Medically treated patients had lower mortality (9.6%) compared with surgically treated patients (32.1%). Hypotension or shock, absence of chest or back pain upon initial presentation, and branch vessel involvement were independent risk factors for increased in-hospital mortality.[20]

In a more recent follow-up study using the IRAD registry, 365 patients with acute type B dissection were categorized according to risk profile into two groups: patients with recurrent or refractory pain or refractory hypertension (group I) and patients without clinical complications at presentation (group II).[42] The in-hospital mortality following medical management was significantly increased in group I compared with group II (35.6% vs. 1.5%; $p = 0.0003$). Multivariable logistic regression analysis confirmed that recurrent or refractory pain or refractory hypertension following medical management was a strong predictor of in-hospital mortality.

In another review of 79 patients treated for acute type B aortic dissection, actuarial survival at 1 month and 8 years was 98.4% and 93.5%, respectively, in patients treated with medical therapy alone.[43] Of the patients who were managed medically, two patients developed subsequent type A dissections, one patient died from a late rupture, and two other patients died from mesenteric ischemia and pneumonia. In a similar study, Onitsuka and colleagues[44] identified the presence of a patent false lumen and a maximum aortic diameter of greater than 40 mm upon initial presentation as predictors of complications during long-term follow-up in a cohort of 76 patients treated medically for acute type B dissections.

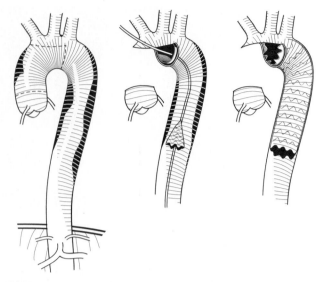

FIGURE 38-6 ■ Antegrade deployment of stent-graft during open repair of type A aortic dissection. (From Pochettino A, Brinkman WT, Moeller P, et al: Antegrade thoracic stent grafting during repair of acute DeBakey I dissection prevents development of thoracoabdominal aortic aneurysms. Ann Thorac Surg 88:482–490, 2009.)

Endovascular Treatment

Type A Dissection

Open surgical repair is the standard of care for the treatment of type A aortic dissections. Fenestrated endografts for aortic arch repair are currently in development, but are not available currently for clinical practice. However, "hybrid" techniques for managing acute aortic arch pathology have been described and are currently in use.[45] Pochettino and colleagues[45] demonstrated comparable results to traditional open surgical repair following antegrade stent graft deployment in the descending thoracic aortic dissection at the time of aortic arch replacement for acute type A dissection (Figure 38-6). Both groups demonstrated equivalent cardiopulmonary bypass times, rates of malperfusion syndrome, rates of stroke, and in-hospital mortality. Resultant false-lumen thrombosis in the thoracic aorta was significantly higher in the stented group (63%) compared with the non-stented group (17%).[43] In a follow-up study at the same institution by Desai and colleagues,[46] 40 patients underwent similar repair of acute type A dissection with antegrade stent-graft placement. The occurrence of postoperative stroke and early mortality were both 15%.[46] No patients developed permanent paraplegia. The long-term results of hybrid therapy for acute type A dissection are not yet known.

Type B Dissection

Endovascular repair for uncomplicated and complicated type B dissections remains a controversial topic, and there is a lack of definitive evidence regarding its use. There are several endovascular devices available for deployment in the thoracic aorta (Figure 38-7). However, in the United States, the current devices are approved by the U.S. Food and Drug Administration (FDA) only for

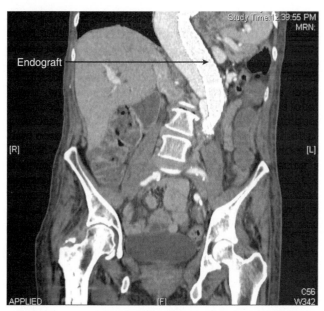

FIGURE 38-7 ■ Computed tomography following endograft deployment in the true lumen for type B aortic dissection.

the treatment of descending thoracic aneurysms and penetrating ulcer. The goals of endovascular therapy for this disease process are:

- Coverage of the entry tear
- False lumen thrombosis
- Reapposition of the true and false lumens
- Improved flow through the true lumen to improve organ perfusion
- Prevention of aneurysmal degeneration
- Avoidance of aortic cross-clamping and thoracotomy

Techniques of Endovascular Repair

Access into the true lumen is usually achieved via the femoral artery either with cutdown or percutaneously. Occasionally, iliac artery access with a conduit is required if the diameter of the femoral arteries is too small for device delivery. Transesophageal echocardiography and intravascular ultrasound (IVUS) can be used to verify placement of the guidewire in the true lumen and localize the location of the entry tear. Depending on which endovascular device is being used, sheath placement in the aortic arch may be required before endograft positioning. A marker pigtail flush catheter is placed into the ascending aorta through contralateral femoral or brachial access. A 260-cm stiff guidewire is then positioned in the ascending aorta and the endograft is advanced to the level of desired deployment. Ideally, 2 cm of seal zone proximal to the entry tear is required to minimize type I endoleak. If coverage of the left subclavian artery is required, carotid-subclavian bypass prior to thoracic endovascular repair is performed in the presence of a dominant left vertebral artery, a patent left internal mammary artery to coronary artery bypass graft, or in patients with a history of arm ischemia. In the emergency setting, left carotid-subclavian bypass is not required and can be performed

postoperatively in symptomatic patients.[47] Balloon angioplasty of the endograft is generally avoided, especially in patients with acute dissections because the risk of retrograde dissection or rupture is high in these patients.

Aortic Remodeling Following Thoracic Endovascular Repair

There is evidence that aortic remodeling occurs following endograft coverage of the dissected true lumen and the proximal intimal tear, and it may decrease the risk of future aneurysmal degeneration.[48] Conrad and colleagues[46] at the Massachusetts General Hospital reviewed their results following 33 thoracic endovascular repair (TEVAR) cases for complicated type B aortic dissection. Postoperative CT images demonstrated partial or complete false lumen thrombosis at 1 year in 88% of patients. Maximal aortic diameters and false-lumen diameters decreased significantly over time ($p = 0.4$ and 0.46, respectively) and true-lumen diameters increased over time ($p = 0.02$) in this patient cohort. Huptas and colleagues[49] demonstrated similar results in their series of 27 patients who underwent TEVAR for type B dissection. In this study, true and false lumen volumes over the entire descending aorta were measured using contrast enhanced CT at baseline and at follow-up (mean, 14 ± 6 months). TEVAR resulted in a continued increase in total true-lumen volume compared with patients who underwent medical therapy alone. Total false-lumen volume also decreased significantly in the TEVAR group; however, no significant change in false-lumen volume was noted in the medical therapy patients.

INSTEAD Trial: Uncomplicated, Chronic Type B Dissection

The first and only published randomized trial comparing TEVAR and medical therapy for uncomplicated type B dissection is the INSTEAD trial.[50] One hundred forty patients with stable, chronic (>14 days) type B dissection were randomized to optimal medical therapy plus stent-graft placement versus optimal medical therapy alone. Patients with acute and complicated type B dissections were excluded from this trial. There was no significant difference in all-cause survival rates between the two groups at 2 years. Survival at 2 years was 97.0% ± 2.0% with medical treatment alone and 94.4% ± 2.7% with TEVAR. Of note, significant aortic remodeling was noted in the TEVAR group compared with the medical therapy cohort. Following TEVAR, 91.3% of patients demonstrated aortic remodeling (with true-lumen recovery and thoracic false-lumen thrombosis) compared with only 19.4% in the medical therapy demonstrating these changes on postoperative CT.

Complicated Acute and Chronic Type B Dissection

In a nonrandomized study by Oberhuber and colleagues,[51] 19 patients underwent TEVAR for chronic type B dissections. Indications for endovascular intervention were: aneurysmal degeneration (>6 cm) and rapid aortic expansion (>1 cm/yr). The primary technical success rate was 94.7%, and there were no in-hospital deaths. Persistent paraplegia occurred in one patient (5.2%). The late reintervention rate was high after maximal follow-up of 124 months (47.3%). Indications for reintervention were: increase in aortic diameter, persistent perfusion of the false lumen, and type I endoleak. These interventions included: distal–proximal stent-graft extension (n = 8), replacement of the aortic arch owing to retrograde dissection (n = 1), and open infrarenal aneurysm repair (n = 1). No late deaths were noted to result from stent-related complications.

Several recent studies have demonstrated favorable results following TEVAR for the treatment of acute, complicated type B dissections. White and colleagues[52] analyzed 1-year outcome data following emergency TEVAR for patients with complicated type B dissections. Indications for repair were malperfusion (71.8%) and rupture (31.8%). In this cohort of 99 patients, the point-estimate mortality rate at 30 days was 10.8% and 29.4% at 1 year, comparing favorably to published studies of open thoracic aortic surgical repair[53,54] and TEVAR[55] for acute, complicated type B dissection.

Verhoye and colleagues[56] performed TEVAR in 16 patients within 48 hours for acute, complicated type B dissection. Early mortality was 25%, but no late deaths were noted. Actuarial survival at 1 and 5 years was 73 ± 11%. Parsa and colleagues[56a] reported a 63% actuarial survival in a similar patient cohort with an aorta-specific actuarial survival of 94%. Thus, TEVAR for the high-risk patient cohort of acute type B dissection appears promising; however, randomized trials are required to provide definitive evidence of its benefit. A summary of modern series' results following TEVAR for type B dissection is presented in Table 38-1.

Endovascular Fenestration

In the setting of acute malperfusion syndrome following acute type B dissection, percutaneous fenestration of the dissection flap is an option for restoration of organ perfusion. Although several different techniques are generally performed, the principles of endovascular fenestration include percutaneous catheterization of the true and false lumina with identification of entry tears or puncture through the dissection flap. Balloon angioplasty is used to enlarge the fenestration and provide improved end-organ perfusion through the true lumen. Aortic stents can be used to expand the true lumen if significant collapse persists following fenestration. If the organ bed perfused by aortic branch vessels is persistently impaired by extension of the dissection flap into the vessel origin, stenting of the orifice can be used to restore flow.

One early series of 40 patients treated with endovascular fenestration for complicated type B dissection demonstrated a successful revascularization rate of 93%.[57] The 30-day mortality was 25%, and five late deaths were noted. At a mean follow-up of 29 months, the remaining 25 patients demonstrated persistent relief of ischemic symptoms. Midulla and colleagues[58] reported a 100% technical success rate in a more recent study following this procedure for 35 patients treated for malperfusion syndrome secondary to dynamic compression. A 34%, 30-day mortality was noted, and thoracic and abdominal aortic diameters were not significantly different after fenestration (mean follow-up, 48 ± 30 months).

Limitations of endovascular fenestration compared with TEVAR include minimal stabilization of associated aneurysmal disease and no direct influence on false lumen thrombosis and aortic remodeling. Recent evidence has demonstrated that TEVAR is associated with redirection of flow back into the true lumen, resulting in organ reperfusion, and may lead to false lumen thrombosis and prevention of aneurysmal degeneration.[59] Thus, primary stent-grafting followed by secondary fenestration is likely the treatment of choice for patients with acute malperfusion syndrome following aortic dissection.

Surgical Management

Type A Dissection

Acute type A dissection is a life-threatening emergency, and urgent surgical repair is indicated for suitable

---

TABLE 38-1   Endovascular Repair of Type B Aortic Dissection: Results of Contemporary Series

Study	Year	Acute or Chronic	Complicated?	No. of Patients	Mean Follow-up (Mo)	Complete False-Lumen Thrombosis (%)	Permanent Paraplegia (%)	Stroke (%)	In-Hospital Mortality (%)	Late Mortality (%)
White et al.[52]	2011	Both	Yes	99	12	NR	9.4	9.4	10.8	29.4
Oberhuber et al.[51]	2011	Chronic	Yes	19	13 (median)	5.3	5.3	0	0	5.3
Parsa et al.	2010	Both	Yes	55	7.1	65	2	0	2	37
Ehrlich et al.	2010	Acute	Yes	32	26	NR	9.4	0	12	19
Nienaber et al.[50] (INSTEAD)	2009	Chronic	No	68	24	91.3	2.9	1.5	2.8	11.1
Feezor et al.[55]	2009	Acute	Yes	33	5.5	75	15	12	21	39
Verhoye et al.[56]	2008	Acute	Yes	16	36	25	6.3	0	25	27
Szeto et al.	2008	Acute	Yes	35	18.3	74.1	2.8	2.8	2.8	6.6
Dake et al.	1999	Acute	Yes	19	13	79	5.2	0	16	0

operative candidates. The IRAD registry reported an overall mortality of 55.9% for patients treated without surgery.[60] Potential complications of untreated type A dissections include: pericardial tamponade, coronary artery obstruction, malperfusion of the great vessels, and rupture. Despite timely surgical intervention, perioperative mortality rates still remain significantly high. Trimarchi and the IRAD investigators[60a] reported a 25.1% in-hospital mortality rate in 526 patients who underwent surgical intervention for acute type A aortic dissection. Among nonsurvivors, 41% of patients died within 48 hours after the beginning of the operation, and mortality in patients with surgical treatment delayed beyond 24 hours was 17.1%.[5] Independent preoperative predictors of operative mortality were: a history of aortic valve replacement, migrating chest pain, hypotension, preoperative cardiac tamponade, and preoperative limb ischemia.

A recent study by Sun and colleagues[61] reported significantly improved results compared with the IRAD registry with a reported in-hospital mortality of 4.67% in 257 patients who underwent surgical treatment for type A disease. Fifteen patients developed postoperative respiratory failure, two patients experienced permanent paraplegia, and two patients had postoperative strokes.

Several different techniques are generally used for the surgical management of acute type A dissection, depending on the presenting anatomic variation. A median sternotomy with total cardiopulmonary bypass is performed with selective use of hypothermic cardiopulmonary arrest and antegrade cerebral perfusion. Replacement of the ascending aorta with resection of the intimal tear can be used for most patients without involvement of the aortic root or aortic valve.[62] Detailed operative strategies for repair of acute type A dissection are beyond the scope of this chapter.

Type B Dissection

Type B dissection is associated with lower overall mortality compared with type A dissection.[6] Patients in stable condition with uncomplicated type B dissections are managed medically with favorable outcomes as described previously, and these treatment protocols have reduced the role of surgery to approximately 15% of cases.[63,64] Complicated type B dissections are accompanied by worsening clinical signs and conditions, which include aneurysmal expansion, aortic rupture, hypotension, signs of visceral and/or limb ischemia, poorly controlled hypertension despite optimal medical treatment, and persistent and refractory pain. Under these circumstances, surgical correction has been the mainstay of treatment.

Trimarchi and colleagues[6] reported an in-hospital mortality of 29.3% for patients requiring surgical treatment for acute type B dissection in a recent review.[6] Preoperative malperfusion was present in 30% of patients, which included 14.5% of patients with mesenteric ischemia or infarction, and 16.9% with limb ischemia. Surgical intervention was indicated for aortic rupture in 23.1% of patients, for visceral ischemia in 23.9%, and for limb ischemia in 15.5%. Preoperative hemodynamic status was the primary factor determining surgical outcome in

this series, whereby patients with severe hypotension and shock on admission or at the time of surgery had a mortality of 60%. The other independent predictor of surgical mortality was age greater than 70 years. Factors associated with favorable outcomes included: radiating pain, normotension at the time of surgery, and reduced hypothermic circulatory arrest time.

A recent review from Baylor University (Houston, Texas) identified 76 patients who underwent surgery for acute type B dissection over a 16-year period.[65] Eight patients required hypothermic circulatory arrest, and 15 patients required left heart bypass. Rupture was a presenting sign in 17 patients (22.4%). Perioperative mortality was 22.4% (17 patients), including 11 patients (14.5%) who died within 30 days of operation. Five patients developed postoperative paraplegia (6.6%), 15 patients (19.7%) required postoperative hemodialysis, and 7 patients required permanent hemodialysis.

The most common indication for surgical treatment in patients with chronic type B aortic dissections is aneurysmal expansion. A study by Estrera and colleagues[66] demonstrated that 50% of patients undergoing repair of thoracic aortic aneurysms had an associated chronic dissection. Zoli and colleagues[67] repaired 104 chronic distal aortic dissections over a 13-year period. Aneurysmal degeneration was the most common indication for surgical repair (73%). Other indications included: rupture (11%), visceral malperfusion (6%), and intractable pain (6%). The reported in-hospital mortality in this series was 9.6%, with 4.8% of patients developing permanent paraplegia. Survival at 1, 5, and 10 years was 78%, 68%, and 59%, respectively. In this patient cohort, the presence of atheroma in the resected aorta and age were independent risk factors for long-term survival.

Surgical Repair of Complicated Type B Dissection

Despite the lack of randomized, controlled trials supporting the unequivocal use of TEVAR for complicated type B dissections, the significant morbidity and mortality associated with surgical repair of this disease process warrants first-line endovascular management. A variety of surgical treatment options exist based on the anatomic variation of the dissection and the patients' clinical presentation. Traditional surgical management of acute type B dissection is complication specific, and the aim is to prevent aortic rupture and relieve malperfusion secondary to obstruction.

When a proximal type B dissection is present, the goal is to close the intimal tear and eliminate flow through the false lumen in order to promote false lumen thrombosis and reestablish flow to compromised critical aortic branches. Traditional surgical correction of proximal, complicated type B dissection involves exposure through a left posterolateral thoracotomy. Total cardiopulmonary bypass and circulatory arrest are rarely required; however, in the study by Bozinovski and Coselli, these techniques were used in 19.7% and 10.5% of patients, respectively.[54] The aortic cross-clamp is usually placed between the left common carotid artery and the left subclavian artery, and can sometimes be placed distal to the left subclavian artery if the intimal tear is more distal in the descending

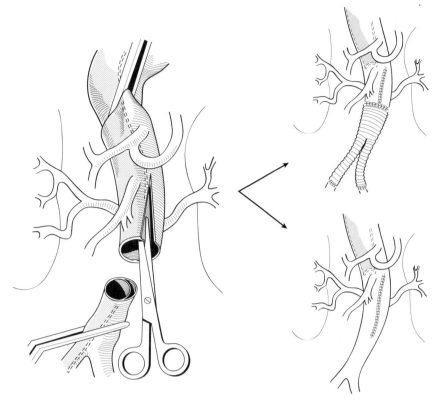

FIGURE 38-8 ■ Different techniques for fenestration and reconstruction of the abdominal aorta following fenestration for dissection. (From Panneton JM, The SW, Cherry KJ, et al: Aortic fenestration for acute or chronic aortic dissection: an uncommon but effective procedure. J Vasc Surg 32:711–721, 2000.)

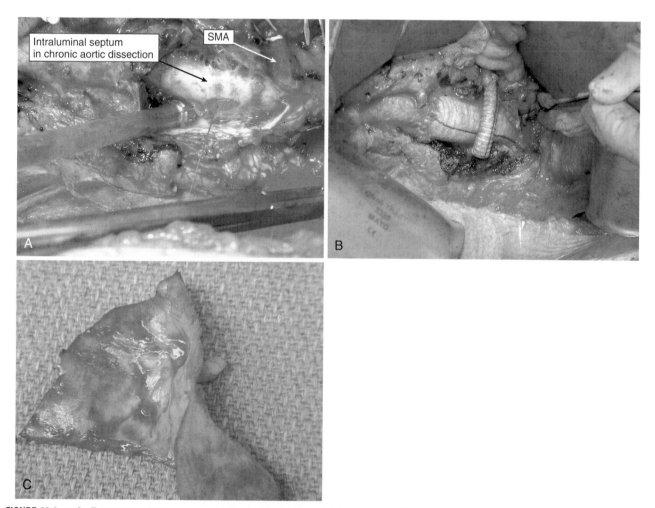

FIGURE 38-9 ■ **A,** Exposure of the septum between the true and false lumina following chronic dissection in the visceral aorta. **B,** Reconstruction following aortic fenestration with interposition graft and renal artery bypass. **C,** Septum removed following aortic fenestration in a chronic aortic dissection. (Photographs courtesy William J. Quinones-Baldrich.)

thoracic aorta. A short, woven Dacron graft can be used for central aortic replacement following resection of the intimal tear. Teflon strips in addition to glue aortoplasty are used to enhance anastomotic integrity. If the repair does not completely remove the entire length of dissected aorta, the septal flap should be taken to the distal aortic wall to reperfuse the true lumen.[52]

When malperfusion persists despite proximal surgical repair or when a more distal dissection is present with clinical evidence of malperfusion, surgical fenestration can be used to restore adequate organ perfusion. The goal of surgical fenestration is to provide free, unobstructed flow and equalization of pressures between the true and false lumina.[68] When the dissection involves the visceral aortic segment, external control of the renal and mesenteric branches is obtained through a left thoracoabdominal or retroperitoneal approach, depending on the extent of the disease process. Following supraceliac clamping, a longitudinal aortotomy can be used to resect the septum between the true and false lumina and inspect the orifices of the visceral and renal arteries. The clamp can be moved to the infrarenal aorta before reconstruction of the infrarenal aorta either with aortoiliac or aortofemoral bypass or primary closure (Figure 38-8). Aortorenal or aortovisceral bypass may be used if static obstruction persists following aortic fenestration (Figure 38-9).

References available online at expertconsult.com.

QUESTIONS

1. Which of the following is true regarding the incidence of aortic dissection?
   a. It occurs more commonly in women
   b. Type B dissections are more common than Type A
   c. Patients with collagen vascular disorders generally present at an earlier age
   d. Aortic dissection is more common in the elderly (> 70 years of age)
   e. The majority of patients with Type A dissection do not need intervention

2. The following are recognized risk factors for aortic dissection:
   a. Uncontrolled hypertension
   b. Ehlers-Danlos Syndrome
   c. Structural abnormalities of the aortic wall
   d. Methamphetamine abuse
   e. All of the above

3. Which of the following is true regarding the pathophysiology of aortic dissection?
   a. Acute Type A dissections tend to occur at the sinotubular junction
   b. Acute Type B dissections tend to occur just proximal to the left common carotid artery
   c. The aortic wall following the false lumen is significantly stronger than the true lumen
   d. The true lumen is always larger than the false lumen
   e. The celiac trunk and the superior mesenteric arteries always arise from the false lumen

4. Regarding the clinical presentation of aortic dissection, which of the following is true?
   a. Pain in the chest, back and abdomen is the most common presenting symptom of acute aortic dissection.
   b. Horner syndrome from compression of the adjacent sympathetic ganglia has been described.
   c. Spinal cord ischemia may occur as a result of Type B dissection
   d. Pulse deficit with or without extremity ischemia in a patient with severe chest and back pain may be indicative of acute aortic dissection.
   e. All of the above

5. Which of the following is true?
   a. Magnetic resonance angiography is the most commonly indicated radiographic examination in patients with acute aortic dissection
   b. Reliable imaging of both the true and false lumens is available with computed tomography angiography (CTA).
   c. Transthoracic echocardiography (TTE) is superior to transesophageal echocardiography (TEE) to image intimal tears in aortic dissection.
   d. Angiography should be obtained prior to CTA even in clinically stable patients.
   e. MRA has poor sensitivity and specificity for aortic dissection.

6. Optimal medical management for Acute Type B dissections includes:
   a. Inpatient admission to an intensive care unit
   b. Central venous pressure monitoring and arterial pressure monitoring
   c. Strict urine output monitoring with a Foley catheter
   d. Intravenous antihypertensive therapy
   e. All of the above

7. Indications for mandatory subclavian artery revascularization following endovascular repair of Type B aortic dissections include:
   a. Patients younger than 30 years of age
   b. A dominant contralateral vertebral artery
   c. A patent left internal mammary artery to coronary artery bypass graft
   d. Patients without evidence of arm ischemia upon presentation
   e. All of the above

8. Which of the following is true regarding the Investigation of STEnt grafts in Aortic Dissection (INSTEAD) trial?
   a. It was the first randomized trial comparing TEVAR and optimal medical therapy for uncomplicated Type B dissection
   b. There was no significant difference between all cause survival rates between the two treatment groups.
   c. Significant aortic remodeling was noted in the TEVAR group
   d. Patients with complicated Type B dissections were excluded from the trial
   e. All of the above

9. Which of the following is true regarding Type A dissection?
   a. Emergent surgical repair is usually required in patients with acute Type A dissection
   b. Endovascular repair with fenestrated stent grafts is the current FDA approved standard of care for treatment of Type A aortic dissections
   c. A preoperative predictor of operative mortality following Type A dissections is preoperative cardiac tamponade.
   d. A and C
   e. All of the above

10. Which of the following is true regarding surgical repair of complicated acute Type B dissection?
    a. The aortic cross clamp is usually placed between the left common carotid artery and the left subclavian artery
    b. Circulatory arrest and cardiopulmonary bypass are not usually required
    c. A woven Dacron graft may be used to replace the aorta following resection of the intimal tear
    d. Teflon strips and glue aortoplasty are techniques which may be used to enhance anastomotic integrity
    e. All of the above.

ANSWERS

1. c
2. e
3. e
4. e
5. b
6. e
7. c
8. e
9. d
10. e

CHAPTER 39

ANEURYSMS OF THE AORTA AND ILIAC ARTERIES

Jerry Goldstone

Aneurysms of the abdominal aorta are common. The incidence (the number of new cases) has been increasing for more than 3 decades, having tripled since 1970. The increased incidence has been noted in the United States and other Western countries; it is due not only to the aging of the population and improved diagnostic methods, but also to an absolute increase in the number of new cases.[1-4] It is estimated, from large national health screening programs, that 1.1 million Americans have this condition—a prevalence of 1.4% in the 50- to 84-year-old population.[5]

Approximately 190,000 new cases are diagnosed and more than 50,000 repairs are performed annually. The incidence and prevalence vary, depending on a number of factors, including the population studied; it is lowest in unselected groups and higher in patient groups with other atherosclerotic lesions (Table 39-1).[5-10] In a study at Massachusetts General Hospital, abdominal aortic aneurysms were found in 2% of 24,000 consecutive autopsies.[6] In a more recent autopsy series from Malmö, Sweden, abdominal aortic aneurysms were found in 4.3% of men and 2.1% of women.[6] This last study, as well as others, was performed on an almost entirely white population, and it is known that aneurysms are most common in white males. Aneurysms were found in 5.9% of male smokers older than 55 years in a U.S. Department of Veterans Affairs (VA) screening program.[8] The prevalence in screening studies from Asian and African countries is much lower, because it is among African and Hispanic Americans (ratio of white to African American is 3.5:1). The male-to-female ratio is 4:1 to 5:1 in the 60- to 70-year-old group, but beyond 80 years old the ratio approaches 1:1. The frequency of aneurysms increases steadily in men older than 55 years, reaching a peak of 5.9% at 80 to 85 years. In women, there is a continuous increase in prevalence after the age of 70 years, reaching a peak of 4.5% at age greater than 90 years. In community screening programs, the prevalence in men 65 to 74 years old ranges from 2.7% to 3.4%, whereas in elderly hypertensive men and women, the prevalence has been reported as high as 10.7% to 12%.[11-13] The increased incidence and prevalence noted over the past 3 decades has occurred in both men and women during a time when the incidence of death from coronary artery and other forms of atherosclerosis has been decreasing.

Abdominal aortic aneurysms, if untreated, are lethal lesions. They have a propensity for sudden rupture leading to death. Unfortunately, the age-specific death rate from ruptured aneurysms has increased along with the incidence. In the United States, approximately 15,000 deaths per year are due to abdominal aortic aneurysm, making it the thirteenth leading cause of death but the tenth leading cause of death in men older than 65 years. The importance of this condition is obvious, in that the proportion of elderly in the population is growing, there is no effective medical therapy, and rupture is a highly lethal event. The only way to reduce the death rate is to identify and treat these lesions before rupture occurs.

There is disagreement about the definition of an aneurysm, and several formulas have been proposed. The ad hoc committee on reporting standards of the Society for Vascular Surgery (SVS) and the International Society for Cardiovascular Surgery (North American chapter) defined an aneurysm as a permanent localized dilatation of an artery with an increase in diameter of greater than 50% (1.5-fold) its normal diameter.[14] This ratio accounts for the normal variability in aortic diameter owing to several factors, including age, sex, and blood pressure. The aortic diameter increases steadily with age. As a result, the infrarenal aortic diameter in a 75-year-old person can vary from 12.4 mm in a small woman to 27.6 mm in a large man.[15] An aortic diameter of 30 mm might not meet the definition of 50% increase in some people, but this value has been chosen as the definition for a number of studies on the natural history of small aneurysms and has been adopted by both the Society for Vascular Surgery and the European Society for Vascular Surgery because it is more than 2 SD above the mean for both men and women.[16,17] The normal sizes of the aorta in adult males and females are listed in Table 39-2.[14,15] Generalized dilatation of an arterial segment is frequently present in patients with aneurysms. When the diameter is increased less than 50% above normal, this is termed *ectasia*, whereas arteriomegaly represents diffuse enlargement of the arterial tree, but not large enough to meet the definition of aneurysm.[18] In some patients with abdominal aortic aneurysms, the entire aortoiliofemoral arterial tree is arteriomegalic or ectatic. Arteriomegaly is an interesting condition caused by a systemic alteration in the elastic components of the arterial wall. It was seen in approximately 5% of nearly 6000 patients undergoing arteriography in one series, and there were discrete aneurysms in at least three different locations in about one third of them. All were men who were approximately 5 years younger than those with solitary aortic aneurysms.[19]

651

TABLE 39-1   Incidence of Abdominal Aortic Aneurysms

Category	Incidence (%)
Autopsy	1.5-3.0
Unselected patients screened by ultrasonography	3.2
Selected patients with CAD	5.0
Selected patients with PVD	10.0
Patients with femoral or popliteal aneurysms	50.0

CAD, Coronary artery disease; PVD, peripheral vascular disease.

TABLE 39-2   Normal Diameter of Human Aorta*

Sex	11th Rib	Suprarenal Aorta	Infrarenal Aorta	Aortoiliac Bifurcation
Male	26.9 ± 3.9	23.9 ± 3.9	21.4 ± 3.6	18.7 ± 3.3
Female	24.4 ± 3.4	21.6 ± 3.1	18.7 ± 3.3	17.5 ± 2.5

Data from Steinberg CR, Morton A, Steinberg I: Measurement of the abdominal aorta after intravenous aortography in health and arteriosclerotic peripheral vascular disease. AJR Am J Roentgenol 95:703, 1965.
*All measurements in millimeters, plus or minus standard error.

Aneurysms of the infrarenal aorta are by far the most common arterial aneurysms encountered in clinical practice. They occur three to seven times more frequently than thoracic aneurysms. Men are affected more than women by a ratio of 4:1.8 Other aneurysms frequently coexist in patients with aortic aneurysms, including common or internal iliac aneurysms (in 20% to 30% of patients) and femoropopliteal aneurysms. Up to 85% of patients with femoral artery aneurysms have an aortic aneurysm. Popliteal aneurysms are also markers of abdominal aortic aneurysms. Aortic aneurysms can be found in approximately 8% of patients with a unilateral popliteal aneurysm, but in up to 60% of patients who have bilateral popliteal aneurysms. In at least one group of patients with carotid atherosclerosis, there was a 10% incidence of abdominal aortic aneurysm, and a 40% incidence of aortic aneurysms was found in another group of patients with tortuous internal carotid arteries.[19,20] Overall, multiple aneurysms occur in 3.4% to 13% of patients with thoracic aneurysms in approximately 12% of those with abdominal aortic aneurysms.[21,22]

SCREENING

There have been several recent large ultrasound-based screening programs involving over 149,000 persons to detect aortic aneurysms.[23,24] Aortic aneurysms were found in 4.9% to 7.6% of ultrasound-screened British men older than 65 years, but only in 1.3% of women. Similar data has been reported from Denmark, Australia, the Netherlands, and Norway. Although most screen-detected aneurysms are small (<4 cm) screening has been shown to be cost-effective and to reduce aneurysm-related, but not all-cause, mortality, at least in men.

Because it is impractical and financially unfeasible to screen all adults, screening programs have been designed based on known aneurysm-related risk factors. Cigarette smoking correlates with the presence of aortic aneurysms, with an 8:1 preponderance of aneurysms in smokers compared with nonsmokers.[25-27] Aortic aneurysms have been detected by ultrasound screening in 8.8% of male smokers older than 65 years who have peripheral vascular occlusive disease. There is also a well-recognized familial component to aortic aneurysms, present in 15% to 25% of cases. The current SVS Guidelines recommend screening for all men 65 years of age or older and for women 65 years and older who have smoked or have a family history of aortic aneurysm. These recommendations are somewhat more inclusive than those of the United States Preventive Services Task Force that did not include women without a family history or men who had never smoked. Nevertheless, this leads to Medicare offering ultrasound screening to men 65 to 75 years old who have smoked at least 100 cigarettes as well as in both men and women of the same age with a family history of aneurysm. It is reasonable to also recommend screening for all first-degree relatives of any patient with this diagnosis, based on the known genetic relationships.[28]

Hypertension is another common accompanying condition, found in up to 40% of patients with aortic aneurysms. These and other associations have implications regarding the cause of aneurysms.

PATHOGENESIS OF AORTIC ANEURYSMS

There are several well-known but uncommon causes of abdominal aortic aneurysm, including cystic medial necrosis, dissection, Ehlers-Danlos syndrome, HIV, and syphilis. More than 90%, however, are associated with atherosclerosis, which has traditionally been considered the primary cause.[29] Although aneurysms and occlusive atherosclerosis share most of the same risk factors (e.g., aging, tobacco use, hypertension, male gender, hypercholesterolemia) and atherosclerosis is uniformly present in the wall of aortic aneurysms, it is believed that several factors in addition to atherosclerosis are involved in aneurysm development.[30-34] One observation that casts doubt on atherosclerosis being the sole cause of aortic aneurysms is that most patients with aneurysmal disease do not have occlusive vascular disease involving the aortoiliofemoral segments. It has been estimated that no more than 25% of aortic aneurysms are associated with significant occlusive disease. Another factor is the negative association of diabetes with aneurysms in contrast to its strong relationship with occlusive vascular disease. In addition, induction of aneurysms in animals fed an atherogenic diet has not been predictable, although regression of experimental atheromas has led to aneurysm formation in monkeys. These plus other observations have led to the concept that atherosclerosis is either a coincidental or a facilitating process rather than the primary cause and that complex biological processes are responsible for the destruction of the media of the aortic wall that characterizes aneurysms.

Mature elastin and collagen are the major structural proteins responsible for the integrity of the aortic wall. Collagen composes approximately 25% of the wall of an atherosclerotic aorta, but only 6% to 18% of an aneurysmal aortic wall. Biochemical studies have shown decreased quantities of both elastin and collagen, but an increased ratio of collagen to elastin in the walls of aneurysms.[35,36] Elastin fragmentation is the initial structural event in aneurysm formation, and elastin depletion is complete early in aneurysm development. This has been correlated with the histopathologic features of a thin, dilated wall with fragmentation of elastin in the media, its replacement by a much thinner layer of collagen (mostly types I and III), loss of smooth muscle cells, and remodeling of the extracellular matrix. This thinned wall usually contains calcium and atherosclerotic lesions, rendering the

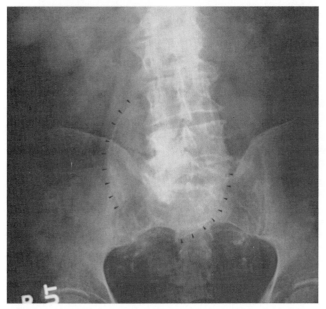

FIGURE 39-1 ■ Plain abdominal radiograph showing large aortic aneurysm with calcified rim *(arrowheads).*

wall brittle. Laminated thrombus lines the lumen, often eccentrically, resulting in a nearly normal flow channel (Figures 39-1 to 39-3; see color plate for Figure 39-3*C*), but possibly making the inner layers of the aortic wall relatively hypoxic. Aneurysms elongate as they dilate, causing them to become bowed and tortuous. It is believed that the weakening and fragmentation of the elastic lamellae is what permits vessels to lengthen excessively and become tortuous. As a result, the failure of elastin to provide sufficient retractive force in both the circumferential and longitudinal directions allows for increased aneurysm diameter and length, respectively.

The aortic wall is composed of lamellar units that consist of collagen (mainly types I and III) and elastin, as well as vascular smooth muscle cells. There are more lamellar units in the thoracic (58) than in the abdominal aorta (40), and there is a further abrupt decrease below the renal arteries (26). This factor is believed to have a role in the predilection for aneurysms to develop in the terminal portion of the aorta combining with the fragmentation of the elastin and the overall thinning of the wall to contribute to its weakening.[27] The large loss of elastin is one of the most consistent biochemical and histochemical findings in human aortic aneurysms.[37,38] A chronic inflammatory cell infiltrate is also prominent. A key unresolved question is what triggers this inflammatory reaction and the subsequent chain of events. Many theories have been proposed, including a reaction to mural atherosclerotic plaque or a latent infectious process (e.g., *Chlamydia pneumoniae* or oral flora).[39-41]

These well-established histologic features have prompted a search for nonatherogenic mechanisms that disrupt collagen and elastin in the aortic wall. Several investigators have found excessive collagenase (matrix metalloproteinase [MMP]-1, -2, -3) activity in the wall of aneurysmal aortas, and others have found increased elastase (MMP-9) activity. These are members of a family of MMPs that are believed to have an essential role in aneurysm formation. MMP-9 is found in abundance in medial smooth muscle cells as well as in inflammatory cells, and

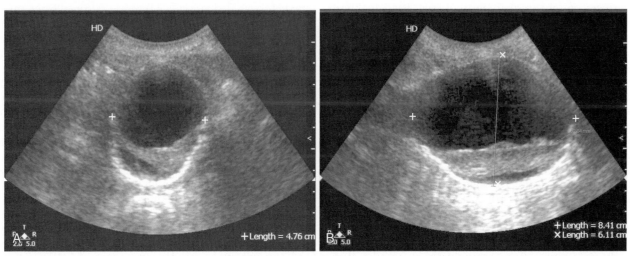

FIGURE 39-2 ■ **A,** B-mode ultrasound scan showing large aortic aneurysm measuring 47 mm in diameter and mural thrombus on posterior wall (transverse view). **B,** B-mode ultrasound scan in the same patient showing large aortic aneurysm (61 mm), mural thrombus, and enlarged flow channel (sagittal view).

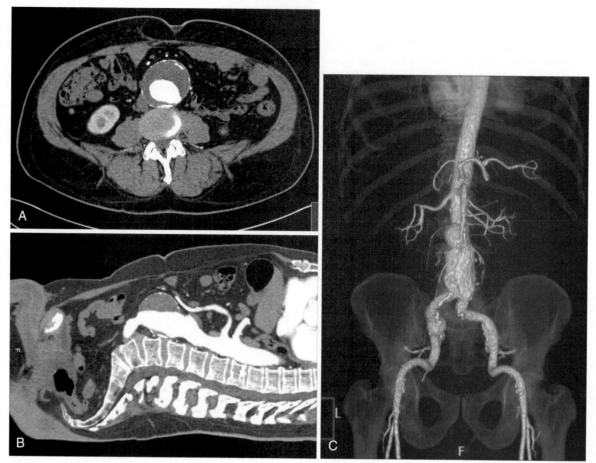

FIGURE 39-3 ■ **A,** Computed tomographic scan of the abdomen showing a large aortic aneurysm with partially calcified wall and abundant mural thrombus (axial view). **B,** Sagittal reconstruction showing the posterior flow channel, superior mesenteric artery, and celiac arteries. **C,** Three dimensional reconstruction, anteroposterior view, showing only the flow channel. Note the irregular aneurysm shape. See Color Plate 39-3.

increased levels have been found in both the aortic wall and serum in up to 50% of patients with aortic aneurysms, but not in those with aortic occlusive disease. These increased serum levels decline to normal after aortic aneurysm repair. Increased activity of other matrix proteases in aneurysmal aortic tissue has also been reported, as has an increased leukocyte-derived elastase in the blood of smokers with aneurysms. Deficiencies in antiproteases, such as several tissue inhibitors of metalloprotease and α_1-antitrypsin, have also been described. α_1-Antitrypsin is one of the most important natural antagonists to elastase and is responsible for the association between chronic obstructive pulmonary disease (emphysema patients with reduced α_1-antitrypsin levels) and increased prevalence of aortic aneurysm and increased rate of rupture. Another factor is the chronic inflammatory infiltrate that occurs in the outer layers of aneurysmal aortas, consisting of macrophages and T and B lymphocytes. There are also increased levels of cytokines, immunoglobulin (Ig) G, and IgM that are not seen in association with aging or with occlusive aortic lesions. These findings may be the explanation for the increased levels of serum inflammatory markers, such as Il-6, C-reactive protein, neutrophil elastase, and others found in patients with aneurysms but not in those with occlusive

disease. These inflammatory cells and cytokines are believed to interact in some as yet unexplained way with the connective tissue cells and matrix proteins in the pathogenesis of aneurysms.[39,40] Most of the research has focused on the aortic media, but the role of the adventitia in aneurysm formation has recently received some interest. Normally, the adventitia is thought to limit maximal aortic diameter. Topical application of elastase to the adventitia leads to aneurysm formation in experimental animals solely owing to degradation of elastin.[42]

Although not all the studies are conclusive, it is generally agreed that an imbalance between aortic wall proteases and antiproteases is an important factor in the pathogenesis of human abdominal aortic aneurysms. This imbalance causes degradation of extracellular matrix and loss of structural integrity of the aortic wall, and it is largely responsible for the extensive remodeling of the aorta that occurs during aneurysm formation.

There is also considerable evidence that there is a genetic susceptibility to aortic aneurysm formation.[43-49] Several investigators have discovered genetically linked enzyme deficiencies that are associated with aneurysms in experimental animals. For example, Tilson and Seashore[45,46] showed that a deficiency in the copper-containing enzyme lysyl oxidase is the cause of aortic aneurysms in a strain of mice. Lysyl oxidase is important in collagen and elastin cross-linking, and this enzyme defect is sex chromosome linked. In addition, several reports of familial clustering of abdominal aneurysms support the notion of a genetic predisposition to this disease. Approximately 20% to 29% of patients with abdominal aneurysms have a first-order relative with the same condition.[49] The age- and sex-adjusted increased risk of having an aneurysm is 11.6 times, according to one report. Female siblings are at particularly high risk. The genetic pattern of increased susceptibility is yet to be completely worked out. Available evidence supports both X chromosome–linked and autosomal dominant patterns of inheritance. Among the mutant suspect genes are the type III collagen gene *(COL3A1)* and the fibrillin gene (on chromosome 15). So-called familial aneurysms do not appear to be anatomically or clinically distinguishable from those with no familial pattern, except that they develop earlier in life, have a decreased male-to-female ratio of 2:1, and appear to have an increased risk of rupture. The clinical implications of these genetic studies, as limited as they are, strongly support the screening of all first-degree relatives of patients with abdominal aortic aneurysms.

Hemodynamic (mechanical) factors may also contribute to aneurysm development. The abdominal aorta is subjected to large pulsatile stresses as a result of its tapering geometry, relatively increased stiffness distally, and the reflected pressure waves from the peripheral vessels. Reductions in the number of elastic lamellae and the virtual lack of vasa vasorum in the media of the distal abdominal aorta may also be factors favoring aneurysmal formation in this segment of the arterial tree, making the aorta structurally less capable of handling the increased hemodynamic stresses that occur there.[32]

In summary, contemporary concepts of aortic aneurysm formation and growth incorporate two distinctly different pathophysiologic processes: (1) elastin fragmentation as the critical structural defect required for aneurysm formation; and (2) collagen deposition, degradation, and remodeling governing aneurysm enlargement. These two processes result in a complex remodeling of the aortic wall. The other factors described previously, including inflammation, smoking, biomechanical wall stress, and genetic predisposition, interact with these processes to produce the clinical features that are so well recognized. Clearly, aortic aneurysm formation is far more complex than passive dilatation owing to age. Therefore these aneurysms should be referred to as *degenerative* or *nonspecific* rather than *atherosclerotic aneurysms*. They account for more than 90% of aneurysms involving the abdominal aorta.

ANEURYSM ENLARGEMENT

Once an aneurysm develops, it tends to enlarge gradually yet progressively. The enlargement rate has been well studied and averages 0.2 to 0.3 cm/yr for small aneurysms (3.0 to 5.5 cm diameter) to 0.3 to 0.5 cm/yr for larger aneurysms.[50] Unfortunately the growth rate is nonlinear, making it impossible to predict the rate of enlargement

of any individual aneurysm. Some aneurysms remain the same size for many years, whereas others enlarge rapidly. Factors associated with more rapid growth include larger initial size, hypertension, pulse pressure, active smoking, and cardiac or renal transplant. Interestingly, diabetes mellitus does not appear to be a factor in aneurysm development or growth. Once an aneurysm develops, regardless of the cause, its enlargement is governed by physical principles, especially Laplace's law, which describes the relationship between the tangential stress (T) tending to disrupt the wall of a sphere, the radius (R), and the transmural pressure (P): $T = PR$. Thus, for a given transmural pressure, the wall tension is proportional to the radius. Once dilatation of the aorta has started, Laplace's law explains why aortic enlargement is enhanced. It also explains why large aneurysms are more prone to rupture than small ones and why hypertension and pulse pressure are important risk factors for rupture. Using Laplace's law, tripling the aortic radius from 2 to 6 cm results in a more than threefold increase in wall tension, and when this tension exceeds the tensile strength of the collagen in the aortic wall, disruption occurs. Although Laplace's law has long been used as the sole explanation for aneurysm enlargement and rupture, it is at best an imperfect explanation because it was derived for perfect cylinders and spheres, and aortic aneurysms do not have uniform shape; it also does not consider the wall thickness, which can be highly variable. In addition, it does not explain why all aneurysms of the same diameter do not rupture or why some small aneurysms rupture and some large ones do not. Aneurysms usually do not rupture at the point of greatest diameter, as would be predicted by Laplace's law. Recent studies using finite element analysis of computed tomography (CT) scan–derived data have measured wall stress and strain patterns and have shown that, in addition to decreased tensile strength, aneurysm walls have increased wall stress, an asymmetrical shape, and a complex radius (actually many radii) of curvature.[51-55] Wall stress varies with shape and thickness, and the points of maximal stress do not necessarily coincide with the location of maximal diameter. They do, however, correspond closely with the location of rupture. Wall stress data might also explain why eccentric and saccular aneurysms have a greater risk of rupture than those with smooth fusiform shapes. The influence of calcification and mural thrombus on stress patterns is uncertain but may be important. These stress analyses have been validated by several investigators and may become a useful method for predicting risk of aneurysm rupture.

There has been wide interest in pharmacotherapy to reduce the rate of enlargement of small aortic aneurysms and thereby reduce rupture risk. β-Blockers have been studied in several randomized clinical trials with disappointing negative results. Similar results have been found with doxycycline and roxithromycin as well as angiotensin-converting enzyme inhibitors. Statins, however, have been found to reduce expansion rate and rupture risk. Unfortunately most of the studies with all these agents were not well designed or had insufficient statistical power to permit definitive conclusions, but it seems prudent for patients with small aortic aneurysms to be taking a statin drug for this purpose.[16,17]

CLINICAL MANIFESTATIONS

Seventy percent to 75% of all infrarenal abdominal aortic aneurysms are asymptomatic when first detected.[56] Detection can occur during a routine physical examination, but most often occurs during an imaging study performed for some other reason (e.g., upper gastrointestinal series, barium enema, intravenous pyelography, lumbosacral spine radiography, or abdominal CT or ultrasound examination). Occasionally, an aneurysm is first discovered during an unrelated abdominal operation.

Abdominal aortic aneurysms can cause symptoms as a result of rupture or expansion, pressure on adjacent structures, embolization, dissection, or thrombosis.[56,57] Compression of adjacent bowel can cause early satiety and even nausea and vomiting. Because the duodenum crosses in front of the aorta, it is the part of the bowel most frequently compressed. Virtually any type of abdominal, flank, or back pain can be caused by an aneurysm. This fact often leads to delays in diagnosis. Chronic abdominal or back pain is the most common symptom, occurring in up to one third of patients. Large aneurysms can actually erode the spine and cause severe back pain, even in the absence of rupture.

The abrupt onset of severe pain in the back, flank, or abdomen is characteristic of aneurysmal rupture or expansion. It is uncertain why pain is produced by an expanding but unruptured (intact) aneurysm. The best explanation is sudden stretching of the layers of the aortic wall, with pressure on adjacent somatic sensory nerves or overlying peritoneum. Tenderness of the palpated aneurysm suggests that abdominal symptoms are arising from the aneurysm, although tenderness by itself is not a reliable indicator of impending rupture. In most surgical series, symptomatic but unruptured aneurysms account for 6% to nearly 40% of cases (average of five series totaling 311 patients: 13.7%).[58] The timing of surgical treatment is made more difficult in these cases. A good-quality CT scan can show no sign of rupture but cannot predict when rupture might occur.

Ruptured aneurysms constitute between 20% and 25% of most series. The presence of an aneurysm is known in 25% to 33% of patients before rupture occurs. The nature of symptoms and their time course vary depending on the nature of the rupture.[58-60] Small tears of the aneurysmal sac can result in a small leak that temporarily seals with minimal blood loss; this is usually followed within a few hours by frank rupture, which produces a catastrophic medical emergency. Rupture most frequently occurs through the posterolateral aortic wall on the left side into the retroperitoneal space; less commonly, it occurs through the anterior wall into the free peritoneal cavity. The incidence of this latter type of rupture is higher than indicated in most surgical series, because most of these patients die before reaching the hospital. Rarely, an abdominal aortic aneurysm ruptures into the inferior vena cava or one of the iliac veins, producing an aortocaval (or aortoiliac) fistula, or it ruptures into the gastrointestinal tract, producing a primary aortoenteric fistula.

The classic clinical manifestations of ruptured aortic aneurysm consist of severe mid or diffuse abdominal pain, shock, and a palpable, pulsatile abdominal mass. The pain may be more prominent in the back or flank, or it may radiate into the groin or thigh. Because the most frequent site of rupture is the left posterolateral wall, pain is more commonly felt on the left side. The pain tends to be severe and steady. The severity of the shock varies from mild to profound, depending on the amount of blood loss. Abdominal distention is common, often preventing palpation of the expected pulsatile abdominal mass. The duration of symptoms can vary from a few minutes to more than 24 hours. Although aneurysm rupture is usually an acute catastrophic event, it can be contained for prolonged periods. These chronic ruptures have masqueraded as radicular compression, symptomatic inguinal hernia, femoral neuropathy, and even obstructive jaundice. It is thought that chronic contained ruptures eventually progress to free ruptures, and they should be treated surgically on an urgent basis.[61]

The pain of an expanding but intact aneurysm may closely mimic that of a ruptured one. It tends to be severe, constant, and unaffected by position. The signs of hypovolemia are absent because hypotension and shock do not usually occur in the absence of actual rupture.

The diverse and nonspecific nature of the pain caused by expanding and leaking aneurysms all too often leads to errors in diagnosis, delays in finally establishing the correct diagnosis, and catastrophic rupture in the midst of a diagnostic procedure. Occasionally, a patient with a contained rupture arrives in the emergency room with angina pectoris from blood loss and reflex tachycardia and is rapidly transported to a coronary care unit without the abdominal examination that would identify the true cause of the chest pain. A similar situation can occur with rupture into the vena cava, with the resulting aortocaval fistula presenting as congestive heart failure. Most diagnostic errors such as these are due to failure to palpate the expansile, pulsatile epigastric mass, or failure to consider ruptured aneurysm as a possibility.

DIAGNOSTIC METHODS

Aortic aneurysms lie against the thoracolumbar spine and project anteriorly in the midline in the epigastrium. Elongated tortuous aneurysms may be located to the right or left or even in the lower quadrants. Careful physical examination can detect most large aneurysms. Except in thin patients, an abdominal aortic aneurysm must be approximately 5 cm in diameter to be detectable on a routine physical examination. As a result, aneurysms are seldom palpated in obese patients unless they are large. The reported accuracy in establishing the correct diagnosis by physical examination alone ranges from 30% to 90%, depending on aneurysm size and body habitus.[62] However, even when an aneurysm is palpable, determination of its size by palpation is imprecise. Obesity, ascites, and lack of patient cooperation can impair aneurysmal detection by physical examination. Conversely, tumors or cystic lesions adjacent to the aorta, unusual aortic tortuosity, and excessive lumbar lordosis can all lead to a diagnosis of abdominal aortic aneurysm when none is present. The expansile nature of a pulsatile mass is a key element in deciding whether it is an aneurysm or a transmitted pulsation from an adjacent tumor.

Although physical examination detects most large aneurysms, more objective methods are necessary to measure size and identify smaller aneurysms. Size determination is especially important because it is the most important predictor of rupture risk and is usually the basis of management decisions. Plain abdominal and lateral spine radiographs can establish the diagnosis of 67% to 75% of abdominal aortic aneurysms by detecting linear calcification of the aortic wall (see Figure 39-1). Unfortunately, accurate determination of maximal aortic size is possible in only two thirds of these cases.

IMAGING MODALITIES

Several imaging modalities are widely available to establish the presence of an aortic aneurysm and accurately determine its size. These modalities include ultrasound, CT, and magnetic resonance imaging (MRI).

Real-time B-mode ultrasound is available in most hospitals and clinics and is the imaging method used in the large aneurysm screening and surveillance studies.[63-65] It uses no ionizing radiation, provides physiologic data as well as structural detail of vessel walls and atherosclerotic plaques, and can accurately measure aneurysm size in longitudinal and cross-sectional directions (i.e., it is three dimensional; see Figure 39-2). Compared with intraoperative measurements, ultrasonic measurements are accurate to within ±5 mm. Many studies have documented the ability of ultrasound to establish the diagnosis (100% sensitivity, 95% to 99% specificity) and accurately determine the size of abdominal and peripheral aneurysms.[62-64] Ultrasound has not been as useful for imaging the thoracic or suprarenal aorta because of the overlying air-containing lung and viscera. Similarly, it has been less reliable in defining the relationship between abdominal aortic aneurysms and the renal arteries. Because ultrasonography can obtain images in longitudinal, transverse, and oblique projections, it can be especially helpful in differentiating a tortuous aorta from an aneurysm. Ultrasound imaging is degraded by obesity, intestinal gas, or barium in the bowel. The overlying bowel gas also interferes with evaluation of the iliac arteries. The major advantages of ultrasound are its wide availability, painlessness, absence of known side effects, lack of ionizing radiation, relatively low cost, and ability to image vessels in multiple planes. These factors make ultrasonography the modality of choice for the initial evaluation of pulsatile abdominal or peripheral masses and for follow-up surveillance of aneurysms to determine increase in size and for screening. In addition, the portability of ultrasound machines is advantageous for the emergency department, where it can quickly establish the presence of an aneurysm in most cases, but it is not nearly as accurate (approximately 50%) in demonstrating rupture.

CT uses ionizing radiation to obtain cross-sectional images of the aorta and other body structures. These images provide detailed information about the size of the entire aorta, including the thoracic portion, so that the extent and size of an aneurysm can be measured accurately. Modern CT scanners using helical (spiral) technology and an increasing number of detectors possess sufficient spatial resolution to allow precise identification of the celiac, superior mesenteric, renal, and iliac arteries and their branches, as well as their relationship to the aneurysm and adjacent organs. Major venous structures, including anomalies, can also be identified.[49] The administration of intravenous contrast allows evaluation of the size of the aortic lumen, the location and status of aortic branch vessels, the amount and location of mural thrombus, and, in the presence of dissection, differentiation of the true lumen from the false lumen (see Figure 39-3; see color plate for Figure 39-3C). Contrast-enhanced CT scans are also useful for assessing the retroperitoneum and can identify retroperitoneal hematoma (aneurysmal rupture), renal abnormalities, and the periaortic fibrosis associated with inflammatory aneurysms[50-53] (Figure 39-4). Metallic surgical clips and orthopedic hardware create artifacts that can interfere with CT interpretation. And although the images are acquired in only one (transverse) plane, three-dimensional reconstructions creating a CT angiogram are now almost universally available. CT provides more information about other abdominal and retroperitoneal structures than does ultrasound. CT scanning has emerged as an excellent technique to image the abdominal aorta and its branches.[54] One of its most helpful aspects is the ability to define the relationship of an aneurysm to the renal artery origins. The multiplaner reconstructions are extremely helpful in clarifying the true anatomic relationships when there is anterior or lateral displacement of the aorta.[55] Scan times are

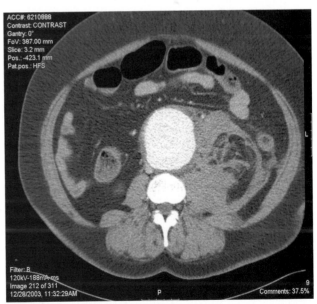

FIGURE 39-4 ■ Computed tomographic scan showing contained rupture of aneurysm into the left retroperitoneal space (axial view). Note the absence of mural thrombus. (From Clayton MJ, Walsh JW, Brewer WH: Contained rupture of abdominal aortic aneurysms: sonographic and CT diagnosis. AJR Am J Roentgenol 138:154–157, 1982 and Weinbaum FI, Dubner S, Turner JW, et al: The accuracy of computed tomography in the diagnosis of retroperitoneal blood in the presence of abdominal aortic aneurysm. J Vasc Surg 6:11–20, 1987.)

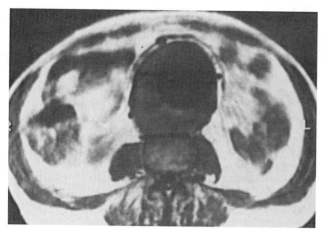

FIGURE 39-5 ■ Magnetic resonance image of a large abdominal aortic aneurysm showing eccentric mural thrombus and flow channel.

extremely short, and slices as thin as 2 to 3 mm can be obtained; this allows three-dimensional reconstruction of the overlapping cross-sectional images, producing a CT angiogram (See Figure 39-3C, see color plate). The reconstructed three-dimensional images can be rotated in space and viewed from any projection. CT angiography (CTA) is an excellent method of determining the often complex relationships among the aorta, its branches, and the aneurysm.[68,69] CT scans require significant radiation exposure and a relatively large volume of intravenously administered contrast material, which limits their usefulness in the presence of severe renal functional impairment. Non–contrast-enhanced images are useful for determining the degree and location of calcification in the aorta and its branch vessels. Overall, CT scans are currently the most useful imaging method for evaluating the abdominal aorta and have nearly obviated the need for catheter aortography in the evaluation of aneurysmal disease. CT is also an almost essential component of the process of determining an aneurysm's suitability for and size of endograft treatment.

MRI has also proved to be a useful modality for the evaluation of aortic disease (Figure 39-5).[71] MRI uses pulsed radiofrequency energy in a strong magnetic field to produce images in longitudinal, transverse, and coronal planes. MRI instruments are not as widely available as ultrasound or CT scanners, and the selection and interpretation of proper scan sequences and images require considerable experience and skill. The spatial resolution has significantly improved, but the presence of implanted metal-containing devices (surgical clips, cardiac pacemakers) or the need for monitoring equipment are contraindications to MRI. Also, MRI studies are more expensive and require more time than either CT or ultrasound. Nevertheless, MRI clearly distinguishes arteries and veins from viscera and other surrounding tissue, and there is excellent agreement between MRI and ultrasound or CT images in determining aortic diameter. MRI is better than ultrasound for demonstrating involvement of branch vessels, especially the renal arteries, with some authors reporting visualization of the renal arteries in more than 90% of cases.[72] Other advantages of MRI over CT are the lack of ionizing radiation, the ability to

obtain multiplane images (now also available with CTA), and the relatively large image field. In addition, MRI does not require the use of nephrotoxic contrast agents to achieve intravascular enhancement; however, paramagnetic contrast agents, such as gadolinium, are routinely used to improve the imaging of vascular structures. MRI machines are able to quantitate blood flow, although this feature is not commonly used clinically, and they can produce multiplanar reconstruction of the images that look like conventional angiograms (magnetic resonance angiography [MRA]). However, adequate visualization of aortic branch arteries is not achieved as frequently with MRA as with CTA, and a significant number of patients cannot undergo MR scanning because of claustrophobia.

Objective documentation of the aortic size should be accomplished with one of these imaging modalities in all patients with suspected abdominal aortic aneurysms. Each method can measure the diameter accurately. An initial scan can be used for comparison with subsequent scans to monitor aneurysmal enlargement. For most routine situations, ultrasonography is the method of choice because of its widespread availability, lower cost, and lack of ionizing radiation.[70] When there is suspicion of suprarenal or thoracoabdominal aortic involvement or dissection, MRI or CT is preferable. For preoperative planning in these complex cases, a multiplanar study with three-dimensional reconstruction (CTA, MRA) is usually necessary to clearly delineate the aneurysm, aortic branch vessels, and neighboring structures. This is especially true if treatment by endografting is being considered. CT and MRI probably have equal capability to demonstrate unexpected features such as venous anomalies, perianeurysmal fibrosis, and horseshoe kidney, although the ureters are not easily identified by MRI. For symptomatic aneurysms, MRI and CT also are better than ultrasound in their ability to identify contained rupture. The limitations of catheter aortography for the diagnosis and evaluation of aortic aneurysms, like those of plain film radiography, are well known. Because the mural thrombus that which is nearly always present tends to reduce the aneurysmal lumen size toward normal, aortography is not a reliable method to determine the diameter of an aneurysm or even to establish its presence. With better imaging methods now routinely available, aortography has little use as a diagnostic method for abdominal aortic aneurysms. However, it may be useful in the preoperative evaluation of selected patients with aneurysms to define the extent of the aneurysm, especially suprarenal and iliac involvement, the associated arterial lesions involving renal and visceral vessels, and distal occlusive lesions (Table 39-3). Although many of these associated lesions are readily detectable and appropriately managed intraoperatively, preoperative identification is useful in planning operative strategy, especially if complex anatomy is suspected. However, in most cases the same information can be obtained with CTA.

Aortography should be performed selectively in patients with aneurysms for the following indications: (1) clinical suspicion of visceral ischemia, (2) occlusive iliofemoral vascular lesions, (3) severe hypertension or

TABLE 39-3 **Angiographically Detected Lesions Associated with Abdominal Aortic Aneurysms**

Findings	No. of Patients	Number (n)	Percent
Suprarenal extension	680	46	6.7
Renal stenosis or occlusion	763	138	18.0
Accessory or multiple renal arteries	680	92	13.5
Celiac or superior mesenteric artery stenosis	628	87	13.8
Iliofemoropopliteal stenosis or occlusion	680	298	43.8
Iliofemoropopliteal aneurysm	680	243	34.7

Collected data from Rich NM, Clagett GP, Salander JM, et al: Role of arteriography in the evaluation of aortic aneurysms. In Bergan JJ, Yao JST, editors: Aneurysms: diagnosis and treatment, New York, 1982, Grune and Stratton, pp 233–241; Gaspar MR: Role of arteriography in the evaluation of aortic aneurysms: the case against. In Bergan JJ, Yao JST, editors: Aneurysms: diagnosis and treatment, New York, 1982, Grune and Stratton, pp 243–254.

impaired renal function in a patient in whom a concomitant renal artery stenosis would be repaired if discovered, (4) suspicion of a horseshoe kidney to delineate renal artery anatomy, (5) suspicion of suprarenal or thoracoabdominal aneurysm, and (6) presence of femoral or popliteal aneurysms. With the evolution and availability of CTA and MRA, it is possible to obtain information similar to that available from aortography with fewer risks. Newer CT scanners with large numbers of detectors (128 or more) perform even faster scans, with improved resolution and better three-dimensional images. Sophisticated three-dimensional reconstructions of CT scans are already available online from commercial vendors, making these sophisticated images available to any provider who can transfer the CT data onto a CD or transmit it electronically to the imaging facility.

RISK OF ANEURYSM RUPTURE

As noted earlier, the majority of abdominal aortic aneurysms are discovered in asymptomatic patients during an evaluation for an unrelated problem. Aneurysms are being discovered at a smaller size than when the original studies on their natural history were first published by Estes, Wright, Szilagyi, and others.[73-75] Most aneurysms detected in screening programs are small (<4 cm), which has permitted the development of new concepts about the natural history of these lesions. Although aneurysms can cause symptoms and serious consequences from thrombosis and distal embolization, rupture is the most important risk, and aneurysm diameter is the most important factor that determines the risk of rupture. In general, the risk of rupture correlates directly with size: the larger the aneurysm, the greater the risk of rupture. For example, the yearly risk of rupture for abdominal aortic aneurysms[5,30,63-65] between 4 and 5.4 cm in size is 0.5% to 1%; this increases to 6% to 10% for aneurysms between 6 and 7 cm and to 19% to 35% for aneurysms larger than 7 cm in diameter.[76-78] Calculated as 5-year rupture rates, these figures become 5%, 50%, and about 95%, respectively. The steepness of the curve plotting these data increases sharply at a diameter of approximately 5 cm, which is the basis for recommendations to defer elective aneurysm repair until a size of 5.0 to 5.5 cm is reached.[79] These data were provided from two randomized, controlled prospective clinical trials that studied survival in patients with asymptomatic abdominal aortic aneurysms that were between 4 and 5.4 to 5.5 cm in diameter: the United Kingdom Small Aneurysm Trial, published in 1998, and the Veterans Administration–sponsored Aneurysm Detection and Management (ADAM) trial.[80-83] These two trials were similar in design, size, and results. The rupture rate for aneurysms in these trials was 0.5% to 1% per year, as noted previously, and neither trial showed a difference in long-term survival, which was the primary end point, between patients allocated to early operation or ultrasonography or CT surveillance. The 6-year survival was similar in both trials, 64% in the U.K. trial and approximately 70% in the ADAM trial. Although 61% of those randomized to surveillance in both studies ultimately underwent aneurysm operation for enlargement or symptoms, long-term survival was not improved by early operation. Furthermore, delaying operation for these small aneurysms was not associated with increased operative or late mortality. These data are consistent with those from older, nonrandomized studies.[82,84,85] For example, population-based data from Rochester, Minnesota, showed a mean enlargement rate for aneurysms less than 5 cm in diameter of only 0.32 cm/year, and after 5 years of observation, no aneurysm smaller than 5 cm had ruptured.[85] Rupture risk may be higher in high-surgical-risk patients, but the ADAM and U.K. trials enrolled mostly good-risk patients. In both series, there was a higher rupture rate among the ineligible (i.e., high-risk) patients than in those randomized.

Other clinical features associated with increased risk of rupture include smoking, chronic obstructive lung disease, hypertension, female gender, transplant recipient, and rapid enlargement (defined as 1 cm/yr or more). Cronenwett and associates[86] showed that chronic obstructive pulmonary disease and systolic hypertension are predictors of increased risk of rupture of small abdominal aneurysms. In a subsequent study, they found that the rate of enlargement of small aneurysms was unpredictable, but either increased systolic or decreased diastolic pressure (i.e., increased pulse pressure) was associated with an increased rate of aneurysm expansion.[87] In this study, there was considerable variability in the rate of aneurysm enlargement, although the average rate of expansion was 0.4 cm/yr in anteroposterior dimensions and 0.5 cm/yr in lateral dimensions. Some data suggest that the expansion rate of small aneurysms can be diminished by β-adrenergic blockade (propranolol), which should lead to a decreased rate of rupture.[88] Unfortunately, this theory was not supported in three randomized clinical trials. Other studies have shown that aneurysms are frequently elliptical rather than round and that aneurysmal expansion is initially more rapid in the lateral direction. It is interesting to recall that the most frequent site of aneurysm rupture is in the lateral wall. In a review of four series, including their own, Cronenwett and coworkers[86] described the outcome of 378 patients with small aortic aneurysms initially treated nonoperatively. After an average follow-up of 31 months, 27% of the patients were alive with intact aneurysms, 29% had died of other causes, 39% had elective aneurysm operations because the aneurysm diameter reached 5 to 6 cm, and 4% had suffered aneurysm rupture or acute expansion leading to emergency operation. Overall, there was a mean 5-year survival of 54% in these patients, somewhat less than the 6-year survival rates of 64% in the U.K. trial and 70% in the ADAM trial.[83,84] In light of these more recent studies, autopsy studies showing high rates of rupture of small aneurysms must be interpreted with caution.[7] Some have shown that 23.4% of aneurysms between 4.1 and 5 cm rupture, and the same is true for up to 10% of aneurysms less than 4 cm in diameter. Data such as these have led surgeons to recommend operation for almost all aortic aneurysms in good-risk patients. However, autopsy studies underestimate aneurysm size owing to the lack of a distending blood pressure, and several more recent studies on living patients demonstrate a rupture rate of approximately 1% per year for aneurysms less than 5 cm in diameter.

There is little debate about the appropriateness of elective aneurysm surgery for patients with large aneurysms (>5.5 cm in diameter) because of the high risk of rupture and the associated mortality when rupture occurs. This is also true in so-called high-risk patients, because most of these patients will die from rupture and not from the conditions that caused them to be considered high risk. Several cohort studies indicate that women have a greater risk of aneurysm rupture at a given size than men; therefore it has been suggested that women be offered definitive treatment at a smaller aneurysm size (i.e., 4.5 to 5.2 cm) than men.[89]

It must be emphasized that although the risk of aneurysm rupture correlates most closely with aneurysm size, and the average rate of aneurysmal enlargement is known (0.4 to 0.5 cm/yr), it is impossible to predict when a small aneurysm will rupture in a given patient.[74] Perhaps the best explanation relates to the fact that aneurysms rupture at points of maximal wall stress, as discussed earlier, and areas of maximal wall stress do not necessarily coincide with areas of maximal diameter.[75,76] Clinical investigations of aneurysm wall stress using finite element analysis of CT-derived data are promising but not widely available. For now, diameter remains the best available predictor of risk of aneurysm rupture. The harmlessness of a small, asymptomatic abdominal aortic aneurysm is deceptive. Some do rupture, but coronary artery disease, and not rupture, is the most frequent cause of death in patients with small aneurysms.

RISKS OF SURGICAL TREATMENT

The natural history of untreated abdominal aortic aneurysms is well documented. This is especially true for

TABLE 39-4	Operative Mortality and Late Survival of Elective Open Surgical Treatment of Abdominal Aortic Aneurysm			
Reference	**No. of Patients**	**Mean Age (Yr)**	**Operative Mortality (%)**	**Cumulative 5-Year Survival (%)**
Levy et al. (1966)[99]	100	64	17	34
Szilagyi et al. (1966)[75]	401	—	15	49
May et al. (1968)[100]	135	—	13	49
Baker and Roberts (1970)[101]	240	63	9	54
Stokes and Butcher (1973)[102]	87	—	3	60
Hicks et al. (1975)[103]	225	67	8	60
O'Donnell et al. (1976)[104]	63	82	5	70
Crawford et al. (1981)[90]	860	66	5	63
Reigel et al. (1987)[105]	499	76	3	66
Bernstein and Chan (1984)[77]	123	71	1	72
U.K. trial (1998)[80]	563	69	5.8	64
Hertzer et al. (2002)[93]	1293	71	1.2	75
ADAM trial (2002)[81]	569	68	1.8	70
Dream trial (2004)[97]	174	69	4.6	Not given

those aneurysms measuring 5.5 cm or less in diameter. Since the first report of successful surgical resection and graft replacement of an infrarenal aortic aneurysm in 1952, many publications have documented the operative and long-term survival after surgical treatment. There has been a steady improvement in operative results for elective operations. Several large, contemporary series have reported operative mortality rates between 0.9% and 5% for university and other large, single medical centers and only somewhat higher rates for community hospitals.[90-106] The 1.8% operative mortality in the ADAM trial from selected VA medical centers compares favorably with these (Table 39-4). Higher mortality rates, ranging from 5% to 8%, have consistently been reported from analyses of large state-wide or national data bases. Lower operative mortality has also been found to be associated with operations performed in high-volume institutions and by high-volume surgeons, although the definitions of high volume are not uniform. The recently published SVS guidelines recommend that elective open surgical repair is best performed at centers with a documented in-hospital mortality of less than 5%. Operative mortality in this range (<5%) justifies elective repair, even for relatively small aneurysms in good-risk patients.

The general improvement in surgical results has occurred despite the fact that more patients are being operated on who are older and have more severe comorbid conditions. Preoperative detection and treatment of significant cardiac disease have been important factors, as have improved anesthetic and critical care management and better perioperative drugs such as β-blockers and statins.

Most of the deaths, even in elective operations, occur in so-called high-risk patients. Unfortunately, there is again no consensus on what constitutes high risk. Chronologic age is not as important as physiologic age in assessing operative risk; therefore patients should not be denied elective operation based solely on age. Even octogenarians can undergo elective aneurysm surgery with low morbidity and mortality rates.[94,95] Most vascular surgeons have successfully treated ruptured aneurysms in patients previously rejected for elective operation because they were considered too old.

The major risks for elective abdominal aortic aneurysm resection are similar to those for other major intraabdominal operations and include adequacy of cardiopulmonary and renal function. High-risk patients are those with unstable angina or angina at rest, cardiac ejection fraction less than 25% to 30%, congestive heart failure, serum creatinine level greater than 3 mg/dL, and pulmonary disease manifested by room air Po_2 of less than 50 mm Hg, elevated Pco_2, or both. A substantial percentage of these high-risk patients will die of ruptured aneurysm and not from the disease that led to their categorization as high risk. With intensive perioperative monitoring and support, aneurysm resection has been performed even in these high-risk patients, with operative mortality of less than 6% by Hollier and colleagues[107] and others.[90,102,103] Therefore, even in high-risk patients, large abdominal aneurysms should be considered for elective treatment if the appropriate support facilities are available. It is in this group, however, that endovascular repair can be expected to offer significant improvement in survival over standard open aneurysm repair. Already in the United States the majority of aneurysm repairs are being treated with this technology; this has resulted in a higher proportion of open repairs being complex, but the anticipated increased morbidity and mortality has not been documented. However, this trend in complexity of open repair could be reversed with more wide-spread use of fenestrated and branched endografts for juxtarenal, pararenal, and suprarenal aneurysms. The consistent findings from clinical trials are that 50% to 60% of patients with abdominal aortic aneurysms are anatomically suitable for endoluminal repair with current commercially available devices and that it can be accomplished with mortality rates equal to or lower than those for open surgical repair. Morbidity rates are clearly lower than those for open surgical repair, hospital stay is shortened, and patient satisfaction and surgeon enthusiasm are high; however, all aortic aneurysms can be treated by open repair. In addition, because of lingering uncertainties about long-term results of endovascular repair, there is uncertainty regarding which patients and which

aneurysms are best treated in this manner. For these reasons, the indications for endoluminal repair should be the same as those for open surgical repair in terms of aneurysm size and expected longevity. Endovascular aneurysm repair is covered in detail in Chapters 40 and 41.

Despite widespread elective aneurysm treatment programs, the incidence of aneurysm rupture has not decreased. A substantial percentage (50%) of patients whose aneurysms rupture die before reaching a medical facility. An additional 24% arrive at a hospital alive but die before a definitive operation can be performed; therefore operative mortality figures underestimate the true significance of aneurysmal rupture. The overall mortality from ruptured aneurysms, as reported in two large community-based studies, ranges from 74% to more than 90%.

The operative results for ruptured aneurysms are not nearly as favorable as those for elective aneurysm repair and generally have not improved greatly over the years.[108-111] Although there are a few series with better results, nearly 50% of patients die after being operated on for rupture. The nature of the rupture influences the results. Less than 10% of patients presenting in shock with free intraperitoneal rupture survive. In contrast, patients in stable condition with small, contained leaks have a better than 80% survival rate. Several authors have reported improved mortality rates (30% to 35%) using endovascular treatment for ruptures, and others have reported no survival advantage.[112,113] The operative mortality at University Hospital Case Medical Center for open repair of ruptured aneurysms over the past 5 years is 27% (unpublished data), which is in the same range as most of the endovascular repair (EVAR) studies. In one study, endovascular treatment of ruptured aneurysms yielded worse outcomes in nonteaching and low-volume EVAR hospitals.[112]

The factors contributing to failure in the treatment of ruptured abdominal aortic aneurysm have been reviewed by Hiatt and associates.[108] The four most important factors were failure to perform elective aneurysmectomy in patients with known aneurysms; errors in diagnosing rupture when it occurred, leading to delay in operation; technical errors committed during the operation (all venous injuries); and undue delays in induction of anesthesia. These are all realistically preventable. Other series have also attempted to identify factors leading to death after aortic aneurysm rupture. Repeatedly, delays in performing surgery and the total volume of blood transfused are found to be important.[109,110] Preoperative cardiac arrest, female gender, age 80 years or older, massive blood loss, and ongoing major transfusion requirements were predictors of 90% to 100% mortality in the series by Johansen and colleagues,[111] which included a highly efficient transport and resuscitation response. Some of the differences in operative mortality among various reports are due in part to inconsistencies in patient categorization or considering all forms of rupture together. Many of these series also fail to separate patients with unruptured but symptomatic aneurysms who undergo emergency operations. The operative morbidity and mortality for this group are intermediate between elective, asymptomatic patients and those with frank rupture, averaging 16% to 19%.[85,114] It has been postulated that the reasons for this increased mortality is the omission of the usual preoperative evaluation and preparation necessitated by the emergency operation as well as institution-based issues related to emergency procedures during nights and weekends.

LATE SURVIVAL

The most common cause of death among patients with large abdominal aortic aneurysm is rupture. The objectives of surgical repair are to prevent rupture and thereby prolong life. Without doubt, surgical repair prevents rupture, but does it prolong life, and what is the long-term outlook for survivors? Several long-term studies using life-table methods have shown 5-year survival rates ranging from 49% to 75% (average, 61%; see Table 39-4).[114-116]

Although these data are far more encouraging than those for the survival of patients not undergoing operation, they do not equal the survival expected for the normal age-matched population. For example, Johnson and coworkers[115] reported a 50% survival of 7.4 years for patients surviving elective operative treatment for abdominal aneurysm, whereas the age-adjusted figure for the U.S. general population was 15.7 years, and that for North Carolina citizens was 14.5 years. These authors could not identify any influence of age on operative mortality as did Hertzer and colleagues (5-year survival of 82% for ages 45-55 years vs. 60% for ages 76 and older),[93] although it affected late mortality as expected. Most of the excess late mortality in most reports could be attributed to coronary artery disease and cancer. This has led some centers to pursue an aggressive coronary evaluation and treatment protocol before elective aortic aneurysm operations.[118]

Several large surveys have shown that the safety of vascular surgical procedures in patients who have had previous coronary revascularization is comparable to that in patients with no evidence of ischemic cardiac disease, but this has not been evaluated by randomized clinical trials.[119-123] It has been estimated that, based on data from the Canadian Aneurysm Study, aggressive cardiac treatment increases the 5-year survival by only 5% to 10%.[124]

Overall, aortic aneurysm repair is durable and approximately 70% of patients survive 5 years. The survival of those treated for rupture is similar. Quality-of-life studies have demonstrated that it is well maintained after either open or endovascular repair.

ASSESSMENT OF CARDIAC RISK

Approximately 30% to 40% of patients with aortic aneurysms do not have clinically evident coronary artery disease (e.g., no angina pectoris or history of myocardial infarction, normal electrocardiogram [ECG], normal exercise stress test result). However, there is a high prevalence (50%) of angiographically documented severe coronary artery disease in patients in whom coronary disease

is clinically suspected (approximately 50% of the total).[118,123] The prevalence is still 20% in patients in whom the traditional clinical indicators of coronary disease are absent. Coronary artery disease is responsible for at least 50% to 60% and is the leading cause of perioperative and late deaths after operations on the abdominal aorta.[125] The incidence of fatal myocardial infarction after elective abdominal aortic aneurysm surgery has been reported to be as high as 4.7%, and nonfatal infarction has been reported in up to 16% of patients. Nonfatal infarction is more common and is associated with significant late cardiac morbidity, which makes it critical to minimize risk of cardiac morbidity. Comprehensive guidelines for perioperative cardiovascular evaluation and care for noncardiac surgery have been published by the American College of Cardiology and American Heart Association and endorsed by the SVS.[128] The SVS has published its own guidelines dealing with this issue.[16,129] Readers are referred to these documents for details.

It is possible to identify high-risk cardiac patients using clinical assessment, exercise stress testing, radionuclide angiography (multiple gated scan), echocardiography, dipyridamole-thallium scanning, continuous portable electrocardiographic Holter monitoring, and coronary angiography. The challenge is deciding which patients need cardiac screening before aneurysm surgery. Patients with active cardiac disease require thorough cardiac evaluation and functional optimization before elective aneurysm repair, either open or endovascular. An ejection fraction less than 30% has been associated with increased cardiac complications in some series, but it does not predict postoperative myocardial infarction or death. Continuous portable ECG monitoring of vascular surgical patients for silent ischemia associated with ST-T segment changes has been shown to correlate with postoperative myocardial infarction in some series, but additional studies are needed to verify the value of this technique. Routine preoperative screening of all aortic aneurysm patients with coronary angiography is not feasible or prudent, even though Hertzer and colleagues[118,119] reported a nearly fivefold increase in operative mortality (5.1%) in aneurysm patients with suspected coronary disease, compared with those with no (1.1% mortality) or corrected (0.44% mortality) coronary artery disease. Late survival was also better in the groups with no or corrected coronary artery disease. Despite these data, no solid evidence has proved that there is decreased perioperative mortality or increased long-term survival among patients undergoing prophylactic coronary revascularization before aortic aneurysm repair. Furthermore, no single means exists to accurately predict perioperative cardiac risk after aortic aneurysmorrhaphy, but this is currently an area of intensive research.

Younger patients without overt cardiac disease with a normal 12-lead ECG and capable of at least moderate physical activity (MET > 4) probably need no additional evaluation. Older patients with active coronary disease need careful cardiac evaluation. The difficult decisions are in patients who fall between these two extremes (approximately 50% of the total), in whom unexpected coronary events still occur.[127] Because the ultimate objective of a cardiac evaluation is to identify and correct dangerous coronary artery lesions, the results of any subsequent intervention (e.g., coronary artery bypass grafting, percutaneous transluminal angioplasty) in the appropriate hospital must be considered and balanced against the relatively low myocardial infarction rates that can be achieved in patients who do not undergo coronary revascularization. Overall, preliminary myocardial revascularization before aortic aneurysm repair is truly necessary in only 10% to 20% of patients.

Several other comorbid conditions are common in patients with aortic aneurysm, including renal, pulmonary, and hematologic diseases and diabetes mellitus. All can lead to morbidity and should be optimized before elective aneurysm repair.

INDICATIONS FOR ABDOMINAL AORTIC ANEURYSM REPAIR

The objectives of surgical treatment of abdominal aortic aneurysm are to relieve symptoms (if present), prevent rupture (thereby prolonging life), and restore arterial continuity. These goals are best accomplished when operations are performed electively under optimal conditions. The natural history of unoperated abdominal aortic aneurysms and the excellent results currently achievable with surgical treatment justify an aggressive diagnostic and therapeutic approach. Thus far, the only way to prevent or delay rupture is surgical treatment. The decision to recommend operation can be difficult and must account for the rupture risk of the aneurysm, the life expectancy of the patient, and the operative risk of the procedure. Several scoring systems have been developed to aid decision making for individual patients.

Emergent operation is indicated for almost all patients with known or suspected rupture, regardless of the size of the aneurysm or age of the patient. There are obvious exceptions to this recommendation. The coexistence of another fatal illness, such as metastatic cancer, or severe dementia with poor quality of life may be sufficient reason for choosing a nonoperative approach. Some reports suggest that patients older than 85 years who are in shock should be selected for nonoperative management because of the high operative mortality in this group; however, some do survive and decisions must be individualized. Emergent or urgent operation is also indicated for symptomatic (abdominal or back pain) aneurysms in the absence of signs of rupture, because it is often impossible to determine whether an aneurysm has in fact ruptured or is just expanding. Although CT and MRI scans can be relied on to detect the presence of periaortic blood in most cases, other more subtle findings, such as a break in the aortic calcium ring or stranding of retroperitoneal fat, may provide clues to an impending rupture. The absence of these findings should not lead to unnecessary delays in operating, because actual rupture can occur at any time. Elective aneurysm repair should be recommended for asymptomatic patients with aneurysms 5.5 cm or larger in diameter, who are acceptable operative risks, and who have an estimated life expectancy of 2 years or more. Elective operation should also be considered for smaller aneurysms, between 5.0

and 5.4 cm in diameter, in good-risk patients, especially if they are hypertensive or live in remote areas where proper medical care would not be readily available should signs and symptoms of rupture develop. Aneurysms between 4 and 5.5 cm in diameter that have shown documented enlargement of more than 0.5 cm in less than 6 to 12 months by serial imaging studies should also be treated surgically. Enlargement at this rate has long been considered a sign of an unstable, changing aortic wall with an increased risk of rupture, but there are few if any published data supporting this concept. In the future, wall stress analyses will hopefully become readily available for use in making surgical decisions. Data from several studies showed that aneurysms in women ruptured at a higher frequency and at a smaller size than in men; therefore it may be appropriate to recommend elective repair at 4.5 to 5.2 cm in women.

High-risk patients (those who are very old or who have nonreconstructible coronary disease, poor left ventricular function with congestive heart failure, renal failure, or severe obstructive lung disease) with small aneurysms should be observed until the aneurysm becomes symptomatic or large. High-risk patients with large aneurysms require thorough evaluation for the condition that puts them in the high-risk category.[107] Frequently, such evaluations fail to substantiate the original degree of presumed risk, and it has been reported that less than 50% of these patients die of the disease for which they were initially denied aneurysm repair. Unfortunately, there is lack of agreement on the definition of these various high-risk categories. It is in these high-risk patients that endoluminal repair may be especially beneficial.

Before the introduction of EVAR, several groups advocated extraanatomic bypass in conjunction with induced thrombosis of the aneurysm in very high-risk patients with large abdominal aneurysms.[130] Thrombosis of the aneurysm, it was argued, would eliminate the risk of rupture, and the extraanatomic bypass would lower operative mortality by avoiding the risks of a major intraabdominal operation and aortic cross-clamping. Unfortunately, nonresective therapy has not been as successful as originally hoped. Operative mortality exceeds 10%, and rupture still occurs in approximately 20% of patients so treated, which is higher than the mortality reported in similar but highly selected groups of patients subjected to conventional aneurysm operations.[92,131,132] Fortunately, this nonresective form of surgical therapy for abdominal aneurysms has been abandoned, even by some of its earlier proponents, and endoluminal stent-grafting has become the treatment of choice for these high-risk patients when they have suitable anatomy.

OPERATIVE TECHNIQUE

Incision and Exposure

There are three options for the incision for abdominal aortic aneurysm operations: full-length midline, wide transverse, and oblique.

The full-length midline incision is the most popular because it provides access to the entire abdominal cavity, including the supraceliac aorta and iliac arteries; it can be made and closed rapidly and has the fewest limitations. For the treatment of suprarenal or pararenal aneurysms, medial visceral rotation provides adequate exposure of the entire suprarenal segment of the abdominal aorta. This maneuver involves mobilization, from lateral to medial, of the left colon, spleen, and pancreas in what is normally an avascular plane. Significant splenic injury requiring splenectomy occurs approximately 25% of the time when this is done, and there is an increased risk of pancreatic injury. Midline incisional hernias occur more frequently after aneurysm repair than after other operations performed through midline incisions, possibly because of the same or similar connective tissue abnormality that is involved in the pathogenesis of aneurysms.

A wide transverse incision extending from flank to flank and curved either above or below the umbilicus, depending on the aortic and iliac pathology, also provides excellent transperitoneal exposure. It is more time-consuming to create and close than a midline incision, but is said to be stronger, although proof of superiority in terms of wound dehiscence is lacking. Transverse incisions are less painful and therefore interfere less with respiratory function postoperatively, because they cut across fewer intercostal nerves.

Both the midline and the transverse incisions offer wide access to the peritoneal cavity and retroperitoneum and its contents. These incisions permit a thorough abdominal exploration that should be performed as a preliminary step in all elective operations, because there is a significant incidence of coexisting intraabdominal pathology, including colon tumors and gallstones.

Retroperitoneal exposure of the aorta can be achieved through an oblique incision extending from the left eleventh intercostal space or tip of the eleventh rib to the edge of the rectus abdominis muscle.[133-135] The patient is placed in a semilateral position, but with the hips allowed to rotate back toward the supine position, which allows access to both femoral arteries. Through this retroperitoneal exposure, the suprarenal and supraceliac aorta can be controlled more easily, but access to the right iliac artery is often limited, especially if the aortic aneurysm is large or if there is a large right iliac aneurysm. Among the advantages of the retroperitoneal approach are less postoperative respiratory compromise, lower intravenous fluid requirements, less intraoperative hypothermia, a shorter period of postoperative ileus, and avoidance in many cases of the need for postoperative nasogastric intubation. Although the perception is that these patients generally fare better than those operated on through a midline incision, when the two incisions were compared in prospective studies, no significant important differences were found.[133-135] One major disadvantage of the retroperitoneal approach is that the contents of the peritoneal cavity are not available for inspection, although an opening in the peritoneum can be made easily if necessary. Another is the occurrence of a postoperative flank bulge that can be particularly annoying to some patients. This is probably due to injury to the intercostal nerve in the line of the incision. The retroperitoneal approach loses most of its advantages when there is a retroaortic left renal vein or left-sided vena cava, because these structures are then in a vulnerable location. Nevertheless, many surgeons prefer this approach for all elective aneurysm operations, especially pararenal and suprarenal types. Some even use it for contained ruptured aneurysms because of the ability to achieve rapid control of the upper abdominal aorta.[136] The retroperitoneal approach is probably preferable in the presence of an inflammatory aneurysm or horseshoe kidney.

The choice of incision is a matter of surgeon preference and patient factors. Factors to consider in making this choice include the extent of the aneurysm, the status of the iliac arteries, the degree of obesity and pulmonary disease, previous abdominal operations, the presence and location of stomas, the necessity to inspect intraperitoneal structures (especially in patients with atypical symptoms), and the speed with which aortic control must be attained. Surgeons should be familiar with all three approaches so that they can take advantage of each when appropriate.

Transperitoneal or retroperitoneal exposure of the aorta through small incisions, with or without laparoscopic assistance, has been used successfully to treat aortic aneurysms by several surgical groups. The special instruments, vascular clamps, and retractors necessary to accomplish this have been developed and are being improved. Turnipseed[137] compared 50 patients who had aortic aneurysms or occlusive disease treated via minimal incisions with 50 similar patients treated using a long midline incision. The minimal incision technique was as safe and effective as the standard incision and was associated with shorter intensive care unit and total hospital stay, less morbidity, and reduced costs. It was more cost efficient than either the standard incision or endoluminal stent-grafting techniques. Completely laparoscopic aneurysm repair has also been performed, and several fairly large series have been reported, with improving results and reduced operative times.[138] Only a few groups have significant experience with the use of robotic devices for aneurysm replacement. With experience, the duration of the procedure has been reduced and the success rate is high.

When midline or transverse incisions are used, the aorta is exposed by an infracolic retroperitoneal incision that should be kept slightly to the right of the midline. The duodenum must be carefully reflected laterally, along with the rest of the small bowel; this requires division of the ligament of Treitz, which should be carefully reapproximated as part of the retroperitoneal closure. The left renal vein usually marks the cephalad extent of the dissection, unless the aneurysm extends to the renal arteries (juxtarenal aneurysm) or involves them (pararenal aneurysm; Figure 39-6). In either of these situations, suprarenal aortic clamping is necessary, and the left renal vein should be thoroughly mobilized so that it can be retracted cephalad or caudad to facilitate adequate exposure of the pararenal aorta.[139,140] It is sometimes necessary to divide the left renal vein; this is usually well tolerated if the left adrenal and gonadal veins are not ligated, but there is an increased risk of sustained elevation in the serum creatinine level, a temporary reduction of left renal function, and increased retroperitoneal bleeding.[141]

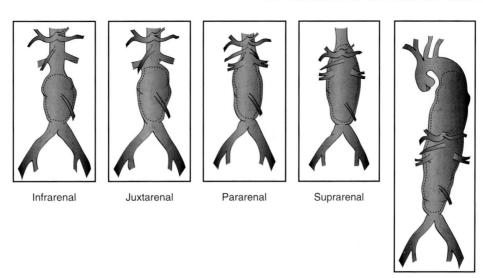

Infrarenal   Juxtarenal   Pararenal   Suprarenal

Thoracoabdominal

FIGURE 39-6 ■ Morphologic classification of abdominal aortic aneurysms. Aneurysms can be classified according to their relationship to the renal arteries as infrarenal, juxtarenal, pararenal, and suprarenal.

Reanastomosis of the transected renal vein avoids these complications, but it is not always necessary.[128]

Distally, the dissection should avoid the fibroareolar tissue overlying the left common iliac artery in men because it contains branch vessels of the inferior mesenteric artery and the autonomic nerves that control sexual function. If the common iliac arteries are relatively normal (i.e., not aneurysmal, stenotic, or heavily calcified), they can be clamped and a straight tube graft can be used for the aortic replacement. Significant disease of the common iliac arteries makes a bifurcated graft preferable. Control of the iliac arteries in these situations is best achieved by mobilizing the external and internal iliac arteries and controlling them individually. Particular care must be taken in this location to avoid injury to the accompanying posterior venous structures and to the ureters, which cross anterior to the common iliac bifurcation. Every effort should be made to ensure antegrade perfusion in at least one hypogastric artery to minimize the risk of postoperative ischemia of the left colon as well as buttock claudication. A majority of reconstructions will require a bifurcated graft with distal anastomoses constructed with the transected common iliac artery. If this is not possible, the distal anastomosis can be made in an end-to-side fashion with the external iliac and the common iliac stump oversewn, thereby permitting hypogastric perfusion in a retrograde fashion. If this is not possible, hypogastric revascularization can be accomplished by a side-arm graft from the iliac limb of the bifurcation graft to the internal iliac. An easier technique is to perform an end-to-end anastomosis between the end of the iliac limb and the hypogastric and then place a graft from the iliac graft limb to the external iliac artery.

Extensive perioperative monitoring is indicated for patients undergoing abdominal aortic aneurysm repair.[142,143] This monitoring contributed significantly to the improved results reported in large series of electively treated patients. Monitoring usually includes continuous recording of the ECG, intraarterial pressure, body temperature, urine output, and central venous or pulmonary artery pressure. In high-risk patients, especially if the aorta will be cross-clamped above the renal arteries, transesophageal two-dimensional echocardiographic monitoring of left ventricular function may be superior to measurements of pulmonary artery pressure for the evaluation of intravascular volume status.[143] Various blood components should be monitored as well, including arterial oxygen and carbon dioxide content and pH, plasma glucose, electrolytes, and coagulation parameters and factors. Monitoring the clotting system is especially important in ruptured aneurysms and in cases in which large volumes of blood and blood products have been infused or a supraceliac clamp has been used. The use of autotransfusion is routine in some places to minimize the need for homologous blood transfusion. Unfortunately, its use was not found to be cost effective in randomized trials. For elective operations, patients should be encouraged to donate their own blood for autologous transfusion in the perioperative period.

Aneurysm Repair

Regardless of the extent of the aortic aneurysm, the proximal graft anastomosis should be made as close as possible to the renal arteries to prevent recurrent aortic pathology. The proximal aortic neck can be evaluated on the preoperative imaging studies to assess diameter, length, and wall characteristics, such as calcification, thrombus and plaque. These features are important in determining where to place the proximal cross clamp, which in turn may influence the choice of incision. Juxtarenal aneurysms extend to the renal arteries but do not involve them. These aneurysms can be repaired with an infrarenal graft, but suprarenal cross clamping is required. In contrast, pararenal aneurysms involve at least one of the renal arteries so that renal revascularization is required for at least one kidney. This procedure requires suprarenal and frequently supraceliac clamping in order to perform the aortic anastomosis and renal artery repair. The degree of disease in the iliac arteries determines the distal extent of the graft. In some series, up to 80% of patients have been treated successfully with a straight tube graft, although in the experience of others, only approximately one third of patients had suitable anatomy for this approach. There does not appear to be a significant incidence of subsequent iliac aneurysm formation when tube grafts are used in the presence of normal-sized or slightly enlarged common iliac arteries (less than 2.5 cm diameter).

The choice of graft material—polyester (knitted or woven) or expanded polytetrafluoroethylene (ePTFE)—is a controversial but relatively unimportant issue. There is no proven superiority of either graft type when used for aortic replacement. Polyester grafts are the most popular and most surgeons prefer knitted grafts because they are easier to handle. Knitted grafts sealed with collagen or gelatin are not porous, do not require preclotting, can bind topically applied antibiotics, and have less bleeding through needle holes than ePTFE. For ruptured aneurysms, nonporous grafts are clearly preferable because of savings in time and interstitial blood loss. Many surgeons routinely use woven polyester or ePTFE grafts for elective aneurysm repair for the same reason.

Systemic heparin is administered almost universally during the occlusive phase of elective aneurysm operations, because most surgeons believe that its use provides added protection from distal thrombosis. The distal clamps should be applied before the proximal aortic clamp to prevent distal embolization. It has been traditionally taught that distal clamps should be applied before the aortic clamp to prevent distal embolization, but recent evidence suggests otherwise because of the risk of renal embolization from reversed and turbulent flow produced by distal occlusion. The aorta is opened longitudinally and either partially or completely transected at the site of the proximal anastomosis. If there is a very short or no infrarenal neck (juxtarenal aneurysm), temporary proximal aortic clamping above the renal arteries is required to accomplish an adequate infrarenal anastomosis (see Figure 39-2). This also requires control of the renal arteries to prevent the entrance of embolic debris. The proximal anastomosis can be done with a continuous or interrupted suture technique; the former is obviously quicker. If the aorta is especially weak or friable, the sutures can be supported with Teflon-felt pledgets or strips.

The distal anastomoses can be end to end or end to side, depending on their location and the status of the common and internal iliac arteries. All mural thrombus and atheroma should be debrided from the aneurysm wall. Several studies have shown a surprisingly high incidence of positive bacterial cultures of this material, ranging from 10% to 40% of patients. The significance of these positive cultures is unknown, but most of them have been due to coagulase-negative *Staphylococcus* species, an organism commonly found in aortic graft infections.[144]

Back-bleeding lumbar vessels can be the source of significant blood loss and should be suture-ligated from within the aortic sac. If the inferior mesenteric artery is patent and actively back-bleeding, it can also be ligated within the aneurysm sac, but if back-bleeding is meager, it should be preserved and reassessed after distal flow is reestablished, especially if internal iliac flow is compromised. Reimplantation of the inferior mesenteric artery is relatively easy to perform, when necessary, with the use of the Carrel patch technique.

All anastomoses should be constructed with permanent synthetic sutures. Braided polyester and monofilament polypropylene or PTFE are the most commonly used. Theoretical fears about late fracture of polypropylene sutures have not been substantiated in clinical practice. If suprarenal clamping is necessary, the clamp should be moved onto the graft and below the renal arteries as soon as possible to minimize renal ischemia after ensuring that the proximal anastomosis is secure. The distal anastomoses can then be constructed as indicated by the iliac artery disease. If the iliacs are severely calcified, it is sometimes easier to control iliac artery back-bleeding by the use of intraluminal balloon catheters and to oversew the common iliac arteries from within the opened aortic or iliac aneurysms. In unusual circumstances, external iliac disease necessitates making the distal anastomosis to the common femoral artery.

Declamping hypotension is now an unusual event in elective aortic aneurysm surgery. It is essential to maintain excellent communication with the anesthesiology team so that depth of anesthesia and blood and fluid replacement can be adjusted in anticipation of lower extremity reperfusion. Although the graft and native vessels are flushed and back-bled before reestablishing distal flow, it is preferable to reestablish flow first into one hypogastric artery to minimize the chance of distal embolization to the leg. Before abdominal closure, adequacy of lower extremity and left colon perfusion should be ensured by direct inspection or noninvasive instrumentation. The graft should be insulated from the overlying bowel by careful closure of the aneurysm sac over the graft. This is sometimes impossible when the aneurysm is small, and in these situations, rotation of a flap of the aneurysm wall or a vascularized omental pedicle can be used to separate the graft from the duodenum.

It is beyond the scope of this chapter to discuss all the technical details that might be encountered during the surgical treatment of an aortic aneurysm. The principles outlined here are generally applicable in most cases. If additional vascular procedures are required, such as renal or visceral artery reconstruction, appropriate modifications in technique are obviously required.[145]

Repair of Ruptured Aneurysm

For ruptured aneurysms, the first priority is to control the hemorrhage by gaining proximal control of the aorta. Resuscitation is best done in the operating room rather than in the emergency department, and it is better to restore blood pressure only to levels sufficient to maintain vital organ function and cerebral perfusion before the induction of anesthesia.[146] It is also better to have the patient prepared and draped, with the surgical team ready to make a rapid entry into the abdomen, before the induction of anesthesia. The induction of anesthesia in these circumstances is often associated with sudden and severe hypotension when the tamponade effects and reflex vasoconstriction are relieved by relaxation of the abdominal wall and the administered anesthetic agents. The practice of proximal aortic control by balloon occlusion using a catheter inserted via a transbrachial or transfemoral approach has been repopularized largely to avoid this phenomenon. The availability of high-quality digital fluoroscopy and endovascular supplies in the operating room makes this feasible. If the rupture is contained, proximal aortic control is best achieved at the level of the supraceliac aorta through the lesser omentum. This requires mobilization of the left lobe of the liver and can be far more difficult than anticipated when there is a large hematoma in the mesentery that pushes the transverse mesocolon and upper abdominal viscera cephalad (see Figure 39-4). The hematoma can then be entered and the clamp is repositioned distally after the aortic neck is identified. The hematoma usually makes this portion of the dissection relatively easy, but caution must be exercised to avoid injury to major venous structures, which is one of the most common causes of excessive hemorrhage and subsequent death. If there is a free intraperitoneal rupture, the aorta can be quickly compressed at the diaphragm with an assistant's hand or a commercial compression device without formally dissecting this area. An infrarenal clamp or an intraluminal occluding balloon catheter should be substituted as soon as possible. After bleeding is controlled, adequate blood and volume replenishment should be achieved before attempting to restore flow to the lower extremities. Heparin is unnecessary and should be avoided in ruptured aneurysms because bleeding and coagulopathy are frequently associated with the shock, hypothermia, and massive blood loss and replacement that occur. The aggressive use of blood and blood products, including platelets and fresh frozen plasma, is essential for the survival of these patients.[147,148]

COMPLICATIONS OF AORTIC ANEURYSM REPAIR

Survival after aortic aneurysm surgery was discussed earlier in this chapter. Operative mortality ranges from 0% to 3% for patients with uncomplicated aneurysms operated on electively to more than 80% for patients with rupture, hypotension, and oliguria. The most frequent cause of death is myocardial dysfunction, usually ischemic in origin.[117,125,126] Overall, 15% to 30% of patients have at least one complication after open surgical repair. Nonfatal myocardial infarction is fairly common even after elective aortic aneurysm repair, occurring in 3.1% to 16% (average, 6.9%) of patients in reported series.[9] The varying incidence is due to different criteria used to define myocardial infarction (e.g., non-ST elevation, troponin leak) and possibly due to different protocols for evaluating and treating coronary artery disease preoperatively.

Several other major complications can occur during or after aortic aneurysm operations. Hemorrhage is a constant threat, most often from injury to iliac or lumbar veins. It can be severe and extremely difficult to control, especially if it involves the left common iliac vein where it passes beneath the right common iliac artery. For this reason, extreme care must be taken when mobilizing and clamping the iliac arteries, especially if they are aneurysmal, in which case they are more likely to be adherent to the underlying veins. Injury to the left renal vein or one of its tributaries is also associated with brisk bleeding. This is particularly likely when there are venous anomalies such as a retroaortic left renal vein or a circumaortic venous collar. These venous anomalies can usually be identified preoperatively if a CT scan has been obtained. Intraoperatively, major venous anomalies should be suspected when, during cephalad dissection of the aortic neck, either a small or no left renal vein is encountered in its usual location crossing anterior to the aorta. Postoperative hemorrhage can occur in any patient, and hemodynamic instability and evidence of continued blood loss should lead to early re-exploration of the abdomen. Nonsurgical bleeding can be minimized by careful monitoring of the coagulation system to provide the basis for administration of platelets, clotting factors, and protamine when appropriate.

Declamping hypotension is not as frequent or severe a problem as it once was. Better understanding of its physiology, more aggressive management of intravascular volume, and better monitoring and anesthetic techniques have all contributed to the reduction in the incidence and seriousness of this problem. The surgeon can help to minimize this condition by giving the anesthesiologist advance notification of plans to restore distal perfusion and then doing it gradually. Instilling vasopressors down the leg before declamping is done rarely. Despite these precautions, declamping hypotension can still be a serious problem, especially in the setting of a ruptured aneurysm in a cold, hypovolemic patient with poor cardiac performance. Gradual restoration of distal flow can minimize the severity of declamping hypotension.

Renal failure is another serious but infrequent complication. At one time, 3% to 12% of deaths after elective abdominal aortic aneurysm operations and an even higher percentage after emergency operations for rupture were attributable to acute renal failure.[149,150] Renal failure or less severe degrees of renal impairment can occur even when there is no hypotension and the proximal aortic clamp is infrarenal in location. The cause of renal dysfunction in these situations is poorly understood but is thought to involve reflex renal vasoconstriction and intrarenal redistribution of blood flow. Atheromatous embolization from clamping or manipulation of the perirenal aorta is also a potential contributing factor, as is temporary suprarenal clamping when it is required. Sometimes, the large contrast load of an aortogram or CT scan obtained 1 or 2 days preoperatively can cause renal dysfunction that only becomes apparent postoperatively. Mannitol or loop diuretics are commonly administered before aortic cross-clamping to increase urine output and prevent renal failure. Although this seems reasonable, studies have shown that intraoperative urine volume does not predict postoperative renal function.[151] Renal failure owing to acute tubular necrosis is much more common after operations for ruptured aortic aneurysms, occurring in 21% of survivors of operation in one series. Unfortunately, the mortality associated with this complication still ranges from 50% to 70%, despite the use of acute hemodialysis and adequate nutritional support.

Technical injury to the bowel or ureters can cause catastrophic infectious complications involving the newly implanted prosthetic graft. This is most likely to occur when there are adhesions from previous operations or the structures are in an unusual position (e.g., the ureters displaced anteriorly and laterally by the aneurysm). Such injuries should be meticulously repaired, and the area should be thoroughly irrigated with antibiotic solution. Ureteral injuries should be repaired and stented. In some situations, nephrectomy is the safest course to avoid possible graft contamination.

Gastrointestinal complications of a functional nature regularly occur after conventional aortic aneurysm surgery. Ileus is the rule for at least 2 to 3 days after transperitoneal surgery. Typically, gastric and colonic ileus persists longer than small bowel ileus. Nevertheless, the use of nasogastric tubes has not been shown to reduce the incidence of early gastrointestinal dysfunction, and they should be able to be removed on the first postoperative morning. Small amounts of liquids can often be safely administered orally beginning on postoperative days 1 or 2. Occasionally, duodenal obstruction persists for longer periods. The presence of hematoma and edema in the vicinity of the proximal anastomosis is thought to contribute to this problem as is improper reconstitution of the ligament of Treitz during the retroperitoneal closure. Postoperative pancreatitis is relatively common, as determined by elevation of the serum amylase and lipase levels, although clinically apparent pancreatitis is unusual. The pancreas can be injured by retractors, however, and a few patients have serious consequences from these seemingly minor injuries.

The most serious gastrointestinal complication is ischemia of the left side of the colon and the rectum. The incidence of ischemic colitis after aortic reconstruction is approximately 2% (range, 0.2% to 10%).[152] It is threefold to fourfold more common after operations for aortic aneurysm than after operations for occlusive disease, and the incidence is several times higher in patients studied prospectively with colonoscopy after sustaining a ruptured aneurysm. Ligation of a patent inferior mesenteric artery in the presence of inadequate collateral circulation to the sigmoid colon and rectum is thought to be an important pathophysiologic mechanism, but the inferior mesenteric artery is already occluded in 40% to 50% of patients with abdominal aneurysms. Improper ligation of the inferior mesenteric artery too far away from the wall of the aneurysm can contribute to this complication by interfering with collateral blood supply to the rectosigmoid.[153] Postoperative hypotension and hemodynamic instability are significant contributory factors. Therefore, as noted earlier, it is important to maintain antegrade perfusion in at least one internal iliac artery after arterial reconstruction for aortic aneurysm. Although most patients with occlusion of both internal iliac arteries and the inferior mesenteric artery have adequate colonic perfusion, postoperative hypotension, bowel distention, and mesenteric vessel compression by hematoma can all contribute to postoperative colonic ischemia.

Postoperative colonic ischemia can involve the mucosa only, which usually causes a transient, mild form of ischemic colitis, or it can involve mucosa and muscularis, which can result in fibrous healing and stricture formation. The most severe and dreaded form is transmural ischemia, which occurs in more than 60% of the reported cases. The clinical manifestations of bowel ischemia depend on its severity. Diarrhea, especially if it is bloody, is one of the earliest manifestations and usually begins within 48 hours of operation. It is an indication for colonoscopy to assess the status of the colonic mucosa. Other findings indicative of bowel gangrene and peritonitis may be present and demand prompt reoperation, resection of all compromised bowel, and creation of appropriate stomas. During bowel resection, efforts should be made to isolate the underlying aortic prosthesis from the surgical field, although this is usually impossible, setting the stage for subsequent prosthetic infection. If the graft becomes grossly contaminated, it should be removed and lower extremity perfusion is restored by axillofemoral bypass. Less severe degrees of colonic ischemia can be managed nonoperatively, although subsequent correction of a colonic stricture may be required. A high index of suspicion of this complication must be maintained to detect and treat it in a timely fashion. Some surgeons routinely perform flexible sigmoidoscopy on the first day after repair of a ruptured aortic aneurysm in order to establish early diagnosis of rectosigmoid ischemia.

The mortality for postoperative colonic ischemia following aortic aneurysm surgery is approximately 50% overall, but increases to 90% when full-thickness colonic gangrene and peritonitis occur. Preoperative evaluation of the blood supply to the colon and intraoperative assessment of colonic perfusion by Doppler or inferior mesenteric artery back-pressure measurements may help to identify patients at highest risk for this disastrous complication so that preventive measures (i.e., inferior mesenteric artery reimplantation) can be taken.[154] Routine inferior mesenteric reimplantation is advocated by some surgeons, but there are no solid data on how often this is really necessary. The SVS guidelines recommend reimplantation of a patent inferior mesenteric artery (IMA) whenever there is an increased risk of colonic ischemia. Such circumstances include poor IMA backbleeding, occlusive lesions of the celiac and superior mesenteric arteries, presence of a large meandering mesenteric artery, inability to restore hypogastric perfusion, and previous rectosigmoid colectomy. Intraoperative and postoperative hypotension, especially if vasopressors are used, exacerbates all these conditions. Even following these guidelines, IMA reimplantation should be necessary in only 5% to 10% of cases.

Paraplegia caused by spinal cord ischemia, a well-recognized complication of thoracoabdominal aneurysm repair, is a rare event after operations confined to the infrarenal aorta, with only slightly more than 50 cases reported. Szilagyi and coworkers[155] noted an incidence of 0.2% in more than 3000 aortic operations, and it occurred tenfold more frequently in patients with ruptured aneurysms. This finding suggests that hypotension is a contributing factor in most cases, although injury to an unusually located arteria magna radicularis (artery of Adamkiewicz) to the spinal cord may be the primary event. Pelvic hypoperfusion associated with internal iliac artery occlusion is an important contributing factor in some patients; this emphasizes again the importance of maintaining perfusion of at least one hypogastric artery. Unfortunately, this complication is not predictable, preventable, or treatable. Spinal fluid drainage and high-dose steroids have been tried with occasional success. Although the severity of the clinical manifestations varies and approximately 50% of affected survivors recover some neurologic function, there is a 50% mortality associated with this complication.

Ischemia of the lower extremities can also occur after aortic aneurysm surgery. This may be the result of embolization of dislodged mural thrombus or atherosclerotic plaque from the aneurysm itself, thrombosis of a downstream vessel due to distal stasis, creation of an intimal flap, or crushed atherosclerotic plaque. The use of heparin during the occlusive phase of aneurysm repair does not prevent embolic events from occurring, but may limit the propagation of thrombus and should prevent the formation of stasis thrombi in the distal vascular beds. Before closing the abdomen, the surgeon must be satisfied with the perfusion status of the lower extremities.

Microembolization can also occur, resulting in small patchy areas of ischemia, usually on the plantar aspect of the feet. Pedal pulses are usually still palpable in this situation. Colloquially, this is known as *trash foot*, and if it is recognized intraoperatively, the passage of small balloon catheters can sometimes retrieve at least some of the atheromatous debris. Lumbar sympathectomy may also be beneficial in limiting or preventing full-thickness tissue loss.

An abdominal compartment syndrome has been recognized as an unusual but important cause of renal and respiratory failure, especially after operations for ruptured aneurysms. Manifested by massive abdominal distention, oliguria, and difficulty maintaining adequate ventilation, it is an indication for prompt reexploration of the abdomen to relieve the intraabdominal pressure. Measurement of airway and urinary bladder pressures can be helpful in deciding to return a patient to the operating room for abdominal decompression. The usual finding is massive visceral edema and blood, and a deliberate abdominal wall hernia must be created for its treatment. This syndrome can be treated by mesh-assisted delayed abdominal closure.

Infection involving the prosthetic graft used to restore aortic continuity occurs in less than 1% to approximately 6% of patients. It is more common after treatment for ruptured than nonruptured aneurysms. It may be associated with graft-enteric fistula, which is more common after surgery for aortic aneurysm than after surgery for aortic occlusive disease. These infections usually become manifest months to years after graft implantation and are discussed in detail in Chapter 56.

UNUSUAL PROBLEMS ASSOCIATED WITH ABDOMINAL AORTIC ANEURYSMS

A number of anatomic and pathologic conditions can complicate the management of abdominal aortic aneurysms and adversely affect the outcome.

Saccular Aneurysms

Almost all abdominal aortic aneurysms are fusiform in shape, but they are often not uniform or round in cross-section and some have flattened areas, blebs, and other asymmetrical features. A small percentage is saccular in shape, involving only a portion of the aortic wall. These aneurysms typically have very thin walls and some are, in fact, pseudoaneurysms. Their etiology is variable, but infection is one of the most important causes. Little is known about the relationship between size and rupture of saccular aneurysms, but there is consensus that these are more likely to rupture and should be treated regardless of size. Treatment must be individualized based upon location and size. A saccular aneurysm arising from a normal caliber aorta may require aortic replacement as required for a fusiform aneurysm.

Venous Anomalies

There are several anomalies of the inferior vena cava and left renal vein that are important in aortic surgery. They were found in 2.8% of nearly 1400 aortic operations in one series and are potential sources of serious, unexpected hemorrhage. Many of these anomalies can be identified on preoperative CT scans.[156] The inferior vena cava may be present entirely on the left side (without situs inversus) or may be duplicated, with one on each side of the aorta. Double vena cava is estimated to occur in up to 3% of patients, but isolated left-sided vena cava occurs in only 0.2% to 0.5%.[157,158] An isolated left-sided vena cava usually crosses obliquely in front of the aorta and may be joined by a short, immobile right renal vein. It can also cross from left to right behind the aorta. These anomalies can be especially troublesome if the aorta is approached retroperitoneally from the patient's left side. These anomalously positioned veins are prone to injury during dissection near the neck of an aortic aneurysm. Sometimes a crossing left inferior vena cava must be divided to enable satisfactory handling of the proximal aortic anastomosis. With a duplicated inferior vena cava, the left-sided one can be ligated if necessary, but care must be taken to ensure that adequate venous drainage of the adrenal gland and left kidney is maintained.

A retroaortic left renal vein, either alone or in association with an anterior vein in the usual location, is another rare anomaly that can lead to exsanguinating hemorrhage if it is injured during dissection or clamping of the aortic neck.[159] The incidence of this anomaly is 1.8% to 2.4% and is the most commonly encountered venous anomaly in some series. As mentioned earlier, when the surgeon cannot find the left renal vein in its usual preaortic location, he or she should assume that it is retroaortic and limit dissection in that area. Great care must be taken when applying the aortic cross-clamp to avoid tearing these posterior veins. If such a vein is injured, transection of the aorta is usually required to expose it well enough to control the bleeding.

Circumaortic venous collar is more common, occurring in up to 8.7% of cases.[160] This anomaly is even more prone to injury because the anterior component can be normal in size, leading the surgeon to disregard the possibility of a second, posterior renal vein.

Inflammatory Aneurysm

Nearly 5% of abdominal aortic aneurysms are associated with a dense, inflammatory, fibrotic reaction involving the aortic wall and the retroperitoneum that incorporates adjacent structures.[161,162] This appears to be a distinct clinicopathologic entity of uncertain cause, although an autoimmune process has been proposed. It is characterized histologically by marked thickening of the adventitia and media (in contrast to other aortic aneurysms, which have a thinned, attenuated medial layer). Both layers are infiltrated with a prominent acute and chronic inflammatory reaction that includes giant cells. The majority of the inflammatory cells are activated T lymphocytes. The desmoplastic inflammatory reaction involves the duodenum in 90% of cases, the inferior vena cava and left renal vein in more than 50%, and the ureters in approximately 25%; it can extend above the renal arteries as well as to the iliac arteries.[163] These aneurysms tend to be large, and most patients are symptomatic (i.e., pain) in the absence of rupture. Despite the extremely thickened wall, these aneurysms can and do rupture. A majority of patients have an elevated erythrocyte sedimentation rate of uncertain significance, and many have elevated C-reactive protein levels and have lost weight. The diagnosis can be suggested based on the CT scan, where the periaortic fibrous tissue can easily be seen obliterating the normal tissue planes around the aorta, and a typical halo effect of this tissue appears after intravenous contrast administration. MRI also shows a characteristic appearance of inflammatory aneurysm consisting of several concentric rings surrounding the aortic lumen. This contrast-enhancing halo represents the highly vascular nature of the inflammatory fibrous tissue. Either of these imaging techniques can establish the presence of an inflammatory aneurysm in a high percentage of cases.

Published reports have pointed out several advantages of the left-sided retroperitoneal approach for these lesions, as discussed earlier, and establishing this diagnosis preoperatively allows the selection of this technique. In cases of ureteric involvement, the ureters are pulled medially and may be obstructed (again, in contrast to other large aneurysms, which tend to push the ureters laterally). At laparotomy, the diagnosis can be established immediately by the unmistakable appearance of a dense, shiny, white, highly vascular reaction in the retroperitoneum, centered over the aortic aneurysm. Once the lesion is recognized, the usual maneuvers of aneurysmorrhaphy should be modified to avoid injury to adherent structures, especially the duodenum. The aorta should be exposed cephalad to the renal vein or at the diaphragm and opened without dissecting the

duodenum off the wall. The advantage of the retroperitoneal technique in this condition is that the aorta is approached from a lateral direction and the left kidney and renal vein are displaced anteriorly, out of harm's way. The duodenum does not have to be mobilized, and the inflammatory tissue, which is mostly anterior, can mostly be avoided. There have been several reports of successful endovascular repair of inflammatory aneurysm using standard patient selection criteria. With either approach, concomitant ureterolysis is seldom necessary because the inflammatory reaction usually resolves postoperatively. Ureteral catheterization can be a useful adjunct, however, and can help to avoid intraoperative ureteral injury. Although the transfusion requirements and operative mortality are slightly higher than for noninflammatory aneurysms, the long-term outlook for these patients is comparable to that for patients with ordinary abdominal aortic aneurysms, and the usual criteria for recommending elective operation should be applied, because these aneurysms can rupture despite their thick anterior wall.[164]

Horseshoe Kidney

Horseshoe kidney occurs in 1 in 400 to 1 in 1000 of the general population. Its association with abdominal aortic aneurysm is rare, but it complicates graft replacement because the kidney mass is usually fused anterior to the aorta, the collecting system and ureters are medially displaced, and there are frequently multiple renal arteries arising from the aorta (including the aneurysmal part), the iliac arteries, or both.[165,166] The renal blood supply is anomalous in 80% of cases and may require some form of surgical correction in most of them.[167] The anomalous fused renal mass is readily apparent on diagnostic imaging studies (CT, MRI, ultrasonography), but if the renal arterial anatomy is not well defined by CTA, preoperative arteriography may be necessary for its proper evaluation. The isthmus of a horseshoe kidney seldom needs to be divided (nor should it be), because the aortic graft can be tunneled behind it. If renal arteries arise from the aneurysm, they can be bypassed or reimplanted into the graft as a Carrel patch. There have been recent reports of successful endovascular repairs of aortic aneurysms in association with horseshoe kidney and favorable renal artery anatomy. The presence of a horseshoe kidney is another situation in which a left retroperitoneal approach is preferable, because it allows easier management of the multiple and accessory renal arteries.

Associated Intraabdominal Pathology and Concomitant Surgical Procedures

Occasionally, there are stenotic atherosclerotic lesions in aortic branches that require surgical correction at the time of aortic aneurysm repair. This most often involves the renal arteries in patients with renovascular hypertension or impaired renal function.[168,169] Rarely, chronic visceral ischemia necessitates concomitant visceral artery repair and aneurysmorrhaphy. In most series, the morbidity and mortality of combined procedures exceed those of elective aneurysm repair alone; therefore caution is urged in the performance of purely prophylactic procedures in this setting.

Malignant tumors, most of them colonic, are unexpectedly found in 4% to 5% of patients undergoing operation for abdominal aneurysm. They are much more common in patients with aortic aneurysms than in those with aortic occlusive disease. Because operating on the colon converts a clean procedure into a contaminated one, with the potential for prosthetic graft infection, the decision regarding how to treat each lesion (aneurysm, colon mass) and the sequence is not easy. It is sometimes difficult to distinguish colon cancer from inflammatory lesions intraoperatively by palpation. In addition, most vascular surgeons do not use a formal bowel preparation for patients undergoing elective aortic aneurysm surgery. For these reasons, unless there are compelling reasons for treating the colon lesion (perforation, obstruction, hemorrhage), the aneurysm procedure should be completed and the colon is left alone. The colon lesion can then be properly evaluated and treated postoperatively. Generally, it is possible to perform an elective colon operation sooner after an aortic aneurysm repair than vice versa, especially if there has been a septic complication (common after colon surgery but rare after aortic surgery). This is another situation for which endovascular repair can provide an excellent option for both surgeon and patient.

The presence of asymptomatic gallstones is a far more common condition that is found unexpectedly in 5% to 20% of patients undergoing aortic surgery. Several series have been published attesting to the safety of concomitant cholecystectomy and aortic repair.[170,171] A major impetus for this philosophy is the purported high incidence of postoperative cholecystitis in patients in whom only the aortic pathology is treated. In the series reported by String,[170] there was only one documented late graft infection in 34 patients who underwent combined procedures. However, the follow-up was rather short, especially considering the usual long interval between aortic grafting and the first manifestations of graft infection. In addition, the incidence of positive cultures from the bile of patients with cholelithiasis is as high as 33%. As with colon lesions, performance of elective cholecystectomy, which could lead to contamination of a newly implanted aortic prosthesis, should not be performed in conjunction with vascular grafting operations.[171,172] The consequences of infection of the aortic graft are so grave that the risk of performing elective cholecystectomy is unjustified. The advent of laparoscopic cholecystectomy has made this less of an issue because of the relatively benign nature of this procedure, which can be performed safely either shortly before or after aortic aneurysm repair, if necessary.

Aortocaval Fistula

Abdominal aortic aneurysms can erode into the inferior vena cava or iliac veins, producing an aortocaval fistula. This occurs in 0.2% to 1.3% of patients with typical, nonspecific abdominal aortic aneurysms.[173,174] The incidence is at least twice as high in cases of ruptured aneurysm. Approximately 5% to 10% of spontaneous aortocaval fistulas occur in conjunction with other entities, such as mycotic aneurysm, Ehlers-Danlos syndrome, and Marfan syndrome. The most frequent site of fistulization is the distal aorta at or just above the confluence of the iliac veins. Almost all aortocaval fistulas are symptomatic, and impaired renal function is common. Hemodynamically, there is typically a hyperdynamic, high-output state (tachycardia, decreased diastolic blood pressure, and cardiac dilatation) that can quickly progress to medically refractory congestive heart failure. Abdominal or back pain is present in more than 80% of patients, and most have a palpable mass; 75% have an audible bruit, but only about 25% have a palpable thrill. Venous hypertension can affect the gastrointestinal and urinary tracts as well as the lower extremities, and this is why swollen legs, lower gastrointestinal tract bleeding, and hematuria are common. As a result, a multitude of diagnostic studies have tried to explain these manifestations.

Despite these protean manifestations, the diagnosis of aortocaval fistula is usually not suggested clinically. Aortography has been the most accurate diagnostic modality, although the fistulas can usually be documented by contrast-enhanced CT, MRI, or even ultrasound scans. The natural history of aortocaval fistula is progressive cardiac decompensation and death. Surgical correction offers the only hope for survival and should be undertaken promptly. A conventional infrarenal aortic aneurysm operation with oversewing of the fistula from within the opened aneurysm sac cures the fistula. Hemodynamic improvement is immediate, and renal function usually recovers rapidly. Nevertheless, reported mortality rates are between 22% and 51%, largely a result of blood loss, cardiac decompensation, and pulmonary embolism.[174]

MYCOTIC AORTIC ANEURYSMS

A mycotic aneurysm is one of infectious but not necessarily fungal origin. The term *mycotic* is derived from the typically mushroom-shaped false aneurysm of the arterial wall. These aneurysms usually occur when a sufficient quantity of bacterial or septic emboli lodges at a point on the intimal surface of an artery to produce a locally invasive infection that becomes a transmural arteritis. Although this can occur in normal arteries, it more commonly affects large, major atherosclerotic vessels and their branches. Septic emboli can also lodge in the vasa vasorum and initiate the infectious, necrotic process in the arterial wall. A third mechanism is arterial invasion from a septic focus adjacent to a major artery (Figure 39-7). Traumatic contamination of an artery has replaced endocarditis as the most common cause, often as a result of drug abuse or even arterial catheterization procedures.[160]

In the largest collective review of mycotic aneurysms, the abdominal aorta was the second most frequent site of involvement (31%), exceeded only by the femoral artery (38%).[158] Chan and associates[176] reported 22 mycotic aortic aneurysms in a series of 2585 patients, an incidence of 0.85%.[161] Coincident with the change in cause, there has been a change in the bacteriology of mycotic aneurysms, with *Salmonella* species declining and *Staphylococcus* species increasing. Together, these are still the

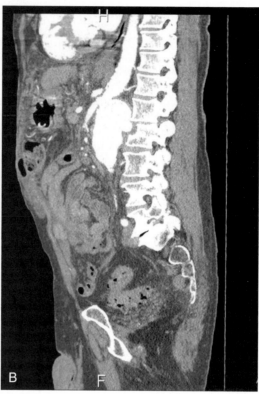

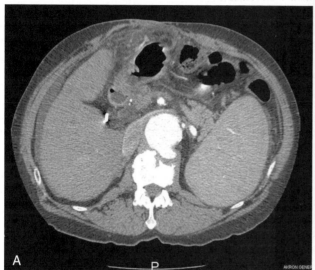

FIGURE 39-7 ■ Computed tomographic scan showing large mycotic aneurysm adjacent to septic process in lumbar vertebral body. **A,** Axial view showing erosion of lumbar vertebral body. **B,** Sagittal reconstruction showing relationship of aneurysm to the superior mesenteric artery.

most frequently cultured organisms from aortic mycotic aneurysms.[162] The predilection for the infrarenal abdominal aorta probably relates to the frequent occurrence of atherosclerotic plaques in this location.

The triad of abdominal pain, fever, and a pulsatile abdominal mass should suggest the diagnosis of mycotic aneurysm. However, many of these aneurysms are small or saccular and not palpable. Usually there is an initial diagnosis of a nonspecific febrile illness of variable duration. Approximately one third have abdominal pain. Leukocytosis is a common finding, but only approximately 50% have positive blood cultures. Mycotic aneurysms are often detected by CT scans performed for the evaluation of undiagnosed fever; they appear as a mass located on one side of the aorta rather than a circumferential enlargement.[160,162] These aneurysms enhance with intravenously administered contrast agent, but the significance of this can be difficult to appreciate. Both CT and catheter angiography demonstrate the characteristic lobulated saccular aneurysm, which may be multiple and contiguous. These are false aneurysms, contained by compressed periaortic tissue. The aneurysm wall tends to be thin and friable and is associated with contiguous lymphadenopathy and obvious inflammation. Blood clot of varying age is present both within and outside the aneurysmal sac, because there is a high incidence of rupture, although it is usually contained. Periaortic abscess may also be present. The opening between the aorta and the aneurysm tends to be irregular or ragged.

Mycotic aneurysms are a fulminant infectious process and must be treated vigorously and promptly.[161,163-165] Control of clinical sepsis does not appear to be necessary before surgical treatment, and delays in operative intervention are associated with aneurysmal rupture. Proper antibiotic therapy must be combined with resection of the infected arterial segments, debridement of all adjacent necrotic tissue, and arterial reconstruction. Control of infection by antibiotics does not prevent rupture of the aneurysm, and excision is mandatory and should be carried out promptly. Many of these aneurysms involve the upper abdominal aorta, where it is not always possible to avoid aortic and branch vessel reconstruction. In situ replacement using femoral veins as the conduit is the safest but most challenging approach when renal or visceral perfusion would be compromised by aortic excision. In situ replacement with an antibiotic-soaked graft has been used successfully if the intraoperative Gram stains are negative and there is no periaortic purulence. It should be followed with at least 6 to 8 weeks of intravenous culture-specific antibiotic therapy and, in the case of *Salmonella* infections, probably lifelong antibiotics. When there is frank periaortic pus or a positive Gram stain of an infrarenal mycotic aneurysm, the safest approach is aortic debridement and ligation and extraanatomic bypass or, for non-virulent organisms, the in situ grafting technique with femoral veins. Recent data indicate that the in situ method is becoming more popular.[175-180] Using these principles, Chan's group

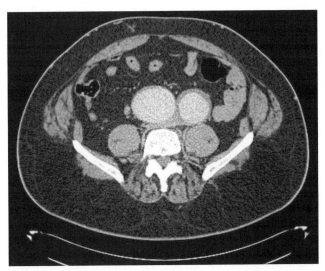

FIGURE 39-8 ■ Computed tomographic scan showing bilateral common iliac aneurysms (axial view).

reported an operative survival rate of 86%, with only one recurrent infection.[176]

ILIAC ARTERY ANEURYSMS

Common iliac artery aneurysms occur in continuity or association with abdominal aortic aneurysms in 16% to 20% of patients but as isolated lesions they are uncommon, accounting for only 1% to 2% of all aneurysms involving the aortoiliac segments and being identified in only 0.03% of autopsies[181-184] (Figure 39-8). The cause in the vast majority of cases is the same as that for nonspecific or multifactorial aortic aneurysms; therefore they occur in association with atherosclerosis in the atherosclerosis-prone age group. However, iliac artery aneurysms can develop during pregnancy in the absence of atherosclerosis, and several other causes have been recognized. Mycotic and traumatic iliac artery aneurysms have been reported, the latter usually after lumbar disk or hip surgery. Other less frequent causes include cystic medial necrosis, dissection, Takayasu disease, Marfan and Ehlers-Danlos syndromes, and Kawasaki disease.

Most isolated iliac aneurysms involve the common iliac (70%) or internal iliac (20%) arteries.[185-186] Isolated external iliac artery aneurysms are extremely rare. Multiple iliac aneurysms occur in the majority of patients, and they are bilateral in approximately 33%. In the series by Richardson and Greenfield,[187] two or more vessels were involved in 67% of patients. Because most of these aneurysms occur in association with atherosclerosis, the average age at diagnosis is around 69 years, and the male-to-female ratio is 7:1. The left and right sides are involved equally.

The clinical presentation of iliac aneurysms is variable and often obscure. Because they are in the pelvis, they are difficult to palpate on physical examination unless they are large. The majority, 50% to 67% in recent reviews, are symptomatic even in the absence of rupture. Symptoms are caused mainly by pressure on adjacent pelvic structures (e.g., urinary tract, lower gastrointestinal tract, lumbosacral nerves, pelvic veins).[188] Thus, lower abdominal, flank, and groin pain is common. Because these are not usually symptoms attributable to the arterial system, delays in diagnosis occur frequently. Diagnosis is usually based on an imaging study looking for the cause of the symptoms or for an unrelated condition. Both CT and ultrasonography are highly reliable for these lesions, and there is excellent correlation between CT and ultrasound measurements.

Many are diagnosed during cardiac catheterization but, as with aortic aneurysms, arteriography can document the presence of iliac aneurysms but frequently underestimates their size because of the presence of laminated thrombus. Other studies that occasionally suggest the diagnosis are barium enema, proctosigmoidoscopy, cystoscopy, and plain radiographs.

Although iliac artery aneurysms are difficult to detect by routine physical examination, large ones can be palpated on abdominal, rectal, or pelvic examination. Common iliac aneurysms are generally more easily felt abdominally, whereas internal iliac aneurysms are more easily felt rectally.

In most reports, iliac aneurysms tend to be large when diagnosed, which probably accounts for the high incidence of symptoms and rupture. In Schuler and Flanigan's collected review, the average size was 8.5 cm, and the incidence of rupture was 51%.[184] In Krupski and coworkers' more recent report, the average size was 5.6 cm, with a 29% rupture rate.[189]

There are no prospective studies of isolated iliac artery aneurysms, but the natural history of large ones appears to be unfavorable. The reported high rate of rupture within a few months of diagnosis probably reflects the aneurysm's large size at the time of discovery. Not surprisingly, operative mortality in patients with ruptured aneurysms ranges from 25% to 56%, with an average of 40%. In contrast, the operative mortality for elective operations is much better, averaging 10% to 11%. The outlook for smaller aneurysms does not appear to be so poor. In Santilli and associates' series of 47 isolated iliac aneurysms, the average size was 2.3 cm, and the only rupture was an aneurysm larger than 5 cm.[190] The average rate of enlargement in that series was 0.12 to 0.26 cm/yr, with larger aneurysms expanding at a greater rate than smaller ones. No patient developed symptoms with an aneurysm smaller than 4 cm. These and other data suggest that isolated common iliac aneurysms smaller than 3 cm can be followed with semiannual ultrasound or CT scans, with minimal risk of symptom development or rupture. Aneurysms 3.5 to 4 cm or larger should be repaired, even if asymptomatic. Symptomatic iliac aneurysms should be repaired regardless of size. The same size guidelines should be used for internal and external iliac aneurysms because so few data are available regarding these uncommon isolated lesions. Common iliac aneurysms associated with aortic aneurysms appear to have the same rupture potential as isolated ones. It is prudent to deal with contiguous common iliac aneurysms larger than 2 to 2.5 cm at the time of aortic aneurysm repair using a bifurcated graft. Smaller-sized iliac arteries can be left in place, allowing tube graft replacement of the aorta, with a very low probability that they will ever enlarge enough to become clinically significant.

The standard treatment for isolated common iliac aneurysms is graft replacement, and because the external iliac artery is almost never aneurysmal, the operation can be confined to the abdomen. Bilateral common iliac aneurysms necessitate the use of an aortoiliac graft configuration. Small internal iliac aneurysms can be treated with catheter-based techniques by injecting coils, plugs, and other thrombogenic materials into the aneurysm and its branches. Alternatively, they can be treated by open endoaneurysmorrhaphy, which can be challenging for large lesions deep in the male pelvis because of difficulty obtaining distal control and controlling back bleeding. These aneurysms should not be treated by simple ligation of the neck because they will remain pressurized via collaterals, enabling further enlargement and potential rupture. The use of stent-grafts has added another option to the treatment of common and external iliac aneurysms and is gaining in popularity with favorable early results.[191] This subject is discussed in more detail elsewhere.

The long-term prognosis of isolated iliac aneurysms after treatment has not been well documented. Nachbur and colleagues[192] reported a 55% 5-year survival rate for patients with ruptured iliac aneurysms. It is reasonable to expect the survival rates to be similar to those for the treatment of aortic aneurysms.

BIBLIOGRAPHY

Bergqvist D: Pharmacological interventions to attenuate the expansion of abdominal aortic aneurysm (AAA)—a systematic review. Eur J Vasc Endovasc Surg 41:663–667, 2011.

Brewster DC, Cronenwett JJ, Hallaett JW, Jr, et al: Guidelines for the treatment of abdominal aortic aneurysms: report of a subcommittee of the Joint Council of the American Association for Vascular Surgery and the Society for Vascular Surgery. J Vasc Surg 37:1106, 2003.
Chaikof EL, Brewster DC, Dalman RL, et al: The care of patients with an abdominal aortic aneurysm: the Society for Vascular Surgery practice guidelines. J Vasc Surg 50:S1–49, 2009.
Fillinger MF, Marra SP, Raghavan ML, et al: Prediction of rupture risk in abdominal aortic aneurysm during observation: wall stress versus diameter. J Vasc Surg 37:724, 2003.
Gadowski GR, Pilcher DB, Ricci MA: Abdominal aortic aneurysm expansion rate: effect of size and beta-adrenergic blockade. J Vasc Surg 19:727, 1994.
Lederle FA, Wilson SE, Johnson GR, et al: Immediate repair compared with surveillance of small abdominal aortic aneurysms. N Engl J Med 346:1437, 2002.
Moll FL, Powell JT, Fraedrich G, et al: Management of abdominal aortic aneurysms. Clinical practice guidelines of the European Society for Vascular Surgery. Eur J Vasc Endovasc Surg 41:S1–S58, 2011.
Rutherford RB, Krupski WC: Current status of open versus endovascular stent-graft repair of abdominal aortic aneurysm. J Vasc Surg 39:1129, 2004.
Santilli SM, Wernsing SE, Lee ES: Expansion rates and outcomes for iliac artery aneurysms. J Vasc Surg 31:114, 2000.
United Kingdom Small Aneurysm Trial participants: Mortality results for randomized controlled trial of early elective surgery or ultrasonographic surveillance for small abdominal aortic aneurysms. Lancet 352:1649, 1998.
United Kingdom Small Aneurysm Trial participants: Long-term outcomes of immediate repair compared to surveillance of small abdominal aortic aneurysms. N Engl J Med 346:1445, 2002.

References available online at expertconsult.com.

QUESTIONS

1. All the following are thought to be involved in the pathogenesis of abdominal aortic aneurysms except:
   a. Heredity
   b. Atherosclerosis
   c. Enzyme imbalance
   d. Smoking
   e. Diabetes mellitus

2. The incidence of abdominal aortic aneurysm is highest among patients with which of the following?
   a. Femoral aneurysm
   b. Aortoiliac occlusive disease
   c. Thoracic aortic aneurysm
   d. Popliteal aneurysm
   e. Isolated iliac artery aneurysm

3. Which of the following statements about the risk of rupture of infrarenal abdominal aortic aneurysms is true?
   a. It increases with increasing size of the aneurysm.
   b. It increases with increasing age of the patient.
   c. It is negligible for aneurysms less than 6 cm in diameter.
   d. It is not affected by blood pressure.
   e. It is related to plasma lipoprotein levels.

4. What is the most common cause of late death following surgical treatment of abdominal aortic aneurysms?
   a. Renal failure
   b. Respiratory failure
   c. Myocardial ischemia
   d. Graft infection
   e. Malignancy

5. What is the true mortality for ruptured abdominal aortic aneurysms, including prehospital deaths?
   a. 15%
   b. 30%
   c. 50%
   d. 60%
   e. 90%

6. During the course of an aortic aneurysm operation from a transperitoneal approach, the surgeon does not see the left renal vein crossing anterior to the aorta. The surgeon should do which of the following?
   a. Extend the dissection farther cephalad to the superior mesenteric artery.
   b. Thoroughly mobilize the neck of the aneurysm.
   c. Carefully preserve the adrenal and inferior mesenteric veins.
   d. Assume the left renal vein is probably congenitally absent.
   e. Take extra care during application of the aortic cross-clamp.

7. Which of the following statements about aortocaval fistulas is true?
   a. They are usually infectious in origin.
   b. They are usually symptomatic.
   c. They usually occur just below the left renal vein.
   d. All of the above
   e. None of the above

8. Which of the following statements about complications of aortic aneurysm repair is true?
   a. Colon ischemia is associated with a mortality rate of about 50%.
   b. Renal failure does not occur if the aortic cross-clamp is totally infrarenal.
   c. Paraplegia occurs only with suprarenal clamping.
   d. Myocardial dysfunction is now an uncommon cause of postoperative death.
   e. The use of autotransfusion devices has greatly reduced the degree of postoperative hemorrhage.

9. All the following statements about inflammatory aneurysms are true except:
   a. They have thick fibrous walls.
   b. They are frequently associated with abdominal tenderness in the area of the aneurysm.
   c. They require CT scanning for definitive preoperative diagnosis.
   d. They frequently rupture.
   e. They are frequently associated with ureteral obstruction.

10. All the following statements about iliac artery aneurysms are true except:
    a. Asymptomatic aneurysms should be at least 2.5 cm in diameter for repair to be indicated.
    b. Most are associated with or are an extension of infrarenal abdominal aortic aneurysms.
    c. Most isolated iliac aneurysms manifest symptoms before rupture.
    d. They may be diagnosed by digital examination of the vagina and rectum.
    e. They are commonly bilateral.

ANSWERS

1. **e**
2. **a**
3. **a**
4. **c**
5. **e**
6. **e**
7. **b**
8. **a**
9. **d**
10. **a**

CHAPTER 40

ENDOVASCULAR REPAIR OF JUXTARENAL (CHIMNEY), INFRARENAL, AND ILIAC ARTERY ANEURYSMS

Grace J. Wang • Jon S. Matsumura • Ronald M. Fairman

In 1991, Parodi and colleagues[1] published a seminal study of patients who underwent abdominal aortic aneurysm repair using an intraluminal, stent-anchored polyester prosthetic graft delivered retrograde from the common femoral artery and revolutionized the field of vascular surgery. While initially considered the preferred modality for patients deemed unfit for open surgery, endovascular aneurysm repair (EVAR) has rapidly evolved as an important alternative, less invasive, and frequently preferred treatment for patients with abdominal aortic aneurysms. The technology has significantly reduced perioperative morbidity and mortality resulting in expanded application, and the wide acceptance by physicians has been the impetus for subsequent device evolution. Since its inception, the technology has undergone multiple iterations, with earlier generation grafts having been abandoned in favor of current endografts with their superior radial force, columnar support as well as additional modes of fixation. There are currently six endografts approved by the U.S. Food and Drug Administration (FDA) and on the market for the treatment of infrarenal abdominal aortic aneurysms (Table 40-1). The endograft consists of a metal stent attached to prosthetic graft material which is housed in a sheath, to allow for intraarterial delivery of the device. Most bifurcated stent-grafts use a modular design, the exception being the Endologix device in which the bifurcated component is deployed in a unibody fashion. The basic differences in construct are outlined in Table 40-1.

PATIENT SELECTION

The introduction of EVAR as a lesser invasive alternative to open aortic aneurysm repair has not changed the indications for repair. Repair is undertaken when abdominal aortic aneurysms reach 5 to 5.5 cm in diameter; however, certain anatomic criteria need to be met for successful EVAR to occur. The most important area of interest is the proximal aortic neck. A cylindrical neck of at least 15 mm in length measured from the renal arteries, with a diameter of 33 mm or less is preferred. In addition, the neck should be relatively free of thrombus and calcification, as these interfere with apposition of the stent graft against the aortic luminal surface. Neck angulation

defined as the angle between the infrarenal aorta and the neck of the aneurysm of greater than 60 degrees can also interfere with the ability to achieve a proximal seal. The distal landing zone has several elements that require evaluation. The aortic bifurcation should be large enough to accommodate both limbs of the bifurcated stent graft; preferentially greater than 22 mm in diameter. The maximal iliac artery diameter must be at least 2 mm smaller than the largest limb size available. Several manufacturers produce iliac limbs with flared diameters, allowing for preservation of the internal iliac artery and this is referred to as the bell-bottom technique. If the common iliac artery is short or aneurysmal and external iliac artery landing is required, internal iliac artery embolization is performed to prevent an endoleak. Typically, unilateral hypogastric artery occlusion is well tolerated. If a patient has bilateral common iliac artery aneurysms, repair should be staged to avoid complications with pelvic ischemia. In practice, discussions with patients about potential hip and buttock claudication, as well as erectile dysfunction, should be undertaken preoperatively. Access for delivery of the device is another important consideration. The diameter of the femoral and iliac vessels must be of sufficient size for traversal of the sheath delivery system. Preoperative assessment of the patient's imaging, as well as careful consideration of the device manufacturer's specifications in regard to outer diameter of the delivery system, will allow the formulation of an access strategy. Alternatively, iliac conduits and retroperitoneal approaches have expanded the application of EVAR beyond traditional femoral approaches, i.e., Iliac artery tortuosity should be routinely assessed, as severe degrees may necessitate adjunctive maneuvers such as brachio-femoral access techniques to straighten and "rail" the system. The ability to navigate difficult anatomy has been greatly improved by modern stiff wires. Any patient whose intestinal circulation is based on the inferior mesenteric artery (in the instance of celiac and superior mesenteric artery occlusions) should also not undergo EVAR. Patients who have accessory renal arteries are not routinely disqualified from EVAR consideration, unless their coverage would likely affect renal function. In patients who have diabetes mellitus and an elevation of their baseline creatinine, covering even small accessory renals may result in deterioration of renal function. Patients who are

TABLE 40-1 **Current Commercially Available Abdominal Aortic Stent-Grafts**

Device Name	Company	Configuration	Max Device Diameter	Min Device Diameter	Fabric	Metal	Active Fixation	Anatomic Fixation
Zenith	Cook	Trimodular	36	22	Woven Dacron	Stainless steel	Suprarenal stent with barbs	
Talent	Medtronic	Bimodular	36	22	Woven Dacron	Nitinol	Suprarenal stent	
Aneurx	Medtronic	Bimodular	28	20	Woven polyester	Nitinol		
Endurant	Medtronic	Bimodular	36	23	Woven polyester	Nitinol	Suprarenal stent with barbs	
Excluder	Gore	Bimodular	31	23	ePTFE	Nitinol	Barbs	
Powerlink	Endologix	Unibody	34 (Cuff)	22	ePTFE	Cobalt chromium	Suprarenal stent on aortic cuff	Deployment at aortic bifurcation

reluctant to undergo the surveillance protocol should not be considered for EVAR, because the need for secondary intervention following EVAR is not insignificant.

ENDOVASCULAR TREATMENT OF JUXTARENAL AORTIC ANEURYSMS

Juxtarenal and *pararenal* are terms used to refer to abdominal aortic aneurysms with an infrarenal neck less than or equal to 1 cm in length. Although these aneurysms would traditionally require an open approach, the drive of industry and technology, as well as a comorbid patient population, have motivated the expansion and use of endovascular approaches for repair. Branched and fenestrated grafts offer a "totally endovascular" solution, but are not currently commercially available in the United States. These specialized grafts are available to patients enrolled in a clinical trial and take 6 to 8 weeks to manufacture, provided the patient meets protocol-defined anatomic and clinical constraints. These endografts are discussed in a separate chapter.

Renal artery stenting via the encroachment or snorkel (or chimney) technique allows preservation of renal blood flow when treating juxtarenal aneurysms with traditional infrarenal stent grafts. This chapter will outline these endovascular approaches to treating juxtarenal aneurysms.

SETTING

Traditionally, endovascular abdominal aortic aneurysm repair has been done in an interventional or catheterization suite. Currently, however, the hybrid operating room with fixed C-arm positioning affords greater flexibility and safety. Alternatively portable C-arm imaging systems are far more sophisticated than when many clinicians began performing EVAR in the mid 1990s. EVAR has been described with regional block, local anesthesia, and general anesthesia, but the authors believe that general anesthesia gives the surgeon maximal control over the

operation with minimal risk to the patient. Having immediate access to an open vascular set is paramount and at times lifesaving should the patient need to be converted emergently. It is also useful if attendant open adjunctive procedures such as femoral-femoral artery bypass grafting, iliac conduit, or local femoral endarterectomy need to be performed. As EVAR is being performed increasingly in much older comorbid patients with less than ideal anatomy, the need for sophisticated operative imaging to optimize precision deployment, as well as a surgical preparedness for potentially catastrophic access issues, underscores the importance of the operating room or hybrid suite in performing these procedures. The outcomes of EVAR for ruptured abdominal aortic aneurysm (AAA) have also been favorable, particularly in institutions where a systematic algorithm ensures that the appropriate endovascular team is alerted when a ruptured aneurysm is identified in the emergency room.[2,3] It is clear that, in this subset of patients, having the ability to convert from an endovascular to an open approach should they rapidly deteriorate is an important consideration. Of paramount importance to the success of every aortic endovascular program is identifying and training a dedicated endovascular team of nurses, operating room scrub technicians, and radiology technologists. For many institutions this will require a major shift in operating room culture.

ENDOVASCULAR STENT GRAFT PLANNING AND PLACEMENT FOR INFRARENAL AORTIC ANEURYSMS

The majority of the case is performed before entering the operating room. Axial imaging is obtained via computed tomography angiography or magnetic resonance angiography provided that the patient does not have renal insufficiency. Three-dimensional reconstructions performed by either Terra Recon (Foster City, Calif.), Vitrea (Vital Images), Leonardo (Siemens), or M2S (Lebanon, N.H.) have become the standard and are used to measure the

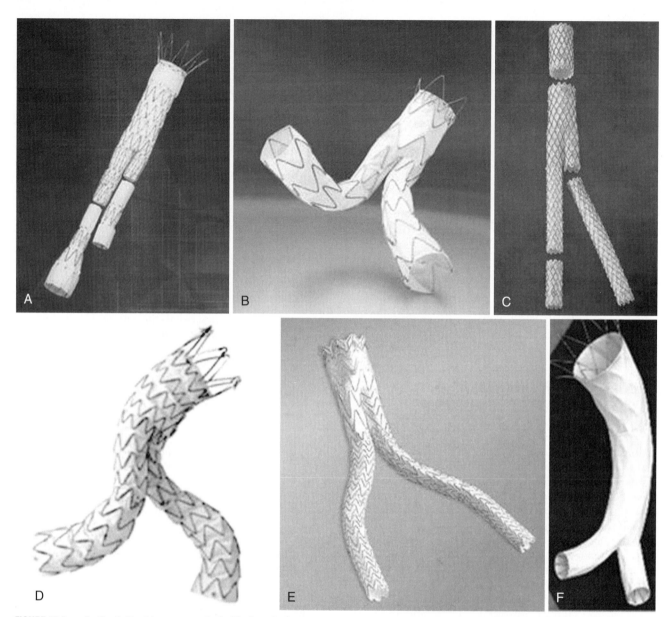

FIGURE 40-1 ■ **A,** Cook Zenith stent graft. **B,** Medtronic Talent stent graft. **C,** Medtronic AneuRx stent graft. **D,** Medtronic Endurant stent graft. **E,** Gore Excluder stent graft. **F,** Endologix Powerlink stent graft.

distance from the lowest renal artery to the aortic bifurcation, the lowest renal artery to the ipsilateral hypogastric artery, and the lowest renal artery to the contralateral hypogastric artery (Figures 40-1 and 40-2). Diameter measurements of the neck and of the common iliac arteries are then performed. It is important at this time to note the extent of neck angulation and rotation of the juxtarenal aorta to optimize accurate endograft deployment. Broeders and Blankensteijn[4] describe a simple technique to optimize imaging prior to endograft deployment. The juxtarenal aorta should be visualized in the sagittal plane to measure the degree of craniocaudad angulation (Figure 40-3). The axial sections are then used to measure the degree of aortic neck rotation (Figure 40-4). These angle calculations should be noted to ensure that the C-arm is orthogonal to the takeoff of the lowest renal artery. The tortuosity of the vessels, the degree of calcification and

any thrombus is also noted. Circumferential thrombus or calcification will prevent complete apposition of the stent graft to the aortic wall and thus compromise the ability to achieve a proximal seal. Using 10% to 20% proximal graft oversizing, the stent-graft devices are typically ordered and delivered in advance of the scheduled case. The stent grafts are housed in relatively large sheaths and obviate either bilateral groin cutdowns or percutaneous access that is later closed with vascular closure devices. After introduction of the delivery system over a stiff wire to the juxtarenal aorta, an aortogram is performed, and under "roadmap" guidance, the main body of the stent graft is positioned and deployed just under the lowest renal artery. Care is taken to insert and deploy the main body of the graft with the contralateral gate deployed in an anterolateral position, which is optimal for subsequent retrograde cannulation. Once the contralateral gate is

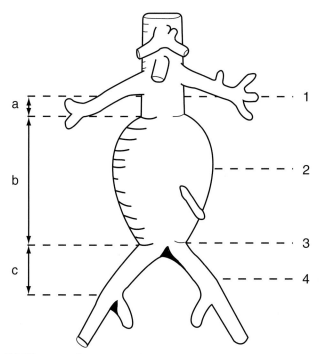

FIGURE 40-2 ■ Schematic of abdominal aortic aneurysm measurements for stent-graft sizing. *a,* Length of neck; *b,* length of aneurysm; *c,* length of common iliac artery; *a + b + c* = distance from lowest renal artery to ipsilateral internal iliac artery; *1,* diameter of aortic neck; *2,* maximal diameter of aneurysm; *3,* diameter of aortic bifurcation; *4,* diameter of common iliac artery.

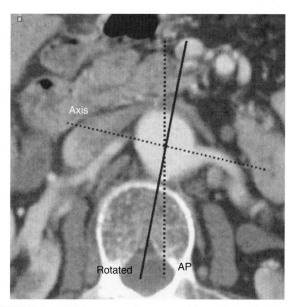

FIGURE 40-4 ■ Axial computed tomographic angiography image demonstrating the axes relative to the aorta in the anteroposterior and rotated projections relative to the axis between the lowest renal artery orifice and the center of the aorta. (From Broeders IA, Blankensteijn JD: A simple technique to improve the accuracy of proximal AAA endograft deployment. J Endovasc Ther 7:389–393, 2000.)

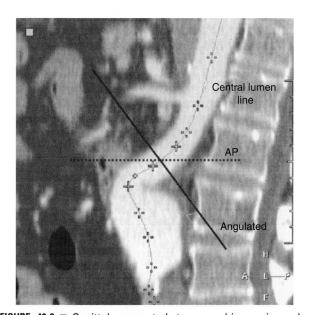

FIGURE 40-3 ■ Sagittal computed tomographic angiography reconstruction demonstrating the central lumen line and the axes relative to the aorta in the anteroposterior and angulated projections. Note that the angulated line is perpendicular to the aortic center line axis. (From Broeders IA, Blankensteijn JD: A simple technique to improve the accuracy of proximal AAA endograft deployment. J Endovasc Ther 7:389–393, 2000.)

deployed, it is cannulated, and efforts are made to ensure that the catheter is indeed within the stent graft and not behind the graft in the aneurysm sac. When deploying devices with separate suprarenal fixation, a magnified aortogram is performed at this time to confirm the location and position of the renal arteries. Cranial obliquity is usually required to ensure that the origin of the lowest renal artery is seen in an orthogonal orientation. Once the suprarenal stent is deployed, the stiff wire is placed up the contralateral limb and a pelvic arteriogram with the C-arm obliqued 15 to 20 degrees to the other side is performed to demonstrate the origin of the contralateral hypogastric artery. The contralateral iliac limb is then deployed taking care to preserve flow to the internal iliac artery. The remainder of the main body or ipsilateral limb is deployed. In an obligate three-piece system, another pelvic arteriogram is performed in the opposite obliquity to demonstrate the takeoff of the ipsilateral internal iliac artery. The junctions are ballooned, and stiff wires are removed before the completion of arteriography to ensure that limb kinking is not a concern. Graft limb kinking is of particular concern in individuals with external iliac landing because of concomitant iliac artery aneurysms or small iliac artery diameters. Any type I or III endoleaks should be addressed in the operating room. Type I endoleaks can be addressed with proximal extensions, large-diameter bare stents, or simple ballooning. Type III endoleaks can be addressed with bridging pieces or repeated ballooning. Type II endoleaks can be observed, as the majority of them resolve with conservative management within 6 to 12 months. Completion arteriography should demonstrate both renal and hypogastric artery patency and good flow down both iliac limbs. In the setting of small calcified aortic bifurcations (<20 mm diameter), adjunctive bilateral kissing balloon angioplasty should be a consideration.

ENDOVASCULAR REPAIR OF COMMON ILIAC ARTERY ANEURYSMS

The majority of individuals with common iliac artery aneurysms have concomitant abdominal aortic aneurysms. If the common iliac artery aneurysm encroaches on the aortic bifurcation such that there is not enough length for a proximal seal, or if they have a concomitant AAA, endovascular aortic stent-grafting is performed simultaneously. Intervention for common iliac artery aneurysms typically occurs when they are 3 to 4 cm in diameter. Endovascular repair involves coil embolization of the ipsilateral hypogastric artery to prevent a type II endoleak. The iliac limb is then deployed into the external iliac artery. Small series have shown that staging embolization of the internal iliac artery in the instances where patients have bilateral common iliac artery aneurysms is better tolerated and results in a lower risk of pelvic ischemia (i.e., colorectal ischemia, buttock claudication, and sexual impotence).[5,6] Iliac branched devices have been developed and are currently under trial investigation in the United States, although initial results abroad are promising.[7] The branched devices allow for preservation of flow to the internal iliac while achieving a distal seal in the external iliac artery. This study reported a secondary patency rate of 87.3% at 22 months.

ENDOVASCULAR REPAIR OF JUXTARENAL AORTIC ANEURYSMS

For some patients with a proximal infrarenal neck length less than 15 mm (the traditional desired neck length for endovascular aortic aneurysm repair), partial renal artery coverage with adjunctive renal artery stenting can be performed.[8] Using either the encroachment technique, where the superior margin of the stent graft is pushed inferiorly by the renal stent, or the snorkel technique, where the stent graft is pushed inward by the renal stent (Figures 40-5 and 40-6), a case series showed that sealing of the aneurysm was possible (no type I endoleak at 1 month follow-up) with a primary assisted patency of renal artery stents of 100%. Transbrachial access is key for the snorkel maneuver, because it is often used when more extensive coverage of the renal artery is required, and the stent is required to run alongside the stent graft before entering the orifice of the artery. The encroachment methods, however, can usually be effectively approached transfemorally.

Encroachment Technique

This technique is used when partial renal artery coverage is needed to achieve a seal. The aortic stent graft is deployed in the usual fashion, with careful attention paid to the relationship between the top of the stent-graft fabric and the lowest renal artery. The optimal degree of

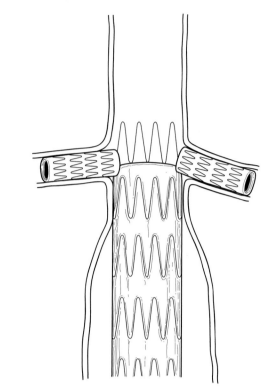

FIGURE 40-5 ■ The encroachment technique during endovascular aneurysm repair. (From Chaikof E, Cambria R: Atlas of vascular surgery and endovascular therapy, Philadelphia, 2013, Elsevier.)

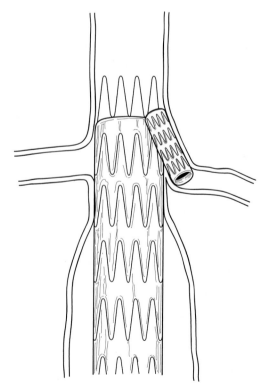

FIGURE 40-6 ■ The chimney technique during endovascular aneurysm repair. (From Chaikof E, Cambria R: Atlas of vascular surgery and endovascular therapy, Philadelphia, 2012, Elsevier.)

angulation and rotation for visualizing the takeoff of the renal artery is then determined. Catheter and wire access of the renal artery is obtained. If a device with a suprarenal stent is used, care is taken to access the base of the triangular stent rather than in between the triangular stents. One recommendation is the use of a combination of a Rosen wire (Cook Medical, Bloomington, Ind.) and a guide catheter system to serve as a platform for performing the renal stent. Balloon-expandable stents are favored in this location because the increased radial force is essential to push the superior margin of the stent-graft inferiorly to preserve renal artery flow.

Snorkel Technique

The snorkel technique is used when complete coverage of the renal artery origin is required to achieve a seal. Brachial access to the renal is performed before stent-graft deployment. A combination of a Rosen wire and a long Destination sheath (Terumo, Somerset, N.J.) as a platform is recommended. The renal stent comes to lie entirely outside the aortic stent graft, parallel to it until it enters the renal artery orifice. Both covered and uncovered stents have been used for this purpose. The length of the stent is usually longer because of the distance along the aortic stent graft, which needs to be traversed before reaching the origin of the renal artery. It is important to maintain balloon support of the renal stent while ballooning the aortic graft, because compression of the stent can occur with this maneuver.

Although the authors admit that the long-term durability of these methods are not known, both techniques effectively lengthen the seal zone while preserving renal blood flow, allowing the use of off-the-shelf stent-grafts for pararenal aneurysm repair. In addition, the authors have been more enthusiastic and aggressive in the use of these endovascular opportunities in much older and frail patients with significant comorbidities.

POSTOPERATIVE COMPLICATIONS

Local

Groin wound complications include hematoma, pseudoaneurysm formation, seromas, and cellulitis. Attention to detail in closing the arteriotomy sites as well as reapproximating the subcutaneous tissues in multiple layers, including the oversewing of lymphatics, can help to avoid the majority of these local wound complications. We and others have endorsed the use of transverse groin incisions.

Systemic

Renal insufficiency can be exacerbated in patients with underlying chronic renal insufficiency and can be overcome with adequate preoperative and perioperative hydration with a bicarbonate solution as well as judicious use of diluted contrast agents in the operating suite. Thromboembolic complications from thrombus-laden aortic necks to the renal arteries following EVAR have been described, but are surprisingly less frequent than anticipated when these procedures are performed with regularity. Patients with short, angulated necks and challenging proximal seal zones who may require adjunctive renal stenting for preservation should be closely monitored for any drop in urine output. If there is any doubt as to whether renal artery flow is compromised, urgent interrogation via duplex or arteriography is required.

Postimplantation syndrome is characterized by low-grade fevers and an elevated white blood count without an obvious infectious source and is thought to be secondary to cytokine release following thrombosis of the aneurysm sac. It is important in these patients to rule out an infectious source as an etiology for these fevers. This syndrome typically is self limiting and lasts 7 to 10 days.

LATE COMPLICATIONS

Late complications following EVAR are largely attributable to endoleak. Figure 40-7 depicts the different types

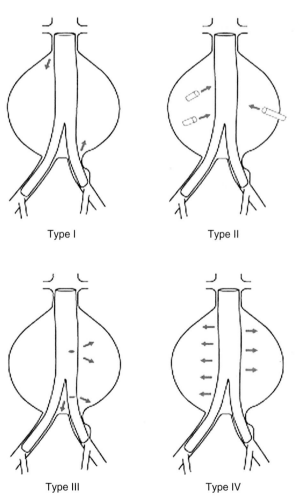

Type I

Type II

Type III

Type IV

FIGURE 40-7 ■ Diagram of the different types of endoleak. Type I endoleaks occur at the proximal (Ia) or distal (Ib) seal zones. Type II endoleaks occur because of back-bleeding from branch vessels such as the lumbar arteries or inferior mesenteric artery. Type III endoleaks are the result of a defect in the graft fabric or lack of intercomponent seal. Type IV endoleaks are due to graft fabric porosity.

of endoleak. The need for secondary intervention following EVAR is not insignificant, with a reported frequency of 10% to 18%.[9] The majority of these interventions can be performed endovascularly (76%), underscoring the importance of regular surveillance for maintenance of successful endovascular repair. Late failure can be categorized as secondary to a change in structure or position of the stent graft, resulting in endoleak or graft thrombosis, or due to a change in aortic anatomy.

Migration is defined as caudal migration of the stent graft by more than 1 cm; this can result in a proximal type I endoleak, which can result in sac pressurization, growth, and rupture if not treated. Proximal device extension, bare metal stent deployment to buttress radial support in the area, or renal artery snorkel or encroachment techniques can be used to achieve a proximal seal again. If the main body of the prior stent-graft is too short for the deployment of a proximal extension, an aorto-uniiliac device can be used, necessitating a femoral-femoral artery bypass and embolization of the contralateral proximal iliac artery with an occlusion device. Type III endoleak from fabric erosion is effectively treated with stent-graft relining or bridging of components to effectively seal the hole. Component separation is likewise treated with relining. When the device pieces are particularly separated in space owing to excessive tortuosity, obtaining wire access through both components may be challenging; transbrachial access with a snare may be useful in this situation. Stent fracture has been noted in follow-up and for the most part is not associated with untoward effects. Proximal extension or relining may be appropriate if fracture results in concomitant migration and endoleak.

Aortic neck dilatation may be another mode of failure following EVAR. Provided that there is a commercial device available to seal the dilated aortic neck, a proximal extension may be deployed to achieve a proximal seal. Distal common iliac artery dilation with a type IB endoleak is retreated with hypogastric artery occlusion and extension to the external iliac artery.

There is consensus that type II endoleaks in the presence of an enlarging aneurysm sac require intervention; these are typically due to a patent inferior mesenteric artery or iliolumbar arteries. Embolization can be performed using coils or *N*-butyl cyanoacrylate glue. The transarterial approach can be used to embolize the inferior mesenteric artery through the superior mesenteric artery from the marginal artery of Drummond. The translumbar approach uses a direct aneurysm sac puncture technique. Regardless of the approach, these endoleaks physiologically behave like arteriovenous malformations, and embolization of the nidus of the endoleak including the inflow and outflow vessels is the optimal approach. Retroperitoneal endoscopic ligation of the lumbar arteries has also been described. Type IV endoleaks are related to porosity of the graft fabric, occur less frequently with current generation stent grafts, and are noted within 30 days of graft implantation. These endoleaks are most commonly observed as a blush of contrast coming through the fabric of the stent-graft on the completion arteriogram before heparin reversal; they usually resolve once graft interstices thrombose. Endotension, or

TABLE 40-2	**Types of Endoleaks and Management Strategies**	
Classification	**Causes of Perigraft Flow**	**Therapeutic Options**
Type I	Inadequate seal of proximal or distal end of endograft	Proximal or distal extension or cuff
	Inadequate seal of iliac occluder plug	Overstenting
		Embolization or glue
		Conversion
Type II	Flow from patent lumbar, middle sacral, or inferior mesenteric artery; hypogastric, accessory renal, or other visceral vessel	Observation
		Coil embolization or glue
		Laparoscopic ligation
		Conversion
Type III	Fabric disruption or tear	Secondary endograft or cuff
	Module disconnection	Conversion
Type IV	Flow from fabric porosity, suture holes (<30 days after graft placement)	Observation
Endoleak of undefined origin	Flow visualized from unidentified source	Observation
		Angiographic investigation

type V endoleak, is defined as elevated sac aneurysm pressure without a clearly defined endoleak. It is generally believed that the etiology is an undetected endoleak or transmission of systemic pressure through thrombus. Endotension is typically detected as continued sac enlargement on computed tomography (CT) scan, but can also be detected by direct aneurysm sac pressure sensors (Cardiomems, Atlanta, Ga.).

A summary of the types of endoleaks and how they are managed is provided in Table 40-2. Should the methods discussed here prove unsuccessful in managing EVAR failure, open conversion and explant should be performed. This has been shown to be possible with acceptable morbidity and mortality in both the elective and emergent setting.[10]

Graft limb occlusion has been estimated between 3% and 7%,[11,12] usually occurs within the first 6 months following EVAR, and is more frequent in patients with aortoiliac occlusive disease, with a small distal aorta (<14 mm), who have tortuous iliacs, or who require external iliac artery landing. Earlier generation stent grafts with unsupported limbs are also at risk for limb kinking.[13,14] The majority of patients exhibit buttock, thigh, or calf claudication. In the majority of instances, the limb can be recanalized with either thrombolysis or surgical thrombectomy techniques, with adjunctive iliac stenting as needed. It is of utmost importance that the etiology and site of the limb kink be identified. Arteriography with oblique orientation can be helpful in providing the views to help identify the problem. In addition, intravascular ultrasound and measurement of pullback pressures may help to identify graft infolding, which might not be noted on arteriography.[15] In patients in whom the limb cannot be reopened, femoral-femoral bypass is performed to revascularize the contralateral leg.

Infection of the aortic stent graft is a rare event, with small case series reporting an incidence of 0.2% to 0.7%.[16] In the largest case series to date, nine patients presented with infected EVAR at a tertiary referral center.[17] All patients underwent complete explants of the stent graft with either preemptive revascularization (axillary-femoral to femoral artery bypass) in five patients or in situ reconstruction with Rifampin-soaked polyester in the other four. Seven of the patients survived to discharge, and the mean follow-up of the surviving patients was 11 months. In this series, the presence of a concomitant aortoenteric fistula was particularly virulent. Two of the three patients with aortoenteric fistula died before discharge. While generally considered a highly morbid condition with mortality rates estimated at 36%,[18] the findings from this study suggest that explantation of infected grafts can be performed with acceptable mortality rate.

POSTOPERATIVE SURVEILLANCE

Postoperative surveillance following EVAR is essential for ensuring success. Postoperative surveillance allows the detection of endoleaks, aneurysm sac expansion, stent fracture, limb kinking, and material fatigue. Initial protocols were adopted from the initial FDA-sponsored trials that recommended CT scans at 1-, 6-, and 12-month intervals and annually thereafter.[19] The frequent use of CT scanning has raised concerns related to the added cost of these studies, as well as cumulative radiation exposure[20,21] and use of nephrotoxic agents. Although ultrasound duplex avoids radiation exposure and the use of contrast dye, concerns have been raised in the past regarding its variable sensitivity in detecting endoleaks.[22] The utility of ultrasound is also limited in obese patients or those with substantial bowel gas. Based on these recent reports, some investigators have proposed that follow-up with duplex as the sole imaging modality is appropriate,

provided there is no endoleak or sac enlargement documented on the first annual CT scan.[23] A significant increase in sac size or a newly diagnosed endoleak would then prompt CT imaging.[24] Omitting the 6-month scan has also been recommended, if CT imaging at 1 month does not identify an endoleak.[23,25] These protocols have been shown to be safe with minimal risk of clinical adverse event.[26] The Society for Vascular Surgery practice guidelines currently recommend contrast-enhanced CT scanning 1 and 12 months during the first year after EVAR.[19] Detection of an endoleak at 1 month would prompt another CT scan at 6 months to evaluate the need for intervention. If neither endoleak nor aneurysm expansion are detected during the first year after EVAR, duplex may be a reasonable alternative. In patients with renal insufficiency, duplex ultrasound in combination with a non-contrast CT scan is a reasonable surveillance strategy. A summary of this management strategy is provided in Figure 40-8. Although the risk of endoleak declines with each negative surveillance CT scan, new endoleaks have been identified as late as 7 years after EVAR,[27] underscoring the importance of lifelong surveillance. The long-term (>20 years) outcome of stent grafts has not been established, and multiple studies reporting the midterm results of EVAR using various devices cite a need for secondary intervention. From the EVAR-1 and EVAR-2 trials, the secondary intervention rates were 7.0% for the Zenith and 9.4% for the Talent grafts at approximately 4 years of follow-up.[28] In the 5-year follow-up study of the patients who underwent Zenith stent-graft repair as part of the pivotal trial, the cumulative risk of conversion, limb occlusion, migration greater than 10 mm, or component separation was 3% or less at 5 years. The cumulative risk of late endoleak was 12% to 15%, accounting for the majority of secondary interventions, and underscoring the importance of continued surveillance long term.[29] While the majority of these secondary interventions can be performed by endovascular means, a minority of patients will require explant of the graft and formal open repair of their aneurysm.

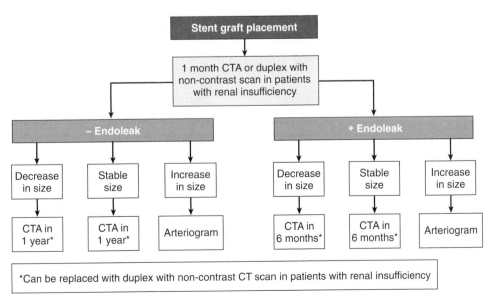

FIGURE 40-8 ■ Surveillance following endovascular repair of abdominal aortic aneurysm.

MIDTERM OUTCOMES

Despite the early perioperative benefits noted with EVAR,[30] randomized trials and population-based studies have shown similar late survival after endovascular and open AAA repair.[31-35] In the DREAM and EVAR-1 trials, there was a 3% reduction in aneurysm-related mortality throughout the follow-up period, but the initial reduction in all-cause mortality was eliminated within 1 to 2 years. The survival curves overlapped by 18 months in randomized control trials and at 3 years in Medicare beneficiaries.[31-33] In addition, EVAR was associated with a greater number of late complications and secondary reinterventions. In the EVAR-1 trial, reinterventions occurred at a rate of 20% at 4 years, compared with 6% for open surgical repair.[32] The DREAM trial showed a higher reintervention rate in the EVAR group at 9 months compared with the open surgical group (hazard ratio, 2.9; 95% confidence interval, 1.1 to 6.2). In a population-based study of 45,660 Medicare beneficiaries, AAA-related intervention was 9.0% following EVAR compared with 1.7% after open repair. AAA-rupture was also slightly higher after EVAR at 1.8% versus 0.5% after open repair. As expected, laparotomy-related complications were more likely in the open repair group (9.7% vs. 4.1%). Giles and colleagues[36] conducted a study in Medicare beneficiaries in an attempt to discern the effect of reintervention on survival. Reintervention and readmission rates were slightly higher after EVAR (7.6% vs. 7.0%). They also found that reinterventions or readmissions accounted for 9.6% of all EVAR deaths and 7.6% of all open repair deaths in the follow-up period. These findings indicate that survival is negatively affected by reintervention or readmission after EVAR and open surgery, which could account for the lack of survival benefit of EVAR over time.

In summary, EVAR has been associated with reduced morbidity, reduced intensive care unit and hospital length of stay, and lower perioperative mortality rates; however, further research is needed to optimize the risk-to-benefit ratio in the long term. Continued improvements in device design, favorable patient and anatomic selection, and imaging capabilities will surely advance this technology and lead to durable endovascular AAA repair.

References available online at expertconsult.com.

QUESTIONS

1. What is the most important anatomic variable for determining a patient's suitability for EVAR?
   a. Proximal aortic neck
   b. Size of iliac vessels
   c. Tortuosity of iliac vessels
   d. Degree of calcification in the aneurysm sac

2. Which type of endoleak is initially managed with continued monitoring?
   a. Type I
   b. Type II with stable or decreased aneurysm sac size
   c. Type II with increased aneurysm sac size
   d. Type III

3. True or false: Patients undergoing EVAR exhibit decreased perioperative morbidity and mortality rates but equivalent long-term survival rates compared with patients undergoing open surgical repair.

4. Which of the following device characteristics can prevent graft migration?
   a. Radial force
   b. Suprarenal fixation
   c. Hooks or barbs
   d. All of the above

5. True or false: Patients with juxtarenal abdominal aortic aneurysms can be treated with EVAR and renal stenting via the encroachment or chimney maneuvers.

6. True or false: Patients undergoing EVAR have a lower rate of secondary intervention compared with the open surgical repair group.

7. The most appropriate postoperative surveillance study is:
   a. Arteriogram
   b. CTA
   c. Abdominal radiograph
   d. Serum creatinine level

8. All the following endografts use a modular system except:
   a. AneuRx
   b. Zenith
   c. Powerlink
   d. Excluder

9. True or false: Most type I endoleaks are treated with immediate surgical conversion.

10. True or false: An occluded superior mesenteric artery and an enlarged inferior mesenteric artery and marginal artery of Drummond preclude endovascular stent graft repair.

ANSWERS

1. **a**
2. **b**
3. **True**
4. **d**
5. **True**
6. **False**
7. **b**
8. **c**
9. **False**
10. **True**

OPEN SURGICAL AND ENDOVASCULAR MANAGEMENT OF RUPTURED ABDOMINAL AORTIC ANEURYSM

Frank J. Veith • Neal S. Cayne • Todd L. Berland • Dieter Mayer • Mario Lachat

A ruptured abdominal aortic aneurysm (AAA) is a relatively common but catastrophic problem that, if untreated, will almost always result in the death of a patient. With treatment, which can consist of open surgical repair or endovascular graft exclusion of the ruptured AAA, many patients will survive and live out their normal lifespan. This chapter will discuss important aspects of the open surgical and endovascular graft repair of ruptured AAAs that have a rupture site in the aorta or common iliac arteries. Because the preoperative, intraoperative, and postoperative management associated with open surgical repair is well known and well standardized, this chapter will stress only crucial and less well-known aspects of these areas of open repair. The remainder of this chapter will then address the history and current status of endovascular treatment of ruptured AAAs, with an emphasis on endovascular aneurysm repair (EVAR) by endograft exclusion of the ruptured AAA. The text will also emphasize key management strategies, technical maneuvers, and adjuncts that are important in achieving optimal outcomes in the very sick patient group with a ruptured AAA.

OPEN SURGICAL MANAGEMENT: KEY POINTS

Crucial Diagnostic Triad

Pain, syncope, and a known or palpable AAA are a crucial diagnostic triad. If a patient has all three elements, he or she should be considered to have a presumptive diagnosis of a ruptured AAA. If open surgical treatment is planned, the patient should be taken immediately to the operating room and prepared for operation. No further diagnostic evaluation is necessary. Although an occasional patient will have another catastrophic problem, most of these patients require a laparotomy anyway. The only exceptions are an acute myocardial infarction and pancreatitis. The former can be suggested because of electrocardiogram findings, the latter because of a high hematocrit and an elevated amylase.

The history of syncope is usually a manifestation of hypovolemia if cardiac causes can be excluded. The

known AAA may be confirmed by history or the presence of a palpable pulsatile mass on physical examination. Although the pain element of the triad is usually in the mid-abdomen or back, it may be in the chest, lower abdomen, flank, or groin. These unusual locations are caused by the pressure of the hematoma, which might not be centrally located and therefore produce unusual pain patterns. One example would be flank and groin pain mimicking a renal or ureteral stone. Another example would be left lower quadrant pain and a mass mimicking diverticulitis.

If a patient only has two elements of the triad, further emergent diagnostic studies with ultrasound or CT scanning are justified. However, a member of the surgical team should be with the patient during these urgent studies in case hemodynamic collapse occurs. The main purpose of these studies is usually just to confirm the presence of an AAA, although occasionally blood can be seen outside the wall of the AAA or other important information can be provided.

Other Diagnoses That Can Be Mimicked By a Ruptured Abdominal Aortic Aneurysm

Other diagnoses that can be mimicked by a ruptured abdominal aortic aneurysm most commonly include a ureteral stone or diverticulitis. Other intraabdominal acute entities such as a perforated ulcer, a small bowel problem, or a pancreatic lesion can be mimicked by a ruptured AAA and its associated hypovolemic shock and abdominal pain. Finally, a ruptured AAA may appear as a myocardial infarction with lower chest pain and nonspecific electrocardiogram changes because of the hypovolemic shock. One of the aspects of a ruptured AAA that can contribute to this diagnostic confusion is the variable time course of the process depending on the variable containment of the rupture by adjacent structures. Another aspect is the variable location of the rupture site and its associated hematoma.

Strategies in Planning Operative Treatment

When the diagnosis of a ruptured AAA is presumed (i.e., three elements of the triad) or confirmed if two elements are present initially, a decision can be made to proceed with operative treatment. Although the patient should be taken immediately to the operating room, other elements or strategies in the treatment are important. The team must be assembled; this includes junior and senior surgeons, nurses, and anesthesiologists. Because these ruptured AAA emergencies often occur at night or on weekends, assembling the team needed to treat them can take some time and organization. However, most operative procedures should not begin and the patient should not be anesthetized until all members of the team are present. While the team is gathering, lines and nasogastric and bladder tubes can be placed, instruments set up, and the abdomen prepared and draped. Only when all personnel are present should the patient be put to sleep, because circulatory collapse is prone to occur when the anesthesia removes the sympathetic compensation that maintains the circulation in the hypovolemic state. Only if the patient's circulation collapses completely should a junior member of the team begin the operation before the whole team is fully assembled and operative preparations are completed. The strategic principle should be to get the patient rapidly to the operating room, but then

proceed deliberately and only anesthetize the patient and begin the operation when everyone and everything is set and in place.

One final strategy that is as effective in open repair management, as it is in endovascular treatment, is the use of hypotensive hemostasis or restricted fluid resuscitation. This strategy curtails bleeding by allowing the patient to be hypotensive throughout the preoperative and intraoperative phases of treatment. This subject will be discussed in greater detail in the endovascular treatment section.

Key Technical Points for Open Repair of Ruptured Abdominal Aortic Aneurysms

Once the abdomen is opened through a short midline incision, the base of the mesentery is inspected; if blood is seen, the diagnosis of rupture is confirmed. The incision is then extended from xiphoid to pubis.

If the area of the infrarenal neck of the AAA is involved with hematoma, supraceliac aortic control should be obtained as shown in Figure 41-1; this is done without direct vision by tearing the lesser omentum with a finger

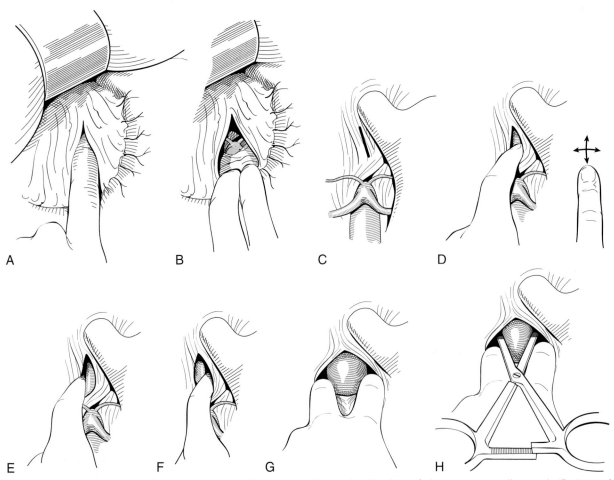

FIGURE 41-1 ■ Technique for occluding the supraceliac aorta without visualization of the structures dissected. (Redrawn from Veith FJ, Gupta S, Daly V: Technique for occluding the supraceliac aorta through the abdomen. Surg Gynecol Obstet 151:648–650, 1980.)

(see Figure 41-1*A*). This process exposes the retroperitoneum above the celiac axis and pancreas (see Figure 41-1*B*). Next, using the gloved index finger and its nail, the posterior peritoneum over the diaphragmatic crura is torn as indicated by the line in Figure 41-1*C*, and the fingertip is pushed through the muscle fibers until the periadventitia of the aorta is encountered (see Figure 41-1*D*). Next, the finger bluntly dissects medially and laterally in the same plane, creating a potential space on both sides of the aorta (see Figure 41-1*E* to *G*). Two fingers are placed in the potential space and pulled caudally (see Figure 41-1*G*). A large curved DeBakey clamp is then placed vertically above the fingers into the space to occlude the aorta (see Figure 41-1*H*). The clamp will be occlusive only if the aorta is freed from the crural fibers anteriorly, medially, and laterally. It is also crucial to have a nasogastric tube in the esophagus during these maneuvers so that this structure can be identified and protected from injury.

Following placement of this clamp, it is essential to minimize the time of supraceliac aortic occlusion (15 to 20 minutes is tolerable) to minimize liver and gut ischemia. To do this, the anterior wall of the AAA is exposed in its most prominent portion away from all venous and other structures. The anterior wall of the AAA is incised, and a finger is placed within the AAA sac to identify the aortic neck. This may be deviated sharply to the right, left or anteriorly because of aortic tortuosity associated with AAAs. With a finger inside to identify the position of the neck, it can gently be dissected bluntly from adjacent structure in the periadventitial plane without injuring major veins. Once dissected anteriorly, medially, and laterally, an infrarenal aortic clamp can be placed and the suprarenal clamp is removed.

The iliac arteries can then be identified from without and clamped with gently placed atraumatic clamps. If they cannot be easily identified by palpation from without, they can be identified from within the lumen by a finger within the AAA sac. Clamps can then be placed on them without further dissection or with minimal dissection.

Clot is then removed from the interior of the AAA. Bleeding lumbar and any other branches are identified and controlled with sutures from within. A prosthetic graft is then sutured in place from within the lumen of the AAA. The posterior walls of the aortic and iliac arteries should never be dissected to prevent damage to other vascular structures. The posterior walls of the aorta and iliac arteries should not be transected to avoid injuries to adherent major veins and minimize bleeding from other vascular structures.

Although controversial, heparin should be administered as soon as aortic clamp control is obtained. All dissection should be minimized in these ruptured AAA repairs to minimize injury to other structures and blood vessels, the position of which can be distorted by the AAA and the hematoma. Otherwise, the repair should be as much like a standard AAA repair as possible. Care should be taken to monitor and treat hypothermia and coagulation defects. Lastly, care should be taken to diagnose and treat abdominal compartment syndrome as detailed in the endovascular section that follows.

ENDOVASCULAR MANAGEMENT

History

Endovascular repair of a ruptured abdominal aortic aneurysm (RAAA) was first performed successfully by Marin and colleagues in 1994.[1] Another case was first reported by Yusuf and colleagues in 1994.[2] Since then, many centers have used EVAR to treat RAAAs with varying results.[3-12] Several groups have developed standardized systems of management in the RAAA setting, have used EVAR whenever possible, and have achieved good results.[3-9] In contrast, other authors have used EVAR for RAAAs more selectively and have reported no better results with EVAR than with traditional open repair (OR).[10-12]

On the basis of these many reports, it is reasonable to say that the comparative efficacy of EVAR and open repair for RAAAs is controversial and that randomized, prospective comparative trials of the two treatment methods are needed with this entity. This chapter will show why this is not the case and why there is sufficient evidence without such trials to demonstrate that RAAAs with anatomy suitable for EVAR should be treated in this way, provided that suitable facilities, equipment, and skills are available.

Theoretical Considerations

EVAR has been used increasingly to treat RAAA and offers many theoretical advantages over OR. It is less invasive, eliminates damage to periaortic and abdominal structures, decreases bleeding from surgical dissection, minimizes hypothermia, and lessens the requirement for deep anesthesia. Because of these potential advantages, together with reports of lower procedural mortality, EVAR has been deemed superior to OR for the treatment of RAAA.[3-9]

A Single-Center Experience

Between April 22, 1994, and January 15, 2008, 57 patients with RAAAs were treated at Montefiore Medical Center in New York. Much of this experience has been reported previously.[4] After an initial experience of EVAR in 12 patients with RAAA, who were deemed unsuitable for OR, showed only a 17% 30-day mortality, the center adopted a policy of using EVAR to treat all ruptured AAA patients with suitable anatomy if appropriate staffing and endografts were available.[4] A total of 45 patients were treated with endografts and 12 with OR. In the patients who underwent EVAR, 25 received surgeon-made endografts and 20 received industry-made modular endografts. The surgeon-made endografts were constructed from a large balloon-expandable stent and a tulip-shaped PTFE graft, placed in an aorto-unifemoral position with contralateral iliac artery occlusion and a femorofemoral bypass.[4] Twelve of the 57 patients with RAAA underwent OR: 10 because their anatomy was unsuitable for EVAR, and 2 because appropriate staff or grafts were not available. Many of the patients treated with EVAR represented prohibitive risks for OR, yet many of these survived exclusion of their ruptured AAA by an EVAR procedure.

EVAR was performed without a preprocedure CT scan in 17 patients. In these patients, intraoperative arteriography using calibrated catheters was used to determine suitability for EVAR and to make measurements for graft sizing. A preprocedure CT scan was obtained in the other 28 patients because of uncertainty in the diagnosis or because the patient was initially admitted to another hospital or service. No differences in outcomes were observed between these two small groups.

Fluids were aggressively restricted and the patient's blood pressure was allowed to fall to 50 mm Hg without fluid administration, or lower if the patient was moving or talking.[4] Although local anesthesia was used in the early phases of most EVAR procedures (placement of catheters, guidewires, and sheaths), general anesthesia was used to prevent motion in order to optimize imaging and allow precise endograft deployment. Large sheath placement and balloon occlusion were used only in the case of cardiovascular collapse, and were required in 10 of 45 patients undergoing EVAR and 3 of 12 undergoing OR. The technique for continuous balloon control of the aorta while deploying a modular endograft has been described by Malina and colleagues.[13] Abdominal compartment syndrome (ACS) was detected in only 3 of the 45 patients undergoing EVAR when they became hypotensive and difficult to ventilate. Laparotomy and evacuation of the hematoma relieved the problem. However, unrecognized ACS probably contributed to fatal multiorgan failure in some patients. Six of the 45 patients treated by EVAR and 1 of the 12 patients treated by OR died within 30 days.

Collected World Experience

Data from 49 centers around the world performing EVAR for RAAAs were collected between July 1, 2002, and January 15, 2009. Data from the 13 centers that were committed to EVAR and performed this procedure on all or almost all patients with RAAA who had suitable aortic neck and iliac artery anatomy were updated to January 15, 2009. These updated data, as well as all the data from the other centers, were reported in November 2009.[14]

Data from 1037 patients with an RAAA or a ruptured aortoiliac aneurysm treated with EVAR show an overall 30-day mortality of 21.2%, which is clearly lower than the rates of 35% to 55% with OR for RAAAs reported in multiple studies.[15] However, many of the centers in the collected experience had limited the use of EVAR to patients in stable condition with RAAA or even those with contained ruptures. Because hemodynamic instability is associated with a higher risk of procedural mortality,[5,7,15] it is invalid to compare procedural mortality with EVAR and OR in this way.

As a result, the updated outcomes for EVAR were examined in the selected group of 13 centers that were committed to performing EVAR to treat RAAA in all patients with anatomy suitable for endograft treatment, including those that were hemodynamically unstable and

those in profound shock.[14] These centers were usually the ones with the greatest experience. Although there was some variability in the approach used in these centers to the treatment of patients with RAAA, most had some degree of standardization and many had a defined protocol. All were experienced in the use of EVAR and endovascular adjuncts for elective treatment of abdominal aneurysm, and all had dedicated endovascular facilities and imaging equipment. The use of EVAR to treat all possible patients with RAAA and suitable anatomy was associated with a favorable 30-day mortality of 19.7% in 680 patients (range, 0% to 32%).[14] During this same period, these same 13 centers performed OR for RAAAs in 763 patients whose anatomy was thought to be unsuitable for EVAR. The 30-day mortality for OR was 36.3% (range, 8% to 49%; $p < 0.0001$ for EVAR vs. OR).[14]

These updated comparative outcome results (30-day mortality 19.7% for EVAR vs. 36.3% for OR from the 13 centers committed to EVAR of as many RAAAs as possible) strongly suggest that EVAR is a superior way to treat RAAAs in patients whose aortic neck and iliac anatomy is suitable for endovascular graft treatment. Additional proof that EVAR is a better treatment for some patients with RAAA is that many patients in this collected experience who were categorically unsuitable or prohibitively high risk for OR survived for many years after EVAR.

Why Are Results Variable?

Several possible reasons might explain the discordant results reported by different authors for treatment of RAAA by EVAR.[3-12] These reasons include strategies, adjuncts, and technical factors that are thought to influence the outcome of EVAR for RAAAs, and which probably account for the favorable outcomes with EVAR in the 13 centers in the collected experience.[14] Some of the key reasons are described in the following sections.

Standard Approach or Protocol

The use of a protocol allows the most effective decision making and treatment of patients in circumstances that often are confusing and stressful.[8,9] Protocols are also important to facilitate education of generalists, emergency department personnel, and others to recognize RAAAs, in order to enable early diagnosis and mobilization of the specialized caregivers best trained to optimize treatment.

Fluid Restriction (Hypotensive Hemostasis)

Fluid resuscitation should be restricted even if the patient becomes hypotensive. Experience has shown that systolic arterial pressures of 50 to 70 mm Hg are well tolerated for short periods and limit internal bleeding and associated loss of platelets and clotting factors.[4,5,9,14,16] It remains to be shown conclusively, however, whether or not pharmacologic lowering of blood pressure is beneficial.[5,9]

Treatment Site

EVAR procedures are optimally performed in a site equipped for excellent fluoroscopic imaging and open surgery, because some patients will require OR or open adjuncts to EVAR.

Anesthesia and Catheter Guidewire Placement

Guidewire placement should be done percutaneously using local anesthesia. This guidewire permits arteriography to define aortic and arterial anatomy, facilitates large sheath and supraceliac balloon placement if needed, and prevents circulatory collapse caused by the induction of general anesthesia. Whether general anesthesia is subsequently required to eliminate motion and improve fluoroscopic imaging in order to permit precise graft deployment remains controversial. Some groups have successfully used local anesthesia supplemented by sedation throughout as an alternative.[3,5,9]

Supraceliac Aortic Sheath Placement and Balloon Control

Most groups use supraceliac aortic sheath placement and balloon control only when there is severe circulatory collapse. In such cases, deflation of the balloon before sealing of the rupture site will result in immediate recurrence of the circulatory collapse. Techniques have therefore been developed to maintain continuous aortic control until the endograft has sealed the leak.[4,5,13,17] Renal and visceral ischemia is minimized by placing secondary balloons within the endograft as the supraceliac balloon is deflated and removed though its supporting sheath.

Endograft Type and Configuration

Both bifurcated and aorto-uniiliac (or femoral) grafts can be used successfully, although some patients have unilateral iliac disease that mandates a unilateral configuration. Modular and unibody grafts have been used successfully in both configurations. An appropriate inventory of suitable grafts and accessories must be stocked sterile in the treatment site and must be available for the procedure and unexpected contingencies.

Abdominal Compartment Syndrome

Abdominal compartment syndrome (ACS) is a major cause of morbidity and mortality after EVAR for RAAA, and a high index of suspicion for this entity should be maintained. Monitoring of bladder pressure has been helpful in early detection of ACS.[5,9] Conservative measures (diuretics, colloid administration, and neuromuscular blockade) may be helpful for minimal elevations in intraabdominal pressure. However, laparotomy and open abdomen treatment (OAT) are required to alleviate the hypotension, high ventilatory compliance, and oliguria that occur with full-blown ACS. Early laparotomy with OAT and suction and sponge dressings may allow survival in otherwise hopeless circumstances when small-bowel and mesenteric edema causes loss of domain for the abdominal viscera.[9] Evacuation of most of the retroperitoneal hematoma is usually not needed with OAT and should usually be avoided to prevent further bleeding and damage to the adjacent structures.

EVAR for Highest-Risk Patients

EVAR is probably most beneficial in augmenting survival when it is used in the highest-risk patients who are unlikely to survive an OR. This category includes patients who are hemodynamically unstable or in profound circulatory collapse, those who have a hostile abdomen, and those unable to receive transfusion. If such patients, particularly those who are hemodynamically unstable, are excluded from EVAR, it is likely that the improved survival that can accrue from this form of treatment would be diminished.[14]

Is a Randomized Controlled Comparison of EVAR and OR needed?

The reduced 30-day mortality after EVAR compared with OR (19.7% vs. 36.3%), together with the survival of many RAAA patients who are prohibitive risks for OR, constitute strong evidence that EVAR is a better way to treat RAAAs in at least some patients, provided that the described strategies, adjuncts, and techniques are used. Accordingly, many believe that there is no need for a randomized controlled comparison of EVAR and OR in patients with RAAA, given the data from the collected experience.[14] If those who believe that such evidence is necessary to confirm the value of EVAR in the RAAA setting wish to perform such trials, these results would be awaited with interest. However, such studies will be difficult to perform in this setting of a morbid and life-threatening condition.

References available online at expertconsult.com.

QUESTIONS

1. True or false: RAAAs can have a variable time course.

2. True or false: The variability in the time course of an RAAA depends on the previous health of the patient.

3. True or false: When performing a laparotomy for an RAAA, the initial incision should be very long.

4. True or false: Supraceliac aortic control can be achieved rapidly without visualizing all involved structures.

5. True or false: Supraceliac aortic control can be achieved by placing the clamp on the aorta with minimal dissection of diaphragmatic fibers.

6. True or false: Abdominal compartment syndrome can occur after open RAAA repair.

7. True or false: Supraceliac aortic balloon control must always be obtained during an EVAR procedure for an RAAA.

8. True or false: Having an established protocol is crucial to achieving optimal results with EVAR for RAAAs.

9. True or false: During open repair of an RAAA, isolation of the proximal neck is often facilitated by opening the aneurysm and inserting a finger in the lumen rather than by dissection of the neck from surrounding structures.

10. What is the best method for detecting abdominal compartment syndrome after EVAR for RAAA?
    a. By symptoms of hypotension, difficulty in ventilation, and organ dysfunction
    b. By feeling abdominal distension
    c. By measuring intragastric pressure
    d. By monitoring bladder pressure
    e. By observing the colonic mucosa

ANSWERS

1. True
2. False. It depends on the degree of containment of the rupture.
3. False. Only when the rupture is confirmed should a long incision be made.
4. True
5. False. Only by isolating the aorta can clamp control be achieved.
6. True
7. False
8. True
9. True, but only with supraceliac clamp control.
10. d

LAPAROSCOPIC AORTIC SURGERY FOR ANEURYSM AND OCCLUSIVE DISEASE: TECHNIQUE AND RESULTS

Ralf Kolvenbach • Catherine Cagiannos

The initial enthusiasm of endovascular procedures to safely exclude abdominal aortic aneurysms is currently reduced because of the significant late failure rate, aneurysm rupture, and costs. With the improved technology, described laparoscopic techniques can be a durable alternative.[1-3]

The outcome of laparoscopic abdominal aortic aneurysm resection can be expected to be similar to the gold standard (i.e., a transperitoneal tube graft repair), because the conventional operation is performed laparoscopically. Total laparoscopic aortic procedures can be performed in patients with occlusive disease as well as in aneurysm cases. The basic principle of a total laparoscopic operation is that the anastomosis is performed with laparoscopic needle holders under pneumoperitoneum.

Total laparoscopic aortic surgery in patients with occlusive disease can be performed routinely in the majority of patients.[1] Since the first total laparoscopic aortic operation, the technique has been refined and can now be used in a patient with an aortic aneurysm.[2,3]

TECHNIQUE

All patients receive the standard preoperative examination required for major aortic surgery. If necessary, coronary angiography and pulmonary function tests are performed. A laxative is given 1 day before the procedure like in bowel surgery. The patient is placed on the operating table on a vacuum bag. When tilting the table to the right, the patient can be positioned almost 70 degrees on the right side (Figure 42-1A). The left hemicolon and the splenic flexure are mobilized medially.

The line of Told is used for orientation to incise the lateral attachments of the sigmoid colon. In many patients, there are adhesions that should be taken down to avoid a postoperative ileus. Incomplete mobilization of the splenic flexure can cause lacerations of the spleen particularly in cases with adhesions after previous surgery. When conversion to a minilaparotomy is required, conventional retractors can cause severe damage of the spleen, necessitating a splenectomy. It is best to avoid any dissection of the ureter, which is only placed laterally when necessary. In most cases, any mobilization of the ureter can be avoided.

The technique of medial mobilization was originally described by Dion and colleagues[3,4] to separate the abdominal contents from the retroperitoneal space. One laparoscopic retractor is required in obese patients. A left hemicolon retrorenal approach with medial mobilization of the left kidney and the ureter is usually preferred (see Figure 42-1B); this permits expeditious exposure of the aorta even in obese patients. This approach can also be used for medial viscero rotation to obtain access to the suprarenal aorta. All three surgeons are standing on the right side of the patient during the entire procedure.

Laparoscopic exposure of the aorta is initiated at the level of the neck of the aneurysm.[3] The left renal vein is one of the first structures we see when dissection is started. The laparoscopic camera stays in port 2 most of the time during exposure of the aorta (Figure 42-2). Especially in patients with occlusive disease, only the site for the anastomosis proximal to the origin of the inferior mesenteric artery is dissected. This exposure technique avoids damage of the lumbosacral nerves adjacent to the aortic bifurcation. During retroperitoneal dissection, the first assistant holds the camera and helps to put the tissue on attention with a grasping clamp (see Figure 42-2).

Lumbar arteries are controlled extra luminally from the left side. When the left-sided lumbar arteries are divided after clipping, the adjacent right-sided lumbar artery can be clipped. Lumbar arteries that are still bleeding after incision of the sac of the aneurysm are stitched with laparoscopic sutures and secured with a titanium clip to save time.[5]

When the sac of the aneurysm is incised and collapsed, most lumbar arteries can expeditiously be identified medially and laterally of the aorta and occluded with a clip. Hernia staplers have also been used to stop bleeding from lumbar arteries.

AORTOILIAC ANEURYSMS

In large iliac or aortoiliac aneurysms, a hybrid procedure is used combining endovascular and laparoscopic techniques.

The hybrid procedure consists of transfemoral balloon occlusion of the right common iliac artery after insertion of an 8-French hemostatic sheath. The left common iliac

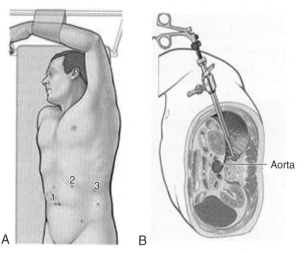

FIGURE 42-1 ■ **A,** Right decubital position of the patient. **B,** Retrorenal exposure of the aorta.

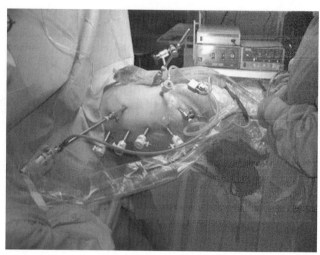

FIGURE 42-3 ■ Table tilted to the right with the monitor standing on the left side of the patient.

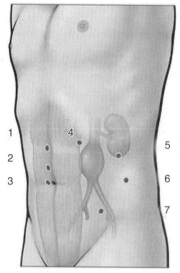

FIGURE 42-2 ■ Placement of trocars.

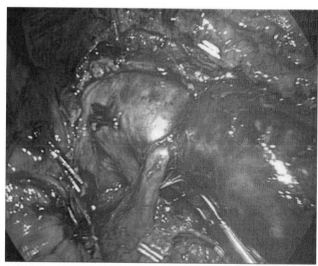

FIGURE 42-4 ■ Suprarenal exposure of the aorta. The left renal artery can be seen. The aorta is prepared for suprarenal clamping.

artery is occluded from within the aneurysm. A balloon catheter is introduced intraabdominally through an 8-French hemostatic sheath inserted directly through the abdominal wall. An average of three endovascular balloons is used in each case. One endovascular balloon is used for occlusion of the hypogastric artery from within.

If possible, at least one distal anastomosis is performed with the iliac bifurcation; this anastomosis is sutured also laparoscopically. In cases with hypogastric artery aneurysms, coil embolization is performed followed by staple occlusion of the common iliac and the proximal external iliac artery and a distal anastomosis with the external iliac artery.

No distal clamps are required when using this technique. Only the infrarenal aorta is clamped using a laparoscopic aortic clamp (Storz Endoscopic Manufacturer, Tuttlingen FRG).

LAPAROSCOPIC ANASTOMOSIS

Laparoscopic dissection and suturing is performed with the surgeon standing on the right side of the patient[5] (Figure 42-3). The transperitoneal left retrorenal exposure of the aorta permits access to the entire suprarenal aorta, permitting subdiaphragmatic cross-clamping (Figure 42-4). In patients with an end–end anastomosis with the proximal aorta, the posterior wall of the aorta is left intact as in open surgery.

In patients with an end–side anastomosis, an aortotomy is performed and the anastomosis is started posteriorly with a 10 cm, 3-0 Prolene suture. A second suture is taken anteriorly and both are tied intracorporally. A laparoscopic nerve hook is useful to put the suture line on attention. Time can also be saved by using two 3-0 Prolene sutures blocked with a pledget at the end as

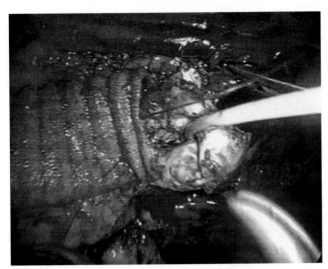

FIGURE 42-5 ■ Balloon catheter occludes iliac artery.

originally described by Coggia.[5] The first assistant can follow the suture with an atraumatic De Bakey clamp covered with a thin rubber layer to avoid any damage to the Prolene thread. The assistant also keeps the operating field dry of blood with the suction device. When the anastomosis is performed, the camera is in the left upper abdomen the entire time (Figure 42-5).

CONVERSION

Reasons for conversion to a minilaparotomy should be outlined already before surgery; these can include an aortic cross-clamping time of more than 2 hours and a total operating time exceeding 4 hours. In theses cases, one can convert to a laparoscopic hand-assist procedure in which the anastomosis is performed under the pneumoperitoneum yet with the nondominant hand of the surgeon inserted into the abdomen.[6-9] Other reasons for conversion are extensive adhesions, excessive calcification, and uncontrollable blood loss. When severe calcification does not permit safe clamping of the iliac artery, a balloon catheter can be inserted through a trocar to block the vessel intraluminally.

Calcification of the iliac arteries was the main reason for technical problems and prolonged cross-clamping time. Combining endovascular techniques with laparoscopic procedures can be an effective way to overcome technical problems. Total laparoscopic tube graft repair is often easier to perform than a distal anastomosis with a calcified common iliac artery[11] (see Figure 42-5).

RESULTS

Between 1996 and 2005, laparoscopic aortic surgery was performed in 638 cases. Among these were 236 total laparoscopic procedures and 402 laparoscopy-assisted operations in which a miniature incision of 6 to 8 cm was used to suture the anastomosis.

In a 4-year period, 131 patients with abdominal aortic aneurysms were operated on using a total laparoscopic approach. A tube graft repair was performed in 55% of patients (72); a bifurcated graft could be implanted in the remaining 59 patients. The mortality was 3%, and major nonlethal complications occurred in 17.5%. Conversion was required in 12 cases (9.1%). After a mean follow-up period of 39 months, 127 patients were still alive and available for a follow-up examination. In 26 total laparoscopic aneurysm cases, patients reported problems related to the operative procedure, such as paraesthesia at the site of the groin incision. The main difference in outcome between laparoscopy assisted operations and total laparoscopic procedures was the incidence of incisional hernias in the assist group. Mortality did not differ significantly (2.4% versus 3.8%).[6-9]

DISCUSSION

How to Start a Laparoscopic Aortic Program

Laparoscopic aortic surgery can be performed only when the surgeon already has basic laparoscopic skills. It does not matter whether these skills come from general surgical procedures or from laparoscopic courses where the basics of laparoscopy are taught. There are not many "minor" laparoscopic vascular operations to begin with, such as laparoscopic cholecystectomy in general surgery. A special laparoscopic vascular course should therefore be part of the training program when starting laparoscopic aortic surgery. Back home, the next step should be a laparoscopic assisted operation that should ideally be a hand-assist case in which in the beginning is much easier, because of the tactile feedback or a case when a minilaparotomy is performed to suture the anastomosis after laparoscopic dissection.[10-19]

Having experience with laparoscopy-assisted operations, the next step is a total laparoscopic procedure in an "ideal" patient with occlusive disease who needs an aortofemoral graft preferably with a proximal end–side anastomosis. A total laparoscopic aneurysm resection should be performed only at the end of the learning curve.[5]

There is a substantial learning curve when starting laparoscopic aortic surgery, but the technique can be mastered by vascular surgeons the same way that complex laparoscopic operations are routinely performed by gastrointestinal surgeons. Finally, the importance of some kind of proctoring by more experienced laparoscopic vascular specialists should not be underestimated.[20-22]

Future Perspectives

The future will show whether stapling devices for the aortic anastomosis will significantly shorten clamping time, further facilitating the procedure as in colorectal surgery. In preliminary clinical trials, an aortic anastomosis could be performed in less than 10 minutes in patients with a tube graft repair (E. Shiffrin, unpublished data). It could also be shown in a clinical study that by combining endovascular and conventional Dacron grafts, ischemia can be reduced, offering the best of both possibilities to the patient.[20,21]

CONCLUSION

Total laparoscopic aortic procedures can be offered to the majority of patients with aortic disease, with excellent long-term results.[15,19-12] There is a steep learning curve, especially for aneurysms. Laparoscopy-assisted

procedures can be performed more expeditiously compared to a total laparoscopic procedure. All patients must be fit for open surgery, especially aneurysm patients. Endovascular aneurysm repair is a truly minimal invasive alternative with reduced surgical trauma. In aneurysm patients, total laparoscopic procedures will have an increasing role in the future when aortic stapling devices become available.[22]

References available online at expertconsult.com.

QUESTIONS

1. Choose the correct answer.
   a. The outcome of laparoscopic aortic procedures is different from open surgery.
   b. The outcome of laparoscopic aortic procedures is similar to conventional aortic surgery.

2. The most common used approach to the aorta is:
   a. transperitoneal
   b. retroperitoneal
   c. transperitoneal, left hemicolic

3. Choose the correct answer.
   a. The left kidney is always mobilized medially.
   b. The left kidney always stays in situ.

4. A combination of laparoscopic and endovascular procedures is most commonly used in:
   a. patients with occlusive disease
   b. patients with Iliac artery aneurysms

5. Several answers are correct.
   Hand-assisted aortic surgery is:
   a. a laparoscopic procedure
   b. a laparoscopic-assisted procedure
   c. a total laparoscopic operation

6. Only one answer is correct.
   Most laparoscopic aortic operations are performed:
   a. with mechanical elevation of the abdominal wall
   b. with the help of pneumoperitoneum

7. Choose the correct answer.
   a. An aortic anastomosis requires a minilapartomy.
   b. An aortic anastomosis can be performed total laparoscopically.

8. Choose the correct answer.
   a. Conversion is always a major complication.
   b. Conversion should be performed at any stage if necessary to avoid complications.

9. Choose the correct answer.
   a. Laparoscopic aortic surgery should always be started with total laparoscopic procedures.
   b. A laparoscopic aortic program should be started with a hand assisted approach.

10. Choose the correct answer.
    a. Staplers can never replace a hand sewn aortic anastomosis.
    b. Without staplers, total laparoscopic procedures will be performed in a few centers only.

ANSWERS

1. **b**
2. **c**
3. **a**
4. **b**
5. **a, b**
6. **b**
7. **b**
8. **b**
9. **b**
10. **b**

CHAPTER 43

SPLANCHNIC AND RENAL ARTERY ANEURYSMS

James C. Stanley • Louis M. Messina • Gerald B. Zelenock

Aneurysms of the visceral branches of the abdominal aorta are being recognized with increasing frequency. More than half of the splanchnic and renal artery aneurysms described in the English-language literature have been reported in the past 25 years. Splanchnic aneurysms are approximately threefold more common than renal aneurysms. Both aneurysm types are best addressed individually because of the marked variability in their biological character and clinical importance.

SPLANCHNIC ARTERY ANEURYSMS

Splanchnic artery aneurysms are an uncommon but important vascular disease (Table 43-1). Nearly 22% of these aneurysms appear as surgical emergencies, including 8.5% that result in the patient's death. The major splanchnic vessels involved with these macroaneurysms, in decreasing order of frequency, are the splenic; hepatic; superior mesenteric; celiac; gastric and gastroepiploic; jejunal, ileal, and colic; pancreaticoduodenal and pancreatic; and gastroduodenal arteries.

The clinical manifestations of splanchnic artery aneurysms have become well defined during the past 3 decades.[1-15] Rupture is the most serious complication of these aneurysms (Table 43-2). In many circumstances, endovascular therapy provides a distinct advantage over conventional surgical therapy.[2,6,9,15-21] Nevertheless, treatment of certain splanchnic artery aneurysms by open operative therapy remains appropriate.[4,8,14,22] The cause, presentation, and management of aneurysms affecting each of the splanchnic arteries deserve separate comment.

Splenic Artery Aneurysms

Splenic artery aneurysms account for 60% of all reported splanchnic artery aneurysms. The frequency of splenic artery aneurysms in the general population approaches the 0.78% incidence noted in nearly 3600 consecutive abdominal arteriographic studies performed for reasons other than suspected aneurysmal disease.[22] Women are nearly fourfold more likely than men to have these aneurysms,[13,23] although in more contemporary times this female predilection appears to be reduced.[24]

Four distinct, preexisting conditions are suspected to contribute to the development of splenic artery aneurysms. The first is medial fibrodysplasia with its derangements and thinning of the vessel's medial smooth muscle.

Although medial fibrodysplasia is commonly recognized as a cause of hypertension secondary to its renal artery involvement, approximately 2% of patients exhibiting this disease have splenic artery aneurysms.[22] In addition, blood pressure elevations in these patients may contribute to aneurysm development. Coexistence of renal artery medial fibrodysplasia and splenic artery aneurysms has been identified only in women.

Second are the effects of increased splenic blood flow and the altered levels of reproductive hormones that accompany pregnancy. Both have deleterious effects on elastin and other matrix proteins in the splenic artery wall. In past decades, approximately 40% of women harboring these aneurysms had completed six or more pregnancies.[22] Given the fact that in contemporary times fewer children are being born to women in Western societies, the frequency of grandmultiparity in women exhibiting these aneurysms has declined to approximately 10%.[24]

Third, portal hypertension with splenomegaly is associated with splenic artery macroaneurysms in nearly 10% to 15% of patients.[25-28] This may result from the higher velocities in splenic blood flow[29-30] as well as elevated estrogen activity associated with advanced cirrhosis. There has been an increased recognition of these aneurysms in patients subjected to orthotopic liver transplantation.[25,27,31,32] These aneurysms are more common in female than male liver transplant patients, and they appear directly related to the severity of the patient's antecedent portal hypertension.[33,34]

Fourth, inflammatory disease, such as chronic pancreatitis, with destruction of the adjacent splenic artery or erosion into a pseudocyst is a less common but important cause of these aneurysms. In contrast, microaneurysms within the splenic panrechyma are most often associated with a generalized inflammatory vasculitis, such as polyarteritis nodosa, and usually are of less clinical relevance than extraparenchymal macroaneurysms.

Trauma, both penetrating and iatrogenic following abdominal operations, is a separate and well recognized cause of splenic artery aneurysms. Blunt trauma is a less frequently encountered etiology, although small intraparenchymal aneurysms commonly evolve from splenic fractures and arterial disruptions within the substance of the spleen.

Many splenic artery aneurysms exhibit arteriosclerotic disease. Although advanced arteriosclerotic changes in these aneurysms may contribute to further aneurysmal

TABLE 43-1   Distribution and Etiology of Splanchnic Artery Macroaneurysms

Aneurysm Location	Frequency within Splanchnic Circulation (%)	Male:Female Ratio	Common Contributing Factors
Splenic artery	60	1:4	Medial degeneration; arterial fibrodysplasia; multiple pregnancies; portal hypertension; pancreatitis with arterial erosion by pseudocysts, trauma
Hepatic artery	20	2:1	Medial degeneration; blunt and penetrating liver trauma; iatrogenic trauma during hepatobiliary procedures
Superior mesenteric artery	5.5	2:1	Infection related to bacterial endocarditis, often associated with nonhemolytic streptococci; medial degeneration
Celiac artery	4.0	1:1	Medial degeneration
Gastric and gastroepiploic arteries	4.0	2:1	Periarterial inflammation; medial degeneration
Jejunal, ileal, and colic arteries	3.0	1:1	Medial degeneration; infection; connective tissue diseases
Pancreaticoduodenal, pancreatic, and gastroduodenal arteries	1.5	4:1	Medial degeneration; abnormal flow as a collateral vessel; pancreatitis-related inflammation

TABLE 43-2   Rupture and Treatment of Splanchnic Artery Macroaneurysms

Aneurysm Location	Frequency of Reported Rupture	Site of Bleeding	Mortality with Rupture	Usual Treatment Options
Splenic artery	2% bland; 10% inflammatory	Intraperitoneal within lesser sac; intragastric with pancreatitis-related inflammatory aneurysms	25% bland and unassociated with pregnancy; during pregnancy 70% maternal, 75% fetal	Endovascular aneurysm obliteration; splenectomy; aneurysm exclusion or excision without splenectomy
Hepatic artery	20%	Intraperitoneal and biliary tract with equal frequency	35%	Endovascular aneurysm obliteration; aneurysmectomy with and without hepatic artery reconstruction
Superior mesenteric artery	10%; thrombosis with dissections relatively common	Intraperitoneal and retroperitoneal; intestinal ischemia with thrombosis	50%	Endovascular occlusion in select cases; aneurysmectomy with superior mesenteric artery reconstruction; ligation if collateral circulation is adequate
Celiac artery	13%	Intraperitoneal	50%	Aneurysmectomy with celiac artery reconstruction; ligation if circulation is adequate
Gastric and gastroepiploic arteries	90%	Intraperitoneal (30%); intestinal tract (70%)	70%	Endovascular aneurysm obliteration; aneurysm excision with involved gastric tissue; ligation if extramural
Jejunal, ileal, and colic arteries	30%	Intestinal tract, intramesenteric and intraperitoneal with equal frequency	20%	Aneurysm excision with involved intestine; ligation if extramural
Pancreaticoduodenal, pancreatic, and gastroduodenal arteries	30% bland; 75% inflammatory	Intestinal tract (85%); intraperitoneal (15%)	20% bland; 50% pancreatitis-related	Endovascular aneurysm obliteration; aneurysm ligation within false aneurysms (pseudocyst-related); pancreatic resection; ligation if extrapancreatic

degeneration, they are considered a secondary event rather than an initiating etiologic process.

Most splenic artery aneurysms associated with arterial fibrodysplasia, multiple pregnancies, or portal hypertension are saccular and occur at vessel branchings (Figure 43-1). These are true aneurysms, not false aneurysms. Discontinuities exist in the internal elastic lamina of normal vessels at branchings, and subsequent alterations in elastic tissue, such as those occurring during late pregnancy, are apt to produce aneurysmal changes at these sites. Aneurysms unrelated to portal hypertension are multiple 20% of the time. Among patients with portal hypertension and cirrhosis undergoing liver transplantation, multiple aneurysms are even more common.[27,33] In

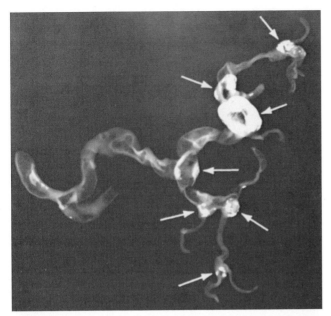

FIGURE 43-1 ■ Multiple splenic artery aneurysms *(arrows)* occurring at each bifurcation of the distal artery (specimen radiograph). Calcific arteriosclerosis is limited to the aneurysms and not the intervening artery. (From Zelenock GB, Stanley JC: Splanchnic artery aneurysms. In Rutherford RB, editor: Vascular surgery, ed 5, Philadelphia, 2000, WB Saunders, p 1371.)

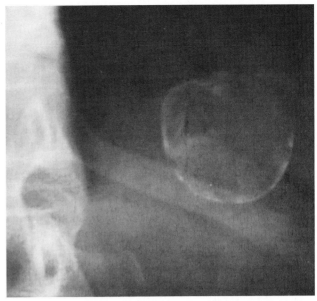

FIGURE 43-3 ■ Splenic artery aneurysms. Radiographic appearance of characteristic signet-ring–like calcifications. (From Zelenock GB, Stanley JC: Splanchnic artery aneurysms. In Rutherford RB, editor: Vascular surgery, ed 5, Philadelphia, 2000, WB Saunders, p 1371.)

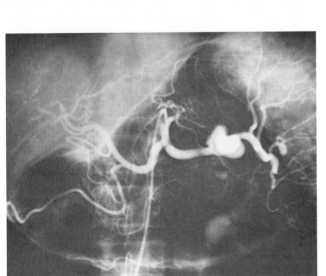

FIGURE 43-2 ■ Solitary splenic artery aneurysm affecting the midportion of the vessel, caused by arterial erosion from a pancreatic pseudocyst. (From Zelenock GB, Stanley JC: Splanchnic artery aneurysms. In Rutherford RB, editor: Vascular surgery, ed 5, Philadelphia, 2000, WB Saunders, p 1372.)

contrast, false aneurysms associated with pancreatitis usually involve the main splenic artery and tend to be solitary (Figure 43-2).

Curvilinear or signet-ring calcifications in the left upper quadrant on radiographs are often evidence of a splenic artery aneurysm (Figure 43-3). However, diagnosis is more likely to follow demonstration of the aneurysm during imaging undertaken for some other disease state. Conventional arteriography, ultrasonography, computed tomography (CT), CT arteriography, and magnetic resonance arteriography are not only useful in recognizing

these lesions, but are often helpful in identifying bleeding aneurysms.

Left upper quadrant or epigastric pain directly referrable to splenic artery aneurysms occurs in a minority of individuals, although some form of abdominal discomfort affects approximately 20% of these patients.[22] In this regard, although nearly half the patients having intact aneurysms in a recent review had abdominal symptoms, in no case were the symptoms attributed to the aneurysm.[24] In contrast, a 1996 review of 83 cases that included many single case reports noted that 46% of patients had abdominal pain and 25% were in shock.[11] The disparity in these publications is attributed to the fact that reviews often summarize spectacular individual case reports that are unlikely to be representative of the usual patient's clinical course.

Initial bleeding from a ruptured splenic artery aneurysm may be contained within the lesser sac. Eventually, free hemorrhage into the peritoneal cavity occurs and causes vascular collapse. This "double-rupture" phenomenon is often referred to in discussions of splenic artery aneurysms but is, in fact, relatively uncommon. Pancreatitis-related aneurysms are often a source of intestinal hemorrhage after erosion of a pseudocyst into an adjacent artery and subsequently into the stomach or pancreatic ductal system.[10,35-37] Arteriovenous fistula formation from rupture of a splenic artery aneurysm into the adjacent splenic vein is a rare but recognized cause of gastrointestinal hemorrhage from esophageal varices resulting from left-sided portal hypertension.[38,39]

The risk of splenic artery aneurysm rupture is related to its cause. Rupture of bland aneurysms has been generally accepted to be approximately 2%.[22] However, the actual rupture risk may be less. In fact, a recent review of

168 patients with these aneurysms reported a rupture rate of zero among those not subjected to surgical therapy.[23] Contrary to earlier misconceptions, rupture is just as likely to occur with a calcified aneurysm in a normotensive patient or in a very old patient. In the past, the mortality accompanying rupture of a bland splenic artery aneurysm in a nonpregnant patient has been reported to be 25%.[13] Rupture of inflammatory pancreatitis-related aneurysms is approximately 20% and is associated with a 40% mortality rate.

Bland aneurysms in liver transplant recipients appear to be nearly twice as likely to rupture as those in other patients.[31,33] Rupture is most likely to occur early in the period after transplantation.[25,27] The mortality following rupture of a splenic artery aneurysm in a liver transplant patient exceeds 50%.

Nearly 95% of reported aneurysms first recognized during pregnancy have ruptured.[40-44] However, these figures are misleading, in that women develop splenic artery aneurysms during the course of repeated pregnancies, and most of these aneurysms are likely to go unrecognized without rupture. Nevertheless, splenic artery aneurysm rupture during pregnancy represents a serious potential threat to the health of the mother and the fetus. Overall maternal and fetal mortality in these cases has generally been accepted to approach 70% and 75%, respectively. Rupture, even when recognized early enough to allow for operative intervention, still carries a reported maternal of 22% and fetal mortality of 16%.[41]

It would seem prudent to undertake elective operative intervention for asymptomatic (bland) splenic artery aneurysms, when the risk of operative death is less than 0.5%. This latter figure represents the product of the 25% open operative mortality and the 2% rupture rate of bland aneurysms. In more contemporary times, the mortality rate accompanying operation for rupture may be less; therefore any elective open surgical or endovascular intervention should be undertaken only when the operative risk is exceedingly low.

Percutaneous transcatheter embolization using various agents, including differing types of particulate matter, coils, and glue (acrylate derivatives), has become preferred over open operative interventions in the treatment of most splenic artery aneurysms (Figure 43-4).* Nevertheless, splenic infarction, delayed rupture of the spleen, inconsistent and transient obliteration of the anuerysm, and migration and erosion with stricture of adjacent viscera are all recognized complications of endovascular therapy.[2,9,24,48-50] Careful follow-up of endovascular-treated patients thus becomes mandatory. Stent-graft exclusion of an aneurysm with maintenance of splenic artery flow may avoid many of the complications attending embolic interventions and is appropriate in select cases.[51-54]

Splenectomy historically has been the most commonly reported open surgical intrevention undertaken for the treatment of splenic artery aneurysms.[11,22] With recognition of the immunologic benefits of splenic preservation,

*References 2, 6, 10, 15, 16, 21, 45-47.

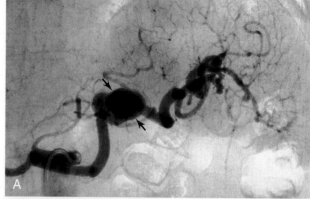
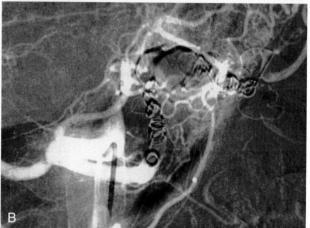

FIGURE 43-4 ■ **A,** Splenic artery aneurysm *(arrows).* **B,** Aneurysmal occlusion following coil embolization. (From Upchurch GR, Jr, Zelenock GB, Stanley JC: Splenic artery aneurysms. In Rutherford RB, editor: Vascular surgery, ed 6, Philadelphia, 2005, Elsevier-Saunders, p 1569.)

even in the aged, simple ligature obliteration or excision of these aneurysms has become preferable to splenectomy when an open surgical procedure is pursued.[55] In select cases, these procedures may be undertaken by a laparoscopic or a robotic approach.[56-58]

Certain inflammatory splenic artery aneurysms embedded in the pancreas may require distal pancreatectomy. Other aneurysms, especially false aneurysms associated with pseudocyst erosion into the adjacent artery, may be most effectively treated by initially incising the aneurysmal sac and ligating the entering and exiting vessels.[36] Pancreatic resection in the former cases depends on the degree of associated pancreatic inflammation and the general condition of the patient.[59]

Hepatic Artery Aneurysms

Hepatic artery aneurysms account for 20% of all reported splanchnic artery aneurysms[60-63]; they appear to be more common in contemporary practice.[11] Men are twice as likely to be affected as women, although gender differences appear to be less significant in more recent times. More than one third of patients with these aneurysms have other splanchnic artery aneurysms.[60] Nontraumatic and nonmycotic aneurysms are most often discovered during the sixth decade of life.

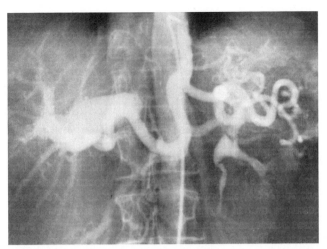

FIGURE 43-5 ■ Large common hepatic artery aneurysm affecting the distal artery at the origin of the proper hepatic artery. (From Zelenock GB, Stanley JC: Splanchnic artery aneurysms. In Rutherford RB, editor: Vascular surgery, ed 5, Philadelphia, 2000, WB Saunders, p 1374.)

Both penetrating and blunt liver injuries have led to a marked increase in the number of reported hepatic artery aneurysms. Many of these lesions have been recognized as small pseudoaneurysms on CT studies obtained in evaluating major abdominal trauma. Traumatic etiologies are a likely reason that almost half of the reported hepatic artery aneurysms are noted in the intrahepatic arterial branches. Iatrogenic false aneurysms secondary to biliary tract and pancreatic operative trauma are well recognized. In particular, pseudoaneurysms associated with percutaneous and therapeutic hepatobiliary procedures are relatively common.[2,11,64]

Connective tissue arteriopathies, such as periarteritis nodosa, have also been incriminated as a cause of occasional macroaneurysms involving the hepatic vessels. Mycotic aneurysms associated with sepsis, often related to intravenous drug abuse and endocarditis, are relatively uncommon in contemporary practice.

Hepatic artery aneurysms are usually solitary; they are extrahepatic in nearly 80% of cases and intrahepatic in 20% (Figure 43-5). Arteriosclerosis is considered a secondary event rather than an actual cause of any of the various types of hepatic artery aneurysms.

Most hepatic artery aneurysms are asymptomatic and are discovered incidentally during imaging for other illnesses.[11,62,63] Nontraumatic hepatic artery aneurysms are occasionally symptomatic, in which case they characteristically produce right upper quadrant and epigastric pain. Acute expansion of hepatic artery aneurysms can cause severe abdominal discomfort, similar to that of pancreatitis. Large aneurysms may cause obstructive jaundice.[65]

The incidence of hepatic artery aneurysm rupture remains ill-defined, but the rupture rate in contemporary times approaches 20%.[7,60] However, bleeding has accompanied more than half of the aneurysms from institutions reporting large numbers of iatrogenic intrahepatic aneurysms.[2] Bleeding from ruptured hepatic artery aneurysms occurs equally into the biliary tract and into the peritoneal cavity. In the case of the former, hemobilia is often

evident, manifested by biliary colic, hematemesis, and jaundice.[66,67] Chronic gastrointestinal hemorrhage is an uncommon but recognized sequela of aneurysm rupture into the biliary tract. Intraperitoneal bleeding is usually associated with false aneurysms caused by periarterial inflammatory processes eroding into the hepatic vessels. Multiple nonarteriosclerotic aneurysms have an apparent greater risk of eventual rupture.[60] The reported overall mortality rate attending aneurysm rupture approaches 35%, although recent experience suggests that mortality is lower.

Endovascular or open surgical treatment is recommended for all symptomatic aneurysms and all asymptomatic saccular hepatic aneurysms exceeding 2 cm in diameter. Smaller expanding intrahepatic aneurysms and pseudoaneurysms of the extrahepatic arteries warrant an earlier intervention.

Percutaneous transcatheter obliteration of hepatic artery aneurysms with balloons, coils, various types of particulate matter, and even thrombin, is often preferred over an open surgical intervention (Figure 43-6).[2,15,64,68-70] Transcatheter embolization may be only transiently successful, and repeated embolization or eventual surgical therapy may be required to adequately treat certain patients. Endovascular stent graft exclusion of select aneurysms avoids some of the limitations accompanying embolization alone.[71-75]

Common hepatic artery aneurysms in the past were usually treated by open ligation, aneurysmectomy, or aneurysm exclusion, without arterial reconstruction.[11,17,61,76] If liver blood flow was compromised after hepatic artery occlusion, a direct vascular reconstruction needed to be undertaken with a prosthetic or autologous graft.[8,9,60] Hepatic ischemia is most likely to accompany treatment of aneurysms involving the proper hepatic artery or its extrahepatic branches and, whenever possible, arterial reconstruction of these vessels is favored following aneurysmectomy.[9,17] Casual ligation of extrahepatic branches to control bleeding from intrahepatic aneurysms may cause liver necrosis, and in this setting hepatic territory resection may be necessary in rare cases.[62]

Superior Mesenteric Artery Aneurysms

Aneurysms of the proximal superior mesenteric artery are the third most common splanchnic artery aneurysm, accounting for 5.5% of these lesions. Men are affected nearly twice as often as women.[77] An infectious etiology associated with bacterial endocarditis was more common in the past.[78-80] Nonhemolytic streptococci account for the majority of mycotic lesions encountered in contemporary practice. Superior mesenteric artery aneurysms may also be related to medial degeneration, periarterial inflammation, and trauma. Arteriosclerosis, when present, is considered a secondary event rather than an etiologic process.

Superior mesenteric artery aneurysms are usually recognized during imaging studies for other diseases. The majority of these aneurysms are asymptomatic. When symptomatic, there is usually an acute expansion, dissection, or rupture of the aneurysm. Rupture affected a little

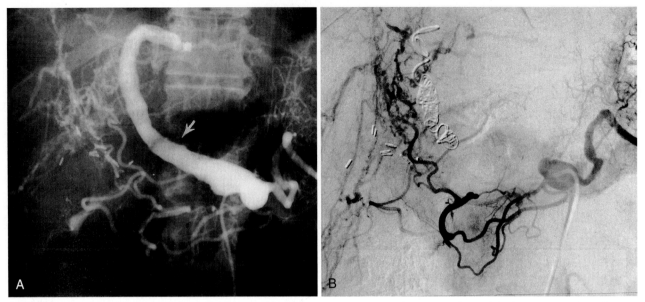

FIGURE 43-6 ■ **A,** Hepatic artery aneurysm with extensive thrombus surrounding the patent channel in the common hepatic artery *(arrow)*. **B,** Postembolization occlusion of aneurysm with reconstitution of distal collateral vessels entering the liver parenchyma. (From Upchurch GR, Jr, Zelenock GB, Stanley JC: Splenic artery aneurysms. In Rutherford RB, editor: Vascular surgery, ed 6, Philadelphia, 2005, Elsevier-Saunders, p 1572.)

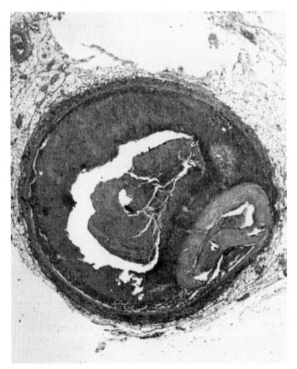

FIGURE 43-7 ■ Superior mesenteric artery aneurysm associated with a dissection compressing the arterial lumen. (From Zelenock GB, Stanley JC: Splanchnic artery aneurysms. In Rutherford RB, editor: Vascular surgery, ed 5, Philadelphia, 2000, WB Saunders, p 1376.)

more than one third of cases reported from a large health care system.[77] However, a rupture rate near 10% is more likely representative of contemporary practice. Mortality approaches 50% with rupture. Aneurysmal dissection is believed more common than rupture (Figure 43-7).[81-84] The unique location of dissecting aneurysms near the origins of the inferior pancreaticoduodenal and middle colic arteries place the distal mesenteric circulation at risk if these vessels become occluded. Thrombosis of the superior mesenteric artery in such cases results in a loss of the usual collateral networks from the adjacent celiac and inferior mesenteric arterial circulations. Occasionally, the latter causes intestinal ischemia with pain suggestive of abdominal angina. Symptomatic, expanding aneurysms and those greater than 2 cm diameter warrant interventional therapy.

Endovascular stent-graft placement has appeal for selected superior mesenteric artery aneurysms.[85-88] Although late complications of thrombosis and infection may accompany endovascular stent-graft therapy, the early morbidity and mortality are much less than what occurs with open surgical procedures. Certainly, obliteration of these aneurysms by coils or direct thrombin injection may be preferred in high-risk patients with discrete aneurysm necks.[77,89]

Open surgical ligation of superior mesenteric artery aneurysms without arterial reconstruction has proved possible in certain cases, especially for aneurysms associated with prior arterial obstruction and an adequate collateral circulation to the midgut structures.[77,90] In fact, ligation has been the most common open surgical means of managing these lesions. If trial clamping results in bowel ischemia, then intestinal revascularization is required.

Celiac Artery Aneurysms

Celiac artery aneurysms account for 4% of all splanchnic artery aneurysms. Men and women appear to be equally affected. Half the celiac artery aneurysms encountered before 1950 were mycotic, although infectious lesions have been relatively uncommon in recent years.[91] Most aneurysms are associated with medial defects. Aortic aneurysms affect nearly 20% of these patients, and nearly 40% have other splanchnic aneurysms. Arteriosclerosis is a frequent finding, but it is considered a secondary process, as in the case of other splanchnic artery aneurysms. Celiac artery aneurysms are usually saccular, affecting the distal trunk of this vessel (Figure 43-8), with some evolving from poststenotic dilatations caused by preexisting occlusive disease or median arcuate ligament entrapment and narrowing of the proximal celiac artery.

Most contemporary celiac artery aneurysms are asymptomatic or are associated with vague abdominal discomfort.[11,91,92] Antemortem diagnosis usually results when these aneurysms are recognized as incidental findings during imaging for other diseases. Rupture reportedly occurs in 13% of these aneurysms, is usually intraperitoneal, and carries a mortality of 50%.[91] Aneurysmal rupture rarely occurs into the gastrointestinal tract. Intervention is warranted for all symptomatic celiac artery aneurysms and those exceeding 2 cm in size.

Endovascular treatment of celiac artery aneurysms is infrequently performed because of the need to occlude the hepatic, splenic, left gastric arteries, and in some cases the inferior phrenic arteries. Nevertheless, successful endovascular therapy of these aneurysms has been reported and has a role, especially in patients at high risk for open surgery.[2,15,93,94]

Open surgical procedures are the most common intervention for celiac artery aneurysms, and are recommended unless prohibitive operative risks exist. Most nonruptured aneurysms can be treated through an abdominal approach, although in the presence of acute expansion or rupture, a thoracoabdominal incision may be favored. Arterial reconstruction of the celiac trunk is preferred following aneurysmectomy,[91,95] although simple aneurysmal exclusion with ligation of entering and exiting branches may be performed in select patients.[11,91,96,97] If the latter is undertaken, the foregut collateral blood flow to the liver must be sufficient to prevent severe hepatic ischemia. When such is not the case, an aorto-celiac or aortohepatic artery bypass is usually undertaken. Successful outcomes of open surgical therapy are greater than 90%.[91]

Gastric and Gastroepiploic Artery Aneurysms

Gastric and gastroepiploic artery aneurysms account for 4% of splanchnic artery aneurysms (Figure 43-9). Gastric artery aneurysms are tenfold more common than gastroepiploic artery aneurysms. Men are twice as likely than women to have these aneurysms. The majority of these lesions affect patients older than 50 years. Most of these aneurysms are solitary and are acquired as a result of either periarterial inflammation or medial degeneration. Arteriosclerosis, when present, is invariably a secondary accompaniment of these lesions. Gastric and gastroepiploic artery aneurysms are usually very small, and a search for them is often tedious if they have not been localized preoperatively by detailed imaging.

Most reported gastric or gastroepiploic artery aneurysms have been symptomatic when initially recognized. In fact, these perigastric aneurysms usually appear as emergencies with few antecedent symptoms.[98-100] Rupture has occurred in more than 90% of reported cases, with gastrointestinal bleeding being twice as common as intraperitoneal hemorrhage. Aneurysm rupture may be catastrophic, as emphasized by the reported 70% mortality of such an event.[13] Given the life-threatening risk of these aneurysms, it is

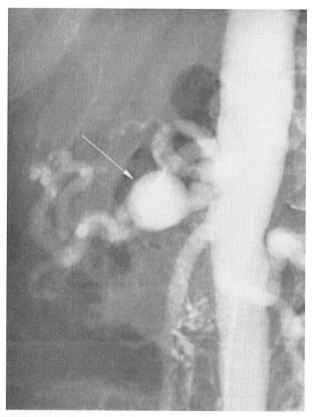

FIGURE 43-8 ■ Celiac artery aneurysm *(arrow)* affecting the distal trunk of the vessel. (From Whitehouse WM, Jr, Graham LM, Stanley JC: Aneurysms of the celiac, hepatic, and splenic arteries. In Bergan JJ, Yao JST, editors: Aneurysms: diagnosis and treatment, New York, 1981, Grune and Stratton, p 407.)

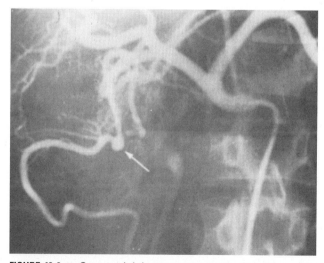

FIGURE 43-9 ■ Gastroepiploic artery aneurysm. Selective celiac arteriogram documenting small saccular aneurysm. (From Zelenock GB, Stanley JC: Splanchnic artery aneurysms. In Rutherford RB, editor: Vascular surgery, ed 5, Philadelphia, 2000, WB Saunders, p 1378.)

recommended that they be treated once the diagnosis is established.

Surgical treatment of gastric and gastroepiploic artery aneurysms does not involve vascular reconstructive surgery. Intramural gastric aneurysms often require excision with the involved portion of the stomach. Extramural aneurysms may be treated by arterial ligation alone, with or without aneurysm excision. In contemporary practice endovascular embolization at the time of arteriographic diagnosis in hemodynamically stable patients is favored over open surgery.[2,5,15,101,102]

Jejunal, Ileal, and Colic Artery Aneurysms

Aneurysms of the jejunal, ileal, and colic arteries account for 3% of splanchnic artery aneurysms. They are usually recognized in patients older than 60 years, with men and women affected equally. Solitary aneurysms are reported in 90% of cases. Those aneurysms affecting the proximal inferior mesenteric artery are often a result of this vessel being subjected to markedly high flow in patients having celiac and superior mesenteric artery occlusive disease.[103] The middle colic artery is the most common site of mediolytic arteritis, a disease of undetermined etiology.[104] Multiple aneurysms tend to evolve as a result of emboli associated with subacute bacterial endocarditis,[105] or from periarteritis nodosa.[106] Arteriosclerosis, present in 20% of these aneurysms, is considered a secondary event rather than a causative process.

Most reported aneurysms affecting these small arteries have been symptomatic, with the majority exhibiting abdominal pain.[103,104,107-109] Nevertheless, many aneurysms are undoubtedly asymptomatic and are recognized as incidental findings during arteriography for other diseases (Figure 43-10). Although the majority of reported

intestinal branch aneurysms have ruptured, actual rupture rates are probably closer to 30%. Aneurysms of ileal branches are most likely to rupture, with jejunal aneurysm rupture being relatively rare. Rupture occurs with near equal frequency into the intestinal tract, mesentery, or mesocolon, as well as the peritoneal cavity, and carries a mortality risk of approximately 20%.

Operations for extraintestinal aneurysms usually entail arterial ligation, with or without aneurysmectomy. Occasional patients will require an arterial reconstruction. Intramural aneurysms or those associated with bowel infarction usually necessitate resection of the involved segment of intestine. In select patients, transcatheter embolization may be undertaken, but intestinal necrosis with acute perforation or later stricture formation is a recognized complication of such therapy.[110-112]

Pancreaticoduodenal, Pancreatic, and Gastroduodenal Artery Aneurysms

Pancreatic and pancreaticoduodenal artery aneurysms account for 2% and gastroduodenal artery aneurysms 1.5% of all splanchnic artery aneurysms, respectively. Most patients with these lesions are older than 45 years. Men are fourfold more likely than women to have pancreaticoduodenal and gastroduodenal artery aneurysms, with this gender difference being more notable in the former than the latter aneurysms. There are two types of these lesions: pseudoaneurysms and true aneurysms. Arteriosclerosis is often present in both aneurysmal types and is considered a secondary process.

Approximately 50% of gastroduodenal and 30% of pancreaticoduodenal artery aneurysms are pancreatitis related (Figure 43-11). Pseudoaneurysms of these arteries are most often a consequence of pancreatitis-associated vascular necrosis or vessel erosion by an adjacent pancreatic pseudocyst (see Figure 43-6).[113-115] Traumatic aneurysms, especially those caused by iatrogenic events, are uncommon and most frequently involve the gastroduodenal artery.[116]

True aneurysms of these arteries exhibit medial thinning and degeneration of elastic tissue. Many evolve as an apparent consequence of excessive blood flow within the pancreaticoduodenal and gastroduodenal

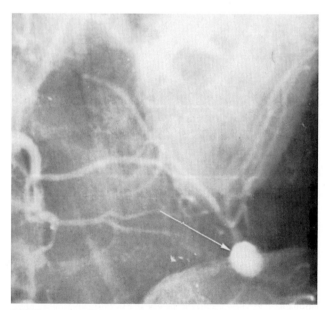

FIGURE 43-10 ■ Ileal artery branch aneurysm *(arrow).* (From Stanley JC, Whitehouse WM, Jr: Aneurysms of splanchnic and renal arteries. In Bergan JJ, Yao JST, editors: Surgery of the aorta and its body branches, New York, 1979, Grune and Stratton, p 505.)

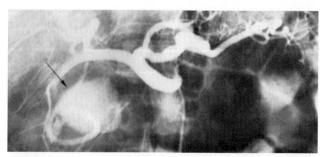

FIGURE 43-11 ■ Gastroduodenal artery aneurysm associated with arterial erosion by a pancreatic pseudocyst in a patient with pancreatitis. (From Eckhauser FE, Stanley JC, Zelenock GB, et al: Gastroduodenal and pancreaticoduodenal artery aneurysms. A complication of pancreatitis causing spontaneous gastroduodenal hemorrhage. Surgery 88:335–344, 1980.)

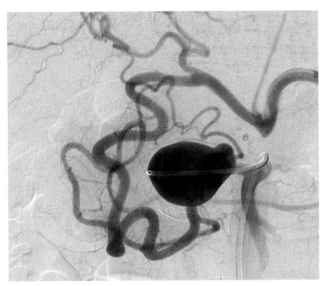

FIGURE 43-12 ■ Inferior pancreaticoduodenal artery aneurysm associated with a celiac artery occlusion.

arteries that are functioning as collaterals to the foregut in patients having celiac artery stenoses or occlusions (Figure 43-12).[117-121] Among the latter individuals, pancreaticoduodenal artery aneurysms are tenfold more common than those affecting the gastroduodenal arteries. Although less well recognized, similar aneurysms of these collateral vessels may develop in the presence of a superior mesenteric artery stenosis.[122]

Most patients with pseudoaneurysms and nearly all those with true aneurysms experience abdominal pain. In the case of pseudoaneurysms, this may also reflect underlying pancreatic disease. Among patients with true pancreaticoduodenal aneurysms and celiac artery stenoses, only one quarter have abdominal discomfort.

Rupture is the most serious complication of these aneurysms. Surprisingly, inflammatory aneurysms carry a risk of rupture of approximately 10%, which occurs into the intestinal tract more often than into the peritoneal cavity or retroperitoneum. Rupture carries a mortality of 20%.

True gastroduodenal and pancreaitocduodenal artery aneurysm rupture affects nearly 35% and 60% of these lesions, respectively. Bleeding from true gastroduodenal artery aneurysms occurs most often into the gastrointestinal tract. Bleeding of true pancreaticoduodenal artery aneurysms occurs most often into the retroperitoneum. Mortality following rupture of true gastroduodenal aneurysms approaches 20%. The overall mortality is less than 10% following rupture of true pancreaticoduodenal aneurysms in patients with celiac artery stenoses.

Endovascular or open operative interventions have been proposed for all but the highest-risk patients with gastroduodenal and pancreaticoduodenal arterial aneurysms.[12,123,124] Despite the fact that the natural history of some aneurysms appears relatively benign,[125] most clinicians favor early treatment of these lesions.

Endovascular embolization is favored as the initial treatment of most true aneurysms and pseudoaneurysms in patients stable enough to be treated electively or semiurgently.* In some cases, stent graft placement may prove to be advantageous.[127] Infection or even late aneurysmal rupture may follow endovascular therapies and such justifies careful long-term follow-up. However, even in critically-ill patients who are unstable, endovascular occlusion of the bleeding aneurysm may be a lifesaving measure that can be followed by a later definitive open procedure.[113,115,117]

Open surgical treatment is most often pursued when endovascular therapy is not technically feasible, when it might result in ischemic organ injury, and in most unstable bleeding patients. Large pancreatitis-related pseudoaneurysms associated with pseudocysts are often treated by open arterial ligation from within the aneurysmal sac rather than extra-aneurysmal arterial ligation. Extensive dissection about the pancreas in this setting is hazardous. Some form of pseudocyst drainage may be needed in many patients. Concurrent or later pancreatic resection to address the underlying pancreatic disease may include distal pancreatectomy or even pancreaticoduodenectomy.[128]

Among patients having the aneurysms and coexistent celiac artery occlusions or stenoses, the affected artery may be part of an essential collateral vessel, and transcatheter embolic occlusion or simple arterial ligation can result in profound foregut ischemia. In these circumstances, open surgery and revascularization of the celiac circulation may be appropriate when treating the aneurysm.[8,117,118,129]

RENAL ARTERY ANEURYSMS

Renal artery aneurysms are an uncommon and controversial vascular disease (Table 43-3). It is likely that complications and clinical importance of these aneurysms have been overestimated in spectacular case reports rather than relying on population-based experiences.[130-131] Discussion of these lesions must consider the differences between true aneurysms and dissections of the renal artery.

True Renal Artery Aneurysms

The incidence of true renal artery aneurysms approaches 0.1%, a figure derived from the 0.09% frequency of these lesions in approximately 8500 patients subjected to arteriographic studies for nonrenal disease.[132] Women are slightly more likely than men to have renal artery aneurysms.[133] Most renal artery aneurysms are saccular (Figure 43-13). Seventy-five percent are located at first- or second-order renal artery bifurcations. Intraparenchymal aneurysms occur in less than 10% of cases.

True renal artery aneurysms are usually caused by a medial degenerative process. The majority of these processes appear to be unrelated to any known systemic vascular disease, perhaps being a reflection of a preexisting congenital defect in the arterial wall elastic tissue. In other instances, this may be a manifestation of medial

*References 2, 5, 6, 10, 115, 118, 126.

TABLE 43-3   **Renal Artery Aneurysms**

Lesion	Male:Female Ratio	Common Contributing Factors	Frequency of Reported Rupture	Mortality with Rupture	Usual Treatment Options
Renal artery aneurysm	1:1.2	Medial degeneration; arterial fibrodysplasia; hypertension	3% bland	10% bland; during pregnancy 50% maternal, 75% fetal	Aneurysmectomy with renal artery reconstruction; endovascular aneurysm obliteration; nephrectomy for ruptured aneurysms
Renal artery dissection	10:1	Blunt abdominal trauma; medial degeneration with arteriosclerosis and fibrodysplasia	Uncommon (thrombosis more common)	Very uncommon	Renal artery reconstruction; nephrectomy for irreparable renal ischemia

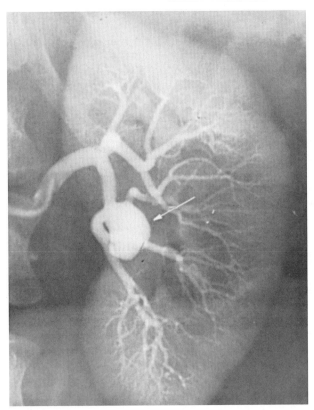

FIGURE 43-13 ■ Saccular renal artery aneurysm *(arrow)* occurring at a segmental branching. (From Stanley JC, Whitehouse WM, Jr: Renal artery macroaneurysms. In Bergan JJ, Yao JST, editors: Aneurysms: diagnosis and treatment, New York, 1981, Grune and Stratton, p 419.)

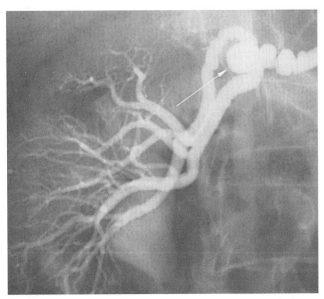

FIGURE 43-14 ■ Renal artery macroaneurysm *(arrow)* affecting the primary bifurcation of a vessel exhibiting medial fibrodysplasia. (From Stanley JC, Whitehouse WM, Jr: Renal artery macroaneurysms. In Bergan JJ, Yao JST, editors: Aneurysms: diagnosis and treatment, New York, 1981, Grune and Stratton, p 420.)

arterial fibrodysplasia (Figure 43-14). That the right renal artery is more likely than the left to develop aneurysms may reflect the fact that fibrodysplastic disease is known to more often affect the right renal artery. Other arteriopathies, such as Ehler-Danlos syndrome, are a relatively uncommon cause of these aneurysms. Arteriosclerosis affects one third of true aneurysms, and is thought to represent a secondary event. Necrotizing arteritides, such as polyarteritis nodosa, are a cause of microaneurysms and an occasional macroaneurysm.[134]

The majority of true renal artery aneurysms are asymptomatic.[133] Nevertheless, aneurysmal expansion or renal infarction from dislodged thrombus may occasionally account for flank and abdominal pain that may mimic renal colic.

An ill-defined relation exists between renal artery aneurysms and elevated arterial blood pressure.[133,135] Occasionally, aneurysmal thrombus may embolize or propagate and occlude a distal artery, thereby producing renal ischemia and renovascular hypertension.[132,136] Computational modeling suggests that deformation of branches adjacent to aneurysms at bifurcations may produce a pressure gradient and also cause renovascular hypertension.[137] It has also been hypothesized that energy dissipation in large aneurysms causes a similar drop in renal blood pressure and results in systematic blood pressure increases because of renin release. Intrinsic stenotic disease adjacent to an aneurysm, not always evident on preoperative arteriograms, is a more likely cause of secondary hypertension in other patients, especially those with renal arterial fibrodysplasia.

Rupture represents the most serious complication of true renal artery aneurysms. It has been suggested that aneurysms less than 1.5 cm in diameter, calcified aneurysms, and those occurring in normotensive patients are not likely to rupture, but this has not proved to be the case. Rupture may be overt into the retroperitoneal and abdominal cavity or covert into an adjacent renal vein. Such events are likely to affect less than 3% of cases.[138]

Overt rupture causes flank pain and often hypotension owing to excessive bleeding. It carries a reported mortality of approximately 10%, but that figure appears less in contemporary practice. Loss of the kidney is greater than 90% with overt aneurysm rupture. Renal artery aneurysm rupture during pregnancy does not appear related to patient age, presence of hypertension, or parity, and it is more life threatening. Rupture during pregnancy is associated with nearly 75% fetal mortality rate and 50% maternal mortality.[138]

Symptomatic patients with possible aneurysmal expansion should be subjected to treatment. Intervention is also recommended for aneurysms coexisting with functionally important renal artery stenoses. Asymptomatic aneurysms 2 cm in diameter and those 1.5 to 2 cm diameter in hypertensive patients justify treatment by experienced interventionists. Aneurysms 1.0 to 1.5 cm in diameter provide a relative indication for elective treatment, but only when a high degree of suspicion exists that they are the cause of refractory renovascular hypertension. Because of the potential for catastrophic rupture during pregnancy, therapy is recommended for all aneurysms in women of childbearing age who might conceive in the future.

Endovascular therapy of true renal artery aneurysms offers an important alternative to open aneurysmectomy.[139-143] Intraparenchymal aneurysms and select aneurysms of the extrarenal arteries can often be effectively treated by catheter interventions. However, endovascular embolic or stent-graft exclusion of extraparenchymal renal artery aneurysms without segmental renal artery occlusion is difficult because of the aneurysm's usual location at arterial bifurcations. Nevertheless, newer multilayered stents and coil embolization facilitated by prior stent placement by experienced interventionists may carry less risk to the patient than an open procedure.

Open surgical therapy of nonruptured renal artery aneurysms is directed at eliminating the aneurysm without loss of the kidney or compromise of normal renal blood flow.[134,144-150] Large aneurysms of the main renal artery or its bifurcation can often be excised with simple primary closure of the artery. Excision of smaller aneurysms may necessitate a vein patch closure or implantation of the involved artery into an adjacent uninvolved artery. In situ renal artery reconstruction with autogenous saphenous vein or internal iliac artery grafts is preferred for most aneurysms coexisting with functionally important stenoses. In other cases, ex vivo repairs may be appropriate. Open surgical treatment of true renal artery aneurysms is successful in more than 90% of cases and provides for improvement of blood pressure control in nearly 50% of patients.[133,144,148]

Renal Artery Dissections

Isolated dissections of the renal arteries, excluding iatrogenic endocatheter-related lesions, are classified as those due to blunt or penetrating trauma or those occurring

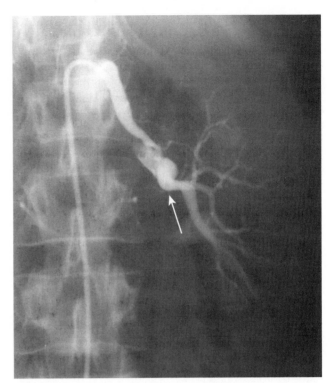

FIGURE 43-15 ■ Renal artery dissection with contrast in the false lumen and a narrowing of the adjacent renal artery.

spontaneously.[151-156] All forms of dissection may be associated with false aneurysm formation (Figure 43-15). Men are nearly tenfold more likely than women to exhibit dissections of the renal artery.[151] The right renal artery is affected with traumatic dissections more than the left. This may be due to increased arterial stretching, especially with deacceleration trauma, because of the greater ptosis and mobility of the right kidney.

Spontaneous dissections involve the renal arteries more than any other muscular artery, and they affect the left renal artery more often than the right.[152] Approximately one third of these dissections are bilateral. Spontaneous dissections are usually related to coexistent arteriosclerotic or fibrodysplastic renovascular disease. They are more common with the latter, being reported in 0.5% of patients with renal artery fibrodysplasia.[152] These dissections usually extend within the outer media; this is in contrast to the subintimal and inner medial location of traumatic dissections. Spontaneous renal artery dissections most often originate in the distal main renal artery and terminate at a first-order branching.

Flank pain, hematuria, and elevated blood pressure are frequent manifestations of both acute spontaneous and traumatic renal artery dissections. Delayed arterial rupture is uncommon. Chronic dissections are usually silent, becoming evident with renovascular hypertension and impaired renal function. Loss of life accompanying an isolated renal artery dissection is very uncommon.

The initial clinical diagnosis was incorrect in nearly 60% of patients with acute renal artery dissections. Prompt diagnosis may improve the outcome of therapy, justifying early arteriographic studies. Criteria for the arteriographic diagnosis of renal artery dissection include: luminal irregularities, with aneurysmal dilatation or saccular dissections associated with segmental stenosis; the predilection of dissections to extend distally to the first renal artery bifurcation; cuffing at branchings, causing a "rolled-down sock" appearance; and variable degrees of reversibility documented by serial studies.

Acute spontaneous dissections involving the distal main renal artery warrant intervention if hemodynamically significant stenoses or occlusions appear responsible for difficult-to-control hypertension or a deterioration in renal function. Some isolated branch dissections may be followed closely without surgical intervention.[157] Kidney parenchymal preservation is of prime importance in patients having spontaneous dissections, particularly because of concomitant contralateral renal artery stenotic disease in half the patients.

Arterial reconstruction using autogenous saphenous vein or hypogastric artery may be complex, and ex vivo repairs are appropriate in select cases. Acute traumatic renal artery dissections associated with blunt injuries usually necessitate emergent arterial reconstruction for kidney salvage, with delayed repairs for chronic dissections being undertaken in the presence of renovascular hypertension or deterioration in renal function. Treatment using endovascular coils and stents has appeal, but still remains an evolving therapy in the management of most acute renal artery dissections.[158,159]

BIBLIOGRAPHY

Abbas MA, Fowl RJ, Stone WM, et al: Hepatic artery aneurysm: factors that predict complications. J Vasc Surg 38:41, 2003.

Fankhauser GT, Stone WM, Naidu SG, et al: The minimally invasive management of visceral artery aneurysms and pseudoaneurysms. J Vasc Surg 53:966–970, 2011.

Graham LM, Stanley JC, Whitehouse WM, Jr, et al: Celiac artery aneurysms: historical (1745–1949) versus contemporary (1950–1984) differences in etiology and clinical importance. J Vasc Surg 2:757–764, 1985.

Ha JF, Phillips M, Faulkner K: Splenic artery aneurysm rupture in pregnancy. Eur J Obstet Gynecol Reprod Biol 146:133–137, 2009.

Henke PK, Cardneau JD, Welling TH, et al: Renal artery aneurysms: a 35-year clinical experience with 252 aneurysms in 168 patients. Ann Surg 234:454–463, 2001.

Latkin RO, Bena JJF, Sarac TP, et al: The contemporary management of splenic artery aneurysms. J Vasc Surg 53:958–965, 2011.

Stanley JC, Fry WJ: Pathogenesis and clinical significance of splenic artery aneurysms. Surgery 76:889–909, 1974.

Stone WM, Abbas M, Cherry KJ, et al: Superior mesenteric artery aneurysms: is presence an indication for intervention? J Vasc Surg 36:234–237, 2002.

References available online at expertconsult.com.

QUESTIONS

1. Which of the following represents the reported ranking of splanchnic artery aneurysms in order of decreasing frequency?
   a. Splenic, hepatic, superior mesenteric, celiac
   b. Hepatic, splenic, celiac, superior mesenteric
   c. Jejunal, celiac, hepatic, splenic
   d. Splenic, hepatic, celiac, superior mesenteric

2. Which of the following statements about splenic artery aneurysms is true?
   a. They are more common in women than men.
   b. They tend to be saccular and occur at vessel branchings.
   c. They may exhibit a "double-rupture" phenomenon.
   d. All of the above

3. Which of the following statements about hepatic artery aneurysms is true?
   a. They account for 20% of reported splanchnic artery aneurysms.
   b. They often present with obstructive jaundice.
   c. Rupture has occurred in 20% of reported cases, with a 50% mortality rate.
   d. They are fourfold more likely to rupture into the biliary tract as into the peritoneal cavity.

4. Which of the following statements about aneurysms of the superior mesenteric artery is true?
   a. They are the fifth most common splanchnic artery aneurysm, accounting for 2.5% of all such aneurysms.
   b. They are frequently mycotic in origin.
   c. They affect women twice as often as men.
   d. Rupture occurred in 12% of reported cases.

5. Which of the following statements about celiac artery aneurysms is true?
   a. They are best treated by simple ligation with or without aneurysmectomy.
   b. They are rarely diagnosed before rupture in contemporary practice.
   c. Mortality is 50% when they rupture.
   d. They affect women four times more often than men.

6. Which of the following statements about jejunal, ileal, and colic artery aneurysms is true?
   a. They are most commonly caused by atherosclerosis.
   b. They affect men 10 times more often than women.
   c. When multiple, they tend to be associated with subacute bacterial endocarditis or periarteritis nodosa.
   d. They carry a 30% risk of rupture.

7. Which of the following statements about renal artery aneurysms is true?
   a. They are demonstrated in 0.1% of patients undergoing angiography for nonrenal indications.
   b. They tend to be fusiform and occur most often in the main renal artery.
   c. They are usually caused by atherosclerosis.
   d. They cause hypertension in approximately 80% of cases.

8. Which of the following statements about ruptured renal artery aneurysms is true?
   a. They usually present with hematuria.
   b. They carry a mortality approaching 10%.
   c. They are most commonly treated by arterial reconstruction.
   d. They are more likely to occur with noncalcified than calcified aneurysms.

9. Renal artery aneurysms may be associated with hypertension due to which of the following?
   a. Obstruction of urine flow in collecting system
   b. Compression of adjacent renal veins
   c. Intrinsic renal artery stenotic disease adjacent to the aneurysm
   d. Contralateral release of renal renin

10. Which of the following statements about spontaneous dissection of the renal artery is true?
    a. It is a common form of renal artery disease.
    b. It occurs most often in women.
    c. It is bilateral in a third of cases.
    d. It rarely requires surgical therapy.

ANSWERS

1. **d**
2. **d**
3. **a**
4. **b**
5. **c**
6. **c**
7. **a**
8. **b**
9. **c**
10. **c**

CHAPTER 44

ANEURYSMS OF THE PERIPHERAL ARTERIES

D. Preston Flanigan

Peripheral arterial aneurysms are distinctly less common than aortic aneurysms but can cause significant morbidity. Although these lesions occasionally lead to death, the most common serious complication is end-organ loss or dysfunction. For the purposes of this chapter, peripheral aneurysms include those of the upper extremity arteries distal to and including the subclavian artery, the lower extremity arteries distal to and including the femoral artery, and the extracranial carotid arteries. Mycotic aneurysms affecting these vessels are also included.

NONMYCOTIC PERIPHERAL ANEURYSMS

Incidence and Cause

Overall, the most common cause of nonmycotic peripheral aneurysms is atherosclerosis; however, depending on location, this is not true for all peripheral aneurysms. In general, all peripheral aneurysms can be considered rare. In descending order, the relative frequency of these aneurysms is popliteal, femoral, subclavian or axillary, and carotid. Reports on distal aneurysms involving the brachial, radial, ulnar, deep femoral, and tibial or peroneal arteries are limited to small series or case reports. Although true aneurysms have been reported in these areas,[1,2] for the most part, forearm, hand, tibial, and peroneal aneurysms are secondary to trauma or are mycotic in origin.[3]

Age and sex distribution are dependent on cause. Atherosclerotic aneurysms tend to occur primarily in men older than 50 years. Aneurysms caused by trauma are also more common in men, but occur at a younger age. Aneurysms secondary to thoracic outlet syndrome are most commonly seen in middle-aged women (75%).

Extracranial Carotid Artery Aneurysms

The rarity of extracranial carotid aneurysms is demonstrated by numerous reports of institutional experience with aneurysm patients. Of 2300 aneurysms reported from Baylor University, only 7 were extracranial carotid aneurysms.[4] In 30 years at Johns Hopkins, only 12 such aneurysms were seen.[5] Only 8 carotid aneurysms were noted by Houser and Baker after obtaining 5000 cerebral arteriograms.[6] The largest single series of patients with true extracranial carotid aneurysms was reported by McCollum and coworkers,[7] who saw 37 such aneurysms over a 21-year period. Zhang and associates[8] reported 66 extracranial carotid aneurysms, 28 of which were true, nonmycotic aneurysms.

Currently, the common carotid artery is affected most often, followed closely by the internal carotid artery. The external carotid artery is rarely involved.[9]

The most common cause of extracranial carotid aneurysms is atherosclerosis. These aneurysms tend to be fusiform and are almost always associated with arterial hypertension. Most of the patients also have evidence of generalized atherosclerosis.[9] Another cause of carotid aneurysm is trauma, both blunt and penetrating.[10] False aneurysms of the carotid artery have occurred after carotid endarterectomy and carotid artery dissections.[11] Rarer causes include cystic medial necrosis, Marfan syndrome, fibromuscular dysplasia, medial arteriopathy, granulomatous disease, radiation, and congenital defects.[10] El-Sabrout reviewed the literature from 1950 through 1995 and found that of 392 carotid aneurysms, reported etiology was as follows: 40% atherosclerotic, 21% pseudoaneurysm, 14% trauma, 12% dissection, 8% fibromuscular disease, 2% infection, and 3% other.[12]

Subclavian and Axillary Artery Aneurysms

Aneurysms of the subclavian and axillary arteries are also rare. In 1982, Hobson and colleagues reviewed the literature on the subject and found only 195 aneurysms in these locations[13]; these account for only 1% of all peripheral aneurysms. Of the 195 cases, 88% involved the subclavian artery. Subclavian and axillary aneurysms are rarely due to atherosclerosis, with this cause accounting for only 15% of the aneurysms. Thoracic outlet syndrome is responsible for the majority of subclavian artery aneurysms (74%), whereas crutch trauma accounts for most axillary artery aneurysms (54%). Other more rare causes have also been reported (Table 44-1).

Forearm and Hand Aneurysms

True aneurysms in the forearm and hand are extremely rare. During a 10-year period, only 10 such patients were treated at the University of Chicago.[2] Half of the true aneurysms in these areas are associated with occupational or recreational trauma. Most forearm and hand aneurysms are false aneurysms secondary to penetrating trauma[3]; most true aneurysms in these locations are secondary to blunt trauma.[14]

Femoral and Popliteal Artery Aneurysms

Femoral and popliteal artery aneurysms are grouped together because of their similar cause, their similar clinical behavior, and their frequent association.

TABLE 44-1	Causes of Subclavian and Axillary Artery Aneurysms		
Cause	Subclavian	Axillary	Total
Thoracic outlet syndrome	127	1	128
Crutch trauma	—	13	13
Atherosclerosis	24	5	29
Pseudoaneurysm	5	2	7
Blunt trauma	2	—	2
Fibromuscular dysplasia	—	2	2
Dissection	—	1	1
Other	13	—	13
Total	171	24	195

Data from Hobson RW II, Isreal MR, Lynch TO: Axillo-subclavian arterial aneurysms. In Bergan JJ, Vito JST, editors: Aneurysms, New York, 1982, Grune and Stratton, pp 435–447.

Aside from trauma and rare degenerative and congenital disorders, femoral and popliteal aneurysms are almost exclusively atherosclerotic in origin.[15,16] Together, these two types of aneurysms account for more than 90% of peripheral aneurysms.[17] Femoral aneurysms may involve the common femoral artery in the groin, but occasionally these aneurysms are limited to the superficial femoral artery. These latter lesions are often seen in patients with arteriomegaly or aneurysmosis.

Dent and colleagues showed an association between popliteal and femoral aneurysms and other aneurysms of atherosclerotic origin.[18] Most commonly, these associated aneurysms are located in the aortoiliac vessels, but more rarely they involve the renal, splanchnic, and brachiocephalic vessels. Among patients with at least one peripheral aneurysm, 83% had multiple aneurysms. Among patients with a common femoral aneurysm, 95% had a second aneurysm, 92% had an aortoiliac aneurysm, and 59% had bilateral femoral aneurysms. Among patients with a popliteal aneurysm, 78% had a second aneurysm, 64% had an aortoiliac aneurysm, and 47% had bilateral popliteal artery aneurysms. Conversely, in a more recent study, the Michigan group has also shown that the incidence of femoral and popliteal aneurysms in men with abdominal aortic aneurysms is 14% (0% in women).[19] Of further importance is that most of the femoral and popliteal artery aneurysms in their series were undetectable by physical examination, therefore underlining the need for ultrasound screening for femoral and popliteal aneurysms in men with abdominal aortic aneurysms. Profunda femoris aneurysms have a 75% incidence of synchronous aneurysms.[1] Patients with peripheral aneurysms are at high risk for the development of future peripheral aneurysms. Dawson showed that in patients with a popliteal artery aneurysm, new peripheral aneurysms were found in 32% of these patients after 5 years and in 49% of these patients after 10 years.[20]

Natural History

As with aortic aneurysms, peripheral aneurysms can be asymptomatic or lead to significant complications. Unlike aortic aneurysms, which tend to rupture, peripheral aneurysms most commonly thrombose or give rise to arterial emboli.

Extracranial Carotid Artery Aneurysms

Central neurologic events are common in these patients. Rhodes and coauthors reported that 13 of the 19 patients with carotid aneurysms reported in the University of Michigan series had amaurosis fugax, transient ischemic attacks, stroke, or vague neurologic symptoms such as dizziness.[9] Most of these symptoms are thought to be secondary to embolization. Cranial nerve compression leads to local neurologic dysfunction and can include facial pain (cranial nerve V), oculomotor palsies (cranial nerve VI), auricular pain (cranial nerve IX), and hoarseness (cranial nerve X). Horner syndrome can also occur from compression of the sympathetic chain. As cervical carotid aneurysms enlarge, they can cause dysphagia, cranial nerve compression, and pain. Hemorrhage has also been seen as a complication of these aneurysms; however, rupture is uncommon.

Subclavian and Axillary Artery Aneurysms

Only 10% of patients with known subclavian or axillary aneurysms are asymptomatic.[13] Good natural history studies are not available, probably because of the small number of patients with this problem. Because 90% of patients are symptomatic at the time of presentation, the likelihood of complications eventually occurring in asymptomatic aneurysms appears to be great. The primary complication seen with subclavian and axillary aneurysms is embolization (68%).[13] Thrombosis and rupture are rare but have been reported.[13,21]

Forearm and Hand Aneurysms

The most common presenting signs and symptoms of aneurysms in the forearm and hand are mass and pain. Distal embolization occurs in approximately one third of these patients.[2]

Femoral and Popliteal Artery Aneurysms

The natural history of unoperated femoral and popliteal aneurysms shows a high incidence of thromboembolic events. Tolstedt and associates reported a 43% rate of thrombosis in conservatively managed femoral aneurysms,[22] and in Cutler and Darling's series,[23] 47% exhibited major complications. In a study of popliteal aneurysms by Szilagyi and colleagues,[15] only 32% of those managed conservatively remained without complications at 5 years. Vermilion and colleagues[16] studied 26 popliteal aneurysms for an average of 3 years and demonstrated that 31% of patients suffered limb-threatening complications, with 2 patients requiring major amputation and 2 patients left with rest pain.[16] Rupture of femoral or popliteal aneurysms has been reported rarely. Deep femoral aneurysms are particularly prone to rupture, with rates of 13% to 45% being reported.[1] Popliteal aneurysms rupture, on occasion, into the popliteal vein.[24] Less catastrophic complications include pain secondary to tibial nerve compression and popliteal vein thrombosis secondary to popliteal vein compression.

Diagnosis

Most peripheral aneurysms can be diagnosed by simple palpation of the artery in question. More sophisticated studies such as ultrasonography, computed tomography (CT) scans, magnetic resonance imaging or angiography, and arteriography augment the diagnosis and allow for better preoperative planning.

Extracranial Carotid Artery Aneurysms

Excluding neurologic findings, the most common physical finding in patients with carotid aneurysms is a palpable pulsatile, submandibular, lateral neck mass or a mass in the tonsillar fossa. The former presentation is most often seen with common carotid aneurysms, whereas presentation in the tonsillar fossa is more often seen with internal carotid artery aneurysms. Because of the variability in the location of the carotid bifurcation, the presentation is only a rough guide to the artery involved. The differential diagnosis includes kinked or redundant carotid arteries, enlarged lymph nodes, salivary gland tumors, branchial cleft cysts, cystic hygromas, and carotid body tumors. When the diagnosis is not clear, carotid duplex scanning and CT angiography is usually diagnostic. Arteriography further aids in elucidating the diagnosis and is required for proper preoperative planning.

Subclavian and Axillary Artery Aneurysms

The most common presenting signs and symptoms of subclavian and axillary aneurysms are secondary to distal embolization (68%; Table 44-2). Other signs and symptoms include tissue loss, claudication, pain, and evidence of brachial plexus compression. When the aneurysm is secondary to thoracic outlet syndrome, it often cannot be palpated. Aneurysms secondary to atherosclerosis tend to be larger and are palpable in two thirds of patients at the time of presentation.[21] A bruit may be present in the subclavian fossa or in the axilla. Small, punctate, cyanotic lesions affecting the fingers and palm that are painful and occur suddenly are often present as a result of distal embolization. Rarely, embolization causes large axial artery occlusion. This event usually requires immediate embolectomy, but can lead to claudication if the initial ischemia does not precipitate the need for immediate medical attention. With chronic small embolization, the distal radial and ulnar pulses might not be palpable owing to buildup of embolic material. Repeated embolization

may be associated with distal digital ulceration or tissue loss and severe pain. Many patients show vague shoulder pain on presentation. Rupture produces severe shoulder pain radiating into the upper arm and lower neck.

When all types of subclavian and axillary aneurysms are considered, only 16% can be palpated.[13] Duplex ultrasound is useful to diagnose subclavian and axillary artery aneurysms, but the bony cage of the thoracic outlet may preclude adequate insonation of proximal subclavian artery aneurysms. CT scanning can also demonstrate subclavian and axillary aneurysms. However, because in most cases the diagnosis should be suggested on the basis of history and physical examination, arteriography is the most useful test because it is also needed for proper planning of the operative procedure.

Forearm and Hand Aneurysms

Forearm, and especially hand, aneurysms are most often diagnosed by palpation of a pulsatile mass. These aneurysms can also be diagnosed by ultrasound or CT scanning, but nonpalpable aneurysms are generally found on arteriography in patients being studied for embolization.

Femoral and Popliteal Artery Aneurysms

The diagnosis of femoral and popliteal aneurysms is often made by palpation because of their superficial nature. Popliteal aneurysms are suspected in any patient in whom the popliteal pulse is widened and easily felt. Diwan and associates,[19] however, found that most femoral and popliteal aneurysms were not detected by physical examination and suggested the routine use of ultrasonography to look for femoral and popliteal aneurysms in men with aortic aneurysms. Femoral and popliteal aneurysms should be considered in any patient with an acute arterial occlusion in the leg or with embolic disease affecting the foot and lower leg. Many popliteal aneurysms are calcified and can be detected by plain radiographs of the popliteal fossa. Both femoral and popliteal aneurysms are easily diagnosed by ultrasonography. CT scanning is particularly accurate in making the diagnosis and is helpful in planning endovascular repair (Figure 44-1). Despite the presence of mural thrombus, arteriography usually confirms the diagnosis and may be necessary for proper

TABLE 44-2	Clinical Findings in Subclavian and Axillary Artery Aneurysms	
Finding	**Number**	**Percent**
Asymptomatic	20	10
Claudication	9	5
Pain	36	18
Brachial plexus palsy	24	12
Tissue loss	20	10
Embolization	136	68

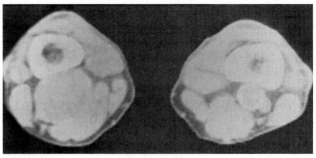

FIGURE 44-1 ■ Computed tomography scan showing an obvious right popliteal artery aneurysm and a smaller left popliteal artery aneurysm.

operative planning. The status of the runoff vessels visualized arteriographically is particularly important for patients with popliteal aneurysms, because there is a direct correlation to early and late graft patency after repair.[25]

Indications for Aneurysm Repair

Unlike aortic aneurysms, for which size is the main determinant of the need for repair, the mere presence of a peripheral aneurysm often suggests the need for repair. As with aortic aneurysms, the decision to repair a peripheral aneurysm must be tempered by the patient's overall medical condition so that the risk of repair is considerably less than the risk of the natural history of the disease.

Extracranial Carotid Artery Aneurysms

The indication for operation in a patient with a cervical carotid artery aneurysm is usually the presence of the aneurysm. Because patients with this condition are rarely seen when asymptomatic, most patients are treated for symptomatic relief or for prevention of recurrent symptoms. The high incidence of cranial nerve compression and central nervous system events in untreated patients (68%)[9] justifies treatment for asymptomatic carotid aneurysms as well. This finding is common in nearly all reported studies, and the point is not a controversial one.[26-28]

Subclavian and Axillary Artery Aneurysms

Generally, the presence of a subclavian or axillary aneurysm is an indication for repair. The natural history suggests that these lesions are both life threatening and limb threatening.[21] As is the case with carotid aneurysms, most patients are symptomatic at the time of presentation and have clear indications for intervention. Some controversy exists regarding the small, fusiform, post-stenotic subclavian dilatation often seen with thoracic outlet compression of the subclavian artery. The natural history of this lesion, if not resected at the time of thoracic outlet decompression, is not well established. In the four patients with subclavian artery aneurysms who had only thoracic outlet decompression, no subsequent thromboembolic events occurred during follow-up.[21]

Femoral and Popliteal Artery Aneurysms

Dawson and colleagues[20] compared operative and nonoperative approaches to 71 popliteal artery aneurysms. Thromboembolic complications developed in 57% of unoperated asymptomatic popliteal aneurysms over a mean follow-up period of 5 years. In aneurysms studied for a full 5 years, the complication rate was 74%. In comparison, operated patients had graft patency and limb salvage rates of 64% and 95%, respectively, at 10-year follow-up. As noted previously, these authors also found a high risk of subsequent aneurysm development in these patients. At 5-year follow-up, 32% of patients had developed additional aneurysms; at 10 years, 49% had new aneurysms.

The report by Dawson and colleagues[20] and those referenced previously in the natural history section strongly support the early surgical treatment of asymptomatic femoral and popliteal aneurysms and underscore the need for careful follow-up of these patients for the development of new aneurysms.

Current recommendations for the treatment of femoral and popliteal aneurysms include aneurysms between 1.5 and 2.0 cm with thrombus and for all aneurysms of 2 cm or greater. This recommendation is based on the high incidence of thromboembolic complications associated with these lesions, as detailed earlier, and the low morbidity and mortality associated with repair.[29]

Treatment

Justification for the treatment of most peripheral aneurysms lies in the high morbidity and mortality of untreated peripheral aneurysms and the low morbidity and mortality of modern treatment modalities. The two primary objectives in the treatment of peripheral aneurysms are exclusion of the aneurysm and restoration of arterial continuity. In most cases, both objectives can be achieved. In some inaccessible aneurysms, however, exclusion alone must be accepted because restoration of arterial continuity may not be possible. Additional goals are to apply treatment methods that will relieve compressive symptoms when present and to minimize the risk of aneurysm enlargement after repair.

Extracranial Carotid Artery Aneurysms

The techniques applied to the management of extracranial carotid aneurysms are ligation (or angiographic occlusion), endoaneurysmorrhaphy, resection with primary anastomosis, resection with graft replacement, or stent-grafting.

The preferred treatment is resection with primary anastomosis or graft replacement. Redundancy of the carotid artery is not uncommon when aneurysm is present. In such cases, resection of the aneurysm with mobilization of the carotid artery and primary anastomosis is sometimes easily accomplished (Figure 44-2). This technique is most applicable to internal carotid artery aneurysms. An alternative technique for flow restoration after resection of an internal carotid artery aneurysm is to divide the distal external carotid artery and perform an end-to-end anastomosis between the proximal external carotid and the distal internal carotid arteries. Aneurysms of the external carotid artery are rare and can be resected without the need to restore arterial continuity. Aneurysms of the carotid bifurcation usually require resection with graft replacement between the common and internal carotid arteries. When the internal carotid is redundant, it can be mobilized and anastomosed end to end to the common carotid artery. In both these latter cases, the external carotid is usually ligated. Aneurysms involving the common carotid artery can usually be treated by resection and primary anastomosis or graft replacement. All these procedures can be performed through a standard neck incision such as that used for carotid endarterectomy.

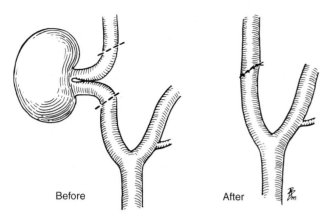

FIGURE 44-2 ■ Method of end-to-end repair of a redundant internal carotid artery after aneurysm resection. (From Trippel OH, et al: Extracranial carotid aneurysms. In Bergen JJ, Yao JST, editors: Aneurysms, New York, 1982, Grune and Stratton, pp 493–503.)

The need for an indwelling carotid artery shunt is no better understood for aneurysm patients than for patients undergoing carotid endarterectomy. If shunting is desired, it can be accomplished in most patients. In patients undergoing resection with primary anastomosis, a shunt can be inserted into the open ends of the arteries to be anastomosed after opening of the aneurysm. If a graft is to be used, the shunt is placed through the graft before performing any anastomosis and is inserted into the arterial ends after opening of the aneurysm.

Aneurysms that involve the distal cervical internal carotid artery are often inaccessible using standard techniques. In some patients, mandibular subluxation or transection allows for the application of the previously mentioned methods of repair.[30] Alternative approaches are often required for high internal carotid lesions, however. In some patients, high-fusiform aneurysms can be treated with aneurysmorrhaphy using an indwelling shunt for flow continuity and as a method of distal arterial control. In some cases, distal lesions must be treated by ligation. Unfortunately, acute occlusion of the internal carotid artery in these patients is associated with high neurologic morbidity. Stroke rates from 30% to 60% have been reported after this procedure, with half of those patients dying as a result of the stroke.[10] This degree of morbidity and mortality clearly approaches that associated with the natural history of the disease.

One way to select patients who may safely undergo carotid ligation is to measure intraoperative carotid stump pressure. The carotid stump pressure can also be measured by temporary balloon occlusion at the time of arteriography using an end-hole balloon catheter.[31] Stump pressures greater than 70 mm Hg appear to be safe for patients undergoing carotid ligation. Because many strokes that occur after carotid ligation manifest hours to days after the procedure, these patients should be maintained on heparin anticoagulation for 7 to 10 days postoperatively.

When stump pressure measurements indicate that carotid ligation is not safe, the performance of an extracranial-to-intracranial bypass using ipsilateral superficial temporal artery has been suggested.[30] Because this procedure is generally necessary only for high internal

carotid lesions, the ipsilateral external carotid artery is usually preserved, thus allowing for adequate inflow into the superficial temporal artery.

More recently, endovascular treatment modalities have become commonplace in some centers.[32-34] Zhou looked at the Baylor experience from 1985 to 1994 and compared it to their experience from 1995 to 2004. All procedures were surgical during the early period, whereas during the later period 70% of procedures were endovascular, consisting of stent-grafts, stents combined with coil embolization, and endovascular occlusion.[34] In some cases, coil embolization of the external carotid artery may be necessary to allow coverage of the entire aneurysm and to prevent endoleak.[35] Endovascular interventions reduce the risk of cranial nerve injury, can be done without general anesthesia, are useful for distal lesions where surgical exposure is difficult, are associated with shorter hospital stays, and have lower morbidity and mortality rates.[34]

Subclavian and Axillary Artery Aneurysms

The surgical approach to subclavian and axillary aneurysms depends on the cause, size, and location of the aneurysm and the status of the distal circulation. Except in cases of small, asymptomatic subclavian artery aneurysms secondary to thoracic outlet (for which thoracic outlet decompression alone may be adequate), the aneurysm should be excluded and arterial continuity should be restored if possible. Proximal and distal ligation of these aneurysms has been reported. Although tissue loss does not usually occur after this procedure, claudication is not uncommon.[21]

When a symptomatic or large asymptomatic subclavian aneurysm is present as a result of thoracic outlet syndrome, repair of the aneurysm should be accompanied by thoracic outlet decompression. Although this combined technique has been reported through an axillary approach, the supraclavicular approach is generally preferred; this allows for safe control of the artery, although the thoracic outlet decompression is more involved. Hobson and colleagues[13] recommended performing the aneurysm repair through the supraclavicular approach combined with a transaxillary approach to the first rib.

Atherosclerotic and traumatic distal subclavian artery aneurysms or pseudoaneurysms can be managed with a supraclavicular approach. When the aneurysm is proximal enough so that proximal control cannot be safely obtained through this approach, a median sternotomy (right side) or a left-sided thoracotomy (left side) is needed, usually in combination with the supraclavicular approach. Midsubclavian lesions can often be managed through a supraclavicular approach with medial clavicular resection or through a trapdoor ministernotomy.

Primary anastomosis is usually not possible, and graft replacement is required. This is most commonly performed as an interposition graft using either saphenous vein or prosthetics. Prosthetics are more commonly used because of the size of the subclavian artery. The vertebral artery should be preserved when possible. In patients with a dominant contralateral vertebral artery, this may not be necessary. High-risk patients with proximal aneurysms who are considered too frail to undergo a major procedure can be treated with distal ligation and axillo-axillary bypass.

More recently, stent-grafting has been applied to carefully selected patients with subclavian aneurysms, but long-term results are not yet known.[36-38] Stent-grafting of the subclavian artery can avoid major surgical procedures. Stent-grafts have been used in the treatment of true and false subclavian artery aneurysms and traumatic subclavian arteriovenous fistulae. Limitations of stent-grafting include short fixation zones and the risk of covering important vessel origins such as the right carotid, the vertebral artery, and the internal mammary artery. Concern has also been raised regarding stent compression in the area of the thoracic outlet.[36-38]

Management of axillary artery aneurysms can often be accomplished through the axillary approach. In many patients, proximal control must be obtained through an infraclavicular approach. With more proximal lesions or lesions involving both the subclavian and the axillary arteries, a combined supraclavicular and infraclavicular approach must be used. Aneurysms involving the axillary artery are often intimately involved with the cords of the brachial plexus, and resection may be hazardous. When symptoms of brachial plexus compression are present, resection and interposition grafting may be indicated. For smaller lesions, however, proximal and distal ligation combined with bypass can be performed, thus avoiding dissection around the brachial plexus. Stent-grafting of the axillary artery has been performed most commonly for traumatic hemorrhage and pseudoaneurysms and has been presented in the form of case reports. No significant series of axillary artery stent-grafting was found in review of the literature.

When subclavian and axillary aneurysms are complicated by embolization and ischemia, revascularization of the arm may be required in combination with aneurysm repair. This is usually accomplished by autogenous vein bypass proximal to the aneurysm to the most appropriate distal artery. In this situation, the aneurysm can be either ligated, if appropriate, or resected. Alternatively, stent-grafting of the aneurysm followed by local bypass of the occluded segments may be possible in some patients.

Forearm and Hand Aneurysms

Aneurysms of the forearm arteries can be treated by ligation if the remaining vessels provide adequate collateral circulation to the hand. More often, however, vein interposition grafting is performed because it is simple to accomplish. Aneurysms of vessels in the hand tend to be less well collateralized, and vein graft repair is usually necessary.[2] Stent-grafting of these small arteries has not been reported.

Femoral and Popliteal Artery Aneurysms

The treatment of true femoral artery aneurysms is usually resection and graft interposition. Because of the size of the common femoral artery, a prosthetic graft is preferred. When the deep femoral artery is involved, the graft may be sewn end to end to the superficial femoral artery, and the origin of the deep femoral artery implanted

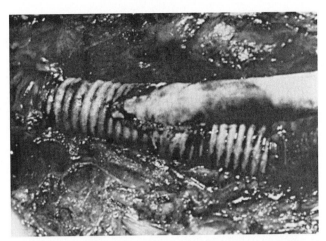

FIGURE 44-3 ■ Concomitant repair of femoral aneurysm followed by prosthetic femoropopliteal bypass.

into the side of the graft. When femoral aneurysms are being treated concomitantly with an inflow or outflow procedure, it is still best, in most cases, to replace the common femoral artery with an interposition graft. Inflow or outflow grafts are then anastomosed to the interposition graft in an end-to-side fashion (Figure 44-3). Femoral artery pseudoaneurysms following femoral artery puncture for catheterization procedures can be treated with ultrasonically guided compression, ultrasonically guided thrombin injection, or open surgical repair. Stent-grafting for common femoral aneurysms is not thought to be advisable. Stents and stent-grafts in the common femoral artery are subjected to significant flexion forces as a result of hip flexion, and there is concern regarding stent fracture and compression. In addition, stents and stent-grafts in this area may complicate future arterial access.

Repair of deep femoral artery aneurysms is dictated by the patency of the superficial femoral artery and by how distally the aneurysm is located in the artery. Approximately 50% of deep femoral aneurysms can be ligated safely, and 50% require the reestablishment of arterial continuity.[1] Treatment has traditionally been interposition or bypass grafting with aneurysm exclusion. Stent-grafting may be possible in some patients depending on individual anatomy.

Treatment of isolated superficial femoral artery aneurysms can be performed by either open surgical repair or endovascular techniques. Open repair is done in the form of aneurysm resection and interposition grafting or by bypass with aneurysm ligation. Proximal isolated superficial artery aneurysms are more surgically accessible, whereas more distal isolated superficial femoral artery aneurysms require more extensive surgical dissection as a result of the artery passing deep to the adductor muscles. Stent-grafting can be applied anywhere along the superficial femoral artery as long as there are adequate fixation points. As with popliteal artery aneurysms, superficial femoral artery aneurysms treated with stent-grafting may be subject to enlargement secondary to endoleaks after the repair.

Likewise, repair of popliteal artery aneurysms can also be accomplished by open surgical repair or stent-grafting

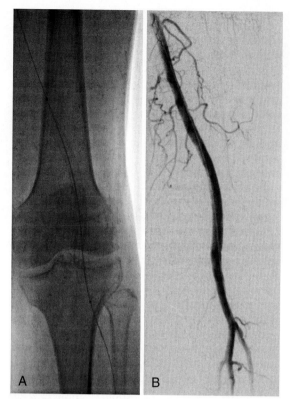

FIGURE 44-4 ■ A, First (proximal) Viabahn stent-graft in place in a patient requiring two stent-grafts for repair of a large popliteal artery aneurysm. **B,** Completed stent-graft repair after placement of second stent-graft.

(Figure 44-4). There has been more experience with stent-grafting of popliteal artery aneurysms than with any other peripheral aneurysm.

Open repair of popliteal artery aneurysms includes aneurysm ligation with above-knee to below-knee bypass through a medial approach, aneurysm resection with interposition grafting usually through a posterior approach, and aneurysmorrhaphy. In some patients, the popliteal aneurysm may extend proximally into the superficial femoral artery. In these patients, the aneurysm is ligated and the proximal anastomosis is made to the common femoral artery or, more commonly, to the mid-superficial femoral artery proximal to the adductor canal. The superficial femoral artery cannot be exposed through a posterior popliteal space approach.

When popliteal aneurysm are large enough to cause symptomatic compression of the surrounding nerve and vein, consideration should be given to resection of the aneurysm with interposition grafting. The risk of damage to these structures is greater, but if resection is not done, many patients remain symptomatic postoperatively. This procedure is best performed through a posterior approach, as long as the aneurysm does not extend into the superficial femoral artery proximally or to the anterior tibial artery takeoff distally and both anastomoses can be safely performed within the limitations of the operative field. Aneurysm resection with interposition grafting has the added benefit of precluding the development of endoleaks that can occur when either aneurysm ligation with bypass or stent-grafting is used. As a general rule, results are better when autogenous vein is used for surgical repair, although polytetrafluoroethylene (PTFE) grafts have shown good results when used as popliteal artery interposition grafts in the presence of good runoff.[39] When extensive chronic embolization leading to obliteration of the outflow tract of the popliteal artery has occurred, bypass to the tibial or peroneal arteries is required. Such bypasses should be performed using autogenous vein.

When patients develop thromboembolic complications of popliteal artery aneurysms, the degree of arterial occlusion is often so great that no outflow vessel is patent. Many of these patients, especially those appearing late, also have thrombosis of the microcirculation. In such patients, bypass is often not possible or is subject to a high failure rate owing to poor runoff. The use of pre-repair thrombolytic therapy provides patent runoff in most of these patients, thereby allowing for successful bypass or stent-grafting.[40] In patients at especially high surgical risk, thrombolytic therapy alone has been used with success.[41,42]

Numerous reports have been published on the use of stent-grafts for the treatment of popliteal artery aneurysms.[43-49] Stent-grafts have also been used successfully in the treatment of ruptured popliteal aneurysms.[50] As more experience has been gained with stent-grafting in the treatment of popliteal artery aneurysms proper indications are being elucidated. Relative contraindications to stent-grafting of popliteal artery aneurysms include extension of aneurysmal disease to the superficial femoral artery or to involve the anterior tibial origin, tortuosity, and large aneurysms with compression symptoms.[51]

Results of Therapy

Because most patients with peripheral aneurysms do not have occlusive disease, the results of reconstructive vascular procedures are usually excellent. In some cases, however, embolization from the aneurysm can lead to obliteration of some or all of the outflow tract, leading to poor results.

Extracranial Carotid Artery Aneurysms

The small number of patients included in reports assessing the results of surgical therapy for carotid aneurysms somewhat hampers the accurate calculation of morbidity and mortality statistics. Most reports, however, indicate that these procedures can be performed with safety. In a study from Michigan that included only atherosclerotic aneurysms, 1 of 19 aneurysm operations resulted in a stroke, which was thought to be due to intraoperative embolization.[9] No operative death occurred. Excision of large and distal aneurysms was associated with an increased incidence of cranial nerve injury. El-Sabrout and Cooley found a similar incidence of 30-day stroke at the Texas Heart Institute for atherosclerotic aneurysms, but the incidence of 30-day stroke was higher (11%) for pseudoaneurysms.[12] Overall in the Texas Heart Institute experience, the 30-day stroke–death rate was 9%. Long-term results of treatment showed that at a mean follow-up of 5.9 years (1.5 months to 30 years), 30% of patients died, but none were procedure related deaths and no late strokes were reported. Lauder and colleagues[52] followed 50 patients who had carotid bypass grafting with saphenous vein, although patients with carotid aneurysms were not included. Cumulative freedom from recurrent stenosis greater than 70% was 86% at 1 year and 83% at 3 years.[52] Most investigators agree that the results of surgery are vastly superior to the natural history of the disease.[9,10,12,26-28]

Long-term results for carotid aneurysm repair using stent-grafts has not been well established. However, Zhou and colleagues[34] showed a decrease in the 30-day stroke–death rate from 14% (1985 to 1994, all treated surgically) to 5% (1995 to 2004, 70% treated with endovascular techniques).[34]

Subclavian and Axillary Artery Aneurysms

The results of surgery for subclavian and axillary aneurysms are similar to those for upper extremity reconstruction for occlusive disease.[21,53] Pairolero and colleagues showed that 18 of 18 patients undergoing aneurysm resection with restoration of arterial continuity retained patent reconstructions during an average of 9.2 years of follow-up,[21] most likely due to the lack of distal occlusive disease. Patients with obliteration of the radial and ulnar arteries, however, have a high failure rate following arm revascularization.[53] This latter point further emphasizes the need for early surgical intervention in these patients. Primary and secondary patency rates as high as 89% and 100% have been reported at 29 months for stent-graft repair of subclavian artery aneurysms.[37]

Forearm and Hand Aneurysms

Both ligation in the presence of adequate collateral circulation and vein graft repair are successful in the treatment of forearm and hand aneurysms. Clark and associates[2] reported 100% patency at 7 years for vein graft repairs in the forearm and hand.

Femoral and Popliteal Artery Aneurysms

When femoral and popliteal aneurysms are treated before complications arise, the results are excellent. The 18 asymptomatic patients with femoral aneurysms in the series by Cutler and Darling[23] all had excellent early and late results (no graft occlusions). However, of the 45 symptomatic patients with femoral aneurysms, 4 had amputations, and 17 remained symptomatic despite therapy.

Therapy for femoral artery pseudoaneurysms has evolved in recent years to include ultrasonically guided compression and thrombin injection. Taylor compared these two approaches and found that compression was successful in 63% of patients, whereas thrombin injection was successful in 93% of patients.[54] Not only was thrombin injection more often successful, but it was associated with less pain and the need for sedation. Neither treatment was associated with complications in Taylor's series[54]; however, iatrogenic arterial thrombosis has been seen with thrombin injection. Taylor attributed the lack of iatrogenic thrombosis in his series to the use of more dilute thrombin (100 U/mL) and slow injection with immediate cessation of the injection once thrombus was first seen. Taylor advised observation for pseudoaneurysms less than 2 cm as spontaneous thrombosis often occurs. Kresowik and colleagues[55] found the incidence of femoral pseudoaneurysm after femoral artery puncture for coronary angioplasty to be 6%. The pseudoaneurysms ranged in size from 1.3 to 3.5 cm and 88% of these thrombosed spontaneously within 4 weeks without the need for further treatment.[55] Femoral pseudoaneurysms larger than 2 cm and those that fail compression and thrombin injection should be surgically corrected.

Harbuzariu and colleagues[56] followed 17 patients with profunda femoris aneurysms, 11 of which were asymptomatic. Fifteen of the profunda femoris aneurysms were treated with bypass grafting. There was no 30-day death, graft thrombosis, or limb loss. Long-term graft patency was 100%.[56]

In a study of 48 popliteal aneurysms, the 5-year patency rate for reconstructions for asymptomatic lesions was 91%, compared with 54% for symptomatic lesions.[57] These differing results were directly related to the status of the tibial runoff vessels. In a series of 51 popliteal aneurysms reported by Shortell and colleagues,[58] results were dependent on the clinical presentation and the status of the runoff vessels. Patients with limb-threatening ischemia had a graft patency rate of 69% at 1 year, whereas all electively performed grafts were patent at 1 year. After 3 years, runoff dictated patency; grafts with good runoff had a patency rate of 89%, whereas poor runoff was associated with a 3-year patency rate of only 30%. Numerous, more recent reports of large series of popliteal aneurysms have confirmed these earlier results.[40,59-62] Huang and colleagues[63] reported on 358 popliteal aneurysms treated with open surgical approaches. Forty percent were asymptomatic, 39% had chronic ischemia, and 21% had acute ischemia. The 30-day thrombosis rate was 1% in asymptomatic limbs, 4% in limbs with chronic ischemia, and 9% in limbs with acute ischemia. There were three deaths and six early amputations, all in the acute ischemia group. Mean follow-up was 5.2 years. Five-year primary and secondary patency rates were 76% and 87%, respectively, with saphenous vein patency being significantly higher than PTFE patency (94% vs. 85%). Five-year limb salvage rate was 97%, but only 85% in the acute ischemia group. Within that group, limbs treated with preoperative thrombolysis had better limb salvage (96%) than those limbs treated with surgery alone (69%). Two percent of limbs required reintervention for enlargement, and all these limbs had been treated with ligation and bypass.[63] The largest domestic series of popliteal aneurysms comes from Veterans Administration-National Surgery Quality Improvement Program (VA-NSQIP) data from Veteran's Administration hospitals. Johnson and colleagues analyzed the database and found 583 operations. Of the patients included, 88% had multiple comorbidities and were American Society Anesthesiologists (ASA) class 3 or 4. Unfortunately the database did not include elements that would allow analysis of aneurysm size, surgical approach, graft material, runoff status, use of thrombolysis, need for tibial artery bypass or endovascular repair. Survival was 97.6% at 1 year and 96.2%

at 2 years. Limb salvage was 99% at 30 days, 97.6% at 1 year, and 96.2% at 2 years. Mortality at 30 days was 1.4%. The main conclusion of the study was that, despite high surgical risk, popliteal aneurysms can be treated with a high rate of success with low mortality and high limb salvage rates.[64]

Because of the vastly inferior results of therapy, once thromboembolic complications have occurred, attention has focused on the reestablishment of runoff preoperatively through the use of thrombolytic therapy.[40] Most reports indicate good success in improving runoff and suggest improved limb salvage when preoperative thrombolytic therapy is used. Varga and coworkers[40] performed a retrospective, multicenter study of 200 popliteal aneurysms and concluded that intraarterial thrombolytic therapy clearly improves preoperative runoff in patients with limb-threatening ischemia.[40] Hoelting and associates[41] described 24 patients with acute ischemia secondary to popliteal artery aneurysm thrombosis. Nine patients were treated with preoperative thrombolysis and underwent successful bypass. Six of these patients achieved complete lysis. For three patients, lysis was incomplete but established sufficient runoff so that successful bypass could be performed. These authors also reviewed the literature and demonstrated an amputation rate of approximately 27% in 455 patients treated with bypass alone, compared with approximately 20% in 14 patients in whom only thrombolytic therapy was used.[41] However, in 30 patients in whom thrombolytic therapy was combined with bypass, no limb was lost. Varga and colleagues[40] suggested that thrombolysis is of value in restoring distal runoff before bypass in the presence of limb-threatening ischemia but not in elective situations. Carpenter reported on seven limbs with popliteal aneurysm thrombosis and complete thrombosis of all runoff vessels.[25] These patients were treated with preoperative thrombolysis, with 100% limb salvage and superior graft patency compared to similar patients not treated with preoperative thrombolysis.

Early treatment of popliteal artery aneurysms with stent-grafts was successful technically, but patency was considerably less than that achieved with bypass and exclusion. Tielliu and coauthors[65] in 2003 reported a 15-month patency rate of 74% for 23 popliteal aneurysms treated with stent-grafting.[65] In 2005, the series was updated with 57 popliteal aneurysms treated (5 emergently) with stent-grafting. At a mean follow-up of 2 years, 21% had occluded. Primary and secondary patency rates were 80% and 90% at 1 year and 77% and 87% at 2 years. Use of postoperative clopidogrel was predictive of success.[66] In 2008, Longrove and colleagues[67] reported a metaanalysis of the literature comparing 37 endovascular with 104 open repairs. Thirty-day graft thrombosis and reintervention were more likely to follow endovascular repair (5% vs. 19%). Hospital length of stay was shorter in the endovascular group. There was no significant difference in long-term primary patency. The authors opined that the only advantage to endovascular repair was a shorter hospital stay. In 2005, Antonello and colleagues[68] reported on the only prospective randomized comparison of open repair versus endovascular repair.[68] This series after 53 popliteal aneurysm repairs showed

early failure. There was no early failure in the open group, whereas the early thrombosis rate in the endovascular group was 9.6%; however, no statistical differences were noted in primary and secondary patency rates at 6 years. Based on their experience, the authors recommended that endograft oversizing of greater than 10% to 15% be avoided, that enough distal popliteal artery be left uncovered by the stent-graft to allow future bypass to the distal popliteal artery if necessary, that overlapping stent-grafts avoid critical flexion points, and that postoperative antiplatelet therapy be used. Contraindications were a distal popliteal artery less than 4 mm, a hypercoagulable state, less than one tibial artery runoff, and a distal neck less than 1 cm. In 2010, Cina[47] reviewed the literature on both open and endovascular repair. Cina found 43 endovascular repairs and 116 open repairs that could be compared. There was no difference in primary patency at 1, 2, and 3 years. For open repair, pooled estimates of 5-year patency was 72%, mortality was 0% to 2%, and the amputation rate was 3.2%. Of 320 endovascular repairs, 30-day patency was 94%, and at 1-year primary and secondary patency rates were 83% and 86%, respectively. Three-year primary and secondary patency was 74% and 85%. The authors concluded that, in the presence of suitable anatomy and good tibial runoff, endovascular repair was not different from open repair. Results from endovascular repair now seem to have exhausted the learning curve. In 2010, Midy and colleagues[46] reported experience with 57 endovascular repairs from three French hospitals.[46] The primary and secondary patency rates were 85.8% and 87.5% at 1 year and 82.3% and 87.5% at 3 years. Limb salvage was 96.5%. Tielliu and colleagues[69] followed 78 Hemobahn and Viabahn stent-grafts for a mean of 50 months and noted a 16.7% incidence of circumferential stent fractures; however, stent fracture could not be shown to adversely affect graft patency.[69]

Since Edwards[70] first described the technique of bypass with aneurysm ligation through a medial approach, it has become the preferred open method of repair. In the vast majority of surgical series described earlier, the Edwards technique was used. However, as experience accumulated with the technique, it became evident that late aneurysm expansion and even rupture could occur. In 2003, Ebaugh and colleagues[71] reported the Northwestern experience with 57 popliteal aneurysms treated with exclusion and bypass grafting. At a mean follow-up of 4.3 years, 32% of aneurysms treated in this manner expanded. The authors hypothesized that type II endoleaks were the cause, but neither graft patency nor contrast filling of the aneurysms on contrast CT scans could be found to correlate with aneurysm expansion. Bellosta and colleagues[72] also assessed late aneurysm expansion after the ligation–bypass technique and found an 8% incidence of postoperative aneurysm expansion in 53 aneurysms followed for a mean of 35 months.

Beseth and Moore reported on 30 popliteal aneurysms in the study at the University of California–Los Angeles that were treated through a posterior approach using a short prosthetic interposition graft.[39] Mean follow-up was 21.5 months. Primary patency, primary assisted patency, and secondary patency were 92.2%, 95.8%, and

95.8% at 1 and 2 years. Limb salvage was 100%. Aneurysms that extended proximal to the adductor canal were excluded from the posterior approach, and all aneurysms had one or more patent tibial artery runoff vessels. The authors noted that their results were comparable to the exclusion–bypass technique, but had the added advantage of allowing aneurysm resection or aneurysmorrhaphy with oversewing of popliteal branches with the elimination of risk for postoperative aneurysm expansion. Kropman and colleagues analyzed 110 popliteal aneurysms treated with either a medial (ligation, bypass) or an endovascular approach.[73] No difference in patency or limb salvage was demonstrated at a mean follow-up of 47 months. Regardless of the surgical approach, the use of vein for reconstruction resulted in significantly better patency (84% vs. 67%). Two patients having the medial approach required reintervention for aneurysm expansion, whereas no patient in the posterior approach required reintervention. Ravn and colleagues[74] analyzed the Swedish Vascular Registry, which resulted in 717 popliteal aneurysms to study. Mean follow-up was 7.2 years. The medial approach was used in 87%, the posterior approach in 8.4%, and an endovascular approach in 3.6%. There was no difference in patency between vein and prosthetic when the posterior approach was used, but there was better patency with vein using the medial approach (90% vs. 72%). Emergency procedures and the use of prosthetic graft were associated with higher amputation rates. Postoperative aneurysm expansion was demonstrated in 33% when the medial approach was used, but in only 8.3% when the posterior approach was used. Zaraca and colleagues[75] found that the posterior approach was possible in 78% of aneurysms using proximal extension beyond the adductor canal as the primary contraindication to posterior repair.

With the appreciation of the significant postoperative aneurysm expansion rate following endografting and the medial approach to ligation and bypass of popliteal aneurysms, the posterior approach is gaining popularity. The technique has excellent patency and limb salvage rates, even with the use of prosthetic graft. It offers the added advantage of decreasing or eliminating the problem with postoperative aneurysm expansion. The few contraindications include aneurysm extension proximal to the adductor canal, less than one vessel runoff, and when distal tibial bypass is required. This author prefers the posterior approach in properly selected patients. Patients with proximal aneurysm extension and the need for distal bypass are best treated with vein bypass. High-risk patients with suitable anatomy can undergo endovascular repair, although the VA-NSQIP data indicate that even high-risk patients can be treated safely with open repair.[64] Fortunately, the results of all three approaches are good and all approaches are acceptable methods of repair in properly selected patients. Patient demand, however, is driving an increasing trend toward endovascular repair.

MYCOTIC ANEURYSMS

Mycotic aneurysms are considered separately because they generally have a different cause, affect arteries in a different distribution, require different treatment, and have poorer outcomes than bland aneurysms. Despite the term, mycotic aneurysms are considered to be any true or false aneurysm that is infected.

Cause

Numerous classifications for mycotic aneurysms have been proposed and are nicely described by Moore and Malone[76] and Wilson and colleagues.[77] Patel and Johnston[78] indicated that the source of infection must be either endogenous or exogenous. Endogenous sources include embolism, septicemia, or direct extension; exogenous sources include trauma and iatrogenic injury. They further suggested that classifications be based on the preexisting status of the artery: normal, atherosclerotic, aneurysmal, or prosthetic. Any classification must consider these factors.[78]

Normal axial arteries are seldom infected primarily, but clumps of bacteria or fungi may lodge in smaller vessels and cause transmural necrosis and aneurysm formation. Normal larger arteries can be infected, however, by organisms lodging in the vasa vasorum. Arteries that are diseased with atherosclerosis or aneurysms, as well as prosthetic grafts, are subject to local invasion by circulating organisms. The process is similar to that described earlier, in that infection leads to arterial wall weakening and subsequent aneurysm formation. Infection may spread to arterial walls from outside the vessel through direct contact with abscesses, wound infections, salivary glands, and the like. Exogenous sources of arterial infections include diagnostic and therapeutic catheterizations, penetrating trauma, and drug abuse. Graft infections may also lead to infected pseudoaneurysm formation, usually as a result of disruption of an anastomosis.

Mycotic aneurysms have been reported in essentially all arteries, and their location is determined primarily by their cause. Those secondary to bacterial endocarditis favor the superior mesenteric artery, followed by the aorta and femoral arteries. Mycotic aneurysms that occur after trauma mostly commonly involve the extremities, whereas those caused by infection of preexisting atherosclerotic aneurysms commonly affect the aorta and the femoral and popliteal arteries. Those secondary to atherosclerosis alone involve the aorta and superficial femoral arteries as well as other common atherosclerotic sites. Those secondary to catheters and drug abuse involve the brachial, radial, and, most commonly, femoral arteries. For unknown reasons, *Salmonella* species favor the infrarenal aorta.

The organisms most commonly involved in mycotic aneurysms differ, depending on the source of the organism. When bacterial endocarditis is the source, *Streptococcus* and *Staphylococcus* species prevail. *Salmonella* species, *Staphylococcus* species, and *Escherichia coli* are the most common organisms causing mycotic aneurysms secondary to bacteremia. Mycotic aneurysms secondary to direct extension of infections are predominantly caused by *Salmonella*, *Staphylococcus*, and *Mycobacterium* species and fungi.[76] *Staphylococcus aureus* and *E. coli* are the most common organisms seen in mycotic aneurysms secondary to trauma (all types).[79]

In the era preceding antibiotic drugs, most mycotic aneurysms were secondary to bacterial endocarditis and syphilis. Today, most mycotic aneurysms are probably secondary to trauma (including drug abuse, surgery, and arterial catheterization). This change is most likely due to the use of antibiotic therapy for endocarditis, the significant decrease in the prevalence of syphilis, the increasing use of diagnostic catheterization, the increase in violent trauma, and widespread drug abuse. These forces have made common femoral artery mycotic aneurysms the most common type currently encountered.

Natural History

Once established, the natural course of a mycotic aneurysm is to enlarge and eventually rupture in most known cases. Occasionally, spontaneous thrombosis may occur, with resolution of the septic process; however, the thrombosed aneurysm may serve as a continuing septic focus. Septic emboli arising from aneurysms are not uncommon and can lead to miliary abscesses and septic arthritis.

Diagnosis

Patients with mycotic aneurysms may show catastrophic illness or insidious disease. Most patients have some combination of fever, malaise, weight loss, chills, night sweats, pain, leukocytosis, positive downstream blood cultures, and elevated sedimentation rate. A history of trauma or a recent infectious disease usually exists. When the aneurysm is superficial, as most peripheral aneurysms are, it can be palpated in 90% of patients.[80] The aneurysm may appear bland, but more commonly shows signs of erythema, warmth, and tenderness. Particularly large aneurysms may also show skin necrosis and risk of imminent rupture (Figure 44-5). Petechial lesions in the skin may be seen distal to the aneurysm when embolization has occurred. Many patients show rupture on presentation.

The diagnosis of mycotic aneurysm is often deduced by combining the history and physical examination findings with test findings. In some patients, the history and physical examination may be sufficient (see Figure 44-5; this patient had a retained polyester chimney left attached to her right femoral artery after removal of an intra-aortic

balloon catheter). In other patients, the diagnosis is made by the finding of sepsis and an aneurysm in a patient in whom no other septic focus can be found.

Ultrasound and CT scans can be used to visualize mycotic aneurysms. CT scans have the advantage of being able to clearly demonstrate surrounding fluid or gas, a finding consistent with infection. Gallium scans and radioactively tagged white cell scans are usually positive with mycotic aneurysms. Arteriography is usually required for preoperative planning, except in emergency situations, and usually demonstrates a saccular aneurysm or pseudoaneurysm (Figure 44-6).

Treatment

The indication for treatment of a mycotic aneurysm is its presence. Antibiotic therapy, guided by culture results when available, should be used in all patients. Antibiotics alone are not sufficient, and surgical removal of the mycotic aneurysm is required in nearly all cases. Basic surgical principles dictate that all infected tissue must be removed and that adequate circulation must remain or be provided, when possible.

Extracranial Carotid Artery Mycotic Aneurysms

As noted earlier, cervical carotid aneurysms are rare, and cervical carotid mycotic aneurysms are extremely rare. In 1988, Jones and Frusha[81] reviewed the English-language literature and found only 23 bacteriologically proven cases. In 1991, Jebara and colleagues[82] noted an additional four cases.

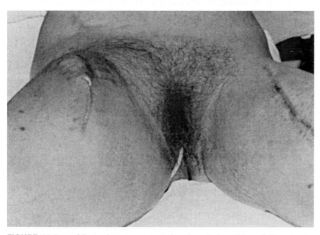

FIGURE 44-5 ■ Mycotic aneurysm in the right side of the groin with overlying skin necrosis and imminent rupture.

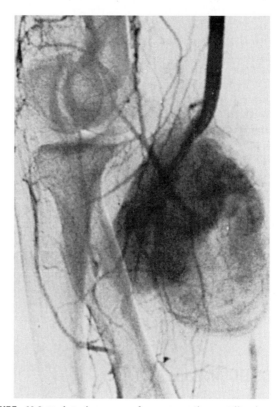

FIGURE 44-6 ■ Arteriogram of a mycotic popliteal artery aneurysm.

Treatment of these lesions requires complete excision of the artery under antibiotic coverage and debridement of all infected tissue. Vascular reconstruction should be avoided, if possible, because reconstruction in an infected field yields less than optimal results.[83] Patients should be selected for arterial ligation based on carotid stump pressure as described earlier. Heparin should be continued for 7 to 10 days postoperatively when ligation is used. If ligation is not safe, reconstruction using autogenous vein is the treatment of choice. In the review by Jones and Frusha,[81] the overall mortality rate was 23%. The mortality rate was 27% in the ligation group, compared with 11% in the grafted group. Extracranial-intracranial bypass has not been reported in these patients.

Subclavian and Axillary Artery Mycotic Aneurysms

Mycotic aneurysms in this area are also rare and are usually the result of trauma or drug abuse. The approach to the subclavian artery depends on the size and on the distal and proximal extent of the aneurysm, as described for bland aneurysms in this location. Complete excision of the aneurysm may be too risky in view of the proximity of the brachial plexus and subclavian vein. Successful treatment with arterial ligation and incision and drainage of the aneurysm has been reported.[84] Proximal subclavian artery ligation usually does not lead to the need for revascularization.

Axillary mycotic aneurysms are usually palpable. The management principles for subclavian mycotic aneurysms generally apply to axillary lesions as well. Axillary artery ligation may be associated with a greater risk of ischemia, however, and extraanatomic bypass may be required in some patients. This can usually be performed in clean tissue planes about the shoulder using autogenous vein.

Forearm and Hand Mycotic Aneurysms

Treatment of mycotic aneurysms in these areas follows the general guidelines for other mycotic aneurysms. Arterial ligation with aneurysm excision is generally all that is required. In the rare situation in which distal ischemia might occur, autogenous revascularization in clean planes is required.

Femoral and Popliteal Artery Mycotic Aneurysms

The treatment of infected groin aneurysms has evolved through several stages. Although most of these lesions are secondary to trauma or drug abuse, the same management principles apply to mycotic groin aneurysms from other causes. Several options are available, including remote bypass followed by aneurysm resection; aneurysm resection followed by remote bypass, if needed; aneurysm resection alone; or aneurysm resection with in situ reconstruction.

Initial obturator bypass followed by aneurysm resection usually requires the use of prosthetic material, because most of these patients are drug addicts whose saphenous veins have been destroyed. Reddy and colleagues showed that this approach was associated with a 100% graft infection rate in drug addicts.[79] In other patients in whom vein is available, this approach is preferred. Buerger and Feldman reported that revascularization is not effective in reducing the amputation rate after aneurysm resection in drug addicts (17% in their series) and may occasionally be a fatal approach.[85] In their series, the same amputation rate was achieved without any deaths when aneurysm excision and ligation alone were used.

Reddy and colleagues[79] obtained a similar amputation rate (19%) with excision and ligation. They reported that excision and ligation of only one of the three femoral arteries in the groin can be performed without limb loss, but that when the common femoral artery is involved, thus necessitating the ligation of all three vessels, the amputation rate is very high. As an alternative in these latter patients, they suggested that immediate autogenous vein reconstruction with sartorius muscle flap coverage be used when adequate debridement can be performed to control sepsis. Using this approach, they reported a 9% amputation rate without mortality. Reddy and colleagues found that even in drug addicts, satisfactory saphenous vein usually exists in the thigh for femoral artery reconstruction. Benjamin and coworkers[86] reported successful treatment of mycotic aneurysms using deep leg veins when larger-sized conduits were required. Ligation and excision with postoperative observation to assess the need for subsequent revascularization did not yield satisfactory results in the Reddy series.[79]

Mycotic aneurysms involving the popliteal artery are uncommon, and few guidelines are provided in the vascular surgical literature. In general, aneurysm excision with in situ autogenous interposition grafting works well. Most of these patients have normal tibial artery runoff, facilitating long-term patency, and the readily available soft tissue coverage afforded by the muscles in the popliteal space facilitates healing of the surgical wound without complications.

BIBLIOGRAPHY

Antonello M, Frigatti P, Battocchio P, et al: Open repair versus endovascular treatment for asymptomatic popliteal artery aneurysm: results of a prospective randomized study. J Vasc Surg 42:185, 2005.

Beseth BD, Moore WS: The posterior approach for repair of popliteal artery aneurysms. J Vasc Surg 43:940, 2006.

Dent TL, Lindenauer SM, Ernst CE, et al: Multiple arteriosclerotic arterial aneurysms. Arch Surg 105:338, 1972.

Hobson RW, II, Isreal MR, Lynch TO: Axillo-subclavian arterial aneurysms. In Bergan JJ, Yao JST, editors: Aneurysms, New York, Grune & Stratton, 1982, pp 435–447.

Huang Y, Gloviczki P, Noel AA, et al: Early complications and long term outcome after open surgical treatment of popliteal artery aneurysms: J Vasc Surg 45:706, 2007.

Lilly MP, Flinn WR, McCarthy WJ, et al: The effect of distal arterial anatomy on the success of popliteal aneurysm repair. J Vasc Surg 7:653, 1988.

Pairolero PC, Walls JT, Payne WS, et al: Subclavian-axillary artery aneurysms. Surgery 90:757, 1981.

Reddy DJ, Smith RF, Elliot JP, et al: Infected femoral artery false aneurysms in drug addicts: evolution of selective vascular reconstruction. J Vasc Surg 3:718, 1986.

Rhodes EL, Stanley JC, Hoffman CL, et al: Aneurysms of extracranial carotid arteries. Arch Surg 111:339, 1976.

Szilagyi DE, Schwartz RL, Reddy DJ: Popliteal arterial aneurysms: their natural history and management. Arch Surg 116:724, 1981.

References available online at expertconsult.com.

QUESTIONS

1. Subclavian artery aneurysms are most commonly caused by which of the following?
   a. Atherosclerosis
   b. Thoracic outlet syndrome
   c. Fibromuscular dysplasia
   d. Trauma

2. What is the most common complication of subclavian artery aneurysms?
   a. Rupture
   b. Pain secondary to nerve compression
   c. Embolization
   d. Thrombosis

3. Most carotid artery aneurysms are identified because of which of the following?
   a. Rupture of the aneurysm
   b. Mass in the neck
   c. Neurologic complications
   d. Swishing sound heard in the patient's ipsilateral ear

4. Which of the following statements is true regarding femoral and popliteal artery aneurysms?
   a. These aneurysms should be repaired only when they become very large and cause pain from adjacent nerve compression.
   b. These aneurysms are rarely associated with other peripheral aneurysms.
   c. These aneurysms are particularly dangerous because of a high incidence of distal embolization or aneurysm thrombosis.
   d. Long-term results of the surgical treatment of these aneurysms are not dependent on the degree of arterial occlusive disease distal to the aneurysm.

5. What is the most common cause of peripheral aneurysms?
   a. Atherosclerosis
   b. Infection
   c. Trauma
   d. Connective tissue disorders

6. Which of the following peripheral aneurysms is most likely to rupture?
   a. Popliteal
   b. Carotid
   c. Deep femoral
   d. Axillary

7. For a patient with ischemia secondary to thrombosis of a popliteal artery aneurysm and occlusion of the popliteal outflow tract, what is the best initial treatment?
   a. Thrombolytic therapy
   b. Thrombectomy and bypass
   c. Observation
   d. Sympathectomy

8. What is the most common cause of mycotic aneurysms?
   a. Trauma
   b. Bacterial endocarditis
   c. Direct extension of adjacent infection
   d. Food poisoning

9. Which of the following statements about popliteal aneurysms is true?
   a. They are frequently bilateral.
   b. They are commonly associated with abdominal aortic aneurysms.
   c. They rarely rupture.
   d. All of the above

10. A 64-year-old man has a 3.4-cm-diameter left popliteal artery aneurysm. The proximal portion of the aneurysm ends 3 cm distal to the adductor tendon. There is 2.5 cm of uninvolved distal popliteal artery. He has three-vessel runoff. He is an acceptable surgical candidate. Which of the following treatments is most likely to successfully treat the aneurysm and result in no need for future treatment of the same aneurysm?
    a. Stent-graft placement
    b. Above-knee to below-knee popliteal to popliteal bypass using saphenous vein coupled with aneurysm ligation through a medial approach
    c. Posterior approach with aneurysm resection and interposition graft using either PTFE or saphenous vein
    d. Above-knee to below-knee popliteal to popliteal bypass with aneurysm ligation using PTFE

ANSWERS

1. **b**
2. **c**
3. **c**
4. **c**
5. **a**
6. **c**
7. **a**
8. **a**
9. **d**
10. **c**

CHAPTER 45

VASCULAR TRAUMA

Brian S. Knipp* • David L. Gillespie

BACKGROUND

"One of the chief fascinations in surgery is the management of wounded vessels." This statement by William Stewart Halstead illustrates the intellectual challenge and physical demands of managing patients with vascular trauma. What it does not capture, however, is the enormity of the difficulties often faced by the surgeon in the setting of severe vascular injury. Severe physiologic derangements secondary to massive hemorrhage, frequent and multiple concomitant injuries, and various priorities vying for primacy create a situation that requires experience, stamina, and sometimes a little luck to yield a positive outcome. This is compounded in some cases by the lack of resources in austere environments, such as battlefields or small community hospitals. The management of these injuries is not for the faint of heart.

The social effects of trauma are substantial; approximately 40 million emergency department visits and 2.6 million hospitalizations result annually from traumatic injuries.[1] Patients younger than 45 years sustain 75% of the total lifetime cost of injury, an aggregate measure of the health care costs and societal costs over the patient's lifetime from all injuries occurring in a given year. Societal costs include lost lifetime productivity, lost wages, and the need for social support such as unemployment wages and workers compensation. In both civilian and combat settings, the incidence of vascular injury is approximately 0.2% to 7% of all injured patients.[2-8] Males represent the overwhelming majority of victims of vascular trauma specifically in nearly all anatomic locations,[9-27] leading some to label vascular trauma as a disease of young males.[28]

It is important to consider both the similarities and differences in civilian and military vascular injury. While many surgical advances have taken place during wartime and we have learned a great deal from these experiences, the degree and pattern of injuries seen in civilian settings are generally different from those seen in military trauma. Among civilian victims, for example, gunshot wounds are responsible for the majority of peripheral vascular injury, stab wounds for a smaller percentage, and the remainder is due to blunt trauma.[10,29] Because most civilian gunshot wounds are generally due to low-velocity

projectiles, the degree of associated trauma is limited, usually involving only venous or neural injury. This is in contrast to military trauma, in which arterial injury usually occurs in the setting of massive extremity involvement, where orthopedic fractures, large soft tissue defects, and nerve and vein injuries are common. This pattern is seen in one third of patients presenting with vascular injury to combat trauma receiving centers; it can also be seen in civilian close-range shotgun blasts. The majority of military traumatic injuries are due to explosive devices (74%), with high-velocity gunshot wounds being responsible for most of the remainder (17%); blunt injury is infrequent.[6,30]

EARLY CONTROL OF HEMORRHAGE

The most common cause of potentially survivable death is uncontrolled hemorrhage, in both the military and civilian settings.[31-35] Patients sustaining major vascular injury exhibit severe physiologic derangements resulting from hemorrhage, tissue hypoxia, and the sequelae of anaerobic metabolism (Figure 45-1). Severe hemorrhage leads to what has been termed the *lethal triad* of hypothermia, coagulopathy, and acidosis. Patients requiring massive transfusions, generally defined as requiring greater than 10 units of packed red blood cells, suffer mortality rates of 20% to 50%.[36] Historically, trauma management algorithms have emphasized crystalloid fluid resuscitation and early administration of packed red blood cells to support cardiac output and tissue-level delivery of oxygen, with administration of plasma and platelets based on subsequent laboratory analysis. However, recent research has called this practice into question. In 2007, Borgman and colleagues[37] reported that the ratio of blood products was related to casualty mortality at a combat support hospital. Subsequent research has documented similar findings in military[38,39] and civilian[40] populations.

The following principles constitute the damage control resuscitation approach to reversal of the lethal triad. The first step is identification of patients who require damage control management, as opposed to the physiologically stable patient who will tolerate definitive treatment of injuries in the initial operative setting. Once the decision is made to pursue a damage control strategy, an assessment of the patient's immediately life-threatening issues must be performed. The basic tenet of damage control surgery is to stop ongoing contamination and hemorrhage and transport the patient as rapidly as possible to

*The views expressed in this chapter are those of the authors and do not necessarily reflect the official policy or position of the U.S. Department of the Navy, U.S. Department of Defense, or the U.S. Government.

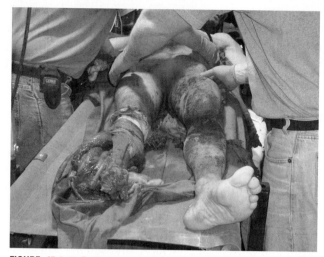

FIGURE 45-1 ■ Patients sustaining multisystem trauma often have significant blood loss, leading to hemodynamic instability, hypothermia, acidosis, and coagulopathy.

a resuscitative environment, such as the intensive care unit, in order to halt progression of the lethal triad. Any large vessel bleeding should be controlled surgically and repaired in an expeditious fashion. Any sources of gross contamination, such as injury to the gastrointestinal tract, should be controlled as well. If possible, vascular continuity should be restored by either an expeditious definitive repair or a temporizing measure, such as a vascular shunt. However, life must take precedence over limb, and if it is impossible to restore blood flow without exposing the patient to severe risk from a prolonged repair, ligation of the artery and management of the ischemic sequelae is preferable to losing the patient through a well-intentioned but overly heroic effort to save a limb. Acidosis should be prevented or treated. Hypothermia, found to be an independent predictor of mortality among combat casualties,[41] must also be prevented or treated. Packed red blood cells are infused along with plasma and platelets in a 1:1:1 ratio, minimizing the use of red cells prior to vascular control and repair, and minimizing the use of crystalloid in general. Finally, new data support the early use of recombinant factor VII.[42] Fibrinogen has been evaluated as part of this protocol and is a predictor of survival; however, a typical unit of fresh frozen plasma has 400 mg of fibrinogen, which supplies the recommended dose if at least a 1:2 ratio of packed red blood cells to plasma is maintained.[39] Additional adjuncts such as tourniquets (which will be discussed in the Extremity Vascular Injury section) and hemostatic dressings such as Quickclot (zeolite powder; Z-Medica, Wallingford, Conn.) or HemCon (chitosan-based bandage; HemCon Medical Technologies, Portland, Ore.) are also used in combat environments to aid in rapid hemostasis. Tourniquet use has been shown to have such sufficient effects on outcome that it has become a part of most prehospital management algorithms in the civilian community.

To address concerns that damage control resuscitation might have a deleterious effect on vascular reconstructions, Fox and colleagues[43] performed a case-control study of battlefield casualties who underwent vascular repair and compared patients treated with a rigorous damage control resuscitation protocol versus conventional crystalloid and nonmatched erythrocyte resuscitation. There was no worse outcome among patients when the coagulopathy was treated. The author's admonition was to "fix the injury, fix it well, and trust that your patient doesn't need to be coagulopathic for the graft to work."[43]

In 1993, Rotondo and colleagues[44] coined the term *damage control surgery*, referring to a limited surgical procedure or set of procedures with discrete, life-saving goals and the intent to defer more definitive repair until further resuscitation has occurred. The quandary of a patient in extremis requiring a further surgical insult to correct a life-threatening injury has been recognized for generations. Debakey and Simeone[2] commented that while some injuries are clearly beyond any repair the patient could tolerate, others are complicated by the physiologic cost to the patient of that repair. Hughes stated in his report on arterial injuries in Korea that "the need for adequate amounts of blood and complete resuscitation in such individuals is stressed … rushing the improperly resuscitated patient to surgery in an attempt to save a limb may possibly result in loss of life."[5] The spectrum of procedures and maneuvers classified as damage control techniques has been growing as experience with this concept broadens, but the basic principles include rapid surgical control of bleeding, control of sources of contamination, and deferral of definitive procedures until the patient is more stable. Damage control options for vascular trauma include tourniquet use, temporary vascular shunting (TVS), ligation, or balloon tamponade.[45-53] These specific techniques will be discussed in later sections. At this point, it is difficult to associate any particular damage control surgery technique with improved outcomes, because the numbers are too small and the confounding variables in patients in extremis are too numerous to achieve statistical power. Taken as a whole, however, damage control for major trauma is associated with improved physiology, increased limb salvage, and decreased mortality.[40,43,45,46]

DIAGNOSIS OF VASCULAR INJURY

The specifics of diagnosis of vascular injury in particular territories will be addressed in later sections, but some basic principles deserve mention now. To start, the examination of the patient with suspected vascular injury should begin with an assessment of mechanism. Blunt injuries have their own pathophysiology and patterns; penetrating injuries present in a different fashion. Once the general mechanism has been assessed, specifics of the injury should be elicited. For blunt trauma, the examiner should develop as thorough an understanding of the injury as possible. For motor vehicle crashes, rate of speed, position of patient in the vehicle, direction of impact, additional forces such as vehicular rollover or patient ejection, or degree of intrusion should be documented. Falls should be investigated for height, position of patient on impact, surface hit, and any obstacles during the fall. Penetrating injury should be classified by weapon: gunshot wound, knife, shotgun, or other type of wounding agent, caliber, muzzle velocity (or at least a general distinction between high-powered and low-powered projectiles), distance from gun to patient, number of wounds, catalog of entry and exit wounds, type and length of knife, or type of shotgun shell used.

Once a thorough history has been elicited, the physical examination should be performed. The examination can be conceptualized from the heart outward. While the examination may be tailored for the specific injury pattern, in general the trunk should be examined for entrance and exit wounds which could suggest the need for thoracotomy. Auscultation of heart and lung sounds will reveal signs suggestive of hemothorax, pneumothorax, or tamponade. Jugular vein examination is also helpful in diagnosing right-sided cardiac outflow obstruction from tension pneumothorax or tamponade. Decreased breath sounds, dullness to percussion, or penetrating injuries to the thorax should prompt placement of thoracostomy tubes. The presence of significant initial bleeding, greater than 1500 mL, or significant ongoing bleeding greater than 200 to 250 mL/h are indications for thoracotomy.

Manual palpation of pulses is the next step. Carotid, subclavian (in the infraclavicular recess), brachial, radial, ulnar, femoral, popliteal, and pedal pulses should be palpated and documented. The use of continuous wave Doppler ultrasound to augment the physical examination is appropriate. In 1971, Lavenson and colleagues[54] evaluated the auscultation of Doppler signals in the distal pulses as a means of extremity pulse assessment, as an extension of the physical examination.[54] The benefit of this technique is that it is both rapid and, if a sphygmomanometer is used in concert, can be quantified as the ankle-brachial index (ABI). The disadvantage, however, is that it is an indirect, blind study and does not exclude vascular injury. ABI has been found to be highly sensitive for clinically significant vascular injury. Patients with ABI greater than 0.9 may be observed, and angiography is reserved for those with ABI less than 0.9.[55]

Significant vascular injury may produce physical findings that should be obvious to a trained examiner. The classic "hard signs" of vascular injury include active hemorrhage, an expanding hematoma, a palpable thrill, a continuous murmur, or the signs of ischemia, namely pain, pallor, pulselessness, paralysis, or poikilothermia. The presence of one or more of these signs is an appropriate indication for operative exploration. Signs suggestive of vascular injury (i.e., the "soft signs") include proximity of a wound to a major vascular structure, a stable hematoma, an ipsilateral neurologic defect, shock, or a report of prehospital hemorrhage from the wound. Consideration must also be given to concomitant injuries, such as orthopedic or neurologic trauma, as the risk of significant vascular injury increases in these settings.

Arteriorraphy has been the gold standard for diagnosis of vascular injury and remains an indispensable tool for the management of vascular trauma. It has a number of indications, including evaluation of the need for surgery, investigation of a suspected injury, and operative planning. It is indicated for blunt trauma with associated fractures, penetrating injury to the chest, zone I and III

cervical injury, multiple pellet wounds, injuries to the forearm or leg, and knee dislocation. In the recent decades, there has been a great deal of effort to identify patients at risk for occult vascular lesions (Figure 45-2). In a series of 538 patients, Conrad and colleagues[56] documented no missed injuries in the setting of a normal physical examination and normal ABI was associated with no missed injuries and concluded that angiography is unnecessary in this population. The limitation of this study was that there was only 51% follow-up of those discharged without further workup.[56] In a series of 507 asymptomatic patients, however, Reid and colleagues[57] documented abnormal arteriograms in 6.7%. In another study, 157 patients with penetrating extremity injuries but no hard signs of vascular injury underwent arteriorraphy; 11% of patients had abnormal arteriograms, of which 27% were major abnormalities.[58] Gillespie and colleagues reported 90 patients with penetrating extremity injuries without hard signs and found 27% to have abnormal arteriograms; all injuries were successfully managed nonoperatively.[59] A critical distinction must be made from a diagnostic standpoint between combat-related and civilian trauma. In combat settings, there is a higher rate of occult injuries found with arteriorraphy than in the civilian literature (45% versus 11%), most of which are associated with normal physical examination, and a higher percentage of these findings require operative or endovascular intervention (10% versus 1%).[60]

With the advent of high-resolution multislice computed tomography scanners, the ability to perform noninvasive arteriorraphy is changing the diagnostic algorithm for vascular injury. A series of 20 patients with combat-related vascular injuries were examined using a 64-slice multidetector computed tomographic angiography (MDCTA). Injuries were identified in 10 of 20 patients (50%) and the study was deemed adequate in 94% of cases. Four patients underwent comparative studies and there were no discordant findings. MDCTA seems to yield sufficiently high resolution images to be useful for the early evaluation of combat casualties. The presence of metallic fragments or orthopedic hardware did not interfere significantly in this report with the value of MDCTA.[61]

Finally, duplex ultrasonography should be considered in general for the diagnosis of vascular injury. Although sensitivity of this modality is variable and it is arguably operator dependent, some vascular territories are highly amenable to duplex examination (e.g., cervical vascular trauma). Its main advantages are relative speed of the study, noninvasive nature, and repeatability in order to follow injuries.[62]

THORACIC VASCULAR INJURY

Vascular injuries involving thoracic vessels are some of the most lethal injuries that patients can sustain. These patients can be divided into three groups. The first group dies immediately at the scene of trauma from rapid exsanguination. The second group becomes unstable en route to medical care, and the majority (>96%) die secondary to multisystem trauma. If patients are able to survive with

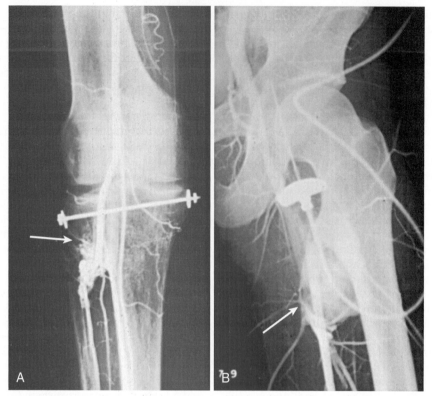

FIGURE 45-2 ■ **A,** Arteriovenous fistula of the anterior tibial artery and vein *(arrow).* Orthopedic repairs were completed previously, without knowledge of the vascular wound. **B,** This large false aneurysm of the deep femoral artery *(arrow)* was diagnosed only by arteriorraphy.

thoracic vascular injuries to medical care, their chance of survival goes up substantially to approximately 70% to 95%, with deaths in this group often being secondary to neurologic injury.[63] These injuries require a significant investment of hospital resources. A recent study identified that patients treated at a level I trauma center had lower mortality from major thoracic vascular injury than at a level II center.[64]

There are a variety of findings suggestive of thoracic great vessel injury. These include hypotension, upper extremity hypertension, intermittent paralysis or focal neurologic findings, inequality of blood pressure or pulses between extremities, external evidence of chest trauma, an expanding hematoma at the thoracic outlet, an intrascapular murmur, a palpable fracture of the sternum or the thoracic spine, or a left-sided flail chest.[63] The initial management of these patients should follow the standard trauma resuscitative pathways. Fluid resuscitation should be minimized for several reasons. If there is a full-thickness vascular injury, minimization of fluid resuscitation and permissive hypotension will help to stabilize early soft-platelet plugs. Any patients with military antishock trousers in place and the suspicion of a proximal vascular injury should have them removed immediately, because this is effectively a distal cross-clamp and can lead to instability of clots and worsened bleeding.[63] If there is blunt injury, aggressive prevention of hypotension helps to avoid propagation of the injury. Finally, concomitant pulmonary contusions or other injuries are common, and minimization of fluid resuscitation will avoid iatrogenic worsening of respiratory status.

In cases of penetrating injury, patients with thoracic vascular injury generally are hemodynamically unstable. Patients with blunt thoracic vascular injury are generally hemodynamically stable, because those who are unstable from this mechanism die in the prehospital setting in almost 100% of cases. This distinction is critical, because a patient with blunt trauma who arrives in stable condition and subsequently turns unstable is most likely bleeding outside of the thoracic cavity.[63]

Penetrating Injury

The most common mechanism of injury to thoracic great vessels is penetrating trauma, responsible for 90% of injuries. In a series of 3823 gunshot wounds or stab wounds to the chest or abdomen, the aorta was injured in 1.6%. Most of these injuries were due to gunshot wounds (69%), with stab wounds (18%) and shotgun wounds (12%) composing the remainder of penetrating thoracic injuries. Whereas thoracic aortic injury was less common than abdominal aortic injury (28% vs. 72%), it was associated with a decreased likelihood of having a recordable blood pressure (27% vs. 71%), increased need for emergency department thoracotomy (EDT, 77% vs. 21%), and decreased survival (8% vs. 24%). Most patients with penetrating injury to the thoracic aorta arrived in shock (83%), with half of these patients demonstrating no recordable blood pressure. Mortality was 81% overall in this cohort, with gunshot wounds having a higher associated mortality (88%) than stab wounds (65%). Predictors of mortality in this series were gunshot wounds, injury to the thoracic aorta as opposed to the abdominal aorta, a nonrecordable blood pressure on admission, and the need for an EDT. Although concomitant injury to other structures occurred in 81% of patients, most commonly the lung, there was no association with mortality.[4]

Plain film radiography in these patients may reveal findings suggestive of great vessel injury, such as mediastinal widening, a foreign body out of focus with other structures indicating possible intracardiac location, a foreign body in close proximity to vascular structures, a confusing missile trajectory suggesting possible missile embolism, or a missile that is altogether missing, which suggests possible distal embolism. Radiopaque markers should be placed at the entrance and exit wounds to delineate missile trajectories.[63]

If the patient is a candidate for an EDT, it is performed by making a left anterolateral thoracotomy in the fourth interspace. A Finochietto rib spreader is placed, oriented with the handle toward the lateral aspect of the wound in case the incision needs to be extended across the midline, and the lung is examined. If there is evidence of lung bleeding, it is either clamped or, if it is central or hilar, the inferior pulmonary ligament is divided and a hilar clamp placed. Alternatively, the lung can be twisted 180 degrees on its hilum to temporarily control bleeding. The pericardium is then grasped anterior to the phrenic nerve and opened longitudinally, delivering the heart. Any obvious injury is sutured with 3-0 polypropylene pledgeted sutures or stapled. Open cardiac massage is then initiated. Finally, a cross-clamp is placed on the aorta. A nasogastric tube should be inserted to assist in differentiation of the aorta from the esophagus, which is not always an easy task in the exsanguinated patient. Any additional sources of bleeding should be controlled with finger tamponade, clamps, or packing, and the patient should be taken immediately to the operating room.

Anatomically, the aortic arch is oriented in an anterior posterior direction, and the left subclavian artery originates off of the aorta in the posterior mediastinum. As a result, it is nearly impossible to obtain rapid proximal control of this artery through a median sternotomy. In a patient with a penetrating injury above or below the left clavicle, the best approach to control the left subclavian artery is through an incision in the third interspace of the left chest. This high anterolateral thoracotomy will allow adequate visualization of the root of the left subclavian artery to gain vascular control. Once bleeding is controlled, the surgeon can explore the injured subclavian artery through standard supraclavicular incision (Figure 45-3).

The most versatile exposure for penetrating thoracic trauma is a left anterolateral thoracotomy through the fourth interspace. It is not an accident that this is the same incision used for the EDT. The left side of the mediastinum including the pericardium and the descending aorta can be accessed through this incision. If this does not provide sufficient access, the incision is extended across the midline via a transverse sternotomy and can be continued into a right anterolateral thoracotomy in the third interspace. This is known as the *clamshell incision* (Figure 45-4). It is a highly morbid procedure, but if it is necessary, the patient is near death and all maneuvers are considered heroic at this point.

In the patient with a known site of injury, alternative incisions may be used. One of the most common approaches to the thoracic cavity is the midline sternotomy. An incision is made vertically from the sternal notch to the xiphoid process down to the sternum. Using blunt dissection, a retrosternal space is established, and a sternal saw is used to divide the sternum longitudinally. The Finochietto retractor is then placed and the thoracic cavity is opened. This affords access to the ascending aorta, the brachiocephalic vein, and the pulmonary artery. The transverse aortic arch may be reached through this incision, although it may require a cervical extension. In order to fully control the innominate artery or the right subclavian artery or vein, the median sternotomy is extended to include a right cervical incision. Extension of the sternotomy into a left cervical incision will provide access to the left common carotid artery. The mid and distal left subclavian artery and vein are more challenging to access and require a left anterolateral thoracotomy in the third or fourth interspace coupled with a left supraclavicular incision (Figure 45-5). Connecting these incisions with a vertical sternotomy is the trapdoor incision, which is discussed often but associated with significant morbidity and risk of causalgia. The descending aorta can be reached, as previously mentioned, through a left fourth interspace anterolateral thoracotomy, but preferentially should be exposed through a posterolateral thoracotomy in the same interspace. Finally, the distal pulmonary veins or the pulmonary hilum can be reached through a posterolateral thoracotomy on the appropriate side.

Penetrating injuries of the anterior wall of the ascending aorta can be repaired with simple interrupted sutures. However, posterior wall or through-and-through injuries of this segment of the aorta will require bypass to correct. Injury in the transverse arch requires extension of the sternotomy into cervical incisions to control the branch vessels. The brachiocephalic vein can be ligated and divided if necessary to improve exposure. If complex repairs are necessary, cardiopulmonary bypass is required.

Injury to the innominate artery from penetrating trauma can occur anywhere along its length. If possible, proximal and distal control through appropriate incisions should be secured and then debridement and repair versus interposition grafting can be accomplished. Injury to the proximal innominate artery is essentially an injury to the ascending aorta (Figure 45-6). This artery is also the most common site of injury for blunt innominate artery trauma (see Figure 45-6) that is essentially an ascending aortic injury. The bypass and exclusion technique is useful in this scenario (Figure 45-7). Before entering the hematoma, the distal innominate artery just proximal to the bifurcation is controlled, clamped, and divided. Collateral flow to the carotid artery is maintained via retrograde flow from the subclavian artery, which fills through collaterals. A prosthetic graft is

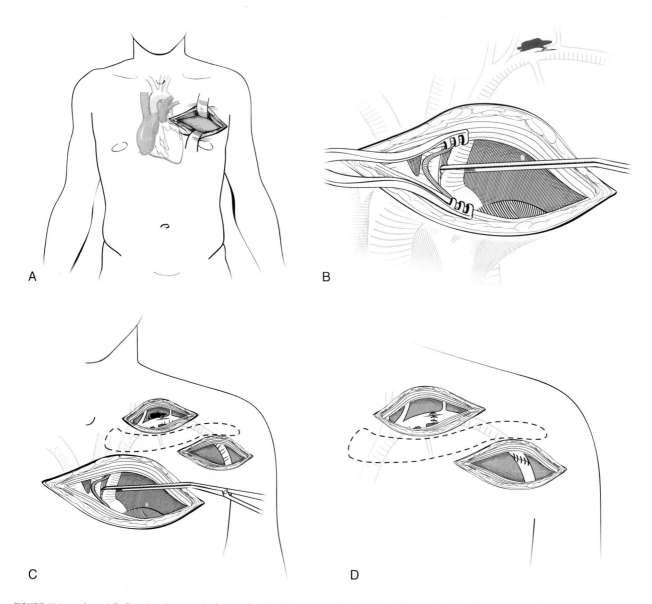

FIGURE 45-3 ■ **A** and **B,** Proximal control of the left subclavian artery is obtained through a left third space anterolateral thoracotomy. **C,** Once proximal control is achieved, distal control can be obtained through an infraclavicular incision, and the wound is exposed through a supraclavicular incision. **D,** The subclavian artery is repaired via the supraclavicular and infraclavicular incisions.

anastomosed to the distal innominate artery. A side-biting Satinsky clamp is placed on the aorta proximal to the origin of the innominate artery, and the graft is anastomosed to the aorta. Finally, the hematoma is entered, the injury is identified, the proximal innominate artery is divided, and the side hole in the aorta is oversewn. If there is a concomitant venous injury, a pericardial patch should be placed between the graft and the venous repair to avoid erosion and fistula formation.

Blunt Aortic Injury

The most common blunt injury in the thoracic cavity is blunt aortic injury (BAI). It was first described by Loren Parmley, a pathologist at Walter Reed Army Medical Center, in a series of 275 autopsies reported in 1958. The mortality in this series was staggering; 14% survived until arrival at the hospital, and 33% of these patients died within 24 hours, 60% by 1 week, and 90% by 4 months.[65] Only 5% of these patients were considered cured.[66] While there were isolated reports of attempts at repair of these lesions during that era, the state of the art was sufficiently primitive that Steinberg made a "plea for conservative treatment" of these patients.[67] These injuries continue to have significant on-scene mortality, with 80% to 90% of victims not surviving the initial insult. In an analysis of the National Trauma Databank, the incidence of BAI was 0.3% of all trauma admissions and represented 8000 deaths per year. Four percent of patients were deceased on arrival to the emergency department, and an additional 19% died during triage efforts.[68] Operative mortality has historically ranged from

15% to 28%,[69] and paraplegia complicated nearly 9% of cases[70] before the advent of alternative treatment modalities. In the initial report by Parmley and colleagues,[65] 57% of cases of BAI were secondary to automobile crashes, and 16% were due to airplane crashes. This remains true today; more than 80% of BAI is due to automobile accidents. In the initial report of the American Association for the Surgery of Trauma multicenter trial of BAI (known as AAST I), patients presented in one of four groups. Eight percent of patients arrived in extremis and suffered 100% mortality, all from rupture of their aorta. The other high-mortality group (9%) were those who arrived in stable condition but suffered rupture of the aorta before surgical repair; again, mortality was 100% in this subset. The most common presentation was

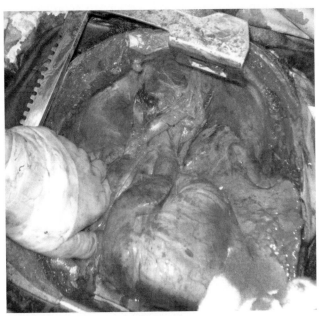

FIGURE 45-4 ■ Clamshell incision. This incision provides extensive exposure to the entire thoracic cavity at the cost of a very morbid procedure.

patients in stable condition (76%) with a mortality rate of 14%, the majority of the deaths being due to nonvascular injuries. Finally, 7% of patients did not undergo operative repair; mortality in this cohort was 52% because the severity of other injuries, primarily central nervous system trauma.[70] Patients with BAI typically have additional injuries to other organ systems. Closed head injury is seen in 30% to 50% of patients, multiple rib fractures in 46%, pulmonary contusion in 38%, major abdominal trauma in 29%, and pelvic fracture in 31%. The mean injury severity score (ISS) on arrival in patients with BAI is 42.[68,70]

The most common finding on plain film chest radiography, by far, is a widened mediastinum, seen in 85% of cases. Other findings include an indistinct aortic knob (24%), a left pleural effusion (19%), and an apical cap (19%). Uncommon findings include fracture of the first or second rib, tracheal deviation, a depressed left bronchus, and nasogastric tube deviation. No radiographic abnormalities are seen, however, in 7% of patients.[70] These cases are likely due to minimal aortic injury, defined as an intimal flap less than 1 cm in size not penetrating to the media. This finding was detected in 8% of Parmley's autopsy cases.[66]

Aortography was the most common diagnostic modality in the AAST I study, with transesophageal echocardiography used in a small subset of patients. However, both of these modalities have been supplanted by MDCTA in the updated report by the AAST, known as the AAST II study. Aortography decreased from 87% to 8% of cases, echocardiography from 12% to 1%, with CTA increasing from 35% to 93% of cases.[71] MDCTA now stands as the modern gold standard diagnostic modality for BAI.[72]

In his autopsy series, Parmley described six types of BAI. The first was an intimal hemorrhage, and the second was an intimal hemorrhage with a laceration. More severe injuries include medial laceration, complete aortic laceration, pseudoaneurysm, or periaortic hemorrhage[65]; 93% of these injuries occur at the ligamentum arteriosum.[72]

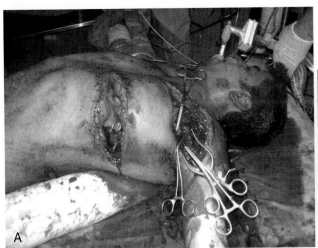
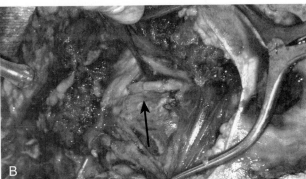

FIGURE 45-5 ■ **A,** Initial proximal control of this left subclavian injury was obtained via an emergency department thoracotomy in the fourth interspace. A supraclavicular incision and claviculectomy allowed access to the wound. **B,** The subclavian artery is repaired with a reversed saphenous interposition graft.

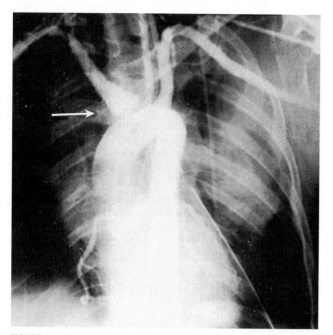

FIGURE 45-6 ■ A load of lumber fell on this patient and produced lung contusions and a wide mediastinum, which prompted the arteriogram. Note the nearly avulsed innominate artery *(arrow)*.

In the AAST I trial, the standard of care for treatment was operative repair if the patient could tolerate the procedure, versus expectant management for those with severe multisystem injury. Clamp and sew was the usual operative approach, and mortality and paraplegia rates were 31% (22% excluding patients presenting in extremis) and 9%, respectively.[70] A paradigm shift has taken place in the last decade, however. Modern treatment of BAI follows three principles. The first is aggressive pharmacologic blood pressure control, the second is appropriate selection and prioritization of repair, and the final is the use of endovascular techniques in an increasingly broad set of indications.

Antihypertensive therapy has been shown to decrease the rate of in-hospital aortic rupture from 12% to less than 2%.[70,73] Intravenous esmolol or labetalol is used to titrate systolic blood pressure to approximately 100 mm Hg with a relative bradycardia. Nitroprusside can be added if additional blood pressure control is needed. While there has been a substantial reduction in the use of pulmonary artery catheters in the last decade, these patients could potentially benefit from catheter-guided titration of pressures and SvO$_2$. Head-injured patients should be considered for intracranial pressure monitoring to optimize cerebral perfusion pressure.[66]

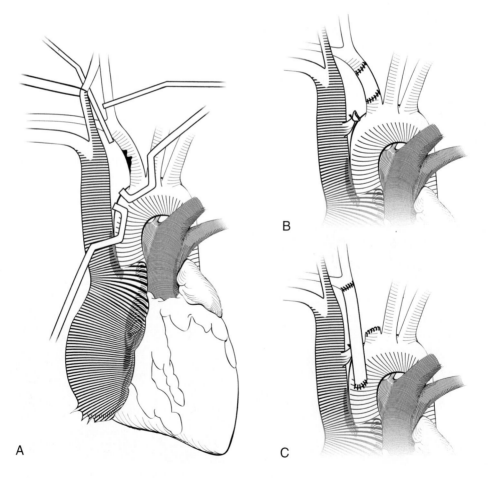

FIGURE 45-7 ■ **A,** Exposure of a proximal innominate injury. **B,** Division of the brachiocephalic vein is frequently necessary to access the innominate artery. **C,** Bypass and exclusion technique provides flow from the ascending aorta to the distal innominate artery.

Prioritization of repair requires a balancing of the degree of injury, the risk of rupture, the ability to aggressively control blood pressure, and the risk to the patient. At one end of the spectrum, minimal aortic injury can be safely followed nonoperatively. In their series of nine patients with minimal aortic injuries, one patient underwent immediate operative repair and two died of other injuries. Of the six remaining patients, three resolved completely. One underwent operative repair demonstrating a healed flap with intimal thickening. The other two were followed clinically.[73a] They concluded that minimal aortic injury does not require operative intervention but should be followed until the injury has healed to rule out progression to a pseudoaneurysm.

Patients with more significant injuries should undergo repair, but their intervention can be delayed if aggressive antihypertensive therapy is instituted. Hemmila and colleagues[73] showed that surgical delays beyond 16 hours did not increase mortality if a strict antihypertensive regimen was followed, but the price was increased intensive care unit and ventilator days. At the University of Michigan, the indications for delayed procedures includes significant associated injuries preventing thoracotomy and single lung ventilation, significant traumatic brain injury preventing use of heparin, other contraindications to anticoagulation, or active infection.[74]

Descending thoracic aortic repair of BAI is still considered by some authors to be the gold standard,[74] although others would argue that endovascular stent-grafts have supplanted descending thoracic aortic repair as the mainstay of therapy, despite the lack of level I data.[69] Historically, a rapid clamp-and-sew has been promoted as the most straightforward repair, although some authors believe that paraplegia rates are higher with this technique than using bypass. A multivariate analysis of risk factors for paraplegia found cross-clamp times greater than 30 minutes and the clamp-and-sew technique to be independently predictive of paraplegia postoperatively.[70] One group proposes the following principles to avoid this dreaded complication: preservation of intercostal vessels intraoperatively when possible, avoidance of the clamp-and-sew technique, use of permissive hypertension postoperatively to improve spinal blood flow, and the use of spinal drains only in highly selected patients.[74]

CERVICAL VASCULAR INJURY

Blunt Cervical Vascular Injury

Incidence and Mechanism of Injury

Several decades ago, blunt cervical vascular injury (BCVI), encompassing injuries to the carotid or vertebral arteries, was thought to be a rare injury relegated to the level of case reports. However, during the 1990s, pioneering work from trauma groups in Memphis and Denver uncovered a much larger incidence of this type of injury than had been previously described. One of the initial reports evaluated 20,349 trauma admissions at the Presley Regional Trauma Center; 67 patients (0.33%) were found to have 87 BCVIs.[75] In a pilot study of all patients

TABLE 45-1	Screening Criteria for Blunt Cervical Vascular Injury
Hard Signs of BCVI	**Signs Suggestive of Occult BCVI**
Hemorrhage from the mouth, ears, nose, or wounds	Severe cervical hyperextension and rotation or hyperflexion if associated with displaced midface or complex mandibular fracture or closed head injury consistent with diffuse axonal injury
Expanding cervical hematoma	Near hanging resulting in anoxic brain injury
Cervical bruit in a patient <50 years old	Seat belt abrasion or other soft tissue injury of the anterior neck resulting in significant swelling or altered mental status
Evidence of cerebral infarction on CT scan	Basilar skull fracture
Unexplained or incongruous neurologic deficit, transient ischemic attack, amaurosis fugax, or Horner syndrome	Cervical vertebral body fracture

From Biffl WL, Moore EE, Offner PJ, et al: Blunt carotid arterial injuries: implications of a new grading scale. J Trauma 47:845–853, 1999.

BCVI, Blunt cerebrovascular injury; *CT,* computed tomography.

undergoing postinjury thoracic aortograms performed at the University of Colorado, 3.5% of patients were found to have a documented BCVI, only half of whom manifested symptoms.[76] Disconcerted by these findings, the trauma surgeons in Denver undertook a prospective study in 249 patients: 40 with symptoms consistent with BCVI and 209 with high-risk features (Table 45-1). This report documented BCVI in 28 (70%) of the symptomatic patients and 57 (27%) of the asymptomatic patients. Injuries included 65 isolated carotid artery injuries, 10 isolated vertebral artery injuries, and 10 combined carotid and vertebral artery injuries.[77] In another report from the same year, their overall incidence was reported at 0.38% of trauma admissions, but was 1.07% among admissions during the time they performed aggressive screening.[78] Contemporary estimates of BCVI incidence is 0.4% to 1.0% of blunt trauma admissions.[79-81] The mechanism of the majority of these injuries is motor vehicle crash, reported in 45% to 82% of series, followed by pedestrian trauma (12%), motorcycle crash (11%), falls (9% to 10%), and assaults (5% to 6%).[75,77,79] Fifty-five percent of patients with BCVI had a lateralizing examination in the University of Michigan series. In the 45% without a lateralizing examination, neurologic findings became evident from 3 hours to 10 days after admission.[79]

Screening

Given the unexpectedly high incidence of BCVI in blunt trauma, investigators began searching for a means of detecting the injury in asymptomatic patients. In the original report from Memphis, circumstances that prompted invasive evaluation with cerebral angiography included cervical soft tissue injury, a neurologic examination incompatible with imaging findings, the development of a neurologic deficit after admission, or the presence of Horner syndrome.[75] In an effort to further elucidate which patients were at risk, the Denver group developed the following criteria. Patients underwent four-vessel cerebral angiography (FVCA) for any of the following: hemorrhage from the mouth, ears, nose, or wounds; expanding cervical hematoma; cervical bruit in a patient younger than 50 years; evidence of cerebral infarction on CT scan, or an unexplained or incongruous neurologic deficit, transient ischemic attack, amaurosis fugax, or Horner syndrome. The group would also screen patients with FVCA for the following: severe cervical hyperextension and rotation or hyperflexion if associated with displaced midface or complex mandibular fracture or closed head injury consistent with diffuse axonal injury; near hanging resulting in anoxic brain injury; or a seat belt abrasion or other soft tissue injury of the anterior neck resulting in significant swelling or altered mental status, basilar skull fracture, or cervical vertebral body fracture.[77] In an effort to standardize practice, the Eastern Association for the Surgery of Trauma (EAST) published recommendations for the screening, diagnosis, and treatment of BCVI. They found no level I evidence. Level II recommendations are to screen for any neurologic abnormality not explained by a diagnosed injury, or blunt trauma associated with epistaxis from suspected arterial source. Level III evidence supports screening asymptomatic patients with blunt head trauma and the following risk factors: Glasgow Coma Scale score of 8 or less, petrous bone fracture, diffuse axonal injury, cervical spine fracture (especially C1-C3 and through foramen transversarium or with subluxation or rotational component), or a Lefort II or III facial fracture.[82] The major hurdle at this point, and the reason behind the efforts to elucidate an at-risk population, is that FVCA still remains the gold standard for diagnosis. The EAST guidelines state that duplex ultrasonography and four-slice or less CT scanners are inaccurate for the detection of BCVI. FVCA is, however, labor intensive, expensive, and invasive. There is a great deal of enthusiasm for the latest generation of MDCTA systems (MDCTA).[77] However, a report from the Memphis group raised a cautionary flag after they found an overall 51% sensitivity with MDCTA in a thorough, prospective study in which all patients underwent both MDCTA and FVCA.[81] At this time, FVCA seems to be the most conservative, safe option for at-risk patients (Figure 45-8).

Findings and Outcomes

The Denver group[77] proposed a grading scale for BCVI in 1999 (Table 45-2). The scale correlates well with mortality and stroke risk and has been used as the basis for treatment recommendations. In a recent report, the overall stroke risk for patients with BCVI was 14% and the in-hospital mortality was 10%.[81] Another report cited 26% in-hospital mortality. Among those who survived to

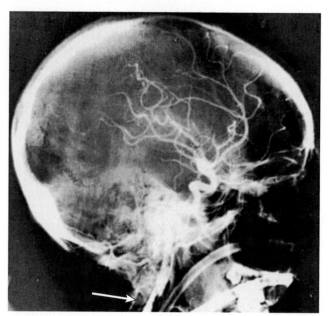

FIGURE 45-8 ■ Area of the internal carotid artery damaged by hyperextension trauma *(arrow)*.

TABLE 45-2	Grading Scale for Blunt Carotid Injury
Injury Grade	**Description**
I	Luminal irregularity or dissection with <25% luminal narrowing
II	Dissection or intramural hematoma with ≥25% luminal narrowing, intramural thrombus, or raised intimal flap
III	Pseudoaneurysm
IV	Occlusion
V	Transection with free extravasation

From Biffl WL, Moore EE, Offner PJ, et al: Blunt carotid arterial injuries: implications of a new grading scale. J Trauma 47:845–853, 1999.

discharge, only 31% were discharged home, whereas 43% were transferred to another inpatient facility such as rehabilitation or skilled nursing.[83] By injury grade, mortality was 0% to 33% for grade I-III lesions, 11% to 60% for grade IV, and 100% for grade V; stroke risk was 3% for grade I, 11% for grade II, 33% for grade III, 44% for grade IV, and 100% for grade V.[78,79,84,85] These findings agree with the early report from the Memphis group, which documented an overall 31% mortality among BCVI patients. They also noted that the mortality was 100% in patients not treated with systemic heparin and that all these deaths were due to stroke, compared to a 20% mortality for those treated with heparin.[75] The location of the lesions was primarily in the cervical internal carotid artery (68%) in the Michigan series; skull base carotid injury occurred in 45%, and intracranial injury occurred in 32%.[79]

Treatment of Blunt Cerebrovascular Injury

The primary treatment for BCVI is anticoagulation. Since the report by Fabian and colleagues[75] in 1996 demonstrated that heparin was the only factor independently predictive of improved neurologic outcomes, anticoagulation has been considered appropriate therapy for most BCVI, with surgery or endovascular treatments considered for specific lesion types. Recommendations from EAST are that heparin should be started without a bolus and should be converted to warfarin (Coumadin) with a goal initial normalized ratio (INR) of 2 to 3 for a period of 6 months.[82] No PTT goal is given in the EAST recommendations, but other authors have recommended a conservative goal of 40 to 50 seconds, especially in patients at high risk for bleeding.[75] There is also literature supporting the equivalence of antiplatelet therapy to anticoagulation in this patient population; in a study of 22 patients with BCVI, there were no differences in neurologic outcome among patients treated with anticoagulation or antiplatelet therapy, but there was a significant decrease in bleeding events with antiplatelet agents.[79] The other general recommendation from EAST is that patients with an early neurologic deficit and an accessible lesion should undergo operation or intervention to restore flow as soon as possible.[82]

Treatment of Grade I Injury

A grade I injury, defined as a luminal irregularity or dissection with less than 25% narrowing of the lumen, is thought to result from stretching of the artery or a direct blow. The pathophysiology is similar to that which produces Horner syndrome, a stretch or blow that disrupts the sympathetic ganglion fibers. Exposure of the thrombogenic subendothelial collagen puts patients at risk for thromboembolic strokes, which occur in approximately 3% of these patients.[78] Over time, 62% of nonocclusive dissections resolve with anticoagulation,[75] which supports the EAST recommendations that these patients be treated with antiplatelet or anticoagulation therapy.[82] However, there are no prospective data supporting the type or duration of therapy, and treatment should be tailored to the patient, the lesion, and comorbid injuries.

Treatment of Grade II Injury

Grade II injury—defined as a dissection or intramural hematoma with luminal narrowing of 25% or more, intramural thrombus, or raised intimal flap—has a 70% risk of progression to grade III or IV despite full anticoagulation; only 10% of these wounds heal. Despite this progression to a higher grade lesion, anticoagulation seems to be protective against stroke and is recommended. It is also recommended that these patients have repeated imaging studies 7 days after the injury to evaluate for progression.[78,82]

Treatment of Grade III Injury

Grade III injuries are pseudoaneurysms that develop secondary to egress of blood into the subadventitial layer and often result from progression of grade II injuries. Pseudoaneurysms pose a risk for rupture and hemorrhage, as well as thromboembolism; they rarely resolve with anticoagulation.[75,78] If the aneurysms are surgically accessible, operative repair is appropriate, although the distal artery may be surprisingly friable and difficult to work with. If the lesion is not surgically accessible, stenting is becoming a preferred treatment. One report initially warned of a 45% occlusion rate following carotid stenting, but these patients were treated with warfarin therapy as opposed to antiplatelet therapy, which has become standard of care for patients with stents until endothelialization is complete.[86] No occlusions were detected by Edwards and colleagues in stented arteries when patients were treated with clopidogrel.[83] The acutely injured artery, however, should not be subjected to angioplasty or stenting within 48 to 72 hours after injury.[78] Consensus opinion seems to be that patients with grade III injuries should be initially given anticoagulants and reimaged at 7 days after the injury. If the pseudoaneurysm persists (or has developed), consider stent placement with or without coil embolization and convert the patient to antiplatelet therapy; heparin and warfarin therapy may be continued or discontinued at the discretion of the surgeon based on the patient's overall risk and catalog of injuries. One final option for high skull-based lesions is an extracranial-intracranial bypass; this is a specialized skill requiring a microvascular neurosurgeon, however, and is not usually available at smaller hospitals.

Treatment of Grade IV and V Injury

Grade IV lesions are occlusions, and grade V injuries are transections. Both are highly morbid and lethal injuries. Some authors believe that outcomes are generally independent of treatment efforts,[79] although others have suggested decreased stroke risk with heparin therapy for grade IV lesions.[78] Interestingly, one center reports treating occlusion of the internal carotid artery in asymptomatic patients after penetrating trauma with embolization to prevent an occluded artery from "reopening" and providing a substrate for distal embolization after vasospasm dissipates.[26] Grade V transections require obtaining proximal and distal control, which can be extremely challenging depending on the location of the injury. Outcomes are miserable; one series reported 100% mortality from this injury.[78]

Penetrating Cervical Vascular Injury

Incidence, Mortality, and Mechanism of Injury

Penetrating injury to the cervical vessels has historically been treated somewhat differently than BCVI, because of differences in pathophysiology, diagnosis, treatment, and outcomes. In a series of 63 patients with combat-trauma–related penetrating neck trauma with suspected vascular injuries, 21 patients underwent ligation or repair in-theater. All patients underwent further evaluation following evacuation, which revealed 12 additional occult injuries and one graft thrombosis that were subsequently repaired. Blast fragments were responsible for the majority of these wounds (79%), with high-velocity gunshot wounds being responsible for the remainder.[87] In civilian trauma, the most common mechanism is a gunshot wound.[20] In a series of 38 civilian gunshot wounds to the internal carotid artery (ICA), 89% of patients had symptoms including neck hematoma (84%), active hemorrhage (32%), and neurologic deficits (26%). Mortality in this series was 19%, primarily because of stroke. The most common associated injury was pharyngeal (39%), which has implications for management of the suture line. The most commonly injured associated vascular structures were the internal maxillary artery (16%), external carotid artery (11%), and vertebral artery (8%). The likelihood of ICA occlusion correlated with the location of injury along the ICA; 20% of injuries of the ICA origin led to occlusion, compared to 29% of injuries below the odontoid process, 73% at the odontoid process, and 100% at the skull base.[26] Rao and colleagues[88] evaluated 76 patients with cervical vascular injuries among 528 patients with penetrating neck trauma. The overall mortality rate was 2.5%; among those with vascular injury, the mortality rate was 16%. Four patients underwent therapeutic embolization of an injured vessel in zones 1 or 3.[88]

Zones of the Neck

In 1969, Monson and colleagues[89] described three zones of cervical trauma with implications for technique of exposure and exploration. Zone 1 encompasses the root of the neck and is defined by the clavicles inferiorly and the cricoid cartilage superiorly. Zone 2 is the midcervical region defined by the cricoid cartilage inferiorly and the angle of the mandible superiorly. Zone 3 is superior to the angle of the mandible.[89]

Diagnosis

Classically, surgical exploration is the diagnostic maneuver used for a zone II wound with hard signs of vascular injury such as intraoral or extraoral bleeding, an expanding hematoma, a palpable thrill or audible bruit, or the loss of carotid pulse with a neurologic deficit. Soft signs in this region, such as a wound with proximity to the carotid artery, a stable hematoma, a carotid-jugular fistula at an unknown level, or the loss of the carotid pulse without a neurologic deficit, should undergo imaging to delineate the injury. It is important to remember that high-energy penetrating missiles can cause blunt injury resulting from cavitation in addition to direct trauma. This type of injury must be considered and treated appropriately. Similarly, zone I injuries should undergo arteriorraphy both for diagnosis and operative planning. Zone III injuries are diagnosed with arteriorrhaphy, which can present therapeutic solutions at the same time if the lesion is in a location not easily surgically accessible.[90] The ability of MDCTA to detect BCVI has been questioned recently; however, MDCTA seems to have better sensitivity for penetrating cervical injury in select patients. Fox and colleagues[87] found that the presence of nearby fragments decreased the sensitivity of this modality and recommended checking a plain film first if MDCT-A is planned. FVCA remains the gold standard. Duplex examination is often limited by the wound, dressing, or injuries to the cervical spine.

Management

The first issue to address with penetrating cervical trauma is airway management. In addition to the usual maneuvers, there are special considerations for active bleeding involving the airway. Proximal compression of the common carotid can be helpful to control bleeding while establishing a protected airway. Intraoral bleeding may be temporized with finger pressure, balloon occlusion, or gauze packing. A contained cervical hematoma may deviate the trachea and elevate the floor of the mouth, making orotracheal intubation challenging or impossible. Nasotracheal intubation is an option if the correct instruments are available, but cricothyroidotomy should be performed expeditiously if it is unavailable or unsuccessful.[90]

There are several damage control options available in the cervical region. Rapid insertion of a balloon catheter such as a Foley into the wound tract, inflation, and outward traction may provide tamponade and temporize bleeding. In zone III, exposure is generally difficult and the ICA may be difficult to compress. One option is to perform an arteriotomy on the common carotid after controlling it with vessel loops, insert a no. 3 or 4 Fogarty embolectomy catheter, and advance and inflate it in a serial fashion until bleeding from the distal ICA abates. This may also be done using angiographic guidance if the patient is in the fluoroscopy suite. An additional advantage of intramural balloon occlusion is that a determination of patient tolerance to ligation can be determined. If the patient manifests a focal neurologic deficit with occlusion, some form of repair should be attempted if possible. Finally, for resistant bleeding high in zone III, packing of the carotid canal with bone wax may allow tamponade for life-saving purposes.[26,90] After hemostasis is achieved with a damage control strategy, the options include: formal high cervical exploration for repair or ligation; arteriographic embolization and stenting; or 48-hour balloon occlusion. The Fogarty balloon is filled with contrast and the patient is monitored for signs of cerebral ischemia. If there is no sign of ischemia, the balloon remains in place until 48 to 72 hours after placement, at which time it is deflated and removed. The patient should be imaged with a crossover angiogram to rule out a pseudoaneurysm above the occlusion. If the patient manifests signs of ischemia, a bypass from the cervical ICA to the petrous ICA is necessary and will require the assistance of a neurosurgeon.[91]

The types of injuries that can be present with penetrating trauma are similar in type and recommended treatment to those for BCVI, although major wall disruption is much more likely. For intramural hematomas, intimal defects, or dissection with preserved distal flow, treatment similar to that for grade I and II BCVI is appropriate, namely heparinization. Stenting may be appropriate to tack down the intima for major dissections. Patients should undergo repeated imaging in 1 to 2 weeks. Pseudoaneurysm with contrast extravasation should be either observed (for small aneurysms) or stented with or without coil embolization. Heparin is risky in this situation given the possibility of rupture[90]; however, antiplatelet therapy should be used if a stent is placed. For occlusions, anticoagulation is recommended to prevent distal propagation or embolization. As previously mentioned, embolization of the thrombosed ICA is recommended.[26] Finally, carotid-jugular arteriovenous fistulae may be asymptomatic if small, but if sufficiently large they can produce high-output heart failure or coma secondary to elevated intracranial pressure. Treatment is with operative repair for lesions in zone II and embolization in zone III.[26,90]

There has historically been controversy regarding the surgical management of the patient with a cervical vascular wound and a neurologic deficit, with concern that revascularization would convert an area of ischemia into hemorrhage. This issue was addressed in 1978 by Liekweg and Greenfield.[92] Among noncomatose patients, 85% of patients with neurologic deficits who are revascularized have positive outcomes versus 50% of those ligated ($p < 0.05$). However, among comatose patients, favorable outcome with repair was seen in 27% versus 25% of patients undergoing ligation (p = not significant).[92] Current practice is to revascularize all patients with penetrating injury regardless of neurologic deficits except for coma. Patients with Glasgow Coma Score less than 8 not related to hypovolemia, hypothermia, or intoxication are likely to have an adverse outcome regardless of management. If the presentation is delayed more than 3 to 4 hours after injury, a CT scan should be obtained. If an ischemic stroke is present, revascularization is contraindicated, because this may convert to a hemorrhagic infarct.[90]

Exposure of these wounds varies by zone of injury. The simplest is zone II, which can be approached with a standard anterior sternocleidomastoid incision similar to that used for a carotid endarterectomy. Injuries to zone I

may require thoracotomy or sternotomy to access the aortic arch and the roots of the great vessels for proximal control. Zone III injuries necessitate a high skull-base dissection. Adjuncts such as mandibular subluxation or osteotomy are occasionally necessary to approach the vessels surgically, and therefore endovascular repairs are ideal if possible in this position. Before clamping the vessel, patients should be systemically heparinized with 100 U/kg. Local heparin flushes with 50 U/mL concentration should be used to irrigate locally to ensure vessels are cleared of thrombi.[90] Patients should also be given anticoagulants if observation is chosen; repeated imaging is mandatory.

Surgical options include ligation, primary repair, bypass graft with autogenous vein (Figure 45-9) or prosthetic graft, patch graft, or external carotid to internal carotid bypass for injuries near the carotid bulb (Figure 45-10). As mentioned previously, Liekweg and

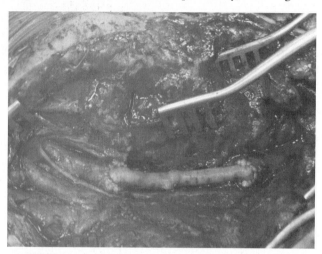

FIGURE 45-9 ■ Repair of a penetrating carotid injury with autogenous vein.

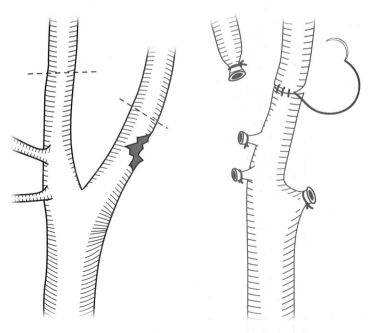

FIGURE 45-10 ■ External to internal carotid artery bypass. The proximal internal and distal external carotid arteries are ligated and the proximal external carotid artery is swung over and anastomosed to the internal carotid artery.

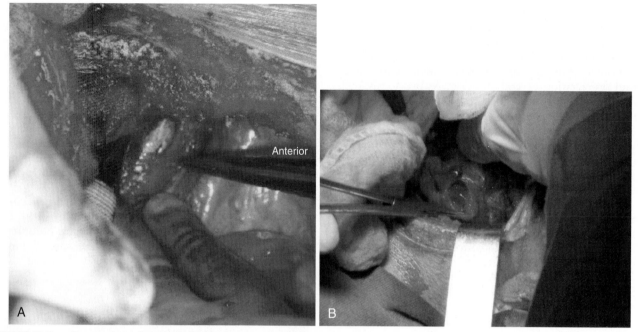

FIGURE 45-11 ■ Penetrating injury to the cervical region should prompt careful examination of the aerodigestive tract for occult injury. **A**, Tracheal injury. **B**, Esophageal injury.

Greenfield[92] demonstrated improved outcomes for revascularization over ligation for noncomatose patients. For comatose patients, they recommend repair only if there is evidence of prograde flow.[92] If bypass grafting is performed, polytetrafluoroethylene (PTFE) is appropriate for common carotid injuries; autogenous vein should be used for ICA repairs given the improved patency rates.[90] As always, prosthetic grafts should be avoided if possible in contaminated wounds.[87] If surgical repair is performed, a careful search should be made for injury to other structures, especially the aerodigestive tract (Figure 45-11). If such an injury is encountered, in addition to repairing it appropriately, the vascular suture line should be isolated by means of interposition of vascularized tissue. The sternocleidomastoid muscle can be detached from its sternal head and rotated to cover the repair. Nonoperative therapy options include angioplasty to tack down intimal flaps and coil embolization and stents for pseudoaneurysms. In patients where observation is selected as the treatment plan, repeated imaging is necessary to ensure resolution of the lesion. In the series by Fox and colleagues,[87] vertebral artery occlusions were safely observed.

ABDOMINAL VASCULAR INJURY

Almost all cases of abdominal vascular injury are caused by penetrating trauma, usually from a gunshot wound. The AAST grading system for abdominal vascular injury is shown in Table 45-3. Associated damage to gastrointestinal organs is common, yielding a lethal combination with an associated mortality rate greater than 50%. One of the problems leading to a high mortality rate is that the symptoms are often not specific. Hypotension and abdominal distension are commonly seen, and distal

TABLE 45-3   American Association for the Surgery of Trauma–Organ Injury Scale for Abdominal Vascular Injury

Grade	Description
I	Unnamed superior mesenteric artery or superior mesenteric vein branches; unnamed inferior mesenteric artery or inferior mesenteric vein branches; phrenic artery or vein; lumbar artery or vein; gonadal artery or vein; ovarian artery or vein; other unnamed small arterial or venous structures requiring ligation
II	Right, left, or common hepatic artery; splenic artery or vein; right or left gastric arteries; gastroduodenal artery; inferior mesenteric artery, trunk, or inferior mesenteric vein, trunk; primary named branches of mesenteric artery (e.g., ileocolic artery) or mesenteric vein; other named abdominal vessels requiring ligation or repair
III	Superior mesenteric vein, trunk; renal artery or vein; iliac artery or vein; hypogastric artery or vein; vena cava, infrarenal
IV	Superior mesenteric artery, trunk; celiac axis proper; vena cava, suprarenal, and infrahepatic; aorta, infrarenal
V	Portal vein; extraparenchymal hepatic vein; vena cava, retrohepatic, or suprahepatic; aorta, suprarenal, subdiaphragmatic

This classification system is applicable for extraparenchymal vascular injuries. If the vessel injury is within 2 cm of the organ parenchyma, refer to specific organ injury scale. Increase one grade for multiple grade III or IV injuries involving >50% vessel circumference. Downgrade one grade if 25% vessel circumference laceration for grades IV or V.

pulse deficits may be appreciated. In planning the exploration of potential abdominal vascular injury, it is best to have sufficient large-bore intravenous access already established, blood or blood products in the room, and the anesthesia team fully prepared for an unstable patient. If there is any sign of renal vascular or parenchymal injury, such as hematuria or an injury tract near the kidneys, a one-shot intravenous pyelogram may be helpful to confirm the presence of a contralateral functional kidney if a nephrectomy becomes necessary.

Once the team is ready, a rapid midline incision is made to enter the abdomen. Blood is evacuated, and the abdomen is packed in all four quadrants rapidly with laparotomy pads. The operation is then temporarily suspended to allow the anesthesia team to catch up with the patient's resuscitation. Once the patient's condition is sufficiently stable, a systematic exploration of the entire abdomen is performed. Proximal and distal control should be obtained for any vascular injury. If retroperitoneal hematomas are seen, a decision must be made about exploration.

The retroperitoneum can be divided into three zones. Zone 1 is the upper midline retroperitoneum, from the aortic hiatus to the aortic bifurcation longitudinally, and laterally from renal hilum to renal hilum. This zone is subdivided into the supramesocolic and inframesocolic regions. Zone 2 is the lateral perinephric area, encompassing the upper lateral retroperitoneum from the renal hilum laterally. Zone 3 is the pelvic retroperitoneum from the aortic bifurcation inferiorly.

The decision to explore a retroperitoneal hematoma is straightforward in penetrating trauma. All Zone 1 and 3 hematomas must be explored. Zone 2 hematomas are selectively explored; if the patient is hemodynamically stable and there is preoperative imaging evidence of a minor renal injury, the hematoma can be left undisturbed. Otherwise, it should be unroofed and explored for penetrating renal injury. Retroperitoneal injuries in blunt trauma should be managed differently. Zone 1 injuries must be explored, as for penetrating trauma. However, except in cases of rapid expansion, pulsatility, or free rupture into the peritoneum, zone 2 and 3 injuries should not be explored.

In zone 1a, the supramesocolic upper midline region, the critical vascular structures are the celiac axis, the superior mesenteric artery (SMA) and vein, the proximal renal arteries and distal renal veins, the supraceliac inferior vena cava, and the portal vein. Access to these structures is gained by dividing the avascular portion of the gastrohepatic ligament and entering the lesser sac. The esophagus is swept laterally away from the liver to allow the diaphragmatic crus to be isolated and divided, yielding access to the supradiaphragmatic aorta. A clamp is then placed on the aorta in this location. The infrarenal aorta is then exposed in the usual fashion and clamped to isolate the zone 1a arterial system; this allows exploration of this region of the retroperitoneum under relative vascular control.

Zone Ib structures include the infrarenal aorta and the infrarenal inferior vena cava. An infracolic hematoma should be approached proximally through the root of the mesocolon to obtain proximal control. These injuries

often involve the pancreas, duodenum, liver, and portal venous system. A left medial visceral rotation (Mattox maneuver) can be used to expose the aorta from the diaphragm to the bifurcation, all the visceral branches, and the left renal branch. Access to the right renal branch and the right common iliac artery is challenging from this exposure.

Left-sided zone 2 structures include the left kidney and its associated artery, vein, and ureter. Access to this area requires a left medial visceral rotation that includes mobilization of the left colon along the white line of Toldt and medial rotation of the spleen and tail of the pancreas. The kidney may be elevated into the field or left in situ. Access to zone 2 on the right requires mobilization of the hepatic flexure and right colon followed by a Kocher maneuver and medial rotation of the duodenum and the head of the pancreas. If this is followed by mobilization of the root of the mesentery, it is known as a Cattell-Braasch maneuver and exposes zone 2 on the right and the entire infrarenal vena cava as well as the majority of the aorta from the SMA inferiorly.

Abdominal Aortic Injury

The aorta is the most commonly injured vessel in the abdomen. Historically, this injury was rarely seen, primarily because patients would not survive to medical care after sustaining aortic trauma. In World War I, Makins reported five cases of aortic injury in the British experience (0.4% of all vascular injuries reported) with a 100% mortality.[92a] This improved slightly in World War II; three aortic injuries (0.1% of vascular trauma) were reported with a 67% mortality.[2] In a series of 470 patients with abdominal vascular injuries reported by Tyburski et al, there were 71 injuries to the aorta (15% of patients); 62% of these injuries involve the pararenal or suprarenal segments of the aorta, which are associated with 92% mortality, compared to 66% in the infrarenal segment.[93] The overwhelming majority of injuries to the aorta are from penetrating trauma, primarily gunshot wounds. Among the approximately 10% of aortic injuries from blunt trauma, motor vehicle crashes are the usual mechanism.[29,94,95]

Patients with abdominal aortic injury are usually in hypovolemic shock; the lethal triad of hypothermia, acidosis, and coagulopathy is commonly seen. Some authors are aggressive with EDT in these patients, but the results are poor and others recommend avoiding EDT in patients with abdominal vascular injury.[94] Clues to the location of injury can be gleaned from the physical examination. Injury above or involving the SMA will produce abdominal pain, pararenal involvement may lead to hematuria, or injury to the infrarenal aorta may manifest as unilateral or bilateral lower extremity ischemia.

Exposure of the suprarenal aorta can be significantly challenging, especially in a patient with multiple organ injury. The most versatile option is the anterior approach. Temporary proximal control is achieved by compression of the aorta against the vertebral bodies at the diaphragmatic hiatus. This can be accomplished most expeditiously with the surgeon's hand; this task should then be given to the assistant so that the surgeon can proceed with dissection. The lesser omentum is then opened through the bare space, the stomach and esophagus are retracted to the left, and the aorta is identified and compressed behind the esophagus. Once further dissection is completed, a clamp may be applied. If additional exposure is required, the celiac axis can be ligated and divided in a young patient; this vessel should be preserved in older patients, however, as the status of the SMA orifice is unknown. An alternative approach to the suprarenal aorta is via a left medial visceral rotation. The white line of Toldt is incised, the splenic flexure and descending colon are mobilized, and the spleen, tail of the pancreas, and stomach are rotated medially. The kidney may be left in situ or rotated up into the midline as well. This will expose the aorta from the diaphragmatic hiatus to the iliac bifurcation, providing access to the celiac axis, the first part of the SMA, the IMA, the left renal artery, and the left iliac artery; access to the right renal and iliac arteries is challenging from this approach. If additional proximal exposure is needed, the left crus of the aortic hiatus can be divided radially at the 2 o'clock position to expose the distal descending aorta. Exposure of the infrarenal aorta is best achieved via an anterior approach unless the abdomen is rather hostile; the transverse colon is elevated, the small bowel is eviscerated to the right, and the ligament of Treitz is divided. The retroperitoneum covering the aorta is then opened, and the left renal vein is identified. The left and right renal arteries are then identified after the left renal vein is retracted superiorly. Great care must be taken to ensure that there is no circumaortic or retroaortic left renal vein before the application of an aortic clamp.

Among patients who survive the initial operation, primary suturing is the most common repair technique (69% to 86%), followed by prosthetic graft in 14% to 23%; 17% to 32% of patients do not survive the operation.[94,95] Small wounds of the aorta can be closed primarily with 3-0 or 4-0 polypropylene sutures. If there are multiple aortic wounds in close proximity, they can be connected surgically to allow for a single closure. If possible, the wound should be closed transversely to prevent stenosis, although up to a 50% luminal narrowing is generally well tolerated and may be addressed at a later date.[96] If there is significant tissue loss to the aortic wall, patch aortoplasty with PTFE or interposition grafting with 12- to 16-mm Dacron woven grafts may be necessary.

Concomitant hollow viscus injury and field contamination is a common problem in aortic trauma.[97] One technique for managing this injury is to use a Dacron graft, as the literature does not support a high-risk of graft infection in young trauma patients. It is wise to thoroughly irrigate the abdomen and protect the graft with an omental pedicle if interposition grafting is performed. The alternative is ligation and delayed extraanatomic bypass.[29] The obvious downside of this approach is the need for two general anesthetic cases, as well as an iatrogenic ischemia-reperfusion insult.

In cases of blunt aortic injury, endovascular strategies may be useful. Chronic dissections are best treated by rigid, balloon-expandable stents, whereas self-expanding stents are better tolerated for acute dissections. The

TABLE 45-4	Representation of the Relative Frequency of Repair Strategies for Celiac Artery Trauma As Reported in the Literature with Associated Reported Mortality			
Repair	**Number Performed**	**Percent**	**Number Deaths**	**Mortality**
Ligation	23	63.9	9 of 16	56.3
Arteriorrhaphy	10	27.8	2 of 9	22.2
Anastomosis	1	2.8	1 of 1	100
Exsanguination	2	5.6	2 of 2	100

obvious advantage of this approach is the avoidance of a retroperitoneal dissection, aortic cross-clamping, and prevents contamination of vascular graft materials in cases of contaminated fields. Yeh and colleagues[98] describe a case report of a ruptured mycotic pseudoaneurysm treated successfully with endovascular exclusion 14 days after the initial injury and primary aortic repair. The field had been contaminated because of multiple enterotomies, leading to the mycotic pseudoaneurysm. This approach avoided a tedious, dangerous dissection through a hostile abdomen in a hemorrhaging patient; the patient survived.[98]

Celiac Artery Injury

Injury to the celiac artery is extremely rare. In a series of 2357 patients who underwent laparotomy for trauma, 13 cases of celiac artery injury were identified for a rate of 0.01%.[99] Overall, there have been 46 cases of celiac artery injury reported in the literature.[95,99-106] All but one have been secondary to penetrating trauma (97.8%). Among the cases in which the type of repair was documented, ligation was the most common procedure (63.9% of cases; Table 45-4). There was an associated mortality of 56.3% among the 16 cases in which outcome was given. Similarly, arteriorrhaphy was performed in 27.8% of cases, with a 22.2% mortality in the nine cases with outcome given. There was only one report of an end-to-end anastomosis (2.8%) with the patient not surviving. Two patients exsanguinated in the operating room. There are no reports in the literature of the use of an intraluminal shunt.

These injuries are commonly associated with zone I retroperitoneal hematomas, although they tend to be evenly distributed between supramesocolic and inframesocolic. There is an average of two nonvascular associated injuries in each case, along with an associated vascular injury in approximately two thirds of cases.[99]

Similar to other retroperitoneal artery injuries, approach to these injuries usually requires either a left or right medial visceral rotation. Dissection of the vessel is challenging because of the dense neurolymphatic plexus surrounding the takeoff of the celiac artery. Once vascular control is established, a decision between ligation and attempted repair is required. Table 45-4 presents the mortality associated with different repair strategies; however, there is likely bias as arteriorrhaphy is generally useful in less devastating injuries. Jurkovich and colleagues[18] documented 29 hepatic artery injuries in their series; the locations were in the common hepatic artery in 6 (20.7%), the proper hepatic artery in 6 (20.7%), the left hepatic artery in 6 (20.7%), and the right hepatic artery in 11 (37.9%). If it is possible to repair the artery expeditiously with a simple lateral repair, the attempt to do so is justified; however, ligation is likely the best approach for more complex injuries. The celiac trunk has a rich collateral circulation; therefore ligation of the splenic and left gastric arteries may be performed without hesitation. Ligation of the common hepatic is relatively safe if the gastroduodenal artery remains patent. Ligation of the proper hepatic artery is higher risk and should not be performed concomitantly with portal vein ligation; an alternative would be to consider a small intraluminal shunt in this position.

Complications of celiac ligation are rare. There are no reports of bowel ischemia, although there is one report of gallbladder necrosis.[106] Because of the usual association with trauma to other vascular and nonvascular structures, rapid consideration of damage control and a planned second look operation are recommended.

Superior Mesenteric Artery Injury

Injury to the SMA is a highly lethal injury because of several factors. It is difficult to access, it supplies a large portion of the gastrointestinal tract, and injury to the SMA is often associated with severe injury to surrounding structures such as small bowel, colon, liver, and pancreaticoduodenal complex. Operative findings include hemoperitoneum, a mesenteric hematoma around the SMA, and bowel ischemia. The management of this injury begins with direct compression of the likely site of trauma, followed by cross-clamping of the aorta proximal to the origin of the SMA. If the injury is retropancreatic, either a left medial visceral rotation or a direct approach by dividing the neck of the pancreas can be used to access the artery. The infrapancreatic SMA can be isolated by direct dissection. It is generally wise to avoid exploration of stable hematomas or those found in blunt trauma cases in the absence of bowel ischemia. Angiography or color-flow Doppler interrogation is helpful to delineate the nature of the injury in questionable cases.

In 1972, Fullen and colleagues[107] presented a classification system of SMA injury, which is presented in Table 45-5. Zone I extends from the takeoff of the SMA to the first branch, the inferior pancreaticoduodenal. This portion of the artery is retropancreatic, increasing the difficulty of access. Zone II extends from the inferior pancreaticoduodenal artery to the middle colic artery. Zone III includes the remainder of the trunk and zone IV represents the segmental branches. Fullen and colleagues[107] also described four grades of ischemia (see Table 45-5). These ischemic grades seem to correlate well with the location of SMA injury.

SMA injuries are rare. No cases of wartime injury to the SMA were presented in any of the landmark papers from Debakey and Simeone, Hughes, or Rich and colleagues.[2,5,108] The most extensive series of patients with SMA injuries in the literature was reported by Asensio and colleagues in 2001.[109] In this study, 13 institutions contributed retrospective data on patients with SMA injuries between 1990 and 1999. A total of 250 patients were reviewed, and many interesting observations were made. First, there was a high mortality rate of 39%. The majority of deaths (71%) occurred in the operating room or within the first 24 hours. Contrary to expectations, there was an even proportion of blunt and penetrating trauma in this series.

Ligation was the most frequent repair option (72%), followed by primary repair (22%). The remainder of patients underwent attempted grafting with either saphenous vein or PTFE. There was only one shunt used in this series. Heparinization was infrequent. There was a high likelihood of associated injuries. Nonvascular injuries included small bowel (64%), colon (43%), liver (28%), duodenum (24%), and pancreas (22%). Other abdominal organs were injured approximately 15% of the time. The biliary tree proper was injured in only 3% of cases.

The most common associated vascular injury was to the superior mesenteric vein (SMV), in 33% of cases. Interestingly, there was no mortality difference whether the vein was ligated or repaired (44.2% vs. 40.0%; $p = 0.916$). In approximately 5% to 10% of cases, other vascular structures were injured. Not surprisingly, the lethal triad of metabolic acidosis, hypothermia, and coagulopathy was frequent, seen in approximately 50% of cases. The most frequent injury-specific complications were gut ischemia (20%) and infarction (15%). Of sixteen attempted graft repairs (10 with vein graft and 6 with PTFE), three failed (19%).

In the patients in this study, there was a correlation between the zone of injury and mortality (Table 45-6)—not a surprising finding, but a fact addressed in only one other study.[110] Mortality did not, however, correlate with the type of repair performed. Also notable was that

TABLE 45-5 Fullen's Anatomic Classification of Superior Mesenteric Artery Injury by Zone and Grade

Zone	Segment of Superior Mesenteric Artery	Grade	Ischemic Category	Bowel Segments Affected
I	Trunk proximal to first major branch (inferior pancreaticoduodenal)	1	Maximal	Jejunum, ileum, right colon
II	Trunk between inferior pancreaticoduodenal and middle colic	2	Moderate	Major segment of small bowel, right colon, or both
III	Trunk distal to middle colic	3	Minimal	Minor segments of small bowel or right colon
IV	Segmental branches, jejunal, ileal, or colic	4	None	No ischemic bowel

TABLE 45-6 Mortality by Type of Surgical Procedure and Fullen's Anatomic Zones (n = 233)

Procedure	Zone I	Zone II	Zone III	Zone IV	Total
Ligation	77% (17/22)	43% (6/14)	26% (6/23)	24% (24/99)	34% (53/158)
Primary repair + interposition vein graft	77% (10/13)	45% (5/11)	33% (4/12)	17% (1/6)	48% (20/42)
Ligation + primary repair + interposition vein graft	100% (2/2)	0% (0/1)	0% (0/1)	0% (0/2)	33% (2/6)
Interposition graft – PTFE	80% (4/5)	100% (1/1)	—	—	83% (5/6)
None of the above	67% (6/9)	43% (3/7)	25% (1/4)	0% (0/1)	48% (10/21)
TOTAL	76% (39/51)	44% (15/34)	28% (11/40)	23% (25/108)	39% (90/233)

From Asensio JA, Britt LD, Borzotta A, et al: Multiinstitutional experience with the management of superior mesenteric artery injuries, J Am Coll Surg 193:354–365, 2001. Reproduced by permission.
PTFE, Polytetrafluoroethylene.

vascular shunting was used only once in this series. Given the combination of extensive physiologic insult from exsanguination and frequent challenging injuries to nearby organs, TVS may be a measure worth investigating, especially in zone I and II injuries. In 1995, Reilly and colleagues[111] reported this technique being successfully used in a 31-year-old trauma patient.

Given these findings, some recommendations for management of these injuries follow. Injury to the SMA should be suspected in patients with early signs of malperfused bowel, especially in the small bowel and ascending colon. Additional signs of SMA injury include a retroperitoneal hematoma, seen in 94% of patients with these injuries in the series by Asensio.[109] The majority of these hematomas arise in the supramesocolic midline, but a significant percentage had retroperitoneal hematomas either in the inframesocolic compartment or zones II or III.

In terms of management, plan to move early to damage control measures. Any evidence of massive blood loss, coagulopathy, shock, or acidosis should prompt temporizing measures or ligation over a definitive repair. Likewise, ligation of the SMV should be considered if the alternative is a lengthy or challenging repair. Be thorough and search for associated injuries as isolated SMA injuries are extremely rare. Expect that heparinization will be contraindicated because of the nature of the patient's injuries. Given the high likelihood of associated pancreatic injury, it is critical to isolate the vascular anastomosis from a pancreatic leak using omentum or other surrounding soft tissues. If a graft to the SMA is planned, it should be taken off the distal aorta to move the anastomosis from the region of the pancreas. Finally, plan for another operation within 24 hours if the patient's condition is stable.

Regarding injuries to the SMA, the discussion of ligation of the artery being preferable to repair in an unstable trauma patient is reminiscent of recommendations for early ligation of extremity arterial injury to minimize mortality in battlefield conditions before and during World War II. There have been tremendous advances in the management of the extremity arterial injury in the past decades, leading to a significant improvement in both survival and limb salvage. The management of SMA trauma, however, lags in terms of survivable options, because of the common presence of associated trauma and the overwhelming physiologic insult this injury

causes. Hopefully further research in both surgical techniques and critical care will yield such improvements for the management of this devastating injury.

Renal Artery Injury

Injury to the renal vein and artery occurs in approximately 6% to 16% of traumatic injuries.[94,112] The largest review of renal artery trauma was a series of 154 cases in which 84% were due to penetrating mechanisms.[113] Knudson and colleagues reported 43 blunt renal vascular injuries over a 16-year period.[114] These two reports comprise the majority of the experience with renal vascular trauma in the literature. Renal trauma tends to occur more frequently on the left than on the right, given the protective effects of the overlying liver and the longer left renal vein, making avulsion injury more likely on the left.[115,116] Sixty percent of injuries are isolated to renal arteries, 30% are related to veins, and 10% are combined arteriovenous injuries.[113] These injuries rarely occur in isolation; up to 75% have other intraabdominal injuries as well.[112,114,117] Spleen, liver, and renal parenchymal trauma are most common.

In a study of 302 abdominal vascular injuries of which 88% were due to penetrating trauma, there were 14 renal artery injuries, 8 of which were isolated injuries, and 34 renal vein injuries, none of which were isolated. The overall mortality rate was 54%, combined arterial trauma mortality was 66.7%, isolated arterial mortality was 37.5%, and renal vein trauma mortality was 55.8%.[94]

Renal vascular injury can occur in several different ways. Vascular stretch and intimal disruption can occur during a deceleration injury, leading to intimal flaps and thrombosis. Vascular compression against vertebral bodies can be caused by compressive injuries, causing thrombosis, avulsion, or spasm.[118] Penetrating injuries account for 4% to 24% of all renovascular trauma and lead to direct disruption of the vascular wall.[119] Overall, 44% of renal vascular injuries are due to thrombosis, 12% avulsion, 7% intimal flaps, 4% lacerations, and 4% vascular spasm.[113]

Workup of the patient with a renovascular injury is challenging. Physical examination is rarely helpful in diagnosis, and delayed presentation is common because the focus is generally on other more apparent life-threatening injuries.[118] Clark and colleagues[113] reported that of 250 blunt renal injuries, 50% did not receive treatment within 3 days because of delayed or missed diagnosis. One major indicator that renal injury may be present is hematuria, either gross or microscopic. Microscopic hematuria was seen in 54% to 89% of patients with renal vascular trauma.[115,119-122] CT scans are useful for the diagnosis of renal vascular trauma; they are able to demonstrate regional or global renal perfusion deficits, perirenal hematomas, or extravasation of contrast.[123,124] One drawback is that they tend to miss intimal flaps.[125] Intravenous pyelography has been the traditional mainstay of diagnosis before the advent of multislice CT scanners. It remains a useful adjunct in that it is portable and can be performed intraoperatively. The absence of the kidney on the image is a sign of severe injury. It is rather nonspecific, which is its major drawback.[118] Yet when used liberally, it has been shown to decrease the time to diagnosis and treatment of renal injury to 6 and 7 hours, respectively.[120] The other major diagnostic modality is arteriorraphy, which is highly sensitive for injuries, including intimal flaps, and is also therapeutic. The drawback is that arteriorraphy is invasive and labor intensive, and in some places it cannot be performed intraoperatively.

Renal salvage is effective in only 25% to 35% of cases. The length of time between injury and reperfusion is a major factor in the outcome of the kidney. Irreversible damage begins occurring at 30 to 90 minutes of warm ischemia time.[121] Relative contraindications to attempted repair include the following: multiple injuries, prolonged ischemic time, hilar injuries, extensive associated arterial injury, and a normal contralateral kidney.[126] The presence of two or more of the listed factors suggests that nephrectomy may be preferable for the patient, especially if there is a normal contralateral kidney. In the case that the injury is bilateral or the patient has only one functional kidney, efforts at repair should be undertaken at longer ischemia times, up to 18 hours.[118] Lock and colleagues reported a 42% success rate with repair; the mean ischemic time for successful repair was 12.3 hours, compared to 26 hours for unsuccessful repairs.[121] In a report by Clark and colleagues,[113] only 15% of unilateral renal vascular injuries were repaired versus 50% of bilateral injuries. In this series, 24% of patients underwent immediate nephrectomy.[113]

There are two situations in which no repair efforts should be undertaken. The first, similar to the minimal aortic injury, is the renal arterial intimal flap. The risk of thrombosis is 1.5% to 4%; in the rare patient who suffers thrombosis, the outcome is poor regardless of whether an intervention is performed.[118,127] The other situation that calls for nonoperative management is an ischemic time greater than 24 hours, unless there is active bleeding, infection, or the patient develops hypertension. Otherwise, the likelihood of renal salvage is virtually nonexistent and the risk to the patient from an operation is not justified.[128]

Renovascular injuries should be considered major vascular injuries.[112] The indications for exploration include a large, expanding perinephric hematoma, displacement of viscera, a palpable thrill, or a known vascular injury. Proximal vascular control should be secured first via transperitoneal exposure of the perirenal aortic segment.

The left renal vein is identified and retracted superiorly to expose the origins of the renal arteries.[118] Once proximal control is secured, a Mattox maneuver is performed to access the left kidney or a wide Kocher maneuver is used to access the right kidney. Distal vascular control can be achieved with fingertip pressure or a balloon catheter. The arterial wall should be debrided gently. Frequent irrigation with heparinized saline to prevent distal embolization is critical. The kidney should be perfused intermittently with iced heparinized saline to maintain viability. Just before completion of the repair, a thrombectomy catheter should be gently passed along the proximal and distal vessel. An associated renal vein injury on the right should be repaired if possible, otherwise the kidney should be removed. Ligation of the right renal vein is incompatible with function of the right kidney. Distal (near the IVC) injuries of the left renal vein can be safely ligated if repair is complex, because venous drainage will occur through the adrenal, gonadal, and posterior lumbar vessels.[118]

As with other arteries, a variety of repair options are available and should be tailored to the situation. Lateral arteriorraphy, primary anastomosis, vein patch, or interposition grafting with PTFE are valid options. Another alternative is the use of segments of resected vessels (e.g., splenic artery if a splenectomy is performed for trauma).[126] If an interposition graft is used, performance of the distal anastomosis first will simplify the procedure, as the proximal anastomosis is technically less challenging. One additional option with renal trauma is ex vivo reconstruction and reimplantation of the kidney. In the 48 renovascular injuries reported by Asensio and colleagues[94] in a series of 302 abdominal vascular injuries, there were 2 primary arterial repairs, 9 arterial ligations, 10 venous repairs, and 17 venous ligations; 10 patients died before repair. Mannitol (1 g/kg) is generally administered after the repair is completed.[118] The definition of successful renal revascularization is the prevention of renal failure in patients with bilateral renal injury or the prevention of renovascular hypertension for unilateral injury.[118] Success rates for repair range from 23% to 38%,[113,115,117,121] and most successful repairs are performed within 3 to 18 hours after the injury.[113,119] Repairs that are more complex than lateral arteriorraphy have a success rate of only 36% compared to 85% for simple repair.[126]

The final option is nephrectomy. This was performed in 47% of 487 cases reviewed by Bongard.[128a] There is controversy over the use of early nephrectomy. Proponents recommend it for all injuries not diagnosed early or amenable to repair, whereas others recommend waiting and performing nephrectomy only in the subset of patients who develop hypertension.[117,121,129] Renovascular hypertension develops in 4% to 50% of nonoperatively treated and 35% of operatively treated patients; most cases appear within the first year.[113,117]

Injury to the Inferior Vena Cava

Injury to the inferior vena cava (IVC) has historically been a highly lethal injury, and contemporary series continue to document significant mortality rates. In 1961,

Ochsner and colleagues reported that 36% of patients sustaining injuries to the IVC would not survive to hospitalization and that 57% of those who made it to the hospital would die.[130] Current estimates of mortality range from 31% to 70%.[17,21-23,25] Predictors of mortality in this patient population include shock, anatomic location of injury, number of associated injuries, and concomitant aortic trauma.[17,21,23,27] The incidence of this injury pattern is low; Netto and colleagues[23] identified caval injuries in 0.2% of all blunt trauma, and Navsaria and colleagues[22] reported caval injuries in 2.3% of patients undergoing trauma laparotomy.

Caval injury is secondary to penetrating trauma in 68% to 96% of cases and is associated with 48% mortality. Of these, gunshot wounds are the most prevalent (75%-94%). Knife wounds are less prevalent (2%-20%) and are associated with infrequent mortality. Shotgun wounds are generally devastating; Rosengart and colleagues[25] cited a 14% incidence in their series of shotgun wounds for penetrating caval injuries with an associated 100% mortality. Blunt injuries are less frequent than penetrating injuries, ranging from 7% to 22%, but are associated with higher mortality (63% in the Rosengart series).[17,21,22,25,27]

The most common preoperative factor associated with mortality is severe or refractory hypotension. In the series by Rosengart and colleagues,[25] patients in shock had a 76% mortality compared with a 30% in patients who were hemodynamically stable preoperatively. Interestingly, the mortality was only 33% for patients who were in shock but responded to fluid resuscitation and maintained hemodynamic stability throughout the operation. Those who were in shock and remained so during the operation had a mortality rate of 86%. Finally, those who were hemodynamically stable and became hypotensive had a mortality of 67%. There were no deaths among patients who were normotensive throughout. The conclusion is that if initial efforts at resuscitation fail, immediate laparotomy and damage control should be instituted given the lethality of these wounds.[25]

Another significant predictor of outcome is the location of the injury. The cava is divided into four zones: the infrarenal vena cava extends from the iliac bifurcation to the renal veins, the suprarenal cava extends from the renal veins to the inferior surface of the liver, the retrohepatic cava extends from the inferior border of the liver to the diaphragmatic hiatus, and the supradiaphragmatic cava extends from the diaphragm to the atriocaval junction. Incidence of infrarenal caval injury ranges from 33% to 54% with mortality ranging from 23% to 41%; these injuries are fairly accessible and amenable to repair or early ligation. Incidence rates for suprarenal caval injuries range from 21% to 33% with 38% to 75% mortality, due to decreased accessibility and the patient being less able to tolerate ligation for damage control. Retrohepatic caval injuries are a major challenge to trauma surgeons. Their incidence is 15% to 27%, and mortality ranges from 66% to 93%.[17,21,25,27] The vena cava in this position is encircled by suspensory ligaments, the diaphragm, and liver parenchyma and accepts the hepatic veins at its superior extent. All potentially lethal wounds of the cava in this location have two things in common: the venous

wound itself and disruption of the supporting tissues that can contain the hematoma. Buckman and colleagues[131] classified these injuries into two types: type A, which is more common, is an intraparenchymal venous injury and predominantly bleeds through a disrupted liver capsule; type B is extraparenchymal, and bleeding occurs through disrupted suspensory ligaments, diaphragm, or both.[131] Access to these injuries is surgically challenging and often leads to exsanguination once the hematoma is unroofed. Finally, suprahepatic caval injuries are fairly rare (8%-10%) with substantial mortality (50%-100%) because of the proximity to cardiac structures and difficulty of exposure.[25,27]

The diagnosis of caval injuries has several pitfalls. In patients who fail to respond or respond only transiently to resuscitation, a caval injury should be suspected in the appropriate clinical setting. The difficulty is that this tenet holds for vascular injuries in other locations as well, and exploration with possible loss of containment is the cost of diagnosis. If the patient responds to resuscitation long enough to undergo CT imaging, the study itself may be misleading. In one series in which six patients with subsequently identified caval injuries underwent preoperative CT scanning, no active extravasation was identified. Other findings suggestive of caval injury are retroperitoneal hematoma centered on the vena cava, irregular vena caval contour, and caval filling defects.[23,132,133] A high degree of suspicion must be present to identify these subtle findings on a trauma scan.

The most common associated nonvascular injuries in order of frequency are liver, small bowel, colon, kidney, and duodenum. The presence of associated vascular injuries is a highly lethal combination; the overall mortality of this pattern is 66%, ranging from 50% to 100% depending on the vessel or vessels injured.[17,22,25]

The surgical approach to patients with caval injury begins with rapid transport to the operating room. The patient should be resuscitated with warm intravenous fluids as they are being prepared for exploration. The initial exposure should be via a long midline incision, with preparation for a midline sternotomy or right thoracotomy if the situation warrants supradiaphragmatic exposure. If a hematoma is seen behind the ascending colon or along the duodenal loop, a caval injury should be suspected. For infrahepatic exposure, a Cattell-Braasch maneuver should be performed. If the injury is suprahepatic, proximal control in the chest necessitates either sternotomy or thoracotomy. In cases of retrohepatic injury, a decision must be made as to whether dividing the suspensory ligaments and medially rotating the liver is likely to improve chances for patient survival or whether the loss of containment will lead to rapid exsanguination; the critical issue is whether the containing structures are intact. If not, there is nothing to be lost by improving exposure, but if they are intact, exposure may cost the patient the one possible chance at containment and survival. Another potential risk of surgical exposure is entrainment of venous air and air embolism. If there is no tamponade of hemorrhage for retrohepatic caval injuries, there are three possible options. It is critical to acknowledge that the patient is in dire straits at this time, and the simplest solution that works should be used.

First, pack the area tightly to "restore, replace, or reinforce the containment structures" of the liver. Another option that has been used, but is almost universally associated with adverse outcomes, is lobar resection; patients in unstable condition rarely tolerate this. Finally, direct repair with or without vascular isolation has been described, but it suffers from the same problems as lobar resection, which is severe mortality.[131] Two techniques have been described to isolate the venous injury in retrohepatic caval trauma: hepatic isolation and atriocaval shunting. Hepatic isolation is performed by placing a supraceliac aortic clamp, followed by a clamp on the proximal and distal IVC, and finally portal triad occlusion with a Pringle maneuver. This technique was originally described by Waltuck and colleagues[134] and Yellin and colleagues.[135] This maneuver may be tolerated if the patient is volume resuscitated (a rare occurrence in retrohepatic caval trauma). If the decrease in venous return causes the patient's condition to become unstable, as it will in hypovolemic patients, consider atriocaval shunt at this point.[21] The atriocaval shunt was first described by Schrock and colleagues in 1968.[136] After sternotomy or right thoracotomy, the right atrium is grasped with a clamp, a purse-string suture placed in the right atrial appendage, a cardiotomy is performed in the middle of the stitch, and a chest tube, at least 32 French in size, or a 9-mm endotracheal tube is placed into the right atrium through the purse-string suture. The tube should be prepared ahead of time with side holes cut to allow adequate blood flow proximal and distal. Rummel tourniquets are used at both ends to secure the shunt in place; alternatively, for the endotracheal tube, the balloon may be inflated to exclude the inferior cava[21] (Figure 45-12).

Once the injury is exposed, hemostasis should be achieved with either fingertip occlusion for small injuries or proximal and distal compression with sponge sticks for larger injuries. A side-biting Satinsky clamp may be used to exclude an injury, or a balloon catheter may be inserted into the cava to control bleeding and allow identification of the wound edges. If possible a simple lateral venorraphy with polypropylene should be performed. However, if the injury is complex or the patient's condition is unstable, ligation may be the best option. Contemporary series cite ligation in 10% to 25% of cases, with mortality rates of 66% to 75%, generally because of the degree of physiologic compromise that leads to ligation. Patients generally tolerate infrarenal ligation reasonably well, but suprarenal ligation, while occasionally necessary as a lifesaving maneuver, is a morbid procedure. Mortality rates for suprarenal ligation are greater than 50%. There is, however, a case report of a patient surviving suprarenal ligation and recovering normal renal function after a limited course of dialysis. Long-term morbidity, such as edema, chronic venous insufficiency, or thromboembolism, is surprisingly infrequent after caval ligation.[22,27]

Patients undergoing caval interruption should be considered for below-knee fasciotomy, which was required in 10 of 13 (77%) survivors of caval ligation in the series documented by Sullivan and colleagues.[27] Indications to perform fasciotomy include: firm and incompressible lower extremity compartments, intraoperative measurement of compartment pressures greater than 25 to

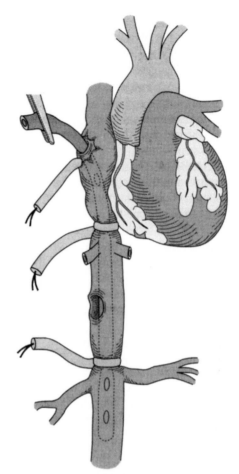

FIGURE 45-12 ■ Transatrial intracaval shunt in place. (From Pachter L, Liang HG, Hofstetter SR: Liver and biliary trauma. In Moore EE, Mattox KL, Feliciano DV, editors: Trauma, ed 2, East Norwalk, CT, 1991, Appleton & Lange, p 450.)

30 mm Hg, combined arterial and venous injury, arterial injury leading to greater than 6 hours of ischemic time, and crush injury.[27]

If the patient is sufficiently stable and the injury is amenable, primary venorraphy is the most expeditious approach to restore venous continuity. This surgical approach is possible in 55% to 73% of cases, with mortality ranging from 30% to 44%.[17,21,25] A high percentage of suprarenal injuries are typically repaired primarily because of the morbidity of ligation. Navsaria and colleagues used lateral repair in 83% of cases of suprarenal injuries compared to 29% of infrarenal injuries.[22]

If the patient's condition is stable and expertise is immediately available, the patient may do well with a complex repair such as a vein patch or prosthetic graft. Reported mortality for these approaches is nearly 100%, however, highlighting the rarity of appropriateness of this approach and the critical requirement of selecting the correct patient.[17] For minimal injuries or contained hematomas, observation in the hemodynamically stable patient is a reasonable plan. Tremendous vigilance is necessary, however, to rapidly diagnose loss of containment. Failure to recognize this complication will likely be fatal to the patient.

In summary, caval injuries are low-pressure wounds that are amenable to local tissue containment in some cases. Evidence of refractory hypotension suggests free rupture, and expeditious vascular control is necessary for survival. It is important to make an early and correct decision about whether to explore a hematoma or to pack and allow it to tamponade, which surgical repair option to consider (and if thinking of anything more complex than a lateral repair, being sure that the patient will tolerate the blood loss and extra operating room time), and how best to expose the injury. Finally, awareness of the potential complications, such as compartment syndrome or venous outflow obstruction, will mitigate the risk to the patient in the postoperative period.

Portal and Mesenteric Venous Injury

Injury to the portal and mesenteric venous system is an uncommon and devastating injury. It occurs in approximately 1 in 1000 trauma admissions, and in approximately 1% of patients requiring laparotomy for trauma.[16,24] Because of the rarity of this injury, few surgeons develop familiarity with the management of this condition, and multi-institutional retrospective reviews are generally required to study the management of this problem.[18] Mortality ranges from 40% to 72%, behind aortic injury and retrohepatic caval injuries for lethality.* Intraoperative uncontrolled hemorrhage is the primary cause of death in these patients, responsible for 38% to 92% of deaths.[11,14,18,24] Fraga and colleagues[16] evaluated the trend in mortality versus time and found worse mortality in the recent era, leading to the concern that this injury may be "too lethal" for current management strategies.[16] Unsurprisingly, the major predictor of mortality is shock, with hemodynamically stable patients sustaining 17% to 43% mortality versus 55% to 91% for patients in shock.[14,16] The degree of injury to the vessel also predicts outcome. Associated injuries, especially vascular injuries, are another significant predictor of outcome.[14,18] The inferior vena cava and the SMA are the most common additional vascular injuries in these patients,[11,14] whereas there is a broad range of associated hollow and solid organ injuries. Jurkovich and colleagues[18] described the most common location of portal vein injuries as being in the hepatoduodenal ligament (in 68% of injuries), facilitating a double Pringle maneuver for isolation. Exploration of these patients is almost always notable for a retroperitoneal hematoma, although its location may be misleading; whereas 73% of hematomas are the midline (zone I), 18% are in zone II, and 9% are in zone III.[11]

There is a variety of surgical options described in the literature for this complex of injuries. The safest approach, however, is to rapidly assess whether there is a straightforward repair option available and whether the patient will tolerate the attempt. If the answer to either question is "no," the best option is ligation. Child[140] performed a series of experiments in 1950 that led to his belief that 80% of humans would tolerate ligation of the portal vein, although it is notable that these experiments

did not account for the massive physiologic derangements of multisystem trauma. It is clearly the best option, however, in a patient in unstable condition.[16] Patients may develop systemic hypotension and portal hypertension that usually resolves over the next week. These patients tend to require aggressive fluid resuscitation, however, to compensate for 50% reduction in sequestered blood volume.[14] Asensio reported an incidence of this syndrome of approximately 5% in patients undergoing SMV ligation.[11] However, if the patient should not develop collateral circulation, another option may become necessary. There is a case report of a delayed interposition graft at 15 hours after initial exploration where the SMV was oversewn, likely with many of the collaterals including the middle colic vein, with a good outcome.[141] It is also recommended that all patients with ligated portomesenteric venous vessels undergo a second look operation at 24 to 48 hours postoperatively.[142] Portal vein ligation has been performed in 0% to 50% of injuries in several major series, with mortality rates ranging from 27% to 100%.[14,16,18,24,137] Stone and colleagues[137] discovered that when they performed portal vein ligation as a last-ditch effort after a failed attempt at reconstruction, the mortality was approximately 60%, whereas when they went to ligation early for clearly nonreconstructible damage, the mortality fell to 15%.[137] Similarly, SMV ligation has been performed in 17% to 60% of cases, with mortality ranging from 15% to 50%.[11,14,16,137,143] It is crucial to note that if the hepatic artery is concomitantly injured, patency must be restored to either the portomesenteric circulation or the hepatic artery, because occlusion of both is incompatible with life.[24]

Primary repair of the portal vein and superior mesenteric vein has been successful in 38% to 100% and 31% to 64% of series, respectively, with mortality rates of 14% to 67% and 29% to 45%, respectively.* Complex repairs such as end-to-end anastomosis, interposition grafts, saphenous vein patches, and portocaval shunts have been attempted with poor outcomes. There are currently no reports of the use of shunts in the portomesenteric circulation for trauma.

The operative approach to the portomesenteric system is through a right medial visceral rotation, which can be extended to a Cattell-Braasch maneuver to achieve full exposure of the retroperitoneum. The top priority is to identify and control the source of hemorrhage. Once exposure is obtained, pressure from packs or the operator's hand should be used to obtain initial control. In most cases, a Pringle maneuver will control vascular inflow, and a double Pringle maneuver will isolate the injury and may allow for a lateral venorrhaphy in the majority of portal venous injuries. Access to the portal-SMV confluence may require division of the neck of the pancreas. Finally, as previously stated, all patients with trauma to this system should be considered for second-look laparotomy in 24 to 48 hours postoperatively.

A variety of postoperative complications have been described. Aside from the previously described sequestration syndrome, other documented complications include

---

*References 11, 14, 16, 18, 24, 137-139.

*References 14, 16, 18, 24, 137, 143.

sepsis and wound infection in nearly 80%,[24] intraabdominal abscess, pancreatitis, thrombosis of the portomesenteric system, hemorrhage, and respiratory failure. This is a challenging patient population to manage, because of to the initial physiologic insult and the commonly associated multiple organ and vascular injuries.

Pelvic Vascular Injury

Injuries to the pelvic vasculature are challenging to manage and tend to be associated with significant morbidity and mortality. One of the major problems with these injuries is their inaccessibility. Fortunately, they are also fairly rare. In World War I, Makins reported a 0.4% incidence of iliac artery injury.[92a] This incidence rose over subsequent conflicts to 1.7% in World War II,[2] 2.3% in Korea,[5] and 2.6% in Vietnam,[108] likely resulting from improvements in initial resuscitation and rapid transport to medical facilities. Current estimates of incidence is 3.5% of patients with significant pelvic trauma (abbreviated injury score [AIS] 3 or 4 pelvic fractures).[13] The mechanism for most pelvic vascular injuries is penetration, ranging from 64% to 95%,[9,144] and the most common mechanism of penetrating injury is the gunshot wound, representing 86% to 91% of penetrating injuries,[9,12,15,41] with a smaller proportion being from stab wounds and blast fragments.

Mortality rates have been reported from 21% to 42%, with higher mortality seen in combined arteriovenous injuries.[9,12,15,41,144] The mortality of these wounds is primarily related to whether the hematoma is contained or free. Haan and colleagues[144] reviewed their 10-year experience with pelvic vascular injury and demonstrated a significant correlation between free rupture of the hematoma and presentation in shock. Shock was the single biggest predictor of mortality in their study, with mortality being 55% if shock was present at admission versus 18% if the patient was hemodynamically stable. In addition, all mortalities in the penetrating trauma cohort and 36% of the blunt trauma cohort who died within the first 24 hours were secondary to refractory shock.[144] Other studies have supported uncontained hemorrhage and shock being responsible for mortality.[9,12,41] Other factors associated with mortality were iliac artery combined with caval injury (incidence 20%, 63%-71% mortality) or aortic injury (incidence 13%, mortality 100%).[9,15,144] Current battlefield studies have shown that protective body armor worn by soldiers was associated with 100% survival among patients with penetrating pelvic vascular injuries.[41] The early use of damage control principles has shown promise of decreasing mortality; of those who underwent an "abbreviated laparotomy," 7% died and 38% underwent a standard laparotomy for trauma.[12]

The clinical presentation of these patients can be misleading, because the vascular examination is normal in two thirds of patients, given the extensive collateral network in the pelvic region, yet hypotension is common.[15] Ryan and colleagues[145] suggested a triad of clinical findings that should alert the astute surgeon to the possibility of penetrating pelvic vascular injury: wounds below the umbilicus, a positive abdominal examination, and hypotension.[145] Other injuries seen in penetrating trauma include small bowel (55%-63%), colon (25%-37%), and renal (26%).[9,12] Alternatively, for blunt trauma, there is a tetrad of common injuries: pelvic vascular injury, pelvic fracture, colon injury, and genitourinary tract injury.[13,144] Upon exploration of patients with pelvic trauma, multiple vascular injuries are commonly encountered. Although retroperitoneal hematomas are common, they are present in zone III in only 53% to 58% of cases, with zone I hematomas occurring in 25% and zone II occurring in 17%.[9,12] The most common injury pattern is isolated venous injury (36% to 51%), with the common iliac vein being the most common venous structure injured (51%). Isolated iliac arterial injury occurs in 24% to 27% of cases, with trauma to the hypogastric artery and its branches being the most common injury (47%). Combined arterial and venous injuries occur in 25% to 38% of cases. In one series, there seemed to be an association between blunt trauma and the presence of arterial injury.[9,12,144]

There are a variety of operative approaches for pelvic vascular injury. The selection of the appropriate technique must account for the nature of the injury, the accessibility of the injury, and the physiologic state of the patient. For patients in unstable condition, damage control alternatives for pelvic arterial injury are shunts and ligation.[12,15,41] Shunting of the pelvic vessels is not a commonly used technique, but there is a case report of bilateral 14-French Argyle shunts being used in a patient in extremis who made an uneventful recovery after subsequent revision with a Dacron graft.[146] Patients who undergo arterial ligation must be watched closely for signs of distal ischemia, which may necessitate revision or extraanatomic bypass to prevent limb loss. Iliac veins and hypogastric arteries and veins can be ligated more safely.[9,41] One author reported the use of a Palma procedure staged after common iliac vein ligation to prevent the development of chronic venous obstructive symptoms with good outcomes.[147] For patients in stable condition, primary repair is ideal for venous injuries and limited arterial injuries. Other alternatives include end-to-end anastomosis, autogenous graft, prosthetic graft, or vein patch.[9,12,41,148]

The key to successful surgical management of these patients is rapid intervention with immediate exposure and securing proximal and distal vascular control. Time from arrival to the operating room should be minimized, as should fluid resuscitation before achieving vascular control. Any patient arriving in shock with signs of pelvic trauma should be assumed to have an uncontained pelvic hematoma, which is true in 78% of cases.[144] Access is via a midline laparotomy, incision of the white line of Toldt, and medial rotation of the left and right viscera. Rapidly achieve finger tamponade if the bleeding is free; if the hematoma is contained, do not disrupt it until proximal and distal control are secured. If it is not clear which vessel is the source of bleeding, perform total pelvic exclusion by clamping, in order, the aorta, the right and left iliac vessels, and finally the IVC.[15] Although rapid packing is appropriate, keep in mind that packing will not work for arterial bleeding, and surgical control is mandatory if the patient is to survive. At this point, a decision is made regarding the stability of the patient. Definitive repair can be undertaken for patients in stable condition. As mentioned previously, primary arteriorrhaphy, end-to-end anastomosis, autogenous graft with vein or hypogastric artery, or prosthetic graft are options. While contamination is a relative contraindication for artificial grafts, contamination did not lead to any graft infections in one series.[12] Another author recommended PTFE for expedited repair despite signs of contamination, although current management trends are moving toward temporary shunting if rapid establishment of vascular continuity is required for patient in unstable condition.[15] If ligation is the bailout option chosen, the window of time when extraanatomic bypass is likely to succeed may be shorter than one would think. In a series of five patients undergoing emergency iliac artery ligation with extraanatomic reconstruction, two of two immediate reconstructions had no complications, whereas of the three reconstructions that were delayed, one patient died and one required ipsilateral lower extremity amputation.[12]

Unusual maneuvers may be necessary to access injuries because of the challenging topology of the pelvis. Some authors have proposed division of the overlying right iliac artery to access the underlying vein, but Asensio and colleagues[9] cautioned against this, recommending that in a patient with severe trauma, adding new injuries is usually not in the best interest of the patient. Division of the inguinal ligament may be necessary to achieve distal control.[12] Finally, in the completely stable patient with isolated pelvic vascular trauma, a preperitoneal approach may be useful and minimally invasive.[148] However, this incision is not extensile and is not recommended for general trauma cases.

Postoperative management of these patients can be challenging and is generally related to the entire constellation of injuries. In addition to the complications of the vascular injury itself, perturbation of pelvic blood flow will interfere with wound healing in the pelvic region and may lead to difficulties with pelvic fractures or injury to local soft tissue structures. Complications directly related to the pelvic vasculature include venous thromboembolism in approximately 7% of patients, chronic venous insufficiency in cases of ligation of iliac veins, amputation in approximately 7%, arteriovenous fistula in 3%, or ischemic complications from thrombosis or stenosis of the repair.[9,12,149] Graft infections have been reported to be rare, which is counterintuitive.[12,15]

In summary, pelvic vascular trauma is a challenging situation that carries significant associated morbidity and mortality. A high index of suspicion must be maintained in patients with unexplained hypotension and physical findings suggestive of pelvic injury despite a reassuring vascular examination. Rapid vascular control and damage control adjuncts may help to decrease the mortality of this injury pattern.

EXTREMITY VASCULAR INJURY

Overview

Injury to the arteries and veins of the extremities is commonly encountered in both military and civilian trauma,

secondary to both blunt and penetrating mechanisms. While there are particular aspects of management that are specific to an anatomic location, there are many general principles that apply to extremity vascular trauma.

Incidence and Mortality

The incidence of extremity vascular injury at ranges from 0.5% to 4% of traumatic injuries; 80% are secondary to penetrating trauma.[150] In a study of all patients admitted over a 2-year period to a level I trauma center, 28 patients with 30 upper extremity arterial injuries were identified for a 0.5% incidence. The most common injury was to the brachial artery (40%), followed by the ulnar (27%), radial (23%), and axillary (10%) arteries. Penetrating injury represented 60% of cases.[151] Similar patterns of frequency in upper extremity arterial injury have been reported by other authors.[19,152] In recent reports of military casualties, extremity vascular injury occurred in 4% to 6% of combat wounded treated at U.S. Air Force and Navy battlefield hospitals.[7,153] The most commonly wounded extremity vessel is the femoral artery and vein.[8,10,30] Among upper extremity injuries, the brachial artery is the most common at approximately 50% of wounds, followed by the axillary artery. The subclavian artery is fairly uncommon, likely because of its protected position within the thorax; trauma to this vessel is usually associated with exsanguination or death from other causes.[152] In a study of femoral and popliteal injuries from Balad, Iraq, femoral injuries were found to be more common (69%); most (51%) were combined arteriovenous injuries.[8] Among 153 combat-wounded soldiers with 218 extremity vascular injuries, femoral arterial trauma was again the most common; 57% of the injuries were arterial, and 50% were venous.[30] Mortality is far lower than that for truncal vascular injury. Estimates of lower extremity vascular injury mortality range from 3% to 9% with elevated injury severity score, low Glasgow Coma Scale score, coagulopathy, two or more hard signs of hemorrhage, and advanced age being predictive of mortality.[8,10] One of the main reasons for decreased mortality is the improved access to the vessel relative to truncal trauma and the ability to use tourniquets.

Tourniquet Use

There has been a resurgence of interest in the use of tourniquets in the combat setting. Historically, there has been concern that tourniquet use for the control of extremity hemorrhage would lead to limb dysfunction or loss with prolonged ischemic times. However, there has been a clear documentation that uncontrolled bleeding from extremity vascular injuries is one of the leading causes of preventable battlefield deaths.[35] This led the U.S. military and other countries to supply tourniquets to combat medics and troops. Evaluation of recent outcomes of tourniquet use has documented several critical points. First, there is a clear decrease in mortality with the early use of tourniquets, especially when applied before the onset of shock.[154-156] Even in cases where the wound was too proximal for the proper placing of the tourniquet (5 cm proximal to the most proximal wound, placed on bare skin), there was a 75% survival rate. In addition, morbidity directly attributable to the tourniquet was rare and reversible. In a series of 232 patients treated with 428 tourniquets on 309 limbs, there were only 4 (1.7%) transient nerve palsies at the level of the tourniquet, all of which resolved subsequently.[156] There was no association of tourniquet duration with other morbidities such as vascular clots, myonecrosis, rigor, pain, fasciotomy, or renal failure.

It is critical that those responsible for placing tourniquets are trained in their use. Proper application of the tourniquet is indicated by both the cessation of bleeding and the absence of a distal pulse. Misplacement of the tourniquet is associated with a 44% mortality. There was an identifiable pattern of clinical deterioration with ineffective tourniquet application: persistent pulse, venous congestion, venous distension, rebleeding after a period of hemorrhage control, expanding hematomas, compartment syndrome, fasciotomy, and death. This pattern was seen in 61% of cases when there was continued bleeding despite application of the tourniquet and in 51% of cases when there was a persistent distal pulse.[156]

It is also critical to use correctly designed tourniquets. The three most commonly used tourniquets in the U.S. military are the Emergency Medical Tourniquet (EMT, Delfi Medical Innovations, Vancouver, B.C.), the Combat Application Tourniquet (CAT, North American Rescue Products, Greer, S.C.), and the Special Operations Forces Tactical Tourniquet (SOFTT, Tactical Medical Solutions, Anderson, S.C.). All three designs were 100% effective in laboratory self-application use,[157] but among actual casualties, the EMT was shown to be 92% effective, the CAT to be 79% effective, and the SOFTT to be 66% effective.[156] The EMT, however, is not a prehospital tourniquet; therefore the U.S. Army issues CAT tourniquets for medics and troops and supplies EMTs for aid stations and higher levels of care. The width of the tourniquet seems to be related to its effectiveness.

A final critical point to effective tourniquet use is maintenance of vigilance. Slippery skin, underlying clothing or padding, or gradual decrease in limb diameter owing to exsanguination can lead to a loose tourniquet and rebleeding. Initial inappropriate application owing to occult wounds can also put the patient at risk. Frequent checks of the tourniquet, with application of additional tourniquets if necessary, are critical for optimal outcomes (Figure 45-13).

Assessment and Diagnosis

Patients with extremity vascular trauma must be assessed using the standard protocols for trauma patients. A rapid assessment of airway and breathing are followed by evaluation of circulation. Any hemorrhage is controlled, ideally with point pressure on the vascular injury, or if that is not possible, tourniquet application. The patient is fully examined while appropriate resuscitation is being performed. Distal pulses on physical examination are documented; the Doppler ultrasound probe can augment this physical examination. A thorough physical examination is critical in the management of these injuries. In a study

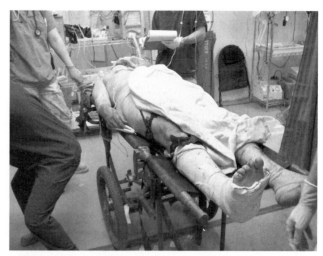

FIGURE 45-13 ■ A soldier arriving in a casualty receiving area in Afghanistan. Note the presence of two tourniquets on the right lower extremity. (Courtesy Sandra Halterman. Used with permission.)

TABLE 45-7   Physical Findings Suggestive of Vascular Injury

Hard Signs Indicating Need for Operative Exploration	Soft Signs Suggestive of Injury, Requiring Further Evaluation
Pulsatile bleeding	History of significant hemorrhage
Expanding hematoma	Injury pattern suggestive of vascular trauma
Palpable thrill	Diminished pulse
Audible bruit	Peripheral nerve deficit
Evidence of ischemia	

of 99 military trauma patients, 36 of 73 (49%) patients with normal physical examinations had angiographic abnormalities, but only 6 (8%) required intervention. Among 26 patients with abnormal physical examinations, 22 (85%) had angiographic findings and 19 (73%) required intervention. Although a normal physical examination does not rule out an injury requiring treatment, it does a good job of picking up the majority of clinically significant vascular injuries. Physical examination findings are classically divided into hard signs and soft signs (Table 45-7). Patients with hard signs should undergo operative exploration if the mechanism is penetrating and the location of injury is apparent. When the site of injury is unclear (e.g., shotgun blast with multiple entry injuries, blunt trauma), preoperative or intraoperative angiography are appropriate. The presence of physical findings suggestive of injury allowed Asensio and colleagues[10] to decrease preoperative angiography to 15% and proceed with expeditious repairs.

If only soft signs are present, the ABI has been shown to be a useful modality to detect occult injuries. If the ABI is less than 0.9, then further diagnostic testing is indicated.[55] If the ABI is normal, then the patient should be followed clinically. If this is impossible (e.g., a patient

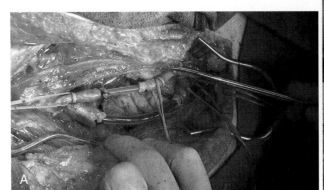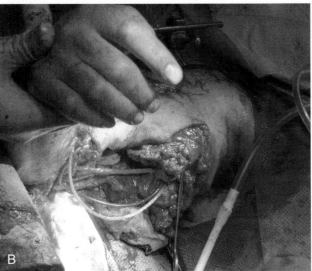

FIGURE 45-14 ■ **A,** Temporary arterial and venous shunts. **B,** A Morgan Lens ocular irrigation catheter (MorTan, Inc., Missoula, MT) was modified to use as a vascular shunt in this patient. (Courtesy Jonathan Eliason and Sandra Halterman. Used with permission.)

with multiple orthopedic injuries making vascular examinations difficult) or the ABI is abnormal, then angiography should be performed. Another subtle sign that should prompt further workup is the "fluctuating pulse examination." Pillay and colleagues[159] presented two cases of such a finding being related to intact external vessel walls, but significant intimal injury with thrombus formation; they postulated that the fluctuations were due to thromboembolism from the site of injury.

Extremity vascular trauma most commonly occurs with associated orthopedic or neurologic trauma. Among 33 patients treated for arterial injury to the upper extremity, the prevalence of concomitant neural or orthopedic injuries was 72%.[160] Others have reported incidences of nerve injury in 13% to 57% and orthopedic injury in 38% to 95%.[8,19,151,161-164] In patients where extremity vascular injury is suspected by mechanism or physical findings, angiography has been the standard diagnostic test. However, new research is suggesting that multislice (32 or 64) CTA may have sufficient sensitivity to detect these injuries. A prospective study of 21 patients with potential extremity vascular injuries, primarily from gunshot wounds, and abnormal ABIs underwent CTA followed by either conventional angiography or operative exploration. CTA had 100% sensitivity for clinically relevant findings; 50% of patients had concomitant orthopedic injuries as well.[163] Vascular surgeons at Walter Reed Army Medical Center evaluated the use of CTA to detect vascular injuries and found that it performed well even in the presence of metallic fragments or external fixators.[61]

Temporary Vascular Shunting

The use of TVS has been used routinely for carotid surgery and has been studied extensively in the past decade for traumatic injuries. In patients requiring damage control surgery, shunts can rapidly provide temporary blood flow to a vascular bed distal to an injury.

Both Javid and Sundt shunts work well in the setting of complex vascular injury, yet many tubular devices can be made to work in austere environments (Figure 45-14). The duration of shunting should be minimized, but shunts are adequate for up to 24 hours without systemic heparinization of the patient.

One report documented the experience of a U.S. Navy surgical unit in Operation Iraqi Freedom.[164] Twenty-seven vascular shunts were placed in patients with a mean ISS score of 18 (range, 9-34) and a mangled extremity severity score (MESS) of 9 (range, 6-11). All patients survived, although three (15%) ultimately required amputation. Six (22%) of the shunts clotted during transport, but they provided an effective perfusion window that allowed the majority of limbs to be salvaged.[164] Other reports from military investigators have documented that 50% to 60% of patients being treated for vascular trauma at forward surgical units have shunts placed; patency rates range from 86% to 96% when the patients arrived at the next echelon of care for definitive surgery.[77,153,165] U.S. Air Force investigators at Balad, Iraq, found that the patency rates for proximal arterial shunts was 86% and 100% for venous shunts; distal shunts (e.g., infrapopliteal) had a poor patency rate of 12%.[165] Although there are no level I data demonstrating improved survival or limb salvage, research by Gifford and colleagues[51] demonstrated a trend toward a decreased amputation rate with TVS in a case-control study using propensity adjustment.[51]

Principles of Surgical Management

When handling extremity vascular injuries, several surgical principles should be noted. A well-executed operation begins before the patient arrives in the operating room. If there are no contraindications such as a closed head injury or active bleeding, the patient should be heparinized if there is evidence of embolization or thrombosis. Second, good communication with other specialists is extremely important. A discussion of plans for vascularized tissue coverage with plastic surgeons will help to guide the surgeon in terms of incision placement and operative plan. One continuing area of controversy is the sequencing of operations if the patient requires vascular repair and orthopedic fixation. Dogmatic adherence to the dictum that the patient has 6 hours to restore blood flow to the extremity before causing irreversible damage has been questioned through a series of animal experiments by the U.S. Air Force. Their results suggest that any duration of lower extremity ischemia leads to notable changes and irreversible changes in function occur after as little as 2 to 3 hours of ischemia.[50,52,166,167] One study demonstrated a trend toward higher fasciotomy rates with orthopedic fixation preceding vascular repair (80% vs. 36%; $p = 0.10$) despite 48% of cases using TVS.[168] In another series, a protocol of initial revascularization was used. Limb salvage was 92%, the fasciotomy rate was 60%, and there were no vascular complications owing to subsequent orthopedic procedures.[169] It is therefore reasonable to perform an initial vascular repair before orthopedic fixation.

The incision should be placed with an eye toward extensibility if needed, meaning that axially oriented incisions are preferred. Inguinal incisions should be longitudinal in case extension above the inguinal ligament or distally is required. Posterior approaches to the popliteal artery are not ideal for trauma; this artery should be approached medially and the incision can be extended proximally or distally.

There are several choices for repair. In a study by Franz and colleagues of 30 upper extremity injuries,[151] 14 (46.7%) were repaired primarily, 8 (26.7%) were ligated, 6 (20.0%) were repaired with saphenous vein graft bypasses, and 2 (6.7%) were repaired with endovascular procedures. In another study of 218 combat-related vascular injuries, 36% were primarily repaired, 34% were repaired with a vein interposition graft, 29% were ligated, and 2% were repaired with a prosthetic graft.[30] If interposition or jump grafts are required, the choice of conduit should be guided by the situation. The traditional teaching is that contralateral saphenous vein is the proper choice, which is appropriate if possible. However, in multiply-injured extremities, finding adequate conduit may be challenging. PTFE provides a rapidly accessible option and can be used if autologous vein is not available or if the patient will not tolerate a long vein harvest; this latter scenario may also argue for TVS. One major concern with prosthetic graft is its use in infected surgical beds. Vertrees and colleagues[170] demonstrated that in patients with limited autologous vein, prosthetic graft can be used temporarily in contaminated wounds in multiple anatomic locations with acceptable short-term patency and an opportunity for later revision.

In general, endovascular approaches may be helpful in certain situations given the availability of equipment and expertise. Pseudoaneurysms, arteriovenous fistulae, and side-branch bleeding are particularly amenable to endovascular repair. Rosa and colleagues[171] report on the use of embolization of a traumatic pseudoaneurysm and arteriovenous fistula for a peroneal artery injury secondary to a fragment wound. Another series reported 10 embolizations of profunda femoris, superior gluteal, and inferior gluteal arterial injuries with good outcomes.[172] In a report from Balad, Iraq, U.S. Air Force investigators reported the first application of endovascular techniques in-theater; 150 diagnostic angiograms were performed and 61% were found to have abnormalities; 47 underwent repair. In 30 cases, the repair was performed surgically, and in 17 the repair was endovascular, including 10 embolizations and 5 stent placements. The technical success rate was 100%.[173]

Finally, completion angiography should be performed in cases of vascular repairs. In a study of 104 patients with penetrating trauma to the femoral (n = 71) and popliteal (n = 33) arteries, completion angiography led to revision of anastomosis in 30%. The amputation rate was 3% amputation among patients in whom completion angiography was performed compared with 18% if it was not performed.[174]

Outcomes

Overall mortality rates vary widely in this population, predictably based on the overall trauma burden. Data from the Balad vascular registry documents an overall 4.3% perioperative mortality rate and 6.6% early amputation rate for all U.S. forces, local nationals, and Iraqi forces treated during a 2-year period for vascular trauma.[7] Similar results were found at the 31st Combat Support Hospital, where a 6% all-cause mortality and a 20% amputation rate was seen; upper extremity limb salvage fared better at 95% than lower extremity at 71%.[30] In a local population of Iraqi nationals treated for vascular injuries, a mortality of 1.5%, early amputation rate of 3.0%, and an overall complication rate of 16% were observed.[175] Asensio and colleagues[10] documented a 3% risk of early amputation with femoral vessel injury, with no late amputations. Their complications included wound infection in 23%, venous thrombosis in 3%, perioperative hemorrhage in 3%, and arterial thrombosis in 1%.[10]

According to Parry and colleagues,[176] patency rates for venous repairs of the lower extremity by an experienced trauma team are approximately 65% to 75%, regardless of the approach: primary repair, autogenous vein graft, or PTFE. Temporary intraluminal shunts have been used successfully in these cases as well.[176] Similar to the pattern seen with TVS, patency rates for venous repairs seems to diminish with distance. Kuralay and colleagues reported that common femoral and superficial femoral veins had patency rates of 100% and 89% at 1 year and 100% and 78% at 6 years, respectively, popliteal repair patency rates were worse (86% at 1 year and 60% at 6 years).[177] To assess the possibility that venous repairs would put patients at a higher likelihood of thromboembolism, Quan and colleagues[178] evaluated 82 patients with 103 named venous vascular injuries. In this series, ligation was performed in 63% and open surgical repair in 27%. Deep venous thrombosis was seen in 15% of ligations and 7% of repairs (p = not significant), embolism was seen in 4.2% of ligations and 3.4% of repairs (p = not significant), and phlegmasia was seen in 2.1% of ligations and 0% of repairs (p = not significant). The conclusion is that

TABLE 45-8   Mangled Extremity Severity Score (MESS)*

Category	Points
Skeletal and Soft Tissue Injury	
Low energy (stab wound, low velocity GSW, simple fracture)	1
Med energy (open or multiple fracture or fracture with dislocation)	2
High energy (high-speed deceleration, high velocity GSW)	3
Very high energy (high-speed trauma with gross contamination)	4
Ischemia (Double for Ischemia Time >6 Hours)	
Pulse reduced or absent, normal perfusion, and capillary refill	1
Pulseless, paresthesias, diminished capillary refill	2
Cool, paralyzed, insensate, numb	3
Shock	
Normotension	0
Transient hypotension <90 mm Hg	1
Persistent hypotension <90 mm Hg	2
Age (Years)	
<30	0
30-50	1
>50	2

GSW, Gunshot wound.
*A score greater than 7 is predictive of amputation.

although venous ligation may be necessary for damage control, repair is safe in terms of thromboembolic complications[178] and may be advantageous in terms of improving limb salvage rates.[51]

Two factors that have been shown repeatedly to predict complications after extremity vascular injury are fracture and MESS[51,179] (Table 45-8). Callcut and colleagues[180] demonstrated in civilian vascular trauma that a MESS of seven or less was associated with a 93% limb salvage rate versus 55% for MESS of eight or more.[180] MESS greater than 7 also correlates well with upper extremity amputation.[181] In addition, this score has been validated for combat-related vascular trauma. MESS was significantly higher in patients treated with amputation versus limb salvage (7.87 ± 1.91 versus 2.44 ± 0.438; $p = 0.001$).[182]

Management of Upper Extremity Arterial Injury

Subclavian Artery

Injuries to the subclavian artery are challenging in several respects. First, the patients are generally critically ill when they arrive because of significant hemorrhage. In a series of 3888 patients with penetrating injuries to the neck or chest, 2% overall were found to have sustained a subclavian vascular injury.[183] Other investigators have documented a subclavian injury rate of 2% to 17% in upper extremity arterial trauma. In a subset of 228 patients with subclavian injuries, 61% died before

arriving at the hospital, and the operative mortality was 16%. The vein was injured in 44%, the artery alone in 39%, and both in 17%. Interestingly, patients with venous injuries had a higher mortality risk than those with arterial injuries.[184] Patients arriving at the hospital alive are most likely to have stable injuries characterized by vessel thrombosis or the formation of a stable hematoma, whereas those with unstable injures tend to die in the prehospital setting.

The most rapid means of damage control for a subclavian injury is to insert a Foley balloon along the missile tract and inflate the balloon while placing the catheter under tension. If this arrests bleeding, clamp the catheter at the skin level with a heavy Kelly clamp.

Exposure of the subclavian artery is challenging. Access to the right subclavian artery requires a median sternotomy and division of the brachiocephalic vein. The thymus may impede access to the innominate artery and should be divided between clamps if encountered. If difficulty is encountered in identifying the root of the innominate artery because of bleeding, opening the pericardial sac may provide a clean field to allow more accurate dissection. Once it is identified, the vagus nerve and its recurrent branch, which wraps around the proximal right subclavian artery, must be identified and preserved. At this point, proximal control of the innominate artery should be possible. If the injury is on the left, a third interspace left anterolateral thoracotomy is necessary to achieve proximal control. To expose the midsubclavian artery, a supraclavicular approach is needed. The clavicular head of the sternocleidomastoid and the omohyoid muscles are divided from the clavicle to expose the subclavian vein and scalene fat pad. The pad is mobilized from lateral to medial until the phrenic nerve is seen on the anterior scalene muscle. The nerve is isolated and retracted to safety, and the anterior scalene muscle is divided as caudally as possible, exposing the artery.[185]

Axillary Artery

Injury to the axillary artery represents approximately 5% to 23% of arterial trauma in most civilian and military series.[19,151,152] Ninety-five percent of these injuries are due to penetrating mechanisms; blunt trauma is uncommon, given the high degree of protection by overlying tissues in this anatomic location; likewise, presentation in hypovolemic shock is rarely due to trauma to this artery. The axillary vein is in close proximity to the artery in this location, however, and there is a fairly high risk of arteriovenous fistula, which can develop from minor vascular trauma in this location. The artery and vein are also in intimate communication with the brachial plexus, especially at the distal extent, making concomitant neurologic injury the rule rather than the exception.

Injury to the axillary artery should be suspected if there is a palpable subclavian pulse felt in the supraclavicular fossa and a weak or absent pulse distally in the brachial artery. Exposure of the axillary artery for trauma can be achieved with the deltopectoral approach. The arm is abducted 30 degrees and externally rotated. An incision is made from the midpoint of the clavicle 5 to 7 cm along the anterior border of the deltoid muscle.

This incision is carried down to the intermuscular groove between the pectoralis and deltoid muscles, containing the cephalic vein. The pectoralis muscle is then retracted medially, and the underlying clavipectoral fascia is divided. The cephalic vein and deltoid muscle are retracted laterally. The third part of the axillary artery is then encountered with the brachial plexus cords surrounding it. Division of the thoracoacromial trunk and the pectoralis minor muscles permits access to the second and first parts of the axillary artery.

Some investigators have evaluated endovascular repair of suitable lesions in the axillosubclavian system. Valentin and colleagues[186] present a case of a traumatic subclavian artery dissection treated successfully with a self-expanding stent. Another report analyzed 46 vascular injuries in 40 patients, which would be suitable for endovascular repair, including pseudoaneurysms, arteriovenous fistulae, first-order branch vessel injury, intimal flaps, and focal lacerations. Relative contraindications to endovascular repair were injury to the third portion of the axillary artery (between the lateral edge of the pectoralis major and the lateral border of the teres major), major venous injury, refractory hypotension, and upper-extremity compartment syndrome with neurologic involvement. Strict contraindications included long segmental injuries, lack of fixation points, and arterial transection. They reported that approximately 50% of the lesions they evaluated would be amenable to endovascular repair.[187]

Brachial Artery

The brachial artery is the most commonly injured artery in the upper extremity, occurring in 40% to 50% of cases.[19,151,152] The most common mechanism is penetrating injury (92%); 53% of these penetrating injuries arise from stab wounds, window glass (24%), or gunshot wounds (20%).[162]

On examination, the absence of an arterial pulse is the most common presentation (88%); weakness of the brachial pulse is found in 12%. Using brachial-brachial indices (with <0.85 being considered abnormal), preoperative index was found to be 0.43 (standard deviation 0.05, range 0.23 to 0.48) in patients with brachial artery injuries. This increased to 0.89 (standard deviation 0.03, range 0.83 to 0.93) postoperatively.[162]

Exposure of the brachial artery is straightforward. With the arm abducted 90 degrees and supported on an arm board, an incision is made in the groove between the biceps and triceps muscle on the medial aspect of the arm. This incision is considered extensile and can be extended proximally or distally as needed. It is important to avoid the basilic vein as the brachial artery is approached; it courses through the subcutaneous tissues just posterior to the brachial groove to the midpoint of the upper arm, where it penetrates the fascia and then runs near the brachial structures. The deep fascia at the inferior border of the biceps muscle is incised and the biceps are retracted anteriorly. The basilic vein is then retracted posteriorly and the brachial sheath is opened. The median nerve is the most superficial structure. It is widely mobilized and gently retracted anteriorly. The artery is then found deep to the median nerve with two veins on either side. The

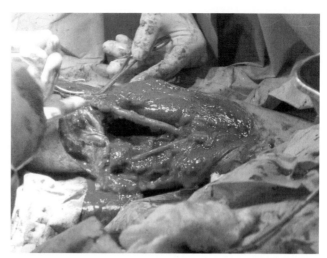

FIGURE 45-15 ■ Saphenous interposition graft of a brachial artery injury.

deepest structure in this sheath is the ulnar nerve. Occasionally, two arteries may be encountered in the sheath; this represents a high bifurcation of the artery and they represent the radial and ulnar arteries.

Exposure of the distal brachial artery in cases of trauma should be performed through a lazy-S–shaped incision placed over the antecubital fossa. The superior longitudinal portion is located along the medial border of the biceps muscle, and the inferior portion is made lateral to the midpoint of the volar forearm for 4 to 6 cm. The basilic vein should be identified and protected, and the medial antecubital nerve should be retracted medially. The bicipital aponeurosis is then divided, exposing the brachial artery. Ligation of two crossing vein branches permits wider exposure of this artery and its bifurcation into the radial and ulnar arteries.

In a report of 49 patients with brachial artery injury, end-to-end anastomosis was the most common technique (57%), followed by interposition vein graft (31%; Figure 45-15), primary repair (10%), and PTFE interposition (2%).[162]

Radial and Ulnar Arteries

Forearm vascular injuries occur in 10% to 50% of cases.[19,151,152] Control of the radial artery at the mid forearm can be accomplished through an incision over the medial border of the brachioradialis muscle, located on a line between the midpoint of the antecubital fossa and the styloid process of the radius. The antebrachial fascia is divided, and the brachioradialis muscle retracted laterally to expose the radial artery. Exposure of the radial artery at the wrist is accomplished by making a longitudinal incision over the radial pulse if one exists, or just lateral to the flexor carpi radialis tendon and extending proximally 3 to 4 cm. The cephalic vein is lateral to the artery and should be preserved in the subcutaneous tissues if possible and retracted laterally. The antebrachial fascia is then incised and the artery exposed. Exposure of the ulnar artery in the wrist is accomplished through a longitudinal incision lateral to the flexor carpi

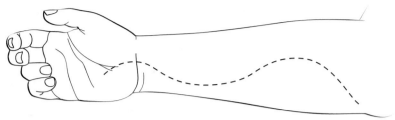

FIGURE 45-16 ■ Forearm fasciotomy incision.

ulnaris tendon. Division of the antebrachial fascia exposes the artery.

Fasciotomy

The forearm fasciotomy is performed by making a long S-type incision on the volar aspect of the forearm. The incision starts distally along the base of the thenar eminence, bends slightly radially at the proximal thenar eminence, then moves directly transverse from radial to ulnar across the wrist, releasing the carpal tunnel. The incision is complete when the median nerve is visualized. The incision then continues along the ulnar aspect of the forearm, looping back radially in the midportion of the forearm (which allows a flap to be created to cover the median nerve if necessary) and again moving in an ulnar direction behind the medial epicondyle. The incision then moves somewhat in the radial direction and finally follows the medial border of the biceps muscle. If the incision has not decompressed the mobile wad on the medial aspect of the flexor compartment, a separate longitudinal incision over this compartment will release it (Figure 45-16). On the dorsal surface, a longitudinal incision is made over the forearm flexor compartment. The dorsal surface of the hand should be decompressed with linear incisions between the extensor digitorum tendons of the second and third and the third and fourth digits. The interossei can then be detached from the metacarpals if necessary to further decompress the hand.[188]

Dente and colleagues[189] reported a series of 37 upper extremity fasciotomies performed in 27 patients. The mechanisms were distributed between penetrating trauma (35%), blunt trauma (24%), and burn injury (14%), of which 80% were due to electrical injuries. Most fasciotomies (89%) were performed at the initial operation and usually were based on clinical assessment. Of the 22% of cases where compartment pressures were checked, the mean pressure was 52 mm Hg, with a range of 40 to 87 mm Hg. In this series, no amputations were required because of a failure to perform fasciotomy.[189] Risk factors for compartment syndrome of the forearm in cases of brachial artery injury include combined arterial injuries, concomitant nerve injury, motor deficits, fractures, and significant blood loss interoperatively.[190]

Outcomes

The overall limb salvage rate in upper extremity arterial injury has been reported to range from 96% to 98% with little or no mortality related to the extremity injury. In the uncommon cases of amputation, early graft failure, compartment syndrome, and associated skeletal and brachial plexus injury were found to be significant predictors of limb loss. Military mechanisms are also significantly associated with risk of amputation.[19,151,152,162] Of 49 brachial artery repairs, 4 thrombosed; 3 were opened successfully and remained patent. The fourth vessel remained occluded, but no amputation was necessary because of collateral blood flow.[162] However, despite maintenance of limb viability, neurologic injury has been found to be the most significant predictor of functional outcome.[160] In the single amputation in one series of brachial artery injuries, the reason for amputation was significant neurologic and orthopedic trauma.[162]

Management of Lower Extremity Arterial Injury

Femoral Artery

The femoral artery is the most commonly injured vessel in the lower extremity. In a report of nearly 2500 wartime vascular injuries from World War II, Debakey and Simeone[2] reported 517 (21%) injuries to the femoral artery. Reports from the Korean war estimated the incidence at 19% to 31%[5,191]; the incidence was 35% in the Vietnam vascular registry.[108] Civilian series cite rates of approximately 70%.[10] Injury to the femoral artery was also the most commonly found peripheral vascular injury in an autopsy series of 6769 cases.[192] Injury at this site is generally considered nonlethal, although postoperative morbidity is high; the complication rate is 23% and the wound infection rate is 15%. The mechanism is primarily penetrating, with gunshot wounds being the most common cause. Associated injuries are frequent: combined arteriovenous trauma is seen in 46%, orthopedic injuries are seen in 22% (generally femur fractures), and femoral nerve injuries are seen in 10%. Distal ischemia is present in 48% of cases, pulses are weak or absent in 43%, and an expanding hematoma is seen in 29%. Soft signs such as delayed capillary refill are less common. The ABI averages 0.92 in these injuries, which is highly misleading.[10]

Surgical treatment of these lesions is similar to other areas. One hundred forty-five combat-related femoral and popliteal injuries were treated primarily with autogenous vein graft (88%). Ligation was rare (5%).[8] In a series of 204 civilian femoral injuries, a reversed

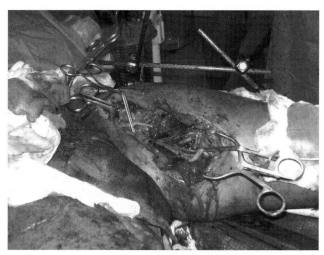

FIGURE 45-17 ■ Extensile exposure permits wide access to the femoral triangle and can be continued proximally or distally depending on the surgical findings.

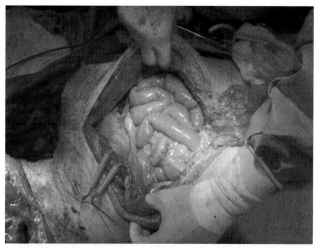

FIGURE 45-18 ■ This patient arrived at a combat casualty receiving hospital with multiple extremity injuries. Proximal control was achieved with vessel loops around the iliac arteries through a laparotomy incision. (Courtesy Sandra Halterman. Used with permission.)

saphenous graft was used in 53%, primary repair in 26%, PTFE interposition in 10%, ligation in 6%, and vein patch in 4%. PTFE was considered a "conduit of choice" for patients in extremis because of its ready availability leading to decreased operative time.[10] Vascular shunting may change this designation.

The surgical approach to the femoral artery should follow the same principles discussed previously (Figure 45-17). The incision should be made longitudinally to allow for extension proximally and distally. An obvious wound or hematoma should be avoided initially until proximal and distal control is achieved. The proximal approach to the femoral artery begins just inferior to the inguinal ligament at approximately midway between the anterior iliac spine and the pubic tubercle. Once the vessel is isolated proximally, it is controlled with a double-looped vessel loop or a clamp. Before occlusion, the patient should be heparinized if possible given the catalog of injuries. If necessary, the inguinal ligament can be divided to achieve more proximal control of the vessel for high injuries. If this maneuver is insufficient to gain control, a low midline laparotomy and intraabdominal control should be secured (Figure 45-18). Once high proximal control is established, clamps can be moved distally in a serial fashion known as "walking the clamps."[193] Distal control of the vessel should occur similarly. Begin by avoiding the zone of injury and moving more proximally. Backbleeding is rarely as problematic as forward bleeding, however, and entry into the wound to achieve distal control can work if necessary. Another option for control of vessels is balloon occlusion either endovascularly from a remote access site or directly through the wound using balloon catheters.

Popliteal Artery

These injuries occur less frequently than femoral artery injuries; however, there is a particular injury pattern associated with the popliteal artery that can be subtle yet devastating. After blunt injury, especially following posterior knee dislocations, the rate of vascular injury is substantial. Of 18 patients in one study with posterior knee dislocations and popliteal artery injury, there were 4 (22%) amputations.[194] Among 1395 popliteal injuries in the National Trauma Data Bank, the incidence was 0.2% of all traumas. Blunt trauma was the mechanism in 61% of cases. The overall rate of amputation was 15%; risk factors for amputation were fracture, complex soft tissue injury, nerve injury, and elevated Abbreviated Injury Scale.[195] Using a protocol of performing angiography in the operating room, investigators at the University of Wisconsin have demonstrated improvement in limb salvage (100% vs. 70%) if angiography is performed in the operating room versus the radiology suite, likely because of the decrease in ischemic time.[180]

The best approach to the popliteal artery is through a large medial incision. The posterior margin of the femur and the tibia are the major landmarks. The saphenous vein should be protected during exposure. An incision is placed along the anterior border of the sartorius muscle. The fascia is incised and the muscle is retracted posteriorly. The vastus medialis is then retracted anteriorly. The fascial bridge connecting the adductor magnus tendon and the semimembranosus muscle is divided, and the neurovascular bundle is exposed. If additional exposure is necessary, the adductor magnus tendon can be divided, allowing more proximal control of the artery. The artery is then controlled below the knee through an incision placed 1 cm behind the posterior border of the tibia. The crural fascia is incised 1 cm posterior to the tibia and opened to the semitendinosus proximally. The medial head of the gastrocnemius is then retracted posteriorly to allow the neurovascular bundle to be approached. If necessary, the semitendinosus, gracilis, and sartorius muscles can be divided for further exposure, but should be repaired at the end of the case for maintenance of knee stability.[196]

In patients with a concern for compartment syndrome, a four-compartment below-knee fasciotomy should be performed. The two-incision technique is technically the easiest and safest approach. A longitudinal incision is made on the lateral leg two fingerbreadths laterally to the tibia. This incision is carried down to the fascia of the muscular compartment. Care is taken to avoid the superficial peroneal nerve. An incision is then made in the fascia of the muscular compartment, and the incision is carried proximally to the tibial tuberosity and distally to 3 to 4 cm from the lateral malleolus. It is vital that once the anterior or lateral compartment is entered, the intermuscular septum is identified to ensure that the other compartment is then decompressed in the same way; a critical mistake is to decompress the same compartment twice, leaving the remaining compartment at high pressure and high risk of myonecrosis, nerve loss, and dysfunction. The second incision is made two fingerbreadths medial to the tibia. In this case, the saphenous vein should be avoided. Both the deep and superficial posterior compartments can be reached easily through this incision. Again, ensure that both compartments are fully released.

Gonzalez and colleagues[197] studied 321 patients with 393 lower-extremity penetrating injuries and found that the most common cause of lower extremity compartment syndrome was due to penetrating injury to the proximal infrageniculate leg. Development of compartment syndrome secondary to thigh injuries occurred only in the presence of surgically significant vascular injury, including injury requiring ligation of the femoral vein.[197] Asensio and colleagues[10] documented a 12% rate of fasciotomy; their indications were the presence of shock, combined arteriovenous injury, or associated fracture requiring external fixators or internal fixation.

Extremity Venous Injury

The repair of venous injury in the extremity has followed in the wake of arterial repair. Whereas in World War II the majority of arterial extremity injuries were ligated,[2] in the Korean War there was a quantum shift in management to vascular repair. The same quantum shift to venous repairs began during the Korean war with reports from Hughes and Spencer documenting the repair of 20 veins, primarily by lateral suture, in order to decrease the postoperative venous stasis.[5,191,198] These efforts were carried forward by Rich and colleagues[199] in Vietnam. Of 110 popliteal venous injuries, 53 were repaired (32 by lateral repair, 15 by end-to-end anastomosis, and 6 by interposition graft), whereas 57 were ligated. The risk of venous hypertension postoperatively was 51% after ligation, compared with 13% after repair. Among patients who were available for follow-up, the patency rate was 92%.[199]

In contemporary reports, the frequency of venous repair strategy still varies widely. Primary repair is reported in 31% to 72% of series, vein grafts in 4% to 12%, prosthetic interposition grafts in 2% to 31%; ligation is still performed in 23% to 63% of injuries.[8,10,30,176,178] The one method that is not included in most reports is patch angioplasty; however, Kuralay and colleagues[177] reported this technique to have superior patency (75%) at 6 years compared with lateral repair (58%), end-to-end anastomosis (43%), and autogenous vein graft (36%).[177]

References available online at expertconsult.com.

QUESTIONS

1. Which of the following is not part of the "lethal triad" of trauma?
   a. Hypoxia
   b. Acidosis
   c. Coagulopathy
   d. Hypothermia

2. Arterial injuries as a result of blunt trauma are especially likely with which of the following injuries?
   a. Shoulder dislocation
   b. Posterior knee dislocation
   c. Midfemoral shaft fracture
   d. Clavicular fracture

3. Which of the following is correct regarding mesenteric vascular injury?
   a. Ligation of the superior mesenteric vein is not compatible with life.
   b. A second-look operation should be planned within 24 hours to assess bowel viability.
   c. Mortality is highest in Fullen Zone IV injuries.
   d. Ligation of the proximal celiac artery is unsafe.

4. A 22-year-old man is admitted with a gunshot wound to the right groin. His leg is pulseless and cool. At exploration, he is found to have extensive soft tissue destruction and a 3-cm defect in the superficial femoral artery. He is hemodynamically stable during the exploration. What is the best strategy at this time?
   a. Replace the missing segment with an appropriately sized PTFE graft.
   b. Replace the missing segment with ipsilateral saphenous vein.
   c. Replace the missing segment with contralateral saphenous vein.
   d. Ligate the proximal and distal ends of the vessel and plan reoperation as indicated if the limb becomes ischemic.

5. A 17-year-old boy incurred a penetrating wound of his left medial thigh during a motor vehicle crash. When examined, he had no ischemia, but moderate swelling surrounded the wound. A continuous murmur was heard in this area. Which of the following clinical features is least likely to be present?
   a. Nicoladoni-Branham sign
   b. Tachycardia
   c. Empty veins
   d. Decreased ankle blood pressure

6. What is the best course of treatment for the patient in question 5?
   a. Admit him for observation, awaiting resolution.
   b. Observe him and measure the ABI every 4 hours.
   c. Schedule MRI of the legs.
   d. Admit him for arteriorraphy.

7. Which of the following are true about cervical vascular injury?
   a. Patients who are comatose with cervical vascular injury should undergo vascular repair.
   b. Angiographic imaging is indicated for all zone II penetrating injuries in the neck.
   c. There are clear level I data for appropriate screening of patients at risk for occult cervical vascular injury.
   d. Patients with documented grade II blunt cervical vascular injury should be anticoagulated or treated with antiplatelet therapy.

8. Which of the following is true about combined portal vein and hepatic artery injury?
   a. Collateral flow to the liver is sufficient to allow for both the portal vein and the hepatic artery to be ligated.
   b. Either the portal vein or the hepatic artery must be repaired for survival.
   c. The patient will require hepatic transplantation.
   d. Both the portal vein and the hepatic artery must be repaired for survival.

9. Which of the following is true in regard to injuries of the inferior vena cava?
   a. Infrarenal injuries carry the best chance for survival.
   b. Posterior injuries usually do not need to be explored.
   c. Posterior injuries cannot be repaired through an anterior venotomy.
   d. Pulmonary emboli occur frequently after repair.

10. Current data supports which of the following about distal extremity ischemia?
    a. Tourniquet use is significantly associated with poor long-term neurologic outcomes.
    b. Functional outcomes are improved with ligation of the vein if arterial ligation is necessary.
    c. Any ischemic time greater than 1 hour has been shown to be associated with diminished limb function in animal studies.
    d. Ischemic times in excess of 6 hours are tolerated if the limb is kept cool.

ANSWERS

1. **a**
2. **b**
3. **b**
4. **c**
5. **c**
6. **d**
7. **d**
8. **b**
9. **a**
10. **c**

CHAPTER 46

ENDOVASCULAR APPROACH TO VASCULAR TRAUMA

Lorraine Choi • Charlie C. Cheng • Zulfiqar F. Cheema • Michael B. Silva, Jr.

The past decade has witnessed the near complete adoption of endovascular techniques as alternative therapies for management of vascular disease in virtually all vascular beds. With advanced training paradigms for practicing vascular surgeons and incorporation of catheter skills at every level of the experience for doctors in training, endovascular therapy has permeated all aspects of the contemporary vascular practice. Clinicians find themselves faced with the real problem of creating training strategies that provide sufficient open surgical experience for the next generation of vascular surgeons.[1]

Interestingly, one area in which endovascular techniques need wider adoption and investigation is in the management of traumatic vascular injuries. In many ways, these techniques are ideally suited for this patient population. These patients need immediate and urgent solutions to complex problems. Traumatic vascular injuries are often life threatening, but open exposure and vascular control take time, can be highly complex, and are associated with significant morbidity, depending on the location of the injury. An endovascular solution for the patient with multiple trauma has the potential to expediently address one of the more immediate life-threatening aspects of the polytrauma, thereby enabling surgeons from other disciplines to proceed in a more stable environment.

Endovascular management of trauma is gaining acceptance. The volume of endovascular repairs of arterial trauma as identified by the National Trauma Data Bank increased twenty-sevenfold between 1997 and 2003. However, open surgical management remains vastly more common for this patient group. The overall utilization rate of endovascular interventions during this time period was only 3.7%.[2] In most other areas of vascular surgical practice, when endovascular alternatives exist and can be determined to be safe, effective, and durable, open surgery is reserved for failures of endovascular therapy.

One explanation for the relatively slow adoption of endovascular techniques in this group of patients may have to do with the specialist in charge of management decisions. Traditionally, trauma surgeons have managed many vascular injuries themselves with varying degrees of involvement with their vascular surgery consultants. Trauma surgeons are more likely to use open vascular techniques than are vascular surgeons. Endovascular training for trauma surgeons needs the same kind of structure that was developed for vascular surgeons over the past 20 years.

Still, successful endovascular treatment of both blunt and penetrating arterial injuries, even in unstable patients, is described regularly in the academic literature. These are principally case reports or small series because of the relatively low incidence of traumatic vascular injuries at any given institution, with an even smaller percentage being managed endovascularly. Long-term follow-up is usually lacking, in part owing to the novelty of these approaches and to the known challenges to outcomes research with trauma patients. For continuous progress to be made in this field, collaboration and data sharing among institutions with prospective database mining and long-term follow-up will be important.

An additional paradigm shift that is occurring naturally is the transition of endovascular procedures from the interventional radiology suite to the hybrid operating room (OR), equipped with state-of-the-art imaging, racks of endovascular tools and the potential for concomitant or staged open surgical procedures. Previously, only hemodynamically stable patients were deemed eligible for angiography, with injury severity score (ISS) for patients undergoing endovascular interventions significantly lower than that of patients undergoing open surgery for arterial injuries (13 vs. 20; $p < 0.001$).[2] With these minimally invasive techniques being more universally available in the same room as the multidisciplinary trauma team, the OR may prove to be where endovascular therapy reaches its true potential in helping to treat vascular injury in the polytrauma patient.

The University of Texas Medical Branch (UTMB) in Galveston is a level 1 trauma center. This chapter introduces tools and training that has been helpful in creating an OR for emergency endovascular surgery as well as an approach to specific injuries. The authors' experience reflects the combined efforts of trauma and vascular services in expanding the use of endovascular techniques for this important patient population.

DEVELOPING AN ENDOVASCULAR TRAUMA PROGRAM

Training

Advanced preparation and team education is essential to optimizing outcomes. It is not possible to address the hypotensive, hemodynamically unstable patient with an operating team that is unfamiliar with the imaging equipment, the power injector, the quick handling of the

260-cm–long wire. The UTMB vascular surgery staff meets twice yearly with the OR staff to review the basic equipment and the most common procedures. Instructional videos on the endovascular suite, the fixed C-arm, and the power injector are available on the perioperative care website for OR staff to review.

Tools

Endovascular equipment should be available and easily visualized in the room where the procedures are performed.

The basic trauma pack should include a 4-French micro-introducer kit (Vascular Solutions, Minneapolis, Minn.), 180-cm angled Glidewire (Terumo, Somerset, N.J.), and a 10-cm, 6-French sheath (Terumo, Somerset, N.J.). All other endovascular tools are in the room and readily accessible; this arrangement is important to avoid circumstances that require the circulating nurse to leave the OR. It is essential that the trauma vascular surgeon have an excellent knowledge of the inventory, including the location of each item, so that support staff can be expeditiously directed to open the exact and appropriate tools requested. Visual inspection by the operating surgeon is important before opening sterile packages to avoid communication errors and limit expensive mistakes.

Vascular Operating Room Table

If not in a fixed-unit endovascular suite, the OR table needs to be C-arm compatible. This usually requires the fixed, radiopaque base to be located at the head or the foot, depending on which portion of the body is of primary radiographic interest. This requirement needs to be communicated to the OR team before transfer of the patient to the OR. The floating vascular bed has a manual device enabling surgeon control of the OR table, diminishing the need for frequent C-arm movements.

Fluoroscopic Imaging Equipment

Whether operating in a hybrid endovascular suite or using a traditional OR with portable C-arm, the surgeon must be trained and adept in the use of the equipment. Special training for the operating surgeons and radiology technicians is required to use the vascular software or advanced C-arm units and regularly scheduled training to review such programs is vital. The software purchased with most advanced imaging equipment is powerful and sophisticated with significant potential for customization. Many users limit their effectiveness and increase exposure risks by failing to invest sufficiently in becoming facile with all aspects of their imaging equipment.

Power Injector

As discussed previously, the surgeon must be familiar with how to load and run the power injector as well as trouble shoot basic problems. Although many studies might not require the use of the power injector, the quality of the images obtained, and thereby the performance of certain procedures such as thoracic stent-grafting, will be curtailed with manual injection.

Wires

In the trauma setting, the surgical assistant may be less familiar with endovascular equipment and it may be beneficial to keep the number of wires to a minimum. Routinely used wires include: a "black" wire (180-cm angled Glidewire, Terumo, Somerset, N.J.), a "green" wire (260-cm Amplatz wire; Cook Medical, Bloomington, Ind.), a "white" wire (260-cm Lunderquist wire; Cook Medical), and a "small" wire (0.014- or 0.018-inch, 260-cm Platinum Plus (Boston Scientific, Natick, Mass.).

Catheters

For nonselective aortic injections, a 65-cm (abdominal) or 90-cm (thoracic), 5-French multi-sidehole catheter such as the Omniflush (Angiodynamics, Latham, N.Y.) or a marker pigtail catheter (Angiodynamics, Latham, N.Y.) can be used. For selective catheterization, the hydrophilic, flexible Glidecath catheters (Terumo, Somerset, N.J.) are versatile. Supplies should include the simple angled, tapered Glidecaths (5 French, 65 cm; 5 French, 100 cm; and 4 French, 120 cm); 5-French, 100-cm Simmons 1 and Simmons 2 shepherd's hook–shaped catheters. For highly selective coil embolization, a microcatheter such as the 0.027 Renegade (Boston Scientific) is useful.

Sheaths

A 6-French sheath is sufficient for diagnostic arteriography and most balloon angioplasty, stent placement, or coil embolization procedures. For efficiency and enhanced imaging, a longer sheath placed with the tip near the area of interest provides support, limits contrast use, and reduces frequent catheter exchanges. As a result, the endovascular armamentarium should include Destination sheaths in lengths of 45, 65, and 90 cm (Terumo, Somerset, N.J.), in 6- to 8-French diameters. Larger diameter sheaths are required for larger stent-graft delivery (9 to 12 French), endograft delivery (18 to 24 French), or use of an aortic occlusion balloon (12 to 14 French). A particular advance is the Gore Dryseal sheath (WL Gore, Flagstaff, Ariz.) that allows a single sheath to be cannulated by multiple devices without loss of valve hemostasis.

Closure Devices

In practice, closure devices are used routinely to reduce access site complications and provide for secure hemostasis and earlier ambulation. For access larger than 8 French, use a "preclose" technique with one or two Proglide suture closure devices (Abbott Vascular, Redwood City, Calif.) or the larger Prostar suture closure device (Abbott Vascular, Redwood City, Calif.).[3] Brachial artery access is usually performed using a 4-French sheath. Use of percutaneous closure devices in the brachial artery, while not standard therapy, is possible[4] and occasionally

TABLE 46-1 Occlusion Balloon Catheters

Balloon	Manufacturer	Sheath Requirement (French)	Diameter Range (mm)	Catheter Length (cm)
Coda balloon	Cook Medical	14	32-40	120
Q50	WL Gore	12	10-50	65
Reliant	Medtronic	12	10-46	100
Berenstein	Boston Scientific	6	11.5	80

indicated. Starclose (Abbott Vascular, Redwood City, Calif.), an extraarterial nitinol clip, has been used on the brachial artery with satisfactory results.[3,4] Successful use of the preclose technique has been described for 14-French venous access as well; it is noteworthy that venous backbleeding from the marker port is less brisk than with arterial access and can be augmented with a Valsalva maneuver. Valsalva maneuver can be also be used effectively to validate the integrity of the closure.[5]

Balloon Catheters

Balloon catheters have two principal applications in trauma: angioplasty of stents or stent grafts in order to ensure their adequate molding to the vessel wall, and temporary occlusion of blood flow for hemorrhage control. In the case of the former, balloons of 5 to 14 mm in diameter, 60 to 80 mm in length, and on 80- and 135-cm long catheters are most frequently used. The aortic occlusion balloon, as described later, is used to maintain cerebral and coronary perfusion in the hemodynamically unstable patient and requires large-bore access. Examples of available occlusion balloons are listed in Table 46-1.

Stents

Self-expanding or balloon-expandable bare metal stents have applications in the treatment of arterial dissection or venous hemorrhage.

Stent Grafts

Fabric-covered stents include:
- The Wallgraft (Boston Scientific) self-expanding stent covered with Dacron polyester, with pullback deployment system
- Viabahn (WL Gore) self-expanding nitinol exoskeleton covered with thin polytetrafluoroethylene (PTFE) with pull-string deployment
- Fluency (Bard, Tempe, Ariz.) self-expanding nitinol with PTFE
- iCast (Atrium medical corporation, Hudson, N.H.) balloon-expandable stainless-steel stent with an encapsulated cover made of expanded PTFE

Endografts

Thoracic endografts for the treatment of aortic transection are produced by Cook, Medtronic, and WL Gore. Many trauma patients are young and have small-diameter aortas that preclude use of devices designed for aneurysm repair. While smaller devices are being produced, extension cuffs have seen modified use for the purpose of excluding thoracic aortic injury. Both abdominal endograft extension limbs and thoracic endografts have been used for inferior vena cava (IVC) injury.

Embolization Elements

Hemorrhage control and vascular occlusion are typically achieved with embolization using coils. Alternative embolization techniques using polyvinyl alcohol (PVA), Gelfoam (Upjohn, Kalamazoo, Mich.) or acrylic copolymer microspheres such as Embospheres and EmboGold (Biosphere Medical, Rockland, Mass.)[6] are not routinely used in patients with active extravasation. Coils come in standard size configurations, such as the platinum-based 0.035-inch Tornado coils (Cook, Bloomington, Ind.) or variable size configurations found in the Vortex coil (Boston Scientific), available in 0.018-, 0.021-, and 0.038-inch diameters.

The Amplatzer (3 to 22 mm; St Jude Medical, St Paul, Minn.) self-expanding nitinol plug is an alternative device with a minimum vessel diameter requirement of 1.42 mm for the smaller plugs, deliverable via a 4-French minimum diameter sheath access. The largest device requires a 7-French sheath. Oversizing of 30% to 50% is recommended.

Anticoagulation

Anticoagulation is individualized. In patients with hypovolemic shock from blood loss of unknown extent and etiology, or in those for whom intracranial injury has not been ruled out, systemic heparin is not initially used. Sheaths and catheters are flushed frequently with dilute heparinized saline. Once the source of hemorrhage is identified and a strategy for management is determined, judicial systemic anticoagulation can be used to limit complications from sheath and device instrumentation in the appropriately selected patient.

INITIAL EVALUATION: RETHINKING THE TRAUMA ALGORITHM

The traditional algorithm of trauma patient management has always included an assessment of hemodynamic stability and the potential benefit of obtaining additional information from imaging, balanced by the possible risk associated with a delay of necessary surgical intervention. In the standard paradigm, the more stable patients are able to undergo primary and secondary surveys as well as radiographs and computed tomography (CT) scans to delineate injuries. The involvement of the vascular surgeon or interventionist is usually after the diagnosis of extremity vascular injury or solid organ injury has already been made. Treatment of the patient's various injuries are prioritized by the trauma team, and repair of the vascular injury is addressed according to severity, occasionally following a period of alternative evaluation and hemodynamic management. The management of patients with these types of identified injuries is described later in this chapter. The patient who requires endovascular imaging and potential intervention is given appropriate intravenous (IV) fluids. It is not infrequent that patients will receive multiple IV contrast loads in their initial 24 hours in the hospital because of multiple CT scans and angiograms. Adequate hydration and bicarbonate solution are useful in reducing contrast-induced kidney complications.

In the traditional trauma paradigm, the unstable patient or patient in extremis will often not survive to undergo evaluation by a vascular surgeon, being managed by standard open surgical techniques in a trauma bay or OR with limited imaging or endovascular capabilities. Exsanguination from noncompressible injury to the torso remains a major cause of death in both military and civilian trauma. The use of endovascular techniques to affect these potentially preventable mortalities has been targeted by the U.S. Department of Defense as an important area for clinical research.[7] After patent airway and breathing are established, the critically ill hypotensive patient may require emergent thoracotomy for proximal control of the aorta before rapid transfer to the OR for emergent laparotomy or thoracotomy to address injury. A growing body of experimental[8,9] and clinical[10,11] evidence supports the placement of an aortic occlusion balloon rather than thoracotomy. Emergency department thoracotomy for penetrating trauma has a survival rate of 8.8%; the procedure, when performed for blunt trauma, has an even more dismal record with survival of 1.4%.[12] Clearly an improved approach is warranted. It is common practice to perform all trauma surgery in a setting that provides as many therapeutic options as possible for patients with potential vascular injuries. By using a hybrid operating suite with advanced imaging, anesthesia support and appropriate trauma personnel involvement, it is possible to simultaneously stabilize, image, and treat many injuries with endovascular techniques or a combination of open and catheter-based surgical alternatives. For example, patients with hypotension can undergo placement of an aortic occlusion balloon under fluoroscopic guidance before induction of general anesthesia, which can often precipitate arrest because of vasodilatory effects of agents used during induction.[7,12]

Technique

A micropuncture system is used to gain access to the vascular system using ultrasound guidance and is then upsized to a 6-French introducer sheath. A 0.035-inch, 260-cm angled Glidewire is then passed into the thoracic aorta under fluoroscopy. Angiographic visualization of the arch anatomy is performed using a pigtail catheter and power injector, if indicated. A Proglide closure device is used to preclose the artery; a 10-cm, 6-French sheath is placed; and an angled Glidecath advanced into the thoracic aorta. The wire is exchanged for an Amplatz wire, and a 12-French sheath is advanced under fluoroscopy. The aortic occlusion balloon is inflated in the descending thoracic aorta[13] until hemodynamics improve with blood products and crystalloid resuscitation. The balloon is then deflated and removed, and additional diagnostic and therapeutic interventions are performed. Alternatively, the contralateral groin is accessed with a 6-French sheath for diagnostic and therapeutic catheter placement, and the aortic occlusion balloon is left in place for intermittent inflation or partial deflation as needed. The Gore Dryseal sheath allows multiple cannulations with devices of varying diameters while limiting leakage from the hemostatic valve, thereby decreasing the need for multiple access sites. When using this technique, however, the fluid-filled valve may decrease the maneuverability of the therapeutic catheter placed alongside the occlusion balloon, complicating the ability to selectively cannulate branch vessels.

MANAGEMENT OF SPECIFIC INJURIES

Physical examination or radiographic imaging will inform the decision to perform arteriography of certain anatomic areas. Table 46-2 summarizes methods of contrast arteriography.

Carotid and Vertebral Artery

The reported incidence of carotid injuries varies widely, ranging between 0.3% and 20%.[14] Blunt trauma to the carotid occurs at 0.1% to 0.45%, with mortality rates as high as 20% to 40%.[15] Penetrating carotid injuries account for approximately 3% of injuries.[16] Vertebral artery injuries are much less common because of bony protection. Clinical findings that support diagnostic workup include mandibular or facial fractures, C2-C3 fractures, neck contusion or laceration, neck hematoma, and mechanism of injury (deceleration). Injuries constitute transection, dissection, thrombosis, pseudoaneurysm, and arteriovenous fistula (AVF) leading to stroke and death.[17] Cervical injuries are initially classified according to their location along the neck in order to facilitate decision-making. Anatomic zones in the neck were initially described by Monson and colleagues[18] and have implications for management of cervical vascular injuries: guiding traditional open surgical alternatives for achieving proximal and distal vascular control. Zone I is located below the cricoid cartilage, zone II is between the cricoid cartilage and angle of the mandible, and zone III injuries occur above the angle of the mandible. Penetrating zone II trauma with hard signs, such as bleeding, expanding hematoma, or loss of carotid pulses and acute neurologic deficits have traditionally mandated immediate surgical exploration without further studies. Classically, proximal control in zone I injuries would

TABLE 46-2 Technical Tips for Arteriography for Trauma

Artery	Placement of Distal Tip of Catheter	Catheter*	Contrast Administration					Image Acquisition	
			Rate (mL/s)	Volume (mL)	Pressure† (psi)	Rise (s)	Injection Delay (s)	Frames Per Second	Image Intensifier Position
Aortic arch	Ascending aorta	90 cm Omniflush‡ or pigtail	20	40	800-1200		1	6	Left anterior oblique
Innominate artery	Innominate artery	100 cm angled Glidecath, Simmons 1 or 2 (Vitek)	5	10	300-500	0.2-0.5	1	4	Right anterior oblique
Right subclavian artery	Proximal right subclavian artery	100 cm angled Glidecath, Simmons 1 or 2	4	8	300-500	0.2-0.5	1	4	Right anterior oblique
Right vertebral artery	Proximal right subclavian artery	100 cm angled Glidecath, Simmons 1 or 2	3	6	200	0.2-0.5	1	4	
Right common carotid artery	Proximal right common carotid artery	100 cm angled Glidecath, Simmons 1 or 2	4	8	300-500	0.2-0.5	1	4	Anteroposterior, lateral, oblique
Left common carotid artery	Proximal left common carotid artery	100 cm angled Glidecath, Simmons 1 or 2	4	8	300-500	0.2-0.5	1	4	Anteroposterior, lateral, oblique
Left subclavian artery	Proximal left subclavian artery	100 cm angled Glidecath, H1	4	8	300-500	0.2-0.5	1	4	
Left vertebral artery	Proximal left vertebral artery	100 cm angled Glidecath, H1	3	6	200	0.2-0.5	1	4	
Axillary artery	Axillary artery	100 cm angled Glidecath	4	12	300-500		1	4	
Brachial artery	Proximal brachial artery	100-120 cm angled Glidecath	4	8	300-500		1	4	
Abdominal aorta	Abdominal aorta at T12/L1	65 cm Omniflush or pigtail	10	30	800-1200		1	4	Anteroposterior
Celiac/superior mesenteric artery origin	Abdominal aorta at T12/L1	65 cm Omniflush or pigtail	10	30	800-1200		1	4	Lateral
Renal artery origin	Abdominal aorta at T12/L1	65 cm Omniflush or pigtail	10	30	800-1200		1	4	Anteroposterior, oblique
Renal artery	Renal artery	Angled Glidecath, Simmons 1, Cobra, Sos	4	8	300-500		1	4	
Celiac axis	Celiac axis, splenic artery, common hepatic artery	Angled Glidecath, Simmons 1, or Cobra	5	15	300-500		1	4	Anteroposterior
Superior mesenteric artery	Superior mesenteric artery	Angled Glidecath, Simmons 1, or Cobra	5	15	300-500		1	4	
Aortoiliac	Abdominal aorta at iliac crests	65 cm Omniflush or pigtail	10	12	800-1200		1	4	
Common iliac artery/hypogastric artery	Distal common iliac artery	65 cm angled Glidecath	5	10	300-500		1	4	Ipsilateral oblique
Common femoral artery/profunda artery	Distal external iliac artery	65 cm angled Glidecath	4	8	300-500		1	4	Contralateral oblique
Popliteal artery/tibial/pedal artery	Distal superficial femoral artery	100 cm angled Glidecath	3	12	300-500		1	4	Oblique

*All catheters are 5 French, with presumptive access from the common femoral artery.
†Injection pressure is for 5 French catheter system.
‡Omniflush (Angiodynamics, Latham, N.Y.); Glidecath (Terumo, Somerset, N.J.); Vitek catheter (Cook, Bloomington, N.Y.); Sos (Angiodynamics, Latham, N.Y.); Cobra (Cook, Bloomington, Ind.).

require a median sternotomy. For patients with an injury in zone III, distal vascular control is difficult without subluxation of the mandible. However, classical limitations in vascular control have evolved with current endovascular solutions. Balloon occlusion of the proximal cervical vessels in the chest can be accomplished via femoral access. Similarly, proximal control can be obtained in zone III injuries with compliant balloons placed in the proximal internal carotid or vertebral arteries. This also provides the opportunity to obtain imaging to better define and potentially manage the cervical vascular injury endovascularly.

Duplex ultrasound can identify dissection as well as pseudoaneurysm. Any abnormal findings, such as turbulent flow, reduced flow velocity, absence of flow, or presence of an echolucent intraluminal lesion, should lower the threshold for further investigation with angiography. CTA has been used for penetrating injuries of the neck, with a 75% sensitivity to diagnose venous vascular injury.[19,20] However, digital subtraction angiography remains the gold standard for carotid artery injuries and offers the opportunity for endovascular therapy. Traumatic carotid lesions amenable to endovascular treatment are intimal dissection, pseudoaneurysm, and AVF.[21-24] External carotid artery injuries have been managed safely with endovascular ligation using coils, N-butyl 2-cyanoacrylate embolization and balloon occlusion for endovascular ligation.[17] Similarly, vertebral artery injuries may be amenable to coiling and balloon occlusion as well as with covered stent deployment, allowing for maintenance of inline flow.[25]

Treatment options for carotid dissections with intact distal flow include surgical repair, endovascular stenting, or observation with repeat diagnostic studies 1 to 2 weeks after the injury. Systemic heparinization in patients without any contraindications is typically indicated and may be all that is required.[16] Open surgical approaches are rare. Uncovered stents may be placed to treat short lesions.[26,27] If the site of entry is identified, an attempt at placement can be considered for even more extended dissections if anticoagulation is contraindicated.

Pseudoaneurysms can result from direct injury or as a sequelae of a maturing dissection. When large, they can expand and cause compressive symptoms, requiring operation or embolization.[28,29] Surgical intervention can be complex, especially for lesions near the skull base, where temporomandibular joint subluxation or vertical ramus osteotomy may be required to obtain adequate exposure. Ligation of the carotid artery carries an associated mortality of up to 44% and neurologic deficit in 100%.[30] Restoration of flow with open repair of the internal and common carotid arteries is associated with persistent neurologic deficit in up to 30% of cases.[30] Covered stents have been used to exclude pseudoaneurysms. Coils have also been used to treat these lesions and, in some cases, both have been applied.[28,29,31] The major risk in treating a pseudoaneurysm in the carotid artery is distal embolization and stroke; however, data on the use of distal protection devices are limited. Stent grafts were placed successfully in 19 patients with penetrating injuries (10 pseudoaneurysms, 9 AVFs). At follow-up, ranging from 1 to 56 months, 14% had stent graft occlusion with one

associated stroke.[32] A literature review of stent-graft placement indicates a 15% postoperative occlusion rate.[33] When stent-graft placement is planned, premedication is done with antiplatelet agents, preferably clopidogrel and aspirin. Traumatic carotid lesions pose a unique challenge with acute, possibly unstable thrombus susceptible to embolization during wire manipulation. Although no specific data exist for it, the use of an embolic protection device may reduce the potential for embolic complications.

Technique

Proximal injuries may require direct cervical exposure for a retrograde approach with the role of the distal protection device played by an internal carotid artery clamp. However, most injuries are approachable from the femoral artery. A 5-French, 90-cm Omniflush catheter is placed in the ascending aorta, and a left anterior oblique aortogram is taken to demonstrate the ostia of the arch vessels. Based on this image, an end-hole catheter is selected for cannulation of the common carotid artery. In uncomplicated arch anatomy, the 5-French, 100-cm angled Glidecath is used. Once the ostium of the carotid artery is engaged, 2 mL of contrast is injected to corroborate position. The 0.035-inch Glidewire is advanced gently into the target artery, and the angled catheter is advanced, with particular care taken not to advance the wire too distally into the internal carotid artery. Carotid angiography is performed in anteroposterior (AP) and lateral positions. Additional oblique views may be needed to properly assess the anatomy and extent of injury. The intracranial circulation is also evaluated with AP and lateral views. Up to 30% of blunt carotid injuries are bilateral, mandating a complete four-vessel angiogram. Once the injury has been defined, the wire is exchanged for the 260-cm Amplatz wire; a 6-French, 90-cm–long Destination sheath (Terumo, Somerset, N.J.) is placed with its tip above the clavicle. A distal embolization protection filter may be placed. Self-expanding bare metal stents or a Viabahn-covered self-expanding stent may be advanced directly over the 0.014-inch filter wire. If coil embolization of pseudoaneurysms is performed in conjunction with distal embolization protection, a 7-French Destination sheath may be used to facilitate advancement of both the filter wire and a 45-French catheter into the common carotid artery. Endovascular occlusion of the severely damaged carotid or vertebral artery has been described. Glue, microbeads, or other liquid agents such as N-butyl 2-cyanoacrylate are not typically used in the common or internal carotid artery, but have been used in the external carotid. Amplatzer plug placement has also been described. The preferred method for hemorrhage control for injury to branches of the external carotid artery uses a 6-French sheath, a 4-French Glidecath, and 0.035-inch embolic coils. Vertebral artery injuries can be treated similarly. Figure 46-1A to C shows management of a traumatic arteriovenous fistula from the vertebral artery to the internal jugular vein treated with placement of a 5 mm × 2.5 cm covered stent.

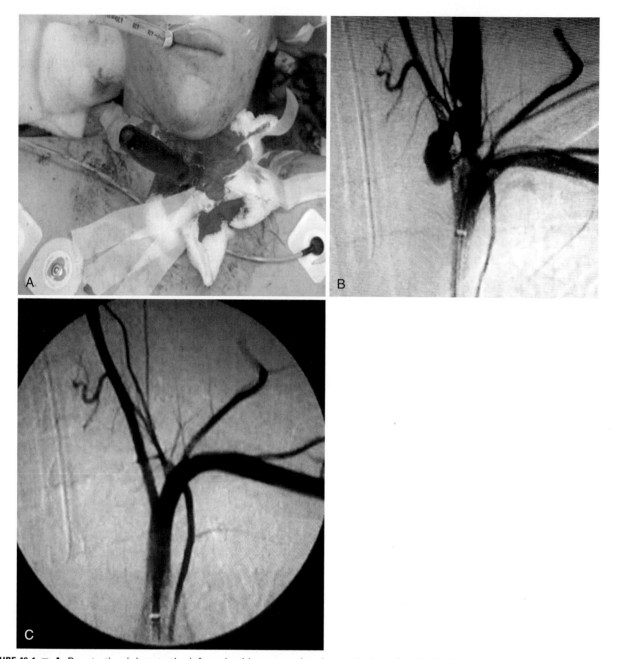

FIGURE 46-1 ■ **A,** Penetrating injury to the left neck without associated neurologic deficit. **B,** Digital subtraction image demonstrates pseudoaneurysm of the left vertebral artery. **C,** Resolution of the pseudoaneurysm following placement of a Viabahn stent (WL Gore, Flagstaff, Ariz.).

Innominate Artery and the Descending Thoracic Aorta

Thoracic Aorta

Only 15% of patients with severe blunt thoracic aortic trauma survive to reach the hospital. Only 50% of those who reach the hospital will ultimately survive the aortic injury.[34] Typically, patients who survive the initial injury have a contained rupture with tissue tamponade and a hematoma that is constrained. When patients convert to free rupture, the mortality rate is 100%. The mechanism of injury involves stress, applied to transition points between fixed and relatively mobile segments of the

aorta. These forces are compounded by sudden internal changes in blood pressure and pulse pressure. Aortic injury of this kind is most often due to a motor vehicle crash (MVC) or a fall, with attendant sudden deceleration. In patients with contained rupture, control of blood pressure and the resultant reduction in sheer forces associated with hypertension and tachycardia is important. Administration of β-blockers, including permissive hypotension, is useful in the initial management of patients with aortic injury and normal or hyperdynamic hemodynamics. The minority of patients (15%-19%) who survive the initial injury and period of transport to the hospital are in various stages of shock because of other concurrent injuries, with systolic blood pressures ranging from 50%

to 98% of normal.[35,36] Both hypotension and hypothermia (body temperature <35°C) are associated with early mortality, with an adjusted odds ratio of 8.54.[35] Major factors contributing to increased mortality include the severity of associated injuries and the timing of repair. The primary initial management of blunt aortic injuries requires early and efficient resuscitation and the treatment of associated injuries.[37,38] Some centers have moved to delayed endovascular repair of stable (without contrast extravasation) blunt aortic injuries in order to treat associated injuries first.[39,40]

The mean ISS of traumatic thoracic aortic transections is 39.[41] Associated injuries, including head injury, pulmonary contusion, long bone injury, and solid organ injury, occur in 90% of blunt aortic traumas. The abdomen and chest have the highest associated injury severity score.[41] Open surgical management of thoracic aortic trauma is complicated by the physiologic stresses associated with single lung ventilation and aortic cross-clamping. Open repair is associated with a mortality rate of 15% to 40% and resultant paraplegia rates of 8% to 20%.

Endovascular management for these injuries has the potential to mitigate some of the risks associated with open surgical alternatives. Thirty-day mortality rates associated with endovascular repair of thoracic aortic injuries have been reported as high as 8.3% with an associated 1-year mortality of 14.4%.[41] Major adverse events associated with endovascular repair include, stroke (10%), respiratory failure (3.3%), and paralysis or paraparesis (1.7%) at 30 days with no additional events recorded at 1-year follow-up.

In the patient with blunt thoracic trauma but in stable condition, CTA with three-dimensional reconstruction is the preferred tool for assessing the injury. The anatomic information obtained aids in planning for access and determining the size of the native aorta and the extent of coverage needed to repair the injury. In the less stable patient, direct evaluation in the hybrid OR with angiographic evaluation and immediate endovascular repair may be warranted.

The early reports of endovascular repair of blunt aortic injury described the use of endovascular cuffs that were designed for proximal extension of infrarenal aortic endografts.[42-44] Currently, appropriately sized thoracic stent-grafts are available for traumatic thoracic aortic injuries made by a number of manufacturers including the Talent graft (Medtronic, Minneapolis, Minn.), the TAG graft (an acronym for thoracic aortic graft; WL Gore), the TX2 graft (Cook, Bloomington, Ind.) and the AneuRx graft (Medtronic, Minneapolis, Minn.). More commonly available grafts, sized for thoracic aortic aneurysm repair, are often too large for the normal-sized aorta of the typical trauma patient. Careful sizing is essential to provide for a satisfactory seal and to prevent infolding.

Technique. General anesthesia is standard. Placement of a spinal catheter is useful for pressure reduction by spinal fluid drainage in patients exhibiting signs of spinal cord ischemia perioperatively. Given the larger size of endovascular devices designed for thoracic aortic

intervention, open exposure of the external iliac arteries may be required to facilitate device delivery and closure. Alternatively, common femoral artery cutdown or percutaneous access using the previously described preclose technique may be performed.[42] An arch aortogram is performed using a marker pigtail catheter. If left subclavian artery coverage is required to obtain a proximal landing zone of 2 cm, the left subclavian artery may be occluded proximal to the vertebral artery, through left brachial artery access using an Amplatzer plug or coils. Retrospective reviews of blunt thoracic injuries have reported subclavian artery coverage rates ranging from 0% to 80%.[43] The issue of carotid-subclavian bypass is controversial. Bypass should be performed for patients with a dominant left vertebral artery, a blind posterior inferior cerebellar artery, or a left internal mammary artery–left anterior descending coronary artery bypass.[44] If more arch is required for an adequate landing zone, then a carotid to carotid bypass can be performed for further debranching.

The major challenge of endograft placement is sizing. Most companies recommend 10% to 15% oversizing of the endograft compared to the native aortic diameter either measured from inner lumen to inner lumen (WL Gore) or outer adventitia to adventitia (Medtronic). In otherwise normal aortas without dilatation or aneurysmal deterioration, the aortic diameter is generally 18 mm. Oversizing can jeopardize both the proximal and distal seal zones secondary to pleating and in-folding of the stent graft; this can lead to displacement and slippage of the stent graft, compromise of luminal flow, or "bird-beaking" of the proximal graft, with resultant endoleak and device fracture. Therefore accurate sizing of the stent-graft to aortic diameter is required. Accurate sizing may be compromised by hypovolemia and an associated reduction of aortic diameter by 30%.[45]

Temporary pacing or pharmaceutical slowing of the heart can be used as an adjunct to assist in accurate placement of the thoracic endograft. The endograft seal zones are postdilated with an aortic balloon. A trilobed balloon that allows for some antegrade flow during balloon inflation is recommended.

Significant morbidity and death have been reported in endovascular repair of thoracic aortic transection associated with iliac artery complications. These injuries might not be recognized until sheath removal (Figure 46-2A). In patients with iliac arteries less than 8 mm in diameter (24 French), whether due to spasm in the young or atherosclerotic disease in the older patient, retroperitoneal exposure of the abdominal aorta or left common iliac artery, with a plan for either direct cannulation or creation of a prosthetic conduit through which the endograft may be delivered, is a safe option.

Innominate Artery

Injury from blunt trauma to thoracic arch branches is rare, encompassing 5% of traumatic vascular injuries, a rate significantly lower than that for penetrating injuries in this region. However, the incidence is likely underestimated because of the high mortality associated with arch injury in the field (80%-90%). The innominate

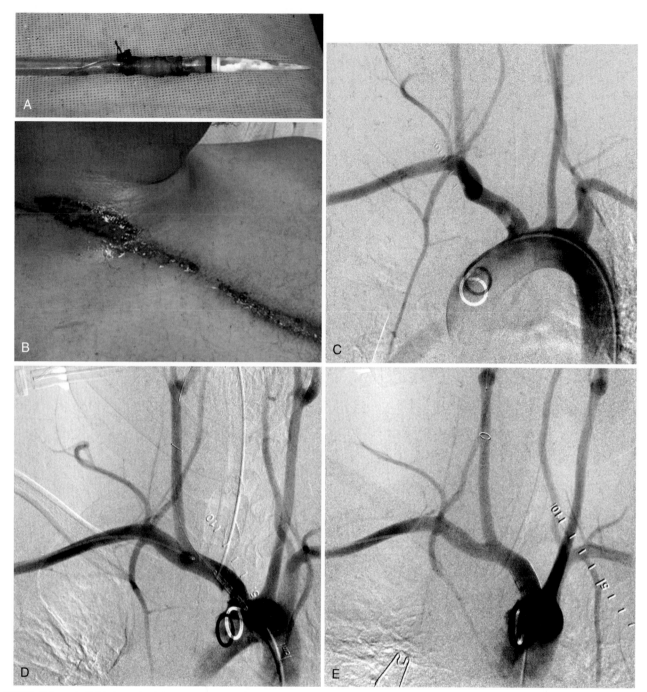

FIGURE 46-2 ■ **A,** Withdrawal of thoracic endograft sheath from a young female trauma patient demonstrates common iliac artery avulsion which was repaired via an interposition graft. **B,** Seatbelt sign in a young male patient after high-speed motor vehicle crash; he complained of right neck, chest, and back pain. **C,** Innominate artery injury was demonstrated via femoral and right brachial accesses. **D,** After deployment of an embolic protection device in the right common carotid artery, an 11-mm Viabahn stent-graft (WL Gore, Flagstaff, Ariz.) was deployed and successfully excluded the lesion **(E).** (**A,** Courtesy T.T. Huynh, MD, Anderson Cancer Center and The Methodist Hospital, Houston, Tex.)

artery accounts for half of all arch vessel injuries, with a mortality ranging from 0% to 24%. The most common mechanism of injury is MVC (88.9%), followed by crush (8.9%) and fall (2.2%). Head-on collisions constitute the majority of MVC-associated innominate artery injuries (72%), followed by side (24%) and rear impacts (4%) at relative velocities greater than 60 mph or with a change in velocity of greater than or equal to 20 mph. Chest compression increases the intramediastinal pressure between the sternoclavicular joint and the vertebral column, pushing the heart posteriorly and to the left to stretch the aortic branches. Hyperextension of the cervical spine and lateral rotation of the head serve to maximize the shear stress at the origin of innominate artery. Key clinical indicators of injury include the seatbelt sign (see Figure 46-2B) and steering wheel imprint as well as dyspnea, dysphagia, interscapular and neck pain, absent upper extremity pulses, neurologic deficit, acute superior vena cava syndrome, pseudocoarctation, presence of a bruit from an arteriovenous fistula, and congestive heart failure. Diagnosis is suspected with widened mediastinum, rib fractures, tracheal or esophageal deviation, and right hemothorax or pneumothorax on chest radiography. The diagnosis can be made on chest CTA, angiography, transesophageal echocardiography (TEE; 86%-92% sensitive), magnetic resonance angiography, and intravascular ultrasound.[15,46-53] Innominate artery injuries are most common at the orifice (81.8%), followed by the distal (9.1%) and midpoint (4.5%) of the vessel, with 2.3% of injuries occurring at two separate parts of the artery. These injuries encompass intimal tears (70%), pseudoaneurysms, and rupture. After efficient and aggressive resuscitation to normotension through femoral venous access, open and endovascular options for repair are considered. The decision for open repair is often predicated on the existence of concomitant injuries mandating thoracic exploration via median sternotomy or trap door thoracotomy. These approaches are inherently morbid, with significant risk of neurologic and respiratory injury.[54-57] In cases without significant related injuries in proximity requiring exploration, endovascular repair can be accomplished with femoral access distant from the field of injury, with less pain, fewer respiratory and neurologic complications, and decreased length of stay.[58,59] Dissection or intimal flap in the innominate artery can be treated with a bare metal or covered self-expanding stent. Pseudoaneurysm and transection or rupture are treated with covered stents. The primary endovascular limitation is the lack of adequate distal landing zone before the artery bifurcates. If necessary, the right subclavian artery can be excluded by the stent-graft with performance of a carotid-subclavian artery bypass, if needed for right arm ischemia. Premedication with clopidogrel and aspirin is ideal when the patient's condition permits, and is continued indefinitely for patients receiving endovascular implants in this location.[60] Although there is a paucity of data on the use of embolic protection devices in traumatic innominate artery injury, it is common to use a device placed within the distal common carotid artery during stent advancement and deployment.

Technique. Percutaneous common femoral artery access is obtained, and arch arteriography is completed using the pigtail catheter. The innominate artery can be cannulated with an angled Glidecath in a type I arch. A type II or III arch may require a Simmons 1 or 2 Glidecath. A 0.035-inch Glidewire is carefully advanced to the lesion, taking care not displace an injury-associated soft thrombus. The wire is exchanged for the Amplatz wire, and the 90-cm, 6-French sheath is advanced to the innominate artery, as space permits, proximal to the lesion. An embolic protection device is then advanced through the lesion and deployed in the distal common carotid artery. A self-expanding stent can be deployed over the filter wire. A covered stent-graft, routinely oversized by no more than 10% for the normal artery, will usually require a 9- to 12-French sheath for diameters greater than 8.5 mm. Postdeployment balloon angioplasty is performed with a compliant balloon, selected to match the vessel diameter (see Figure 46-2C to E).

Subclavian-Axillary-Brachial

Penetrating injuries of the subclavian and axillary arteries are far more common than blunt lesions. Of the 93 cases of subclavian artery injury reported by Graham and associates,[46,61] only two were related to blunt trauma. Blunt injury accounts for only 3% of subclavian and 1% of axillary artery traumatic injuries.[46] Surgical exploration and control may require a median sternotomy with periclavicular incisions for proximal and distal right subclavian artery control. A left lateral thoracotomy with additional periclavicular incisions may be required for adequate exposure of left subclavian artery injuries.[62] These anatomic approaches may entail substantial tissue edema, risk for neurologic injury, and significant blood loss, and they are associated with mortality rates between 3% and 33%. Absolute indications for angiogram at the initial evaluation of injuries to this region are absence of pulses, persistent shock despite resuscitation, and copious intrathoracic bleeding. Relative indications include injury with associated brachial plexus palsy, fractured clavicle and concomitant fracture of the first three ribs, supraclavicular contusion with or without hematoma, and soft tissue injury of the neck and upper extremity.[62]

A recent series published by du Toit and colleagues[63] demonstrated the feasibility of endovascular approaches to subclavian and axillary arterial injuries. Ten patients with penetrating injuries (n = 9 gunshot wounds; n = 1 stab wound) were treated with stent-graft deployment. No deaths, amputations, or procedure-related morbidities were noted, and short-term follow-up of 7 months demonstrated no evidence of stenosis or occlusion. Xenos and colleagues[64] recently compared their open versus endovascular experience of subclavian and axillary artery injuries, noting significantly less blood loss and procedure time with the endovascular cohort, and no difference in patency rates of the repairs at 1 year. Long-term patency rates are unknown.[64] Lacerations, intimal flaps, vessel occlusion, pseudoaneurysm, AVFs, and avulsion of branches can be treated with covered stents. Potential contraindications to this approach include the lack of adequate proximal landing zone, limited on the right by the common carotid artery and bilaterally by the vertebral and internal mammary arteries. In patients undergoing an open procedure, endovascular balloon occlusion and hemorrhage control may be useful.[65]

Technique

It is possible to attain both femoral and retrograde percutaneous brachial access using an ultrasound guided micropuncture technique. For a dissection or intimal flap, it is imperative to cannulate the true lumen. Once guidewire traversal has been achieved and true lumen continuity verified, the stent-graft can be advanced from either direction. Accurate positioning can be verified by puff contrast angiography from a catheter advanced from the other access (Figure 46-3A to F).

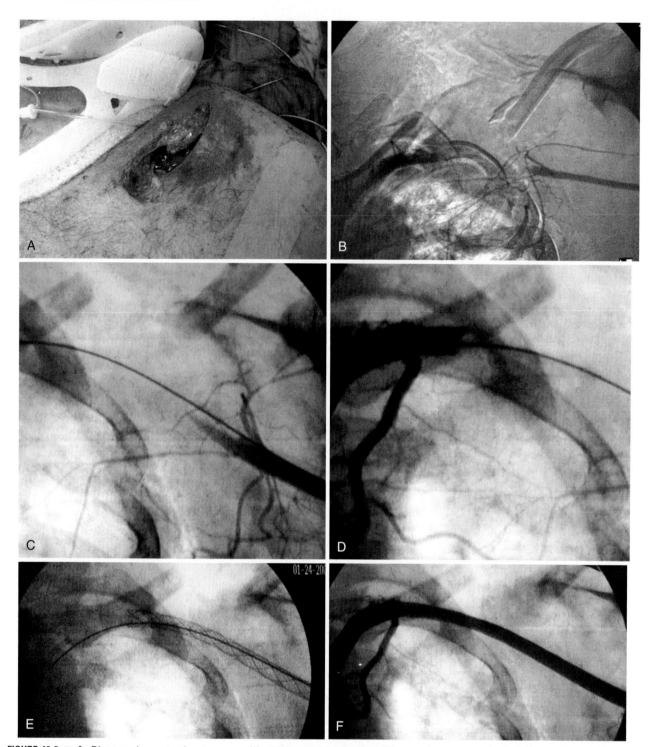

FIGURE 46-3 ■ **A,** Blunt and penetrating trauma with clavicular fracture and **(B)** complete transection of the left subclavian artery demonstrated by arteriogram via femoral and brachial artery approaches. **C,** After a hydrophilic wire is passed from the proximal to the **(D)** distal segment, **(E)** a Wallgraft (Boston Scientific, Natick, Mass.) is deployed with **(F)** restoration of arterial continuity.

Injury to the distal axillary, brachial artery, or distal branches often occurs in the setting of open injury. When distal signals are present, it is common practice to ligate the thrombosed or frankly bleeding branch. When restoration of flow is needed in the presence of an open wound, bypass is performed with tunneling away from the open wound. In the setting of polytrauma, with unstable patients, an endovascular approach can provide rapid hemostasis without ligation, restoring flow. The MVC victim in Figure 46-4*A* suffered intracranial, pelvic, and extremity trauma. His brachial injury (see Figure 46-4*B*) was temporized efficiently with placement of a covered stent-graft (see Figure 46-4*C*).

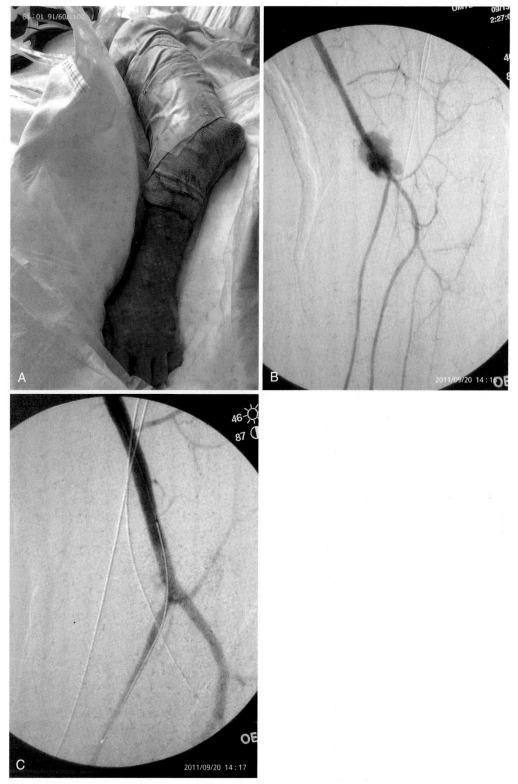

FIGURE 46-4 ■ **A** and **B,** This polytrauma patient suffered left arm fractures with left brachial artery injury. **C,** Left brachial artery injury excluded with a Viabahn stent-graft (WL Gore, Flagstaff, Ariz.).

Chest Wall

Trauma to the chest wall, both blunt and penetrating, represents a significant challenge. Often, thoracotomy for hemothorax caused by internal mammary or intercostal artery injury will not be at the correct intercostal level to visualize the injury, which can be particularly elusive in large patients. Coil, Gelfoam, and PVA particle embolization of internal mammary and intercostal arteries has been described for primary therapy of hemothorax,[66,67] persistent or recurrent hemothorax after thoractomy,[66] or arterial bleeding into the chest wall.[68] Injuries described have included blunt[66-68] and penetrating[66] trauma as well as iatrogenic injury.[67]

Technique

A descending thoracic aortic angiogram with a pigtail catheter is performed with delayed visualization of the contrast outflow. If a bleeding intercostal is identified, it is cannulated using a 5-French angled Glidecath. Selective angiography is performed to delineate the anatomy, such as spinal branches arising from the intercostal artery of interest. A microcatheter is then used for placement of

coils as close to the area of injury as possible. If selective angiography of the intercostal artery fails to reveal a bleeding source, the ipsilateral internal mammary artery is studied because of the anterior anastomotic connections between the internal mammary and the intercostal arteries. If the internal mammary itself has been identified as the bleeding source, the subclavian artery is cannulated using the 5-French angled Glidecath or Simmons 1 catheter. The internal mammary artery is cannulated using the 0.014-inch wire. The microcatheter is advanced, and embolization is performed using appropriately sized microcoils. Figure 46-5*A* to *C* demonstrates the use of both coil embolization and covered stent deployment to manage active bleeding in a patient with an injury to the

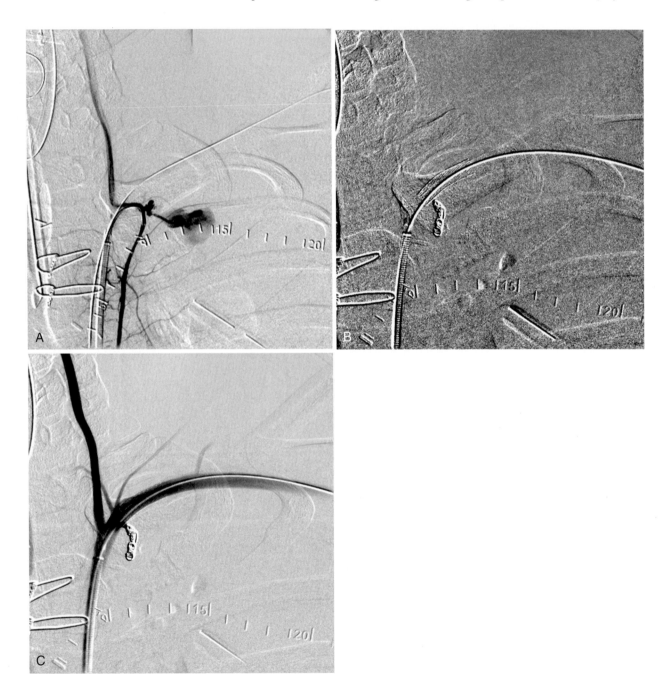

FIGURE 46-5 ■ **A,** Penetrating injury to the left internal mammary artery, with rapidly expanding hematoma. **B** and **C,** Injury resolved with coiling of the internal mammary artery and left subclavian artery Viabahn stent-graft (WL Gore, Flagstaff, Ariz.) placement.

left subclavian artery at the origin of the left internal mammary artery.

Splenic Trauma

The spleen is the second most commonly injured organ after the liver, with splenic injury occurring in 32% of abdominal trauma.[69] It is most often seen in blunt abdominal trauma, such as MVCs, sports, and assaults. Blunt splenic trauma is associated with other intraabdominal organ injuries in 36.5% of cases.[70] The management of splenic injury has undergone evolution. In the past, operative management with splenectomy was the standard of care for patients with high-grade injury or contrast extravasation on CT scan. With increasing awareness of the importance of splenic function and lifelong risk of postsplenectomy sepsis, a trend toward spleen conservation with partial resection, mesh splenography, and coagulation techniques emerged.[71,72] Today, most splenic injuries can be treated with nonoperative management. A review of literature from 1995 to 2006 by Raikhlin and colleagues[73] showed the overall success of nonoperative management to be 86% to 100%. However, failure may still occur, requiring surgical intervention; this risk of failure has been shown to increase with the severity of splenic injury. In 2000, the multi-institutional study of the Eastern Association for the Surgery of Trauma reported failure rates of nonoperative treatment for each grade of splenic injury from the American Association for the Surgery of Trauma (AAST).[74] The failure rate for Grade I was 4.8%, Grade II was 9.5%, Grade III was 19.6%, Grade IV was 33.3%, and Grade V was 75.0% for an overall rate of 10.8%.

In our Trauma center, ultrasound is used to rapidly assess the abdomen for internal injuries. The Focused Abdominal Sonography for Trauma (FAST) is the method of choice for detecting free fluid; it has largely replaced diagnostic peritoneal lavage in trauma centers. It can be performed at the same time as ongoing resuscitation efforts with minimal disruption. FAST has a sensitivity of 90% for detecting hemoperitoneum, but has low sensitivity for detecting splenic injury itself.[75] For hemodynamically stable patients, CT scan should be used routinely regardless of FAST results, with up to 29% of CT-proven splenic injury without detectable hemoperitoneum on FAST.[76] CT scan is the most accurate test to diagnose and grade splenic injury,[77] and may reveal additional injuries that change the treatment plan and outcome of trauma patients.[78] Positive CT findings include active contrast extravasation in the splenic parenchyma, subcapsular space or in the peritoneum.[79]

Transarterial embolization of splenic injuries was first described by Sclafani in 1981.[80] Since then, embolization has been shown to increase the success rate of nonoperative management by achieving hemostasis and reducing the incidence of delayed rupture. Controversy exists regarding the indication for embolization in splenic injuries. Current indications reported in the literature include CT findings of active contrast extravasation, vascular injury, high-grade parenchymal injury, and large hemoperitoneum.[74,81-83] A more aggressive approach has been described in which angiography is considered for any patient with splenic vascular injury or active bleeding on CT.[84] All patients with high-grade (AAST grades III to V) injuries for whom nonoperative management is attempted also undergo splenic angiography. Results of this algorithm include successful nonoperative management of more than 80% of grade IV and V injuries.[83] Other studies have also shown the efficacy of splenic embolization in high-grade splenic injuries.[74,85]

The spleen can be embolized by either proximal splenic artery embolization or selective distal embolization.[80,81,83] Proximal artery embolization results in decreased blood flow and perfusion to the entire spleen to allow for hemostasis, while preserving the organ via sufficient collateral flow from the short gastric arteries. This is the endovascular equivalent to suture ligation of the splenic artery. In contrast, distal embolization involves only the injured smaller, blood vessels that are usually within the splenic parenchyma. Distal embolization almost always results in segmental splenic infarct, whereas proximal embolization results in smaller, more peripheral infarction.[86] Based on scintigraphy, several small studies have shown preservation of splenic function after both proximal and distal embolization.[87] Proximal main artery embolization is usually used for diffuse bleeding or multivessel injury when time is of the essence. Selective distal embolization is used for one or few focal bleeding vessels. Currently, there is no literature supporting the use of proximal embolization over distal embolization, and the technique should likely be individualized.

The largest study to report complications after splenic embolization was the Western Trauma Association multi-institutional trial.[81] In a total of 140 patients, major complications occurred in 19% of patients, most commonly blood loss. Half of these patients required a splenectomy because of persistent bleeding. Splenic infarct was reported in 21%. Most cases of splenic infarction are asymptomatic and can be followed conservatively. However, some may develop fever and require further workup to elaborate a possible infectious etiology. Incidence of abscess is 3%, which may be amenable to percutaneous drainage.

Technique

Following AP and lateral abdominal aortograms with a flush catheter, a Simmons 1 Glidecath is used to select the splenic artery. An angled Glidewire is advanced distally into the splenic artery and the catheter is advanced over the wire. The Glidewire is then exchanged for an Amplatz wire. The short, femoral 6-French access sheath is then replaced with a 6-French, 60-cm Destination sheath. Embolization can then be performed via the 5-French angled Glidecath with 0.035-inch coils, or, if distal embolization is selected, the microcatheter can be telescoped through the 5-French Glidecath for the delivery of microcoils (Figure 46-6A to C).

Hepatic Trauma

The liver is the most commonly injured organ in abdominal trauma,[69,88,89] and it is frequently associated with splenic injury.[90] Similar to other solid abdominal organ

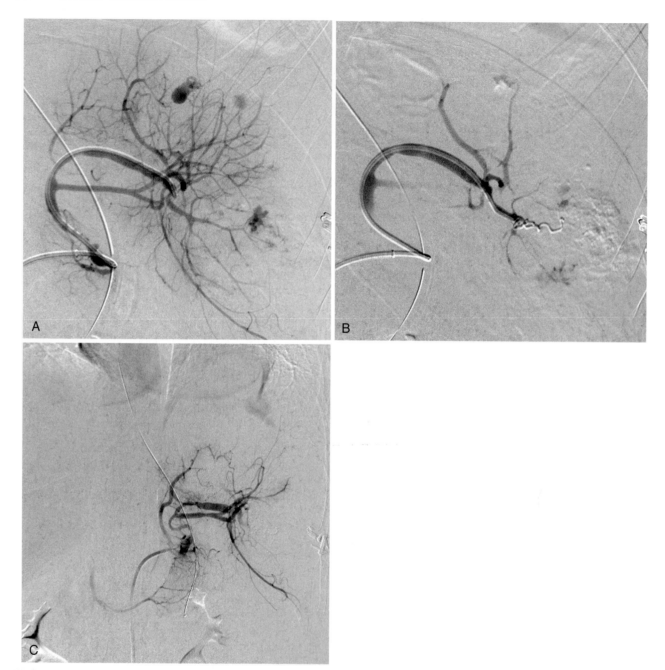

FIGURE 46-6 ■ **A,** Digital subtraction image of selective splenic angiogram demonstrates area of injury in a blunt trauma victim. **B** and **C,** Resolution of bleeding after coil embolization. Splenic preservation was achieved.

injuries, there is a trend toward nonoperative management over the past 2 decades. Nonoperative management of blunt hepatic injuries was found to be successful in 85% to 98.5% of hemodynamically stable patients, regardless of the grade of injury or degree of hemoperitoneum.[91,92] Bleeding complications are infrequently encountered (3.5%); active extravasation in liver injury is seen less often than splenic injury (9.1%). Delayed bleeding is rare.[91,94,96] Bleeding from blunt hepatic injuries, in contrast to splenic hemorrhage, may be worsened by surgical intervention. It has been suggested that the primary reason for the decrease in hepatic-related mortality over time is the parallel shift toward nonoperative

management.[93] Surgical intervention is primarily reserved for those patients with hemodynamic instability unresponsive to resuscitation.

The initial imaging modality is the bedside ultrasound; however, regardless of FAST examination results, most hemodynamically stable patients undergo CT scan. CT scan accurately grades liver injury and demonstrates the location of intrahepatic or extrahepatic bleeding. Active hepatic hemorrhage is suggested by "blush," or pooling of intravenous contrast material within the liver parenchyma. A classification of CT scan findings to predict clinical outcome after hepatic injury was described by Fang and colleagues.[94] They found that the presence of pooling of contrast material within the peritoneal cavity indicated active and massive bleeding. These patients showed rapid deterioration of hemodynamic status, and most of these patients required emergent surgery. Pooling of contrast material within ruptured hepatic parenchyma indicated active bleeding; however, close monitoring and emergent angiography could be performed safely. Deterioration of hemodynamic status in these patients usually required prompt surgical intervention. Finally, intraparenchymal pooling of contrast material with an intact liver capsule indicated a self-limited hemorrhage. These patients had a high possibility of successful nonoperative treatment.

The use of embolization for the management of blunt hepatic trauma was first described in 1977.[95] Currently, it is used as a valuable adjunct to nonoperative management, and early embolization is an effective way to control bleeding in even high-grade hepatic injuries. Embolization can be used early following initial CT scan findings of active arterial bleeding, postoperatively following damage control laparotomy, or in a delayed fashion, outside the window of initial resuscitation period.[96] It is effective in both blunt and penetrating hepatic injuries.[97,98] There is increasing experience with the use of embolization in the management of hemodynamically unstable patients with high-grade hepatic injuries. Asensio and colleagues[99] reported improved mortality rates of 8% and 22% for grades 4 and 5 hepatic injuries, respectively. These patients with complex hepatic injuries underwent surgery, early packing, and postoperative embolization. Recently, Monnin and colleagues[100] reported a success rate of 93% in the management of hemodynamically unstable patients with hepatic injuries.

Technique

Following AP and lateral abdominal aortogram with a flush catheter, a 5-French Simmons 1 Glidecath is used to select the celiac axis and common hepatic artery. When sufficient purchase has been gained using the angled Glidewire and Glidecath, the wire is exchanged for the Amplatz wire. The 6-French access sheath is replaced with a 6-French 60-cm–length Destination sheath. Embolization can then be performed via the 5-French angled Glidecath for 0.035 coils, or, if distal embolization is selected, the microcatheter can be telescoped through the 5-French Glidecath for the delivery of smaller micro coils (Figure 46-7A to C).

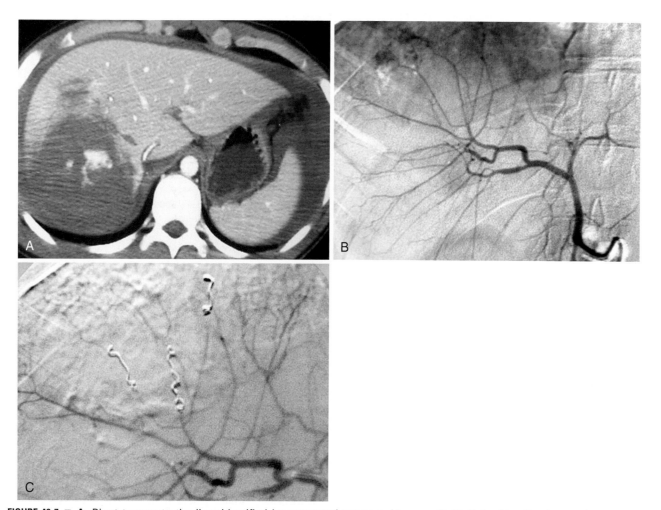

FIGURE 46-7 ■ **A,** Blunt trauma to the liver identified by computed tomographic scan. **B,** Digital subtraction image demonstrates hepatic artery branch injuries. **C,** Coil embolization successful.

Visceral Vessel Injury

The use of selective angiography and coil embolization of branches of the celiac trunk and superior mesenteric artery in the setting of gastrointestinal bleeding is well established. There are no cases of endovascular treatment of mesenteric bleeding secondary to penetrating trauma in the English-language literature. Isolated injury to the mesentery following blunt trauma, identified by CT scan, has been effectively treated with coil embolization,[101-103] and might not require bowel resection.[101,102]

Technique

A 6-French sheath is placed via femoral approach using ultrasound guidance and a micropuncture technique. AP and lateral abdominal aortograms at the level of T12 via a flush catheter are obtained, providing visualization of the celiac axis, superior mesenteric artery, and renal artery origins. Selective catheterization of the celiac axis is accomplished with a Glide Simmons 1 catheter. Selective catheterization of the superior mesenteric artery is then performed. Once the source of the bleeding branch is identified, the Glidewire and Glidecath are advanced until sufficient purchase is obtained; the Glidewire is then exchanged for the 260-cm Amplatz wire. A 6-French, 45- or 60-cm–long sheath is advanced into the proximal artery. The 5-French angled Glidecath and the microcatheter are advanced into the distal artery. Coils are delivered via the microcatheter. Just before withdrawal of the Glidecath, a small volume of methylene blue can be injected to help identify the area at risk in the event that laparotomy or laparoscopic evaluation is required (Figure 46-8A and B).

Renal Injury

Urologic injuries occur in less than 5% of all trauma patients and in only 10% of patients with penetrating trauma. However, approximately 80% of genitourinary injuries involve the kidney, with 90% caused by blunt trauma. Conservative, nonoperative management can be used to treat the majority of urologic injuries, resulting in a low nephrectomy rate. This rate is further decreased with adjunct endovascular intervention. The National Trauma Data Bank reported 9002 renal injuries during 2002 to 2007. Only 2% required angiography; of these, 47% underwent concomitant transarterial embolization.[104]

FAST examination is performed to evaluate for perirenal fluid collections or bladder injury. Hemodynamically stable patients undergo CT scan. Active extravasation of contrast is a reliable indication for embolization.[105] Technical success for embolization is high, even in high-grade injuries with vascular avulsion and shattered kidney (grade IV and V).[106-108] Brewer and colleagues[108] described nine patients with grade V renal injury secondary to blunt trauma. These patients were hemodynamically unstable, but did not require surgery for other intraabdominal injuries. Technical success with complete resolution of active extravasation on angiography was achieved in all patients, and none required further intervention. Embolization can also be used to treat iatrogenic renal injury incurred during percutaneous and interventional procedures.[109,110]

The effect of transarterial embolization on renal parenchyma and function was evaluated by Chatziioannou and colleagues[111]; they showed that the immediate, postembolization area of ischemic parenchyma was

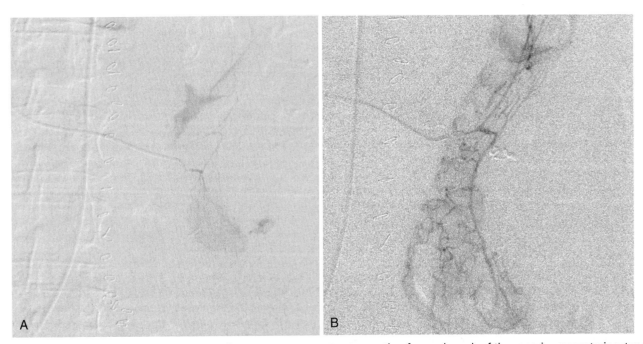

FIGURE 46-8 ■ **A,** Super-selective arteriogram demonstrates contrast extravasation from a branch of the superior mesenteric artery in a patient with hemoperitoneum of occult source. **B,** Microcoils delivered via microcatheter in the gastroduodenal artery with excellent results.

11.7% (range, 0%-30%), which was reduced to 6% (range, 0%-15%) on follow-up (mean, 12 months; range, 5%-23%). Serum creatinine level returned to preembolization levels in all patients 1 week after the procedure and at the latest follow-up.[111] Poulakis and colleagues[112] reported similar findings of improved area at risk and preserved function over time, with the initial parenchymal ischemic area measuring 0% to 20% (mean, 9%). At 6 months, the area of perfusion deficit was estimated at 0% to 10% (mean, 5%).[112] The serum creatinine concentration returned to preinjury values within 10 days. These techniques have been used safely in renal transplant allografts with iatrogenic AVF from renal biopsy. Loffroy and colleagues[109] reported minimal renal parenchymal loss and no midterm deterioration of allograft function. Morita and colleagues[107] reviewed glomerular filtration rates using dynamic scintigraphy to assess differential renal function in grade IV blunt renal injuries and found that the function of the injured kidney was preserved in all patients.

Hotaling and colleagues[104] investigated national patterns of diagnostic angiography and embolization after blunt and penetrating renal trauma using the National Trauma Data Bank. The initial success rate for the procedure was low, with 100% failure in the grade IV and V renal injuries. However, secondary intervention improved the success rate to 88.3%. AAST renal grade was associated with an increased risk of transarterial embolization failure and the need for repeated intervention. However, initial and repeated attempts for these high-grade injuries prevented nephrectomy in 78% to 83% of these patients. Penetrating trauma was also found to be more likely associated with percutaneous treatment failure (relative risk, 3.04; 95% confidence interval, 1.60-5.79). The authors concluded that embolization for AAST grade IV to V injuries should be done with caution, with close observation after the initial embolization attempt. The role of diagnostic arteriography and embolization in grades I to III awaits consensus.

Technique

AP abdominal aortography at the level of T12 with visceral runoff is performed, and the renal artery with contrast extravasation is identified. The flush catheter is exchanged over wire for a Simmons 1 Glidecath, and this catheter is used for selective catheterization of the renal artery. Over a Glidewire, the Simmons 1 catheter is advanced into the middistal renal artery. The Glidewire is exchanged for an Amplatz wire. A 45- or 60-cm, 6-French Destination sheath is placed, with the tip of the sheath in the main renal artery. Selective renal angiography is performed. An angled Glidecath and Glidewire are used for super-selective catheterization of the bleeding artery. Embolization using 0.038 platinum coils can be performed via the Glidecath. If the bleeding artery is small in caliber, a Renegade catheter is advanced through the Glidecath into the end artery, and embolization is performed using microcoils.

Aortoiliac Injury

The majority of endovascular repairs to the traumatic abdominal aorta are done in delayed fashion, days to years after the occurrence of the injury. Blunt traumatic injuries have been addressed with commercially available endografts.[113]

Endovascular treatment of acute retroperitoneal hemorrhage secondary to penetrating trauma has been described in case reports. The endovascular approach to ruptured abdominal aortic aneurysm has demonstrated the feasibility of this approach in the emergency setting.[114] García-Gimeno and colleagues[115] reported on a hemodynamically stable patient following an epigastric gunshot wound found to have supraceliac aortic transection; it was repaired using a Talent 30 × 28 mm aortic cuff (Medtronic, Minneapolis, Minn.).[115] The patient then underwent laparotomy to treat gastric and hepatic injuries and was without signs of infection or graft migration at 9 months. Hussain and colleagues[116] reported a retroperitoneal hematoma with aortic pseudoaneurysm identified by CT scan the day after an exploratory laparotomy to address bowel and liver injuries following stab wounds. The injury was treated with a 28 mm × 3 cm aortic cuff (WL Gore) via a right common femoral artery exposure with positive outcome at 2 years. Both of these patients, with multiple injuries, were administered 5000 units of heparin during endograft placement. Yeh and colleagues[117] described endovascular repair for a ruptured pseudoaneurysm of the infrarenal aorta that occurred 2 weeks after the initial laparotomies for gunshot injury involving the duodenum, colon, aorta, and superior mesenteric vein.[117] The original aortic injury was treated with pledgeted suture repair and became infected. Open repair attempt failed because of postoperative adhesions. The mycotic pseudoaneurysm was excluded using a Zenith 18 × 55 mm aortic endograft limb (Cook, Bloomington, Ind.). At 1-year follow-up, the patient was doing well without infectious issues. These limited studies suggest an important role for endograft repair of aortoiliac injury in the setting of abdominal contamination from bowel injury and merit further investigation.

Technique

In hypotensive patients, an aortic occlusion balloon can be placed as described previously. Provided the patient is stable, aortoiliac arterial injury can be assessed via a percutaneous 6-French sheath, introduced under ultrasound and fluoroscopic guidance. The Omniflush catheter is introduced to obtain the initial aortogram and pelvic views. Adequate visualization of the internal iliac artery origins usually requires oblique views. If the injury to treat is a dissection, cannulation of the true lumen can be a challenge. A contralateral approach or tandem access via the brachial artery may be helpful to access the true lumen.

If aortic injury is identified, two Proglide closure devices are deployed to preclose the 18- to 22-French arteriotomy required for an aortic cuff or endograft. After this is completed, an exchange catheter is carefully inserted into the aorta, and a Lunderquist wire is placed in the descending thoracic aorta. The appropriate sheath for the endograft is advanced over this stiff wire under fluoroscopy. Depending on the area of injury requiring coverage and the diameter of the native aorta, cuffs, covered stents, endograft limbs or complete bifurcated devices may be utilized. It is important to consider that the use of a bifurcated endograft may be complicated in these patients, secondary to difficulty in cannulating the contralateral limb in a normal-sized aorta. If an isolated iliac injury is identified, a self-expanding covered stent-graft is the preferred treatment.

Inferior Vena Cava and Iliac Veins

Traumatic injury to the IVC, particularly the retrohepatic IVC, remains a lethal problem with poor operative solutions.[118,119] Experimental data[120] and a limited number of case reports[121-125] support the use of endografts and stent grafts within the vena cava. Castelli and colleagues reported successful use of the Excluder (WL Gore) for the treatment of an injury to the ileocaval bifurcation following an MVC.[121] The bifurcated device (31 to 14 mm × 15 cm) was deployed via left common femoral vein exposure and percutaneous right common femoral vein access with success. Laparotomy was not required despite hypotension and significant blood loss. Long-term durability is unknown because the patient died of other injuries.[124] Sam and colleagues[122] reported the exclusion of a blunt trauma–induced IVC injury at the level of the third lumbar vertebrae (L3), using two aortic cuffs (28.5 mm × 3.3 cm). The IVC diameter was estimated during a Valsalva maneuver, with oversizing of 10% to 15%. The patient was maintained on anticoagulation, and the endograft was patent at 14 months.[122] De Naeyer and Degrieck[125] use a 44-mm Talent thoracic endoprosthesis (Medtronic, Minneapolis, Mich.) to repair an L3 injury that occurred intraoperatively. This injury was initially controlled with two Talent balloons inserted into the IVC above and below the injury. Postoperatively, this patient was prescribed warfarin and had a patent graft at 18 months.[125] Erzurum and colleagues[124] reported the successful treatment of a retrohepatic IVC injury with two AneuRx (Medtronic, Santa Rosa, Calif.) cuffs (28 mm × 3.75 cm) with 6-month patency. Finally, Watarida and colleagues[123] treated a blunt trauma victim with retrohepatic IVC rupture with a homemade stent-graft with multiple holes created to allow flow from the hepatic veins (30 mm × 5 cm Gianturco Z stents × 2, Cook, Bloomington, Ind.; 24-mm Hemashield Dacron graft, Hemashield, Oakland, N.J.). The patient received warfarin and his follow-up at 18 months demonstrated graft patency.

These reports demonstrate that endovascular techniques can be used to treat unstable patients whose IVC injuries are known to respond poorly to open surgery. Four of these patients did not require laparotomy,[121-123,125] while the fifth injury occurred during laparotomy for retroperitoneal sarcoma resection.[124] Sizing may be a challenge; the diameter of the devices used in these reports ranged from 24 to 44 mm. Postoperative anticoagulation appears to be the consensus. Aortic occlusion

balloons may provide instrumental control of venous hemorrhage before definitive endovascular repair.

Balloon occlusion has been described as an adjunct during laparotomy. Right internal jugular vein access and left common femoral vein access were used to advance two 27-mm balloons for proximal and distal control of a gunshot wound to the juxtahepatic IVC, allowing for visualization of the injury for suture repair.[126] An intra-operative injury to the left common iliac vein during open repair of left common iliac aneurysm was controlled via aortic occlusion balloon placed at the distal IVC via an introducer sheath in the right saphenous vein, and another placed in the more proximal (peripheral) left common iliac vein via left common femoral vein exposure. This control of venous hemorrhage allowed suture repair of the iliac vein.[127]

Stent-graft placement has been performed for exsanguinating hemorrhage that is unresponsive to hypogastric artery embolization after pelvic fracture.[128] Eleven of 25 patients who failed to respond to pelvic embolization underwent transfemoral venography with nine iliac vein injuries identified. The mean ISS of these patients was 45.8, significantly higher than the ISS mean of the pelvic fracture cohort. Three of these patients underwent endovascular stent placement and survived.[128] Zieber and colleagues reported on two patients with iliac vein injury who presented with hypotension and leg swelling.[129] After negative pelvic arteriography results, antegrade venograms demonstrated the injuries to the common iliac and the external iliac veins. Both injuries were successfully treated with 14 × 50 mm Wallgraft endoprosthetics (Boston Scientific).

Technique

Access is obtained using ultrasound guidance and micro-puncture technique, and a 6-French sheath is placed in the ipsilateral common femoral vein. Venography is performed. If venous hemorrhage is identified and balloon tamponade is warranted, a 12-French sheath is placed to allow the use of a large occlusion balloon. The preclose technique can be used.[5] Both groins and the right internal jugular area should be prepared into the field, in the event that secondary access is needed for above and below control of the injured vein and for device delivery. For IVC trauma, the trauma stock should contain aortic cuffs, thoracic endografts, and bifurcated devices in sizes that will allow clinicians to address an appropriate injury as needed, whether as an adjunct to open surgery or for an endovascular-only solution.

Pelvic Injury

Traumatic injury to the pelvis accounts for 6% to 8% of all trauma deaths. Pelvic arterial rupture is associated with a 50% to 75% mortality rate.[130,131] Significant bleeding can also occur from disruption of pelvic veins. Bleeding from lateral compression, vertical shear, and combined injury mechanisms are often associated with arterial trauma. Open surgical intervention of a zone III retroperitoneal hematoma is not indicated. In a patient in unstable condition, with pelvic injury and hematoma formation, angiographic inspection of the internal iliac arteries and coil embolization may be useful. Matalon and associates have demonstrated an 85% to 94% success rate using endovascular techniques in obtaining hemostasis in posttraumatic arterial injuries to the pelvis.[132]

A multidisciplinary approach to the management of pelvic trauma is essential to hemorrhage control. Expert management of transfusion requirements, coagulopathy, hypothermia, and acidosis are best handled by an engaged anesthesiologist while trauma and endovascular surgeons work on the source of hemorrhage. Active hemorrhage, indicated as a blush on CTA in the stable patient, is often from branches of the internal iliac artery. Endovascular techniques can be used to embolize the specific bleeding branches or a more proximal artery for multiple sources of hemorrhage. Unilateral or bilateral internal iliac artery embolization may be necessary in the patient with significant ongoing hemorrhage.

Technique

Contralateral femoral access from the suspected bleeding site of injury is preferred. A 5-French Omniflush or pigtail catheter can then be used to perform abdominal and pelvic angiography to delineate bleeding sources (Figure 46-9). A 45-cm, 6-French sheath is advanced into the internal iliac artery, and a 100-cm, 5-French Glidecath is used to inspect various branches. Embolization is performed with coils. Any other smaller or chemical embolization agent is likely to be ineffective secondary to ongoing extravasation and vessel disruption. It is common

to place coils both in the distal bleeding branches and in more proximal branch points to securely control hemorrhage. Coils can be placed through either a 0.018- or 0.035-inch system based on the size of the vessel. Distal embolization of small branch bleeders (1-3 mm) are performed with the 0.018-inch system via the Renegade microcatheter placed through the 5-French Glide catheter and Destination sheath. More proximal embolization of larger branches is completed with the 0.035-inch system (4- to 12-mm coils) through the 5-French nontapered Glidecath. After treatment of the contralateral internal iliac artery, the Destination sheath is withdrawn into the ipsilateral external lilac artery for selection of the ipsilateral hypogastric artery with the Glidecath and Glidewire. The Destination sheath can be advanced over the Glidecath or the sheath's dilator into the proximal hypogastric artery, and then the artery can be treated as on the contralateral side.

Lower Extremity Injuries

In the patient with lower-extremity trauma (blunt or penetrating), assessment begins with a physical examination and measurement of ankle-brachial indices. For asymmetrical or abnormal pulse examinations, significant hematomas, neurologic impairment, or any abnormality in ankle-brachial indices, an imaging study is indicated. Duplex ultrasonography or CTA may be helpful in identifying the area and extent of vascular injury, but angiography is preferred because it provides a means for both diagnosis and therapeutic intervention. Hard signs of

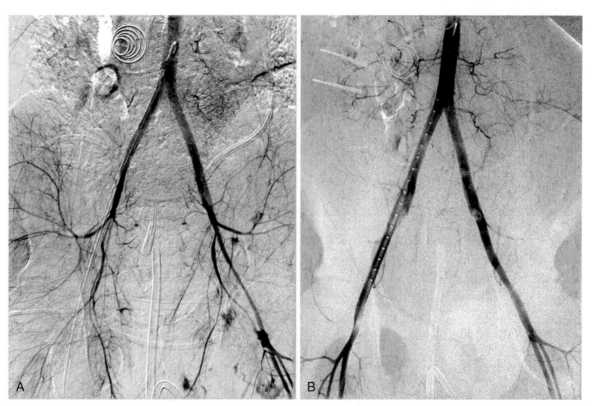

FIGURE 46-9 ■ **A,** Digital subtraction image of a motorcycle crash victim demonstrates multiple injured branches of bilateral hypogastric arteries. **B,** Bilateral coil embolization of the proximal hypogastric arteries.

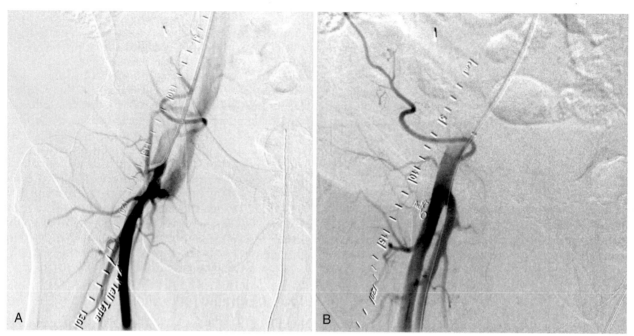

FIGURE 46-10 ■ **A,** Symptomatic arteriovenous fistula between the profunda femoris artery and the common femoral vein. **B,** Resolution of fistula, leg swelling and claudication with coil embolization.

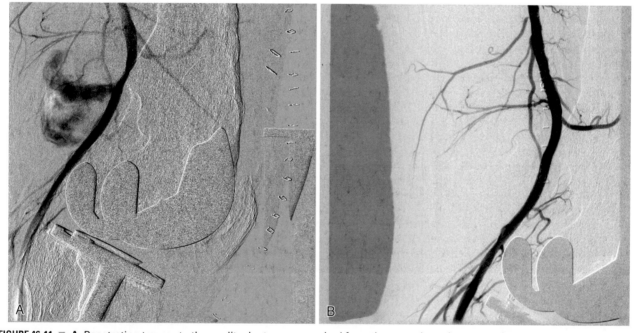

FIGURE 46-11 ■ **A,** Penetrating trauma to the popliteal artery approached from the contralateral common femoral artery. **B,** Successful exclusion of the injury with a Viabahn stent placement (WL Gore, Flagstaff, Ariz.).

injury mandating action include rapidly expanding hematoma or signs of acute arterial injury, such as loss of distal Doppler signals, sensory deficit, or motor impairment not explained by musculoskeletal damage. Whereas exploration was the only surgical option previously, it is now possible to manage the majority of extremity traumatic vascular injuries using a combination of covered stent deployment and coil embolization techniques.

For delayed injuries following trauma, or for iatrogenic complications such as pseudoaneurysm and arteriovenous fistula of the common or deep femoral artery

following percutaneous catheterization, or injuries sustained during orthopedic hardware placement, endovascular management is the first-line approach. Open surgical alternatives are reserved for failures of endovascular techniques (Figures 46-10, 46-11).[1,134,135]

Technique

For infrainguinal injuries, the best approach uses the standard "up and over" technique, which enables selection of the superficial femoral artery or the profunda artery more easily than with an antegrade femoral approach. After placement of a 10-cm, 6-French sheath, the contralateral common iliac artery is selected with an Omniflush catheter and the wire placed in the superficial femoral artery or profunda. The catheter is exchanged for a 100-cm, 5-French angled Glidecath. Oblique views may be useful for adequate imaging of the profunda femoris artery origin. The wire is exchanged for the Amplatz wire and then a 45-, 60-, or 90-cm Destination sheath is selected depending on the location of the injury. The tip of the sheath should be as close as possible to the injury. For branch vessel hemorrhage, the standard coil embolization techniques described previously are used. For transected arteries, intimal injuries, and arteriovenous communications, covered stents are used. With the 0.018 Viabahn system, covered stents of 5 or 6 mm in diameter and lengths of 2.5 to 15 cm can be delivered through a 6-French sheath; these diameters are appropriate for the majority of extremity arterial injuries. For larger arteries, 7- and 8-mm covered stents can be delivered through a 7-French sheath.

For hybrid procedures, a 4- to 5-mm balloon can be placed proximal to the injury; this may assist in hemostasis and decrease the dissection needed for proximal control.

CONCLUSION

Endovascular techniques have influenced all aspects of the contemporary vascular practice, allowing for alternatives to open surgical management of vascular diseases in every vascular bed. Currently, the management of traumatic vascular injuries does not yet rely on endovascular techniques to the same degree. With the wider availability of hybrid operating suites and adoption of trauma protocols that take advantage of their utility, reliance on traditional open surgical techniques in the trauma patient will likely evolve as has been seen in all other aspects of vascular surgery. Endovascular tools and techniques expand the ability to creatively manage vascular disease and injury. Further work will be required to assess the safety, efficacy, and durability of these procedures in this important population of patients.

SELECTED REFERENCES

Dake MD, White RA, Diethrich EB, et al: Report on endograft management of traumatic thoracic aortic transections at 30 days and 1 year from a multidisciplinary subcommittee of the Society for Vascular Surgery Outcomes Committee. J Vasc Surg 53:1091–1096, 2011.
  Data from five physician-sponsored investigational device exemption clinical trials from 2000 to 2008 on outcomes of patients with traumatic thoracic aortic transections treated with endovascular grafts. An important model of the collaborative efforts of data collection which will be necessary for meaningful evaluation of the techniques described in this chapter.
Demetriades D, Velmahos GC, Scalea TM, et al: Operative repair or endovascular stent/graft in blunt traumatic thoracic aortic injuries: results of a AAST multicenter study. J Trauma 64:561–570; discussion 570–571, 2008.
  18 major trauma centers enrolled 193 patients in a 26-month study period for this important, non-randomized prospective study. Findings include decreased blood loss and mortality for endovascular repair patients, a substantial device-related complication rate, and decreased risk of complications for endovascular patients treated at high-volume centers.
Haan JM, Biffl W, Knudson MM, et al: Splenic embolization revisited: a multicenter review. J Trauma 56:542–547, 2004.
  Four major trauma centers participated in this retrospective review; computerized tomographical scan findings as well as concomitant injuries were among the baseline variables captured in an effort to delineate complications of splenic embolization and predictors of technique failure.
Rasmussen TE, Woodson J, Rich NM, et al: Vascular trauma at a crossroads. J Trauma 70:1291–1293, 2011.
  An articulate summary of the challenges facing vascular, general, trauma and military surgeon training in vascular injury in the current environment of increasing endovascular treatment of vascular disease and changing training paradigms.
Stannard A, Eliason JL, Rasmussen TE: Resuscitative endovascular balloon occlusion of the aorta (REBOA) as an adjunct for hemorrhagic shock. J Trauma 71:1869–1872, 2011.
  A step-by-step description describing aortic occlusion balloon placement and removal illustrates the specific endovascular training needed for the modern trauma surgeon.
White R, Krajcer Z, Johnson M, et al: Results of a multicenter trial for the treatment of traumatic vas-cular injury with a covered stent. J Trauma 60:1189–1195; discussion 1195–1186, 2006.
  Multicenter, prospective study focusing on covered stent graft use in traumatic injury to the subclavian, iliac and femoral arteries.

References available online at expertconsult.com.

QUESTIONS

1. What is the minimum sheath size for an aortic occlusion balloon?
   a. 12 French
   b. 14 French
   c. 16 French
   d. 18 French
   e. 22 French

2. 0.018 coils can be deployed via:
   a. 5 French simple curved catheter
   b. 5 French double curved catheter
   c. Microcatheter
   d. Any size sheath or catheter
   e. None of the above

3. Clinical findings that support diagnostic workup of carotid or vertebral artery injuries include all of the following except:
   a. Alcohol intoxication
   b. Mandibular or facial fracture
   c. Cervical spine injuries at level C2-C3
   d. Neck contusion, laceration or hematoma
   e. Deceleration mechanism of injury

4. Treatment options for carotid dissections with intact distal flow include:
   a. Open surgical repair
   b. Bare metal or covered stent placement
   c. Anticoagulation
   d. Observation
   e. All of the above

5. Thoracic endograft placement for blunt aortic injury is associated with:
   a. 30-day mortality 15% to 40%
   b. 30-day stroke risk of 10%
   c. Paraplegia risk of 8% to 20%
   d. Subclavian artery coverage in 90% of cases

6. Carotid-subclavian artery bypass should be performed after thoracic endograft coverage of the left subclavian artery for all of the following except:
   a. Dominant left vertebral artery
   b. Blind posterior inferior cerebellar artery
   c. Left internal mammary artery–left anterior descending coronary artery bypass
   d. Left hand dominance

7. Covered stent placement for subclavian artery injury:
   a. Is not recommended in penetrating trauma due to infection risk.
   b. Is associated with up to 5% limb loss due to poor long-term patency rates.
   c. May be contraindicated by inadequate proximal landing zone if injury occurs close to the right common carotid artery, bilateral vertebral or internal mammary arteries.
   d. Is associated with increased blood loss, longer procedure times and decreased patency compared to open repair.

8. Regarding splenic embolization:
   a. Proximal splenic artery embolization leads to segmental splenic infarction.
   b. Distal splenic artery embolization results in peripheral infarction.
   c. Distal splenic artery embolization is associated with increased rates of splenic preservation compared to proximal splenic artery embolization.
   d. Complications of splenic embolization include persistent bleeding, splenic infarction, and abscess.
   e. Splenic arteriography is indicated for AAST Grade I-II splenic injury, with open repair reserved for Grades III and higher.

9. Regarding hepatic trauma:
   a. CT findings that should prompt open exploration and packing over arteriography include blush or pooling of intravenous contrast in the hepatic parenchyma.
   b. Coil embolization is more successful in treating blunt hepatic injury than penetrating injury.
   c. Hemodynamically unstable patients have been successfully treated with coil embolization, often in combination with surgical exploration.
   d. Mortality rates of AAST Grade IV-V injury remain in excess of 40%.

10. Which of the following statement is true for pelvic arterial injury?
    a. Pelvic arterial injury is associated with 20-38% mortality rate.
    b. Coil embolization of bilateral hypogastric arteries is indicated in unstable patients.
    c. Endovascular management of pelvic arterial injury has a 29% to 50% success rate, but is favored over open exploration due to its minimally invasive nature.
    d. Zone III retroperitoneal injury are best treated with retroperitoneal exploration and packing.

ANSWERS

1. **a**
2. **c**
3. **a**
4. **e**
5. **b**
6. **d**
7. **c**
8. **d**
9. **c**
10. **b**

SECTION 5

VENOUS DISEASE

CHAPTER 47

Venous Thromboembolic Disease

Thomas W. Wakefield · Danielle N. Campbell · Andrea Obi · Peter K. Henke · Jordan Knepper · John Rectenwald · Frank Vandy

Venous thromboembolic disease (VTE), which includes both deep venous thrombosis (DVT) and pulmonary embolism (PE), is very common. Although the etiology of acute venous thrombosis is defined by Virchow triad of hypercoagulability, stasis, and endothelial injury, it is clearly a multifactorial process influenced by many other conditions. The acute thrombotic process must be managed appropriately to relieve edema and pain, to prevent death from PE, and to avoid reoccurrence and the long-term sequelae of postthrombotic syndrome, which is estimated to occur in 30% of patients over 8 years. In addition to compression and ambulation, there are a number of pharmacologic treatment options: unfractionated heparin, low-molecular-weight heparin, and vitamin K antagonists, such as warfarin (Coumadin). Many new and alternative agents are becoming available and may require less rigorous monitoring. Length of anticoagulation typically ranges from 3 to 6 months for a first-time event, although certain inherited thrombophilias warrant life-long therapy. In other cases, surgical placement of inferior vena cava (IVC) filters may be indicated to prevent further propagation of PE. The current chapter is divided into sections encompassing discussions on all of these topics, including pathophysiology of venous thrombosis, anticoagulants including the new agents, length of anticoagulation for VTE treatment, vein wall abnormalities after DVT, diagnosis and treatment of superficial thrombophlebitis, and a discussion about inferior vena caval interruption.

PATHOPHYSIOLOGY OF VENOUS THROMBOSIS

Venous thrombosis is governed by the three principles of Virchow triad: hypercoagulability, stasis, and endothelial injury. Activation of coagulation appears to be critical in the pathogenesis of DVT. Although the hemostatic system is continuously active, thrombus formation is ordinarily confined to sites of local injury by a precise balance between activators and inhibitors of coagulation and fibrinolysis. A prothrombotic state may result either from imbalances in the regulatory and inhibitory systems or from activation exceeding antithrombotic capacity.[1] Regardless of etiology, most venous thrombi originate in areas of static, low blood flow, often behind valve pockets.[2] Furthermore, many risk factors for acute DVT are associated with immobilization and slow venous flow, and several mechanisms have been advanced to explain the

role of stasis in thrombogenesis. For example, in comparison to pulsatile flow, static streamline flow is associated with profound hypoxia at the depths of the venous valve cusps and may induce endothelial injury.[3] Under basal conditions, the endothelium provides a vasodilatory and local fibrinolytic environment. In this setting, coagulation, platelet adhesion, platelet activation, inflammation, and leukocyte activation are inhibited.[4] After a disturbance of the endothelium, a prothrombotic and proinflammatory state occurs and is defined by vasoconstriction, activated platelets, and upregulation of cellular mediators to recruit inflammatory cells to the site of endothelial damage.[4] Individually, stasis, endothelial injury, and activated coagulation factors may be insufficient to provoke thrombosis.[5] However, when localized in regions of stasis, and incited by endothelial disruption, the coagulation cascade allows activated factors to rapidly intensify the thrombotic stimulus leading to platelet aggregation, coagulation factor localization, and fibrin formation.[5,6] Thus, thrombosis appears to be a multifactorial phenomenon, with convergence of several pathologic factors often required to produce a thrombotic event.[7]

The pathophysiology of venous thrombosis is a cyclical event, amplified by the associated inflammatory process.[8] With inflammation, there is an increase in tissue factor, platelet reactivity, fibrinogen, phosphatidylserine expression on membrane surfaces, and PAI-1 (inhibiting fibrinolysis) and a decrease in thrombomodulin (and thus a decrease in the activity of protein C).[9] Cell adhesion molecules allow leukocyte transmigration, and selectins are intimately involved in this process. Venous stasis and ischemia result in upregulation of P-selectin, and this localizes microparticles, which are prothrombotic, to the area of evolving thrombosis.[10,11] The role of the inflammatory cell adhesion molecule P-selectin in thrombosis is critical. Recent data suggest that elevated levels of soluble P-selectin combined with a clinical examination favoring DVT has a positive predictive value for diagnosing DVT far exceeding that of D-dimer.[11a,11b]

Epidemiology

The incidence of recurrent, fatal, and nonfatal VTE has been estimated to exceed 900,000 cases annually in the United States.[12] VTE has been estimated to occur with an incidence of approximately 1 per 1000 adult patients annually.[13] This figure is supported by the 35-year population-based Rochester Epidemiology

Project database of Olmstead County, Minnesota, which demonstrated an overall average age- and sex-adjusted annual incidence of VTE of 122 per 1,000,000 person-years.[14] This landmark study also demonstrated higher age-adjusted rates in men compared with women (134 vs. 115 per 100,000 patients, respectively). First-time, or incident, VTE cases are estimated to occur in approximately 250,000 white individuals annually in the United States.[15] However, there is a difference in ethnic groups diagnosed with VTE. African Americans demonstrate greater than a 25% increased incidence in first-time VTE compared with whites (103 vs. 141 per 100,000 patients). Conversely, the incidence of first-time VTE in both Hispanic and Asian or Pacific Islanders is significantly lower than in whites (62 vs. 104 per 100,000 patients; 29 vs. 104 per 100,000 patients, respectively).[16,17] Nevertheless, the issue of VTE is not isolated to the United States. Recent estimates across the European Union have totaled nearly 700,000 cases of DVT, 435,000 cases of PE, and 543,000 fatalities.[18]

Although estimated incidences of VTE in both the community and hospital have been well documented, individuals at risk for VTE have been less well studied. Substantial differences have been noted in the distribution of risk factors between inpatients and outpatients.[19] Extrapolating hospital inpatient data on the estimated 38 million patients discharged in 2003, 31% were considered to be at risk for VTE secondary to either major surgery or a medical illness.[20] Although the incidence of VTE is multifactorial varying with the population studied, use of thromboprophylaxis, the intensity of screening, and the diagnostic test used, specific risk factors have been significantly associated with increasing VTE. Patients at highest risk are exemplified in the critically ill and trauma patients in whom bleeding risks prohibit thromboprophylaxis, and immobility contribute up to a greater than 80% DVT rate in specific populations.[21] Risk stratification for VTE based on a number of individualized patient specific clinical attributes was initially proposed and validated by Caprini.[22] In a large, single-center study, a modified Caprini risk assessment tool was applied to patients undergoing general surgery, associating higher scores with an increased incidence of VTE.[23] Currently, electronic order entry to mandate a modified Caprini risk assessment tool should be performed for all hospitalized patients (Figure 47-1). Recognition of patients at high risk for VTE is a critical part in its prevention. In the next section, risk factors for VTE will be discussed in detail.

Risk Factors

Age

A higher incidence of VTE has consistently been associated with advanced age. In a community-based study of phlebographically documented DVT, the yearly incidence of DVT increased progressively from almost 0 in childhood to 7.65 cases per 1000 in men and 8.22 cases per 1000 in women older than 80 years, with the incidence of DVT increasing thirtyfold from 30 to 80 or more years of age.[24] Similarly, Hansson and colleagues found that the objectively documented thromboembolic events in men increased from 0.5% at 50 years of age to 3.8% at 80 years.[25]

Immobilization

Immobilization promotes venous stasis and is a major risk factor for VTE. The prevalence of lower extremity DVT in autopsy studies parallels the duration of bed rest, with DVT occurring in 15% of patients dying after 0 to 7 days of bed rest as opposed to 79% to 94% of those dying after 2 to 12 weeks.[26] Preoperative immobilization is associated with postoperative DVT, contributing a twofold higher risk.[27] Patients with extremity paresis have a threefold higher risk for DVT and PE independent of hospital confinement.[28]

Travel

Despite the questionable importance of prolonged travel as a risk factor for VTE, in 2001 the World Health Organization acknowledged an association between air travel and VTE.[29] Lapostolle and coworkers observed that over an 86-month period, 56 of 135.3 million airline passengers had severe PE. The frequency of PE in those who traveled more than 5000 km was 150-fold higher than those who traveled less than 5000 km.[30] Paganin and associates observed a high incidence of VTE in patients with risk factors for DVT who traveled long distances. These investigators concluded that low mobility during flight was a modifiable risk factor for PE and that those with additional risk factors should increase their mobility.[31]

History of Venous Thromboembolism

Approximately 23% to 26% of patients with acute DVT have a previous history of DVT, and histologic studies confirm that acute thrombi are often associated with fibrous remnants of previous thrombi in the same or nearby veins.[19,32,33] Depending on sex and age, population-based studies have demonstrated that recurrent thromboembolism develops in 1 of every 11 to 50 persons with a previous episode of thromboembolism, with the risk for recurrent thromboembolism being higher in patients with idiopathic DVT.[34,35]

Obesity

The evidence supporting obesity as a risk factor remains equivocal. In postmenopausal women, a body mass index of greater than 25 to 30 kg/m[2] has been associated with significantly increased risk.[36,37] Some investigators have reported obesity to be associated with a twofold greater risk for postoperative DVT,[38] but multifactorial analysis by others has not shown obesity to constitute an independent risk.[39] Obesity was not an independent risk factor for DVT in the Olmsted County study[40] and has not been proved to be a risk factor for the development of DVT after stroke.[41] Obesity has been found to be a risk factor, however, for recurrent DVT.[40,42]

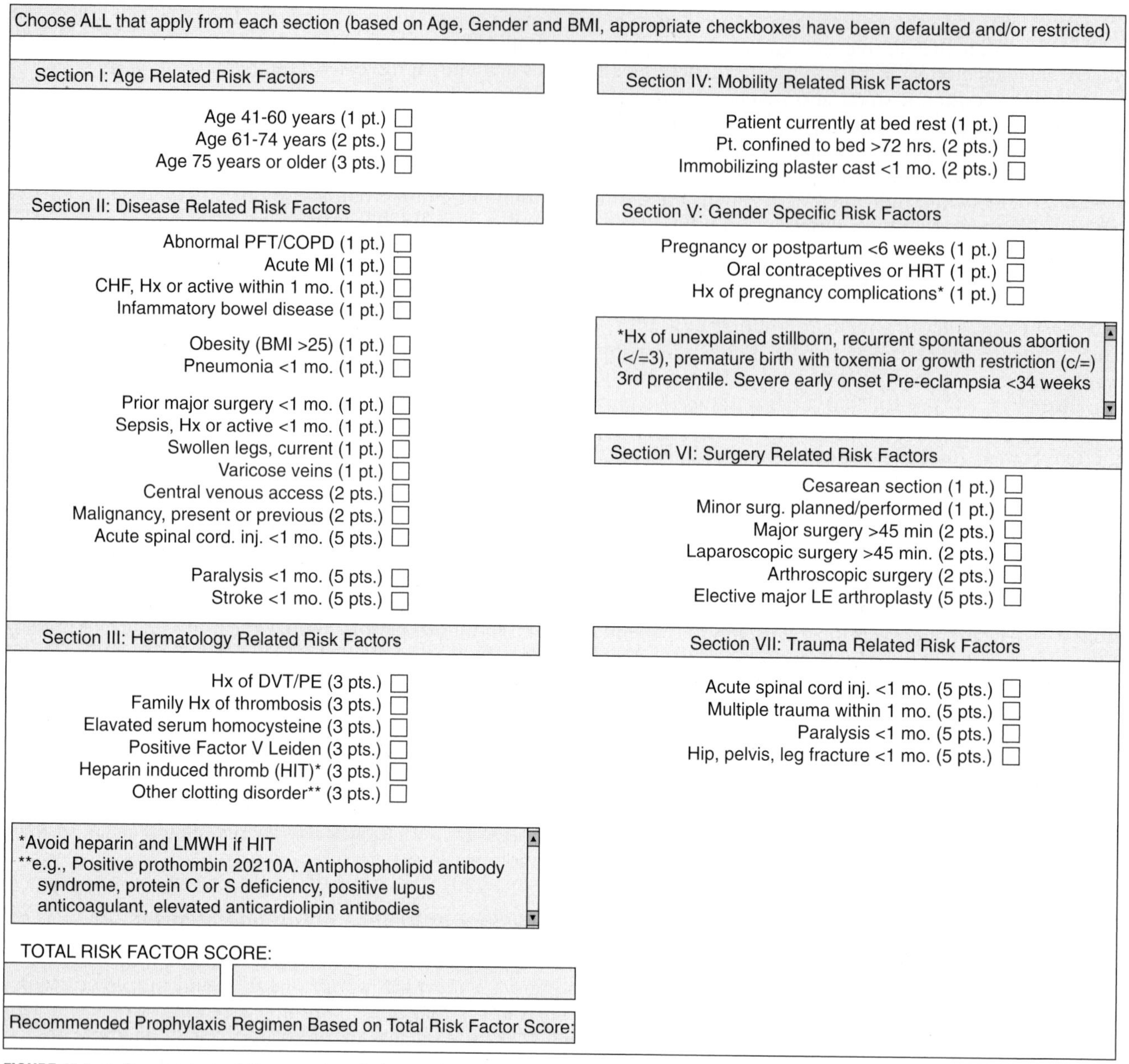

Choose ALL that apply from each section (based on Age, Gender and BMI, appropriate checkboxes have been defaulted and/or restricted)

Section I: Age Related Risk Factors	
Age 41-60 years (1 pt.)	☐
Age 61-74 years (2 pts.)	☐
Age 75 years or older (3 pts.)	☐

Section II: Disease Related Risk Factors	
Abnormal PFT/COPD (1 pt.)	☐
Acute MI (1 pt.)	☐
CHF, Hx or active within 1 mo. (1 pt.)	☐
Inflammatory bowel disease (1 pt.)	☐
Obesity (BMI >25) (1 pt.)	☐
Pneumonia <1 mo. (1 pt.)	☐
Prior major surgery <1 mo. (1 pt.)	☐
Sepsis, Hx or active <1 mo. (1 pt.)	☐
Swollen legs, current (1 pt.)	☐
Varicose veins (1 pt.)	☐
Central venous access (2 pts.)	☐
Malignancy, present or previous (2 pts.)	☐
Acute spinal cord. inj. <1 mo. (5 pts.)	☐
Paralysis <1 mo. (5 pts.)	☐
Stroke <1 mo. (5 pts.)	☐

Section III: Hermatology Related Risk Factors	
Hx of DVT/PE (3 pts.)	☐
Family Hx of thrombosis (3 pts.)	☐
Elavated serum homocysteine (3 pts.)	☐
Positive Factor V Leiden (3 pts.)	☐
Heparin induced thromb (HIT)* (3 pts.)	☐
Other clotting disorder** (3 pts.)	☐

*Avoid heparin and LMWH if HIT
**e.g., Positive prothombin 20210A. Antiphospholipid antibody syndrome, protein C or S deficiency, positive lupus anticoagulant, elevated anticardiolipin antibodies

Section IV: Mobility Related Risk Factors	
Patient currently at bed rest (1 pt.)	☐
Pt. confined to bed >72 hrs. (2 pts.)	☐
Immobilizing plaster cast <1 mo. (2 pts.)	☐

Section V: Gender Specific Risk Factors	
Pregnancy or postpartum <6 weeks (1 pt.)	☐
Oral contraceptives or HRT (1 pt.)	☐
Hx of pregnancy complications* (1 pt.)	☐

*Hx of unexplained stillborn, recurrent spontaneous abortion (</=3), premature birth with toxemia or growth restriction (c/=) 3rd precentile. Severe early onset Pre-eclampsia <34 weeks

Section VI: Surgery Related Risk Factors	
Cesarean section (1 pt.)	☐
Minor surg. planned/performed (1 pt.)	☐
Major surgery >45 min (2 pts.)	☐
Laparoscopic surgery >45 min. (2 pts.)	☐
Arthroscopic surgery (2 pts.)	☐
Elective major LE arthroplasty (5 pts.)	☐

Section VII: Trauma Related Risk Factors	
Acute spinal cord inj. <1 mo. (5 pts.)	☐
Multiple trauma within 1 mo. (5 pts.)	☐
Paralysis <1 mo. (5 pts.)	☐
Hip, pelvis, leg fracture <1 mo. (5 pts.)	☐

TOTAL RISK FACTOR SCORE:

Recommended Prophylaxis Regimen Based on Total Risk Factor Score:

FIGURE 47-1 ■ Screenshot of the mandated electronic order entry associated venous thromboembolism risk assessment that must be completed on each patient before additional order entry.

Malignancy

Approximately 20% of all first-time VTE events are associated with malignancy.[43] Either DVT or PE will develop in an estimated 1 in 200 individuals with malignancy, a fourfold higher risk than in those without malignancy.[28] Considering all-cause in-hospital mortality for cancer patients, one in seven will die of PE.[44] Correlation with location of the tumor reveals that the highest rates of VTE are associated with pancreatic malignancies, followed by kidney, ovary, lung, and stomach malignancies.[45] Venous compression secondary to tumor growth, cancer-associated thrombocytosis, immobility, indwelling central lines, and chemotherapy or radiation therapy are all risk factors that increase the likelihood of developing VTE.[46] Furthermore, as many as 90% of patients with cancer have abnormal coagulation parameters, including increased levels of coagulation factors, elevated fibrinogen or fibrin degradation products, thrombocytosis, and elevated levels of circulating prothrombotic microparticles.[47-49]

Surgery

All components of Virchow triad may be present in surgical patients: perioperative immobilization, transient changes in coagulation and fibrinolysis, and the potential for gross venous injury. In addition, surgery constitutes a spectrum of risk that is influenced by patient age, coexistent thrombotic risk factors, type of procedure, extent of surgical trauma, length of the procedure, and duration of postoperative immobilization.[50,51] Approximately half of postoperative lower-extremity thrombi detected by ^{125}I-labeled fibrinogen scanning develop in the operating room, and the remainder occur over the next 3 to 5 days.[52] However, the risk for development of DVT does not end uniformly at hospital discharge. In one study, 51% of the thromboembolic events that occurred in patients undergoing gynecologic surgical procedures occurred after initial discharge.[53] Similarly, up to 25% of abdominal surgery patients have been noted to have DVT within 6 weeks of discharge.[54]

Trauma

Despite improvements in trauma care and thromboembolism prophylaxis, DVT remains a significant source of morbidity and mortality in injured patients. In modern venographic series the incidence of DVT in the trauma patient is 58%.[21] Recent trauma was the second most common risk factor for thromboembolism in the Olmsted County study by Heit and associates and was associated with a nearly thirteenfold increase in risk.[55] As with postoperative DVT, several pathophysiologic elements may be responsible for the high incidence of DVT in trauma patients. Immobilization by skeletal fixation, paralysis, and critical illness are obviously associated with venous stasis, whereas mechanical injury is important after direct venous trauma and central venous cannulation. Less appreciated is the hypercoagulable state after depletion of coagulation inhibitors and components of the fibrinolytic system.[56,57]

Inherited Thrombophilia

Resistance to activated protein C was initially described by Dahlbach and associates in 1993.[58] Subsequent studies from the Leiden University Hospital in the Netherlands revealed a mutation in the gene for factor V conferring resistant to cleavage by activated protein C.[59,60] The factor V Leiden mutation has an autosomal dominant mode of inheritance and is at least tenfold more common than other inheritable defects.[61,62] In a study of 4047 Americans, the carrier frequency of the mutation was 5.3% for whites, 2.2% for Hispanic Americans, 1.25% for Native Americans, 1.2% for African Americans, and 0.45% for Asian Americans, with no significant gender difference.[63] The relative risk for first-time DVT is increased sevenfold in those who are heterozygous for the factor V Leiden mutation. However, the relative risk is increased eightyfold in individuals who are homozygous for the mutation.[64]

The prothrombin G20210A mutation, first described by Poort and associates in 1996, was demonstrated in 28 families with a documented history of VTE.[65] Characterized by a transition from guanine to adenine at the 20210 nucleotide on the prothrombin gene, risk for VTE in the presence of the prothrombin G20210A mutation is threefold higher in heterozygotes than in wild type, and the presence of homozygosity further increases this risk.[66] Although prothrombin G20210A is rare in individuals of Asian or African descent, additional investigations have shown that in those with spontaneous DVT, the incidence of the mutation may range from 7% to 16%, depending on the patient population studied.[67,68]

Protein C is a vitamin K–dependent serine protease that inhibits the coagulation system by inactivating factors Va and VIIIa.[69] In a study of 10,000 healthy blood donors, the observed prevalence of inherited protein C deficiency was 1.45 per 1000.[70] In a study of 2132 patients with VTE, 3.2% were found to have protein C deficiency.[71] It is estimated that individuals who are heterozygous for protein C deficiency have a sevenfold higher risk for the development of VTE than the general population.[72]

Protein S is a vitamin K–dependent cofactor for the protein C–mediated inactivation of factors Va and VIIIa. Inheritance of protein S deficiency is autosomal dominant, and it is more common than protein C deficiency. The incidence of protein S–associated VTE has been reported to be 5% to 7%, with the prevalence in the general population being 0.13%.[71,73,74] It is estimated that individuals who are heterozygous for protein S deficiency have an 8.5-fold higher risk for the development of VTE than the general population does.[75]

Antithrombin inhibits thrombin as well as factors Xa, IXa, XIa, and XIIa.[76] Antithrombin deficiency is inherited in an autosomal dominant fashion. The majority of patients are heterozygous because homozygote patients usually die in utero. The incidence of VTE associated with antithrombin deficiency has been reported to be 0.5% to 3%, with a prevalence in the general population of 0.2%.[71,76] However, it is estimated that individuals who are heterozygous for antithrombin deficiency have a twentyfold higher risk for the development of VTE than in the general population.[77]

Pregnancy

The incidence of VTE in the pregnant population is sixfold to tenfold greater than in nonpregnant controls.[78] VTE accounts for approximately 10% of all maternal deaths.[79] Studies that diagnosed DVT with venography, Doppler ultrasonography, or ventilation-perfusion scans for evaluation of clinically suspected thromboembolism have suggested an incidence of 0.029% to 0.055%.[80] The risk for thrombosis appears to be twofold to threefold greater during the puerperium, with the highest incidence found after cesarean section.[7,81-81b] DVT in pregnancy has been attributed to impaired venous outflow secondary to uterine compression, and up to 97% of reported thromboses have been isolated to the left leg.[81a] Furthermore, pregnancy is associated with a transient hypercoagulable state because of increases in levels of fibrinogen; von Willebrand factor; and factors II, VII, VIII, and X.

Oral Contraceptives and Hormonal Therapy

Case-control and population-based studies have established the use of oral contraceptives as an independent risk factor for the development of DVT. Most studies have reported odds ratios of 3.8 to 11.0 for idiopathic thrombosis,[82-85a] with an unweighted summary relative risk of 2.9 in 18 controlled studies.[83] Approximately one quarter of idiopathic thromboembolic events in women of childbearing age have been attributed to oral contraceptives.[84] The risk of hospital admission for a thromboembolic event, including cerebral thrombosis, has been estimated to be 0.4 to 0.6 per 1000 for oral contraceptive users versus 0.05 to 0.06 for nonusers.[82,86,87] Estrogenic compounds also increase the risk for VTE when used for suppression of lactation,[88] in the treatment of carcinoma of the prostate, and as postmenopausal replacement therapy.[89] Several studies have now reported a twofold to fourfold higher risk in women taking hormone replacement therapy.[36,37,89-91] This increased risk is greatest during the first year of treatment.[36,91]

Central Venous Catheters

The use of central venous cannulation for hemodynamic monitoring, infusion catheters, and pacemakers has been associated with a rising frequency of DVT. This is particularly true for upper extremity thrombus, with as many as 65% being related to central venous cannulation.[92] Although the incidence of symptomatic thrombosis may be low, studies using objective surveillance have reported thrombosis to occur at a mean incidence of 28% after subclavian cannulation.[93] This risk also extends to femoral venous catheters; ipsilateral thrombosis develops in 12% of patients undergoing placement of large-bore catheters for trauma resuscitation.[94]

Inflammatory Bowel Disease

Clinical series have reported VTE to complicate inflammatory bowel disease in 1.2% to 7.1% of cases.[95,96] Patients with Crohn disease have incidence rates of 31.4 and 10.3 per 10,000 person-years for DVT and PE, respectively. Ulcerative colitis was reported as having incident rates of 30.0 and 19.8 per 10,000 person-years for DVT and PE, respectively. Such thromboses frequently occur in young patients, are more common with active disease, and may affect unusual sites such as the cerebral veins.[95,96]

Systemic Lupus Erythematosus

In patients with systemic lupus erythematosus (SLE), lupus anticoagulant is present in 34%, and anticardiolipin antibodies are present in 44%, as compared with 2% for lupus anticoagulant and 0% to 7.5% for anticardiolipin antibodies in the general population.[97] Among patients with SLE, those with lupus anticoagulant have a sixfold higher risk for VTE, whereas those with anticardiolipin antibodies have a twofold greater risk.[98] The incidence of arterial or venous thrombosis is 25% in patients with lupus anticoagulant and 28% in patients with anticardiolipin antibodies.[97] The relationship between antiphospholipid antibodies and thrombosis is much less clear in non-SLE disorders.

ANTICOAGULANTS, INCLUDING THE NEW AGENTS

There are many pharmacologic options in current use for the treatment and prevention of venous thromboembolism (VTE). These medications include unfractionated heparin (UFH), low-molecular-weight heparin (LMWH), direct Xa inhibitors (anti Xa drugs), direct thrombin inhibitors (anti IIa drugs), and vitamin K antagonists (VKAs).[99] UFH and directed thrombin inhibitors (such as argatroban and bivalirudin, which will not be discussed because they are not indicated for routine use) are used intravenously, requiring invasive administration and monitoring of dose effect. The LMWHs such as enoxaparin, and the pentasaccharide fondaparinux[100] require subcutaneous administration but do not require monitoring. VKAs (e.g., warfarin) are the only oral anticoagulant approved by the U.S. Food and Drug Administration (FDA) for VTE. However, the use of VKAs requires frequent monitoring, and they have many interactions with medications and foods. Finally, some of these anticoagulants (e.g., UFH, LMWH) have known compounds capable of reversing their anticoagulant effects.[101] In addition, new agents for treatment are undergoing testing, such as apixaban, rivaroxaban (Table 47-1), dabigatran, and edoxaban.

TABLE 47-1 Characteristics of Traditional and New Anticoagulants

	VKA	LMWH	Heparin	Fondaparinux	Apixaban	Rivaroxaban	Dabigatran
Route	PO	SQ	IV/SQ	SQ	PO	PO	PO
Frequency	QD	bid or qid	Infusion bid or tid	bid or qid	bid	qd	bid or qd
VTE prophylaxis data	Yes	Yes	Yes	Yes	Yes	Yes	Yes
VTE treatment data	Yes	Yes	Yes	Yes	Ongoing	Yes	Yes
Reversibility	Vitamin K, FFP	Partially with protamine	Protamine, short half-life	No	No/Unknown	No/Unknown	Novoseven
Food interactions	Many	No	No	No	None apparent	None apparent	None apparent

VKA, Vitamin K antagonists; *LMWH,* low-molecular-weight heparin; *PO,* by mouth; *SQ,* subcutaneously; *IV,* intravenously; *bid,* twice per day; *qd,* one time per day; *tid,* three times per day; *VTE,* venous thromboembolism; *FFP,* fresh frozen plasma.

Low-Molecular-Weight Heparins

There are many LMWHs in clinical use; enoxaparin, dalteparin, and tinzaparin are approved for use in the United States.[102] The class of LMWHs are defined most notably as being a more specific inhibitor to factor Xa than factor IIa, and the average molecular weight of the compound is 30% less than UFH.[103] Clinical trial data has nearly unanimously revealed that LMWHs are as effective if not more effective than unfractionated heparin with their safety profile at least equivalent.[103]

A limitation to LMWH use is in those patients with renal dysfunction (creatinine clearance less than 30 mL/min). In these cases, effects are not predictable and safe dosing is difficult because LMWHs have the majority of their elimination by the kidneys.[102] In addition, in an obese patient or another patient whose dosing appears complicated, anti-Xa activity can be measured to titrate therapeutic effect.[102] The half-life of LMWH is longer, and as such may not be ideal for a high-risk patient with bleeding concerns, but in most other patient groups the LMWHs are viable and in many cases the current preferred method of anticoagulation for VTE.

Fondaparinux

Fondaparinux is a pentasaccharide that is in current use for the prevention and treatment of VTE with a subcutaneous delivery. Similar to LMWHs, fondaparinux is derived from UFH. It is based on the pentasaccharide moiety of the heparin molecule that selectively inhibits factor Xa via antithrombin, and it exhibits no endothelial or protein binding and is not thought to produce thrombocytopenia.[102] Fondaparinux has been approved for VTE prophylaxis in total hip, total knee, and hip fracture patients, in extended prophylaxis of hip fracture patients, in abdominal surgery patients, and for the treatment of DVT and PE.[104,105]

Apixaban

Apixaban is an oral, direct factor Xa inhibitor by Bristol-Myers Squibb. The ADVANCE-1 study compared apixaban with a prophylactic dose twice daily of enoxaparin in total knee replacement patients. The bleeding rates were significantly lower in the apixaban group, but major bleeding rates were similar between compounds and they did not show noninferiority.[106] The ADVANCE-2 trial compared apixaban with 40 mg daily of enoxaparin in the same population, concluding that apixaban was not inferior to the 40 mg daily of enoxaparin in VTE prophylaxis.[107] ADVANCE-3 showed that apixaban compared with 40 mg daily of enoxaparin in hip replacement patients was not inferior in VTE prevention, while the bleeding events were not significantly different.[108]

Rivaroxaban

Rivaroxaban is an oral, direct factor Xa inhibitor sponsored by Bayer.[109] RECORD-1 showed superiority of rivaroxaban and nonsignificantly different major bleeding events when comparing extended duration anticoagulation to 30 days for VTE prohpylaxis.[109,110] The

RECORD-2 trial examined extended duration rivaroxaban compared with standard short-term enoxaparin at 40 mg daily in patients undergoing hip replacement and again showed rivaroxaban to be superior.[111] The RECORD-3 trial studied the same dosages, but both treatments were 14 days in duration in patients who had undergone knee replacements. This trial showed noninferiority of rivaroxaban with a similar safety profile.[112] The RECORD-4 trial compared rivaroxaban (10 mg daily) to enoxaparin (30 mg twice per day) patients with knee replacements and again showed noninferiority with rivaroxaban with no statistical significant increase in bleeding.[113]

The EINSTIEN trial evaluated rivaroxaban versus standard anticoagulation in the treatment of acute DVT for standard duration.[114] The primary outcome was recurrent VTE. The results indicated that rivaroxaban is statically not inferior to standard therapy in the treatment of acute DVT, without increased bleeding risk. The EINSTIEN group also added a continued treatment group to compare rivaroxaban with placebo for an additional 6 to 12 months after completion of their prescribed anticoagulation course. This study demonstrated a significant decrease in recurrent VTE, but there were four clinically significant bleeds in the treatment group and none in the placebo group, which did not reach statistical significance.[114]

Dabigatran

Dabigatran is an oral, direct thrombin inhibitor introduced by Boehringer Ingelheim (Ingelheim, Germany).[115] Uniquely, dabigatran has some reversal with recombinant activated factor VII.[115]

The RE-MODEL trial was a VTE prophylaxis trial following total knee replacement. The trial showed that dabigatran was not inferior to daily enoxaparin at 40 mg once per day.[116] The RE-NOVATE trial in a hip replacement population also showed noninferiority.[117] The RE-MOBILIZE trial showed dabigatran was inferior to 30 mg enoxaparin twice daily for postoperative VTE prophylaxis.[118]

The RE-COVER trial compared dabigatran to therapeutic anticoagulation VKAs (internal normalized ratio [INR] 2.0 to 3.0) in the treatment of acute VTE for 6 months. Dabigatran was not inferior in the 6-month rate of VTE recurrence and with similar bleeding rates. This important study showed that dabigatran can be effective in longer-term anticoagulation and had a similar safety profile to warfarin without the need for laboratory monitoring.[119] Dabigatran is FDA approved for stroke and thromboembolism prevention in atrial fibrillation patents after similar effectiveness to warfarin was seen in the RE-LY trial.[120]

Edoxaban

Edoxaban is another oral factor Xa inhibitor that has been developed by Daiichi Sankyo (Tokyo, Japan). Edoxaban is currently being investigated in a series of phase III studies, from VTE prophylaxis in major orthopedic surgery to stroke prevention in atrial fibrillation. Early results for some earlier trial are promising.

Future Anticoagulants

In addition to these anticoagulants, there are other promising compounds currently in preclinical development. One such example is soluble P-selectin/PSGL-1 inhibitors. In a series of nonhuman primate studies using a model of proximal venous thrombosis, inhibition of P-selectin or its ligand PSGL-1 was similar to LMWH in preventing and treating DVT.[121] The P-selectin inhibitors reduce inflammation and therefore reduce thrombosis without inhibition of the coagulation cascade with less bleeding risks. Future clinical trials with these compounds are likely.

Oral anticoagulants provide an alternative to parenteral anticoagulants and VKAs and appear to have data to support their use in practical clinical situations without significant increase in bleeding risk.

LENGTH OF ANTICOAGULATION FOR VTE TREATMENT

Therapy for deep venous thrombosis is undertaken with the goals of reducing risk of pulmonary embolism, preventing extension of thrombus, and preventing thrombus recurrence. Immediate systemic anticoagulation should be achieved, as the risk of recurrent venous thromboembolism is significantly increased if anticoagulation is not therapeutic within the first 24 hours. In cases of suspected pulmonary embolism, this may necessitate heparinization before completion of diagnostic testing. Confirmation of DVT with duplex imaging is rapid and as a result usually precedes anticoagulation.[122,123]

Heparin

Historically, initial systemic anticoagulation has been undertaken with UFH with a loading dose of 80 U/kg and infusion rate adjusted to achieve activated partial thromboplastin time to 2 to 2.5 times normal. However, because of decreased rates of thrombotic events, decreased bleeding complications, decreased mortality (in cancer patients), and improved pharmacokinetic profile, LMWH is preferred over UFH for the initial treatment of acute DVT in most cases.[123] LMWHs are dosed in a weight-based fashion and rarely require monitoring, except in circumstances such as renal failure, pregnancy, and morbid obesity. LMWH can be given subcutaneously once or twice daily with equal efficacy on an outpatient basis.

Vitamin K Antagonists

Oral administration of VKAs (warfarin being most common) is begun shortly after initiation of heparin therapy, because several days are usually required to bring the prothrombin time to an INR of 2.0 to 3.0. When initiating warfarin therapy, it is preferable to use a maintenance dose rather than a loading dose to avoid suppression of protein C. VKAs block the γ-carboxylation of several clotting factors, and prolongation of the prothrombin time beyond the range suggested is associated with a high incidence of bleeding complications. Nonhemorrhagic side effects are uncommon but include skin necrosis, dermatitis, and a syndrome of painful erythema in areas with large amounts of subcutaneous fat. Most changes are reversible if the drug is stopped, and the administration of fresh frozen plasma usually restores the prothrombin time. After an episode of acute DVT, anticoagulation should be maintained for a minimum of 3 months; some investigators favor 6 months for thrombi in the larger veins or after a second thromboembolic event. Many drugs alter the pharmacodynamics of warfarin by altering its metabolic clearance, rate of absorption, or inhibition of vitamin K–dependent coagulation factor synthesis or by altering other hemostatic factors. Phenylbutazone, sulfinpyrazone, disulfiram, metronidazole, and trimethoprim-sulfamethoxazole all potentiate the action of warfarin.[124] Therefore, regular monitoring of prothrombin time is essential. In addition, levels of concurrent medications should be monitored, because warfarin may compete for binding sites, thus altering plasma levels of these drugs. Some foods that have high levels of vitamin K, such as broccoli, green leafy vegetables, and green teas, are also known to alter the effects of warfarin. Oral anticoagulants are teratogenic and should not be used during established or planned pregnancy. In a pregnant patient, LMWH is the drug of choice, and for long-term management, subcutaneous self-administration should be taught. This regimen allows a normal delivery and can be continued postpartum.

Duration of Anticoagulation

Anticoagulation following an episode of DVT should be continued until the benefits of preventing recurrent venous thromboembolism no longer outweigh the risks of anticoagulation.[125] The major risks of recurrence depend on the patients risk factors for VTE and whether the initial episode has been appropriately treated.[126] Major patient risk factors include reversible risk factors such as previous 1-month history of major surgery (general anesthesia longer than 30 minutes), or hospitalization longer than 3 days or cast immobilization of the lower extremity. In general, the greater the provoking risk factor, the lower the risk of DVT once anticoagulation therapy is stopped.[127] Patients with modifiable risk factors should be treated for 3 to 6 months for a proximal (iliofemoral) or 6 to 12 weeks for a distal DVT. Shorter durations of therapy are associated with double the risk for recurrent DVT or PE within the next year.[128-130]

Patients with nonreversible risk factors include those with cancers and inherited molecular thrombophilias. Patients with cancer have an increased risk of recurrence and major bleeding complications compared with all other causes of DVT.[131] Vomiting, malnutrition, and liver dysfunction, common among cancer patients, makes achieving consistent anticoagulation goals with oral VKA therapy challenging. Several randomized studies have been conducted comparing LMWH to oral VKA in this particular subset of patients; because of decreased mortality from bleeding complications and decreased risk of recurrence, initial treatment with LMWH is recommended with grade 1A evidence.[132-134] These patients should be maintained on LMWH for the first 3 to 6 months and continued on anticoagulation until the cancer resolves.

Among patients with a thrombosis at an age younger than 40 years, a strong family history of VTE (two or more symptomatic relatives) or thrombosis at unusual locations, screening for hereditary thrombophilias is indicated.[135] Screening of unselected individuals is not useful in predicting recurrence and should not guide therapy.[127,136] Selected patients with clinically significant thrombosis and genetic defect may be maintained on anticoagulation indefinitely with periodic reassessments of the risk-to-benefit ratio of continuing oral VKA therapy. Heterozygote carriers of factor V Leiden and prothrombin 20210 gene mutations have only a modest risk of recurrence and should be treated according to standard recommendations.[69] However, an individual who is a heterozygote carrier of both traits has an increased risk of VTE events and should be considered for lifetime anticoagulation.[137]

Patients with DVT in the absence of any identifiable risk factors are said to have an idiopathic DVT. Compared to patients with a reversible risk factor, recurrent VTE events are much more common in this patient population (≤3% vs. 10% at 1 year).[138] Kearon and colleagues[139] studied patients with unprovoked DVT, comparing 3 months of anticoagulation with indefinite anticoagulation. They demonstrated a 95% relative risk reduction in recurrence in patients receiving indefinite anticoagulation, but with a trend toward an increased risk of nonfatal major bleeding ($p = 0.09$). Because longer durations of anticoagulation reduced DVT recurrence but were associated with increased bleeding risk, Ridker and colleagues[140] studied long-term subtherapeutic anticoagulation. The PREVENT investigators randomized patients after completing their full course of VKA anticoagulation (3 to 6 months) to either placebo or subtherapeutic VKA therapy (target INR of 1.5-1.9). At 2.1 years of follow-up, patients receiving indefinite subtherapeutic anticoagulation had a 62% relative risk reduction of recurrent DVT (14.6 vs. 5.5%; $p < 0.001$).

Three months of anticoagulation therapy is sufficient to decrease the risk of recurrent thrombosis related to the initial DVT. However, once therapy is discontinued, the risk for recurrence rises dramatically, with 30% to 50% of patients experiencing a recurrence at 10 years.[141,142] Male gender, elevated D-dimer, incomplete resolution of DVT, body mass index of 30 kg/m² or greater and postthrombotic syndrome are all associated with increased likelihood of recurrence.[143] Additional anticoagulation therapy beyond 3 months is useful at preventing further episodes of recurrence not related to the initial event. Following the initial 3 to 6 months of therapy, all patients should be evaluated for long-term anticoagulation therapy.[139] Similarly, patients with a recurrent VTE are at increased risk of additional episodes. In patients with a second DVT who were treated with 6 months of therapy, 20.7% experienced recurrent thrombosis, compared to 2.6% of patients treated indefinitely with anticoagulation.[144] In high-risk patients, the risks of major bleeding during prolonged therapy (1.1% per patient-year), should be periodically weighed against the benefits

of continuing anticoagulation. Advanced age (older than 75 years), history of gastrointestinal hemorrhage, noncardioembolic stroke, renal or hepatic disease, concomitant antiplatelet therapy, and poor control of anticoagulation increase the risk of bleeding complications.[126]

Two additional tests may be used to guide length of anticoagulation in selected patients. Follow-up duplex ultrasound screening identifies patients with residual thrombus. These patients have a twenty-fivefold greater risk of recurrence compared with patients who demonstrated recanalization of veins.[142] A recent study demonstrated a 35% decrease in recurrent VTE events when duration of anticoagulation was guided by ultrasound evidence without any increase in bleeding complications.[145] A second, better validated parameter is the D-dimer level, measured 1 month after completion of a standard oral VKA course. Patients with elevated D-dimer levels are prothrombotic and should continue to receive anticoagulation therapy.[146]

Fibrinolysis

Great interest has been shown in the use of fibrinolytic agents to activate the intrinsic plasmin system. Tissue-type plasminogen activator, streptokinase, and urokinase are effective, although they are associated with a high incidence of hemorrhagic complications. Ten percent of patients treated with streptokinase suffer allergic reactions, from urticaria to anaphylaxis. In addition, streptokinase offers no advantage over heparin in the treatment of recurrent venous thrombosis or thrombosis that has existed for more than 72 hours. Lytic agents are contraindicated in postoperative or posttraumatic patients and may be associated with an increased risk of pulmonary embolism.

Regional lysing with specialized catheters may be used to deliver recombinant tissue-type plasminogen activator directly to the thrombus. This technique can result in early thrombus resolution, with long-term valve preservation and a reduced incidence of postthrombotic syndrome.[147-151] Mewissen and colleagues[152] reported outcomes from a registry of patients with DVT treated with lytic therapy. Acute thrombosis completely lysed in 34% of cases, but at the expense of bleeding in 11% (but with a minimum of intracranial bleeding). One-year primary patency was 60%. Venous stents were used adjunctively in 104 of 473 patients. Other small studies have demonstrated the potential benefits of regional thrombolysis with improvements in vein patency[153,154] and in the prevention of venous reflux.[153]

Surgical Therapy

Thrombectomy directly removes thrombi from the deep veins of the leg. Despite early efficacy, venographic follow-up often shows rethrombosis. However, when creation of an arteriovenous fistula is added to the procedure, patency is improved. Long-term follow-up is necessary to determine the incidence of postthrombotic syndrome, although small studies have demonstrated excellent efficacy.[154,155] In the United States, this procedure is usually reserved for limb salvage in the presence of phlegmasia cerulea dolens and impending venous gangrene, although there are certainly cases in which surgical thrombectomy should be considered.

VEIN WALL ABNORMALITIES AFTER DEEP VENOUS THROMBOSIS

Chronic venous disease (CVD) encompasses mild varicosities to disabling ulcers, which occasionally can progress to limb loss.[156,157] The underlying pathophysiology is related to venous injury, valve damage, and obstruction; all of which culminate as venous hypertension when in the upright position.[158] Venous hypertension leads to end organ damage, namely the skin and dermis. The sine qua non is hyperpigmentation, corona phlebectatica, lipodermatosclerosis, or frank ulceration of the limb.[159] Once skin changes occur, dermal fibrosis and inflammation are present histologically.[157] Factors involved include leukocyte activation with adhesion and emigration through the basement membrane with release of fibrotic growth factors and proteases. Dysregulation of iron may exacerbate this process.[160]

Postthrombotic syndrome (PTS) is a chronic sequelae of DVT, and typical symptoms include pain, heaviness, swelling, and cramping of the leg, which are generally worsened by standing and exercising.[158] In advanced cases, venous ulceration occurs, causing additional pain and disability and increasing the cost of treatment.[161,162] Postthrombotic morbidity has been reported to occur in 25% to 46% of patients following anticoagulation alone for acute DVT.[8,158] The severity of PTS manifests relatively early after DVT and usually neither worsens nor improves, highlighted by a prospective multicenter cohort of 387 patients with acute DVT.[9,163] Variables that predicted more severe postthrombotic morbidity included: severity of venous symptoms at 1 month; iliofemoral location; recurrent ipsilateral DVT; high body mass index; older age; and female gender.[163] Thus, calf vein thrombosis is less often associated with PTS. Vein valve reflux plays a role in PTS, both in the affected deep segments and the superficial system.[164]

Definition of Postthrombotic Syndrome and Diagnosis

Unlike arterial diseases, PTS is more difficult to quantify. Expert consensus for PTS definition is the Villalta score, combining patient limb symptoms and signs in a graded scoring system[165] (Box 47-1). The higher the score, the greater the severity of PTS (e.g., a score of greater than 15 suggests severe PTS). This system also allows for an evaluation of change in severity of disease over time.

The Clinical Etiologic Anatomic Pathophysiology (CEAP) score is used for objectively characterizing chronic venous disease[166] (see Box 47-1). The parameters in this system include clinical features of the limb, etiology, anatomy, and pathophysiology. While useful, this static measure does not reflect quality-of-life issues or functional status. The Venous Clinical Severity Score (VCSS) is also useful to capture the disability and functional aspects of PTS over time.

BOX 47-1 Villalta Scale CEAP: Classification Scales for Postthrombotic Syndrome

SYMPTOMS
- Heaviness
- Pain
- Cramps
- Pruritus
- Paresthesias

SIGNS
- Pretibial edema
- Induration
- Hyperpigmentation
- New venous ectasia
- Redness
- Pain of calf compression
- Ulceration (receives a score of 15)

EACH FACTOR RECEIVES A RANGE of 0 TO 3 (0 = NONE; 3 = SEVERE)
- Mild: 5 to 9
- Moderate: 10 to 14
- Severe: 15 or greater

CLINICAL
- 0 = None
- 1 = Telangiectasis
- 2 = Varicosities
- 3 = Edema
- 4 = Pigmentation, lipodermatosclerosis
- 5 = Healed ulceration
- 6 = Ulcer

ETIOLOGY
- Congenital
- Primary
- Secondary

ANATOMIC DISTRIBUTION
- Superficial
- Deep
- Perforator
- Combination

PATHOPHYSIOLOGY
- Reflux
- Obstruction
- Combination

SEVERE: > (CEAP class)

Adapted from Kahn SR, Partsch H, Vedantham S, et al: Definition of post-thrombotic syndrome of the leg for use in clinical investigations: a recommendation for standardization. J Thromb Haemost 7:879–883, 2009; and Eklof B, Rutherford RB, Bergan JJ, et al: Revision of the CEAP classification for chronic venous disorders: consensus statement. J Vasc Surg 40:1248–1252, 2004. *CEAP,* Clinical etiologic anatomic pathophysiology.

Duplex ultrasound is the standard for quantifying venous reflux and location, as well as documenting thrombotic obstruction, but imaging per se is neither part of the definition of PTS nor correlated with severity. Similarly, CT venography and magnetic resonance venography can delineate thrombotic obstruction, but are not routinely used outside of planning for interventions or defining proximal iliac or IVC thrombosis.[167]

Prevention of Postthrombotic Syndrome by Preventing Deep Venous Thrombosis

Primary Deep Venous Thrombosis

The most effective way to decrease PTS occurrence is to prevent DVT. When DVT occurs, rapid treatment with evidence-based therapies is indicated. It is clear that surgical patients are at high risk for VTE and prophylaxis is often underprescribed.[168] All surgical patients should have a VTE risk assessment, and excellent guidelines exist.[169] Recently, Bahl and colleagues[170] have shown the utility of the Caprini risk assessment tool. Among vascular patients, those undergoing aortic surgery have the highest risk of postoperative DVT,[171,172] but are also at risk for bleeding. Mixed data exist for the true incidence of postoperative VTE in vascular surgery patients, ranging from 2% to 20%, depending on how it was diagnosed.[169] Therefore patients at high risk (e.g., prior VTE, family history, active malignancy) should receive both pharmacologic and mechanical prophylaxis. For others, such as carotid surgery, no prophylaxis outside of ambulation is usually needed.[173]

Recurrent Deep Venous Thrombosis

Recurrent DVT is both etiologic and a consequence of the damaged vein wall, and it is a major factor for PTS.[158,163] The quality of early anticoagulation for acute DVT significantly affects the likelihood of recurrence. Hull and colleagues[174] reported that subtherapeutic anticoagulation early in the course of patient management (the first 24 hours) increased the risk of recurrent venous thromboembolic events fifteenfold (24.5% vs. 1.6%; $p < 0.001$).

Anticoagulation is typically LMWH or factor Xa inhibition followed by oral VKAs (e.g., sodium warfarin [Coumadin]).[169] A reduction in postthrombotic morbidity (including reduction of venous ulcers) with the use of LMWH was recently published by Hull and colleagues,[175] supporting the advantage of LMWH in the early management of acute DVT. Similarly, LMWH as compared with warfarin showed benefit in deep vein recanalization, and a trend toward less PTS.[176] How the newer anticoagulants will factor into PTS prevention requires study.

Identifying Patients at Risk of Recurrent Deep Venous Thrombosis

Determining who is at increased risk of recurrent DVT (and hence PTS) is important for balancing prevention of recurrent DVT (and decreased PTS risk) against bleeding. New management paradigms may help to determine who is at risk for recurrent DVT at 3 to 6 months after incident DVT, including: imaging the deep venous system for residual thrombus (or wall abnormality) and identifying patients with elevated D-dimer levels, which reflects active thrombus metabolism. Patients

identified by one or both of these methods would then be offered extended continued anticoagulation (see previous discussion in this chapter).

Prandoni and colleagues[144] evaluated patients with venous duplex imaging for residual thrombus (abnormal vein wall) at the time anticoagulation was discontinued. They demonstrated a nearly threefold increase in recurrent DVT in patients with residual abnormality compared to those with a normal venous duplex. However, these criteria need further study because others have not replicated the findings.[177] Using D-dimer as a blood test to evaluate thrombus activity, Eichinger and colleagues[178] and Palareti and colleagues[179] demonstrated that elevated D-dimer levels following termination of oral anticoagulation identified patients who faced a threefold increased risk of recurrence during the next 2 years. Furthermore, extending anticoagulation in those with a significantly elevated D-dimer was associated with a marked reduction in recurrence. Future studies will define these two adjuncts and their role in DVT recurrence management.

Compression and Ambulation for Acute Deep Venous Thrombosis to Decrease Postthrombotic Syndrome

Initial treatment of acute DVT with effective leg compression and ambulation is essential. Randomized trials have demonstrated the value of 30 to 40 mm Hg ankle-gradient stockings in the management of acute DVT.[180,181] Randomized trials with applied compression and ambulation early in the course of treatment have shown significantly reduced progression of thrombus length and volume, reduced pain, and reduced edema.[182,183] There is no evidence that new PEs occur, while there is a significant (50%) reduction of PTS at two years. Indeed, immobility may increase the risk of PE.[184] Early data also suggest that structured exercise may decrease PTS.[185]

Active Thrombus Removal to Decrease Postthrombotic Syndrome

Whereas anticoagulation reduces thrombus propagation, the risk of PE, and the risk of recurrent DVT, it does not affect the natural consequences of venous obstruction and valvular destruction that result in ambulatory venous hypertension. Patients with extensive DVT, defined as those with iliofemoral venous occlusion, are at increased risk of PTS[163,186,187]; therefore it makes sense that eliminating thrombus will reduce postthrombotic morbidity.[188] Removing the thrombus will also potentially reduce the risk of recurrence. Strategies of active thrombus removal have been recognized by the 2008 American College of Chest Physicians (ACCP) Consensus Conference,[126] including options for operative venous thrombectomy and catheter-directed thrombolysis. An ongoing National Institutes of Health–sponsored multi-institutional trial called the ATTRACT Study will answer this question: is active thrombus removal plus best medical therapy superior to best medical therapy for iliofemoral DVT? The primary outcome measure will be development of PTS at 2 years, as well as

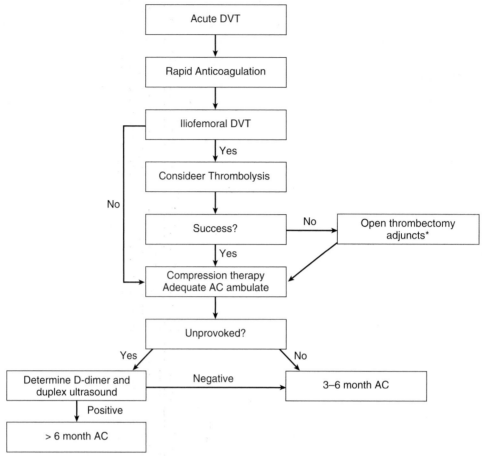

FIGURE 47-2 ■ Algorithm of recommended therapy for acute venous thromboembolism to decrease postthrombotic syndrome. *Adjuncts = webectomy; venoplasty; AV fistula. *AC,* Anticoagulation.

bleeding occurrence. A suggested treatment algorithm is shown in Figure 47-2.

Other Consideration for Postthrombotic Syndrome

Pharmacologic Interventions

Although no pharmacologic agents specifically treat PTS, several agents may have potential benefit. Daflon (micronized purified flavanoid fraction) is available in Europe and is effective for chronic venous insufficiency.[189] Pentoxifylline has been shown to be of benefit for CVI symptoms and venous ulcer healing.

Deep System Reconstruction

Native valve reconstruction procedures are less effective in patients with postthrombotic syndrome compared to those with primary venous insufficiency.[157] Prosthetic valves for the venous system have undergone limited experimental evaluation.[190] The risk of thrombosis and durability of these bioprosthesis is still uncertain. Furthermore, whether valves can reduce venous hypertension in the setting of long-segment postthrombotic vein wall damage is not clear.

Biomarkers

An active area of research involves biomarkers to stratify patients at risk of PTS after DVT. Several biomarkers correlate with surrogate measures of PTS—namely, intercellular adhesion molecule-1 (ICAM-1), interleukin 6, and C-reactive protein.[191] Preliminary studies on humans also suggest alteration in MMP levels in acute DVT and nonresolution a risk for PTS.[192] Larger studies will be necessary to determine their sensitivity and specificity in relation to clinical PTS. Ideally, a biomarker panel could be drawn at the time of diagnosis of DVT, and if predictive of PTS, these patients might be best served by active thrombus removal and increased compression strength and duration.

Endothelial Protection

In humans, it is likely that the endothelium is damaged after DVT, and the healing response and function of the endothelium is critical to prevent rethrombosis. The recent JUPITER trial suggests a benefit of HMG-CoA reductase inhibitors (statins) in patients at modest cardiac risk also reducing incident VTE.[193] It is interesting that the risk reduction for DVT (but not PE) was of similar magnitude to the reduction in arterial cardiovascular events. It is still unknown whether statins may decrease PTS in the long term. Although speculative, statins may reduce perioperative DVT risk.

DIAGNOSIS AND TREATMENT OF SUPERFICIAL THROMBOPHLEBITIS

Superficial vein thrombophlebitis (SVT) is characterized by a painful erythematous and palpable cordlike structure, usually involving the lower extremities but capable of affecting any superficial vein in the body. SVT has traditionally been managed with compression support, nonsteroidal antiinflammatory drugs (NSAIDs), and lower extremity elevation. However, SVT may coexist with DVT, propagate, and rarely cause PE.[194-198] Anticoagulant therapy appears to be the treatment of choice when there is above-knee SVT with deep venous system involvement. However, the best treatment without DVT if the thrombus approaches the saphenofemoral junction is controversial. In addition, with the new data on the effectiveness of fondaparinux in the treatment of SVT,[199] the treatment of routine SVT may need to be reassessed.

In a prospective epidemiologic study including 844 patients with symptomatic SVT, 210 (24.9%) had concomitant DVT upon enrollment. Of the 600 patients without DVT followed for 3 months, 58 (10.2%) developed thromboembolic complications, including 3 (0.5%) with pulmonary embolism, 15 (2.8%) with DVT, 18 (3.3%) with extension, and 10 (1.9%) with recurrence of SVT. These events occurred despite the use of anticoagulant treatment with LMWH 374 (62.9%) at therapeutic and 216 (36.7%) at prophylactic dose for 10 to 17 days. Almost all patients (584; 97.7%), received elastic compression stockings. Risk factors for complications at 3 months were male sex, history of DVT or PE, previous cancer, and absence of varicose veins.[200]

The incidence of SVT has been reported to occur in approximately 125,000 people per year in the United States.[201] Others estimate that this number could be even higher than that of DVT, which has been reported at 56 to 160 per 100,000 people per year.[202] Lower extremity veins are most commonly involved, followed by upper extremity veins.[203] Approximately 54% to 65% of the reported cases affect females, with an average age 58 to 65 years old.[200,204,205] The presence of varicose veins is the most frequent predisposing risk factor for SVT, being seen in approximately two thirds of patients.[200] Other risk factors associated with nonintravenous line–associated SVT include immobilization, trauma, postoperative states, older age (>60 years), obesity, tobacco use, history of DVT or SVT, pregnancy and the puerperium, autoimmune disease, use of oral contraceptives or hormonal replacement therapy, and hypercoagulability.[200,204-206] Thrombophilic disorders may be associated with SVT as a significant or presenting clinical sign.[207] In patients with ascending or worsening thrombosis despite initial treatment, hypercoagulable testing should be considered.[208,209] Malignancy is a risk factor for SVT, affecting 13% to 18% of patients.[197,210] Although lower in frequency, SVT developing in nonvaricose veins may be associated with

a risk of malignancy (4.8% of 42 cases), nonneoplastic disease (9.5% of 42 cases), or thrombophilia (48% of 42 cases).[211] The overall recurrence of SVT is 18% over an average observation period of 15 months and is equally frequent in varicose and nonvaricose veins. Deep venous reflux increases the recurrence to 33%, and hypercoagulable states increase recurrence rates to 42% over the same time period.[212]

The clinical diagnosis of SVT usually involves pain, a firm palpable cord with inflammation, tenderness, surrounding erythema, and edema.[213,214] Duplex ultrasound of the affected extremity should be performed to rule out extension into the deep venous system or concomitant DVT.[208,213] Complete thrombophilia workup, although not routinely performed, may be indicated in selected patients with recurrent primary thrombophlebitis or a strong family history. The workup is similar to that obtained for patients with DVT. Screening for underlying diseases, including malignancy or vasculitis, should be performed if indicated including: mammography and colonoscopy, and chest radiograph if the patient is a smoker.[213]

A renewed interest for this disease has arisen because of the significant association with the deep venous system and possible pulmonary embolism, especially if the phlebitis extends toward the level of the saphenofemoral junction.[195,198,215] Several therapeutic approaches have been proposed including surgical ligation or vein stripping, elastic stockings, NSAIDs to reduce pain and inflammation, and variable doses of UFH or LMWH followed by oral anticoagulant therapy. However, there is no general consensus on optimal treatment. It seems clear that the treatment for SVT should be tailored accordingly to its location, the presence or absence of concomitant DVT, and any associated infectious process. SVT in the main trunks of either the great saphenous or small saphenous vein may have the highest risk of extension into the deep venous system, thus requiring aggressive treatment such as LMWH at therapeutic dose for a period of 2 weeks.[198] On the other hand, other locations may be associated with a lower risk of extension, thus warranting less aggressive treatment such as compression stockings and NSAIDs.[216] Traditionally, the treatment for primary SVT localized in tributary veins and the distal great saphenous vein includes ambulation, warm soaks, compression, and NSAIDs.[207,215] If the patient presents risk factors for extension to DVT, pharmacologic treatment with LMWH at prophylactic dose for a period of 4 weeks should be considered.[216] Clearly, if there is concomitant DVT with SVT, then the patient needs to be treated for the DVT. Based on the recent data regarding fondaparinux, one must consider daily treatment for 45 days for patients with symptomatic superficial thrombophlebitis at least 5 cm long and at least 3 cm distal to the saphenofemoral junction at a dose of 2.5 mg/day subcutaneously.

Studies have been performed comparing different approaches for the medial treatment of SVT. Compared with NSAIDs, LMWH over a 7-day period has been found to be better regarding persistence of signs and symptoms both 1 week and 2 months after diagnosis.[217] In a second study of patients with documented acute symptomatic superficial vein thrombosis of the legs, the incidence of deep and superficial venous thromboembolism by day 12 was significantly reduced in all active treatment groups (LMWH and NSAIDs) compared to placebo, with a trend that remained in favor of the active treatments for DVT and SVT combination at 3 months of follow-up.[218] No major bleeding or heparin-induced thrombocytopenia was observed in any treatment group. There was a trend in favor of LMWH relative to NSAIDs. Prophylactic LMWH was equivalent to bodyweight therapeutic LMWH once daily for 1 month in another study, in which the cumulative rate of SVT progression and venous thromboembolism complications did not differ between groups after 3 months of follow-up.[219]

Prophylactic intravenous UFH was used as a comparator treatment in two studies. The first study in 562 patients with SVT with large varicose veins without systematic disorders treated patients with elastic compression alone, compression plus early surgery (flush ligation or complete stripping), compression plus standard heparin or LMWH, or compression plus warfarin only.[220] At 3 to 6 months, the incidence of superficial thrombus extension was greater in the elastic compression and saphenous vein ligation groups ($p < 0.05$), with no significant differences in DVT incidence at 3 months. A second study compared high- versus low-dose intravenous UFH.[221] With 6-month follow-up, patients with high-dose UFH had better results than those with low-dose UFH.[221] There was no major bleeding or heparin-induced thrombocytopenia in either group.

LMWH has been compared with saphenofemoral disconnection for the treatment of proximal great saphenous vein thrombophlebitis in a prospective, randomized clinical study.[222] In this study, 84 consecutive patients with a diagnosis of proximal thrombophlebitis alone were divided into two comparable groups treated with: saphenofemoral disconnection under local anesthesia with a short hospital stay (n = 45) or enoxaparin (1 mg/kg bid) on an outpatient basis for 4 weeks (n = 39). Thirty patients in each group completed the study requirements. Follow-up was at 1, 3, and 6 months. In the surgical group, two patients (6.7%) presented complications of the surgical wound, one (3.3%) had thrombophlebitis recurrence and two (6.7%) developed nonfatal pulmonary embolism over 6 months. In the medical group, there was no progression of the thrombosis to the deep venous system or pulmonary embolism; there were two cases (6.7%) of minor bleeding and three cases (10%) of thrombophlebitis recurrence. Although the study found no statistically significant difference between the two groups, the LMWH group had a significant socioeconomic advantage and confirmed the efficacy of LMWH treatment in resolving symptoms and signs and preventing DVT and PE.

Twenty-four studies involving 2469 patients were included in a Cochrane review.[216] Both LMWH and NSAIDs significantly reduced superficial thrombophlebitis extension or recurrence by approximately 70% compared to placebo, whereas surgical treatments improved local symptomatic relief from pain. As in a previous review of the literature, surgical treatment with ligation of the great saphenous vein at the saphenofemoral junction allows for superior symptomatic relief of pain,

whereas medical management with anticoagulants appears to be superior for minimizing complications and preventing subsequent DVT and PE.[223] Finally, in the CALISTO study, fondaparinux was given over 31 to 45 days (along with graduated compression stockings) to patients with SVT of at least 5 cm length.[199] There was a significant improvement in those treated with fondaparinux compared with placebo in composite end points of death, PE, DVT, and extension or recurrence by both days 47 and 77, suggesting that this therapy should be considered in these patients. Regarding the latest ACCP guidelines, prophylactic or intermediate doses of LMWH for 4 weeks are recommended as a grade 2B recommendation.[126] As an alternative, oral vitamin K antagonists (INR 2-3) overlapped with 5 days of heparin or LMWH and continued for 4 weeks is given a grade 2C recommendation. Medical treatment is recommended over surgical treatment. Finally, it is likely that less extensive SVT requires only symptom control with oral or topical NSAIDs, although fondaparinux for 45 days now has support in the literature for thrombophlebitis at least 5 cm in length.

INFERIOR VENA CAVAL INTERRUPTION

Because of the general lack of prospective, randomized data for IVC filter use, the use of IVC filters has been driven primarily by their relatively low complication rate, ease of placement, and the fact that a mechanical barrier to prevent PE makes intuitive sense. However, adequate anticoagulation whenever possible is the cornerstone of effective treatment of DVT and PE, and physicians must remember that an IVC filter does not treat existing DVT and PE, but only prevents further significant PE. Unfortunately, not all patients can be safely or effectively anticoagulated, and it is this patient population that benefits from placement of IVC filters. The indications for IVC filter placement can be generally classified into three types: absolute or classic indications, accepted relative indications, and extended indications for IVC filter placement (Box 47-2). Of the indication for IVC filters, the classic indications for placement are the least controversial. These indications require the presence of DVT or PE and either a significant bleeding complication directly related to anticoagulation, an underlying contraindication to anticoagulation, or a failure of anticoagulation to prevent PE or DVT. When considering a failure of anticoagulation as an indication for filter placement, it is important to differentiate between a failure of therapeutic anticoagulation to prevent a PE or DVT from a failure to adequately achieve therapeutic anticoagulation (INR <20; activated partial thromboplastin time <50 seconds) who subsequently develops a DVT or PE.

Accepted relative indications for IVC filter placement also require the presence of DVT or PE and are more controversial than the classic indications. Relative indications include a history of massive PE with residual DVT in a patient without cardiopulmonary reserve enough to tolerate an additional PE as well as patients that have required a pulmonary thrombectomy for PE. Patients with preexisting severe pulmonary hypertension or

ABSOLUTE (CLASSIC)

Presence of DVT or PE plus one of the following:
- Bleeding complication related to anticoagulation
- Contraindication to anticoagulation
- Failure of anticoagulation to prevent DVT or PE

ACCEPTED (RELATIVE)

Presence of DVT or PE plus one of the following:
- Chronic PE with residual DVT and no cardiopulmonary reserve
- Previous pulmonary thrombectomy for PE
- Preexisitng severe pulmonary hypertension or right heart failure
- Free-floating iliocaval thrombus
- Significant fall risk

EXTENDED

Does not require the presence of DVT or PE:
- Prophylactic (prevention of PE; e.g., trauma, long bone or pelvic fractures)
- High-risk immobilized patient (e.g., paraplegia)
- Preoperative patient with multiple risk factors for DVT

IVC, Inferior vena cava; *DVT,* deep venous thrombosis; *PE,* pulmonary embolism.

significant right heart failure and DVT may also benefit from an IVC filter placement if they have a significant DVT. Patients with free floating iliocaval thrombus with long, free floating tails and those at significant fall risk are also believed to be appropriate candidates for IVC filter placement.

Extended indications for the use of IVC filters remain the most controversial and least supported by the medical literature. In contrast to the absolute and relative indications for IVC filter placement, the extended indications do not require the presence of DVT or PE. This indication encompasses the placement of IVC filters for prophylactic purposes (prevention of PE). Patients that frequently undergo filter placement for these indications include trauma patients at high risk of DVT or PE and patients with closed head injury, spinal cord injury, or long bone and pelvic fractures. Other high-risk immobilized patients such as those with paraplegia, and preoperative patients with multiple risk factors for DVT, such as patients undergoing bariatric surgery, frequently undergo filter placement for this indication.

Inferior Vena Cava Filter Devices

The Greenfield filter remains the standard to which all other filters are compared. The cone-shaped Greenfield filter was developed more than 30 years ago to prevent pulmonary embolism while maintaining caval patency, preventing lower extremity venous stasis, and facilitating lysis of the embolus. A 20-year review of the Greenfield Filter Registry revealed a 4% rate of recurrent embolism and a caval patency rate of 95%.[224,225] A 30-year review indicated that the long-term results became more

favorable as experience accumulated with the smaller-profile versions of the device. The high caval patency rate makes it possible to position the filter above the renal veins when thrombus extends into the inferior vena cava or in young women with childbearing potential. A long-term follow-up study of patients with suprarenal filters demonstrated the safety and efficacy of such placements.[226,227] The complications of filter insertion range in severity from minor wound hematoma resulting from early resumption of anticoagulation to potentially lethal migration of the device into the pulmonary artery or right ventricle, as documented initially with the bird's nest filter and more recently with the Recovery nitinol filter (Bard). Filter fracture and embolization of the device or fragments of the device have been problematic for some filters despite several generations of redesign.[228] These filters are generally retrievable and frequently manufactured from nitinol and have led to an FDA Alert letter suggesting that "implanting physicians and clinicians responsible for the ongoing care of patients with retrievable IVC filter consider removing the filter as soon as protection from PE is no longer needed."[229] The most common complication with the original stainless steel Greenfield filter was misplacement, which occurred in 7% of cases. This rate fell to 4% when the use of a guidewire became standard. With the titanium and percutaneous stainless steel devices, the misplacement rate is less than 1%. When the filter is misplaced into a renal or iliac vein, it poses no regional problem, but there is no protection from pulmonary embolism. A second filter can be placed in the appropriate location. Follow-up has shown that filters misplaced in the right ventricle or pulmonary artery need not be retrieved unless an arrhythmia or tricuspid insufficiency develops. When obesity precludes fluoroscopy, intravascular ultrasonography can be used to identify the renal veins and guide filter placement. Bedside placement using either surface or intravascular ultrasonography has also been recommended for patients at risk during transport to the radiology suite, such as severely injured trauma patients. Furthermore, this method may prove to be more cost effective because it frees staff and leaves the interventional suite available for procedures generating greater revenue. Pulmonary embolism has occurred in 2% to 4% of cases after filter placement and may be caused by a source of thrombus outside of the filtered flow, such as the upper body veins or the right atrium. Recurrent embolism is an indication for inferior venacavography to evaluate the filter for possible attached thrombus. This finding is rare and can be managed either by thrombolytic therapy if the amount of thrombus is small or by placement of a second filter in the suprarenal vena cava. Secondary infection of a captured thrombus within a Greenfield filter has been produced in the laboratory, but it was possible to sterilize the filter and thrombus with a 2-week course of antibiotic therapy.[230] Although the FDA identifies septic embolism as a contraindication to filter insertion, our experience does not support that recommendation.[231] The capture of a very large embolus within a filter may suddenly occlude the vena cava, with a precipitous fall in blood pressure. In a patient with known prior pulmonary embolism, this event can be mistaken for recurrent pulmonary embolism, with disastrous results if vasopressor therapy is administered. The basic distinction between functional hypervolemia of caval occlusion and right ventricular overload from recurrent pulmonary embolism can be made at the bedside by measuring the central venous pressure and arterial oxygen tension and observing for jugular venous distension. The response to volume resuscitation for a patient with sudden vena caval occlusion should be dramatic improvement.

Favorable experience with the Seldinger technique for percutaneous introduction of catheters and devices led to a variety of innovative vena caval filter devices. Three devices—the bird's nest filter (Cook, Bloomington, Ind.), the Simon nitinol filter (Bard Peripheral Vascular, Tempe, Ariz.), and the Vena Tech device (B. Brown, Bethlehem, Pa.)—gained popularity during the 1990s.[232-234] Retrievable filters have dominated the market since 2003.

Retrievable Optional Filters

It is important to realize that the basis for the retrievable filter design has been driven by the publication of the 2- and 8-year results of the PREPIC trial.[235,236] The PREPIC study, the only long-term randomized study of caval filter placement in the prevention of PE, had its 2-year results published in 1998. In this multi-institutional trial, 400 patients with venographically confirmed acute proximal DVT were randomized to treatment with anticoagulation (LMWH for 8 to 12 days and a vitamin K antagonist for at least 3 months) alone versus anticoagulation and a permanent caval filter. At 12 days, there were two PEs in the filter group (1.1%) versus nine PEs in the nonfilter group (4.8%; $p = 0.03$). At 2 years, there were 6 PEs in the filter group (3.4%) and 12 PEs in the nonfilter group (6.3%; $p = 0.16$). The incidence of recurrent DVT was 37 (20.8%) in the filter group and 21 (11.6%) in the nonfilter group ($p = 0.02$).[235] These 2-year results suggested that caval filters provided significant additional short-term protection from PE compared with anticoagulation, and that this benefit seemed to wane over time and was associated with an increased risk of recurrent DVT. The 8-year results of the PREPIC trial, published in 2005, showed that there were 9 PEs in the filter group (6.2%) versus 24 PEs in the nonfilter group (15.1%; $p = 0.08$). The filter group had 57 patients with DVT (35.7%) versus 41 (27.5%) in the nonfilter group ($p = 0.042$). The incidence of PTS was similar: it was observed in 109 (70.3%) filter patients and 107 (69.7%) nonfilter patients at 8 years. Mortality was also similar: 103 filter patients had died, compared with 98 nonfilter patients.[236] These results showed that at 8 years, vena cava filters reduced the risk of PE while increasing the incidence of DVT, and without effect on the incidence of the postthrombotic syndrome or on survival. Since the initial publication of the PREPIC trial in 1998, there has been increased interest in filters designed to provide the option of retrieval. In fact, the six filters introduced into the market have been retrievable optional filters: the G2 and Eclipse filters (Bard Peripheral Vascular), Gunther Tulip and Celect filters (Cook), OptEase (Cordis, Miami, Fla.), and the Option filter (Argon Medical, Athens, Tex.; Figure 47-3). Interestingly, the Recovery filter was taken off the market in 2005 for problems with filter fracture and embolization. Filter migration was also problematic for this particular filter. Since 2005, this filter has gone through two additional adaptations, the G2 (Generation 2) and most recently it has been reintroduced in an electropolished version called the Eclipse. The Recovery, G2, and now the Eclipse are manufactured from nitinol and retain the two trapping levels of the original nitinol filter, but with an innovative change to the proximal level that allows less disturbance of the blood flow. Not surprisingly, the G2 filter has been associated with similar fracture and migration issues as the original Recovery filter.[228] The advantage of these filters appears to be the length of time it can remain in the vena cava and still be safely recovered. However, ease of retrieval requires less secure fixation, which may explain early reports of movement with this device. The Gunther tulip filter (Cook) is a conical device with a smaller volume attached to the vena cava by four rather than six hooked legs; however, according to the FDA's adverse event reporting site, it has been associated with migration. The profile is 8 French, and retrieval is facilitated by the presence of a hook at the apex. Millward and coworkers[237] published results that suggest that few are actually removed, despite this option. Retrieval of the Gunther tulip filter is approximately 90% at approximately 2 months and the difficulty of retrieval the filter increases with increased incorporation of the filter into the vena cava over time.[238] A modified version of the Gunther tulip filter, the Celect filter (Cook) has been developed and is associated with greater success of retrieval even after longer vena caval indwell.[239] The TrapEase filter (Cordis) has a unique cone-on-cone design that traps emboli against the wall of the vena cava. Although effective for clot capture, the TrapEase has been reported to produce vena caval obstruction leading to renal failure, limb loss, and death. A recent prospective, randomized study confirmed a higher rate of symptomatic IVC thrombosis in comparison with the Greenfield filter.[240] The device has a low delivery profile and is available without hooks (the OptEase Filter), offering the option of retrieval.[241,242] The most recent device to receive FDA approval is the Option filter (Argon Medical Devices) in 2010. This device capitalizes on the conical design and is made of nitinol. It is deployed through a 6.5-French delivery system. It has a nonspecific window of retrieval and is purported to be retrievable after prolonged periods of indwell time in the vena cava. This filter appears promising. It remains important to remember that this latest step in the evolution of vena caval filters, the development of retrievable optional filters, is based on a single study and lacks a solid body of confirmatory evidence to support its safety and efficacy. It is important to note that although the PREPIC trial stands as the only prospective, randomized trial examining the long-term effects of IVC filters, no additional study has been performed to confirm these results.

The features that make a device retrievable—lack of endothelial incorporation and flexible hooks—are also the features that make it less secure as a permanent device. More information on patient outcomes after filter removal is necessary to determine whether the concept of retrieval, with its added risk and cost, is appropriate.

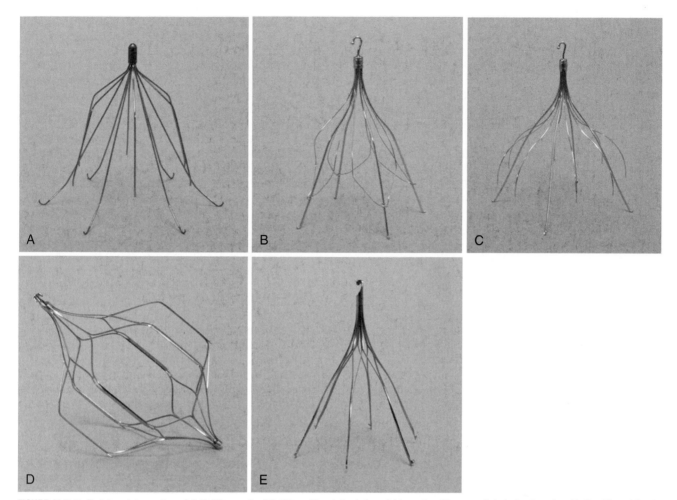

FIGURE 47-3 ■ Retrievable optional IVC filters. **A,** G2 Filter (Bard Peripheral Vascular, Tempe, Ariz.). **B,** Gunther Tulip Filter (Cook, Bloomington, Ind.). **C,** Celect Filter (Cook). **D,** OptEase Filter (Cordis, Miami, Fla.). **E,** Option Filter (Argon Medical, Athens, Tex.).

Classical indications for the use of IVC filters are unlikely to be altered, but further study to determine the most appropriate indications for filter placement, especially in the case of relative and extended indications, is warranted. The current trend in IVC filters is clearly weighted in favor of further development of retrievable IVC filters despite the limited data to support their use. Regardless of the current questions surrounding the use of retrievable filters, it is clear that the use of IVC filters in appropriately selected patients saves lives and will remain an important tool in the armamentarium of clinicians in the treatment of DVT and PE.

References available online at expertconsult.com.

QUESTIONS

1. Which of the following are significant risk factors for venous thromboembolism?
   a. Age, immobilization, Caucasian race
   b. History of DVT, malignancy, malnutrition
   c. Surgery, obesity, malignancy, inflammatory bowel disease
   d. Central venous catheters, hypertension, hyperlipidemia, pregnancy

2. In the treatment algorithm for VTE, which of the following would be appropriate?
   a. Rapid anti-coagulation should be considered for only iliofemoral DVT.
   b. Catheter-directed thrombolytic therapy should be considered for an acute extensive iliofemoral DVT.
   c. Rapid anticoagulation is initiated not only to prevent further extension of clot, but also to help break down any existing thrombus.
   d. Open thrombectomy should be considered before thrombolysis.

3. A limitation of LMWH is that:
   a. LMWH is eliminated by the kidneys, making safe dosing difficult with renal dysfunction (defined at CrCl < 30 mL/min)
   b. LMWH is as effective as unfractionated heparin, but the safety profile is not well defined.
   c. LMWH is a more specific inhibitor of factor Xa, which cannot be measured and titrated to therapeutic effect.
   d. LMWH has a shorter half-life and is not ideal for high-risk patients with bleeding concerns.

4. Which of the following inherited thrombophilias is associated with the greatest increase in risk for VTE (in the heterozygous form)?
   a. Factor V Leiden
   b. Prothrombin G20210A
   c. Protein C deficiency
   d. Antithrombin deficiency

5. After an episode of acute DVT, anticoagulation should be initiated for:
   a. 6 to 12 weeks
   b. 3 to 6 months
   c. Indefinitely
   d. Until the etiology of the DVT can be determined and reversed

6. New management paradigms in determining who is at increased risk of recurrence (and PTS) at 3 to 6 months after incident DVT include which of the following?
   a. Imaging of the deep venous system for evidence of residual thrombus
   b. Identifying patients with elevated C-reactive protein
   c. Identifying patients with elevated D-dimer levels
   d. Both *a* and *c*

7. Which of the following is true regarding superficial vein thrombophlebitis (SVT)?
   a. Duplex ultrasound of the affected extremity to rule out extension to the deep venous system is not indicated.
   b. A complete thrombophilia work-up is almost always indicated.
   c. Regardless of location, SVT never warrants treatment with therapeutic doses of LMWH, although treatment with a 30- to 45-day course of fondaparinux may be beneficial if the lesion is greater than 7 cm in length.
   d. The clinical diagnosis usually involves pain, a firm palpable cord with inflammation, tenderness, surrounding erythema, and edema.

8. PTS is a chronic sequelae of DVT with typical symptoms including pain, heaviness, swelling, and cramping of the leg, worsened by standing and exercising. Which of the following are true regarding PTS?
   a. It is defined by the Clinical Etiologic Anatomic Pathophysiology (CEAP) score, with parameters including clinical features of the involved limb, etiology, anatomy, and pathophysiology.
   b. PTS is defined by duplex ultrasound imaging, with resulting imaging that correlates to disease severity.
   c. PTS is defined by the Villalta score, combining patient limb symptoms and signs into a graded scoring system, with a score greater than 15 suggesting severe disease.
   d. Severity of disease is inversely related to body mass index, female gender, older age, iliofemoral location, or recurrent ipsilateral DVT.

9. In addition to anticoagulation, the initial management of acute DVT includes early ambulation and effective leg compression with 30 to 40 mm Hg ankle-gradient stockings. Randomized trials have shown which of the following?
   a. Significant reduction in PTS.
   b. There is some evidence of increased incidence of PE with lower extremity compression.
   c. There is no evidence that PTS is significantly reduced with these therapies.
   d. These therapies are minimally effective at reducing thrombus length and volume, but may improve the patient's subjective evaluation of pain.

10. In what percentage of patients does a PE occur with an IVC filter in place?
    a. Less than 1%
    b. 2% to 4%
    c. 6% to 8%
    d. Greater than 10%

ANSWERS

1. **c**
2. **b**
3. **a**
4. **d**
5. **b**
6. **d**
7. **d**
8. **c**
9. **a**
10. **b**

CHAPTER 48

Thrombolysis for Deep Venous Thrombosis and Pulmonary Embolism

Anthony J. Comerota

Thrombolytic therapy for venous thromboembolism represents a valuable option for the management of patients with extensive venous thromboembolic disease, iliofemoral venous thrombosis, and pulmonary embolism (PE), which alter hemodynamics and cause pathologic myocardial stretch or cellular damage. This chapter will address those patients. Specifically, in patients with deep venous thrombosis (DVT), iliofemoral DVT presents with the most severe acute morbidity, and these patients suffer the most severe long-term postthrombotic sequelae.

Patients with massive PE defined by sustained hypotension and those with submassive PE characterized by right heart strain are those who would benefit most by eliminating the acute obstruction of right ventricular outflow.

There is a common theme in treating both extensive venous thrombosis and large pulmonary emboli, and that is restoring hemodynamics. In the lower extremity, the goal is to avoid venous hypertension (ambulatory venous hypertension), and in the cardiopulmonary circulation, the goal is to correct cardiopulmonary hemodynamics and avoid chronic thromboembolic pulmonary hypertension.

ACUTE ILIOFEMORAL VENOUS THROMBOSIS

It may be instructive to begin with a summary of a 22-year-old woman who was referred with severe venous claudication. As a high school student, this patient was the state champion in the 400-meter and 800-meter runs. She was awarded a full college scholarship as a member of a Big Ten women's track team. Three months after starting to take oral birth control, she developed an extensive iliofemoral venous thrombosis. She was hospitalized, treated with low-molecular-weight heparin and converted to warfarin. Her leg remained swollen, and her acute symptoms of venous claudication never resolved. Her symptoms limited her activity; she could no longer participate as a member of the track team and had difficulty with sustained walking. She lost her athletic scholarship and, because of family finances, could not remain in college. The result was a part-time job paying minimum wage.

Acute obstruction of the single channel outflow from the lower extremity (common femoral, external iliac, and common iliac veins) leads to high compartment and venous pressures. Qvarfordt and colleagues[1] reported compartment pressures in patients with iliofemoral DVT who subsequently underwent venous thrombectomy. These patients had high compartment pressures, which is a surrogate for venous pressure upon presentation. Following thrombus removal and restoration of venous outflow, compartment pressures returned to normal.

The pathophysiology of chronic venous disease is venous hypertension, specifically ambulatory venous hypertension. It is known that venous valve function and luminal obstruction are the two main components leading to ambulatory venous hypertension. However, it is this author's opinion that obstruction is far more important than valvular dysfunction in producing severe venous hypertension and the most debilitating form of chronic venous disease.

In a study evaluating venous hypertension by measuring arm-foot pressure differential, Labropoulos and colleagues[2] showed that patients with postthrombotic obstruction of the iliofemoral venous system had the highest venous pressures (highest arm-foot pressure differential).

Anticoagulation alone for iliofemoral DVT reduces the risk of pulmonary embolization and reduces the extension of thrombus. Unfortunately, obstruction of the venous outflow channel remains, producing significant venous hypertension. Figure 48-1 is a photograph of a man who had iliofemoral DVT treated with anticoagulation alone 3 months earlier. Despite therapeutic anticoagulation and wearing 30- to 40-mm ankle-gradient compression stockings, he suffered with venous claudication, swelling of the lower extremity, and skin discoloration in the lower leg, with the ascending phlebogram showing extensive deep venous obstruction. Another ascending phlebogram (Figure 48-2) of a patient with severe postthrombotic morbidity and venous ulceration 10 years after anticoagulation alone for iliofemoral DVT shows the extensive amount of venous obstruction. The day following the phlebogram, the patient underwent a classic Linton procedure. The operative photograph of his postthrombotic femoral vein demonstrates the fibrotic obstruction with webbing and synechiae that occur in these patients, causing much more anatomic obstruction to venous return than can be appreciated on the phlebogram.

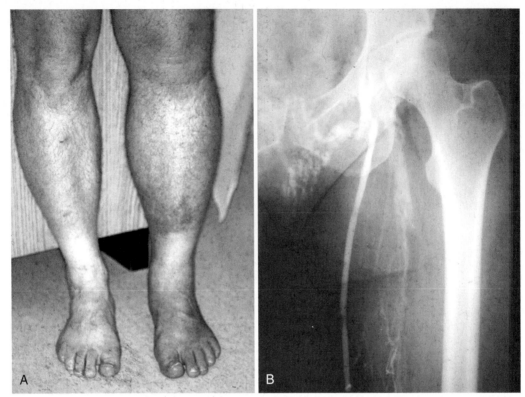

FIGURE 48-1 ■ **A,** The lower extremities of a patient suffering iliofemoral deep venous thrombosis 3 months earlier treated with anticoagulation alone. **B,** The associated ascending phlebogram demonstrating extensive deep venous obstruction. The saphenous vein is patent, but it too is obstructed at the saphenofemoral junction.

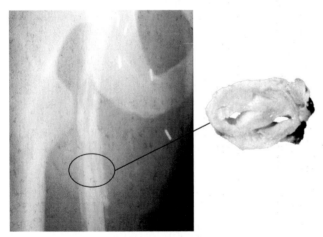

FIGURE 48-2 ■ Ascending phlebogram of a patient treated for iliofemoral DVT with anticoagulation alone 10 years earlier. A noninvasive vascular laboratory test measuring maximal venous outflow was normal. The ascending phlebogram was read by the radiologist as "tree-barking appearance of chronic venous disease with no evidence of obstruction." The specimen demonstrates a cross-section of the femoral vein just below the profunda femoris vein after the patient had a classic Linton procedure. One can see extensive luminal obstruction with typical recanalization channels.

NATURAL HISTORY STUDIES

Natural history studies of patients with acute DVT treated with anticoagulation alone have revealed a number of important principles. Meissner and colleagues[3] followed patients with acute DVT with sequential venous duplex examinations. Some patients had the good fortune to lyse their thrombus during the first few months of observation, whereas in others the thrombus remained. Their observations demonstrated that when thrombus lysed early (within 60-90 days), patients were likely to retain normal valve function. However, valve reflux occurred in patients whose thrombus did not lyse. In longer term follow-up studies, these authors demonstrated that patients who did not have early lysis had a significantly higher recurrent DVT rate.[4]

Kahn and colleagues[5] performed a prospective analysis of 387 patients with acute DVT. Their intent was to evaluate postthrombotic syndrome following acute DVT. These authors found that patients with iliofemoral DVT had the most severe postthrombotic morbidity (odds ratio [OR], 2.23; $p < 0.001$). They also found that the patients' clinical condition at 1 month was the best predictor of long-term outcome ($p < 0.001$).

A number of authors have followed patients with iliofemoral DVT who were treated with anticoagulation alone.[6,7] These patients uniformly suffered with chronic venous disease. Within 5 years, 15% developed venous ulceration and up to 40% had venous claudication. The patients' quality of life was significantly diminished.

One frequently overlooked observation is that recurrent DVT is more frequent in patients with iliofemoral DVT than in patients with femoropopliteal DVT.[8] This is likely due to the large burden of thrombus that remains in the venous system following anticoagulation alone.

VENOUS THROMBECTOMY

The purpose of this is not to address operative venous thrombectomy. The principles of restoring patency, normalizing venous pressures, and long-term benefits are well illustrated by the randomized trial performed by Plate and colleagues.[9-11] The Scandinavian investigators randomized patients with iliofemoral DVT to venous thrombectomy plus arteriovenous fistula followed by anticoagulation or anticoagulation alone. A careful follow-up at 6 months, 5 years, and 10 years demonstrated significant benefits in patients who underwent venous thrombectomy. Patients randomized to thrombectomy had improved patency, lower venous pressures, less leg swelling, and fewer postthrombotic symptoms compared with anticoagulation alone. These data illustrate the benefit of eliminating obstruction to venous drainage from the leg to the vena cava. The details of contemporary operative venous thrombectomy have been recently reviewed by Comerota and Gale.[12]

CATHETER-DIRECTED THROMBOLYSIS

All drugs currently used for thrombolytic therapy are plasminogen activators. As a result, clot dissolution occurs as a result of plasminogen being activated, resulting in the production of plasmin, which is the active clot dissolving enzyme. Plasminogen circulates as an inactive zymogen. In the systemic circulation, free plasminogen circulates as GLU-plasminogen. When thrombosis occurs, plasminogen binds to fibrin and is altered, forming LYS-plasminogen, which is more susceptible to activation by a plasminogen activator. Alkjaersig and colleagues[13] demonstrated that the basic mechanism of clot lysis by plasminogen activators is the activation of fibrin-bound plasminogen within the thrombus to form plasmin, which is the active enzyme that dissolves the clot. If plasmin escapes into the systemic circulation, it is instantaneously neutralized by α-2-antiplasmin or, secondarily, α-2-macroglobulin. Low doses of plasminogen activators are neutralized in the systemic circulation by plasminogen activator inhibitors. Pharmacologic doses of plasminogen activators persist in the circulation because they supersaturate circulating plasminogen activator inhibitors.

Systemic thrombolytic therapy is an inefficient method of treating acute DVT. A relatively small amount of systemically infused plasminogen activator will contact the thrombus to activate fibrin-bound plasminogen. The results of studies evaluating systemic thrombolytic therapy for acute DVT have been disappointing and generally are associated with higher than acceptable bleeding complications and lower than acceptable success rates.[14] It is understandable that techniques for delivering the plasminogen activator into the thrombus, thereby maximally activating fibrin-bound plasminogen and minimizing the systemic delivery of the plasminogen activator, will be associated with greater success rates and fewer bleeding complications.

Numerous reports have demonstrated good outcomes of catheter-directed thrombolysis (CDT) for acute DVT. Most of these reports (20 limbs or more) are listed in Table 48-1, which also includes pharmacomechanical techniques used as adjuncts to CDT. In general, when patients with acute DVT are treated with catheter-based techniques, success rates in the range of 75% to 90% can be anticipated. The rate of bleeding complications ranges from 5% to 11%. Fortunately, serious distant bleeding is uncommon and intracranial bleeding is a rarity. Most bleeding complications are localized to the venous access site, and reports surfacing in the past 7 years generally report bleeding complications as 5% or less. Symptomatic pulmonary embolization during infusion is uncommon, and fatal PE is rare.

An interesting report by Chang and coauthors[15] documented the benefit of intrathrombus bolus dosing of recombinant tissue plasminogen activator (rt-PA) in a small group of patients (10 lower extremities with acute DVT), which has been recently updated. The pulse-spray technique was used to infuse 50 mg of rt-PA delivered intrathrombus by catheter infusion on a daily basis. Patients underwent the pulse-spray technique, returned to their rooms, and were brought back the following day for complete phlebographic evaluation and additional treatment if necessary. Patients were treated for a maximum of four sessions of pulse-spray thrombolysis. Significant or complete lysis was achieved in 11 of 12 extremities, and 1 had 50% to 70% lysis. Although the average dose of rt-PA was 106 mg, bleeding complications were minor and in no patient did the hematocrit drop more than 2%. This small patient sample draws attention to the importance of high-pressure pulse-spray infusion into the thrombus by demonstrating that lysis will continue long after the treatment session ends if the rt-PA is bound to the plasminogen within the clot. It also raises the question of whether one needs the full 50-mg dose. Patients may have responded equally as well to a smaller dose of rt-PA delivered in a larger volume of solution.

The National Venous Registry[16] reported a large cohort of patients treated with lytic therapy for acute DVT. Seventy-one percent of these patients had iliofemoral DVT and 25% had femoropopliteal DVT. It is interesting to note that patients with iliofemoral DVT seem to have had better and more durable results than patients with femoropopliteal DVT.

Patients treated in the National Venous Registry were treated with intrathrombus infusion of urokinase via CDT. In the group with acute first-time iliofemoral DVT, 65% had complete clot resolution. There was an important correlation ($p < .001$) of thrombosis-free survival with the results of initial therapy. At 1 year, 78% of patients with initially complete clot resolution had patent veins, and only 37% of patients had less than 50% lysis. In the patients with first-time iliofemoral DVT who initially had successful thrombolysis, 96% of the veins remained patent at 1 year. Initial lytic success also correlated with valve function at 6 months. Thirty-eight percent of patients with less than 50% thrombolysis had normal valve function, whereas 72% with complete lysis retained normal valve function ($p < 0.02$).

TABLE 48-1 Studies of Catheter-Directed Thrombolysis for Acute Deep Venous Thrombosis

Reference	Patients (Limbs)	Intervention	Results			Complications			
			Significant/ Complete Resolution (%)	Partial Resolution (%)	No Resolution (%)	Bleeding		PE	Death from Rx (%)
						Minor (%)	Major (%)		
Semba et al., 1994[53]	21 (27)	CDT with UK, angio/stenting	18 (72)	5 (25)	2 (8)	1 (4)	0 (0)	0	0
Semba et al., 1996[54]	32 (41)	CDT with UK, angio	21 (32)	9 (28)	2 (6)	0 (0)	0 (0)	0	0
Verhaeghe et al., 1997[55]	24	CDT with rt-PA, stenting	19 (79)	5 (21)	0 (0))	0 (0)	6 (25)	0	0
Bjarnason et al., 1997[56]	77 (87)	CDT with UK, angio/stenting, thrombectomy	69 (793)	0 (0)	18 (21)	11 (14)	5 (6)	1	0
Mewissen et al., 1999[16]	287 (312)	CDT with UK, stenting, systemic lysis	96 (31)	162 (52)	54 (17)	15 (28)	54 (11)	6	2 (<1)
Comerota et al., 2000[57]	54	CDT with UK or rt-PA, thrombectomy	14 (26)	28 (52)	6 (11)	8 (15)	4 (7)	1	0
AbuRahma et al., 2001[58]	51	CDT with UK or rt-PA, stenting	15 (83)	0	0	3 (17)	2 (11)	0	0
			1 (3)	0	0	3 (9)	2 (6)	2 (6)	0
Vedantham et al., 2002[24]	20 (28)	CDT with UK, rt-PA, or rPA, thrombectomy, stenting	23 (82)	0	0	0	3 (14)	0	0
Elsharawy and Elzayat, 2002[20]	35	CDT with SK, angio/stenting	13 (72)	5 (28)	0 (0)	0	0	0	0
			2 (12)	8 (47)	7 (41)	0	0	0	
Grunwald and Hofmann, 2004[59]	74 (82)	CDT with UK, tPA, or rPA, angio/stenting	54 (73)	26 (32)	0	6 (8)	4 (5)	0	0
Laiho et al., 2004[60]	32	CDT with rt-PA or systemic lysis with rt-PA	8 (50)	5 (31)	0	4 (25)	2 (13)	2 (13)	0
			5 (31)	8 (50)	0	6 (38)	1 (6)	5 (31)	0
Vedantham et al., 2004[61]	18 (23)	CDT with reteplase plus mechanical thrombectomy	7 (31)	12 (52)	4 (17)		1 (6)	0	0
Bush et al., 2004[62]	20 (23)	Pharmacomechanical thrombectomy with reteplase, UK, and rt-PA, angio/stenting	15 (65)	8 (35)	0	2	0	0	0
Sillesen et al., 2005[23]	45	CDT with rt-PA, angio/stenting	42 (93)	0	0	4 (8)	0	1 (2)	0
Jackson et al., 2005[63]	28	CDT with UK or rPA, stenting	5 (18)	20 (72)	0	2 (7)	0	0	0

Study	No. of patients (limbs)	Treatment								
Ogawa et al., 2005[64]	24	CDT with UK or CDT with UK plus IPC	0 (0)	10 (100)	0	0	0	0	0	0
Kim et al., 2006[65]	37 (45)	CDT with UK or CDT + PMT	5 (36)	9 (64)	0	0	0	0	0	0
			21 (81)	3 (11)	2 (8)	1 (4)	2 (7)	1 (4)	1 (4)	0
			16 (84)	3 (16)	0	0	1 (5)	1 (5)	0	0
Lin et al., 2006[25]	93 (98)	CDT with rPA, rt-PA, or UK, angio/stenting or PMT with rPA, rt-PA, or UK, angio/stenting	32 (70)	14 (30)	5 (11)	2 (4)	1 (2)	0	0	0
			39 (75)	13 (25)	4 (8)	2 (4)	0	0	0	0
Cynamon et al., 2006[66]	24	Pharmacomechanical thrombectomy, CDT, angio/stenting	12 (50)	12 (50)	0	0	2 (8)	0	0	0
Protack et al., 2007[67]	69	CDT with UK, tPA, Retavase, pulse-spray, mechanical thrombectomy, stenting, IVC filters	40 (63)	19 (30)	4 (6)	0	0	0	0	0
Arko et al., 2007[68]	30	Pharmacomechanical thrombectomy with tenecteplase	Not reported							
Martinez et al., 2008[69]	52	CDT with rt-PA or ISPMT with rt-PA	19 (70)	8 (30)	0	6 (27)	1 (4)	0	0	0
Parikh et al., 2008[27]	47 (53)	CDT using ultrasound-accelerated catheter with UK, rPA, tPA, and tenecteplase; adjunctive PTA, stenting, mechanical thrombectomy, arteriovenous fistula	23 (92)	2 (8)	0	5 (19)	1 (4)	0	0	0
			37 (70)	11 (21)	5 (9)	0	2 (4)	0	0	0
Rao et al., 2009[70]	43	Pharmacomechanical thrombectomy in patients with contraindication to lysis	95% based on >50% lysis				2 (4)		0	0
Baekgaard et al., 2010[30]	101 (103)	CDT with rt-PA, stenting, stockings, anticoagulation	82% had patent veins with no reflux at 6-year follow-up		8 (8)	5 (5)	1 (1)		0	0
Gasparis et al., 2009[31]	23	Pharmacomechanical thrombectomy, CDT	14 (61)	9 (39)	0	1	0		0	0
Enden et al., 2009[21]	50	CDT, angio/stenting	24/50 (48)	20/53 (38)	4 (8)	2	1		0	0
Kim et al., 2009[71]	26 (29)	Single-session pharmacomechanical thrombectomy with UK	24 (83)	5 (17)	0	0	0		0	0

PE, Pulmonary embolism; *Rx*, prescription drug; *CDT*, catheter-directed thrombolysis; *UK*, urokinase; *angio*, angioplasty; *rt-PA*, recombinant tissue plasminogen activator; *rPA*, recombinant plasminogen activator; *SK*, streptokinase; *IPC*, intermittent pneumatic compression; *PMT*, pharmacomechanical thrombolysis; *ISPMT*, isolated segmental pharmacomechanical thrombolysis; *IVC*, inferior vena cava; *tPA*, tissue plasminogen activator.

A quality-of-life (QOL) study was performed to assess whether lytic therapy altered QOL in patients with iliofemoral DVT.[17] A cohort-controlled study in the institutions participating in the National Venous Registry was performed. Patients with iliofemoral DVT treated by CDT were compared with a contemporary cohort of patients with the same extent of DVT and from the same institutions who were treated with anticoagulation alone. All patients treated with anticoagulation alone were candidates for lytic therapy; however, the choice of treatment was determined by physician preference. Patients were evaluated with a validated QOL questionnaire that was used to query patients at 16 and 22 months following acute treatment.[18] Ninety-eight patients were evaluated; 68 were treated with CDT and 30 were treated with anticoagulation alone. The results demonstrated that CDT was associated with better QOL than anticoagulation alone. QOL was directly related to thrombolytic success. Patients who had a successful lytic outcome reported a better Health Utilities Index, improved physical functioning, less stigma of chronic venous disease, less health distress, and fewer postthrombotic symptoms. Not surprisingly, patients in whom CDT failed had outcomes similar to those treated with anticoagulation alone. A subsequent single-center observational study demonstrated that QOL following CDT for iliofemoral DVT directly correlated with success of clot lysis.[19]

A small, randomized trial performed by Elsharawy and Elzayat[20] compared CDT with anticoagulation alone. CDT resulted in significantly better patency and valve function at 6 months. Enden and colleagues[21] reported preliminary results from an ongoing trial of 200 patients randomized to CDT with tPA versus anticoagulation alone with low-molecular-weight heparin followed by warfarin. The preliminary report included approximately half of the projected 200 patients. The primary outcome of this study was patency of the iliofemoral venous segment at 6 months and the incidence of postthrombotic syndrome at 2 years. Preliminary observations indicate significantly better patency in patients randomized to CDT compared to those treated with only anticoagulation. The study has not yet matured to the point of commentary on postthrombotic morbidity.

PATIENT EVALUATION AND TECHNIQUE

Patients with iliofemoral DVT have a large thrombus burden and appear to have a greater stimulus to thrombosis than most other patients with acute infrainguinal DVT. It appears warranted that a search for an underlying etiology should occur. Asymptomatic pulmonary emboli are present in at least 50% of these patients. It would seem appropriate to identify asymptomatic pulmonary emboli early, because up to 25% will subsequently become symptomatic, manifesting as pleuritic chest discomfort once the inflammatory pulmonary process or parenchymal infarct reaches the pleural surface.[22] If the PE is not recognized at presentation, clinicians may mistakenly assume that the subsequent pleuritic symptoms are due to a new PE resulting from failure of treatment. A spiral computed tomographic (CT) scan of the chest

with contrast evaluates the pulmonary vasculature for PE and other thoracic pathology. The CT scan is then extended to the abdomen and pelvis to identify the proximal extent of thrombus and to evaluate for abdominal or pelvic pathology. This process has been an important addition to the evaluation of these patients, because previously undiagnosed pathologies have been found with surprising frequency. Evaluation of the brain, chest, abdomen, and pelvis is recommended. Renal cell carcinoma, adrenal tumors, retroperitoneal lymphoma, pulmonary adenocarcinoma, hepatic metastases, iliac vein aneurysms, vena caval atresia, and asymptomatic abdominal aortic aneurysms have all been identified. Hematologic evaluations for an underlying thrombophilia are selectively performed, although it may be more useful to obtain a thrombophilia workup in young, female, first-degree relatives of childbearing potential than in the patient being treated.

The technique of CDT has evolved. The preferred approach is through an ultrasound-guided popliteal puncture with antegrade passage of an infusion catheter. Patients who have distal popliteal vein and tibial vein thrombosis are also treated with a second catheter passed with ultrasound guidance into the posterior tibial vein at the ankle. Adjunctive mechanical techniques are frequently used to shorten the duration of lysis and to speed clot resolution.

The dose and volume of the plasminogen activator has also evolved. Because the activation of fibrin-bound plasminogen is not a dose-dependent phenomenon, its exposure to the plasminogen activator appears to be the most important factor. The volume of lytic solution has increased over the years with a corresponding decrease in the concentration (dose) of the plasminogen activator. It is now preferable to increase the volume of lytic infusion to 80 to 100 mL/h. The larger volume is intended to saturate the thrombus, thereby exposing more fibrin-bound plasminogen to the plasminogen activator. The dose of rt-PA is generally 1 mg/h. If two catheters are used, the dose is increased to 1.5 to 2 mg/h split between the catheters.

Phlebograms are usually repeated at 12-hour intervals and are used to monitor the success of lysis, reveal the need for additional interventions, and reposition the catheters if necessary. Vena caval filters are not routinely used but are recommended for patients with free-floating thrombus in the vena cava. A retrievable filter can be used in patients for whom only temporary protection is required.

Following successful thrombolysis, the venous system is examined with completion phlebography. If an underlying stenosis exists, which is frequently observed in the left common iliac vein where it is compressed by the right common iliac artery, the vein is dilated and stented as necessary. It is important to use a stent of adequate diameter. The common iliac vein frequently requires a 14- to 16-mm stent, and the external vein requires a 12- to 14-mm stent. The addition of intravascular ultrasonography has improved the evaluation of iliac compression and the precision of stent deployment. Residual areas of stenosis must be corrected to achieve long-term success, otherwise the patient faces a high risk of rethrombosis.

PHARMACOMECHANICAL THROMBOLYSIS

Although good results have been achieved with CDT, treatment times are often unacceptably long; therefore bleeding risk and cost associated with therapy are unacceptably high. A recent report of extensive DVT treated with CDT alone demonstrated a 93% success rate.[23] These patients were generally treated within 7 days of symptom onset. It would be expected that lysis could be achieved efficiently in these patients, because they represented a true acute DVT; however, treatment times for CDT alone averaged 71 hours. This duration of acute care is logistically difficult, if not impossible, for many practitioners and many medical centers. The associated cost is high because patients receiving lytic therapy are generally monitored in intensive care units; therefore techniques to speed lytic success will be important for efficient and effective patient care.

ENDOVASCULAR MECHANICAL THROMBECTOMY

Mechanical techniques alone or in combination with thrombolysis have been developed to more rapidly clear the venous system. Vedantham and associates[24] evaluated the effectiveness of mechanical thrombectomy alone or in combination with pharmacologic thrombolysis in 28 limbs of patients with acute DVT. They evaluated multiple devices. Venographic scoring was performed at each step of the procedure. Twenty-six percent of the thrombus was removed by mechanical thrombectomy alone, whereas adding a plasminogen activator solution to the mechanical technique (pharmacomechanical) removed 82% of the thrombus. Mechanical thrombectomy (rheolytic technique) alone was highly successful when removing intraprocedural thrombus, which is usually gelatinous and not cross-linked by factor XIII. The average infusion time was approximately 17 hours per limb, and 14% of patients had major bleeding complications.

RHEOLYTIC THROMBECTOMY

Lin and colleagues[25] reported their 8-year experience with pharmacomechanical thrombolysis using a rheolytic thrombectomy catheter. Of their 98 patients, 46 received CDT alone and 52 underwent pharmacomechanical thrombolysis using the AngioJet catheter (Medrad, Minneapolis, Md.). Their observations demonstrated that the pharmacomechanical technique was associated with significantly fewer phlebograms, shorter intensive care unit stays, shorter hospital stays, and fewer blood transfusions. Bleeding complications were not different between the two groups. A smaller patient group treated by rheolytic thrombectomy was reported by Kasirajan and associates,[26] who demonstrated that mechanical thrombectomy alone was less effective than the combined pharmacomechanical technique.

ULTRASOUND-ACCELERATED THROMBOLYSIS

Parikh and colleagues[27] reported an initial clinical experience with ultrasound-accelerated thrombolysis in 53 patients treated for acute DVT with the EKOS EndoWave system (EKOS, Bothell, Wash.). Both upper- and lower-extremity DVT patients were included as well as use of a variety of lytic agents. This makes a comparison with other reports difficult, because axillosubclavian DVT responds more quickly than lower-extremity venous thrombosis.

Complete lysis (≥90%) was observed in 70% of patients and overall lysis (complete or partial) in 91%. The median infusion time was 22 hours and 4% of patients had major complications, which were essentially puncture site hematomas. It was the authors' impression that, compared with historical controls, treatment times and dose of lytic agents were reduced with ultrasound-accelerated thrombolysis compared with CDT using the drip technique alone.

ISOLATED SEGMENTAL PHARMACOMECHANICAL THROMBOLYSIS

The Trellis catheter (Covidien, Mansfield, Mass.) is a double-balloon catheter that is passed through the thrombus with the proximal balloon inflated above the clot and the distal balloon inflated to isolate a segment of the venous system. Between these two balloons, a plasminogen activator is infused and a dispersion wire causes the interballoon segment of the catheter to assume a spiral configuration. The catheter is then activated and spins at 3500 rpm for 15-20 minutes. Liquefied and fragmented thrombus can be aspirated and treatment success can be evaluated by repeated segmental phlebography. If thrombus is resolved, the catheter is repositioned and additional thrombosed segments are treated. If residual thrombus persists, a second treatment is done or a repeated treatment of another appropriate intervention (e.g., rheolytic thrombectomy, ultrasound-accelerated thrombolysis, balloon angioplasty, stenting) is performed.

Martinez and coworkers[28] reviewed 52 consecutive limbs treated for iliofemoral DVT, the first 27 with CDT alone and the following 25 with isolated segmental pharmacomechanical thrombolysis (ISPMT) plus CDT when necessary. Thrombus burden and treatment outcomes were quantified. Ninety-three percent of the patients were treated with rt-PA. Venoplasty and stenting were used to correct underlying stenoses, and all received long-term therapeutic anticoagulation. Sixteen of the 27 limbs treated with CDT required adjunctive mechanical techniques to clear the thrombus, such as the AngioJet, ultrasound-accelerated lysis, or pulse-spray techniques, whereas only 7 of the limbs treated with ISPMT had additional mechanical techniques. A larger percentage of the thrombus was removed with ISPMT than with CDT. Complete lysis (≥90%) was achieved in

11% of the limbs of CDT patients as opposed to 28% of the limbs treated by ISPMT ($p = 0.077$). Treatment time was shorter (23.4 vs. 55.4 hours; $p < 0.001$) and the rt-PA dose was lower (33.4 vs. 59.3 mg; $p = 0.009$) with ISPMT. Hospital and intensive care unit length of stay was no different, which appeared to be a result of underlying patient comorbid conditions. Only 18% of the limbs had complete lysis following the use of the ISPMT catheter alone. Bleeding complications occurred in 5% of patients undergoing CDT alone and 5% of patients treated with ISPMT.

PHARMACOMECHANICAL TECHNIQUES AND VEIN VALVE FUNCTION

An important question regarding pharmacomechanical techniques is whether the mechanical manipulation of thrombus inside a vein adversely affects vein valve function. Vogel and colleagues[29] recently reported their observations in 69 limbs of 54 patients treated with either CDT alone (n = 20) or pharmacomechanical thrombolysis (n = 49). There was a tendency toward better thrombus resolution with the pharmacomechanical techniques. There was no difference in valve function between the groups; 53% of patients treated with pharmacomechanical thrombolysis had vein valve reflux greater than 1 second versus 65% treated with CDT ($p = 0.42$). An interesting observation was that of the patients with unilateral iliofemoral DVT; 31% had valvular reflux. The best predictor of reflux in the treated limb was reflux in the nontreated contralateral limb. Pharmacomechanical thrombolysis does not adversely affect valve function compared with CDT alone.

OUTCOMES OF CATHETER-BASED INTERVENTION FOR ILIOFEMORAL DEEP VENOUS THROMBOSIS

Contemporary results of CDT, using the drip technique alone or by adding PMT, have improved patient outcomes. Baekgaard and colleagues[30] reported 103 patients followed for 6 years after CDT for iliofemoral DVT. Eighty-six percent of patients at 6 years had patent veins and normally functioning valves.

Grewal and colleagues[19] performed a QOL evaluation on patients undergoing CDT for iliofemoral DVT. The question they posed was whether patient QOL is related to the degree of successful lysis. They found a direct correlation indicating that the better the success of lytic therapy, the better the patient's QOL. In a smaller study, Gasparis and colleagues[31] also found that patients enjoying successful thrombolysis for iliofemoral DVT had a good QOL.

Comerota and colleagues[32] reported a direct correlation of postthrombotic morbidity with residual thrombus following CDT (Figure 48-3). The greater the amount of residual thrombus, the worse the postthrombotic syndrome as measured by the validated Villalta scale. The better the clot resolution, the lower the Villalta scale.

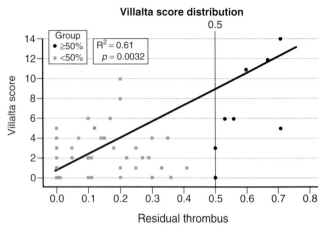

FIGURE 48-3 ■ A graph of the Villalta score versus residual thrombus in patients treated with catheter-directed thrombolysis (CDT) for iliofemoral deep venous thrombosis. There is a direct correlation of the severity of postthrombotic morbidity with residual thrombus at the completion of CDT.

Patients who had 90% or more clot resolution essentially had no postthrombotic morbidity (Figure 48-4).

As mentioned earlier, the large thrombus burden of iliofemoral DVT is associated with significantly higher recurrence rates compared to patients with infrainguinal DVT alone.[8] It has been our observation that patients treated with CDT for extensive venous thrombosis had a low incidence of recurrence. This was studied by Aziz et al,[33] who recently reported that patients with iliofemoral DVT who were treated with CDT or pharmacomechanical thrombolysis had lower than expected recurrence rates. They also showed residual thrombus at the end of lysis correlated with recurrence. Patients with more than 50% residual clot had a significantly higher recurrence rate than patients with less than 50% clot. It appears evident that residual thrombus is in large part responsible for recurrent thrombosis.

Summary

Extensive DVT is associated with severe postthrombotic morbidity. One can restore venous hemodynamics to near normal or normal with successful thrombus removal. Pharmacomechanical techniques have increased treatment success, decreased treatment time, and reduced dose of plasminogen activator. Successful thrombus removal improves QOL, reduces or eliminates subsequent postthrombotic morbidity, and appears to reduce the risk of recurrence.

ATTRACT TRIAL

The ATTRACT trial (Acute Venous Thrombosis: Thrombus Removal with Adjunctive Catheter-directed Thrombolysis) promises to offer the most important information of any study to date regarding the value of a strategy of thrombus removal. This prospective randomized trial funded by the National Institutes of Health (NIH) examined patients with acute proximal

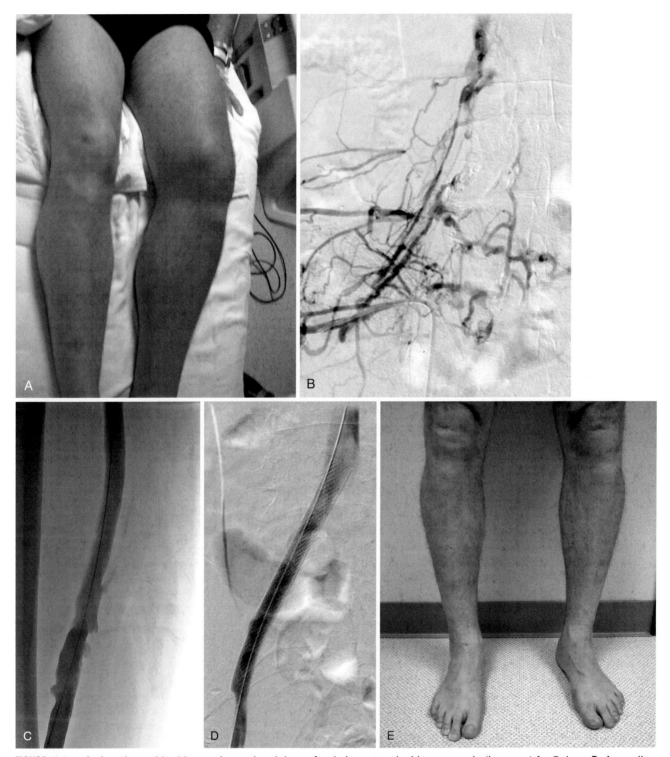

FIGURE 48-4 ■ **A,** A patient with phlegmasia cerulea dolens after being treated with enoxaparin (Lovenox) for 7 days. **B,** Ascending phlebogram shows extensive thrombotic obstruction of the iliofemoral venous system. **C,** Following pharmacomechanical thrombolysis and CDT, patency and valve function were restored to the patient's femoral vein and **(D)** iliac venous system. Stenting was required to correct an underlying iliac vein stenosis. **E,** Twelve-month follow-up demonstrates a normal physical examination, and noninvasive evaluation demonstrated patent veins with normal valve function.

DVT treated with a catheter-based strategy of thrombus removal plus anticoagulation versus anticoagulation alone.

Among the questions to be answered by the ATTRACT trial are:

1. Is thrombus removal better than anticoagulation alone?
2. Is there differential benefit in patients with iliofemoral DVT versus femoropopliteal DVT?
3. How does treatment affect QOL?

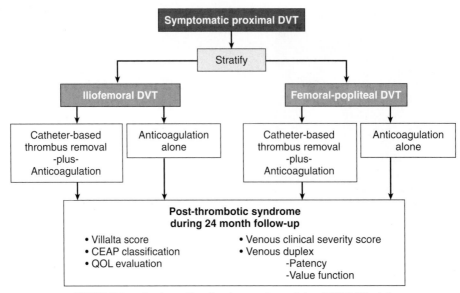

FIGURE 48-5 ■ Basic outline for the conduct of the ATTRACT trial.

4. Is degree of clot lysis correlated with benefit (morbidity)?
5. How is valvular reflux and residual obstruction correlated with postthrombotic morbidity?
6. Is pharmacomechanical thrombolysis better than CDT with the drip technique alone?
7. Is percutaneous intervention cost effective?

There is a broad consensus that the ATTRACT trial addresses a clinical research question of major importance to patients, physicians, and national health care systems.

Approximately 700 patients with symptomatic proximal DVT will be randomized to either CDT plus standard anticoagulation or standard anticoagulation alone. Patients will be stratified by extent of their DVT (iliofemoral versus femoropopliteal; Figure 48-5). Approximately 60 clinical centers in the United States are participating. The primary outcome measure is the cumulative occurrence of the postthrombotic syndrome at 24 months. Patients between the ages of 16 and 75 years who have symptomatic proximal DVT involving the iliac, common femoral, or femoral veins will be included. The symptom duration is limited to the first 2 weeks, and patients are required to have a life expectancy of 2 or more years.

All patients will be treated with standard therapeutic anticoagulation and receive 30- to 40-mm Hg ankle-gradient compression stockings. During follow-up, patients will be assessed for the postthrombotic syndrome using the validated Villalta scale, severity of leg pain, QOL, and the Venous Clinical Severity Score. Objective assessment of vein patency and venous valve function will be performed with venous duplex examinations.

The ATTRACT trial has the potential of answering the key questions of whether thrombus removal should be attempted during management of acute proximal DVT and whether there are differential outcomes in patients with iliofemoral versus femoropopliteal DVT.

This will be the largest prospective randomized database correlating postthrombotic QOL to objective measures of chronic venous disease and physiologic measures of venous valve function. This trial can potentially quantify the benefits of thrombus removal, provide new insight into postthrombotic chronic venous disease (and its avoidance), and integrate a cost analysis of treatment paradigms.

PULMONARY EMBOLISM

When managing patients with acute PE, it is instructive to answer the question: "What is the goal of therapy?" Appropriate goals of therapy are: (1) restore cardiopulmonary hemodynamics in those patients in whom it is deranged, (2) avoid recurrent PE, and (3) avoid chronic thromboembolic pulmonary hypertension with its associated morbidity and mortality. It is known that chronic thromboembolic pulmonary hypertension is associated with recurrent PE, a younger age of onset, large perfusion defects, and idiopathic PE.[34]

Pulmonary emboli large enough to cause right ventricular dysfunction are associated with a sixfold increase in hospital mortality and a 2.4-fold increase in 1-year mortality.[35]

The NIH-sponsored trials[36,37] of patients with PE randomized the patients to systemic thrombolytic therapy versus anticoagulation alone. Unfortunately, the entry criteria included anyone with a documented PE; however, cardiopulmonary hemodynamics were not measured. All patients had arteriographically confirmed PE and had arteriographic and lung scan follow-up. Despite these limitations, results from the NIH trials demonstrated that lytic therapy rapidly improved arteriogram and lung scan resolution of pulmonary emboli compared to patients treated with anticoagulation alone ($p < 0.05$). Thrombolytic therapy reduced pulmonary artery pressures and right atrial pressures ($p < 0.05$). However, bleeding complications were 46% with lytic therapy, which is unacceptably high but likely due to the multiple interventions performed in these patients. Twenty-seven percent of the patients treated with anticoagulation alone had bleeding complications. There was no difference in mortality between the two groups; however, the majority of patients would not be expected to die if treated with anticoagulation alone and, importantly, mortality was not considered a primary endpoint. The NIH studies were not designed to evaluate mortality.

At 1-year follow-up, patients treated with lytic therapy had normal pulmonary capillary blood volumes, and their oxygen diffusing capacity was 93%.[38] Patients treated with anticoagulation alone had a significantly reduced pulmonary capillary blood volume, and their oxygen-diffusing capacity was only 72% ($p < 0.05$).

At 7-year follow-up, surviving patients from the NIH PE trials underwent right heart catheterization.[39] There was a significant reduction in pulmonary artery pressures both at rest and at exercise in patients treated with lytic therapy, and pulmonary vascular resistance was significantly lower both at rest and with exercise in patients who had been treated with lytic therapy. This resulted in several important clinical benefits; namely, fewer patients developed DVT or recurrent PE who had been treated with lytic therapy and there were significantly fewer patients in the lytic therapy group who suffered with congestive heart failure.

Goldhaber and colleagues[40] performed a randomized trial of patients with acute PE to evaluate early functional benefit. One hundred one patients were randomized to either rt-PA (100 mg over 2 hours) or anticoagulation alone. Outcome measures were right ventricular function and recurrent PE. Patients who were randomized to rt-PA had significantly improved right ventricular function at 24 hours ($p = 0.005$), their end diastolic area was less ($p = 0.01$), they had improved pulmonary perfusion ($p = 0.0001$), and there was a strong trend toward a reduction in recurrent PEs at 14 days ($p = 0.06$). Jerjes-Sanchez and colleagues[41] designed a study to assess whether thrombolytic therapy would improve survival in patients with massive PE. Patients with massive PE (PE causing hypotension) were randomized to streptokinase plus heparin or heparin alone. The ethics committee terminated the trial after eight patients were randomized. Four patients receiving heparin alone died, whereas four patients receiving streptokinase plus heparin survived. The committee believed that it was unethical to continue the trial.

Konstantinides and colleagues[42] showed in a multicenter European registry of thrombolytic therapy versus anticoagulation for PE that there was a significantly lower 30-day mortality rate in PE patients who received lytic therapy versus anticoagulation alone (4.7% vs. 11.1%; $p = 0.016$). These investigators found that primary lysis was the only independent predictor of survival on multivariate analysis. In a follow-up randomized trial of lytic therapy versus anticoagulation, the anticoagulation group had greater hemodynamic deterioration and required more salvage measures compared with the patients randomized to thrombolysis.[43]

PATIENT SELECTION

Observational studies have demonstrated the importance of abnormal cardiopulmonary hemodynamics, abnormalities on echocardiography,[44] and biomarkers indicating ventricular stretch[45] and myocardial damage.[46] Echocardiography has become a helpful tool in the evaluation of patients with PE. Poor prognostic indicators on echocardiography in patients with PE include right ventricular thrombus, right ventricular hypokinesis, right ventricular dilation, pulmonary hypertension, tricuspid insufficiency, ventricular septal deviation, and a patent foramen ovale.

A metaanalysis of right ventricular dysfunction in patients with PE demonstrates a high short-term mortality from PE (12%-14%) in patients with right ventricular dysfunction compared to <1% in patients who have a normally functioning right ventricle.[44] Longer-term observations have also correlated mortality with right ventricular dysfunction, increasing mortality sixfold to thirteenfold in patients with right ventricular dysfunction versus those with a normally functioning right ventricle. Therefore, based on the observed natural history of PE that reduces right ventricular function, it would appear that this subset of patients should be considered as candidates for thrombolysis.

A systematic review of elevated pro-beta natriuretic polypeptide (BNP) in PE was performed by Klok and colleagues.[45] They found that, in patients with an elevated pro-BNP, there was a significant increase in right ventricular dysfunction (OR, 38.6; $p = 0.00001$), adverse clinical outcomes (OR, 6.8; $p = 0.00001$), and death (OR, 6.5; $p = 0.002$). Likewise, PE causing pathologic myocardial stretch is associated with increased morbidity and mortality and should be considered for lytic therapy.

Myocardial damage as a result of PE can be measured with troponins. A troponin-1 greater than 0.03 µg/L was a significant predictor of mortality.[46] Konstantinides and colleagues[47] showed a linear correlation of increased troponin with death, systemic complications, and recurrent pulmonary emboli. Troponin can be considered another biomarker of hemodynamically significant PE, which would benefit from a treatment strategy designed to eliminate the PE causing obstruction to right ventricular outflow.

It is our practice to assess patients with PE clinically, with echocardiography and with the biomarkers pro-BNP and troponin. In general, patients who are on the borderline of stable hemodynamics (tachycardia but normal blood pressure) and have suboptimal oxygenation, abnormal cardiac echo, and elevated pro-BNPs and troponins would be considered for thrombolytic therapy (Figure 48-6).

The American College of Chest Physicians in 2008 recommended that all patients with PE should undergo rapid risk stratification (grade 1C).[48] They further suggested that patients with hemodynamic compromise and no contraindication to lytic therapy receive thrombolytic therapy (grade 1B). They also suggested that additional selected patients without hypotension at low risk of bleeding receive thrombolytic therapy (grade 2B). They

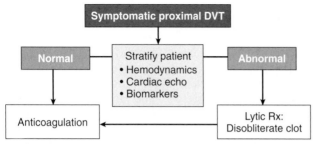

FIGURE 48-6 ■ An algorithm for the approach to managing patients with symptomatic pulmonary embolism.

TABLE 48-2	**Results of Rheolytic Pulmonary Thrombectomy**		
Parameter	Pretreatment	Posttreatment	p Value
sBP (mm·Hg)	119	145	0.02
Heart rate	101	84	0.02
sPAP (mm Hg)	54	44	0.048
dPAP (mm Hg)	21	16	0.02
PVR	758	637	0.004
PaO₂/FiO₂	169	325	0.001
Miller score	17.9	11.8	0.0003

Data from Chauhan MS, Kawamura A: Percutaneous rheolytic thrombectomy for large pulmonary embolism: a promising treatment option. Catheter Cardiovasc Interv 70:121–128, 2007.
sBP, Systolic blood pressure; *sPAP*, systolic pulmonary artery pressure; *dPAP*, diastolic pulmonary artery pressure; *PVR*, pulmonary vascular resistance; *PaO₂*, partial pressure of oxygen; *FiO₂*, fraction of inspired oxygen.

went on to suggest that in compromised patients who are unable to receive lytic therapy, interventional catheter techniques are recommended (grade 2C). Since the publication of the 2008 guidelines, technology has improved considerably, increasing the success rates of direct catheter-based treatment and reducing the rates of complications.

CATHETER-BASED INTERVENTION FOR PULMONARY EMBOLISM

Catheter-based intervention for large pulmonary emboli is becoming more popular, with observations of rapid improvement following fragmentation or dissolution of proximal pulmonary emboli.

Tajima and coauthors[49] reported 25 patients with hemodynamically important pulmonary emboli who were treated with a modified rotating pigtail catheter. After embolic disruption, 13 mg of rt-PA was injected into the affected pulmonary arteries followed by manual clot aspiration. All patients survived and their clinical status improved. After treatment, arteriography showed improved pulmonary perfusion that resulted in a significant reduction in the Miller score and a 30% decrease in the mean pulmonary artery pressure ($p < 0.01$).

Combining rheolytic thrombectomy with an infusion of a plasminogen activator solution would seem to be an effective approach. Zeni and colleagues[50] treated 17 patients with the AngioJet device, 10 of whom also received an infusion of reteplase. Immediate angiographic improvement with relief or symptoms occurred in 16 of 17 patients. Heart block, which is a potential complication of this technique, occurred in one patient in whom procedure was terminated. Fifteen patients survived the initial hospitalization. Two were lost to follow-up and the remaining 13 were still alive 19 months later, more than would have been expected based on their natural history if treated with anticoagulation alone.

Fourteen patients with significant pulmonary emboli (10 with massive PE) who were ineligible for systemic thrombolysis or operative embolectomy were treated with rheolytic thrombectomy by Chauhan and Kawamura.[51] Five of the 14 patients also received catheter-based pulse-spray fibrinolytic treatment. One patient died as a result of sustained cardiogenic shock, and posttreatment hemoptysis developed in one patient. Successful treatment was observed in 12 of 14 patients (Table 48-2). During a mean follow-up of 9 months, all

survivors reported significant improvement in symptoms without recurrent PE. Margheri and colleagues[52] reported early and long-term results of rheolytic thrombectomy in patients with acute PE. Eight patients had severe, 12 had moderate, and five had mild hemodynamic compromise. Successful treatment as demonstrated by significantly reduced pulmonary artery obstruction, improved perfusion, and reduced Miller indices ($p < 0.001$) was achieved in all patients. Four of the 25 patients died during hospitalization. Twenty of the 21 remaining patients were alive after a mean 61-month follow-up. Although mechanical pulmonary embolic fragmentation is possible in high-risk patients and reduces pulmonary artery pressure, administration of pulsed plasminogen activator solution into the thrombus during fragmentation is likely to result in better short- and long-term benefit. Small doses (5-10 mg) diluted into relatively large volume and infused into the embolus are unlikely to cause bleeding complications, yet offer the opportunity of clot dissolution after fragmentation as a result of the plasminogen activator penetrating the thrombus and binding to fibrin-bound plasminogen (LYS-plasminogen).

Gratifying results have been observed in a smaller group of patients with massive PE treated with rheolytic thrombectomy (Figure 48-7). Pulse-spray fibrinolytic infusion during mechanical fragmentation of the thrombus rapidly restores cardiopulmonary hemodynamics and pulmonary perfusion and improves oxygenation.

These catheter-based techniques are new and, to date, all reports are anecdotal and retrospective. However, in view of the morbidity of hemodynamically important pulmonary emboli, a skilled interventionist can use these techniques to reduce hospital mortality and the long-term morbidity of large pulmonary emboli.

SUMMARY

Patients with extensive VTE, namely those with ilio-femoral DVT and massive or submassive PE, should be considered for strategies of thrombus removal. Thrombolytic therapy delivered by intrathrombus infusion is more effective than systemic infusions by virtue of

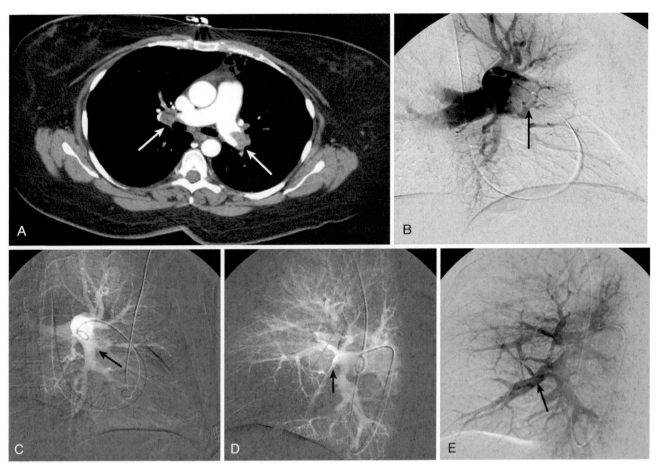

FIGURE 48-7 ■ **A,** Computed tomographic scan showing bilateral submassive pulmonary emboli in a patient with active gastrointestinal bleeding. **B,** A direct pharmacomechanical intervention was performed using the AngioJet catheter (Medrad, Minneapolis, Md.), showing the large left-sided pulmonary embolism (PE), **(C)** posttreatment perfusion of the left lung, and **(D)** obstructing PE of the right lung with **(E)** posttreatment perfusion. The patient's hemodynamics and oxygenation rapidly stabilized.

activation of fibrin-bound plasminogen. Contemporary outcomes of CDT for iliofemoral DVT demonstrate a marked reduction in postthrombotic morbidity and preliminary observations that recurrent DVT is reduced.

Patients with PE who are appropriately stratified, such as those with an enlarged right ventricle, abnormal echocardiogram, increased pro-BNP, and increased troponins, also appear to have better short- and long-term outcomes when treated with lytic therapy and catheter-based techniques to disobliterate the large central embolus.

As technology improves, delivery of plasminogen activators to the clot and the addition of mechanical manipulation of the thrombus speeds resolution. Randomized trials are necessary to establish these treatment modalities with confidence, and whenever possible, patients should be entered into randomized trials. However, absent a randomized trial, patient stratification and good clinical judgment should guide therapy, and with central venous or pulmonary obstruction, generally a strategy of thrombus removal is favored.

References available online at expertconsult.com.

QUESTIONS

1. Which of the following statements regarding iliofemoral DVT is true?
   a. Iliofemoral DVT is associated with the highest risk of postthrombotic morbidity, exceeding the risk imposed by ipsilateral recurrent DVT.
   b. Patients with femoropopliteal DVT have the same resting and hyperemic venous pressures as those with iliofemoral DVT.
   c. Natural history studies show that approximately 40% of patients with iliofemoral DVT suffer serious postthrombotic morbidity.
   d. There are no level 1 data supporting either venous thrombectomy or catheter-directed thrombolysis for the management of patients with iliofemoral DVT.

2. Which of the following statements is true regarding postthrombotic syndrome?
   a. The underlying pathophysiology of the postthrombotic syndrome is ambulatory venous hypertension.
   b. Ambulatory venous hypertension is caused by venous valve reflux, venous luminal obstruction, or both.
   c. The combination of venous valve reflux and luminal obstruction produces the highest ambulatory venous pressure and the most severe postthrombotic syndrome.
   d. All of the above.

3. Which of the following statements regarding postthrombotic syndrome is the most accurate?
   a. Patients with venous obstruction suffer the most severe postthrombotic syndrome.
   b. Venous obstruction is reliably identified by noninvasive maximal venous outflow studies.
   c. Noninvasive diagnostic tests for venous obstruction are more reliable than those for venous valvular incompetence.
   d. Luminal obstruction is reliably diagnosed by ascending phlebography.

4. *Phlegmasia Cerulea Dolens* is a term often used to categorize some patients with acute DVT. Which of the following statements is correct?
   a. It is reserved for patients who have impending venous gangrene.
   b. It is seen only with patients with iliofemoral DVT.
   c. It refers to all patients with a painful, swollen limb having bluish discoloration.
   d. Fasciotomy is the most important step in management following therapeutic anticoagulation.

5. Which of the following statements is most correct in the management of patients with iliofemoral DVT?
   a. Approximately 50% of patients with iliofemoral DVT have asymptomatic PE.
   b. If a patient with DVT is found to have a PE, all patients should have a vena caval filter inserted prior to venous thrombectomy or catheter-directed thrombolysis.
   c. If catheter-directed thrombolysis is chosen to treat the patient, a much higher dose of lytic agent should be infused to dissolve the pulmonary embolus.
   d. Following catheter-directed thrombolysis, a repeat CT scan of the chest should be performed to assess the status of asymptomatic pulmonary embolus.
   e. All of the above
   f. None of the above

6. A 62-year-old gentleman presents with a painful, swollen left leg with bluish discoloration. You are discussing a catheter-based strategy of thrombus removal with the patient. Which of the following pieces of information will you give the patient?
   a. He has a 90%-100% chance of serious postthrombotic morbidity if treated with anticoagulation alone.
   b. If pharmacomechanical thrombolysis is used instead of a catheter drip technique, treatment times will be shorter, the dose of plasminogen activator will be less, and overall success rate will be improved.
   c. It is important to persist with treatment to remove as much clot as possible as postthrombotic morbidity is related to the amount of residual thrombus at the end of catheter-directed thrombolysis.
   d. The ACCP 12 guidelines do not recommend catheter-directed thrombolysis for iliofemoral DVT.
   e. All of the above

7. Which of the following statements regarding the ATTRACT trial is correct?
   a. It is the largest randomized trial to date addressing catheter-directed thrombolysis versus anticoagulation alone for acute DVT.
   b. It stratifies femoropopliteal DVT versus iliofemoral DVT.
   c. It will evaluate the efficacy of pharmacomechanical techniques versus a catheter-based drip technique alone.
   d. It will answer quality of life and cost effectiveness questions.
   e. All of the above

8. You are called to see a 48-year-old woman in the emergency room who is short of breath, has a P02 on room air of 88%, a heart rate of 100, and a BP of 126/70. A CT scan of the chest with contrast demonstrates large bilateral PE. A cardiac echo demonstrates an RV/LV ratio of 1.0. The patient and her family have numerous questions about her acute management and how it relates to her long-term outcome. You tell them the following:
   a. She has a submassive PE and is much more likely to suffer chronic thromboembolic pulmonary hypertension than most patients with PE.
   b. Systemic thrombolysis with rt-PA is associated with more rapid return of normal cardiopulmonary hemodynamics than anticoagulation alone.
   c. Nonrandomized trials have demonstrated significant survival advantage to lytic therapy.
   d. The randomized NIH PE trials have shown significant advantage in restoring normal cardiopulmonary hemodynamics and reduction in congestive heart failure over the long term if lytic therapy was used.
   e. All of the above

9. Which of the following is true regarding risk assessment in patients with pulmonary emboli?
   a. The ACCP 12 recommends that patients with an abnormal echocardiogram undergo thrombolytic therapy.
   b. Troponin elevation reflects excessive myocardial stretch.
   c. Elevated pro-beta natriuretic polypeptide (pro-BNP) in PE patients reflect myocardial damage.
   d. None of the above
   e. All of the above

10. Catheter-based intervention for PE:
    a. Is not recommended
    b. Is associated with cardiac tamponade secondary to ventricular perforation.
    c. Offers no advantage over systemic thrombolysis
    d. None of the above
    e. All of the above

11. Which of the following statement regarding aspirin in the use of patients with venous thromboembolism is correct?
    a. Aspirin should not be used for DVT prophylaxis in any patient.
    b. Randomized trial data demonstrate that aspirin significantly reduces recurrent venous thromboembolism when used following a full course of anticoagulation.
    c. Aspirin augments the inhibition of activated factor Xa.
    d. All of the above
    e. None of the above

ANSWERS

1. **a**
2. **d**
3. **a**
4. **c**
5. **f**
6. **e**
7. **e**
8. **e**
9. **d**
10. **d**
11. **b**

CHAPTER 49

SURGICAL MANAGEMENT OF CHRONIC VENOUS OBSTRUCTION

Nitin Garg • Peter Gloviczki

Reconstruction of the occluded iliofemoral vein or the inferior vena cava (IVC) may be required in patients with post-thrombotic venous occlusion and who exhibit signs and symptoms of chronic venous insufficiency (CVI). Reconstruction of large veins may also be needed in patients with acute traumatic or iatrogenic venous injuries or in those who undergo excision of primary or metastatic malignant tumors invading the IVC or the iliac veins. May-Thurner syndrome (occlusion or stenosis of the left common iliac vein resulting from compression by the overriding right common iliac artery) is a cause of acute or chronic left iliac vein obstruction that is likely much more frequent than previously thought.[1] It can be responsible for CVI in up to one third of the patients with CVI.

Endovascular treatment for iliocaval obstruction has progressed rapidly, and venous stenting is currently the primary choice for treatment of benign iliac, iliofemoral, or iliocaval venous occlusions in patients who fail conservative compression therapy. In the last 2 decades, results of open surgical reconstructions have improved, and symptomatic patients who are not candidates or who fail endovascular reconstructions can be treated with venous bypasses to relieve venous outflow obstruction.[2] A thorough preoperative evaluation to identify significant venous outflow obstruction in these patients is essential.

ETIOLOGY

Venous outflow obstruction can be the result of primary venous disease, like May-Thurner syndrome,[3] or it can be the result of a previous acute deep venous thrombosis (DVT). Uncommon causes include retroperitoneal fibrosis; iatrogenic, blunt, or penetrating trauma; placement of IVC filter, congenital venous anomalies such as deep vein agenesis or hypoplasia, and benign or malignant tumors. May and Thurner observed secondary changes, such as an intraluminal web or spur, in the proximal left common iliac vein in 22% of 430 autopsies. The most frequent primary malignant tumor originating from large veins is venous leiomyosarcoma; secondary tumors invading the vena cava include adenocarcinoma or liposarcoma. Renal carcinoma may extend into the IVC, and the tumor thrombus in some patients may reach all the way into the right atrium, although invasion of the wall of the IVC is rare. Congenital suprarenal caval occlusion can occur because of webs or caval coarctation that may also develop with associated hepatic vein occlusion (Budd-Chiari syndrome).[4,5]

PATHOPHYSIOLOGY

During the acute phase of DVT, the thrombus in the vein activates the inflammatory cascade, which in turn promotes partial lysis of the thrombus and leads to recanalization. However, these processes are also responsible for damage to the vein wall and to the venous valves, leading to chronic obstruction and valvular incompetence. If collateral venous circulation in occlusion is inadequate, ambulatory venous hypertension develops because of a functional venous outflow obstruction. In postthrombotic syndrome (PTS), deep reflux and obstruction of multiple venous segments often coexist.

PRESENTATION

Limb swelling and pain during and after exercise that is relieved with rest and leg elevation (venous claudication) is the typical presentation of patients with chronic venous obstruction owing to previous DVT, PTS, or obstruction of common iliac veins (May-Thurner syndrome).[6] Patients with obstruction may also have symptoms similar to those associated with primary valvular incompetence, such as varicosity, edema, skin changes, or venous ulcers; however, claudication and edema are usually more severe with venous obstruction, and relief with limb elevation is not as pronounced.

Depending on the extent of the collateral circulation, patients with outflow obstruction will have pain, swelling, and heaviness of the limb, and the most severe forms of venous obstruction can interfere with the viability of the limb. Obstruction alone can also result in skin changes and venous ulcerations. In the Mayo Clinic, experience with 64 venous reconstructions performed in 60 patients with benign disease, mean duration of symptoms was 6 years (Table 49-1).

CLINICAL EVALUATION

Detailed medical history may establish the diagnosis of primary, secondary, or congenital venous problems. Adequate history should address previous DVT or

TABLE 49-1	Clinical Symptoms in 60 Patients Undergoing Venous Reconstructions for Benign Disease at the Mayo Clinic

Symptom	n (%)
Venous edema	56 (94%)
Venous claudication	54 (90%)
Edema and claudication	50 (84%)
Healed ulceration	8 (13%)
Active venous ulcers	12 (19%)

From Garg N, Gloviczki P, Karimi KM, et al: Factors affecting outcome of open and hybrid reconstructions for nonmalignant obstruction of iliofemoral veins and inferior vena cava. J Vasc Surg 53(2):383–393, 2011.

thrombophlebitis, previous abdominal or pelvic interventions, trauma, tumor or symptoms of malignancy, personal or family history of thrombophilia, medication history (particularly oral contraceptive pills), smoking, obstetric history, and a family history of venous disorders (most patients with varicose veins would be able to relate to their parents' or grandparents' disease).

An abdominal mass or lymphadenopathy can provide a clue to venous compression and outflow obstruction. Perineal, vulvar, or groin varicosities can be seen in iliac vein obstruction or internal iliac vein or gonadal vein incompetence causing pelvic congestion syndrome. Scrotal varicosity may be a sign of gonadal vein incompetence, left renal vein compression between the superior mesenteric artery and the aorta (Nutcracker syndrome) or, occasionally, IVC lesions or renal carcinoma.

INVESTIGATIONS

Duplex Scanning

Venous duplex scanning should be performed in all patients with symptoms of CVI to help to define the location, cause, and severity of the underlying problem. The test is safe, noninvasive, cost-effective, and reliable and is recommended as the first diagnostic test for all patients with suspected CVD.[7-9] Duplex scanning is excellent for evaluation of both infrainguinal venous obstruction and valvular incompetence.[10]

The four components that are essential in a complete duplex scanning examination for CVD are visibility, compressibility, venous flow, and augmentation. Typical appearance of a postthrombotic vein at duplex scanning is that of a thickened, hardly compressible vessel with damaged, incompetent valves and variable degrees of venous flow owing to partial recanalization. Asymmetry in flow velocity, lack of respiratory variations in venous flow, and waveform patterns at rest and during flow augmentation in the common femoral veins indicate proximal obstruction. Obesity and bowel gas may prevent good visualization of the common hepatic veins and the IVC with ultrasound.

Plethysmography

Venous plethysmography is rarely used, but it is a useful tool that provides information on venous function in patients with CVI and is a complementary examination to duplex scanning. Plethysmography quantifies venous reflux and obstruction and has been used to monitor venous functional changes and assess physiologic outcome of surgical treatments.[11,12] These studies are especially helpful in patients with suspected outflow obstruction but normal duplex findings or in those suspected of having venous disease because of calf muscle pump dysfunction, but no reflux or obstruction noted on duplex scanning. Air or strain gauge plethysmography is designed to evaluate the global leg hemodynamics by measuring reflux, obstruction, and calf muscle pump function. Decreased vein wall compliance in patients with PTS may interfere with proper evaluation of calf muscle pump function.

Computed Tomography and Magnetic Resonance Venography

Early venous disease (C1-2) rarely requires advanced imaging studies than duplex ultrasonography. Computed tomography and magnetic resonance imaging have progressed tremendously in the last decade, and they provide excellent three-dimensional imaging of the venous system. Both modalities are suitable for identifying pelvic or iliac venous obstruction in patients with lower limb varicosity, when proximal obstruction or iliac vein compression (May-Thurner syndrome) is suspected.[13] Venous phase examination will help to identify any obstructing mass or tumor and provides sufficient information in most patients about venous anatomy, obstruction, or stenosis.

Contrast Venography and Hemodynamic Studies

Ascending or descending (or both) contrast venography for CVI is performed only selectively in patients with deep venous obstruction, postthrombotic syndrome, thrombotic or nonthrombotic pelvic vein obstruction (May-Thurner syndrome), pelvic congestion syndrome, nutcracker syndrome, vascular malformations, venous trauma, or tumors or if invasive treatment is planned. Descending venography is used to study associated venous valve incompetence with Valsalva maneuver is classified to grade the severity of reflux (grade 1 to 4: 1 = to upper thigh; 2 = to distal thigh; 3 = popliteal reflux; 4 = reflux to tibials and perforators).[14,15] This test has been much less frequently used in recent years. Ascending venography is performed in a standing position to evaluate patency of the superficial or deep venous system, or both. Ascending venography is useful as a map of the deep veins of the limb; it defines the sites of obstruction and images the collateral venous circulation and the patterns of preferential flow.

Contrast venography is routinely used in CVD to perform endovenous procedures, such as angioplasty or venous stenting or open venous reconstructions. A pressure gradient across iliofemoral obstruction at rest in the supine patient (3 mm Hg) or 10 mm Hg after exercise is indicative of functional venous obstruction. Exercise consists of 10 dorsiflexions of the ankles or 20 isometric contractions of the calf muscle. Arm or foot venous pressure test and ambulatory venous pressure measurement in a dorsal foot vein are additional tests that can be performed. Detailed descriptions and techniques for these tests are provided in the consensus statement.[16]

Intravascular Ultrasound

Recent assessment of patients with iliofemoral venous occlusion suggested that intravascular ultrasound (IVUS) is useful for evaluation of patients with suspected or confirmed iliac vein obstruction. IVUS can be used in veins with obstruction without occlusion to assess the venous wall morphology and mural thickness, identify trabeculations and recanalization, frozen valves, and external compression. Some of these lesions, as emphasized by Neglen and Raju,[13] are not seen with conventional contrast venography; IVUS provides measurements in assessing the degree of stenosis. In addition, IVUS confirms the position of the stent in the venous segment and the resolution of the stenosis.[13]

Laboratory Evaluation

Selective patients, based on their history, with recurrent DVT, thrombosis at a young age, or thrombosis in an unusual site, should undergo screening for thrombophilia.[9]

TREATMENT

Conservative Management

Symptoms of chronic deep venous obstruction should be first treated with compression therapy and local wound care of venous ulcerations, if there are any. Compression is recommended in addition to lifestyle modifications that include weight loss, exercise, and elevation of the legs whenever possible. The rationale of compression treatment is to compensate for the increased ambulatory venous hypertension. Pressures to compress the superficial veins in supine patients range from 20 to 25 mm Hg, whereas in the upright position, pressures of 35 to 40 mm Hg have been shown to narrow the superficial veins, and pressures higher than 60 mm Hg are needed to occlude them.[17] Ambulatory compression techniques and devices include elastic compression stockings, paste gauze boots (Unna boot), multilayer elastic wraps, dressings, and elastic and nonelastic bandages and nonelastic garments. Pneumatic compression devices, applied primarily at night, are also used in patients with refractory edema and venous ulcers.[18] Compression garments result in variable degrees of success and mandate strict patient compliance, which in a hot climate can be both distressing and difficult. Patients with persistent disabling symptoms, such as venous claudication, severe swelling, and nonhealing or recurrent ulcers not responding to conservative treatment, should be considered for endovascular or open surgical reconstruction.

Endovascular Treatment

Iliac or iliocaval stenting has become the primary treatment for chronic nonmalignant venous occlusions. Early and midterm results of endovascular techniques, most frequently using self-expandable stents, such as angioplasty and stenting, have been good. Techniques and results are discussed further in Chapter 50.

Hybrid Reconstruction

In patients with common femoral vein obstruction and proximal disease, conventional venous stenting is frequently not possible. Endovenous recanalization and stent placement, however, can be combined in selected cases with femoral vein endophlebectomy and patch angioplasty, using bovine pericardial patch. Balloon angioplasty and stenting is performed before or at completion of the patch angioplasty. Jugular vein access is obtained for retrograde recanalization as an alternative to or in combination with femoral access. The stent is extended proximally to the healthy vein and across the inguinal ligament distally. With recent experience, the distal end of the stent can be extended into the venous patch.[2] Others have reported good patient outcomes with the hybrid technique, using saphenous vein patch for closure.[19]

Open Surgical Treatment

Patients who are not candidates or who fail endovascular reconstructions can be treated with venous bypasses to relieve symptomatic venous outflow obstruction. Venous reconstruction is also performed in patients who undergo excision of malignant tumors invading the vena cava or iliac veins.

Saphenopopliteal Bypass

First described independently by May and Husni, saphenopopliteal bypass is indicated for femoral or proximal popliteal vein obstruction. The great saphenous vein (GSV), which most commonly is the major outflow from the leg via collaterals in these patients, is exposed above the knee joint, and a direct anastomosis is performed between the GSV and popliteal vein (end to side). Alternatively, a free vein conduit can be used if the ipsilateral GSV is not suitable.

Crossover Saphenous Vein Transposition (Palma Procedure)

Patients with symptomatic unilateral iliac vein obstruction are candidates for Palma procedure (Figure 49-1). With this technique, the contralateral saphenous vein is used for a crossover bypass to decompress venous congestion in the affected limb. The common femoral vein on the affected side is exposed first through a 6- to 8-cm long longitudinal groin incision. The collateral veins should be preserved if possible. The great saphenous vein of the contralateral leg is dissected through a 3- to 5-cm incision made in the groin crease, starting just medial to

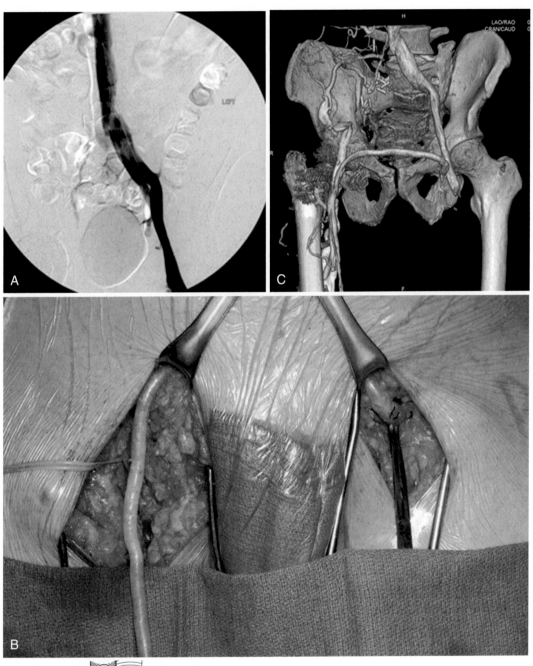

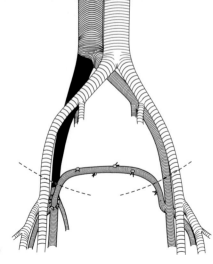

FIGURE 49-1 ■ Palma procedure in a 38-year-old male with postthrombotic syndrome. **A,** Chronic right iliofemoral obstruction after multiple failed attempts at endovenous recanalization. **B,** A right-to-left femoral vein bypass with left GSV (Palma procedure). **C,** Follow-up computed tomographic venogram at 2 months. **D,** Schematic representation of the procedure. (**A-C,** From Garg N, Gloviczki P, Karimi KM, et al: Factors affecting outcome of open and hybrid reconstructions for nonmalignant obstruction of iliofemoral veins and inferior vena cava. J Vasc Surg 53:383–393, 2011. **D,** Redrawn with permission from Mayo Clinic Foundation.) See Color Plate 49-1.

the femoral artery pulse. Tributaries of the saphenous vein are ligated and divided, and the saphenous vein is mobilized in a length of 10 to 12 cm. A short, second upper-thigh incision is made to dissect a 20- to 25-cm long portion of the saphenous vein. The vein is ligated distally, and it is divided proximal to the ligature and pulled up to the groin incision. Alternatively, endoscopic harvesting of the saphenous vein can also be performed, although this likely results in increased vein wall damage that could affect patency.

It is essential to free the saphenofemoral junction completely and dissect at least the anterior wall of the common femoral vein around the saphenous vein so that there is no kink or buckle when the saphenous vein is pulled into the suprapubic tunnel. A kink is unavoidable in some patients with a low saphenofemoral junction. Excision of the saphenous vein with a 2-mm cuff from the common femoral vein and reanastomosis to the femoral vein with running 6/0 polypropylene suture, after turning the junction upward 180 degrees, is the way to solve this problem. Before tunneling, a small Satinsky clamp is placed on the common femoral vein to allow distension of the saphenous vein and the saphenofemoral junction under gentle pressure using heparinized papaverine-saline solution. The vein is then tunneled subcutaneously in the suprapubic space over to the contralateral side using an aortic clamp to ensure a large tunnel without any constriction of the graft whatsoever. Saphenous vein graft in morbidly obese patients is not recommended because of the high chance of external compression of the vein. The common femoral vein is cross-clamped with small vascular clamps or bulldogs, and the vein is opened longitudinally in a length of approximately 2 cm. End-to-side anastomosis is performed between the saphenous vein and ipsilateral common femoral vein. This anastomosis can be spatulated onto the ipsilateral GSV if the femoral or deep femoral veins are diseased and the GSV is the predominant outflow in the affected leg. The anastomosis between the saphenous vein and the femoral vein is performed with running 6/0 polypropylene suture. A vein at least 5 mm in diameter is required to achieve a satisfactory result and provide high venous flow to treat the basic problem of poor venous emptying in these patients.

Although few large series have been reported, overall patency of Palma grafts in nine series ranged between 70% and 83% at 3 to 5 years.[4] Results were better in patients who had no or minimal infrainguinal venous disease in those with May-Thurner syndrome without previous deep vein thrombosis. We observed a 70% primary and a 78% secondary patency rate at 5 years in 25 Palma vein grafts.[2] Endoscopic vein harvest was associated with decreased primary, but not secondary patency rates.

Crossover Femoral Venous Prosthetic Bypass

An externally supported 10- to 12-mm diameter polytetrafluoroethylene (PTFE) graft is used if the GSV is

inadequate, less than 5 mm in diameter, or of poor quality (Figure 49-2). Similar to the autologous femoral suprapubic bypass, the femoral veins are exposed bilaterally, the ePTFE graft is positioned in the subcutaneous suprapubic tunnel, and an end-to-side anastomosis is performed to the common femoral veins at each side. A distal arteriovenous fistula (AVF) on the affected side is routinely added to the procedure using a 4- to 5-mm PTFE graft for the fistula between the PTFE graft and the superficial femoral artery. Sottiurai[20] recommended cutting out a small window rather than just making a longitudinal cut in cross-femoral graft at the hood of the femoral anastomosis to optimize inflow and decrease intimal hyperplasia of the AVF.

Variable patency rates of expanded PTFE (ePTFE) grafts in this location have been reported and range between 0% and 100%.[21] In the authors' experience, the secondary patency of these bypasses is only 50%, and preference still should be given to saphenous crossover grafts.

Femorocaval or Complex Bypass

Long bypasses from the femoral vein to the IVC have poor results because of the hemodynamics of flow across the femoral vein. Most of these patients also have extensive postphlebitic changes in the femoral and distal veins, making these procedures technically challenging and prone to failure because of poor inflow. Patients with bilateral disease or those with obstruction of suprarenal or suprahepatic IVC, who have failed endovascular intervention, are evaluated for a complex reconstruction using either a bifurcated or tube graft with a contralateral jump graft.

For in-line reconstruction of iliocaval or caval occlusions, an ePTFE graft with external support is the preferred conduit. Short, large-diameter (12-mm) grafts are used most frequently; a diameter of 12 to 14 mm is used for iliocaval bypasses and at least 10 mm for femorocaval bypass. The upper portion of the infrarenal IVC at and immediately distal to the renal veins is best approached transperitoneally through a midline incision, reflecting the ascending colon medially and mobilizing the duodenum using the Kocher maneuver. The low IVC just above the iliac bifurcation is well approachable through a right flank incision retroperitoneally (Figure 49-3). If the occlusion is limited to the right common iliac vein, the same incision is used to expose the external iliac vein for the distal anastomosis. Inflow is obtained from the iliac vein, exposed via a flank incision or femoral vein, through a standard groin incision. The graft is tunneled under the ureter. If a femorocaval graft is placed, the graft is tunneled under the inguinal ligament. To all grafts originating from the femoral vein and to most long iliocaval grafts, an arteriovenous fistula is added at the groin (see Figure 49-3).

The use of autologous vein for femoroiliac or femorocaval reconstruction is also an option. Because of a relatively small size, saphenous vein in this location can be used only rarely. If short segment of the common femoral or iliac vein has to be reconstructed, a better size match is a spiral saphenous vein graft, prepared using the

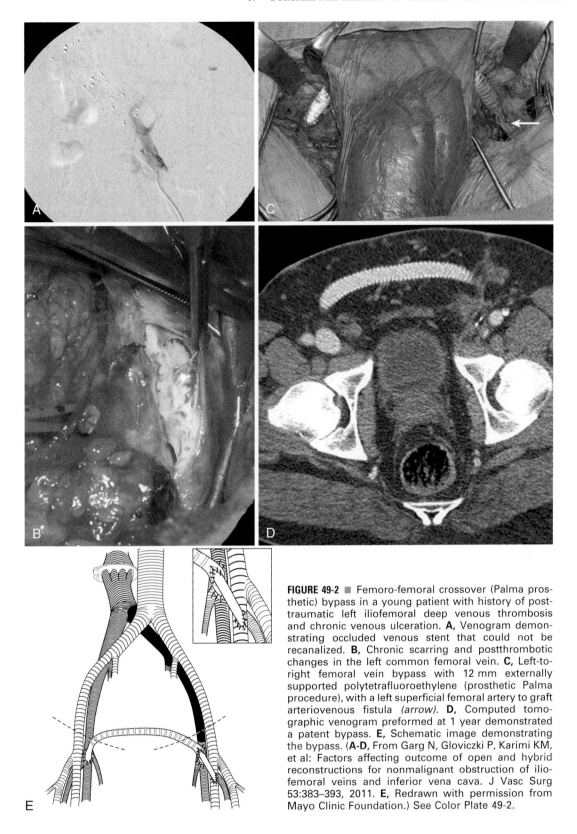

FIGURE 49-2 ■ Femoro-femoral crossover (Palma prosthetic) bypass in a young patient with history of posttraumatic left iliofemoral deep venous thrombosis and chronic venous ulceration. **A,** Venogram demonstrating occluded venous stent that could not be recanalized. **B,** Chronic scarring and postthrombotic changes in the left common femoral vein. **C,** Left-to-right femoral vein bypass with 12 mm externally supported polytetrafluoroethylene (prosthetic Palma procedure), with a left superficial femoral artery to graft arteriovenous fistula *(arrow).* **D,** Computed tomographic venogram preformed at 1 year demonstrated a patent bypass. **E,** Schematic image demonstrating the bypass. (**A-D,** From Garg N, Gloviczki P, Karimi KM, et al: Factors affecting outcome of open and hybrid reconstructions for nonmalignant obstruction of iliofemoral veins and inferior vena cava. J Vasc Surg 53:383–393, 2011. **E,** Redrawn with permission from Mayo Clinic Foundation.) See Color Plate 49-2.

contralateral saphenous vein (Figure 49-4). The excised vein is opened longitudinally, the valves are excised, and the graft is wrapped around a 28- or 32-mm argyle chest tube. The edges are approximated with running 6/0 polypropylene sutures or with stainless steel

nonpenetrating vascular clips. The internal or external jugular veins are other conduits that can be considered for venous reconstruction. The femoral vein is also an alternative for reconstruction of abdominal veins, although morbidity of removing this vein in many of

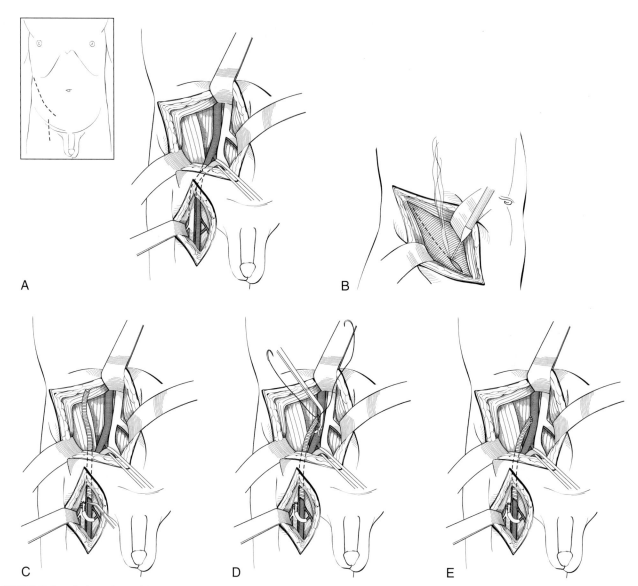

FIGURE 49-3 ■ **A,** Location of the incisions of a right femorocaval bypass. The common femoral vein and the proximal saphenous vein is exposed through a 6- to 8-cm vertical incision at the groin. **B,** The distal inferior vena cava is exposed retroperitoneally through a right oblique anterolateral flank incision, transecting the abdominal muscles and the transversalis fascia. The ureter is retracted medially. **C,** The femoral arteriovenous fistula is performed first in this case with a large tributary of the saphenous vein and the femoral artery. The distal anastomosis is performed in an end-to-end fashion between the common femoral vein and the 10-mm externally supported polytetrafluoroethylene graft. The graft is tunneled under the inguinal ligament **D,** The anastomosis between the graft and the inferior vena cava is performed in an end-to-end fashion using 5/0 polypropylene suture. Air is carefully flushed from the graft before removing the clamp from the inferior vena cava. **E,** Completed femorocaval bypass with a sapheno-femoral arteriovenous fistula. (Redrawn by permission of Mayo Foundation for Medical Education and Research. All rights reserved.)

these patients with underlying thrombophilia or post-thrombotic syndrome is high and other options are recommended. Cryopreserved saphenous or femoral vein has also been reported for venous reconstruction, but long-term patency of these grafts for venous replacement has been poor.

Experience with femorocaval or iliocaval PTFE bypass grafts for benign disease has been limited. Long-term patency of 77% was reported in one series published by Sottiurai.[20] A 5-year primary and secondary patency of 31% and 57%, respectively, was also observed for femoro-infrahepatic IVC bypasses.[2]

Femoroiliac or Iliocaval Bypass

The iliac vein is exposed via a flank incision, and femoral vein is exposed through a standard groin incision as detailed previously. In cases with common iliac vein occlusion, infrahepatic vena cava is used as outflow, exposed through a midline incision or the right flank incision. These short bypasses have a hemodynamic advantage because of the length and high flow. An externally supported 10- to 14-mm PTFE graft is preferred for these bypasses. Among 17 patients who underwent a short bypass, 5-year primary and

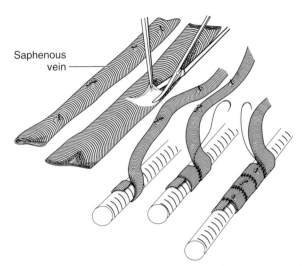

Saphenous vein

FIGURE 49-4 ■ Technique to prepare a spiral saphenous vein graft. The vein is opened longitudinally, venous valves are excised, and the vein is wrapped around a 28- or 32-French argyle chest tube. Vein edges are approximated using running 6/0 polypropylene sutures, with interrupted stitches after each circle to minimize purse stringing. Alternatively, nonpenetrating vascular clips can be used for this purpose. (Redrawn by permission of Mayo Foundation for Medical Education and Research. All rights reserved.)

secondary patency of 63% and 86% was observed, respectively.[2]

Inferior Cavoatrial Bypass

Patients with symptomatic short membranous occlusion of the IVC or longer congenital or acquired narrowing (caval coarctation) without or with hepatic venous outflow obstruction (Budd-Chiari syndrome) can be treated with cavoatrial bypass when attempts at percutaneous angioplasty or stenting have failed. The largest experience for the treatment of Budd-Chiari syndrome comes from the Asian countries, and multiple modalities have been described to treat associated caval occlusion. Some of the preferred techniques include membranectomy, endovenectomy with patch angioplasty, cavocaval bypass, and mesoatrial bypass with or without caval limb.[5,22] Results of these techniques are encouraging, with greater than 85% long-term success in appropriately selected patients. Recent data suggest significantly better outcomes with mesoatrial caval bypass compared with mesocaval bypass,[23] and originating one limb from the superior mesenteric vein has higher patency rates compared with the splenic vein.[24]

The suprahepatic inferior vena cava or right atrium is approached through an anterolateral right thoracotomy (Figure 49-5). The pericardium is opened anterior to the phrenic nerve. If the membranous occlusion is short and is located to this area, a short PTFE interposition graft can be performed from this exposure. If the occlusion extends distal to the hepatic veins, the abdomen is entered through the same thoracotomy, transecting the diaphragm circumferentially and mobilizing the liver forward and medially. Division of the triangular and the

right coronary ligament will help mobilization of the liver. The adrenal gland and the kidney are left in their bed, and dissection is moved more medially. Excellent exposure of the suprarenal IVC can be achieved through this approach. If the distal anastomosis has to be made more distally, a separate right subcostal or midline incision can be performed as described previously.

For a cavoatrial bypass, an end-to-side anastomosis to the IVC is performed, and the graft is routed under the liver parallel to the IVC. The graft is then anastomosed end to side to the suprarenal IVC or the lower portion of the right atrium. Partially occluding clamps are used to perform the anastomosis, and cardiopulmonary bypass is not needed. Traumatic or iatrogenic occlusions can also be managed by this technique. The use of a 16- to 20-mm externally supported PTFE graft is recommended.

The reported clinical success rate with cavoatrial grafts is approximately 77%, with a perioperative mortality of 3% and 2-, 5-, and 10-year patency rates of 86%, 78%, and 57%, respectively.[21,25]

Inferior Vena Cava Reconstruction following Excision of Malignant Tumors

Primary venous leiomyosarcoma or secondary tumors invading the vena cava are the most frequent indications. Most renal carcinomas that extend into the vena cava do not invade the wall of the vessel, and the tumor thrombus can frequently be removed from the IVC without the need for venous reconstruction. Partial excision of a chronically dilated cava in most of these cases permits resection of up to 50% of the caval circumference with primary closure. For wider excision of the wall, PTFE or bovine pericardial patch are options for reconstruction. Attention must be paid to avoid tumor embolization to the right atrium, and extension of the tumor thrombus into right atrium may mandate cardiopulmonary bypass and circulatory arrest to permit safe removal.

The incision for resection of primary IVC tumors is transperitoneal, usually midline or right subcostal. Hepatic tumor resection may require a right thoracolaparotomy (Figure 49-6). The infrahepatic IVC is exposed as described before. PTFE grafts (14 to 20 mm) with external support provide excellent patency of the reconstructed suprarenal or infrarenal inferior vena cava, because inflow is usually excellent and there is no associated iliac vein thrombosis. Short, 8- or 10-mm–wide, externally supported PTFE grafts can also be used to reconstruct the renal veins if nephrectomy for treatment of the tumor does not have to be performed.

A venovenous bypass between the IVC or iliac vein and the axillary or internal jugular vein using a mechanical (Bio-Medicus, Medtronic, MN) pump is only rarely needed in patients with poor cardiac function who cannot maintain a systolic blood pressure greater than 100 mm Hg when both the IVC and the hepatic veins are occluded for an anastomosis. When resection of the retrohepatic suprarenal vena cava has to be performed, the proximal anastomosis is performed first to allow early restoration of hepatic venous outflow (see Figure 49-6C, D). A femoral AVF is usually not required because of the excellent venous inflow.

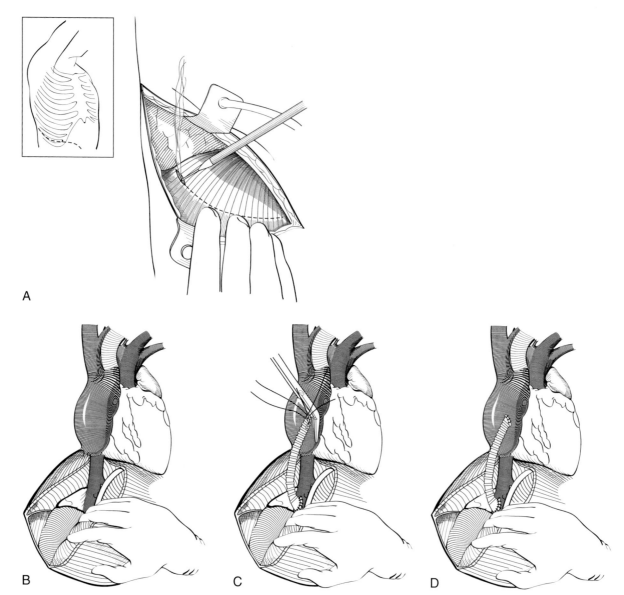

FIGURE 49-5 ■ Cavoatrial bypass for suprarenal caval occlusion. **A,** The thorax is entered through the eighth intercostal space performing an anterolateral thoracotomy. The costal arch is sharply divided through the eight and ninth ribs but the abdomen is not entered. The inferior pulmonary ligament is divided and the diaphragm is circumferentially incised and the abdomen is entered. **B,** The triangular and right coronary ligament is divided and the right lobe of the liver is mobilized medially and anteriorly. **C,** The suprarenal inferior vena cava is dissected and partially cross-clamped. A 14- or 16-mm externally supported polytetrafluoroethylene (PTFE) graft is anastomosed first to the cava, then to the right atrium. Air is carefully flushed before opening up flow in the graft. **D,** Completed cavoatrial PTFE bypass. (Redrawn by permission of Mayo Foundation for Medical Education and Research. All rights reserved.)

Perioperative complications are frequent (43%) and operative mortality, because of the associated liver resection, can be high (7%). Graft patency is excellent at 93% at 3 years.[26] Survival in many patients, however, is limited because of recurrent local tumor or distant metastases. Nevertheless, aggressive surgical management may offer the only chance for cure or palliation of symptoms for patients with primary or secondary IVC tumors. Caval reconstruction can result in significant improvement of the quality of life in these patients even if their survival is short owing to the underlying malignant disease.

SPECIAL CONSIDERATIONS

Endophlebectomy

Postthrombotic femoral veins frequently have multiple lumens due to partial recanalization of the thrombus. Excision of the organized and fibrotic thrombus will enlarge the lumen, although the exposed collagen in the media of the vein wall is more thrombogenic than the intact venous wall. Still, careful endophlebectomy will improve inflow to a great extent; attention, however, must be paid to avoid injury to the thin residual venous

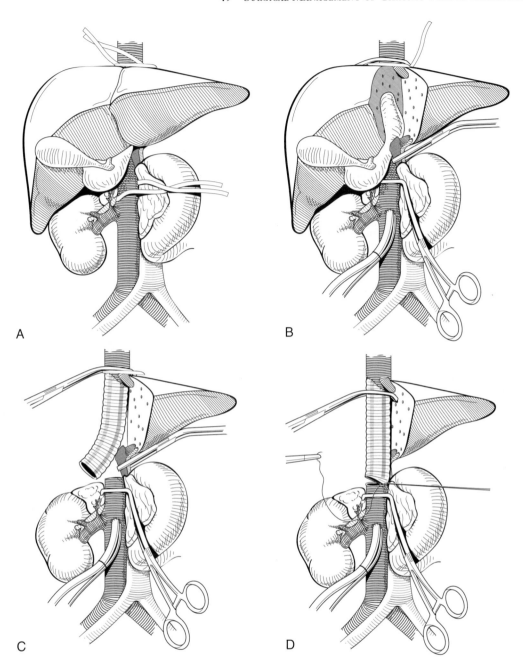

FIGURE 49-6 ■ Technique for polytetrafluoroethylene graft replacement of the suprarenal inferior vena cava for right hepatic lobe malignancy and caval invasion. **A,** Suprahepatic and suprarenal vena cava isolation and division of the right hepatic artery and portal vein branches. **B,** Hepatic vascular exclusion with a Pringle maneuver is used to complete resection of the liver, tumor, and retrohepatic vena cava. Venovenous bypass via an infrarenal cannula and centrifugal pump is used if necessary. **C,** Proximal caval anastomosis is performed first to minimize hepatic ischemia. **D,** The suprahepatic caval clamp is transferred across the graft after acid metabolites have been flushed from the liver. Distal caval anastomosis is then completed. (Redrawn by permission of Mayo Foundation for Medical Education and Research. All rights reserved.)

wall. In patients who have localized high-grade stenosis of the common femoral vein, this operation alone is sufficient to improve venous outflow. This procedure has also been performed combined with deep venous valve transplantation in patients with PTS. The defect is closed with a patch using a segment of the saphenous vein or bovine pericardium. The endophlebectomized segment can also be used to improve inflow for iliocaval stenting (see hybrid reconstructions) or for a cross-femoral or femorocaval bypass. In a series of patients who underwent endophlebectomy, early results showed 77% primary patency of the operated segments at 8 months and a 93% secondary patency rate.[27]

Arteriovenous Fistula

Caval reconstructions or short iliocaval grafts, including prosthetic bypasses do not need an adjunctive temporary

AVF to maintain patency, except in cases of poor inflow and distal anastomosis at the level of common femoral vein. Even in these distal cases, the additional benefit provided by AVF to prevent early thrombosis is questionable.[2]

Prevention of Complications

In general, large vein reconstructions for benign disease are performed in good surgical candidates only, with a low risk of systemic complications. Of the local, nonvascular complications, wound infection, hematoma, and lymphatic leaks (fistula, lymphocele) are the most frequent. Atraumatic surgical technique, antibiotic prophylaxis, and standard surgical principles are helpful in prevention. Intraoperative air embolism, especially during caval reconstruction, is a potentially fatal complication and can be prevented by meticulous flushing of the grafts before reestablishment of the circulation and passive Valsalva maneuver (30 mm Hg), in addition to Trendelenburg position before release of the proximal clamp.

DVT and pulmonary embolism are serious systemic vascular complications. During a series of 64 procedures performed for nonmalignant disease, there was no mortality and no pulmonary embolism.[2] Although early graft thrombosis rate was high (20%), and reinterventions were needed, 96% of the patients left the hospital with a patent graft after open surgical bypass. Perioperative anticoagulation with heparin and warfarin, the use of elastic stockings, intermittent pneumatic compression pumps, and early ambulation help to prevent thromboembolic complications, which are fortunately rare. Local vascular complications are specific to venous reconstructions and include graft stenosis or thrombosis, perioperative bleeding, graft infection, and injury to the surrounding vascular and nonvascular structures.

Anticoagulation

Grafts placed in the venous system have a higher rate of thrombosis than arterial grafts because of a low venous flow. Presence of thrombophilic disorders and thrombogenic surface of any prosthetic graft increases the risk of graft failure. Infrainguinal venous obstruction and valvular incompetence further decrease inflow to the graft, and it is a major contributing factor to failure. For these reasons, perioperative anticoagulation is indicated in patients undergoing reconstructive venous surgery for deep venous obstruction.

The patient is fully heparinized during reconstruction, and protamine is avoided at the completion of the procedure. Unfractionated heparin infusion is started immediately in the postoperative period. Complete postoperative systemic heparinization is achieved by 48 hours, and full-dose low-molecular-weight heparin is continued subcutaneously for another 3 to 5 days, given simultaneously with warfarin. The incidence of postoperative bleeding has been between 5% and 10%, mainly as a result of anticoagulation. Warfarin is continued indefinitely in most patients with prosthetic grafts and in all with a known underlying coagulation abnormality.

Follow-up and Reinterventions

Duplex scan on the first postoperative day or contrast venography is performed to confirm graft patency. Stenosis or thrombosis is corrected immediately after recognition. If thrombosis occurred in a graft without fistula, thrombectomy is done with addition of a fistula. Graft stenosis discovered during surveillance in the late postoperative period is treated first with angioplasty or venous stenting. Late graft thrombosis is treated with thrombolysis, angioplasty, and stenting. Surgical revision is usually limited to patch angioplasty of the stenotic portion of the graft, although occasionally aneurysmal dilation of the saphenous crossover graft may also need surgical correction. On long-term follow-up, approximately half of the patients require some kind of reintervention. More than 60% of the patients had no venous claudication and no or minimal swelling on long-term follow-up.

References available online at expertconsult.com.

QUESTIONS

1. What is the first line of management of chronic iliac vein obstructions?
   a. Compression therapy and lifestyle changes
   b. Balloon angioplasty
   c. Venous stent placement
   d. Femoro-caval bypass

2. A 40-year-old male with past history of left iliofemoral DVT and recurrent ulcerations despite compression therapy presents with large lower extremity varicosities and great saphenous vein reflux. No infrainguinal venous obstruction is obvious on duplex scan. What would you recommend?
   a. High ligation and great saphenous vein stripping
   b. Endovenous ablation of the saphenous vein
   c. Endovenous ablation and stab phlebectomies
   d. CT or MR venogram of the abdomen and pelvis

3. What is the minimum diameter of the great saphenous vein that is acceptable for a cross femoral bypass (Palma procedure)?
   a. 3 mm
   b. 7 mm
   c. 5 mm
   d. 6 mm

4. In which of the following patients is a cross femoral venous bypass (Palma procedure) ill advised?
   a. Morbidly obese
   b. Hypercoaguable disorder
   c. Recurrent ulceration
   d. Previous failed venous stenting

5. An adjunctive femoral AV fistula improves patency of femorocaval prosthetic bypasses.
   a. True
   b. False

6. A Palma procedure using autologous saphenous vein has the best chance of long-term patency in patients with
   a. Isolated unilateral iliac vein obstruction
   b. Multilevel obstruction
   c. Severe infrainguinal obstruction
   d. Failed previous iliac vein stent

7. In patients requiring resection of the inferior vena cava for invasion by a malignant tumor, up to 50% of the circumference of the vena cava can be resected with primary closure.
   a. True
   b. False

8. A femoral arteriovenous fistula is frequently needed in patients who undergo segmental replacement of the inferior vena cava, invaded by a malignant tumor.
   a. True
   b. False

9. Postprocedure antiplatelet therapy has been conclusively shown to reduce thrombotic events in venous bypasses.
   a. True
   b. False

10. Patients with prosthetic graft for venous replacement require life-long anticoagulation in most cases.
    a. True
    b. False

ANSWERS

1. **a**
2. **d**
3. **c**
4. **a**
5. **a**
6. **a**
7. **a**
8. **b**
9. **b**
10. **a**

CHAPTER 50

Endovascular Repair of Chronic Venous Obstruction

Seshadri Raju

Percutaneous endovenous stenting has emerged as a powerful new technique to treat chronic venous obstructions. Stenosis and chronic total occlusions (CTOs) are amenable to endovascular correction.[1-4] The technique is minimally invasive, safe, and effective and does not preclude open correction in case of failure. The technique can be applied in the geriatric subset and others with comorbidities that would normally preclude open procedures. Intravascular ultrasound (IVUS) diagnostics have revealed that obstruction is present in a broader spectrum of chronic venous disease (CVD) than previously imagined.[5] Furthermore, stent correction of obstruction alone in combined obstruction–reflux appears to yield good symptom relief even when the reflux component remains uncorrected[6]; this suggests that the pathophysiologic importance of obstruction has been underestimated.[7] These observations suggest a broad, dominant role for stent usage in highly symptomatic CVD patients which signifies a major therapeutic paradigm shift in the management of advanced CVD.

PATHOPHYSIOLOGY

Postthrombotic etiology for chronic venous obstruction is well established. With the use of IVUS, it has become clear that nonthrombotic iliac vein lesions (NIVLs) are a common feature among "primary" CVD patients with advanced symptoms as well.[5] The lesions occur at arterial crossover points over the vein (Figure 50-1). Intraluminal webs and strictures are often present and are thought to result from pulsatile trauma of intimately associated artery.[8] Other less common causes of chronic venous obstruction include tumors, retroperitoneal fibrosis and radiation injury. Inferior vena cava (IVC) filters are also emerging as a significant cause of iatrogenic caval-iliac obstruction; some models appear to be more prone to this development than others.[9]

Postthrombotic disease often involves multiple venous segments, but symptom production appears to be mainly related to the iliac vein segment because of poor collateral potential in this venous segment.[10] Natural collateral pathways based on embryology appear to develop rapidly in obstructions of other venous segments, particularly in femoral vein obstructions and to a lesser extent in caval obstructions. These collateral pathways may exist already in putative form, becoming functional when straight-line flow faces higher resistance than in the quiescent collaterals.[11] The process is just the reverse of that seen

in venous stenting when collaterals disappear instantaneously with clearance of obstruction. The profunda femoris vein is an embryologic collateral and often becomes visible on venography within a few hours after onset of femoral vein thrombosis. CTO lesions of the IVC are sometimes an incidental finding in asymptomatic patients.[10] In contrast, pelvic vein collaterals that appear impressive on venography are often functionally inadequate, and the patient continues to be symptomatic.[12] Some postthrombotic iliac vein lesions develop a tough perivenous sheath that restricts the vein and retards collateral development. Such diffuse iliac vein stenosis, first noted by Rokitanski in autopsy studies, appears as a patent but smaller caliber iliac vein on venography. The reduction in lumen size is clearly evident on IVUS examination, but is easily missed on venography (Figure 50-2). Focal iliac vein lesions may be impervious to routine venography as well.[13] For these reasons, a symptomatic iliac vein lesion may remain occult, whereas the more obvious femoral vein occlusions are readily apparent. The latter are seldom the main source of symptoms, however, and a diligent search for the culprit lesion in the iliac veins is in order.

The discovery of a high incidence of NIVL in symptomatic CVD cases with IVUS and relief of symptoms with venous stenting has highlighted pathophysiologic peculiarities of these lesions. First, these lesions are widely prevalent in the asymptomatic population, with a gross prevalence of up to 30% in autopsy studies[14] and up to 66% with more sensitive modern imaging techniques.[15] With IVUS, the lesions are found in greater than 90% of patients with advanced symptoms.[5] These are characteristics of *permissive pathology*, which is widely prevalent in human disease. Patent foramen ovale (PFO), with an incidence of approximately 25% in the asymptomatic general population, becomes symptomatic in a small fraction with onset of paradoxic embolus. Not surprisingly, PFO is invariably found in patients with paradoxic embolus. Other examples of permissive or secondary pathologies include obesity or diabetes, diabetes or neuropathy, carotid plaque or transient ischemic attack, ureteric reflux or pyelonephritis, *Helicobacter pylori* or peptic ulcer, and acid reflux or asthma. In case of silent iliac vein obstructions, a number of secondary events may trigger onset of symptoms (Box 50-1). A postthrombotic iliac vein lesion related to a remote thrombotic event can also remain silent for years or decades before symptoms are precipitated by a later trigger event (Figure 50-3). A general principle in treating these complex pathologies is

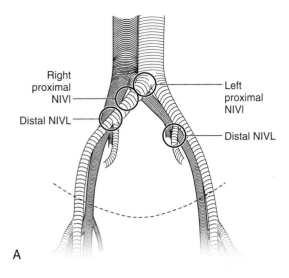

A

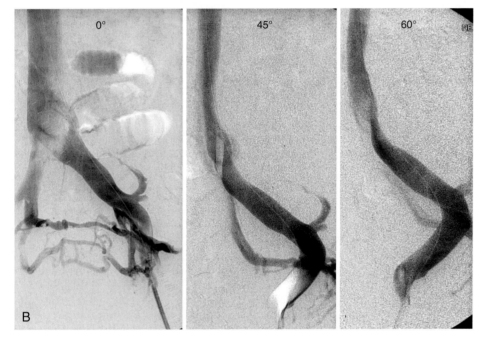

FIGURE 50-1 ■ A, The pathologic anatomy of a nonthrombotic iliac vein lesion (NIVL). The classic left-sided proximal lesion is related to abrupt crossing of the left iliac vein by the right iliac artery. Coursing lazily across the vein, the right iliac artery may be related to the proximal or distal NIVL, or both. The left hypogastric artery crossing may be related to the left distal NIVL. The hypogastric veins have been omitted to reduce clutter. **B,** The proximal NIVL appears as a translucent area on venography in frontal projection. The tight stenosis is clearly visible in 60-degree projection. Collaterals seen in this case are present only in one third of cases.

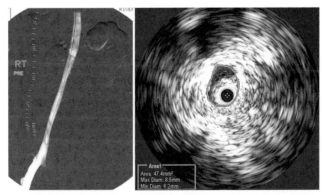

FIGURE 50-2 ■ Diffuse postthrombotic stenosis may not be recognized on venography *(left).* It is clearly visible on intravascular ultrasound (IVUS) examination *(right).* Cross-section area by IVUS planimetry measured 47 mm² (normal ≥160 mm²).

BOX 50-1	Secondary Insults That May Precipitate Symptoms in the Presence of a Silent Iliac Vein Lesion

- Trauma
- Infection (cellulitis)
- Reflux
- Deep venous thrombosis
- Joint surgery
- Orthostasis and poor calf pump (elderly)
- Obesity
- Edematogenic medications (many cardiovascular drugs)
- Postmenopausal hormonal changes
- Lymphatic damage and vein disease itself or from cancer, chemotherapy, radiation, or surgery

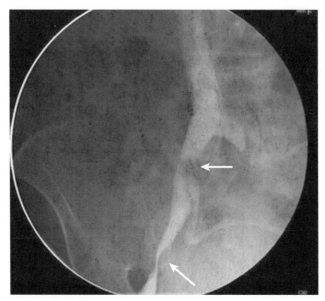

FIGURE 50-3 ■ The postthrombotic iliac vein lesion shown here is likely a result of deep venous thrombosis related to a motor vehicle crash when the patient was in her twenties. There was onset of leg swelling when the 80-year-old patient suffered a fibular fracture after a fall. Stent placement resolved the swelling.

to address the permissive pathology first, which usually provides definitive cure. The experience with iliac vein obstructions has been similar. In cases of combined obstruction and reflux, iliac vein stenting alone has provided effective symptom remission even when associated reflux was quite severe and remained untreated.[6] In an analysis of 528 limbs that underwent iliac vein stenting for obstruction, severe reflux (reflux segment score ≥3) was present in 58% and axial reflux in 42% that remained uncorrected. Cumulative ulcer healing and clearance of dermatitis were 54% and 81%, respectively, at 5 years. No difference was noted between limbs with severe residual reflux and limbs with no reflux or less severe reflux. Venous pathologies uniquely respond to partial correction with symptom remission. For example, in combined superficial and deep reflux, correction of superficial reflux alone may provide symptom relief. In axial reflux, repair of a single valve may suffice.[16] Valve reconstruction of a refluxive valve below an obstructed venous segment has been shown to be effective.[17] With the advent of stent technology, repair of obstruction has become much easier than correction of reflux, which still requires open surgery. The satisfactory therapeutic response to partial pathologic correction means that a stepwise treatment paradigm starting with the simplest and minimally invasive techniques can be pursued; more complex or open treatment modalities can be reserved until later if there is recurrence of symptoms. The satisfactory clinical relief obtained with correction of chronic venous obstruction has suggested that in terms of pathophysiology, obstruction is as important as reflux, which has been the focus for the last 3 centuries.[18] IVUS-proven iliac vein obstruction occurs in isolation without associated reflux in 27% to 36% of CVD patients with advanced symptoms.[5,6]

Venous ulceration appears to occur most commonly with combined obstruction and reflux, and only rarely with a single pathology of either obstruction or reflux.

There is an intimate relationship between venous and lymphatic systems in genesis as well as function. Lymphatic dysfunction can be demonstrated in approximately 30% of patients with advanced CVD.[19] Lymphoscintigraphic delay in node visualization appears to be a defect in the precollectors at the microcirculatory level; the form and function of large collector lymphatics are apparently preserved. The precise nature of the damage to the precollectors is unknown, but is presumed to be related to the overloaded lymphatic transport imposed by venous dysfunction.

CLINICAL FEATURES

Clinical presentation of chronic venous obstruction is often indistinguishable from that attributed to reflux alone or in combination. Venous obstruction can manifest in the entire spectrum of clinical classes represented in CEAP. All age groups, both sexes (women more often) and both sides (left more often) are affected. Advanced clinical manifestations of pain, swelling, or skin changes have a high likelihood of being associated with venous obstruction with or without reflux, as already outlined. These clinical features can occur alone or in combination. Some aspects of clinical presentation associated with iliac vein obstruction deserve special commentary.

Limb pain usually has strong orthostatic (standing or seated) features. It is typically diffuse over the limb (differing from pain localized to varices), although pain may be predominant in one region such as calf or shin. The character of the pain may vary from "bursting," "shooting," or "heaviness." No overt pain is present, but soreness to touch or contact is present in some individuals. Restless legs and cramps are common. Pain is relieved by elevation or ambulation, both of which reduce venous pressure. Stockings, when properly used, provide relief. Many of these pain-relieving maneuvers have become habitual in long-standing disease, and leading questions are necessary to elicit the information. Many patients routinely sleep with their legs on pillows, for example, and may not offer this information unless specifically asked. Atypical pain presentation is not uncommon, such as when pain occurs at night while the patient is recumbent. Patients often get up and "walk off" the nocturnal pain. In some patients, venous limb pain can mimic claudication, with difficulty going long distances or climbing stairs without intermittent rest. A special form of orthostatic venous pain (venous hypertension syndrome) occurs in approximately 10% of patients and is often missed because the limb looks entirely healthy with no venous signs. Venous pain disproportionate to clinical signs of venous disease is usually due to iliac vein obstructions.

Limb swelling occurs more commonly and more extensively with iliac vein obstructions than with superficial or deep reflux alone. With saphenous reflux, swelling is usually intermittent and confined to the ankles. With extensive deep venous reflux, swelling may advance to involve the leg, but is confined to below the knee and is generally only mild to moderate in severity. Massive limb swelling is invariably due to iliac vein obstruction. Recurrent cellulitis of the limb usually indicates the presence of iliac vein obstruction.

Venous dermatitis and ulceration are most commonly the result of a combination of deep venous reflux and obstruction. However, in a small subset of isolated saphenous reflux, venous dermatitis or ulceration can be present if the saphenous vein is large in size (often >10 mm).

Iliac vein thrombosis is a special form that can propagate distally, prompted by an underlying NIVL-type lesion.[20] Recurrent venous thrombosis is a recognized cause of onset of symptoms in postthrombotic syndrome.[21] The etiology of iliac vein obstruction (i.e., NIVL vs. postthrombotic) cannot be determined in most cases by clinical features alone, except when there is a clear history of prior deep venous thrombosis.

INVESTIGATIONS

Standard investigative techniques have poor sensitivity to iliac vein obstruction. Routine duplex technique does not provide adequate color flow images of the iliac vein. A new technique described by Labropoulos and colleagues[22] offers better visualization and velocity metrics, but its accuracy has not been determined. Presence of reflux, even severe reflux (multisegment or axial), does not rule out the presence of iliac vein obstruction or the opportunity for symptom remission with stent correction, as already outlined. Absence of reflux or trivial reflux (reflux in only one or two segments, nonaxial reflux, or reflux in a small saphenous vein) in the context of severe presentation does suggest iliac vein obstruction. It is well established that routine venography, even through the transfemoral route, is only approximately 50% sensitive to iliac vein obstructive lesions in frontal projections.[6] The accuracy of modern imaging techniques such as high-resolution computed tomography or magnetic resonance imaging in detecting iliac vein lesions remains undetermined. No hemodynamic tests have adequate sensitivity to detect iliac vein obstruction. Exercise femoral vein pressures, outflow fraction measurement and arm/foot pressure measurement can be useful when positive, but do not rule out obstruction because of their low sensitivity. Using a combination of these techniques and transfemoral venography, it is possible to predict the presence of an iliac vein obstruction with approximately 80% accuracy.[6] IVUS examination, a morphologic method, remains the most reliable technique in detecting iliac vein obstruction at present.[23] Because of the high diagnostic yield with this method in symptomatic patients, it remains the preferred diagnostic modality at the present time. Stent correction of the detected stenosis can be performed concurrently with prior consent.

TECHNIQUE OF STENT PLACEMENT

Venous stenting differs from arterial stenting in significant respects (Box 50-2). Modification of the

BOX 50-2   Venous Stenting Technique Is Different from Arterial Technique

- Balloon angioplasty does not work because the lesion is fibrous, and recoil is the rule.
- Large-caliber stents approximating natural lumen size is necessary to normalize distal venous pressure; patency alone is not enough.
- Stents should be extended into the inferior vena cava, otherwise the choke band at the iliac-caval junction will squeeze the stent distally causing recurrence.
- Venous stents (braided) can be extended across the inguinal ligament without erosion or fracture.
- Iliac veins are intolerant of residual lesions; the cause is residual or recurrent symptoms.
- Extensive stenting is often required; veins are very tolerant of metal load (no thrombosis).
- Intravascular ultrasound is mandatory for good results.

endovascular technique learned in arterial practice is essential for symptom relief.

The optimal access point is midthigh where the femoral vein is posterolateral to the artery. The midthigh access offers close proximity to the lesion and antegrade maneuvers while allowing adequate room above the sheath to deploy the stent below the inguinal ligament if necessary. Access through the internal jugular vein or the popliteal vein is farther removed from the lesion and the latter has the additional disadvantage of prone positioning required in an increasingly obese population. Large-sized (10 or 11 French) sheaths are used. Access complications have been rare with the routine use of sealant devices.

After an optional on-table venogram (omitted in renal dysfunction), IVUS examination is performed and the presence of an obstructive lesion is confirmed. IVUS planimetry provides accurate measurement of even irregular stenosis, which is common in iliac veins. The proximal common iliac vein where the artery crosses over is the classic site for nonthrombotic obstruction. Obstructive lesions near the hypogastric vein orifice occur more frequently,[5] however, and are sometimes impervious to IVUS examination. Gentle balloon sizing of this location is necessary to identify such lesions. Minor lesions are commonly present behind the inguinal ligament. In postthrombotic disease, these compression points from arterial or ligamentous structures are particularly prone to fibrosis, because thrombus resolves poorly at these locations.[20] In severe postthrombotic disease, the entire iliac-femoral segments may be involved.

Large-caliber balloons appropriate for the anatomic site are used. Size 16 mm for the common iliac vein and 14-16 mm for the external iliac and common femoral veins are commonly used in normal-sized adults. Iliac vein obstructions are fibrous and recoil is universal after balloon dilatation alone. Stent placement is therefore universally required. Large-caliber stents oversized by 2 mm for the location are deployed under fluoroscopy with generous overlap between stent stack members. The slight oversizing allows later hyperdilatation in case of stent compression or in-stent restenosis.[24] The preferred upper landing site is distal vena cava at the level of the top of L 4 vertebral body. This will extend the stent 3-5 cm into the distal IVC. Without such extension, stents placed at the iliac-caval junction are 'squeezed' distally by the fibrous band at the location causing recurrence.[25] 'Jailing' of the contralateral iliac vein has not been a problem; adequate contralateral flow through and around the stent is the rule. All significant lesions (>50%) should be corrected in continuity without short skip areas. Currently, stents in the majority of patients are extended from the distal inferior cava to the common femoral vein (Figure 50-4). Infrainguinal deployment has not resulted in stent fractures, erosions or stent thrombosis.[26] Metal load from extensive stent stack length does not appear to adversely affect patency.[10] Leaving uncorrected residual lesions has often been responsible for residual or recurrent symptoms.[24] IVUS is used extensively during the procedure to identify lesions, determine optimal landing sites for the stent, and ensure proper apposition between stent stack members after postdilatation. Concurrent venography during the procedure has shown that IVUS is far superior to venography alone in guiding stent placement. Furthermore, the patient and the operator are spared avoidable radiation exposure.

BILATERAL STENT PLACEMENT

About 20% of CVD patients in advanced clinical classes have bilateral disease. If the disease is severe in both limbs, bilateral stenting using the 'double barrel' technique is optimal (Figure 50-5A).[27] Unilateral stenting is recommended when the opposite limb has only mild manifestations. Contralateral symptom improvement has been observed after unilateral iliac vein stenting in some

cases, presumably because collateral load is removed. Contralateral limb symptoms may advance over time, however, due to disease progression. In that event, sequential bilateral stenting may be required. The double barrel technique does not work well when done sequentially

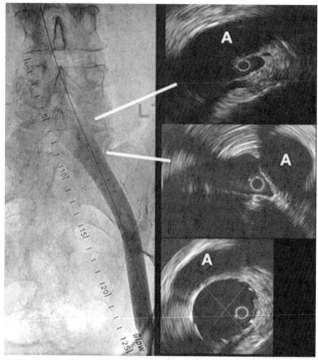

FIGURE 50-4 ■ The venogram on the left appears grossly normal. Note the absence of collaterals. However, intravascular ultrasound (IVUS) examinations at indicated locations show significant stenosis. The IVUS image at the bottom *(right)* shows normal lumen after stent placement.

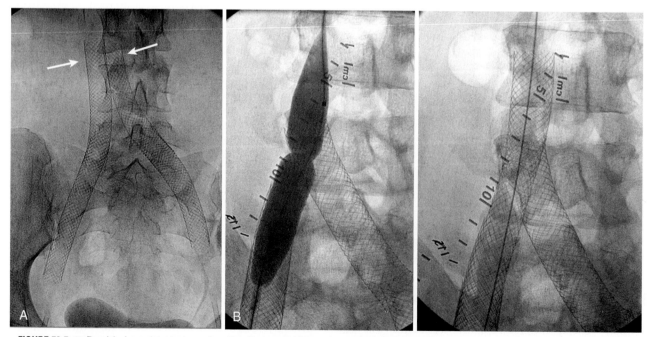

FIGURE 50-5 ■ Double-barrel technique for simultaneous bilateral stenting **A**. Fenestration technique for sequential stenting **B**.

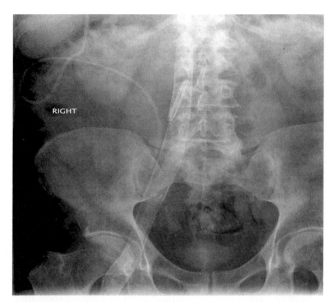

FIGURE 50-6 ■ Stent across inferior vena cava filter that was compacted by balloon dilation. Note stent extension below the inguinal ligament. Stent fractures, erosions, or thrombosis do not result from stent extension across the groin crease.

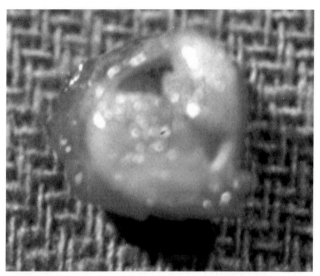

FIGURE 50-7 ■ Transverse section of a postthrombotic vein. The guidewire is threaded through these small channels in the trabeculated vein during the recanalization procedure. See Color Plate 50-7.

after a long interval. The stiffer, older stent tends to compress the newer, more compliant stent. A fenestration technique must be used (see Figure 50-5B).[27]

INFERIOR VENA CAVA FILTERS

Previously placed IVC filters pose a special technical problem during iliac vein stent placement. Some makes of filters may be associated with stenosis of the vena cava at the implantation site. This can be assessed by IVUS examination during the procedure. If no stenosis is found, the iliac vein stent can be safely placed below the filter. If the filter site is stenotic (>50%), the stent should be extended across after compacting the filter by repeated balloon dilatations (Figure 50-6).[28] Temporary filters that are not retrieved as intended may be associated with a higher incidence of stenosis or thrombosis of the IVC.

RECANALIZATION OF ILIAC-CAVAL CHRONIC TOTAL OCCLUSIONS

Recanalization of iliac-caval chronic total occlusions involves manipulating a guidewire through the CTO segment.[4] Unlike in CTO arterial lesions, postthrombotic venous occlusions are not a solid core but are traversed by recanalized channels (Figure 50-7, see color insert). Even dense trabeculations can be crossed with patience (80% procedure success). CTO lesions that appear long on venography may be relatively short because of poor contrast opacification of the segment above the lesion. A recanalization attempt is worthwhile despite a daunting venographic appearance. An angled-tip, 5- or 6-French catheter with hydrophilic coating is used to direct the guidewire through the CTO segment without straying into branches or collaterals. A long

sheath (45-55 cm) is often required to provide additional rigid support for guidewire passage. Perforations that can occur during the maneuvers are innocuous, unlike in arterial stenting, because of the low venous pressure and the constraining influence of perivenous fibrosis and fascial sheaths. The guidewire can be withdrawn, and the procedure can be resumed without ill effects. Proper reentry into the vena cava above the obstruction should be confirmed by advancing the guidewire into the right atrium, venography, or IVUS examination. The next step is to enlarge the guidewire tract to normal luminal size for the location. A 7-French hydrophilic-coated sheath with obturator (Shuttle Sheath, Cook Medical, Bloomington, Ind) is used first to enlarge the tract and allow easy balloon catheter passage. The recanalized channel should be dilated to sizes appropriate for the anatomic location as specified previously; this is essential for adequate peripheral venous decompression. Dilating a CTO fibrous cord to such large sizes may seem hazardous, but it has not proved to be threatening in practice. There has been only one instance of significant bleed (contained hematoma requiring transfusion) in more than 167 recanalization procedures. Slightly oversized stents (by one or two sizes) are placed with generous overlap in the recanalized channel. Stent compression in the dense fibrous channel is a common feature in recanalization procedures (Figure 50-8). The slight oversizing allows for hyperdilation if it occurs. IVUS is distinctly superior to venography in confirming luminal adequacy of the stented recanalized channel.

ANTICOAGULATION

Low-molecular-weight heparin at a prophylactic dosage is routinely used immediately before the procedure and for 1 or 2 days afterward. Intraoperatively, bivalirudin (75 mg) is administered intravenously. Long-term

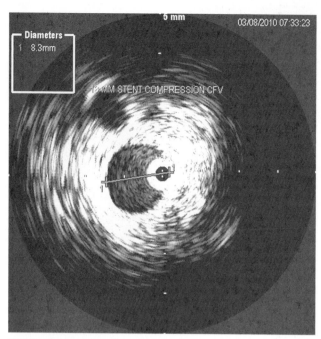

FIGURE 50-8 ■ Stent compression by perivenous fibrosis is unique to venous stenting. An 18-mm stent has been compressed to 8.3 mm.

anticoagulation is not necessary for nonthrombotic cases and postthrombotic patients with previous provoked thrombosis. Aspirin (81 mg daily) is used for stent maintenance in these patient sets. Long-term warfarin anticoagulation is recommended for the following patient groups: thrombophilia, recurrent venous thrombosis, unprovoked deep venous thrombosis, and in complex stenting procedures (e.g., IVC recanalizations).

STENT SURVEILLANCE

Stent imaging, using the technique described by Labropoulos and colleagues,[22] has become the standard for monitoring stent patency. Transfemoral venography can be used in selected cases when duplex findings are equivocal.

Stent patency is monitored the day after the procedure, at 6 weeks, at 6 months, and at yearly intervals thereafter. More frequent monitoring is required in postthrombotic cases,[3] particularly CTO recanalizations in the first 3 months after the procedure, as stent occlusions occur most often in this subset. Residual or recurrent symptoms are an indication for stent imaging outside the routine intervals.

REINTERVENTIONS

Residual or recurrent symptoms indicate stent malfunction or new or missed lesions.[24] Obstructive lesions that cause residual or recurrent symptoms are due to lesions within the stent stack or in the outflow–inflow tracts immediately adjacent to the stent.

Approximately 25% of stent placements will require reinterventions in the succeeding years. The nature of the problem is often evident on duplex imaging or venography. However, discrete focal lesions may be impervious to these techniques. IVUS examination may ultimately be required to identify and correct the problem.

In nonthrombotic cases, the distal NIVL lesion near the hypogastric vein orifice can be missed, even on IVUS examination, and is often the source of symptoms when the original stent placement was confined to the common iliac vein. Less often, a residual uncorrected lesion behind the inguinal ligament is present. Inadequate stent extension into the IVC during the original procedure often leads to local stent migration distally, resulting in recurrent stenosis at the iliac-caval junction.

In postthrombotic cases, lesions at the inflow or outflow site to the stent may be the cause of symptoms. Diffuse postthrombotic stenosis of the IVC is easily missed on venography alone, unless routine IVUS measurements are taken. A peculiar form of new stenosis that develops late after stenting involves the external iliac vein (i.e., de novo stenosis), the nature of which remains unknown.

Intrastent lesions regardless of the original pathology fall into two catagories: (1) stent compression by anatomic fibrous bands in nonthrombotic cases and by postthrombotic fibrous tissue in thrombotic cases and (2) in-stent restenosis. The latter appears to have two forms, a soft variety lined by layered thrombus owing to sluggish flow and a hard variety more similar to the one seen in arterial stenting. Both types appear to have an affinity for the external iliac vein. In either cases of in-stent restenosis, associated lesions below or above the stent that might have been contributory should be corrected by stent extensions. High-pressure (16 atm) balloon dilatation yields satisfactory resolution in clearing in-stent restenosis; it is much less effective in stent compression.

MORBIDITY

Percutaneous stent placement is associated with low morbidity, with good tolerance by the geriatric set and even by those with comorbidities that would preclude open procedures.[3] There has been no procedure-related mortality in more than 2000 stent placements. Lower back pain is a common complaint immediately post-procedure (25% of patents), but is generally easily controlled by nonsteroidal antiinflammatory drugs and supportive measures on an outpatient basis. The incidence of post-stent DVT (<30 days) is 1.5%. The incidence of pulmonary embolism has been 0.02%.

OUTCOME

Cumulative secondary patency for primary and postthrombotic limbs with a separate curve for CTO recanalizations are shown in Figure 50-9. Stent thrombosis is an extreme rarity among nonthrombotic limbs after venous stenting.[3] Stent thrombosis is nearly exclusive to

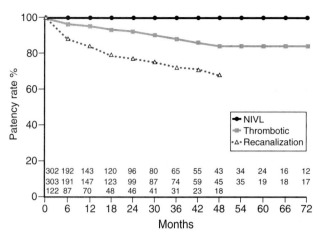

FIGURE 50-9 ■ Cumulative secondary stent patency rates for nonthrombotic and thrombotic limbs. Patency after chronic total occlusion recanalization is shown separately. Stent thrombosis is extremely rare in nonthrombotic limbs.

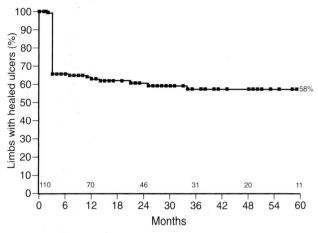

FIGURE 50-11 ■ Cumulative ulcer healing after iliac vein stent placement. A large number of limbs were censored because of follow-up loss soon after stent placement before the ulcers had a chance to heal. There is little ulcer recurrence after healing, yielding a flat curve.

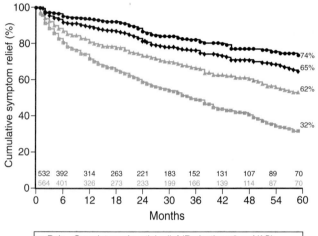

FIGURE 50-10 ■ Cumulative improvement in pain and swelling after iliac vein stent placement. Partial improvement in pain (≥3/10 VAS) and partial swelling relief (≥1 grade) are shown separately from complete relief.

completely relieved of pain. Many patients are able to tolerate residual swelling if the pain component is relieved. Swelling relief is less than pain relief. Approximately one third of patients were completely relieved of swelling long-term. Cumulative healing of venous stasis ulcerations is shown in Figure 50-11. There was cumulative ulcer healing of 58% at 5 years. Quality of life (CIVC) shows improvement in every category and in the overall score.

CONCLUSION

Iliac vein stenting has emerged as a powerful new minimally invasive technique for treatment of a wide spectrum of advanced venous disease. The procedure is safe and effective. As a result, it can be applied to a wider spectrum of patients, including those of advanced age and with comorbidities, which is not possible with traditional open techniques. Its efficacy even in patients with severe uncorrected reflux has focused new attention on the relative pathophysiologic importance of venous obstruction vis-á-vis reflux in chronic venous disease.

References available online at expertconsult.com.

postthrombotic limbs, particularly the CTO subset. Among 464 postthrombotic limbs, there were 31 stent thromboses; 7 were reopened by thrombolysis.

Pain relief and swelling improvement are shown in Figure 50-10. Nearly two thirds of patients were

QUESTIONS

1. "Primary" NIVL iliac vein obstruction is due to
   a. Prior resolved thrombus
   b. Predominantly ontogenic
   c. Traumatic
   d. Endothelial hypertrophy
   e. Vascularized proliferation

2. Post-thrombotic iliac vein lesions are commonly
   a. Focal
   b. Diffuse (Rokitanski type)
   c. Segmental
   d. Poorly collateralized
   e. All of the above

3. With modern imaging, NIVL's are found in:
   a. 20% of the population
   b. 66% of the population
   c. 90% of symptomatic patients
   d. <10% of the population

4. The sensitivity of venography for iliac vein obstruction is
   a. 72%
   b. ≈ 50%
   c. 100% in NIVL
   d. 30%
   e. Increased by reactive hyperemia

5. Iliac vein obstruction without reflux occurs in
   a. 27-36% of CVD patients
   b. Very rare
   c. 58% of CVD patients
   d. Only post-thrombotic disease
   e. Exclusively NIVL

6. The incidence of lympocintographic abnormalities in chronic venous diseases is
   a. <5%
   b. >75%
   c. extremely rare
   d. ≈ 30%
   e. Unknown

7. Preferred technique of correcting iliac vein obstructions:
   a. Angioplasty
   b. Large caliber self-expanding stents
   c. Short balloon dialatable stents
   d. Large caliber covered stents
   e. 8-10 mm stent to restore flow

8. Recanalization of chronic total occlusions is technically achieved by
   a. Subintimal guidewire passage
   b. Subadvential guidewire passage
   c. Passage through collaterals
   d. Passage through trabeculae

9. A major complication of venous stenting and recanalization procedures is
   a. Hemorrhage
   b. New intimal hyperplasia, higher than in arterial stenting
   c. Stent thrombosis requiring effective anticoagulation
   d. Pulmonary embolism in ≈ 10% of cases
   e. None of the above

10. Venous stenting has been shown to
    a. Heal venous ulcers
    b. Completely relieve venous pain in the majority of patients
    c. Improve leg swelling
    d. All of the above
    e. Only b and c are correct

ANSWERS

1. **c**
2. **e**
3. **b**
4. **b**
5. **a**
6. **d**
7. **b**
8. **d**
9. **e**
10. **d**

CHAPTER 51

ETIOLOGY AND MANAGEMENT OF CHRONIC VENOUS INSUFFICIENCY: SURGERY, ENDOVENOUS ABLATION, AND SCLEROTHERAPY

Kenneth K. Kao • David A. Rigberg

The term *chronic venous insufficiency* (CVI) encompasses a spectrum of symptoms such as edema, skin changes, or ulceration, which are attributed to functional abnormalities of the venous system and venous hypertension.[1] Varicose veins alone are not considered evidence of CVI unless they are associated with other symptoms.[2] CVI is a common problem, with more than 2 million adults in the United States suffering from advanced venous disease, 150,000 new cases diagnosed each year, and an estimated cost of half a billion dollars annually for their care.[3,4] In the Edinburgh vein study, more than 1500 subjects were screened with a questionnaire, physical examination, and duplex ultrasound.[5] CVI prevalence closely correlated with sex and age, with rates of 21.2% and 12% in men and women greater than 50 years of age, respectively. The most common symptoms of CVI include pain, sensations of heaviness, swelling, aching, restless legs, cramps, itching, tingling, throbbing, and tired legs. Of these symptoms, those significantly correlated with worsening grade of CVI included heaviness, swelling, aching, and itching.[2] The Bonn Vein Study examined more than 3000 people from the general population and found signs of CVI, including edema in 13.4%, skin changes in 2.9%, and healed or active ulceration in 0.6% or 0.1%, respectively.[6]

ANATOMY

Standardized nomenclature of lower extremity venous anatomy was published by Caggiati and colleagues in 2002,[7] and this terminology should be adopted to provide uniform description and treatment of CVI. The venous system can be considered as three interconnected groups: (1) superficial veins, which lie above the fascia and drain both the skin and subcutaneous tissue; (2) deep veins, which lie below the fascia and drain the leg musculature; and (3) perforating veins (PVs), which penetrate the fascia and connect the deep and superficial systems. These veins have bicuspid valves that are found at the termination of major tributaries, with increasing numbers found more distally in the venous tree.[8] The superficial veins are usually involved with CVI and include the great

and small saphenous veins. The great saphenous vein connects to the femoral vein at the saphenofemoral junction; a valve lies at this junction in 94% to 100% of individuals, and this is the most common site for clinically significant reflux.[9] The great saphenous vein has approximately six valves and branches into an anterior branch and posterior arch below the knee. The small saphenous vein runs along the calf, has 7 to 10 valves. Although the anatomy has much variation, it usually connects to the deep system at the popliteal vein via the saphenopopliteal junction.[9]

There are more than 150 PVs in the lower extremity; however, only four groups are clinically significant, and they may be found within the foot, medial and lateral leg, and thigh.[10] These perforators directly empty into the deep venous system or indirectly via venous sinuses of the lower leg. The thigh and calf perforators contain one to three valves and provide a pathway for blood to flow from the superficial to deep venous system. In contrast, perforating veins in the foot direct blood from the deep to superficial systems.[10] The medial lower leg perforators include the paratibial (or Sherman and Boyd) and posterior tibial (or Cockett) PV. Paratibial PV direct blood from the posterior arch and great saphenous vein to the posterior tibial veins, whereas posterior tibial PV connect the posterior accessory great saphenous vein with the posterior tibial veins. The medial thigh PV includes the inguinal and femoral canal (Dodd) perforators, and these connect the great saphenous vein with the superficial femoral vein at the groin or proximal to the knee, respectively.[7]

The deep veins run with their similarly named arterial counterparts and are subfascial structures. The number of valves increases distally, with one valve at the external iliac-common femoral junction, one valve at the saphenofemoral junction, three valves in the proximal superficial femoral vein, two valves in the distal superficial femoral and popliteal veins, and numerous valves in the anterior and posterior tibial veins as well as the peroneal veins.[8,10] Venous sinuses are present in the deep compartments of the lower extremity, with both gastrocnemius and soleal sinuses. Although these muscular venous sinuses are valveless, they empty into adjacent valved veins and are the principle collecting system within the calf.[8]

PATHOPHYSIOLOGY

The physiology of venous return is useful in understanding the signs, symptoms, and treatments available for venous disease. Resting venous pressure is a function of capillary inflow, valve function, outflow obstruction, and muscle pump action. Approximately 90% of blood return occurs through the deep venous system through muscular contraction of the foot, calf, and thigh.[11] Under normal conditions, postcapillary venous pressure ranges between 12 and 18 mm Hg. However, in the dependent lower extremity, hydrostatic pressures can range from 30 to 100 mm Hg.[12] Contraction of the calf can generate pressures as high as 250 mm Hg, with a resultant ejection fraction of 65%.[13] Clinically it has been demonstrated that after walking 7 to 12 steps, lower-extremity venous pressure is reduced from 100 mm Hg to a mean of 22 mm Hg.[14] With intermittent muscle pump action (in the presence of competent valves), the deep veins empty, and the resting venous pressure is reduced. During muscular relaxation, venous pressure slowly rises secondary to capillary inflow as well as emptying from the superficial venous system via perforators. Thus, the valves serve to compartmentalize the hydrostatic column of blood and prevent reflux.[15]

Valvular dysfunction reduces venous emptying and contributes to venous hypertension through pathologic retrograde flow. In addition, in the presence of incompetent perforator valves, increased pressure may be transmitted back to the superficial venous system.[12] Venous hypertension can also lead to dilation of the venous segment below the malfunctioning valve, resulting in subsequent failure of the valve at this level. This simple pathology explains why patients with CVI consistently report that their symptoms are minimized in the morning, before getting out of bed. In the supine position, the effect of gravity is essentially eliminated from the venous system, thus minimizing pressure gradients across the valves. Large varicosities, essentially branches of refluxing veins that have been chronically under high pressure, may all but disappear with leg elevation.

The underlying etiology of venous disorders may be congenital, primary, or secondary. Primary venous disorders pertain to pathology without a precipitating event and involve structural and biochemical changes of the venous wall, whereas secondary disorders occur after an event, such as an acute deep venous thrombosis (DVT). According to the North American subfascial endoscopic perforator surgery (SEPS) registry, CVI results from primary venous disease in 70% of the population and from a postthrombotic state in 30%.[16] The pathogenesis of primary valve dysfunction is not entirely clear; however, connective tissue defects involving both the cellular and extracellular matrix have been identified. Multiple investigators have documented smooth muscle cell proliferation and infiltration, increased numbers of fibroblasts, and atrophied vasa vasora.[17-19] The composition of varicose veins has been found to have reduced total elastin content,[20] variations in both the content and types of collagen, and alterations in the activity of matrix metalloproteinases as well as their tissue inhibitors.[18,21,22] These changes in venous composition are thought to compromise the structural integrity of the vein wall, resulting in venous dilatation and the development of valvular incompetence, with reflux as a consequence.[23]

With secondary venous disorders, a deep venous thrombus can trigger an inflammatory response, which creates vein wall injury. The direct apposition of thrombus against the vein wall has been shown to activate leukocytes, upregulate activity of matrix metalloproteinases, and promote fibrosis.[24] In addition, recanalization of the vein is often incomplete with only 55% of patients demonstrating complete resolution of DVT within 6 to 9 months.[25] The resulting hemodynamic abnormality is thus one of both reflux and obstruction.[26]

The interaction of venous anatomy and physiology has yet to completely explain the clinical manifestations of CVI. Venous ulceration is not clearly colocalized with perforating veins, and single lesions may be associated with multiple levels of valvular incompetence within the superficial, deep, or perforating systems.[27] Despite these minor discrepancies, chronic venous hypertension typically has physical signs concordant with the severity of the underlying disease. Prolonged venous hypertension creates a hydrostatic profile that favors edema formation because of the transudation and exudation of macromolecules and fluid.[28] Hyperpigmentation can result from hemosiderin deposits within dermal macrophages after extravasated red blood cells are broken down.[29] Early signs of advanced disease are corona phlebectatica: numerous, fine intradermal veins overlying the medial or lateral aspects of the foot found in a fan-shaped pattern.[1] With more severe venous disease, fibrosis of the skin and subcutaneous tissue, known as lipodermatosclerosis, results secondary to localized, chronic inflammation.[1] Atrophie blanche is a localized, atrophic, white area of skin surrounded by dilated capillaries or hyperpigmentation, and is also a sign of severe CVI.[1] Venous ulceration is the most advanced form of venous disease and manifests as a full-thickness defect in the skin, with greater than 75% of lesions localized to the medial aspect of the ankle, about the distribution of the posterior arch.[27]

CLASSIFICATION

Given the panoply of signs and symptoms, the classification and treatment of CVI suffered from tremendous heterogeneity. A consensus statement regarding chronic venous disorders was released at the American Venous Forum in 1994, which proposed a standardized categorization of chronic venous disorders based on both the clinical classification and severity of disease.[11] The CEAP system was later updated in 2004 with seven categories of clinical manifestations (C), four etiologic categories (E), four categories of anatomic distribution (A), and four basic pathophysiologic categories (P)[1] (Table 51-1). The subgroups that describe the clinical manifestations include: class 0, no visible or palpable signs of venous disease (i.e., symptoms only); class 1, telangiectasias or

TABLE 51-1   Classification of Chronic Venous Insufficiency

C-Clinical Class	Characteristics
0	No visible or palpable signs of venous disease
1	Telangiectasias or reticular veins
2	Varicose veins (diameter of 3 mm or more)
3	Edema
4a	Pigmentation or eczema
4b	Lipodermatosclerosis or atrophie blanche
5	Healed venous ulcer
6	Active venous ulcer
A,S	Asymptomatic, symptomatic

The CEAP system considers the clinical class, etiology (congential, primary and secondary), anatomy (superficial, perforator or deep) and pathophysiology (reflux, obstruction or both). The clinical classes are listed above. Each clinical class is characterized by the presence or absence of symptoms (A or S).

reticular veins; class 2, varicose veins; class 3, edema; class 4, skin changes due to venous disease; class 5, skin changes with healed ulceration; and class 6, skin changes with active ulceration. The etiologic classification includes congenital, primary, secondary (post-thrombotic), or without any venous cause. Anatomic classification includes superficial, perforator, or deep veins, as well as no identifiable venous location. Finally, the basic pathophysiologic classification describes reflux, obstruction, both reflux and obstruction, or no venous pathophysiology identifiable.

In the CEAP revision, the following example is offered. A patient has painful swelling of the leg, varicose veins, lipodermatosclerosis, and active ulceration. Duplex scanning shows great saphenous vein reflux above and below the knee, incompetent calf perforator veins, and axial reflux in the femoral and popliteal veins. There are no signs of postthrombotic obstruction. Classification according to basic CEAP: C6s, Ep, Aspd, Pr.[1] Of note, physician-derived CEAP scores have been demonstrated to predict both symptom severity and patient-reported quality of life.[30]

DIAGNOSIS

The Society for Vascular Surgery (SVS) and the American Venous Forum (AVF) released practice guidelines for the care of patients with CVI.[31] The workup for CVI starts with a complete history and physical examination. There is a fair amount of variation in the presenting symptoms for the condition, but there are common elements in the history that are of great use in securing the diagnosis. Symptoms include pain, sensations of heaviness, swelling, aching, restless legs, cramps, itching, tingling, throbbing, and tired legs.[2] One of the hallmarks of CVI is symptom progression throughout the day, particularly when the patient has been standing for prolonged periods of time. This is true for subjective

complaints such as heaviness and fatigue, as well as more objective signs like swelling and engorged varicosities. Many patients, after determining this for themselves, will have learned to elevate their legs or have even started wearing compression stockings. Symptoms that occur during and after exercise, and improve with rest and leg elevation, may be indicative of venous claudication.[32] The history may also establish whether the etiology is primary, secondary, or congenital. The presence of prior DVT, history of a hypercoagulable state or any other factors that predispose patients to thrombosis (e.g., oral contraceptives, pregnancies, smoking), and family history of CVI or thrombotic disorders should be elicited.

The physical examination is useful not only for arriving at the diagnosis of CVI, but also for determining the pattern of disease. Patients should be examined standing, with attention paid to the presence of varicosities, palpable cords, tenderness, thrills, bruits, or pulsatility. The presence of telangiectasia, leg swelling, induration, hyperpigmentation, corona phlebectatica, lipodermatosclerosis, atrophie blanche, or ulceration must be carefully noted.[31] CVI can certainly coexist with peripheral arterial disease; therefore the pedal pulses must be checked and documented. The saphenous veins themselves should be sought, and if they can be seen or felt, their size and depth should be noted. For patients with numerous varicosities, a diagram can be drawn or a digital photograph taken. Swelling is best documented by taking measurements of the leg below the knee and at the ankle. The time of day of the measurements should be recorded as well, for there can be considerable variation as was previously described. Finally, one must record the presence of any varicosities that have eroded, or appear to be on the verge of eroding, through the skin. When this occurs, the bleeding can be impressive, and patients should be instructed on how to dress their leg if this occurs.

The anatomic pattern should be established, with an attempt to determine whether signs are localized to the superficial, deep, or perforator systems; this can be accomplished with duplex ultrasonography.[31] This modality is more accurate than continuous-wave Doppler ultrasound, as B-mode imaging can help to identify anatomic points of obstruction or turbulence and to determine directionality of flow.[12] The SVS/AVF clinical practice guidelines describe four components of the examination: visibility, compressibility, venous flow, and augmentation.[31] In addition, confirmation of valvular incompetence should be performed in the upright position using one of the following methods. A Valsalva maneuver will increase intraabdominal pressure, and should be performed in conjunction with duplex assessment of the common femoral vein or the saphenofemoral junction. Alternatively, manual or cuff compression and release of the limb distal to the point of examination can be performed to evaluate the more distal veins.[31] Many noninvasive vascular laboratories have a protocol for CVI, and the clinician should always specify why the venous examination is being ordered. The study should include all the elements of a DVT study as well as examination of the great and small saphenous veins. Notation should be made whether reflux occurs spontaneously, and it is useful to document the presence of reflux with the patient in a standing position. The recommended cutoff value for reflux is 1 second in the femoral and popliteal veins, whereas it is 500 ms for the great saphenous, small saphenous, tibial, deep femoral, and perforating veins.[31] However, many health insurers require greater times; therefore the actual time should be carefully recorded in the study. The sizes of the saphenous veins are needed as well, and these structures should be measured at the level of the saphenofemoral junction, the mid thigh and just below the knee (for great saphenous vein [GSV]), and at the popliteal space and ankle (for small saphenous vein [SSV]). These size measurements should also be performed with the patient in a standing position. Larger varicosities should be examined as well, and reflux should be reported if present. As with the saphenous veins, the sizes of the branches need to be recorded in the study. Finally, perforator veins need to be noted in the study. Those with an outward flow of duration greater than 500 ms or a diameter greater than 3.5 mm, which are associated with a healed or open venous ulcer, are considered pathologic, but these perforators should be noted even in the absence of localized disease.[31]

The basic CEAP system, described earlier, should be used to determine the class, etiology, anatomy, and pathophysiologic classification of CVI.[1] An adjunct evaluative instrument, the revised Venous Clinical Severity Score (VCSS) released by Vasquez and colleagues, should also be incorporated to document the severity of CVI.[33] It generates a score based on (1) patient-reported intensity of pain or other discomfort, (2) severity of varicose veins, (3) severity of lower extremity edema, (4) degree of skin pigmentation, (5) extent of inflammation, (6) distribution of induration, (7) number of active ulcers, and (8) duration of active ulceration.[33] In conjunction, these instruments will provide unambiguous classification and a means of serial assessment for patients with CVI.

TREATMENT

For most patients, the diagnosis of CVI is secured with the history, physical examination, and duplex ultrasonography. The initial therapy for the vast majority of patients with mild venous insufficiency is conservative treatment with (1) compression, (2) leg elevation, and (3) nonsteroidal antiinflammatory drugs (NSAIDs). Compression therapy exists in various forms, including elastic stockings, Unna boot, elastic wraps, and pneumatic compression devices, and is recommended to reduce ambulatory venous hypertension. While supine, superficial venous pressures range from 20 to 25 mm Hg; whereas while standing, pressures can be measured as high as 100 mm Hg.[12] In the upright position, applying pressures greater than 60 mm Hg is required to occlude the superficial veins, whereas 35 to 40 mm Hg of pressure has been demonstrated to narrow them.[34] In a study of more than 100 patients, treatment with 30 to 40 mm Hg stockings in patients with CVI, described as CEAP clinical classes 0 to 6, resulted in improvement of pain, edema, skin changes, and overall well-being at 16 months.[35] However, a recent systematic review of

TABLE 51-2 Compression Stocking Options

Pressure	Clinical Situation
15-20 mm Hg	Mild edema, mild varicosities, aching legs
20-30 mm Hg	Advanced aching/fatigue, moderate edema, DVT prophylaxis
30-40 mm Hg	Established CVI, advanced edema, post thrombotic state
40-50 mm Hg	Severe edema, open venous ulceration
≥50 mm Hg	Severe edema not responsive to lesser pressures, severe post thrombotic syndrome

DVT, Deep venous thrombosis; CVI, chronic venous insufficiency. Graded compression stockings are available in a range of pressures. Venous indications for the pressures are listed above. They are also available in various lengths, from knee-high up to panty hose. Consideration should be given to the likelihood that the patient will wear the garments; a knee-high stocking is more beneficial if the patient uses it than a more restrictive appliance that is avoided.

compression stockings for uncomplicated varicose veins found that although compression therapy provided symptomatic relief, there was no evidence for prevention of varicose vein recurrence or cessation of disease progression.[36] The SVS/AVF Guideline Committee currently suggests stockings with an ankle pressure of 20 to 30 mm Hg for treatment of symptomatic varicose veins.[31] With more significant CVI, compression therapy is the standard of care. A systematic review of graded compression for venous ulcers confirmed that this modality improves the healing of ulcers, with greater effectiveness found with higher levels of compression.[37] Most patients with typical CVI symptoms are prescribed stockings of 20 to 30 mm Hg, with different levels of compression available for various indications (Table 51-2). The length of the garment depends on the patient's pattern of disease and the location of tender varicose branches. Typically, a stocking that is knee-high will suffice, and patients will more consistently use garments of this length instead of longer, more restrictive stockings.

As mentioned previously, many patients determine on their own that elevation is beneficial in alleviating their symptoms. As part of their conservative treatment, the physician should encourage the patient to find time to elevate his or her legs at intervals throughout the day. Many patients find that they are able to continue exercise regimens if they elevate their legs for a period of time directly following these activities. For patients with continued aching and pain, NSAIDs can be helpful, and are considered an integral part of first-line conservative therapy. Additional adjuvant conservative therapy may consist of weight loss when appropriate.

Throughout the course of conservative treatment, the physician must follow the progress of the patient and note any effects of the therapy. The therapy itself can have diagnostic implications. For example, a patient who has no benefit from compressive therapy may have a different etiology for their symptoms. If a patient tries but is unable to tolerate the compression stockings, this must be clearly documented in the medical record. Patients are occasionally wary of reporting a beneficial effect of compression, because they may be under the false impression that if their stockings are helpful, they will not receive any further therapy. Although most health insurers require a trial of compression therapy usually in the range of 6 weeks to 6 months, patients will usually qualify for treatment if there is an appropriate definitive therapy available.

Patients with CVI secondary to GSV or SSV incompetence may be treated with open surgery or endovenous ablation. The classic high ligation and stripping of the GSV or SSV involved division of the GSV at the junction with the common femoral vein, along with all its tributaries, and removal with a vein stripping device.[38] The incompetent vein is removed from the circulation so that passive reflux of venous pressure down the leg does not occur. However, with stripping from the groin to the ankle, saphenous nerve injury frequently occurs, and the technique has been modified to remove the vein from the groin to the knee only.[39] Additional refinements such as stab phlebectomy for varicose veins in the calf and transilluminated powered phlebectomy have made the procedures for branch removal less invasive.[40,41]

More recently, endovenous techniques have replaced open surgical treatment of CVI. These procedures essentially reproduce the effects of high ligation and stripping of the saphenous veins, are done in a minimally invasive fashion, and are routinely performed in an office setting with local anesthesia. All endovenous ablation works by thermal destruction of the vein. Direct thermal injury results in endothelial destruction, denatured collagen in the media, and both fibrotic and thrombotic venous occlusion.[31] The source of heat generation is either a laser fiber (endovenous laser therapy [EVLT]) or a radiofrequency generator (radiofrequency ablation [RFA]). Both of these sources of energy produce high, focused temperatures. As a result, normal body temperature can be maintained within 5 mm of an RFA catheter that is 120° C at its surface or a laser fiber with a temperature of 1000° C. This method prevents extended thermal damage to the vein and surrounding tissues (particularly the skin and adjacent nerves) during treatment. The principles of therapy are the same for both modalities and for treatment of both the GSV and SSV. Initially, there must be confirmation that the vein is refluxing, enlarged (greater than 4 to 5 mm with patient standing), no greater than 1.5 cm, and not excessively tortuous (which precludes catheter advancement). The vein is accessed under ultrasound guidance, usually 5 to 10 cm below the knee, and a sheath is placed in the vein. A laser fiber or RFA catheter is then advanced through the sheath under ultrasound and positioned 2 to 3 cm from either the saphenofemoral or saphenopopliteal junction. This portion of the case is done under great care, because inadvertent placement of the catheter too close to the deep system can cause damage to the deep veins. The target vein is then surrounded with tumescent anesthetic. This solution is composed of saline, lidocaine, epinephrine, and bicarbonate, and it accomplishes three goals: (1) anesthesia of the target area, (2) the prevention of thermal injury via a heat sink, and (3) compression of the target vein. The GSV is located between layers of fascia, and the fluid can be administered between these layers such that the

vein is both surrounded and depressed away from the skin to a minimal depth of 2 cm. The bed is than placed in a steep Trendelenburg position to further empty the target vein, and the energy is applied while the physician provides external pressure over the segment of vein being treated. For the RFA, segments of 7 cm of vein are treated for 20 seconds, and then the catheter is backed up in a retrograde fashion. For the EVLT, there is continuous withdrawal of the catheter at a rate of 1 to 2 mm/s for the first 10 cm, and 2 to 3 mm/s for the remaining distance. The process of actual thermal ablation is rapid, and on the order of 90 to 120 seconds for both modalities. The sheath and catheter are removed, and the patient's leg is wrapped with an ace bandage for 48 hours. Patients are encouraged to ambulate in the immediate post procedural time, but also to elevate their legs following light activities. Strict bed rest is discouraged, because it could theoretically lead to thrombotic complications.

Follow-up in most practices includes physical examination of the treated leg and a duplex ultrasound examination of treated vein and the saphenofemoral junction within 48 to 72 hours. For the GSV, the ideal finding is an occluded GSV with a maintained epigastric vein (Figure 51-1). Complications include bruising and hematoma formation (usually associated with the injection of the tumescent anesthetic), paresthesias secondary to nerve injury, and rarely thermal injury to the skin. As stated earlier, a more serious complication of endovenous thermal ablation is extension of a thrombus from the GSV into the deep venous system; this has been reported with an incidence as high as 16% of procedures,[42] although in most series this number is less than 1%. Lawrence and colleagues[43] established a classification system for the level of proximal endovenous closure of

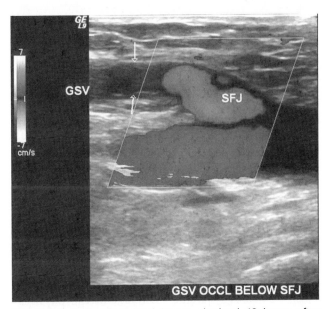

FIGURE 51-1 ■ An ultrasound image obtained 48 hours after endovenous ablation of the great saphenous vein (GSV) is shown. The GSV is occluded, as evidenced by the lack of color flow. The saphenofemoral junction is patent, and clearly there is no involvement with the common femoral vein (blue flow on scan). See Color Plate 51-1.

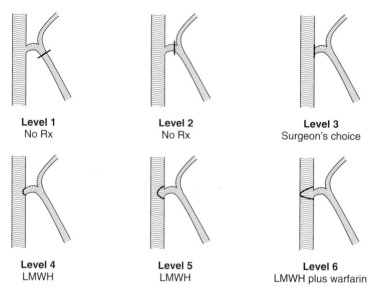

Level 1	Level 2	Level 3
No Rx	No Rx	Surgeon's choice

Level 4	Level 5	Level 6
LMWH	LMWH	LMWH plus warfarin

FIGURE 51-2 ■ Classification of closure level and treatment algorithm.

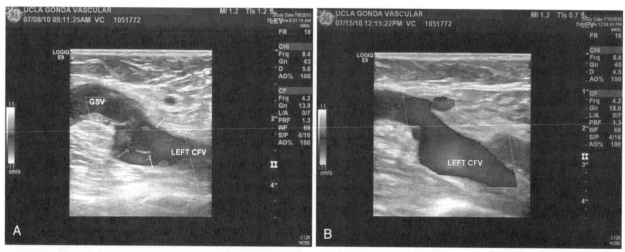

FIGURE 51-3 ■ **A,** Initial scan after radiofrequency ablation demonstrates thrombus extending into the common femoral vein. This patient was given enoxaparin (Lovenox), and the scan was repeated 1 week later. **B,** Note the complete retraction of the thrombus and patency of the epigastric vein on the follow-up scan. Lovenox was stopped after the second scan demonstrated an appropriate level of closure. Of note, most patients with level 4 and 5 closures do not have postprocedure symptoms that differ from patients with closure levels of 3 or less. See Color Plate 51-3.

the GSV and proposed a standardized treatment algorithm for thrombus extension. Closure levels were graded from levels 1 to 6 based on the extent of thrombus extension into the femoral vein, in proximity to the epigastric vein, as follows (Figure 51-2): (1) below the epigastric vein, (2) flush with the orifice of the epigastric vein, (3) flush with the saphenofemoral junction, (4) bulging into the common femoral vein, (5) past the saphenofemoral junction and adherent to the adjacent wall, and (6) into the common femoral vein—consistent with DVT. Levels 1 to 2 require no postoperative treatment, level 3 can be managed at the discretion of the physician with either observation and repeated duplex ultrasound or with low-molecular-weight heparin (LMWH), levels 4 to 5 warrant treatment with LMWH until thrombus retraction is observed, and level 6 demands systemic anticoagulation for 3 months. Of the 500 patients studied,

99.6% had successful occlusion of the GSV; however, 2.6% were found to have a thrombus of level 4 or greater. The authors noted that a significantly higher rate of thrombus extension occurred in patients with a history of DVT or with a GSV diameter greater than 8 mm.[43] Although progression to true DVT and even pulmonary embolism have been reported, the thrombus following endovenous ablation is really better thought of as endovenous heat-induced thrombus than DVT, because the behavior of this thrombus tends to follow a more self-limited course than does conventional DVT (Figure 51-3).

Long-term studies of RFA using first-generation devices have revealed occlusion rates of 87% at 1 and 5 years after the procedure in more than 1200 treated limbs.[44] They identified three types of anatomic failures, including: (1) nonocclusion owing to primary treatment failure, (2) recanalization after an initially successful ablation, and (3) groin reflux involving an accessory vein. In patients with any type of failure, they still reported improvement of pain, fatigue, and edema in 70% to 80% of limbs. This clinical symptom improvement was even greater (85% to 94% of limbs) in patients with anatomic success. The authors noted that catheter pullback speed and body mass index were significant risk factors for anatomic failure, and those with type II or III failures were prone to recurrent varicose veins.[44] A more recent report using a newer device describes occlusion rates of 99.6% at 3 days, 3 months, and 6 months, with sustained improvements in Venous Clinical Severity Scores.[45] Long-term results of EVLT reveal similar outcomes. In a study of 499 limbs, 98.2% demonstrated immediate successful GSV occlusion, and closure similarly persisted at 2 years (93.4%).

TREATMENT OF BRANCHES AND PERFORATORS

Many patients with CVI have large, symptomatic varicosities. During a duplex examination, an astute clinician will note that a large varicose vein branching from the saphenous system can essentially siphon off the majority of refluxing flow. In this situation, the GSV appears enlarged down the level where the branch joins it. The GSV can all but disappear below this level, while the branch, now running superficial to the saphenous fascia, attains a very large size. Phlebectomy is often performed in combination with saphenous vein ablation in order to address both the varicosities and eliminate the etiological source of reflux. These branches, if straight, can be accessed directly and treated with endovenous ablation. However, these branches are usually tortuous and must be treated using an alternate modality. For larger branches, Muller microstab phlebectomy works well.[46] Tumescent local anesthesia is injected about the veins, 2- to 3-mm incisions are made adjacent to the varicosity, and a hook-shaped instrument is inserted and used to grasp the vein and to lift it above the level of the skin. The branch is then gently rotated to disrupt the connections to the surrounding tissues, and gentle traction is continued until the vein avulses. Pressure is held over the site for several minutes, and a compression dressing avoids the formation of a hematoma. Transilluminated powered phlebectomy (TIPP) is an alterative technique that uses an endoscopic device with a fiber-optic light source and irrigation pump, and an endoscopic tissue dissector. A randomized trial comparing stab phlebectomy and TIPP for local avulsion of varicose veins found that patients who underwent TIPP had significantly fewer incisions; however, they reported increased bruising, prolonged pain at 6 weeks, and reduced early postoperative quality of life.[47] In contemporary venous practice, TIPP has become less commonly used.

Although the pathophysiologic role of incompetent perforating veins in the development of venous ulceration has been established, the indications for their ablation are unclear. Historically, to ablate these veins, large operations were required to access the subfascial anatomy.

Several minimally invasive techniques are now used, including SEPS, percutaneous ablation, RFA, EVLT, and sclerotherapy. SEPS involves balloon dissection and CO_2 insufflation to access the subfascial space. A paratibial fasciotomy is necessary to identify medial perforating veins, and endoscopic clips or a harmonic scalpel can be used to ligate perforating veins. The North American SEPS Registry described the results from 17 medical centers in the United States and Canada for patients with CVI. VCSS was significantly improved in most patients, and cumulative ulcer healing was 88% by 1 year and 95% by 2 years.[48] In subgroup analysis, they also examined patients who underwent SEPS without saphenous vein ablation. They still identified significant improvements in clinical scores, but also identified significantly reduced cumulative ulcer healing at 1 year (78%) and 2 years (88%). A systematic review of outcomes in patients undergoing treatment for CVI by SEPS (both with and without saphenous vein ablation) similarly described healing of ulcers in 88% of treated limbs, with 13% recurrence at a mean of 21 months. However, the authors qualified their recommendations because of the study's inability to discern the contribution of saphenous vein closure or compression therapy.

More recent data suggest a demonstrable connection between the treatment of incompetent perforator veins and venous ulcer healing. In a study looking at recalcitrant venous ulceration, patients who underwent ablation of their perforator veins had a 90% healing rate, and this was in patients undergoing intensive wound care both before and after their perforator treatment.[49] Additional studies with detailed mapping of the wound healing process have confirmed these findings.[50]

SCLEROTHERAPY

Another alternative for the treatment of both varicose branches and smaller spider and reticular veins is sclerotherapy. In this treatment, the vein is injected with a detergent solution (e.g., polidocanol, sodium morrhuate, sodium tetradecyl sulfate), osmotic sclerosant (e.g., hypertonic saline), or alcohol agent (e.g., chromated or nonchromated glycerin). The material damages the endothelium in the target vessel and exposes subendothelial collagen fibers, leading eventually to obliteration.[31] Hypertonic saline is used in a concentration of 23.4% and results in osmotic dehydration of endothelial cells followed by cell death. Polidocanol is the most commonly used agent and is injected in concentrations between 0.6% to 3% depending on the size of the vein. Sodium tetradecyl sulfate (STS) is used in concentrations of 0.125% to 3% in a similar fashion. These agents are injected intraluminally, starting proximally, with a maximum volume of 1 mL per site, and no more than 20 injections per session.[51] A multicenter, randomized trial comparing 0.5% polidocanol and 1% STS for the treatment of telangiectasia and reticular veins, demonstrated superiority of polidocanol in terms of effectiveness and patient satisfaction.[52] Sclerotherapy has been used primarily for closure of spider veins or telangiectasia, but foam sclerotherapy has been found to be a safe and effective method to treat varicose veins. A ratio of 1 part STS or polidocanol to 4 parts air is mixed, using a three-way stopcock connected to two syringes.[53] The veins are injected starting with the saphenous trunk, followed by varicose and perforating veins, and a maximum of 20 mL is injected per session. After both liquid and foam sclerotherapy, patients are then instructed to wear 30- to 40-mm Hg graduated compression stockings for 1 to 2 weeks. A multicenter, randomized trial was conducted to compare 3% polidocanol in foam or liquid forms, for treatment of primary varicose veins because of an incompetent GSV.[54] They reported elimination of reflux in 69% and 27% of patients who underwent foam or liquid sclerotherapy, respectively. These procedures can also be performed under ultrasound guidance, and there are advocates of using foam sclerotherapy for treatment of everything from the refluxing saphenous veins and their associated branches to perforator veins and spider veins. At this time, insurance coverage varies widely, with many plans denying use of sclerotherapy because of the lack of a randomized prospective trial demonstrating rates of venous closure commiserate with that achieved by endovenous ablation.

CONCLUSIONS

CVI is a common condition with underappreciated clinical sequelae. Newer technologies allow the modern clinician to approach this disorder with an array of minimally invasive therapies that are especially useful in a patient population that is frequently young, working, and active. Developing a practice to care for CVI requires the clinician to develop the skills to interpret venous duplex scans, both for diagnosis and during treatment. An understanding of the pathophysiology behind the disorder allows the clinician to appropriately diagnose and treat CVI with techniques that are both acceptable to the patients and successful in correcting the disorder.

References available online at expertconsult.com.

QUESTIONS

1. Which of the following situations is most closely associated with EHIT?
   a. History of superficial thrombophlebitis
   b. Reflux in both the superficial and deep systems
   c. Double treatment with laser or radiofrequency catheter along entire length of vein
   d. 18 mm diameter of saphenous vein at level of saphenofemoral junction
   e. Use of oral contraceptive pills

2. Which of the following statements is true?
   a. There is greater anatomic variation at the saphenofemoral junction than the saphenopopliteal junction.
   b. The vein of Giacomini provides a direct connection between the greater saphenous vein and the deep system of the thigh.
   c. There are no valves in the popliteal veins.
   d. Perforator vein flow should be superficial to deep in normal flow conditions.
   e. The posterior and anterior arch veins typically arise above the knee.

3. Which of the following is true regarding the CEAP classification system?
   a. CEAP class 3 represents edema.
   b. CEAP 4b represents eczema
   c. The etiologic classification includes congenital as a criterion.
   d. CEAP class 2 requires varicose veins greater than 2 mm in size.
   e. Patients with healed ulcers are CEAP class 5.

4. Which of the following is a component of treatment for reflux disease?
   a. Leg elevation
   b. Compression stockings
   c. Manual massage of the lower extremities
   d. Non-steroidal anti-inflammatory agents
   e. Endovenous ablation.

5. With regard to endovenous ablation, the role of tumescent anesthesia is:
   a. not needed with EVLT
   b. only needed when treating the entire length of saphenous vein
   c. to deaden sensory nerves running inside the saphenous vein
   d. helpful for draining blood from the saphenous vein
   e. not needed if adequate Trendelenburg position is attained.

6. A post endovenous ablation scan demonstrates a level 2 closure. This patient:
   a. needs a follow up scan within a week.
   b. needs to start low molecular weight heparin and then Coumadin.
   c. should have a hypercoaguable work up initiated.
   d. needs no further treatment.
   e. should be placed on periprocedural lovenox if the contralateral leg is treated.

7. Which of the following regarding perforator veins is true?
   a. Refluxing perforator veins are a common cause of CEAP class 2 disease.
   b. Treatment always requires open surgical ligation.
   c. Perforator reflux should be dealt with before saphenous reflux.
   d. Foam sclerotherapy is more effective than laser for treating perforator reflux.
   e. Perforator treatment is usually indicated in patients with CEAP 5 or 6 disease.

8. Which of the following is not a consideration when planning endovenous ablation?
   a. Use of compression stockings
   b. Depth of the target vein
   c. Ability of patient to tolerate epinephrine containing tumescence.
   d. Tortuosity of target vein
   e. Age of patient

9. Which of the following has not been reported following endovenous ablation?
   a. Sural nerve injury
   b. Arterial thrombosis
   c. Acute suppurative thrombophlebitis
   d. Pulmonary embolism
   e. Skin burns

10. Which of the below agents is a detergent used for sclerotherapy?
    a. Glycerin
    b. Hypertonic saline
    c. Polidocanol
    d. Doxycycline
    e. Lidocaine

ANSWERS

1. **d**
2. **d**
3. **a**
4. **c**
5. **d**
6. **d**
7. **e**
8. **e**
9. **b**
10. **c**

CHAPTER 52

PORTAL HYPERTENSION

David A. Rigberg • Hugh A. Gelabert

Portal hypertension and variceal hemorrhage are important clinical problems in which vascular surgeons may still have a significant interest and concern. New developments have altered the once-familiar face of this disease, with endoscopic and endovascular approaches having replaced what was once a disease process treated predominantly with open surgical procedures. Orthotopic liver transplantation has also found a vital role in essentially curing this process in appropriately selected patients.

For a surgeon to have a role in treating these patients, it is of paramount importance to have a clear understanding of the effects of underlying liver disease, the pathophysiology of portal hypertension, and the management of these problems. The goal of this chapter is to provide a solid basis for determining the cause of hepatic disease, understanding the presentation, and managing portal hypertension.

DEFINITION

Portal hypertension is a condition in which the circulation of blood in the portal venous system is impeded, resulting in an increase in portal venous pressure. Elevation of the portal venous blood pressure results in a series of physiologic alterations, including ascites, hypersplenism, and variceal hemorrhage. Normal portal venous pressure is between 5 and 10 mm Hg. Portal hypertension is said to be present when portal pressure is elevated above 15 mm Hg. Clinically significant portal hypertension exists when the portal pressure is elevated more than 10 mm Hg above systemic pressure as measured at the inferior vena cava (corrected portal pressure).

The natural history of patients with portal hypertension differs, depending on the cause of the condition and the stage of presentation. The patient's ability to withstand the stress of hemorrhage or surgery largely depends on the functional hepatic reserve.

PATHOGENESIS

Physiologically, portal hypertension results from either an increase in the portal blood flow (rare) or an obstruction to the outflow of blood from the portal circulation (common). Obstructions to the portal circulation have been classified anatomically based on their location relative to the hepatic sinusoids. Accordingly, the obstruction may be presinusoidal, sinusoidal, or postsinusoidal.

Presinusoidal and postsinusoidal obstructions have been subclassified as intrahepatic or extrahepatic (Box 52-1).

Extrahepatic Presinusoidal Obstruction

Presinusoidal extrahepatic obstruction is most commonly due to thrombosis of the portal vein. Although less common than other forms of obstructive portal hypertension, portal vein thrombosis occurs in a significant number of children. It can occur in adults, but the causes are remarkably different between children and adults.

Portal vein thrombosis in children occurs as a complication of an infectious process such as omphalitis and appendicitis (most common causes). In adults, the most common cause of portal vein thrombosis is a gradual and relentless decrease in the portal blood flow secondary to the high resistance in the hepatic circulation caused by cirrhosis. Other causes in adults include pancreatitis, hypercoagulable states or tumor thrombus, and mechanical obstruction of portal venous flow. The last may be the result of malignant invasion, lymphadenopathy, or caudate lobe compression. Hypercoagulable conditions may result from polycythemia, cancer, or hypovolemia. Sepsis can lead to portal vein thrombosis by several mechanisms: low-flow states, hypovolemia, and activation of the coagulation system.

Intrahepatic Presinusoidal Obstruction

Most causes of intrahepatic presinusoidal obstructive portal hypertension relate to fibrosis and compression of the portal venules, with subsequent restriction of portal flow. Included among these diseases are congenital hepatic fibrosis, sarcoidosis, chronic arsenic exposure, Wilson disease, hepatoportal sclerosis, primary biliary cirrhosis, schistosomiasis, and myeloproliferative disorders.

Schistosomiasis is the most common cause of portal hypertension in third-world countries. Deposition of ova in the portal vein walls results in a granulomatous inflammatory reaction, which in turn results in fibrosis and portal flow restriction. Hepatic function is preserved in the early stages, but later stages of this disease are characterized by advanced cirrhosis and loss of hepatic function.[1] Myeloproliferative disorders such as myelosclerosis and myeloid leukemia occasionally lead to presinusoidal hypertension by virtue of the deposition of primitive cellular material infiltrating the portal zones.[2] Sarcoidosis causes portal hypertension by two mechanisms: sarcoid

PRESINUSOIDAL

Extrahepatic: portal vein thrombosis
  Omphalitis
  Pancreatitis
  Trauma
  Malignancy
  Polycythemia
  Periportal lymphadenopathy
Intrahepatic
  Biliary atresia
  Schistosomiasis
  Sarcoidosis
  Arsenic toxicity
  Congenital hepatic fibrosis
  Myeloproliferative disorders
  Primary biliary cirrhosis
  Hepatoportal sclerosis

SINUSOIDAL

Cirrhosis
Toxic hepatitis
Fatty metamorphosis

POSTSINUSOIDAL

Intrahepatic
  Cirrhosis
  Postnecrotic
  Portal
  Hemochromatosis
Veno-occlusive disease
Extrahepatic
  Budd-Chiari syndrome
  Hepatic vein webs
  Malignant obstruction
  Oral contraceptives
  Pregnancy
  Plant alkaloids
Cardiac causes
  Congestive heart failure
  Constrictive pericarditis

INCREASED BLOOD FLOW: ARTERIOVENOUS FISTULAS

Splenic artery to splenic vein
Hepatic artery to portal vein

---

granulomas within the portal vein leading to obstruction, and increased portal blood flow.

Hepatic function is usually preserved in the early stages of these diseases. In later stages, significant hepatic impairment may result from progressive cirrhosis. Hemodynamic characteristics are similar to those of extrahepatic portal vein obstruction: low hepatic wedge pressure and elevated portal venous pressure.

Intrahepatic Sinusoidal and Postsinusoidal Obstruction

Sinusoidal portal hypertension may be the sequela of alcoholic hepatitis, viral hepatitis, or toxic hepatitis. Although pure sinusoidal obstruction is relatively rare, it is frequently part of a combined sinusoidal and postsinusoidal obstructive picture. As such, it is the most common cause of portal hypertension in the United States and is estimated to be the tenth leading cause of death. Postsinusoidal obstruction is seen most commonly in cases of alcoholic liver disease, postnecrotic cirrhosis, or hemochromatosis. As would be expected in these diseases, hepatic function is usually significantly impaired.

Two mechanisms account for the portal hypertension in these patients. First is the mechanical obstruction of the portal blood flow by the regenerating hepatic nodules and cirrhotic bands within the damaged liver. These changes may extend beyond the confines of the hepatic sinusoids, accounting for the presence of presinusoidal, sinusoidal, and postsinusoidal distortion of the hepatic architecture. The second element is an increase in the splanchnic perfusion, in part attributed to the genesis of multiple arteriovenous shunts and collateral channels. One third of portal blood flow may bypass functional hepatocytes through these channels.[3] The clinical correlate of this increased blood flow is the hyperdynamic state that typifies cirrhosis: elevated cardiac output and a diminished systemic resistance.[4]

The portal hemodynamic characteristics of these diseases usually consist of elevated hepatic wedge pressure along with elevated portal vein pressure. Because most of these diseases directly affect hepatocytes, hepatic function is frequently impaired, even in the early stages of disease. These patients frequently have poor hepatic reserve and decompensate with each bleeding episode. Selection and timing of interventions are important aspects of their management.

Extrahepatic Postsinusoidal Obstruction

Postsinusoidal hepatic vein obstruction is usually the result of thrombosis in the hepatic veins. Although the cause of most cases is unknown, a number of associated diseases have been identified. Membranous webs of the hepatic veins, malignancies (hepatomas, renal carcinomas, adrenal carcinomas), trauma, pregnancy, contraceptive use, acute alcoholic hepatitis, veno-occlusive disease, and *Senecio* species (ragwort) toxicity may all result in hepatic vein thrombosis.[5] Constrictive pericarditis and chronic congestive heart failure may also cause postsinusoidal obstruction.

Budd-Chiari syndrome is the result of hepatic venous occlusive disease and is characterized by massive ascites, esophageal varices, variceal hemorrhage, hepatic failure, and death. Chiari disease is due to primary hepatic vein ostial occlusion. The clinical progression after hepatic vein occlusion may be fulminant or gradual. Hepatic failure is the result of chronic congestion and ischemia from impaired hepatic blood flow. The factors that determine the rate of progression are not well understood. Angiography is essential in establishing the diagnosis; it identifies the presence of thrombus and its location.[6,7]

The fulminant course is marked by rapid development of ascites, fatigue, and jaundice. In addition, elevated liver enzymes and prothrombin time indicate hepatocellular damage. Patients who do not improve with anticoagulation should be considered for either shunting or liver transplantation.

The more gradual presentation may have many similar features, such as ascites and chronic fatigue, but hepatic function is preserved to a greater degree. Hypersplenism and variceal hemorrhage may be more prominent features in these patients.

An initial trial of anticoagulation may allow endogenous fibrinolysis to resolve the venous thrombosis. Patients whose course is gradually progressive and who have intact hepatocellular function should be considered for portal decompression by a portacaval, mesocaval, or mesoatrial shunt. Shunt selection is dependent on the patient's anatomy, as defined by angiography. When the Budd-Chiari syndrome leads to deterioration of hepatic function, as demonstrated by abnormal liver function tests, hepatic transplantation is the procedure of choice.[8]

Arteriovenous Fistulas

As a cause of portal hypertension, arteriovenous fistulas are relatively rare. Most fistulas are either traumatic or splenic. Traumatic arteriovenous fistulas may occur as a consequence of transhepatic biliary manipulations or as a result of penetrating trauma. Splenic fistulas may be associated with splenic artery aneurysms, sarcoidosis, Gaucher's disease, myeloid metaplasia, or tropical splenomegaly. Women of childbearing age are at greatest risk. The portal hypertension results initially from increased flow in the portal circulation. At later stages, fibrosis, along with secondary obstruction of the presinusoidal spaces, exacerbates the portal hypertension.

DIAGNOSIS

The diagnosis of portal hypertension rests on demonstrating increased portal venous pressure or the anatomic evidence of this increased pressure. In practical terms, the diagnosis of portal hypertension is made by identifying signs of elevated portal venous pressure in a patient with a history that supports these findings.

The signs of elevated portal venous pressure include the presence of esophageal varices, splenomegaly, ascites, or abdominal wall collaterals. Ascites, splenomegaly, and abdominal wall collateralization may be apparent on physical examination. Esophagogastric endoscopy is currently considered the most reliable means of identifying gastroesophageal varices.

Signs of underlying hepatic disease include spider angiomas, palmar erythema, gynecomastia, muscle wasting, loss of pubertal hair growth, and testicular atrophy. Encephalopathy, asterixis, fetor hepaticus, and fatigue may also be noted in patients with chronic hepatic insufficiency. The presence of liver disease is not conclusive evidence that the patient has significant portal hypertension.

Historical support for the diagnosis of portal hypertension includes identification of any of the diseases that are known to lead to portal hypertension (e.g., alcohol ingestion, hepatitis, hepatotoxins). The duration of such problems is also important in substantiating the diagnosis of portal hypertension. Both alcoholic toxicity and viral hepatitis lead to cirrhosis and usually portal hypertension, but the time between the onset of these insults and the development of hypertension may be 10 years or more.

Adjunctive means of demonstrating portal hypertension include angiography and hemodynamic measurements. Neither is essential to making the diagnosis; both are supportive. Angiography may reveal both splenomegaly and collateralization in the portal region and the gastroesophageal axis. In addition, angiography may provide information regarding the direction of portal blood flow (hepatopetal or hepatofugal).

Hemodynamic measurement of the portal circulation is most commonly accomplished by transjugular venous catheterization and measurement of the wedge hepatic vein pressure.[9] This technique is able to record the pressure in the hepatic veins and the hepatic sinusoids. Elevations of the wedge pressure reflect elevations in the portal venous pressure. False-negative results may be encountered in patients with presinusoidal obstruction and in cases of catheter malfunction. Normal hepatic venous pressure is essentially the same as the right atrial pressure (0 to 5 mm Hg); portal venous pressure is approximately 2 to 6 mm Hg higher than hepatic venous pressure. A gradient greater than 10 mm Hg is considered abnormal.

Other methods of measuring portal venous pressure have been developed but have largely been abandoned because of the increased risk associated with them. These tests include direct cannulation of the portal vein (requires surgical exposure), percutaneous transhepatic portal venous catheterization, transjugular portal vein catheterization, and percutaneous splenic pulp pressure measurement.[10]

The most recent development in assessing the portal circulation is the application of noninvasive ultrasonography. Duplex scanning has been used to establish patency and measure the direction and velocity of portal blood flow. Information gathered from this technique identifies portal vein thrombosis, hepatopetal and hepatofugal flow, and portal hypertension.[9-12] Bolondi and associates[13] documented high sensitivity and specificity with these techniques.

DIAGNOSTIC EVALUATION

Laboratory Testing

The initial step in evaluating most patients is to assess their serum chemistries. Specific attention should be placed on testing the liver enzymes (serum glutamic-oxaloacetic transaminase [SGOT], serum glutamic-pyruvic transaminase [SGPT], lactate dehydrogenase [LDH], alkaline phosphatase) and hepatic synthetic function (prothrombin time and serum albumin). Information from these two sets of tests identifies patients who are suffering from acute hepatocellular damage and those who have had sufficient damage to reduce the liver's ability to synthesize essential proteins. This represents two distinct gradations of hepatic dysfunction. The first is indicative of an acute insult; the second represents the degree of hepatic dysfunction. The presence and degree of abnormalities in liver function tests correlate with

TABLE 52-1 Classification of Portal Hypertension Patients as Prognosticator of Survival

Child Classification

	Risk		
Criteria	Good	Moderate	Poor
Bilirubin (mg/dL)	<2.0	2.0-3.0	>3.0
Albumin (mg/dL)	>3.5	3.0-3.5	<3.0
Ascites	Absent	Easily controlled	Poorly controlled
Encephalopathy	Absent	Minimal	Advanced
Nutrition	Excellent	Good	Poor

Pugh Classification

	Points Scored for Increasing Abnormality*		
Criteria	1	2	3
Albumin (mg/dL)	>3.5	2.8-3.5	<2.8
Bilirubin (mg/dL)	1.0-2.0	2.0-3.0	>3.0
Ascites	Absent	Slight	Significant
Encephalopathy	Normal	1 or 2	3 or 4
Prothrombin time (seconds prolonged)	1-4	4-6	>6

*5 or 6 points for class A encephalopathy; 7 to 9 points for class B encephalopathy; 10 to 15 points for class C encephalopathy.

outcome: the more abnormal the test results, the worse the prognosis.[14,15]

Abnormal liver function tests combined with physical findings and historical data form the basis for classifying patients with portal hypertension. The Child classification or, more recently, the combined Child-Pugh classification serves as a prognosticator of survival in cirrhotic patients who undergo both emergent and elective surgery (Table 52-1).[16]

Additional laboratory investigations should include a determination of serum ammonia and a complete blood count (CBC)—white blood cells (WBCs), red blood cells (RBCs), and platelets. Serum ammonia may be elevated in cases of severe hepatic dysfunction and coma. It correlates loosely with mentation but may serve as an indicator of a treatable cause of encephalopathy, hyperammonemia.[17]

The CBC detects the presence of anemia and hypersplenism. Anemia in cirrhotic patients can result from a number of causes other than hemorrhage. Chronic malnutrition is a particularly important cause of anemia in these patients. Although splenomegaly is present in virtually all portal hypertensive patients, hypersplenism may not develop until later in the course of the disease. The size of the spleen does not correlate directly with either the degree of portal hypertension or the severity of hypersplenism, but an enlarged spleen is found in virtually all patients with portal hypertension and hypersplenism.[18] Hypersplenism is defined principally in terms of splenic sequestration and destruction of platelets and WBCs. This leads to significant depressions in the platelet and WBC counts. Platelet counts less than 50,000/mm³ and WBC counts less than 2000/mm³ support this diagnosis.

Upper Gastrointestinal Endoscopy

Endoscopy plays a pivotal role in the management of portal hypertensive patients. For both diagnostic and

therapeutic reasons, endoscopy should be one of the first tests performed. Endoscopy identifies not only the presence of varices, but also the source of bleeding in patients with hemorrhage.

The diagnosis of portal hypertension can be established by noting the presence of varices. The size, appearance, and location of the varices may significantly affect the patient's management. Endoscopy also notes the presence of other sources of bleeding in portal hypertensive patients, such as hypertensive gastropathy, gastritis, gastric ulceration, duodenal ulceration, gastric mucosal lacerations (Mallory-Weiss tears), or esophageal ulcerations. Because of the variety of possible bleeding lesions and the significant differences in the management of these lesions, patients admitted for hemorrhage must undergo upper gastrointestinal endoscopy on each admission. As many as 40% to 60% of patients with documented varices have associated gastritis or peptic ulcer disease.[19] In patients with esophageal and gastric varices, the gastric varices have been documented as the site of bleeding in up to 18%.[20]

Liver Biopsy

The role of liver biopsy in the preoperative evaluation of portal hypertensive patients has been a focus of controversy. The goal of liver biopsy in this setting is to identify those patients who have active hepatitis. In alcoholic patients, this is most commonly denoted by the presence of Mallory bodies, which signifies acute hyaline necrosis. Mallory bodies may also be seen in patients with Wilson disease, cholestasis, and primary biliary cirrhosis. The reason for identifying patients with acute hepatic necrosis is that these patients are thought to be at increased risk of dying during shunt surgery.

Mikkelsen and others noted an operative mortality of 69% in elective shunt cases and 83% in emergent cases in the presence of acute hyaline necrosis.[20,21] Other authors have contested whether acute alcoholic hepatitis alters survival.[14,22] Finally, it should be noted that Mallory bodies disappear when patients abstain from alcohol and the liver recovers from the insult.[23]

The current recommendation is that patients suspected of having acute hepatitis and who are candidates for elective shunt surgery should undergo percutaneous liver biopsy. If Mallory bodies are identified, consideration should be given to postponing the elective operation to give the liver time to recover. This must be carefully balanced against the risk of recurrent hemorrhage and the likelihood of the patient's compliance.

Duplex Scanning

Duplex scanning is finding greater application in the evaluation of portal hypertensive patients. In patients who are being considered for portacaval shunting or hepatic transplantation, the duplex scan is frequently sufficient to document portal vein patency. Duplex scanning determines both the patency of the portal vein and the direction of portal venous blood flow. This is the minimal anatomic information required to proceed with these operations. The combination of color-flow imaging and duplex scanning has improved the accuracy and extended the diagnostic abilities of duplex scanners.[11]

Angiography

Preoperative anatomic definition is essential for optimal surgical management, particularly when peripheral shunts are being considered. If possible, angiography should be performed on all patients who are to undergo elective shunting procedures. Techniques that are of primarily historical interest include splenoportography[24] (introduction of radiopaque material into the spleen), umbilical vein catheterization, and transhepatic percutaneous portal venography.[21-30]

Currently, the vast majority of portal angiography is performed by selective cannulation of the celiac and superior mesenteric arteries, as well as observation of the venous phase of these angiograms. Additional studies that should be obtained include an injection of the renal veins and a hepatic wedge angiogram and pressure recording. The combination of these studies is commonly referred to as a *liver package*.

The goal of these studies is to delineate the major portal tributaries—the splenic vein, the superior mesenteric vein (SMV), and the portal vein itself—and their relation to the renal vein. An additional goal of the liver package is to measure the hepatic wedge pressure and visualize the hepatic sinusoidal circulation. These last two elements are helpful in confirming the presence of portal hypertension, estimating the severity of the hypertension, and determining the cause of the elevated pressure. Low hepatic wedge pressure (<10 to 12 mm Hg) in a patient with variceal hemorrhage should prompt a careful search for evidence of portal vein thrombosis.[31] The wedge hepatic vein catheter allows determination of the morphology of the sinusoids and the direction of blood flow (Figure 52-1). The wedge hepatic venogram in cirrhotic patients demonstrates irregular sinusoids with multiple scattered filling

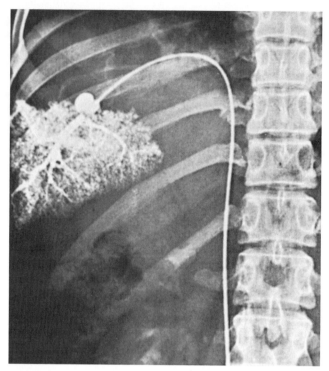

FIGURE 52-1 ■ Abnormal wedged hepatic venogram demonstrating a coarse, mottled parenchymal pattern consistent with cirrhosis.

defects. Retrograde portal vein filling indicates hepatofugal flow.[24]

Delineation of the portal tributary anatomy is essential in planning an elective portal decompressive procedure, because the choice of procedure is limited by the patient's anatomy. The angiographic findings correlate with the degree of cirrhosis. In early cirrhosis, no definite angiographic abnormalities are present. As cirrhosis becomes more severe, one sees the development of collateral pathways, dilatation of the hepatic artery, and pruning of intrahepatic portal vein branches (Figure 52-2). In advanced cirrhosis, reversal of flow in the portal vein may be detected.

COMPLICATIONS

Esophageal Varices

Esophageal varices develop in approximately 30% of cirrhotic patients. Of those who have upper gastrointestinal bleeding at presentation, approximately 30% bleed from varices. The other 70% bleed from chemical gastritis, hypertensive gastritis, ulceration, erosions, mucosal tears, and neoplastic growth. Of the cirrhotic patients who bleed from esophageal varices, 5% to 15% have massive hemorrhage that is difficult to control. The mortality of these patients—bleeding to death from esophageal varices—is approximately 30% to 50%.

The pathogenesis of esophageal varices centers around the development of collateral circulatory pathways for blood exiting the portal circulation. The impetus for the development of these collaterals is the difference in pressure between the portal system and the systemic venous

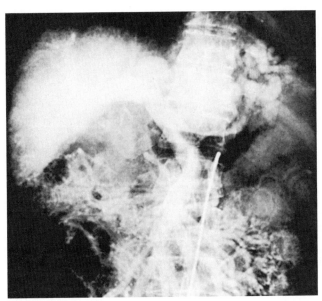

FIGURE 52-2 ■ Venous phase superior mesenteric angiogram demonstrating superior mesenteric, portal, and dilated coronary veins.

circulation. Several major collateral networks have been described in cirrhotic patients: the coronary-esophageal veins, the umbilical vein, the hemorrhoidal veins, and the retroperitoneal veins (veins of Retzius). Each of these venous systems may develop into significant collateral networks.

Any blood vessel that is attenuated and distended under supranormal pressures is at risk of disruption and bleeding. The addition of mechanical trauma or chemical irritation may increase the likelihood of bleeding. Consequently, any of the collaterals that develop because of portal hypertension may bleed. Hemorrhoidal vessels, intestinal varices, and stomal varices have all been documented as bleeding sites in cirrhotic patients. The mechanical and chemical irritants that bathe the gastro-esophageal region result in esophagitis, attenuation of the mucosal layers, and disruption of the varices. When the increased blood pressure within the varices is combined with periodic exacerbations of this pressure by activities that increase the intraabdominal and intrathoracic pressure (e.g., coughing, retching), the risk of bleeding from esophageal varices is significantly increased. The elevation of portal pressure results in dilatation of all these collateral pathways (Figure 52-3).

Several attempts have been made to predict the risk of hemorrhage from esophageal varices. Characterization of the severity of portal hypertension on the basis of corrected sinusoidal pressure has not correlated with subsequent hemorrhage. Factors that predict the risk of bleeding include the size of the varices, the Child class of the patient, and the presence of erosions on the varices (red-dot signs).[32-36]

Encephalopathy

Although not usually considered a life-threatening complication of hepatic failure, encephalopathy can have a profoundly disabling effect on patients. The clinical manifestations of encephalopathy are varied and cover a spectrum from mild inattention to frank coma. The most commonly used system of staging encephalopathy classifies patients from stage I through stage IV. Progression begins with mild personality alterations and occasionally with asterixis or clonus in stage I. Stage II may be characterized by drowsiness, sometimes with mild confusion. Stage III is typified by stupor and obtundation. Coma is the hallmark of stage IV. Electroencephalography is not specifically diagnostic, characteristically showing only slow wave activity, primarily in the frontal regions.[37]

The mechanism by which liver failure leads to coma is not clearly understood. Several agents have been postulated as encephalopathic, especially in the presence of a diseased liver. Ammonia, nitrogenous amines, increased false neurotransmitters, decreased true neurotransmitters, and an increased ratio of aromatic to branched chain amino acids are the most likely candidates.

Elevated ammonia levels have several significant repercussions. First, they elevate glucagon levels. This in turn stimulates gluconeogenesis, which produces more ammonia. In addition, the gluconeogenesis leads to elevated insulin levels, which promotes catabolism of branched chain amino acids. This ultimately leads to increased levels of straight chain amino acids such as phenylalanine, tyrosine, and methionine. An elevated ratio of straight chain to branched chain amino acids drives neutral amino acids past the blood-brain barrier. The cerebral uptake of these neutral amino acids is possible because ammonia stimulates brain glutamine synthesis, allowing rapid equilibration of brain glutamine for straight chain neutral amino acids. These same neutral amino acids may act as false neurotransmitters and are thought to produce encephalopathy.[38]

The treatment of encephalopathy is based on reduction of ammonia levels and supplementation of branched chain amino acids. Lactulose and neomycin reduce ammonia uptake from the gut by altering the intestinal pH, reducing the number of intestinal bacteria, and reducing intestinal transit of protein. Other agents such as levodopa have been used, with mixed results, in improving encephalopathy.[39]

Ascites

Ascites is a common symptom of portal hypertension. Up to 80% of these patients may have some degree of ascites. The mechanism by which ascites develops is a combination of hemodynamic, physiologic, and metabolic factors. The hemodynamics of the portal circulatory system in the face of cirrhosis is driven primarily by the increased portal venous pressure. In such a state, Starling forces tend to drive fluids out of the vessels and into the interstitial space. Compounding this problem is the low oncotic pressure that characterizes many cirrhotic patients by virtue of their hypoalbuminemia. Finally, many of these patients chronically register a relatively low effective intravascular volume, which in turn triggers the renal aldosterone-renin-angiotensin system and, perhaps, an additional natriuretic hormone. These changes then produce a state in which the patient retains free water and salt, both of which aggravate the ascites. The net

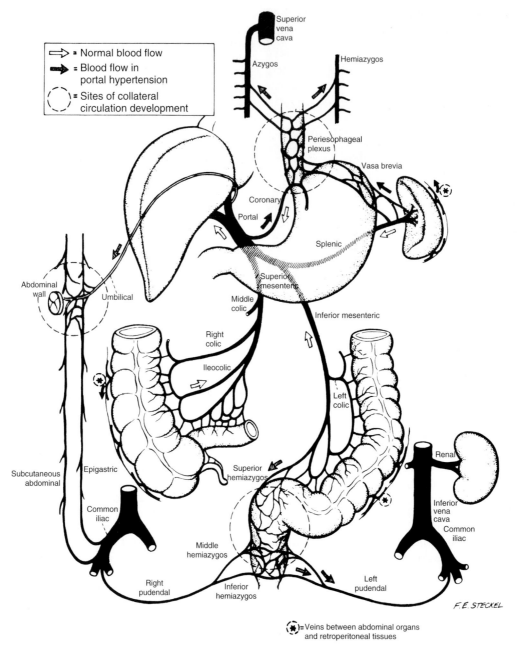

FIGURE 52-3 ■ Schematic diagram of collateral venous pathways. (From Sedgwick CE, et al: Portal hypertension, Boston Little Brown, 1967.)

effect is the translocation of fluid from the intravascular space to the interstitial space and the abdominal cavity.

The compensatory mechanism that normally counteracts the accumulation of interstitial and peritoneal fluid is primarily the lymphatic system. In a cirrhotic patient, the lymph flow is frequently increased. Ascites accumulates when the ability of the lymphatics to reabsorb this fluid is overwhelmed.

The cornerstone of the management of ascites is restriction of salt intake and judicious use of diuretics. These measures control the vast majority of ascitic patients. In only 5% of cases can ascites be considered intractable, and other means of addressing the ascites are required.

MEDICAL THERAPY

General Medical Care

Medical care is based on evaluating and defining the cause of the liver disease. The first step is to address any factors related to the cause of the liver disease that are amenable to change (e.g., stopping alcohol consumption). The second step is establishing the patient's current state of health and hepatic function: defining the presence of portal hypertension, splenomegaly, ascites, or varices. An assessment of the hepatic disease and the degree of hepatic deterioration helps in predicting the eventual course of the patient. The next step involves maintenance of nutrition, supplementation of vitamins and minerals, and avoidance of salt (especially in ascitic patients).

Management of Acute Complications

The management of acute complications is a highly specialized area in the care of these patients. The most common problem that requires urgent care is hemorrhage. The significance of hemorrhage in these patients is difficult to understate. Hemorrhage may be associated with up to 70% mortality, depending on the cause and severity of the liver disease and the degree of decompensation of the patient at the time of presentation. Furthermore, the risk of a second hemorrhage within 1 year may be as high as 60%.[16]

The essential steps in caring for a cirrhotic patient with an upper gastrointestinal hemorrhage include establishing peripheral venous access, volume-resuscitating the patient, and determining the source of bleeding. This is best accomplished by upper gastrointestinal endoscopy. As mentioned previously, between 40% and 60% of cirrhotic patients with known varices who have an upper gastrointestinal hemorrhage are not bleeding from their varices.[40]

If the patient is bleeding from an esophageal varix or hypertensive gastritis, several specific steps are taken promptly. First, the rate of bleeding is assessed. Second, the patient must be adequately resuscitated. Third, the patient must be prepared for a possible therapeutic intervention.

Assessing the rate of bleeding is essential. The assessment is based largely on the progressive change in the patient's vital signs, mentation, and perfusion during the course of resuscitation. A nasogastric tube also provides information about continued bleeding. Emergency endoscopy may provide insight into whether the patient is suffering a massive hemorrhage or is bleeding at a moderate rate. The change in the patient's hematocrit is not necessarily the best indicator of bleeding because there may be a significant lag between the bleeding episode and the subsequent drop in hematocrit.

Patients with relatively minor bleeding episodes frequently stop bleeding spontaneously. The few patients who are actively bleeding at the time of admission almost always respond to an infusion of octreotide. The key to managing these patients is to avoid overloading them with fluid and salts, because this may precipitate rebleeding with further decompensation.

Patients with moderate bleeding rates stand a reasonable chance of having their bleeding stopped without surgical intervention. These patients frequently respond to infusions of octreotide, emergency sclerotherapy, or balloon tamponade.

Patients who bleed massively may require more advanced intervention, often in addition to octreotide and balloon tamponade. Emergent endoscopy is frequently impaired by the massive bleeding. Subsequent steps include angiographic embolization, percutaneous attempts to create an intrahepatic shunt (transjugular intrahepatic portosystemic shunt [TIPS]), or emergency surgical shunting.

The fluids used in resuscitation vary with the severity of the hemorrhage. Patients with minor bleeds may be resuscitated with intravenous crystalloid solutions. In patients with more severe hemorrhages, it may be necessary to supplement this with infusions of albumin. In severe hemorrhages, it is necessary to infuse both packed RBCs and fresh frozen plasma. Occasionally, infusions of other blood components are required, such as platelets or cryoprecipitate, but this is relatively rare. The goal of resuscitation is to maintain the patient at a level at which vital organs can be perfused while the bleeding source is addressed. Indicators of a successful resuscitation include the ability of the patient to produce urine, maintain acid-base balance and display clear mentation.

Preparation of these patients for possible therapeutic interventions includes cleansing of the gastrointestinal tract, stabilization of the blood volume, identification of the bleeding source, and administration of blood components as needed to allow the proposed interventions.

SPECIFIC MEASURES FOR THE CONTROL OF ACUTE HEMORRHAGE

Protein and Gut Lavage

Hemorrhage into the gastrointestinal tract poses a significant risk of encephalopathy, particularly in patients with bleeding varices. The combination of a large protein load in the intestinal tract and poor hepatic function frequently results in encephalopathy. The intestinal tract must be cleansed of the blood and any other nitrogenous substances by a combination of enemas and oral cathartics or gastric lavage.

The upper gastrointestinal tract should be laved with the aid of a large-bore tube (e.g., Ewald tube) to remove the clotted blood from the stomach. The rest of the tract is cleansed at the appropriate time by the administration of lactulose and neomycin by mouth. Neomycin and lactulose are given to alter the intestinal absorption of ammonia. Neomycin is a relatively nonabsorbable antibiotic; it destroys urease-producing bacteria and thereby decreases ammonia production. Lactulose is converted by lactase-containing intestinal bacteria into lactic acid and acetic acid, thus decreasing the intraluminal intestinal pH. The lower pH ionizes ammonia into ammonium (NH_4^+), which is less able to diffuse through the colonic mucosa. Lactulose also promotes diarrhea, cleansing the intestine of its contents.[17,41,42]

Vasopressin

Vasopressin (Pitressin) should no longer be considered first-line therapy in the management of active bleeding varices. However, information from its use has provided significant insights into the early management of variceal bleeding. The drug is specifically directed at slowing and stopping variceal hemorrhage. It has been recognized since 1917 for its vasoconstrictive effects and its ability to decrease portal pressure.[43] Vasopressin is a naturally occurring nonapeptide that demonstrates general vasoconstrictive effects, with particular efficacy in the splanchnic bed. This splanchnic vasoconstriction leads to decreased portal flow. Vasopressin is also known to diminish cardiac output by an average of 14% and heart rate by 11%. This, in turn, reduces hepatic blood flow by approximately 44% and wedge hepatic vein pressure by 11%. As much as a 23% reduction in the gradient between hepatic venous pressure and wedge vein pressure has been documented.[44]

A consequence of the vasoconstrictive effects of vasopressin is the potential exacerbation of cardiac ischemia. To counter these ischemic effects, a number of pharmacologic agents have been used in conjunction with vasopressin.[44-46] Isoproterenol, when administered with intravenous vasopressin, results in an equivalent reduction of portal vein pressure but maintenance of cardiac output.[45] Sublingual nitroglycerin plus vasopressin has been shown to reduce the deleterious effects of vasopressin alone while preserving the decrease in portal vein pressure.[44,47] In the course of a controlled trial, Gimson and associates[48] noted that nitroglycerin may reverse some of the cardiac suppressive effects of vasopressin, as well as enhance the portal hypotensive effects.

Intravenous vasopressin should be used before balloon tamponade. It stops variceal bleeding in at least 80% of cases. The initial dose is 0.2 to 0.4 units/min. If bleeding does not cease with the initial dose, the dose may be increased up to 1 unit/min.

Somatostatin and Octreotide

Because of its fewer side effects and equal efficacy compared with vasopressin, octreotide has become the agent of choice in managing acute variceal hemorrhage. Somatostatin is a tetradecapeptide derived from the hypothalamus that has demonstrated an ability to decrease splanchnic blood. Octreotide is a synthetic octapeptide analog of somatostatin. It has a longer half-life than somatostatin (100 minutes vs. 2 to 3 minutes). Both have been demonstrated to be as effective as vasopressin for the control of acute bleeding, with fewer complications.[49] Hemodynamic studies indicate that somatostatin decreases the portal venous pressure gradient.[42,50] Randomized studies have shown equal efficacy between the two, and metaanalysis has demonstrated no survival benefit. Somatostatin has been repeatedly shown to have fewer side effects than vasopressin.[49,51]

Octreotide is effective in reducing and halting variceal hemorrhage in 80% of cases. Intravenous octreotide should be used before, and along with, balloon tamponade. It should be started before endoscopy. The initial dose of octreotide is a bolus infusion of 50 μg. This is followed by an infusion of 50 μg/h. As with vasopressin infusions, the octreotide infusion should be continued over a 3-day period. After this period, the drug should be gradually discontinued.[46]

Data have been mixed regarding somatostatin and related agents, but several studies demonstrated decreased blood loss when these drugs are used. For example, a metaanalysis comprising 12 trials (1452 patients) showed an overall decrease in transfusion requirements of 1 unit of blood per patient.[52] Mortality, rebleeding, and need for balloon tamponade were not decreased. As the authors concluded, the transfusion requirements are significant,

but it is not evident that there is any clinical benefit in saving a single unit of blood.

Terlipressin is a synthetic vasopressin analog that can be given intermittently as an injection, unlike vasopressin, which must be administered as an intravenous drip. In comparison with vasopressin, no significant differences in outcome were shown in a metaanalysis of 20 studies comprising 1609 patients.[53] It is not clear whether this drug will become a front-line treatment agent. In summary, because these drugs are easy to administer, have relatively safe profiles, and may be effective, many centers use them routinely for bleeding varices. Additional support for their use comes from a recent update of a Cochrane Database review demonstrating that vasoactive drugs appeared to work well when sclerotherapy was not readily available. The therapy was also found to be associated with few risks.[54]

Propranolol

Propranolol, a beta-blocking drug, has been found to be useful in controlling chronic portal hypertension and reducing the risk of recurrent bleeding from esophageal varices. Its action is thought to be mediated on the basis of reduced cardiac output, reduced systemic pressure, and subsequent reduction in portal venous pressure.

Evidence of its efficacy in the reduction of recurrent bleeding has been mixed. Burroughs and colleagues[55] compared propranolol with placebo and found no significant difference in rebleeding or survival. Fleig and colleagues[56] randomized 70 patients to sclerotherapy or propranolol and found no difference in the rebleeding rate or survival; however, propranolol decreased the size of the varices significantly after 3 months of treatment. In a prospective, controlled study of 79 patients, Lebrec and associates[57,58] noted that after 3 months, 2.6% of patients maintained on propranolol had recurrent gastrointestinal tract bleeding, compared with 66% maintained on a placebo drug. Similar findings have been reported by others.[59] Poynard and coauthors analyzed 127 patients treated with propranolol and found five factors that were associated with rebleeding: (1) hepatocellular carcinoma, (2) lack of persistent decrease in heart rate, (3) lack of abstinence from alcohol, (4) lack of compliance, and (5) prior history of rebleeding[60] More recently, Schepke and associates[61] compared propranolol therapy to band ligation in primary prophylaxis of varices in high-risk patients, noting that there were no differences in bleeding between these treatments. More recent data suggest that sclerotherapy is more effective in this regard, reducing the risk of a first variceal bleeding episode to 5% versus a cohort receiving propranolol alone, which had a risk of 20%.[62]

Propranolol has been specifically used as maintenance therapy to decrease the risk of recurrent esophageal variceal bleeding in patients with portal hypertension. Its use in acute bleeding episodes has not been studied.

Balloon Tamponade

Balloon tamponade is a technique that uses compression by an intragastric balloon to stem the bleeding of esophageal and gastroesophageal varices. The technique dates to the early 1950s, when Linton, Nachlas, Sengstaken, and Blakemore developed the tubes that now bear their names.

All these tubes work on the same principle, tamponade of varices. The design variations include the presence of one or two balloons for compression of the stomach alone or the esophagus and stomach (Linton-Nachlas vs. Sengstaken tube) and the presence of adjunctive ports for aspiration of the stomach and esophageal secretions (Sengstaken-Blakemore vs. Edlich modification or Minnesota tube).[63,64] The Sengstaken-Blakemore tube is probably used more often because it can compress both esophageal and gastric varices, whereas the Linton-Nachlas tube can compress only gastric varices.

The Sengstaken-Blakemore tube can be passed through either the mouth or the nose. Passage of this tube must be performed carefully and precisely to prevent complications. The manufacturers recommend that the gastric balloon be inflated with a low volume of air (250 mL) and that an abdominal radiograph be taken to ensure that the gastric balloon is on the stomach before full inflation (with 750 mL of air). This should avoid the problem of fully inflating the gastric balloon in the esophagus, where it could tear open the esophageal wall.

Once the gastric balloon is inflated, it is taped to the facemask of a football helmet with approximately 1 kg of pressure. The gastric and esophageal ports are connected to intermittent low Gomco suction. The position of the gastric balloon is checked periodically to ensure that migration into the esophagus has not occurred. If bleeding does not cease with gastric balloon inflation and tension, the esophageal balloon is inflated to 24 to 45 mm Hg pressure. If bleeding ceases with the Sengstaken-Blakemore tube insertion, it is left inflated for 24 hours. After this period, the esophageal balloon should be deflated. Twenty-four hours later, the gastric balloon is deflated. If bleeding does not recur, the tube is deflated and left in place. It should be removed after an additional day.[63] Esophageal variceal tamponade results in cessation of hemorrhage in 45% to 92% of cases.[65-68] Bleeding recurs shortly after the Sengstaken-Blakemore tube is deflated in 24% to 42% of cases, however, and cannot be controlled in 33% to 37% of cases.[65,66] The incidence of recurrent bleeding after a second period of balloon control is 40%.[67]

This tube has been associated with significant complications: gastroesophageal tears, ulceration, and perforation. Pulmonary complications include aspiration pneumonia and asphyxia from tracheal intubation. Conn and Simpson reported a complication rate of 41% and a mortality rate of 20%.[69] More commonly, the incidence of major complications is in the range of 4% to 9%.[65-67]

SURGICAL SHUNT CORRECTION

Shunt Nomenclature

The anatomic naming of shunts is based on elements of the shunt. Thus, the principal shunts are portacaval, mesocaval, and splenorenal. The first portion of the name denotes the donor vessel, and the second portion denotes the recipient vessel. A portacaval shunt may be either a side-to-side or an end-to-side portacaval shunt. Similarly, a splenorenal shunt may be either a proximal or a distal splenorenal shunt. The principal advantage of this system is that it allows a clear, descriptive means of labeling an operation. This system is probably the most widely used shunt nomenclature.

The taxonomic nomenclature is derived from both physiologic and anatomic considerations. These names are ingrained in the lexicon of surgery and should be understood. The two principal sets of names are central and remote and selective and nonselective. A central shunt is one constructed in the region of the porta hepatis, or at the center of the portal confluence. Included among these are the various portacaval shunts. The term is used to distinguish shunts that involve the portal vein itself from those that are remote from the portal vein, such as splenorenal and mesocaval shunts. The distinction has regained some usefulness in the context of distinguishing shunts that are recommended for potential liver transplant candidates.

Selectivity of a shunt refers to its effect on the portal venous blood flow. Selective shunts preserve the flow of mesenteric blood through the portal vein to the liver while decompressing esophageal varices. Nonselective shunts drain all portal blood flow into the vena cava. The selective shunts include the distal splenorenal shunt (DSRS) and the coronary-caval shunts. Nonselective shunts include the end-to-side portacaval shunt, side-to-side portacaval shunt, mesocaval shunt, and proximal splenorenal shunt. Currently, the term *selective shunt* is nearly synonymous with a DSRS.

Many shunts are still associated with the names of their proponents. Included are the Warren shunt (DSRS), Linton shunt (proximal splenorenal), Clatworthy shunt (mesocaval shunt using the inferior vena cava [IVC]), Drapanas shunt (mesocaval shunt using a Dacron interposition graft), Inokuchi shunt (coronary-caval), and Sarfeh shunt (portacaval polytetrafluoroethylene [PTFE] interposition graft).

Prophylactic Shunting

Proponents of prophylactic shunting argued that variceal hemorrhage could be prevented by creating a shunt in patients with varices before they had the opportunity to bleed. Four prospective, controlled studies addressed this issue.[19,21,70,71] These four early studies were similar in design. The patients were divided between medical and surgical treatment and were followed for recurrent bleeding, development of encephalopathy, and survival.

The Boston Interhospital Liver Group (BILG) allocated 45 patients to the medical group and 48 to the surgical group. At 1-, 3-, and 5-year intervals, there was no difference in survival; at 5 years, the survival rate was 50%. Encephalopathy was likewise equal (21%).[72] The Department of Veterans Affairs (VA) study demonstrated a 45% incidence of encephalopathy after shunting, almost twice that of medical therapies. It was disconcerting that the 5-year survival after shunting (51%) was less than with medical therapy (64%).[19] Similarly, the experience of the Yale group demonstrated decreased survival after shunting, with an increased incidence of encephalopathy.[73,74]

Indications for prophylactic variceal decompression have also been studied by the Cooperative Study Group of Portal Hypertension in Japan. By comparing only nondecompressive transection procedures and selective shunts, this group found no difference in survival rates at 2 years and suggested that in certain patients, prophylactic procedures may be indicated.[21] It should, however, be noted that these patients were primarily nonalcoholic, and the applicability of these results has been widely debated in the United States.

These studies demonstrated that prophylactic shunts do not benefit patients with asymptomatic varices. Although the incidence of variceal hemorrhage is virtually eliminated, these patients tend to suffer from hepatic encephalopathy and die of hepatic failure. Encephalopathy is increased following portacaval shunting, and long-term survival may in fact be decreased by a shunt procedure. These results are not surprising, in that only 30% of patients who have varices bleed, and the decreased incidence of death from bleeding may be offset by the operative mortality of a shunt procedure, as well as by the effects of subsequent hepatic encephalopathy.

Therapeutic Shunting

The efficacy of portosystemic shunting has been studied with prospective, randomized clinical trials. Four such trials were performed in the United States and France to evaluate the fundamental question of whether therapeutic shunts prolong survival and maintain the quality of life compared with conventional medical therapy.[75-78]

The VA study, begun in 1961, followed the survival of 155 selected patients over a 5.5-year period. Although 78 patients were randomized to the surgical group, only 67 actually received shunts. Operative mortality following therapeutic portacaval shunts was 8%. Recurrence of variceal bleeding was 7% in the surgical group and 65% in the medical group. Encephalopathy occurred with approximately equal frequency in both groups, but was more severe in the shunted group. The long-term survival rate at 5 years was 57% in the shunt group and 36% in the medical group. The increase in long-term survival was not, however, statistically significant.[70]

In the BILG study,[72] patients underwent end-to-side portacaval shunt, side-to-side portacaval shunt, or medical therapy. The long-term survival was better in the shunt group than in the medically treated group, but this difference was not statistically significant. On the basis of both the VA and the BILG studies, Conn concluded that, despite the lack of statistical significance, therapeutic portacaval shunts prolong the mean duration of life in cirrhotic patients who have suffered from variceal hemorrhage.[79]

Researchers at the University of Southern California published a 12-year follow-up of a prospective, randomized study comparing end-to-side portacaval shunts with medical therapy. There were 190 episodes of bleeding in the group receiving medical therapy, compared with 11 in the surgical group. Encephalopathy of a moderate to severe degree occurred in 35% of shunt patients. A 5-year life-table analysis revealed a 44% survival rate among patients treated with shunts and a 24% survival rate among those treated medically. This difference was not statistically significant, however.[21]

Rueff and associates, in a study at the Hôpital Beaujon in Clichy, France, compared therapeutic end-to-side portacaval shunts with medical therapy.[78] The long-term survival was 47% in the shunt group and 56% in the medical group. The diminished long-term survival in the shunt group is unique to this study and may be due to the high operative mortality (19%, compared with 13% for the BILG study and 8% for the VA study). Encephalopathy was equally common in the medical and surgical groups, with an incidence of 40%. As in the other studies, it tended to be more severe and chronic in the shunt group, however. Recurrent bleeding occurred in 8% of the shunt group and in 72% of the medical group.

The most compelling conclusion drawn from these studies is that they failed to demonstrate a survival advantage. Portacaval shunts are clearly superior in preventing recurrent variceal bleeding. Encephalopathy is not more common in patients undergoing portacaval shunting, but it tends to be more severe and chronic than in medically treated patients.

Emergency Portacaval Shunting

Portacaval shunting on an emergency basis is no longer widely performed because of the reported high mortality. Despite this risk, it has proved highly efficacious in its ability to stop bleeding and prevent recurrent bleeding.[80] Orloff and colleagues[81] continued to advocate the portacaval shunt in the acute setting, and they achieved a 4-year actuarial survival of 69%. Interestingly, this same group reported actuarial survivals of 99% at 5 years and 97% at 10 years when all patients (those bleeding acutely and those operated on for recurrent bleeds) were considered.[82] Villeneuve and coworkers also supported the use of this shunt in acutely bleeding patients who have mild to moderate liver disease and in whom other forms of treatment have failed.[83] In general, emergency surgical intervention is performed less frequently as nonsurgical options become more effective.

Common Portosystemic Shunts

Nonselective Shunts

Portacaval Shunts. Both end-to-side and side-to-side portacaval shunts are nonselective and cause diversion of portal flow into the systemic circulation. The only specific indication for the portacaval shunt is esophageal variceal hemorrhage. Intractable ascites was once treated with a side-to-side portacaval shunt, but this technique has been discarded in favor of peritoneovenous shunting and TIPS.[84,85]

The question of whether an end-to-side or a side-to-side portacaval shunt is more effective is still debated. An end-to-side portacaval shunt is certainly not indicated in the presence of Budd-Chiari syndrome, because the portal vein serves as a decompressive outflow tract for intrahepatic portal blood. Uncontrolled studies comparing end-to-side with side-to-side shunts indicate that the side-to-side shunt is associated with a lower surgical mortality in patients with poor hepatic function.[86] Others find the side-to-side portacaval shunt to be more technically demanding. Encephalopathy has been shown to be somewhat more common in side-to-side than in end-to-side portacaval shunts.[87] Investigators previously found that in addition to allowing total diversion of portal venous flow, the side-to-side shunt may create a siphon effect, permitting egress of hepatic arterial blood through the portal vein rather than the hepatic vein. This may be an explanation for the increased incidence of encephalopathy with side-to-side portacaval shunts.

End-to-Side Portacaval Shunt. Two approaches have been described: the midline incision and the right subcostal incision. After the abdomen has been entered, the duodenum is mobilized medially to expose the IVC. The dissection is carried up along the IVC to the level of the first hepatic vein under the liver. The portal vein should be exposed by rotating the bile duct and hepatic artery using a vein retractor or peanut sponges. The division of the portal vein should be done after it has been securely clamped (proximally and distally) and the hepatic portion of the vein suture-ligated.

A Satinsky clamp is placed at the appropriate point on the vena cava, and an ellipse of cava is removed to allow anastomosis. Pressure in the portal vein should be measured to document the adequacy of the decompression and to detect any unobserved technical problems. A 50% reduction in portal venous pressure should be expected after the shunt is completed.[88,89]

Arterialization of End-to-Side Portacaval Shunts. In an attempt to reduce the morbidity of end-to-side portacaval shunts, a variety of measures have been used to maintain portal perfusion of the liver. Portal vein arterialization refers to the anastomosis of an arterialized conduit to the hepatic end of the portal vein. Various arteries have been used for this purpose, including the right gastroepiploic artery, splenic artery, and saphenous vein grafts from the hypogastric artery or aorta.

Side-to-Side Portacaval Shunt. The side-to-side portacaval shunt is technically more difficult than the end-to-side shunt. The initial approach is similar to the end-to-side shunt; a longer segment of the vena cava is exposed and circumferentially dissected so that it can be lifted out of its bed. The portal vein must also be exposed for a greater length, because a 4-cm segment is necessary for the anastomosis. Portal pressures are measured before the shunt is performed. After applying the vascular clamps, an elliptic segment measuring approximately 2 cm is excised from the IVC and portal vein directly opposite each other. Again, mesenteric venous pressure measurements should reflect a 50% reduction in portal vein pressure.[88]

Portacaval H-Graft. An alternative to the side-to-side portacaval shunt is the portacaval H-graft. Technically easier than the side-to-side shunt, the large-diameter (16 to 20 mm) H-graft effectively prevents variceal rebleeding, but encephalopathy occurs frequently. Building on this experience, Sarfeh and colleagues[90] systematically reduced portacaval H-graft diameters and found that an 8-mm PTFE graft combined with portal

collateral ablation effectively prevented rebleeding, maintained hepatic perfusion, and reduced encephalopathy. The 5-year cumulative late patency rate was 97%.

Mesocaval Shunts. In 1955, Clatworthy and associates devised a new portosystemic shunt procedure involving division of the IVC above its bifurcation and anastomosis of the proximal cava to the side of the SMV.[91] The portosystemic shunt procedure has been particularly successful in children with extrahepatic portal vein thrombosis. In adults, massive lower extremity edema has limited its usefulness. Because of the extensive dissection necessary to expose the vena cava, a number of alternative graft materials have been used, including cadaveric IVC, iliac vein, PTFE, and Dacron, which is currently favored.[92-96]

There has been considerable debate about whether portal perfusion (hepatopetal flow) is maintained by mesocaval shunts. Drapanas and colleagues[97] documented continued hepatopetal flow in 44% of their patients. Others have noted, however, that portal perfusion can persist only if there is partial or total H-graft occlusion.[98] Misinterpretation of angiographic studies may also be attributable to the phenomenon of portal pseudoperfusion, as explained by Fulenwider and coauthors.[99] Overall, H-graft mesocaval shunts are considered nonselective shunts.

Clinical Role of Mesocaval Shunts. The primary application of the interposition H-graft mesocaval shunt is for the urgent control of massive variceal hemorrhage. This graft is technically easier to perform than a portacaval or a selective shunt and is frequently indicated in the emergency management of variceal hemorrhage.[100] In the case of previous surgery in the right upper quadrant, a portacaval shunt of any type is especially challenging and is usually contraindicated. If a selective shunt is contraindicated, a mesocaval shunt may be a good alternative. This is true in patients with significant ascites. Other factors that favor mesocaval shunting include extensive periportal fibrosis, a large overriding caudate lobe, an obliterated portal vein, extreme obesity, and Budd-Chiari syndrome.[101]

Interposition Mesocaval H-Graft. The operation, as described by Drapanas and coauthors in 1975, remains essentially unchanged to this day.[97] The transverse mesocolon is elevated superiorly, and the small intestine is retracted inferiorly. At the root of the small intestine mesentery, the peritoneum is opened transversely to expose the superior mesenteric vessels. An important goal is to preserve as many branches of the SMV as necessary to preserve intestinal venous flow. After the SMV is isolated, the anterior surface of the vena cava is exposed through the right transverse mesocolon. Only dissection sufficient to permit the use of a Satinsky clamp on the vena cava is required. Once the vena cava is partially isolated, the third and fourth portions of the duodenum must usually be mobilized to allow the duodenum to ride above the graft. Failure to do this may cause obstruction of the occasional low-lying duodenum or occlusion of the interposed graft.

The graft length should be only 3 to 6 cm to minimize kinking of the prosthesis. Anastomosis is performed in the posterior surface of the vein, with a continuous suture of 5-0 polypropylene (Prolene [Ethicon, Sommerville, New Jersey]). With the clamps removed, the graft should distend quickly. In most instances, a palpable thrill should be present. Post-shunt pressures are then measured in the SMV; if the shunt is functioning properly, there should be at least a 50% reduction of pressure with the shunt open.

Clinical Results. Sarr and colleagues[102] published a series of 33 patients who underwent the mesocaval C-shunt procedure. There was a 24% operative mortality rate (all Child class C nonelective cases), an 8% rebleed rate, and a 46% incidence of encephalopathy. However, there were no graft thromboses.

The average incidence of encephalopathy after a mesocaval graft is approximately 25%.[101,103] The reported incidence of encephalopathy ranges from 9% to 45%.[96,100] Late graft occlusion is caused by excessive layering of thrombus, possibly aggravated by perigraft scarring, leading to kinking and constriction.[98] The incidence of shunt occlusion ranges from 4% to 24%.[97,98,105-108] Rebleeding occurs in approximately 14% of mesocaval shunts (range, 12% to 16%). One third of these cases may be related to occlusion of the graft.[100] Overall, the mortality is approximately 15%. The cumulative long-term mortality ranges from 28% to 57%. The long-term mortality is probably dependent on the state of liver function rather than the type of shunt.

Mortality related to mesocaval H-shunts is not significantly different from that for other types of shunts and is dependent on the patient's Child classification. Initial hospital mortality is related to the urgency of surgery, significant elevation of SGOT or bilirubin, or the presence of encephalopathy.[98]

Proximal Splenorenal Shunts. Currently of historical interest only, the nonselective splenorenal shunt, or Linton shunt, was first developed by Blakemore and Lord in 1945 using a Vitallium tube.[74] Linton and coworkers[109] advocated this shunt in the years that followed and considered it the operative procedure of choice for the correction of portal hypertension. Early reports of noncontrolled studies suggested a decreased incidence of encephalopathy with this shunt compared with the portacaval shunt.[110] This finding, however, has not been substantiated. Other investigators failed to demonstrate significant differences between central splenorenal and portacaval shunts in regard to encephalopathy or long-term survival. In fact, some reports noted an increased incidence of thrombosis associated with the central splenorenal shunt.[1,111]

Splenorenal Shunts. Portacaval shunts suffer from two significant problems: progressive hepatic failure and progressive, occasionally disabling, encephalopathy. These problems are thought to be due to the diversion of portal blood from the liver. In an attempt to avoid the complications of total diversion of portal flow, the DSRS, or Warren shunt, was developed in the late 1960s.[112]

This operation is based on the principle of compartmentalization, as discussed by Malt.[1] The portal-azygos system and the portal-splanchnic system can be surgically

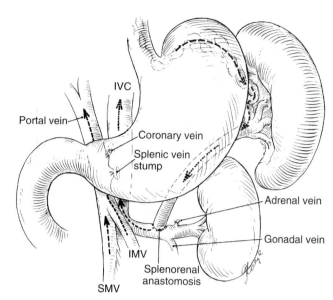

FIGURE 52-4 ▪ Illustration of the selective distal splenorenal shunt. *IMV,* Inferior mesenteric vein; *IVC,* inferior vena cava; *SMV,* superior mesenteric vein.

separated into parallel and independent hemodynamic units. Thus, decompression of the portal-azygos system can be accomplished without reducing the portal-splanchnic system perfusion pressure or blood flow.[1,101] Therefore one should be able to decompress esophageal varices and prevent hemorrhage without diverting the hepatopetal flow of the portal-splanchnic blood. In principle, this is accomplished in two steps. First, by disrupting the coronary vein and right gastroepiploic vein, blood flow into the esophageal variceal system is reduced. Second, by anastomosing the distal splenic to the left renal vein, without performing a splenectomy, blood is able to freely drain from the esophageal varices through the short gastric into the lower-pressure systemic circulation (Figure 52-4).

The theoretical benefit of the DSRS includes preservation of hepatic perfusion and function, with consequent prolongation of survival and lower risk of disabling encephalopathy. The search for evidence of this benefit has led to the creation of several randomized trials. Five trials compared the DSRS and portacaval shunts. Three trials compared the DSRS with best nonsurgical management and sclerotherapy.

Distal Splenorenal Shunt versus Other Shunts. The DSRS was compared with the end-to-side portacaval shunt in three randomized studies by Langer and colleagues in Toronto,[113] Resnick and coworkers in the Boston–New Haven trial,[114] and Harley and associates at the University of Southern California Medical Center[115] (Figure 52-5). Langer's group reported a 14% incidence of post-shunt encephalopathy in the selectively shunted patients, but a 50% incidence in the end-to-side portacaval group. There was no difference in long-term survival.[113] Preliminary data from Resnick's group indicated no substantial difference between the two operations in regard to either encephalopathy or long-term survival. It should be noted, however, that the follow-up period was

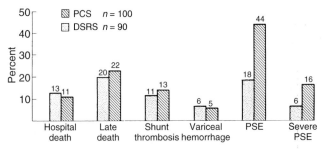

FIGURE 52-5 ■ Combined experience of the distal splenorenal shunt (DSRS) versus the portacaval shunt (PCS). *PSE,* Portosystemic encephalopathy. (Data from randomized trials by Rikkers and colleagues,[116] Langer and colleagues,[113] Reichle and colleagues,[106] and Harley and colleagues[115] and their respective colleagues.)

relatively short.[114] Harley and associates randomized 54 patients between the two shunts and failed to demonstrate any superiority of one over the other in regard to encephalopathy or survival. They did, however, experience an unusually high rate of rebleeding with the DSRS (27%).[115]

A study in Atlanta compared the DSRS with nonselective shunts, most commonly interposition mesorenal shunts.[116,117] The operative mortality was similar for the two groups: 12% for the DSRS and 10% for nonselective shunts. Early postoperative angiography demonstrated persistent hepatopetal flow in 88% of the DSRS patients, but in only 5% of the nonselective shunt patients. Corresponding to this were quantitative measurements of hepatic function, maximal rate of urea synthesis, and the Child class, which were similar to preoperative values in the DSRS group but greatly decreased in the nonselective group. The incidence of encephalopathy correlated with preservation of hepatopetal blood flow. Patients with hepatopetal flow suffered no encephalopathy; patients with hepatofugal flow experienced a 45% incidence of encephalopathy. Overall, encephalopathy occurred in 27% of the DSRS group and 52% of the nonselective group (*p* < 0.001). Recurrent variceal hemorrhage occurred in 4% of selective and 8% of nonselective shunts. Although survival was similar for the two groups, it appears that the quality of survival was improved in the DSRS group.

Zeppa's group[118] demonstrated that the 5-year survival of patients with nonalcoholic cirrhosis after DSRS was 89%, compared with 39% in the alcoholic cirrhotic group. It should be noted that improved survival in nonalcoholic cirrhotic patients was also suggested by another group,[117] but other investigators have contested this point.[19] In addition, a number of other unmatched studies have demonstrated excellent results with the DSRS.[119-127] A combined review of the literature comparing mesocaval H-grafts to DSRSs unequivocally demonstrated the latter to be superior in decreasing the incidence of both encephalopathy and recurrent hemorrhage.[100]

Splenopancreatic Disconnection. Because of the results of trials indicating that, with the passage of time, the DSRS gradually becomes a nonselective shunt, Warren modified the operation. In 1986, he and his coauthors proposed that the DSRS procedure include complete dissection of the splenic vein and division of the splenocolic ligament (splenopancreatic disconnection).[128]

In theory, this should reduce the pancreatic sump or siphon effect—the tendency of pancreatic branches of the splenic vein to progressively enlarge and serve as an outflow collateral for the portal mesenteric circulatory system. This modification was intended to prolong and preserve the selective quality of the DSRS. Clinically, Warren's group found that this modification preserved postoperative portal perfusion in alcoholic cirrhotic patients better than the DSRS alone.[128] It also considerably extended the magnitude of the operation.

Indications for Distal Splenorenal Shunt. The principal indication for a DSRS is to prevent recurrent variceal hemorrhage that is not controllable with sclerotherapy. The specific strengths of the DSRS include its lower incidence of encephalopathy and its anatomic remoteness from the porta hepatis. For these reasons, it is considered the shunt of choice in patients who require elective shunting and have no specific contraindications to the DSRS. The most important of these contraindications is the presence of significant ascites, which in practice means ascites that is difficult to control by the administration of diuretics. In addition, patients should have an adequately sized patent splenic vein. Some authors consider the presence of hepatofugal portal blood flow to be a contraindication to the DSRS. In cases of portal hypertension owing to extrahepatic portal vein thrombosis, the DSRS has been demonstrated to be effective in preventing recurrent hemorrhage.[124] Finally, although the DSRS has been performed as an emergency procedure, it is not widely considered the shunt of choice in these circumstances because of the relative difficulty of the operation.

Surgical Technique: Distal Splenorenal Shunt. The technique used for the DSRS is essentially the method described by Warren and Millikan.[129] The first goal of this operation is to anastomose the distal splenic vein to the left renal vein. The second goal is to disconnect the portal-azygos system from the splanchnic-venous system. A bilateral subcostal incision provides optimal exposure. The splenic vein may be approached either through the lesser sac or from below the transverse mesocolon. Most surgeons use the lesser sac approach. As part of this approach, the right gastroepiploic vein is divided, but the short gastric veins are carefully preserved. The pancreas is identified, and the peritoneum covering its inferior border is incised. Careful blunt dissection of the retroperitoneal tissue allows the pancreas to be rotated anteriorly and exposes the splenic vein. The splenic vein dissection is the most delicate portion of this operation; it should be carried out to the point of confluence with the SMV. The left renal vein is located by incising the posterior parietal peritoneum in the lesser sac just superior to the fourth position of the duodenum. Often, the ligament of Treitz must be incised and the duodenum reflected inferiorly to locate the vein. Dividing the adrenal vein may allow better mobilization of the renal vein. To prepare the anastomosis, the splenic vein is occluded with vascular clamps and transected close to its junction with the SMV. The stump is ligated with a suture ligature to decrease the incidence of portal vein thrombosis secondary to traumatic manipulation of the splenic vein stump.[90] A partial occluding clamp is placed on the left renal vein, and the anastomosis is performed.

After completing the devascularization and the spleno-renal anastomosis, measurements are made of the superior mesenteric, renal, and splenic veins. Superior mesenteric (portal) pressures should not be altered if a total portal-azygos disconnection has been performed. Splenic vein pressure will be decreased by 60% to 70%. If this pressure fails to fall, intraoperative angiography should be used to demonstrate a technically sound anastomosis.[33]

Results: Patency and Portal Perfusion. The maintenance of portal perfusion in the early postoperative period has been documented in more than 90% of patients.[110,115,116,127] The principal question regarding this operation, however, is one of durability: how long does the benefit of the DSRS last? It has been shown that the incidence of early partial portal vein thrombosis may be as high as 22%, and that of complete portal vein occlusion 6%. When followed over a 6-month period, most nonocclusive portal vein thromboses resolve spontaneously.[130] A 10-year follow-up by Warren and coworkers of the DSRS group revealed that 75% had persistent portal perfusion at 10 years.[127] Patients who were demonstrated to have portal perfusion at 3 years maintained this until the conclusion of the study at 7 years.[117,121]

The DSRS has several advantages over other nonselective shunts: it preserves portal flow to the liver, it maintains hepatotropic perfusion, it permits the metabolism of toxic metabolites, and it maintains a high portal perfusion pressure in the intestinal venous bed, decreasing the absorption of toxic substances.[67] It is the best procedure to perform under elective conditions in a patient with hepatopetal flow. Child classes A and B patients under emergent conditions also benefit from selective shunts. It should be noted that the DSRS has not been clearly demonstrated to improve survival by itself, but when used in conjunction with judicious sclerotherapy, it appears to provide the best chance of survival to these patients.

Current Indications for Shunt Procedures

As noted, shunting operations are performed infrequently since the advent and proliferation of TIPS procedures. In a recent report by Orug and coauthors,[131] less than 1% of patients with portal hypertension at their institution over a 9-year period underwent open shunt procedures. In a multicenter study of bleeding varices, 3.3% of patients underwent open procedures.[132] The need for repeated intervention is the primary disadvantage of TIPS compared with open operations, but even this aspect can be improved with the use of covered stents (discussed later). Nonetheless, one of the compelling reasons for choosing an open shunt over a TIPS procedure continues to be the lack of access for follow-up. Wong and coworkers[133] reported on their use of splenorenal shunts in patients with poor access to follow-up care in the South Pacific. They concluded that open procedures can be performed safely and are appropriate when tertiary care centers are not easily available. The other clinical scenario in which open shunts continue to be

performed is when other methods fail to control variceal hemorrhage, particularly in Child class A patients. Interestingly, if one considers the available data, open procedures could be recommended in many low-risk Child class A and B patients.[134] A recent metaanalysis examined shunts versus TIPS in the setting of bleeding varices in Child class A and B patients. There were fewer shunt failures and longer survival in the shunted patients than in the TIPS patients.[135] Indeed, in properly selected patients, surgical portocaval shunts may offer not only a small survival benefit, but may do so at essentially a very modest increase in cost.[136] However, the trend in clinical practice is clearly otherwise. Finally, the effectiveness of emergency portacaval shunts in the setting of bleeding has recently been reported by Orloff and colleagues.[137] In comparison to sclerotherapy, which achieved long-term control of bleeding in only 20% of patients, emergency shunting was successful in 100% of patients. Patients undergoing the shunting procedures also had increased survival rates up to 15 years out from the initial intervention.[137]

NONSHUNT SURGICAL PROCEDURES

Emergency portosystemic shunting results in an operative mortality of approximately 47%.[15] Furthermore, in the presence of certain clinical laboratory test results, including an SGOT greater than 300 units/L, or the presence of ascites or other determinants of Child class C status (e.g., bilirubin >6 mg/dL, hyaline necrosis, severe muscle wasting), a portosystemic shunt is almost sure to result in death. Because of this, numerous nonshunting surgical procedures have been developed.

Splenectomy

Based on Banti's theory that the diseased spleen caused portal hypertension and ascites, splenectomy was one of the first operations proposed for the treatment of Banti's syndrome (splenomegaly, hypersplenism, and ascites, often accompanied by esophageal varices). The use of splenectomy in this setting was largely due to its advocacy by Osler, a great admirer of Banti's work. It was not until 1936, when Rousselot reviewed the experience at Columbia University in New York, that the failings of this operation were noted: a significant incidence of recurrent hemorrhage after splenectomy and the consequent loss of the splenic and portal veins, which would preclude possible shunt surgery.[138] In 1940, Thompson was able to demonstrate statistically that splenectomy was of value only to those patients with isolated splenic vein thrombosis[139]; this continues as an indication for splenectomy and can be performed as either an open or laparoscopic procedure.[140] Finally in 1945, Pemberton and Kiernan[141] reported a 54% incidence of recurrent variceal hemorrhage with splenectomy alone.

Collateralization

Development of collateral pathways between the portal circulation and the systemic circulation was the goal of several procedures. Omentopexy, introduced by Talma in 1898, produces collateral pathways by suturing the omentum to the peritoneum.[141a] Another collateral-promoting operation was the transposition of the spleen into the thorax.[142,143] Like omentopexy, its goal was to allow the development of large venous collateral pathways between the portal venous system and the systemic venous circulation. Unfortunately, these collateral pathways were never able to adequately decompress esophageal varices. Thus, the patients were doomed to repeated hemorrhage.

Ablation

Perhaps the most successful devascularization procedure was that developed by Suguira and Futagawa in Japan.[144,145] Because of the significant risk of encephalopathy, shunt procedures were abandoned in favor of an extensive periesophagogastric devascularization accompanied by esophageal transection. The procedure is performed via separate thoracic and abdominal incisions; in poor-risk patients, a two-stage procedure is indicated. The esophagus is devascularized from the gastroesophageal junction to the left inferior pulmonary vein. The vagus nerve is carefully preserved. At the level of the diaphragm, the esophagus is partially transected, leaving only the posterior muscular layer intact. Esophageal varices are occluded, not ligated, by oversewing each with interrupted sutures. The esophageal muscle is closed, but the mucosa is not sutured. The abdominal operation is performed through a separate midline incision and includes splenectomy, devascularization of the abdominal esophagus and proximal stomach, and pyloroplasty and fundoplication.

The early results of this operation, as reported by Suguira and Futagawa,[144] were excellent. The authors reported an overall operative mortality of 4.6%, and the emergency operative mortality was 20%. Varices were eradicated in 97% of patients, and recurrent bleeding occurred in only 2.5%. Their long-term survival was 84%. A follow-up report by the authors on 276 patients indicated equally good survival rates, with excellent control of variceal bleeding and no encephalopathy.[146] In a later report, they analyzed their results according to the patients' Child classification. They found that in class C patients, both operative mortality and long-term survival were discouraging. For classes A and B patients, the results were very good, with combined (A, B, and C) 15-year survival as high as 72%.[147]

Reports by Suguira's group have been confirmed by others in Japan, as well as by selected investigators in the United States.[148] A number of other reports have suggested the use of esophageal transection procedures in the management of selected patients with poor hepatic reserves (Child class C patients). The end-to-end anastomosis (EEA) stapler has made this a relatively simple procedure, but the possibility of esophageal perforation and leakage still makes the procedure a considerably risky one. Overall, these studies demonstrate that esophageal transection should be considered a reasonable option in the management of acute hemorrhage in a debilitated patient with both gastric and esophageal varices.[149-153]

TRANSJUGULAR INTRAHEPATIC PORTOSYSTEMIC SHUNT

The TIPS has become a commonly used technique for controlling variceal hemorrhage. This has had a dramatic effect on the performance of operative shunting procedures, despite the fact that TIPS has been used clinically only since 1988. Over the last few years, the indications for TIPS have expanded, although these applications have not always been backed by randomized trials. Recent developments in TIPS research, most notably the use of covered stents, have improved the patency of TIPS and will most likely lead to even more widespread use of this procedure.

Rosch and colleagues demonstrated 30 years ago that intrahepatic portacaval shunts could be created in a minimally invasive fashion.[154] Palmaz and colleagues applied his stent to this type of procedure, leading to prolonged patency of these shunts in animal models.[155] After its initial application in human subjects, there was a rapid expansion in its application, so that a large number of interventionists became skilled in this technique. Most major medical centers now perform TIPS.

TIPS can be performed with conscious sedation and is frequently carried out in interventional suites. Ultrasonography should be done before the procedure to document the patency of the portal vein and assess the need for a peritoneal tap. Most interventionists minimize the amount of ascites before performing TIPS so that the liver is not "floating" in the abdomen. Access is ideally attained via the right internal jugular vein, which provides the most direct route for cannulation of right hepatic vein branches. Wedged venogram and portal pressures are obtained, and a portal vein branch is then punctured. There are a number of commercially available devices for advancing through the liver parenchyma to the portal vein; the Rosch-Uchida transjugular liver access set (Cook Surgical, Bloomington, Ind.) is used at my institution. These devices combine a cutting needle with an aspiration port and are usually designed to fit a 10-French sheath. Portal access is confirmed by aspirating blood during needle advancement. A guidewire is advanced so that the hepatic and portal circuits are in continuity. Finally, the track is balloon-dilated and stented. At the end of the procedure, pressure measurements can be repeated to confirm that the portal-systemic gradient is less than 12 mm Hg. A completion venogram must also be obtained to assess stent placement and to ensure that varices are no longer filling.

TIPS for acute variceal bleeding stops the hemorrhage in more than 90% of patients.[156] This compares favorably with endoscopic sclerotherapy in many series, including at least eight prospective, randomized trials.[157,158] However, most studies have shown a decreased rate of rebleeding with TIPS versus sclerotherapy. Rosch and Keller[159] reported a 5.6% rebleeding rate at 3 months' follow-up, compared with the 20% to 30% usually seen following endoscopic therapy. As with rebleeding following other therapies, a significant number of patients (25% to 30%) will have a different, nonvariceal lesion as the hemorrhage source. Confirmation of the source is thus extremely important.

When the bleeding is from varices, it is almost invariably associated with improper function of the shunt. As with other vascular conduits, short-term problems are usually technical in nature, whereas those developing later are related to neointima formation. Although TIPS can be revised to control the bleeding, one of the chief criticisms of these shunts is the need for repeated interventions.[160] In fact, the primary patency of TIPS is approximately 40% at 1 year, but secondary patency approaches 90%.[161]

Despite the benefit in preventing rebleeding, TIPS is considered a second-line procedure after sclerotherapy owing to several factors, most notably the increased incidence of hepatic encephalopathy (approximately 50% vs. 20%). In addition, for patients whose bleeding is controlled by sclerotherapy, there is no survival benefit with TIPS.

It is clear that TIPS has replaced open surgical shunt procedures for most Child classes B and C patients. This is underscored by the fact that it is not uncommon for a surgical resident to finish his or her training without performing a single shunting procedure. Interestingly, in the largest prospective trial comparing TIPS and surgical shunts (8-mm prosthetic H grafts), TIPS was found to have higher rates of death, rebleeding, and treatment failure.[162] This trial, as well as an additional 4 years of follow-up, was published by Rosemurgy and colleagues[162] and evaluated 35 patients in each arm, pairing them based on their Child class. A comparison of the rates of post-treatment encephalopathy generally favored surgery as well. These data are in agreement with that in the meta-analysis by Clark cited in the shunt section of this chapter.

TIPS has been applied in several other clinical situations. One broad category is as a bridge to hepatic transplantation. Theoretically, the procedure leaves the porta hepatis unperturbed and allows for easier subsequent operation. Some have argued that TIPS actually accelerates liver failure in patients awaiting transplantation.[163] However, several studies support the use of TIPS in this setting, particularly as a means for improving patients' general condition, sometimes with decreased blood loss at the time of surgery.[164-168] One technical note of importance is placement of the distal end of the stent well above the IVC so that it does not interfere with the transplant itself or cause damage to the portal vein.

Another application of TIPS has been for the management of refractory ascites. There are numerous retrospective trials documenting the effectiveness of TIPS in this setting, but only a few randomized trials. In a randomized study by Rossle and coauthors,[169] TIPS was shown to be more effective than paracentesis in controlling refractory ascites. In a study by Lebrec and coworkers,[170] TIPS was shown to benefit Child class B patients with ascites but was of no help in class C patients, in whom it had little effect on ascites and increased mortality.[170] In a more recent review of randomized trials, Saab and associates,[171] using clinical registries, found that TIPS reduced ascites reaccumulation better than paracentesis at 3- and 12-month follow-up.[171] Encephalopathy was more common in the TIPS group,

but all other variables analyzed were equal. Finally, Rosemurgy and colleagues[172] performed a randomized, prospective trial comparing TIPS and peritovenous shunts. They concluded that TIPS was more beneficial in patients unless they had only a very short life expectancy. Siegerstetter and colleagues[173] reported retrospectively on the benefits of TIPS in treating refractory hydrothorax.

TIPS has also been used with some success in the treatment of Budd-Chiari syndrome. There are several small studies investigating its use in this setting. Perello and coauthors[174] managed 13 such patients with TIPS and found that 11 were doing well after a follow-up of 4 years. Interestingly, many of the patients' TIPS were no longer patent but did not require treatment owing to the absence of signs of portal hypertension. Blum and coauthors[175] reported on 12 Budd-Chiari patients who underwent TIPS.[175] Two of the patients had fulminant hepatic failure and died, but the remaining 10 had resolution of their ascites. In a larger series, Rossle and colleagues reported on 35 patients receiving TIPS for Budd-Chiari syndrome.[176] The cumulative 1- and 5-year survival rates without transplantation in this group were 93% and 74%, respectively, suggesting that TIPS will continue to evolve as a treatment for this disease.

One additional application of TIPS has been for hepatorenal syndrome. Brensing and colleagues[177] reported an improvement in renal function in these patients compared with nonshunted patients. Other studies also support the use of TIPS in this setting.[178] Recently, Wong and colleagues[179] demonstrated prospectively that TIPS can be used in conjunction with a protocol of midodrine, octreotide, and albumin to improve renal function in type 1 hepatorenal syndrome.

As mentioned previously, the main drawbacks of TIPS are the poor primary patency and the need for repeated interventions to maintain the shunt. It has been shown in animal studies that the use of covered stents improves the patency of TIPS, and there are now human data to support this contention. Otal and associates[180] used PTFE-covered nitinol stents in a recent series of 20 patients and reported primary and secondary patency rates of 80% and 100% at 387 days (as opposed to 58% primary patency at 1 year for uncovered stents reported in the literature).[180] Rossi and coworkers[181] reported 1-year primary patency rates of 83.8% with these stent-grafts, and Maleux and associates[182] reported only a single occlusion after 56 TIPS procedures using PTFE-covered stents at a mean follow-up of 246 days (range, 3 to 973 days). A more recent metaanalysis of PTFE-covered stents versus bare metal stents for use in TIPS demonstrated not only improved patency for the covered stents, but also a trend toward increased survival. No concomitant increase in encephalopathy was noted.[183]

TIPS has also been used successfully in patients who have already undergone orthotopic liver transplantation (OLT). King and coauthors[184] recently reported on a series of OLT patients who went on to develop either variceal bleeding or refractory ascites. The patients with a pre-TIPS model for end-stage liver disease (MELD) score of less than 15 essentially did as well as a control group (i.e., non-OLT) of patients undergoing TIPS for the same indications. However, with a MELD score greater than 15, patients in the OLT group did poorly.[184]

ORTHOTOPIC LIVER TRANSPLANTATION

With the advent of liver transplantation as an established modality for patients with end-stage liver failure, the role of nontransplantation procedures (shunt surgery in particular) has been the subject of considerable debate. Currently, the best transplant survival rates are generally more favorable than those of Child class C patients after the best care with a combination of sclerotherapy and shunting. This issue has been the subject of two reports from Iwatsuki and colleagues[185,186] at the University of Pittsburgh Liver Transplant Unit. These reports described the survival of 302 patients who had bleeding esophageal varices. According to the authors, these patients were all ranked as Child class C in regard to hepatic function. Their survival was reported in a life-table format as 79% at 1 year, 74% at 2 years, and 71% at 5 years. The authors then compared these results with shunt survival as reported in the medical literature and concluded that in Child class C patients with bleeding varices, liver transplantation should be considered the treatment of choice, assuming that the patients are reasonable transplant candidates.

Our experience at the University of California–Los Angeles, has revealed that transplantation affords superior survival to Child class C patients (Table 52-2). In a series of 761 patients operated on between January 1986 and December 1991, 77 underwent portosystemic shunting as their initial procedure, and 684 underwent hepatic transplantation. Of the patients receiving transplants, 86% were Child class C, whereas only 16% of the shunt patients were class C. Despite this, 15% of shunt patients eventually required liver transplantation for progressive hepatic deterioration. Furthermore, the 5-year survival for the shunt group was 64%, in contrast to 73% for the transplant patients. Similar 5-year survival data in excess of 75% were recently published by Roberts and associates,[187] reflecting patients' studies through 1999. These data support the impression that portosystemic shunting is an appropriate therapy for Child classes A and B patients, but that class C patients who are reasonable candidates are best managed by liver transplantation.

Further complicating the issue is the effect of a prior shunt operation on a subsequent transplant operation. It

has been reported that patients who must receive a liver transplant after having a portacaval shunt have considerably greater blood loss, longer operative procedures, increased morbidity, and higher mortality.[188] The portacaval shunt is a particularly troublesome procedure to overcome, because the performance of a successful liver transplantation requires dissection through the scarred tissues about the portal structures, disconnection of the shunt, and reconstitution of the normal caval anatomy; only then can the liver transplant operation begin. This is in contrast to peripheral shunt operations, such as the mesocaval shunt or the DSRS. Although these shunts have an effect on the transplantation procedure, they are not as difficult to manage as the central shunts are. In the case of a mesocaval shunt, the shunt must be disconnected or occluded before the transplant operation is completed, or the new liver may be deprived of portal nutrient blood flow. A similar problem can arise with the DSRS, although because of the nature of this shunt, the siphon effect (drainage of portal blood through peripancreatic collaterals into the shunt) is usually relatively minor, and the shunt frequently does not require dismantling.

In any consideration of the role of shunting versus liver transplantation, the essential factors are the underlying cause of the hepatic disease, the current stage of hepatic dysfunction, and the expected progression (the natural and treated history) of the hepatic disease. Assuming that the patient is a reasonable transplant candidate and that the liver disease is approaching the end stage (Child class C), transplantation should be strongly considered. If the patient requires an emergent procedure to control bleeding before undergoing transplantation, all efforts should be made to provide a peripheral shunt. If the patient is not a transplant candidate, treatment should consist of the best therapy available: sclerotherapy supported by either esophageal transection with devascularization or shunting.

VARICEAL SCLEROTHERAPY

Esophageal variceal sclerotherapy was introduced by Crafoord and Frenckner in 1939.[189] These authors reported a single patient who underwent rigid endoscopic sclerotherapy to prevent further variceal bleeding. With the upsurge in the variety of surgical procedures for variceal hemorrhage in the 1940s, however, sclerotherapy was soon forgotten. Once it was recognized that therapeutic portacaval shunts, with their inherent operative mortality and risk of encephalopathy, were not the ultimate surgical procedure, attention was redirected toward less invasive, more direct methods of treatment, and there was renewed interest in sclerotherapy after the results of several controlled trials.

The first major review of sclerotherapy was by Johnston and Rodgers in 1973.[190] In 117 patients, bleeding was initially controlled in 92%, and the hospital mortality per admission was 18%. The average time to recurrence of variceal hemorrhage was 10 months. This group, however, made no attempt to perform sequential variceal sclerotherapy and recommended a shunt for long-term variceal control.

TABLE 52-2 **Results of Portosystemic Shunting and Liver Transplantation from January 1986 to December 1991***

	No. of Patients	Child Class C (%)	5-Year Survival
Portosystemic shunt	77	16	64
Liver transplantation	684	86	73

*University of California–Los Angeles, experience. Distal splenorenal shunts constituted 50% of shunt operations; 15% of shunt patients eventually underwent liver transplantation because of deterioration of hepatic function.

TABLE 52-3 **Sclerotherapy versus Medical Management (Control)**

Study	Follow-up (Mo)	Sclerotherapy			Control		
		No. of Patients	Rebleed (%)	Percentage Surviving (Yr)	No. of Patients	Rebleed (%)	Percentage Surviving (Yr)
Terblanche and colleagues[198]	60	37	43*	45 (5)	38	73	45 (5)
Paquet and Feussner[193]	9-52	93	48	36 (2)	97	54	25 (2)
Westaby and colleagues[197]	3-60	56	55*	60 (4)	60	80	31 (4)
Korula and colleagues[200]	3-35	63	44*	60 (2)	57	70	56 (2)
Soderlund and Ihre[199]	12-48	57†	49 (2)	50†	34 (2)		

*There was a significant decrease in transfusion requirements in the sclerotherapy group, as well as fewer rebleeding episodes per patient-month if followed up.
†Overall recurrent hemorrhage was 3.6 times more frequent in the control group.

Endoscopy is necessary to confirm the presence of varices and differentiate those that are actively bleeding from those that have ceased to bleed. The use of sclerotherapy to stop acute bleeding at the time of initial endoscopy has been advocated as the treatment of choice.[191,192] Urgent or emergent sclerotherapy is used in many institutions after stabilization with balloon tamponade or after failure of conservative supportive therapy and somatostatin. Several controlled trials have compared sclerotherapy with medical management with the Sengstaken-Blakemore tube in the acute setting.[193-197] Three studies demonstrated a significantly lower early rebleeding rate,[193-195] and all the studies supported the use of sclerotherapy for acute bleeding. Only Paquet and Feussner demonstrated significantly improved overall survival with sclerotherapy.[193]

The ability of sclerotherapy to prevent recurrent variceal hemorrhage and improve long-term survival with extended treatment has been examined in numerous controlled trials (Table 52-3).[196-200] When sclerotherapy was performed to eradicate all varices and compared with conservative medical management, sclerotherapy patients had fewer recurrent bleeds[196,198] and improved long-term survival.[197] Terblanche and colleagues[198] were able to demonstrate complete eradication of varices in 95% of sclerotherapy patients; however, they could not demonstrate a significant difference in survival, and varices recurred in more than 60% of the sclerotherapy patients.[198]

Only since 1984 has sclerotherapy been systematically compared with portosystemic shunts in the management of variceal hemorrhage. Cello and associates[201,202] compared the portacaval shunt to sclerotherapy in Child class C patients, showing greater rebleeding, increased rehospitalization, and higher blood transfusion requirements in the sclerotherapy group, with 40% of sclerotherapy patients ultimately requiring surgical therapy. However, they were unable to demonstrate any significant difference in survival (Table 52-4). The authors concluded that in high-risk patients, sclerotherapy and portacaval shunting are equal in the acute setting, but one must consider shunt surgery if varices are not totally obliterated.

The DSRS has been compared with endoscopic sclerotherapy for the long-term management of variceal bleeding in three controlled trials (Table 52-5). Warren

TABLE 52-4 **Sclerotherapy versus Portacaval Shunt in Management of Variceal Hemorrhage**

	Sclerotherapy (n = 32)	Shunt (n = 32)	p Value
Rebleed rate (%)	50	19	<0.009
Encephalopathy (%)	13	13	NS
Surgery not required	7 (22%)	—	—
Long-term cost	$23,000	$28,000	NS
18-month survival (%)	28	13	NS

NS, Not significant.
Data from Cello J, Grendell J, Crass R, et al: Endoscopic sclerotherapy versus portacaval shunt in patients with severe cirrhosis and variceal hemorrhage, N Engl J Med 311:1589-1594, 1984.

TABLE 52-5 **Sclerotherapy versus Distal Splenorenal Shunt in Long-Term Management of Variceal Hemorrhage***

	Sclerotherapy	DSRS	p Value
Warren and colleagues[203]			
No. of patients	36	35	
Rebleed rate (%)	53	3	<0.05
Portal perfusion (%)	95	53	<0.05
Patients requiring surgery	10	(28%)	
2-yr survival (%)	84	59	<0.01
Rikkers and colleagues[205]			
No. of patients	30	27	
Rebleed rate (%)	57	19	0.003
Encephalopathy (%)	7	16	
2-yr survival (%)	61	65	NS
Teres and colleagues[204]			
No. of patients	55	57	
Rebleed rate (%)	37.5	14.%	<0.02
Encephalopathy (%)	8	24	<0.05
2-yr survival (%)	68	71	NS

*All controlled trials.
DSRS, Distal splenorenal shunt; NS, not significant.

and coworkers[203] showed that although early mortality was the same, there was a higher rebleeding rate with sclerotherapy, and one third of the patients failed treatment and required surgery.[203] Treatment with sclerotherapy resulted in significant improvement in liver function when successful, with less encephalopathy and improved survival when backed up by surgical therapy for patients with uncontrolled bleeding. Therefore the improved survival in the sclerotherapy group actually represents a combination of sclerotherapy and surgical therapy. Teres and colleagues[204] found no difference in early and long-term mortality, nor did Rikkers and coworkers.[205] However, the rebleeding rate was greater in patients who had sclerotherapy, and encephalopathy rates were higher in shunt patients in the study by Teres and colleagues.[204]

In 1989, Burroughs and associates[206] concluded a prospective, randomized study comparing staple transection with sclerotherapy for emergency control of variceal bleeding. They found no difference in overall mortality and improved control of bleeding with esophageal transection compared with a single injection, but there was a similar incidence of hemorrhage after three injection treatments. Teres and colleagues[207] randomized cirrhotic patients with uncontrolled bleeding to portacaval shunt or staple transection in low-risk patients and staple transection or sclerotherapy in high-risk patients. Survival was similar in the two groups. In the low-risk patients, portacaval shunt had a greater hemostatic effect but a greater incidence of encephalopathy. In high-risk patients, sclerotherapy and staple transection had similar rebleeding rates and survival, but fewer complications were observed in the sclerotherapy group. The authors therefore recommended staple transection for low-risk patients and sclerotherapy for the initial management of high-risk patients. Although a consensus has not yet been reached, sclerotherapy may represent an appropriate alternative ablative procedure in selected patients with hepatic dysfunction.[207-214]

More recently, interest has increased in an alternative endoscopic technique, variceal banding. This has the advantage of avoiding the caustic agents required for sclerotherapy. In comparison studies, the rates of efficacy in halting bleeding are similar between the two techniques. There is debate whether the incidence of complications with banding is reduced compared with sclerotherapy. Clearly the same major complications attend both techniques: recurrent bleeding, as well as esophageal ulceration and perforation.[214]

Endoscopic variceal sclerotherapy and variceal banding have the distinct advantages of no risk of portal vein thrombosis, good control of variceal hemorrhage, and easy accessibility for repeat sclerotherapy. There is no question that in patients with acute variceal bleeding who have had a prior splenectomy or a portosystemic shunt that has failed, endoscopic therapy is indicated. Because of the high mortality associated with emergency shunting procedures, variceal sclerotherapy in conjunction with octreotide is indicated in the acute management of variceal hemorrhage. Recurrent variceal hemorrhage is likely if follow-up routine sclerotherapy is not performed; therefore sclerotherapy should be considered an adjunctive therapeutic management tool for the acute control of variceal bleeding rather than definitive treatment.

TREATMENT PLAN FOR VARICEAL HEMORRHAGE

When a patient has an upper gastrointestinal tract hemorrhage and the history and physical examination suggest esophageal varices in association with hepatic disease, a preset treatment plan should be followed (Figure 52-6). It is important to remember that time is of the essence in these patients, and delays to consider, define, and formulate a plan of action may jeopardize the patient's life. The initial care of a bleeding portal hypertensive patient should be as routine as the initial care of a trauma patient, following the *ABC*'s. Special variations are implemented because of the underlying hepatic disease and the associated risks.

Initial laboratory studies should include a CBC, electrolytes, blood typing, and crossmatching. Additionally, determinants of liver function, including bilirubin, SGOT, LDH, SGPT, prothrombin time, partial thromboplastin time, albumin, total protein, and alkaline phosphatase, should be obtained. Nasogastric tubes must be placed in all patients; if blood is present in the stomach, then gastric lavage and emergency endoscopy are indicated. This allows verification of the source of the hemorrhage and emergent sclerotherapy, if required.

Initial fluid management is crucial. Treatment with fluids and blood products should be directed at maintaining adequate tissue perfusion. Resuscitation should include packed RBCs and fresh frozen plasma, as needed. Cryoprecipitates and calcium may be required in cases of massive bleeding. It is generally preferable to resuscitate with a combination of crystalloid and blood components (albumin and packed RBCs) rather than with saline only. Thiamine should be administered to prevent Wernicke encephalopathy. Propranolol or diazepam (Valium) may be required for the symptoms of alcohol withdrawal.

If the bleeding does not stop during resuscitation and transfusion, octreotide should be administered intravenously and repeated sclerotherapy should be performed. Balloon tamponade may be especially helpful at this juncture. If the patient fails to stop bleeding after injections and balloon tamponade, emergent intervention is indicated. Depending on the institution's resources, the patient should be considered for a TIPS, portosystemic shunt, or esophageal transection with devascularization. If the patient is a potential liver transplant candidate, a peripheral shunt (DSRS or mesocaval) should be performed. The choice of TIPS or surgical shunt should probably be based on the local expertise and ability of the managing physicians.

Once bleeding is controlled, patients with relatively good hepatic function (Child class A or B) should undergo long-term sclerotherapy until varices are obliterated. If this is successful, the patient should continue to be observed, and no further intervention need be planned. If the patient has breakthrough bleeding from noncompliance, gastric varices, or hypertensive gastritis and is an

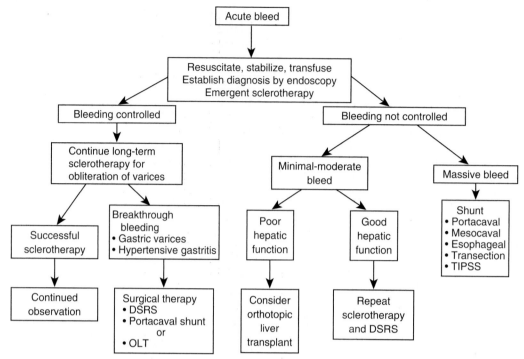

FIGURE 52-6 ■ Protocol for the management of variceal hemorrhage. *DSRS,* Distal splenorenal shunt; *OLT,* orthotopic liver transplantation; *TIPSS,* transjugular intrahepatic portosystemic stent-shunt.

appropriate candidate for an elective shunt, a preoperative evaluation should be done (angiography, duplex scan) and a shunt is performed.

Patients with poor hepatic function should be considered for transplantation if they meet the appropriate criteria. While the patient is awaiting orthotopic liver transplantation, a peripheral shunt may be necessary as a bridge. Child class C patients with marked muscle wasting and obvious hyaline necrosis have a prohibitively high operative mortality rate and should undergo endoscopic sclerotherapy followed by transplantation. If this technique is not available, esophageal transection with or without the EEA stapler and ligation of portal-azygos collateral pathways is indicated, although the mortality can be expected to be greater than 60%.

MANAGEMENT OF ASCITES

Ascites predisposes portal hypertensive patients to potentially lethal complications, including renal failure, peritonitis, variceal hemorrhage, pleural effusions with respiratory insufficiency, abdominal wall hernias, anorexia, and generalized malaise. In most patients, ascites can be controlled with a restricted-salt diet and a diuretic regimen. However, a subgroup (5%-10%) of ascites patients have refractory ascites, and this is associated with increased mortality.[215] Treatment options for these patients include paracentesis, TIPS, peritoneovenous shunting, or OLT. Paracentesis can be an effective strategy, particularly when large volume paracentesis can be tolerated.[216] When this treatment modality is not successful or practical, TIPS may provide an attractive

alternative.[169] A return of ascites should prompt a diagnostic work up for a TIPS stenosis or occlusion.

Although rarely performed, peritoneovenous shunting can also be used for the treatment of ascites. In 1974, LeVeen and colleagues introduced the peritoneovenous shunt.[217] This device consists of a Silastic tube that runs from the peritoneum to the superior vena cava. It is controlled by a one-way valve so that a pressure gradient of 5 cm H_2O suffices to transfer the ascitic fluid from the abdomen to the intravascular space. The Denver shunt, a variation of the LeVeen shunt, incorporates a pump in line with the shunt and is implanted into the subcutaneous tissues in the chest wall. Its proposed benefit is the ability to clear the shunt of debris by using the pump mechanism.[122]

Although promising innovations, both of these shunts are dogged by complications. Early complications include congestive heart failure (from the infusion of ascitic fluid) and disseminated intravascular coagulation (DIC).[218] Coagulation values tend to improve after the first postoperative week, possibly related to diminished ascitic flow into the venous system.[219] If clinically apparent DIC develops, the only definitive treatment is shunt ligation. Because of the host of complications accompanying these shunts, they are rarely performed today.

The final option for the management of refractory ascites is OLT, which is performed as a definitive treatment in this situation. However, data evaluating the role OLT for ascites are actually lacking. Ascites is not considered in the MELD score; therefore it is unclear how patients transplanted in this clinical scenario ultimately do.

SUMMARY

The management of portal hypertension and its sequelae of ascites, encephalopathy, and recurrent variceal hemorrhage continue to be significant challenges to clinicians. Its cause and pathogenesis have been well described. Alcoholic cirrhosis resulting in intrahepatic sinusoidal and postsinusoidal obstruction continues to be the most common cause.

Long-term survival depends on rapid control of hemorrhage and institution of the most appropriate care for the patient according to the nature and severity of the hepatic disease. A patient who has variceal hemorrhage should be resuscitated quickly. Endoscopy should be performed to establish the source of gastrointestinal bleeding, followed by sclerotherapy. Initial management should include intravenous vasopressin followed by balloon tamponade. Angiography or duplex Doppler studies should be performed in patients being considered for shunting. Emergent shunt surgery should be avoided if possible, because the mortality is excessive.

Selective shunt procedures (e.g., DSRS), although they do not extend long-term survival, produce less encephalopathy and stop bleeding. Patients should be considered for elective shunting if they cannot be controlled with sclerotherapy and have relatively good hepatic function (Child class A or B). Child class C patients and "unshuntable" patients are best treated with nonshunt procedures or transplantation. Esophageal variceal sclerotherapy provides effective control of acute variceal hemorrhage; however, if it is unsuccessful after several attempts, a portal-azygos devascularization procedure should be performed. Ultimately, the survival of these patients depends on the degree of hepatic function. Patients with end-stage liver disease should be considered for liver transplantation.

Encephalopathy is a consequence of hepatic failure. It may be ameliorated by a medical regimen of neomycin, lactulose, and a low-protein diet. Ascites can usually be managed with salt restriction and diuretics. In a patient with intractable ascites, a peritoneovenous shunt provides effective control.

Determining the best treatment for patients with portal hypertension relies on the recognition that the hepatic disease dictates the progression of liver failure. Depending on the stage of hepatic dysfunction, different options are available. In deciding how best to manage a particular patient, it is necessary to keep in mind that the goal is not merely survival but also quality of life.

References available online at expertconsult.com.

QUESTIONS

1. A 35-year-old woman with a history of viral hepatitis and cirrhosis, status postcholecystectomy, has a clinical presentation of variceal hemorrhage unresponsive to medical therapy. Which surgical procedure is indicated if sclerotherapy fails?
   a. End-to-side portacaval shunt
   b. Side-to-side portacaval shunt
   c. H-graft mesocaval shunt
   d. EEA abdominal esophageal transection
   e. Distal splenorenal shunt

2. A 10-year-old boy with a history of omphalitis experiences his first episode of variceal hemorrhage. Which is the most appropriate therapy?
   a. Distal splenorenal shunt
   b. Medical regimen
   c. Variceal sclerotherapy
   d. End-to-side portacaval shunt
   e. H-graft mesocaval shunt

3. Specific contraindications to peritoneovenous shunts include all of the following except:
   a. Hepatic necrosis
   b. Bilirubin greater than 6 mg/dL
   c. Hepatorenal syndrome
   d. Infected ascitic fluid
   e. Prothrombin time prolonged more than 4 seconds

4. Which of the following statements about prophylactic portacaval shunts is true?
   a. They prolong longevity
   b. They decrease encephalopathy
   c. They have a greater than 50% recurrent hemorrhage rate
   d. They are associated with a prohibitively high operative mortality
   e. They are not indicated

5. The Budd-Chiari syndrome may be treated by all of the following except:
   a. Anticoagulants
   b. Side-to-side portacaval shunt
   c. End-to-side portacaval shunt
   d. Mesoatrial shunt
   e. Mesocaval shunt

6. Technical considerations in favor of performing a distal splenorenal shunt include which of the following?
   a. Cavernomatous transformation of the splenic vein
   b. Acute hyaline necrosis
   c. Splenic vein greater than 4 mm in diameter
   d. Intractable ascites
   e. Hepatopetal flow

7. Which of the following statements regarding sclerotherapy is false?
   a. Percutaneous transhepatic coronary vein occlusion is associated with a 20% portal vein thrombosis rate.
   b. Sclerotherapy should not be used in the acute setting because of high mortality.
   c. Sodium morrhuate and ethanolamine oleate are appropriate sclerosing agents.
   d. Repeated sclerotherapy is necessary for control of hemorrhage.
   e. Esophageal ulcerations usually resolve spontaneously without sequelae.

8. Which of the following is an advantage of selective shunts?
   a. Continued portal perfusion
   b. Gastric and esophageal varix decompression
   c. No greater incidence of shunt thrombosis than with portacaval shunts
   d. Decreased incidence of encephalopathy
   e. All of the above

9. A 40-year-old man has hematemesis and hypotension. What initial diagnostic measures should be performed after stabilization?
   a. Superior mesenteric arteriography
   b. Splenoportography
   c. Esophagogastroscopy
   d. Celiac angiogram with venous phase
   e. Upper gastrointestinal series

10. What is the most common site of obstruction causing portal hypertension in the Western world?
    a. Portal vein (thrombosis)
    b. Extrahepatic postsinusoidal
    c. Intrahepatic presinusoidal
    d. Intrahepatic sinusoidal and postsinusoidal
    e. Extrahepatic presinusoidal

11. A 40-year-old man with cirrhosis is determined to be Child class A; his bleeding has been controlled with sclerotherapy and vasopressin. What is the most appropriate treatment plan?
    a. Emergency shunt surgery
    b. Warren shunt
    c. Mesocaval shunt
    d. TIPS procedure
    e. Periodic sclerotherapy

ANSWERS

1. c
2. b
3. c
4. e
5. c
6. e
7. b
8. e
9. c
10. d
11. e

CHAPTER 53

LYMPHEDEMA

Andrew K. Kurklinsky • Thom W. Rooke

Lymphedema is an important topic for vascular surgeons for three reasons. First, it is highly common. Estimates vary, but hundreds of thousands of patients in the United States have lymphedema,[1] and hundreds of millions are affected worldwide according to the World Health Organization.[2] Second, even the best surgeons may have patients who develop lymphedema after operations involving the limbs or trunk. Third, lymphedema may be confused with venous disease or other vascular anomalies that are typically referred to vascular surgeons. For these reasons, vascular surgeons are likely to encounter patients with lymphedema.

PATHOGENESIS

Fluid, proteins, and various soluble substances extravasate from the capillaries into the interstitial space.[3] This fluid is removed through venous capillaries and lymphatic vessels, which provide equilibrium between the amount of fluid released into the interstitium and that removed from it. Fluid transported by the lymphatic vessels carries macromolecules and is rich in protein, increased concentrations of which raise osmotic pressure of the tissues by binding fluid in the interstitium.[4] Interstitial fluid is called *lymph fluid* once it enters the lymphatic vessel. If the flow of lymphatic fluid through the lymphatic vessels is hindered, it accumulates in the tissues producing edema.

Normal lymphatic vessels exhibit spontaneous regular rhythmic contractions that pump fluid centripetally. This process is independent of hydrostatic pressure, muscle contractions, or external pressure in healthy individuals. These mechanisms become important for maintaining fluid flow when lymphatic vessels are damaged. Various insults may produce a range of lymphatic vessel abnormalities, such as total obstruction of lymphatic trunks in erysipelas, vessel wall changes in staphylococcal dermatitis or after trauma. Progressive stages of lymphedema are marked by increasing abnormalities of the lymphatic vessel contractions leading to stasis and increased tissue pressure.[5]

Lymphedema occurs when interstitial fluid accumulates because of lymphatic obstruction or reflux (or rarely from extreme overproduction of lymph fluid). Over time, inflammatory alterations in connective tissues marked by altered cytokine production, accumulation of plasma proteins, and fibrous proliferation with deposition of collagen lead to dermal fibrosis. The brawny or woody texture of lymphedema (Figure 53-1) is thought to be caused by chronic inflammation associated with the excessive interstitial protein trapping that overwhelms intrinsic neutrophil and macrophage proteases.[6] Paradoxically, the protein concentration of the interstitial fluid in the swollen arm of patients with breast cancer-related lymphedema is lower than that in the contralateral arm, and correlates negatively with the degree of swelling. In addition to mechanical obstruction and inflammation, other factors, including impaired capacity for lymphangiogenesis causing a reduced number of collaterals and lymphovenous communications, may contribute to lymphedema formation.[7]

CAUSES

Lymphedema may be either primary or secondary, resulting from either the failure of lymphatics to develop normally or from the degeneration and loss of lymphatics over time. Primary lymphedema may occur shortly after birth (heritable forms include Milroy disease),[8,9] around the time of puberty (lymphedema praecox),[9] or rarely during adulthood (lymphedema tarda).[10] Phenotypic characterization of the genetic defects has been possible for some forms of primary lymphedema.[11] More than 30 mutations in vascular endothelial growth factor receptor-3 (VEGFR3 or FLT4) have been identified for Milroy disease. Because of incomplete penetrance, presence of these mutations results in lymphedema in 64% to 90% of all patients. In this condition, skin lymphatics are abundant but are nonfunctional.[11] In lymphedema-distichiasis, the mutation is in *FOXC2* with penetrance of 94% to 100%.[12] The characteristic double row of eye lashes is present at birth, while lymphedema onset is delayed until puberty. Lymphedema-distichiasis may also include another disease variant known as *lymphedema-ptosis syndrome*.[11] Hypotrichosis-lymphedema-telangiectasia syndrome is due to mutation in *SOX18*.[13] Isolated pubertal-onset primary lymphedema (Meige disease) does not have an identified genetic defect. Many complex syndromes, such as Hennekam, Aagenaes (cholestasis-lymphedema syndrome), microcephaly-chorioretinopathy-lymphedema, Mucke, Noonan, Turner, Prader-Willi, neurofibromatosis type I (von Recklinghausen), lymphedema-hypoparathyroidism, Klippel-Trenaunay-Weber, and yellow nail syndromes, include lymphedema as a clinical feature.[11,14,15]

In practice, clinical grading of lymphedema (Table 53-1) is commonly used based on the physical condition of the affected tissues.[16,17] Volumetric documentation and bioimpedance technologies improve diagnostic precision and may help to detect subclinical disease.[18,19]

Secondary lymphedema is much more common than the primary form and can result from anything that leads to the destruction of lymphatic vessels or nodes.[10] In the United States and other developed countries, most cases are secondary to surgical interventions and radiation treatment, usually related to cancer.[20] Incidence ranges 9% to 41% after axillary lymph node dissection, although it decreased to 4% to 10% with sentinel node biopsy.[21] It remains to be seen whether new surgical approaches[22,23] will become widely accepted and lead to reduction of the associated rates of lymphedema. Other common causes include trauma, surgery, radiation therapy (leads to lymphatic sclerosis), invasion of the lymphatic system by tumor, recurrent infections or lymphangitis (usually caused by streptococci or, less often, staphylococci) that obliterate the vessels, and certain parasites. Worldwide, filariasis necessitated treatment in nearly half a billion people (primarily in tropical countries) in 2009 and thus is the most common cause of lymphedema.[2] The most common filariae are *Wuchereria bancrofti* and *Brugia* species.[24] Although most of these are tropical organisms, some *Brugia* species are found in North America. Many

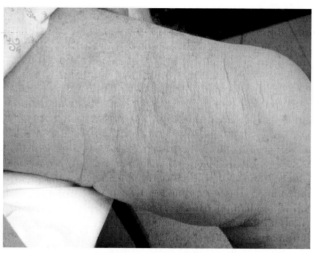

FIGURE 53-1 ■ Skin changes in lymphedema. Protein accumulation within the interstitial space produces "brawny" induration of the skin. The resulting "orange-peel skin" is a common clinical finding in chronic lymphedema.

other conditions, including autoimmune diseases, pregnancy, illegal drug injections, and factitial injuries may produce lymphedema.[25-28] Risk factors for lymphedema development include weight gain or obesity, trauma, history of malignancy, family history of lymphedema, travel to the endemic geographic areas.[18]

DIAGNOSIS

Lymphedema is often suspected or diagnosed on clinical grounds. Age, an appropriate history describing the circumstances leading to the onset of edema, and the presence of comorbid conditions help to discern primary and secondary lymphedema cases. In some variants of primary lymphedema, family history along with characteristic phenotypical traits may facilitate the diagnosis.[11]

Lymphedema is usually confined to a single upper or lower limb, although involvement of multiple limbs (including hemihypertrophy) is possible. Local pressure may cause a pitting indentation of the skin in early lymphedema, but it is less prominent than in venous edema. As tissue induration progresses, the pitting becomes less notable.

Lymphedema is typically worse at the distal end of the extremity. However, swelling may be compartmentalized in some cases (with sparing of the most distal parts of the extremity) thus challenging the somewhat simplistic traditional "stopcock hypothesis" of impeded lymphatic flow.[7] When it affects the lower limb, the feet and toes are rarely spared (Figure 53-2) unlike in lipedema, in which feet are characteristically spared.[29] Indeed, chronic toe edema leads to remodeling changes that produce the "squaring" of the toes (or "boxcar toes") classically seen in lymphedema. **Stemmer sign** is a classic feature of lymphedema and denotes the inability to pinch the skin on the dorsum of the second digit of the foot. Venous prominence and "ski-jump toenails" are found in Milroy disease, a form of primary lymphedema. In lymphedema-distichiasis venous varicosities, ptosis, cleft palate, congenital heart disease, spinal extradural cysts, and other abnormalities are also commonly found.[11] Verrucous or papillomatous skin changes are common; these wartlike lesions can lead to unnecessary biopsies in some cases. In extreme cases, particularly those produced by tropical filariae, the limb may take on a grotesque appearance associated with massive edema, fibrosis, and verrucous

TABLE 53-1	**Stages of Lymphedema**			
Stage	Fibrosis	Pitting	Elevation	Skin
0 (latent or subclinical condition)	None	None	No effect	No change
1 (early protein rich fluid accumulation)	None or minimal	May be present with pressure	Reduces edema	No change
2 (initial fibrosis development)	Moderate	May be present	Minimal to no reduction	Early changes
3 (marked fibrosis)	Substantial	None to minimal	No reduction	Marked trophic changes

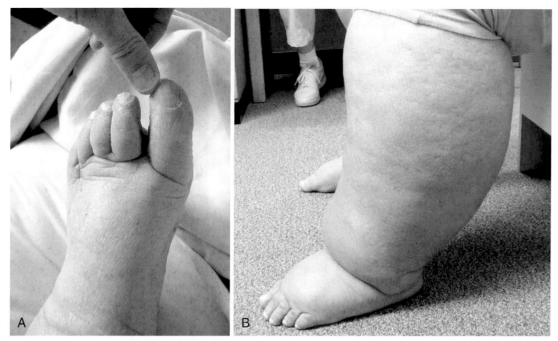

FIGURE 53-2 ■ Clinical findings in lymphedema. **A,** Typical "swollen sausage" appearance of the toes. Lymphedema is usually most severe in the distal limb. **B,** When lymphedema involves the leg, the toes and feet are almost always affected.

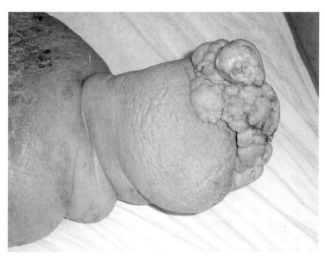

FIGURE 53-3 ■ End-stage changes in lymphedema. Wartlike (verrucous) skin changes are commonly seen in advanced cases of chronic, long-standing lymphedema.

changes (Figure 53-3). This appearance is commonly called *elephantiasis.*

It may be necessary to rule out other problems that can cause limb swelling, especially venous occlusion. This is particularly problematic when limb swelling occurs after an operation such as mastectomy or pelvic surgery (Figure 53-4), during which lymph nodes and vessels may have been damaged or removed (producing lymphedema) and veins may have been injured or thrombosed (producing venous edema). Both qualitative and quantitative assessments of lymphedema are useful.[21]

Duplex ultrasound scanning and venography will help to assess possible contribution of venous pathology to

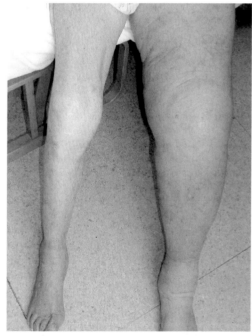

FIGURE 53-4 ■ Lymphatic versus venous disease. This man developed progressive left leg edema following radical prostatectomy. In this case, the disease is the result of both lymphedema and venous obstruction. The left limb has a perioperative iliofemoral deep venous thrombosis and secondary lymphedema from surgical disruption of the nodes and lymphatics.

edema. Cross-sectional imaging with computed tomography (CT) or magnetic resonance imaging (MRI) may be appropriate to look for enlarged, tumor-filled lymph nodes or other lesions, such as nonmalignant masses and fluid collections, which can produce lymphatic

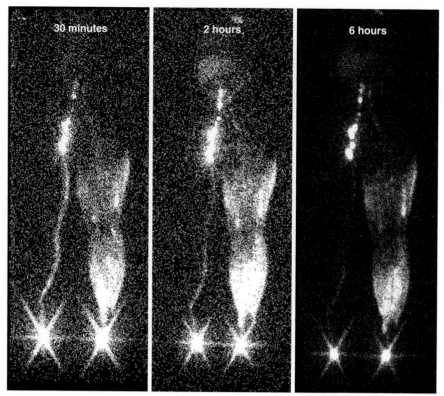

FIGURE 53-5 ■ Lymphoscintigram (anterior view) in patient with left leg secondary lymphedema obtained 30 minutes, 2 hours, and 6 hours after injection of radionuclide shows significant uptake asymmetry. Isotope quickly reaches ilioinguinal lymph nodes via a single lymphatic channel on the right. Marked dermal backflow is noted on the left without reaching the ilioinguinal lymph nodes. By 6 hours, isotope transit from the injection site is completed on the right; dermal backflow persists on the left.

obstruction. In addition, CT may reveal characteristic honeycomb appearances of the tissues. MRI can help to differentiate the cutaneous edema of lymphedema from other types of limb swelling, including lipedema and phlebedema.[30-33] Additional methods of assessment include CT lymphography, fluorescent microlymphangiography,[34] dual-emission x-ray absorptiometry, and biphotonic absorptiometry.[16]

The two tests used to assess lymphatic patency are lymphangiography and lymphoscintigraphy. They provide both anatomic and functional information. Lymphangiography involves cannulation of a distal lymphatic vessel via a surgical incision.[35] Contrast dye is injected into the cannulated vessel, and x-ray images are obtained. The study provides a detailed view of the lymph vessels and nodes. It is now used rarely because it is painful, technically difficult to perform, and in some cases may cause sterile lymphangitis and worsen lymphatic obstruction.[36] In addition, the necessary equipment is no longer manufactured.[37] Lymphoscintigraphy involves the subcutaneous injection of a radiolabeled colloid into the distal extremity.[38] The colloid travels through lymphatic vessels and nodes, and its flow can be assessed using traditional nuclear imaging cameras. In normal subjects, transport to the abdominal level occurs in 1 hour or less. When lymphatic obstruction is present, the colloid never ascends the lymphatics but instead becomes trapped in the interstitial spaces of the distal limb, producing a dermal

backflow pattern. Delayed transport or dermal backflow patterns identify limbs with lymphatic obstruction[4,39,40] (Figure 53-5).

Many scales exist and precision of lymphedema grading depends on the purposes (clinical vs. research) and varies in terms of time and cost.[41] Quantification of lymphedema is clinically meaningful and is commonly performed by simple circumferential measurements at 4-cm intervals using a measuring tape. The more sophisticated methods include volumetry, optoelectronic volumetry (perometry),[42] quantitative lymphoscintigraphy,[43] and bioimpedance spectroscopy.[19] Tonometry measures resistance of tissues to compression.[44] No single standard of lymphedema severity assessment exists, and the choice of specific methods varies among institutions.

Several immunohistochemical markers can aid the examination of the lymphatic system.[45,46] However, there is a scarcity of basic research of the lymphatic system, at least partially owing to the lack of animal models.[47-49]

In addition to venous disease, there are other conditions that can mimic the clinical appearance of lymphedema. Myxedema associated with thyroid dysfunction, cardiac or renal failure, hypoproteinemia, and chronic dependency can resemble lymphedema or aggravate otherwise mild cases of lymphedema.[50] Obesity (including morbid obesity and lipedema) is frequently seen in conjunction with lymphedema or is mistaken for it.

RATIONALE FOR TREATMENT

Lymphedema is almost never life-threatening; the goals of treatment are to improve limb function, reduce pain, improve cosmesis, and prevent long-term complications. Lymphedema is generally an incurable, chronic disease that often requires life-long care.[16] Natural history of the disease is characterized by progression both in terms of the amount of lymphedema and its grades. This progression is slower for primary cases compared to secondary ones, and slower for arms than for legs. In general, secondary lymphedema cases are marked by accelerated fibrosis.[17] Adverse psychological effects of lymphedema can be significant.

The rationale for therapy directed at pain relief, functional improvement, or appearance seems obvious. Therapy intended to prevent future complications is less intuitive but often is of greater importance. Limbs with lymphedema are at risk for numerous problems, including increased susceptibility to injury, infections such as cellulitis or lymphangitis (Figure 53-6; both of which lead to progressive destruction of lymphatics and increasing edema), and tumor formation (particularly angiosarcoma or Stewart-Treves syndrome).[51] It may be difficult to appreciate the importance of lymphedema treatment for the prevention of complications in patients with no limb pain, no functional impairment, and no cosmetic concerns. However, the ensuing complications can be devastating when patients develop cellulitis or lymphangitis that ravages the remaining lymphatics and leaves the limb dysfunctional with severe lymphedema. Even more devastated are the patients who develop angiosarcoma, a condition that usually leads to rapid loss of the limb and life (5-year survival time, 10% to 16%; mean survival, 19 to 31 months).[52-55]

It is easy to conclude that a young, healthy patient with severe, disabling, painful, cosmetically disfiguring lymphedema warrants treatment. Other decisions may not be

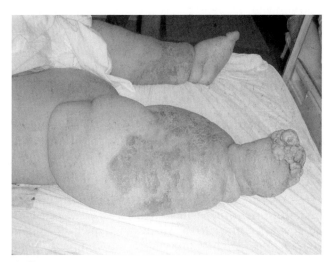

FIGURE 53-6 ■ Complications of lymphedema. A limb with lymphedema is highly susceptible to cellulitis and other infections. The causative agents are usually streptococci or staphylococci.

so easy. What about the young woman whose swelling is so mild that she notices it only when she tries to wear tight jeans, or the patient whose lymphedema is caused by obstruction of lymph nodes due to metastatic cancer, or an elderly patient with significant lymphedema? In these instances, the costs of treating lymphedema (given the mild symptoms, bad prognosis, or advanced age) must be weighed against the likely benefits.

Unfortunately, cost-benefit determinations can be extremely challenging. Cost is determined not only by the dollars spent on therapy, but also by less tangible factors such as the time devoted to therapy (which may be substantial), the inconvenience of certain treatment measures (e.g., wearing stockings or wraps all day), and the emotional challenge of having to incorporate regular treatment sessions into one's lifestyle. The benefits of therapy are likewise often subjective. How much better does the patient feel or function after treatment? How much better does he or she look? There is no one right answer; therefore therapy must be individualized for each patient. Differences in treatment rationale and patient demographics define the variety of institutional practices.

GOALS OF THERAPY

The goals of therapy may seem obvious—to reduce the size of the limb and thus to minimize functional impairment, pain, cosmetic disfigurement, and the chance of long-term complications. But how much fluid has to be removed from a lymphedematous limb to achieve these goals, and what degree of reduction is feasible? Is it a rational goal to make the limb as close to perfect as possible? Beyond a certain point, aggressive treatment compared with less intensive treatment, although producing further limb size reduction, may actually become disadvantageous to the patient by compromising the patient's ability to participate in regular daily activities or to hold down a job. Thus "better" lymphedema therapy may paradoxically decrease the patient's quality of life.

Even in this era of evidence-based medicine, lymphedema treatment remains more art than science. Effective therapy is often a balancing act—the more aggressively the edema is controlled, the more intense (and often lifestyle-altering) the treatment is. It is important to recognize that the patient and the physician may have vastly different ideas about the ultimate goals of therapy. Realistic outcomes should be communicated to the patient, and the patient's individual preferences and expectations should always be carefully considered.

TREATMENT OPTIONS

There is no universal consensus on the best approaches to lymphedema treatment and protocols vary among institutions. Attempts have been made by the International Society of Lymphology and by the International Union of Phlebology to amalgamate the spectrum of these diverse diagnostic and treatment approaches in consensus documents.[16,56]

For resolution of edema, either fluid production and sequestration should be decreased or fluid removal should be enhanced. Conservative therapy is traditionally the preferred initial approach.[57] However, improving microsurgical techniques may eventually lead to their wider and earlier application.[58]

The use of pharmacologic methods in lymphedema is limited. Diuretics are generally not recommended because of the risk of increased fibrosis and worsening fluid accumulation. They may be adjunctive in patients with certain comorbidities (e.g., cardiac or renal failure, prolonged dependency) that aggravate their lymphedema. Benzopyrones (coumarins) are thought to increase proteolysis by macrophages; they used to be touted as drugs that can help patients with lymphedema.[59,60] Lack of evidence to support these early claims of beneficial effects[61] and links to hepatotoxicity[62] caused these drugs to fall out of favor. Nutritional supplements have not shown to be effective.[18]

In practical terms, because lymphedema appears to be largely the result of impaired interstitial fluid removal, most treatment modalities aim to enhance fluid drainage. Evacuation of the excessive fluid from the extremities affected by lymphedema can be accomplished by maximizing the evacuation through the remaining lymphatic vessels. Alternatively, new conduits for lymphatic outflow can be created to replace defective ones.

The mainstay of conservative therapy is complex decongestive lymphatic therapy (DLT) based on the principles developed by Vodder and Foldi.[57,63,64] In 1936, Emil Vodder, a massage practitioner who initially did not realize he was trying to manipulate lymphatic flow, presented his method of light-pressure massage, called *manual lymph drainage* (MLD), in Paris.[64] In the 1980s, Foldi incorporated MLD into a multidisciplinary approach of complex decongestive therapy for lymphedema.[57,65,66] This approach encompasses several treatment modalities, including a special form of massage (manual lymphatic drainage), physical therapy, compression garments, and external sequential pneumatic compression devices (lymphedema pumps). It is geared toward augmenting the contractility of lymphatic vessels and increasing lymphatic flow through cutaneous lymphatics, thus improving lymphatic fluid evacuation from deeper tissues. Randomized controlled studies have been performed, some demonstrating 40% to 60% decrease in the excess limb volume. However, follow-up is generally limited and the results on individual level are highly variable, which may be due to the differences in the stages of the disease in these patients.[18]

Lymphedema compression pumps[67,68] have been used for decades and evolved over time to include a range of single and multi-chamber models. Some of the newer pumps encase the trunk and limbs and use scores of individually inflatable chambers that can be programmed to mimic lymphatic massage. The newest generation of pumps may indeed offer the best of both worlds (Figure 53-7). Some lymphatic pumps are designed to inflate at a certain moment during the cardiac cycle (cardiac-gated), although it is not clear whether this provides an additional benefit. Lymphatic pumps are used for several short sessions per day or for prolonged periods. The

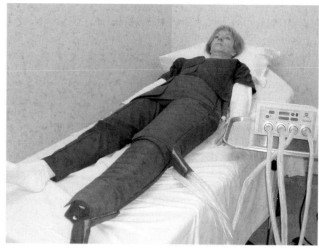

FIGURE 53-7 ■ Pumps for lymphedema. This pump is coupled to a "body cuff" containing scores of inflatable chambers. By sequentially activating each cell in a predetermined order, the pump can be programmed to simulate lymphatic massage.

applied pressure varies depending on the model (generally 60 to 100 mm Hg) and the concern about potential additional tissue damage, especially with high-pressure systems, may not be a real problem.[69,70] Several clinical trials demonstrated efficacy of the lymphatic pumps in reducing lymphedema, especially in the early postprocedure period, and the effects seem to be greater in combination with DLT.[71-75]

Gravity can be used to improve passive drainage through limb elevation and is helpful especially in the early stages of lymphedema.[16] A special lymphedema sling[76] or foam wedges can be used for these purposes.

Surgical approaches are generally classified into ablative (debulking) and physiologic operations that aim to restore lymph flow. Traditionally, the first report of a debulking procedure is attributed to Charles in 1912,[77] although the credit may actually belong to Baldwin in 1910.[78] Charles's procedure underwent modifications by Sistrunk and Thompson.[21,79-82] These interventions are rarely used now given the significant associated morbidities. Liposuction is an effective debulking alternative when lymphovenous shunts cannot be created. In therapy, it can disrupt residual lymphatics resulting in exacerbation of lymphedema, but in clinical reports using lymphoscintigraphy it did not cause further compromise of lymph kinetics.[83-85]

Physiologic operations are becoming more popular and may be more effective in the earlier stages of lymphedema.[21] They aim to improve drainage of the trapped lymph into other lymphatic basins or into veins. Omentum flaps have been used in the past in the hope that their rich lymphatics might provide lymphatic shunting.[86] Microvascular lymph node transfer was expected to provide a substrate from which new lymphatic vessels could sprout.[87,88] These procedures, however, are without objective evidence of efficacy. Lymphaticolymphatic bypass procedures may be more promising, with initial lymphatic patency demonstrated by lymphoscintigraphy and volume reduction maintained at 3 years after the operation. Interposition vein grafting has been performed between the proximal and distal lymphatic vessels.[89-93] Preliminary results of lymphaticoventricular bypass are promising in breast cancer patients with upper extremity lymphedema.[21,94] Microvascular surgical techniques continue to improve.[95,96]

Once a limb has been optimally reduced, its smaller size must be maintained. This maintenance almost always involves elastic compression, sometimes with foam padding underneath the wraps. Both high-stretch and low-stretch wraps have their advocates. Whenever possible, patients are encouraged to use compression stockings. Stockings generally have a superior cosmetic appearance to wraps and can be worn all day without the need for constant rewrapping or readjustment. It is generally recommended that pressures be 30 to 40 mm Hg, although compression of 50 to 60 mm Hg (or more) may be necessary to adequately control edema. Indeed, physiologic studies suggest that the compression bandages may raise lymphatic pressures to 40 to 70 mm Hg and that sequential intermittent pneumatic compression devices may be producing a similar effect. Massage and active foot movements are also effective in the earlier lymphedema stages; these therapies are futile in the last stage of lymphedema when nearly all lymphatic transport has ceased.[5,97] Various nonelastic compression devices with static pressure gradient can also be used for the maintenance of the limb size.[98] Pumps and massage can also be incorporated into a regular maintenance program to keep the limb at a reduced size and, in some cases, a combination of modalities is best. As noted earlier, expensive, highly aggressive, time-consuming programs may not be necessary for every patient. Use of specific treatment modalities and specific protocols depends on the patient's preference, availability of the treatment methods, financial resources afforded, and access to care. In general, the simplest maintenance program that reasonably controls edema is usually the best. Practitioners must resist the temptation, often egged on by industry sources and advertising, to prescribe aggressive, expensive, or inconvenient therapies for every lymphedema patient.

In addition to the specific edema reduction measures just described, there are adjuvant therapies that may be useful in selected patients. An appropriate diet, particularly one that helps the patient lose weight and control obesity, can be valuable. Many patients with lymphedema report that their edema worsens with a high salt intake; avoiding salt, therefore, could make the edema easier to manage. Exercise is useful in most patients with lymphedema, not only for controlling obesity but also for promoting lymphatic drainage. Concerns exist regarding the safety of weightlifting exercises in lymphedema patients, although recent studies suggest that graduated weight lifting exercises are not only safe, but may provide additional reduction benefits.[99-102] Antibiotics may be useful in patients with recurrent episodes of cellulitis.[103] It is prudent for lymphedema patients to keep penicillin or a first-generation cephalosporin on hand at home to start therapy at the first sign of cellulitis. If patients have frequent episodes, prophylactic therapy (typically 1 week out of every month) may be useful.[103] In rare cases, chronic antibiotic therapy may be necessary.

The newest focus of research in the therapy of lymphedema includes gene therapy, such as the use of the adenovirally introduced vascular endothelial growth factor in animals.[104,105] Blockade of transforming growth factor has been shown recently to promote lymphangiogenesis in animal studies.[106]

Lymphedema clinics now exist in several centers. The approaches and treatment modalities vary. Although there is no consensus regarding the best treatment approach, patient-centered treatment offers results that are tailored to the individual patient's clinical situation and social needs.

References available online at expertconsult.com.

QUESTIONS

1. Which of the following statements is true?
   a. Lymphedema is rare in the United States.
   b. Lymphedema affects up to 500 million people worldwide.
   c. Modern surgical techniques that are carefully applied allow one to completely avoid lymphedema.
   d. Lymphedema is always easy to distinguish from other causes of swelling.

2. Which of the following statements is true of lymphatic vessels?
   a. Unlike veins, they do not contain valves.
   b. They are characterized by constant slow flow of the lymphatic fluid.
   c. They may cause lymphedema only when they become obstructed.
   d. The fluid contained within lymphatic vessels is rich in proteins and other macromolecules.

3. What is the correct term for primary lymphedema that develops around the time of puberty?
   a. Lymphedema praecox
   b. Milroy disease
   c. Secondary lymphedema
   d. Lymphedema tarda

4. Secondary lymphedema is not caused by which of the following?
   a. Tumor
   b. Trauma
   c. Mutation in the *FOXC2* gene
   d. Infection

5. The most common cause of lymphedema worldwide is which of the following?
   a. Autoimmune disease
   b. Pregnancy
   c. Filarial disease
   d. Cellulitis

6. The clinical features of classic, chronic lymphedema do not include which of the following?
   a. Very soft, easily pitting edema
   b. Verrucous skin changes
   c. Square toes
   d. Swelling of the foot or hand

7. Which of the following modalities may be helpful in counseling families of patients with primary lymphedema?
   a. Computed tomography scan
   b. Genetic consultation
   c. Lymphoscintigraphy
   d. Magnetic resonance imaging

8. Which of the following statements is true of lymphangiography?
   a. It usually gives poor-quality images.
   b. It is technically difficult to perform.
   c. It is less likely to injure the lymphatic vessels than is lymphoscintigraphy.
   d. All of the above

9. What is the least common reason for treating lymphedema?
   a. To improve cosmetic appearance
   b. To improve mobility of the limb
   c. To alleviate pain
   d. To prevent the occurrence of future problems

10. What is the conventional initial treatment approach to lymphedema?
   a. Complex decongestive lymphatic therapy
   b. Debulking operation
   c. Liposuction
   d. Coumarin pharmacotherapy

ANSWERS

1. **b**
2. **d**
3. **a**
4. **c**
5. **c**
6. **a**
7. **b**
8. **b**
9. **c**
10. **a**

CHAPTER 54

HEMODIALYSIS AND VASCULAR ACCESS

Madhukar S. Patel • Juan Carlos Jimenez • Samuel E. Wilson

Direct access to the vascular system for the delivery of medications and for the removal of life-threatening endogenous or exogenous chemicals from the circulation is one of the foundations of modern clinical practice. In broad terms, vascular access includes any form of cannulation of arteries or veins. This chapter reviews the historical aspects; provides a practical consideration of percutaneous cannulation, autogenous fistulas, and internal arteriovenous fistulas; and discusses the prevention of complications and the outcome for each type of vascular access.

Temporary access to the venous system for the infusion of drugs or the transfusion of blood products has been a common practice for well over 300 years. Sir Christopher Wren, the great seventeenth-century English architect, is generally credited with developing an instrument for intravenous therapy in 1656, which was used for injecting drugs (opium and crocus metallorum) into the veins of dogs.[1] It consisted of a cannula made from a goose quill with a pointed tip which permitted penetration of the skin and underlying vein. In 1663, Robert Boyle described and published Wren's experiments and was the first person to extend intravenous infusions to humans, using prison inmates in London as subjects.[2]

The development of long-term cannulation of the circulatory system, however, was spurred by the introduction of a practical hemodialysis machine by Kolff in the mid 1950s.[3] Initial enthusiasm for hemodialysis was blunted by the major technical problems associated with the need for repeated vascular access. Having to perform a cutdown on the artery and vein for each dialysis session, and then ligating these vessels at the termination of each procedure, essentially limited early hemodialysis to short-term therapy for acute renal failure. In 1960, the development of the Scribner arteriovenous shunt afforded relatively safe long-term access to the circulation,[4] and repeated hemodialysis for the treatment of chronic renal failure became a reality.

As shown in Figure 54-1, the number of individuals requiring vascular access for hemodialysis continues to rise. By the end of 2008, there were nearly 550,000 people in the United States with end-stage renal disease (ESRD) from all causes, including more than 110,000 who received a diagnosis that year.[5] In what appears to be an ongoing trend, the number of patients using hemodialysis increased approximately 3.5-fold between 1988 and 2008.[5] Figure 54-2 demonstrates the number of vascular access device insertions from 1995 to 2010.[6] Of note, the number of prosthetic access grafts inserted decreased while the number of arteriovenous fistulas increased. These changes are in line with the guidelines favoring fistulas published by the National Kidney Foundation's Kidney Disease Outcomes Quality Initiative and the National Vascular Access Improvement Initiative known as the Fistula First Breakthrough Initiative (FFBI).[6] Specifically, the FFBI has supported an increase in the prevalence of national arteriovenous fistula rates from approximately 32% in 2003 to 55% in 2010.[6] During this same period, there has been a decrease in chronic central venous catheter use rates.[6] It should be noted, however, that the incident rate of central venous catheter (CVC) use in new hemodialysis patients remains to be high at over 80% in 2009.[6]

SHORT-TERM HEMODIALYSIS ACCESS

The external arteriovenous shunt described by Quinton and colleagues[4] in 1960 consisted of a loop of silicone rubber tubing lying on the volar aspect of the forearm connecting two cannulas placed in the radial artery and a nearby wrist vein (Figure 54-3). Although quickly and widely adopted as a practical means of providing access in chronic renal failure patients, three major disadvantages to the long-term use of external shunts became apparent: (1) high risk of infection because of the likelihood of bacterial contamination at the tubing's entrance sites in the skin; (2) frequent clotting owing to the small diameter of the silicone rubber and intravenous conduits; and (3) restriction of the patients' daily activities, such as bathing, by the external appliance and the extra care necessary to prevent dislodgment or infection. Consequently, patency rates of external shunts were very low.[8]

Although acute hemodialysis was once conducted primarily with external shunts, these have now been replaced by percutaneously placed central venous catheters.[9] This technique allows preservation of the vascular sites best suited for later construction of subcutaneous arteriovenous fistulas. The usual indications for hemodialysis by percutaneous venipuncture are (1) acute renal failure in which only a short course of dialysis is required; (2) immediately after surgery, while awaiting maturation of an internal fistula in patients with chronic renal failure; (3) patients with poorly functioning transplants who have thrombosed arteriovenous fistulas; (4) patients needing urgent transfer from peritoneal dialysis; and (5) treatment of poisoning.

Short-term dialysis needs are met through the percutaneous introduction of a catheter into a central vein

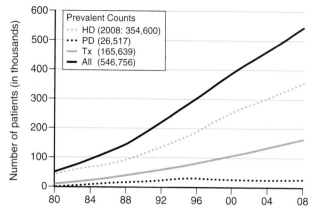

FIGURE 54-1 ■ Number of treated end-stage renal disease patients in the United States by treatment modality, 1980 to 2008. (From the U.S. Renal Data System, USRDS 2010 Annual Data Report: Atlas of Chronic Kidney Disease and End-Stage Renal Disease in the United States, National Institutes of Health, National Institute of Diabetes and Digestive and Kidney Diseases, 2010, Bethesda, Md.)

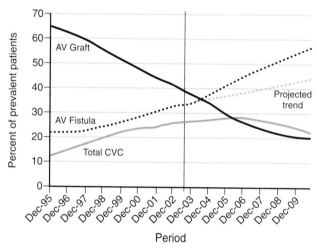

FIGURE 54-2 ■ Percent prevalence of arteriovenous (AV) grafts, AV fistula, and total CVC use in the United States, December 1995 to December 2009. Trend represents projection forward of AV fistulas use before the Fistula First Breakthrough Initiative. (From 2010 Fistula First Breakthrough Initiative Annual Report. Available at http://www.fistulafirst.org/AboutFistulaFirst/FFBIData.aspx. Accessed May 22, 2011.)

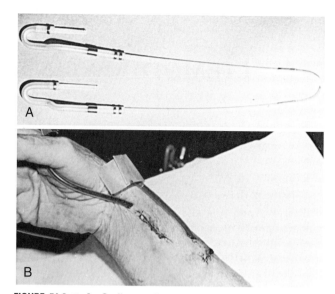

FIGURE 54-3 ■ **A,** Scribner shunt apparatus. **B,** Radiocephalic Scribner shunt in place.

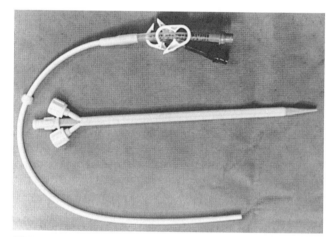

FIGURE 54-4 ■ Percutaneous hemodialysis catheter with Dacron cuff and oval dilator and sheath.

(Figure 54-4). The catheters are usually introduced via the Seldinger technique over a guidewire and can last up to several months.[10] The catheter may be changed over a guidewire and the tip is cultured. Any drainage from the cutaneous entry site should also be routinely cultured. Thrombosis is prevented by continuous low-dose heparin infusion or an intermittent injection of heparin every 12 hours. Patients in stable condition can be given the option of going home with the catheter in place and receiving intermittent heparin injections for outpatient dialysis. Interestingly, patients with these indwelling catheters have a 40% incidence of moderate to severe ipsilateral subclavian vein stenosis on angiography.[11] Placement of the catheter in the internal jugular vein is associated with less stenosis.

Central venous catheters are usually placed via the internal jugular and subclavian veins into the superior vena cava; this involves the usual risk of a percutaneous puncture of a major vein.[12] The femoral vein may also be used if the previously mentioned veins are not patent and the catheter tip usually resides in either the common iliac vein or inferior vena cava; however, because of the risk of pelvic venous thrombosis, indwelling catheters in this location for a prolonged period should be avoided. Although the incidence of catheter sepsis is generally low, one series reported a 28% incidence of infection in catheters left in position more than 4 weeks.[13] With adherence to standard antiseptic protocols, a catheter-related bloodstream infection rate below one episode per 1000 catheter days is possible, even without the use of antimicrobials.[14]

Long-term use of percutaneous vascular access is becoming a more common form of chronic hemodialysis in patients with no other site for hemodialysis. Using a silicone dual-lumen catheter with a Dacron cuff, a 65% 1-year catheter survival rate and an 18.5-month median length of catheter use have been reported.[15] Although thrombotic complications occurred in 46% of patients, the use of thrombolytic therapy was successful in restoring catheter function more than 95% of the time. Catheter exit site infection in 21% of patients and bacteremia in 12% of patients were the other principal complications.

AUTOGENOUS ARTERIOVENOUS FISTULA

The autogenous arteriovenous fistula, usually constructed by joining a superficial vein to an adjacent peripheral artery at the level of the wrist or in the mid forearm, remains the most dependable type of long-term vascular access. One long-term prospective study demonstrated a useful patency rate for first-time fistulas of 90% at 1 year and more than 75% at 4 years.[16] In addition, revision of a failing fistula can extend its longevity. An autogenous arteriovenous fistula may be unsatisfactory, however, in patients (especially those with diabetes) with advanced atherosclerotic changes extending into the radial artery or in patients whose veins are too small, fragile, or thin walled for repeated needle punctures.

Radiocephalic Arteriovenous Fistula

The subcutaneous autogenous arteriovenous fistula was initially described by Brescia and coworkers in 1966.[17] Readily accepted by nephrologists and surgeons, the Brescia-Cimino fistula, constructed of the patient's own vessels, largely overcomes the disadvantages of infection and early clotting found with external arteriovenous fistulas. After formation of the fistula, arterial pressure is transmitted directly into the contiguous veins, resulting in dilatation and development of a hypertrophied muscular wall (Figure 54-5). This "arterialization" of the veins can take up to 6 weeks before vessels of sufficient size and wall thickness have developed to tolerate repeated venipuncture. During this postoperative period, hemodialysis may be accomplished using peripherally placed central venous catheters.

Before the operation, the superficial arm veins, preferably in the nondominant arm, are distended and

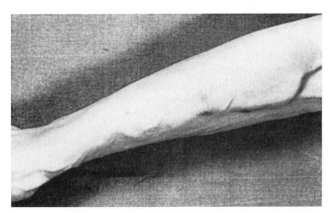

FIGURE 54-5 ■ View of dilated forearm veins following construction of a Brescia-Cimino radiocephalic fistula.

examined using a tourniquet applied to the upper arm to produce venous engorgement. All suitably sized veins are marked with an indelible pen. This is done so that if the fistula of choice fails immediately after construction, these markings can aid the surgeon in identifying other possible fistula sites. The ulnar and radial artery pulses are palpated, and if there is any uncertainty about their adequacy, the systolic pressure in each is measured with a Doppler probe. An Allen test, which predicts the ability of ulnar artery to support adequate circulation of the hand, should be performed to prevent symptomatic steal. The patient makes a fist and the examiner applies digital compression to the wrist, occluding both arteries; this is followed by pallor of the elevated and opened hand. Release of compression over the ulnar artery returns the hand's appearance to normal if the blood supply is sufficient. In addition to visual inspection, many surgeons perform duplex examination of both arms to find the most suitable veins. In fact, the routine use of ultrasound vessel mapping has been recommended.[18] In one study, ultrasound vessel mapping changed the preoperative plan in approximately 23% of patients.[18]

Local infiltration anesthesia using 0.5% to 1% lidocaine is usually satisfactory for construction of autogenous arteriovenous fistulas in the forearm or antecubital fossa. Although general anesthesia may be required in an extremely apprehensive or potentially uncooperative patient, a report on the effect of different types of anesthesia on blood flow during construction of a fistula showed that general anesthesia significantly decreases mean arterial blood pressure compared with local infiltrative anesthesia or regional block.[19] In addition, brachial plexus block (supraclavicular approach) significantly increases brachial artery blood flow compared with local anesthesia. If available, an axillary block is an ideal anesthetic for vascular work in the forearm.

The arm is prepared in standard fashion, abducted at a right angle from the body on an arm board, and aseptically draped. For a Brescia-Cimino fistula, an oblique or longitudinal incision is made midway between the radial artery and the cephalic vein at the wrist. An adjacent 4- to 5-cm length of cephalic vein is dissected free of surrounding subcutaneous tissue. Its tributaries are ligated, freeing it further so that it lies adjacent to the radial artery without kinking or twisting. A 2- to 3-cm length of the radial artery, found under the deep fascia of the forearm, is also isolated from surrounding structures. The distal cephalic vein is divided, and its proximal segment is approximated to the radial artery in an end-to-side fashion using 6-0 monofilament suture.

Four different anastomotic connections of artery and vein have been used (Figure 54-6), and each has its advantages and disadvantages:

1. Side-to-side anastomosis, with a fistula opening approximately 1 cm long, was the first procedure used. Technically, this is an easy anastomosis to construct and produces the highest fistula blood flow.[20] It is also the most likely fistula to be associated with venous hypertension of the hand.[21] This complication is moderated by the presence of venous valves that prevent reversal of venous blood flow in the hand, at least in the early months.

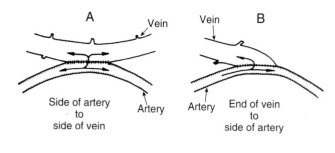

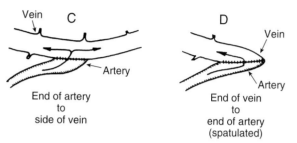

FIGURE 54-6 ■ Four anastomotic options for autogenous arteriovenous fistula construction.

2. Vein end–to–arterial side anastomosis also decreases turbulence if constructed properly and results in the highest proximal venous flow with minimal distal venous hypertension.[22] It is more technically difficult to construct than the side-to-side fistula, and fistula flow overall is somewhat decreased. If a branch vein is present, opening the inner aspect of the Y creates a generous oval patch to join to the side of the radial artery.

3. Arterial end–to–vein side anastomosis minimizes turbulence and distal steal of blood but may result in slightly lower fistula flows because it is subject to twisting of the artery during construction.

4. End-to-end anastomosis produces the least distal arterial steal and venous hypertension but has the lowest fistula flow of the four configurations.[23]

Proximal and distal control of the two vessels is gained by the application of small vascular clamps or a fine silicone rubber sling. The inability to pass a 3-mm or larger coronary dilator into the outflow vein has been associated with poor fistula maturation in our experience. The vessels are anastomosed in the desired configuration with 6-0 polypropylene sutures, with knots placed outside the lumen. One must ensure that when approximating the artery and vein, spiral rotation of these vessels does not occur. Before the anastomosis is finally closed, a check is made by gently passing a coronary artery dilator to detect any stenosis. This technique is especially useful to alleviate proximal arterial vasospasm in young patients. Hydrostatic dilatation with heparin-treated saline of a marginally small vein may aid in maintaining early patency.[24] Any bleeding from the anastomotic site should first be controlled by simple pressure with a gauze swab for several minutes. Immediate suture repair can produce further bleeding sites and narrowing of the anastomosis.

Upon conclusion, the artery and vein should lie without twists or kinks. A thrill should be easily felt over the fistula and propagated for a moderate distance along the proximal venous channel. A transmitted pulse without a thrill suggests an outflow obstruction or a clotted fistula. In this case, the proximal vein may be probed and inflated with a Fogarty catheter (avoiding intimal damage by not inflating the balloon during manipulation of the catheter) or carefully dilated with bougies. If these maneuvers do not produce a strong thrill and the fistula is technically satisfactory, construction of the fistula at another, more proximal site should be considered. On occasion, however, the appearance of a bruit and thrill is delayed until the veins dilate and blood flow increases, especially when no outflow obstruction can be demonstrated.

Following discharge, the patient is instructed to keep the arm elevated for 24 hours and to avoid sleeping on the arm. Avoidance of constricting dressings, sphygmomanometer cuffs, and tight clothing is mandatory. Any swelling usually resolves over subsequent weeks. Generally, 4 to 6 weeks allows for adequate venous maturation for use. Puncturing the vessels before they are arterialized is often associated with hematoma formation, because the dilated veins are thin walled during the first few weeks.[21] Although exercise of the forearm by squeezing a rubber ball to increase fistula flow and promote maturation of the arterialized veins has been advocated by some,[24] others have reported that it has no benefit.[25] Once the fistula is ready for cannulation, the buttonhole or constant-site technique should be considered in patients who self-cannulate.[26]

Brachiobasilic and Brachiocephalic Arteriovenous Fistulas

Brachiobasilic (with vein transposition) and brachiocephalic arteriovenous fistulas may be used to achieve upper extremity vascular access after failure of a more distal extremity arteriovenous fistula or if the cephalic vein at the distal forearm or wrist is inadequate. Patency rates of 80% at 3 years have been reported at these sites for chronic hemodialysis vascular access.[27]

Construction of the brachiocephalic fistula (Figure 54-7B) is preferred before brachiobasilic placement. The cephalic vein lies in a more superficial and accessible anatomic location on the anterolateral aspect of the arm compared with the basilic vein. The use of a transverse incision distal and parallel to the antecubital crease is recommended. Often a median antecubital vein, which drains into the cephalic vein, can be used and adds additional vein length for a tension-free anastomosis. Because more proximal vein diameters tend to be greater, brachiocephalic fistulas have a shorter time to maturity and longer primary patency when compared to radiocephalic fistulas.[28] Attempts at more distal construction (Brescia-Cimino) should be performed whenever possible because upper arm access sites are limited.

The brachiobasilic fistula (see Figure 54-7C) is constructed by identifying the basilic vein just anterior to the medial epicondyle of the humerus. Because of the deeper and more medial location of the basilic vein, this access site is usually avoided during phlebotomy and

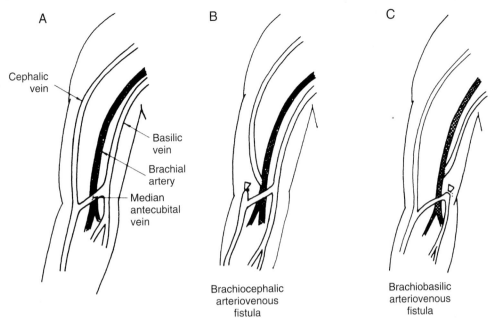

Cephalic
vein

Basilic
vein

Brachial
artery

Median
antecubital
vein

Brachiocephalic
arteriovenous
fistula

Brachiobasilic
arteriovenous
fistula

FIGURE 54-7 ■ Normal anatomy **(A)** and brachiocephalic **(B)** and brachiobasilic **(C)** autogenous arteriovenous fistulas.

venipuncture. However, its location usually requires relocation in a subcutaneous tunnel running down the anterior aspect of the arm. If adequate basilic vein diameter (3 mm) is present distal to the elbow crease, the vascular anastomosis should be constructed in this location to maximize vein length for superficialization. This operation can be performed in one stage (vein mobilization, superficialization, and anastomosis) or two stages (anastomosis with delayed superficialization). Advantages of the two-stage approach include the ability to determine fistula maturation prior to vein mobilization, which requires a longitudinal incision in the upper arm, prolonged operative time, and increased postoperative pain. If a short basilic vein is present, length can be added for superficialization with either prosthetic polytetrafluoroethylene (PTFE) or autogenous (e.g., Artegraft, cryopreserved vein) conduits. Care must be taken during mobilization to avoid injuring the cutaneous nerves to the forearm, which lie adjacent to the vein. The proximal end of the vein remains in continuity with the axillary vein. The brachial artery is isolated in the antecubital fossa, and the end of the relocated vein is anastomosed to the anterior aspect of the artery in an end-to-side fashion at this level.

VASCULAR GRAFTS (BRIDGE FISTULAS)

Successful long-term management of chronic renal failure frequently means that the patient outlives the usefulness of several serially constructed vascular access routes. When an autogenous arteriovenous fistula is no longer feasible, the use of a prosthetic conduit to form a bridge arteriovenous fistula is the best alternative. Arteriovenous grafts can be placed between almost any suitably sized superficial artery and vein. After implantation,

these easily palpable conduits can be readily punctured by a needle; however, if possible, this should be delayed for about 2 weeks until the prosthesis has been incorporated into the patient's subcutaneous tissue. Early puncture without careful hemostasis after needle removal may result in leaking of blood from the puncture site and formation of a perigraft hematoma.[29]

The prosthetic material selected for the conduit in an arteriovenous bridge graft is anastomosed end to side to the recipient artery and vein. If the two anastomoses are situated close to each other, the conduit takes on a U-shaped configuration; if they are separated by some distance, the conduit may lie straight or in a gentle curve. The conduit courses subcutaneously, allowing an adequate length for hemodialysis access.

Sites for Arteriovenous Prosthetic Grafts

Bridge arteriovenous grafts can be constructed at almost any location where suitably sized arteries and veins are surgically accessible. For patient comfort, ease of handling during hemodialysis, and safety, however, the majority are constructed in the upper extremity or occasionally in the thigh.

In the upper extremity, bridge arteriovenous grafts can be satisfactorily constructed between the radial artery and an antecubital fossa vein, between the brachial artery (in the antecubital fossa before its branching) and either the adjacent cephalic or basilic vein (U configuration loop), and between the brachial artery and the axillary vein (Figure 54-8). Construction of an upper-extremity bridge fistula is often more technically demanding than the creation of a femoral fistula, and its long-term patency is not as high.[30,31] This is generally attributed to the larger vessels and greater blood flow in the thigh. The risk of infection and distal limb ischemia is less in fistulas

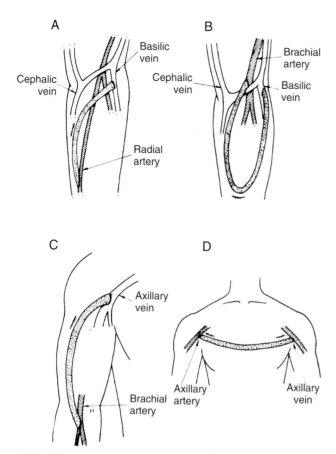

FIGURE 54-8 ■ Upper extremity bridge arteriovenous fistulas.

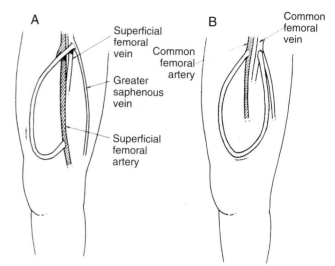

FIGURE 54-9 ■ Lower extremity bridge arteriovenous fistulas.

constructed in the upper extremity,[29] however, and this is the preferred site. Patients with claudication or an ankle arterial pressure less than 80% of that at the wrist might not be suitable for thigh fistulas, because the proximal steal of blood through the fistula is likely to increase ischemia in the leg.[32] Therefore upper extremity fistulas are particularly well suited for elderly patients with significant atherosclerosis in the lower extremities. Obese patients in whom perspiration or dermatitis involving the groin skinfolds may increase the likelihood of infection should have an arm fistula. Incontinence is a relative contraindication for implantation of the graft in the upper thigh.

The arterial anastomosis in the lower extremity should be to the superficial femoral artery, immediately proximal to either the adductor canal or its more cephalad portion (Figure 54-9A). If the superficial femoral artery is occluded, the common femoral artery may be used (see Figure 54-9B), with the understanding that if it becomes infected and ligation is subsequently necessary, leg ischemia may ensue. At times, patency of a short segment, including the origin of the superficial femoral artery, can be reestablished and used for the arterial anastomosis. The venous anastomosis is made to the proximal saphenous, common, or superficial femoral vein.

Historically, the site selected for the initial placement of an arteriovenous graft was in the forearm, from the distal radial artery to the cephalic or basilic vein in the antecubital fossa.[33] The graft was anastomosed in an end-to-side fashion to the distal radial artery, tunneled along the lateral aspect of the forearm, and then anastomosed end to side to the largest vein in the antecubital fossa. In positioning the graft, one had to ensure that the patient's arm would rest comfortably when receiving hemodialysis.

Currently, more common vascular access sites in the upper extremity include brachiocephalic or brachiobasilic loop fistulas in the forearm and brachioaxillary fistulas in the upper arm. Loop fistulas placed in the forearm allow a large area of graft to be available for needle puncture, whereas the brachioaxillary fistula, which curves over the lateral aspect of the upper arm, has several sites for venous anastomosis on the axillosubclavian segment. Upper extremity loop grafts have also been found to have significantly higher patency rates at all time intervals than do straight upper extremity grafts.[34] Upper-extremity procedures can be performed using an axillary nerve block or local infiltration anesthesia with sedation.

Arteriovenous grafts in the thigh are usually constructed with the patient under a spinal or general anesthetic, although in cooperative patients, a local infiltration technique can be used. Placing the arterial origin of the conduit just proximal to the adductor canal portion of the superficial femoral artery is often advisable so that if a vascular complication should cause occlusion of the artery, adequate collateral channels will provide filling of the popliteal segment. The end-to-side arterial anastomosis should be oblique, and the graft should leave the artery at an angle to minimize turbulence. The venous anastomosis is also performed in an end-to-side fashion and as obliquely as possible. This method is used to counteract any purse-string effect of the suture, as well as buildup of fibrin and fibrous tissue at the venous anastomosis, which commonly causes late graft thrombosis. A vascular steal phenomenon, with reversal of flow in the distal superficial femoral artery, is common in bridge fistulas in the lower extremity and can lead to symptoms of limb ischemia.[35] Fortunately, most patients with steal do not have symptoms, because dialysis patients are often fairly inactive.

The femorosaphenous bridge fistula is curved subcutaneously over the lateral aspect of the thigh and anastomosed to the proximal saphenous vein. The caudal portion of the saphenous vein may be ligated to prevent retrograde venous flow, although venous hypertension in the lower extremity is not a problem with a patent iliofemoral system. Another lower-extremity access configuration is the loop fistula placed in the groin from the common femoral or very proximal superficial femoral artery to the femoral vein. The high blood flow rate (>1000 mL/min) can lead to a significant increase in cardiac output. The possibility of limb loss in the event of infectious complications and the increased risk of infection make this site less desirable.[35]

With the longer survival of chronic hemodialysis patients, the surgeon may be asked to evaluate a patient who requires vascular access but whose extremity access sites have all been expended. In this circumstance, a more central location, such as a bridge arteriovenous fistula placed between the axillary artery on one side and the axillary vein on the other side, has been used successfully.[36] The grafts are of fairly large diameter, so they are easy to cannulate; flow is reported to be excellent, and despite the location of the access site on the anterior chest wall, patients adapt promptly.[37] The major drawback of central access sites is that when complications occur, they are serious and more difficult to manage.

Materials for Prosthetic Arteriovenous Bridge Grafts

Both biological and prosthetic materials have been used in the creation of arteriovenous bridge fistulas for hemodialysis since this modality was introduced in 1969.[38] Although saphenous vein, bovine heterografts, human umbilical vein, cryopreserved homografts, and Dacron velour grafts have all been tried during the last 4 decades, only expanded PTFE grafts have had an extended period of observation. Although one report on the use of autologous tissue-engineered vascular grafts in high-risk patients demonstrated primary patency in 78% of patients 1 month after implantation and 60% of patients 6 months after implantation, larger trials are needed to better determine the safety and efficacy of these grafts.[39]

Since its initial introduction as an alternative material for the creation of arteriovenous bridge fistulas in 1976,[40] expanded PTFE has become the most commonly used material. Much of its popularity stems from the fact that it is easy to handle, requires no preclotting, is widely available, has a long shelf life, and has relatively high patency rates with secondary revisions. PTFE bridge fistulas are consistently reported to have 12-month secondary patency rates of more than 70%.[41] In a large comparative clinical study comprising 187 graft placements, 36-month patency rates of PTFE grafts were significantly greater than those of bovine heterografts (62% vs. 24%).[42] Forty-eight–month patency rates of 43% to 60% have been reported.[43,44] However, multiple procedures for revision are usually required to maintain patency, with one study reporting an average of one operation for revision required every 1.1 years (range, 1 to 16 revisions per graft).[45]

Thrombosis of the conduit is a relatively common event in PTFE bridge fistulas, with figures ranging from 7% to 55%.[43,44] Endovascular techniques such as thrombolysis, percutaneous mechanical thrombectomy, and angioplasty allow for reestablishment of graft flow and function. Surgical revision with Fogarty thrombectomy and patch angioplasty of the stenotic outflow vein is also effective.[44] Infection of PTFE is not uncommon, with one report of 80 AV grafts monitored for 30 months showing an overall incidence of infection of 19%, with 67% of these infections occurring during the initial 4 months of use.[46] Of the infected grafts, 73% required excision, and the remainder were treated successfully with antibiotics. The most common type of graft infection today occurs at needle puncture sites. Pseudoaneurysm at needle puncture sites develops in approximately 5% of fistulas.[43]

Recently, heparin-bonded ePTFE grafts have been introduced in reports of increased patency compared with conventional ePTFE grafts.[47] The long-term advantages and complications of heparin-bonded ePTFE grafts are not yet known.

PEDIATRIC VASCULAR ACCESS

Maintenance of chronic vascular access in children is a formidable task for vascular surgeons, with their small vessels and arterial vasospasm being a major limiting factor. Although many of the principles and techniques are the same as for adults, certain aspects of the placement of long-term central venous catheters for total parenteral nutrition (discussed later) and the creation of hemodialysis access sites are sufficiently different to warrant discussion.

Dialysis (either hemodialysis or peritoneal dialysis) with subsequent renal transplantation is the preferred therapeutic regimen for ESRD in children. Transplantation is usually attempted as quickly as possible, because in general, children tolerate dialysis poorly; they frequently develop severe growth retardation (not reversible by transplantation), failure of maturation, renal osteodystrophy, and psychosocial problems.[48,49] In addition, long-term hemodialysis is, at best, difficult in children younger than 10 years and is extremely difficult in those younger than 5 years.

Short-term hemodialysis in children can be performed in a variety of ways with good results. Newborn or premature infants can be dialyzed via direct cannulation of the umbilical vessels using a 5- or 8-French catheter. Single-cannula hemodialysis can be used in older children in whom the superior or inferior vena cava has been cannulated with either the Seldinger technique or direct venous cutdown.[49]

Long-term vascular access for hemodialysis in children weighing less than 20 kg can be accomplished by placing a central venous catheter, inserted as described previously.[50] When external access is used, the recommended blood flow rate should be at least 3 to 5 mL/kg/min in most patients.[51] In addition, creation of an autogenous arteriovenous fistula between the brachial artery at the elbow and an antecubital vein using microsurgical techniques has been done in children weighing between 10 and 23 kg, with excellent results.[52,53]

For long-term hemodialysis access in children weighing more than 30 kg, an internal form of access, either autogenous fistula or bridge fistula, should be attempted. For children weighing 20 to 30 kg, the type of access attempted must be individualized according to the size of their vessels. Long-term access in children weighing greater than 20 kg should be seriously considered when transplant wait list times are anticipated to be greater than 1 year.[51] A Brescia-Cimino autogenous arteriovenous fistula can be created in children weighing more than 30 kg without much difficulty, and with patency rates of approximately 80% at 12 months. The use of microsurgical techniques enhances the patency rate, especially in children with small vessels.[53] Bridge fistulas of PTFE have also been used in children, with acceptable patency rates.

The usual types of complications and their rates of occurrence with both autogenous and bridge fistulas in children approximate those in adults. However, one of the most common complications of hemodialysis in small children is convulsions, occurring in up to 30% of patients.[54] This is probably the result of two factors: the use of overly efficient dialysis and the greater sensitivity of children to changes in osmolality. Convulsions can probably be avoided by tightly regulating the efficiency of the dialysis procedure based on the child's body weight. One major disadvantage of the use of internal vascular access fistulas in children is the physical and psychological pain of repeated needle punctures, which may require much time and counseling to overcome.

VASCULAR ACCESS COMPLICATIONS

Infection

Infection causes 15% to 36% of all deaths in dialysis patients, exceeded only by cardiovascular disease.[55] It also accounts for 20% of inpatient hospital admissions in these patients.[55] Many of the systemic infections encountered in these patients are direct complications of infection at the site of hemodialysis access. Two large dialysis centers found an incidence of 0.11 septic episodes per patient-dialysis-year related specifically to the vascular access site.[56] This represented more than 73% of the total number of septic episodes encountered.

The elevated rate of sepsis associated with hemodialysis vascular access sites is partially due to the deficient immune defense mechanisms in patients with chronic renal failure and the consequent increase in infection risk.[57] The bacterial phagocytic and killing ability of polymorphonuclear leukocytes also decreases by nearly 50% in patients with chronic renal failure.[58] Lymphocytes in chronic renal failure exhibit suppressed cellular immunity, and inhibition of lymphocyte transformation, which is unaffected by dialysis, has been detected.[59] In addition, the serum of uremic animals contains a nondialyzable inhibitor of the mixed lymphocyte reaction, which is probably a glycoprotein and distinct from either α-macroglobulin or immune complexes.[60] The actual ability of the animal to produce antibodies when antigen

stimulated, however, does not appear to be depressed in chronic renal failure.[61]

In addition to alterations in host defense mechanisms, other factors contribute to the increased propensity of patients to develop infection when requiring long-term hemodialysis. Poor healing of surgical wounds is a recognized consequence of renal failure and may result in wound infections. Measurement of the bacterial colonization rate of patients receiving hemodialysis revealed that 62% of these patients carried *Staphylococcus aureus* in their oropharynx or nasopharynx or on the skin, and 65% of those patients with positive cultures developed infections in their hemodialysis access sites.[62] Furthermore, 30% of the dialysis staff carried *S. aureus*, whereas only 11% of normal controls had positive cultures. In the same study, more than 70% of all infections encountered were caused by *S. aureus*. In a separate study, it was found that the 12-week mortality for patients with *S. aureus* bloodstream infections was 20.2% and for those with non-bloodstream infections was 15.7%.[63] Strict antisepsis is the best means to prevent *S. aureus* colonization and reduce the risk of vascular access site infection.[64] In a prospective evaluation of patients undergoing hemodialysis at multiple outpatient facilities, it was noted that patients with AV grafts, tunneled catheters, and temporary catheters had a significantly higher risk of developing infection than those with native AV fistulas.[65] Specifically, patients with AV grafts had a 2.2-fold higher risk, patients with tunneled catheters had a 13.6-fold higher risk, and patients with temporary catheters had a 32.6-fold higher risk.[65]

Although infection of an autogenous arteriovenous fistula is unusual, it can occur. Repeated puncture of the fistula can result in formation of a hematoma that can subsequently become infected by skin microflora. The method of cannulation can also affect the incidence of infectious complications in autogenous fistulas.[66] A quality improvement study comparing infectious complications following conversion to buttonhole cannulation concluded that with stringent adherences to a protocol for the buttonhole technique, as well as appropriate education and training, this technique is associated with a decrease in infectious morbidity.[66] In addition, the anastomotic site of the fistula itself can become infected, resulting in an endovasculitis with subsequent septicemia and metastatic abscess formation. Treatment generally consists of therapeutic courses of appropriate antibiotic agents coupled with local measures such as drainage of a perifistular abscess from an infected hematoma. Rarely, the fistula anastomosis may have to be dismantled, and the vessels are ligated in the presence of an infection-induced anastomotic pseudoaneurysm.

AV grafts placed for vascular access are susceptible to multiple sources of infection. Contamination from skin flora can occur during implantation and is more frequent when the fistula is placed in the thigh than when it is located in the upper extremity. In part, this is caused by the greater difficulty in preparing a sterile surgical field on the medial thigh and inguinal skinfold.[67,68] Direct inoculation of the graft by needle puncture through inadequately prepared skin also occurs, as well as inoculation of hematomas, resulting in perigraft abscess formation.

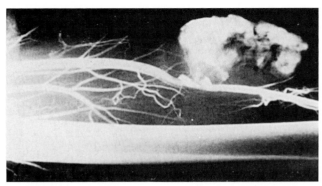

FIGURE 54-10 ■ Angiogram demonstrating disruption of an infected bridge fistula anastomosis.

The type of material in AV grafts also affects the infection rate, with autogenous saphenous vein fistulas demonstrating few, if any, infections and biological conduits (human umbilical vein graft, bovine heterograft) being particularly susceptible to aggressive infections; synthetic conduits are also susceptible to infection by low-virulence organisms.[69] The newly implanted prosthesis is particularly susceptible to infection; however, tissue incorporation and neointima formation confer increased resistance to infection.[70] A 2-week delay in initiating hemodialysis using AV grafts allows tissue incorporation of the prosthesis and development of a neointima. Disruption of an infected graft anastomosis (Figure 54-10) can occur at any time during the course of a prosthetic infection and does not appear to be influenced by incorporation.[69]

Treatment of an established infection of a conduit is excision of the prosthetic material. Attempts at in situ sterilization using antibiotics or povidone-iodine irrigation have not been reliably successful. A possible exception would be infection surrounding an autogenous saphenous vein prosthesis, for which treatment with antibiotics has been reported.[71] After excision of the infected access site, several days should elapse before placing a new access, for control of any associated bacteremia.

Given that the type of vascular access is a risk factor for developing infection, one means of decreasing this complication is through avoidance of access types that carry relatively higher infection rates. Specifically, avoiding or minimizing the use of central venous catheters will decrease the number of overall vascular access related infections.[55] In addition, regimens aimed at preventing this complication should always be practiced, including perioperative antibiotic administration. Randomized, prospective, double-blind studies have consistently shown the protective role of perioperative antibiotics in vascular surgery.[72,73] This finding was confirmed in a study of vascular access surgery, in which the perioperative use of a cephalosporin in a randomized, double-blind setting resulted in a significant decrease in postoperative wound infection rates, including cellulitis.[74] Vancomycin is highly effective in the prevention of vascular access graft infections, especially in the pediatric population.[75] In addition, the use of aseptic technique by the dialysis staff and the patient is required to prevent infection at the site of hemodialysis access.

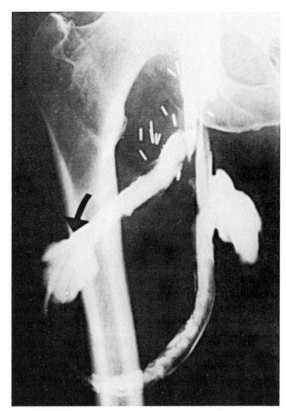

FIGURE 54-11 ■ Angiogram demonstrating extravasation of blood and hematoma formation *(arrow)* following too early use of a bridge fistula.

Thrombosis

The most frequent complication encountered in vascular access surgery is thrombosis of the fistula or shunt. The likelihood of thrombosis depends on multiple factors, including the type of shunt or fistula constructed, the site of the arteriovenous anastomosis, the prosthetic material used, and the adequacy of the patient's vessels. Thrombosis at the access site can occur at any time after construction. Early thrombosis, usually defined as occurring within the first month, is generally due to technical factors, whereas late thrombosis, occurring after 1 month, is usually caused by continuing trauma to the access site by needle puncture, outflow stenosis, or external pressure.

Lack of adequate venous runoff is the primary cause of early failure of distal access sites.[76] In the operating room, this can be recognized soon after completion of the final anastomosis by the absence of pulse, bruit, or palpable thrill. Ascertaining the patency and adequate diameter of the runoff vessel by using a Fogarty embolectomy catheter or coronary artery dilators can guard against this setback. Narrowing of the lumen of the artery or vein during construction or catching the back wall of the vessel while suturing can result in immediate clotting. Thrombosis in the early postoperative period may also be due to compression of the fistula by a hematoma; it can result from inadequate hemostasis during the procedure or early puncture of the fistula, with subsequent extravasation of blood (Figure 54-11). Excessive pressure

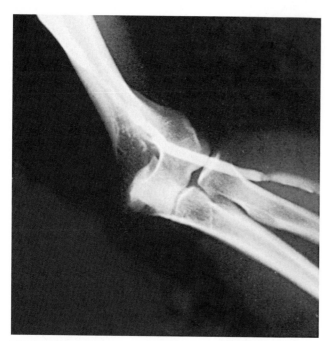

FIGURE 54-12 ■ Angiogram demonstrating stenosis near a venous anastomosis.

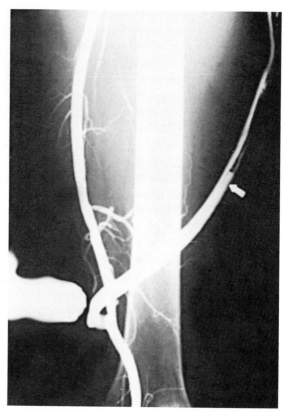

FIGURE 54-13 ■ Angiogram showing partially occluding thrombus *(arrow)* in a lower extremity bridge fistula.

over the needle puncture site after a hemodialysis run may also result in fistula thrombosis. In each of these situations, early reexploration, with evacuation of any hematoma and thrombectomy of the fistula, often results in salvage of the fistula.[77] Endovascular techniques may be helpful in dissolving thrombosis with lytic therapy, mechanical thrombectomy, and improvement of outflow by transluminal angioplasty and stenting.

Thrombosis of a vascular access site may be due to repeated trauma from needle punctures, with subsequent fibrosis and narrowing. In AV grafts, a needle-induced flap tear of the prosthetic wall can cause late thrombosis.

Outflow obstruction resulting from stenosis at the site of venous anastomosis is a relatively frequent cause of thrombosis in older AV grafts and may be heralded by a gradual increase in the venous return pressure measured during hemodialysis. The combination of forceful pulsation throughout the fistula and a loud bruit at the venous end strongly suggests the development of outflow obstruction, which can be confirmed by angiography or duplex scanning (Figures 54-12 and 54-13). True vessel aneurysmal dilatation from repeated needle punctures has also been reported as a major cause of late thrombosis in autogenous fistulas.[76] In addition, cigarette smoking significantly increases the likelihood of thrombosis and late occlusion of arteriovenous fistulas and should be avoided if possible.[78]

Fistula thromboses were treated successfully with thrombectomy, restoring flow in more than 80% of fistulas in one report.[79] This same study, however, indicated that approximately 70% of successfully thrombectomized fistulas reclotted within 6 months. This was thought to be due to unsuspected anatomic lesions and technical imperfections, which can be demonstrated with

angiography.[80] Aggressive outflow revision, directed by angiography at the time of thrombectomy, has resulted in 6-month patency rates greater than 70%.[79]

Because elevated venous return pressure during dialysis is a very sensitive indicator of significant venous stenosis,[81,82] we strongly recommend some type of imaging of the fistula as soon as an elevation in venous return pressure is noted. Although fistula angiography remains the gold standard, noninvasive methods of assessing fistula flow are more convenient. Doppler ultrasound examination of the fistula can diagnose partial or complete thrombosis, aneurysmal dilatation, or perifistular hematoma with exceptional accuracy.[83,84] Ultrasound imaging should probably be the initial investigative technique in cases of suspected fistula malfunction. If differences in angiography, Doppler ultrasound, or physical examination are noted, the use of intravascular ultrasound (IVUS) can be considered because it has been noted to be more sensitive than angiography in detecting intraluminal thrombus and dissection.[85,86] Extensive studies on the use of IVUS for hemodialysis access management are lacking, however, and it remains a demanding modality in regards to expense and time required.[86] If recognized before thrombosis, venous runoff stenosis can often be corrected with percutaneous transluminal dilatation with stenting (Figure 54-14).[87] Results of a recent prospective, multicenter, randomized, controlled trial, comparing balloon angioplasty alone to balloon angioplasty with placement of a stent graft in 190 patients with a prosthetic arteriovenous graft with venous anastomotic stenosis

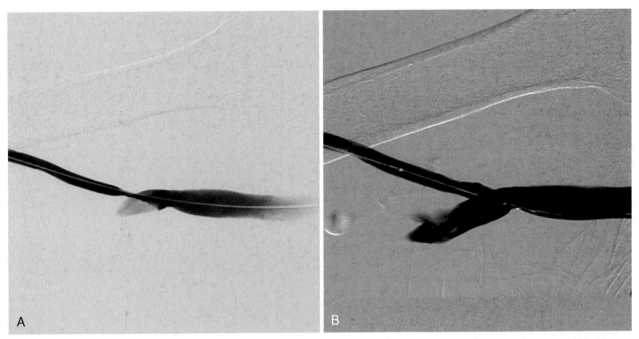

FIGURE 54-14 ■ Angiogram demonstrating venous stenosis **(A)** and correction with the placement of a stent **(B)**. (Courtesy Russell A. Williams.)

showed that percutaneous revision with a stent-graft offers significantly greater 6-month primary patency of the treatment area (51% vs. 28%).[87] In addition, those patients randomized to receive balloon angioplasty plus a stent-graft had significantly less restenosis (defined as stenosis >50% of diameter) at 6 months (28% vs. 78%).[87] It is thought that the addition of a self-expanding stent graft helps to prevent postangioplasty elastic recoil as well as growth of neointimal tissue and may decrease turbulent flow and tangential stress that could potentially lead to stenosis.[87] Disadvantages of stent-grafts within arteriovenous access sites include the risk of infection and proximal stent migration.

If acute thrombosis has already occurred, thrombolytic agents may be successful in clearing the fistula of thrombus. In one series using streptokinase, 52% of thrombosed fistulas were restored to function without surgical intervention, and another 21% had restoration of flow but required surgical correction of an underlying problem thereafter.[88] Another group was successful in restoring function in more than 65% of cases using urokinase.[89] The use of fibrinolytic agents in this manner appears to be most successful when the cause of failure is thrombosis secondary to hypotension or excessive compression of fistula puncture sites after dialysis. Combination therapy involving thrombolysis and mechanical thrombectomy has been noted to increase clot clearance and decrease procedure time.[90] Fistula failure associated with excessive proliferation of neointima does not respond nearly as well and usually requires surgical revision.

In an effort to counteract the thrombogenic tendency of vascular access fistulas, prophylaxis against thrombosis has been attempted with mixed results. One investigative group reported a highly significant reduction in fistula thrombotic episodes with low-dose aspirin therapy

(160 mg/day).[91] Another group reported the successful establishment and maintenance of arteriovenous fistulas in nonuremic individuals by the use of aspirin and low-dose heparin therapy.[92] A randomized, double-blind, placebo-controlled trial evaluating the effect of extended release dipyridamole and aspirin on primary unassisted graft patency found that treatment, compared with placebo, led to a significant but modest improvement in the absence of increased bleeding.[93] Specifically, the effect was noted to be equivalent to a delay of 6 weeks in the median time to loss of primary patency.[93] It is thought that the antiproliferative activity of dipyridamole may account for this improvement.[93]

Hemodynamic Complications

The principal hemodynamic complications of an arteriovenous fistula are congestive heart failure; peripheral vascular insufficiency, or steal phenomenon; and venous hypertension. The physiologic responses associated with an arteriovenous fistula for hemodialysis include a decrease in total systemic vascular resistance; an increase in cardiac output, with increases in heart rate and, somewhat later, stroke volume; an increase in venous pressure and venous return to the heart; and reversal of flow in the artery distal to the site of the fistula when the diameter of the fistula opening exceeds the diameter of the feeding artery.[22,23,94] In addition, a significant decrease in subcutaneous tissue oxygen tension to levels less than 30 mm Hg occurs.[95]

Depending on the diameter of the arteriovenous communication and the size of the artery feeding it, the venous return to the heart from an arteriovenous fistula increases proportionately. This increase leads to a variable increase in cardiac output and work of the heart, which can be significant enough to lead to cardiomegaly and congestive heart failure and has been found to lead to a subsequent increase in the vasodilatory hormone, atrial natriuretic peptide, because of an increase in atrial stretch.[96] Fistula flow as low as 20% to 25% of the resting cardiac output has resulted in heart failure.[97] Because the mean blood flow rate through distal (radiocephalic) upper extremity autogenous or bridge fistulas has been measured in one report as 242 ± 89 mL/min, high-output heart failure is unusual but does occur.[98,99] In the same report, resting flow rates from more proximal upper extremity fistulas based on the brachial artery were noted to more than double, averaging 641 ± 111 mL/min. Similarly, bridge fistulas placed in the thigh arising from the superficial femoral artery had resting flow rates of 592 ± 134 mL/min; therefore congestive heart failure is much more likely to result from a more proximally located fistula.

Initial blood flow through an autogenous arteriovenous fistula for hemodialysis is too low to cause heart failure, except in patients who already have severely compromised cardiac function.[99] With dilatation of the venous outflow system, shunted blood flow through the fistula can increase greatly. One group of investigators, using echocardiographic evaluation of cardiac performance, suggested that creation of any hemodialysis vascular access fistula causes a significant time-related cardiac decompensation compared with normal controls.[100] Echocardiographic assessment may also be useful preoperatively to identify patients with poor contractility, as manifested by changes in the mean velocity of fiber shortening, ejection fraction, and left ventricular or septal wall hypertrophy.[101] Abnormal studies may warn the clinician of a propensity toward future development of heart failure and lead to creation of the smallest and, if possible, most distal arteriovenous fistula compatible with adequate access.

When congestive heart failure arises from a high-flow arteriovenous fistula, operative correction is possible. In order to help select patients who are more likely to benefit from permanent closure of their arteriovenous fistula, temporary manual occlusion followed by measurement of hemodynamic parameters can be conducted.[102,103] Patients who may benefit from permanent closure often respond to temporary manual occlusion with a decreased pulse rate or a significant increase in total peripheral resistance and mean arterial blood.[102,103] Although revision of the fistula by narrowing the arterial anastomosis or construction of a completely new fistula may be done to correct the problem, the simplest corrective procedure is banding of the existing fistula by suturing a small cuff (1 cm wide) of synthetic material (Dacron, PTFE) around the prosthesis of a bridge fistula or the main venous outflow tract of an autogenous fistula. An electromagnetic flowmeter can be placed around the vein proximal to the fistula and banding cuff, and continuous flow is recorded. When the fistula flow is within the range of 300 to 400 mL/min, the banding cuff is securely sutured.

Patients who are identified preoperatively as being at risk for access-induced congestive heart failure (e.g., older patients or those with existing cardiac dysfunction)

and who require an AV graft should have either a tapered or a stepped conduit placed. The diameter of the arterial end of these grafts is 4 mm, so that when they are placed in the patient (with the smaller end anastomosed to the artery), flow through the graft is somewhat reduced, thereby lessening the risk of congestive heart failure.

Arterial insufficiency, or steal syndrome, in patients with vascular access for hemodialysis was originally described as occurring in Brescia-Cimino fistulas with side-to-side anastomoses because of reversed blood flow in the distal radial artery.[104] An area of very low resistance is formed on the venous portion of the anastomosis so that the blood flow tends to course through the palmar arch from the ulnar to the radial side and steals flow from the muscles and soft tissues of the palm and fingers.[105] The syndrome is characterized by pain on exertion of the musculature of the hand, and the hand often appears cold, clammy, and pale. Severely symptomatic radial artery steal is rare, with one large study reporting only 8 of 444 patients who had 516 Brescia-Cimino fistulas constructed for hemodialysis (1.6%) developing significant steal symptoms,[106] although up to 80% of patients with Brescia-Cimino fistulas have mild, asymptomatic arterial steal documented by a significant decrease in thumb blood pressure.[107] Steal syndrome has also been described in 6.4% of 357 patients with upper extremity bridge fistulas, one third of whom required fistula ligation to preserve function of the hand, whereas the other two thirds were successfully managed with surgical narrowing of the arterial side of the fistula.[108] Surgical correction of radial steal from a side-to-side autogenous fistula has been accomplished by ligation of the radial artery immediately distal to the fistula, which converts the side-to-side anastomosis to an arterial end-to-side anastomosis.[105]

Arterial insufficiency has also been noted with the use of AV grafts in both the upper extremity[29] and the lower extremity[32] as a result of steal from the high-flow fistulas. When steal becomes symptomatic with AV grafts, restriction of arterial inflow (by placing a clip on the graft at the arterial end) to decrease fistula flow often causes these patients to become asymptomatic.[30] In rare cases, the entire fistula may have to be dismantled, or, if this is the only route for access, arterial ligation with distal revascularization using saphenous vein bypass results in restoration of satisfactory perfusion ("DRIL" procedure).

Arterialization of the venous system proximal to an arteriovenous fistula results in venous hypertension and, if the venous valves are incompetent, retrograde venous flow. Noted most frequently with side-to-side Brescia-Cimino fistulas and, to a lesser extent, reverse arteriovenous fistulas, retrograde venous hypertension is marked by distal extremity edema, distention of superficial veins, and pigmentation of the skin (Figure 54-15). Ulceration and neuralgias can also occur in long-standing cases.[109,110] Surgical correction is obtained by ligation of the vein immediately distal to the fistula, converting the side-to-side anastomosis of the Brescia-Cimino fistula to a functional venous end-to-side anastomosis, and converting the bridge fistula to a functional end-to-end anastomosis.

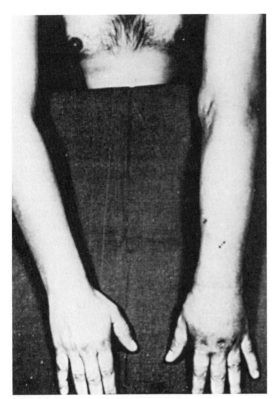

FIGURE 54-15 ■ Left upper extremity edema caused by venous hypertension from a Brescia-Cimino fistula.

Intimal Hyperplasia

Progressive venous stenosis occurring as a consequence of vascular access fistula placement is a recurring problem leading to thrombosis and multiple revisions or replacement of fistulas in patients requiring long-term hemodialysis. Indeed, it is the main drawback associated with prosthetic conduits. Although the stenosis may be related to the technical performance of the anastomosis, it is mainly attributable to chronic changes known to occur in the runoff veins of arteriovenous fistulas. The development of intimal myointimal hyperplasia can result from focal endothelial trauma caused by the shearing effect of blood flow at the site of the venous anastomosis.[111,112] In addition, venous hypertension in the runoff vessels of an arteriovenous fistula causes intimal lipid deposition, further compounding the situation.[113] Segmental stenosis of autogenous fistulas and bridge fistulas constructed using biological conduits has also been noted to occur from fibrosis and intimal hyperplasia secondary to the trauma of repeated needle punctures.[114]

Early detection of potential access dysfunction is recommended in efforts to increase patency rates. Monthly monitoring of access sites should be performed via physical examination by a qualified examiner.[7] Surveillance using direct flow measurements, physical findings, or duplex ultrasound is preferred for fistulas.[7] Similar surveillance methods are preferred for grafts, with the substitution of direct or derived static venous dialysis pressures for physical findings.[7] In regard to diagnostic testing, referrals should be based on trend analysis rather than isolated abnormal values.[7] In addition, other indications for diagnostic testing include the following: access

flow rates less than 400 to 500 mL/min in fistula, access flow rates less than 600 mL/min in grafts, venous segment static pressure ratios greater than 0.5 in grafts or fistula, or arterial segment static pressure ratios greater than 0.75 in grafts.[7]

Surgical correction of the stenotic area can be accomplished with patch angioplasty at the site of an anastomosis, by placing an extension of the graft around a long stenotic area or by locating the venous anastomosis in a new vein. The use of percutaneous transluminal balloon angioplasty has been advocated for dilatation of stenotic segments in failing arteriovenous fistulas and shunts.[115] Using the Seldinger technique to gain access to the fistula, a noncompliant angioplasty balloon is placed at the site of the stenosis under fluoroscopic control, and the stenosis is dilated twice for 30 seconds each time. Before catheter removal, an angiogram is obtained, and the dilatation is repeated if greater than 30% residual stenosis is present. Using this technique, an initial success rate of 95% has been achieved.[115] Patency, however, is shorter than that achieved by surgical outflow correction. Other modalities of correction, such as brachytherapy, have also been evaluated.[116] A randomized, double blind, multicenter, pilot study of patients with patent but dysfunctional PTFE access grafts demonstrated a potential benefit in primary patency using endovascular radiation following angioplasty, but additional larger studies are needed.[116]

Aneurysm Formation

Aneurysmal dilatation of AV graft conduits depends on the material used. True aneurysm formation occurs primarily in biological materials (saphenous vein, bovine heterograft, human umbilical vein graft) and has been attributed to degeneration over time of the graft material itself.[29] Early PTFE grafts were also prone to true aneurysm formation from nodal fracture and a gradual stretching of the PTFE fibrils[117]; however, with an increase in the wall thickness of PTFE grafts, this is no longer a problem. Excessive aneurysmal enlargement of the fistula is best treated by parallel placement of a new conduit of synthetic material. Pseudoaneurysm formation secondary to trauma at the site of needle punctures can occur with any of the materials used for AV grafts (Figure 54-16). If no infection is apparent, treatment consists of local suture repair of the defect in the graft material. Somewhat larger defects may require excision of the defect and the interposition of a small segment of new graft material. Asymptomatic aneurysms, though unsightly, may be safely observed unless skin breakdown or thrombosis occurs.[118] Repair should be considered when an aneurysm effects fistula use or significantly interferes with the patient's quality of life.[118] Skin erosion overlying a pseudoaneurysm with associated bleeding is a surgical emergency, and access revision should be performed immediately to avoid life-threatening hemorrhage.

Central Venous Occlusion

Occlusion of the axillosubclavian veins or the superior vena cava in patients undergoing hemodialysis for ESRD

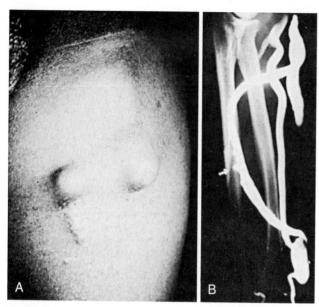

FIGURE 54-16 ■ **A,** Pseudoaneurysm formation at needle puncture sites of a hemodialysis fistula. **B,** Angiogram demonstrating multiple pseudoaneurysms *(arrow)* at needle puncture sites of a bridge fistula.

via percutaneous catheters is a common occurrence. Over time, a central dialysis catheter can injure the endothelium of the large vein, resulting in thrombus formation, fibrosis, and eventually total occlusion. Nearly 5% of patients undergoing chemotherapy by peripherally placed central venous access devices developed symptomatic axillosubclavian vein thrombosis[119]; it is likely that more were asymptomatic. In dialysis patients, the proportion of symptomatic patients is increased to 12% because of the augmentation of venous flow in the upper extremity.[120] After catheter insertion, the time to development of thrombosis can be short, with venograms detecting partial thrombus formation in 30% and complete occlusion in 6% of patients by 6 weeks; 10% of patients had total occlusion by 12 weeks.[121]

The diagnosis of central venous occlusion is suggested on clinical grounds by swelling of the entire upper extremity, particularly if there is a rapid onset of edema after arteriovenous correction in that extremity. Subcutaneous collateral vein formation, venous aneurysms, and skin breakdown are often seen later. Dialysis personnel may report increased recirculation or elevated venous return pressure; however, somewhat surprisingly, most arteriovenous fistulas and access grafts continue to function even with central vein occlusion. Confirmation can be obtained with greater than 90% reliability using duplex ultrasonography, which detects occlusion by imaging the thrombus and showing an absence of spontaneous flow, no respiratory phasic flow, and an incompressible vein with increased collaterals.[122]

Initial treatment for acute central venous thrombosis is anticoagulation to prevent clot extension and potential pulmonary embolus. For most patients, clot lysis followed by percutaneous transluminal angioplasty and stenting is the first method to consider. Initial success can be expected in more than 75% of patients, with resumption of successful dialysis in more than 50%.[120]

Cumulative patency rates of 70% at 2 years can be expected after salvage in this manner, although patency seems to decline rapidly thereafter.[123] If intervention is unsuccessful in a symptomatic patient, relocation of the access site may eliminate symptoms if there is a well-developed collateral circulation. A surgical approach is possible in selected patients with a limited segment of occlusion. The surgical options include transposition of the internal jugular vein to the axillary vein ("turndown" procedure), axillary-to-jugular PTFE bypass, and crossover bypass using a PTFE graft to the other axillary vein. The first technique has been used successfully in appropriate anatomic occlusions; however, there is minimal experience with the other two methods. In patients with right atrial clot formation, those with catheter removal and subsequent thrombectomy have been noted to have lower mortality (0%) than those with removal and anticoagulation (33%), removal of the catheter only (40%), or no treatment (100%).[124]

Because central venous catheters cannot be avoided entirely in hemodialysis, the prevention of potential problems should be actively pursued. Techniques include limiting the duration of indwelling percutaneous catheters to approximately 6 weeks whenever possible and minimizing the use of Dacron-cuffed, tunneled, long-term catheters. A subclavian vein catheter has a higher incidence of thrombosis than one laced through the internal jugular vein, although thrombosis associated with this insertion site certainly occurs. It is important to position the tip of the catheter in the superior vena cava at the right atrial junction because there is an increase in axillosubclavian vein thrombosis when the catheter tip resides in the brachiocephalic or subclavian vein. Patients who have had a catheter in place for more than 3 weeks should have routine screening duplex ultrasonography of the axillosubclavian veins performed before a permanent access site is chosen.

VASCULAR ACCESS FOR TOTAL PARENTERAL NUTRITION OR CHEMOTHERAPY

Surgically created arteriovenous fistulas can be used to obtain vascular access for reasons other than hemodialysis. Several reports have found that chronic total parenteral nutrition (TPN) can be administered using arteriovenous fistulas that remain patent up to 7 years.[125,126] The advantages are a low incidence of infection and longevity of the access site. The primary disadvantage is that the patient must undergo a significant operation to establish vascular access. The use of autogenous arteriovenous fistulas for the delivery of chemotherapeutic agents and plasmapheresis has also been reported.[127,128] Bridge arteriovenous fistulas have been used; however, one series reported a significantly higher complication rate for bridge fistulas compared with Silastic right atrial catheters (48% vs. 19%) for chemotherapy use.[129]

Despite these reports on the use of arteriovenous fistulas for chemotherapy and TPN, the more common method used to deliver these therapeutic modalities is a

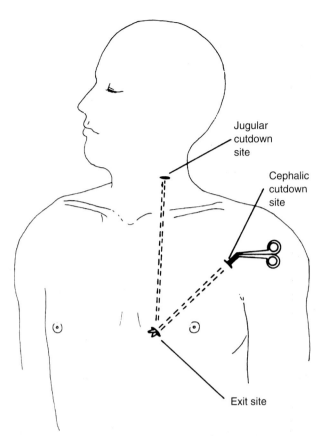

FIGURE 54-17 ▪ Position of subcutaneous tunnel exit site for an upper body Broviac or Hickman catheter.

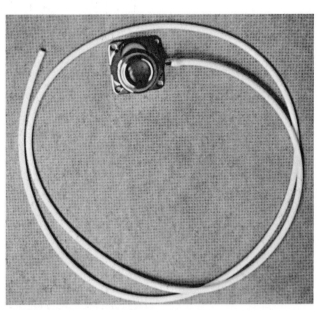

FIGURE 54-18 ▪ Implantable port showing the reservoir with a self-sealing septum and the silicone catheter.

chronic indwelling central venous catheter. For a number of years, the accepted method for central venous cannulation involved percutaneous catheterization with a polyethylene catheter. The propensity of percutaneously placed polyethylene catheters to develop infection and thrombosis and the inherent danger of the technique used to place these catheters led to the development of specialized large-bore catheters that are less reactive and less thrombogenic.

The Broviac[130] and Hickman[131] central venous catheters are made of soft, radiopaque silicone material; they are 90 cm long and have a small Dacron felt cuff 30 cm from the external end. The only difference is that the Broviac catheter has an internal diameter of 1 mm, and the Hickman catheter's internal diameter is 1.6 mm. Each catheter consists of a relatively thin-walled intravascular segment and a thicker-walled extravascular portion. A smaller, pediatric-sized Broviac catheter is also available, as are double-lumen catheters in various sizes. These catheters are placed via direct venous cutdown into the cephalic (Figure 54-17), external jugular, or greater saphenous vein, and the extravascular portion of the catheter is tunneled through the subcutaneous tissue to separate the skin exit site from the venotomy site. Fibrous tissue ingrowth into the Dacron cuff located in the subcutaneous tunnel serves to anchor the catheter and presents an effective barrier to the migration of microorganisms from the skin into the venous system along the outer surface of the catheter. For further protection against infection, some catheters have an additional cuff positioned in the subcutaneous tunnel between the Dacron cuff and the skin exit site. As a consequence, the sepsis rate with these catheters is relatively low.[132,133]

Innovations in central venous access include the introduction of the Groshong catheter and implantable ports. Unlike either the Hickman or the Broviac catheters, the Groshong catheter has no clamps, comes without the hub attached, and possesses a unique two-way valve. This valve is designed to remain closed when the catheter is not in use, and it opens either outward for fluid infusion or inward for blood draws. This design requires significantly less maintenance by either the patient or the health care worker, with only a single 5-mL saline flush being recommended once a week when the catheter is not in use. One group has suggested that less frequent flushing is needed if a heparinized saline solution is used.[134]

Implantable ports (Figure 54-18) are central venous access devices that consist of a subcutaneously implantable reservoir containing a self-sealing septum that can withstand more than 2000 needle punctures. They are connected to a silicone rubber catheter with an internal diameter ranging from 1 to 1.6 mm. The reservoir body, which can be constructed of plastic, stainless steel, or titanium, is placed in a subcutaneous pocket over the anterior chest or abdomen in an easily palpable location and is accessed with a Huber needle for either blood withdrawal or drug delivery. These implantable ports have the advantage of requiring little daily care and therefore interfere less with the patient's normal activities. In addition, implantable ports have a catheter-related sepsis rate of 3% and a 1% incidence of thrombosis, compared with a 15% rate of catheter-related sepsis and a 22% incidence of thrombosis in external central venous catheters.[135] A prospective comparison demonstrated that external shunts have 0.13 exit site infections and 0.03 bacteremic episodes per 100 catheter-days, compared with 0.06 pocket infections and no bacteremic episodes

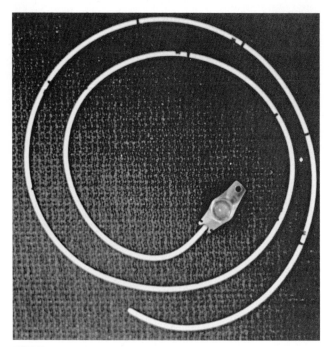

FIGURE 54-19 ■ Peripherally inserted central catheter line, which is placed via an antecubital vein.

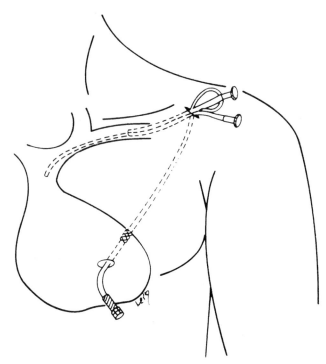

FIGURE 54-20 ■ Placement of a Silastic catheter by percutaneous subclavian venipuncture.

per 100 catheter-days for implantable ports.[136] A newer subcutaneous port is the peripherally inserted central catheter line shown in Figure 54-19. A polyurethane catheter is placed via an antecubital vein and threaded into the superior vena cava. Its primary advantage is ease of insertion; the procedure can be performed at the bedside. The placement of any central venous catheter for TPN or chemotherapy is always considered an elective, sterile, operative procedure. Thus, hypovolemia and any electrolyte abnormalities should be corrected before catheter placement. Adequate lighting, instruments, assistance, and aseptic techniques are absolute prerequisites for the safe insertion of the catheter. The internal jugular vein is preferred for long-term patency and can be located with Doppler imaging. In patients requiring long-term central venous catheterization who have had numerous previous catheters placed, preoperative duplex ultrasonography or venography may be required to verify the patency of the vena cava (superior or inferior), the subclavian or iliac vein, or their tributaries.

In most hospitals, Broviac or Hickman catheter insertion is performed in the controlled environment of the angiographic suite, where radiography or fluoroscopy is available to confirm the proper position of the catheter tip before skin closure. The central vein is punctured using ultrasound guidance. A guidewire is inserted through the needle, thus allowing the needle to be removed. An incision is then made in the chest wall at the proposed site of catheter exit. The catheter is then tunneled to the site of venous access, and a vein dilator and peel-away sheath are placed over the guidewire under fluoroscopic guidance. The guidewire and dilator are then removed and the Broviac or Hickman catheter is introduced into the vein through the peel-away sheath. The sheath is withdrawn and peeled apart, leaving the

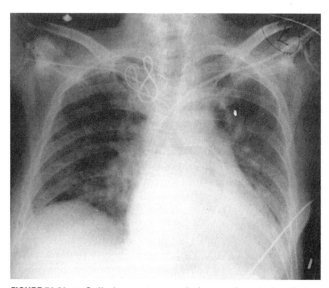

FIGURE 54-21 ■ Coiled percutaneously inserted central catheter.

catheter in place. Radiographic verification of catheter position is obtained, and wound closure and catheter care are performed as for standard Broviac or Hickman catheter placement (Figure 54-20).[137] The catheter is fixed to the skin at the exit site with a monofilament suture, which is removed 7 to 14 days later, after fibrous ingrowth into the Dacron cuff has occurred. Povidone-iodine ointment and a sterile dressing are applied to the exit site, and the loop of redundant catheter is taped to the body wall. The catheter may be either heparin-locked or immediately connected to an intravenous infusion set.

Although malposition of the catheter (Figure 54-21) is the most common complication of direct venipuncture,[137] any of the complications seen with standard central venous catheter placement are possible. These complications include pneumohemothorax, arterial laceration or perforation, arteriovenous fistula formation, brachial plexus or other nerve injury, air or catheter embolism, and lymphatic fistula formation.[12]

Once they are properly inserted and positioned, Broviac and Hickman catheters can be left in place for more than 1 year, with an average duration of more than 2 months.[132,133] Because of the chronic nature of the underlying diseases in patients who require long-term catheterization, multiple insertions were necessary in 13% of patients in one study.[132] The primary complications of Broviac and Hickman catheter use are sepsis, thrombosis, and dislodgment of the catheter; in two series comprising 199 catheter placements, these complications occurred in 12%, 5%, and 3.5% of cases, respectively.[132,133] Central vein thrombosis as a result of long-term catheterization can also occur, but infrequently.

BIBLIOGRAPHY

Hodges TC, Fillinger MF, Zwolak RM, et al: Longitudinal comparison of dialysis access methods: risk factors for failure. J Vasc Surg 26:1009–1019, 1997.
National Kidney Foundation: K/DOQI Clinical practice guidelines for vascular access. Am J Kidney Dis 48(Suppl 1):S176–S247, 2006.

References available online at expertconsult.com.

QUESTIONS

1. After construction of a radiocephalic autogenous fistula, which configuration is associated with the lowest incidence of venous hypertension?
   a. Arterial side–to–vein side anastomosis
   b. Vein end–to–arterial side anastomosis
   c. Arterial end–to–vein side anastomosis
   d. Brachiobasilic side-to-side anastomosis
   e. None of the above

2. The highest 1-year primary patency rate in vascular access procedures has been achieved with which of the following?
   a. PTFE bridge fistulas
   b. Autogenous saphenous vein bridge fistulas
   c. Scribner shunts
   d. Autogenous arteriovenous fistulas
   e. Percutaneous double-lumen Silastic catheters

3. Early postoperative hemodynamic changes that may be encountered soon after construction of a proximally located, high-flow arteriovenous fistula for hemodialysis include all of the following except:
   a. Increased stroke volume
   b. Reversal of flow in the distal artery when the fistula opening exceeds the diameter of the feeding artery
   c. Increased cardiac output
   d. Increased heart rate
   e. Decreased total systemic resistance

4. Which of the following is not a complication of percutaneous subclavian central venous catheterization?
   a. Hemopneumothorax
   b. Catheter embolism
   c. Brachial plexus injury
   d. Lymphatic fistula formation
   e. All are possible complications

5. Correction of localized venous anastomotic stenosis can be accomplished by all of the following except:
   a. Patch angioplasty of the outflow anastomosis
   b. Extension bypass graft to a more proximal vein
   c. Percutaneous transluminal dilatation and stent
   d. Relocation of the venous anastomosis to an adjacent vein
   e. Restoring arterial inflow

6. Which of the following is a characteristic of venous runoff stenosis?
   a. It may be related to the shearing effect of blood flow on intima at the anastomotic site.
   b. It develops as early as 6 months after graft placement.
   c. It is most often seen after construction of prosthetic arteriovenous fistulas.
   d. It manifests as an increase in venous return pressure during dialysis.
   e. All of the above

7. The potential benefits of implantable ports over percutaneous central venous catheters for the delivery of chemotherapy include all of the following except:
   a. Lower catheter-related sepsis rate
   b. Lower incidence of thrombosis
   c. Requires little daily care
   d. Interferes less with the patient's normal activities

8. Vascular access in children weighing less than 10 kg may be reliably accomplished by each of the following except:
   a. Percutaneous central vein catheterization
   b. Forearm PTFE bridge fistula
   c. Creation of a brachial artery–to–antecubital vein autogenous fistula
   d. Direct cannulation of umbilical vessels if the patient is a newborn

9. Increased risk of infection in a prosthetic arteriovenous graft for hemodialysis can be related to all of the following except:
   a. Poor aseptic technique during needle puncture
   b. High colonization rate of dialysis patients and dialysis staff with *Staphylococcus aureus*
   c. Decreased chemotactic response of polymorphonuclear leukocytes in uremia
   d. Decreased bacterial phagocytosis in uremic patients
   e. All of the above

10. In regard to thrombosis of the axillosubclavian vein after percutaneous dialysis catheter placement, which of the following is correct?
    a. Diagnosis can be made reliably only with venography.
    b. It rarely occurs after internal jugular placement.
    c. It is not a source of pulmonary emboli.
    d. It may be treated with percutaneous transluminal dilatation and stent in many patients.
    e. It occurs only after the catheter has been in place for more than 3 months.

ANSWERS

1. **b**
2. **d**
3. **a**
4. **e**
5. **e**
6. **e**
7. **b**
8. **b**
9. **e**
10. **d**

COMPLICATIONS IN VASCULAR SURGERY

CHAPTER 55

Neointimal Hyperplasia

Melina R. Kibbe • Ted R. Kohler • Wesley S. Moore

The development of strategies designed to suppress neointimal hyperplasia after peripheral vascular interventions has become increasingly important in light of the current enthusiasm for less invasive but more locally injurious percutaneous therapies. Nearly all vascular interventions are prone to the development of neointimal hyperplasia because manipulation of the arterial wall induces some form of endothelial cell injury. This injury initiates a cascade of events that ultimately results in neointimal hyperplasia and limits the durability of these vascular interventions. Some vascular interventions are more prone to the development of neointimal hyperplasia; these include prosthetic bypass and arteriovenous grafts.[1] However, percutaneous balloon angioplasty with or without stenting, endovascular atherectomy, vein bypass grafting, and endarterectomy are all susceptible to this process.[2-5] Thus peripheral vascular interventions will remain temporary and palliative rather than durable and potentially curative unless effective treatment of neointimal hyperplasia can be achieved.

Neointimal hyperplasia results from a complex cascade of events that involves all three layers of the arterial wall as well as circulating blood elements. Much has been learned about this process in the past decade that has changed the way neointimal hyperplasia is viewed and has opened up new strategies for therapeutic development. The classic description of neointimal hyperplasia resulting from proliferation and migration of vascular smooth muscle cells (VSMC) from the media to the intima, along with deposition of the extracellular matrix after endothelial cell injury, no longer accurately represents the pathophysiologic changes that occur during this injury process.[6,7] It is now recognized that the adventitia as well as resident and circulating stem and progenitor cells play a large role in this process. Furthermore, in addition to the well-described role of cytokines and growth factors that are secreted from platelets and leukocytes at the site of injury, reactive oxygen species and adipokine have been shown to be intimately involved in the regulation of this process. This chapter summarizes the current concepts regarding the pathology and pathophysiology of neointimal hyperplasia.

PATHOLOGY

Neointimal hyperplasia can be described as the abnormal continued proliferation of cells and connective tissue elements that occurs at sites of arterial injury. During the first decade of the 20th century, Carrel and Guthrie[8] noted that "within a few days after the operation, the stitches placed in making the anastomosis became covered with a glistening substance similar in appearance to the normal endothelium." This early description of arterial healing most likely represents the normal response of an artery to injury. Neointimal hyperplasia, in contrast, is more likely the result of an exaggeration of this response through the inability to control, or the continued stimulation of, this normal regenerative process.

Lesions of neointimal hyperplasia are firm and homogeneous upon gross examination. They look smooth, shiny, and subendothelial. These lesions were often referred to as *myointimal hyperplasia*, initially highlighting the thought that the medial VSMC is the origin of the proliferating tissue. However, given that it is now recognized that multiple cell types contribute to the neointimal mass, the term *neointimal hyperplasia* or *intimal hyperplasia* is more commonly used today. Assessment of neointimal lesions using intravascular ultrasound has supported the notion that the majority ($\approx$90%) of lesions are homogeneous in appearance. However, with advances in technology, such as intravascular optical coherence tomography, it appears that up to 40% of lesions may be heterogeneous in nature.[9] Pathologic histologic examination of neointimal lesions reveals mainly stellate cells surrounded by a clear fibromyxomatous stroma and connective tissue. These stellate cells contain smooth muscle–like features and stain positively for actin and sulfated glycosaminoglycans.[10,11] These appear to originate from several different sources, including the media; the adventitia (i.e., fibroblasts); the endothelium; and resident and circulating stem cells. Cellular proliferation begins within 24 hours of injury and is one of the hallmarks of neointimal hyperplasia. However, proliferation, migration, phenotypic differentiation, cellular infiltration, and extracellular matrix deposition all occur, resulting in wall thickening that continues to develop over several weeks (Figure 55-1).[12]

PATHOPHYSIOLOGY

The classic description of the arterial injury response by both Clowes and Ross involves damage to the vascular endothelium and exposure of the underlying VSMC to circulating blood elements.[6,7,13-15] This exposure of the subendothelial arterial wall elements triggers the activation of myriad cellular and enzymatic events. The underlying internal elastic lamina and VSMC are exposed to circulating blood elements. Platelets immediately

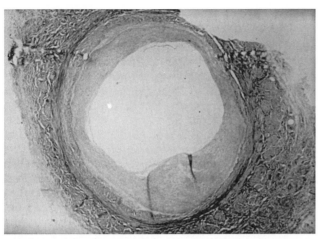

FIGURE 55-1 ■ Photomicrograph of a failed infrainguinal autogenous vein bypass graft showing a large amount of hyperplastic intimal proliferation (Verhoeff-van Gieson stain; original magnification x20).

TABLE 55-1 **Proliferating Cell Number/mm²
after Arterial Injury**

Time Point	Media	Adventitia
Noninjured	0.2	0.1
4 hours	42	286
8 hours	37	510
12 hours	38	531
24 hours	369	82
48 hours	972	691
72 hours	930 (29%)	1164 (53%)
7 days	576 (14%)	1424 (41%)
14 days	420 (13%)	810 (23%)
30 days	22 (0.4%)	75 (2%)

Modified from Couffinhal T, Dufourcq P, Jaspard B, et al: Kinetics of adventitial repair in the rat carotid model. Coron Artery Dis 12:635–648, 2001.

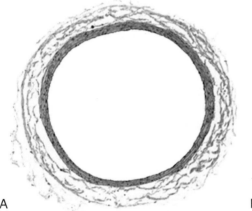
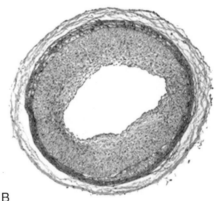

FIGURE 55-2 ■ **A,** Cross-section of a rat carotid artery. **B,** Cross-section of a rat carotid artery 2 weeks after balloon injury. See Color Plate 55-2.

aggregate and adhere to the site of injury.[16] An inflammatory response follows, with the infiltration of neutrophils, macrophages, and leukocytes.[17,18] Twenty-four hours after injury, under the influence of growth factors and cytokines, medial VSMC convert from a contractile to a synthetic phenotype and begin to proliferate.[19] VSMC migrate to the neointima, where they continue to proliferate for up to 8 weeks.[6,20,21] Concurrently, endothelial cell regeneration occurs through the stimulation of basic fibroblast growth factor (bFGF) within 24 hours after injury and can continue for 6 to 10 weeks.[22] Finally, transforming growth factor beta (TGF-β) stimulates extracellular matrix deposition.[23,24] The culmination of these events results in the formation of neointima hyperplasia (Figure 55-2).

The classic arterial injury response just described includes no mention of the adventitia. However, the adventitia is now thought to be one of the main driving forces in the development of neointimal hyperplasia. Investigators have characterized the proliferative response after arterial injury in rat and pig arteries.[25,26] Common

to both is that the proliferative response in the adventitia, compared with the intima and media, is much greater at almost all time points. Although 1.5-fold to twofold more proliferation has been reported in the adventitia compared with in the media in rat carotid arteries (Table 55-1), nearly sevenfold more proliferation has been reported in the adventitia than in the media in pig coronary arteries.[25,26] Furthermore, upon examination of early time points, proliferation has been found to occur in the adventitia before the media at time points as early as 4 hours (see Table 55-1).

The development of neointimal hyperplasia in vein grafts bears a similarity to neointimal hyperplasia after arterial injury, but it differs in that there are fewer medial cells that respond and there is an additional response to increased wall tension. Prominent features in rodent models of vein grafting include extensive early denudation of the endothelium and smooth muscle cell layers, attachment of leukocytes and platelets to the subendothelial matrix, and elaboration of cytokine and growth factor products by these cells. This results in the

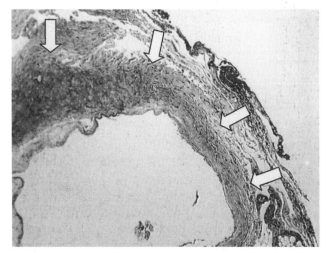

FIGURE 55-3 ■ Trichrome-elastin stain of a 72-hour-old vein graft. The luminal side is depicted on the bottom edge of this tissue section. There is evidence of endothelial and smooth muscle cell denudation, with adherence of leukocytes and platelets.

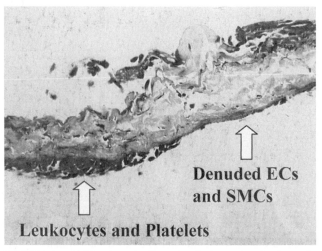

FIGURE 55-4 ■ Trichrome-elastin stain of a 2-week-old vein graft. *Arrows* denote the region of the external elastic lamina, within which resides the neointima. Many of the nuclei visualized in the neointima proved to be macrophages when stained with ED-2 macrophage stain (not depicted). *ECs*, Endothelial cells; *SMCs*, smooth muscle cells.

activation, migration, and proliferation of vein graft adventitial myofibroblasts to form a neointima.[27-32] Pathologically, the trauma resulting from surgical manipulation and exposure of the vein graft to arterial pressure and flow results in nearly complete denudation of the endothelium and loss of the smooth muscle cell layers within the first 24 hours (Figure 55-3). Early after denudation, attachment of leukocytes and platelets occurs. Macrophage infiltration dominates the early inflammatory changes observed with vein graft pathobiology. This prominent inflammatory response peaks during the first 2 weeks of vein graft adaptation, which exceeds the response observed in models of arterial injury (Figure 55-4). Stark and Hoch elegantly demonstrated that by inhibiting macrophage activity early in this inflammatory process, a significant reduction in neointimal hyperplasia was achieved.[29,31]

Vein graft neointimal changes persist and can progress despite re-endothelialization, in contrast to arterial neointimal proliferation, which tends to halt its progression upon restitution of the endothelial cell layer. It is believed that the ongoing neointimal thickening associated with vein graft neointimal hyperplasia is an adaptive response to arterial pressure and flow.[33] Wall thickening is greater in regions of low shear (e.g., at the inner wall of a curve). Neointimal hyperplasia results in wall thickening, which decreases wall stress to more physiologic levels. These hyperplastic changes were described by Carrel and Guthrie[34] when vein grafts were first examined histologically. They referred to this process as "arterialization." It is now known that this arterialization process involved phenotypic transformation of the vein cells to an arterial phenotype, as indicated by the loss of ephrin-B4. Wall thickening can be accentuated at valve cusps, perhaps because of local flow abnormalities; at the anastomoses, where shear and wall tension are greatest; and at sites of clamp injury. Hemodynamically significant lesions caused by intimal hyperplasia usually occur after the first month

and are rare after a year. After that time, vein grafts can develop lesions similar to atherosclerosis.

In addition to the processes just described, which involve platelets, inflammatory cells, VSMC, adventitial fibroblasts, and the extracellular matrix, there is now an understanding of the contribution of resident and circulating stem cells to the development of neointimal hyperplasia, as well as the role of reactive oxygen species in regulating many of these processes. Several mechanisms are likely responsible for stimulating these responses, including mechanical changes, such as turbulence and compliance mismatch, and complex interactions between these different cells. Thus, a complex view has emerged that involves the synergistic action of several biological pathways. The remainder of this section reviews, separately, the experimental basis for the hypothesized involvement of each of these systems.

Hemodynamic and Mechanical Factors

A wide variety of hemodynamic and mechanical factors, including high- and low-flow velocities, high and low wall shear stress, and mechanical compliance mismatch, have been implicated in the formation of intimal hyperplasia.[35-37] The effects of flow velocity on the subsequent development of intimal hyperplasia have been studied in a variety of models. In general, low blood velocity tends to favor the development of neointimal hyperplasia. For example, in a canine carotid vein interposition model, segments with low-flow velocities developed significantly thicker intimal layers[38]; however, there are exceptions to this rule. In a high-flow renal artery–to–vena cava anastomosis, significant intimal thickening was documented by electron microscopic examination 3 months after formation.[39] Similar intimal lesions have also been noted in arteriovenous fistulas (AVF) constructed for hemodialysis access.[40] This may be a result of the compliance mismatch noted between the arterial and venous systems. In a monkey iliac AVF model, 6 months after construction no increase in intimal thickening occurred on the experimental side.[41] In that study, although flow rate and velocity were markedly increased on the side of the AVF, the calculated wall shear stress was equal on both sides. This equality of shear stress, despite a significant difference in flow velocities, was the result of a twofold increase in the vessel lumen diameter. The vessel wall regulates its diameter to produce a physiologic level of shear stress at the lumen. The endothelium regulates diameter by producing both vasoconstrictors such as endothelin, and vasodilators such as nitric oxide (NO). These factors also affect VSMC proliferation and when chronically present, cause remodeling of the vessel to maintain the new diameter without vasoactivity.

In other primate studies, arteriovenous flow has been shown to inhibit neointimal thickening in highly porous polytetrafluoroethylene (PTFE) grafts.[42] Return to normal flow causes thickening of these lesions. In a rodent model of arterial injury, low flow caused increased intimal hyperplasia.[43] These and many other studies demonstrate that intimal hyperplasia is increased by low shear and inhibited by high shear. Regions of low wall shear stress also may stimulate intimal proliferation by increasing the time for lipid transport.[35,38] The results of postmortem studies have shown that early atherosclerotic lesions occur more commonly in areas of low wall shear stress.[44] In the carotid artery, atherosclerosis starts at the outer wall of the bulb, where shear forces are low and oscillating.[45,46]

Compliance mismatch is also an important hemodynamic factor in the production of anastomotic intimal hyperplasia.[47] Compliance is defined as the percentage of radial change per unit pressure and is a useful index of vessel wall distensibility to a pressure force. Although experimental and clinical studies have shown that conduits with compliance values approaching that of the native artery have better patency, none of these studies controlled for differences in graft surfaces. In one study, femoropopliteal autografts made from glutaraldehyde-treated carotid arteries had better patency when fixation produced a more compliant graft.[48] However, other studies have shown that the creation of stiffer, less compliant grafts by treating arteries with glutaraldehyde results in markedly diminished patency rates.[47,49] Although the compliance of a vein graft at the time of implantation is similar to that of a native artery, according to the results of one study the compliance values actually remained within the normal range for a median follow-up of 33 months.[50] Textile and fabric prostheses, in contrast, are relatively noncompliant. Furthermore, 4 months after implantation, a significant loss of compliance is noted in both polyester fabric and PTFE grafts.[51]

For this reason, some authors have suggested imposing a short interposition of autogenous vein between the native artery and prosthetic grafts.[52] These modifications are largely intended to decrease the compliance mismatch between the prosthetic graft and the native artery. They include vein cuffs, vein patches, vein boots, and AVF at the distal anastomosis (Figure 55-5).[53] A prospective randomized trial to examine the efficacy of Miller vein cuffs in improving lower extremity PTFE graft

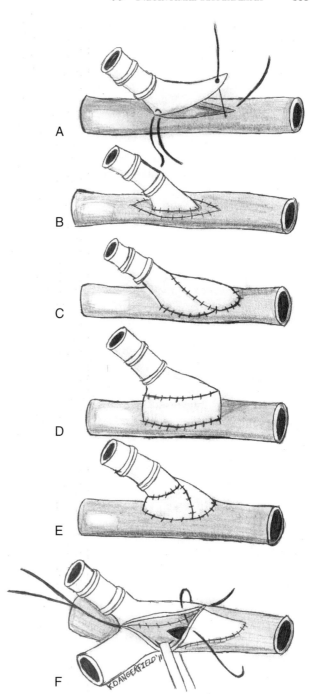

FIGURE 55-5 ■ Surgical techniques using vein interposition for creation of distal anastomoses. **A,** Standard end-to-side anastomosis; **B,** Linton patch; **C,** Taylor patch; **D,** Miller cuff; **E,** vein boot; and **F,** arteriovenous fistula.

patency showed that vein cuffs did not improve patency rates in bypasses to the above-knee popliteal artery.[54] However, cuffed below-knee popliteal artery grafts had a 45% 3-year patency rate versus a 19% patency rate in uncuffed grafts ($p = 0.018$).[55] Similarly, the use of vein patches, such as those developed by Taylor and Linton, at the distal anastomosis yields better long-term patency rates versus prosthetic material alone.[56,57] Although there have been no randomized, prospective trials to date, retrospective reviews have demonstrated improved patency of vein-patched PTFE versus PTFE alone when used for below-knee bypasses. Taylor and colleagues reported a 5-year primary patency of 54% for 83 infrapopliteal PTFE grafts using his vein patch modification.[56] Although there is no control arm to this study, previously reported patency rates with PTFE alone are significantly worse.[1] A review of 145 patients who had undergone either above- or below-knee bypasses using autologous vein, unmodified PTFE, and Linton patch–modified PTFE found that above-knee bypasses had no statistical difference in 1- and 3-year patency rates between the three groups.[58] However, the cumulative patency rates for 1, 3, and 5 years after below-knee bypasses were 93%, 75%, and 75% for the autologous vein group (n = 30); 74%, 52%, and 42% for the unmodified PTFE group (n = 37); and 93%, 93%, and 93% for the Linton patch–modified PTFE group (n = 16), respectively. They speculated that the improved results over unmodified PTFE bypass grafts were a result of improved compliance mismatch between the prosthetic graft and the targeted native artery. The study was limited by the small number of Linton patch–modified PTFE grafts used compared with the autologous vein and PTFE groups. Finally, a retrospective analysis of outcomes of patients with AVF-modified PTFE grafts versus PTFE alone to the infrapopliteal arteries showed that the 2-year patency rates were significantly better for grafts with the AVF modification (23% vs. 5% for the PTFE alone grafts, $p < 0.05$).[59] The AVF, originally described by Ascher and colleagues, is created by first mobilizing an adjacent vein and transecting it.[60] The vein is then anastomosed to the artery in an end-to-side fashion. A veinotomy is created near the AVF and the ePTFE is anastomosed, creating the AVF modification at the distal anastomosis (see Figure 55-5). Despite these surgical improvements, patency rates remain poor, especially when the distal outflow is at or below the level of the popliteal artery, primarily as a result of the formation of neointimal hyperplasia.

Platelets

Platelets have long been known to play a central role in the reaction of a vessel wall to injury. To date, most research in this area has focused on the activation of platelets by the injured endothelium as the major factor in the development of intimal hyperplasia. Denudation of the arterial wall exposes the subendothelial matrix, which leads to adherence and subsequent activation of platelets. The luminal surface quickly passivates by adsorption of plasma proteins, limiting the period of platelet aggregation to less than 24 hours. Platelet adherence requires the interaction of subendothelial collagen, a platelet membrane glycoprotein receptor (GP Ib), plasma von Willebrand factor, and fibronectin. After adherence, platelets undergo a morphologic change, stretching to cover the exposed surface. Activated platelets release adenosine diphosphate and activate the arachidonic acid pathway to release thromboxane A2. Both of these factors lead to platelet aggregation. Recruitment of platelets requires the rapid expression of the platelet membrane receptor complexes GP IIb and GP IIIa, both of which promote platelet aggregation through the binding of circulating fibrinogen. Platelet adhesion and granule release also lead to a parallel acceleration of the coagulation cascade. This activation of clotting pathways, combined with high local concentrations of fibrinogen mediated by binding to the GP IIb/IIIa complex, creates a fibrin protein network that further stabilizes the aggregated platelet plug. Once platelet aggregation is initiated by the pathways mentioned earlier, its further formation is actively inhibited by an intact endothelium. Thus, a damaged endothelium not only initiates platelet activation but also impairs its inhibition.

Platelet-derived growth factor (PDGF) is secreted along with other granule constituents, including platelet factor 4, thromboglobulin, and thrombospondin. PDGF is a cationic protein with a molecular weight of 28 to 31 kDa. It comprises two subunits (α and β). Physiologically, PDGF functions as both a chemoattractant and a mitogen for VSMC and fibroblasts. Because it binds with high affinity to VSMC, some have suggested that PDGF may attract the VSMC from the media into the intima, bind to them, and stimulate their proliferation. Interestingly, evidence has shown that the platelet may not be the only source of this protein. PDGF (α and β subunits) is produced by human umbilical vein and saphenous vein endothelial cells. In fact, a large increase in PDGF production can be measured in injured endothelial cells. Also, both α-subunit and β-subunit messenger RNA (mRNA) have been noted in fresh endarterectomy specimens obtained during carotid surgery.[61] VSMC themselves also produce PDGF-like activity in response to arterial injury, and VSMC from human atheroma contain mRNA for the PDGF α subunit.[62] Taken together, these findings may explain how proliferation continues after re-endothelialization occurs. PDGF may be released by both platelets and endothelial cells, causing the activation and migration of VSMC and myofibroblasts, which then secrete additional PDGF, leading to proliferation. Finally, demonstrating the importance of PDGF to the arterial injury response, inhibition of PDGF using antibodies or antisense oligonucleotides in animal models of arterial injury has been shown to inhibit neointimal hyperplasia by 60% to 80%.[63-65]

Inflammatory Cells

Inflammatory cells are intimately involved in the arterial response to injury. Electron microscopic studies after balloon catheter intimal injury show that leukocytes attach to the de-endothelialized surface of an arterial lumen within minutes.[17,18,66] This includes polymorphonuclear neutrophil (PMN), monocytes, and lymphocytes. In addition to adhering to the damaged endothelium, these cells even penetrate it in some instances. These adherent leukocytes are paramount to the secretion of many cytokines and growth factors that influence the subsequent events in neointimal hyperplasia (Table 55-2).[67-69] The central role of leukocyte chemotaxis in the arterial injury response has been demonstrated through several novel models of inflammation. One model that supports the role of inflammation in the development of

TABLE 55-2 **Cellular Sources of Growth Factors and Cytokines Involved in the Arterial Response to Injury**

Growth Factor/ Cytokine	Leukocytes	Monocytes/ Macrophages
IGF-1		X
PDGF		X
TGF-α		X
TGF-β	X	X
VEGF	X	X
EGF		X
FGF		X
TNF-α	X	X
IL-1β	X	X
IL-4	X	
IL-6		X
IL-8	X	X
IL-10		X
IL-18	X	X
MCP	X	X
IGF-1		X
PDGF		X

Adapted from Mitra AK, Del Core MG, Agrawal DK: Cells, cytokines and cellular immunity in the pathogenesis of fibroproliferative vasculopathies. Can J Physiol Pharmacol 83:701–715, 2005.
IGF, Insulin-like growth factor; *PDGF,* platelet-derived growth factor; *TGF,* transforming growth factor; *VEGF,* vascular endothelial growth factor; *EGT,* epidermal growth factor; *FGF,* fibroblast growth factor; *TNF,* tumor necrosis factor; *IL,* interleukin; *MCP,* macrophage chemoattractant protein.

neointimal hyperplasia consists of delivering leukocyte-derived myeloperoxidase in the presence of its substrate hydrogen peroxide (H_2O_2). The infusion of myeloperoxidase and H_2O_2 into an isolated rat common carotid artery without mechanical injury elicited the development of neointimal hyperplasia.[70]

In another model, an endotoxin-soaked thread was placed on half of a rat femoral artery to produce an inflammatory response.[71] This technique consistently caused a significant leukocyte infiltration, which occurred only on the treated side of the vessel. Histologic examination performed 14 days later revealed nonuniform neointimal lesions in which proliferating VSMC were located exclusively on the side of the lumen adjacent to the treated half of the arterial wall. Clearly, these animal models suggested a strong association between inflammation and neointimal hyperplasia. The mechanisms controlling this relationship are a target for therapeutic intervention.

PMN adhesion to the surface of endothelial cells is controlled by several complex glycoproteins located on the surface of both endothelial and white blood cells. Together, these binding molecules constitute a sophisticated communication system. Two endothelial cell adhesion molecules involved in neutrophil binding have been well characterized: endothelial leukocyte adhesion molecule-1 (ELAM-1) and intercellular adhesion molecule-1 (ICAM-1). ELAM-1 is either unexpressed or remains intracellular in the inactive endothelial cell. However, after activation by a variety of different cytokines, this adhesion complex is rapidly induced and appears on the membrane surface of the stimulated endothelial cell. ICAM-1 is located in small amounts on the surface of inactive endothelial cells. After activation by either injury or a variety of stimulating agonists, the expression of this binding complex is significantly increased. ICAM-1 is the binding ligand for the CD11a/CD18 receptor on the leukocyte membrane.

Histochemically, the adhesion molecules located in the surface membranes of the white blood cells responsible for leukocyte binding to endothelial cells can be separated into three related heterodimers. Each of these heterodimer protein complexes are composed of an α and a β subunit. The α subunit differs among the three glycoprotein complexes (CD11a, CD11b, or CD11c), whereas the β subunit remains constant (CD18). The CD11a/CD18 complex is found on the surface of all white blood cells and mediates the attachment of unstimulated PMNs to stimulated endothelial cells. This binding probably occurs through an interaction with the ICAM-1 receptor that, as mentioned, is expressed on the luminal surface of activated or injured endothelial cells. The binding of the CD11a/CD18 complex to the ICAM-1 receptor may also play a role in the cytokine-induced transendothelial migration of PMNs. The CD11b/CD18 adhesion complex is referred to as either "Mac-1" or the "C3b complement receptor." This glycoprotein has been implicated in the adhesion of chemotactically stimulated PMNs and controls several cellular functions such as aggregation and cytotoxicity. The third heterodimer complex, CD11c/CD18, exists on both PMNs and monocytes, but its role in binding to endothelial cells remains undetermined.

During inflammatory states, the attachment of PMNs to the involved endothelium is greatly increased, primarily because of the upregulation and enhanced expression of the binding glycoproteins described earlier. A variety of substances are capable of stimulating this enhanced PMN adherence. Interleukin (IL) 1, tumor necrosis factor-α, lymphotoxin, and bacterial endotoxins (lipopolysaccharide) all increase the production of both ELAM-1 and ICAM-1 on the surface of affected endothelial cells. In addition, PMN activation can be stimulated by several substances that are released secondary to inflammation. Examples include the complement factors C5a and C3b, which stimulate PMN chemotaxis and phagocytosis, respectively. Likewise, PMN adhesion and chemotaxis can also be stimulated by interleukin-1, xanthine oxidase, PDGF, and the lipid mediators leukotriene B and platelet-activating factor. Finally, tumor necrosis factor-α is an important mediator of PMN phagocytosis and can lead to increased lysosomal enzyme release.

After activation and adhesion to the damaged vessel lumen, leukocytes migrate into the arterial wall. In one study, 42 days after a denuding injury, leukocytes were shown to penetrate the arterial media and were seen deep within the hyperplastic lesions.[72] Several different mechanisms trigger this leukocyte migration. VSMC and macrophages elaborate potent chemotactic factors for leukocytes, which could sustain continued leukocyte recruitment.[73] Supporting this notion, serum containing medium that was conditioned from VSMC stimulated leukocyte migration. Other chemotactic agents for

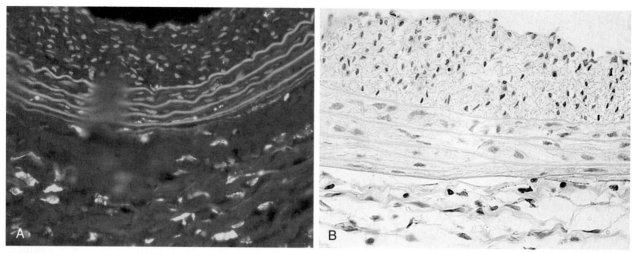

FIGURE 55-6 ■ Arterial cross sections of immunohistochemical staining for **(A)** monocytes/macrophages *(red staining)* and **(B)** lymphocytes *(brown staining)* 2 weeks after arterial balloon injury in the rat carotid artery. Note that the majority of infiltrates are found in the adventitia. See Color Plate 55-6.

leukocytes include PDGF and, in some reports, factors released by fibroblasts. VSMC removed from atherosclerotic plaques expressed ICAM-1, suggesting a possible connection between these medial cells and leukocyte recruitment and activation.

The mechanism by which leukocytes may initiate the formation of intimal hyperplasia after penetrating the injured arterial wall remains unknown. Again, several pathways have been suggested. After a denuding endothelial injury and the deposition of inflammatory cells, a variety of inflammatory products may be elaborated. These include chemotactic factors, growth factors, complement components, and enzymes. One of the most studied substances is monocyte- and macrophage-derived growth factor (MDGF). MDGF is a well-known stimulator of VSMC and fibroblast proliferation. This growth factor is similar and may be identical to PDGF. Thus, the stimulation of VSMC proliferation is one mechanism by which inflammatory cells may contribute to the formation of neointimal hyperplasia. A second possibility involves the production of lysosomal degradation enzymes. Activated leukocytes secrete several potent proteases capable of degrading collagen, basement membranes, and other important extracellular structural proteins. One example of a PMN-derived enzyme that has been implicated in peri-inflammatory extracellular damage is myeloperoxidase. Liberation of these destructive enzymes into the wall of an injured vessel may weaken the extracellular matrix. This "loosening" of the vessel wall may facilitate the migration of VSMC from the medial layer toward the lumen. Finally, leukocytes may act directly at sites of vessel injury to extend endothelial injury. PMNs can produce oxygen-free radicals through the action of the (nicotinamide adenine dinucleotide phosphate [NADPH]) oxidase system present on their membranes. The toxic substances elaborated by these activated PMNs, including superoxide anion, hydrogen peroxide, and hydroxyl radicals, can damage endothelial cells and alter capillary permeability. With PMN activation, marginally injured endothelial cells

bordering a lesion may be destroyed, increasing the magnitude of the damage to the vessel wall. This further exposure of the subendothelial layer allows more platelet cell adherence, aggregation, and activation, as well as the recruitment of more leukocyte mediators and thus the stimulation of a continued cycle of inflammatory injury.

In addition to luminal entry, the adventitia has been recognized as an important site of inflammation after arterial injury (Figure 55-6). The accumulation of B cells, T cells, and macrophages in the adventitia has been documented in numerous studies.[74-77] Okamoto and colleagues[78] characterized macrophage localization to the adventitia after porcine coronary artery angioplasty and which receptors are important to their recruitment. Macrophages present in the adventitia were significantly increased at day 1 after injury, peaked at day 3, and then slowly decreased back to baseline at day 14. Interestingly, the number of adventitial macrophages was larger than the number found in either the media or the intima. In addition, macrophage accumulation preceded cell proliferation by 48 to 72 hours. Remarkably, they also found that macrophages had a nearly twentyfold greater presence than neutrophils. Early and sustained expression of E-selectin, P-selectin, and VCAM-1 by the vasa vasorum indicated that these receptors were important in allowing the macrophages to localize to the adventitia. Macrophages have also been noted to phenotypically differentiate into myofibroblasts after arterial injury and contribute to the development of neointimal hyperplasia.[79] Bayes-Genis and coworkers[79] demonstrated that 14 days after arterial injury to the pig coronary artery, 42% of the neointimal cells expressed the macrophage-specific antigen SWC3, and 9% of the cells co-expressed SWC3 and alpha smooth muscle actin (αSMA). Finally, macrophage localization and activation has been found to rely on angiotensin II (Ang II)–induced upregulation of CCL2 and IL-6. Tieu and associates was recently able to quantify the degree to which Ang II increases the macrophage population in the adventitia and found a 5.3-fold increase in populations of mice treated with Ang II.[80] They also documented the importance that CCL2 plays in Ang II–induced macrophage localization because the absence of CCR2, a CCL2 receptor, in CCR2[-/-] mice significantly attenuated adventitial macrophage accumulation. The cytokine IL-6 was shown to be important to the activity of Ang II because IL-6[-/-] mice adventitia did not show the same propensity to recruit macrophages as the IL-6[+/+] mice after Ang II stimulation.

Growth Factors

The stimulation of cellular proliferation is the final common pathway of all postulated mechanisms, leading to the development of intimal hyperplasia. The view that the vascular wall is a complex integrated organ, complete with its own endogenous local autocrine system, is gaining increasing support. In this theory, neointimal hyperplasia is postulated to result from an imbalance of these local hormonal systems. This could be caused by an excess of stimulatory molecules; alternatively, cellular proliferation may result from the absence or reduction of inhibitory hormones.

Angiotensin II, PDGF, and MDGF are all examples of growth factors believed to be involved in the formation of hyperplastic neointimal lesions; each has been reviewed in detail earlier. bFGF, a smooth muscle cell mitogen that is not secreted, is released from damaged VSMC and acts in an autocrine fashion to stimulate proliferation of adjacent, viable cells. This mitogen is largely responsible for the proliferative response after balloon injury.[6] Denudation of endothelium with a fine wire that does not damage the endothelium results in much less VSMC activation.[81] Lindner and associates[19] observed that administration of bFGF after an injury increased VSMC proliferation from 11.5% to 54.8%. Their finding of an equivalent increase in proliferation after wire loop injury demonstrates that bFGF can act as a mitogen for undamaged medial cells. bFGF administered to normal, nondenuded arteries has no effect on VSMC growth. bFGF is also a potent stimulator of endothelial cells and, accordingly, stimulates angiogenesis. After arterial injury, bFGF is important for stimulating endothelial cell growth to completely cover injured regions that would normally remain denuded. Cuevas and colleagues demonstrated that the direct local infusion of bFGF into either normal adventitia or injured media results in proliferation of both vasa vasorum and VSMC.[82]

TGF-β is mostly known for its role in stimulating extracellular matrix deposition. More recently, however, it is now understood to have a role in negatively regulating endothelial cell activation, VSMC migration, and macrophage and lymphocyte accumulation.[83] Early studies demonstrated that TGF-β was expressed after arterial injury.[24] Furthermore, application of TGF-β to the arterial wall using gene therapy or intraluminal delivery stimulated the development of neointimal hyperplasia.[23,84,85] Inhibition of TGF-β using antibodies inhibited neointimal hyperplasia.[86-88] These early studies focused on the stimulation of procollagen and fibronectin, as well as effects on remodelling. However, identification of SMAD3 because the downstream target of TGF-β has

shed more light on the precise role of TGF-β. SMAD3 knockout mice exhibited significantly more neointimal hyperplasia after injury compared with the wild type controls. Specifically, they exhibited more cellular proliferation, and bone marrow transplantation studies revealed that the neointima that developed in the SMAD3 knockout mice was derived from resident cells, not circulating cells.[89]

Renin-Angiotensin System

The classic view of the regulatory function of the renin-angiotensin system is that it is primarily an endocrine-based system designed for the homeostatic control of hemodynamic and electrolyte balance. In response to low perfusion pressures, renin is released by renal tissue and circulates in the plasma, where it cleaves angiotensinogen, produced by the liver, into angiotensin I. Angiotensin I is converted into active Ang II by angiotensin-converting enzyme (ACE), located primarily in the pulmonary vasculature. Finally, Ang II exerts its homeostatic hemodynamic effects via specific Ang II receptors located in peripheral vascular arterial beds. This traditional view of the renin-angiotensin system has been revised, and a much more complex concept has emerged. In this new description, the primary site of Ang II production is not the pulmonary vasculature but rather local sites within the affected tissues themselves. This portion of the entire renin-angiotensin axis has been referred to as the *tissue renin-angiotensin system.*

The concept that active Ang II in the vascular wall is synthesized locally, and not delivered via the systemic circulation, was originally suggested by Swales and Thurston.[90] In this report, the authors noted that the amount of angiotensin antiserum required to inhibit endogenous angiotensin effects in sodium-loaded rats could not be explained solely on the basis of systemic production. In addition, several investigators had noticed residual renin-like activity after bilateral nephrectomy in animal studies.[91] More convincing evidence for the existence of a locally active vascular renin-angiotensin system, operating independently of the classic systemic circuit, has been provided by several studies. Angiotensinogen mRNA, the only known precursor to the angiotensin peptides, has been detected in several extrahepatic vascular tissues, including the aorta.[92,93] Immunohistochemical studies have demonstrated renin in cells throughout the vascular wall.[94] Both VSMC and endothelial cells can synthesize renin in vitro.[95,96] Also, mRNA coding for renin has been identified in human VSMC.[91,97] Finally, ACE is located primarily on the luminal surface of vascular endothelial cells.[98] Thus, the normally functioning vascular wall possesses all the necessary components for the independent local production of Ang II.

The physiologic function of locally produced Ang II is an area of continued controversy. Ang II receptors have been identified on vascular endothelial cells, VSMC, and circulating platelets.[91,99-101] Ang II stimulation of endothelial cell–bound receptors leads to the secretion of prostacyclin and possibly endothelium-derived relaxant factor.[102,103] Both of these substances cause VSMC quiescence and relaxation. Activation of the angiotensin receptors located directly on the VSMC themselves causes the opposite effect. Campbell-Boswell and Robertson[104] reported that Ang II stimulates the proliferation of human VSMC in vitro. Geisterfer and associates[105] found that the protein content of these VSMC increased by 20% when stimulated by Ang II for 4 days. Further, this stimulation was abolished by the Ang II receptor antagonist saralasin. Finally, the Mas protooncogene, located on the surface of medial VSMC, increased mitogenic activity when stimulated and has been identified as a functional Ang II receptor.[106] Therefore, one explanation for the physiologic function of a locally active renin-angiotensin system is the autocrine balance of vascular wall metabolic activity and tone.

This view has led many investigators to study the effect of the local production of Ang II on the subsequent development of intimal hyperplasia. In this hypothesis, denudation of the arterial endothelium disrupts the balance of the local renin-angiotensin system and allows the anabolic and mitogenic effects of Ang II on the medial VSMC to proceed unchecked. Another possible mechanism for the promotion of hyperplastic neointimal growth by the local production of Ang II involves the activation of platelet metabolic pathways. As mentioned previously, human platelets possess specific binding sites for Ang II, and platelet activation and the subsequent release of PDGF may play a role in the development of neointimal hyperplasia.[101] In a 1990 study by Swartz and Moore,[107] Ang II enhanced both collagen-induced platelet aggregation and the production of thromboxane A2. Finally, the expression of PDGF by activated VSMC is upregulated in the presence of Ang II.[108]

Coagulation and Fibrinolytic Pathways

Products of coagulation pathways participate in the development of neointimal hyperplasia in complex and diverse ways. Formation of a fibrin matrix in an area of endothelial damage helps stabilize the aggregating platelet plug. Many substances released by organizing thrombus can affect VSMC growth and migration. Among thrombin's many actions, it is a VSMC mitogen. The locally active vascular fibrinolytic system allows VSMC to detach from the surrounding matrix and migrate to the intima. Several molecules participate in this activity, including plasmin, the active end product of the tissue plasminogen-plasmin system. Other important components of this system include the precursor plasminogen and its main endogenous activators: urokinase plasminogen activator (u-PA) and tissue plasminogen activator (t-PA). The catalytic action of these proteases is inhibited in vivo by the plasmin inhibitors α_2-antiplasmin, α_2-macroglobulin, and a group of related plasminogen activator inhibitory proteins.

Several studies link plasmin to VSMC migration. First, circulating plasminogen is a relatively large protein that is normally prevented from entering the medial layer by an intact endothelium. However, after endothelial damage, this protein diffuses readily.[109] Once present in the extracellular medial layer, plasminogen converted into plasmin directly degrades several matrix proteins and activates other collagenases.[110] VSMC express plasminogen activator activity in tissue culture and are a likely source of this enzyme locally in the vessel wall.[111,112] In an in vivo model of arterial repair, Clowes and associates[27] demonstrated that VSMC contain increased levels of both u-PA and t-PA. These plasminogen activators act synergistically and their secretion depends on the functional state of the VSMC. During cellular proliferation, u-PA is the major product, whereas during migration, t-PA expression predominates. These experimental observations suggest that injury to the endothelium allows the local penetration of plasminogen and chemotactic substances elaborated from activated platelets and leukocytes into the arterial wall. The conversion of extracellular plasminogen into plasmin by VSMC degrades the structural matrix proteins. This process may be enhanced by the presence of leukocyte-derived enzymes. Finally, activation of VSMC by the elaborated growth and chemotactic factors initiates migration of these cells through the weakened arterial wall. The direction of migration is determined automatically by the gradient of plasminogen and mitogenic activity, which is highest adjacent to the endothelial defect.

Nitric Oxide

Nitrous oxide (NO) is a small, gaseous molecule normally produced in endothelial cells and serves to protect the vascular health of the vessel wall. NO was originally described as endothelium-derived relaxing factor by Furchgott and Zawadzki[113] in 1980. It is a small, diffusible molecule with a very short half-life that is produced from L-arginine by one of three different enzymes—endothelial nitric oxide synthase (eNOS), neuronal nitric oxide synthase (nNOS), or inducible nitric oxide synthase (iNOS). Although these isoforms share a number of similarities, they are also clearly distinct. They all require the cofactors NADPH, FAD, FMN, heme, and tetrahydrobiopterin to catalyze the reaction.[114] In general, however, eNOS and nNOS are constitutively expressed enzymes and NO production is regulated predominantly by intracellular Ca^{2+} fluxes that permit calmodulin binding, which activates the enzymes.[114] In contrast, iNOS is transcriptionally regulated and is not normally produced by most cells.

NO has been shown to possess many different vasoprotective properties that serve to protect the artery against the development of neointimal hyperplasia. It has been shown to inhibit platelet aggregation, inhibit leukocyte chemotaxis and adherence, inhibit VSMC and adventitial fibroblasts proliferation and migration, stimulate VSMC apoptosis, inhibit endothelial cell apoptosis, and stimulate endothelial cell growth (Figure 55-7).[115-122] NO is also a potent vasodilator. By stimulating soluble guanylate cyclase and leading to increased cyclic guanosine monophosphate release, NO regulates basal vasomotor tone.[123,124] All these properties of NO serve to maintain vascular homeostasis by affecting all the key components in the injury response.

Endothelial cell injury results in loss of NO given that endothelial cells are the main source of constitutive NO production. This loss of NO after vascular injury is pivotal to the development of neointimal hyperplasia.

Several investigators have demonstrated this in animal models. Rudic and coworkers[125] studied eNOS knockout mice and found that these mice developed significantly more neointima after carotid artery ligation than their wild type partners. Fischer and associates[126] used a different approach: They performed the balloon injury to the rat carotid artery, but in some animals they administered a NO synthase inhibitor—N-nitro-l-arginine—in the drinking water. Two weeks after injury, the animals exposed to the NO synthase inhibitor developed 30% more neointimal hyperplasia. Mayr and coworkers[127] evaluated the effect of iNOS deletion on vein graft intimal hyperplasia. They found that autologous vein grafts implanted into the carotid artery of iNOS knockout mice developed twofold more vein graft intimal hyperplasia compared with the wild type controls.

More recently, NO has also been shown to be an important regulator of progenitor cell involvement in the development of neointimal hyperplasia after arterial injury (see Stem Cell section). Using an animal model of hind-limb ischemia, Aicher and colleagues[128] originally described that eNOS knockout mice had impaired endothelial progenitor cell (EPC) mobilization. Shortly

thereafter, Iwakura and coworkers,[129] and later Wegiel and coworkers,[130] demonstrated impaired recruitment of EPC in eNOS-deficient mice after arterial injury, and this was associated with impaired re-endothelialization and greater neointimal hyperplasia. Using a mouse vein-graft model, Mayr and coworkers[127] demonstrated impaired regeneration of endothelial cells in the vein graft of iNOS knockout versus wild type mice. They also showed that the iNOS knockout mice expressed less VEGF and had fewer microvessels in the adventitia compared with the wild type controls, suggesting that the vasa vasorum in the adventitia may be important to the development of vein graft intimal hyperplasia. Zhang and colleagues[131] evaluated the contribution of Sca1+ progenitor cells in eNOS knockout mice using the carotid artery ligation model. They reported increased stromal cell–derived factor-1α (SDF-1α) expression, a chemokine known to regulate hematopoietic progenitor cell mobilization, increased circulating Sca1+ cells, and increased Sca1+ cells in the adventitia 1 week after carotid artery ligation in eNOS knockout versus wild type control mice. These data correlated with increased adventitial proliferation and neointimal hyperplasia. Together these studies demonstrate a role for NO in regulating progenitor cell recruitment after arterial injury, but the effects may differ according to the progenitor cell type and the injury model being used.

Solidifying the role of NO in the arterial injury response, many investigators have shown that supplementation of NO at the site of injury prevents the development of neointimal hyperplasia. These forms of NO-based approaches have included systemic delivery of L-arginine or NO donors, inhalational NO, local application of NO donors or NO-releasing polymers/gels, NO-releasing prosthetic materials, and gene therapy of one of the NOS enzymes.[132-147] Demonstrating the potency of NO, simple periadventitial application of the diazeniumdiolate NO donor PROLI/NO, a short-acting NO donor, inhibited the development of neointimal hyperplasia by 91% when applied to the carotid artery after balloon injury (Figure 55-8).[141] In addition, it

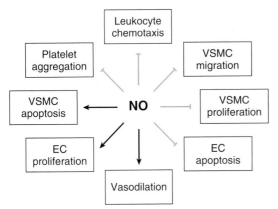

FIGURE 55-7 ■ Schematic of the vasoprotective effects of nitric oxide. *EC,* Endothelial cell; *VSMC,* vascular smooth muscle cell.

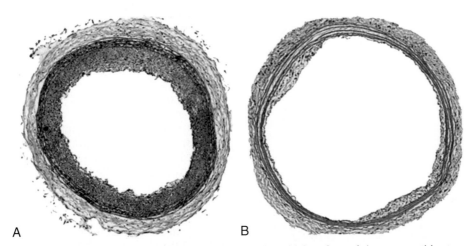

A   B

FIGURE 55-8 ■ The nitric oxide donor PROLI/NO applied to the periadventitial surface of the rat carotid artery after balloon injury inhibits the development of neointimal hyperplasia at 2 weeks. **A,** Rat carotid artery cross section after balloon injury; **B,** rat carotid artery cross section after balloon injury and application of PROLI/NO. See Color Plate 55-8.

appears that these effects are mostly caused by NO and less by its metabolites nitrite or nitrate.[148] Although NO demonstrated potent inhibitory effects on cellular proliferation and inflammation, nitrite and nitrate only inhibited inflammation in a normoxic animal model of neointimal hyperplasia.

Reactive Oxygen Species

Reactive oxygen species (ROS) are recognized as important contributors to the pathophysiology of neointimal hyperplasia. The precursor for all ROS is $O_2^{\cdot-}$, which can be produced from NADPH oxidase (NOX), the mitochondrial respiratory chain, lipoxygenases, xanthine oxidase, cytochrome p450, and uncoupled eNOS.[149] However, in the vasculature, the predominant source of $O_2^{\cdot-}$ production is from stimulation of the NOX enzymes.[150,151] Seven different homologs of the NOX family exist, but only four have been identified in the vasculature: NOX1, NOX2, NOX 4, and NOX5. Once $O_2^{\cdot-}$ is formed, it is rapidly dismutated by superoxide dismutase (SOD) to H_2O_2, which in turn is metabolized by catalase, peroxiredoxin, or glutathione peroxidase to oxygen and water (Figure 55-9). $O_2^{\cdot-}$ can also react with NO to form peroxynitrite ($ONOO^-$) or it can react with iron to form hydroxyl radical ($^{\cdot}OH$). Both superoxide and hydrogen peroxide have been shown to be involved in regulating endothelial cell function, VSMC apoptosis, VSMC and fibroblast migration, VSMC and fibroblast proliferation, and inflammation after arterial injury.[149,152-159] However, the more direct role of oxidative stress has been borne out through the use of animal models of arterial injury and bypass grafting.

Several animal models have demonstrated a more direct role for ROS after vascular injury. One of the first suggestions of the importance of ROS to the arterial injury response was a study by Laurindo and colleagues[160] in 1991 that showed that infusion of SOD inhibited neointimal growth after balloon angioplasty in dogs. Subsequently, Nunes and coworkers[161,162] demonstrated that high levels of superoxide were detectable after balloon injury, even 14 days after injury in pigs, and that administration of vitamins C and E affected vascular remodeling in association with reducing superoxide production. Azevedo and associates[163] characterized the oxidative stress after balloon injury in rabbits. They reported a marked increase (100-fold induction) in superoxide production immediately after injury, with a slow decline to baseline levels 4 weeks after injury. This increase in superoxide levels correlated with cellular proliferation and a decrease in the glutathione/oxidized glutathione ratio, a marker of reduced/oxidized glutathione. Similarly, Souza and coworkers[164] characterized oxidative stress after injury in a balloon injury model in rabbits with comparable results and suggested that the redox imbalance is likely caused by NOX. Shi and coauthors[165] showed that balloon injury of porcine coronary arteries resulted in an increased production of O_2^- and specifically an increased expression of the NOX subunits p47phox and p67phox in the adventitial fibroblasts, but not in the media. Dourron and coauthors[166] more directly demonstrated the importance of ROS production in the development of neointimal hyperplasia. They delivered an adenoviral vector carrying a NOX inhibitor periadventitially to rat common carotid arteries after balloon catheter injury. The NOX inhibitor resulted in a significant reduction of distension-induced ROS production. Furthermore, subsequent analysis of the intima:media area ratio showed significant attenuation in neointimal development in the group in which NOX had been inhibited compared with controls. Other investigators have found reduced ROS after arterial injury with different antioxidants. NOX inhibitors, genetic NOX deletions, or xanthine oxidase inhibitors have been shown to decrease the formation of neointimal hyperplasia.[166-171] Investigators have also overexpressed SOD using adenoviral-mediated delivery of SOD or treatment with a SOD mimetic to attenuate the formation of neointimal hyperplasia.[172-174] Thus it is clear that oxidative stress is intimately involved in regulating the arterial response to injury.

Given the importance of the NOX enzymes to the vasculature and the arterial injury response, special mention of each family member is warranted.[150] NOX1 is expressed in endothelial cells, VSMC, and adventitial fibroblasts. NOX2 is found in the cells throughout the arterial wall except in VSMC from large arteries. NOX4 is present in all three cell types and is much more abundant than the other NOX enzymes. NOX5 is present in at least endothelial cells and VSMC, but because it is not present in rodents, less is known about it. With respect to function, NOX1 appears to stimulate VSMC proliferation and inflammation and is upregulated after vascular injury, and lack of NOX1 through knockout mice is associated with less neointimal hyperplasia.[167] NOX2 may have more of a role in affecting blood pressure, inflammation, and atherosclerosis. The unique feature of NOX4 is that it is thought to be responsible for basal superoxide production. However, recent reports have suggested that NOX4 is distinct from the other NOX enzymes in that it produces mainly basal hydrogen peroxide, not basal superoxide, and that the other

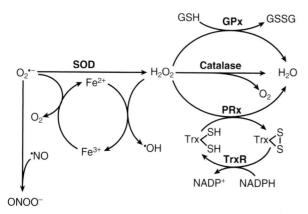

FIGURE 55-9 ■ Schematic of superoxide ($O_2^{\cdot-}$) metabolism. *GSH,* Gluthathione; *GSSG,* oxidized glutathione; *GPx,* glutathione peroxidase; *H₂O,* water; *O₂,* oxygen; *Trx,* thioredoxin; *NADPH,* nicotinamide adenine dinucleotide phosphate; *NADP+,* dihydrophyrimidine dehydrogenase; *Fe²⁺,* iron II; *Fe³⁺,* iron III; *SOD,* superoxide dismutase; *ONOO⁻,* peroxynitrite; *NO,* nitric oxide; *TrxR,* thioredoxin reductase; *H₂O₂,* hydrogen peroxide.

enzymes produce superoxide that is then converted to hydrogen peroxide.[175,176] Haurani and colleagues[154] discovered something unexpected when myofibroblasts were transfected with NOX4/p22. Initially, they hypothesized that overexpression of NOX4/p22 would increase Ang II-induced production of H_2O_2. Interestingly, their data showed the opposite. Transfection and overexpression of NOX4/p22 led to a reduction in the migratory capacity of myofibroblasts after treatment with Ang II compared with empty-vector transfection (46% decrease vs. 192% increase, respectively). The hypothesis postulated by the authors to explain these data included the unique ability of H_2O_2 to downregulate NOX4. They postulated that elevated levels of exogenous NOX4 exert negative feedback on endogenous NOX4 mRNA, or that the protein produced by the NOX4 mRNA has a negative feedback effect on the mRNA itself. Thus, from these data, it is clear that each of the NOX isoforms is intimately involved in regulating some aspect of the arterial injury response.

Stem and Progenitor Cells

Human stem cell research is a relatively new and exciting field that until recently has not included a lot of investigation involving cells residing in the vasculature. However, with the description of the EPC, the appreciation of the multipotency of the vascular pericyte, and the discovery of the resident adventitial stem cells, a more in-depth look into the world of the vascular stem cell is underway. The first vessel wall resident cell to be identified as possessing progenitor cell properties was the pericyte.[177] Pericytes, which incompletely surround the endothelial cells of the microvasculature and share the same basement membrane and numerous junctions with endothelial cells, have traditionally been described and characterized by their supportive role. These cells play an important role in the development of capillaries through the regulation of the surrounding endothelial cells. However, it has now been demonstrated that pericytes can differentiate into multiple different cell types depending on the stimuli, which include adipocytes, chondrocytes, osteoblasts, VSMC, macrophages, and fibroblasts.[178-181] By having this pluripotent ability, pericytes may serve as a reservoir of precursor cells, giving rise to cells of multiple different lineages.

Further investigation has revealed that progenitor cells are not limited to the pericytes within the vascular wall. In fact, in the past several years it has become apparent that the vascular wall, and specifically the adventitia, is an active site of recruitment of circulating stem and progenitor cells. Hematopoietic stem cells (HSC), mesenchymal stem cells (MSC), and EPC have all been shown to contribute to the formation of the neointima after arterial injury, resulting in a paradigm shift of what occurs in the arterial wall after injury.[182-185] Sata and colleagues[182] and Han and colleagues[186] were the first investigators to independently demonstrate, using bone marrow–irradiated mice transplanted with labeled or sex-specific bone marrow, that bone marrow–derived cells constituted approximately 50% to 60% of the neointima after injury. Some cells stained positive for CD31 and others stained positive for αSMA. Taking this one step further, Wang and coauthors[187] studied the response to injury in mice deficient in stem cell factor (SCF) or c-Kit, both important molecules for stem cell signaling. Interestingly, they found a near complete lack of neointima in these mice after arterial injury compared with wild type controls, confirming the importance of stem cells to the formation of the neointima. Further studies by Tanaka and coauthors[188] demonstrated that the degree of incorporation of bone marrow–derived cells into the neointima was dependent on the type of injury model used, with the wire-mediated injury resulting in the largest percentage of bone marrow–derived cells in the neointima. Thus, although it is now clear that stem and progenitor cells are mobilized and recruited to the site of arterial injury and undergo phenotypic differentiation to endothelial or VSMC, much remains to be learned about forces regulating these processes.

Tigerstedt and coworkers[189] characterized the involvement of precursor cells in the arterial injury response. After rat arterial injury, there was a fivefold increase in adventitial cells that preceded the formation of the neointima. This was accompanied by a fourfold increase in the adventitial microvasculature, which peaked at day 14. The cytoskeletal marker vimentin, which stains VSMC, fibroblasts, and myofibroblasts, stained mostly positive in the adventitia at days 3 to 4; thereafter, the staining declined in the adventitia and shifted to the neointima. Flk-1 staining, a stem cell marker, was noted in the first cells, which localized to the neointima and adventitia. By day 14, all layers of the vascular wall expressed flk-1, with the greatest intensity seen in the neointima. These findings support the assertion that cells in the adventitia are activated or recruited very early in the injury response and contribute to neointima formation. To further characterize the adventitial cell types contributing to neointima formation, outgrowth assays were performed from aortic explants. Cells from these outgrowth assays coexpressed markers of multiple cell lineages including VSMC, endothelial cells, and myofibroblasts, and a high percentage of these cells was also positive for the stem cell markers flk-1, Sca1, and CD34. Thus, these data suggest that stem and progenitor cells contribute significantly to the development of neointimal hyperplasia after arterial injury.

An interesting study by Shoji and associates[190] described a mechanism by which human MSC block macrophage involvement with neointimal hyperplasia. Human MSC were injected into the left ventricle of rats immediately, 6 days, and 13 days after ligation of the left common carotid artery. The ligated arteries were then harvested at 7, 14, and 28 days after ligation. Assessment of the human MSC incorporation into the resulting neointimal lesion revealed an absence of transplanted stem cells despite a significant reduction in the size of the neointima. Monocyte recruitment into the neointima decreased by 30% ($p < 0.05$). In addition, human MSC–treated rats exhibited 44% less monocyte chemoattractant protein-1 (MCP-1), a protein responsible for the mobilization and targeting of monocytes ($p < 0.05$). The authors argue that human MSC, although not incorporated into neointimal lesions, exert vasoprotective properties by limiting the activation of circulating monocytes after vascular injury.

The adventitia is also home to resident adult pluripotent cells, including Sca1+ cells, CD34+ cells, and pericytes. Passman and coworkers[191] found that Sca1+ cells, which are integral to the developing artery, are present in adult arteries in the adventitia, near the media/adventitia interface. In an effort to determine how the adventitial Sca1+ cells are targeted to, and maintained within, the adventitia, they identified a layer of sonic hedgehog protein (Shh) located between the media and the adventitia. Shh is known to be important in the retention of other progenitor cell populations in areas such as the skin, nervous system, and lymphoid tissue.[192-194] Shh knockout mice were also found to have significantly fewer adventitial Sca1+ cells compared with wild type mice. In a quiescent state, adventitial Sca1 cells do not express VSMC or endothelial cell markers in vivo. However, these cells can readily differentiate into VSMC or endothelial cells in vitro depending on the stimulus.[191,195] For example, Hu and coworkers[195] demonstrated the presence of progenitor cells within the adventitia of the aortic root in an atherosclerotic mouse model, the apolipoprotein E knockout mice. These cells were found to express a number of markers characteristic of progenitor cells, including stem cell antigen–1 (Sca-1), c-Kit, and CD34. Similar cells were notably absent from the media and intima. Sca-1–positive cells carrying the *LacZ* gene were then transferred to the adventitia of vein grafts in these atherosclerotic mice. *LacZ*-positive cells were subsequently found to populate the intimal atherosclerotic lesions of the vein grafts. This study has far-reaching implications and suggests that resident adventitial stem cells may play an important role in the development of neointimal hyperplasia.

Finally, Zengin and coauthors[196] recently identified the presence of resident adventitial CD34+ cells in the wall of adult human arteries. These cells were located in the same zone as the Sca1+ cells described before, at the media/adventitia interface, and demonstrated the potential to differentiate into endothelial cells and contribute to the vasa vasorum. Thus, it is clear that the adventitia contains a vasculogenic zone of pluripotent cells capable of differentiating into a variety of cell types.

Adiponectin and Periadventitial Adipose Tissue

Adiponectin is a small, 30-kDa protein produced by periadventitial adipose tissue. It belongs to a class of compounds called adipokines and can be found systemically in the plasma in concentrations between 3 and 30 μg/mL.[197,198] In general, adipokines increase as a person's adiposity increases (i.e., obese individuals produce more adipokines). Interestingly, this is not the case with adiponectin. In fact, the level of adiponectin is inversely related to the amount of adipose tissue in a person.[199] Low levels of adiponectin have been linked to the development and progression of obesity-related diseases, including type 2 diabetes and hypertension.[200-203] In addition, adiponectin levels have been linked to the severity of peripheral artery disease. Higher levels of adiponectin are associated with better ankle-brachial indices and improved symptom-free walking distances.[204] Given its relationship with arterial disease, adiponectin has recently garnered more attention as to what role it plays in the vasculature.

Adiponectin has already been shown to have numerous beneficial effects on the endothelium. It stimulates endothelial cell proliferation and inhibits endothelial cell apoptosis (i.e., programmed cell death), both important in attenuating the progression of arterial disease.[205,206] Repair of damaged endothelium involves the recruitment and differentiation of circulating EPC. Shibata and coauthors[207] showed that adiponectin influences the degree to which EPC are used: adiponectin knockout mice show attenuated activity of EPC, whereas adenovirus-mediated adiponectin overexpression restored the activity level of EPC. In addition, adiponectin has been shown to be a chemoattractant for EPC to the endothelium and induces EPC to differentiate. NO, which exhibits numerous vasoprotective properties, has also been shown to be regulated in part by adiponectin. Adiponectin modulates the production of NO by upregulating the phosphorylation, and thus activation, of eNOS.[205,208,209] Thus, adiponectin has been shown to be a protector of the vascular endothelium: it increases endothelial cell proliferation and migration, increases the activation and chemotaxis of EPC, and increases the local concentration of NO.

Further supporting the vasoprotective role of adiponectin, Takaoka and coworkers[210] recently demonstrated that adiponectin produced by periadventitial adipose tissue, and not systemic adiponectin, is an important regulator of neointimal hyperplasia. First, the ability of periadventitial adipose tissue to inhibit neointima formation was established. Wild type mice underwent femoral artery injury after removal of the periadventitial adipose tissue. Neointimal hyperplasia was markedly increased in the wild type mice after adipose removal. This was attenuated if subcutaneous adipose tissue was transplanted back to the adventitia of the injured artery. This demonstrates that local adipose tissue inhibits neointimal hyperplasia. Second, Takaoka and coauthors demonstrated that this protective effect was, in fact, caused by locally produced adiponectin. They did so by studying neointimal hyperplasia in the setting of adiponectin knockout mice. At 4 weeks after femoral artery injury, wild type mice showed significantly less neointimal hyperplasia development than the adiponectin knockout mice. Perivascular application of an adiponectin donor (i.e., adiponectin gel) caused a significant reduction in neointimal hyperplasia development compared with adiponectin delivered subcutaneously and in adiponectin knockout mice. Together, these data demonstrate the important role of adiponectin in limiting the formation of neointimal hyperplasia after arterial injury.

In a subsequent study, Takaoka and colleagues[211] demonstrated a 66% decrease in adiponectin expression in periadventitial adipose tissue 24 hours after balloon injury of rat iliac arteries ($p < 0.05$). This was accompanied by an increase in proinflammatory adipocytokines: a twofold increase in TNF-α, a twofold increase in MCP-1, and a tenfold increase in IL-6 ($p < 0.05$). TNF-α appeared to be the driving force behind the subsequent increases in MCP-1 and IL-6 because these increases were attenuated in TNF-α knockout mice. Further investigation demonstrated that TNF-α acted on adiponectin levels through MCP-1 because postinjury decreases in adiponectin were attenuated in MCP-1 knockout mice. Immunofluorescent staining revealed that the ultimate source of postinjury TNF-α was from infiltrating periadventitial macrophages, with a minority of TNF-α deriving from the adipocytes themselves. Neointimal hyperplasia development was reduced in TNF-α knockout mice. Neointimal severity was then restored by supplying the TNF-α knockout mice with a periadventitial infusion of TNF-α, elegantly confirming the importance of TNF-α to neointimal growth. Thus, regulation of the arterial injury response extends into the periadventitial tissue, creating a pro-inflammatory milieu that promotes the growth of the neointima.

Vasa Vasorum

The vasa vasorum consists of a network of microvascular channels that supply oxygen and nutrients to the vessel wall. These conduits consist of a lumen lined by endothelial cells surrounded by smooth muscle cells. This architecture allows its caliber to be modified by vasodilatory compounds. In addition to delivering nutrients, the vasa vasorum can act as a port of entry for different circulating cell types into the adventitia. Monocytes, progenitor cells, and cytokines can take advantage of the branching vasa vasorum to enter the adventitia and participate in the reaction caused by arterial injury.

Studies have shown that arterial injury alters the adventitial density of the vasa vasorum. Kwon and coauthors[212] were one of the first to describe the neovascularization that occurs in the adventitia after balloon angioplasty. To induce arterial injury and neointima formation, they used a porcine model of coronary artery balloon angioplasty. After 28 days, the animals were sacrificed and the arteries were perfused with a radiopaque liquid polymer, MV-122. Microscopic three-dimensional computed tomography reconstruction was then used to image the arteries. The authors found that the density of the vasa vasorum per square millimeter was increased 66% in the vessel wall of injured arteries versus in uninjured controls ($p < 0.01$), but the overall percentage of vessel wall composed of vasa vasorum decreased 30% after injury ($p = 0.018$). There was a strong, direct relationship between the number of vasa vasorum and intimal thickness, but it was unclear from this study whether increased vasa vasorum number was a cause or effect of the thickness of the neointima. A well-developed vasa vasorum network present soon after injury could promote neointimal growth by serving as a better route through which monocytes and other inflammatory cells invade the vascular wall. However, an increase in vasa vasorum density after injury could reduce adventitial hypoxia, a potent inducer of neointimal hyperplasia. Supporting the latter is a study by Mayr and associates[127] of vein graft intimal hyperplasia in iNOS knockout versus wild type mice. Although they found that iNOS knockout mice

developed greater vein graft intimal hyperplasia, they also noted that the iNOS knockout mice exhibited a lower density of vasa vasorum, as indicated by CD31 staining, in the adventitia compared with the wild type mice. Thus, from these data it appears that injury increases vasa vasorum arborization in the vessel wall, but the effect this has on neointimal hyperplasia is less clear because density may be more important than absolute number.

The transcription factor nuclear factor-κB is known to be important to the development of neointimal hyperplasia early after arterial injury because inhibition of NF-κB attenuates neointimal growth.[213-217] A recent study by Damrauer and colleagues[218] sought to identify the role of NF-κB in vasa vasorum neovascularization after arterial injury. Irradiated rats underwent bone marrow transplant with cells ubiquitously expressing green fluorescent protein (GFP). Neointimal hyperplasia was then induced by performing balloon injury of the common carotid artery, after which the rats were transfected with A20, a compound known to inhibit NF-κB. There was a significant reduction in CD31 expression, an endothelial cell marker, in arteries transfected with A20 versus arteries transfected with an empty vector. The endothelial cells present in the adventitia sometimes expressed GFP, indicating that some were derived from the bone marrow. Importantly, although the presence of endothelial cells was reduced in the adventitia, the rate of re-endothelialization of the vessel lumen, necessary for arterial recovery from injury, actually accelerated. The endothelial cells repopulating the endothelium were GFP negative, indicating that they did not originate in the bone marrow. The authors were able to conclude that inhibition of NF-κB affected the layers of the vessel wall differently, with the adventitia exhibiting a marked reduction in neovascularity and the endothelium exhibiting an increase in the rate of re-endothelialization. This may be explained in part by an inability of the adventitia to recruit circulating endothelial cell precursors, which may serve as the building blocks for vasa vasorum angiogenesis.

A study by Misra and coworkers[219] investigated the influence of hypoxia on murine adventitial fibroblasts in vitro. Mouse fibroblasts were grown under hypoxic conditions (3% O_2) or normoxic conditions (20% O_2) for 24, 48, and 72 hours. They found that hypoxic conditions cause acceleration in fibroblast differentiation into myofibroblasts as evidenced by an increase in the expression of αSMA, a myofibroblast marker. Cell lysates were then collected and the proteins concentrated by immunoprecipitation. Western blot analysis was then performed to assess the level of expression for hypoxia-induced factor 1α (HIF-1α) and matrix metalloproteinase 2 (MMP-2). HIF-1α is a transcription factor upregulated under hypoxic conditions and affects the expression of many genes. One such gene is for MMP-2, an enzyme that degrades the extracellular matrix and eases the migration of myofibroblasts from the adventitia to the media. Misra and coworkers showed that hypoxia leads to an increase in HIF-1α and MMP-2 at 24, 48, and 72 hours. They concluded that hypoxia acts as a driving force behind neointimal growth by stimulating fibroblast differentiation, increasing HIF-1α levels, and increasing expression of MMP-2. This study implies that adventitial hypoxia is optimal for neointimal growth.

CONCLUSION

It is apparent that the arterial injury response represents a complex interplay of events that culminates in the formation of neointimal hyperplasia. It can no longer be viewed as a simple proliferative response of the medial VSMC to the intima under the stimulation of growth factors and cytokines released from platelets and leukocytes. Instead, all three layers of the arterial wall are involved, with the adventitia playing a much more important role than was appreciated originally, given that the adventita is the portal of entry for many cells through the vasa vasorum, contains adiponectin, and prominently expresses NOX4. The cell types involved in the arterial injury response include both resident and circulating cells, and these include platelets, leukocytes, endothelial cells, VSMC, adventitial fibroblasts, as well as stem and progenitor cells. Finally, reactive oxygen species have also been shown to play a prominent role. By gaining a better understanding of the pathophysiology of neointimal hyperplasia, targeted therapies can be developed to prevent restenosis after vascular interventions.

References available online at expertconsult.com.

QUESTIONS

1. The origin of the proliferating cells found in neointimal hyperplastic lesions includes all of the following except:
   a. Adventitial fibroblasts
   b. Macrophages
   c. Progenitor cells
   d. Vascular smooth muscle cells
   e. All of the above

2. Which hemodynamic force has been implicated as a contributing factor in the development of intimal hyperplasia?
   a. Vessel wall compliance
   b. High shear stress
   c. Flow velocity
   d. Low shear stress
   e. All of the above

3. Which surface membrane receptor regulates vascular smooth muscle cells' accumulation of low-density lipoprotein (LDL)?
   a. Glycoprotein receptor Ib
   b. High-affinity LDL receptor
   c. Glycoprotein receptor IIb/IIIa
   d. Low-affinity LDL receptor
   e. High-affinity high-density lipoprotein receptor

4. Platelet aggregation is stimulated by which of the following?
   a. Adenosine triphosphate
   b. Platelet-derived growth factor
   c. Adenosine diphosphate
   d. Low-density lipoprotein
   e. Prostacyclin

5. Angiotensin-converting enzyme is located primarily on the membrane surface of which of the following?
   a. Platelets
   b. Neutrophils
   c. Fibroblasts
   d. Vascular endothelial cells
   e. Macrophages

6. Nitric oxide is constitutively expressed in the vasculature in which cell type?
   a. Platelets
   b. Neutrophils
   c. Endothelial cells
   d. Vascular smooth muscle cells
   e. Adventitial fibroblasts

7. Which of the following NOX enzymes directly produces hydrogen peroxide?
   a. NOX1
   b. NOX2
   c. NOX3
   d. NOX4
   e. NOX5

8. Which of the following has been shown to be a resident progenitor cell in the arterial wall, just external to the external elastic lamina?
   a. Pericytes
   b. Sca1+ cells
   c. flk+ cells
   d. CD34+ cells
   e. CD31+ cells

9. In the vasculature, adinonectin stimulates:
   a. Platelet aggregation
   b. Leukocyte chemotaxis
   c. Endothelial cell proliferation
   d. Vascular smooth muscle cell proliferation
   e. Adventitial fibroblast proliferation

10. Arterial injury has been shown to alter which characteristic of the vasa vasorum?
   a. Absolute number of vasa vasorum
   b. Density of the vasa vasorum
   c. Percentage of the vessel wall consisting of the vasa vasorum
   d. a and b
   e. a, b, and c

ANSWERS

1. **e**
2. **e**
3. **b**
4. **c**
5. **d**
6. **c**
7. **d**
8. **b**
9. **c**
10. **e**

CHAPTER 56

PROSTHETIC GRAFT INFECTION

Christopher J. Abularrage • Niren Angle • Julie Ann Freischlag

The development of prosthetic biomaterial devices has made it possible to treat conditions that otherwise would have resulted in significant morbidity and mortality. Examples of such clinical conditions include but are not limited to aortic aneurysms, hemodialysis access in patients in whom autologous fistulas are not possible, and infrainguinal bypass for limb ischemia. The advent of the use of prosthetic conduits has also resulted in the problem of prosthetic graft infection. The morbidity associated with infected prosthetic vascular grafts is considerable and can be catastrophic, resulting in limb loss, sepsis, and possibly death. This chapter examines the cause, diagnosis, and management of prosthetic graft infection.

INCIDENCE

Prosthetic graft infection is relatively uncommon, with a reported incidence ranging from 0.2% to 5%. There are few prospectively obtained data analyzing the true incidence of prosthetic graft infection, but a survey of retrospective data with extended follow-up suggests that graft infections are influenced by the implant site, the indications for operation, and the host's defense status, as manifested by the patient's comorbid disease. A prospective, multicenter Canadian study of repair of unruptured abdominal aortic aneurysms revealed a graft infection rate of 0.2%.[1] Szilagyi and colleagues' analysis of 2145 patients undergoing a variety of vascular reconstructions, including aortofemoral, aortoiliac, and femoropopliteal reconstructions, revealed an overall graft infection rate of 1.5%.[2] The insertion of a prosthetic graft in the femoropopliteal or femorotibial position has a higher rate of infection, ranging up to 5% in some reports.

The last decade has seen a sharp rise in the number of aortic aneurysms treated with endovascular grafts, and although it is relatively early, reports of endovascular prosthesis infection are already available. Although access for implanting these devices and other intravascular grafts is less invasive, it appears that the incidence of aortic endograft infection may be around 1%.

An emergency operation (e.g., for a ruptured abdominal aortic aneurysm) carries a higher rate of infection than does an elective operation. The consequences of an infected prosthesis are also different, depending on the location of the graft. The mortality rate is higher with an infected aortic prosthesis, and the risk of limb loss is highest with lower extremity graft infection. A graft infection can manifest months to years after implantation, and this insidious presentation may provide clues to the biology of graft infection.

MICROBIOLOGY

Insight into the cause of vascular graft infections can be gained by examining the microorganisms most commonly recovered from infected grafts. Although any microorganism can potentially cause a graft infection, Staphylococcus aureus is the most prevalent bacterium.[3] S. aureus is responsible for 25% to 50% of vascular graft infections, based on anatomic location. Over the last 15 to 20 years, Staphylococcus epidermidis has increasingly been identified as the responsible pathogen for a significant proportion of graft infections, predominantly the late-appearing, indolent type.

Graft infections are labeled as early (occurring less than 4 months after implantation) or late (occurring more than 4 months after implantation). Early-appearing graft infections are most commonly caused by more virulent organisms, including S. aureus. Coagulase-positive strains elaborate toxins that result in a vigorous host inflammatory response. Late-appearing graft infections are caused by less virulent gram-positive bacteria such as S. epidermidis. This organism is indolent and normally harbored in natural skin. It has the ability to adhere to prosthetic material and to secrete a glycocalyx biofilm that insulates the bacterium. Over time, this biofilm induces an inflammatory response that results in perigraft inflammation, which is seen clinically as perigraft fluid. This organism is fastidious in its attachment and is not easily isolated. S. epidermidis graft infections appear to have a sterile exudate, resulting in poor graft incorporation. Rarely do patients have a leukocytosis. This innocuous presentation has led many to view S. epidermidis infections as inflammatory allergic responses rather than bacterial graft infections.[4] Bergamini and colleagues[5] demonstrated that ultrasonication is required to physically separate S. epidermidis from the graft surface in order to culture it. In addition, broth culture yielded a higher rate of recovery than did agar plating. Bacterial recovery, which was only 30% when plated on agar media, rose to 72% in broth media. The combination of ultrasonication and broth culture resulted in a positive culture in 83% of cases in this report.

Other microorganisms such as fungi and gram-negative bacteria can also result in graft infections. Gram-negative bacteria such as Pseudomonas species, Escherichia coli, Enterobacter species, and Proteus species are highly virulent and result in dramatic clinical manifestations, such as anastomotic disruption and frank hemorrhage.[6] These organisms are able to secrete potent proteases, which account for the tissue disruption that results in artery-graft disruption. Gram-negative infections also induce a substantial host inflammatory response that contributes to the disruption. *Pseudomonas* species infection is most commonly associated with graft disruption and hemorrhage. Severely immunosuppressed patients are also vulnerable to fungal graft infections, an otherwise rare clinical entity in the general population.

CAUSE AND PATHOPHYSIOLOGY

The fundamental question in regard to the cause of prosthetic graft infections is: when does exposure to the infection-causing microorganisms occur? The three major potential mechanisms that can result in prosthetic graft colonization and subsequent infection are the following:

1. Intraoperative contamination
2. Hematogenous spread of bacteria
3. Direct contamination of graft by infection emanating from the skin, soft tissue, gastrointestinal tract, or genitourinary tract

Although all these factors can result in a graft infection, the last mechanism listed is the least common.

Intraoperative Contamination

The host is the most significant source of bacterial contamination resulting in surgical site infection. The resident microflora, usually referred to as the *indigenous microflora*, consists of a complex mixture of microbial species ranging from nonpathogenic saprophytes to pathogens. Endogenous bacteria are a more important source of surgical site infection than exogenous bacteria.

The patient's endogenous flora from a site close to the prosthetic bed—especially from a colonized site, such as the skin or gut—is a common source of graft infection. Most of the intertriginous areas of the body, such as the axillae, groin, and interdigital spaces of the foot, contain large numbers of eccrine sweat glands and harbor large bacterial populations.[7] Thus, prosthetic grafts placed in the groin have a well-characterized propensity to develop *S. aureus* infection. *S. aureus* bacteria from the groin area may contaminate only the wound, or they may also contaminate the graft surface if it is inadvertently dragged across the skin. The lymphatics in the groin may be contaminated at the time of surgery, especially if the patient has an open infected wound in an extremity. These lymphatics can also be a source of intraoperative graft infection. It is exceedingly rare for bacterial contamination to originate from the surgical team, from the graft, or from surgical instruments. The surgeon's hands are seldom a major source of wound contamination.[8]

Bacteria can be present in diseased vessels or in the thrombus lining an aortic aneurysm.[9] Van der Vliet and colleagues[10] cultured the contents of the aneurysms of 216 patients and then followed the patients for more than 3 years. Positive cultures were found in 55 patients (25.5%); however, only 4 graft infections occurred (1.9%). Three of these four patients had positive cultures, but only two patients had the same organism as the original cultures. The authors concluded that bacteria in aneurysm contents have no demonstrable link to subsequent graft infections. A prospective study demonstrated that in patients undergoing peripheral vascular bypass surgery, 41% had positive arterial tissue cultures, 68% of which were coagulase-negative Staphylococcus.[11] Subsequent graft infections were not reported; therefore the significance of the cultures is intriguing but unclear.

Hematogenous Spread

Seeding of an indwelling prosthesis by hematogenous spread of bacteria is potentially important; the frequency with which this occurs is unknown. In experimental animals, infusion of 10 million organisms of *S. aureus* immediately after implantation of a prosthetic aortic graft resulted in a 100% incidence of graft infection.[12,13] Later studies demonstrated a lower incidence of graft infection with a longer time after implantation, suggesting that graft incorporation and the development of a pseudointima may provide some protection.[14,15] Vulnerability to infection from bacteremia has been documented as late as 1 year after implantation, with 30% of aortic grafts becoming infected after a single bacterial infusion at that time.[11] The anatomic difference between the infected and noninfected grafts was the presence of a complete neointimal lining. Parenteral antibiotics significantly reduced the incidence of graft infection, particularly when culture-directed therapy was applied to a remote infection. The significance of remote infection is unclear, but it suggests that transient bacteremia associated with, for example, dental procedures or colonoscopy may account for very late infections.

Direct Contamination

This category is the most easily diagnosed and the least common. The development of an intraabdominal abscess from a variety of clinical conditions can directly infect a recently placed aortic graft. Similarly, failure of the skin incision to heal after an operation places the underlying graft at significant risk of bacterial contamination and subsequent infection. For these reasons, it is prudent to avoid any operation on the gastrointestinal tract at the time of insertion of an aortic prosthetic graft. The exception to this is the performance of a cholecystectomy, but this too is done only after the graft is inserted and the retroperitoneum is closed over the graft.

PREVENTION

The best way to avoid graft infection is to prevent it in the operating room and during the postoperative period. It has been shown that patients who are hospitalized for any length of time have an alteration in their cutaneous microflora.[16] It is unclear whether this is caused by the underlying illness or by antibiotics. The preoperative stay, if any, should be as short as possible to avoid colonization with resistant bacteria. Prophylactic antibiotics have been shown to decrease the incidence of wound infections that could lead to graft infections. Most authors recommend the administration of a first-generation cephalosporin approximately 30 to 60 minutes before incision, with a scheduled dose continued for the first 24 hours. If the operation lasts an extended length of time, additional doses should be administered to maintain adequate circulating levels. There is no evidence to support the continuation of prophylactic antibiotics until indwelling lines, such as central venous or urinary bladder catheters, are removed. The prolonged use of postoperative antibiotics may even be detrimental, because the patient can develop antibiotic-associated colitis or other resistant-organism infections.

Meticulous surgical technique is important in preventing wound and graft infections. The graft must be handled carefully and should not be allowed to contact the patient's skin. Adhesive drapes are commonly used to aid in preventing such contact, although there are no studies demonstrating a reduced incidence of wound or graft infection with the use of adhesive drapes, with or without iodine impregnation. If the adhesive plastic drape is separated from the skin during the operation, however, the infection rate increases.[17,18] Simultaneous gastrointestinal procedures should be avoided to prevent intraoperative contamination. If an unplanned enterotomy occurs, graft implantation should be postponed, if possible. Dead space in surgical wounds should be minimized with the least possible amount of suture material. Irrigation of the peritoneal cavity is routine, but it can lead to washout of macrophages and opsonins. Irrigation should be used to remove all blood from the peritoneal cavity, because blood acts as an adjuvant for bacterial proliferation. If irrigation of a wound is performed, every effort should be made to evacuate the fluid.

In an effort to decrease the rates of graft and wound infections, certain authors have soaked gelatin-impregnated grafts with rifampin.[19,20] This technique was associated with a decrease in the risk of groin wound infection, but showed no benefit in the rates of subsequent graft infection. Therefore, preoperative soaking of grafts in rifampin or other antibiotics is not indicated as a primary preventative measure.

DIAGNOSIS

Graft infections can result in limb loss, systemic sepsis, and sometimes death, even in the setting of correct diagnosis and treatment. In modern reports, the mortality from aortic graft infections still ranges from 20% to 30% in experienced hands. For these reasons, prompt diagnosis is essential to avoid or minimize complications. Accurate diagnosis requires that the surgeon be aware of the subtle manifestations of graft infection. Every attempt should be made to confirm or exclude the diagnosis, either by imaging or by operative exploration. The consequences of a missed diagnosis in this setting can be catastrophic.

Clinical Presentation

The clinical presentation of graft infection can be subtle and is influenced by the anatomic location of the graft. An infection of an infrainguinal graft frequently appears as cellulitis, soft tissue infection, drainage tract, or pseudoaneurysm. The clinical presentation of an extracavitary graft infection is usually not subtle. An intraabdominal graft infection may appear as systemic sepsis or as an ileus or abdominal distension, with or without tenderness. Occasionally, an aortic graft infection can result in an aortoenteric fistula, the first sign of which is a herald bleed. A patient with upper gastrointestinal bleeding and an aortic graft must be presumed to have an aortoenteric fistula until proved otherwise (Figure 56-1).

Early graft infections can manifest with fever, leukocytosis, and purulent drainage from the graft site. Splinter hemorrhages may be present distally. Blood cultures may be positive if taken in the distal arterial circulation downstream from the graft infection. A late graft infection, usually caused by an indolent organism such as

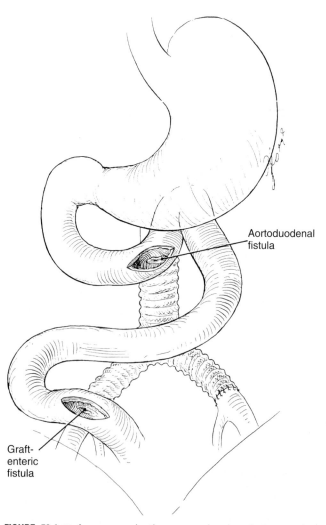

Aortoduodenal fistula

Graft-enteric fistula

FIGURE 56-1 ■ A communication may develop between the bowel lumen and the graft. Hemorrhage may be due to a direct communication between the aorta and the bowel (aortoenteric fistula) or from vessels in the bowel wall that have been eroded by the prosthetic graft (enteroparaprosthetic fistula).

S. epidermidis, appears as a healing complication such as a seroma, pseudoaneurysm, or late graft thrombosis with no anatomic reason. Systemic signs of illness, such as fever, are usually not present.

Laboratory Studies

A leukocytosis with a left shift and an elevated erythrocyte sedimentation rate often accompany graft infection, but their lack of specificity limits their usefulness. Late-appearing perigraft infections with *S. epidermidis* may have none of these laboratory abnormalities. The diagnosis of a prosthetic graft infection often depends on a preponderance of the evidence, not merely on one positive data point. An indolent infection commonly presents with a mild leukocytosis, without a significant left shift, and an elevated erythrocyte sedimentation rate. The diagnosis, however, depends more on imaging and the lack of any other explanation for the aforementioned findings.

Imaging

Imaging plays an important role in the diagnosis of prosthetic graft infection. The particular imaging modality used depends on the site being investigated and the information desired. Computed tomography (CT), angiography, ultrasonography, nuclear medicine, and magnetic resonance imaging (MRI) constitute the diagnostic armamentarium for the evaluation of potential graft infection.

Computed Tomography

CT scanning is probably the most sensitive and reliable imaging test for the diagnosis of graft infections. Perigraft fluid collections, perigraft gas, anastomotic aneurysms, and distortion of tissue planes are all findings suggestive of graft infection and are all well visualized by a contrast-enhanced CT scan (Figure 56-2). Presence of

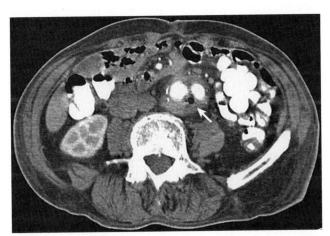

FIGURE 56-2 ■ Postoperative computed tomographic scan of a patient who underwent abdominal aortic aneurysm repair showing air within the aneurysm sac *(arrow),* consistent with graft infection. (From Abularrage CJ, Deaton DH: Vascular surgery. In Ho VB, Reddy GP, editors: Cardiovascular imaging, Philadelphia, 2011, Elsevier.)

gas or fluid around a graft more than 6 to 8 weeks after implantation is definitely abnormal and is presumptive evidence of graft infection.

O'Hara and coworkers published a study examining the natural history of periprosthetic air after abdominal aortic surgery.[21] Twenty-six consecutive patients undergoing elective aortic aneurysm repair had CT scans performed at 3, 7, and 52 days postoperatively. Perigraft air was seen in 65% of patients in the first week following operation. All patients with periprosthetic air had spontaneous resolution, as demonstrated by late CT scanning obtained a mean of 52 days postoperatively (range, 21 to 85 days).

CT-guided aspiration of perigraft fluid is advocated by some as a reliable test that offers a good yield and provides material for Gram stain and culture. However, CT-guided aspiration of perigraft fluid is rarely indicated; once it has been demonstrated that the graft has fluid around it after 6 to 8 weeks, the appropriate treatment is graft excision and reconstruction, with the rare exception of a patient too frail to undergo a major operation.

Ultrasonography

A duplex ultrasound scan is an excellent initial test for the identification of upper and lower extremity graft infections. It is not as accurate in identifying aortic pseudoaneurysms because of the difficulty of imaging owing to bowel gas. It is extremely useful and reliable for the interrogation of femoral and lower extremity sites. Perigraft fluid is easily diagnosed, as is an anastomotic pseudoaneurysm in an infrainguinal bypass; ultrasound scanning can also distinguish between the two. Ultrasonography is quick, portable, and noninvasive. The accuracy of the test depends on the technician's expertise, but in skilled hands, it is informative and reliable.

Magnetic Resonance Imaging

MRI is a useful modality for identifying perigraft fluid because of its ability to distinguish fluid from tissue by recognizing differences in signal intensity between T1- and T2-weighted images. The efficacy of this test was highlighted in a study by Olofsson and colleagues[22] in which 18 patients suspected of having an aortic graft infection underwent preoperative MRI. Twelve patients also underwent CT scanning. MRI successfully identified 14 of 16 patients who were found to have an aortic graft infection at the time of operation, whereas CT was accurate in only 5 of 12 patients. It has been shown that there is only mild enhancement on T2-weighted images in grafts undergoing normal incorporation, whereas infected perigraft tissue demonstrates increased signal intensity.[23] The role of MRI role in the diagnosis of aortic graft infections may become more prominent, but it is not routinely used for this purpose.

Angiography

Angiography delineates intraluminal and extraluminal blood flow, but is unable to assess for extraluminal gas or fluid collections. It is therefore not useful for identifying

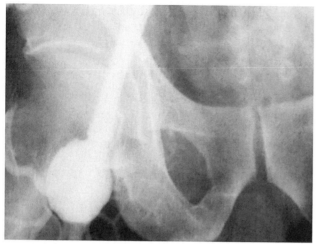

FIGURE 56-3 ■ Graft infection was first manifested by the development of a false aneurysm.

graft infections, and CT and MRI are considered the tests of choice. Angiography can identify graft pseudoaneurysms (Figure 56-3), but these results are not diagnostic per se. Arteriography is used in this context not for the diagnosis of prosthetic graft infection, but to determine the options for arterial reconstruction. It is important to be careful in terms of timing the arteriogram with the CT scan, because both involve a contrast load; this is a consideration in a patient with renal insufficiency.

White Blood Cell Scanning

^{67}Ga- or ^{111}In-labeled white blood cell scanning is highly sensitive for graft infection. An ^{111}In-labeled leukocyte or IgG scan is reliable and offers an advantage over ^{67}Ga scanning because there is minimum nonspecific bowel uptake, resulting in a high target-to-background ratio and better results.[24] ^{111}In-labeled leukocyte IgG scanning has been used by LaMuraglia and colleagues[25] with impressive results. In 10 patients with positive scans, graft infection was confirmed at operation at the same site. Of the 15 patients with negative scans, the only one who had a false-negative result was a patient with an aortoduodenal fistula. The advantage of IgG scanning is that preparation is easier because the patient's own blood is not required for the test and the tracer has a longer half-life.

Gastrointestinal Endoscopy

Endoscopy is a vital diagnostic tool in the evaluation of upper gastrointestinal tract bleeding.[26] A patient with an aortic prosthesis and upper gastrointestinal bleeding must be suspected of having an aortoenteric fistula until proved otherwise. The initial test for this diagnosis is upper gastrointestinal endoscopy, which should be performed expeditiously once the diagnosis of aortoenteric fistula has been considered. The examination must be performed cautiously. The finding of an adherent blood clot in the duodenum confirms the diagnosis, and the patient should be taken immediately to the operating

room. If endoscopy does not reveal any pathology, such as bleeding varices, gastritis, or a stomach or duodenal ulcer, an aortoenteric fistula may still be present but not seen. There are some who prefer to examine only the first and second portions of the duodenum; if this part of the study is negative, a presumptive diagnosis of aortoenteric fistula is made. Others prefer to use a smaller endoscope and actually examine the third and possibly the fourth portions of the duodenum; however, this requires endoscopic expertise and a low threshold for operative exploration should the study be equivocal.

MANAGEMENT OF GRAFT INFECTION: GENERAL PRINCIPLES

Preoperative Preparation

A patient with ongoing hemorrhage, a patient in hemorrhagic shock from an anastomotic rupture, or a patient with an aortoenteric fistula is managed according to the standard principles of resuscitation. In these categories of patients, there is not much time for preoperative planning, diagnosis, or adjuvant therapy.

Fortunately, most patients with graft infections do not appear emergently, and adequate time is available for diagnostic tests and optimization of conditions for a potentially extensive operation. The patient and family must understand that treatment may involve a very demanding operation, both physiologically and psychologically. The patient's cardiac and pulmonary status must be evaluated and optimized. Hemodynamic volume status must be optimized. Antibiotic coverage must be initiated to contain the graft infection and prevent progression to sepsis or septic shock. Routine total parenteral nutrition should not be used preoperatively in these patients. In a prospective, randomized trial, the only patients who benefited from preoperative total parenteral nutrition were those who were severely malnourished, as evaluated by the Subjective Global Assessment.[27] Glycemic control is essential, because hyperglycemia causes suppression of neutrophil function; this is one of the factors that predisposes a diabetic patient to infectious complications. Appropriate imaging studies are performed to evaluate possible options for extraanatomic revascularization or for autogenous in situ reconstruction; these can include CT scan, MRI, and angiography.

Antibiotic Therapy

Preoperative administration of culture-specific antibiotics is ideal. If the infecting organism is not known, broad-spectrum antibiotics, in doses adequate to reach minimal inhibitory concentration, are administered. Some authorities advocate irrigation of tissues with topical antibiotic solution, although its usefulness is questionable.[28] Subsequent therapy with antibiotics should be tailored to culture results. The appropriate duration of antibiotic therapy is unclear. One group advocated at least a 2-week duration of systemic antibiotic therapy.[29] Patients treated with at least 6 weeks of parenteral antibiotics had significantly better outcomes than those treated for 2 weeks or less.

More recently, antibiotic loaded beads have been used in conjunction with serial irrigation and debridement in an effort to sterilize groin wounds and preserve infected lower extremity grafts.[30] The beads are left in place or changed during debridement until the intraoperative wound cultures have no bacterial growth, at which time soft tissue or muscle flap coverage is obtained. Graft preservation was only attempted in those wounds with early graft infections and nonresistant gram-positive species, a group that represented 18% of their patient population. After an average of 2.5 antibiotic bead replacements, sterile wounds were achieved in 90% with a 2-year recurrent graft infection and mortality rate of 10%.[31]

Revascularization

Removal of an infected graft usually mandates some revascularization procedure. Reilly and colleagues and Trout and associates[32] conclusively showed that a staged operation, with initial revascularization followed by graft excision in 1 to 2 days, is associated with significantly less morbidity and mortality. The overall mortality rate was 53% (40 of 75) if graft excision preceded extraanatomic bypass and 17% (5 of 29) if bypass preceded graft excision. The physiologic stress on the patient is probably decreased with a staged approach, and performing the revascularization before the graft excision obviates the need for systemic heparinization, possibly enabling more radical debridement. Throughout this period, systemic antibiotic therapy is continued.

The ideal conduit is autogenous vein or endarterectomy-treated artery, because they obviate the need for extraanatomic bypass. If a prosthetic conduit is chosen for an extraanatomic bypass, polytetrafluoroethylene (PTFE) is preferable to Dacron. Experimental evidence indicates that PTFE is more resistant to bacterial colonization than are other prosthetic conduits[33]; this was validated in a clinical retrospective analysis that discovered a lower infection rate for PTFE compared with Dacron.[34] Towne and coworkers[35] suggested that aortic grafts infected with the low-virulence S. epidermidis may, under strict selection criteria, be safely treated with an in situ PTFE prosthetic graft. Over a 9-year period, 28 patients were treated with in situ PTFE grafts for aortoiliofemoral graft infections with S. epidermidis. At a mean follow-up of 4.5 years, there was no mortality, and all grafts remained patent. Two patients had recurrent infection in the proximal limb of the old graft. These data suggest that in carefully selected patients, in situ replacement with PTFE may be safe and effective.

Graft Excision

A general principle is that if a suture line is involved in the infectious process, this is an absolute indication for removal of the entire infected graft. Any equivocation on the issue of an infected anastomosis inevitably leads to eventual rupture and hemorrhage. Many authorities have advocated conservative treatment consisting of drainage, debridement, and systemic and local antibiotic coverage for the management of perigraft infection, usually limited to inguinal and infrainguinal graft infections. Calligaro and colleagues[35] have been the leading proponents of graft preservation and have been successful in more than 70% of cases. Towne and associates[36] reported on their treatment of 20 infected grafts, 14 of which were aortofemoral grafts. In the 14 aortofemoral grafts, only the femoral limbs were excised; the proximal incorporated segment was left in situ. An interposition PTFE graft was used to replace the explanted segment. Subsequent graft ultrasonication revealed that 17 of 20 grafts grew S. epidermidis, one grew coagulase-positive Staphylococcus species, and two grafts grew both. All the surgical incisions healed, and graft patency was 100%. There was no limb loss. The authors concluded that biofilm graft infections can be safely treated with in situ replacements. This group recently reported its experience with aortic graft infections, comparing the treatment of 30 consecutive patients. The mean interval from implantation to manifestation of infection was 5.5 years. Complete graft excision with bypass in clean, uninfected planes was performed in 15 patients, and partial or complete graft salvage or in situ graft replacement was performed in 15 patients. The investigators found that perioperative and long-term mortality was no different between the two groups. However, this study is limited by the fact that the sample size was small, raising the possibility of a type II error; also, because it was a retrospective analysis, randomization of the patients did not occur. The authors concluded that in selected patients, local resection of infected graft segments is an acceptable option.

Patients must be carefully selected for attempted graft preservation. The graft anastomosis cannot be involved with infection, and the patient should not demonstrate any systemic signs of sepsis. Tissue coverage of the debrided area can be achieved with a rotational flap or a free flap.[37] Seify and colleagues[38] examined 22 patients who underwent a total of 26 muscle flaps for infected prosthetic graft salvage. Poor prognostic indicators of graft preservation included exposure of the arterial anastomosis, infection occurring more than 1 month postoperatively, methicillin resistant bacteria, and Pseudomonas species infection. The risk of hemorrhage from anastomotic rupture is significantly higher with these infections. The optimal treatment for an infected graft in the presence of these poor indicators remains excision of the entire infected graft, with reconstruction through uninfected tissue planes, preferably with autogenous tissue.

More recently, vacuum-assisted closure (VAC) therapy without muscle flap coverage has been advocated in early (<30 days) for the treatment of vascular groin infections. One study examined 14 Szilagyi II and 12 Szilagyi III infections and found no difference between the two groups.[39] Furthermore, there was no difference in the outcomes between those with and without exposed grafts. Two groins in the Szilagyi III group had treatment failures, including one bleed from the anastomotic heel and one reinfection 117 days after the debridement. They concluded that aggressive operative debridement with VAC therapy results in minimal morbidity, limb preservation, and excellent survival.

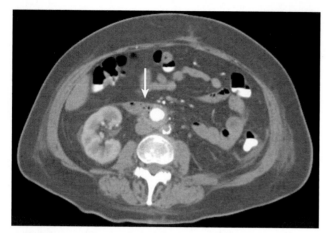

FIGURE 56-4 ■ Aortoenteric fistula *(arrow)* resulting from erosion of the proximal anastomosis into the duodenum.

Aortoenteric fistulas, particularly aortoduodenal fistulas, require complete excision of the graft and closure of the duodenal wall defect (Figure 56-4). There is no role for in situ replacement of the graft in the treatment of patients with this entity. Although less extensive procedures have been attempted, the data clearly show that complete graft excision and, if necessary, placement of an extraanatomic bypass is clearly superior. Less extensive procedures are associated with a higher rate of fistula recurrence and death. The graft must be completely excised and the defect in the duodenum is oversewn. Given that the best treatment consists of graft excision, closure of the enteric defect, and extraanatomic bypass, the sequence of these procedures becomes important. In an actively bleeding patient or one in whom the diagnosis has been made at celiotomy, graft excision must precede extraanatomic bypass. It is often difficult to determine whether a patient needs a remote bypass in such a setting; therefore the safest approach is to perform immediate revascularization in the majority of cases.

Debridement

Blowout and late hemorrhage from the proximal aortic stump may occur in some patients after successful excision of the graft. This is most likely due to residual infection in the bed of the graft in the perigraft and para-aortic tissues. The debridement must be generous enough to ensure eradication of all infected tissue. The aorta must then be oversewn in two layers, if possible, with polypropylene sutures. If the infecting organism is of low virulence, removal of the graft is usually all that is necessary. With a more virulent organism, aggressive debridement is a must.

TREATMENT OF SPECIFIC GRAFT SITE INFECTIONS

Aortic Grafts

When one is faced with an aortic graft infection, a few fundamental points must be addressed. One has to

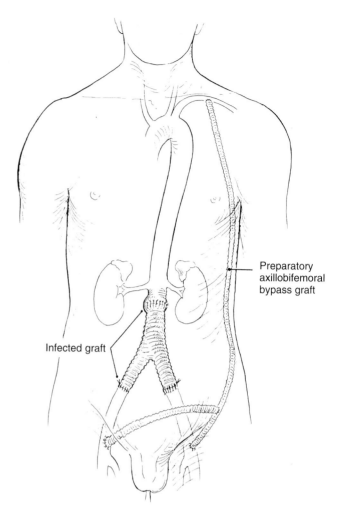

FIGURE 56-5 ■ Before removing an infected intraabdominal prosthetic graft, perfusion of the lower extremities is established by an axillobifemoral bypass graft. This technique provides uninterrupted perfusion of the lower limbs and reduces the morbidity associated with ischemic changes that occur when reconstitution of flow is delayed until after the aortic graft has been removed.

determine whether the aortic graft was performed for aneurysmal or occlusive disease. If the graft was placed for aneurysmal disease, it will be an end-to-end anastomosis; if the graft was placed for occlusive disease, the configuration of the anastomosis may be end-to-end or end-to-side. The distal implantation site has to be addressed as well: if the graft goes down to the femoral vessels, revascularization is a bit more involved than if the distal anastomosis is to the iliac arteries.

Aortoiliac and Aortic Interposition Grafts

Aortoiliac graft infections can be treated by preliminary axillobifemoral bypass through uninfected tissue planes, followed by aortic graft excision (Figure 56-5). This staged approach is associated with significantly less morbidity than the traditional mode of treatment and is currently considered the gold standard therapy. The distal anastomoses can be constructed at both common femoral arteries, because the distal limbs of the aortic graft are confined to the abdomen. This operation can be followed immediately by graft excision; alternatively, graft excision can be performed 1 to 2 days later.

For aortic graft excision, celiotomy is performed, and the aortic graft is isolated. Although systemic heparin is indicated for the axillofemoral bypass, the advantage of the staged operation is that no anticoagulation is necessary during the aortic graft excision. If the procedures are done consecutively, the heparin should be reversed before the aortic graft is approached. Careful dissection in the abdomen is performed, and the graft is separated from adherent bowel and viscera. Once the entire graft is exposed, proximal control is obtained at the supraceliac aorta, particularly if there is a proximal anastomotic aneurysm. The iliac arteries distal to the anastomoses are similarly isolated, and control is obtained. The entire graft is then excised, and the aorta is debrided back to normal, healthy-appearing tissue. The aortic stump is then closed with locking monofilament sutures. The distal aorta and iliac arteries are similarly closed. Perigraft tissue that may be infected is carefully but completely debrided. Closed suction drains may be placed. Care is taken to avoid injury to the ureters, and placement of ureteral stents is often indicated. If debridement is necessary above the renal arteries, it should be performed without compromise. The renal arteries are then revascularized by antegrade bypasses from one or two of the branches of the celiac axis, such as the hepatic or splenic arteries. Perfusion of the pelvic circulation is maintained by retrograde flow from the axillofemoral bypass through the external and internal iliac arteries. If the distal anastomoses are to the external iliac arteries and require excision, perfusion to at least one internal iliac artery should be maintained by means of a bypass.

An alternative method of revascularization has been advocated and popularized by Clagett—namely, complete autogenous reconstruction with superficial femoral vein as the conduit.[40] The superficial femoral vein is a large-caliber vein that can be used to reconstruct the aortoiliac or aortofemoral system in a variety of configurations. The advantage of this approach is that the reconstruction is completely autogenous, thereby avoiding the need for extraanatomic bypass and its poor long-term patency rate. There is a finite complication rate, and the most troublesome complication is compartment syndrome. Approximately one in four patients will need fasciotomy. However, this operation is an excellent option for reconstruction of the infected aortoiliac or particularly aortofemoral prosthesis.

Another autogenous conduit is cryopreserved arterial homografts. In one of the largest studies examining 57 in situ revascularizations of the abdominal aorta using cryopreserved arterial homografts, 30-day mortality was found to be 9% with the majority of deaths caused by sepsis-related multi-organ system failure.[41] The 3-year freedom from revascularization and postoperative survival were 89% and 81%, respectively. The authors concluded that the cryopreserved arterial homografts decreased the risk of recurrent infection, early thrombosis, late graft failure, and amputation compared to extraanatomic bypass with prosthetic conduits. Cryopreserved arterial homografts are prone to long-term degeneration

because of an immune response or imperfections in the cryopreservation methods, and continued surveillance for anastomotic breakdown is necessary. Postoperative immunosuppression following implantation of cryopreserved arterial homografts may decrease the risk of degeneration; however, the risks of immunosuppression in the setting of infection must be weighed in this clinical scenario.

In-line, rifampin-soaked prosthetic grafts with omental coverage and antibiotic suppression have been advocated by the group from the Mayo Clinic for the treatment of aortic graft infection.[42] In patients treated for aortoenteric fistulae, graft reinfection occurred in 4% of patients with a 1- and 5-year survival of 85% and 59%, respectively. All deaths in the follow-up period were not graft related. These results are exceptional considering the severe illness of this specific group of patients.

A prospective, randomized trial in the United Kingdom attempted to define the role of the rifampin-bonded prosthesis in extraanatomic bypass grafts by studying whether they resulted in a decreased risk of graft infection compared with controls.[43] Two hundred fifty-seven patients were randomized at 14 vascular centers to either rifampin-bonded grafts or regular collagen-impregnated grafts. There was no significant difference in the incidence of graft infection on early follow-up (1 month). The 2-year follow-up of these patients was reported in 2000.[44] Disappointingly, the infection rate was 4.5%, with six infections in the rifampin-bonded group and four infections in the nonbonded group. There was no significant difference in the rate of graft infection or mortality between the two groups. The authors in the discussion stated that despite studies on almost 3000 patients, there was no convincing evidence that rifampin bonding decreases the incidence of prosthetic extraanatomic graft infection. This finding is in contradistinction to the treatment of aortic graft infections with in-line rifampin-soaked grafts.

Silver-coated prosthetic conduits represent another option for treatment of infected aortic grafts. The silver is thought to inhibit bacterial colony formation on the prosthetic graft. Pupka and colleagues[45] compared silver-coated grafts to arterial homografts with and without immunosuppression. Postoperative morbidity and mortality was 7% and 11% in the silver-coated group, 16% and 8% in the arterial homograft with immunosuppression group, and 35% and 23% in the arterial homograft without immunosuppression group. There was a statistically significant difference in morbidity between the silver-coated and arterial homograft without immunosuppression groups; however, there were no statistically significant differences between the three groups in terms of mortality.

A recent systematic review and metaanalysis has questioned whether extraanatomic bypass and subsequent graft excision should remain the standard treatment of aortic graft infection. Becquemin and colleagues[46] examined 37 clinical studies and compared amputation, conduit failure, reinfection, and early and late mortality between extraanatomic bypass and in-line rifampin-bonded prosthetic, cryopreserved allografts, and autogenous venous reconstruction.[46] Rifampin-bonded prosthetic grafts were associated with the fewest amputations, conduit failures, and early mortalities, whereas autogenous vein was associated with the lowest risk of reinfection. Late mortality was lowest in the autogenous vein and cryopreserved allograft groups. When examining combined outcomes, extraanatomic bypass was associated with statistically inferior outcomes compared to each of the other groups.

Aortobifemoral Grafts

Although the treatment principles for aortofemoral graft infections are fundamentally the same as those stated previously, the issue of revascularization is more troublesome. This is actually a situation in which the neoaortoiliac system, with the superficial femoral vein as the conduit, represents an attractive option for reconstruction. However, the distal femoral anastomoses of an aortofemoral graft may preclude the attachment of distal limbs of an extraanatomic bypass to the common femoral artery. Therefore, if a prosthetic bypass via an extraanatomic route is to be used, the distal anastomosis of the extraanatomic bypass must be at the profunda femoris artery, the superficial femoral artery, or the popliteal artery. If the graft was performed for occlusive disease in an end-to-side fashion, it may be possible to excise the graft and repair the aortotomy primarily, relying on flow through the native vessels to the lower extremities. Although the native vessels are undoubtedly diseased, there may be adequate flow to avoid the need for immediate revascularization. This issue is best assessed preoperatively, because an intraoperative assessment of the adequacy of flow can result in the graft's being excised first, with subsequent extraanatomic bypass if the flow through the native vessels is inadequate. This would be a return to the traditional method of treating infected aortic grafts, which is an approach that results in increased morbidity.

If the graft infection is localized to the groin and the proximal and distal anastomoses are not involved, graft preservation can be attempted (Figure 56-6). This is done by draining the abscess, aggressively debriding the perigraft tissues, and ensuring tissue coverage.[34] Patients selected for graft preservation must meet all the previously mentioned criteria. Contraindications to graft preservation techniques include an occluded graft, the presence of sepsis, or a virulent organism, particularly *Pseudomonas aeruginosa*. Patients treated with graft preservation should be closely monitored in a controlled setting, not in a department designed for routine nursing care.

The use of muscle flaps in the treatment algorithm of infected graft preservation not only provides coverage in the presence of a large soft tissue defect, but can also provide better vascularized tissue to transport antibiotic therapy. While the majority of complicated muscle flaps, including rectus femoris, rectus abdominis, and gracilis rotational flaps, are performed by cosmetic surgeons, the Sartorius muscle flap is a common flap performed by vascular surgeons. This flap is based on segmental vessels that feed the muscle from the medial side. The muscle is divided from its attachment to the iliac spine, mobilized laterally, and then rotated medially onto the graft.

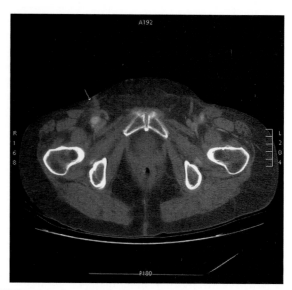

FIGURE 56-6 ■ Computed tomography (CT) scan of a patient with an aortobifemoral bypass graft and chronic occlusion of the right limb of the bypass. The patient had one episode of pulsatile right groin bleeding. CT scan showed perigraft stranding in the right groin and edema tracking to the skin, suggestive of graft infection *(arrow)*.

If the femoral anastomosis is involved with the infection, that graft limb should be excised. The limb can be approached by means of an ipsilateral retroperitoneal exposure (Figure 56-7). If the retroperitoneal portion of the graft is well incorporated, proximal control can be obtained at that level, and the graft limb can be excised. All ligation sites should be covered with viable tissue. The graft-artery anastomosis is excised and the artery is debrided. The femoral arteriotomy is then closed with patch angioplasty, preferably with autologous tissue. If a portion of the common femoral artery at that level must be debrided or excised, an attempt should be made to perform an end-to-end anastomosis of the superficial femoral artery to the deep femoral artery to maintain retrograde perfusion of the pelvis. If the proximal anastomosis is involved, the entire graft must be excised according to the principles elucidated earlier.

An extraanatomic bypass is then fashioned, depending on the need for revascularization of the limb. If only the unilateral limb is excised, the limb can be revascularized by tunneling via a retropubic route or through the obturator canal or by medial tunneling of a femorofemoral bypass (Figure 56-8). The choice of the vessel for distal bypass depends on the condition of the native vasculature. The bypass conduit has to be routed through clean, uninfected territory (Figure 56-9). If the entire graft must be excised, an extraanatomic bypass originating from the axillary artery must be fashioned and anastomosed to the deep femoral artery, the superficial femoral artery, or the popliteal artery (Figure 56-10). Although some practitioners advocate the use of ring-reinforced PTFE grafts to aid in the prevention of external compression of the graft, there is no evidence that this has any merit.

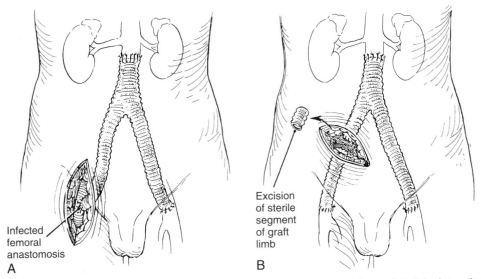

FIGURE 56-7 ■ Through a retroperitoneal approach, the sterility of the proximal portion of the graft limb is determined. **A,** The sterile graft above is isolated from the area of infection at the groin by excision of a segment of graft and obliteration of the communicating tissue planes between the two areas. **B,** The distal portion of the graft limb is then removed from below after the clean procedure has been performed in the retroperitoneal space and the wound has been closed.

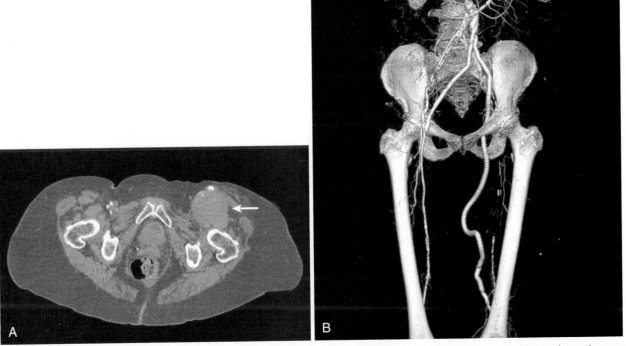

FIGURE 56-8 ■ **A,** Left femoral pseudoaneurysm *(arrow)* due to late graft infection and anastomotic rupture in a patient who previously had an aortobifemoral bypass and left femoropopliteal bypass for rest pain. At the time of surgery, the left limb of the aortobifemoral graft was approached from a retroperitoneal incision and was found to be well incorporated. **B,** Therefore an obturator bypass was performed from the left limb of the aortobifemoral bypass to the distal aspect of the previous femoropopliteal bypass with immediate excision of the infected segments. See Color Plate 56-8.

Femoropopliteal Bypass Grafts

An infected femoropopliteal bypass graft must be excised in its entirety (Figure 56-11). The same principles apply, including radical debridement of infected tissue, debridement of the artery to healthy viable tissue, and closure of the artery with monofilament suture. The viability of the limb determines the need for immediate versus delayed revascularization. Should immediate revascularization be needed, it is ideally performed with

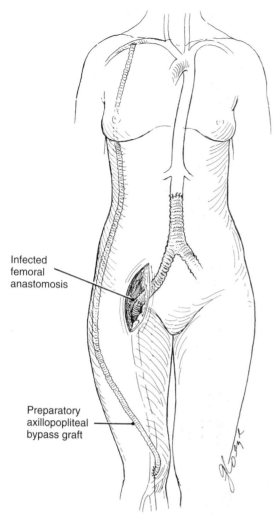

FIGURE 56-9 ■ Perfusion of an ischemic extremity in the presence of sepsis in the ipsilateral groin is achieved with an axillopopliteal bypass graft. Care is taken to bring the graft wide of the groin through unaffected tissue planes.

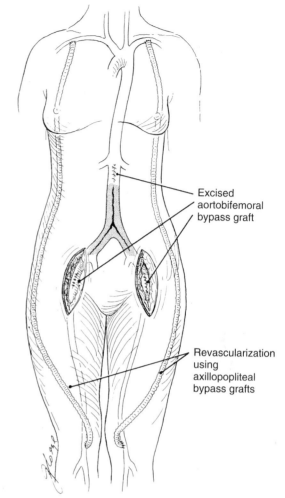

FIGURE 56-10 ■ Ischemia of the lower extremities, caused by a return to dependence on the native circulation after the removal of an infected aortic graft, can be successfully managed by bilateral axillopopliteal bypass grafts.

autogenous vein, and only if the anastomosis is not done in an infected area. Revascularization is performed with adherence to the same principles outlined earlier, with the route of the graft through clean, uninfected tissue.

An alternative is to perform a semiclosed endarterectomy of the superficial femoral artery. In the modern era, the technique of subintimal angioplasty allows successful recanalization without the insertion of a foreign body. A more commonly used conduit for bypass in an infected field is cryopreserved cadaver vein graft or cadaver arterial graft. The advantage of the cadaver vein is its ease of handling, its resistance to infection, and appropriate size matching to the artery. Its principal disadvantages are the significant cost and the poor medium- and long-term patency rates.

Endovascular Stent-Grafts

The overall incidence of aortic endograft infection is approximately 0.2% to 1.2%, and seems to be lower than the incidence after open aortic reconstruction. The diagnosis can also be uncertain, especially soon after graft

insertion. There is a well-described postimplantation inflammatory profile of fever and leukocytosis. Velasquez and colleagues[47] reported on their first 12 patients who underwent endovascular repair with Dacron-covered stent-grafts. A majority of those patients had fever (body temperature >101.4° F [38.5° C]), leukocytosis, and CT evidence of perigraft air. All patients became afebrile with resolution of their leukocytosis, and none had any evidence of graft infection on follow-up. As a result, it appears that the early postimplantation inflammatory profile does not represent evidence of graft infection.

The cause of endograft infection is similar to that of open grafts. Graft infection can occur at the time of implantation or as a consequence of hematogenous seeding. This is especially important because approximately 11% of patients will require secondary interventions for graft related complications.[48] As a result, preoperative antibiotics are indicated at the time of initial endograft implantation and when performing percutaneous procedures in such patients.

One of the largest studies to examine aortic endograft infections found 12 infections in 1431 procedures.[49]

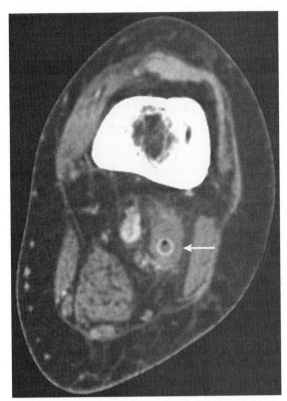

FIGURE 56-11 ■ Axial image from computed tomographic angiography shows a thrombosed lower extremity bypass with intraluminal air and surrounding fluid collection *(arrow)* consistent with graft infection. (From Abularrage CJ, Deaton DH: Vascular surgery. In Ho VB, Reddy GP, editors: Cardiovascular imaging, Philadelphia, 2011, Elsevier.)

Endograft infections were more common after an emergency procedure (0.56% vs. 2.79%; $p = 0.002$). No significant difference was found between those treated with an endovascular abdominal aortic aneurysm repair and those treated with a thoracic endovascular aortic

aneurysm repair. Over the study period, 3 of the 12 patients died (25%), of whom 2 had been treated with antibiotic therapy without graft excision. Although this difference did not reach statistical significance, conclusions regarding the success of nonoperative management should be limited because of the small sample size.

Operative mortality of infected endograft excision is substantial and can be as high as 25%,[50] possibly because many endografts are performed in patients at high risk for open repair. Treatment is similar to open graft infection, with excision and extraanatomic or in situ reconstruction. Antibiotic therapy without graft excision can be performed in poor-risk patients who have a good initial response to parenteral antibiotics.[51] Long-term antibiotic suppression is indicated, and recurrent signs of sepsis should mandate conversion.

CONCLUSIONS

The underwhelming success of traditional modes of managing graft infections has spurred experimentation with alternative methods, such as selective graft preservation, antibiotic and silver-bonded grafts, and the use of autogenous vein for reconstruction in situ. The current understanding of graft infection and its causes and treatment is inchoate. Although evolution in the management of graft infection is ongoing and encouraging, the most fruitful endeavor may be an enhanced understanding of the pathophysiologic factors that predispose certain patients to develop graft infection. The interaction of a foreign body with the host and the subsequent response of the host determine the clinical outcome. With a better understanding of this interaction and the disparate responses of different hosts, a more successful attempt at immunomodulation may reduce the incidence of graft infection and its considerable morbidity and mortality.

References available online at expertconsult.com.

QUESTIONS

1. Which of the following organisms is most likely to cause graft anastomotic disruption and hemorrhage?
   a. *Staphylococcus epidermidis*
   b. *Pseudomonas* species
   c. *Candida* species
   d. All of the above

2. Which of the following statements regarding perigraft air or fluid in the setting of a prosthetic graft is not true?
   a. Perigraft air 3 months after placement of the graft should raise concern of a graft infection.
   b. Ultrasonography or CT is an acceptable imaging technique for the diagnosis of perigraft fluid.
   c. Graft infections manifesting as perigraft fluid can be appropriately treated by percutaneous drainage of the fluid and long-term antibiotics.
   d. The great majority of patients have complete resolution of perigraft air by approximately 8 to 12 weeks following implantation.

3. Which of the following statements regarding *Staphylococcus epidermidis* graft infections is true?
   a. *S. epidermidis* infections manifest most commonly with sepsis and hemorrhage.
   b. Revascularization for *S. epidermidis* graft infections may be performed with in-line PTFE grafts.
   c. Routine Gram stain and culture of the graft are usually adequate for establishing the diagnosis.
   d. Extended (>24 hours) perioperative coverage with antibiotics is more effective at preventing graft infections compared with a single preoperative dose.

4. The options for reconstruction of an infected aortofemoral bypass graft include all of the following except:
   a. Axillobifemoral bypass
   b. Autogenous reconstruction with autogenous superficial femoral vein
   c. Cryopreserved allograft
   d. Collagen-impregnated Dacron graft

5. Which of the following statements regarding prosthetic graft infection is true?
   a. Grafts involving the femoral artery have a higher rate of infection than grafts anastomosed to the iliac arteries.
   b. An emergency operation (e.g., for a ruptured abdominal aortic aneurysm) carries an equivalent rate of infection as an elective operation.
   c. The surgeon is the principal and most likely source of the organism infecting the prosthesis.
   d. The mortality of an operation to treat prosthetic aortic graft infection approaches 75% to 80%.

6. Examples of extraanatomic bypass include all of the following except:
   a. Obturator bypass
   b. Axillopopliteal bypass
   c. Femorofemoral bypass
   d. Neoaortoiliac system involving superficial femoral vein

7. Which of the following is not a clinical presentation of graft infection?
   a. Pseudoaneurysm
   b. Recurrent graft thrombosis
   c. Hemorrhage
   d. Malaise, fever, weight loss
   e. Neointimal hyperplasia at the proximal anastomosis

ANSWERS

1. **b**
2. **c**
3. **b**
4. **d**
5. **a**
6. **d**
7. **e**

CHAPTER 57

NONINFECTIOUS COMPLICATIONS IN VASCULAR SURGERY

Glenn C. Hunter • Alex Westerband

Complications after aortoiliac and peripheral arterial reconstruction often develop and progress rapidly to produce disastrous consequences, including major organ failure or loss of limb or life.

These complications may be the result of technical errors, the extent of the pathologic process, or one or more frequently associated diseases. A timeworn surgical principle applies, especially to vascular surgery: "A complication not anticipated is sure to be experienced." There are currently fewer and more complex open operative procedures being performed by surgeons who lack the suitable training to undertake these operations. Since the introduction of endovascular aneurysm repair (EVAR), the number of patients undergoing open aneurysm repair (OAR) requiring suprarenal clamp placement and adjunctive renal and/or visceral grafts has increased from 6% to 44% and 12% to 44% respectively. Patients undergoing OAR also have a higher incidence of renal vein division (4% to 11% vs. 18%), iliac artery aneurysms (25% vs. 42%), and occlusive disease (12% vs. 20%). Adjunctive renal and/or visceral grafts were required in only 1.9% of patients with infrarenal clamp placement. Although OAR with suprarenal clamp placement can be performed with relatively low mortality rates in major academic centers (0.8% to 6.1%), early recognition and treatment of complications is essential if mortality rates are to be maintained in this range in the future.[1-4] The primary problems reviewed in this chapter are perioperative bleeding, thrombosis, acute renal injury and failure, spinal cord ischemia, operative embolization, iatrogenic ureteric injury and obstruction, bowel obstruction and intraabdominal compartment syndrome (ICS), chylous ascites, graft deterioration, anastomotic false aneurysms, incisional hernias, and postoperative lower extremity lymphoceles and edema.

AORTOILIAC SURGERY

Complications of aortoiliac arterial reconstruction are similar regardless of whether the procedure is for abdominal aortic aneurysmal or occlusive disease.

Perioperative Bleeding

Operative Bleeding

Operative bleeding may occur during dissection of the major vessels from failure to secure hemostasis or from difficulties encountered while sewing in the graft. Venous tears are the most common cause of intraoperative bleeding and usually result from injury to unrecognized venous anomalies and during mobilization of the aorta and iliac arteries from the inferior vena cava (IVC) and iliac veins. The inferior mesenteric, left renal, adrenal, gonadal, and lumbar veins are all at risk of injury during dissection or retractor placement to expose the infrarenal aorta when undertaking aortic bypass procedures for occlusive or aneurysmal disease (Figure 57-1).[5] A thorough understanding of the anatomy, and familiarity with the characteristics of major venous anomalies and careful operative dissection, are essential to avoid this complication.[6] Venous anomalies can involve the infrarenal, renal, or suprarenal segments of the IVC. Infrarenal segment anomalies include agenesis of the IVC, a left-sided IVC (0.2% to 0.5%), and duplicate IVCs (1% to 3%). Either of these anomalies may be associated with a right or, rarely, left retrocaval ureter. When present, the proximal ureter is dorsal to the IVC and, inferiorly, runs between the vena cava and the aorta. In rare instances, a double right vena cava has been observed. Anomalies of the renal segment of the IVC include a retroaortic renal vein (1.7% to 3.4%; Figure 57-2) and circumaortic venous rings (Figure 57-3), in which the retroaortic segment is located in a more caudal position relative to the preaortic segment. Anomalies of the suprarenal segment of the IVC are extremely rare and associated with either azygos or hemiazygos continuation and absence of the hepatic venous segment.[7]

The distal IVC and iliac veins are most vulnerable at the level of the posterolateral aspect of the aortic bifurcation in the area of tight adherence of the aorta and common iliac artery to the adjacent wall of the vena cava and right iliac vein. Complete separation of these structures by circumferential dissection is generally unnecessary, because temporary occlusion can usually be achieved by clamp control more distally or with intraluminal balloon occlusion catheters. If the IVC or one of the iliac veins is inadvertently lacerated, bleeding should be controlled by gentle finger pressure or sponge stick tamponade, and the venous laceration closed with interrupted pledgeted Prolene sutures. Application of clamps is hazardous and may enlarge the rent in the vein.

The left renal vein should be routinely identified early during dissection of the aorta above an aneurysm or proximal to the area of major aortic occlusive disease. The caudal border of the left renal vein should be clearly defined so that this structure can be easily retracted

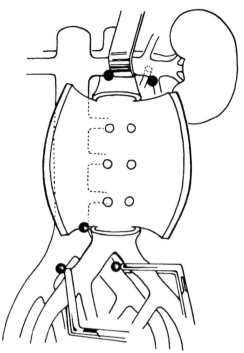

FIGURE 57-1 ■ Sites of venous injury. (From Downs A: Problems in resection of aortoiliac and femoral aneurysms. In Bernhard VM, Towne JB, editors: Complications in vascular surgery, New York, 1980, Grune and Stratton, p 68.)

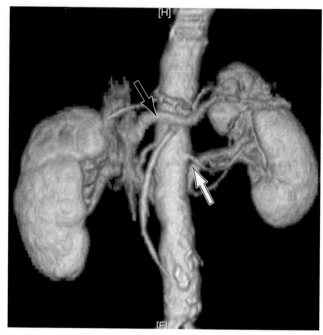

FIGURE 57-3 ■ Magnetic resonance imaging reconstruction of a circumaortic renal vein *(black arrow)*. Note the caudal position of the posterior branch *(white arrow)*.

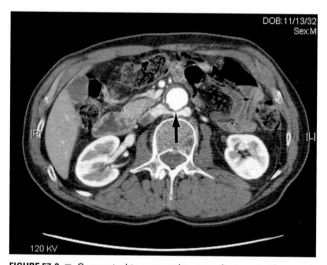

FIGURE 57-2 ■ Computed tomography scan demonstrating a retroaortic left renal vein *(arrow)* in a patient with an abdominal aortic aneurysm.

cephalad. Division of its adrenal, gonadal, or lumbar branches enhances its mobility and improves exposure. Careful consideration should be given to ligation of these branches if division of the renal vein is contemplated to improve exposure in patients with large or inflammatory aneurysms. Failure to find the left renal vein in its usual position suggests its aberrant location behind the aorta (see Figures 57-2 and 57-3), where it may be readily injured during circumferential dissection of the infrarenal aorta preparatory to application of an occluding clamp.[5,6,8,9]

An arteriovenous fistula (AVF) involving the aorta or iliac arteries is an uncommon complication of spontaneous aneurysm rupture into an adjacent vein (about 80% of cases) or of penetrating injury to these major vessels (20%). Aortocaval fistula (ACF) has also been reported after EVAR.[10,11] The incidence of this complication is quite low; it occurs in less than 1% of all aneurysms and in 3% to 4% of ruptured aneurysms.[12-15] The presence of an ACF should be suspected by a continuous bruit over the aneurysm associated with the sudden onset of abdominal pain, lower extremity venous hypertension, oliguria, hematuria, and congestive heart failure. If suspected, the diagnosis of an ACF or iliac AV fistula can be confirmed by color Doppler imaging, computed tomography (CT) scanning, magnetic resonance imaging (MRI), or digital subtraction angiography (DSA). Before the routine use of preoperative imaging studies to evaluate patients with abdominal aortic aneurysms (AAA), the presence of an ACF or ilioiliac AV fistula remained undetected in 25% to 44% of patients undergoing open AAA repair. The patient with an ACF should be rapidly medically optimized before being taken to the operating room. Cardiac catheterization is rarely necessary except in cases of diagnostic uncertainty. The initial medical management should include admission to the intensive care unit (ICU), placement of hemodynamic monitoring lines and catheters, and the use of ACE inhibitors and diuretics. Sufficient blood and blood products should be available because intraoperative bleeding may be profuse. The fistula may sometimes be unsuspected intraoperatively because of its small size or its being obscured by the laminated thrombus within the aneurysm, with it becoming apparent only when sudden massive venous hemorrhage occurs within the lumen of the aorta during

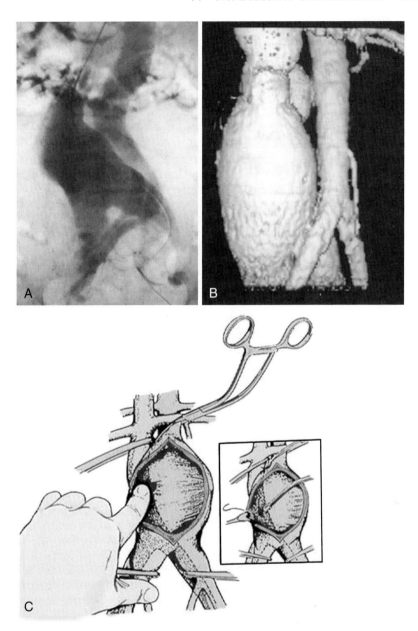

FIGURE 57-4 ■ **A,** Abdominal angiogram showing filling of the vena cava from an aortic aneurysm. **B,** Magnetic resonance angiogram showing a traumatic aortocaval fistula. **C,** The fistula orifice is exposed through the aneurysm and controlled by simple digital occlusion of the hole into the inferior vena cava. The fistula is closed with a simple over-and-over suture from within the aneurysmal sac. A clear and unencumbered field is provided by rapid aspiration and autotransfusion of blood pouring into the aneurysmal sac from the cava.

evacuation of the laminated thrombus from the aneurysmal sac.[16] In all patients undergoing AAA repair without preoperative imaging studies, it is wise to palpate the IVC for the presence of a thrill, indicating an ACF, before opening the aneurysm sac to evacuate the laminated thrombus. If a fistula is suspected, the inferior vena cava should be occluded with a sponge stick or a clamp adjacent to the neck of the aneurysm before the aneurysm is occluded and opened, to prevent embolism of clot or air to the lungs.[13] No attempt should be made to separate the aneurysm wall from the IVC at the fistula site.

Occlusion of the fistulous defect by direct finger pressure over the fistula, followed by proximal and distal caval compression with sponge sticks or insertion of balloon occlusion catheters, are among the maneuvers used to control the venous bleeding so that the defect can be visualized and closed with polytetrafluoroethylene (PTFE) pledget sutures (92%) or patch angioplasty (8%) from within the aortic sac (Figure 57-4).[17,18] Intraoperative bleeding from iliac AVFs is often more difficult to control because of their location deep within the pelvis, the size of the defect, and the intimate relationship between the vein and artery. Elective balloon catheter occlusion or placement of a covered stent to occlude the defect in the femoral vein before entering the aneurysm may control venous bleeding and permit closure of the defect without massive blood loss. Autotransfusion is a useful adjunct in the management of ACF and iliac fistulas.[12] Surgical treatment of ACF includes intraaneu-rysmal closure of the defect and reconstruction of the aorta with a tube or a bifurcated graft. Although endo-vascular repair with an aortic stent-graft may be the optimal method of treating ACF and iliac AVFs with suitable anatomy, rupture of an enlarged aneurysm sac into the IVC after EVAR is a recognized cause of ACF. Open repair, relining the endoprosthesis, or percutane-ous closure of the defect with an Amplatzar VSD muscle plug are among the therapeutic options available for treating patients with ACF after EVAR.[19-21] Prophylactic placement of an IVC filter is rarely necessary. Complica-tions of surgical repair, including excessive intraoperative blood loss, myocardial infarction, respiratory failure, stroke, colonic ischemia, paraparesis, and renal failure, occur in 39% of patients. Mortality rates, ranging from an average of 34% (6% to 71%) have seen a decline to 12% in the most recent report by Davidovic and coworkers.[17] Myocardial infarction and multiple-system organ failure remain the major cause of mortality. Long-term survival after repair is greater than 90%.[18]

Arterial bleeding usually arises from the lumbar, anomalous renal, inferior mesenteric arteries or posterior aortic wall during circumferential dissection or after the aneurysmal sac has been opened.[22-24] Lumbar vessel injury can be avoided in aneurysm surgery by limiting the dis-section to the anterior surface of the aorta and by suture ligation of the lumbar orifices from within the aneurys-mal sac after the aneurysm has been opened and the thrombus evacuated.[15] Precaval location of the right renal artery (5%) and multiple renal arteries (30% to 40%) should be identified. The inferior mesenteric artery should also be suture-ligated from the interior or close to the wall of the aneurysm (if there is pulsatile backflow) to avoid injury to mesenteric collaterals. The posterior aortic wall is often heavily calcified or attenuated in patients with AAA. Calcified plaque at the site of the proposed anastomosis may require an endarterectomy, which further attenuates the aortic wall. The pre-emptive use of a Teflon buttress will reduce the risk of bleeding from tears at the anastomotic suture line from the place-ment of sutures in a fragile aortic wall. When anasto-motic bleeding is encountered, the aorta should be clamped briefly while additional sutures, frequently with PTFE pledgets, are placed to control the bleeding and avoid further tears in the aortic wall. In patients with unfavorable aortic tissues, the use of biological tissue glues may sometimes be helpful. These agents are not a substitute for careful hemostasis, however, and their use is associated with more frequent reoperation for bleeding and the potential for infection.[25,26] Reinforcement of the aortic anastomosis with a cuff of graft material is another option.

Continued intraoperative bleeding may result from failure to reverse or discontinue anticoagulants or plate-let inhibitors preoperatively or the administration of too large a dose of heparin. The massive blood transfusion requirements during repair of thoracoabdominal or rup-tured abdominal aneurysms results in the dilution of coagulation factors and platelets. In patients undergoing repair of pararenal aneurysms or the need for supraceliac clamping to facilitate repair, unrecognized fibrinolysis may be the cause of continued bleeding. Only rarely is the bleeding caused by an unrecognized congenital coagulation factor deficiency. The cause of the coagu-lopathy is often difficult to determine intraoperatively. Because of the higher mortality rates associated with increased intraoperative blood loss and the delay in obtaining the results of laboratory studies, it is recom-mended that blood, fresh frozen plasma (FFP), and platelets be administered concomitantly to improve the survival rate of these patients. If supraceliac clamping is anticipated or repair of a thoracoabdominal aneurysm is being undertaken, the transfusion of FFP should be started before clamp placement. Antifibrinolytic agents such as aminocaproic acid (Amicar) or tranexamic acid should be considered if activation of the fibrinolytic pathway is suspected. It should be noted, however, that there are no prospective data available for the clinical use of these agents in vascular surgery patients.[27,28]

Postoperative Bleeding

Bleeding in the immediate postoperative period usually comes from suture lines, inadequately ligated lumbar vessels, or the inferior mesenteric vein. This is mani-fested by a continuing need for blood replacement and the development of a retroperitoneal hematoma. This can be identified by palpating the flank—usually the left—which loses its normal soft concavity and becomes distended and tense. When aortic or iliac suture line bleeding is rapid, shock is more obvious, and the patient complains of severe backache similar to the pain of a ruptured aortic aneurysm. Postoperative hemorrhage is treated by immediate return to the operating room for identification and control of the bleeding site under fully monitored general anesthesia. The surgeon should search for the potential bleeding site when blood volume and pressure are at the patient's normal level before closing the retroperitoneum over the aortoiliac reconstruction.

Prevention of this complication requires thorough inspection of the intraabdominal anastomoses and the periaortic area, with special attention given to the orifices of the lumbar or anomalous renal vessels, the inferior mesenteric artery, and the ligated or over-sewn stumps of the aorta or iliac vessels.

Hypothermia and acidosis are correctable causes of persistent coagulopathy and postoperative bleeding. Prevention of hypothermia by using heating blankets, increasing room temperature, and infusing adequate volumes of warm blood and fluids to optimize cardiac output are essential. An activated clotting time (ACT) is done and specimens sent for a platelet count, fibrinogen, prothrombin time (PT), and partial thromboplastin time (PTT); these tests may not be helpful in the acute setting. Fibrinogen is the first clotting factor to fall in this situa-tion and should be replaced. A platelet count of ≥100,000 should not negate the need for platelet infusion because the platelets may not be functional. Congenital coagula-tion factor deficiency is rare and can usually be ascer-tained by careful preoperative history and evaluation.[29] Preliminary screening studies do not reliably identify the need to search for precise factor deficiencies and direct their replacement before and during surgery.

Intraoperative monitoring of the ACT before and after heparin administration is the most effective means of identifying variations in the individual response to intraoperatively administered unfractionated heparin and to determine the adequacy of its reversal before closing the abdomen.[29] Proper management of bleeding caused by congenital or acquired deficiencies requires repeated monitoring of pertinent coagulation parameters during and immediately after the operative procedure.

The rising number of cardiac and peripheral percutaneous and endovascular interventions being performed has resulted in antiplatelet agents' being administered to increasing numbers of patients. It is not uncommon for patients undergoing coronary or peripheral vessel angioplasty or stenting to receive a combination of drugs, including aspirin; clopidogrel; heparin; glycoprotein (GP) IIb/IIIa inhibitors such as abciximab, eptifibatide, and tirofiban; and direct thrombin inhibitors such as bivalirudin. Emergency surgical procedures to control bleeding from retroperitoneal hemorrhage or expanding groin hematomas from cannulation sites can be associated with significant perioperative blood loss into the thigh or retroperitoneum.[30-33]

Although thromboelastography may be a useful adjuvant to therapy, it is not universally available. Discontinuation of the antiplatelet agent or anticoagulant therapy and delay of surgery when feasible is sometimes the preferred option. However, should emergency intervention be required, red blood cells, FFP, fibrinogen concentrate, and platelets should be infused. Cryoprecipitate and specific factor replacement should be reserved for patients with specific coagulation factor defects.

Initially approved for treating patients with hemophilia who had antibodies inactivating factor VIII and IX, recombinant activated factor VII (rFVIIa) is used extensively in patients with massive bleeding from surgery or trauma and may be beneficial in patients undergoing rAAA repair. Recombinant activated factor VIIa binds locally to tissue factor at the site of vessel injury, generating small amounts of thrombin sufficient to activate platelets. The activated platelet surface membranes form a template on which rFVIIa directly or indirectly mediates further activation of the coagulation pathway, ultimately generating more thrombin and the conversion of fibrinogen to fibrin. Recombinant factor VIIa also stabilizes clot by activation of a thrombin-mediated fibrinolysis inhibitor. Clinical studies in patients undergoing prostatectomy, liver transplantation, noncoronary cardiac surgery, and trauma have shown that rFVIIa minimizes operative blood loss and reduces transfusion requirements. A major concern with the use of this agent is the risk of thrombosis. The incidence is believed to be low because of the dilution of coagulation factors in patients from massive blood loss.[34,35]

It is estimated that there are approximately 2.5 million patients on long-term vitamin K therapy and 40% of the U.S. population over 40 years of age is on antiplatelet therapy. The need for temporary interruption of these therapies for surgical and other invasive procedures is therefore not infrequent.[36] In a recent study, approximately 15% of patients on long-term vitamin K therapy required a major surgical procedure within a 4-year

follow-up period.[37] Recommendations for the discontinuation of vitamin K and antiplatelet agents preoperatively or preprocedurally must be balanced with the risk of thrombotic occlusion of recently placed stents or stent-grafts, the type of surgery including the risk of hemorrhagic complications, and the pharmacodynamic/-kinetic profile of the therapy used to reverse the vitamin K therapy.

Neilipovitz and colleagues, using decision analysis, showed that the continued use of aspirin in vascular surgery patients reduces perioperative mortality, despite a 2.5% increase in hemorrhagic complications[33] The antiplatelet effects of clopidogrel persist for 7 to 10 days so this drug should be discontinued 1 week before surgery. These recommendations are based on observations from case studies of patients undergoing coronary artery bypass grafting who received aspirin and clopidogrel or aspirin and placebo.[38] Patients receiving both drugs had a higher rate of major postoperative bleeding (9.6% vs. 6.3%), reoperation (9.8% vs. 1.6%), and blood transfusion (3.0 units vs. 1.6 units) compared with patients receiving aspirin and placebo. The effects of GP IIb/IIIa inhibitors on platelets are quite variable. The antiplatelet effects of eptifibatide are usually abated within 8 hours of cessation of therapy in patients with normal renal function. Abciximab has a biological half-life of 8 hours, but its effects on the surface of circulating platelets can be detected for up to 2 weeks after discontinuing the drug.[30]

The risk of hemorrhage and thromboembolism varies with the international normalized ratio (INR) in patients on vitamin K therapy. With INR ratios between 2 and 3, the relative risk of hemorrhagic events is 2.7 compared with 21.8 at INR ratios between 3 and 5. The risk of thromboembolism increases significantly with low INR; compared with INR ratios between 2 and 3, the relative risk of thromboembolism associated with INR below 2 was 3.5; within the range of 2 to 3, there is still a higher risk of thromboembolic than hemorrhagic events (2.6%/year vs. 1.4%/year). Patients with mechanical heart valves or chronic atrial fibrillation and those at high risk of recurrent deep vein thrombosis who are on long-term vitamin K therapy should have the vitamin K agonist reversed and receive bridging low-molecular-weight heparin (LMWH). Therapeutic options for acute reversal of vitamin K agonists include: vitamin K, FFP, prothrombin complex concentrate (PCC), and, possibly, rFVIIa. PCC is obtained from plasma; 60 mL of PCC is equivalent to 1500 mL of FFP, reducing volume requirements.[39]

Thrombosis

Graft thrombosis in the early postoperative period is almost invariably caused by technical problems (Figure 57-5) that usually occur at the distal anastomoses.[40-42] These include an elevated intimal flap, narrowing of the artery at the anastomotic suture line, failure to remove clot adherent to the inner wall of the graft before completion of the anastomosis, twisting or kinking in the retroperitoneal tunnel, compression of the femoral limb of the graft by the inguinal ligament, unrecognized inflow disease, or inadequate runoff secondary to

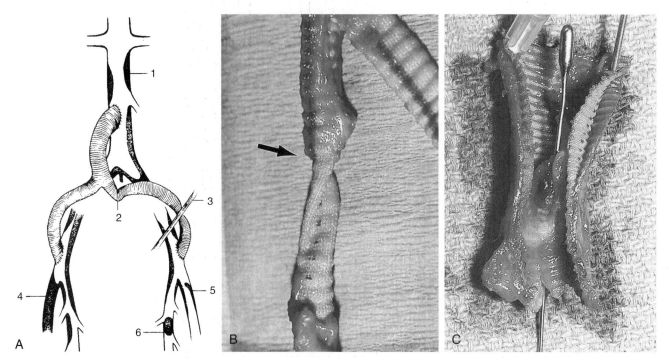

FIGURE 57-5 ■ **A,** Aortic mechanical factors that may cause early thrombosis of aortofemoral graft: *(1)* aortic anastomosis distal to obstructing atherosclerosis at the subrenal level; *(2)* kinking of the graft limb caused by placement of the proximal anastomosis low on the aorta, with an overly long aortic graft segment; *(3)* compression by the inguinal ligament; *(4)* inadequate runoff caused by occlusion of the superficial femoral artery and severe stenosis of the deep femoral artery; *(5)* elevation of the distal intima; *(6)* peripheral embolization or thrombosis. **B,** Operative picture demonstrating a twist in the right limb *(arrow)* of an aortobifemoral graft. **C,** Fibrointimal ingrowth resulting in occlusion of the limb of a bifurcation graft. (**A,** From Bernhard VM: The failed arterial graft: lost pulses and gangrene. In Condon RE, DeCosse JJ, edtors: Surgical care, Philadelphia, 1980, Lea and Febiger, p 155.)

unappreciated iliac, deep femoral, superficial femoral, or infrapopliteal disease. Rarely, thrombosis after aortofemoral bypass or aneurysm replacement is caused by hypercoagulability from inadequate doses or resistance to heparin, antithrombin III deficiency, protein C or S deficiency, a mutation in factor V Leiden or prothrombin genes, homocystinemia, anticardiolipin antibodies, heparin-induced thrombocytopenia (HIT) and thrombosis, or stasis caused by reduced cardiac output.[43-46]

The adequacy of pulsatile blood flow through the graft or endarterectomy should be evaluated in the operating room before the incisions are closed, by palpation of the graft and the arteries immediately distal to the anastomoses and by direct inspection of the pedal circulation beneath the drapes and palpation of distal pulses. If necessary, noninvasive measurements such as Doppler flow or pulse-volume recording tracings can be obtained intraoperatively.[40,41,47-49] Intraoperative completion angiograms or color-flow Doppler imaging should be obtained in all patients who have had extensive reconstructive procedures of the common femoral, superficial femoral, or deep femoral arteries to ensure the adequacy of the repair. Noninvasive studies should be performed routinely in the recovery room when pulses cannot be felt distal to the repair or when the anticipated improvement in circulation has not occurred. Objective information obtained from these easily performed studies is particularly valuable in the immediate postoperative period, when patients are frequently hypothermic and peripherally vasoconstricted. Detection of unsatisfactory graft function

mandates immediate direct evaluation of the involved anastomoses before wound closure or prompt return to the operating room if graft flow subsequently deteriorates.

An ACT should be obtained and additional systemic heparin given as necessary. This is especially important if protamine has been given at the initial operation. Treatment of immediate postreconstructive thrombosis consists of thorough inspection of the intraluminal aspect of the involved anastomosis. This is best accomplished through an incision in the distal end of the graft or by takedown of the anastomosis to directly view the intima and the runoff vessels adjacent to the arteriotomy. Effective revision may require stabilization of an elevated plaque, extension of an iliac limb to the common femoral artery, or patch angioplasty of a deep or proximal superficial femoral stenosis. Complementary bypass from the femoral to the popliteal or infrapopliteal vessels is only infrequently required when runoff through the deep femoral artery is inadequate.[50,51] The lie of the graft should always be inspected throughout its length to ensure that there is no kinking, twisting, or external compression within the retroperitoneal tunnel.

Prevention of early graft thrombosis depends on an accurate evaluation of the distal runoff bed by preoperative noninvasive hemodynamic testing and imaging; computed tomography angiography (CTA), magnetic resonance angiography (MRA), or DSA. The iliac artery, rather than the femoral, should be palpated throughout its length before the selection of this vessel as the site for distal anastomosis. The orifices of the runoff vessels should be inspected and calibrated with dilators. Special attention should be given to the deep femoral orifice, which often requires endarterectomy or extension of the graft over its orifice when the distal anastomosis is performed at the common femoral level. Tacking sutures may be required to prevent distal intimal dissection. Finally, technical perfection in the performance of anastomoses is mandatory to avoid narrowing of the runoff vessels.

The widespread use of unfractionated and LMWH has resulted in an increased frequency of HIT, reported to occur in 5% of patients receiving unfractionated heparin and in 0.5% receiving LMWH. The heparin/platelet factor 4 (PF4) complex generates predominantly IgG and to a lesser extent IgM and IgG antibodies, which activate prothrombotic platelet microparticles, resulting in platelet consumption, increased thrombin generation, and the risk of venous and arterial thrombosis. A milder form of HIT that is neither immune-mediated nor prothrombotic occurs more often in patients receiving heparin. Heparin-induced thrombocytopenia with thrombosis (HITT) should be suspected when the platelet count decreases by more than 50% from baseline or drops to 150,000 or less in patients receiving heparin therapy. Thromboembolic complications usually become evident between 5 and 14 days after heparin therapy and can involve the deep veins of the lower extremity, the pulmonary arteries, and major cerebral veins. Arterial thrombotic complications may involve the lower extremities and the coronary, mesenteric, renal, or cerebral arteries. When HITT is encountered intraoperatively, the surgeon has to act without confirmatory tests. If HITT

is suspected, owing to the presence of "white clots" or unexplained intraoperative thrombosis, blood should be drawn immediately for diagnostic confirmation and a specimen of the thrombus sent to the laboratory for a touch prep to confirm the predominance of platelets in the clot. The administration of all unfractionated heparin should be discontinued and the ACT normalized with protamine if heparin has been administered recently.[52-54]

Laboratory confirmation of HITT using the PF4/polyanion immunoassay is specific if strongly positive but has low specificity (owing to IgM, IgG, and nonspecific antibodies) if the enzyme-linked immunosorbent assay is weakly positive. The platelet serotonin release assay is more specific if there is >80% serotonin release. The principles of treatment include discontinuation of all heparin, administration of direct thrombin inhibitors such as argatroban, lepirudin, or bivalirudin to maintain the PTT between 1.5 times and 3.0 times baseline. Prophylactic platelet transfusions should be avoided. Because warfarin may predispose to microvascular thrombosis in patients with acute HITT receiving direct thrombin inhibitors, it should be reversed with vitamin K if a dose has already been given and should be reintroduced only when the platelet count is >150 × 104/L.

Thrombosis caused by the progression of downstream atherosclerosis or anastomotic intimal hyperplasia (AIH) is the most frequent late complication of aortoiliac and aortofemoral procedures.[55,56] The impaired outflow through the external iliac artery or the branches of the common femoral usually manifests as unilateral limb ischemia (Figure 57-6).[57-63] Anastomotic intimal hyperplasia causes stenosis, usually at graft-artery interface of the distal anastomosis: occlusion occurs when flow

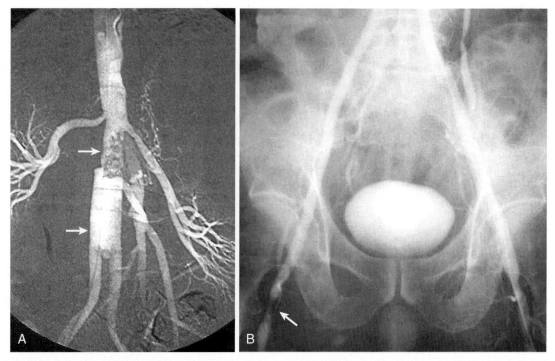

FIGURE 57-6 ■ **A,** Digital subtraction angiogram demonstrating progression of atherosclerosis above an aortofemoral graft. The graft is placed well below the renal arteries and the body of the graft is too long. **B,** High-grade stenosis caused by intimal hyperplasia at the distal limb of an aortofemoral graft.

diminishes sufficiently to result in stasis thrombosis.[62] The majority of patients initially treated with aortofemoral bypass have stenosis/occlusion of the superficial femoral artery at the time of the primary procedure. Therefore, an adequate lumen at the origin of the deep femoral artery is the most significant factor in ensuring long-term patency of these grafts.[48,56,58,61,63] Underestimating the severity of outflow disease at the time of primary reconstruction is an important cofactor in progressive atherosclerosis that increases susceptibility to late graft limb occlusion.[64] Despite an adequate primary procedure, progression of femoral or infrapopliteal atherosclerotic disease is more likely to occur in patients with continued exposure to atherogenic risk factors, particularly patients who continue to smoke.[57,64] Impaired inflow is the second most common cause of late postrevascularization thrombosis. Although it is four to nine times less frequent than impaired outflow, it is the most common cause of simultaneous bilateral postreconstructive lower limb ischemia after aortoiliac or femoral surgery.[56,59,64] The most common mechanism is obstruction from progressive infrarenal aortic atherosclerosis proximal to the site of previous repair (see Figure 57-5A). This is usually the consequence of placing the proximal anastomosis too low on the aorta (i.e., at or below the inferior mesenteric artery; see Figure 57-6A). The area between this site and the renal arteries is an active site of progressive atherosclerosis.[48] Likewise, after aortoiliac endarterectomy, late occlusion is more likely if the proximal infrarenal aorta is not included in the endarterectomy.[65] The use of an end-to-end rather than an end-to-side aortic anastomosis may be associated with fewer thrombotic failures, although this has not been clearly defined. Superior hemodynamic flow characteristics, the absence of competitive flow, less chance of embolization from the host aorta, and less angulation of the limbs as they arise from the body graft have been cited as the advantages of the end-to-end aortic anastomosis.[48,65]

Angulation of the graft limb at the bifurcation may produce kinking because of failure to pull the graft limb out to full length before the distal anastomoses are performed or excessive length of the graft body, resulting in too wide a bifurcation angle (see Figure 57-5B). Inadequate retroperitoneal tunneling of the graft limbs may promote thrombosis as a consequence of extrinsic compression from the mesentery of the sigmoid colon or the recurrent portion of the inguinal ligament (see Figure 57-5C).[64]

Less frequent causes of late thrombosis of aortoiliac and femoral reconstructions include accumulation of mural thrombus and false aneurysms. Mural thrombus develops when the graft diameter is significantly larger than the outflow artery. The flow pattern of the larger graft adjusts itself to the smaller outflow artery, leaving a peripheral layer of slowly moving blood that clots to form the mural thrombus. The normal, smooth, firmly adherent fibrous neointima becomes lined with a thick, gelatinous, loosely adherent mural thrombus that reduces the functioning lumen to the diameter of the outflow vessel. Fragmentation with distal embolization or progressive narrowing of the graft lumen with secondary acute thrombotic occlusion may then occur.[62] Anastomotic

false aneurysms, although relatively rare causes of late limb ischemia, may also produce peripheral embolization or thrombosis of the aneurysm and the adjacent vessel lumen.[64] Finally, aortoiliac and femoral reconstructions can progress suddenly to thrombosis from percutaneous catheter interventions, cardiac embolization or decreased cardiac output secondary to myocardial infarction or congestive heart failure. Rarely, no apparent cause for late thrombosis can be identified, implicating thrombogenicity of the graft surface or degeneration and disruption of the neointima.

The diagnosis of late thrombosis is suggested by the sudden or progressive recurrence of symptoms, a decrease or loss of previously present distal pulses, and a concomitant reduction in ankle pressure indices, Doppler flow, or pulse-volume recording waveform. The degree of ischemia after thrombosis of a reconstruction is usually more severe than before the primary revascularization procedure.[56,59] The frequency of late thrombosis increases from 5% to 10% in the first 5 years to 20% to 30% at 10 years.[48,63,66-68] Therefore, routine and long-term follow-up of these patients at regular intervals is required to monitor the adequacy of graft function. If significant stenosis can be demonstrated before complete thrombosis, surgical correction is simplified. When either abrupt or gradual change is apparent, prompt imaging studies should be performed to determine the status of the graft, the anastomoses, the inflow, and the runoff bed.[47,69]

The severity of recurrent ischemia may range from minimal to severe claudication to rest pain to pregangrene, depending on the extent of compensating collaterals and the vigor of the patient's normal activity. Imaging studies are required to determine whether further surgery is feasible and to guide the surgeon in the selection of the most appropriate reoperative or interventional procedure, considering the patient's age, health status, and level of activity.[57,64]

Correction of late thrombosis requires preoperative delineation of the underlying anatomical problem, followed by appropriate corrective maneuvers.[64,70] The occlusion of one limb of an aortoiliac bifurcation graft is usually caused by overlooked or progressing disease in the external iliac and femoral arteries. Thrombolytic therapy may be useful in delineating the artery involved by the progression of atherosclerosis. Balloon catheter angioplasty with stenting is not usually indicated because of the extent of the disease or location beneath the inguinal ligament. One reliable solution consists of retroperitoneal exposure of the occluded limb, balloon catheter thrombectomy, and graft extension to the femoral level. Femorofemoral bypass is an alternative if the donor iliofemoral inflow is satisfactory, especially in a high-risk patient. Axillofemoral bypass may be required if neither of the preceding methods is feasible.[6,50]

The most commonly encountered situation is a thrombosed aortofemoral graft limb with impaired outflow. Inflow can usually be restored by the use of catheter-based thrombolysis, or surgical or percutaneous graft thrombectomy using a balloon thromboembolectomy catheter or mechanical thrombectomy device with or without regional lytic agents (Figure 57-7).[70] A

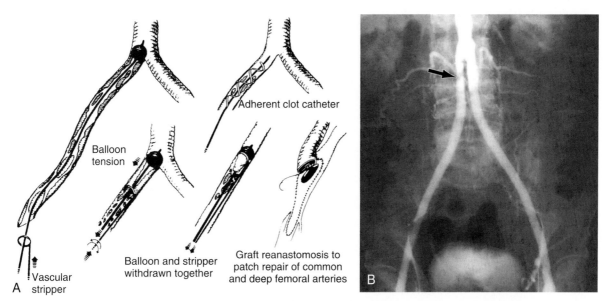

FIGURE 57-7 ■ **A,** A ring endarterectomy stripper is used in conjunction with a balloon catheter or adherent clot catheter to remove thrombus and pseudointima adherent to the wall of an occluded limb of an aortofemoral graft. The cleared graft limb is then sutured to the common or deep femoral outflow after patch angioplasty. **B,** Intraoperative arteriogram demonstrating residual thrombus *(arrow)* in the proximal right limb of an aortobifemoral graft after attempted thrombectomy. (**A,** From Bernhard VM: Late vascular graft thrombosis. In Bernhard VM, Towne JB, editors: Complications in vascular surgery, ed 2, New York, 1985, Grune and Stratton, p 193.)

thromboendarterectomy stripper or adherent clot catheter is often required to complete the extraction of adherent clot and old pseudointima. The Fogarty occlusion catheter is passed through the ring of the stripper into the patent aortic portion of the graft, and its balloon is fully inflated and pulled down to occlude the proximal end of the limb to control bleeding and prevent crossover embolization. The stripper is passed back and forth and rotated around the catheter within the occluded graft limb up to the distended balloon to scrape thrombus from the graft wall. Thereafter, the balloon is deflated just enough to permit its tight withdrawal through the graft limb along with the stripper and detached thrombus (see Figure 57-7). Use of the Fogarty adherent clot catheter obviates the need for the thromboendarterectomy stripper. The patient is systemically heparinized (100 to 125 U/kg) during all these maneuvers.

Thrombectomy is usually combined with a profundoplasty of varying extent to provide outflow. However, femoropopliteal or femorodistal bypass may be required, depending on the extent and location of outflow disease (Figure 57-8).[50,51,70,71] If an occluded graft limb cannot be reopened by thrombectomy, a femorofemoral graft can be inserted. Replacement of the graft limb is another alternative but is technically more difficult. Endovascular options include thrombus removal by catheter aspiration, thrombus dissolution with hydrodynamic catheters such as the Cordis Hydrolyser, the BSIC Oasis and Angiojet systems: mechanical clot destruction combined with tissue plasminogen activator (TPA) (Trellis Device) or some of the newer mechanical devices. These mechanical therapeutic modalities are often combined with the use of thrombolytic agents.[72] Percutaneous thrombectomy is more frequently used to treat lower extremity graft or native arterial occlusions. The use of these mechanical and aspiration thrombectomy catheters to treat aortofemoral limb occlusion is limited to small series and isolated case reports.[73]

If an entire bifurcated graft is thrombosed, a problem at the proximal anastomosis such as low placement of the graft with progression or unrecognized proximal disease, kinking, or anastomotic aneurysm, or cardiac embolization is a likely cause. Imaging with CTA, MRA, or DSA is required to identify proximal progression of disease. If no proximal problem can be demonstrated, thrombectomy with either a balloon or an adherent clot catheter can be attempted but is usually not successful. The alternatives are to replace the original prosthesis or insert an axillobifemoral bypass. The latter procedure is less technically demanding and less hazardous and is the reoperation of choice in a physiologically compromised patient.[70] When groin scarring is especially intense, bypass to the mid-deep femoral artery simplifies the outflow repair of the reoperative procedure by avoiding a tedious and hazardous dissection in the area of a previous femoral anastomosis.[74]

Endovascular treatment of this complication may be feasible in selected patients by establishing inflow with covered stents or stent grafts after dissolution or removal of the thrombus. An aggressive attitude toward reoperation after thrombotic failure of aortoiliac reconstruction is warranted, especially if the patient will derive sustained benefit from long-term patency and improved limb function.[70] Operative morbidity and mortality rates are low. Reoperative mortality rates of 3% and cumulative 3-year patency rates of 68% to 75% have been reported.[56,70] Judicious use of extraabdominal approaches has contributed significantly to reduced reoperative morbidity and mortality.[64]

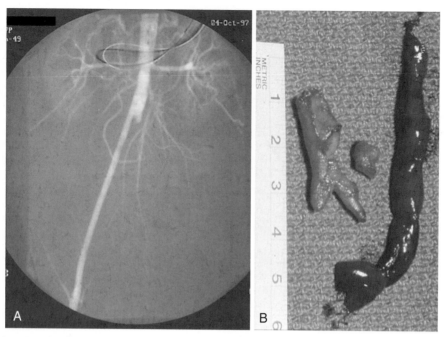

FIGURE 57-8 ■ **A,** Angiogram of the occluded limb of an aortofemoral graft. **B,** The operative specimen demonstrating the thrombus and plaque removed from the proximal superficial femoral and profunda femoris arteries. See Color Plate 57-8.

Lytic Therapy for Graft Thrombosis

Whereas thrombectomy has been the treatment of choice in the management of occluded aortofemoral and femoropopliteal bypass grafts, incomplete removal of thrombotic material and the difficulties associated with reoperation have led to the evaluation of direct intra-arterial infusion of thrombolytic agents, either preoperatively or intraoperatively, for the management of this problem.[75] The potential benefits of lytic therapy include delineation of the cause of the graft thrombosis (most commonly distal occlusion caused by intimal hyperplasia or progression of disease) and, as a consequence, shorter operation time, reduced blood loss, ease of extracting any residual thrombus, and reduced wound complication rate. Potential disadvantages and complications of thrombolytic therapy include the need for monitoring in an intensive care unit, delay in surgical intervention, and risk of bleeding or renal impairment from the contrast load required for frequent angiographic evaluation. Further, mechanical thrombectomy for aortofemoral graft limb occlusion is at least as effective as clot lysis and adds little to the operative procedure required to restore outflow.

Kuhn and colleagues,[76] in a series of 129 patients with acute and subacute occlusions of native arteries (77) and bypass grafts (55), reported recanalization with r-tPA thrombolysis in 73.6% of cases. There was no statistically significant difference in primary therapeutic success rates between native arteries and bypass grafts. The morbidity rate was 31% (minor complications, 20.2%; major complications, 10.9%), and the mortality rate was 2.3%. Twenty-seven patients required radiologic and surgical interventions within 12 months, with a limb salvage rate after primary successful recanalization of 89.5%.[76] Successful lysis, which does not appear to be affected by the duration and cause of the graft thrombosis, can be achieved in 50% to 90% of occluded prosthetic graft limbs, 50% to 77% of saphenous veins, and 38% to 71% of prosthetic grafts.[77-82]

The thrombolytic agents used clinically are recombinant thrombolytic peptides represented by recombinant tissue plasminogen activator (r-tPA) that enzymatically break down cross-linked fibrin strands within the thrombus by converting plasminogen to plasmin. The three recombinant thrombolytic peptides that are clinically relevant are alteplase (r-tPA), reteplase (r-PA), and tenecteplase (TNK). r-PA and TNK have been structurally modified from native r-tPA to increase their half-life and fibrin specificity. TNK possesses a longer half-life, improved fibrin specificity, and increased resistance to plasminogen activator inhibitor and has been shown to have a better safety profile compared with t-PA in patients with acute myocardial infarction (MI). A meta-analysis of studies comparing thrombolysis with surgical intervention concluded that peripheral catheter-directed intraarterial thrombolysis (PIAT) resulted in higher limb salvage rates and lower mortality rates than surgical intervention. Limb salvage rates at 30 days in patients receiving PIAT were 93% compared with 85.5% with surgery. These higher limb salvage rates were maintained at 6- to 12-month follow-up (89% vs. 73%). Mortality at 30 days was 4% for PIAT compared with 15% for surgical patients. This trend in mortality rates was maintained at the 6- to 12-month follow-up (8% vs. 29%), respectively.[83-85]

Infusion of the thrombolytic agents is usually accomplished by a multi–side-hole catheter or an infusion wire placed so that it covers the extent of the thrombus. There are multiple dosage regimens advocated for the use of these agents. Usually a loading dose followed by a continuous infusion is given: t-PA at 0.25 to 10 mg/h, r-PA at 0.25 to 1 U/h, and TNK at 0.25 to 0.5 mg/h. Heparin in a dose of 300 to 500 U/h is usually administered through the access sheath to prevent pericatheter thrombosis.[86-90]

Patients are monitored carefully in the ICU for evidence of bleeding. Blood is drawn for hemoglobin, hematocrit, platelet count, fibrinogen, PT, and aPTT every 6 hours. After successful lysis, the underlying lesion is treated with either catheter-based techniques or surgery. Long-term anticoagulation with warfarin is usually indicated.

Bleeding, the major complication of lytic therapy, occurs after 7% to 48% of infusions.[80,91] The most common sources of bleeding are angiography or venous puncture sites, the interstices of prosthetic grafts, and systemic bleeding at remote sites. Central nervous system bleeding is the most lethal complication. Bleeding from a groin arterial puncture site may also result in femoral pseudoaneurysm or retroperitoneal hematoma, which may compress the femoral nerve within the iliac fascia or in the thigh. The resulting femoral neuralgia, reported to occur in up to 30% of patients, may persist for as long as 1 year.[92,93] Rarely, a femoral nerve palsy develops in patients; this may be extremely debilitating, especially in patients with claudication or amputation of the contralateral limb. There is some evidence that the risk of bleeding may be higher with t-PA than with either r-PA or TNK.

The most important determinant of the long-term success of lytic therapy is the presence of a lesion correctable by surgical revision or balloon catheter dilatation.[94] Such lesions responsible for the occlusion can be identified in approximately 21% to 30% of patients with 86% to 89% patency at 1 year compared with 37% of a similar number of grafts without correctable lesions.[94]

The results of three prospective studies comparing the efficacy of intraarterial thrombolysis and surgery in patients with lower limb ischemia reported successful catheter placement in 72%, clot dissolution in greater than 70%, and limb salvage at 1 year in greater than 80%.[76,95-97] In a study of 114 patients with acute lower limb ischemia of less than 7 days' duration who were randomized to either thrombolytic therapy or surgery, Ouriel and colleagues achieved clot dissolution in 70% and observed equivalent limb salvage rates (82%) and improved patient survival (82% vs. 58%) in the patients receiving thrombolytic therapy at 1 year.[95] They attributed the improved survival in the thrombolytic group to the more frequent occurrence of cardiopulmonary complications in the patients undergoing surgery. In a subsequent study, Ouriel and associates randomized 213 patients with acute limb ischemia of less than 14 days' duration to either recombinant urokinase or surgery.[96] Clot lysis was achieved in a similar number of patients (71%) but there was no difference in either mortality rate (14% vs. 16%) or amputation-free survival rate (75% vs. 65%) between the two groups at 1 year. In the Surgery versus Thrombolysis for Ischemia of the Lower Extremity (STILE) trial,[97] the efficacy of rt-PA and urokinase was compared with that of surgery in 393 patients with limb ischemia of less than 6 months' duration. Failure of catheter placement occurred in 28% of patients. Patients with ischemia of less than 14 days' duration receiving

lytic therapy had lower amputation rates than did surgical patients, whereas patients with ischemic symptoms of more than 14 days' duration fared better with surgery. The results of these studies suggest that in selected patients, thrombolytic therapy may be a useful adjunct or alternative to surgical therapy. However, long-term patency rates of 28% to 37% of thrombolysed grafts are clearly inferior to those obtained with surgery.[94,98] Thrombolytic therapy may be extremely valuable in patients with limb-threatening ischemia secondary to thrombosed popliteal aneurysm. Thrombolysis may improve the chances of achieving long-term patency and limb salvage.[99]

Reteplase differs from alteplase both in its structure and biochemical composition and in its lower affinity for thrombin. McNamara reported a 34% incidence of bleeding in a series of 40 patients treated with t-PA compared with 3% among those receiving r-PA at doses of 2 to 8 mg/hour.[100] Even reducing the dosage of t-PA to 0.5 to 1 mg/hour was still associated with a 25% incidence of bleeding requiring transfusion.

In all cases, the risks and benefits of the use of lytic therapy in the treatment of patients with graft limb occlusions must be evaluated carefully.

The relatively low incidence of complications, improved technique of administration, and efficacy of thrombolytic agents have reduced the need for urgent surgical thrombectomy in patients with noncritical limb ischemia. Successful lytic therapy readily identifies the cause of the graft limb occlusion and may allow a less extensive repair. In addition, lytic therapy may reduce the risk of wound and graft complications and reduce the incidence of reperfusion edema and compartment syndrome associated with extensive redo procedures.

Mechanical Thrombectomy

Mechanical thrombectomy devices that theoretically permit rapid revascularization of an ischemic extremity using minimally invasive techniques are gaining in popularity. The use of mechanical energy to cause fragmentation, dissolution, and aspiration of thrombus is appealing. These devices can be classified broadly into (1) aspiration thrombectomy catheters that remove the thrombus by steady manual suction through a large-lumen aspiration catheter; (2) pull-back thrombectomy catheters that withdraw the thrombus with a balloon catheter or basket into a trapping device, allowing the clot to be removed; (3) recirculation thrombectomy devices that ablate the thrombus by hydrodynamic vortices, which pulverize the thrombus into microscopic fragments; (4) nonrecirculation thrombectomy devices, which macerate the thrombus mechanically into fragments that are larger than those produced by recirculation catheters; and (5) energy-assisted devices that use ultrasound, laser, or radiofrequency to lyse the thrombus or enhance the effects of pharmacologic agents.[101] Several of these devices are currently being evaluated clinically, with complete angiographic success reported in approximately 50% of patients and partial success in an additional 27%.[102] Concomitant lytic therapy or balloon angioplasty is often a necessary adjunct.

The most extensively studied device is the AngioJet rheolytic thrombectomy system, which is approved for peripheral arterial and coronary applications.[103] The Trellis thrombectomy system uses a 7-French drug dispersion catheter with proximal and distal occlusion balloons. Oscillation of the dispersion wire and infusion of a lytic agent allow both mechanical fragmentation and lytic dissolution of the clot. Chief limitations of the current devices include catheter size and working length, the possibility of fluid overload, hemolysis, and cost effectiveness. The major treatment limitation of these devices is their lack of efficacy against organized thrombotic or embolic material.[72,73,104]

Atheroembolism

Preoperative Embolism

Atherothrombotic debris is present to varying degrees in most atherosclerotic arteries but especially in the distal aorta. Protruding atheromas of the aortic arch and descending aorta have assumed increasing importance as potential sites for embolization during catheter manipulation in the aorta for cardiac catheterization, carotid stenting placement of thoracic endografts, or bypass surgery.[105] Embolization may also occur spontaneously or with the use of anticoagulants and thrombolytic therapy.[106] Readily detectable by transesophageal echocardiography, lesions >0.5 cm are most likely to be associated with embolic events.[107,108] Evidence of spontaneous embolization has also been demonstrated at autopsy studies, but the incidence appears to be low (0.3% to 0.7%).[109,110] The effects of spontaneous embolization may be exacerbated by dislodgement of atheromatous debris during intraoperative manipulations.

Intraoperative Embolism

Variable amounts of atherothrombotic material may be dislodged and carried to a downstream territory as a consequence of manipulation during arterial dissection and clamp placement.[34,89,90] After cardiac operative procedures, 66% of emboli lodge in the gastrointestinal (GI) tract and 48% lodge in the kidneys. Visceral embolization occurs in 40.9% of patients undergoing aortic reconstruction with the "Shaggy" aorta syndrome.[111] Embolization may also occur on reestablishment of circulation owing to the accumulation of fresh thrombus in the temporarily static column of blood above or below the clamps if it is not carefully evacuated before circulation is restored. In the immediate postoperative period, atheroembolism should be suspected if the blotchy areas of discoloration of the skin of the abdominal wall and extremities and toes and impaired renal function do not improve with warming and optimization of cardiac output. A nonspecific systemic response characterized by fever, eosinophilia, elevated erythrocyte sedimentation rate (ESR) and highly specific C-reactive protein (hsCRP) may accompany an embolic episode.

Larger emboli lodging in major vessels can usually be retrieved with a balloon thrombectomy catheter. Smaller embolic particles that cannot be retrieved will be flushed

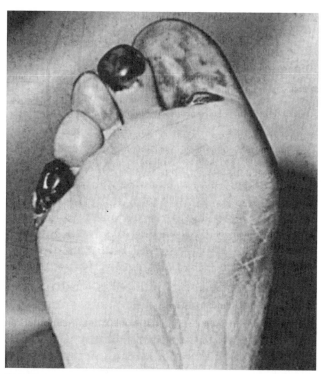

FIGURE 57-9 ■ Atheroembolic ischemic lesions of the toes. (From Eastcott HHG: Complication of aortoiliac reconstruction for occlusive disease. In Bernhard VM, Towne JB, editors: Complications in vascular surgery, New York, 1980, Grune and Stratton, p 59.)

into end arteries of the feet or toes, leading to the "trash foot" syndrome.[5,47,108,112] The end result is the appearance of patchy areas of painful skin gangrene at these sites (Figure 57-9). This may be a minor and self-limited problem, or it may produce extensive gangrene of all the digits and the forefoot, leg, buttocks, and rarely the abdominal wall.

Prevention is key because it is frequently difficult or impossible to treat this complication. Careful review of preoperative imaging studies will determine the site of clamp placement. A variety of technical maneuvers has been used to prevent or minimize operative embolization.[5] Unnecessary and overly vigorous handling of vessels before the application of clamps should be avoided. Effective preclamping heparinization, monitored by intraoperative measurement of the ACT, reduces stasis thrombus formation above the proximal clamp and in the sluggish circulation distally. In patients with suspected or demonstrable atheromatous debris within the aorta on CT scans, the distal clamps should be applied to the common femoral or iliac arteries before proximal occlusion to avoid downstream displacement of debris when the aortic clamp is placed. The proximal clamp may need to be placed at the level of the diaphragm if the pararenal segment of the aorta appears to be involved. The lumen of the aortic prosthesis should be thoroughly aspirated to remove blood and debris after testing the proximal suture line, and efforts should be made to prevent the accumulation of blood within the prosthesis while distal iliac or femoral anastomoses are being performed. Vigorous antegrade flushing of the proximal vessel and retrograde flushing from the distal arteries as the last few stitches are being placed in an anastomosis, before the restoration of circulation, is the most reliable maneuver to ensure that retained debris and clot are effectively removed.[112]

Treatment depends on the severity of embolization. Minor patchy areas of cyanosis or necrosis can be observed, with spontaneous recovery anticipated. More extensive involvement with threatened viability of the distal foot requires attempted removal of embolic material with small Fogarty balloon catheters passed into the distal vessels through the patent popliteal artery. Distal intraarterial infusion of r-tPA may be applicable in selected patients. Occasionally, when there is severe ischemia of a single or multiple digits, lumbar sympathectomy or amputation may be necessary. Low-dose corticosteroids may offer short-term benefit in patients with acute or subacute renal failure with systemic symptoms but have no favorable effect on long-term renal outcome.[113,114] Statins, which stabilize atherosclerotic plaques and potentially improve outcomes, should be offered to all patients. Whether intensive lipid-lowering statin therapy for 3 to 6 months before surgery in patients at known risk of embolization will prove beneficial is presently unknown.[115]

Declamping Hypotension

A sudden decrease in blood pressure should be anticipated after removal of the aortic clamp to restore flow to one or both extremities after aortoiliac reconstruction.[116-119] The cause is hypovolemia resulting from incompletely replaced blood loss and fluid sequestration during surgery, compounded by a variable degree of preoperative dehydration that is usually present.[120] Contributing factors are peripheral vasodilatation secondary to limb ischemia during the period of aortic occlusion and a decrease in cardiac output caused by a sudden return of acidic blood and other vasoactive metabolites to the central circulation on restoration of limb perfusion. The major consequences are significant reduction in coronary perfusion, which may promote myocardial injury, especially in patients with significant coronary artery disease, and temporary renal ischemia, which may contribute to renal failure. Prevention is preferable to treatment after a hypotensive insult has already occurred and depends on adequate hydration and effective restoration of intravascular volume during the procedure, and especially before clamp release.[118-120] Effective volume replacement requires careful monitoring of blood loss and accurate estimation of the extracellular fluid shifts caused by sequestration and loss from evaporation. The extent of intravascular depletion is directly related to the duration of intraperitoneal and retroperitoneal exposure during surgery.

The most reliable guide to ensuring adequate volume replacement without circulatory overload is the use of a Swan-Ganz catheter to monitor left-heart filling pressures and myocardial performance.[120] Cooperation between the surgeon and the anesthesiologist is essential during the critical moments before clamp release. Left atrial filling pressures should be optimized before release of the clamps. The arterial pressure must be continuously observed while blood flow is slowly restored to the extremities by gradual release of the clamps until full flow can be tolerated without hypotension. Finally, when a bifurcated graft is inserted, it is best to complete the anastomosis to one limb and restore its circulation immediately so that lower body perfusion can be resumed with the least amount of delay; this avoids washout acidosis and reduces declamping hypotension.

Acute Renal Failure

Renal impairment in patients undergoing abdominal aortic surgery is an important cause of morbidity and mortality and can range in severity from acute renal injury (ARI) to acute renal failure (ARF). Acute renal injury, manifest by the occurrence of albuminuria (93%) and proteinuria (22%) in patients undergoing aortic surgery is the mildest form of impairment. Albuminuria usually occurs before cross-clamping and peaks between 0 and 6 hours after declamping. Acute renal dysfunction according to the RIFLE criteria (Risk, Injury, Failure, Loss of renal function, and End-stage renal disease) defined as an increase in serum creatininte (sCR) of 50% from baseline or oliguria of less than 0.5 mL/kg/h for 6 hours may progress to acute renal failure manifest as a 200% increase in sCR and oliguria of less than 0.5 mL/kg/h for 24 hours or anuria.[121]

The reported incidence of ARF after elective aortic aneurysmectomy is 1% to 8%, with a mortality rate of 40%. However, if the aneurysmectomy is emergent, the reported incidence of ARF is 8% to 46%, with a mortality of 57% to 95%.[122,123] The major cause of ARI is reduced renal perfusion resulting from decreased cardiac output, decreased blood volume, and dehydration. A contributing factor is renal cortical vasospasm produced by infrarenal application of the aortic clamp, which stimulates the renin-angiotensin mechanism.[124,125] Other promoting factors include: underlying renal artery stenosis; suprarenal aortic cross-clamping (which totally eliminates renal perfusion); ischemia reperfusion injury; ligation of the left renal vein; intraoperative embolization; older age; hypertension; and drugs such as diuretics, β-blockers, calcium antagonists, nephrotoxic antibiotics, nonsteroidal antiinflammatory drugs, cyclooxygenase 2, and angiotensin-converting enzyme inhibitors.[126] Cholesterol embolization to the kidneys may originate from debris and clot accumulating proximal to the aortic clamp or from manipulation of the juxtarenal aorta.[123,127] Preoperative contrast (CTA, DSA) and endovascular catheter manipulations may produce a mild to moderate degree of renal dysfunction, which can be compounded by blood loss, hypotension, and dehydration during the operative procedure. Renal artery obstruction may be produced by displacement of large atherosclerotic plaques, thrombus, or dissection at the orifices of the renal arteries when an aortic clamp is applied. Myoglobinemia can occur after restoration of circulation to limbs that have been severely ischemic for an extended period. Finally intraabdominal hypertension or intraabdominal compartment syndrome (ICS), especially in patients with ruptured aneurysms, must be considered.

Although the consequences of ischemic injury to the kidney are complex, injury to the tubules, especially the S3 segment of the proximal tubule and the thick ascending limb of the loop of Henle, is central to the development of oliguria.[128] Obstruction of the tubular lumen by cellular debris and casts results in a reduction of the ultrafiltration pressure and sequestration of tubular fluid within obstructed tubules, in addition to back-leakage of fluid into the interstitium.[129]

The critical issue in ARF is prevention, which is related primarily to the maintenance of an effective circulating blood volume and adequate hydration in the immediate perioperative period.[123,130] It is essential that the patient be well hydrated and have a good urinary output at the commencement of surgery. Any significant extracellular fluid volume deficits should be restored the evening before surgery, especially if CTA, DSA, or mechanical bowel preparation has recently been performed. The sCR level should be measured after procedures requiring contrast administration, and if a decrease in renal function is identified, surgery should be delayed, if possible. Central filling pressures should be monitored perioperatively to ensure that volume replacement is optimal in relation to cardiac output and myocardial performance.[120] It is appropriate to give mannitol and commence an infusion of renal-dose dopamine (2 to 3 µg/kg) just before cross-clamping the aorta to promote an osmotic diuresis and reduce the effects of renal cortical vasospasm.[124] Bicarbonate is given to alkalinize the urine if there is any question of significant contrast-related nephrotoxicity or myoglobin washout from renewed perfusion of limbs that have undergone prolonged ischemia. Renal insufficiency is a significant complication of surgical procedures requiring cross-clamping of the thoracic or suprarenal aorta. Currently, a number of therapeutic maneuvers including preoperative statins, n-acetylcysteine, heme-oxygenase, ischemic preconditioning, fluid loading, renal cooling, calcium-channel blockers, atrial natriuretic peptide, endothelin antagonist and fenoldopam are being evaluated in cardiac patients to determine their efficacy in reducing the incidence of ARF. The data regarding renal protection in vascular surgery patients are conflicting and have been extrapolated primarily from patients undergoing cardiac surgery procedures.[131-137]

During dissection required to gain proximal control of large infrarenal or juxtarenal aneurysms, the left renal vein and its branches are vulnerable to injury. Access to this portion of the aorta is facilitated by division of the left renal vein close to its origin from the IVC, thus preserving the tributaries and reducing renal venous congestion if the vein cannot be re-approximated at the completion of the aortic anastomosis.[138] In the past, this maneuver was viewed as one of little long-term consequence. However, Huber and coworkers[139] and Abu Rahma and associates[140] demonstrated increased sCR concentrations in patients who had renal vein ligation. Whether the renal dysfunction after renal vein ligation is solely a consequence of the resultant increased venous pressure or develops from a combination of venous hypertension and transient ischemia from intraoperative suprarenal clamp placement, which is required

more frequently than with infrarenal clamp placement (11% vs. 18%), is not yet clear. Nonetheless, it is prudent to repair the renal vein if there is congestion of the left kidney and reanastomosis can be accomplished without undue tension or prolongation of the procedure.[1,138,141,142]

Renal arteries should be dissected free and temporarily clamped in patients with aortic occlusion and thrombus that extends up to the renal orifices. The quality of the renal pulses must be evaluated and the blood flow assessed by Doppler color-flow imaging after restoration of circulation through the aorta in any patient who has had significant juxtarenal aortic manipulation.

Postoperatively, the continued retroperitoneal and intraperitoneal sequestration of extracellular fluid requires replacement with lactated Ringer solution, within the limits imposed by left-heart filling pressures, to ensure adequate renal output.[23] Volume replacement should be reduced after the second postoperative day to prevent fluid overload from the mobilization of large volumes of sequestered extravascular fluid. The urinary output is monitored continuously and should be maintained at or above 0.5 mL/kg/h. The specific gravity is determined frequently, and the blood urea nitrogen and sCR are measured daily for 2 or 3 days to determine the quality of renal function. Diuretics should not be given until intravascular volume has been fully restored. A rise in sCR, the standard marker used to detect ARF does not allow for the early diagnosis of ARI because of a lack of specificity for ARI; poor correlation with glomerular filtration rate; and the influence of age, sex, body mass index, hydration, and nutrition. Several biomarkers are currently being investigated in patients undergoing cardiac surgery to improve the detection of early renal dysfunction. Cystatin C, kidney injury molecule-1 (KIM-1), N-acetyl β-D-glucosaminidase (NAG), and neutrophil gelatinase–associated lipocalin (NGAL) are among the early detectable biomakers in the serum and urine of patients with ARI. However, correlation of individual markers with glomerular filtration rate is variable, and a combination of markers may by required to improve the sensitivity of these molecules in the early diagnosis of ARI.[121,143] At the onset of ARF, urinary specific gravity increases (>1.015) and sodium and urea decrease. Once tubular necrosis occurs, the urine becomes isothenuric; the urinary sodium, fractional excretion of sodium, and urea increase to greater than 20 mml/L, greater than 1%, and greater than 35%, respectively; and the ratio of blood urea nitrogen (BUN)-to-creatinine ratio falls from 20:1 to 10:1.[128] If ARF is diagnosed, fluid replacement should be restricted to maintain central filling pressure in the normal range. Dialysis is used aggressively to control excess volume and relieve azotemia and hyperkalemia.[123,144] Intravenous hyperalimentation or parenteral nutrition should be instituted early in the clinical course of patients with ARF to minimize protein catabolism.[145]

Renal artery stenosis or impaired renal function is frequently present in patients undergoing aortic reconstruction for occlusive and aneurysmal disease. The liberal use of CTA, MRA, and DSA before surgery is recommended to identify renal anomalies, renal artery stenoses, or suprarenal extension of an aneurysm so that appropriate alterations in operative management can be planned. Often, renal revascularization can be accomplished by balloon angioplasty and stenting, along with operative or endovascular correction of the aortic disease. In this setting, patients often have impaired renal function, and the large volume of contrast agents used for imaging studies or intervention may result in additional nephrotoxicity. The preoperative administration of n-acetylcysteine has been shown to reduce contrast-related ARF from 12% to 2% to 4%.[146,147] A cautionary note regarding the use of n-acetylcysteine in the immediate perioperative period: Wijeysundera and coworkers have shown that its use is associated with greater transfusion requirements in patients undergoing cardiac surgery procedures.[133] Additional maneuvers to reduce the risk of renal ischemia include the use of temporary renal perfusion with cold lactated Ringer solution containing heparin, mannitol, and methylprednisolone.[123] Postoperatively, a renal perfusion scan or aortography should be performed immediately if total renal shutdown occurs because this suggests a renal artery occlusion. This requires immediate reoperation to restore kidney circulation. The use of statins in the early postoperative period has been shown to lower the incidence of AKI in cardiac surgery patients. Welten and associates, in a study of 2170 patients undergoing lower extremity bypass or abdominal aortic surgery, demonstrated that early statin use increased the odds of recovery if renal function deteriorated postoperatively.[148,149] In addition, statin use was also associated with improved long-term survival irrespective of changes in renal function.

Intestinal Ischemia

Intestinal ischemia may complicate aortic bypass or endarterectomy for occlusive disease, but the majority of cases involve the colon and follow aneurysmectomy.[150,151] Almost all reported instances of intestinal ischemia following aortic surgery are a result of arterial obstruction or hypotension; venous ischemia is extremely rare.[152] Small bowel ischemia occurs in 0.15% of cases.[150] The clinical presentation of ischemic colitis occurs in 0.2% to 10% of aortic procedures and most commonly involves the rectosigmoid area.[150] Data from the Swedish Vascular Registry showed a frequency of transmural colon necrosis of 7.3% and 2.8% in patients undergoing repair of ruptured AAA with and without preoperative hypotension; 23% of deaths were associated with colonic ischemia. The overall mortality rate for patients with colon ischemia is approximately 50% and approaches 90% for transmural colon involvement.[153]

The cause of bowel ischemia is interruption of the primary or collateral arteries to the bowel wall or operative atheroembolization.[150,151] Two sets of vessels are critical to colon perfusion: (1) The inferior mesenteric artery and its left colic branch, which connect with the superior mesenteric artery through the arc of Riolan and, to a lesser extent, the marginal artery of Drummond, and (2) the superior rectal branch of the inferior mesenteric artery, which connects with the middle and inferior rectal branches of the hypogastric vessels, thus connecting the visceral and systemic circulations.[154] The former connection is referred to as the "meandering mesenteric artery,"

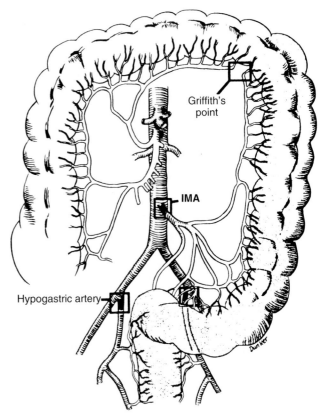

FIGURE 57-10 ■ Lack of marginal artery continuity at the splenic flexure (Griffith's point), with inferior mesenteric artery (IMA) and hypogastric artery occlusions predisposing to left colon ischemia. (From Ernst CB: Colon ischemia following abdominal aortic reconstruction. In Bernhard VM, Towne JB, editors: Complications in vascular surgery, New York, 1980, Grune and Stratton, p 383.)

especially when it becomes enlarged as a collateral to compensate for superior or inferior mesenteric artery obstruction.[155] This vessel is present in approximately two thirds of healthy people and can be seen on angiography in 27% to 35% of patients who have aneurysmal or occlusive disease.[156] Areas of deficiency in this normal anatomic relationship are at Griffith's point at the splenic flexure and in the collateral vessels of the rectosigmoid (Figure 57-10).

Obstruction of the primary arteries supplying the viscera makes viability of the bowel dependent on this collateral circulation. Occlusion of the orifice of the inferior mesenteric artery is frequently associated with aneurysmal disease and obstructive aortic atherosclerosis, thus placing the burden of bowel circulation on collaterals from the superior mesenteric artery and the hypogastric vessels. Severe obstruction or occlusion of the superior mesenteric artery is compensated for by branches from the celiac artery and retrograde flow from the inferior mesenteric artery through the left colic and middle colic arteries. Hypogastric obstruction requires collateral flow from branches of the inferior mesenteric artery. When this source is also impaired, colon circulation must depend on more tenuous connections between the arch of Riolan and the marginal artery and the distal branches of the hypogastric, which in turn take their blood supply from the parietal circulation.

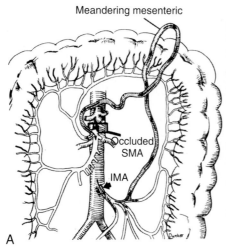
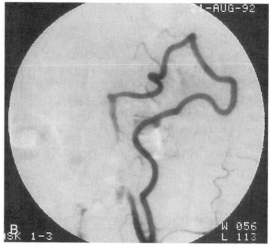

FIGURE 57-11 ■ **A,** When the superior mesenteric artery (SMA) is occluded, meandering mesenteric blood flow is from the inferior mesenteric artery (IMA) to the SMA. Meandering mesenteric sacrifice under these conditions predisposes to small bowel as well as colon ischemia. **B,** Selective visceral angiogram demonstrating a meandering mesenteric artery. (**A,** From Ernst CB: Colon ischemia following abdominal aortic reconstruction. In Bernhard VM, Towne JB, editors: Complications in vascular surgery, New York, 1980, Grune and Stratton, p 385.)

A critical loss of blood flow to an intestinal tract that is dependent on this extensive collateral network may occur if a patent inferior mesenteric artery is ligated during aortic surgery. Collateral flow may be further compromised by ligating the inferior mesenteric artery peripherally rather than flush with the aortic wall because this may occlude the connection between the left colic and superior rectal arteries. Failure to ensure perfusion through at least one hypogastric may promote colon ischemia if this is the primary supply in the absence of the inferior mesenteric artery or effective collateral flow from the meandering artery. Loss of the inferior mesenteric artery or the meandering artery produces right colon and small bowel ischemia when these viscera depend on retrograde flow because of superior mesenteric arterial occlusion (Figure 57-11). The large hematoma associated with a ruptured aneurysm may compress significant collateral vessels, which may explain the high incidence of colon ischemia in this circumstance.[156] Furthermore, angiography is almost never available before repair of a ruptured aneurysm, and the surgeon has no precise information regarding intestinal circulation to allow the design of an operative procedure that will conserve or augment colon perfusion. Prolonged hypotension and the use of vasopressors may exacerbate the effects of preexisting occlusive disease. Recently Djavani and coworkers have demonstrated a correlation between raised intrabdominal pressure and colonic hypoperfusion in patients with ruptured AAA.[157] A relatively unrecognized cause of mesenteric ischemia is cardiopulmonary bypass. Abdominal complications after coronary artery bypass occur in <1% of patients. Acute mesenteric ischemia accounts for 10% to 67% of these complications, with mortality rates of 70% to 100%.[158] Preexisting visceral occlusive disease, cardiac or aortic arch embolization, use of an intraaortic balloon, postoperative renal failure, female gender, duration of cardiopulmonary bypass, and cross-clamp times are important contributing factors.[159]

Depending on the severity of ischemia and the thickness of the bowel wall involved, three forms of ischemic colitis are recognized. Type I is mucosal ischemia, which is transient and mild. Type II, with mucosal and muscularis involvement, reflects more severe ischemia that may result in healing with fibrosis, scarring, and stricture. Type III is transmural ischemia, which produces irreparable damage with gangrene and bowel perforation.[160]

The clinical manifestations of intestinal ischemia immediately after aortic surgery are often masked by incisional discomfort and other problems that may explain abdominal pain, tenderness, fever, an elevated white blood cell count, and fluid sequestration. Findings that suggest the presence of intestinal ischemia and progressing infarction of the colon include progressive distention, sepsis, increasing peritoneal signs, and unexplained metabolic acidosis. The most common clinical presentation is diarrhea—either brown liquid or bloody—which occurs in 65% to 76% of patients with intestinal ischemia.[154,161] Although the onset may occur as long as 14 days after operation, diarrhea usually appears within 24 to 48 hours after surgery.[154] Bloody diarrhea has been reported to be a more ominous prognostic sign than nonbloody diarrhea; however, some investigators have noted no correlation between extent of ischemic injury and presence of bloody diarrhea.[162]

Postoperative *Clostridium difficile* colitis may mimic ischemic colitis. Therefore, in critically ill patients who develop fever, abdominal distension, diarrhea, and leukocytosis after emergency aortic procedures, stool specimens for culture and for *C. difficile* toxin should be obtained and endoscopic evaluation of the colon performed. Appropriate oral antibiotic therapy (metronidazole or vancomycin) should be instituted if the diagnosis of *C. difficile* is confirmed.[163,164]

Because of the high mortality rate associated with transmural colonic ischemia (80% to 100%), early diagnosis is the key to effective management. The diagnosis

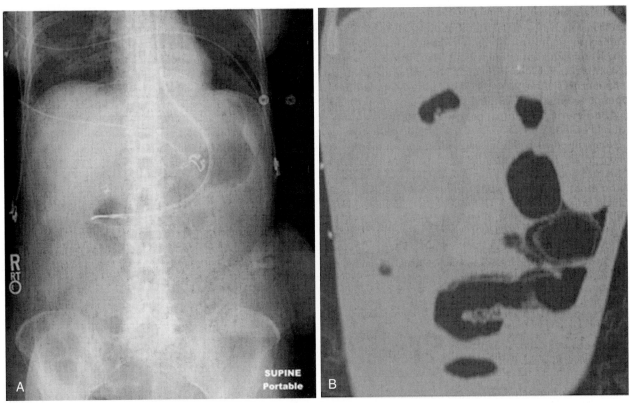

FIGURE 57-12 ■ A, Plain abdominal radiograph showing air in the wall of the colon. **B,** CT scan showing dilatation of the sigmoid colon and edema of the bowel wall, which is characteristic of colonic ischemia.

depends on a high index of suspicion and the prompt performance of endoscopy with the flexible sigmoidoscope or colonoscope.[163] In a prospective study of 100 patients undergoing aortic reconstructive procedures, Zelenock and associates[165] observed a 3% incidence of endoscopic colonic ischemia. Adjunctive procedures were used in 12% of these patients, compared with 4% in earlier studies from their institution. Sigmoid colon pH monitoring begun before surgery and continued postoperatively has been used with some success by Björck and Hedberg to identify patients at risk for ischemic colitis.[166] They found that a sigmoid colon pH below 6.86 for 9 to 12 hours had a sensitivity of 100% and a specificity of 97% for predicting ischemic colitis. When sigmoid colon acidosis below 7.10 pH was reversed within 2 hours, no major complications developed, but when it was prolonged, 8 of 10 patients developed major complications. Further evaluation of sigmoid colon pH monitoring appears warranted before its widespread application. The occurrence of ischemic colitis without left colon involvement is rare enough that endoscopy to 40 cm is usually sufficient to establish the diagnosis.[150] Once ischemic colitis is detected, endoscopy should be terminated to avoid perforation. Mild changes of ischemic colitis consist of submucosal hemorrhage and edema that is usually circumferential. Pseudomembranes, erosions, and ulcers indicate more advanced ischemia. A yellowish-green, necrotic, noncontractile surface indicates gangrene.[154] Repeated endoscopy, every other day by the same individual, is required to document resolution or progression of the process. In a recent report, Acosta and

colleagues demonstrated elevated D-dimer concentrations in patients with acute mesenteric ischemia.[167] This elevation was especially helpful in female patients with atrial fibrillation. Wider application of this test to other causes of acute mesenteric ischemia awaits validation.

Patients under observation for intestinal ischemia are managed by frequent re-examination; serial endoscopy; sigmoid colon and gastric intramucosal pH monitoring; monitoring of blood gases and serum lactate levels, white blood cells and D-dimers, urine output, and fluid requirements; institution of broad-spectrum antibiotic coverage; and bowel rest with nasogastric suction. Intramucosal pH measurements are not readily available and serial endoscopy may result in bowel perforation. Plain radiographs may demonstrate a nonspecific ileus, dilated loops of bowel, or thumb printing; intramural or portal vein gas are rarely seen and usually indicate late-stage disease. Computed tomography scans may show vascular occlusion, intramural gas, free air or intraperitoneal fluid, and infarcts in the kidneys liver and spleen (Figure 57-12). CTA is also helpful in diagnosing nonocclusive mesenteric ischemia. If the colon appears distended, either clinically or radiographically, it should be decompressed by the gentle insertion of a rectal tube because increased intraluminal pressure may further compromise colon blood flow.[154,166] If sustained intraabdominal hypertension (IAH) is present (>20 mm Hg), the patient should be treated with muscle relaxants or abdominal decompression. Optimum fluid management remains controversial. Balogh and colleagues compared two different fluid regimes in trauma patients (500 mL and 600 mL/

min/m^2) and concluded that over-aggressive resuscitation doubled the risk of IAH, abdominal compartment syndrome, organ dysfunction, and death. Although no similar studies have been done in patients with ruptured AAA, there is some evidence that resuscitation with large volumes of isotonic crystalloids increases the risk of complications.

Improvement of the patient, as evidenced by diminishing diarrhea, improvement in vital signs, clinical examination, laboratory values, and resolution of the ischemia documented by endoscopy, permits continuation of nonoperative management.[150] Reversible ischemic lesions should improve within 7 to 10 days.[160,168] Continuing clinical evidence of ischemia beyond 2 weeks requires operative intervention because this usually reflects a walled-off perforation with local peritonitis.[154] Finally, progression of intestinal ischemia during the period of observation, identified by deteriorating clinical signs and symptoms, requires prompt celiotomy. Surgery for transmural ischemic colitis requires resection of nonviable bowel, end-colostomy, and formation of a Hartmann's pouch or resection of the rectum, if involved.[169]

Prevention of intestinal ischemia depends on an appreciation of the potential for this complication and the institution of appropriate steps to either avoid injury to the collateral circulation of the colon or augment circulation to the bowel as part of the aortic reconstructive procedure.[170] Spiral CTA or MRA is frequently used preoperatively to evaluate the abdominal aorta and its visceral branches. This technique permits multiple views of complex aortic lesions, reflects the true diameter of aortic aneurysms, and may alleviate the need for angiography.[171,172] Identification of a patent inferior mesenteric artery with retrograde flow through a large meandering artery that is functioning as a collateral pathway for an obstructed superior mesenteric artery requires preservation of flow through the inferior mesenteric; this orifice is spared by constructing an end-to-side aortic anastomosis or by reimplanting the inferior mesenteric onto the side of an aortic graft using a variation of the Carrel patch technique.[150]

Bypass to the superior mesenteric artery should also be considered.[170] A large, meandering artery with flow from the superior mesenteric toward the sigmoid and rectum in the presence of inferior mesenteric artery occlusion is strong evidence of adequate collateral supply to the bowel.[155] Ischemic colitis is unlikely under these circumstances if this collateral is not impaired by surgery. The status of the hypogastric vessels should be identified on the aortogram or other imaging study so that arterial reconstruction can be designed to maintain flow through at least one of these arteries by direct revascularization or by retrograde perfusion from a femoral anastomosis, especially if a patent inferior mesenteric artery must be ligated.[168]

Measurement of the inferior mesenteric artery backpressure during aortic reconstruction may be a useful guide to the need for restoration of flow to the inferior mesenteric artery.[168] A mean pressure greater than 40 mm Hg and an inferior mesenteric artery–systemic pressure ratio greater than 0.4 indicate satisfactory collateral circulation without the need for mesenteric arterial repair.

Intraoperative duplex ultrasonography in patients undergoing visceral artery repair allows prompt correction of underlying technical defects.[173]

Thorough mechanical preparation of the bowel before aortic surgery reduces the fecal burden to which the potentially ischemic bowel is exposed.[150] During aortic surgery, every effort should be made to prevent injury to the mesenteric vessels. Undue traction on the left colon mesentery should be avoided. When inferior mesenteric ligation is required, this should be carried out by suture ligature within the aortic lumen or immediately adjacent to the aortic wall to avoid injury to its ascending and descending branches.[150] Finally, the presence of Doppler flow signals over the base of the bowel mesentery and the serosal surface of the colon suggests that adequate collateral circulation is present.[161] Absence of a flow signal after reconstruction suggests the need to restore perfusion through the inferior mesenteric artery or through some other major collateral vessel. The association of severe visceral and aortic occlusive disease in younger female patients is accompanied by high mortality and morbidity rates. The severe weight loss resulting from celiac and superior mesenteric artery occlusive lesions makes complete revascularization a hazardous undertaking. In these individuals, a combination of endovascular treatment of the visceral occlusive disease before aortic revascularization may decrease the early morbidity and mortality rates, as well as improve long-term survival.[174]

Gastrointestinal Complications

Gastrointestinal complications occur in 6% to 21% of patients undergoing elective procedures and in 27% of those undergoing emergent aortic procedures. This complication is associated with a prolonged ICU stay and increased mortality (48%) from multisystem organ failure. Paralytic ileus, mechanical small bowel and duodenal obstruction, acute pancreatitis, upper GI bleeding, *C. difficile* enterocolitis, acute cholecystitis, chylous ascites, colonic and rectal ischemia, and liver failure are among the GI complications described. This discussion will be limited to paralytic ileus and mechanical small bowel and duodenal obstruction, the most common problems encountered. The increase in intraoperative blood loss and postoperative fluid requirements associated with these complications accounts for the prolonged requirement for mechanical ventilation and the occurrence of renal failure. Intraoperative hypotension, gastric hyperacidity, visceral embolization, hematoma, sac seroma, superior mesenteric artery syndrome, bowel wall edema, adhesions, and a compromised collateral blood supply are among the etiologic factors contributing to the development of GI complications after aortic surgery. Paralytic ileus is the most common cause of delayed return of small bowel function after abdominal aortic procedures. Small obstruction (SBO) is reported to occur in approximately 2.9% of patients undergoing aortic reconstruction for AAA (n = 818) or occlusive (n = 657) disease within 4 to 28 (mean, 6) days postoperatively. The incidence of SBO after aortic surgery is much lower than the 9.5% reported after nonvascular abdominal operations, although almost 50% of the patients reported by Ellozy had undergone a previous abdominal operation. Duodenal obstruction after AAA repair is rare, with only 16 cases reported in the English literature. The presentation is often delayed, with symptoms occurring 8 to 60 days (mean, 13.3) postoperatively. Surgeons must maintain a high level of suspicion to anticipate possible GI complications. Symptoms include increased nasogastric tube output, nausea, bilious vomiting, abdominal pain, distension, hematemesis, hematochezia, diarrhea, fever, leucocytosis, and a decrease in hematocrit level. Diagnostic tests should include plain abdominal and chest radiographs; CT scanning; upper GI endoscopy; and laboratory monitoring of hemoglobin, hematocrit, white blood cells, amylase and lipase, BUN, sCR, and electrolytes. Early postoperative SBO requiring surgical intervention carries significant morbidity, including abdominal and wound sepsis, fistula formation, wound disruption, and persistent obstruction. Therefore, a 1- to 2-week trial of conservative therapy in these patients is reasonable. Patients with obstruction lasting longer than 2 weeks almost always require operative relief of the obstruction.

Fluid and electrolytes should be replaced, a nasogastric tube reinserted, and nutrition provided. In the series reported by Siporin and colleagues, 18 of 44 (41%) patients with SBO required reoperation (lysis of adhesions, 18; bowel resection, 2) within 6 to 30 days (mean, 14.2) of the initial aortic procedure, whereas only 13% of the nonvascular patients required re-exploration: one required small-bowel resection.[175-180] Conservative treatment with nasogastric decompression is recommended in all patients initially in the absence of bowel ischemia or perforation. Operative relief of the obstruction is indicated in patients with obstruction lasting longer than 2 weeks or if complications ensue. The mortality rate ranges from 0% to 5%. There were no bowel infarctions, small bowel fistulas, or late graft infections in the aortic patients undergoing laparotomy for bowel obstuction.

Abdominal Compartment Syndrome

Intraabdominal compartment syndrome (ICS) is defined as an increase in intraabdominal pressure (IAP) greater than atmospheric pressure (IAP >20 mm Hg or bladder pressure >30 mm Hg) with the new onset of organ dysfunction. In vascular patients, ICS is most commonly encountered with intraperitoneal or contained retroperitoneal AAA rupture after open surgery or EVAR. Sometimes ICS may occur after mesenteric revascularization for ischemic bowel or massive retroperitoneal bleeding in patients on anticoagulants. The increase in intraabdominal pressure is exacerbated by massive fluid resuscitation and positive end-expiratory pressure ventilation (PEEP). Physiologically, an increase in IAP causes elevation of the diaphragm, resulting in a decrease in lung capacity and compliance and respiratory compromise. The associated decrease in venous return, compounded by hypotension, reduces cardiac output and increases peripheral resistance, resulting in impaired

renal, hepatic, and mesenteric perfusion; an increase in bacterial translocation from the gut; and raised intracranial pressure, which, if uncorrected, results in the increased morbidity and mortality in these patients. Ischemia of the abdominal wall results in edema and decreased compliance, further exacerbating the effects of ICS. Direct measurement of IAP is possible but increases the risk of infection. The indirect method requires emptying the bladder and instilling 50 to 150 mL of saline; the drainage tubing is clamped and a needle attached to the pressure transducer is inserted above the clamp and the pressure determined. If the bladder pressure exceeds 20 mm Hg, the pressure should be monitored hourly. A bladder pressure of greater than 30 mm Hg is diagnostic of ICS.

In patients at high risk for postoperative ICS, leaving the abdomen open (OA) at the completion of the initial surgery should be considered. Several options including suture or sequential towel clip closure of the skin; use of a Bogota bag silo; fascial interposition of an absorbable, biological, or nonabsorbable mesh; and use of a vacuum pack or wound vac dressing are available to manage the OA. A short course of a neuromuscular blocking agent may decrease fascial edge retraction and be a useful adjunct to negative pressure devices and conservative measures. Neuromuscular blockade decreases IAP; however, once the paralysis wears off, the IAP returns to baseline levels. Once ICS is diagnosed, decompressive laparotomy and creation of an OA as outlined above is undertaken. Patients with an acute increase in IAP (25 mm Hg) without acute organ dysfunction should also be considered for prophylactic decompressive laparotomy. Postoperatively, efforts should be focused on correcting the oxygen and energy debt, hypothermia, and coagulopathy. As the visceral edema resolves, the abdomen is closed either primarily or with biological or nonabsorbable mesh. The survival of patients with ruptured AAA treated with OA and delayed fascial closure is 50% compared with 27% when the fascia is closed primarily.[157,181,182] Djavani and associates reported 0% mortality and 0% left colon ischemia in patients with ruptured AAA (rAAA) and normal IAPs compared with 22% and 44%, respectively, when the IAP was >21 mm Hg.[157] Patients reoperated for ICS had a mortality rate of 84%.[183]

Abdominal Wall Hernias

The relationship between AAA and abdominal wall hernias (AWHs) is well recognized. However, the prevalence of AAA in patients undergoing inguinal hernia repair remains controversial. In a study of men greater than 55 years of age undergoing inguinal hernia repair, Antoniou and colleagues[184] detected AAA in 8.1% in the hernia group and 3.9% in controls. In subjects with aortic diameters greater than 4.0 cm, the prevalence was 5.1% in the hernia group compared with 1.5% in those without inguinal hernias. In contrast, Andersen and Shiralkar detected only 2 AAAs (3%) in a prospective evaluation of 70 men older than 65 years undergoing inguinal hernia repair.[185] Midline, paramedian, oblique, and transverse incisions are commonly used to expose the abdominal aorta.[186-190] Although transverse incisions are associated with the lowest complication rate, their use is often limited to patients with pulmonary insufficiency. Despite the reported benefits of oblique incisions, a significant number of complications, including long-lasting wound pain and bulging in 11% to 23% of patients and incisional hernias in 7%, have been reported.[189,191] Presumably, the diffuse bulging is caused by muscle atrophy resulting from a combination of factors, including division of the intercostal nerves, incision-related muscular injury, and reduced blood supply. Gardner and colleagues were able to decrease the incidence of bulging from 11% to 0.03% by preserving the 11th intercostal nerve.[192]

The incidence of midline ventral hernias ranges from 10% to 37% and is more common in patients undergoing aortic repair of AAA than those having surgery for occlusive disease. Takagi and associates reported a 3-fold increased risk in both inguinal and incisional hernias in patients with AAA compared with those with occlusive disease.[191,193,194] CT scans and MRI are used with increasing frequency to diagnose the discontinuity of the fascial layers with protrusion of the abdominal viscera because clinical examination may underestimate the prevalence of incisional hernias. The prevalence of incisional hernia detected by CT was 22% at 24 months compared with 8% detected clinically.[195] Two distinct types of defects can be identified. Focal periumbilical defects are almost invariably the result of poor technique. The diffuse bulging associated with lateral retraction of the recti is far more commonly observed in patients with incisional hernias after undergoing aortic aneurysmal resection than aortofemoral bypass for occlusive disease (Figure 57-13). Several studies have found no difference in the incidence of the usual risk factors—age, chronic obstructive pulmonary disease, diabetes, smoking, wound infection, length of ICU stay, and amount of blood transfused—between patients who developed incisional hernias and those who did not.

Mass suturing of the musculoaponeurotic layers of the abdominal wall using monofilament or braided suture is the most frequently used technique to close midline incisions. A meta-analysis of the method of abdominal wound closure after AAA repair, concluded that the ideal suture for abdominal fascia closure was a running nonabsorbable monofilament suture. Also, a suture length–to–wound length ratio greater than 4 reduces the incidence of incision lesions.[196,197] It cannot be overemphasized that careful suture technique with placement of bites 2 cm from the edge and 1 cm apart is essential if this complication is to be prevented. The prophylactic placement of a polypropylene mesh has been shown by Bevis and coauthors to reduce the incidence of incisional hernias without increasing the rate of complications in patients undergoing elective AAA repair.[198] Whether these data can be verified in larger series and the prophylactic use of mesh proves cost effective remain to be determined.

Primary repair using monofilament nonabsorbable suture is appropriate for closure of small periumbilical defects. Surgical or laparoscopic repair using prosthetic mesh is usually necessary to repair large defects in the upper abdomen.[199,200] The incidence of seromas and recurrence rates remain high. The relationship among AWH, AAA, and circulating proteases and their inhibitors is currently being investigated.

Chylous Ascites

Chylous ascites, issuing from a damaged cisterna chyli and its tributaries at the root of the mesentery, is a rare complication of aortic reconstruction and performance of a Warren shunt.[201] In a review of the literature, Pabst and coauthors found that approximately 75% of cases occurred after AAA resection, 19% after aortic reconstruction for occlusive disease, and the remaining 7% after resection of infected aortic grafts.[202] Interruption of

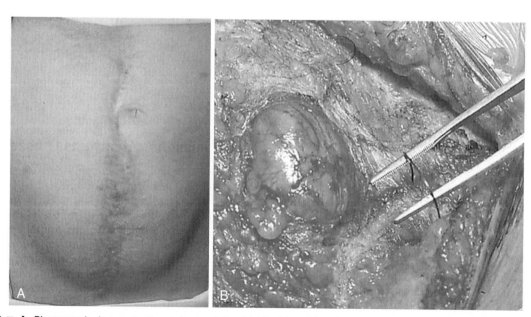

FIGURE 57-13 ■ **A,** Photograph demonstrating a large abdominal incisional hernia in a patient after repair of an abdominal aortic aneurysm. **B,** Operative photograph demonstrating the intact sutures adjacent to the fascial defect. See Color Plate 57-13.

the lymphatics and chylous ascites are not invariably related because the lymphatics are often interrupted during aortic operations without apparent sequelae.[201,203] Patients with chylous ascites typically present within 2 or 3 weeks of aortic repair with anorexia and progressive abdominal distension. Chylous ascites can result in nutritional imbalance, immunologic deficit, and respiratory dysfunction. Ascites is usually evident on physical examination and can be confirmed by abdominal radiography, ultrasonography, or CT scanning. Abdominal paracentesis reveals a milky fluid, with a high lymphocyte count and lipid content, which is bacteriologically sterile. The ascitic fluid is usually contained within the abdomen. Leakage of ascites to the outside through a defect in the incision increases the fluid and protein loss and heightens the risk of infection. Such a leak should be repaired surgically or laparoscopically under sterile conditions and prophylactic antibiotic coverage. Methods used to identify the site of the leak include lymphoscintigraphy, lymphangiography, direct opacification of the thoracic duct with oral fat emulsion observed by CT, and injection of Evans blue dye. The reliability of these tests in identifying the location of the leak or fistula remains unestablished.[204]

The management of chylous ascites includes abdominal paracentesis, a low-fat diet rich in medium-chain triglycerides, and total parenteral nutrition. However, repeated paracentesis may result in the loss of large amounts of protein and lipid that cannot quickly be replaced. An additional risk is that of line-related sepsis. In patients who do not respond to repeated paracentesis, a peritoneal venous shunt, in addition to diet control or total parenteral nutrition, may relieve the ascites. Whether the use of octreotide or fibrin glue accelerates the resolution of ascites remains unclear.[205] Surgical or laparoscopic ligation may be necessary in resistant cases.[201,202] Recurrence of ascites after surgical repair is rare.[206]

Spinal Cord Ischemia

Spinal cord ischemia occurs most frequently during repair of thoracic and thoracoabdominal aneurysms but is sometimes encountered during resection of AAA and, rarely, after aortoiliac bypass for ischemia.[126,207,208] The overall incidence of this complication has been reported to be 0.26% open AAA repair and 0.21% higher after endovascular aneurysm repair and is tenfold after the repair of rAAA than after elective aneurysm resection.[208-210] In a review of series of more than 100 patients undergoing open repair for rAAA, Peppelenbosch and coauthors found an incidence of spinal cord ischemia of 1.2% (0% to 2.8%), with a mortality rate of 46.9% (35.6% to 65.2%).[211] The incidence of spinal cord ischemia after thoracic aortic reconstruction is in the range of 1% to 10%, depending on the extent of the lesion repaired. Patients undergoing thoracic endovascular aortic aneurysm repair (TEVAR) after prior AAA repair have a 12.5% risk of spinal cord ischemia compared with 1.7% for those without prior AAA repair.[212]

The upper level of the neurologic deficit was found to be T10 to L2 in 39 of 44 patients (88.6%) reviewed at the Henry Ford Hospital.[209] Postoperative mortality was directly related to the severity of paraplegia. When the neurologic deficit was complete initially, involving both sensory and motor function, 76% of the patients died; there were only two complete neurologic recoveries and one partial recovery. By contrast, when the initial deficit was only partial motor or sensory loss, 24% died and some degree of recovery was noted in all but one patient.[208,213,214]

In the report of spinal cord ischemia by Peppelenbosch and colleauges, 72.7% of the patients presented with hemodynamic shock and 38.2% required suprarenal clamp placement during rAAA repair; 42% of the patients had complete infarction of the spinal cord, 33% had anterior spinal artery syndrome, and the remaining 21% had varying degrees of cord involvement. The diagnosis was often delayed and made within 3.2 ± 5.2 days after surgery.

The major cause of spinal cord ischemia is interruption of flow through the great radicular artery of Adamkiewicz, which is the major source of supply to the anterior spinal artery at the lower end of the cord.[207,215] The great radicular artery is a major branch of the posterior division of one of the intercostal vessels, arising between T8 and L1. On occasion, it may originate from a lumbar branch of the infrarenal aorta. The anterior spinal artery itself is long and has rather poor collateral contributions from the posterior spinal arteries or from the radicular arteries derived from more proximal intercostal vessels. Because the spinal cord is only tenuously supplied in its lower portion by vessels other than the great radicular artery, embolization or injury to this vessel during aortic reconstruction may lead to some degree of cord infarction. The effectiveness of collateral pathways may be further compromised by hypotension, especially in patients with ruptured aneurysms; prolonged clamp placement; ligation or occlusion of the hypogastric, lumbar, or sacral arteries; and retrograde dissection from the aortic anastomosis occluding intercostal arteries. The placement of a high aortic clamp for temporary control of a ruptured aneurysm, however, does not clearly correlate with the incidence or severity of spinal cord ischemia.[208]

Until recently angiography was the most frequently used imaging modality to visualize the artery of Adamkiewicz in patients with thoracoabdominal aneurysms. The relatively low visualization rates of 43% to 86% with angiography has led to the more frequent use of CTA and MRA to evaluate these patients. MRA has detection rates of 67% to 100% compared with 18% to 100% with CTA.[216-218] The very low incidence of spinal cord ischemia after operations of the infrarenal aorta and the frequent use of CTA and MRA in the evaluation of patients with AAA render angiographic visualization impractical and potentially dangerous.[140,215-217] Moreover, the occurrence of this complication remains unpredictable and may not be preventable in association with infrarenal aortic reconstruction. Monitoring of somatosensory evoked potentials during thoracic surgery has been shown to correlate with cord ischemia.[219] These abnormal findings have been reversed by temporary shunting and implantation of intercostal vessels into the thoracic aortic graft. Practical application of this

Techniques for Preserving Internal Illiac Blood Flow

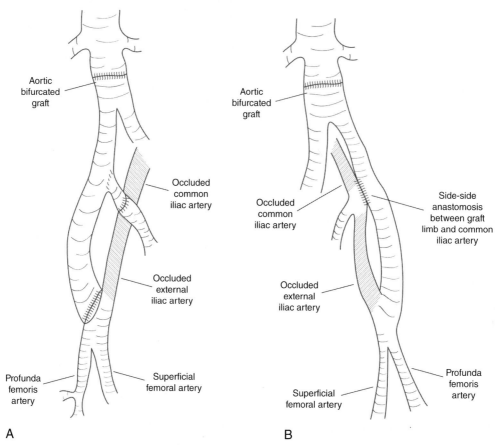

FIGURE 57-14 ■ Techniques for internal iliac revascularization in patients with external and common iliac occlusion. **A,** Interposition graft. **B,** Endarterectomy and side-side anastomosis.

technique to abdominal aortic surgery is undergoing continued investigation.[219-222]

Although there are no data to identify specific preventive measures, it is prudent to avoid prolonged high aortic clamping unless absolutely necessary, to maintain cord perfusion pressure by avoiding systemic hypotension, and to prevent stasis thrombosis in collateral vessels by effective heparinization. Suturing a patch of posterior aortic wall with its intercostal vessel orifices into a window cut out of the graft has been recommended for thoracoabdominal aneurysms.[126] Finally, it is important to ensure pelvic perfusion through one or both hypogastric arteries to maximize collateral contribution to the spinal cord (Figure 57-14).[223] The diagnosis of spinal cord ischemia is made clinically and confirmed by CT and MRI.

When ischemic injury to the spinal cord occurs, treatment is palliative and supportive.[208] Several drugs including steroids, rosuvastatin, cilastozol, angiotensin ll receptor blockade, and oxygen-free radical scavengers are being investigated to limit the extent of or prevent neurologic damage after aneurysn repair.[224-227]

Ureteral Injury and Obstruction

The ureters are immediately adjacent to the operative field and may be easily injured during dissection and arterial repair.[228] This is especially important in patients with large iliac and hypogastric aneurysms or when there is increased adherence to vascular structures in the presence of an "inflammatory" aneurysm or retroperitoneal fibrosis.[229] Nachbur and associates, in a study of 220 patients with asymptomatic aneurysms evaluated with CT scanning, observed 20 cases of ureteral obstruction.[230] In 8 patients, ureteral obstruction was associated with inflammatory aneurysms; in the remaining 12, it was associated with abdominal aortic, common iliac, and hypogastric atherosclerotic aneurysms. A thorough knowledge of the anatomic relationships of the ureters at the level of the iliac bifurcation is essential. Sometimes, multiple ureters may be present or they may be in an aberrant position, owing to congenital anomalies. Although intravenous pyelography and sonography have been used as first-line studies, contrast-enhanced CT and MRI are the most reliable diagnostic modalities. A preoperative contrast-enhanced CT scan is especially indicated in reoperative aortoiliac surgery to identify postoperative changes in the ureteral anatomy or demonstrate possible injury incurred during the initial surgery.

Direct injury to the ureter can best be avoided by keeping the dissection close to the iliac artery at the point where the ureter normally crosses the common iliac bifurcation in transit to the bladder. This is especially important during the blind development of the retroperitoneal tunnel for aortofemoral bypass. The ureter should be elevated away from the iliac vessels so that the graft will lie dorsal to it. Inadvertent passage of the graft ventral to the ureter may cause it to be compressed between the graft limb and the underlying iliac artery, producing hydroureter and hydronephrosis. The incidence of ureteral obstruction after aortic grafting in one prospective study was 2%.[231] However, the ureter may be entrapped in perigraft scar, even if it is placed in its proper position ventral to the prosthesis.[228]

Both ureters should be demonstrated before closing the retroperitoneum. The right ureter must be carefully protected during retroperitoneal closure because this structure can easily be caught up in the suture line. Iatrogenic ureteral injuries sustained during placement or revision of a vascular graft should be repaired primarily. Although renal salvage is possible when the diagnosis is delayed, nephrectomy is often necessary if there has been extensive contamination of the graft.[232] Sometimes, an intraoperative ureteral injury is overlooked, and the diagnosis is delayed for days or weeks. Once recognized, placement of a percutaneous nephrostomy tube may be associated with a shorter hospital stay and lower infection rate than with open repair.[233,234]

Ureteral obstruction was present in 57% of patients with idiopathic retroperitoneal fibrosis (IRF) reported by Kermani and coauthors.[235] Retroperitoneal fibrosis may be idiopathic (2/3) or secondary (1/3) to drugs (e.g., alkaloids, dopamine agonists, β-blockers, hydralazine, and analgesics); malignancy (carcinoma of the prostate, colon, or breast; lymphoma, carcinoids); infection; renal trauma; hemorrhage; and radiation or chemotherapy. Retroperitoneal fibrosis with encasement of the ureters also accompanies inflammatory aortic aneurysms.[235-237] The fibrotic encasement of IRF is usually concentrated at the aortic bifurcation. Ureteric obstruction may also occur after open or endovascular AAA repair and is the most common cause of hydronephrosis after aortic surgery. Postoperative hydronephrosis can be categorized as early (occurring within 6 months) or late (after 6 months). Temporary asymptomatic hydronephrosis can be detected on CT scans in 12% to 30% of patients, and mild to moderate permanent ureteral dilatation is seen in 2% to 14% of patients undergoing aortic surgery. The fibrosis is usually secondary to bleeding; excessive dissection, ligation, or devascularization of the ureter; or pseudoaneurysm formation. Ureteral obstruction is believed to be more common when the limb of the graft is tunneled anterior to the ureter. However, hydronephrosis secondary to anterior graft placement occurs in only 30% of cases. The majority of patients have a clinical presentation within 1 year of the procedure, but delayed presentation up to 14 years has been reported. Approximately 30% of patients manifest with symptoms, including pain, recurrent bouts of urinary tract infection, azotemia, or hematuria.[238-240]

Wright and associates reported a 35-year experience with 58 ureteral complications in 50 patients undergoing aortoiliac reconstructions.[241] Two of the six patients with ureteral obstruction treated before, or in conjunction with, repair of the aneurysm developed graft complications (1 graft limb thrombosis and 1 graft infection). The remaining 44 patients had 46 complications, including hydronephrosis (42), ureteral leaks (3), and ureteral necrosis (1). Twenty-four patients had 36 graft complications, including anastomotic aneurysm (19), graft limb thrombosis (8), graft infection (6), and aortoenteric fistula (3). Twenty-nine of the 44 patients underwent graft or ureteral operations, or both, with a mortality rate of 21%.

The status of the ureters should be carefully evaluated in patients with inflammatory aortic aneurysms with retroperitoneal fibrosis. Hydronephrosis recognized preoperatively should be treated with ureteral stent placement to decompress the obstruction and facilitate ureteral identification during repair. In a systematic review of open surgical repair (OSR) versus EVAR of inflammatory AAA, Paravastu and colleagues[242] reported regression of the periaortic fibrosis in 73% of the OSR patients compared with 65% in the EVAR group. Forty-five patients undergoing OSR and 29 undergoing EVAR had preoperative ureteric obstruction, which regressed postoperatively in 69% and 38% of patients, respectively. Inflammation progressed in 1% and 4%, respectively. The authors suggest that OSR may be the preferred treatment in patients with hydronephrosis. Postoperative hydronephrosis detected by ultrasonography or CT can initially be followed expectantly because it often resolves on its own. Only 12 of the 58 patients reported by Wright and coworkers required surgical intervention for progressive hydronephrosis.[241] The selective use of balloon dilatation, stents, and antibiotics in conjunction with operative repair is essential if the high incidence of graft complications is to be reduced (Figure 57-15).

Impotence

The loss of ability to achieve or maintain an erection adequate for satisfactory coitus may be a result of psychogenic or vasculogenic causes. Current evidence suggests that up to 80% of cases have organic causes,[5] which are subdivided into vasculogenic, neurogenic, and hormonal etiologies. Vasculogenic etiologies represent the largest group, with arterial or inflow disorders being the most common.[243]

Eighty percent of patients who have aortoiliac occlusive disease have significant erectile dysfunction (ED).[244] Among the contributing factors are age, hypertension, diabetes, smoking, alcohol abuse, lipid disorders, heart disease, β-blockers, ACE inhibitors, and urologic and liver disease. Medications account for up to 25% of cases. In a survey of sexual function after elective open (EO), ruptured open (RO), and endovascular AAA repair, the prevalence of ED was 27% (EO), 63% (EVAR), and 45% (RO) preoperatively, and postoperatively was 58%, 76%, and 67%, respectively.[245,246] Approximately 25% of patients will have iatrogenic ED if appropriate technical modifications are not used. Therefore, careful evaluation of penile erectile function by history, noninvasive techniques, and angiography should be included in the preoperative evaluation before elective aortic surgery.[247,248] This will determine whether there is normal sexual function that should be preserved or whether

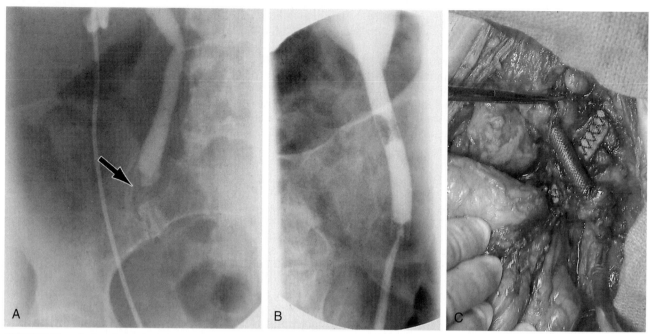

FIGURE 57-15 ■ **A,** A stricture is present in the distal ureter as it crosses over the limb of an aortofemoral graft *(arrow)*. **B,** After dilatation of the stricture, a stent was placed. **C,** Erosion of the ureter by the stent resulted in a 3-cm defect in the ureter and exposure of the limb of the graft.

there is already an established pattern of impotence that might be relieved by altering pelvic blood flow. This information provides valuable insights into the possible psychogenic and cultural factors contributing to an existing problem and gives the surgeon an estimate of the importance of sexual function to the patient. Such preoperative information may alter the type of aortic operation planned.

Preoperative evaluation of erectile function includes nocturnal tumescence studies. The absence of tumescence during an adequate sleep study is strong evidence of organic impotence. Documentation of normal erections during rapid eye movement sleep establishes the psychogenic basis of the patient's ED. Unfortunately, the failure to achieve erection is often qualitative rather than complete, making tumescence studies less discriminating between organic and psychogenic impotence.[244,248]

If organic impotence is suspected, the next step is noninvasive vascular testing. At present, the most reliable measurement is the penile systolic pressure and the penile-brachial index (PBI).[244] Kempczinski and Birinyi found that age had a deleterious effect on the PBI independent of sexual potency.[244] Patients younger than 40 years had a mean PBI of 0.99 compared with a PBI of 0.74 for equally potent men older than 40. This difference was statistically significant. By contrast, impotent men older than 40 had a mean PBI of 0.58, also a statistically significant difference. Despite the significant differences in PBI measurements in these three groups, there is poor correlation between PBI and the degree of ED.[248,249] Although a low PBI is not sufficient to establish the diagnosis of vasculogenic impotence, the finding of a PBI greater than 0.8 confirms the adequacy of penile blood flow and suggests that a vasculogenic cause is extremely unlikely.[244]

Neurogenic impotence is commonly a result of neuropathy secondary to diabetes mellitus, or it may follow autonomic nerve injury from genitourinary or abdominopelvic surgery. This diagnosis is often one of exclusion, but abnormal pudendal nerve velocity studies (sacral latency testing) and abnormal cystometrography (the anatomic pathways in micturition and erection being similar) can implicate this cause.[244,250]

The diagnosis of endocrinologic impotence requires measurement of thyroid function and serum levels of testosterone and other associated hormones. Finally, a thorough medication history is required.[250]

Preoperative angiography is useful in identifying the patency of the hypogastric vessels and their contribution to pelvic perfusion. Unfortunately, angiographic findings correlate poorly with the patient's erectile function.[244] Selective injections to identify the flow through the pudendal vessels into the penis may be required to more accurately assess patients with primarily vasculogenic impotence.[244]

Although the findings on preoperative angiograms correlate poorly with erectile function, preservation of adequate perfusion into at least one hypogastric artery appears to be a vital component in minimizing iatrogenic impotence.[244] When possible, direct antegrade perfusion of the internal iliac artery should be ensured. This may require thromboendarterectomy of the hypogastric orifice. Sometimes angioplasty, stenting, or operative endarterectomy of the orifices of one or both hypogastric arteries will improve erectile function. If both external iliac arteries are occluded or stenotic, and bypass into the common femoral arteries is anticipated precluding retrograde iliac flow, the proximal aortic anastomosis should be constructed end to side when feasible to preserve pelvic blood flow. When proximal aortic disease is extensive (requiring an end-to-end proximal anastomosis) and impaired penile perfusion has been diagnosed by preoperative, noninvasive testing, it may be necessary to reimplant the hypogastric artery into one limb of an aortobifemoral graft or add a jump graft to one hypogastric artery to improve pelvic inflow (see Figure 57-14).[244,250] Finally, careful flushing of the graft in both directions before completion of the final suture line is important to prevent embolization of small particles into the pelvic arteries. DePalma and colleagues[251] reported spontaneous erectile function in 58% of patients with impotence undergoing aortoiliac reconstruction compared with 27% after microvascular procedures.

Retrograde Ejaculation

Ejaculatory dysfunction is not uncommon after aortic surgery. Earlier series reported an incidence of 30% to 75%, but in more contemporary series, the incidence ranges from 3% to 9%.[252,253] This lower incidence is clearly the result of both an increased awareness of the anatomy controlling ejaculation and improved surgical technique. Emission and closure of the bladder neck to ensure antegrade ejaculation are dependent on innervation by postganglionic fibers of the lumbar sympathetic nerves arising from T11 to L3. The loss of one or both functions as a result of dissection in the region of the aortic bifurcation results in dry ejaculation.[254,255]

Careful preservation of the sympathetic-parasympathetic plexus overlying the aorta and its bifurcation and maintenance of blood flow through the hypogastric and pudendal arteries are the important factors in preventing retrograde ejaculation and impotence in men undergoing elective aortic surgery.[247,253,256] Dissection should be carried down to the aortic wall on its right anterolateral surface and the para-aortic structures gently retracted to the left to avoid trauma to the nerves contained within these tissues (Figure 57-16). During aneurysm resection, the inferior mesenteric artery should not be dissected free but should be controlled by suture ligature from inside the aorta after the aneurysm has been opened to avoid disruption of nerve fibers at the junction of the inferior mesenteric artery with the aorta (see Figure 57-16). There should be minimal division of the longitudinal periaortic tissues to the left of the infrarenal aorta, and the nerve plexuses that cross the left common iliac artery should be spared.[244,256] The limbs of bifurcated grafts should be routed within the lumens of the common iliac arteries in patients undergoing aneurysm resection to avoid external dissection and minimize injury to perivascular nerve fibers.

Anastomotic False Aneurysm

False aneurysms can develop at any anastomotic site. They are almost invariably associated with prosthetic rather than autogenous tissue suture lines.[257-263] The most common sites of occurrence are femoral anastomoses after placement of aortofemoral bypass grafts.[258,260,263] Femoral anastomotic aneurysms (FAAs) develop in approximately 3% of all femoral anastomoses and in 6% to 8.7% of patients undergoing aortofemoral

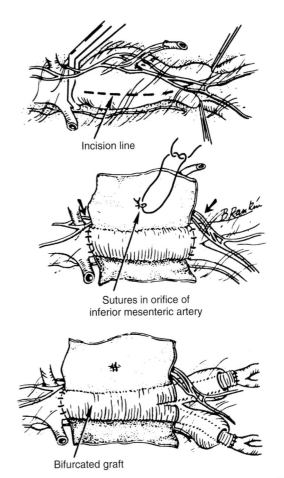

Incision line

Sutures in orifice of
inferior mesenteric artery

Bifurcated graft

FIGURE 57-16 ■ Approaches to abdominal aortic and aortoiliac aneurysm. The sac is left intact and sutured over an inlay graft. (From DePalma RG: Impotence as a complication of aortic reconstruction. In Bernhard VM, Towne JB, editors: Complications in vascular surgery, New York, 1980, Grune and Stratton, p 437.)

bypass. In 3.4% of patients, FAAs may be bilateral or recurrent; aortic anastomotic aneurysms occur in 2.9% of patients.[257,260,262,264] Pathologically, there is a partial separation of the graft from the arterial wall. The perianastomotic fibrous tissue prevents immediate hemorrhage and forms a capsule around the hematoma that gradually expands, owing to the pressure transmitted from the arterial lumen. The fibrous capsule may rupture, with rapid, painful enlargement of the mass, or it may erode the overlying skin to produce infection and external hemorrhage. In the abdomen, false aneurysms are prone to erode into adjacent bowel, forming aortoenteric fistulas.[263,265,266] Because blood flow within the pseudoaneurysm is static, its lumen becomes partially filled with thrombus, which may embolize.[257,263] The luminal distortion produced by the pseudoaneurysm and its thrombus may also cause occlusion of a graft limb.[263]

In the immediate postoperative period, the integrity of all vascular anastomoses is entirely dependent on suture material alone. With time, a prosthesis-artery junction is maintained by the integrity of the suture material and also by external fibrous bonding caused by scarring.[267] The important factors involved in the development of an anastomotic false aneurysm include arterial wall weakness,[262] endarterectomy at the anastomotic site,[268] compliance mismatch between the graft and host artery,[269,270] dilatation of the graft material,[266,271] prosthetic deterioration or an actual flaw in the graft material,[272] increased tension at the anastomotic site because of insufficient length of the prosthesis,[272] uneven tension on the anastomosis as a result of beveling of the end of the graft,[267] and deterioration of suture material, which is extremely rare.[273]

Pseudoaneurysm is occasionally caused by underlying infection, although this is seldom identified.[260,263] When infection is the causative factor, a purulent perigraft exudate is usually, but not always, present. The lack of incorporation of the graft into the surrounding tissue may be the only sign of an infection. Therefore, during repair of any pseudoaneurysm, its wall and contents should be routinely cultured by aerobic and anaerobic techniques.

Recognition is usually quite simple at groin anastomoses, where a large, pulsatile, and sometimes tender mass becomes apparent to both the patient and the examining physician. In a series of a 142 FAAs (76% for A-I occlusive disease, 24% for AAA) reported by Demarche and associates, the presenting features included a painless pulsatile mass (64%), acute leg ischemia (19%), a painful pulsatile mass (8%), hemorrhage (7%), pseudo-postphlebitic edema (0.01%), and microemboli of the toes (0.01%).[274] Skourtis and coauthors reported 11 cases of rupture and 4 cases with thromboembolic complications in their series of 49 cases.[275] False aneurysms developing in the retroperitoneum at an aortic or iliac anastomosis rarely become palpable and go unnoticed until rupture produces pain and shock or erosion occurs in an adjacent loop of bowel, with gastrointestinal hemorrhage.[276] Sometimes, false aneurysms are identified during routine CT scanning or angiography for some other vascular or unrelated problem. Ultrasonography, CTA, and MRA are reliable methods for evaluating grafts and anastomoses for dilatation and pseudoaneurysm formation and the presence of infection.[277] Angiography is seldom indicated except to delineate the distal runoff vessels.[276] If fluid is detected surrounding the graft, it should be aspirated under sterile conditions and sent for culture.

Retroperitoneal false aneurysms should be repaired as soon as they are identified to avoid rupture or bowel erosion.[261,265,276] Unfortunately, these complications are frequently the first indication that a false aneurysm is present. When there is no evidence of infection, the suture line defect can be dissected free and repaired either directly or by the interposition of fresh graft material. Endovascular treatment of thoracic, para-anastomotic aortic, iliac, and femoral pseudoaneurysms is an attractive alternative to surgery in patients with favorable anatomy.[278-280] Lagana and colleagues were able to treat 30 false aneurysms, 13 at the aortic anastomosis and 17 at the distal iliac anastomosis of patients who underwent previous aortoiliac reconstructive surgery with endovascular techniques with primary and secondary success rates of 81% and 91%, respectively at 1 year.[281] In general, FAAs should be repaired as soon as they are identified. However, false aneurysms that are small (<2.5 cm), stable, and asymptomatic may be observed

first, especially if the patient is at increased risk for reoperation.[260,262,263] If surgery is delayed, re-examination at frequent intervals is mandatory so that repair can be carried out when expansion is evident but before complications develop.

When infection or visceral erosion has taken place, the graft must be removed entirely, the aorta and iliac vessels closed, and the extremities revascularized. Management of this problem is discussed in detail elsewhere in this text.

Surgical repair of an FAA is usually performed through the site of the original incision. Dissection is carried down to the graft wall proximally so that it can be controlled with a circumferential tape. Further dissection is then carried distally along the graft to define the anastomosis, the aneurysmal bulge, and the branches of the common femoral artery. It is usually difficult and tedious to dissect out the major branches of the artery at the anastomotic site. When extensive scarring is encountered, further dissection may be abandoned, and the patient is given intravenous heparin. The graft is then clamped and disconnected from the aneurysm, and branch control is achieved by the insertion of balloon occlusion catheters into the lumens of the major branches.[261] The anastomotic site is surveyed carefully to identify the cause of the pseudoaneurysm. The distal frayed end of the graft at the anastomosis is resected, and the edges of the artery are trimmed back to healthy tissue. To avoid tension at the new anastomosis, a short piece of new graft material is usually required to connect the proximal end of the old prosthesis with the freshened arterial orifice. The diameter of the interposed graft segment generally should not exceed 8 mm, to more closely approximate the size of the outflow tract rather than the larger inflow prosthetic limb.[271] Unless retrograde flow up the external iliac artery must be preserved, it is best to convert the femoral anastomosis from end to side to end to end.[261] Before repairing the anastomosis, the orifices of the superficial and deep femoral arteries should be inspected so that significant stenoses can be repaired by endarterectomy or patch angioplasty to ensure adequate runoff. Madiba and coworkers[282] treated 25 femoral anatomotic aneurysms with an interposition graft (15), re-suture (6), tube graft, (1), crossover graft (1), graft-popliteal bypass (1), and ligation (1). There were no deaths or recurrences in the 49-month follow-up period. Wound infection occurred in two patients and occlusion of the opposite limb occurred in one. Endovascular repair of FAA is also an option in selected patients.[283] In a review by Demarche and colleagues, overall mortality for repair of FAA was 2.7% and 20% in patients with infected FAA. Results are distinctly better if this lesion is repaired electively rather than emergently.[262,263] Emergent procedures are associated with increased mortality (46.6%), whereas elective operation resulted in high patency rates and no mortality.[275]

Recurrent Anastomotic Aneurysm

Repair of FAAs remains durable in approximately 80% of patients; however, recurrent FAAs develop in a small percentage of patients. The recurrence rate of anastomotic femoral false aneurysms after initial repair has been reported to range between 5.7% and 19%.[267,271,284] Factors predisposing to recurrent FAA include graft dilatation, local wound complications, cigarette smoking, and previous repair of an FAA in a woman.[271,284] Although there appears to be an inverse relationship between atherosclerotic heart disease and recurrent FAA, the significance of this observation is difficult to explain. Furthermore, factors that have been implicated in the development of primary FAAs (e.g., hypertension, smoking, diabetes, suture material, type of graft, performance of an endarterectomy) have not been related to the development of recurrent FAAs. Recurrent FAAs are subject to the same complications as primary FAAs, including rupture, thrombosis, and peripheral embolization.

Repair is indicated in good-risk patients with recurrent FAAs larger than 2 cm. For those smaller than 2 cm, management includes careful follow-up, especially if coexisting medical problems make surgical intervention risky. The principles of repair are similar to those for primary FAAs and include careful dissection of the distal outflow vessels, use of graft material approximately the size of the outflow vessel, and conversion from end-to-side to end-to-end anastomosis.[271,284]

Infrainguinal Arterial Reconstruction

Femoropopliteal and femoroinfrapopliteal bypasses are the most commonly performed procedures for revascularization of the lower extremity below the inguinal ligament. Specific problems related to endarterectomy of the superficial femoral, popliteal, or deep femoral arteries are reviewed in the discussion of these procedures. The basic principles of infrainguinal bypass are similar to those for aortoiliac reconstruction, with the following significant differences: the vessels involved are smaller, and the length of the bypass conduit is greater, with a consequent increase in the incidence of early and late thrombosis; vein grafts rather than prostheses are used for the majority of procedures; and there is a tendency for less severe systemic complications owing to the more peripheral and less traumatic nature of the operative procedure.

Bleeding

Major blood loss or hemorrhage is not a frequent complication during this surgery but may become a problem in the immediate postoperative period. Ali and coauthors[285] reported a 3% incidence of hemorrhage associated with femoropopliteal veingrafts within 1 hour to 180 days after the procedure. The most common sources are the anastomoses, insecure ligatures on branches of a vein graft, laceration of the vein wall by instruments in the in situ technique, blind disruption of small vessels encountered during blunt dissection of thigh and leg tunnels, inadequate hemostasis during dissection of the major vessels, incomplete reversal of heparin anticoagulation, and oozing from antiplatelet medication.[286] In the immediate postoperative period, bleeding usually appears as wound swelling of the extremity, and the severity of hypotension, if present, mirrors the extent and rapidity

of hemorrhage. Prompt return to the operating room is required to control the source of bleeding and to evacuate the hematoma, which may interfere with healing and promote infection. Wound hemorrhage that occurs after 48 to 72 hours is frequently caused by uncontrolled infection or poor healing at anastomosis sites.[286] However, hemorrhage may occur later in the immediate postoperative period in patients who have been maintained on anticoagulants or in whom fibrinolytic agents have been infused for graft thrombosis within 10 days to 2 weeks of surgery.[287] The management of bleeding after lower extremity bypass requires treatment of the underlying cause and replacement of blood and coagulation factors and the restoration of platelet function. In patients undergoing infrainguinal revascularization, intraoperative blood transfusion is associated with a higher risk of mortality and pulmonary and infectious complications.[288] Long-term graft patency has been shown to be significantly reduced in patients in whom wound hemorrhage develops in the immediate postoperative period.[286]

Thrombosis

The most common significant complication of infrainguinal bypass or endarterectomy is thrombosis of the reconstruction. In the early postoperative period (±30 days), thrombosis is usually related to technical factors (Figure 57-17).[47,69,289,290] The most common of these is imprecise construction of the anastomotic suture line, resulting in stenosis or elevation of a distal intimal flap that obstructs flow; this is especially important at a distal anastomosis to a small-caliber tibial or peroneal vessel. A prosthetic or reversed saphenous vein graft may become twisted when drawn through the thigh tunnel. Kinking or entrapment may occur, owing to compression by nerve trunks or other tissues crossing the tunnel, or by tracking the graft inappropriately in relation to the adductor muscles of the thigh or the medial head of the gastrocnemius. Vein graft stenosis may be produced by a branch ligature placed too close to the main saphenous trunk. For reversed saphenous vein grafts, factors leading to early thrombosis are vein diameter less than 3.5 to 4 mm, thick-walled vein, marked varicosities, and evidence of previous phlebitis.[291,292] In the in situ saphenous vein bypass, technical factors causing early thrombosis are platelet deposition at sites of endothelial damage from improper intraluminal instrumentation, missed valves or incomplete cusp lysis, diversion of flow by significant fistulas, venospasm, and torsion or kinking of the proximal or distal-free segments of the vein. Atherosclerotic disease in the inflow or outflow arteries that was inadequately evaluated before surgery is another significant cause of graft thrombosis. Other technical errors include inadequate heparinization, improper flushing of the arterial system before restoration of graft flow, and clamp injury to the inflow or outflow vessels or the bypass conduit.[69,293] Nonmechanical causes of early thrombosis are decreased cardiac output, arterial vasospasm, and hypercoagulability.[69,294]

Thrombosis that occurs from 1 month to 1 year after implantation is most frequently caused by degenerative changes in the graft itself or at an anastomosis.[289,290,295,296]

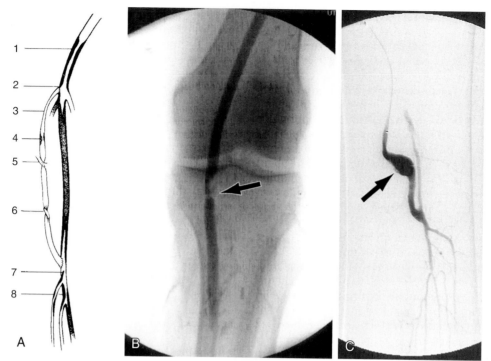

FIGURE 57-17 ■ **A,** Mechanical factors underlying early thrombosis of femoropopliteal and femorotibial grafts: *(1)* Stenosis of iliac inflow; *(2)* stenosis of proximal anastomosis produced by suturing a small vein to a thick-walled femoral artery; *(3)* proximal vein graft <4 mm in diameter; *(4)* recanalized saphenous phlebitis; *(5)* external compression tissue bands in tunnel; *(6)* graft twist; *(7)* elevation of distal intima; *(8)* inadequate runoff. **B,** Stenosis and platelet deposition *(arrow)* in a below-knee saphenous vein graft. **C,** Aneurysmal dilatation *(arrow)* of a saphenous vein graft proximal to a stenosis in a patient with distal embolization. (**A,** From Bernhard VM: The failed arterial graft: lost pulses and gangrene. In Condon RE, DeCosse JJ, editors: Surgical care, Philadelphia, 1980, Lea and Febiger, p 156.)

In reversed saphenous vein bypass, thrombosis is usually caused by fibrosis of a valve or fibrotic changes in the vein graft wall as a result of injury during harvest and preparation before insertion.[69,290,291] These intrinsic vein graft defects are more common in the narrow proximal portion of reversed vein grafts.[290] In in situ saphenous vein bypass grafts, stenoses of the conduit have been reported at the mobilized upper or lower ends of the graft caused by fibrous dysplastic lesions and in the midportion as the result of thickening around a valve cusp.[297] For all types of arterial bypasses, intimal hyperplasia at or just beyond the distal anastomosis may be produced by turbulent flow secondary to alteration of the arterial stream at the junction of graft and artery,[62,298-300] a compliance mismatch,[269,301] and the interplay of platelets and other blood factors at anastomoses.[302] Intimal hyperplasia may also be a consequence of clamp injury to the graft or artery incurred at the time of surgery.[290]

Thrombosis occurring after 1 to 2 years is most frequently caused by progressive atherosclerosis in the arteries proximal or distal to the arterial repair.[290,291,295,303,304] Arterialized venous conduits in an atherosclerotic patient tend to become atherosclerotic themselves[304]; this appears to apply only to reversed, not in situ, vein bypass grafts.[297,305] Giswold and coworkers showed that continued smoking, hemodialysis, hypercoagulable states, and early duplex surveillance failure are independent factors associated with vein graft occlusion.[304] Pedal bypass for previous graft occlusion was also independently predictive of poor graft patency at 1 year.[306]

There is a higher incidence of thrombosis when prosthetic conduits are used, especially when they are carried below the knee to the distal popliteal or infrapopliteal vessels.[244,292,307-310] Thrombosis after vein grafting appears to level off between 1 and 2 years, whereas it is progressive in prosthetic grafts.[290,308] The specific causes of prosthetic thrombosis are the absence of a true intima, with its antithrombotic characteristics; the tendency to develop progressive intimal hyperplasia, usually at the distal anastomosis because of the complex interactions between the more rigid prosthetic graft and the arterial wall; and the greater likelihood of kinking of prosthetic materials as they cross the knee joint. Thrombosis may also occur as a consequence of false aneurysm formation, which is more frequent with prostheses than with vein grafts. Hooded grafts, vein cuffs, and patches have been used at the distal anastomoses of prosthetic grafts to improve their patency. Patency rates range from 37% to 57% for below-knee prosthetic grafts.[311-314]

Heparin bonded to Dacron and PTFE grafts has been used to reduce the incidence of prosthetic graft thrombosis. In a prospective, randomized comparison of heparin-bonded Dacron (HBD) and PTFE (predominantly above knee) bypasses, Devine and colleagues reported primary and secondary patency rates of 46% and 47% for HBD compared with 35% and 36% for PTFE, respectively, at 5 years.[315] In a prospective comparison of Propaten (HBPTFE) with standard PTFE for femoropopliteal bypass, the investigators observed a 37% reduction in the overall risk of primary graft failure with

HBPTFE. Primary and secondary patency rates were 86.4% and 88% and 79.9% and 81% for HBPTFE grafts and PTFE grafts, respectively at 1 year.[316] In a multicenter comparison of saphenous vein (SV) and HBPTFE grafts in the treatment of critical limb ischemia in diabetics, Dorigo and colleagues reported primary, assisted primary, and secondary patency rates at 48 months of 63.5%, 69%, and 69.6% for SV compared with 46.3%, 47.3%, and 57.5% for HBPTFE, respectively.[317] Limb salvage and amputation free-survival rates for SV and HBPTFE were 75.4% and 82.4% and 59.9% and 64.4%, respectively. Thrombosis in a bypass graft may involve only the graft itself, without loss of flow in the segments of the vessel proximal and distal to the points of anastomosis. Under these circumstances, the leg will return to its previous degree of ischemia, assuming there has been no significant change in the inflow or outflow vessels and collateral pathways. If thrombosis extends beyond the anastomosis into the popliteal and infrapopliteal arteries, however, ischemia will invariably be more severe, and the limb may become acutely nonviable unless circulation can be restored.[47]

When a reversed vein graft becomes thrombosed in the immediate postoperative period, the intima and muscularis suffer prolonged anoxic injury because of a loss of nutritive blood flow from the lumen, in addition to the absence of normal graft wall perfusion through the vasa vasorum, which was disrupted during vein graft harvest.[295] The vein thus becomes a less satisfactory conduit, even though flow can be restored within a few hours. This is reflected in the reduced long-term patency of those vein grafts that have undergone thrombosis and initially successful thrombectomy.[290,298]

In the case of late or neglected thrombosis of a vein conduit, either reversed or in situ, the vein tends to undergo irreversible changes. The vein wall becomes thick and edematous, and the lumen becomes stringlike. Thrombus usually cannot be removed by any means, and dilatation of the vein by a balloon catheter may result in splitting of the wall.[297]

In the immediate postoperative period, hypothermia and peripheral vasospasm may make clinical evaluation unreliable. However, noninvasive tests permit the identification of thrombosis at the earliest possible moment.[49,318,319] Therefore, quality of graft flow and overall limb circulation should be evaluated by noninvasive hemodynamic techniques, as well as by clinical observation intraoperatively, immediately after completion of the reconstruction, and at frequent intervals in the early postoperative period.[68,320] Doppler waveform analysis, duplex imaging, ankle pressure indices, and pulse-volume recordings provide reliable objective information. Surgical re-intervention should be carried out immediately in the event of obstructed graft flow to limit propagation of thrombus into distal vessels and minimize the period of ischemia in the limb and the wall of a vein graft.

Beyond the immediate postoperative period, patients with infrainguinal arterial reconstruction, especially with vein grafts, should continue to be examined at regular intervals at least every 3 to 4 months for 12 to 18 months and every 6 months thereafter. A history of worsening claudication, the recognition of reduced distal pulses, and the development of new bruits over the graft or its anastomoses are important findings that should be documented at each visit. In addition, noninvasive hemodynamic tests, including duplex scanning, should be performed; they provide quantitative and objective information and can identify impending thrombosis in the absence of symptoms or clinical findings.[318,320-322] Any evidence of decreasing graft function signals the need for prompt angiography to identify the problem before thrombosis occurs.

Correction of abnormalities within the graft or in the vessels adjacent to a failing graft should be carried out as soon as reduced perfusion has been identified.[318] When possible, intervention should occur before thrombosis has taken place or in the early postthrombotic period, when mechanical obliteration or lytic therapy is most effective. Delay of an aggressive surgical approach may be required in patients who are poor operative risks. Anticoagulants may prevent thrombosis in the presence of progressing stenosis if surgery must be delayed. However, once occlusion has occurred, the longer the thrombus has been present, the less effective recanalization attempts will be.

Areas of isolated stenosis within the graft, at an anastomosis, or in the inflow or outflow arteries can be successfully managed by percutaneous balloon angioplasty.[287] These fibrous vein graft lesions are often difficult to dilate and may require the use of cutting balloons and high-pressure balloons often inflated from 10 to 20 atm. Primary, primary assisted, and secondary patency rates of 38%, 58%, and 84%, respectively, at 24 months after balloon angioplasty have recently been reported by Eisenberg and colleagues.[323] If this technique is not satisfactory, a direct surgical approach at the site of the stenosis is indicated.[47,290] Vein patch angioplasty can usually be accomplished with relative ease to relieve stenosis of the graft itself or at an anastomosis (see Figure 57-17). If the proximal segment of a reversed saphenous vein graft is too narrow, it can be widened (Figure 57-18). Progressive disease in the inflow vessels requires a jump graft from the lower end of the original graft to a patent distal popliteal or infrapopliteal artery to bypass the obstruction.[290]

When thrombosis has already occurred and is recent, the graft lumen may be restored by mechanical extraction of the thrombus with a balloon thromboembolectomy catheter or mechanical devices such as the Trellis or AngioJet devices; prosthetic grafts are more amenable to this procedure than are vein grafts.[47,290,324] Thrombectomy of a fresh reversed saphenous vein graft usually requires exposure of both anastomoses. A transverse incision is made at the distal, wider end of the graft so the thrombus at that level can be removed and the internal aspect of the distal anastomosis viewed directly (Figure 57-19). A second incision over the proximal anastomotic vein hood or partial takedown of the proximal suture line is required for passage of balloon thromboembolectomy catheters and for vigorous forward flushing because retrograde manipulations will be impeded by valves (Figure 57-20). Prosthetic graft declotting can sometimes be accomplished through a single distal graft opening if the thrombosis is recent. The thoroughness of thrombus

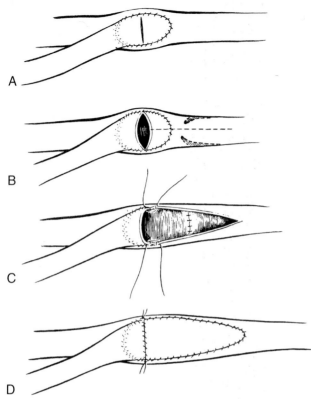

FIGURE 57-18 ■ Technical sequence for inspection and repair of distal anastomosis of femoropopliteal or femorotibial graft. **A,** Transverse incision in a wide "cobra head" overlying the distal anastomosis facilitates thrombus extraction, visualization of the internal aspect of the suture line, and close without stenosis. **B** and **C,** When the distal intima is elevated, the arteriotomy is extended beyond the areas of injury, redundant intima is removed, and the cut edge is secured with tracking sutures. **D,** Closure of the defect with a vein patch. (From Bernhard VM: The failed arterial graft: lost pulses and gangrene. In Condon RE, DeCosse JJ, editors: Surgical care, Philadelphia, 1980, Lea and Febiger, p 160.)

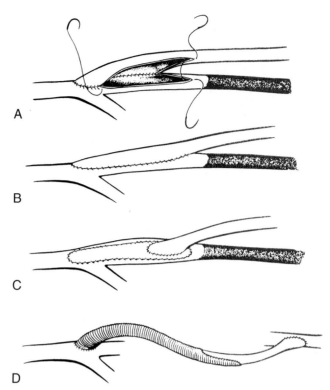

FIGURE 57-19 ■ Techniques for revision of the femoral anastomosis to avoid stenosis caused by a narrow vein and thick arterial intima. **A,** The proximal superficial femoral artery is incised to match the long incision in the vein graft; the vein graft incision is carried distally until the vein diameter is at least 4 mm. **B,** Completion of anastomosis. **C,** Alternative technique using a vein patch to increase the diameter of the artery; the vein graft is then anastomosed to the patch. **D,** Composite vein–Dacron graft is another solution when the available saphenous vein is too short. (From Bernhard VM: The failed arterial graft: lost pulses and gangrene. In Condon RE, DeCosse JJ, editors: Surgical care, Philadelphia, 1980, Lea and Febiger, p 165.)

removal is determined by the vigor of flow through the graft from the proximal to the distal end, which also suggests that there is no inflow obstruction. Operative angiography under fluoroscopic guidance is required after declotting of either venous or prosthetic grafts to confirm the thrombus has been extracted completely, to view both anastomoses, to evaluate the entire length of the intervening graft to identify areas of stenosis that need to be repaired, and to reevaluate the inflow and the runoff bed.[325]

The direct intraarterial infusion of thrombolytic agents is an alternative to balloon catheter thrombectomy in a patient who has no sensory or motor deficits and no signs of impending muscle necrosis.[80,287,297,326,327] Thrombolytic therapy has been successfully applied to vein grafts, prostheses, and endarterectomized segments at all levels of the lower extremity arterial system. The endothelial lining of vein grafts and of small runoff vessels is spared the trauma of mechanical thrombectomy, which may be an important factor in restored vein graft function long term. Although effective lysis can be accomplished several weeks after an occlusion has occurred,[75,328] best results with this form of therapy are usually achieved

within hours or days of thrombosis.[329] The technique of percutaneous intraarterial thrombolytic therapy is discussed elsewhere in this book.

As soon as the clot has been effectively cleared from the graft by lytic therapy, angiographic investigation of the entire length of the graft, both anastomoses, the inflow, and the runoff bed is required to identify the cause of graft failure, which must be corrected to avoid reocclusion. In the interim between lytic recanalization and correction of the causes of graft thrombosis, patients must be effectively anticoagulated to forestall rethrombosis.[75] It is important to recognize that although lytic recanalization of occluded grafts can be achieved, thrombolytic therapy alone suffices in only a minority of patients. Graft stenoses or deterioration of inflow or runoff vessels must be identified and corrected to achieve long-term patency and limb salvage.[80,318,328,330]

Several reports indicate that intraoperative fibrinolytic therapy is an effective adjunct to catheter or mechanical thrombectomy in select cases when residual clot in the distal artery threatens the success of thrombectomy.[331-333] The use of intraoperative fibrinolytic agents has not been associated with significant bleeding complications.[331,332]

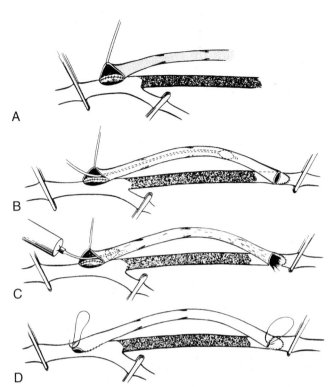

A

B

C

D

FIGURE 57-20 ■ Partial detachment of the proximal anastomosis and graft thrombectomy. **A,** Partial takedown of the proximal suture line. **B,** Passage of a Fogarty catheter to the distal end of the graft and retrograde extraction of clot. **C,** Vigorous flushing of the thrombectomized graft with heparinized Ringer lactate solution. **D,** Resuture of the proximal anastomosis and distal transverse venotomy. (From Bernhard VM: The failed arterial graft: lost pulses and gangrene. In Condon RE, DeCosse JJ, editors: Surgical care, Philadelphia, 1980, Lea and Febiger, p 161.)

Graft thrombosis that is old or that cannot be reopened by mechanical or lytic therapy requires a secondary bypass procedure if the limb is in jeopardy or if claudication is truly incapacitating. Autogenous vein is preferable to prosthetic material, especially for bypasses to the infrapopliteal arteries. When the saphenous vein is not available for reoperation, lesser saphenous and arm veins, when available, are preferable to prosthetic conduits. The long-term results with prosthetic material are poor when used for secondary bypass, whereas arm veins have been shown to have long-term patency rates nearly equal to those of saphenous vein.[334]

It is important to emphasize the need to search for nonmechanical reasons for decreased graft flow, such as diminished cardiac output or hypercoagulability, especially when no other causes of thrombosis can be identified. Curi and associates reported a 13% incidence of diverse hypercoagulable states in this patient population.[335] Failure to identify and correct the reason for graft occlusion usually suggests a poor prognosis, because the underlying cause has not been removed.[71] However, thrombosis in PTFE grafts may occur for no apparent reason other than presumed platelet adherence to a relatively thrombogenic surface. For this reason, antiplatelet therapy in the immediate postoperative period is indicated.[302,336] Long-term anticoagulation with warfarin sodium should be considered in patients who have recurrent thrombosis for no apparent reason.

Reoperation to maintain extremity circulation is worthwhile because prolonged limb salvage can be achieved in 40% to 60% of patients undergoing four or more reoperative procedures.[290] The best results after reoperation for failure of an infrainguinal reconstruction are achieved in patients who require only a vein patch to relieve a stenosis that is repaired before thrombosis takes place.[290,320] For example, Whittemore and associates achieved a 19% 5-year patency rate after thrombectomy and patch angioplasty of thrombosed femoropopliteal vein grafts, a 36% 5-year patency rate after secondary autogenous vein bypass, and an overall 50% long-term limb salvage rate.[290] However, vein patch angioplasty of a stenotic graft or anastomotic lesion before thrombosis occurred yielded an 86% 5-year patency rate. For 72 early and late occlusions of PTFE femoropopliteal grafts that placed the limb in jeopardy, Veith and colleagues reported a 5-year graft patency rate of 37% and a 5-year limb salvage rate of 56% in patients undergoing reoperation.[337] PTFE femoropopliteal bypasses appear to be unusual in that thrombectomy alone, even when delayed up to 30 days after thrombosis, can sometimes restore long-term patency. The success rate for reoperation for thrombosis of PTFE grafts to infrapopliteal arteries is considerably lower than that for femoropopliteal bypasses. Brumberg and colleagues in a study of 131 infrainguinal prosthetic bypasses (44 above-knee, 27 distal popliteal, and 59 tibial/pedal) reported that treatment with warfarin sodium was associated with a patency rate of 89% in patients with an INR in the therapeutic range compared with 55% in patients who were subtherapeutic or nonanticoagulated. Warfarin in the therapeutic range augmented the patency of low-flow grafts, which occluded more frequently than higher-flow grafts (46% vs. 13%).[338]

Wound Complications

Major wound complications after lower extremity bypass grafting to the tibial or pedal vessels are not often reported but may jeopardize the success of these procedures. The reported incidence of significant wound complications after autogenous and prosthetic infrainguinal bypass grafting ranges from 7.5% to 34%.[339-342] In a prospective study of 77 inguinal incisions, Kent and coworkers reported a 10% incidence of wound complications; however, complications occurred in 44% of 79 distal (popliteal or tibial) incisions.[343] More recently Turtiainen and colleagues[339] reported a 34% incidence of surgical wound complications and 27% incidence of surgical wound infections in patients undergoing aortoiliac and infrainguinal revascularization. Independent predictors for wound infection were infrainguinal surgery, obesity, and an angiography injection site within the operative area. Predisposing factors include age, female gender, obesity, diabetes mellitus, renal failure, anemia, postoperative anticoagulation, steroid therapy, ipsilateral limb ulceration or infection, and severity of ischemia. Technical factors, including the length and placement of the incision, prolonged retraction, location of the distal anastomosis, and technique of wound closure, may all influence the ultimate healing of these incisions.[340-344] In a recent analysis of 9932 patients undergoing lower extremity revascularization, O'Hare and colleagues found no significant differences in wound complications or return to the operating room for graft-related complications between patients with renal insufficiency and those without.[345] The amputation rate at 1 year, however, was significantly higher (29% vs. 10%) in patients on dialysis than in those with normal renal function.[346] The use of a continuous incision increases the risk of wound hematoma or seroma and, if it is not positioned directly over the saphenous vein, elevation of a large posterior flap, which is likely to become devascularized. The two parallel incisions required to mobilize the artery and vein for in situ grafting to the dorsalis pedis artery risk necrosis of the intervening skin bridge. Wound complications range from erythema, hematoma/hemorrhage and superficial necrosis of the margins to infection of the deeper layers with exposure of the graft. Gram-positive cocci and mixed bacterial flora are frequently cultured from these wounds.[340-343] In a report by Turtiainen and colleagues, staphylococcal species were cultured from 66% of the infected wounds and in 29% cultures were negative.

Several steps help to prevent wound complications after infrainguinal bypass procedures. Preoperative mapping of the course of the saphenous vein with duplex ultrasound minimizes the likelihood of creating a large posterior flap. The use of skip incisions and leaving skin bridges may be of value in some patients. Isolation of necrotic or ulcerative skin lesions of the foot before preparation of the skin limits contamination of the operative field. In patients undergoing in situ vein bypasses, valve incision with the LeMaitre valvulotome and detection of side branches with Doppler ultrasound, angiography, or angioscopic guidance (when available) and ligation of side branches through small incisions, may obviate the need for long continuous incisions and, as a consequence, reduce the incidence of wound complications.[347-349] A metaanalysis of 4953 patients showed a significant reduction in wound complications from 13% in open vein harvest (OVH) to 3% with endoscopic saphenous vein harvest (EVH).[350] The severity of postoperative pain and hospital length of stay is also reduced. Suture repair of side branch avulsions was required 3 to 5 times more often with EVH than with OVH. There is also some concern regarding thermal spread from the coagulation of the side branches; the detrimental effects of CO_2 and the formation of microthrombi in the collapsed saphenous vein caused by the pressurized tunnel. Damage to the endothelial lining evidenced by reduced calcium mobilization, nitric oxide production, and esterase activity has also recently been demonstrated with EVH.[351,352] A comparison of the 1753 subjects who had EVH with 1247 subjects who had OVH in the Prevent IV trial showed that patients with EVH had higher rates of vein-graft failure (46.7% vs. 38%) at 12 and 18 months. Patients were not randomized for harvest technique and no details of the harvest technique are provided.[353] Compared with open surgery, endoscopic saphenous vein harvest has been shown by Illig and colleagues to be associated with fewer overall wound complications (34% vs. 20%), as well as fewer class II and class III wound complications.[354] Review of the currently available data

and analysis of our own cases has led to limiting the use of EVH for infrainguinal bypass in patients who have an increased risk factors for wound complications: morbid obesity, poorly controlled diabetes, and renal failure and transplant. If a continuous incision is used, careful placement of the incision, meticulous hemostasis, and careful skin closure also reduce the incidence of wound complications. Once a wound complication has occurred, however, the treatment should be tailored to the severity of infection. Wound erythema with minimal necrosis of the wound margins usually responds to appropriate antibiotics and local wound care. More extensive wound infection and necrosis require extensive débridement and, often, skin grafting, muscle transfers, or myocutaneous-free flaps. Rarely, an exposed vein graft ruptures, requiring removal of the graft and placement of a new conduit routed through uninvolved sites. If this is not feasible, amputation may be necessary.

GRAFT SURVEILLANCE

Vein Grafts

When implanted in the arterial system, vein grafts undergo a series of morphologic adaptive changes that include thickening of the wall, anastomotic intimal hyperplasia, valvular stenosis, dilatation, aneurysm formation, and atherosclerosis as a response to arterial blood pressure.[304] The saphenous vein may be used in situ or reversed when used for infrainguinal bypass procedures. The merits of one technique over another remain a topic of considerable debate. Proponents of the in situ technique emphasize the theoretical benefits of better endothelial preservation and compliance characteristics, but there is limited objective evidence to support this assumption. In actuality, the in situ technique may entail more manipulation and damage to the intima from the use of valvulotomes.

Graft failure within the first 30 days is usually a result of fibrin platelet thrombus, retained valves, twists, unrecognized AVFs, or technical problems with the anastomoses; this occurs in up to 3% to 10% of grafts.[355,356] Careful intraoperative assessment of the entire length of the graft with Doppler spectral analysis or angiography is essential if these early complications and subsequent stenosis are to be avoided.[348,349] An unsuspected technical problem (e.g., stenosis, stricture, platelet thrombus, tunneling error) may produce thrombosis or be the source of a subsequent graft stenosis. Platelet thrombi occur at the sites of valve incision or splits in the intima along the length of the vein. Exploration of these sites, with careful removal of any thrombotic material and repair by patch angioplasty or replacement of the damaged vein segment, is often necessary.

Intraoperative duplex scanning of infrainguinal vein bypass grafts has been shown to identify problems that require revision in 10% to 27% of procedures (arm or spliced vein, 27%; in situ saphenous vein, 16%, nonreversed saphenous vein, 13%; reversed saphenous vein, 10%.[357] Bush and coworkers reported a 10% incidence of competent valves in the presence of "normal" operative angiograms.[358] Controversy remains regarding the efficacy of duplex ultrasound surveillance after infrainguinal vein bypass. The 2007 Inter-Society Consensus for the Management of Peripheral Arterial Disease document (TASC II) recommended a clinical surveillance program consisting of an interview for new symptoms of limb ischemia; limb examination with palpation of the proximal graft and outflow vessel pulses; and measurement of resting and, if possible, postexercise ankle-brachial indices (ABIs). Testing is begun in the immediate postoperative period and repeated at 6-month intervals for at least 2 years.[359]

Duplex imaging of the bypass was not recommended on the basis of a European multicenter, randomized, controlled clinic trial (Vein Graft Surveillance Trial [VGST]) that found no clinical benefit for routine duplex testing after femoral-distal vein bypass grafting; at 18 months, graft patency, amputation rate, and quality of life assessment were similar. Davies and coauthors[360] found no differences in primary, primary assisted, and secondary patency rates between clinical (69%, 76%, and 80%) and duplex (67%, 76%, and 79%) surveillance of vein grafts despite a higher incidence of stenosis in the clinical group (19% vs. 12%). The authors conclude that intensive surveillance did not show any additional benefit in terms of limb salvage but did incur additional cost.[360] The optimal surveillance program to detect bypasses at risk for imminent occlusion continue to evolve but should include both a clinical assessment for new or changes in limb ischemic symptoms, measurement of ankle and/or toe systolic pressures, and duplex ultrasound imaging of the bypass graft. The majority of lesions detected by duplex surveillance by Tinder and Bandyk[357] were asymptomatic, progressed in severity on subsequent scans, and amenable to treatment with endovascular techniques. The finding of low graft flow during intraoperative assessment or at a scheduled surveillance study predicts failure, and if associated with an occlusive lesion, a graft revision can prolong patency. The frequency of testing to detect the failing bypass should be individualized to the patient, the type of arterial bypass, and the results of prior duplex imaging. A peak systolic velocity 300 cm/s and peak systolic velocity ratio across the stenosis greater than 3.5 correlates with greater than 70% stenosis and is an indication for repair. Recently Shrikhande and colleagues questioned the validity of the aforementioned criteria for tibial bypasses and suggested a velocity ratio of greater than 2.0 as indicative of a greater than 70% stenosis. However, tibial graft stenoses accounted for only a small number of the lesions evaluated and validation of these findings await the results of studies with larger numbers of patients undergoing tibial bypasses. Johnson and coauthors,[361] using intraoperative duplex scanning, detected lesions requiring revision in 15% (96/626) of infrainguinal bypasses. The lesions detected included 82 vein/anastomotic stenoses, 17 vein segments with platelet thrombus, and 5 low-flow grafts. The revision rate was highest for arm and lesser saphenous vein bypass grafts (27%) compared with reversed saphenous vein bypass grafts (10%); nonreversed translocated saphenous vein (13%) and in situ saphenous vein bypass grafts (16%).[361] A normal initial intraoperative imaging scan, or one performed after revision, was associated with a thrombosis rate of 0.2% at 30 days, whereas 21% of bypass grafts with a residual or unrepaired stenosis by duplex or low flow required a corrective procedure for thrombosis. Ferris and associates[362] found that despite normal completion angiography, early graft velocity abnormalities could be detected in 26% of 224 grafts. Fifty-two percent of these lesions required correction, 38% resolved, and the remaining lesions were revised at a later date. When conducted appropriately, a graft surveillance program should reduce the incidence of unexpected graft failure to less than 3% per year.[357]

Beyond the initial postoperative period, approximately one third of infrainguinal vein grafts develop stenoses that may predispose to thrombosis. Reoperation to correct such defects before graft occlusion permits salvage of the grafts and prevents recurrent ischemia. Unfortunately, between 20% and 40% of grafts occlude without warning or with recently recorded normal ankle pressure indexes.[363] Because of these grafts' propensity to fail, every attempt should be made to detect obstructive changes within the graft, at anastomoses, or in the inflow or runoff vessels before occlusion occurs.

A hemodynamically significant graft stenosis can be detected during carefully executed duplex scanning of the graft. The exact criteria mandating graft revision to prevent graft thrombosis remain controversial. Our observations suggest that when the peak systolic velocity progresses to 350 cm/s or more, or the velocity ratio is 3.5 or more, the graft is at significant risk of failure.[364] These threshold criteria may seem high compared with other published criteria, and larger surveillance studies are necessary to resolve this remaining controversy. Other important parameters are a decreased graft velocity of less than 45 cm/s and a fall in the ABI of greater than 0.15 (Figure 57-21).[364] The former is particularly suggestive of a more proximal lesion, whereas the latter, if isolated, may be indicative of an outflow lesion or a missed graft stenosis on duplex scan. Nonetheless, these abnormal values warrant immediate attention, which may consist of closer follow-up, further evaluation, or immediate intervention, as dictated by the information obtained. After revision or an initial bypass procedure, the patient is seen every month for 1 year and every 6 months thereafter.[363,365]

The majority of vein-graft stenotic lesions respond to endovascular interventions. Use of a cutting balloon in conjunction with a high-pressure balloon may be necessary to achieve optimal results. Repeat interventions are not infrequent and are associated with excellent technical success rates. However, primary and secondary patency rates of 33% ± 7% and 63% ± 7% at 2 years suggest that surgical repair should be considered after early endovascular failure. Surgical repair with patch angioplasty or replacement of a segment of vein offers good long-term results.[366]

Functional failure of patent infrainguinal bypass grafts manifested by extension of necrosis or failure to control infective processes in the foot occurs in 2% to 4% of cases for reversed vein grafts, up to 7.5% for in situ vein grafts, and 8.1% to 9.5% for PTFE grafts.[367-369] Amputation may be required unless graft extension to an additional tibial or pedal vessel is possible. An alternative may

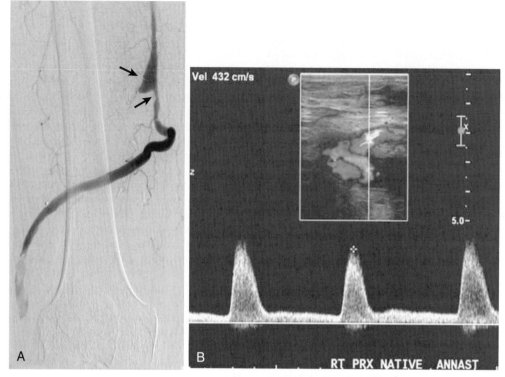

FIGURE 57-21 ■ Vein graft stenosis. **A,** Digital subtraction angiogram demonstrating a high-grade proximal stenosis of an arm vein femoropopliteal graft. **B,** Duplex scan demonstrating increased velocities at the origin of the graft. See Color Plate 57-21.

be microvascular free flap transfer of healthy muscle to cover a persistent defect that usually involves exposed tendons, bones, or joints. Simons and colleagues, in an analysis of lower extremity bypasses for critical limb ischemia from the Vascular Study Group of Northern New England database, reported that 10% of patients with patent grafts met criteria for the composite end points of clinical failure: tissue loss and rest pain (7.4%) and major amputation (2.7%) at 1 year.

Dialysis-dependent renal failure and the preoperative inability to ambulate independently were the significant predictors of clinical failure on multivariate analysis.

Graft Dilatation

With the increased life expectancy of patients undergoing aortofemoral and femoropopliteal bypass grafting, continued surveillance to detect deterioration in the graft material or complications resulting from the implantation of prosthetic devices is becoming more important. Although florid rupture of Dacron grafts and dilatation of PTFE grafts have been nearly eliminated by improvements in manufacturing techniques of the former and by increasing the wall thickness of or applying an external wrap around the latter, deterioration in prosthetic grafts still occurs.

Dacron Grafts

The true incidence of dilatation is unknown because patients with apparently well-functioning grafts, as evidenced by palpable distal pulses or normal ankle pressure indexes on follow-up examinations, are seldom evaluated

unless a problem such as an anastomotic aneurysm or acute occlusion of a graft limb supervenes. Textile grafts initially dilate approximately 15% to 20% after implantation. This is believed to be caused by yarn slippage and is accompanied by a small decrease in tensile strength, which then stabilizes but may continue throughout the life of the graft. Three factors are believed to contribute to dilatation of Dacron grafts: (1) a flattening of the crimp when the graft is subjected to arterial pressure; (2) an increase in diameter and a decrease in length caused by rearrangement of textile structure (i.e., the lighter the graft fiber, the greater the porosity and the more likely it is to dilate); and (3) an increase in diameter and length because of deformation of the graft material.[266,370-373] Dilatation is more likely to occur in knitted rather than woven grafts.[372] Berman and coworkers reported mean dilatation of 49.2% ± 4% for knitted Dacron prostheses, 28.5% ± 3% for woven Dacron grafts, and 20.6% ± 1.9% for PTFE grafts from their preimplantation diameter using CT (Figure 57-22).[373] Although prosthetic rupture and anastomotic aneurysm formation have been reported in patients with dilated grafts, the natural history of such grafts left in place is presently unknown, although Stollwerck and colleagues reported no complications in their series of dilated Dacron grafts that were followed for up to 6 years.[266,271,374-377]

Nevertheless, removal of a grossly dilated graft or lining it with an endograft may be prudent in asymptomatic low-risk patients. In practice, dilated segments of grafts associated with anastomotic aneurysms are replaced. Care should be taken to use a graft corresponding to the diameter of the outflow vessel, and no attempt

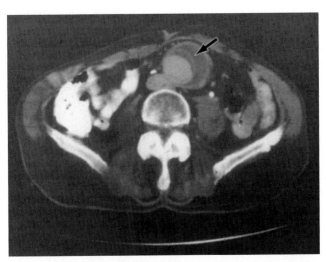

FIGURE 57-22 ■ Abdominal computed tomography scan demonstrating a dilated graft *(arrow)* and the surrounding thrombus from an aortic anastomotic aneurysm. (From Hunter GC, Bull DA: The healing characteristics, durability, and long-term complications of vascular prostheses. In Bernhard VM, Towne TB, editors: Complications in vascular surgery, St Louis, 1991, Quality Medical Publishing, p 65.)

should be made to match the diameter of the interposition graft to that of the dilated implanted graft.

Umbilical Vein

Umbilical vein has been used as a substitute for saphenous vein, with a 5-year patency rate of approximately 45%.[378] Dardik and colleagues, in a series of 756 glutaraldehyde-stabilized umbilical vein grafts (UVGs) implanted over a 7-year period, identified aneurysmal change in 7 grafts (1%) in the entire series.[379,380] The incidence of such aneurysms increased over time, from 1.2% at 4 to 6 years to 7.7% at 6 to 8 years. In a recent report of 211 consecutive femoropopliteal bypass operations with human umbilical vein (HUV; 65 above knee and 146 below knee), Neufang and colleagues[381] reported primary, primary assisted, and secondary patency rates of 54%, 63%, and 76%, respectively, after 5 years; limb salvage was achieved in 92%. There were no significant differences in patency between above- and below-knee anastomoses. Segmental aneurysmal degeneration occurred in six grafts (0.03%), with operative reintervention in three cases.[381] In an evaluation of 283 grafts implanted over a 10-year period, Dardik and colleagues reported no aneurysms. Neufang and colleagues more recently reported a 7% incidence of aneurysmal dilatation of HUV grafts patent beyond 3 years; 3.5% required repair.[381,382] Because of the small but definite risk of continued deterioration of these grafts, it is recommended that HUV grafts be monitored with noninvasive surveillance and an angiogram performed if dilatation is detected.[379,380]

Polytetrafluoroethylene

PTFE grafts do not dilate significantly over time and are only infrequently associated with anastomotic pseudoaneurysms. In a study of 99 consecutive patients undergoing open surgical treatment of AAA with tube grafts, Stollwerck and colleagues observed dilatation of the midgraft segment of 1% ± 5% (ePTFE/Gore), 10% ± 9% (polyester/Braun), and 7% ± 8% (polyester/Vascutek) at discharge, which increased to 19% ± 21% (ePTFE/Gore), 33% ± 22% (polyester/Braun), and 23% ± 19% (polyester/Vascutek) after 6 years. Graft patency was 100% and no graft-related failures or ruptures occurred.[377] Because of its resistance to dilatation, PTFE remains the material of choice for open and endovascular repair of anastomotic aneurysms and possibly for aortofemoral bypass.[383,384]

Edema

Some degree of lower extremity edema accompanies the majority of successful infrainguinal arterial reconstructions and saphenous vein harvesting for coronary artery bypass grafting (CABG). The incidence of unilateral limb swelling ranges from 70% to 100% after femoropopliteal bypass grafting and from 8.9% to 41% after CABG. At 3 months, 56% of patients with leg swelling after CABG had improved: in 23% swelling persisted beyond 2 years.[385] Endoscopic vein harvest is associated with a lower incidence of edema than occurs with the minimally invasive or OVH method (12% vs. 28% at 7 days, 6% vs. 19% at 3 months.[71,386] Although the most important factor in the development of edema appears to be lymphatic interruption at the inguinal, thigh, and popliteal areas during the lower extremity arterial reconstruction, the high incidence seen in cardiac patients suggests that other etiologic factors may be operative. Microcirculatory derangements that exist in the ischemic limb, such as loss of arteriolar autoregulation, loss of the orthostatic vasoconstrictor reflex, capillary recruitment, and focal capillary endothelial injury, all seem to contribute to this lymph-related edema by increasing the net flux of interstitial fluid into the lymphatic system, accounting for the 32% increase in limb volume compared with the nonoperated leg reported by Haaverstad and coworkers.[387] Venous thrombosis has been shown to be an infrequent cause of postreconstruction edema (Figure 57-23).[388-391]

The severity of the edema increases in relation to the severity of pre-bypass ischemia. It is less frequent after aortoiliofemoral reconstruction, presumably because there is less limb lymphatic disruption.[348]

Technical modifications to minimize inguinal and popliteal lymphatic injury during infrainguinal arterial reconstruction may reduce the incidence of postoperative edema.[392] Endoscopic vein harvest, use of a transverse versus vertical incision, and single-layer wound closure are among the technical factors associated with less edema.[393] Edema after lower extremity bypass procedures can be reduced by the use of elastic support stockings (18 mm Hg), bed rest, elevation, and diuretics. Intermittent compression has not been shown to be effective in controlling edema.[394] Fortunately, in most instances, postreconstructive edema is self-limited and improves or disappears during the first few postoperative months. However, the swelling may persist in approximately 10% of patients for up to 1 year.[71]

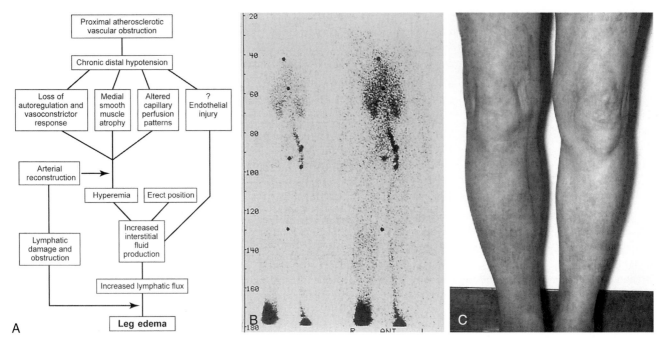

FIGURE 57-23 ■ **A,** Schematic overview of the factors involved in postoperative lower extremity edema after femorodistal reconstruction. **B,** Lymphoscintigram showing decreased uptake of the radionuclide tracer in the swollen right lower extremity. **C,** Patient after femoropopliteal bypass grafting. (**A,** From Schubart PJ, Porter JM: Leg edema after femorodistal bypass. In Bergan JJ, Yao JST, editors: Reoperative arterial surgery, New York, 1986, Grune and Stratton, p 328.)

Lymphoceles and Lymph Leaks

The accumulation of lymph after groin surgery usually appears as an asymptomatic mass without evidence of overlying inflammation. The incidence of lymphoceles and lympho-cutaneous fistulas was 1.2% per incision in a retrospective study reported by Tyndall and colleagues.[395] The highest incidence was seen after aorto-femoral bypass (8.1%) for aneurysmal disease and isolated femoral procedures (5.3%) in previously operated groins, with the lowest frequency seen after femoropopliteal/tibial bypasses (0.5%). The diagnosis of a groin lymphocele is confirmed clinically and with duplex scanning. Aspiration of the fluid under sterile conditions should only be considered if there is suspicion of infection. If the lymphocele is small and located some distance from the incision, it can be followed expectantly. Should the lymphocele fail to resolve spontaneously, increase in size, communicate with the incision, or begin to leak, it should be explored and treated as in patients with lymph leaks.

Drainage of lymphatic fluid from the groin incision is a relatively infrequent complication of arterial reconstruction. In the series reported by Kent and associates, a seroma/lymph leak occurred in 4% of the patients with groin incisions who were evaluated prospectively.[343] The leak appears as a persistent, clear, watery drainage through the wound after the first few postoperative days or as the onset of drainage when the patient resumes ambulation.[71] The frequent presence of bacteria in the lymphatic channels draining ulcerative or gangrenous lesions of the extremity may lead to graft infection and anastomotic disruption. Lymphatic leakage results from transected and unligated lymphatic channels and lymph nodes in the groin wound. Possible contributing factors include poor wound edge and tissue layer approximation and subcutaneous fat necrosis.[71] Ligation of the tissues rather than dissection with diathermy cautery during exposure of the femoral vessels is thought to reduce the risk of this complication. Nonoperative treatment of lymphorrhea includes bed rest and leg elevation to reduce lymph flow while allowing the lymphatics to heal. Wound care must be meticulous, and systemic prophylactic antibiotics should be administered to reduce the risk of secondary infection.[71] If the wound continues to drain for more than 2 to 3 days, the patient should be returned to the operating room and the wound explored. Manual massage of the thigh, the preoperative injection of isosulfan blue dye, or lipiodol or radiolabeled isotopes into the foot several hours before surgery are useful adjuncts in identifying and potentially sealing the leak site.[396,397] The divided lymphatic channels are suture-ligated and the wound is closed in layers over suction drainage, with care being taken to separate the drain from the prosthesis. This technique controls wound drainage and decreases the risk of secondary infection of the lymphatic cavity.[398,399] The reported experience with early wound reexploration suggests shortened hospitalization and a reduction in the incidence of graft infection. There have been anecdotal reports of the successful use of negative pressure suction devices such as wound vacs to control lymph leaks from groin wounds. Whether the routine application of fibrin glue to the femoral lymphatics before wound closure provides an added advantage remains unanswered.

References available online at expertconsult.com.

QUESTIONS

1. Venous bleeding is the more commonly encountered source of intraoperative bleeding because:
   a. Duplication of the inferior vena cava is present in 1% to 3% of patients.
   b. Veins are often adherent to adjacent arteries.
   c. Venous pressure is lower than arterial pressure.
   d. Circumferential mobilization is always necessary to obtain proximal and distal control.

2. Which of the following statements regarding aorto-caval arteriovenous fistulas are true?
   a. Common presenting symptoms include: hematuria, pedal edema and congestive heart failure, abdominal murmur.
   b. They occur in 10% of patients with ruptured aneurysms.
   c. Complete mobilization from the aorta is always required.
   d. Cardiac catheterization is always performed because of congestive heart failure.

3. A 75-year-old patient presents with recurrent left lower extremity claudication and an absent left femoral pulse 5 years after undergoing an aortobi-femoral bypass. The most likely cause of the aortic graft limb occlusion is:
   a. Presence of a hypercoagulable state.
   b. Progression of atherosclerosis at the proximal anastomosis.
   c. Angulation of the graft or compression by the inguinal ligament.
   d. Fibrointimal hyperplasia or atherosclerosis obstructing the profunda femoris artery.

4. Which of the statements are true regarding acute renal failure after infrarenal aortic repair?
   a. Prompt intraoperative volume replacement with fluid and blood is not beneficial.
   b. The mortality rate ranges from 57% to 95%.
   c. Intraoperative embolization and infrarenal clamping are the only causative factors.
   d. Biomarkers are routinely used to distinguish between acute renal injury and acute renal failure.

5. Which of the following statements about postoperative intestinal ischemia are true?
   a. Clinical signs and symptoms: plain abdominal radiographs and CT scans have improved diagnostic accuracy.
   b. Ligation of the inferior mesenteric artery (IMA) should always be done some distance from the aortic wall.
   c. An elevated serum lactate and normal D-dimer are diagnostic of mesenteric ischemia in the postoperative period.
   d. An IMA backpressure of 20 mm Hg and an index of 0.20 confirm the adequacy of flow through the IMA.

6. Twenty-four hours after repair of an abdominal aortic aneurysm, an 80-year-old patient demonstrates low blood pressure, decreasing urine output, increasing ventilatory pressures, and mental confusion. You suspect intraabdominal compartment syndrome. Which of the following interventions may be the most beneficial?
   a. Increase the fluid infusion rate and add vasopressors to improve the blood pressure.
   b. Increase PEEP to improve the oxygenation.
   c. Monitor intraabdominal pressure and open the abdomen if the bladder pressure exceeds 30 mm Hg.
   d. Consult the gastroenterologist to perform immediate endoscopy.

7. Which of the following statements about spinal cord ischemia after infrarenal aortic repair are true?
   a. Interruption of the blood supply to the spinal cord between T-7 and L-3 is the usual cause.
   b. The mortality rate is decreased if patient is paraplegic from the onset.
   c. Abnormalities during monitoring of spinal cord evoked potentials are diagnostic.
   d. Spinal cord ischemia occurs in 0.23% of patients undergoing infrarenal aortic repair.

8. Two weeks after repair of an abdominal aortic aneurysm, a 65-year-old patient presents with complaints of malaise, loss of appetite, increasing abdominal girth, and extremity edema. Which of the following studies would be most appropriate to confirm the diagnosis?
   a. Obtain an immediate CT scan of the abdomen.
   b. Maintain the patient on a high protein, high fat diet.
   c. Abdominal paracentesis and biochemical analysis of fluid.
   d. Obtain a cardiology consult, give Lasix, replace potassium and infuse albumin.

9. Which of the following statements regarding lower extremity edema after femoropopliteal bypass or saphenous vein harvest are true?
   a. It is always associated with venous thrombosis.
   b. Ankle edema after saphenous vein harvest in patients undergoing coronary artery bypass is rare.
   c. It occurs in 70% to 100% of patients after femoropopliteal bypass.
   d. It is unrelated to the severity of preexisting limb ischemia.

10. A patient presents with clear fluid draining from the left groin 10 days after an iliofemoral bypass. All of the following statements regarding lymphatic groin leak are true except:
  a. It is more common after femoropopliteal than aortic reconstructions.
  b. It may be preventable by careful ligation of lymphatic channels in the groin, application of fibrin glue, and multilayered wound closure.
  c. Apply a wound vac device.
  d. Admit to hospital for bed rest, culture of the fluid, and empiric antibiotics therapy.

ANSWERS

1. **b**
2. **a**
3. **d**
4. **b**
5. **a**
6. **c**
7. **d**
8. **c**
9. **c**
10. **a**

CHAPTER 58

MANAGEMENT OF COMPLICATIONS AFTER ENDOVASCULAR ABDOMINAL AORTIC ANEURYSM REPAIR

Margaret W. Arnold • Daniel Silverberg • Sharif H. Ellozy

Endovascular abdominal aortic aneurysm repair (EVAR) for abdominal aortic aneurysms (AAAs) has gained wide acceptance since it was first reported in 1991.[1] Randomized controlled trials have shown decreased short-term morbidity and mortality when compared with open controls.[2,3] Refinements in device design, such as the development of lower-profile delivery systems, and improvements in preoperative imaging for procedure planning and device sizing have reduced the complications associated with EVAR. However, as with any therapy, the potential for complications exists. This chapter reviews the common short- and long-term complications of EVAR, as well as their prevention and management options.

It is useful to classify complications of stent grafting according to their temporal occurrence. Early complications may be related to difficulty with percutaneous access, the passage of the device, failure at a seal zone, or accidental coverage of a side branch such as the renal artery. Late complications are most often related to endoleaks, but can include other entities such as limb occlusion, degeneration of the proximal neck, device fatigue, graft infection, and rupture.

EARLY COMPLICATIONS

Access

In order for EVAR to be considered as an option for a patient, the access vessels (the femoral and iliac arteries) must be fully evaluated and deemed to be of adequate caliber and acceptable tortuosity to accommodate the device and the delivery system. Challenges related to the access vessels can result in significant perioperative morbidity and potential mortality.[4,5]

As device delivery profiles have decreased in size, fully percutaneous endovascular aneurysm repair (P-EVAR) has gained popularity as a technique. Most authors report using percutaneous closure for up to 24-French sheaths. A recent systematic review of all articles published from January 1991 to July 2009 on P-EVAR found an overall access related complication rate of 4.4% (95% confidence interval, 3.5 to 5.3). Increased incidence of access related complications were associated with larger sheath size and obesity.[6]

Major complications of the percutaneous approach are due to failure to adequately close the femoral arteriotomy. These complications include retroperitoneal hemorrhage and femoral artery pseudoaneurysm formation. In most cases, the failure is immediately obvious and open repair of the femoral artery is performed. One study examined 279 femoral arteries that were accessed percutaneously with an immediate failure rate of 6%.[7] The midterm follow-up data on this group showed 3 of 156 (1.9%) having late complications: a femoral artery dissection and 2 pseudoaneurysms.[8]

Relative contraindications to percutaneous repair, which may be associated with a higher rate of complication, include: circumferential or anterior calcifications of the femoral arteries, small access vessel size, severe groin scarring, femoral bifurcation above the inguinal ligament, and large groin pannus.[9] A high puncture site can be associated with hemorrhage on mobilization, whereas a low puncture site can be associated with vessel occlusion. Ultrasound guidance can be a useful adjunctive technique to find the optimal puncture site and avoid potential complications.

Iliac Artery Complications

Iliac artery rupture during passage of the device can lead to significant blood loss; if not controlled expeditiously, it can be potentially lethal. Fortunately, with the quality of current computed tomography (CT) imaging, it is possible to anticipate the majority of access problems. Technologic improvements including smaller sizes and hydrophilic coating make endografting accessible to more patients. However, while the delivery profile of abdominal aortic endografts has been decreasing in size, the smallest endograft approved by the U.S. Food and Drug Administration still requires an 18-French sheath, and typically the size requirements range from 20 to 25 French. As such, depending on the device, the iliac arteries should have a minimal luminal diameter of 7 to 9 mm. Apart from diameter, other anatomic factors need to be considered, such as the extent of calcification and tortuosity (Figure 58-1). In general, if only one of these factors is marginal, transfemoral delivery can be attempted. However, if more than one factor is marginal, an alternative access such as an iliac conduit should be considered.

Two classes of conduits have been described: open and endovascular. Open conduits are typically performed through a retroperitoneal incision. It is the authors' preference to construct this conduit under combined spinal-epidural anesthesia. A 10-mm crimped Dacron graft is

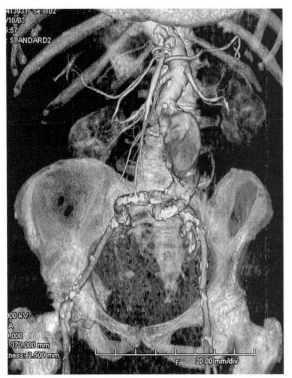

FIGURE 58-1 ■ Challenging iliac access vessels. Note the calcification and severe tortuosity. (From Moore WS, Ahn SS: Endovascular surgery, ed 4, Philadelphia, 2011, Saunders.) See Color Plate 58-1.

sewn in an end-to-side fashion to the distal common iliac artery, and the graft is clamped distally. The graft can then be punctured and used analogously to a native vessel to allow for delivery of the device. After delivery of the device, the graft can simply be ligated, or it can be tunneled down to the groin and anastomosed to the femoral artery to treat any significant iliac occlusive disease. An open conduit also maintains perfusion to the ipsilateral internal iliac artery (Figure 58-2).

Endoluminal conduits consist of a balloon-expandable stent sewn to a thin-walled, 8-mm PTFE graft. The PTFE is predilated at the tip to an appropriate diameter (the diameter of the common iliac artery at the seal zone), sewn to an appropriately sized balloon-expandable metal stent, and then crimped onto a balloon sized for the iliac seal zone (Figure 58-3*A, B*). The balloon, stent, and PTFE graft are then back-loaded into a sheath (typically 16 to 18 French), and an angioplasty balloon (typically 6 mm by 2 cm) is used to form a tapered tip for the delivery system. This conduit can be placed using only local anesthesia if necessary. The endoluminal conduit is delivered transfemorally after judicious pre-dilatation of the iliac arteries. Once the stent is in the common iliac artery, the sheath is withdrawn, the stent is expanded, and the PTFE is then dilated to at least 10 mm throughout its entire length down to the groin. At this point, the endoluminal conduit can be accessed in a fashion similar to a native vessel to allow for delivery of the device (see Figure 58-3*C, D*). Upon completion of the procedure, the PTFE is anastomosed to the femoral artery. The benefit of an endoluminal conduit is that it obviates a retroperitoneal incision in a patient with a hostile abdomen. In addition, in patients with circumferential iliac calcification, the conduit does not need to be sutured

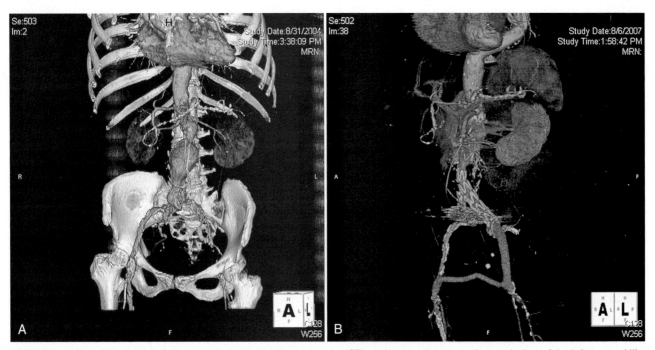

FIGURE 58-2 ■ Open iliac conduit **A,** Preoperative computed tomography (CT) angiogram demonstrating occlusion of the left external iliac artery, with tortuosity, stenosis, and calcification seen on the right. **B,** Follow-up CT angiogram after repair with an aorto-uniiliac device delivered via a left common iliac conduit. The conduit was then anastomosed to the left common femoral artery, and a femoro-femoral bypass was performed. (From Moore WS, Ahn SS: Endovascular surgery, ed 4, Philadelphia, 2011, Saunders). See Color Plate 58-2.

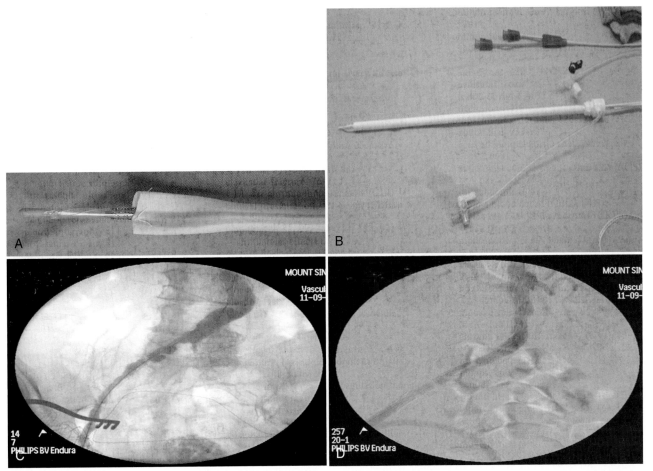

FIGURE 58-3 ■ Endoluminal conduit **A,** Balloon-expandable stent sewn to an expanded polytetrafluoroethylene graft. **B,** Endoluminal conduit in its delivery sheath. **C,** Predeployment angiogram demonstrating occlusion of the left common iliac and right internal iliac arteries, with a stenosed and calcified right iliac system. **D,** Completion angiogram after delivery of an aorto-uniiliac device through the endoluminal conduit. (From Moore WS, Ahn SS: Endovascular surgery, ed 4, Philadelphia, 2011, Saunders.)

to the artery. Disadvantages include the fact that the ipsilateral internal iliac artery needs to be covered. Variations of the endoluminal conduit have been described, such as placement of a commercially available self-expanding stent graft in the iliac artery prior to delivery of the stent graft.[10]

Despite adequate planning, access vessel rupture can occur (Figure 58-4). Two conditions are necessary to allow for a safe outcome. First, prompt recognition of the rupture is mandatory. Any unexplained hypotension intraoperatively should be investigated with a retrograde injection of contrast through the iliac artery. Second, it is absolutely essential to maintain wire access. This allows for placement of a compliant aortic occlusion balloon to control hemorrhage. As the balloon is compliant, it can be inflated in the common iliac artery just proximal to the site of rupture to allow for continued perfusion of the contralateral iliac artery. At this point, a decision can be made as to how to repair the iliac rupture. If the device has already been delivered, an extension limb or a commercially available stent graft can be deployed over the site of rupture. There are several types available (Viabahn, Fluency, Atrium) and the delivery systems range in size from 7 to 11 French. If the rupture is not amenable to repair with a stent-graft, then a retroperitoneal incision

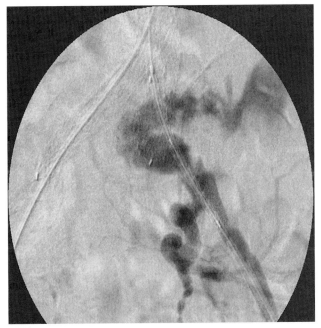

FIGURE 58-4 ■ Retroperitoneal rupture after dilatation of left iliac limb. (From Moore WS, Ahn SS: Endovascular surgery, ed 4, Philadelphia, 2011, Saunders.)

can be made in a controlled fashion, and either direct repair of the artery or placement of an open iliac conduit can be performed at this time.

A small-caliber, calcified distal aorta may present access problems as well, especially when a bifurcated device is planned. A narrow lumen in the distal aorta might not allow full deployment of the main device, making access of the contralateral gate difficult. If possible, partial deployment of the device with constraint of the iliac limb can be performed. Then, after cannulation of the contralateral gate, the device can be fully deployed. This will hopefully prevent jailing out the contralateral gate. Once the aneurysm is excluded, judicious post-dilatation of the iliac limbs should be performed to eliminate any stenoses. An alternative strategy is to use an aorto-uniiliac device.

Acute Neck Complications

While access vessel issues are responsible for the majority of acute complications, the long-term success of endovascular aneurysm repair (EVAR) is ultimately dependant on the seal zone at the proximal neck. A recent study by AbuRahma and colleagues[11] found that aortic neck length of less than 10 mm correlated with an increased rate of both early and late type 1 endoleaks.[11] In addition to length, three other anatomic characteristics of the proximal neck determine suitability: angulation, shape, and the extent of mural thrombus (Figure 58-5). In general, long, straight necks with minimal thrombus are ideal. Preoperative assessment with three-dimensional CT angiography is essential in assessing these characteristics. Center-line reformatted images can provide an accurate assessment of neck length, shaded surface reconstructions can give an accurate view of the angulation and shape of the neck, and orthogonal reconstructions allow for accurate diameter measurements and assessment of the extent of mural thrombus. If one anatomic factor is unfavorable, one can consider attempting EVAR. However, if multiple factors are unfavorable, the likelihood of long-term failure increases significantly.[12]

The choice of device may contribute to the success or failure of the proximal seal zone. Advances in device design such as suprarenal fixation, increased graft flexibility, and an increased range of sizes have allowed endografts to be used in a broader range of patients. However, there are no definitive data proving superiority of any one graft over another.[13] The clinician should base their choice of device on several factors, such as diameter, conformability, trackability, and precision of deployment. In addition, the importance of operator familiarity with the device cannot be overemphasized.

Accurate sizing and placement of the device is essential. Angiography from multiple projections should be performed to identify the true origin of the lowest renal artery. Three-dimensional reconstruction technology can allow for optimal determination of gantry angulation prior to the procedure. The entire length of suitable neck should be used to allow for durable fixation of the stent graft. If a proximal type I endoleak is present after placement of the main device, several maneuvers may be helpful. It is the authors' practice to complete deployment of the contralateral limb before addressing the proximal leak. This provides additional column strength to the device before any salvage maneuvers are undertaken. At this point, the cause of the endoleak needs to be determined. If the device is too low, then placement of an extension cuff is generally the first step. Occasionally, the device abuts the lowest renal but does not cover the entire length of neck on the opposite wall due to neck angulation. In this case, a second cuff may be helpful, as it may position itself in a different fashion once the main body is in place (Figure 58-6).

If a proximal endoleak persists despite coverage of the entire available neck, then the mechanism of the endoleak needs to be determined. Occasionally the device may be correctly sized and positioned, but it does not seal because of conformability issues. Should this be the case, a large balloon expandable stent may help seal the endoleak. Care should be taken when inflating the stent so as not to overdilate the aortic neck (Figure 58-7). It should be noted that the durability of a balloon expandable stent deployed inside a commercially approved device has not been rigorously studied.

Accidental coverage of a renal artery can be a challenging complication. Other authors have described pulling the devices downward using either an aortic occlusion balloon or a wire and a catheter pulled over the device bifurcation and grasped from both femoral arteries.[14] These maneuvers can be challenging to perform with any amount of control. Should there be any residual renal lumen, it is the preference of the authors to simply stent the renal arteries to maintain patency. As with most endovascular interventions, the key is to establish wire access. Brachial access can be particularly helpful, because the stent grafts cover the inferior aspect of the renal ostium. Low-profile systems are preferable (Figure 58-8). Long-term salvage of renal function after accidental renal artery coverage is possible.[15,16]

In addition, other authors describe using the "snorkel" or "chimney" technique as a means to prevent occlusion of the renal artery during endograft deployment. In this method, a brachial approach is used to deploy a stent in the renal artery prior to endograft placement. The stent ends up running parallel to the endograft to provide inflow to the renal artery[17] (Figure 58-9). The maneuver requires a skilled practitioner, but has been shown to have good results in small series.[18,19]

LATE COMPLICATIONS

Endoleak

Endoleaks are defined as any persistent perfusion seen inside the aneurysm sac. They are classified by their point of origin (Table 58-1). The incidence of endoleak has been reported to be from 15% to 50%.[20-22] The majority of these endoleaks are type II, resulting from retrograde filling of the sac via patent side branches. In the absence of sac enlargement, most clinicians believe that these endoleaks are benign and do not warrant intervention. Type I or III endoleaks, however, are believed to convey systemic pressure to the aneurysm sac. Patients with type I or III endoleaks are believed to be at risk of rupture,

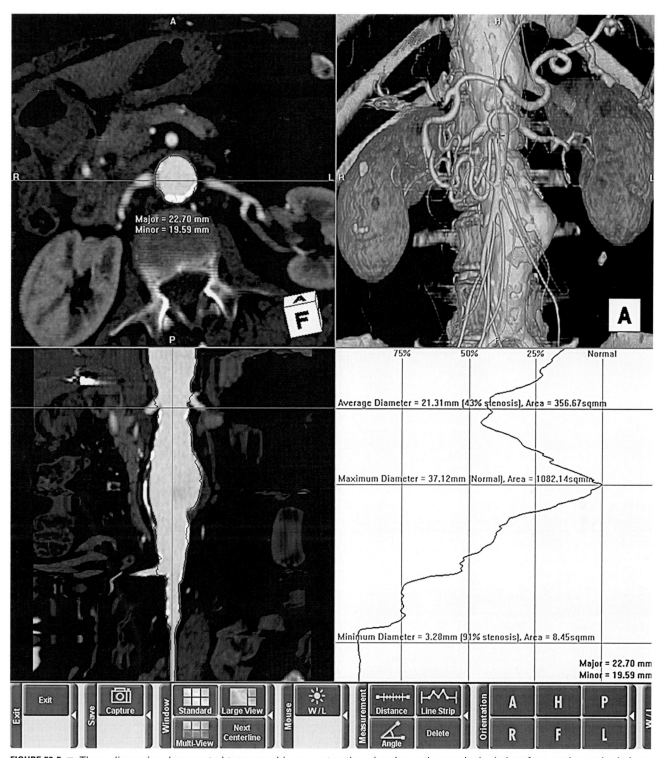

FIGURE 58-5 ■ Three-dimensional computed tomographic reconstruction showing orthogonal, shaded surface, and stretched views of the abdominal aorta.(From Moore WS, Ahn SS: Endovascular surgery, ed 4, Philadelphia, 2011, Saunders.) See Color Plate 58-5.

and the presence of one of these endoleaks mandates correction. Any patient with an enlarging sac and a persistent type II endoleak should be investigated further, because of the possibility that this could represent an unappreciated type I endoleak.

Accurate characterization of an endoleak is the key to its management. CT angiography is the most common

form of surveillance after EVAR, and it is highly sensitive for the presence of an endoleak. However, CT angiography is a static study, and does not demonstrate direction of flow. This is of clinical significance, because type I endoleaks often show flow in patent aortic side branches. The flow is antegrade, in contrast to the retrograde flow seen in type II endoleaks. As such, CT angiography

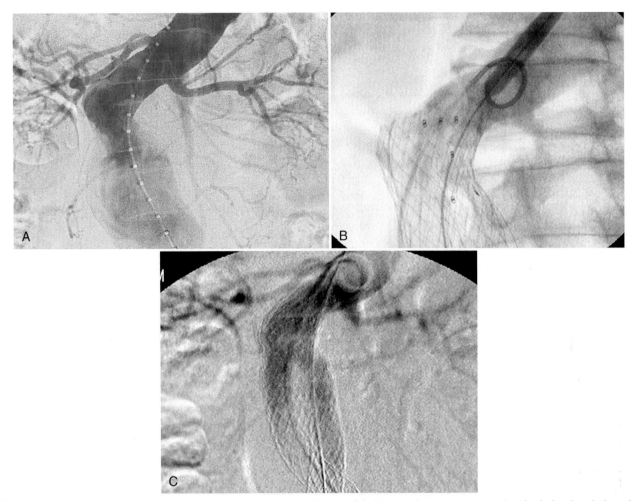

FIGURE 58-6 ■ **A,** Angled neck. **B,** Deployment of the main body. The graft is low on the greater curve despite being just below the left renal on the lesser curve. This is primarily due to the stiffness of the device preventing it from conforming to the neck angulation. **C,** Deployment of a proximal cuff allows for better coverage on the greater curve. (From Moore WS, Ahn SS: Endovascular surgery, ed 4, Philadelphia, 2011, Saunders.)

TABLE 58-1	Endoleak Classification
Endoleak Type	**Point of Origin**
I	Proximal or distal seal zone
II	Patent aortic side branch (inferior mesenteric artery or lumbar arteries)
III	Failure of device integrity (fabric tear or junctional leak)
IV	Endotension (enlarging sac with no demonstrable endoleak)

might not always differentiate between type I and II endoleaks. A dynamic study, such as conventional angiography or time-resolved MR angiography, is needed to tell the direction of flow in the endoleak.

Conventional angiography can be both diagnostic and therapeutic in the management of endoleaks. Flush aortography, selective injection of the superior mesenteric and both internal iliac arteries, and interrogation of the seal zones may be needed to define the nature of the endoleak. The type of treatment depends entirely on the character of the endoleak. Should the sac enlargement be due to a type II endoleak, embolization at the time of angiography can be performed. Access to the sac can be gained typically in one of two ways: either via a microcatheter through the superior mesenteric artery and the marginal artery into the inferior mesenteric artery or via direct translumbar puncture. Both methods have their advantages, but it should be kept in mind that a translumbar puncture cannot definitively define the origin of an endoleak, as it will only demonstrate the outflow from the sac. Therefore a transfemoral angiogram needs to be performed first for diagnostic purposes. Once a catheter has been introduced into the aneurysm sac, a variety of embolic agents, such as coils or glue, can be used (Figure 58-10).

Delayed failure of the proximal seal zone is perhaps the most challenging complication of endovascular stent grafting. If the endoleak is demonstrated to be a proximal type I endoleak, then the determination needs to be made as to whether this can be salvaged with another endovascular device or whether the patient will require open conversion. The same anatomic criteria for endovascular suitability exist for a revision as they do for a primary repair: length, shape, angulation, and

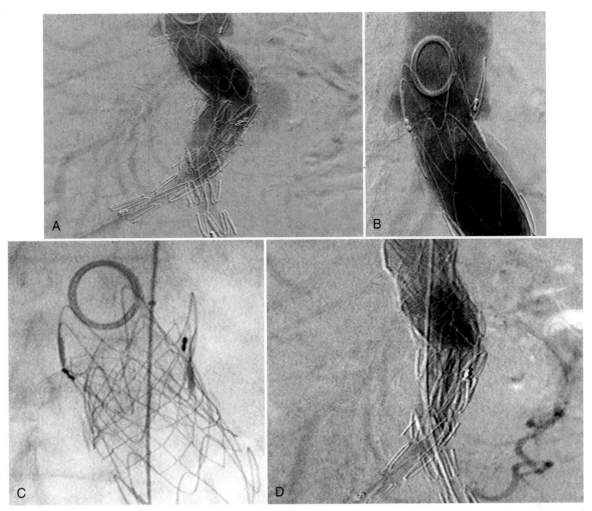

FIGURE 58-7 ■ Neck irregularity treated with a large balloon expandable stent. **A,** Proximal type I endoleak noted despite adequate position and sizing of the graft. **B,** Poor apposition of the graft against the aortic wall calcification. Note the calcification in the wall. **C,** Improved device apposition against the wall after stent placement. **D,** Resolution of the proximal type I endoleak. (From Moore WS, Ahn SS: Endovascular surgery, ed 4, Philadelphia, 2011, Saunders.)

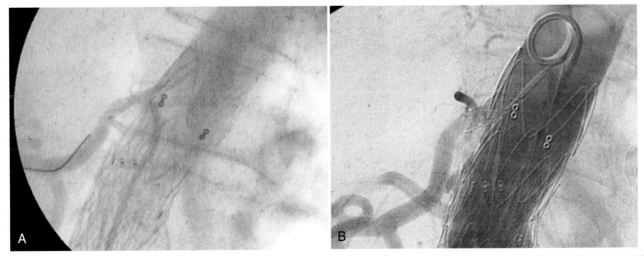

FIGURE 58-8 ■ **A,** Significant of a single renal artery by stent graft fabric. Renal wire access has been obtained using a brachial approach. **B,** Completion angiography after stent deployment demonstrates a widely patent renal artery. (From Moore WS, Ahn SS: Endovascular surgery, ed 4, Philadelphia, 2011, Saunders.)

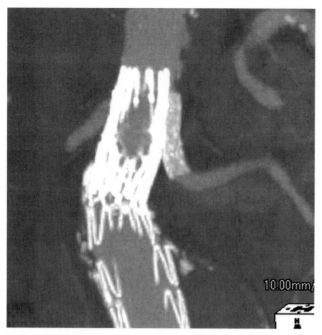

FIGURE 58-9 ■ Left renal artery "snorkel" stent running parallel to the main body component of an aortic stent graft. (From Hiramoto JS, Chang CK, Reilly LM, et al: Outcome of renal stenting for renal artery coverage during endovascular aortic aneurysm repair, J Vasc Surg 49:1100-1106, 2009.)

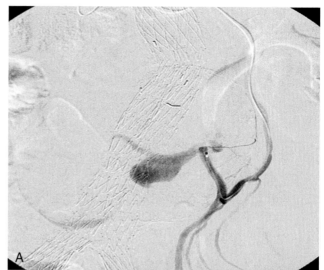

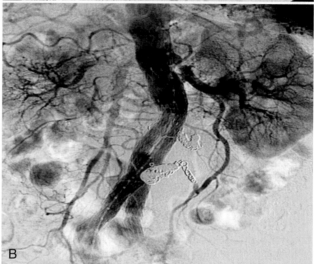

FIGURE 58-10 ■ A, Type II endoleak through a patent inferior mesenteric artery. The microcatheter was advanced into the sac through the superior mesenteric artery via the arc of Riolan. B, Completion angiogram after embolization of the sac with microcoils demonstrates no further endoleak. (From Moore WS, Ahn SS: Endovascular surgery, ed 4, Philadelphia, 2011, Saunders.)

presence of thrombus in the neck. Review of the original, pretreatment images can be useful in determining further therapy. If the original device was undersized or misdeployed, then repeat endovascular repair may be feasible. However, if the original films demonstrate circumferential thrombus in the neck, or if the device failed despite adequate sizing and deployment, endovascular revision is likely to fail. In addition, the presence of a device in the aneurysm may complicate access issues, as it can make passage of a secondary device more difficult. Two approaches have been typically used for endovascular salvage: placement of a proximal cuff or conversion to an aorto-uniiliac device with a femoro-femoral bypass. Although the placement of a cuff is simpler, it relies on a seal between the old device and the new device for long-term fixation. This seal may be difficult to achieve if there is significant angulation in the neck. The aorto-uniiliac repair is more labor intensive, because the goal is to reline the entire aorta from the renal arteries to the iliac seal zone and it requires creation of a femoro-femoral bypass (Figure 58-11). However, it does not depend on the integrity of the old device or on a seal between the old and the new device. In the authors' institutional experience, aorto-uniiliac repairs seemed to be more durable.[23] The use of a device with a suprarenal stent should be considered when revising proximal failures.

Distal type I endoleaks can be easily treated with internal iliac artery embolization and extension of the limb to the external iliac artery. This can usually be performed percutaneously with the use of a closure device.

Type III endoleaks can often be salvaged endovascularly by relining the stent-graft because the seal zones are still intact. Although rare, fatigue and junctional failures can be seen with all devices[24] (Figure 58-12). It is essential to characterize the site of failure in order to correct it. If the endoleak is junctional, then simply placing a limb to bridge the leak typically solves the problem. If, however, the problem with device integrity is in the body of the graft, then the entire device needs to be excluded. This usually requires an aorto-uniiliac device with a femoro-femoral bypass, because a second bifurcated device cannot be placed inside the first.

Branched or Fenestrated Endografts

The use of branched or fenestrated endografts has allowed practitioners to offer EVAR to more patients, but it has also resulted in an increased source of endoleaks and increased need for secondary procedures.[25] One study

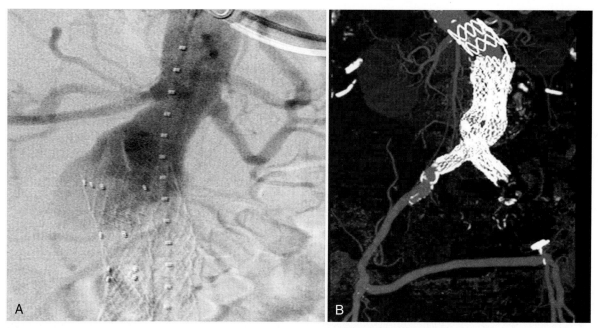

FIGURE 58-11 ■ **A,** Delayed proximal type I endoleak. Note that the device is sitting in the aneurysm sac. **B,** Computed tomographic reconstruction after conversion to an aorto-uniiliac device with a femoro-femoral bypass. (From Moore WS, Ahn SS: Endovascular surgery, ed 4, Philadelphia, 2011, Saunders.)

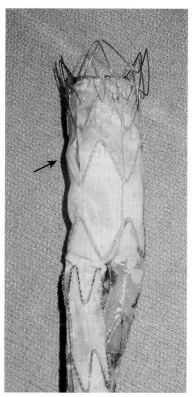

FIGURE 58-12 ■ Fabric tear noted at explant. (From Moore WS, Ahn SS: Endovascular surgery, ed 4, Philadelphia, 2011, Saunders.)

followed 107 patients who underwent either fenestrated or branched endografting or both from 2001 to 2010. The investigators found that 26.2% of these patients developed complications requiring 34 secondary procedures (six repeated interventions). The complications

included limb graft stenoses or thromboses, in-stent visceral vessel stenoses or occlusion, as well as type 1 and 3 endoleaks.[25] In addition, a retrospective review from a multicenter group in France reported reinterventions in 12 of 134 patients who had undergone fenestrated endografting.[26]

Limb Occlusion

Iliac limb occlusion after endovascular stent graft occurs with a reported incidence of 3% to 7% of patients. The risk factors for limb occlusion include extension of the limb to the external iliac, extensive calcification, the use of unsupported graft limbs, kinking of the graft limbs, and small caliber vessels.[27-29] The clinical presentation can vary from an incidental finding on surveillance CT to an acutely ischemic, threatened limb, depending on the collateral circulation. Important collaterals around the area of occlusion include the internal iliac artery and the profunda femoris (Figure 58-13).

The management of an iliac limb occlusion depends on the acuity of the ischemia and the underlying anatomic defect. Certain authors have described endovascular approaches to limb occlusion. Catheter directed thrombolysis and thrombectomy will reveal any contributing stenosis. This can then be managed with angioplasty and stenting.[27] This strategy offers the potential benefit of a completely percutaneous approach. However, in the acutely ischemic patient, it may take several hours to restore perfusion. An additional concern is that it may be difficult to correct the anatomic cause of the occlusion. An alternative approach, generally favored by the authors, is to simply perform a femoral-femoral bypass. This avoids the risks of thrombolysis, and allows for rapid restoration of perfusion. Long-term patency of the femoral-femoral bypass in this setting is very good.[30]

Graft Infection

Endovascular stent-graft infection is a rare but potentially lethal complication. It can arise in the setting of an aortoenteric fistula or come about because of contamination of the graft. Graft infection may be suspected if air is seen in the aneurysm sac on CT more than 1 month out from the initial implantation, or if the patient develops inflammatory findings around the aneurysm with systemic signs of infection. When feasible, the treatment of choice is graft excision with extraanatomic bypass and debridement of all infected tissue (Figure 58-14).

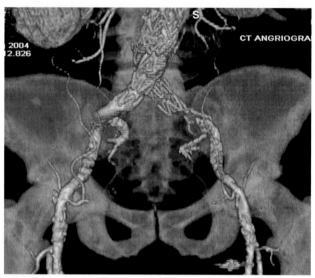

FIGURE 58-13 ■ Occlusion of the left iliac limb with reconstitution at the level of the iliac bifurcation via pelvic collaterals. (From Moore WS, Ahn SS: Endovascular surgery, ed 4, Philadelphia, 2011, Saunders.)

Open Conversion

Under certain circumstances, an endovascular repair must be converted to an open repair to prevent severe patient morbidity or mortality. A recent systematic review found that of the 14,289 AAA patients who underwent endovascular repair, 279 (1.9%) required late conversion with a mortality rate of 10%.[31] They found that the most frequent cause for late open conversion was aneurysm expansion either with or without diagnosed endoleak, migration, or stent-graft disconnection.[30] Open conversion after failed endovascular repair can be facilitated with several techniques. Positioning of the proximal clamp is determined by the presence or absence of suprarenal stents. If there are bare stents across the renal arteries, an initial supraceliac clamp can be placed until the device is out, and then the clamp can be moved into the infrarenal position. Balloon occlusion catheters, deployed either transfemorally or transbrachially, can be helpful in patients with challenging anatomy. Some authors have even described deploying the catheters directly through the indwelling stent graft. Care should be taken in removing the device to prevent damage to the aorta at the pararenal segment. If the suprarenal stents are embedded in the wall of the aorta, a sterile wire cutter can be used to leave the wires in situ. Distally, the iliac arteries and the device limbs can be clamped directly. Vascular clamps with Fogarty inserts can facilitate occlusion of the stent graft limbs. If the distal seal is intact, the iliac limbs do not need to be removed. The limbs can be transected, and an end-to-end anastomosis can be fashioned to the limbs using the native iliac as an external pledget. Despite the increased complexity of repair in the setting of a failed stent graft, some authors have reported good long-term outcomes.[32]

CONCLUSIONS

The key to managing complications in endovascular aneurysm repair is anticipation and case selection. The

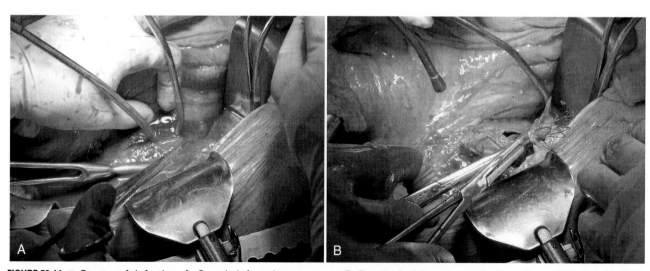

FIGURE 58-14 ■ Stent-graft infection. **A,** Grossly infected sac contents. **B,** Removal of the stent-graft. (From Moore WS, Ahn SS: Endovascular surgery, ed 4, Philadelphia, 2011, Saunders.)

most serious acute complications are related to access vessels, and these are typically predictable. The liberal use of conduits in challenging cases allows for safe endovascular repair. Close surveillance after repair, with the use of dynamic imaging in equivocal cases, allows for early identification and safe treatment of late complications. Precise imaging is key in determining whether endovascular revision of failed stent grafts is possible. Should the patient need open conversion, balloon occlusion catheters, Fogarty vascular clamps, and sterile wire cutters can significantly simplify the operation.

References available online at expertconsult.com.

MISCELLANEOUS TOPICS

CHAPTER 59

THE DIABETIC FOOT

Ronald Belczyk • Lee C. Rogers • George Andros

Diabetes is a growing epidemic in the United States and around the world. The 2011 National Diabetes Fact Sheet estimates that 26 million children and adults in the United States have diabetes, representing 8% of the U.S. population. An additional 79 million have prediabetes but nevertheless may be susceptible to the full range of its complications. Diabetes complications, which include cardiac disease, stroke, hypertension, blindness, renal disease, neuropathy, and amputation, consume more than 30% of U.S. health care expenditures.[1]

Many are surprised to learn that foot disorders, such as ulceration, infection, and gangrene, are the leading causes of hospitalization in patients with diabetes mellitus. Approximately 15% to 20% of persons with diabetes will be hospitalized with a foot complication at some time during their lifetime. Ulcerations are commonly painless and therefore perceived by the patient to be innocuous. Amputations are preceded by a foot ulcer in more than 85% of cases. The final steps on the pathway to major amputation are ischemia and severe infection. The effect of these concurrent factors can make major emergency amputation a life-saving procedure.

More than 80% of nontraumatic lower limb amputations occur in patients with diabetes. Current estimates place the number of amputations in the United States at 80,000 per year. Direct and indirect costs in medical care, hospitalizations, and disability accruing in the wake of the diabetic foot constitute a significant portion of the federal health care budget. This pandemic collectively represents a health care calamity and a crushing financial burden. These figures make it imperative that our society and our profession do more to achieve the twin linked goals of ulcer healing and amputation prevention.

NEUROPATHY

Peripheral neuropathy is one of the most common long-term complications of diabetes, affecting up to 50% of patients by the tenth year of the diagnosis. It typically manifests as a mixture of sensory, motor, and autonomic involvement. The pathogenesis of diabetic neuropathy results from metabolic and vascular disorders that affect nerve blood flow and vascular endothelial function.[2]

Patients are usually divided into two groups: painful neuropathy or painless neuropathy. Painful neuropathy occurs in 15% of cases, with patients complaining of burning, lancinating pain, or allodynia. Various treatments exist to treat the symptoms of painful neuropathy, including antidepressants and anticonvulsants, which modulate neurotransmitters in the central nervous system. Other treatments for pain including surgical decompression, infrared light therapy, or vitamins are unproven. Painful neuropathy usually becomes painless in 2 to 3 years; therefore treatments for pain can be reduced or even eliminated at that time. Painless neuropathy or sensory neuropathy would seem to be preferable to the painful variety; however, it is this type of neuropathy that leads to the ulcerative complications in the diabetic foot. There are no accepted treatments to reverse sensory neuropathy in diabetes, and clinicians should not be lured into marketing traps by vitamin companies or surgical decompression enthusiasts who are without credible evidence to support their claims. A minority of patients have a syndrome with characteristics that are both painful and painless. In addition, ischemic rest pain symptoms induced by lower extremity arterial insufficiency in diabetes can often be difficult to distinguish from neuropathy.

A neurologic examination should be done to evaluate sensory and motor function in all patients with diabetes. Loss of protective sensation (LOPS) is a more severe form of diabetic neuropathy that increases the risk for ulceration. It is most readily revealed by applying pressure on selected dorsal and plantar areas of the foot with a deformable Semmes-Weinstein monofilament (SWMF) (Figure 59-1).[2]

If the patient is unable to feel 10 g of pressure exerted by a SWMF, they have met the criteria for LOPS. Patients should be screened annually for neuropathy. The nerve function profile of Boulton and colleagues provides a useful and reproducible baseline that has been validated as predictive of ulceration.[3,4]

Because diabetic neuropathy affects all three divisions of the peripheral nervous system, the motor signs are sometimes subclinical but can lead to disabling disease progression manifested by muscular atrophy, fasciculation, and weakness. Intrinsic muscle weakness of the foot, once it becomes pronounced, leads to digital contractures and secondary metatarsal-phalangeal instability. The extrinsic muscles gain mechanical advantage over the intrinsic, which results in an unstable foot, prominent metatarsal heads, plantar callus formation, and ulceration. The sensory distribution is predominately of the feet and to a lesser extent the hands. Rather than following specific nerve trunks, the pattern is one of a stocking or glove. Motor neuropathy produces a pronounced clinical finding that is obvious on even cursory examination while the medical history is obtained; interosseus muscle wasting of the hands is evident, sometimes dramatically so.

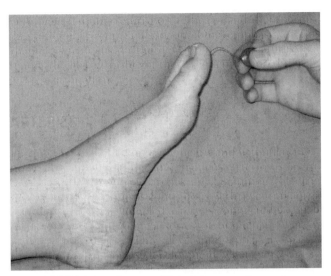

FIGURE 59-1 ■ Semmes-Weinstein monofilament.

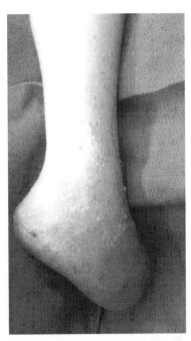

FIGURE 59-2 ■ Severe equinus contracture after transmetatarsal amputation.

Autonomic neuropathy interrupts control of arterial and capillary flow to the feet and tissues, resulting in decreased sudomotor function and dry feet, anhidrosis, noncompliant skin, and, ultimately, fissuring and painful cracking of the skin. Deep heel cracks and fissures are a common manifestation of autonomic neuropathy. This process results in an "auto-sympathectomy," which explains why surgical ablation of the lumbar sympathetic trunk provides no benefit for diabetic ulceration. The stage is thus set for bacterial penetration and clinical infection. Autonomic control of vascular smooth muscle can also be affected, which leads to hyperemic states and possibly contributes to the development of Charcot destruction. The importance of neuropathy in diabetic foot ulceration is best encapsulated by the words of Dr. Paul Brand, considered "the patron saint of the diabetic foot."[4a] He wisely observed: "If the patient walks into your clinic with a diabetic foot ulcer and does not limp, he has neuropathy. For that reason alone the doctor should always observe the patient as he/she walks."

ULCERATION

Evaluation

A review of the clinical examination reports reveals that doctors at all levels of training who see patients for foot ulceration often fail to describe the appearance, size, and location of the lesion, or the state of infection in the presenting complaint. Patients should remove their socks and shoes during routine clinical evaluations.

The size, depth, and location of ulcers should be measured at the first examination and serially documented thereafter to track progression. The use of photographs to document ulcer size and location is recommended. Clinical findings of infection, such as the presence of malodor, exudate, and erythema, are obvious, but in diabetics, clinical manifestations can also be subtle. Clinical signs may help elicit the bacterial pathogen. Malodorous drainage suggests an anaerobic infection; creamy, yellow

pus indicates a *Staphylococcus* species infection; and thin, watery drainage on a green base may herald infection with *Pseudomonas* species. Probing the depth of the ulceration with a metal probe can reveal involvement of tendon sheaths, open fascial planes, or abscess formation. Because of LOPS, this procedure rarely elicits patient complaint.

The evaluation should also identify common deformities and biomechanical abnormalities that contribute to the ulcer. For instance, ill-fitting footwear can cause ulcers to develop on the dorsum of toes, interdigitally, or on the lateral aspect of the foot. Ulcerations located on the dorsal aspect of toes may be related to contracted digits in a shallow toe box. Ankle equinus contracture, defined as ankle dorsiflexion of less than 10 degrees, causes increased pressure of the plantar forefoot and midfoot, leading to calluses and ulceration. Patients with amputations or shortened foot are susceptible to ankle equinus because the ankle flexors overpower the extensors (Figure 59-2).[5]

The Charcot foot rocker bottom deformity increases pressure at the apex of the deformity, usually at the midfoot, leading to mid-foot collapse and to the characteristic ulcer (Figures 59-3 and 59-4).

The plantar ulcerations that arise with increased ankle flexion and plantar pressure are not usually amenable to correction with footwear; the Achilles tendon is best dealt with by tendo-Achilles lengthening (TAL) or operative lengthening of the gastrocnemius muscle.[6]

Ulcer Classification

The established systems to stratify the severity of foot ulceration are based on the size of ulceration (area and volume), location, tissue loss, presence of infection, and

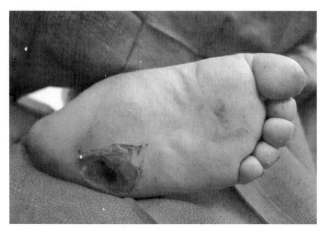

FIGURE 59-3 ■ Plantar lateral ulceration from Charcot deformity.

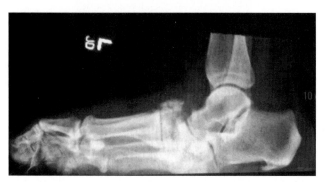

FIGURE 59-4 ■ Radiograph corresponding to Figure 59-3.

the anatomic and hemodynamic state of the arterial circulation. Three diabetic ulcer classification systems are widely used: the University of Texas (UT) classification, PEDIS, and Wagner grading.[7,8] The UT and PEDIS classifications were developed specifically for the diabetic foot. Wagner grades were first described for the foot known or presumed to be dysvascular but are now applied to all etiologies of lower extremity ulcerations.[9] The UT system appears to be a better predictor of ultimate wound outcome, is often used in wound centers, and has been validated. The Wagner classification is based on the depth of penetration, the presence of osteomyelitis, or the extent of gangrene. A major shortcoming of Wagner grading is that the presence of ischemia is not specified in the consideration of the earlier stages. Because most ulcers fall into either grade I or II, the Wagner system inadequately differentiates the etiologic factors that underlie the majority of lesions. Finally, there is the (P)erfusion, (E)xtent, (D)epth, (I)nfection, (S)ensation or PEDIS classification developed by the International Consensus on the Diabetic Foot, which was devised initially as a research tool because of its relative complexity (Table 59-1).

Ulcer stratification continues to loom as a major problem. Without an effective system around which investigators can find agreement and consensus, our ability to compare patient populations, understanding disease severity, and improving effectiveness of treatment will remain an unattainable goal.

CHARCOT FOOT

Charcot neuroarthropathy was first described in tabes dorsalis in syphilis. It is now most commonly associated with diabetes but could occur as a result of any neuropathy.[10] The International Task Force on the Charcot Foot stated the condition is primarily a disease of unopposed inflammation in the foot, leading to increased vascularity and bone resorption. It is a chronic and most often progressive disease of bone and joints. Common features include joint dislocation, pathologic fractures, and severe destruction of the pedal architecture, resulting in debilitating deformity, increased risk of ulceration, and increased risk for major amputation from complications of ulceration. It can lead to disability and premature retirement. The task force recommended classifying Charcot foot as active or inactive, depending on whether inflammation was present.[11]

The most important factor in early detection and the potential to alter the outcome of patients with Charcot foot comes from retaining a high clinical suspicion in patients with the important risk factors. It can be precipitated by seemingly minor trauma. The clinical signs most associated with the disease are an erythematous, hot, and edematous foot. When these clinical findings predominate, it is easy to understand why Charcot can be mistaken for, and is treated as, a deep infection. Approximately 50% of patients have pain with their Charcot foot, which complicates its diagnosis because it is a syndrome caused by neuropathy. The diagnosis is often missed and thus delayed. The characteristic rocker bottom deformity is a late sign of the disease.[12]

Plain radiographs meant to find subtle changes or subluxations should be the initial diagnostic procedure. Magnetic resonance imaging (MRI) or bone scintigraphy can confirm the diagnosis in some cases, but usually clinical suspicion is enough to make the presumptive diagnosis and begin treatment because the consequences of undertreatment or no treatment can be devastating.

There is consensus that the cornerstone of management of acute Charcot foot is early immobilization and offloading. Judicious use of a total contact cast (TCC) or removable cast walker, crutches, walkers, knee walkers, wheelchairs, or bed rest may be appropriate in this setting (Figure 59-5).[13,14]

Immobilization for 4 to 6 months or more may be necessary until inflammation of the extremity becomes quiescent. Skin temperatures are generally 8° F to 10° F (−13.3° C to −12.2° C) hotter on the affected side. Skin temperatures are used to determine when the inflammation finally becomes inactive. In general, a difference of 4° F or less is considered normal. Adjuvant use of bisphosphonates or low-intensity ultrasound bone stimulation has proved ineffective. Prolonged bracing with Charcot Restraint Orthotic Walkers (CROWs) may be necessary for long-term protection.

ULCER MANAGEMENT

After adequate ulcer evaluation, wounds are managed with nonsurgical or surgical strategies.

TABLE 59-1 Table of Ulcer Classification Systems

System	Classifications	System	Classifications
Wagner	Grade 0: Impending skin lesion, presence of predisposing bony deformity, or healed ulcer Grade 1: Superficial skin ulcer that does not involve subcutaneous tissue Grade 2: Full-thickness ulcer that exposes bone, tendon, ligaments, or joint capsule Grade 3: Full-thickness ulcer with presence of osteitis, osteomyelitis, or abscess Grade 4: Gangrenous digit Grade 5: Gangrene severe enough to necessitate foot amputation	PEDIS P: Perfusion E: Extent or size D: Depth or tissue loss I: Infection S: Sensation or neuropathy	1. Wound lacking purulence or inflammation. Uninfected. 2. Presence of more than two manifestations of inflammation (purulence or erythema, pain, tenderness, warmth, or induration), but any cellulitis or erythema extends less than 2 cm around the ulcer, and infection is limited to the skin or superficial or subcutaneous tissues; no other local complications or systemic illness. Mild infection. 3. Infections as grade 2 in a patient who is systemically well and metabolically stable but who has one or more of the following: cellulitis extending >2 cm, lymphangitic streaking spread beneath the superficial fascia, deep-tissue abscess, gangrene, and involvement of muscle, tendon, joint, or bone. Moderate infection. 4. Infection in a patient with systemic toxicity or metabolic instability (e.g., fever, chills, tachycardia, hypotension, confusion, vomiting, leukocytosis, acidosis, severe hyperglycemia, or azotemia). Severe infection.

University of Texas diabetic foot wound classification system	Grade 0: No open lesions; may have deformity
	  A: Without infection or ischemia
	  B: With infection
	  C: With ischemia
	  D: With infection + ischemia
	Grade 1: Superficial wound not involving tendon, capsule, or bone
	  A: Without infection or ischemia
	  B: With infection
	  C: With ischemia
	  D: With infection + ischemia
	Grade 2: Wound penetrating to tendon or capsule
	  A: Without infection or ischemia
	  B: With infection
	  C: With ischemia
	  D: With infection + ischemia
	Grade 3: Wound penetrating to tendon or capsule
	  A: Without infection or ischemia
	  B: With infection
	  C: With ischemia
	  D: With infection + ischemia
	Grade 4: Wound penetrating to bone or joint
	  A: Without infection or ischemia
	  B: With infection
	  C: With ischemia
	  D: With infection + ischemia		

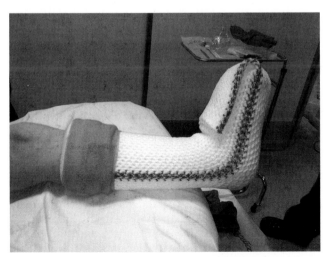

FIGURE 59-5 ■ Typical total contact cast.

Nonsurgical

Nonsurgical treatments include topical wound agents, dressings, and hyperbaric oxygen therapy (HBOT). Topical wound agents and dressings historically served as methods for infection control. Today, a myriad of dressing options is available to assist with moisture, exudate, and bacterial control, as well as with delivery of growth factors. Bioengineered tissues containing living fibroblasts can be applied to a well-vascularized, uninfected ulcer and improve granulation tissue and lead to wound closure. Once infection has been eradicated, potentially harmful topical agents, like povidone iodine, should be diluted or avoided and wounds should remain moist to limit tissue desiccation.

Offloading is an essential complement to all forms of therapy. Offloading assists with ulcer healing by decreasing mechanical stress, shear, and trauma. Patient compliance, however, is often problematic because patients in many cases do not have pain and are not aware that repetitive trauma is occurring. Although the TCC has been reported as the gold standard for offloading, it is not widely used given the difficulty and time required for application and the potential complications. There are other alternative offloading devices and strategies such as non–weight-bearing with crutches, walkers, or wheelchairs, or bed rest. However, attempting to keep patients at least partially weight-bearing with removable cast walkers, knee walkers, half shoes, and prescription accommodative shoes is the goal.

The rationale for HBOT for diabetic ulceration is presumed cellular proliferation and angiogenesis. The patient is placed in a single or multiplace compression chamber set at 2 to 3 atm of pressure and inhales 100% oxygen, thereby dramatically increasing the oxygen partial pressures in tissues. Under normal atmospheric pressure, erythrocyte hemoglobin is essentially saturated while little oxygen is transported by blood plasma. Oxygen transport by plasma is significantly increased using HBOT. Reported effects of increased oxygenation include enhancing antibacterial effects, increasing fibroblast activation, upregulation of growth factors, promotion of collagen synthesis, mobilization of stem/progenitor cells from the bone marrow, and angiogenesis. Specific indications for HBOT include wounds with deep soft tissue infection, necrotizing infection, compromised skin grafts and flaps, and refractory osteomyelitis. Topical HBOT has not been shown to be of any clinical benefit.

Surgical

The diabetic foot has several surgical indications. When infection or gangrene is present, urgent operative therapy should be considered to remove infected or devitalized tissue. If a chronic wound fails to respond to therapy after 4 to 6 weeks, surgery to achieve wound closure may need to be considered.

Diabetic foot surgical interventions fall into one of four classes: elective, prophylactic, curative, and emergent. Elective surgery is composed of procedures for deformities in the absence of neuropathy or ulcerations. Prophylactic surgery includes procedures for the prevention of ulceration in patients with diabetes and neuropathy, but without a wound. Curative procedures are used to heal ulcers in neuropathic diabetic patients. Emergent procedures are performed in the setting of acute infection or ischemia. The risk of postoperative infection increases as the classes progress from elective to emergent (Table 59-2).[15]

Surgical debridement is advisable for diabetic foot wounds. It can be performed by scalpel, curette, or hydrosurgery using the Versajet (Smith and Nephew, London, U.K.). After debridement, a large soft tissue defect can remain. The use of negative pressure wound therapy (NPWT) leads to granulation of wounds with large soft tissue defects while controlling exudate and infection. NPWT works by causing microdeformational forces on the cells that stimulate division and replication. The goal of NPWT is not necessarily to heal wounds but to provide a granular wound bed level with the surrounding tissue. At this point, techniques to close the wound should be used.

When diabetic ulcerations are located on the foot and ankle over bony prominences where there is limited mobility of skin or lack of available tissue, and the surface is involved in a weight-bearing location, wound coverage can be challenging. Reconstruction should cover defects with tissues similar to lost ones while minimizing donor site morbidity. Methods include bioengineered living tissue and acellular matrices, skin grafts, local skin flaps, fasciocutaneous flaps, and muscle flaps. Acellular matrices often serve as a temporary scaffold upon which granulation tissue forms. This tissue prepares the wound for definitive closure with autologous skin grafting or bioengineered living tissue. Often skin grafts and flaps are required because of extensive loss of skin and soft tissue. Excessive skin tension can occur with primary closure, which can lead to skin necrosis and a dehisced wound; these complications can be avoided with meshed split thickness skin graft (STSG) or by using NPWT over incisions. STSG should be avoided whenever possible over weight-bearing areas because plantar skin must withstand the mechanical stress of weight-bearing and footwear. NPWT serves not only as a bolster over STSG or acellular matrices but also controls exudation and accelerates graft incorporation. NPWT is typically used over grafts continuously for 3 to 5 days and then discontinued.

Below-the-ankle amputations in diabetic patients are considered successful outcomes if they result in capable, balanced, plantigrade walking on a foot that is capable of limiting the formation of ulcers. Partial foot amputations including digit and partial ray amputation are often the end result of debridement initially performed to control infection. Secondary closure may be the final step in a series of staged procedures. In the presence of an acute infection, an open amputation achieves drainage, debrides necrotic tissue, and allows for infection to be treated with antibiotics before definitive closure or amputation revision. Definitive closure of the wound is delayed until vascularity is optimized. The preferred location of amputation level is the lowest level that would heal with the most functional remaining foot.

Forefoot amputations are desirable because they preserve length, which preserves maximal mobility and function; the transmetatarsal amputation (TMA) is a case in point. More proximal partial foot amputations such as at the Lisfranc joint or Chopart amputation at the talonavicular and calcaneocuboid joints require adjunctive procedures to maintain a balanced foot (Figures 59-6 and 59-7).

Because energy expenditure for walking is inversely proportional to the length of the remaining limb, below-the-knee amputation (BKA) is preferred to above-the-knee amputation (AKA). Healing of BKAs in diabetic patients is expected to occur in more than 90% of cases. Often, patients have similar peripheral arterial disease on the contralateral and as a consequence they do not tolerate aggressive rehabilitation after a major amputation. Moreover, there is a high contralateral amputation and mortality rate in patients with peripheral artery disease (PAD). Ultimately, the optimal level for a healed and

TABLE 59-2 Classes of Foot Surgery With Clinical Examples

Class	Definition	Clinical Example
Elective	Correction of deformities without neuropathy or ulceration	
Prophylactic	Prevention of ulceration in patients with diabetes and neuropathy without a wound	
Curative	Procedures to heal ulcers in neuropathic patients	
Emergent	Presence of acute infection or ischemia	

functional amputation is determined by assessing the host and vascular status and the extent of the soft tissue defect and infection in the involved extremity. With proper planning, function can be optimized after amputation.

Calcaneal, or heel, ulcers are commonplace and present an enormous challenge to the treating physician, especially when they become infected and develop underlying osteomyelitis. Curettage and debridement may be successful when osteomyelitis of the calcaneus is limited. However, in cases with severe ulceration with or without osteomyelitis, a calcanectomy, which involves removing part or all of the calcaneus, may successfully preserve limb length. Because it provides a more functional limb mechanically with less morbidity and mortality, a calcanectomy is a viable alternative to BKA. This procedure is particularly helpful for the subset of patients who are convalescent, such as those after hip fracture or hip replacement and those predisposed to heel decubitus ulceration. An MRI can be performed to visualize the extent of the bone infection. A partial calcanectomy is preferred when the anterior portion of the calcaneus is not infected, with total calcanectomy reserved for cases in which osteomyelitis involves the majority of the calcaneus.

INFECTION

Infection is a major factor in the pathogenesis of the acute diabetic foot and one of the most common reasons for hospital admissions in patients with diabetes. The infection that complicates an ulcer is a common precursor of

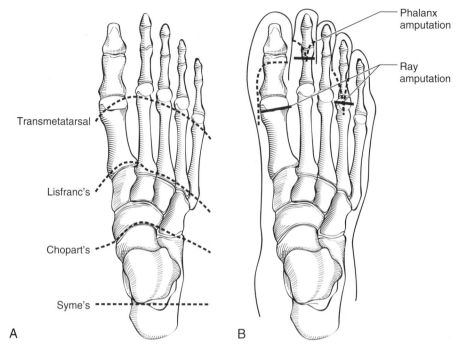

Transmetatarsal

Lisfranc's

Chopart's

Syme's

Phalanx amputation

Ray amputation

A

B

FIGURE 59-6 ■ Schematic drawing of dorsal foot with levels of amputation.

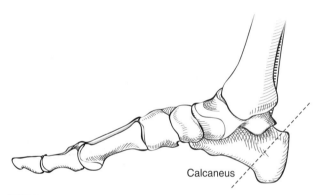

Calcaneus

FIGURE 59-7 ■ Schematic drawing of lateral foot with levels of amputation.

limb loss. Abrasions, heel fissures, calluses, ingrown toenail, or puncture wounds are all common portals of bacterial entry. Diabetes has been described as an immunosuppressed condition caused by impaired leukocyte function and migration.

Infection has been divided clinically as limb-threatening or non–limb-threatening based on the extent of the cellulitis as well as other signs. Failure to quickly identify a limb-threatening infection, such as a deep space abscess or necrotizing fasciitis, can often result in extensive soft tissue loss or amputation. A non–limb-threatening infection has less than 2 cm of erythema surrounding the ulcer without deep spread or systemic signs. A limb-threatening infection can be defined by deep ulcerations with involvement of joint or bone, cellulitis extending beyond 2 cm from the ulcer perimeter, lymphangitis, or systemic toxicity.

Infection can cause thrombosis of small arterioles or in the end arteries of the digits, with resulting impairment of regional perfusion and progression to gangrene. Such thrombi are commonly seen in the pathology specimens of amputated digits and feet. Both macro- and micro-PAD impair the local delivery of antibiotics, oxygen, and leukocytes to infected areas.

In diabetes, infection is purely a clinical diagnosis manifested by infection, swelling, erythema, pain, fever, lymphadenopathy, malodorous drainage, and gangrene. The depth and extent of the infection may be disguised because the patient cannot mount a local or systemic inflammatory reaction in response to the foot infection. Although many routine laboratory tests are often normal, even in severe diabetic foot infections, the blood glucose is usually strikingly elevated and resists insulin control until the infection is controlled. Erythrocyte sedimentation rate and C-reactive protein measurements are sensitive but not specific for infection. Radiographs should be ordered to look for subcutaneous gas. Sometimes MRI or bone scintigraphy is needed to examine for osteomyelitis.

Diabetic foot infections have long been considered to be polymicrobial because three to five organisms are commonly cultured. This occurs when cultures of ulcers are taken from the skin surface and ulcer sinuses. Surface bacterial sampling correlates poorly with deep tissue cultures and actual pathogenic organisms. Correctly identifying the bacteria responsible for clinical infection depends on the technique of obtaining the culture specimen. Notwithstanding the importance of proper deep cultures, it should be emphasized that clinically uninfected ulcers should not be routinely cultured unless done as part of an infection control surveillance protocol. One should cleanse and debride the lesion before obtaining specimens. Tissue specimens are then obtained from the debrided wound and sent for qualitative and quantitative analysis to direct treatment. Bone biopsy is valuable for establishing the diagnosis of osteomyelitis but primarily for determining the pathogenic organisms and determining the antibiotic susceptibility. Blood cultures should be reserved for patients with a severe infection.

The diagnosis of osteomyelitis is suspected when there is a deep or extensive ulceration, especially if it is located over an osseous prominence or joint. Ulcers through which bone can be seen or palpated have been reported to be complicated by osteomyelitis. The probe-to-bone test (PTB) is a widely used diagnostic test in the clinical setting for evaluation of diabetic patients with foot wounds. Palpation of bone with a metal probe is a simple bedside procedure whose reliability has been predicated on a single study that postulated if the probe can reach the bone, then infectious bacteria can as well. Grayson and coworkers calculated that the PTB test had a sensitivity of 66%, specificity of 85%, and positive predictive value of 89%.[16] However, this finding was not substantiated by Lavery and coauthors, who observed that Grayson's patients had a high pretest probability of osteomyelitis.[17] In a clinic-based population, the PTB was only 50% predictive.

The Infectious Diseases Society of America (IDSA) stratifies diabetic foot infections by severity—uninfected, mild, moderate, and severe—and provides antibiotic recommendations for each clinical scenario (Table 59-3).[18,19]

This classification was validated and is predictive of hospitalization and amputation. It also helps determine the type of treatment needed. Mild infections are predominantly caused by gram-positive pathogens, and moderate and severe infections are typically polymicrobial. Methicillin-resistant *Staphylococcus aureus* (MRSA) is a growing problem in diabetic foot infection. It should be considered in mild infections and covered in moderate or severe infections until sensitivities are reported. Risk factors for MRSA include previous history of MRSA, multiple antibiotic use, and recent hospitalization or institutionalization.

An acute diabetic foot infection requires prompt and aggressive treatment to prevent progression of the infection and reduce the potential for amputation. Management strategies usually include a combination of surgical drainage or debridement and antibiotics. The antibiotic choice for diabetic foot infections depends on the severity and the likelihood of MRSA. For mild infections, a first generation cephalosporin, penicillin derivative, or clindamycin could be used. In general, mild infections can be treated on an outpatient basis. Moderate and severe infections require initial broad-spectrum coverage with MRSA coverage. These are most often treated in the hospital with a combination of intravenous antibiotics. Acceptable choices included piperacillin/tazobactam, ertapenem, moxifloxacin combined with vancomycin, or linezolid. A single-agent, broad-spectrum anti-MRSA option is tigecycline.

The appropriate duration of antibiotic therapy depends on the severity of the infection and the response of the host. For uncomplicated mild infections, 14 days should be sufficient. For moderate and severe infections, up to 21 days is indicated. After amputation, if the infection (including osteomyelitis) is completely removed, only 14 days of coverage is needed, for soft tissue involvement. In cases of osteomyelitis, 6 to 8 weeks of therapy is standard, but there is no evidence to support that recommendation.

Acute infection is the most common indication for emergent surgical procedures, usually in the form of sharp debridement or incision and drainage. Abscess drainage with excisional debridement of all necrotic tissue, eschar, slough, hypertrophic callus, and even bone is necessary to prevent tracking of pus along tendon sheaths into deep foot spaces. Pulsatile lavage with generous volumes of irrigant helps in controlling infection. In general, acute abscesses and infections are left open for at least a few days after drainage to be certain that no undrained collections remain. They are then revised and closed only when clean.

CIRCULATION

Vascular disease associated with neuropathy—so-called diabetic neuroischemia—may be the underlying pathophysiologic mechanism for the majority of diabetes-related comorbidities, complications, and major amputations in Western countries. Atherosclerosis in diabetics often occurs at a younger age, is more rapidly progressive and widespread, and tends to be more diffuse than segmental. The leading cause of death in the diabetic patient is heart disease, with approximately more than half of elderly diabetes patients also having hypertension. Risk

TABLE 59-3 ISDA Guidelines

Route and Agent(s)	Mild	Moderate	Severe
Dicloxacillin	X		
Clindamycin	X		
Cephalexin	X		
Trimethoprim-sulfamethoxazole	X	X	
Amoxicillin/clavulanate	X	X	
Levofloxacin	X	X	
Cefoxitin		X	
Ceftriaxone		X	
Ampicillin/sulbactam		X	
Linezolid (with or without aztreonam)		X	
Daptomycin (with or without aztreonam)		X	
Ertapenem		X	
Cefuroxime (with or without metronidazole)		X	
Ticarcillin/clavulanate		X	
Piperacillin/tazobactam		X	X
Levofloxacin or ciprofloxacin with clindamycin		X	X
Imipenem-cilastatin			X
Vancomycin and ceftazidime (with or without metronidazole)			X

ISDA, Infectious Diseases Society of America.

of stroke in diabetic patients is two to four times higher than in nondiabetic patients.

The characteristics that distinguish diabetic macrovascular PAD include Mönckeberg's sclerosis and severe and diffuse infrapopliteal stenosis, while commonly maintaining patency of the paramalleolar arteries and part or all of the plantar arch. Internal iliac artery and deep femoral artery disease resemble the pruning of a tree. In very advanced cases, the arterial calcification affects the intima as well as the media. Although not often described, the adherence of the intima to the media may be fragile, and when an arteriotomy is made for bypass operation, the intima may peel away from the underlying vessel. This occurrence may make the anastomosis of a graft to the artery difficult to accomplish. This problem is best managed by either resecting the loose intimal flap or if the artery is not calcified, securing it with fine transmural "tacking sutures." Diabetic patients tend to have fewer aortoiliofemoral (AIF) atherosclerotic stenotic lesions than do nondiabetic persons who smoke, and they also tend to develop more proximal disease. When diabetic patients do develop AIF plaques, the plaques may resemble coral reefs and the arteries become "unclampable" when during bypass procedures. The development of occlusive disease below the knee enlarges the collateral arteries around the knee and in the upper leg. Disease at this level is rarely associated with symptoms of intermittent claudication of the calf because the site of occlusion does not impair calf muscle perfusion, whereas superficial femoral artery occlusion requires that popliteal artery perfusion is by way of collaterals. It has also been suggested that claudication pain is reduced as a result of diabetic neuropathy. Elderly diabetic patients with advanced arterial disease are often not very active and seldom walk adequate distances to induce claudication symptoms. Clinical problems are usually associated with ankle pressures below 80 mm Hg. At lower arterial perfusion pressure, infection or gangrene may be the initial complication. Because of the multifactorial neuroischemic etiology of diabetic foot ulcers, ankle brachial indices (ABIs) greater than 0.50 are commonplace with diabetic gangrene, whereas atherosclerotic gangrene is more often associated with ABIs less than 0.40. It is this finding that renders the concept of "critical limb ischemia" not applicable to diabetic patients at risk for amputation; the fate of the limb, but not necessarily the circulation, may be critical.

Arterial lesions are equally likely to occur in type 1 and type 2 diabetes, but on average they tend to worsen with the increasing duration of the disease. Sustained severe hyperglycemia is believed to be the mechanism through the production of advanced glycation end products (AGEs) of plaque formation and progression. It is important to bear in mind that the deterioration of a diabetic foot ulcer and the need for urgent treatment is rarely the result of a sudden loss of macrocirculation but is far more likely to occur because of microvascular thrombosis, endothelial dysfunction, and, most often, progressive infection. Thus, the relative lack of perfusion may be insufficient as the sole or major cause of ulceration but may be severe enough to prevent healing.

Arterial Calcification

The most obvious clinical consequence of diabetes-induced arterial wall calcification is that the arteries become incompressible when a blood pressure cuff is applied to the ankle. This causes the measurements of ankle systolic pressure to be spuriously high so the usefulness of this technique for clinical diagnosis is lost. The circulatory effects are less well understood because there is no practical clinical tool for measuring blood flow through the rigid tubes to the foot and calf. Likewise there are no clinically developed methods for assessing the loss of arterial compliance. Arterial systolic flow velocity is known to increase, as is mean pressure, whereas the loss of compliance decreases the capacitance of the arterial system and diastolic flow volumes.

Plain radiographic imaging demonstrates calf and foot artery calcification and should be performed routinely in diabetics with foot ulcers, preferably in the standing and "unloaded" positions. At least one quarter of patients who have had type 2 diabetes for 10 years have radiographic evidence of arterial calcification; this should not be taken as a sign of arterial occlusion because most patients have palpable pedal pulses. Noninvasive ultrasonographic screening for PAD using ABI (discussed later) determinations is recommended. The American Diabetes Association advises screening in diabetic patients older than 50 years of age. All patients with nonhealing ulcerations or evidence of ischemia should undergo vascular diagnostic testing.

Noninvasive Vascular Testing

Various noninvasive tests can provide preliminary information regarding probable location, and severity of arterial obstructions can be correlated with clinical examination, the need for angiography, and the establishment of a baseline for serial follow-up. The noninvasive tests can help clarify the contribution of vascular disease in patients with underlying neuropathy. Some have proposed the planning and execution of distal (paramalleolar) bypasses using ultrasonic techniques alone.

Although studies have shown that there are distinctive features to diabetic macro-PAD, it was long believed that the arterial lesion responsible for ischemia involved "small vessels" that were distal and intrapedal and hence not amenable to repair. This notion has been repeatedly disproved.

Ankle and Toe Brachial Indices

Lower extremity systolic Doppler arterial pressures and waveform analysis obtained at the common femoral artery, superficial femoral artery, popliteal artery above and below the knee, and ankle arteries, as well as at toe levels are the gold standard for noninvasive vascular examination of patients with peripheral vascular disease. Using a handheld Doppler and blood pressure cuff, the ABI is obtained by comparing the higher brachial systolic pressure with the highest ankle pressure. If there is no significant disease at rest, then the ABI is 1 to 1.2. Worsening PAD is inversely proportional to ABI decreases. An ABI less than 0.6 is indicative of inadequate perfusion to heal an ulceration on the foot. Often this is a result of multilevel disease and necessitates invasive testing. An ABI less than 0.3 indicates severe ischemia, which portends ischemic rest pain and gangrene. Postexercise measurements can be compared with resting measurements in selected patients. Patients with plantar ulcerations and unstable Charcot deformities, postamputation patients, or those with severe cardiac disease may not tolerate the physical stress necessary to obtain postexercise ABIs.

The arteries of patients with medial wall calcification may be partially or completely noncompressible, which can falsely elevate the ABI. In general, the ABIs are helpful; however, more than 40% of diabetic patients with foot ulcers may have falsely elevated ABIs (>1.4) that may be masking an ischemic foot. In severe cases, occlusive compression is not possible, even at 300 mm Hg. Although the noncompressible ABI is devoid of diagnostic utility, it has well-validated, prognostic value because it is associated with increased mortality from cardiac disease or stroke.

In diabetic patients, the measurement of the toe-brachial index (TBI) may be more useful because the digital vessels are less frequently affected by calcific atherosclerotic disease. Toe blood pressure in the range of 25 to 45 mm Hg is a good indicator of the healing potential of ulcers and limited (digital) amputations in the diabetic foot.

Doppler waveform analysis is an important aspect of lower extremity arterial disease, especially in diabetic patients with noncompressible vessels. Monophasic waveforms suggest arterial occlusive disease, even in the presence of normal Doppler pressures. A triphasic waveform reinforces the likelihood of a vessel with normal elasticity.

Transcutaneous Partial Pressure of Arterial Oxygen

Transcutaneous partial pressure of arterial oxygen ($TcPO_2$) measurement has been used to evaluate skin perfusion and is widely used in Western Europe. It is helpful for patients with foot ulcers who may be prone to impaired tissue oxygenation from microangiopathy. As with ultrasonic evaluation, $TcPO_2$ is also used to monitor response to revascularization. Transcutaneous oxygen measurement does not produce false readings when calcified vessels are present. A value greater than 30 mm Hg is predictive of circulation adequate for healing. Toe pressures of at least 40 mm Hg are better predictors for healing than the ABI or $TcPO_2$.

Laser Doppler

Laser Doppler velocimetry also provides information about blood flow in skin capillaries. The laser emits a light source that penetrates through the skin to a depth of 1.5 mm and is reflected from the moving red bloods cells within the surface capillaries. Doppler shift of the reflected light is measured, expressed in millivolts, and is proportional to the velocity of blood flow. The values reported for wound healing range from 40 to 125 mV. Although less frequently used in the United States, it is widely applied for diagnosis and screening in Asia.

ARTERIAL IMAGING

If the quality of perfusion is uncertain and revascularization is contemplated, then Doppler imaging (duplex) and/or angiography should be performed. Angiography, preferably with selective arterial catheterization, is considered the gold standard for assessment of the diabetic patient with peripheral vascular disease because Doppler imaging is compromised by the commonly occurring arterial calcification.

Precise imaging of arterial circulation is the cornerstone of successful revascularization of the ischemic extremity in diabetic patients. Arterial imaging is challenging in these patients for at least four important reasons: (1) The occlusive lesions are often multisegmental; (2) there is a predilection for the infrapopliteal arteries that reduces the amount of contrast material reaching the pedal arteries and these are frequently our distal anastomotic sites; (3) the occlusive lesions and the arterial wall itself are often calcified and despite subtraction techniques may be difficult to image; and (4) patients with ischemic complications frequently have underlying renal insufficiency, which limits the amount of iodinated contrast that can be given. Many strategies for renal protection in the presence of renal insufficiency have been promulgated but current studies suggest that they are of limited benefit. Other complications of angiography are discussed elsewhere.

Computerized Tomographic Arteriography

Computerized tomographic arteriography (CTA) is a noninvasive method that has the potential to produce high-quality images of the arterial anatomy, especially when 1-mm "cuts" and three-dimensional reconstruction techniques are used. Disadvantages include reconstruction-based artifacts and difficulty in differentiating calcified stenosis from total occlusions. Patients with multisegment disease may have slow transit of contrast and require additional contrast and secondary acquisitions, resulting in a higher radiation dose and a larger volume of contrast. Whether an endovascular or open approach is contemplated, a repeat imaging study, even one limited in scope, is usually required so that many surgeons will bypass the CTA and go directly to catheter-based arterial imaging.

Magnetic Resonance Angiography

Magnetic resonance angiography (MRA) has several advantages including its noninvasive nature, the production of images not obscured by calcification, and the ability to image arteries not seen with digital subtraction angiography (DSA). The use of special views and coil placement improves image quality and aids in localizing calcification (maximum intensity projection [MIP] views) so that anastomotic placement is facilitated.

Disadvantages include nontherapeutic options, increased risk of nephrogenic systemic fibrosis with gadolinium dyes, large volume of dye, spatial resolution affected by patient motion or breathing, contrast dye flow dependent on cardiac output, and severity of occlusive disease. If perfusion is too slow, then filling of all vessels will not be obtained and late opacified arteries will be contaminated with contrast enhancement of adjacent veins.

Contrast Angiography

High-quality arteriography using digital subtraction techniques has added greatly to our ability to identify candidates for revascularization and is essential before performing bypass or angioplasty. Selective angiography of infrainguinal arteries has gained increased application because of the distal location of the diabetic occlusive lesions and increased use of interventional techniques for treating below-the-knee disease. In fact, the advancement of below-the-knee angioplasty has strengthened the commitment to accurate selective arteriography of the pedal circulation. The popliteal and more distal vessels can be accessed from the contralateral common femoral artery by going over the aortic bifurcation or by direct antegrade ipsilateral puncture and catheterization. If an intervention is being considered, the antegrade approach is preferable.

Selective imaging obviously has the disadvantages associated with all catheter-based procedure but its benefits make it the preferred imaging technique for the management of the diabetic foot with neuroischemia.[20,24] Resolution is outstanding and, even with small contrast volumes, slow injection rates or dilute contrast high quality is possible by using image stacking, as is used in CO_2 arteriography. Combined CO_2 angiography of the larger, more proximal arteries is common, with dilute iodinated contrast injections selectively into infrapopliteal arteries and image stacking to create a hybrid arteriography technique. Using this hybrid technique, even when we acquire three views of the calf ankle and foot arteries, which we consider to be the minimum number of imaging projections, seldom are more than 20 mL of iodinated contrast required. Selective arteriography is the gold standard of infrapopliteal imaging, but MRA can supplement it in certain circumstances. Although most ischemic ulcers result from chronic occlusions, occasionally arterial thrombosis may be "subacute" (less than 6 to 8 weeks in duration). Iodinated contrast may not find its way to the patient but hypoperfused and unopacified paramalleolar arteries unless there is sufficient time to form adequate collateral at the ankle and foot. In this circumstance, we have found that arteries that do not "light up" with iodinated contrast will be seen on MRA. If the foot "looks too good" to be without demonstrable ankle and foot arteries, we will use MRA before giving up on possible revascularization. The ability of drugs and infusions to mitigate contrast-induced nephropathy remains controversial so we limit contrast volume by relying on hybrid angiography. If the patient has normal aortic, femoral, and popliteal pulses without bruits and duplex-derived triphasic flow velocity profiles, we will eschew imaging of the proximal arteries and limit our scope of imaging to below the adductor tendon or even the infrapopliteal arteries.

REVASCULARIZATION

The ulcerated neuroischemic diabetic foot presents unique and complex challenges to the vascular surgeon. Selecting the type of intervention—endovascular versus open surgical approaches—to restore perfusion is often considered a trade between short-term risk and longer-term efficacy. Challenges include the risks inherent to revascularization procedures such as creating another wound, exposure to cardiovascular risk, prolonged hospitalization, and further protein-calorie depletion in patients who are already frail and have limited life expectancy. Specifically for the intervention it is important to assess the patient's severity of ischemia, level of occlusive disease, availability of conduit, and ability to have a functional limb after revascularization.

At initial assessment, the patient's ischemia needs to be assessed. Patients with severe ischemia characterized by pain at rest, dependent rubor, infection, and soft tissue loss need more aggressive treatment than those with mild ischemia. The method and durability of the planned procedure should be appropriate for the anatomic level and severity of the occlusive disease and for the extent of tissue loss. Patients with proximal PAD are more easily treated with endovascular approaches than are those with infrapopliteal disease. Patients with infrapopliteal disease often need a surgical bypass and the surgeon needs to assess all available conduits and target vessels. An autogenous vein is more reliable in terms of long-term patency for distal bypass. Some patients may not have an available autogenous conduit because of small vein size, thrombosis, or prior harvest. Patients with available conduit but poor target vessels have a poor prognosis for healing from revascularization. Another consideration for revascularization is the patient's level of function once the ulcer is healed. Patients with a lack of motivation and/or strength, poor mental capacity, inadequate plantar skin, and compromised biomechanics may not be candidates for revascularization, and the risks of surgery should be weighed against the patient's willingness to strive to retain the affected limb. Typically less severe ulcers need a smaller boost in their perfusion, whereas larger, more severe ulcers, regardless of acuity, will need more perfusion for a longer period of time to achieve durable healing. Deciding on the necessity for a distal bypass is a clinical matter sometimes assisted by preoperative testing. Even in the presence of palpable pedal pulses, the perfusion may be insufficient to heal established foot ulcerations. Only by performing arteriography is it possible to be certain that no revascularization procedures are required to advance the wound healing process.

There are at least a dozen endovascular techniques for achieving revascularization among patients with infrainguinal occlusive disease, including percutaneous transluminal angioplasty (PTA) with or without stents or using bare, drug-eluting, or covered stents; subintimal angioplasty; cutting balloon PTA; cryoplasty; brachytherapy;

laser angioplasty; or atherectomy. It seems plausible that when there are such seemingly disparate options for treating a solitary problem, none work sufficiently and the results do not compare favorably at this time with the results of open surgery for patients with chronic limb ischemia. Diabetic patients undergoing endovascular therapy are more likely to have higher rates of technical failure and restenosis of the femoropopliteal and crural arteries. Whether to perform infrainguinal angioplasty or stenting to treat proximal lesions and enable the use of a more distal inflow anastomotic site is a matter open for discussion. In general, this practice is avoided to ensure that the inflow is secure; in addition, it is preferable not to operate on patients who are receiving clopidogrel, which frequently includes patients with stents. Moreover, in some instances the proximal intervention may augment the foot perfusion enough to obviate the need for the more distal revascularization. Endoluminal techniques for management of infrapopliteal lesions are dealt with elsewhere, as are techniques for the surgical procedures to revascularize the limb to the knee level. What follows is a presentation of arterial procedures commonly performed for foot ulceration not described elsewhere in this volume.

Thromboendarterectomy (TEA) occupies a unique position in revascularization of the ulcerated neuroischemic diabetic foot. There appears to be a disease pattern in which the common femoral artery (CFA) is densely calcified with the plaque extending to just above the inguinal ligament. A strong pulse can be felt low in the iliac fossa immediately above the inguinal ligament. A TEA is performed through a limited groin incision from the CFA extending retrograde up the external iliac artery (EIA) for 8 to 10 cm and onto the DFA and also the superficial femoral artery (SFA) if they are patent. This boosts pedal perfusion so the foot becomes warmer and

if the ulcers are small and relatively superficial, healing can be achieved. Experience has shown that this unique lesion is not amenable to endoluminal revascularization techniques.

Surgical revascularization of the lower extremity using bypass grafts to distal target arteries is an established, effective therapy for advanced ischemia. An ulcerated, severely ischemic limb in a diabetic patient offers some specific challenges; however, numerous studies demonstrate that the outcomes of vein bypass surgery in this population are excellent and define the standard of care. Technical factors, such as conduit and inflow–outflow artery selection, are foremost in determining clinical success. An adequate caliber, good quality greater saphenous vein is the optimal graft for distal bypass in the leg. Alternative veins perform acceptably in the absence of the great saphenous vein, whereas prosthetic and other nonautogenous conduits have markedly inferior outcomes. Graft configuration (reversed, nonreversed, or in situ) seems to have little effect on outcome. Shorter grafts have better patency. Inflow can be improved by surgical or endovascular means if necessary, and distal-origin grafts (e.g., those arising from the superficial femoral or popliteal arteries) can perform as well as those originating from the CFA. Likewise, distal anastomoses should be placed as proximally as possible on the paramalleolar artery; above-ankle targets are preferred to those on the foot if the artery in between is free of disease. The selected outflow vessel should supply unimpeded runoff to the foot, conserve conduit length, and allow for adequate soft tissue coverage of the graft and simplified surgical exposure. There are reports of extended clinical success with bypass grafts extending to isolated crural arteries.[22,23,25,26] This is to be expected because pedal bypasses are normally "isolated" because the primary pedal arch is seldom intact (Figure 59-8).

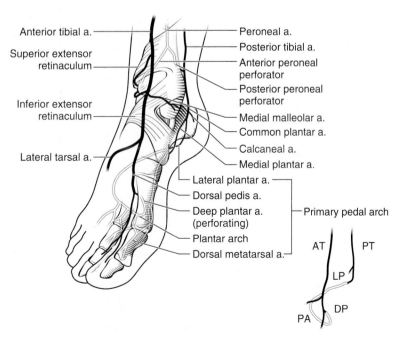

FIGURE 59-8 ■ Arterial circulation of the foot.

Although bypasses to crural infrapopliteal arteries are often feasible, these vessels may be calcified so extensively that it is preferable to extend the grafts to paramalleolar artery distal anastomotic sites. Similarly, choosing crural arteries as the inflow sites for pedal grafts carries with it the risks attendant to sewing to calcified arteries. Use of heavily calcified arteries for distal bypass insertion sites has been possible with techniques such as crushing the involved artery and redilating it before establishing graft flow. Pneumatic occlusion of the arteries using a sterile thigh cuff and intraluminal occlusion (Flo-Rester; Synovis

Surgical Innovations, St. Paul, Minn.) prevents back-bleeding and creates a dry field for suture placement. In almost every case, we select the below-knee popliteal artery or an even more proximal artery for inflow. We prefer to situate grafts in deep orthotopic tunnels, as well as use subcutaneous tunnels, particularly between the midcalf and the ankle. Whatever revascularization method is ultimately used, it must be selected on a case-by-case basis because there are not evidence-based guidelines that show a generalizable advantage of one approach over another. The significance of end-stage renal disease

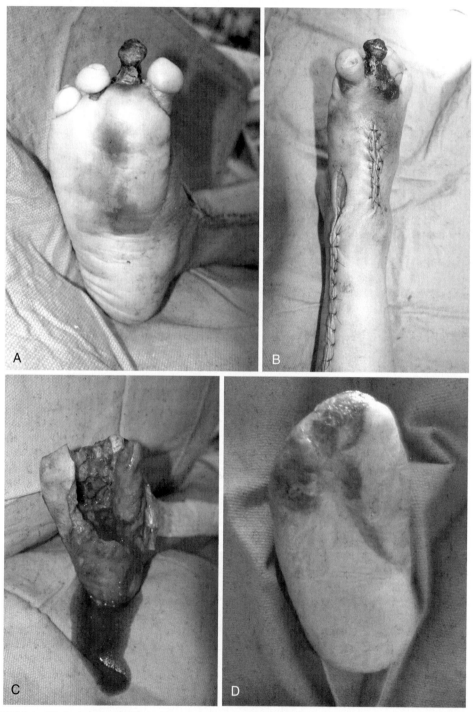

FIGURE 59-9 ■ Clinical example illustrating team approach and typical interventions. See Color Plate 59-9.

as a predictor of worse procedure and limb salvage outcomes must be emphasized when selecting therapeutic options and during discussions with patients and their families. The combination of long-standing diabetes and end-stage renal disease exerts a potent effect on the effort and financial cost expended to salvage a foot.

Graft surveillance is indicated for distal bypasses similar to those placed more proximally. The standard methods are described elsewhere.

TEAMS TO PREVENT AMPUTATIONS

Although it is generally understood that medical teams benefit patients, their advantage is abundantly clear when preventing diabetic amputations.[27,28] If a patient has an acute myocardial infarction, the only specialist needed would be a cardiologist. However, with an acute diabetic foot, a vascular surgeon, podiatrist, diabetologist, infectious disease specialist, orthopaedic surgeon, and any number of other specialists including those involved with rehabilitation who can work together as a cohesive team, are needed. Rogers and Bevilacqua described how organized programs reduced amputations by 72% over one year in a county hospital in the United States.[29] The same has been observed in the United Kingdom,[30] Brazil,[31] Italy,[32] Finland,[33] Australia,[34] India,[35] and the Netherlands.[36] Multidisciplinary protocols are important to know which team member performs what service and in what order (Figure 59-9; see color plate).[29]

In a widely cited report, Rogers and associates[37] describe the "Toe and Flow" team consisting of podiatrists and vascular surgeons as the irreducible minimum for the central structure of the team. They proposed levels of specialist centers based on resources and competence, similar to a classification for trauma centers. The levels of diabetic foot care were classified as: A, basic; B, intermediate; and C, center of excellence.

Collaboration works best when the centers are located in hospitals. Frequently, consultants may be needed in the unit or emergencies occur that require assistance. Quick access to vascular and orthopedic imaging and an operating room are necessary. Having the right tools and team are important, but limb salvage is a philosophy that each member of the team should embrace. Moderate and severe infections are a true emergency and require urgent management, which usually involves surgery and hospitalization with the help of surgeons, podiatrists, and infectious disease specialists.[38] Ischemia should be managed urgently by a vascular surgeon to prevent further soft tissue loss and improve the likelihood of wound healing. After ischemia and infection are managed, the pressure should be relieved from the feet by a podiatrist or physical therapist. Any wound needs regular debridement by a surgical specialist, after which wound closure is eventually performed by a surgeon, podiatrist, or plastic surgeon.

On the basis of these data and reports, the system is of equal importance in achieving limb salvage as in any other factor. By merging their complementary skill sets, improving communication, and optimizing the decision making process, teams effectively shorten the process of diagnosis, treatment, and healing. We have adopted the philosophy that optimal care will enable the patient to walk out of the hospital, even if they did not walk in.

References available online at expertconsult.com.

QUESTIONS

1. Why are patients with amputations or shortened feet susceptible to ankle equinus?
   a. Ankle flexors overpower extensors
   b. Decreased lever arm of the foot to control ankle motion
   c. Ill-fitting shoes
   d. Hypertrophy of the ankle joint capsule

2. The International Task Force on the Charcot Foot recommended classifying Charcot foot as active or inactive depending on having the presence of:
   a. Joint dislocation
   b. Edema
   c. Ulceration
   d. Inflammation

3. Which of the following amputations results in a more functional lower extremity?
   a. Chopart's
   b. Transmetatarsal
   c. Lisfranc's
   d. Syme's

4. Mild diabetic foot infections not suspicious for MRSA can be initially treated with
   a. Trimethoprim-sulfamethoxazole
   b. Cephalexin
   c. Amoxicillin-clavulanic acid
   d. Clindamycin

5. Why can the toe-brachial index (TBI) be more useful in determining vascularity in the diabetic limb compared to the ankle-brachial index (ABI)?
   a. Distal vessels provide a better overall picture of the foot's vascularity.
   b. Toe vessels are less affected by calcific atherosclerosis.
   c. Ankle vessels have a higher pressure gradient.
   d. Microvascular disease is more common than macrovascular disease.

6. In the diabetic foot, an amputation may be preceded by an ulcer in up to _____ of cases.
   a. 20%
   b. 35%
   c. 55%
   d. 85%

7. Diabetic neuropathy affects which pathways?
   a. Sensory, motor only
   b. Sensory, autonomic only
   c. Sensory, motor, autonomic
   d. Motor and autonomic only

8. All of the following may contribute to ulceration except:
   a. Ankle DF > 10 degrees.
   b. Contracted digits in a shallow toe box.
   c. Rocker bottom shaped foot.
   d. Repetitive trauma.

9. Charcot arthropathy _____.
   a. is a direct result of Diabetes Mellitus
   b. occurs due to unopposed inflammation leading to increased vascularity and bone resorption.
   c. is associated with microtrauma and pathologic fracture
   d. B and C only
   e. A, B, and C

10. HBOT Indications involve all of the following except:
    a. Necrotizing infection.
    b. Acute osteomyelitis.
    c. Refractory osteomyelitis.
    d. Compromised skin flaps and grafts.

ANSWERS

1. **a**
2. **d**
3. **b**
4. **b**
5. **b**
6. **d**
7. **c**
8. **a**
9. **d**
10. **b**

CHAPTER 60

THE WOUND CARE CENTER AND LIMB SALVAGE

Peter F. Lawrence • Steven Farley

Knowledge about the management of wounds has evolved into a distinct subspecialty requiring knowledge of normal and nonhealing wound physiology, products to accelerate wound healing, and new therapies for the treatment of recalcitrant wounds. Many subspecialties, such as vascular surgery, plastic surgery, podiatry, and primary care, share a role in managing wounds in the community. Current literature and research regarding wound healing often is published outside of traditional surgical or medical journals, so that many vascular surgeons are not familiar with up-to-date best practices

In many institutions, vascular surgeons are the primary consultant for the management of wounds. This new role in managing wounds has occurred because few other physicians are trained in the evaluation and treatment of wounds.

One of the most common clinical presentations for patients with peripheral arterial disease (PAD) is a nonhealing ischemic wound. Although revascularization may be required for limb salvage, the meticulous management of the primary wound after the surgery determines the success of limb salvage, as well as the time that it will take for a patient to return to function. Wound care after revascularization may be required for months or even years and a nonhealing wound can lead to limb loss, even if revascularization has been successful.

Patients with PAD who have limb-threatening ischemia often have diabetes. Not only are lower extremity ulcers common in diabetics, but they may also develop during the course of treatment. Diabetic wounds require specific management and often are managed by the vascular surgeon.

In the process of limb salvage, vascular surgeons create surgical wounds in ischemic limbs by harvesting vein conduit and exposing distal vessels. These newly created wounds occasionally result in graft exposure, infection, or delay the return to normal activity. Knowledge about the methods of minimizing the risk of creating wounds in ischemic limbs and the management of them is the province of vascular surgery.

Other surgical specialties, whose physicians used to be trained in wound healing, no longer receive training in contemporary wound management and wound healing. The training they receive in wound care is often based on outmoded concepts of wound care. Consequently, the specialist with the most exposure to nonhealing wounds, the vascular surgeon, has become the local expert in wound healing.

NORMAL WOUND HEALING

Wound healing is a complex process, the details of which we are only beginning to understand. Ideally, wound healing involves a well-organized, multifaceted series of events beginning after the actual event of wounding and ends with the formation of mature scar tissue (Figure 60-1). The acute wound is caused by external trauma, and acute wounds heal within a predictable time frame by progressing through orderly phases. Chronic wounds, however, do not follow this predictable course of events and may be the result of or impeded by internal events. However, correction of the internal problem does not always guarantee that the wound will heal in a timely fashion. Health care providers are just now beginning to comprehend the complex cellular and biological abnormalities that are inherent in the wound that has failed to heal.

Much of the latest research on wound healing involves investigation of the effects of various cytokines, growth factors, proteinases and their regulators and how they control the process of wound healing (Figure 60-2). To understand the effect of these substances on the chronic wound, the normal healing process of the acute wound must be understood. In acute wounds, the healing process begins with tissue injury and progresses predictably through the four phases of wound healing: hemostasis, inflammation, proliferation, and remodeling. These stages of healing, while occurring in a predictable manner, can overlap and can last for months.

Acute Wounds

Hemostasis

At the time of the initial injury, platelet activation and vasoconstriction occur after injury to the endothelium. Platelet aggregation, vasoconstriction, and clot formation begin the process of hemostasis. A number of soluble mediators are released by the platelets, including platelet-derived growth factor (PDGF), insulin-derived growth factor 1 (IGF-1), epidermal growth factor (EGF), fibroblast growth factor (FGF), and transforming growth factor-β (TGF-β). These mediators are responsible for initiating the healing process. Growth factors stimulate proliferation of wound cells, act as chemotactic agents, and regulate the differentiated functions of wound cells.[1] Neutrophils and macrophages are recruited to the

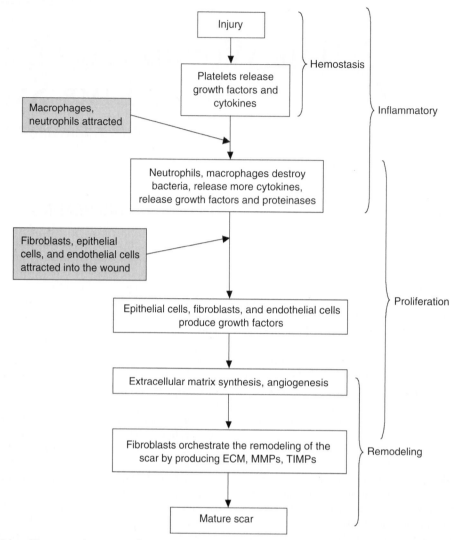

FIGURE 60-1 ■ The normal process of wound healing is complex and involves a series of phases that overlap.

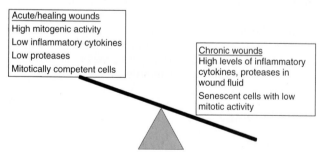

FIGURE 60-2 ■ Balance of healing and nonhealing factors in wounds. (Adapted from Schulz GS, Sibbald G, et al: Wound bed preparation: a systemic approach to wound management, Wound Rep Reg 11:1-28, 2003.)

injured site, attracted by the chemotactant release by the platelets.

Inflammation

Aggregated platelets begin to degranulate and mediators are released that help form the fibrin clot. Initially in the inflammatory phase, there is significant vasodilation, increased capillary permeability, complement activation, and migration of polymorphonuclear neutrophils (PMN) and macrophages to the site of the wound. The antimicrobial defense and removal of devitalized tissue is initiated by the macrophages and PMNs. As they engulf and destroy bacteria, proteases are released, including elastase and collagenase, which begin the degradation process of the damaged extracellular matrix (ECM) components.

Along with their role in defense and debridement, macrophages and neutrophils induce the formation of granulation tissue by secreting growth factors that stimulate fibroblast proliferation (PDGF), collagen synthesis (TGF-β), and new blood vessel formation (FGF). The cytokine IL-B stimulates the proliferation of fibroblasts, and TNF-α and IL-1β stimulate fibroblasts to synthesize matrix metalloproteinases (MMPs).

Proliferation

The proliferative phase begins as the number of inflammatory cells in the wound bed decreases. The synthesis of growth factors continues in the wound bed but is taken over by the fibroblast, endothelial cells, and keratinocytes. Keratinocytes synthesize TGF-β, TGF-α, and IL-1. Fibroblasts secrete IGF-1, bFGF, TGF-β, PDGF, keratinocyte growth factor and connective tissue factor. Endothelial cells produce b-FGF, PDGF, and vascular endothelial growth factor. The process of cell migration and proliferation continues as the process of new capillary formation and synthesis of ECM components are begun.

Fibrin and fibronectin form a provisional wound bed matrix. New collagen and elastin and proteoglycan molecules that form the initial scar are synthesized by fibroblasts. Proteases have an essential role at this point. No integration of the newly formed matrix with the dermal matrix can occur until the damaged proteins in the existing matrix are removed. Neutrophils, macrophages, fibroblasts, epithelial cells, and endothelial cells secrete proteases. Key proteases include collagenases, gelatinases, and stromelysins, which are all members of the matrix MMP super family, and neutrophil elastase, a serine protease.

In the wound bed, cell proliferation and formation of new extracellular matrix is continuing and is sustained by a dramatic increase in the vascularity of the wound bed. The epidermal layer is reformed by the proliferation and migration of epithelial cells across the highly vascularized ECM.

Remodeling

Once the initial scar is formed, the synthesis of ECM continues for several weeks. The newly healed red, raised scar changes over the course of weeks to months to a scar that is less red and may be barely visible. At the cellular and molecular level, the breakdown of the ECM components reaches a balance with the process of synthesis of ECM, allowing remodeling to occur. The increased concentration of fibroblasts and capillaries present in the early phase of healing declines, primarily through apoptosis. In the final remodeling phase, tensile strength reaches a maximum of 80% of the initial strength, as cross-linking of collagen fibrils plateaus.

Chronic Wounds

In contrast to the acute wound, the chronic wound does not heal in a predictable fashion. Lazarus and colleagues[2] defines the chronic wound as one in which the normal process of healing has been disrupted at one or more points in the phases of hemostasis, inflammation, proliferation, and remodeling. Chronic ulcers are characterized by defective remodeling of the ECM, a failure to epithelialize, and prolonged inflammation.[3-5] In the chronic wound, fibroblasts do not readily respond to growth factors such as PDGF-β and TGF-β; this failure to respond is hypothesized to be due to a form of cellular senescence. Hyperproliferation at the wound margin interferes with normal cellular migration across the wound bed, probably because of inhibition of apoptosis within the fibroblasts and keratinocyte cells.[6,7]

The phases of wound healing are replete with factors that have played important roles in the progression of

wound healing; therefore any alteration in one or more of these components may interfere with the healing progression. Growth factors such as PDGF, EGF, bFGF, and TGF-β are present in the chronic wound, but the levels remain constant, rather than displaying the variation seen in normal acute wound healing. The proinflammatory cytokines such as IL-1, IL-6, and TNF-α remain elevated in chronic wounds, when compared with the normal, acute wound, where a dramatic decrease is seen during healing, because there is a reduction in the inflammatory state.[8]

Several studies have shown that chronic wounds stall in the inflammatory phase of wound healing process.[9-11] The inflammatory phase in wound healing is most often associated with an increased amount of exudate, postulated to be from infection, heavy colonization, or from reaction to increased necrotic tissue in the wound bed. The amount and character of fluid produced by the chronic wound can severely impede and even reverse the healing process.[12-15]

Studies investigating chronic wounds effluent have provided increasing evidence that the cellular and molecular environments are substantially altered in chronic wounds. Bucalo and colleagues[16] collected exudate from venous ulcers and examined the effects of chronic wound fluid on the proliferation of dermal fibroblast, microvascular endothelial cells, and keratinocytes in culture. This study found that not only is wound fluid cytotoxic, it inhibited or failed to stimulate the proliferation of dermal fibroblasts, endothelial cells, and keratinocytes. Fluid from acute wounds, in contrast, has been found to stimulate fibroblast proliferation.[17] Proteases in chronic wound fluid have also been shown to degrade growth factors such as PDGF and TGF-1.[18,19]

MMPs are a necessary component of the wound healing process and have an important role in cell migration and modification of the ECM. If the regulation of these protease molecules is disrupted, excessive MMP production may lead to degradation of the ECM, preventing cellular migration and attachment, and ultimately causing tissue destruction.[20] It has been shown that levels of MMP activity are significantly elevated in a high percentage of chronic wounds when compared to acute wounds, suggesting dysregulation in chronic wounds (Figure 60-3). The activity of these proteases decreases consistently in patients whose ulcers progress from a nonhealing to healing phase.[21]

The chronic wound can also be heavily colonized or infected by bacteria that can substantially increase the amount of exudate. Thus, a copious amount of exudate produced by the chronic wounds, whatever its cause, can be a barrier to healing.[15,16,22,23]

ASSESSMENT OF WOUND HEALING CAPABILITY

With the recognition that there are altered cellular and molecular processes at play in the chronic wound has come the realization that wound management must focus on both the wound and the patient as a whole. The goal of wound management is to attain a healthy,

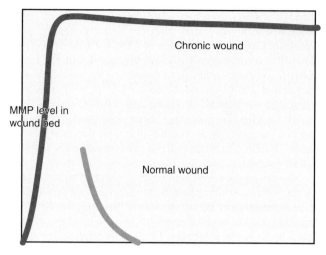

FIGURE 60-3 ■ Matrix metalloprotein levels in wound fluid remain high in patients with chronic nonhealing wounds, whereas they recede in the normal wound.

TABLE 60-1	Documentation of Wound Characteristics
Category	**Observation to be Documented**
Wound size	Length, width, depth, area, volume Undermining presence, location, measurement
Appearance	Granulation tissue; slough, necrotic, eschar; friability
Exudate	Amount, color, type (serous, serosanguineous, sanguinous, purulent), odor
Wound edge	Presence of maceration, advancing epithelium, erythema, even, rolled, ragged

well-vascularized, granulating wound bed. For this to happen, factors that can impede healing must be addressed. The way in which chronic wounds are viewed and managed should be based on a model that is both different from the acute wound paradigm and representative of the complex nature of nonhealing wounds.[24]

Wound bed preparation has become part of the standard nomenclature in wound healing. The concept of wound bed preparation is the management of a wound in order to accelerate endogenous healing or to facilitate the effectiveness of other therapeutic measures. The main barriers to healing in a chronic wound are necrotic tissue, high bioburden, increased exudate, and altered composition of exudate. The goal of wound bed preparation is to remove or reduce these barriers to promote healing, using ongoing debridement, reduction of bacterial burden in the wound bed, and management of exudate.

Patient Assessment

Identification of patient factors that would act as an impediment to healing is an essential component of the healing paradigm. The presence of diabetes, renal disease, heart disease, or liver disease can have detrimental effects of wound healing. Autoimmune diseases such as scleroderma, rheumatoid arthritis, vasculitis, or lupus erythematosus will deter wound healing. Systemic steroids, immunosuppressant medications, and nonsteroidal anti-inflammatory drugs will also interfere with the healing wound.

The nutritional status of the patient is an overlooked factor in wound healing. Protein calorie malnutrition can have devastating effects on the integrity of the body and on any wounds the patient might have. Protein calorie malnutrition is defined as insufficient intake of both protein and calories. In protein calorie malnutrition, morbidity and mortality increases as a result of the proportionate decline in body weight.[25] A decrease in

lean body mass of greater than 10% is associated with compromised wound healing, despite therapeutic interventions. Once depletion of lean body mass reaches 30%, the wound becomes a secondary issue as the body seeks to restore and replenish lost muscle.[26] Correction of any nutritional deficit should begin at the first visit and be maintained throughout the wound healing process. Assessment of dietary intake, including vitamin supplementation, is a necessary part of any wound healing assessment. Appetite stimulants, such as megestrol (Megace), may be helpful. If assessment shows moderate to severe protein calorie malnutrition, supplementation with oxandrolone has been shown to be beneficial to facilitate restoration of lean muscle mass.[27]

Assessment of Wound Characteristics

Accurate assessment of the wound and classifying the etiology of the wound must be accomplished before instituting a plan of care. Significant harm can occur if an incorrect treatment strategy is implemented; for example, active pyoderma gangrenosum should not be debrided and ischemic wounds should not be compressed. Information from the patient regarding the wound should be obtained if possible. How long has the wound been present, how did it start, what has been the progression, and how much pain exists? What aggravates or relieves the pain? What are the associated diseases, such as peripheral arterial or coronary artery disease, type 1 or 2 diabetes, rheumatoid arthritis?

Assessment of the wound includes the location, size, depth, and color of the wound bed (Table 60-1). A cotton swab has been shown to accurately gauge the depth and involvement of deep structures. The depth of a wound can be used to predict the likelihood of healing without extensive debridement of tendon or bone. The most common classification system of diabetic lower extremity wounds is the Wagner system, which grades the depth from superficial skin involvement to deep, involving tendon and bone.

These variables should be photographed, measured, and recorded. The amount and type of exudate should also be assessed. Associated signs such as callous surrounding the ulcer, skin changes in the gaiter (ankle) distribution, peripheral neuropathy, and ischemic (trophic) changes should also be noted and recorded.

Diagnostic Studies for the Nonhealing Wound

There are three questions that need to be answered with diagnostic studies. First, what is the depth of the wound? Depth determines treatment, because involvement of deep structures such as tendon or bone reduces the likelihood of healing without removal of the deep tissue and increases the risk of the ascending infection along tendon sheaths. Subfascial infection is particularly worrisome in diabetic patients who have reduced sensation of the foot and reduced ability to fight infection. The simplest test of depth is to probe the wound to determine whether tendon or bone is involved. This inexpensive and simple method has been shown to be as reliable as more expensive tests in determining the presence of osteomyelitis. Other tests such as plain radiograph and bone scan have less sensitivity and specificity than a magnetic resonance imaging (MRI) scan (Figure 60-4). All these tests have false negatives and positives, so that surgical exploration is often necessary to determine the presence of deep infection and osteomyelitis, as well as to debride and culture the wound.

Second, is the wound infected? The differentiation between colonization, cellulitis, abscess, and osteomyelitis is critical for optimal wound management. Wound culture identifies the organisms and need for topical, oral, and intravenous antibiotics. Colonization often is reflected by a wound culture that has multiple skin organisms. In colonization, there are no clinical signs of infection, such as erythema, swelling, and pain. Tissue biopsy and culture quantitates the number of organisms and determines whether the organisms are merely on the surface of the wound or whether they are present in the deep tissue, which implies an invasive infection and the need for more vigorous treatment. Plain film of the bone in a patient with osteomyelitis becomes positive in the late stages, long after osteomyelitis is established, whereas MRI scan has been shown to be reliable for determining osteomyelitis and detects early signs, such as changes in marrow intensity, periosteal reaction, and cortical erosion.

Third, is the limb ischemic, and does it have adequate blood flow to heal the wound? Adequate tissue oxygenation must be present for wound healing. Oxygen is available bound to hemoglobin and dissolved in plasma. In chronic wounds, plasma dissolved oxygen can be adequate for wound healing, assuming that perfusion of the tissue is satisfactory.

Assessment of the large vessel vascular supply is a critical component of the examination. A palpable pulse indicates a blood pressure of greater than 80 mm Hg in the foot and 70 mm Hg in the hand.[28] If a pulse is not easily palpable, use of a vascular laboratory examination is essential. Doppler waveforms and ankle-brachial index (ABI) as well as plethysmography (Figure 60-5) can be used with transcutaneous pressure of oxygen ($TcPO_2$) and skin perfusion pressure to determine the adequacy of blood supply. In patients with falsely elevated "stiff" arteries (high ABI with poor Doppler signals), pulse volume recordings, Doppler waveforms, and toe pressures are more reliable.

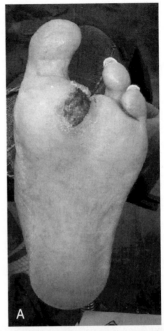

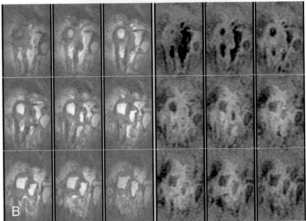

FIGURE 60-4 ■ **A,** A foot with a superficial ulcer needs further diagnostic studies to determine the depth. **B,** Magnetic resonance imaging scan of the foot can show the depth of the wound and evidence of osteomyelitis when it is not clinically apparent.

Normal acute wounds usually have oxygen tensions ($TcPO_2$) of 60 to 90 mm Hg, whereas chronic nonhealing wounds are most often associated with varying degrees of hypoxia because of low oxygen tension and poor blood perfusion. A tissue oxygen tension of greater than 40 mm Hg is adequate for wound healing. Tissue oxygen levels of less than 20 mm Hg in the wound bed are usually associated with failure to heal. When there is inadequate blood flow or perfusion pressure for wound healing, then treatment must be directed at increasing the perfusion by revascularization.

TREATMENT OF NONHEALING WOUNDS

Elimination of Edema

Edema reduces microvascular blood flow and the clearance of bacteria and protein from the wound. It

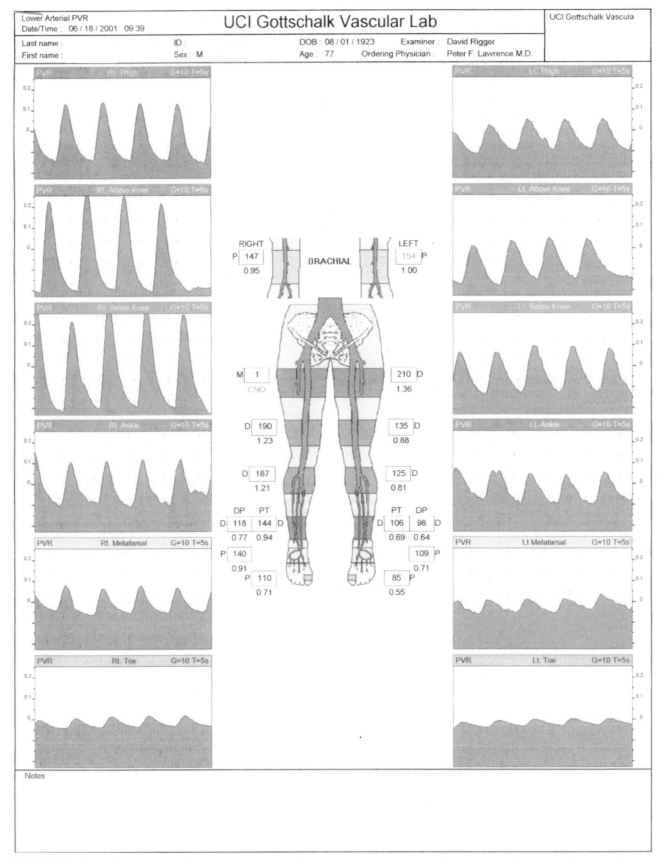

Lower Arterial PVR
Date/Time : 06 / 18 / 2001 09:39

FIGURE 60-5 ■ Physiologic studies of the lower limb are useful to determine the likelihood of wound healing. An ankle-brachial index (ABI) greater than 0.6 and biphasic or triphasic Doppler waveforms suggests a high likelihood of healing, whereas an ABI less than 0.4 and monophasic waveforms makes the likelihood of healing low. See Color Plate 60-5.

eliminates or reduces the likelihood of healing, and other management is often futile until edema is eliminated. The most challenging wounds are those with edema and ischemia, because patients with limb ischemia often place the limb in a dependent position to relieve ischemic rest pain. Prolonged dependency increases the limb edema and reduces perfusion, which paradoxically lead to an additional need for dependency. In ischemic limbs, the best method to reduce edema is to elevate the limb above the heart. Compression using sequential devices (e.g., Lymphopress, wraps [Unna boot or Profore], or support hose at 20 to 40 mm Hg pressure) should be limited to patients with a documented normal ankle brachial index of greater than 0.80 (Figure 60-6).

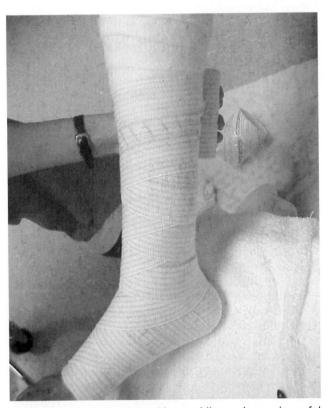

FIGURE 60-6 ■ Compression with a multilayered wrap is useful to reduce edema, if there is adequate perfusion. An ankle-brachial index greater than 0.8 or an ankle pressure greater than 80 mm Hg is recommended to use three- or four-layer wraps, because they create 30-40 mm Hg of pressure.

Debridement

The presence of necrotic tissue in a wound is the most obvious marker of a chronic wound. Reestablishing the balance of cytokines, proteases, and growth factors should be the focus of wound treatment. Efficient removal of devitalized tissue (necrotic burden) is an essential step in chronic wound management. The underlying pathogenic abnormalities in chronic wounds cause a continual buildup of necrotic tissue, and regular debridement is necessary to reduce the necrotic burden and achieve healthy granulation tissue. Debridement of devitalized tissue reduces tissue damage and destruction, removes bioburden, and exposes dead space that can harbor bacteria. Debridement can be accomplished in several different ways (Table 60-2), and the method chosen should be dictated by the condition of the wound and the skill of the practitioner, as well as the patient situation.

Autolytic Debridement

Autolytic debridement uses the body's own natural enzymes to dissolve necrotic tissue within the wound and occurs spontaneously to some extent in all wounds. The macrophages and endogenous proteolytic enzymes liquefy and spontaneously separate necrotic tissue and eschar from healthy tissue. Autolytic debridement is most effective in a moist wound environment. Dressings most commonly used for this method include hydrogels and hydrocolloids, both of which can produce a more effective environment for destruction and phagocytosis of the necrotic tissue. Dressings that are occlusive or semiocclusive facilitate contact between the necrotic tissue and the enzymes within the wound. This method of debridement is selective with little discomfort, but it is often slow. If there is not improvement in the wound bed within 72 hours, another method of debridement should be used. This method is inappropriate for a wound that has a significant amount of necrotic debris or is heavily infected.

Enzymatic Debridement

Enzymatic debridement uses the application of topical agents to the surface of the wound, which chemically disrupts or digests devitalized extracellular proteins present in wound. There are two main preparations

TABLE 60-2 Selecting Methods of Wound Debridement

Characteristic	Debridement Method			
	Autolytic	Surgical	Enzymatic	Mechanical
Rapidity of debridement action	4	1	2	3
Tissue specificity	3	2	1	4
Exudate	1	4	2	3
Infection	3	1	4	2
Cost	4	1	3	2
	1	4	2	3

Adapted from Sibbald RG, Williamson D, Orsted HL, et al: Preparing the wound bed—debridement, bacterial balance, and moisture balance. Ostomy Wound Manage 46(11):14–22, 24–28, 30–35, 2000.
1, Most appropriate; *2,* appropriate; *3,* somewhat appropriate; *4,* least appropriate.

used in enzymatic debridement: collagenase (Santyl) and papain urea (Accuzyme). Collagenase is a partially purified preparation of collagenase derived from *Clostridium histolyticum*. Collagenase has been shown to have specificity for collagen types I and II. It cleaves glycine in endogenous collagen and digests collagen, but is not active against keratin, fat, or fibrin. Papain urea is composed of papain (from papaya fruit) mixed with a chemical agent, urea. Papain digests necrotic tissue by liquefaction of fibrinous debris, but is inactive against collagen. Urea is an activator for the papain. Urea also digests nonviable protein, making it more susceptible to proteolysis. Studies have demonstrated that the combination of papain urea is approximately twofold more effective than the enzyme alone.

Álvarez and colleagues showed that the papain urea product achieved a better wound response than did collagenase, but there was not a significant difference in wound closure between the two groups.[28a] Some patients complain of burning when the papain urea is applied, and this may limit its use in some patients.

Mechanical Debridement

Mechanical debridement is a nonselective method of removing necrotic tissue from the wound using mechanical force. This method can damage healthy tissue in the wound bed and at the margins of the wound, and it can be extremely painful for the patient. Wet-to-dry dressings are the simplest method of mechanical debridement but require frequent dressing changes, and therefore result in increased costs because of increased nursing time. Wet-to-dry debridement involves covering a wound with saline moistened gauze and allowing it to dry. It is then removed, and the necrotic tissue that has adhered to the dressing is removed. This method is nonselective and painful because it lifts away viable tissue as well. Strings from the gauze can be left behind in the wound bed, creating further inflammatory reaction to the presence of a foreign body. Wet-to-wet dressings maintain a moistened dressing until removal and accomplish the same results with less destruction of viable tissue.

Pressurized irrigation involves the application of streams of water at a high or low pressure to wash away bacteria, foreign matter, and necrotic tissue from the wound, but bacteria may be driven even further into soft tissue with this technique.

Whirlpool therapy uses powered irrigation and can be effective at loosening and removing surface debris, bacteria, necrotic tissue, and exudate from the wound. This technique works well for necrotic wounds in the inflammatory phase, but it is inappropriate for granulating wounds with fragile endothelial and epithelial cells that may be damaged or removed by the circulating water. There is also the possibility spreading waterborne infection.

Biosurgical Debridement

Biosurgical debridement involves the use of maggots to remove nonviable tissue from a wound bed. This technique uses sterile maggots applied to the wound bed, covered with a dressing. The maggots then digest necrotic material from the wound bed without damaging the healthy tissue. Maggots also demonstrate the ability to consume bacteria, decreasing the patient's risk of developing infection. The precise mechanism by which the maggots debride the wound and promote healing is not clear. It is speculated that the pH of the wound is changed by the maggots, increasing a bacteriostatic effect. It is thought the maggots also secrete proteolytic enzymes that enhance protein degradation. Despite their effectiveness and encouraging reports on wound healing, some patients complain of increased pain with maggot therapy, and some patients are uncomfortable with use of maggots on their wounds.

Sharp Debridement

Surgical (or sharp) debridement is the fastest way to remove devitalized tissue. Removing dead tissue decreases bacterial burden in the wound bed. Use of the scalpel to remove senescent cells converts a chronic wound into an acute wound within a chronic wound and has been shown to increase the healing rate of diabetic neurotrophic foot ulcers.[29] The major problem with this form of debridement is that viable and nonviable tissue may be removed. This method can also be painful, but the use of topical or local anesthetic (eutectic mixture of local anesthetics [EMLA] cream) can alleviate the discomfort.

TREATMENT OF INFECTION

The presence of bacteria in the wound bed can be categorized as contamination, colonization, critical colonization, or infection. Contamination is the presence of nonreproducing bacteria in the wound bed; they do not interfere with healing. Colonization is the presence of reproducing bacteria in the wound bed; they are adherent to the surface of the wound, but do not impede wound repair. Critical colonization is a step between colonization and infection; replicating bacteria are present in the wound and interfere with wound healing, but do not show the typical signs of infection. Treatment is necessary to rid the wound of the bioburden. The infected wound will show the signs of delayed healing as well as increased pain, an increased amount of exudate, and a change in the color of the wound bed to friable, red granulation tissue or the absence of granulation tissue, along with odor and purulence. Treatment strategies include sustained release silver dressings, or slow released iodine formulations such as cadexomer iodine, along with systemic antibiotics.

Chronic wounds are usually colonized with at least three species of microorganisms.[30] The concentration of bacteria necessary to impede healing of open wounds is controversial; however, 1×10^5 organisms per gram of tissue have historically been associated with impaired healing.[31,32] The type and pathogenicity of the organisms in a wound bed may be a better predictor of the risk of infection than simply the number. Some combinations of bacteria act synergistically to enhance the virulence of a previously benign organism.[32]

Another important factor in infections is the biofilm that is present on some bacteria that can contribute to delayed healing. Biofilm occurs when some bacteria proliferate; they form microcolonies that become attached to the wound bed, secreting a glyocalyx sheath of biofilm that protects the microorganism from systemic antimicrobial agents.[33]

Treatment of an infected wound should begin without delay. Antibiotics are useful to prevent the spread of infection in the soft tissue beyond the wound, but repeated use of antibiotics in patients with chronic wounds can lead to the development of resistant organisms. Therefore systemic antibiotics should be used judiciously and should be avoided unless infection is established.[34] The use of antiseptic agents is useful in the treatment of the infected wound and may be essential.[35] Topical cadexomer iodine and nanocrystalline silver target the bacteria at the cell membrane, cytoplasmic organelle, and nucleic acid level; this combination of actions means that development of resistant bacteria is improbable. Cadexomer iodine is a formulation of cadexomer beads that absorb a significant amount of exudate while slowly releasing iodine into the tissues in a concentration low enough to be bactericidal but not cytotoxic. Cadexomer iodine has been shown to be effective against *Staphylococcus aureus* and methicillin-resistant *S. aureus*, and vancomycin-resistant enterococcus.[36,37] Nanocrystalline silver dressings provide an antibacterial dressing that has been shown to be effective in partial- and full-thickness wounds. The silver is slowly released into the wound bed and maintains an effective antimicrobial barrier for up to 7 days. Nanocrystalline silver is effective against a number of pathogens, including methicillin-resistant *S. aureus* and vancomycin-resistant enterococcus.

MANAGEMENT OF THE EXUDATE

Traditionally, dry wounds have been promoted as optimal for wound healing by avoiding bacterial overgrowth; however, the wound-healing community has long recognized that wounds heal faster in a closed, moist environment. Eaglestein and colleagues[38] showed that experimentally induced wounds healed 40% faster in a closed, moist environment, compared with wounds left exposed to the air.[38] A moist environment has also been shown to facilitate epithelial migration, maintain optimal

temperature, decrease pain, and provide a better cosmetic result; however, excess exudate in a chronic wound has an adverse effect on wound healing.[39] The buildup of wound fluid must be managed to minimize the negative biochemical factors. On the other hand, excessive desiccation slows migration of epidermal cells and limits epidermal regeneration.[40] Therefore the choice of dressings must be made with the goal of controlling exudate while maintaining optimal wound bed moisture.

DRESSING THE NONHEALING WOUND

Wound dressings are all designed with a specific purpose in mind; many serve more than one purpose. The wound, the patient, and their multiple needs should be considered when choosing a dressing (Box 60-1). Optimal wound care decision making focuses on the need for moist dressings, which will maintain the healing environment at the optimum moisture. The Agency for Health Care Policy and Research published guidelines in 1994 for the selection of dressings (Table 60-3).

Hydrogels provide a high level of moisture (70% to 90% water), which is contained in insoluble polymers.[41] Hydrogels are the best choice for dry, sloughy wounds with minimal to moderate levels of exudate. Gels need to be reapplied every 24 to 72 hours because they are not antibacterial; they are nonadherent and soothing. Wound gels facilitate autolytic debridement.

Hydrocolloids provide an occlusive dressing for the wound bed, forming a matrix gel on contact with the

---

BOX 60-1 Principles for Wound Dressings

Wound dressing should:
- Debride necrotic tissue
- Identify and eradicate infection: reduce wound contamination
- Obliterate dead space
- Absorb excess drainage
- Maintain moist wound environment while keeping peri-wound skin protected
- Provide thermal insulation
- Protect the wound from bacteria and trauma
- Promote wound healing

TABLE 60-3 Selection of Dressings for Chronic Wounds

Dressing	Eschar	Slough-Dry	Slough-Moist	Pink/Red, Wet	Pink, Healthy Granulation, Epithelialization
Hydrogels	++	+++			+++
Hydrocolloids	+	++	++		++
Film dressings			++		++
Calcium alginate			+	++	
Foam			++	++	
Enzymes	+++	+++			+
Antimicrobial (silver, cadexomer iodine)			+++	+++	

wound exudate. Hydrocolloids are suited to autolytic debridement for mild to moderately exudative wounds, but care should be taken to avoid maceration of the healthy epidermis. Mild antibacterial activity is present within hydrocolloids because of the lowered pH. Occlusion is achieved with foam or a film-sheet backing with adhesive, which can cause an allergic reaction in some patients.[42,43]

Film dressings are ideal in the later stage of wound healing, when there is no significant exudate. The dressings are permeable to water and oxygen while maintaining impermeability to bacteria and water. Foam dressings are appropriate for sloughy, moderately to heavily exudative wounds. Foams come in many forms and sizes. All provide thermal insulation, high absorbency, and a moist environment. Most have a polyurethane backing to prevent excess fluid loss. Hydrofibers are considered in the category with foam dressings, although visually they are quite different. Hydrofibers are highly absorbent and have good tensile strength. Both foams and hydrofibers can be worn for up to 1 week, are easy to cut to the size and shape of the wound, and do not shed fibers in the wound bed.[44]

Alginates are best used on heavily exudative wounds. They form a gel upon contact with the exudate, promoting a moist wound healing and autolytic debridement. They are made from brown seaweed. After debridement, they donate calcium to the wound bed, facilitating hemostasis. Silicone dressings are among the first products engineered specifically for painless removal of the dressing from the wound. Silicone dressings have a hydrophobic soft silicone layer that prevents the dressing from adhering to the wound surface. They maintain contact with the wound bed, allowing exudate to pass through and be absorbed while also allowing antimicrobials or biologically active properties of other dressings to interact with the wound bed.

GROWTH FACTORS

Much of the latest research in wound healing has focused on the development, use, and effect of various cytokines and growth factors on the wound bed. The only growth factor approved by the U.S. Food and Drug Administration (FDA) and readily available is PDGF, in the form of becaplermin (Regranex). Becaplermin is approved for use in neuropathic ulcers. In 1995, Steed[45] reported that becaplermin gel improved healing rates in diabetic foot ulcers in 48%, as opposed to 25% of patients in the control group. Other studies have not shown similar results in neuropathic foot ulcers, but the 100-µg/g dose had 50% complete closure within the prescribed time compared with 35% of the placebo group.[46] Studies examining becaplermin for use in other types of ulceration, such as pressure ulcers, have not met with the same degree of success.[47] Recently, the use of autologous platelet-rich plasma (PRP) has been used in orthopedic, maxillofacial, and plastic surgery. PRP is an autologous concentration of human platelets in a small volume. Because it is a concentration of platelets, it is also a concentration of seven fundamental protein growth factors

proved to be actively secreted by platelets to initiate all wound healing. These growth factors include the three isomers of PDGF (PDGF-αα, PDGF-ββ, and PDGF-αβ), two of the numerous transforming growth factors-β (TGF-β1 and TGF-β2), vascular endothelial factor, and epithelial growth factor.[48] PRP, because it is suspended in a small amount of plasma, also contains fibrin and fibronectin, which are cellular adhesion molecules. It is known that degranulation of the platelet with the release of growth factors initiates and facilitates the healing cascade. The active secretion of these growth factors is initiated by the clotting of blood and begins within 10 minutes. More than 95% of the growth factors are secreted within 1 hour; therefore the PRP must be developed in the anticoagulated state and should be used within 1 hour.

The literature has been mixed about the results of PRP. PRP in maxillofacial, orthopedic and cosmetic surgery has been associated with positive results.[49] After the initial use of PRP-related growth factors, the platelets synthesize and secrete additional growth factors for the remaining 7 days of their life span.[50-57] Recently, PRP has been used in wound healing. Knighton and colleagues[58] evaluated the use of PRP in patients with wounds of various etiologies; wounds healed in 15% of controls and 81% of patients treated with platelet concentrate. Patients who had failed to heal in the control arm were then treated with PRP, and all patients had epithelialization in an average of 7.1 weeks.[58] Currently, there are two office devices used to develop PRP that have been cleared by the FDA: the Smart PreP (Harvest Technologies, Plymouth Mass.) and the Platelet Concentration Collection System (Implant Innovations, West Palm Beach, Fla.).

TISSUE TRANSFER

Autologous tissue transfer has been used for many years to cover tissue defects; however, the use of autologous tissue creates another tissue defect at the donor site, requires anesthetic, and creates additional pain. Tissue substitutes arose from the need to treat large burns with insufficient donor skin for grafting.[59] This work has extended to wound care, and now there are several choices of skin substitutes. The purpose of a skin substitute is to provide a temporary dressing that is biologically active and accelerates skin tissue regeneration and wound healing by stimulation of recipient wound bed growth factors and skin cells.[60] Significant progress has been made over the last 10 years in expanding from a simple synthetic material to products that have increasing structural and biochemical complexity. Many skin substitutes now closely approximate the biochemical and cellular composition and behavior found in the dermal and epidermal structures. The commercially bioengineered skin consists of sheets of biomaterial matrix containing allogenic cells, which are typically derived from neonatal foreskin, a convenient tissue source with the added advantages of having a higher content of putative keratinocyte stem cells, vigorous cell growth and metabolic activity, and minimal antigenicity.[61,62] The skin substitutes approved for use in vascular and diabetic ulcers

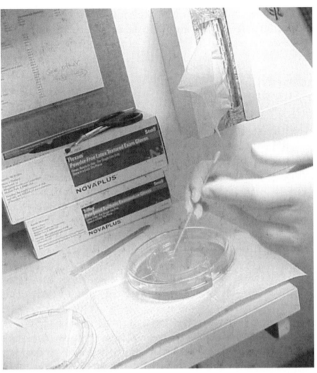

FIGURE 60-7 ■ Apligraft is a skin and dermal substitute that can be useful in the coverage of chronic wounds once adequate perfusion has been restored.

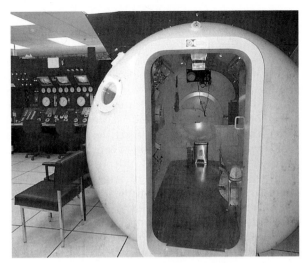

FIGURE 60-8 ■ A hyperbaric chamber can improve wound healing in chronic wounds that show a low TCPO₂ that increases to greater than 30 mm Hg when 100% oxygen is given to the patient.

include Dermagraft (Smith and Nephew, Largo, Fla.), which is a cryopreserved human fibroblastic derived dermal substitute that is approved for treatment of diabetic foot ulcers of greater than 6 weeks' duration. Fibroblasts are isolated from neonatal tissue and then cultured on a bioabsorbable polyglactin mesh for a 3-week period. During incubation the cells secrete matrix proteins, including human dermal collagen, and soluble factors to create a human protein containing three-dimensional matrix that can be used as a dermal replacement.[63,64] Marston reported an increase in complete healing with Derma graft (30% vs. 18%).[65] Another study examining Dermagraft in diabetic foot wounds of long duration showed increased healing at week 12 (71% vs. 14%) compared with saline-soaked gauze–treated control group.[66] The product must remain frozen prior to use and requires thawing and rinsing prior to placement.

Apligraf (Organogenesis Inc, Canton, Mass.) is a bilayered, living skin construct developed to provide multiple functions, similar to human skin (Figure 60-7). Functions include providing a barrier against mechanical damage and infection, producing structural and regulatory substances (e.g., growth factors or cytokines), and interacting with the underlying tissue to promote more effective wound repair.[67] Apligraf assimilates allogeneic cultured human skin cells from neonatal foreskin in a full-thickness skin construct that contains both epidermal and dermal layers. The well-differentiated epidermal layer is formed of living human keratinocytes; the dermal layer is formed of living human fibroblasts that are dispersed in a type I bovine-derived collagen matrix.[68,69] Apligraf is approved

for use in venous ulcers and diabetic foot ulcers.[70] The pivotal Apligraft (Organogenesis Inc, Canton, Mass.) study provided to the FDA for approval in diabetic foot ulcers was done by Veves and colleagues.[71] This multicenter trial of healing rates of neuropathic, diabetic, plantar foot ulcers had a 56% complete wound closure at 12 weeks, compared with 38% of control patients.[71]

Hyperbaric Oxygen Therapy

Oxygen composes 21% of the earth's atmosphere. When administered at higher concentrations, oxygen is technically an inhaled drug. The hyperbaric chamber is a delivery system that can deliver oxygen in super-physiologic concentrations, well beyond what is possible at normobaric pressures (Figure 60-8). Unquestioned, absolute indications for hyperbaric treatment are mechanical problems such as decompression illness, crush injuries, or gas embolism. Hyperbaric treatment in conjunction with oxygen can shrink bubble sizes and more quickly dissolve nitrogen bubbles back into the blood stream. A second category of absolute indications are related to oxidative respiration such as carbon monoxide and cyanide toxicity, which compete for hemoglobin binding and mitochondrial activity.

However, controversy surrounds the benefit of the temporary delivery of high concentrations of oxygen to wound beds. Hyperbaric therapy is expensive and time consuming, and it should be seen as an advanced therapy for problem wounds. Considering these factors combined with the historical and current unscientific use of hyperbaric oxygen for a host of medical problems such as dementia or multiple sclerosis, there is still skepticism surrounding HBOT.

Patients with problem wounds compose a majority of the patients who undergo modern HBOT. More specifically, approximately 80% of patients undergoing

HBOT receive treatment for wounds—40% radiation-associated and another 40% diabetes-associated. In other wounds, modern hyperbaric centers mainly treat wounds and are available for occasional emergency indications. Contraindications to HBOT include untreated pneumothorax and ongoing treatment with several chemotherapies, such as bleomycin or doxorubicin (Adriamycin). Relative contraindications include severe COPD with air trapping, poorly compensated CHF, history of claustrophobia, seizure disorders, history of ear surgery, or retinal surgery.

Central to the evaluation of patients with chronic wounds is tissue oxygenation. Using transcutaneous oxygen sensors, the partial pressure of oxygen at the skin can be measured. $TcPO_2$ testing needs to be done by certified technologists under controlled conditions to achieve meaningful results. In general, a $TcPO_2$ of greater than 40 mm Hg is associated with wound healing. Patients with a $TcPO_2$ less than 40 mm Hg are given a normobaric 100% oxygen challenge. An increase in 50% or a $TcPO_2$ greater than 100 mm Hg represents a positive oxygen response and identifies patients who can benefit from hyperbaric oxygen. Currently, HBOT is approved by CMS for wound treatment in patients with chronic refractory osteomyelitis, failing or threatened skin flaps (including amputation flaps), diabetic foot wounds involving the bone (Wagner stage III), and radiation-associated wounds.

Vacuum-Assisted Closure

Vacuum-assisted closure (VAC) relies on negative pressure or a vacuum to promote wound healing; it has gained increased acceptance in the management of a wound with a heavy exudate and edema that cannot be controlled by conventional methods of wound care. Use of the VAC requires adequate limb perfusion (ABI > 0.6) and absence of osteomyelitis and active infection. A portable device is available that can create negative pressure and collect drainage from the wound, while reducing edema. During therapy, negative pressure facilitates contraction of the wound. Large wounds often reduce in size dramatically over a relative short time span. The positive experience of physicians and nurses with the VAC has led to increasing use of it for large wounds in swollen limbs with adequate perfusion.

New Therapies for Nonhealing Wounds

Some wounds remain recalcitrant despite the established wound care approaches discussed above. Oral or intravenous steroids are often used for vasculitic ulcers that do not respond to conventional treatment, and occasionally colectomy is required to heal pyoderma gangrenosum in a patient with ulcerative colitis. Currently, there are nonapproved options for the nonhealing wound, including use of the Art Assist, an intermittent pneumatic leg compression device used for intermittent claudication that augments limb blood flow, intravenous PGE or PGI2 prostaglandin infusion, and oral sildenafil (Viagra). Although none of these therapies have been demonstrated by level 1 evidence

to close wounds, they are occasionally used when the only alternative is an amputation or a prolonged, open, dysvascular wound.

ORGANIZATION OF A WOUND CARE PROGRAM

A critical component of optimal wound care is an integrated program in which continuity can be provided from the hospital to the ambulatory clinic to home health care. Nurses, physicians, access to all subspecialties, and a facility with equipment and dressings are necessary for optimal wound care and a successful wound care program.

Personnel

The key component to a successful wound care program is personnel. Because wound problems often need treatment more than once per week, a typical physician's office is unable to provide the environment for an excellent wound care program. Nurses and physicians with expertise in wound management must be available every day to heal recalcitrant wounds, and they must be available for consultation with home health and visiting nurse services.

The core of most wound care programs is a complement of nurses with training in wound care. Their expertise must include the ability to assess changes in the status of the wound, training to mechanically debride the wound, and knowledge of optimal dressings for different clinical situations. Nurses provide continuity of care for most patients who have wounds, because physicians often rotate coverage of wound centers and are not available daily. This applies particularly to vascular surgeons, who may be in the operating room for an entire day and are unavailable to patients on some days of the week.

Specialists who have special expertise in the management of patients with dysvascular or nonhealing wounds are an important component of all wound care centers. Plastic surgery, orthopedic surgery, podiatry, endocrinology (diabetes), nephrology, infectious disease, rheumatology, and cardiology are the specialties are most often asked to provide help with the management of this group of patients with many risk factors and comorbidities.

Facility

The optimal wound center has dedicated rooms used to treat patients with wounds. These rooms are designed for patients who are often not ambulatory and have special needs. Rooms dedicated for wound care need ready access to a variety of debriding instruments, wound care products, and dressings. Diagnostic facilities, such as plain radiography, foot MRI, and CT scans are optimally located close to the wound care center, for patient ease. A treatment room for debridement of wounds is also useful. The most expensive capital expense for wound care, hyperbaric therapy, is not necessarily needed within the center, because a small percentage of wound care patients need hyperbaric therapy, but it should be readily accessible. Other capital equipment that is often useful includes a multichamber mechanical compression device (e.g., Lympha Press) and a platelet concentrator for PRP.

REVASCULARIZATION IN PATIENTS WITH A NONHEALING WOUND

Dysvascular patients with nonhealing wounds present a unique challenge to the vascular surgeon, because the process of revascularization, which is often necessary, is frequently associated with creation of another wound, exposure to cardiovascular risk, prolonged hospitalization, and further protein calorie depletion. To determine the need for revascularization, a systematic approach must be taken to this complex group of patients. There are several questions that should be asked to determine the best approach for dysvascular patients with a nonhealing wound:

First, how ischemic is the limb? Patients with mild or moderate ischemia, without rest pain, dependent rubor, or infection may be treated less urgently than those with more advanced ischemia. In addition, the method of revascularization does not require the same degree of durability as a patient who would need revascularization for limb ischemia, even if the nonhealing wound were not present.

Second, what is the level of the disease? Patients with proximal PAD of the iliac arteries are much more easily treated with revascularization procedures than those with distal, infrapopliteal disease. In addition, distal revascularization procedures often are less durable and require an incision in the ischemic limb for either conduit harvest or exposure of the vessels.

Third, what conduit is available? For a distal bypass in an ischemic limb that requires long-term patency, the ideal conduit is autogenous vein. Patients who do not have conduit because of prior harvesting, small size, or prior thrombosis have more limited options.

And last, will the patient have a functional limb if the ulcer is healed with revascularization? To be functional, the patient must have the motivation and strength, adequate plantar skin, and biomechanics to walk. If it is unlikely that the patient will use a revascularized limb, the risks and complexity of the procedure must be weighed against the patient's desire for a cosmetic, nonfunctional limb.

Options for Revascularization

Nonrevascularization

In the presence of mild ischemia, a trial of optimal wound care is a reasonable approach in some patients. Traumatic toe and pressure wounds, particularly in diabetics, that are superficial and not associated with severe preexisting ischemia may heal with relief of pressure, optimal wound care, and patience. Although these wounds might not heal at the rate of a patient without ischemia, if there is otherwise no indication for

revascularization, then a trial of wound care may be the best option. Veith and colleagues[72] showed that a significant number of mildly dysvascular patients healed ulcers without revascularization, using a program of bed rest and wound care.

Angioplasty

Angioplasty is an attractive option for a patient with a dysvascular, nonhealing wound, because it rarely causes additional tissue trauma, which occurs with surgical vessel exposure and vein harvest. Angioplasty alone can often improve perfusion enough to heal a wound. Proximal lesions (iliac and aortic) are optimal for angioplasty and stenting. As the hemodynamically significant disease occurs more distally, the durability of angioplasty and stenting is reduced, although recent reports have shown excellent early patency and results comparable to bypass.[73] In the superficial femoral artery, the type of lesion (TASC A, B, or C, which is a classification system[74] for the length, extent, and degree of calcification of the lesions), determines the likelihood of initial and long-term success. For infrapopliteal disease, Chandra and colleagues[75] recommend angioplasty as the optimal procedure to improve blood flow and heal ischemic ulcers in limbs that do not otherwise require revascularization.

Bypass

Bypass is the standard treatment for patients with limb ischemia and a nonhealing wound. Although an extensive discussion of the alternative techniques and conduits is beyond the scope of this chapter, certain principles should be applied when deciding on a revascularization procedure.

First, limit distal incisions. Kalra and colleagues[76] advise surgeons to limit distal incisions by harvesting more proximal veins and tunneling them distally, to avoid foot and ankle incisions in dysvascular limbs (Figure 60-9; see color plate). In situ bypasses should be performed with a closed technique, if technically feasible.

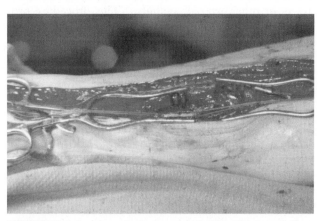

FIGURE 60-9 ■ Incisions that are made in the distal part of an ischemic limb are at significant risk for wound complications of infection or dehiscence. An alternative is to harvest a more proximal vein and tunnel it distally. See Color Plate 60-9.

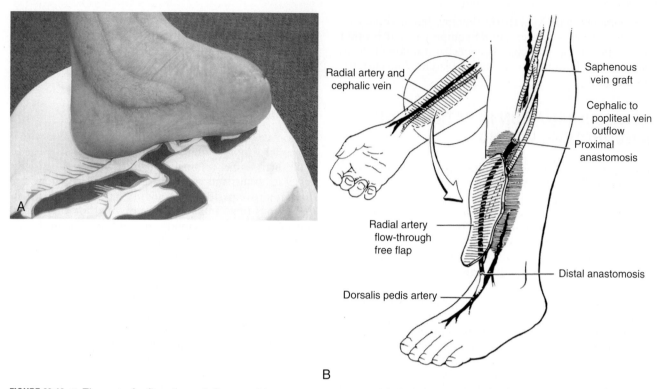

Radial artery and
cephalic vein

Saphenous
vein graft

Cephalic to
popliteal vein
outflow

Proximal
anastomosis

Radial artery
flow-through
free flap

Distal anastomosis

Dorsalis pedis artery

A

B

FIGURE 60-10 ■ The use of a flow-through flap provides an autogenous conduit for bypass with skin and fat to cover a wound with a large skin defect. This patient received a radial flow-through flap to cover a large medial ankle wound. The bypass was from the mid-calf posterior tibial artery to the inframalleolar posterior tibial artery. A transmetatarsal amputation was also performed. See Color Plate 60-10.

The LeMaitre valvulotome, as well as other commercially available valvulotomes, perform the valvulotomy without an incision to expose the vein. Treiman and colleagues[77] reported on the management of wound complications in a small series of patients who developed incision complications post distal bypass, as well as alternatives to maintain patency of the exposed graft.

Second, use tissue transfer procedures. The patient with advanced ischemia, who needs both limb revascularization and closure of a large wound, can often have both accomplished with a flow-through flap, using the radial artery or other arterial conduits.[78] This procedure provides a conduit for revascularization with an elliptical flap of attached, vascularized tissue (Figure 60-10; see color plate). The radial artery usually matches the size of the distal foot vessel and is optimal for this procedure. If a long conduit is needed for the proximal anastomosis, then saphenous vein can be spliced to the radial artery, although the proximal radial artery anastomosis can usually be placed in a proximal tibial or peroneal artery. Vascularized skin and subcutaneous tissue can then be used to cover large ulcers and skin defects. Other flaps, which can be anastomosed to a vein conduit, can even provide fascia to reconstruct the Achilles tendon, if needed.

Third, use prosthetic or cryopreserved conduit for ulcer healing. If a dysvascular, nonhealing wound cannot be healed with wound care or angioplasty, then a conduit with good short-term patency but poor long-term patency can be used to temporarily provide increased blood supply to heal the wound.[79,80] This alternative should be used only if the rest of the limb does not need long-term revascularization. These grafts often require anticoagulation to maintain patency, and they are at increased risk for graft infection.

CONCLUSION

Wound care and revascularization in the dysvascular patient are inextricably intertwined if limb salvage is to occur. Vascular surgeons are the common link in diagnosing, treating, and coordinating care. To achieve an optimal patient outcome, vascular surgeons must be familiar with the principles of wound healing, the alternatives for wound bed preparation, and the techniques for revascularization in the ischemic limb.

References available online at expertconsult.com.

QUESTIONS

1. What defines a wound as chronic?

2. What does proper documentation of wound characteristics include?

3. What are the basics in the treatment of nonhealing wounds?

4. How is a chronic wound defined as infected versus colonized?

5. True or False: Hyperbaric oxygen has a broad role in managing chronic wounds.

6. True or False: Wound healing is promoted by creating a dry environment rather than a moist one.

7. True or False: The management of chronic wounds requires a significant infrastructure including nursing, home health, and multiple specialists including podiatry, plastic surgery, vascular surgery, and endocrinology.

8. Diagnostic studies used to evaluate patients with chronic wounds include:
   a. Ankle brachial index
   b. Venous insufficiency studies
   c. X-ray
   d. $TcPO_2$
   e. MRI
   f. All of the above

9. True or False: Tissue transfer is widely available, can heal most wounds, and is low cost.

10. Current indications for hyperbaric oxygen therapy for chronic wounds include:
    a. Refractory osteomyelitis
    b. Diabetic foot ulcer
    c. Radiation-associated wounds
    d. Failing skin flaps or threatened skin grafts
    e. All of the above

ANSWERS

1. **Wound healing that does not occur in a predictable fashion. The normal processes of healing involving hemostasis, inflammation, proliferation, and remodeling are interrupted.**
2. **Precise description of wound size, appearance, exudate, and the wound edges**
3. **Elimination of edema through leg elevation and compression, débridement of nonviable tissue, treatment of infection, management of the exudate, and dressing the wound**
4. **Wounds can be categorized as contaminated, colonized, or infected. Wound infection is often a clinical finding, including increasing pain, exudate, odor, and wound changes. Wound infection is defined by 1×10^5 organisms per gram.**
5. **False**
6. **False**
7. **True**
8. **f**
9. **False**
10. **e**

CHAPTER 61

Spine Exposure: Operative Techniques for the Vascular Surgeon

Matthew M. Nalbandian

Surgery is the standard treatment for a multitude of benign and malignant disease processes of the spine. The anterior approach to the spinal column is important in degenerative disk disease, neural decompression, resection of neoplasms, trauma, infection, and congenital anomalies.[1-4] Safe access to the spine is paramount to performing successful spinal procedures. Although orthopedic surgeons and neurosurgeons have been responsible for many surgical advances in spine surgery, access to the spine is often provided by vascular surgeons, general surgeons, urologists, or spine surgeons. With increasing frequency, vascular surgeons are the primary surgeons for anterior spine exposure owing to their skill and experience in retroperitoneal surgery. The operative techniques involved in retroperitoneal aortoiliac surgery can be modified to perform spine surgery. An experienced team approach to spine exposure can reduce intraoperative complications.[1]

The level of involvement by vascular surgeons varies by institution. Generally, vascular surgeons perform exposure of the lower thoracic, lumbar, and sacral spine levels. Thoracic surgeons are often involved in upper thoracic exposure, and the cervical spine is the domain of spine surgeons. The morbidity of the anterior approach has been reported to range from 10% to 30%.[1,2] Periprocedure complications can include iatrogenic vascular, visceral, genitourinary, and neurologic injuries.[1-4]

As new spinal prosthetic devices are developed and the indications for surgical repair broaden, there will be a growing demand for surgeons who can provide access to the spine. Vascular surgeons should have this skill in their armamentarium, much as they have developed skill in endovascular procedures. This chapter discusses the vascular surgeon's role in the surgical exposure of the lower thoracic, lumbar, and sacral levels.

APPROACH TO THE THORACOLUMBAR JUNCTION

Lower thoracic and upper lumbar spine exposure is most commonly indicated for scoliosis, infection, and tumor. The anterior approach to the thoracolumbar junction generally provides access between T10 and S1. The extent of exposure is guided by the need for extraction and fixation of the spine. Most cases require access to one normal spinal level above and below the area of disease. This is a difficult exposure owing to the simultaneous entry into the thoracic cavity and retroperitoneal space.

Patient Position

Patients undergoing thoracolumbar exposures require general anesthesia and appropriate monitoring for comorbidities. The patient is placed in the lateral decubitus position. A right lateral decubitus position with a left-sided approach is preferred to avoid the liver and injury to the inferior vena cava. Most patients are positioned at a 90-degree angle to the table, although 45 to 60 degrees may be preferred in some cases.

An axillary roll is placed under the dependent axilla, and the arms are extended straight across the upper chest, with the upper arm supported. The dependent leg is flexed at the knee, and the other leg is straight and supported by pillows. The kidney rest is elevated, and the table is flexed. A beanbag or tape secures the patient's hips and shoulders to the table.

Operative Exposure

The rib space to be entered depends on the level of interest. In general, a curvilinear incision is made in the ninth or tenth interspace for access to the lower thoracic spine. The incision starts in the midaxillary line and extends anteriorly and inferiorly toward the umbilicus (Figure 61-1A). It is important to preserve the intercostal neurovascular bundle at the inferior aspect of the rib. Resection of the costal cartilage facilitates the exposure. The external oblique, internal oblique, and transversus abdominis muscles are divided. A plane is developed between the diaphragm and retroperitoneal space along the costal attachment of the diaphragm. Care must be taken with the diaphragm, which originates from the upper lumbar vertebrae, arcuate ligaments, and twelfth ribs and attaches to the lower six ribs and xiphoid. Dividing the diaphragm circumferentially minimizes injury to the phrenic nerve (see Figure 61-1B); this is facilitated with a reticulating intestinal stapler, which reduces bleeding from the diaphragmatic edge and aids in reapproximation of the diaphragm during closure. Use of a Finochietto or Omni retractor for rib separation maximizes visualization. An Omni retractor provides access to the vertebral bodies while protecting vital structures. The Omni post

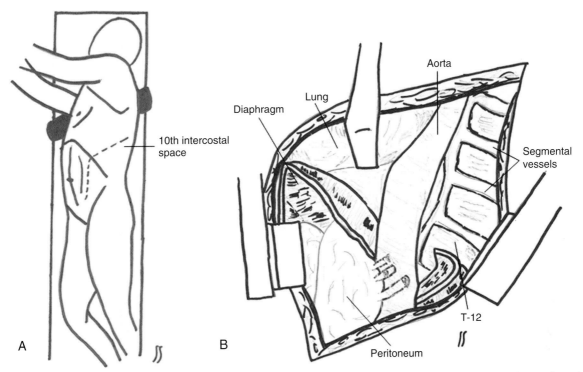

FIGURE 61-1 ■ Thoracolumbar spine exposure. **A,** Thoracoabdominal incision via the tenth intercostal space. **B,** Circumferential division of the diaphragm with exposure of the thoracic cavity and retroperitoneal space.

is generally attached to the right side of the table for a left-sided approach. The Omni retractor is positioned across the incision. A wide retractor is placed anteromedially to retract the peritoneum, ureter, and kidney in a medial position. This retractor will serve to protect these structures along with the aorta during vertebral manipulation by the spine surgeon. Three separate right-angle retractors are placed to retract the lung superiorly, the psoas muscle posteriorly, and the iliac vessels inferiorly. Placement of the retractors in these positions ensures adequate exposure and aids in the prevention of inadvertent injuries.

Using blunt dissection, the retroperitoneal space is developed in a retronephric extraperitoneal plane. The retroperitoneal space is entered laterally. The kidney is mobilized anteromedially, along with the peritoneal contents and ureter. The peritoneal sac is dissected free anteriorly, laterally, and finally medially. The aorta and ureter are protected anteromedially. The psoas muscle is identified, and the attachments are mobilized posteriorly off the vertebrae, allowing access to the spine. Segmental vessels are ligated and divided between nonabsorbable ties. Care must also be taken to ligate the iliolumbar vein at the lower lumbar level. Surgeons must be aware of the sympathetic chain, which is lateral to the spine and medial to the psoas muscle. Injury to the sympathetic chain in the lower lumbar spine can result in retrograde ejaculation in men. A spinal needle is inserted into the disk space, and a radiograph is taken to confirm the appropriate vertebral level.

Closure of this exposure begins with reapproximation of the diaphragm. Under direct vision, a chest tube is placed. The ribs are reapproximated, and the thoracic muscles are closed in layers. The retroperitoneal contents should fall into their normal anatomic position. The transversalis fascia and oblique muscle and fascia are reapproximated. The subcutaneous tissue is reapproximated, and the skin is closed. The chest tube is removed when there is no air leak, and the output is less than 150 mL over a 24-hour period.

Complications

Complications of the thoracolumbar approach to the spine can include thoracic, vascular, visceral, neurologic, and urologic injuries. The most common postoperative complications include wound infection, bleeding, pneumonia, and persistent air leak. Care should be taken to avoid iatrogenic, diaphragmatic, and ureteral injuries. Sympathetic chain injuries may also occur and can result in retrograde ejaculation. Bowel injuries result from violation of the peritoneum. In addition, extremity pulses should be assessed preoperatively and postoperatively to ensure that there was no injury, thrombosis, or embolus during arterial manipulation.

LUMBOSACRAL SPINE EXPOSURE: ANTEROLATERAL APPROACH

The lumbosacral region of the spine can be accessed via the more traditional anterolateral exposure or the increasingly common pure anterior exposure. The anterolateral approach allows simultaneous exposure of

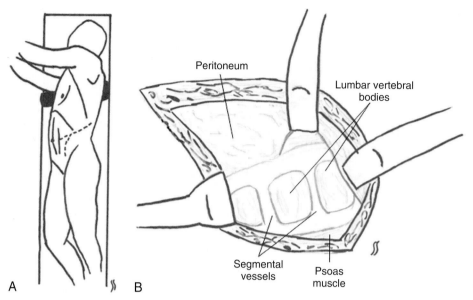

FIGURE 61-2 ■ Anterolateral lumbosacral spine exposure. **A,** Anterolateral lumbosacral incision from the quadratus lumborum to the lateral border of the rectus muscle. **B,** Anteromedial retraction of the peritoneum and kidney, lateral retraction of the psoas, and exposure of the segmental vessels for ligation.

multiple levels in the lumbar spine. Depending on which level needs to be exposed, the incision may be placed between the eleventh or twelfth rib and the superior aspect of the iliac crest.

Patient Position

Similar to the thoracolumbar approach, the patient is positioned in a modified lateral decubitus position with the right side down to avoid the liver and injury to the vena cava. The hips are rotated 45 degrees. The upper and lower extremities are positioned in a similar fashion to the thoracolumbar approach (Figure 61-2*A*). The kidney rest is elevated, and the table is flexed to increase exposure between the lower ribs and the iliac crest.

Operative Exposure

An oblique incision is made over the eleventh rib from the lateral border of the quadratus lumborum to the lateral border of the rectus abdominis muscle for L1 and L2 exposure (see Figure 61-2*A*). For L3 to L5, a similar incision is made off of the twelfth rib. Electrocautery is used to divide the subcutaneous tissue, fascia, external and internal oblique, transversus abdominis, and transversalis fascia. The retroperitoneal space is entered laterally.

An Omni retractor is used to facilitate the exposure and is positioned on the table as described previously in the thoracolumbar approach. In a similar fashion, a wide retractor is used to retract the peritoneum and kidney medially while protecting the peritoneum, aorta, and ureter. However, in the lumbosacral approach, one right-angle retractor is used to retract the diaphragm superiorly. The remaining two right-angle retractors are used

to retract the psoas muscle posteriorly and the iliac vessels inferiorly.

The peritoneal sac is swept off the anterior and lateral aspects of the abdominal wall, taking care not to violate the peritoneum. The peritoneum and kidney are reflected anteriorly. The peritoneum is dissected off the posterior rectus sheath, and the peritoneum is swept medially off the psoas muscle with Gerota's fascia. The ureter should fall anteriorly with the peritoneum. The iliac vessels are exposed and protected. The psoas muscle is elevated bluntly off the lumbar vertebrae and retracted posteriorly. The lumbar segmental vessels are ligated as needed for exposure (see Figure 61-2*B*). Care should be taken to ligate the iliolumbar vein when dissecting the L4 to L5 level; this avoids avulsion of the vein during retraction. A spinal needle is inserted into the disk space, and a radiograph is taken to confirm the appropriate vertebral level.

Closure is performed with reapproximation of the transversalis fascia, oblique muscle, and fascia in layers. The subcutaneous tissue and skin are reapproximated. If the pleura is violated during the exposure, it may be necessary to place a red rubber catheter into the chest cavity to remove air. The defect in the pleura is then closed while the catheter is removed. It is helpful to have the anesthesiologist perform a breath hold after inflating the lungs to minimize air in the chest cavity. If there is any uncertainty about a pneumothorax, a chest tube should be placed.

Complications

Perioperative complications are similar to those described for the thoracolumbar approach to the spine. In addition, injury to the intercostal nerves innervating the oblique muscles can result in weakness of the oblique muscles, resulting in a bulge overlying the incision. The intercostal nerves innervating these muscles are usually at the level of the internal oblique muscles. Limiting the use of cautery in this layer of muscle may be helpful in minimizing this injury. These nerves come off posteriorly; therefore great care should be taken when approaching this area of the incision. Care should be taken to avoid injury to the diaphragm, blood vessels, ureter, and sympathetic chain. Inadvertent entry into the pleural space can result in pneumothorax or lung injury. Violation of the peritoneum can result in unrecognized visceral injuries. As in the thoracolumbar approach, preoperative and postoperative extremity pulses should be obtained to evaluate for an arterial inury, thrombosis, or embolus.

LUMBOSACRAL SPINE EXPOSURE: ANTERIOR APPROACH

The anterior approach has become the preferred technique for access to the lumbosacral spine. It provides adequate exposure while minimizing large dissections and allowing for a cosmetically acceptable result. In general, L3 through S1 can be exposed safely using this technique; however, in some patients with favorable anatomy, L2 through S1 can be approached.

Patient Position

The patient is placed in a supine position with the arms extended laterally or secured across the chest. For exposure of L5 to S1, a transverse incision is made 2 to 3 cm above the symphysis pubis. An L4 to L5 exposure can be performed with a transverse incision midway between the umbilicus and the symphysis pubis. Alternatively, a small infraumbilical midline incision can be used; this is usually more cosmetically appealing because only a portion of the incision is seen above the patient's waist. This incision allows greater exposure in difficult cases. An L3 to L4 exposure can be obtained with a transverse incision 1 cm above the umbilicus or through a midline incision. The midline incision is again preferred for the reasons previously mentioned (Figure 61-3A).

Operative Exposure

The skin incision is carried down to the level of the rectus fascia. Using electrocautery, a subcutaneous flap is created superiorly to the left of the umbilicus and inferiorly down to the symphysis pubis. Next, a paramedian fascial incision is made to the left of the linea alba. This fascial incision is extended superiorly to the left of the umbilicus and inferiorly to the symphysis pubis. For high lumbar exposures, this fascial incision may extend as much as 3 cm beyond the umbilicus.

The medial border of the left rectus muscle is dissected off the linea alba throughout the length of the fascial incision (see Figure 61-3B). Using a Richardson retractor, the rectus muscle is elevated, and the space between the rectus muscle and the posterior rectus fascia is developed laterally to expose the transversalis fascia; this is incised with Metzenbaum scissors throughout the

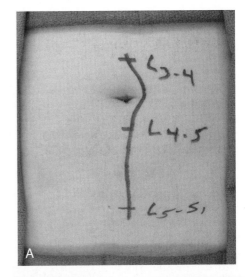

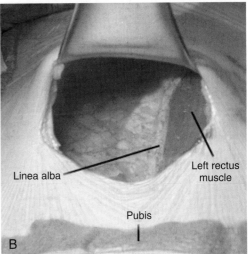

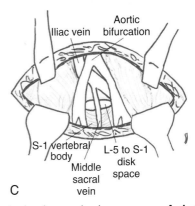

FIGURE 61-3 ■ Anterior lumbosacral spine exposure. **A,** Anterior transverse incision placed between the symphysis pubis and umbilicus, depending on the vertebral level. **B,** Intraoperative view of the left rectus muscle and linea alba. **C,** Anatomic relation of the iliac vessels to the vertebral bodies at the lumbosacral level.

length of the fascial exposure. A retroperitoneal plane is developed laterally along the psoas muscle. The ureter is identified and mobilized medially along with the peritoneum. Care must be taken to avoid injury to the blood supply to the ureter. Exposure is facilitated with retraction of the rectus muscle laterally and the peritoneal contents medially using a total of four renal vein retractors. Care must be taken to avoid entering the peritoneum. If this occurs, the defect should be repaired immediately with an absorbable suture.

For exposure of L5 to S1, a combination of sharp and blunt dissection exposes the medial edge of the left iliac artery and vein. The middle sacral vessels are identified. In order to mobilize the iliac vessels, the middle sacral artery and vein are ligated and divided. The lateral renal vein retractors are then repositioned to retract the left iliac artery and vein in a lateral position. The medial vein retractors are repositioned over the disk space to retract the peritoneum and ureter in a medial position. The retractors also serve to protect these structures and the sympathetic chain.

Additional dissection of the iliac vessels may be required to expose the width of the disk spaces. Care must be taken to preserve the ureter and its blood supply. With the renal vein retractors in this position, the L5 to S1 disk space can be accessed easily (see Figure 61-3C).

Using the same initial approach, the L4 to L5 and L3 to L4 disk spaces can be dissected. Exposure of the L4 to L5 disk space requires more extensive dissection of the lateral edge of the left iliac artery and vein. The iliolumbar vein is ligated and divided. The venous anatomy in this region can be highly variable. In the author's experience, multiple iliolumbar veins can be seen approximately 25% of the time. There can be as few as zero and sometimes more than three (Figure 61-4). The medial retractors are repositioned to retract the iliac vessels, peritoneum, and ureter in a medial position. The lateral retractors are repositioned to retract the left rectus muscle in a lateral position. The retractors also serve to protect these structures and the sympathetic chain. With gentle blunt dissection, the soft tissue overlying the disk space is dissected, allowing complete exposure of the disk space. Exposure of the L3 to L4 disk space requires the same approach. However, the segmental vessels at the L4 vertebral body often need to be ligated and divided. The medial retractors are repositioned to retract the iliac vessels, aorta, peritoneum, and ureter medially, whereas the lateral retractors keep the left rectus muscle in a lateral position. Again, the retractors will protect these structures and the sympathetic chain.

A spinal needle is inserted into the disk space, and a radiograph is taken to confirm the appropriate vertebral level. Closure involves reapproximation of the transversalis fascia, anterior rectus fascia, subcutaneous tissue, and skin.

Complications

There are several perioperative complications that can result from the anterior approach to the lumbosacral spine. These complications are similar to those described in the section on anterolateral exposure to the lumbosacral spine. Injury to the iliac vessels is a potentially life-threatening complication. If this occurs, more extensive exposure is usually necessary to repair the injury; this most often involves an injury to the iliac vein. Small venous injuries are often best treated with topical hemostatic agents and direct pressure. If bleeding is not controlled and suturing the vein is required, several steps should be considered. Direct pressure should be applied to the injured site to immediately control bleeding. Alerting anesthesiologist and the operating room staff that there is a possibility of blood loss should be done. This will allow the operating room team to prepare for any major blood loss that may arise during the repair of the blood vessel. If the bleeding is significant, it is helpful to increase the exposure by making the incision larger. Proximal and distal control can often be obtained by using a sponge on a sponge stick, which should allow the surgeon to place sutures into the bleeding vessels. If necessary, formal control with clamps and vessel loops should be used if the maneuvers listed previously do not work. Venous injuries can be difficult to manage, and the surgeon should seek assistance from colleagues when necessary to perform these types of repairs.

Arterial bleeding is much less common and can usually be treated with simple suture repair. As in all the approaches, pulses should be obtained preoperatively and postoperatively to evaluate for injury, thrombosis, or embolus of the iliac artery during retraction. If an arterial injury is encountered, the proper steps should be taken to identify and correct the injury identified. Care must be taken to avoid injury to the ureter. The ureter should be identified and retracted medially, along with the peritoneum, to avoid iatrogenic injury during the spine manipulation. Finally, identification of the sympathetic plexus and use of bipolar cautery minimizes damage to the sympathetic nerves at the lower lumbar vertebrae, reducing the risk of retrograde ejaculation.

LUMBOSACRAL SPINE EXPOSURE: NINETY DEGREE APPROACH

Over the last several years, technology in the spine surgery field has evolved to allow surgeons to perform spinal fusions through a far lateral or 90-degree approach with minimally invasive techniques. This approach is useful for patients who have a "hostile abdomen" in which an anterior or anterolateral approach could be problematic secondary to scarring. In addition, this technique allows surgeons to perform anterior column spinal fusions at all lumbar levels from L1 to L5. Because L5 to S1 is usually below the iliac crest, this technique is not used for an L5 to S1 fusion.

Patients who undergo 90-degree lateral approaches at higher lumbar levels (L1-L4) tend to have lower requirements for pain medication and faster postoperative recoveries. This technique can be performed from the right or left side, which allows patients with previous anterior spinal fusions to undergo additional anterior column spinal fusions with less risk of bleeding from adhesions of the iliac vessels.

Patient Position

Patients are placed in a right or left lateral decubitus position at 90 degrees to the operating room table. The patient's arms are extended out in front and supported

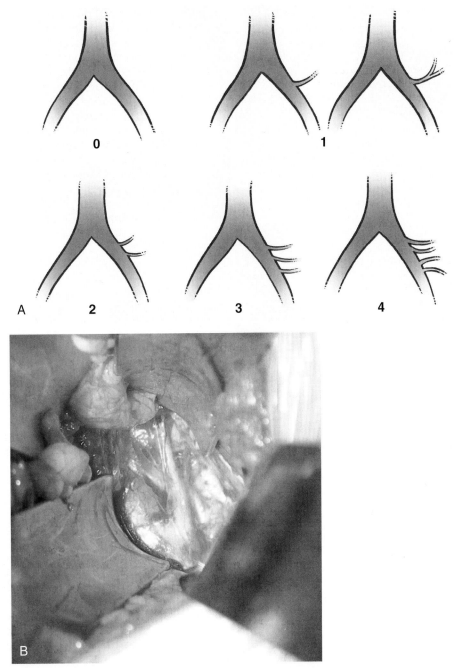

FIGURE 61-4 ■ Variability in iliolumbar veins during spine exposure. **A,** Classification of iliolumbar veins seen on the lateral side of the iliac vein. **B,** Intraoperative photograph of a type 1 iliolumbar vein that branches immediately after its origin from the iliac vein.

appropriately. An axillary roll is placed under the dependant axilla. The patient's knees are flexed with pillows between both legs. All pressure points are padded, and the patient is secured to the table. Silk tape is used across the lower portion of the iliac crest and chest to secure the patient. Because fluoroscopy is going to be used during the surgery, it is difficult to use other supporting devices that are not radiolucent. The table is then flexed to open up the space between the lower ribs and the iliac crest.

Intraoperative fluoroscopy is then used to identify the appropriate disc space. Initially an anterior posterior radiograph is taken to insure that the endplates are

aligned correctly and the disk space is straight. It may be necessary to tilt the table to the left or right a few degrees to ensure that the anteroposterior alignment of the spine is correct. Next, a lateral radiograph is taken with an instrument on the patient's side to identify the appropriate level. A sponge stick can be used for this portion of the positioning; the tip of the sponge stick is placed at the most anterior portion of the spine (Figure 61-5*A*). From this radiograph, it is possible to mark the anterior and posterior limits of the spine on the patient's side with a marking pen (see Figure 61-5*B*). If one level is to be exposed, make a longitudinal incision connecting the

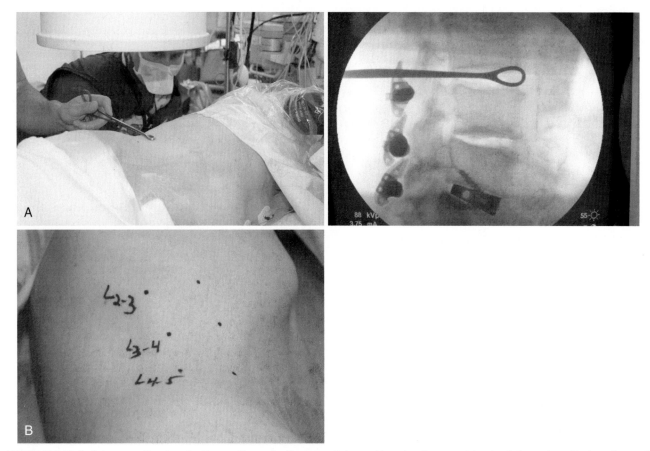

FIGURE 61-5 ■ **A,** Intraoperative localization radiograph. Sponge stick marking the front and back of the spine. **B,** Anterior and posterior limits of the spine.

anterior and posterior portion of the spine that was previously marked. If two adjacent levels are to be exposed, make a vertical incision through the center of the marked disk spaces.

Operative Exposure

An incision is made through the skin either vertically or longitudinally, depending on how many levels are being exposed. Subcutaneous tissue is then divided down to the external oblique fascia. The external oblique fascia is then opened. At this point, a Kelley clamp is preferred to bluntly separate the external oblique muscle fibers, internal oblique muscle fibers, and the transversalis muscle fibers. This manuever minimizes injury to the intercostal nerves. Hand-held Wylie retractors are then used to retract the oblique muscles anteriorly and posteriorly. The peritoneal contents and ureter are dissected bluntly. These structures are swept anteriorly, allowing access into the retroperitoneal space. The psoas muscle is now visualized at the base of the incision. Depending on the size of the psoas muscle and its location relative to the spine, one can either go through the psoas muscle fibers or retract them posteriorly to visualize the disk space. In patients with a large psoas muscle, it is preferable to separate the psoas muscle along its fibers to visualize the disk space. Once the disk space is seen, retractors are used

to keep the psoas muscle fibers retracted anteriorly and posteriorly. In addition, the peritoneal contents and ureter will be retracted anteriorly. Depending on whether a right- or left-sided approach is used, the vena cava or aorta will also be retracted slightly in an anterior direction. Because of their normal anatomic position, little if any manipulation of the aorta or vena cava is required with this technique. This technique can be especially useful in patients with calcified vessels or retroperitoneal scarring that need an anterior column spinal fusion. Once the disk is exposed, a spinal needle is inserted into the disk and a radiograph is taken to confirm that the appropriate level has been dissected. Closure of the incision is performed by closing the fascial layers, subcuataneous tissue, and skin.

Complications

Complications to the 90-degree approach are similar to the other spine approaches. Great care must be taken with positioning the patient and appropriate padding of pressure points to avoid any neuropraxia. Injury to the peritoneal contents is also possible during its manipulation. Vascular injury, although possible, is less common secondary to the normal anterior position of the blood vessels relative to the lateral side of the spine; however, caution is warranted because every patient's anatomy can be different. Arterial and venous injuries would be treated in a manner similar to those described previously. Ureteral injury is also possible with this technique; therefore care must be taken to identify the ureter and take appropriate precautions to avoid any injury to the ureter. Intercostal nerve injuries must also be avoided to prevent muscle weakness and bulging over the incision. Limiting the use of cautery and using blunt dissection through the oblique muscles will minimize this complication. Finally, preoperative and postoperative pulse examination should be performed to evalaute any arterial complication.

CONCLUSION

Over the last 10 years, the role of the vascular surgeon has undergone significant changes. Many procedures that are now routinely performed by vascular surgeons were once the domain of other medical specialists. As a result, vascular surgeons often find that they have not necessarily been formally trained to perform all these procedures. Spine access surgery is certainly not familiar to most vascular surgeons, but their experience with thoracoabdominal and retroperitoneal aortic surgery makes them adept at spine exposure. In addition, the most common complication of hemorrhage from iliac artery and vein injuries is usually treated by vascular surgeons. Therefore it is incumbent on vascular surgeons to be proactive in the treatment and care of spine patients. By taking a team approach to spine surgery, vascular surgeons can aid in minimizing the morbidity and mortality of these procedures. Vascular surgeons need to embrace this surgical procedure to ensure safe and effective treatment of spine surgery patients.

References available online at expertconsult.com.

QUESTIONS

1. Spine surgery is performed for which of the following disease processes?
   a. Degenerative disk disease
   b. Infection
   c. Neoplasm
   d. All of the above

2. Which of the following spine levels are typically exposed by vascular surgeons?
   a. Lumbar
   b. Sacral
   c. Lower thoracic
   d. All of the above

3. In general, spine surgeons require access to which vertebral level?
   a. Only the affected vertebral body
   b. One normal level above and below the affected vertebral body
   c. Two normal levels above the affected vertebral body
   d. One level below the affected vertebral body

4. In a thoracolumbar vertebral exposure, to avoid phrenic nerve injury, the diaphragm is divided in what manner?
   a. Radially
   b. The diaphragm is not divided.
   c. Circumferentially
   d. Axially

5. In relation to the spine, the psoas muscle lies in what direction?
   a. Lateral
   b. Anterior
   c. Medial
   d. Superior

6. In the anterolateral approach to the lumbar spine, the peritoneum and kidney are reflected in what direction?
   a. Posterolaterally
   b. Inferiorly
   c. Anteromedially
   d. Superiorly

7. What structure is divided to facilitate exposure of the L-4 vertebral level?
   a. Sacral artery
   b. Hypogastric vein
   c. Sympathetic chain
   d. Iliolumbar vein

8. Injury to the sympathetic chain can result in which of the following?
   a. Reflex sympathetic dystrophy
   b. Retrograde ejaculation
   c. Sensory deficit of scrotum
   d. Impotence

9. Iatrogenic injury that can result from the anterior lumbosacral approach includes which of the following?
   a. Ureteral injury
   b. Hemorrhage
   c. Thrombosis
   d. All of the above

10. In an anterior lumbosacral approach to the spine, the space developed for exposure is made in which location?
    a. Posterior to the rectus muscle
    b. Anterior to the rectus muscle
    c. Transperitoneally
    d. Transthoracically

ANSWERS

1. **d**
2. **d**
3. **b**
4. **c**
5. **a**
6. **c**
7. **d**
8. **b**
9. **d**
10. **a**

CHAPTER 62

Carotid Sinus Stimulation: Background, Technique, and Future Directions

Karl A. Illig • John D. Bisognano

Hypertension affects more than 65 million people in the United States and is one of the most important risk factors for stroke, heart attack, vascular disease, and death. Cardiovascular risk is estimated to double with each 20 mm Hg increment above 115 mm Hg of systolic pressure.[1,2] Unfortunately, and despite intensive public health efforts and generally effective pharmacologic therapy, control remains poor,[3] in part because adding more antihypertensive medications after a certain point causes side effects to increase while efficacy plateaus (Figure 62-1). In addition, even optimally treated patients who demonstrate perfect compliance can remain significantly hypertensive. A reasonable estimate of those with truly resistant hypertension is 3 to 4 million Americans, and an additional 25 million escape treatment altogether (Figure 62-2).

One of the major physiologic systems affecting blood pressure (BP) is the carotid sinus baroreflex arc. Increased pressure causes the cells at the sinus to stretch, which directly causes increased glossopharyngeal afferent activity and leads to three downstream effects: cardiac inhibition (decreased stroke volume and heart rate), vascular smooth muscle inhibition (vasorelaxation), and increased renal sodium and water excretion (Figure 62-3).[4] This system is responsible for the acute hypotension and bradycardia sometimes seen after carotid endarterectomy, because the sinus is stretched after removal of plaque.

HISTORY

The history of device-based therapy for hypertension has been summarized recently.[5] As early as 1958, it was reported that electrical stimulation of the carotid sinus nerve in normotensive dogs produced an acute decrease in BP,[6] and similar findings were reported in several animal models of hypertension shortly thereafter.[7] Following the original animal model report, it was demonstrated that direct electrical stimulation of the carotid sinus in humans (undergoing neck dissection for cancer) had the same results.[8]

These findings led to more thorough investigation in humans. A single case was reported in 1966 of a 40-year-old man with a BP of 260/165 mm Hg despite four medications. Bilateral stimulation (2.5 V) produced a sustained drop in pressure to 150/90 mm Hg. The device consisted of electrodes at the sinuses connected to a generator placed beneath the pectoralis muscle. The leads were subcutaneously tunneled, and the generator could be turned on or off by placing a magnet over the device, but no further modification could be performed.[9] The first series was reported in 1967 Seymour Schwartz; he described a mean BP decrease of 48 mm Hg in eight patients, six of whom reduced their BP medications.[10] Further clinical benefit was demonstrated by at least one other group around this time.[11] Unfortunately, this treatment came at the wrong time. Most setups at this time required external power sources and communication and were therefore bulky and impractical for long-term use. In addition, pharmacologic therapy dramatically improved in this era, making the problem less acute. As a result, this concept was essentially forgotten for the remainder of the century.

This phenomenon was reevaluated largely through a large body of work by Thomas Lohmeier, a physiologist at the University of Mississippi. In a large series of animal experiments,[4,12] he was able to reconfirm that this effect was real and reproducible, was effective in normotensive as well as hypertensive (sodium-loaded and obesity models) canines and, most importantly, was sustainable (Figure 62-4). This work led to the formation of a company (CVRx, Minneapolis, Minn.) whose sole aim was to resurrect this concept using twenty-first–century technology. To date, five discrete trials have been completed or are underway to investigate this effect.

BaroReflex Activating System Study

The BaroReflex Activating System Study (BRASS) was a proof-of-concept trial performed in Switzerland in 2003. Eleven patients undergoing carotid endarterectomy were tested by direct carotid sinus stimulation, and a mean systolic BP drop of 18 mm Hg was observed at a maximum of 4.4 V.[13] The BRASS showed that this effect was reproducible in relatively normotensive humans and that clinically feasible levels of current delivered unilaterally via a small metal electrode could lower BP.

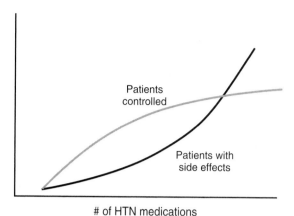

FIGURE 62-1 ■ Graph illustrating the relationship between increasing numbers of antihypertensive medications (*x* axis) and effects. As the number of medications increases, there is a plateau effect for efficacy but an increase in side effects. (Courtesy CVRx, Minneapolis, Minn.)

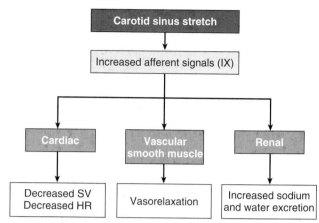

FIGURE 62-3 ■ Schematic diagram of the baroreflex receptor arc. (Modified from Illig KA, Bisognano J: Carotid stimulation for hypertension, Shelton, Conn, 2010, People's Medical Publishing House.)

FIGURE 62-2 ■ Proportions and numbers of Americans in various stages and categories of treatment for hypertension. (Courtesy CVRx, Minneapolis, Minn. Derived from Cushman WC, Ford CE, Cutler JA, et al: Success and predictors of blood pressure control in diverse North American settings: the Antihypertensive and Lipid-Lowering treatment to prevent Heart Attack Trial (ALLHAT), J Clin Hypertension 4:393-404, 2002; and Hajjar I, Kotchen TA: Trends in prevalence, awareness, treatment, and control of hypertension in the United States, 1988-2000, J Am Med Assoc 290:199-206, 2003.)

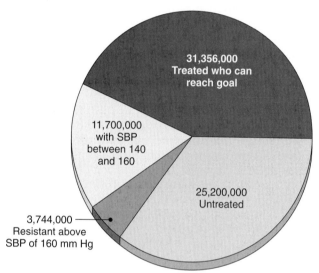

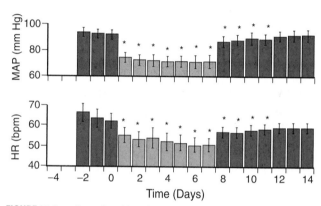

FIGURE 62-4 ■ Sustained (>7 days) blood pressure and heart rate response to carotid sinus stimulation in normal canines. *Gray shaded bars* denote stimulation; an *asterisk* denotes a significant drop. (From Lohmeier TE, Irwin ED, Rossing MA, at al: Prolonged activation of the baroreflex produces sustained hypotension, Hypertension 43:306-311, 2004.)

Device-Based Therapy in Hypertension Trial

The Device-Based Therapy in Hypertension Trial (DEBuT-HT) was the initial controlled feasibility trial of the commercially available, clinically practical device. Patients with resistant hypertension (systolic BP > 160 mm Hg despite three medications, one of which included a diuretic) underwent bilateral carotid sinus exposure and lead placement. Electrodes were tunneled subcutaneously and attached to a pulse generator implanted in the chest wall (Figure 62-5). Forty-five patients were enrolled in this trial, which was performed in Europe starting in 2006. Eighteen patients have completed 4 years of therapy, and the results of this cohort were recently presented at the 2010 European Society of Hypertension's twentieth annual meeting in Oslo, Norway, and published in abstract form.[14] Blood pressure response has been sustained, and reductions are impressive: mean reduction in systolic pressure is 53 ± 9 mm Hg, diastolic pressure is reduced 30 ± 6 mm Hg, and heart rate is reduced 5 ± 2 beats/min (Figure 62-6). Encouragingly, patients have been able to decrease their antihypertensive medications by approximately one third (5 ± 1.3 medications at onset to 3.4 ± 1 medications at 4 years). DEBuT-HT, which continues to follow patients over time, confirms that this system is clinically practical and shows an impressive, sustained effect.

Rheos Feasibility

Formal testing of the Rheos System (CVRx, Inc, Minneapolis, Minn.) began in 2006. A total of 16 patients (10 in the United States) were implanted in the phase II feasibility trial. The trial was primarily focused on safety and feasibility, which were both shown to be acceptable.[12]

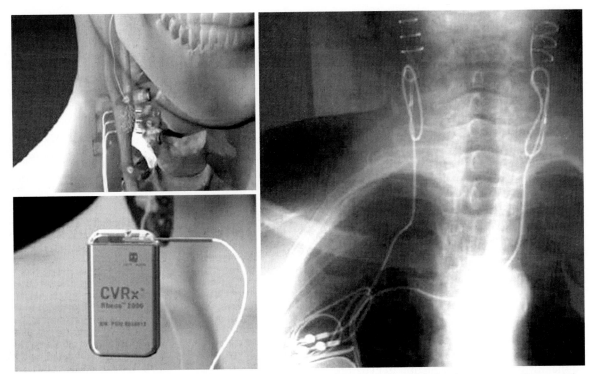

FIGURE 62-5 ■ Illustration of Rheos System implantation for the DEBuT-HT study. *Upper left,* Leads are wrapped around the carotid sinus bilaterally. *Lower left,* Pulse generator (before implantation) and electrode. *Right,* Plain radiograph of patient following implantation. Current practice is to bring the contralateral lead across the neck rather than the chest to allow for future sternotomy. (Courtesy CVRx, Minneapolis, Minn. From Illig KA, Bisognano J: Carotid stimulation for hypertension, Shelton, Conn, 2010, People's Medical Publishing House, pp 25-34.)

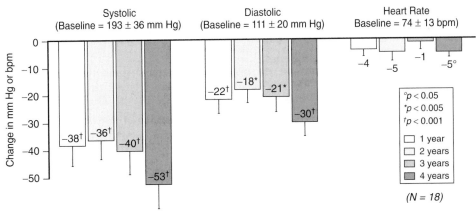

FIGURE 62-6 ■ Graphic results for 18 of 45 patients enrolled in the DEBuT-HT study who have reached 4 years of stimulation. These results are achieved in the context of a decrease in medication. (Adapted from Kroon A, Schmidli J, Scheffers I, et al. Chronically implanted system: 4-year data of Rheos DEBuT-HT study in patients with resistant hypertension, J Hypertension 28:278, 2010.)

Results have generally been combined with those from the DEBuT-HT and the Rheos Pivotal Trial as appropriate; however, after 12 months of therapy, mean systolic ambulatory pressures have fallen from 171 to 157 mm Hg, and patients spend 20% more time with systolic BPs less than 140 mm Hg.[15] No injury to or midterm abnormalities of the carotid arteries have been identified.[16]

Rheos Pivotal Trial

The Rheos Pivotal Trial is a phase III prospective randomized trial approved by the U.S. Food and Drug Administration (FDA) and designed to prove efficacy in a blinded, randomized, controlled fashion. The device itself, implantation technique, and trial eligibility (systolic BP greater than 160 mm Hg despite three medications, one being a diuretic) are the same as for the DEBuT-HT and the Rheos Feasibility trial. Patients undergo implantation, and the device is turned off for 4 weeks to allow healing. Next, patients are randomized in a 2:1 ratio (study sites and investigators are blinded) to "on" or "off" for the next 6 months, then all patients are "on" for months 7 to 12. The major study endpoints are differences in BP after the 6-month randomization period between those receiving therapy and those whose devices are off, an improvement in BP at 12 months in patients whose devices had been off, and an overall improvement at 12 months versus enrollment baseline in the entire cohort.[17]

Enrollment was completed in late 2009, with 322 patients treated (55 roll in, 265 randomized). Unblinding occurred in late 2010, and the results have recently been published.[18] Initially "on" and "off" groups were similar at baseline, having mean systolic BPs of 179 ± 22 and 176 ± 22 mm Hg, respectively, diastolic BPs greater than 100 mm Hg despite taking an average of 5.2 ± 2 medications. After initial discussions with the FDA, endpoints had been decided to be the percentage of patients achieving a response of 10 mm Hg or greater, rather than the absolute BP response. After the first 6 months, 54% of the "on" group showed such a response; however, 46% of the "off" group did as well, illustrating the interaction of the Hawthorne effect combined with a fairly small goal. This difference, at 7.7%, fell below the a priori target of a 20% response rate; however, after 12 months of therapy (all patients being "on" for at least 6 months), sustained improvement was seen in 88% of patients, well above the a priori target of 65% ($p < 0.001$). Six months of device therapy led to a 40% reduction in hypertensive crises and a 23% reduction in overall hypertension-associated adverse events ($p < 0.001$). Implantation and therapy were well tolerated, with a 4.4% permanent nerve injury (much of it from periincisional numbness) being the most significant complication. Long-term device-related adverse events, at 13%, fell below the a priori target of 28% ($p < 0.001$). A manuscript describing these results is currently (mid-2011) in the review process.

Interestingly, absolute BP comparisons are not yet available because the company is complying closely with the reporting criteria agreed upon with the FDA at the start of the trial. However, the percentage of patients whose systolic BP decreased to less than 140 mm Hg is illustrative (Figure 62-7). After the first 6 months, 42% of those receiving stimulation fell below this goal, whereas only 24% of those in the "off" group did so ($p < 0.005$). At 12 months of therapy, approximately 52% of patients (who started with a mean systolic BP of approximately 178 mm Hg) were below this target. Finally, post hoc analysis shows that mean systolic BP drop at 6 and 12 months is 26 and 35 mm Hg, respectively.

Narrowly interpreted in light of a priori agreed-upon categorical endpoints (the percentage of patients that achieved a drop in systolic BP of 10 mm Hg or greater), the goal of a 20% improvement was not seen. However, 80% of patients as a whole responded, 54% met this goal, and mean BP fell 35 mm Hg; the outcome was negative because more patients in the "off" group did better than expected under care by the "hypertension professionals" involved in this study. The overall experience (combined with the reduction of 50 mm Hg at 4 years seen in the DEBuT-HT cohort) and low adverse event rate is interpreted by most to be encouraging enough to continue aggressive investigation. The device has CE approval and is being used clinically in Europe, which will provide additional data as experience accumulates.

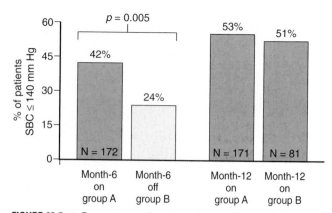

FIGURE 62-7 ■ Percentage of patients in the Rheos Pivotal Trial whose systolic blood pressure (SBP) is less than 140 mm Hg. *Left,* 172 patients *(shaded column)* undergoing stimulation (group A) versus 81 *(white column)* without activation (group B) after 6 months. *Right,* All patients at 12 months. (Adapted from Bisognano J, Sica D, Nadim M, et al: Results from the Rheos pivotal trial. Oral presentation, Sixtieth Annual American College of Cardiology Annual Meeting, New Orleans, 2011.)

Heart Failure

A somewhat unexpected benefit of this therapy is a reduction in ventricular mass and improved diastolic function,[19,20] which raises the possibility that this therapy could be effective for diastolic (preserved ejection fraction) heart failure, an entity for which there is no good pharmacologic therapy.[21] Echocardiograms were obtained in a subgroup of patients within the Pivotal Trial, which showed in aggregate multiple beneficial effects on cardiac function after chronic therapy, including a significant reduction in left ventricular mass[18,19] (Figure 62-8). The HOPE 4HF (Health Outcomes Prospective Evaluation for Heart Failure with Ejection Fraction >40%) is a prospective randomized trial exploring the effect of baroreflex activation therapy to treat diastolic heart failure. This trial is in its preliminary stages and has an enrollment goal of 500 patients.

Pitfalls

At least two major pitfalls exist in the minds of surgeons. First is frustration with not being able to reduce the BP to any arbitrary level, as might seem theoretically feasible. The obvious answer is that not all patients are the same and that many different interrelated systems work together to regulate BP (and the Rheos system only targets one of them). In fact, it probably is possible to lower pressure to any degree, but at a cost of increasing voltage. This not only creates a short battery life, but also results in extraneous stimulation (motor as well as sensory) of tissues in the vicinity of the electrodes. It should be noted that the "average" BP response in a drug that gains FDA approval for hypertension is in the range of 7 to 10 mm Hg; therefore systolic BP reductions of 35 mm Hg at 1 year and 50 mm Hg at 4 years in the Rheos and DEBuT-HT trials, respectively, are

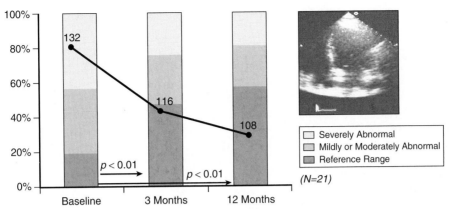

FIGURE 62-8 ■ Reduction in left ventricular mass index (LVMI) in 21 patients undergoing carotid sinus baroreflex stimulation. LVMI fell from 139 g/m² baseline to 114 g/m² after 12 months of therapy. The proportion of patients with normal function rose from 19% to 58%, and those with severely abnormal function fell from 42% to 19%. (From Bisognano JD, de Leeuw P, Bach DS, et al: Improved cardiac structure and diastolic flow velocities in early-stage heart failure with chronic treatment using an implantable device: results from European and United States trials of the Rheos system, J Am Coll Cardiol 53:A188, 2009.)

reassuring. It is likely that future improvements in this device and related technology will serve to increase its efficacy.

The second issue is that of sustainability and habituation. As alluded to earlier, most surgeons' initial impression is that this effect will last only hours to a day or so based upon experience with carotid endarterectomy. It is clear from the data, however, that habituation does not occur, at least to 4 years of therapy. The obvious inference is that the habituation seen after carotid endarterectomy occurs at the level of the glossopharyngeal nerve's response to stretch; the nerve will stop firing after 1 day or so. However, the brain's and body's response to glossopharyngeal nerve activity evidently does not habituate (see Figure 62-3). As a result, if it is possible to artificially produce continuous nerve activity by means of electrical stimulation, the efferent effects will continue.

Surgical Technique

Given current technology, the most critical step in implanting this device is to ensure that it is placed so that electrical stimulation is applied to the most sensitive portion of the carotid sinus—a "sweet spot" that is surprisingly difficult to localize. In practice, this entails 20 to 40 minutes of mapping, providing stimulation at various points (often a few millimeters apart) and noting BP response over the following 1 to 3 minutes. This effect is strongly blunted by most inhalation anesthetics; therefore proper anesthesia technique (in these severely hypertensive patients) is critical.

A detailed anesthetic protocol can be found elsewhere.[12] In brief, anesthetic management is divided into three stages, the middle of which is essentially intravenous general anesthetic alone.

Stage one consists of typical intravenous induction followed by maintenance of anesthesia with inhalation agents. This stage is performed only during the beginning of the procedure itself and is helpful for smooth induction and initial cutaneous stimulation in these very hypertensive patients. Once the skin incision is made and cutaneous stimulation is complete, stage two begins. At this point all inhalation anesthetics other than nitrous oxide are stopped, and general anesthesia is maintained using intravenous agents. These agents are primarily titrated to lack of movement and vital signs, but maintaining bispectral index (BIS) monitor levels between 40 and 60 has been found to allow anesthesia, analgesia, and amnesia while maintaining carotid sinus reactivity. The carotids are usually exposed by 15 to 20 minutes after skin incision, and this timing is usually long enough to allow inhalation agents to wash out of the system. The optimal situation at this point is a relatively high (approximately 150 mm Hg) stable BP, allowing room for electrical stimulation to cause a decrease, but ensuring that the electrical stimulation is the only variable being applied. Finally, stage three applies to the phase after mapping is completed. Tunneling and pocket formation are noxious stimuli and baroreflex sensitivity is not as critical; therefore conventional inhalation anesthesia is resumed until awakening.

Currently, Rheos implantation requires bilateral exposure with full circumferential carotid sinus exposure and mapping, but hardware and implantation techniques have evolved significantly.

The procedure is performed using general endotracheal anesthesia, primarily because of the need for bilateral circumferential carotid exposure along with control of BP. This area of the body is clean, but because a long-term mechanical device is to be implanted (with generator changes anticipated as well), the patient should wash thoroughly the night before surgery with a surgical prep sponge.

After anesthesia is induced (with further management detailed previously), the patient is positioned with the back elevated approximately 30 degrees, and a towel roll is placed vertically on the upper back. The head is extended in midline position, and a Mayo stand is placed symmetrically over the head to about the level of the nose to allow draping without dislodging the endotracheal tube. The entire neck to above the jaw line, including ear lobes, as well as the chest, especially the right side, is

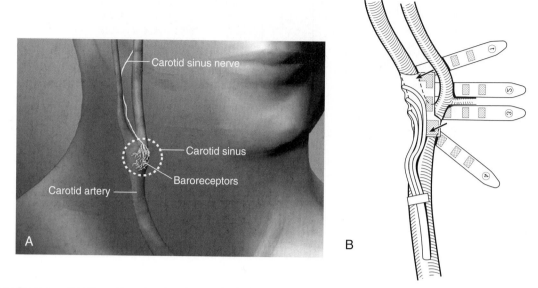

FIGURE 62-9 ■ Right carotid bifurcation showing the method of wrapping the existing lead (used in all trials to date) around it. *Thick arrows* indicate the area between external and internal carotid arteries, which should not be dissected or manipulated to preserve afferent nerve integrity. *Small arrows* indicate the suture pads that are used to ensure secure fixation. (Courtesy CVRx, Minneapolis, Minn.)

prepared with Betadine and sterilely draped. Iodoform drapes are used to achieve a thorough seal around all towel edges, because a prosthetic implant is to be placed.

Both carotid bifurcations are exposed. We have found it most useful to conduct bilateral simultaneous limited exposure with the head in neutral position, but others perform each exposure and mapping in staged sequential fashion. The carotid bifurcation is circumferentially mobilized, with the critical point being that no dissection at all should occur between the internal and external carotid. In other words, the mass consisting of the internal and external carotid combined with undisturbed tissues between should be encircled as one large unit (Figure 62-9). The entire carotid bifurcation should be dissected completely free posteriorly for full circumferential control, with the superior thyroid left intact as a useful anchor point. It is important not to use lidocaine anywhere near the carotid sinus to preserve reactivity for mapping.

At this time, attention is paid to the first side only. The head is turned slightly away from this side, and contralateral dissection is halted. When dissection is complete, the carotid stimulation electrode is placed around the carotid bifurcation (see Figure 62-9). The "fingers" are brought around in whatever way they seem to lie best. Typically, two fingers are above the superior thyroid and two are below. The active area of the electrode lies within the area delineated by the three wires and must be placed on the carotid sinus, which is not evident by visual inspection. In practice, the fingers are wrapped around the carotid bulb mass, and a best guess is made as to where the sinus is. The lead is then attached to the pulse generator, and testing is commenced at 3 to 4 V.

When the "sweet spot" is found, BP response will be obvious, although this might take 60 to 180 seconds. The basic plan is to locate the site at which electrical

stimulation produces the greatest and most reliable BP drop. If only a small response is seen, pressure must reequilibrate before the next spot is tested; this process can take 5 minutes or slightly longer. One useful technique is known as *trolling*; once the best spot in a macroscopic sense is found, the current is left on and the lead is shifted slightly to determine whether any additional benefit can be obtained.

When the site of optimal stimulation is found, the fingers are sutured in place using 6-0 Prolene passed through the reinforced suture pads (see Figure 62-9). It is important to ensure perfect apposition between the electrodes and the wall of the carotid sinus for best electrical contact; the fingers can be wrapped snugly enough to be under slight tension. This process has not been found to be associated with stenosis[16] or any adverse clinical events. Finally, residual excess material is trimmed free. At this point, strain relief loops are fashioned in the leads themselves (see Figure 62-5, radiograph) and the attachment pads used to anchor them to the sternocleidomastoid muscle. A similar process is followed on the contralateral side.

Leads early in the implant experience were tunneled down to the chest wall and then across to the pocket, but this situation poses obvious problems in the event that median sternotomy is someday required. The U.S. Rheos trial investigators universally tunneled the contralateral (usually left side) lead across the neck, superficial to the trachea, and then (usually with a counterincision) both leads are brought over the clavicle to the implantable pulse generator (IPG) pocket. Rheos IPGs have somewhat arbitrarily been placed on the right side to avoid confusion with pacemakers. On the rare occasion that the patient is a right-handed hunter, the pocket should be placed on the left side. The IPG is best tolerated if placed subfascially and well secured to the pectoralis major with

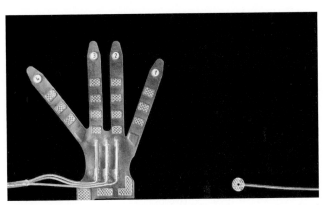

FIGURE 62-10 ■ Existing lead *(left)* versus next-generation lead *(right;* currently available in Europe). (Courtesy CVRx, Minneapolis, Minn. From Bisognano J, Sica D, Nadim M, et al: Results from the Rheos pivotal trial. Oral presentation, Sixtieth Annual American College of Cardiology Annual Meeting, New Orleans, 2011.)

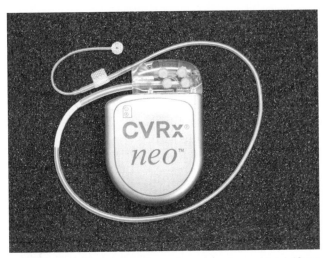

FIGURE 62-11 ■ Next-generation pulse generator and lead. (Courtesy CVRx, Minneapolis, Minn.)

permanent sutures, and enough dissection and loose area should be created medially to allow the leads to exit straight out from the IPG and thus avoid kinking.

The next generation of leads is currently available and is being used in Europe. The new leads are significantly smaller, measuring approximately 1 mm (Figure 62-10), and because the current path is less constrained, the "sweet spot" is functionally much larger. Experience with humans and animals suggests that unilateral stimulation works well in most patients, and the next-generation IPG is smaller than the original device (Figure 62-11). It is anticipated that all these factors will allow implantation using local anesthetic only via a unilateral, small incision.

The device must still be placed on the adventitia; percutaneous, endoscopic, and even transvenous and transarterial placement have all been considered, but are not sufficiently refined to allow clinical use.

WHAT COMES NEXT?

At this point the original technology is close to 10 years old. Rapid advances can be expected in all phases of this system, including smaller generators with more efficient batteries, better recipes for stimulation, less invasive implant strategies, and perhaps internal feedback (e.g., more current is delivered when pressure is high, and less when it is low). Currently, almost every patient has received bilateral implants while under general anesthesia. If unilateral stimulation were shown to be effective, even direct surgical implantation could be performed using local anesthesia.

In addition to heart failure,[21] several other applications of this technology come to mind. Permanent or temporary use of this device can ensure dramatic BP response in the short term, and thus could conceivably be used in emergency situations when BP control is needed (e.g., preeclampsia or acute aortic dissection). In addition, survival after medically treated type B aortic dissection is highly dependant on long-term BP control. The Rheos device could be used in this situation to ensure control in patients who will not comply with medication as well as those who do but are resistant to it.

SUMMARY

To date, more than 400 patients worldwide have undergone implantation of the Rheos carotid stimulator system, with acceptably low morbidity and mortality. In the cohort of patients treated longest (4 years), sustained reductions in systolic BP of approximately around 50 mm Hg have been documented. In addition, treatment has been shown to have favorable effects on ventricular hypertrophy and diastolic function, and trials are underway to further explore this effect and the overall utility of this strategy in diastolic heart failure. Formal results of the Rheos Pivotal Trial are needed before the device can be approved and used in the United States, but it has already received European approval (CE mark) and is being used in clinical practice. Both theory and early empiric results are exciting, and this technology may represent a significant advance in the care of this difficult group of patients.

References available online at expertconsult.com.

QUESTIONS

1. For each 20 mm increase in SBP over 115, cardiac risk:
   a. Increases by 10%
   b. increases by 25%
   c. increases by 100% (doubles)
   d. increases by 200% (triples)

2. Truly resistant hypertension is estimated to occur in:
   a. No one
   b. thousands of Americans
   c. several million Americans
   d. essentially every patient with hypertension

3. Stimulation of the glossopharyngeal nerve is caused by:
   a. carotid sinus stretch
   b. tachycardia
   c. tumors
   d. dehydration

4. Continuous electrical stimulation of the glossopharyngeal nerve in dogs produces hypotension that can be maintained for:
   a. only a few seconds
   b. less than an hour
   c. 12 to 18 hours
   d. at least a week

5. Electrcal stimulation of the carotid baroreflex is accomplished by stimulation of the:
   a. Internal carotid artery
   b. Carotid sinus
   c. External carotid artery
   d. Glossopharyngeal nerve itself

6. Side effects of carotid sinus stimulation could theoretically include:
   a. bradycardia
   b. tachypnea
   c. hypertension
   d. jaw claudication

7. Baroreflex stimulation has also been shown to be associated with:
   a. preeclampsia in vulnerable subjects
   b. mitral regurgitation
   c. renal hyperplasia
   d. reduction in ventricular mass

8. Baroreflex stimulation has been shown to lower systolic blood pressure by:
   a. only 1 to 3 mm
   b. 5 to 10 mm
   c. 30 to 50 mm
   d. 50 to 100 mm

9. In America, baroreflex stimulation is currently (late 2012):
   a. usable only within a clinical trial
   b. usable only for heart failure
   c. useful only in animal models
   d. approved for use in patients with severe hypertension

10. Voltage needed to see meaningful blood pressure drop is in the order of:
    a. a few millivolts
    b. 1 to 6 volts
    c. 30 volts (low wattage)
    d. 30 volts (high wattage)

ANSWERS

1. **c**
2. **c**
3. **a**
4. **d**
5. **b**
6. **a**
7. **d**
8. **c**
9. **a**
10. **b**

CHAPTER 63

BUILDING AN OUTPATIENT INTERVENTION SUITE

Samuel S. Ahn • Hwa Kho

Technological advances in minimally invasive treatments for vascular diseases in the past decade have made it clinically acceptable to perform many peripheral endovascular interventional procedures on an outpatient basis. In recognition of that development, Centers for Medicare and Medicaid Services (CMS) has, since 2006, steadily increased the types of interventional procedures it allowed physicians to perform on an outpatient basis in the physician office setting, thus making it potentially viable economically for vascular surgeons to operate their own intervention suites in their offices.

INCENTIVES

There are three powerful incentives for vascular surgeons to consider building their own intervention suite. The first is quality of the patient experience. The vascular surgeon has much more control over the patient experience, from scheduling of the procedure time, to the environment, to the amount of time with the patient before and after the procedure. By doing the intervention in the office, the vascular surgeon can make the environment much more comfortable and less intimidating to the patient. The surgeon can schedule treatments quickly without having to compete for room time with other physicians at the hospital.

The second incentive is productivity. Without having to travel to and from the hospital and having to wait for the operating room or catheterization room to be ready, the vascular surgeon can make much more efficient use of their time. The typical vascular surgeon wastes a lot of time waiting for procedures scheduled ahead of them to finish and for rooms to be cleaned before they can begin their procedures at the hospital. With an intervention suite in their office, the surgeon can see many more patients in a day.

Finally, in the face of declining professional fees, office-based procedures offer vascular surgeons an opportunity to increase their revenues by capturing the higher global fees that CMS and many other insurance companies pay for office-based procedures. A global fee is the fee that CMS and other payers pay to the physician for providing a service in the physician's office. The fee reimburses the physician for professional services and the technical expenses of providing that service. The latter is equivalent to the technical fees that hospitals and ambulatory surgery centers receive for procedures performed in those facilities. The global fee can be substantially higher than the professional fee, sometimes tenfold higher. The physician will incur more expenses for procedures performed in the office, which will have to be paid from this global fee. However, by managing the intervention suite well, the vascular surgeon has the opportunity to generate a higher income.

CONSIDERATIONS

Financial

Appealing as the incentives are, the vascular practice needs to carefully analyze whether the fixed and incremental expenses of having an intervention suite in the physician office makes financial sense before deciding to build one.

The first question is whether the office has a sufficient number of cases that could be handled in an outpatient setting. How many cases are currently handled elsewhere, such as in hospitals and surgery centers, that can be transferred to the office intervention suite? What are these cases and how much would they reimburse? What is the payer mix? Will the payers reimburse at the global fee rate? Medicare and most commercial payers will reimburse a global fee. However, Medicaid would only pay the professional fees for many interventional procedures in the office setting. Some health management organizations may also refuse to pay a global fee.

Although an interventional procedure in the physician's office may reimburse much more than the professional fee that the vascular surgeon would get in a hospital for doing the same procedure, it is important to remember that the physician's office has to pay for supplies, which can be expensive, for staffing (including nurses, scrub technicians, and x-ray technicians), for equipment, and for other variable and fixed expenses.

Unless the practice has sufficient volume and the right type of cases and payer mix to cover the overheads, and is able to manage its supplies and other expenses efficiently, the intervention suite could easily become an untenable financial burden. It is important to make a careful and realistic financial projection before proceeding with the implementation.

Location

The intervention suite should be within 5 miles of, and ideally adjacent to, a major hospital in the event that a patient needs to be admitted. Such events should be rare, but as with any intervention, the physician needs to have a contingency plan for possible complications. This is usually not an issue because most vascular practices are located near a hospital.

Space

The more space the practice can allocate to the intervention suite, the easier it will be to configure the space to work efficiently for the physicians and patients. At a minimum, the intervention suite needs:

- An angiography room with at least 600 ft², but ideally about 1000 ft² (Lead-lined walls may be needed depending on the radiation pattern of the fluoroscopy machine, the size of the room, the adjacent spaces, and use of the fluoroscopy machine. The practice needs to consult a medical physicist on the actual requirements.)
- One or more recovery rooms measuring at least 100 ft²
- One or more pre-op rooms measuring at least 100 ft²
- Storage area for supplies (This area should ideally be inside the intervention room, or easily accessible from it. At least 100 ft² will be required.)

In addition, spaces for reception area and work areas or offices for staff and physicians are necessary if the practice does not already have them.

The practice needs to consider how the patients flow through the facility and plan for adequate clearance in regard to doors and corridors, bearing in mind that patients may be moved on stretchers from the pre-op room to the intervention room and from the intervention room to the recovery room. The practice also needs to plan for nonambulatory patients arriving and departing the facility, and in particular access for emergency vehicles.

If a practice already has existing space that could be converted into an intervention suite, the build-out cost could be minimal. On the other hand, building a whole new facility could easily cost hundreds of thousands of dollars.

Equipment

The basic equipment for the intervention suite includes the following:

- Fluoroscopy unit
- Imaging table
- Backup power supply
- Defibrillator
- Crash cart
- Anesthesia cart
- Ultrasound scanner
- Patient monitors
- Stretchers
- Sterilizer
- IV stands
- Stainless steel tables
- Lead aprons
- Bovie
- Power injector
- Operating room lights

The most expensive and important piece of equipment is the fluoroscopy unit and imaging table. A portable C-ARM is usually sufficient. It should have the appropriate vascular software package, and ideally, a 15-inch image intensifier. Because the physicians will be using this critical piece of equipment for many years, it is better to acquire one that provides superior clinical functions and user experience than to let price be the driving factor in deciding on a model. By buying some refurbished equipment when possible, the practice could equip the entire intervention suite for approximately $500,000 or less.

Supplies

The practice will want to stock 1 to 2 weeks worth of supplies (e.g., guidewires, catheters, balloons, stents, pharmaceuticals, disposables). Most of the more expensive devices such as balloons and stents may be obtained from the suppliers on consignment. The practice does not have to pay for a consigned item until it is used; therefore the practice should try to get as many items on consignment as possible.

The decision on which devices to get depends on the types of cases the practice plans to perform as well as the physicians' personal preferences. It is important for the physicians to be involved in making these decisions because they know best what they need and are most comfortable using.

Managing and keeping track of the supplies is a time-consuming yet critical function. A working intervention suite stocks more than 1000 unique devices. A single balloon could come in six different permutations of sizes. Just one missing device could compromise the outcome of a case. It is important to be able to discover quickly what is in the inventory at any time and be able to track all the supplies used in each case. There are inventory management systems that provide for utilization tracking through use of barcode readers. The practice should invest in one to help manage its inventory. Initial cash outlay for supplies will typically be $50,000 to $100,000, assuming that most of the expensive devices can be obtained on consignment.

Staffing

The number of staff members required to operate and support the intervention suite depends on the case volume. However, these are some of the key roles that will need to be filled:

- Circulating nurse (registered nurse [RN] or higher)
- Recovery nurse (RN or higher)
- Nurse manager
- Scrub technician
- X-ray technician

The nurse manager's role is to oversee the day-to-day clinical operations of the intervention suite, enforce policies and procedures, and oversee compliance with federal and state regulations covering operation of the intervention suite. In a small practice, this role could be played by one of the physicians. However, in a busy practice, it is essential to have one person, ideally a nurse, be dedicated full time to this role.

In addition to the clinical staff, the practice may need to hire additional clerical and administrative staff to help with the increased workload needed to support the operations of the intervention suite, such as ordering and managing supplies, coding, and billing. An alternative to hiring and training new employees is to outsource some of these functions to third parties.

MANAGING AN OUTPATIENT INTERVENTION SUITE

Once the intervention suite has been built, equipped, stocked with supplies, and staffed, long-term success requires attention to the following issues.

Patient Safety

Any intervention procedure carries a level of risk to patient safety. In an outpatient setting in the physician's office, physicians are on their own in handling any adverse event. There is little room for errors, and every procedure has to be close to perfection.

Potential complications include:

- Groin access problem
- Contrast-induced renal failure
- Contrast allergy
- Blood transfusion
- Urinary retention
- Malignant arrhythmia
- Myocardial infarction
- Vascular rupture
- Infection
- Acute thrombosis
- Thromboemboli
- Airway problem
- Respiratory failure
- Congestive heart failure

However, with appropriate policies and procedures, training, and adoption of defensive intervention techniques, it is possible to reduce the risks and mitigate potential complications.

Policies and Procedures

It is important to have written policies and procedures to cover all aspects of operating the intervention suite and to ensure that all staff members and physicians are trained and understand the policies and procedures. These policies and procedures should proactively define the risks that the practice is willing to take and define the contingency plans for handling emergencies.

A key policy to successfully operating the intervention suite is patient selection. Decide what risks the practice is prepared to tolerate, and implement the appropriate patient selection criteria. For example, the practice may implement the policy to perform procedures on patients only if they meet the following criteria:

- American Society of Anesthesiologists (ASA) classification 1 to 4
- Baseline creatinine ≤ 2.0 mg/dL
- Potassium <5 mmol/L
- Not morbidly obese

Patients will follow a standard preoperative evaluation procedure and should be accepted for treatment only if they meet these and other criteria. By establishing clear policies, the practice can avoid performing risky procedures in the intervention suite. In general, the practice should adapt the protocols that would have applied in a hospital setting, such as preoperative evaluation, intraoperative procedure, and postoperative care.

Accreditation

The development of appropriate and useful written policies and procedures and the training of staff members and physicians are extremely time-consuming tasks, and the tendency is to ignore them. This is also true of many other best practices that should be implemented in operating the intervention suite.

It is, therefore, useful for the practice to voluntarily undergo the Accreditation Association for Ambulatory Health Care (AAAHC) or The Joint Commission (TJC) accreditation process for the intervention suite. AAAHC or TJC accreditation is usually not required to operate the intervention suite in the physician's office setting. However, these accreditations provide useful guidance and templates for best practices, both in terms of patient safety and organizational governance. The process of qualifying for accreditation is labor intensive, but it is well worth the effort in providing the practice with a high-quality frame of reference for best practices and in enforcing the discipline in the practice to adhere to those standards.

Defensive Intervention Techniques

With little room for errors and few resources for handling adverse events compared with a hospital setting, the physician needs to develop and adopt defensive techniques to prevent potential problems as much as possible. For example, the use of ultrasound guidance to locate the puncture site for every intervention is highly desirable. Although insurance payers might refuse to reimburse for the use of ultrasound guidance (and it might not be medically necessary), the reduction in error with ultrasound guidance makes its use one of the keys to reducing complications in the intervention suite.

Similarly, the use of a closure device in every case is highly recommended. Closure devices can be expensive and are not separately reimbursable with most procedures, but their effectiveness in reducing recovery time and complications justifies their use in the intervention suite.

Actual Experience with Complications

A recent study[1] examined the complication rates of 2040 consecutive endovascular cases performed in intervention suites in the author's offices in Dallas and Los Angeles between April 2006 and October 2010. The data come from a total of five vascular surgeons in the Dallas office and three vascular surgeons in the Los Angeles office.

Indications for the procedures were peripheral vascular disease, chronic venous insufficiency, end-stage renal disease, varicose veins, ulcers, stenosis of arteries and veins outside the periphery, vertebrobasilar insufficiency, thrombophlebitis, malfunctioning access, atherosclerosis with claudication or ischemic rest pain, and thoracic outlet syndrome. Hypertension was present in approximately 39% of the patients, diabetes was present in 20%, and coronary artery disease was present in 23%. The vast majority of these patients were ASA classification I, II, or III, but 6% were class IV. The patient population was 57% female and 43% male, with an average age of 59.6 ± 16.0 years SD and a range of 15 to 107 years. The case mix is shown in Table 63-1. Table 63-2 shows the complications encountered.

TABLE 63-1	Procedures Performed in Intervention Suites: April 1, 2006 to October 25, 2010
Procedure	**Number**
Diagnostic angiogram	491
Angioplasty	514
Angioplasty with stent	469
AVF declot	102
RFA	320
Central venous access	118
Coil embolization	9
Other*	17
TOTAL	2040

AVF, Arteriovenous fistula; *RFA*, radiofrequency ablation.
*Consists of 1 great saphenous vein ligation, 2 inferior vena cava filter retrievals, and 14 laser ablations.

TABLE 63-2	Complications Encountered in 2040 Consecutive Procedures*
Complications	**Number**
Groin access problem	0
Contrast induced renal failure	0
Malignant arrhythmia	0
Myocardial infarction	0
Vascular rupture	0
Infection	0
Acute thrombosis	0
Airway problem	0
Respiratory failure	0
Congestive heart failure	0
Thromboemboli	1
Contrast allergy	1
Hematoma	7
Unresponsiveness	2
Ischemia resulting from puncture	1
Electrocariograph changes requiring admission	1
Transition to open procedure	1
Torn femoral vein	1
Penile bleeding	1
TOTAL	16

*Performed from April 1, 2006 to October 25, 2010 in the author's outpatient intervention suites in Dallas, Tex. and Los Angeles, Calif.

A total of 16 complications were encountered out of 2040 consecutive procedures, representing a complication rate of 0.78%. Seven of these patients required immediate transfer to a hospital, and three were sent for elective admission for observation. There was no mortality.

This complication rate of 0.78% compares favorably to complications encountered in hospital settings[1] and demonstrates that, with proper policies and procedures and defensive intervention techniques, the physician office–based outpatient intervention suite is a safe and effective setting to provide endovascular treatments.

Supply Management

Having the right device at the right time makes all the difference between a successful outcome and a failed intervention. It is expensive and operationally challenging to adequately stock a large array of devices in anticipation of the physician's need during an intervention. From a business perspective, the practice wants to tie up as little capital as possible by keeping a low inventory level; however, clinically it is desirable to keep as much inventory as possible in case something is needed.

Keeping an appropriate balance and ensuring the intervention room is adequately stocked at all times is a full-time job in a busy practice. This is a job that is difficult to do without having a good computer system in place to manage the inventory. The computer system should be able to record receipt of supplies, track usage, and report on what is in the inventory in real time. It should be able to identify items that fall below established par levels so that those items can be replenished in a timely basis.

In addition, and importantly from the business perspective, the computer system should be able to itemize the supplies used for each case and the total cost of the supplies for that case to the practice. This information is essential to monitoring costs and providing feedback to the physicians on the costs of their choice of devices. Staffing and supplies are the top two expenses in a case, and keeping supply expenses low is essential to the financial health of the intervention suite.

Coding and Billing

The intervention suite is probably the single most expensive cost center for the practice, and it could easily derail the practice's cash flow if revenue from it is inadequate or delayed through poor coding and billing. Medicare and most major payers take approximately 3 weeks to pay a clean claim after they have received it. It is imperative to code the procedures fully and correctly, with adequate documentation for optimal reimbursement and to submit the claim as quickly as possible.

Interventional endovascular procedures can be challenging to code. A single procedure could involve dozens of codes with complex coding rules. The coding process is typically a bottleneck in getting the claims out quickly. Most physicians are not able to code competently, and good interventional coders are hard to find. However, there are good computer systems that can facilitate or automate the coding process. Using such a system could help to submit a clean claim within a couple of days of the procedure instead of weeks, which can help to ensure a healthy cash flow.

CONCLUSIONS

Introducing an outpatient intervention suite to the vascular practice is a major project that affects almost all aspects of the organization. There will have to be new staff members; new responsibilities; new business, administrative, and clinical priorities; and changes to the way the physicians practice medicine to turn it into a successful enterprise. Managing an intervention suite well on a day-to-day basis requires a whole new set of operational knowledge and skills that the practice will have to acquire. One option for the practice to consider is to outsource some of these operational tasks to third parties and concentrate on its core competencies in providing patient care.

The number one priority is, of course, to ensure that patient care and safety are not compromised. As a result, it is important to have good policies and procedures, training, and adherence to those policies and procedures by both staff and physicians. Voluntary compliance with AAAHC or TJC requirements and guidelines will help to enforce discipline and provide external validation.

Experience has shown that with proper management, an outpatient intervention suite based in the physician's office can provide safe and effective patient care. It can be a highly rewarding and satisfying experience for patients and physicians. For the patients, it provides convenience, a more comfortable environment, and a more intimate interaction experience with physicians and nursing staff members. For the physicians, there is the satisfaction of being able to schedule treatments promptly, being more productive with their time, and getting a better financial return for their services.

References available online at expertconsult.com.

Page numbers followed by "f" indicate figures, "t" indicate tables, and "b" indicate boxes.